# Prostate and Other Genitourinary Cancers

# Cancer
## Principles & Practice of Oncology

**10**th edition

# Prostate and Other Genitourinary Cancers

## Cancer
### Principles & Practice of Oncology
### 10th edition

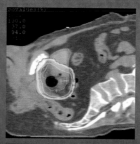
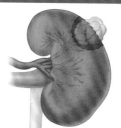
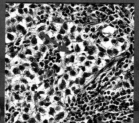
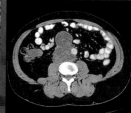

## Vincent T. DeVita, Jr., MD

Amy & Joseph Perella Professor of Medicine
Yale Comprehensive Cancer Center and Smilow
   Cancer Hospital at Yale-New Haven
Professor of Epidemiology and Public Health
Yale University School of Public Health
New Haven, Connecticut

## Theodore S. Lawrence, MD, PhD

Isadore Lampe Professor and Chair
Department of Radiation Oncology
University of Michigan
Ann Arbor, Michigan

## Steven A. Rosenberg, MD, PhD

Chief, Surgery Branch, National Cancer Institute, National Institutes of Health
Professor of Surgery, Uniformed Services University of the Health Sciences
School of Medicine
Bethesda, Maryland
Professor of Surgery
George Washington University School of Medicine
Washington, District of Columbia

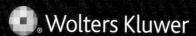
. Wolters Kluwer

Philadelphia · Baltimore · New York · London
Buenos Aires · Hong Kong · Sydney · Tokyo

*Acquisitions Editor:* Julie Goolsby
*Senior Product Development Editor:* Emilie Moyer
*Editorial Assistant:* Brian Convery
*Production Project Manager:* David Orzechowski
*Marketing Manager:* Rachel Mante Leung
*Senior Designer:* Stephen Druding
*Illustration Coordinator:* Jennifer Clements
*Illustrator:* Jason McAlexander, Electronic Publishing Services, Inc.
*Manufacturing Coordinator:* Beth Welsh
*Prepress Vendor:* Absolute Service, Inc.
*Prepress Vendor Project Manager:* Harold Medina

9  8  7  6  5  4  3  2  1

Printed in China

**Library of Congress Cataloging-in-Publication Data**

Names: DeVita, Vincent T., Jr. 1935- , editor. | Lawrence, Theodore S.,
     editor. | Rosenberg, Steven A., editor
Title: Cancer : principles & practice of oncology. Prostate and other
     genitourinary cancers / [edited by] Vincent T. DeVita, Jr., Theodore S.
     Lawrence, Steven A. Rosenberg.
Other titles: Prostate and other genitourinary cancers
Description: Philadelphia : Wolters Kluwer Health, [2016] | Contained in:
     Devita, Hellman, and Rosenberg's cancer. 10th edition. [2015]. | Includes
     bibliographical references and index.
Identifiers: LCCN 2016005137 | ISBN 9781496333971
Subjects: | MESH: Prostatic Neoplasms | Urogenital Neoplasms
Classification: LCC RC280.P7 | NLM WJ 762 | DDC 616.99/463–dc23 LC record available at
http://lccn.loc.gov/2016005137

**Gregory P. Adams, PhD**
Associate Professor, Developmental
  Therapeutics Program
Director of Biological Research and
  Therapeutics
Fox Chase Cancer Center
Philadelphia, Pennsylvania

**Bharat B. Aggarwal, PhD**
Professor of Cancer Research
Professor of Cancer Medicine
  (Biochemistry)
Chief, Cytokine Research Laboratory
Department of Experimental
  Therapeutics
The University of Texas MD Anderson
  Cancer Center
Houston, Texas

**Shirin Arastu-Kapur, PhD**
Associate Director
Biology at Onyx Pharmaceuticals
South San Francisco, California

**Alan Ashworth, FRS**
Professor and Chief Executive
The Institute of Cancer Research
London, United Kingdom

**Sharyn D. Baker, PharmD, PhD**
Associate Member
Pharmaceutical Sciences Department
St. Jude Children's Research Hospital
Memphis, Tennessee

**Alberto Bardelli, MD**
Laboratory of Molecular Genetics
Institute for Cancer Research and
  Treatment
University of Torino Medical School
Candiolo, Italy

**Susan E. Bates, MD**
Head, Molecular Therapeutics Section
Developmental Therapeutics Branch
Center for Cancer Research
National Cancer Institute
Bethesda, Maryland

**Stephen B. Baylin, MD**
Professor of Oncology
Professor of Medicine
Johns Hopkins University School of
  Medicine
Deputy Director of the Cancer Center
Baltimore, Maryland

**Andrew Berchuck, MD**
Professor and Director
Gynecologic Oncology Program
Division of Gynecologic Oncology
Department of Obstetrics and
  Gynecology
Duke Cancer Institute
Duke University Medical Center
Durham, North Carolina

**Leslie Bernstein, MS, PhD**
Professor and Director
Division of Cancer Etiology
Department of Population Sciences
Beckman Research Institute
City of Hope Dean for Faculty Affairs
City of Hope National Medical Center
  and the Beckman Research Institute
Duarte, California

**Bryan L. Betz, PhD**
Assistant Professor
Department of Pathology
University of Michigan
Technical Director
Molecular Diagnostics Laboratory
University of Michigan Health System
Ann Arbor, Michigan

**Lawrence H. Boise, PhD**
Professor
Winship Cancer Institute of Emory
  University
Departments of Hematology/Medical
  Oncology and Cell Biology
Emory School of Medicine
Atlanta, Georgia

**Danielle C. Bonadies, MS, CGC**
Director, Cancer Genetics Division
Gene Counsel, LLC
New Haven, Connecticut

**Hossein Borghaei, MS, DO**
Associate Professor
Chief, Thoracic Medical Oncology
Fox Chase Cancer Center
Philadelphia, Pennsylvania

**Otis W. Brawley, MD, FACP**
Chief Medical Officer
American Cancer Society, Inc.
Atlanta, Georgia

**Dean E. Brenner, MD**
Kutsche Family Professor of Internal
  Medicine
Professor of Pharmacology
University of Michigan Comprehensive
  Cancer Center
Ann Arbor, Michigan

**Christopher B. Buck, PhD**
Investigator
Head, Tumor Virus Molecular Biology
  Section
Laboratory of Cellular Oncology
Center for Cancer Research
National Cancer Institute
Bethesda, Maryland

**Tim E. Byers, MD, MPH**
Associate Dean for Public Health Practice
Colorado School of Public Health
Associate Director for Cancer Prevention
  and Control
University of Colorado Cancer Center
Aurora, Colorado

**A. Hilary Calvert**
Professor
Gynecologic Oncology
University College Hospitals (UCLH)
London, United Kingdom

**Daniel J. Canter, MD**
Vice Chairman
Department of Urology
Urologic Institute of Southeastern
  Pennsylvania
Einstein Healthcare Network
Associate Professor, Urologic Oncology
Fox Chase Cancer Center
Philadelphia, Pennsylvania

**Gayun Chan-Smutko, MS, CGC**
Senior Genetic Counselor
Center for Cancer Risk Assessment
Massachusetts General Hospital
Boston, Massachusetts

**Cindy H. Chau, PharmD, PhD**
Scientist
Medical Oncology Branch
Center for Cancer Research
National Cancer Institute
National Institutes of Health
Bethesda, Maryland

**Arul M. Chinnaiyan, MD, PhD**
Director, Michigan Center for
  Translational Pathology
S.P. Hicks Endowed Professor of
  Pathology
Investigator, Howard Hughes Medical
  Institute
American Cancer Society Research
  Professor
Professor of Urology
Ann Arbor, Michigan

**Edward Chu, MD**
Professor of Medicine and Pharmacology
  & Chemical Biology
Chief, Division of Hematology-Oncology
Deputy Director, University of Pittsburgh
  Cancer Institute
University of Pittsburgh School of
  Medicine
Pittsburgh, Pennsylvania

**Jessica Clague, PhD, MPH**
Assistant Research Professor
Division of Cancer Etiology
Department of Population Sciences
Beckman Research Institute
City of Hope National Medical Center
Duarte, California

**M. Sitki Copur, MD, FACP**
Medical Director of Oncology
Saint Francis Cancer Treatment Center
Grand Island, Nebraska
Professor, Department of Medicine
Division of Hematology Oncology
Adjunct Faculty
University of Nebraska Medical Center
Omaha, Nebraska

**Douglas M. Dahl, MD, FACS**
Associate Professor of Surgery
Harvard Medical School
Chief, Division of Urologic Oncology
Department of Urology
Massachusetts General Hospital
Boston, Massachusetts

**Hari A. Deshpande, MD**
Associate Professor of Medicine
Yale University School of Medicine
Section of Medical Oncology
Yale New Haven Hospital
New Haven, Connecticut

**Khanh T. Do, MD**
Senior Clinical Fellow
Division of Cancer Treatment and
  Diagnosis
National Cancer Institute
National Institutes of Health
Bethesda, Maryland

**James H. Doroshow, MD**
Director, Division of Cancer Treatment
  and Diagnosis
Deputy Director for Clinical and
  Translational Research
National Cancer Institute
National Institutes of Health
Bethesda, Maryland

**Jason A. Efstathiou, MD, DPhil**
Assistant Professor
Department of Radiation Oncology
Massachusetts General Hospital
Harvard Medical School
Boston, Massachusetts

**Charles Erlichman, MD**
Professor, Department of Oncology
Deputy Director, Clinical Research
Peter and Frances Georgeson Professor of
  Gastroenterology Cancer Research
Mayo Clinic
Rochester, Minnesota

**Adam S. Feldman, MD, MPH**
Assistant Professor of Surgery
Harvard Medical School
Assistant in Urology, Department of
  Urology
Massachusetts General Hospital
Boston, Massachusetts

**Steven A. Feldman, PhD**
Staff Scientist
Director, Surgery Branch
Vector Production Facility
National Cancer Institute
Bethesda, Maryland

**Felix Y. Feng, MD**
Assistant Professor, Department of
  Radiation Oncology
Chief, Division of Translational
  Genomics
University of Michigan Health System
Ann Arbor, Michigan

**William Douglas Figg, Sr., PharmD, MBA**
Senior Investigator and Head of the
  Clinical Pharmacology Program
Clinical Director, Center for Cancer
  Research
Head of the Molecular Pharmacology
  Section
Medical Oncology Branch
Center for Cancer Research
National Cancer Institute
National Institutes of Health
Bethesda, Maryland

**Antonio Tito Fojo, MD, PhD**
Medical Oncology Branch and Affiliates
Head, Experimental Therapeutics Section
Senior Investigator
Center for Cancer Research
National Cancer Institute
Bethesda, Maryland

**Larissa V. Furtado, MD**
Assistant Professor
Department of Pathology
Assistant Director
Division of Genomics and Molecular
  Pathology
University of Chicago
Chicago, Illinois

**Sheryl G. A. Gabram-Mendola, MD, MBA, FACS**
Surgeon-in-Chief
Grady Memorial Hospital
Emory University School of Medicine
Deputy Director
Georgia Cancer Center for Excellence
Director, AVON Comprehensive Breast
  Center at Grady
Director, High Risk Assessment Program
Winship Cancer Institute of Emory
  University
Georgia Cancer Coalition Distinguished
  Cancer Scholar
Atlanta, Georgia

**Jared J. Gartner, DO**
Biologist, National Cancer Institute
Surgery Branch
National Institute of Health
Bethesda, Maryland

**Scott Nicholas Gettinger, MD**
Associate Professor of Medicine
Thoracic Oncology Program
Developmental Therapeutics
Yale Cancer Center
New Haven, Connecticut

**Matthew P. Goetz, MD**
Associate Professor of Pharmacology
Associate Professor of Oncology
Mayo Clinic
Rochester, Minnesota

**Sarah B. Goldberg, MD, MPH**
Assistant Professor of Internal Medicine
Medical Oncology
Yale Cancer Center
Yale University School of Medicine
New Haven, Connecticut

**Leonard G. Gomella, MD, FACS**
The Bernard W. Godwin Professor of
  Prostate Cancer
Chairman, Department of Urology
Associate Director
Jefferson Kimmel Cancer Center
Clinical Director, Jefferson Kimmel
  Cancer Center Network
Thomas Jefferson University
Philadelphia, Pennsylvania

**Steven D. Gore, MD**
Yale University School of Medicine
New Haven, Connecticut

**Ellen R. Gritz, PhD**
Professor and Chair
Department of Behavioral Science
The University of Texas MD Anderson
   Cancer Center
Houston, Texas

**José G. Guillem, MD, MPH**
Department of Surgery
Memorial Sloan-Kettering Cancer Center
New York, New York

**Douglas Hanahan, PhD**
Director
Swiss Institute for Experimental Cancer
   Research (ISREC)
Lausanne, Switzerland

**Lyndsay N. Harris, MD, FRCP(C)**
Diana Hyland Chair in Breast Cancer
Director, Breast Cancer Program
Seidman Cancer Center
University Hospitals Case Medical Center
Professor of Medicine
Division of Hematology and Oncology
Case Western Reserve University
Cleveland, Ohio

**James G. Herman, MD**
Johns Hopkins University
Baltimore, Maryland

**Jay L. Hess, MD, PhD**
Professor, Department of Pathology
Carl V. Weller Professor and Chair
Professor, Department of Internal
   Medicine
University of Michigan Health System
Ann Arbor, Michigan

**Christopher J. Hoimes, DO**
Assistant Professor
UH Case Medical Center
Department of Medicine-Hematology
   and Oncology
Cleveland, Ohio

**Vanessa W. Hui, MD**
Department of Surgery
Memorial Sloan-Kettering Cancer Center
New York, New York

**Carolyn D. Hurst, BSc, MSc, PhD**
Senior Postdoctoral Research Fellow
Section of Experimental Oncology
Leeds Institute of Cancer and Pathology
St. James's University Hospital
Leeds, United Kingdom

**Christopher J. Kirk, MD**
Vice President of Research
Onyx Pharmaceuticals, Inc.
South San Francisco, California

**Margaret A. Knowles, PhD**
Head, Section of Experimental Oncology
Leeds Institute of Cancer and Pathology
St. James's University Hospital
Leeds, United Kingdom

**James N. Kochenderfer, MD**
Investigator, Experimental Transplantation
   and Immunology Branch
National Cancer Institute
National Institutes of Health
Bethesda, Maryland

**Manish Kohli, MD**
Associate Professor of Oncology
Department of Oncology
College of Medicine
Mayo Clinic
Joint Appointment, Department of
   Urology
Mayo Clinic
Rochester, Minnesota

**Shivaani Kummar, MD, FACP**
Head, Early Clinical Trials Development
Office of the Director
Division of Cancer Treatment and
   Diagnosis
National Cancer Institute
Bethesda, Maryland

**Brian R. Lane, MD, PhD**
Associate Professor, Department of
   Surgery
Michigan State University College of
   Human Medicine
Betz Family Endowed Chair for Cancer
   Research
Spectrum Health Cancer Program
Grand Rapids, Michigan

**Theodore S. Lawrence, MD, PhD**
Isadore Lampe Professor and Chair
Department of Radiation Oncology
University of Michigan Health System
Ann Arbor, Michigan

**Richard J. Lee, MD, PhD**
Assistant Professor, Department of
   Medicine
Harvard Medical School
Assistant Physician, Division of
   Hematology and Oncology
Massachusetts General Hospital
Boston, Massachusetts

**W. Marston Linehan, MD**
Chief, Urologic Oncology Branch
Center for Cancer Research
National Cancer Institute
Bethesda, Maryland

**Scott M. Lippman, MD**
Director, Senior Associate Dean, &
   Associate Vice Chancellor
Cancer Research and Care
Chugai Pharmaceutical Chair
Professor of Medicine
University of California, San Diego
Moores Cancer Center
La Jolla, California

**Mats Ljungman, PhD**
Professor, Departments of Radiation
   Oncology and Environmental Health
   Sciences
Translational Oncology Program
University of Michigan Medical School
Ann Arbor, Michigan

**Christopher J. Logothetis, MD**
Principle Investigator
Genitourinary Medical Oncology
The University of Texas MD Anderson
   Cancer Center
Houston, Texas

**Carlos López-Otín, PhD**
Professor, Department of Biochemistry
   and Molecular Biology
Universidad de Oviedo
Principality of Asturias, Spain

**Charles L. Loprinzi, MD**
Regis Professor of Breast Cancer Research
Department of Oncology
Mayo Clinic
Rochester, Minnesota

**Yani Lu, PhD**
Assistant Research Professor
Division of Cancer Etiology
Department of Population Science
Beckman Research Institute of the City
   of Hope
Duarte, California

**Xiaomei Ma, PhD**
Associate Professor, Department of
   Chronic Disease Epidemiology
Yale University School of Public Health
New Haven, Connecticut

**Ellen T. Matloff, MS, CGC**
President & CEO
Gene Counsel, LLC
New Haven, Connecticut

**Susan T. Mayne, PhD**
C.-E.A. Winslow Professor of
   Epidemiology
Chair, Department of Chronic Disease
   Epidemiology
Yale University School of Public Health
Associate Director for Population
   Sciences
Yale Cancer Center
New Haven, Connecticut

**Howard L. McLeod, PharmD**
Medical Director, DeBartolo Family
   Personalized Medicine Institute
Senior Member, Division of Population
   Sciences
H. Lee Moffitt Cancer Center
Tampa, Florida

**M. Dror Michaelson, MD, PhD**
Associate Professor of Medicine
Harvard Medical School
Clinical Director, Urologic Oncology
Massachusetts General Hospital Cancer
    Center
Boston, Massachusetts

**Karin B. Michels, ScD, PhD**
Associate Professor
Obstetrician/Gynecologist
Epidemiology Center
Department of Obstetrics, Gynecology
    and Reproductive Biology
Brigham and Women's Hospital
Harvard Medical School
Boston, Massachusetts

**Jeffrey F. Moley, MD**
Chief, Section of Endocrine and
    Oncologic Surgery
Professor of Surgery
Washington University School of
    Medicine
St. Louis, Missouri

**Meredith A. Morgan, PhD**
Research Assistant Professor
Department of Radiation Oncology
University of Michigan
Ann Arbor, Michigan

**Jeffrey A. Norton, MD**
Professor, Department of Surgery
Chief, Section of Surgical Oncology and
    Division of General Surgery
Department of Surgery
Stanford University Hospital
Stanford, California

**Richard J. O'Connor, PhD**
Associate Member, Department of Health
    Behavior
Division of Cancer Prevention and
    Population Sciences
Roswell Park Cancer Institute
Buffalo, New York

**Peter J. O'Dwyer, MD**
Professor of Medicine
Abramson Cancer Center
University of Pennsylvania
Philadelphia, Pennsylvania

**Lance C. Pagliaro, MD**
Professor, Department of Genitourinary
    Medical Oncology
The University of Texas MD Anderson
    Cancer Center
Houston, Texas

**Howard L. Parnes, MD**
Chief
Prostate and Urologic Cancer Research
    Group
Division of Cancer Prevention
National Cancer Institute
Rockville, Maryland

**Giao Q. Phan, MD, FACS**
Associate Professor
Division of Surgical Oncology
Massey Cancer Center
Virginia Commonwealth University
Richmond, Virginia

**Yves Pommier, MD, PhD**
Chief, Laboratory of Molecular
    Pharmacology
Head, DNA Topoisomerase/Integrase
    Group
Center for Cancer Research
National Cancer Institute
Bethesda, Maryland

**Edwin M. Posadas, MD, FACP, KM**
Medical Director, Urologic Oncology
    Program
Assistant Professor, Department of
    Medicine
Samuel Ochsin Comprehensive Cancer
    Institute
Cedars-Sinai Medical Center
Los Angeles, California

**Sahdeo Prasad, PhD**
Cytokine Research Laboratory
Department of Experimental
    Therapeutics
The University of Texas MD Anderson
    Cancer Center
Houston, Texas

**Lee Ratner, MD, PhD**
Professor Departments of Medicine and
    Molecular Microbiology
Co-Director, Medical & Molecular
    Oncology
Washington University School of
    Medicine
Barnes-Jewish Hospital
St. Louis, Missouri

**Brian I. Rini, MD, FACP**
Professor of Medicine
Lerner College of Medicine
Department of Solid Tumor Oncology
Cleveland Clinic Taussig Cancer Institute
Glickman Urological Institute
Cleveland, Ohio

**Paul F. Robbins, PhD**
National Institutes of Health
Bethesda, Maryland

**Matthew K. Robinson, PhD**
Assistant Professor, Developmental
    Therapeutics Program
Fox Chase Cancer Center
Philadelphia, Pennsylvania

**Steven A. Rosenberg, MD, PhD**
Chief, Surgery Branch, National Cancer
    Institute, National Institutes of Health
Professor of Surgery, Uniformed Services
    University of the Health Sciences
School of Medicine
Bethesda, Maryland
Professor of Surgery
George Washington University School of
    Medicine
Washington, District of Columbia

**M. Wasif Saif, MD, MBBS**
Director, Gastrointestinal Oncology
    Program
Leader, Experimental Therapeutics
    Program
Tufts Medical Center
Tufts University School of Medicine
Boston, Massachusetts

**Yardena Samuels, PhD**
Knell Family Professorial Chair
Department of Molecular Cell Biology
Weizmann Institute of Science
Rehovot, Israel

**Charles L. Sawyers, MD**
Investigator, Howard Hughes Medical
    Institute
Chair, Human Oncology and
    Pathogenesis Program
Memorial Sloan-Kettering Cancer Center
New York, New York

**Peter T. Scardino, MD**
Chairman, Department of Surgery
The David H. Koch Chair
Memorial Sloan-Kettering Cancer Center
New York, New York

**Howard I. Scher, MD**
Chief, Genitourinary Oncology Service
Member and Attending Physician
Department of Medicine
Memorial Sloan-Kettering Cancer Center
Professor of Medicine
Weill Cornell Medical College
New York, New York

**Laura S. Schmidt, PhD**
Principal Scientist
Leidos Biomedical Research, Inc.
Frederick National Laboratory for Cancer
    Research
Frederick, Maryland
Urologic Oncology Branch
National Cancer Institute
National Institutes of Health
Bethesda, Maryland

**Peter G. Shields, MD**
Deputy Director, Comprehensive Cancer
    Center
Professor, College of Medicine
James Cancer Hospital
The Ohio State University
Columbus, Ohio

**Alex Sparreboom, PhD**
Associate Member, Department of
Pharmaceutical Sciences
St. Jude Children's Research Hospital
Memphis, Tennessee

**Irene M. Tamí-Maury, DMD, DrPH, MSc**
The University of Texas MD Anderson
Cancer Center
Houston, Texas

**Randall K. Ten Haken, PhD, FAAPM,
FInstP, FASTRO, FACR**
Professor, Associate Chair, and Physics
Division Director
Department of Radiation Oncology
University of Michigan Medical School
Ann Arbor, Michigan

**Kenneth D. Tew, PhD, DSc**
Chairman and John C. West Chair in
Cancer Research
Cell and Molecular Pharmacology
Medical University of South Carolina
Charleston, South Carolina

**Benjamin A. Toll, PhD**
Associate Professor of Psychiatry
Yale University School of Medicine
Yale Comprehensive Cancer Center
Program Director, Smoking Cessation
Service
Smilow Cancer Hospital at Yale-New
Haven
New Haven, Connecticut

**Edouard J. Trabulsi, MD, FACS**
Associate Professor, Department of
Urology
Kimmel Cancer Center
Jefferson Medical College
Director, Division of Urologic Oncology
Thomas Jefferson University
Philadelphia, Pennsylvania

**Brian B. Tuch, PhD**
Associate Director, Translational
Genomics
Onyx Pharmaceuticals
South San Francisco, California

**Robert G. Uzzo, MD**
Professor and Chairman, Department of
Surgery
Fox Chase Cancer Center
Temple University Health System
Philadelphia, Pennsylvania

**Christine M. Walko, PharmD, BCOP**
Clinical Pharmacogenetic Scientist
DeBartolo Family Personalized Medicine
Institute
Applied Clinical Scientist, Division of
Population Science
H. Lee Moffitt Cancer Center and
Research Institute
Tampa, Florida

**Graham W. Warren, MD, PhD**
Associate Professor
Vice Chair for Research in Radiation
Oncology
Department of Radiation Oncology
Department of Cell and Molecular
Pharmacology
Hollings Cancer Center
Medical University of South Carolina
Charleston, South Carolina

**Robert A. Weinberg, PhD**
Member, Whitehead Institute for
Biomedical Research
Department of Biology
Massachusetts Institute of Technology
Director, Ludwig Center for Molecular
Oncology
Whitehead Institute for Biomedical
Research
Cambridge, Massachusetts

**Louis M. Weiner, MD**
Director, Lombardi Comprehensive
Cancer Center
Professor and Chair, Department of
Oncology
Francis L. and Charlotte G. Gragnani
Chair
Georgetown University Medical Center
Washington, District of Columbia

**Walter C. Willett, MD, DrPH**
Professor and Chair, Department of
Nutrition
Harvard School of Public Health
Boston, Massachusetts

**Herbert Yu, MD, PhD**
Professor and Director
Cancer Epidemiology Program
Associate Director for Population
Sciences and Cancer Control
University of Hawaii Cancer Center
Adjunct Professor, Department of
Chronic Disease Epidemiology
Yale School of Public Health
Honolulu, Hawaii

**Stuart H. Yuspa, MD**
Chief, Laboratory of Cancer Biology and
Genetics
Center for Cancer Research
National Cancer Institute
Bethesda, Maryland

**Michael J. Zelefsky, MD**
Chief, Brachytherapy Service
Department of Radiation Oncology
Memorial Sloan-Kettering Cancer Center
New York, New York

**Anthony L. Zietman, MD**
Jenot and William Shipley Professor of
Radiation Oncology
Department of Radiation Oncology
Massachusetts General Hospital
Harvard Medical School
Boston, Massachusetts

# CONTENTS

## PART IV

# Cancer Prevention and Screening

## PART V

# Cancers of the Genitourinary System

## PART I

# Principles
# of Oncology

# 1 The Cancer Genome

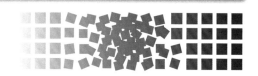

Yardena Samuels, Alberto Bardelli, Jared J. Gartner, and Carlos López-Otin

## INTRODUCTION

There is a broad consensus that cancer is, in essence, a genetic disease, and that accumulation of molecular alterations in the genome of somatic cells is the basis of cancer progression (Fig. 1.1).[1] In the past 10 years, the availability of the human genome sequence and progress in DNA sequencing technologies has dramatically improved knowledge of this disease. These new insights are transforming the field of oncology at multiple levels:

1. The genomic maps are redesigning the tumor taxonomy by moving it from a histologic- to a genetic-based level.
2. The success of cancer drugs designed to target the molecular alterations underlying tumorigenesis has proven that somatic genetic alterations are legitimate targets for therapy.
3. Tumor genotyping is helping clinicians individualize treatments by matching patients with the best treatment for their tumors.
4. Tumor-specific DNA alterations represent highly sensitive biomarkers for disease detection and monitoring.
5. Finally, the ongoing analyses of multiple cancer genomes will identify additional targets, whose pharmacologic exploitation will undoubtedly result in new therapeutic approaches.

This chapter will review the progress that has been made in understanding the genetic basis of sporadic cancers. An emphasis will be placed on an introduction to novel integrated genomic approaches that allow a comprehensive and systematic evaluation of genetic alterations that occur during the progression of cancer. Using these powerful tools, cancer research, diagnosis, and treatment are poised for a transformation in the next years.

## CANCER GENES AND THEIR MUTATIONS

Cancer genes are broadly grouped into oncogenes and tumor suppressor genes. Using a classical analogy, oncogenes can be compared to a car accelerator, so that a mutation in an oncogene would be the equivalent of having the accelerator continuously pressed.[2] Tumor suppressor genes, in contrast, act as brakes,[2] so that when they are not mutated, they function to inhibit tumorigenesis. Oncogene and tumor suppressor genes may be classified by the nature of their somatic mutations in tumors. Mutations in oncogenes typically occur at specific hotspots, often affecting the same codon or clustered at neighboring codons in different tumors.[1] Furthermore, mutations in oncogenes are almost always missense, and the mutations usually affect only one allele, making them heterozygous. In contrast, tumor suppressor genes are usually mutated throughout the gene; a large number of the mutations may truncate the encoded protein and generally affect both alleles, causing loss of heterozygosity (LOH). Major types of somatic mutations present in malignant tumors include nucleotide substitutions, small insertions and deletions (*indels*), chromosomal rearrangements, and copy number alterations.

## IDENTIFICATION OF CANCER GENES

The completion of the Human Genome Project marked a new era in biomedical sciences.[3] Knowledge of the sequence and organization of the human genome now allows for the systematic analysis of the genetic alterations underlying the origin and evolution of tumors. Before elucidation of the human genome, several cancer genes, such as *KRAS*, *TP53*, and *APC*, were successfully discovered using approaches based on an oncovirus analysis, linkage studies, LOH, and cytogenetics.[4,5] The first curated version of the Human Genome Project was released in 2004,[3] and provided a sequence-based map of the normal human genome. This information, together with the construction of the HapMap, which contains single nucleotide polymorphisms (SNP), and the underlying genomic structure of natural human genomic variation,[6,7] allowed an extraordinary throughput in cataloging somatic mutations in cancer. These projects now offer an unprecedented opportunity: the identification of all the genetic changes associated with a human cancer. For the first time, this ambitious goal is within reach of the scientific community. Already, a number of studies have demonstrated the usefulness of strategies aimed at the systematic identification of somatic mutations associated with cancer progression. Notably, the Human Genome Project, the HapMap project, as well as the candidate and family gene approaches (described in the following paragraphs), utilized capillary-based DNA sequencing (first-generation sequencing, also known as Sanger sequencing).[8] Figure 1.2 clearly illustrates the developments in the search of cancer genes, its increased pace, as well as the most relevant findings in this field.

### Cancer Gene Discovery by Sequencing Candidate Gene Families

The availability of the human genome sequence provides new opportunities to comprehensively search for somatic mutations in cancer on a larger scale than previously possible. Progress in the field has been closely linked to improvements in the throughput of DNA analysis and in the continuous reduction in sequencing costs. What follows are some of the achievements in this research area, as well as how they affected knowledge of the cancer genome.

A seminal work in the field was the systematic mutational profiling of the genes involved in the RAS-RAF pathway in multiple tumors. This candidate gene approach led to the discovery that *BRAF* is frequently mutated in melanomas and is mutated at a lower frequency in other tumor types.[9] Follow-up studies quickly revealed that mutations in *BRAF* are mutually exclusive with alterations in *KRAS*,[9,10] genetically emphasizing that these genes function in the same pathway, a concept that had been previously demonstrated in lower organisms such as *Caenorhabditis elegans* and *Drosophila melanogaster*.[11,12]

In 2003, the identification of cancer genes shifted from a candidate gene approach to the mutational analyses of gene families. The first gene families to be completely sequenced were those that

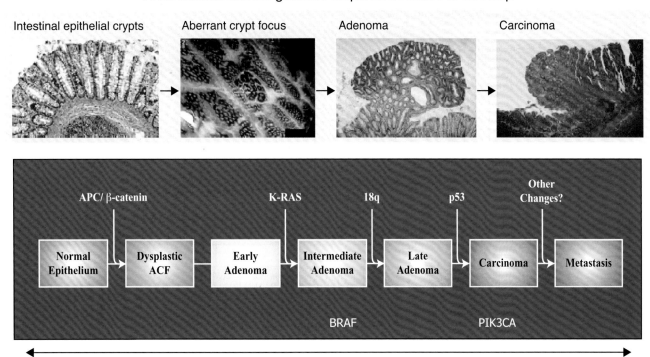

Figure 1.1 Schematic representation of the genomic and histopathologic steps associated with tumor progression: from the occurrence of the initiating mutation in the founder cell to metastasis formation. It has been convincingly shown that the genomic landscape of solid tumors such as that of pancreatic and colorectal tumors requires the accumulation of many genetic events, a process that requires decades to complete. This timeline offers an incredible window of opportunity for the early detection, which is often associated with an excellent prognosis, of this disease.

involved protein[13,14] and lipid phosphorylation.[15] The rationale for initially focusing on these gene families was threefold:

- The corresponding proteins were already known at that time to play a pivotal role in the signaling and proliferation of normal and cancerous cells.
- Multiple members of the protein kinases family had already been linked to tumorigenesis.
- Kinases are clearly amenable to pharmacologic inhibition, making them attractive drug targets.

The mutational analysis of all the tyrosine-kinase domains in colorectal cancers revealed that 30% of cases had a mutation in at least one tyrosine-kinase gene, and overall mutations were identified in eight different kinases, most of which had not previously been linked to cancer.[13] An additional mutational analysis of the coding exons of 518 protein kinase genes in 210 diverse human cancers, including breast, lung, gastric, ovarian, renal, and acute lymphoblastic leukemia, identified approximately 120 mutated genes that probably contribute to oncogenesis.[14] Because kinase activity is attenuated by enzymes that remove phosphate groups called phosphatases, the rational next step in these studies was to perform a mutation analysis of the protein tyrosine phosphatases. A mutational investigation of this family in colorectal cancer identified that 25% of cases had mutations in six different phosphatase genes (*PTPRF, PTPRG, PTPRT, PTPN3, PTPN13,* or *PTPN14*).[16] A combined analysis of the protein tyrosine kinases and the protein tyrosine phosphatases showed that 50% of colorectal cancers had mutations in a tyrosine-kinase gene, a protein tyrosine phosphatase gene, or both, further emphasizing the pivotal role of protein phosphorylation in neoplastic progression. Many of the identified genes had previously been linked to human cancer, thus validating

the unbiased comprehensive mutation profiling. These landmark studies led to additional gene family surveys.

The phosphatidylinositol 3-kinase (*PI3K*) gene family, which also plays a role in proliferation, adhesion, survival, and motility, was also comprehensively investigated.[17] Sequencing of the exons encoding the kinase domain of all 16 members belonging to this family pinpointed *PIK3CA* as the only gene to harbor somatic mutations. When the entire coding region was analyzed, *PIK3CA* was found to be somatically mutated in 32% of colorectal cancers. At that time, the *PIK3CA* gene was certainly not a newcomer in the cancer arena, because it had previously been shown to be involved in cell transformation and metastasis.[17] Strikingly, its staggeringly high mutation frequency was discovered only through systematic sequencing of the corresponding gene family.[15] Subsequent analysis of *PIK3CA* in other tumor types identified somatic mutations in this gene in additional cancer types, including 36% of hepatocellular carcinomas, 36% of endometrial carcinomas, 25% of breast carcinomas, 15% of anaplastic oligodendrogliomas, 5% of medulloblastomas and anaplastic astrocytomas, and 27% of glioblastomas.[18–22] It is known that *PIK3CA* is one of the two (the other being *KRAS*) most commonly mutated oncogenes in human cancers. Further investigation of the *PI3K* pathway in colorectal cancer showed that 40% of tumors had genetic alterations in one of the *PI3K* pathway genes, emphasizing the central role of this pathway in colorectal cancer pathogenesis.[23]

Although most cancer genome studies of large gene families have focused on the kinome, recent analyses have revealed that members of other families highly represented in the human genome are also a target of mutational events in cancer. This is the case of proteases, a complex group of enzymes consisting of at least 569 components that constitute the so-called human degradome.[24] Proteases exhibit an elaborate interplay with kinases and

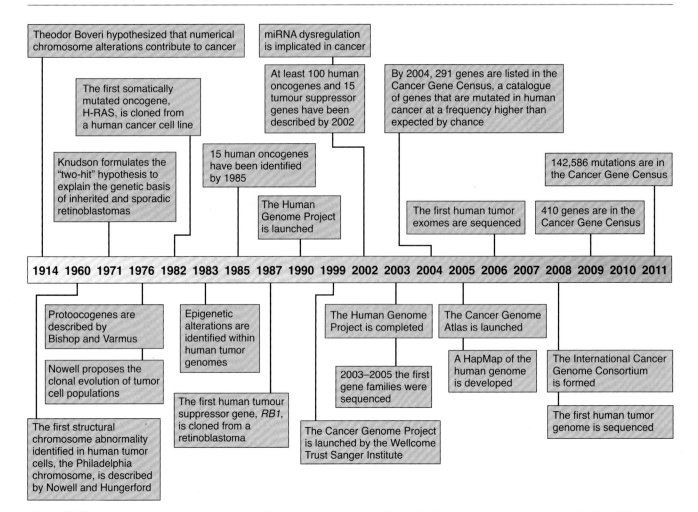

**Figure 1.2** Timeline of seminal hypotheses, research discoveries, and research initiatives that have led to an improved understanding of the genetic etiology of human tumorigenesis within the past century. The consensus cancer gene data were obtained from the Wellcome Trust Sanger Institute Cancer Genome Project Web site (http://www.sanger.ac.uk/genetics/CGP). (Redrawn from Bell DW. Our changing view of the genomic landscape of cancer. *J Pathol* 2010;220:231–243.)

have traditionally been associated with cancer progression because of their ability to degrade extracellular matrices, thus facilitating tumor invasion and metastasis.[25,26] However, recent studies have shown that these enzymes hydrolyze a wide variety of substrates and influence many different steps of cancer, including early stages of tumor evolution.[27] These functional studies have also revealed that beyond their initial recognition as prometastatic enzymes, they play dual roles in cancer, as assessed by the identification of a growing number of tumor-suppressive proteases.[28]

These findings emphasized the possibility that mutational activation or inactivation of protease genes occurs in cancer. A systematic analysis of genetic alterations in breast and colorectal cancers revealed that proteases from different catalytic classes were somatically mutated in cancer.[29] These results prompted the mutational analysis of entire protease families such as matrix metalloproteinases (MMP), a disintegrin and metalloproteinase (ADAM), and ADAMs with thrombospondin domains (ADAMTS) in different tumors. These studies led to the identification of protease genes frequently mutated in cancer, such as *MMP8*, which is mutated and functionally inactivated in 6.3% of human melanomas.[30,31]

The mutational status of caspases has also been extensively analyzed in different tumors because these proteases play a fundamental role in the execution of apoptosis, one of the hallmarks of cancer.[32] These studies demonstrated that *CASP8* is deleted in neuroblastomas and inactivated by somatic mutations in a variety of human malignancies, including head and neck, colorectal, lung, and gastric carcinomas.[33–35] Other large protease families

whose components are often mutated in cancer are the deubiquitinating enzymes (DUB), which catalyze the removal of ubiquitin and ubiquitin-like modifiers of their target proteins.[36] Some DUBs were initially identified as oncogenic proteins, but further work has shown that other deubiquitinases, such as CYLD, A20, and BAP1, are tumor suppressors inactivated in cancer. *CYLD* is mutated in patients with familial cylindromatosis, a disease characterized by the formation of multiple tumors of skin appendages.[37] A20 is a DUB family member encoded by the *TNFAIP3* gene, which is mutated in a large number of Hodgkin lymphomas and primary mediastinal B-cell lymphomas.[38–41] Finally, the *BAP1* gene, encoding an ubiquitin C-terminal hydrolase, is frequently mutated in metastasizing uveal melanomas[42] and in other human malignancies, such as mesothelioma and renal cell carcinoma.[43]

## Mutational Analysis of Exomes Using Sanger Sequencing

Although the gene family approach for the identification of cancer genes has proven extremely valuable, it still is a candidate approach and thus biased in its nature. The next step forward in the mutational profiling of cancer has been the sequencing of exomes, which is the entire coding portion of the human genome (18,000 protein-encoding genes). The exomes of many different tumors—including breast, colorectal, pancreatic, and ovarian clear cell carcinomas; glioblastoma multiforme; and medulloblastoma—have been analyzed using Sanger sequencing. For the first time, these large-scale analyses allowed researchers to describe and understand the genetic complexity of human cancers.[29,44–48] The declared goals of these exome studies were to provide methods for exomewide mutational analyses in human tumors, to characterize their spectrum and quantity of somatic mutations, and, finally, to discover new genes involved in tumorigenesis as well as novel pathways that have a role in these tumors. In these studies, sequencing data were complemented with gene expression and copy number analyses, thus providing a comprehensive view of the genetic complexity of human tumors.[45–48] A number of conclusions can be drawn from these analyses, including the following:

- Cancer genomes have an average of 30 to 100 somatic alterations per tumor in coding regions, which was a higher number than previously thought. Although the alterations included point mutations, small insertions, deletions, or amplifications, the great majority of the mutations observed were single-base substitutions.[45,46]

- Even within a single cancer type, there is a significant intertumor heterogeneity. This means that multiple mutational patterns (encompassing different mutant genes) are present in tumors that cannot be distinguished based on histologic analysis. The concept that individual tumors have a unique genetic milieu is highly relevant for personalized medicine, a concept that will be further discussed.

- The spectrum and nucleotide contexts of mutations differ between different tumor types. For example, over 50% of mutations in colorectal cancer were C:G to T:A transitions, and 10% were C:G to G:C transversions. In contrast, in breast cancers, only 35% of the mutations were C:G to T:A transitions, and 29% were C:G to G:C transversions. Knowledge of mutation spectra is vital because it allows insight into the mechanisms underlying mutagenesis and repair in the various cancers investigated.

- A considerably larger number of genes that had not been previously reported to be involved in cancer were found to play a role in the disease.

- Solid tumors arising in children, such as medulloblastomas, harbor on average 5 to 10 times less gene alterations compared to a typical adult solid tumor. These pediatric tumors also harbor fewer amplifications and homozygous deletions within coding genes compared to adult solid tumors.

Importantly, to deal with the large amount of data generated in these genomic projects, it was necessary to develop new statistical and bioinformatic tools. Furthermore, an examination of the overall distribution of the identified mutations allowed for the development of a novel view of cancer genome landscapes and a novel definition of cancer genes. These new concepts in the understanding of cancer genetics are further discussed in the following paragraphs. The compiled conclusions derived from these analyses have led to a paradigm shift in the understanding of cancer genetics.

A clear indication of the power of the unbiased nature of the whole exome surveys was revealed by the discovery of recurrent mutations in the active site of *IDH1*, a gene with no known link to gliomas, in 12% of tumors analyzed.[46] Because malignant gliomas are the most common and lethal tumors of the central nervous system, and because glioblastoma multiforme (GBM; World Health Organization grade IV astrocytoma) is the most biologically aggressive subtype, the unveiling of *IDH1* as a novel GBM gene is extremely significant. Importantly, mutations of *IDH1* predominantly occurred in younger patients and were associated with a better prognosis.[49] Follow-up studies showed that mutations of *IDH1* occur early in glioma progression; the R132 somatic mutation is harbored by the majority (greater than 70%) of grades II and III astrocytomas and oligodendrogliomas, as well as in secondary GBMs that develop from these lower grade lesions.[49–55] In contrast, less than 10% of primary GBMs harbor these alterations. Furthermore, analysis of the associated *IDH2* revealed recurrent somatic mutations in the R172 residue,

which is the exact analog of the frequently mutated R132 residue of *IDH1*. These mutations occur mostly in a mutually exclusive manner with *IDH1* mutations,[49,51] suggesting that they have equivalent phenotypic effects. Subsequently, *IDH1* mutations have been reported in additional cancer types, including hematologic neoplasias.[56–58]

## Next-Generation Sequencing and Cancer Genome Analysis

In 1977, the introduction of the Sanger method for DNA sequencing with chain-terminating inhibitors transformed biomedical research.[8] Over the past 30 years, this first-generation technology has been universally used for elucidating the nucleotide sequence of DNA molecules. However, the launching of new large-scale projects, including those implicating whole-genome sequencing of cancer samples, has made necessary the development of new methods that are widely known as next-generation sequencing technologies.[59–61] These approaches have significantly lowered the cost and the time required to determine the sequence of the $3 \times 10^9$ nucleotides present in the human genome. Moreover, they have a series of advantages over Sanger sequencing, which are of special interest for the analysis of cancer genomes.[62] First, next-generation sequencing approaches are more sensitive than Sanger methods and can detect somatic mutations even when they are present in only a subset of tumor cells.[63] Moreover, these new sequencing strategies are quantitative and can be used to simultaneously determine both nucleotide sequence and copy number variations.[64] They can also be coupled to other procedures such as those involving paired-end reads, allowing for the identification of multiple structural alterations, such as insertions, deletions, and rearrangements, that commonly occur in cancer genomes.[63] Nonetheless, next-generation sequencing still presents some limitations that are mainly derived from the relatively high error rate in the short reads generated during the sequencing process. In addition, these short reads make the task of de novo assembly of the generated sequences and the mapping of the reads to a reference genome extremely complex. To overcome some of these current limitations, deep coverage of each analyzed genome is required and a careful validation of the identified variants must be performed, typically using Sanger sequencing. As a consequence, there is a substantial increase in both the cost of the process and in the time of analysis. Therefore, it can be concluded that whole-genome sequencing of cancer samples is already a feasible task, but not yet a routine process. Further technical improvements will be required before the task of decoding the entire genome of any malignant tumor of any cancer patient can be applied to clinical practice.

The number of next-generation sequencing platforms has substantially grown over the past few years and currently includes technologies from Roche/454, Illumina/Solexa, Life/APG's SOLiD3, Helicos BioSciences/HeliScope, and Pacific Biosciences/PacBio RS.[61] Noteworthy also are the recent introduction of the Polonator G.007 instrument, an open source platform with freely available software and protocols; the Ion Torrent's semiconductor sequencer; as well as those involving self-assembling DNA nanoballs or nanopore technologies.[65–67] These new machines are driving the field toward the era of third-generation sequencing, which brings enormous clinical interest because it can substantially increase the speed and accuracy of analyses at reduced costs and can facilitate the possibility of single-molecule sequencing of human genomes. A comparison of next-generation sequencing platforms is shown in Table 1.1. These various platforms differ in the method utilized for template preparation and in the nucleotide sequencing and imaging strategy, which finally result in their different performance. Ultimately, the most suitable approach depends on the specific genome sequencing projects.[61]

Current methods of template preparation first involve randomly shearing genomic DNA into smaller fragments, from which

**TABLE 1.1**

## Comparative Analysis of Next-Generation Sequencing Platforms

| Platform | Library/Template Preparation | Sequencing Method | Average Read-Length (Bases) | Run Time (Days) | Gb Per Run | Instrument Cost (U.S.$) | Comments |
|---|---|---|---|---|---|---|---|
| Roche 454 GS FLX | Fragment, mate-pair Emulsion PCR | Pyrosequencing | 400 | 0.35 | 0.45 | 500,000 | Fast run times High reagent cost |
| Illumina HiSeq 2000 | Fragment, mate-pair Solid phase | Reversible terminator | 100–125 | 8 (mate-pair run) | 150–200 | 540,000 | Most widely used platform Low multiplexing capability |
| Life/APG's SOLiD 5500xl | Fragment, mate-pair Emulsion PCR | Cleavable probe, sequencing by ligation | 35–75 | 7 (mate-pair run) | 180–300 | 595,000 | Inherent error correction Long run times |
| Helicos BioSciences HeliScope | Fragment, mate-pair Single molecule | Reversible terminator | 32 | 8 (fragment run) | 37 | 999,000 | Nonbias template representation Expensive, high error rates |
| Pacific Biosciences PacBio RS | Fragment Single molecule | Real-time sequencing | 1,000 | 1 | 0.075 | NA | Greatest potential for long reads Highest error rates |
| Polonator G.007 | Mate pair Emulsion PCR | Noncleavable probe, sequencing by ligation | 26 | 5 (mate-pair run) | 12 | 170,000 | Least expensive platform Shortest read lengths |

NA, not available.

Data represent an update of information provided in Metzker ML. Sequencing technologies—the next generation. *Nat Rev Genet* 2010;11:31–46.

a library of either fragment templates or mate-pair templates are generated. Then, clonally amplified templates from single DNA molecules are prepared by either emulsion polymerase chain reaction (PCR) or solid-phase amplification.[68,69] Alternatively, it is possible to prepare single-molecule templates through methods that require less starting material and that do not involve PCR amplification reactions, which can be the source of artifactual mutations.[70] Once prepared, templates are attached to a solid surface in spatially separated sites, allowing thousands to billions of nucleotide sequencing reactions to be performed simultaneously.

The sequencing methods currently used by the different next-generation sequencing platforms are diverse and have been classified into four groups: cyclic reversible termination, single-nucleotide addition, real-time sequencing, and sequencing by ligation (Fig. 1.3).[61,71] These sequencing strategies are coupled with different imaging methods, including those based on measuring bioluminescent signals or involving four-color imaging of single molecular events. Finally, the extraordinary amount of data released from these nucleotide sequencing platforms is stored, assembled, and analyzed using powerful bioinformatic tools that have been developed in parallel with next-generation sequencing technologies.[72]

Next-generation sequencing approaches represent the newest entry into the cancer genome decoding arena and have already been applied to cancer analyses. The first research group to apply these methodologies to whole cancer genomes was that of Ley et al.,[73] who reported in 2008 the sequencing of the entire genome of a patient with acute myeloid leukemia (AML) and its comparison with the normal tissue from the same patient, using the Illumina/Solexa platform. As further described, this work allowed for the identification of point mutations and structural alterations of putative oncogenic relevance in AML and represented proof

of principle of the relevance of next-generation sequencing for cancer research.

## Whole-Genome Analysis Utilizing Second-Generation Sequencing

The sequence of the first whole cancer genome was reported in 2008, where AML and normal skin from the same patient were described.[73] Numerous additional whole genomes, together with the corresponding normal genomes of patients with a variety of malignant tumors, have been reported since then.[56,63,74–86]

The first available whole genome of a cytogenetically normal AML subtype M1 (AML-M1) revealed eight genes with novel mutations along with another 500 to 1,000 additional mutations found in noncoding regions of the genome. Most of the identified genes had not been previously associated with cancer. However, validation of the detected mutations did not identify novel recurring mutations in AML.[73] Concomitantly, with the expansion in the use of next-generation sequencers, many other whole genomes from a number of cancer types started to be evaluated in a similar manner (Fig. 1.4).[87]

In contrast to the first AML whole genome, the second did observe a recurrent mutation in *IDH1*, encoding isocitrate dehydrogenase.[56] Follow-up studies extended this finding and reported that mutations in *IDH1* and the related gene *IDH2* occur at a 20% to 30% frequency in AML patients and are associated with a poor prognosis in some subgroups of patients.[79,80,88] A good example illustrating the high pace at which second-generation technologies and their accompanying analytical tools are found is demonstrated by the following finding derived from a reanalysis of the first AML whole genome. Thus, when improvements in sequencing

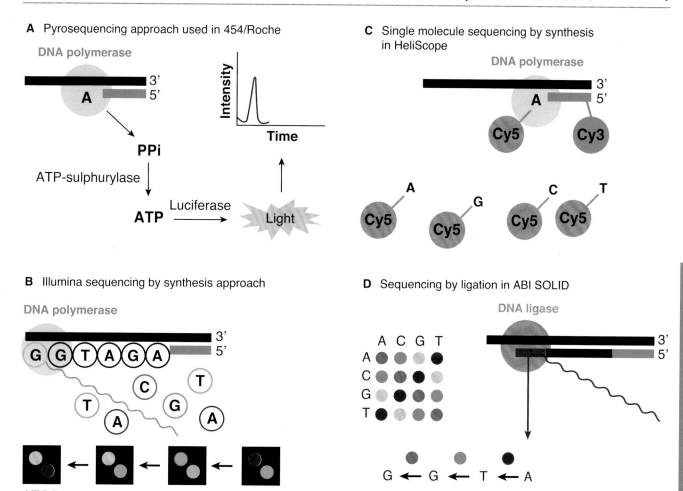

**A** Pyrosequencing approach used in 454/Roche

**B** Illumina sequencing by synthesis approach

**C** Single molecule sequencing by synthesis in HeliScope

**D** Sequencing by ligation in ABI SOLID

**Figure 1.3** Advances in sequencing chemistry implemented in next-generation sequencers. **(A)** The pyrosequencing approach implemented in 454/Roche sequencing technology detects incorporated nucleotides by chemiluminescence resulting from PPi release. **(B)** The Illumina method utilizes sequencing by synthesis in the presence of fluorescently labeled nucleotide analogs that serve as reversible reaction terminators. **(C)** The single-molecule sequencing by synthesis approach detects template extension using Cy3 and Cy5 labels attached to the sequencing primer and the incoming nucleotides, respectively. **(D)** The SOLiD method sequences templates by sequential ligation of labeled degenerate probes. Two-base encoding implemented in the SOLiD instrument allows for probing each nucleotide position twice. (From Morozova O, Hirst M, Marra MA. Applications of new sequencing technologies for transcriptome analysis. *Annu Rev Genomics Hum Genet* 2009;10:135–151.)

techniques were available, the first AML whole genome (described previously), which identified no recurring mutations and had a 91.2% diploid coverage, was reevaluated by deeper sequence coverage, yielding 99.6% diploid coverage of the genome. This improvement, together with more advanced mutation calling algorithms, allowed for the discovery of several nonsynonymous mutations that had not been identified in the initial sequencing. This included a frameshift mutation in the DNA methyltransferase gene *DNMT3A*. Validation of *DNMT3A* in 280 additional de novo AML patients to define recurring mutations led to the significant discovery that a total of 22.1% of AML cases had mutations in *DNMT3A* that were predicted to affect translation. The median overall survival among patients with *DNMT3A* mutations was significantly shorter than that among patients without such mutations (12.3 months versus 41.1 months; p <0.001).

Shortly after this study, complete sequences of a series of cancer genomes, together with matched normal genomes of the same patients, were reported.[56,78,83,84] These works opened the way to more ambitious initiatives, including those involving large international consortia, aimed at decoding the genome of malignant tumors from thousands of cancer patients. Thus, over the last 2 years, many whole genomes of different human malignancies have been made available.[74–76]

In addition to direct applications of next-generation sequencing technologies for the mutational analysis of cancer genomes, these methods have an additional range of applications in cancer research. Thus, genome sequencing efforts have begun to elucidate the genomic changes that accompany metastasis evolution through a comparative analysis of primary and metastatic lesions from breast and pancreatic cancer patients.[77,81,82,85] Likewise, massively parallel sequencing has been used to analyze the evolution of a tongue adenocarcinoma in response to selection by targeted kinase inhibitors.[89] Detailed information of several of these whole genome projects is found in the following paragraph.

The first solid cancer to undergo whole-genome sequencing was a malignant melanoma that was compared to a lymphoblastoid cell line from the same individual.[83] Impressively, a total of 33,345 somatic base substitutions were identified, with 187 nonsynonymous substitutions in protein-coding sequences, at least one order of magnitude higher than any other cancer type. Most somatic base substitutions were C:G > T:A transitions, and of the 510 dinucleotide substitutions, 360 were CC.TT/GG.AA changes, which is consistent with ultraviolet light exposure mutation signatures previously reported in melanoma.[14] Such results from the most comprehensive catalog of somatic mutations not only provide

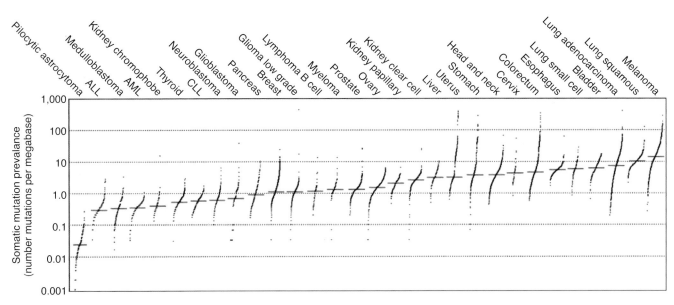

**Figure 1.4** The prevalence of somatic mutations across human cancer types. Every *dot* represents a sample, whereas the *red horizontal lines* are the median numbers of mutations in the respective cancer types. The vertical axis (log scaled) shows the number of mutations per megabase, whereas the different cancer types are ordered on the horizontal axis based on their median numbers of somatic mutations. ALL, acute lymphoblastic leukemia; AML, acute myeloid leukemia; CLL, chronic lymphocytic leukemia. (Used with permission from Alexandrov LB, Nik-Zainal S, Wedge DC, et al. Signatures of mutational processes in human cancer. *Nature* 2013;500:415–421.)

insight into the DNA damage signature in this cancer type, but can also be useful in determining the relative order of some acquired mutations. Indeed, this study shows that a significant correlation exists between the presence of a higher proportion of C.A/G.T transitions in early (82%) compared to late mutations (53%). Another important aspect that the comprehensive nature of this melanoma study provided was that cancer mutations are spread out unevenly throughout the genome, with a lower prevalence in regions of transcribed genes, suggesting that DNA repair occurs mainly in these areas.

An interesting and pioneering example of the power of whole-genome sequencing in deciphering the mutation evolution in carcinogenesis was seen in a study in which a basallike breast cancer tumor, a brain metastasis, a tumor xenograft derived from the primary tumor, and the peripheral blood from the same patient were compared (Fig. 1.5).[85] This analysis showed a wide range of

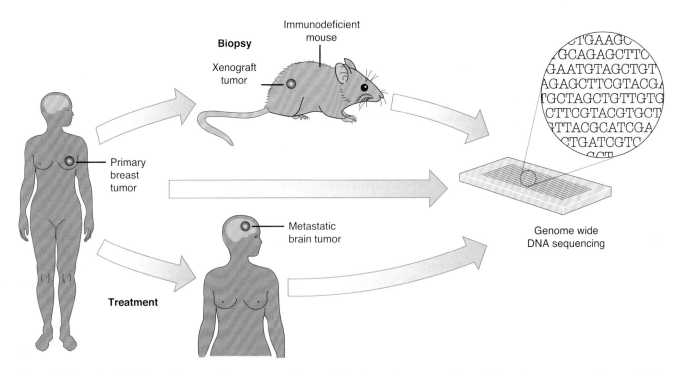

**Figure 1.5** Covering all the bases in metastatic assessment. Ding et al.[85] performed a genomewide analysis on three tumor samples: a patient's primary breast tumor; her metastatic brain tumor, which formed despite therapy; and a xenograft tumor in a mouse, originating from the patient's breast tumor. They find that the primary tumor differs from the metastatic and xenograft tumors mainly in the prevalence of genomic mutations. (With permission from Gray J. Cancer: genomics of metastasis. *Nature* 2010;464:989–990.)

mutant allele frequencies in the primary tumor, which was narrowed in the metastasis and xenograft samples. This suggested that the primary tumor was significantly more heterogeneous in its cell populations compared to its matched metastasis and xenograft samples because these underwent selection processes whether during metastasis or transplantation. The clear overlap in mutation incidence between the metastatic and xenograft cases suggests that xenografts undergo similar selection as metastatic lesions and, therefore, are a reliable source for genomic analyses. The main conclusion of this whole-genome study was that, although metastatic tumors harbor an increased number of genetic alterations, the majority of the alterations found in the primary tumor are preserved. Interestingly, single-cell genome sequencing of a breast primary tumour and its liver metastasis indicated that a single clonal expansion formed the primary tumor and seeded the metastasis.[90] Further studies have confirmed and extended these findings to metastatic tumors from different types, including renal and pancreatic carcinomas.[91]

The importance of performing whole-genome sequencing has also been emphasized by the recent identification of somatic mutations in regulatory regions, which can also elicit tumorigenesis. In a study reviewing the noncoding mutations in 19 melanoma whole-genome samples, two recurrent mutations in 17 of the 19 cases studied within the *telomerase reverse transcriptase (TERT)* promoter region were revealed.[92] When these two mutations were investigated in an extension of 51 additional tumors and their matched normal tissues, it was observed that 33 tumors harbored one of the mutations and that the mutations occurred in a mutually exclusive manner. These two mutations generate an identical 11 bp nucleotide stretch that contains the consensus binding site for E-twenty-six (ETS) transcription factors. When cloned into a luciferase reporter assay system, it was shown that these mutations conferred a two- to fourfold increase in transcriptional activity of this promoter in five melanoma cell lines. Although this alteration is much more frequent in melanoma, it is also present in other cancer types because 16% of the cancers listed in the Cancer Cell Line Encyclopedia harbor one of the two *TERT* mutations. In combination, these *TERT* mutations are seen in a greater frequency than *BRAF*- and *NRAS*-activating mutations. They occur in a mutually exclusive manner and in regions that do not show a large background mutation rate, all suggesting that these mutations are important driver events contributing to oncogenesis. Further supporting this was another recent study that identified these same two mutations in the germ line of familial melanoma patients.[93]

As the *TERT* promoter mutation discovery shows, regions of the genome that do not code for proteins are just as vital in our understanding of the biology behind tumor development and progression. Another class of non–protein-coding regions in the genome are the noncoding RNAs. One class of noncoding RNAs are microRNAs (miRNA). Discovered 20 years ago, miRNAs are known to be expressed in a tissue or developmentally specific manner and their expression can influence cellular growth and differentiation along with cancer-related pathways such as apoptosis or stress response. miRNAs do this through either overexpression, leading to the targeting and downregulation of tumor suppressor genes, or inversely through their own downregulation, leading to increased expression of their target oncogene. miRNAs have been extensively studied in cancer and their functional effects have been noted in a wide variety of cancers like glioma[94] and breast cancer,[95] to name just a few.

Another class of noncoding RNAs (ncRNA) are the long noncoding RNAs (lncRNA). These RNAs are typically greater than 200 bp and can range up to 100 kb in size. They are transcribed by RNA polymerase II and can undergo splicing and polyadenylation. Although much less extensively studied when compared to miRNAs for their role in cancer, lncRNAs are beginning to come under much more scrutiny. A recent study of the steroid receptor RNA activator (SRA) revealed two transcripts, a lncRNA (SRA) and a translated transcript (steroid receptor RNA activator protein

[SRAP]), that coexist within breast cancer cells. However, their expression varies within breast cancer cell lines with different phenotypes. It was shown that in a more invasive breast cancer line, higher relative levels of the noncoding transcript were seen.[96] Because this ncRNA acts as part of a ribonucleoprotein complex that is recruited to the promoter region of regulatory genes, it has been hypothesized that this shift in balance between both noncoding and coding transcripts may be associated with growth advantages. When this balance was shifted in vitro, it led to a large increase in transcripts associated with invasion and migration. The results of this study highlight the importance of the investigation into the roles of ncRNA in tumor development or progression and confirm again that the study of coding variants is not sufficient in determining the full genomic spectrum of cancer.

It must be also noted that the recent analysis of whole genomes of many different human tumors has provided additional insights into cancer evolution. Thus, it has been demonstrated that multiple mutational processes are operative during cancer development and progression, each of which has the capacity to leave its particular mutational signature on the genome. A remarkable and innovative study in this regard was aimed at the generation of the entire catalog of somatic mutations in 21 breast carcinomas and the identification of the mutational signatures of the underlying processes. This analysis revealed the occurrence of multiple, distinct single- and double-nucleotide substitution signatures. Moreover, it was reported that breast carcinomas harboring *BRCA1* or *BRCA2* mutations showed a characteristic combination of substitution mutation signatures and a particular profile of genomic deletions. An additional contribution of this analysis was the identification of a distinctive phenomenon of localized hypermutation, which has been termed *kataegis*, and which has also subsequently been observed in other malignancies distinct from breast carcinomas.[87]

Whole-genome sequencing of human carcinomas has also allowed for the ability to characterize other massive genomic alterations, termed *chromothripsis* and *chromoplexy*, occurring across different cancer subtypes.[97] Chromothripsis implies a massive genomic rearrangement acquired in a one-step catastrophic event during cancer development and has been detected in about 2% to 3% of all tumors, but is present at high frequency in some particular cases, such as bone cancers.[98] Chromoplexy has been originally described in prostate cancer and involves many DNA translocations and deletions that arise in a highly interdependent manner and result in the coordinate disruption of multiple cancer genes.[99] These newly described phenomena represent powerful strategies of rapid genome evolution, which may play essential roles during carcinogenesis.

## Whole-Exome Analysis Utilizing Second-Generation Sequencing

Another application of second-generation sequencing involves utilizing nucleic acid "baits" to capture regions of interest in the total pool of nucleic acids. These could either be DNA, as described previously,[100,101] or RNA.[102] Indeed, most areas of interest in the genome can be targeted, including exons and ncRNAs. Despite inefficiencies in the exome-targeting process—including the uneven capture efficiency across exons, which results in not all exons being sequenced, and the occurrence of some off-target hybridization events—the higher coverage of the exome makes it highly suitable for mutation discovery in cancer samples.

Over the last few years, thousands of cancer samples have been subjected to whole-exome sequencing. These studies, combined with data from whole-genome sequencing, have provided an unprecedented level of information about the mutational landscape of the most frequent human malignancies.[74–76] In addition, whole-exome sequencing has been used to identify the somatic mutations characteristic of both rare tumors and those that are prevalent in certain geographical regions.[76]

Overall, these studies have provided very valuable information about mutation rates and spectra across cancer types and sub-types.[87,103,104] Remarkably, the variation in mutational frequency between different tumors is extraordinary, with hematologic and pediatric cancers showing the lowest mutation rates (0.001 per Mb of DNA), and melanoma and lung cancers presenting the highest mutational burden (more than 400 per Mb). Whole-exome sequencing has also contributed to the identification of novel cancer genes that had not been previously described to be causally implicated in the carcinogenesis process. These genes belong to different functional categories, including signal transduction, RNA maturation, metabolic regulation, epigenetics, chromatin remodeling, and protein homeostasis.[74] Finally, a combination of data from whole-exome and whole-genome sequencing has allowed for the identification of the signatures of mutational processes operating in different cancer types.[87] Thus, an analysis of a dataset of about 5 million mutations from over 7,000 cancers from 30 different types has allowed for the extraction of more than 20 distinct mutational signatures. Some of them, such as those derived from the activity of APOBEC cytidine deaminases, are present in most cancer types, whereas others are characteristic of specific tumors. Known signatures associated with age, smoking, ultraviolet (UV) light exposure, and DNA repair defects have been also identified in this work, but many of the detected mutational signatures are of cryptic origin. These findings demonstrate the impressive diversity of mutational processes underlying cancer development and may have enormous implications for the future understanding of cancer biology, prevention, and treatment.

## SOMATIC ALTERATION CLASSES DETECTED BY CANCER GENOME ANALYSIS

Whole-genome sequencing of cancer genomes has an enormous potential to detect all major types of somatic mutations present in malignant tumors. This large repertoire of genomic abnormalities includes single nucleotide changes, small insertions and deletions, large chromosomal reorganizations, and copy number variations (Fig. 1.6).

Nucleotide substitutions are the most frequent somatic mutations detected in malignant tumors, although there is a substantial variability in the mutational frequency among different cancers.[60] On average, human malignancies have one nucleotide change per million bases, but melanomas reach mutational rates 10-fold higher, and tumors with mutator phenotype caused by DNA mismatch repair deficiencies may accumulate tens of mutations per million nucleotides. By contrast, tumors of hematopoietic origin have less than one base substitution per million. Several bioinformatic tools and pipelines have been developed to efficiently detect somatic nucleotide substitutions through comparison of the genomic information obtained from paired normal and tumor samples from the same patient. Likewise, there are a number of publicly available computational methods to predict the functional relevance of the identified mutations in cancer specimens.[60] Most of these bioinformatic tools exclusively deal with nucleotide changes in protein coding regions and evaluate the putative structural or functional effect of an amino acid substitution in a determined protein, thus obviating changes in other genomic regions, which can also be of crucial interest in cancer. In any case, current computational methods used in this regard are far from being optimal, and experimental validation is finally required to assess the functional relevance of nucleotide substitutions found in cancer genomes.

For years, the main focus of cancer genome analyses has been on identifying coding mutations that cause a change in the amino acid sequence of a gene. The rationale behind this is quite sound because any mutation that creates a novel protein or truncates an essential protein has the potential to drastically change the cellular environment. Examples of this have been shown earlier in the chapter with *BRAF* and *KRAS* along with many others. With the advancements in next-generation sequencing, larger studies are able to be conducted. These studies give the power to detect mutations occurring in the cancer genome at a lower frequency. Interesting to note is that these studies are leading to the discovery that recurrent synonymous mutations occur in cancer. Previously believed to be merely neutral mutations that maintain no functional role in tumorigenesis, these mutations were largely ignored, but a recent study shows[105] that simply dismissing these mutations as silent may be premature.

In a review of only 29 melanoma exomes and genomes, 16 recurring synonymous mutations were discovered. When these mutations were screened in additional samples, a synonymous mutation in the gene *BCL2L12* was discovered in 12 out of 285 total samples. The observed frequency of this recurrent mutation is greater than expected by chance, suggesting that it has undergone some type of selective pressure during tumor development.[105] Noting that *BCL2L12* had previously been linked to tumorigenesis, the mutation was further evaluated for its functional effect, with the finding that it led to an abrogation of the effect of a miRNA, leading to the deregulated expression of *BCL2L12*. BCL2L12 is a negative regulator of the gene p53, which functions by binding and inhibiting apoptosis in glioma.[106] Accordingly, the dysregulation observed in *BCL2L12* led to a reduction in p53 target gene expression.

Small insertions and deletions (*indels*) represent a second category of somatic mutations that can be discovered by whole-genome sequencing of cancer specimens. These mutations are about 10-fold less frequent than nucleotide substitutions, but may also have an obvious impact in cancer progression. Accordingly, specific bioinformatic tools have been created to detect these *indels* in the context of the large amount of information generated by whole-genome sequencing projects.[107]

The systematic identification of large chromosomal rearrangements in cancer genomes represents one of the most successful applications of next-generation sequencing methodologies. Previous strategies in this regard had mainly been based on the utilization of cytogenetic methods for the identification of recurrent translocations in hematopoietic tumors. More recently, a combination of bioinformatics and functional methods has allowed for the finding of recurrent translocations in solid epithelial tumors such as *TM-PRSS2–ERG* in prostate cancer and *EML4–ALK* in non–small-cell lung cancer.[108,109] Now, by using a next-generation sequencing analysis of genomes and transcriptomes, it is possible to systematically search for both intrachromosomal and interchromosomal rearrangements occurring in cancer specimens. These studies have already proven their usefulness for cancer research through the discovery of recurrent translocations involving genes of the *RAF* kinase pathway in prostate and gastric cancers and in melanomas.[110] Likewise, massively parallel paired-end genome and transcriptome sequencing has already been used to detect new gene fusions in cancer and to catalog all major structural rearrangements present in some tumors and cancer cell lines.[63,111–113] The ongoing cancer genome projects involving thousands of tumor samples will likely lead to the detection of many other chromosomal rearrangements of relevance in specific subsets of cancers. It is also remarkable that whole-genome sequencing may also facilitate the identification of other types of genomic alterations, including rearrangements of repetitive elements, such as active retrotransposons, or insertions of foreign gene sequences, such as viral genomes, which can contribute to cancer development. Indeed, a next-generation sequencing analysis of the transcriptome of Merkel cell carcinoma samples has revealed the clonal integration within the tumor genome of a previously unknown polyomavirus likely implicated in the pathogenesis of this rare but aggressive skin cancer.[114]

Finally, next-generation sequencing approaches have also demonstrated their feasibility to analyze the pattern of copy number

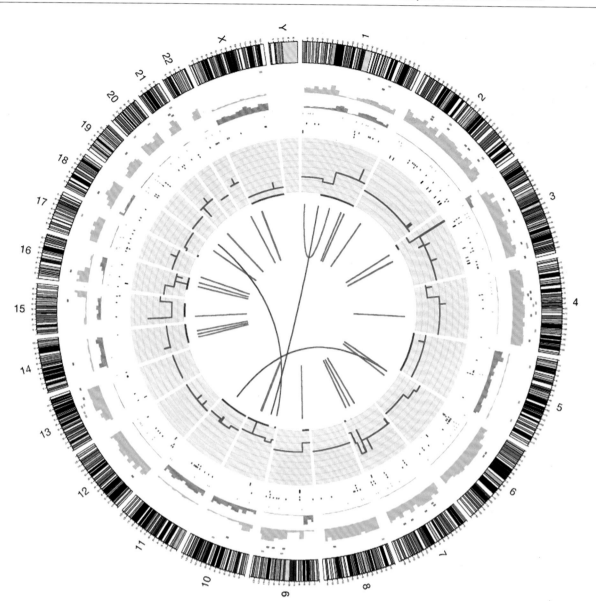

**Figure 1.6** The catalog of somatic mutations in COLO-829. Chromosome ideograms are shown around the *outer ring* and are oriented pter–qter in a clockwise direction with centromeres indicated in *red*. Other tracks contain somatic alterations (*from outside to inside*): validated insertions (*light green rectangles*); validated deletions (*dark green rectangles*); heterozygous (*light orange bars*), and homozygous (*dark orange bars*) substitutions shown by density per 10 megabases; coding substitutions (*colored squares: silent in gray, missense in purple, nonsense in red, and splice site in black*); copy number (*blue lines*); regions of loss of heterozygosity (LOH) (*red lines*); validated intrachromosomal rearrangements (*green lines*); validated interchromosomal rearrangements (*purple lines*). (From Pleasance ED, Cheetham RK, Stephens PJ, et al. A comprehensive catalogue of somatic mutations from a human cancer genome. *Nature* 2010;463:191–196.)

alterations in cancer, because they allow researchers to count the number of reads in both tumor and normal samples at any given genomic region and then to evaluate the tumor-to-normal copy number ratio at this particular region. These new methods offer some advantages when compared with those based on microarrays, including much better resolution, precise definition of the involved breakpoints, and absence of saturation, which facilitates the accurate estimation of high copy number levels occurring in some genomic loci of malignant tumors.[60]

## PATHWAY-ORIENTED MODELS OF CANCER GENOME ANALYSIS

Genomewide mutational analyses suggest that the mutational landscape of cancer is made up of a handful of genes that are mutated in a high fraction of tumors, otherwise known as *mountains*, and most mutated genes are altered at relatively low frequencies, otherwise known as *hills* (Fig. 1.7).[29] The mountains probably give a high selective advantage to the mutated cell, and the hills might provide a lower advantage, making it hard to distinguish them from passenger mutations. Because the hills differ between cancer types, it seems that the cancer genome is more complex and heterogeneous than anticipated. Although highly heterogeneous, bioinformatic studies suggest that the mountains and hills can be grouped into sets of pathways and biologic processes. Some of these pathways are affected by mutations in a few pathway members and others by numerous members. For example, pathway analyses have allowed for the stratification of mutated genes in pancreatic adenocarcinomas to 12 core pathways that have at least one member mutated in 67% to 100% of the tumors analyzed (Fig. 1.8).[45] These core pathways deviated to some that harbored one single highly mutated gene,

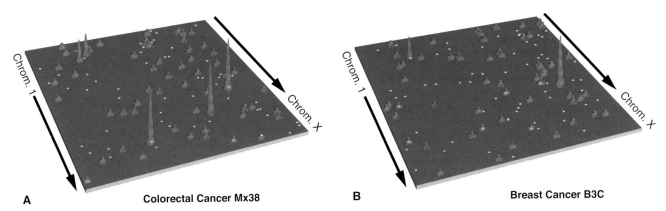

**A** Colorectal Cancer Mx38  **B** Breast Cancer B3C

**Figure 1.7** Cancer genome landscapes. Nonsilent somatic mutations are plotted in a two-dimensional space representing chromosomal positions of RefSeq genes. The telomere of the short arm of chromosome 1 is represented in the rear left corner of the *green plane* and ascending chromosomal positions continue in the direction of the arrow. Chromosomal positions that follow the front edge of the plane are continued at the back edge of the plane of the adjacent row, and chromosomes are appended end to end. Peaks indicate the 60 highest ranking CAN genes for each tumor type, with peak heights reflecting CaMP scores. The *dots* represent genes that were somatically mutated in the individual colorectal (Mx38) **(A)** or breast tumor (B3C) **(B)**. The *dots* corresponding to mutated genes that coincided with hills or mountains are black with white rims; the remaining *dots* are white with red rims. The mountain on the right of both landscapes represents *TP53* (chromosome 17), and the other mountain shared by both breast and colorectal cancers is *PIK3CA* (upper left, chromosome 3). (Redrawn from Wood LD, Parsons DW, Jones S, et al. The genomic landscapes of human breast and colorectal cancers. *Science* 2007;318:1108–1113. Reprinted with permission from the American Association for the Advancement of Science).

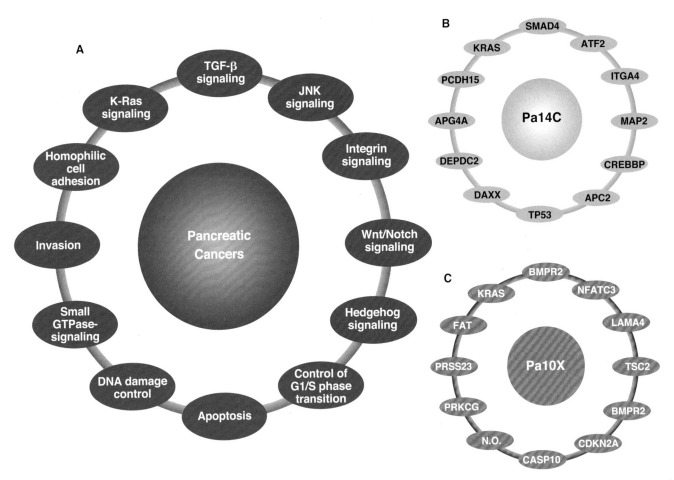

**Figure 1.8** Signaling pathways and processes. **(A)** The 12 pathways and processes whose component genes were genetically altered in most pancreatic cancers. **(B,C)** Two pancreatic cancers (Pa14C and Pa10X) and the specific genes that are mutated in them. The positions around the circles in **(B)** and **(C)** correspond to the pathways and processes in **(A)**. Several pathway components overlapped, as illustrated by the BMPR2 mutation that presumably disrupted both the SMAD4 and Hedgehog signaling pathways in Pa10X. Additionally, not all 12 processes and pathways were altered in every pancreatic cancer, as exemplified by the fact that no mutations known to affect DNA damage control were observed in Pa10X. NO, not observed. (Redrawn from Jones S, Zhang X, Parsons DW, et al. Core signaling pathways in human pancreatic cancers revealed by global genomic analyses. *Science* 2008;321:1801–1806. Reprinted with permission from the American Association for the Advancement of Science).

such as in *KRAS* in the G1/S cell cycle transition pathway and pathways where a few mutated genes were found, such as the transforming growth factor (TGF-β) signaling pathway. Finally, there were pathways in which many different genes were mutated, such as invasion regulation molecules, cell adhesion molecules, and integrin signaling. Importantly, independent of how many genes in the same pathway are affected, if they are found to occur in a mutually exclusive fashion in a single tumor, they most likely give the same selective pressure for clonal expansion.

The idea of genetically analyzing pathways rather than individual genes has been applied previously, revealing the concept of mutual exclusivity. Mutual exclusivity has been shown elegantly in the case of *KRAS* and *BRAF*, where a *KRAS*-mutated cancer generally does not also harbor a *BRAF* mutation, because *KRAS* is upstream of *BRAF* in the same pathway.[9] A similar concept was applied for *PIK3CA* and *PTEN*, where both mutations do not usually occur in the same tumor.[23]

With the ever expanding amounts of genetic information being gathered, the ability to search for common pathways being affected in cancer is increasing. One new pathway that is beginning to emerge is the glutamate-signaling pathway. Glutamate dysregulation has been implicated in a number of cancers. In a study of pancreatic duct adenocarcinoma (PDAC), it was seen that glutamate levels were significantly higher in the tissue of individuals with chronic pancreatitis (CP) and PDAC when compared to normal pancreas tissue.[115] It was also observed that the increased glutamate levels led to proinvasion and antiapoptotic signaling through the activation of AMPA receptors.

Also in this regard, and through the use of whole-exome sequencing, it has been recently shown that the glutamate receptor gene *GRIN2A* is highly mutated in melanoma. The finding that many of these mutations are nonsense has suggested that *GRIN2A* is a novel tumor suppressor. Additional genes in the glutamate pathway have also found mutated in melanomas.[116] Pathway analyses and statistical testing on the whole-exome data have also revealed the glutamate signaling pathway to be dysregulated. These results have been further corroborated in another study reporting mutations in the metabotropic glutamate receptor GRM3[117,118] in melanoma. A functional analysis of mutations found in *GRM3* in melanoma tumor samples has shown an increased activation of MEK1/2 kinase, increased migration, and anchorage-independent growth.[117]

## Passenger and Driver Mutations

By the time a cancer is diagnosed, it is comprised of billions of cells carrying DNA abnormalities, some of which have a functional role in malignant proliferation; however, many genetic lesions acquired along the way have no functional role in tumorigenesis.[14] The emerging landscapes of cancer genomes include thousands of genes that were not previously linked to tumorigenesis but are found to be somatically mutated. Many of these changes are likely to be *passengers*, or neutral, in that they have no functional effects on the growth of the tumor.[14] Only a small fraction of the genetic alterations are expected to drive cancer evolution by giving cells a selective advantage over their neighbors. Passenger mutations occur incidentally in a cell that later or in parallel develops a *driver* mutation, but are not ultimately pathogenic.[119] Although neutral, cataloging passengers mutations is important because they incorporate the signatures of the previous exposures the cancer cell underwent as well as DNA repair defects the cancer cell has. In many cases, the passenger and driver mutations occur at similar frequencies and the identification of drivers versus the passenger is of utmost relevance and remains a pressing challenge in cancer genetics.[120–122] This goal will eventually be achieved through a combination of genetic and functional approaches, some of which are listed as follows.

The most reliable indicator that a gene was selected for and therefore is highly likely to be pathogenic is the identification of recurrent mutations, whether at the same exact amino acid position

or in neighboring amino acid positions in different patients. More than that, if somatic alterations in the same gene occur very frequently (mountains in the tumor genome landscape), these can be confidently classified as drivers. For example, cancer alleles that are identified in multiple patients and different tumors types, such as those found in *KRAS*, *TP53*, *PTEN*, and *PIK3CA*, are clearly selected for during tumorigenesis.

However, most genes discovered thus far are mutated in a relatively small fraction of tumors (hills), and it has been clearly shown that genes that are mutated in less than 1% of patients can still act as *drivers*.[123] The systematic sequencing of newly identified putative cancer genes in the vast number of specimens from cancer patients will help in this regard. However, even if examining large numbers of samples can provide helpful information to classify drivers versus passengers, this approach alone is limited by the marked variation in mutation frequency among individual tumors and individual genes. The statistical test utilized in this case calculates the probability that the number of mutations in a given gene reflects a mutation frequency that is greater than expected from the nonfunctional background mutation rate,[29,124] which is different between different cancer types. These analyses incorporate the number of somatic alterations observed, the number of tumors studied, and the number of nucleotides that were successfully sequenced and analyzed.

Another approach often used to distinguish driver from passenger mutations exploits the statistical analysis of synonymous versus nonsynonymous changes.[125] In contrast to nonsynonymous mutations, synonymous mutations do not alter the protein sequence. Therefore, they do not usually apply a growth advantage and would not be expected to be selected during tumorigenesis. This strategy works by comparing the observed-to-expected ratio of synonymous with that of nonsynonymous mutation. An increased proportion of nonsynonymous mutations from the expected 2:1 ratio implies selection pressure during tumorigenesis.

Other approaches are based on the concept that driver mutations may have characteristics similar to those causing Mendelian disease when inherited in the germ line and may be identifiable by constraints on tolerated amino acid residues at the mutated positions. In contrast, passenger mutations may have characteristics more similar to those of nonsynonymous SNPs with high minor allele frequencies. Based on these premises, supervised machine learning methods have been used to predict which missense mutations are drivers.[126] Additional approaches to decipher drivers from passengers include the identification of mutations that affect locations that have previously been shown to be cancer causing in protein members of the same gene family. Enrichment for mutations in evolutionarily conserved residues are analyzed by algorithms, such as SIFT (sorting intolerant from tolerant (SIFT),[127] which estimates the effects of the different mutations identified.

Probably the most conclusive methods to identify driver mutations will be rigorous functional studies using biochemical assays as well as model organisms or cultured cells, using knockout and knockin of individual cancer alleles.[128] Unfortunately, these methods are not well suited to the analysis of the hundreds of gene candidates that arise from every large-scale cancer genome project. In conclusion, it is fair to say that sequencing cancer genomes is only the beginning of a journey that will ultimately be completed when the thousands of the newly discovered alleles are annotated as being the drivers of this disease. A summary of the various next-generation applications and approaches for their analysis is summarized in Figure 1.9 and Table 1.2.

## NETWORKS OF CANCER GENOME PROJECTS

The repertoire of oncogenic mutations is extremely heterogeneous, suggesting that it would be difficult for independent cancer genome initiatives to address the generation of comprehensive

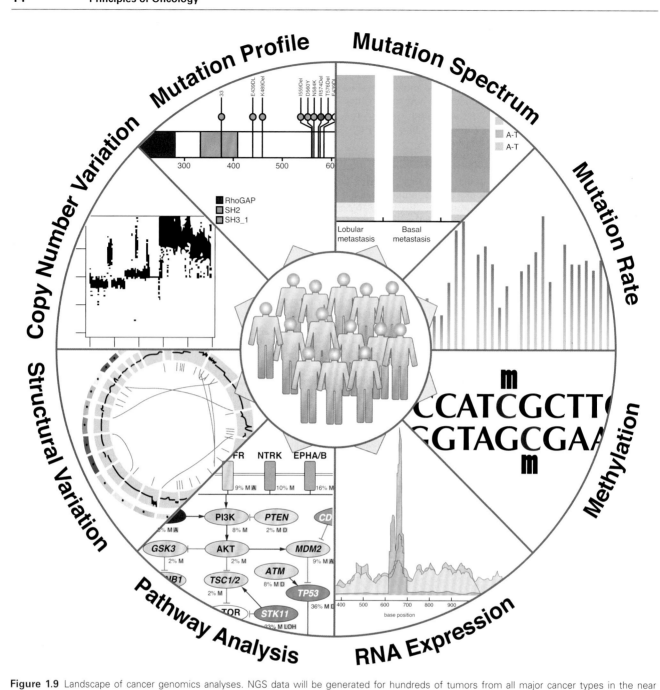

**Figure 1.9** Landscape of cancer genomics analyses. NGS data will be generated for hundreds of tumors from all major cancer types in the near future. The integrated analysis of DNA, RNA, and methylation sequencing data will help elucidate all relevant genetic changes in cancers. (Used with permission from Ding L, Wendl MC, Koboldt DC, et al. Analysis of next-generation genomic data in cancer: accomplishments and challenges. *Hum Mol Genet* 2010;19:R188–R196.)

catalogs of mutations in the wide spectrum of human malignancies. Accordingly, there have been different efforts to coordinate the cancer genome sequencing projects being carried out around the world, including The Cancer Genome Atlas (TCGA) and the International Cancer Genome Consortium (ICGC). Moreover, there are other initiatives that are more focused on specific tumors, such as that led by scientists at St. Jude Children's Research Hospital in Memphis, and Washington University, which aims at sequencing multiple pediatric cancer genomes.[129]

TCGA began in 2006 in the United States as a comprehensive program in cancer genomics supported by the U.S. National Institutes of Health (NIH). The initial project focused on three tumors: GBM, serous cystadenocarcinoma of the ovary, and lung squamous carcinoma. These studies have already generated novel

and interesting information regarding genes mutated in these malignancies.[134] On the basis of these positive results, the NIH announced an expansion of the TCGA program with the aim to produce genomic data sets for at least 20 to 25 cancers during the next few years.

The ICGC was formed in 2008 to coordinate the generation of comprehensive catalogs of genomic abnormalities in tumors from 50 different cancer types or subtypes that are of clinical and societal importance across the world.[130] The project aims to perform systematic studies of over 25,000 cancer genomes at the genomic level and integrate this information with epigenomic and transcriptomic studies of the same cases as well as with clinical features of patients. At present, there are a total of 69 committed projects involving at least 16 different countries coordinated by

---

**TABLE 1.2**

**Computational Tools and Databases Useful for Cancer Genome Analyses**

| Category | Tool/Database | URL |
|---|---|---|
| Alignment | Maq[a] | http://maq.sourceforge.net |
| | Burrows-Wheeler Aligner (BWA)[b] | http://bio-bwa.sourceforge.net |
| Mutation calling | SNVMix[c] | http://www.bcgsc.ca/platform/bioinfo/software/SNVMix |
| | SAMtools[d] | http://samtools.sourceforge.net |
| | VarScan[e] | http://varscan.sourceforge.net |
| | MuTect[f] | http://www.broadinstitute.org/cancer/cga/mutect |
| Indel calling | Pindel[g] | http://gmt.genome.wustl.edu/pindel/current/ |
| Copy number analysis | CBS[h] | http://www.bioconductor.org |
| | SegSeq[i] | http://www.broadinstitute.org/cgi-bin/cancer/publications/pub_paper.cgi?mode=view&paper_id=182 |
| Functional effect | SIFT[j] | http://sift.jcvi.org/ |
| | PolyPhen-2[k] | http://genetics.bwh.harvard.edu/pph2 |
| Visualization | CIRCOS[l] | http://mkweb.bcgsc.ca/circos |
| | Integrative Genomics Viewer (IGV)[m] | http://www.broadinstitute.org/igv |
| Repository | Catalogue of Somatic Mutations in Cancer (COSMIC)[n] | http://www.sanger.ac.uk/genetics/CGP/cosmic |
| | Cancer Genome Project (CGP)[o] | http://www.sanger.ac.uk/genetics/CGP |
| | dbSNP[p] | http://www.ncbi.nlm.nih.gov/SNP |
| | Gene Ranker[q] | http://cbio.mskcc.org/tcga-generanker/ |

[a] Li H, Durbin R. Fast and accurate short read alignment with Burrows–Wheeler transform. *Bioinformatics* 2009;25:1754–1760.
[b] Li H, Durbin R. Fast and accurate long-read alignment with Burrows–Wheeler transform. *Bioinformatics* 2010;26:589–595.
[c] Goya R, Sun MG, Morin RD, et al. SNVMix: predicting single nucleotide variants from next-generation sequencing of tumors. *Bioinformatics* 2010;26:730–736.
[d] Li H, Handsaker B, Wysoker A, et al. The Sequence Alignment/Map format and SAMtools. *Bioinformatics* 2009;25:2078–2079.
[e] Koboldt DC, Chen K, Wylie T, et al. VarScan: variant detection in massively parallel sequencing of individual and pooled samples. *Bioinformatics* 2009;25:2283–2285.
[f] Cibulski K, Lawrence MS, Carter SL, et al. Sensitive detection of somatic point mutations in impure and heterogeneous cancer samples. *Nat Biotechnol* 2013;31:213–219.
[g] Ye K, Schulz MH, Long Q, et al. Pindel: a pattern growth approach to detect break points of large deletions and medium sized insertions from paired-end short reads. *Bioinformatics* 2009;25:2865–2871.
[h] Venkatraman ES, Olshen AB. A faster circular binary segmentation algorithm for the analysis of array CGH data. *Bioinformatics* 2007;23:657–663.
[i] Chiang DY, Getz G, Jaffe DB, et al. High-resolution mapping of copy-number alterations with massively parallel sequencing. *Nature Methods* 2009;6:99–103.
[j] Ng PC, Henikoff S. Predicting deleterious amino acid substitutions. *Genome Res* 2001;11:863–874.
[k] Idzhubei IA, Schmidt S, Peshkin L, et al. A method and server for predicting damaging missense mutations. *Nature Methods* 2010;7:248–249.
[l] Krzywinski M, Schein J, Birol I, et al. Circos: an information aesthetic for comparative genomics. *Genome Res* 2009;19:1639–1645.
[m] Robinson JT, Thorvaldsdóttir H, Winckler W, et al. Integrative Genomics Viewer. *Nat Biotechnol* 2011;29:24–26.
[n] Forbes SA, Bhamra S, Dawson E, et al. The catalogue of somatic mutations in cancer (COSMIC). *Curr Protoc Hum Genet* 2008;Chapter 10:Unit 10.11.
[o] Futreal PA, Coin L, Marshall M, et al. A census of human cancer genes. *Nat Rev Cancer* 2004;4:177–183.
[p] Sherry ST, Ward MH, Kholodov M, et al. dbSNP: The NCBI Database of genetic variation. *Nucleic Acids Res* 2001;29:308–311.
[q] The Cancer Genome Atlas Research Network. Comprehensive genomic characterization defines human glioblastoma genes and core pathways. *Nature* 2008;455:1061–1068.
Based on Meyerson M, Stacey G, Getz G. Advances in understanding cancer genomes through second generation sequencing. *Nature Rev Genet* 2010;11: 685–696, Table 2.

PRINCIPLES OF ONCOLOGY

the ICGC. All of these projects deal with at least 500 samples per cancer type from cancers affecting a variety of human organs and tissues, including blood, the brain, the breast, the esophagus, the kidneys, the liver, the oral cavity, the ovaries, the pancreas, the prostate, the skin, and the stomach.[130]

All of these coordinated projects have already provided new insights into the catalog of genes mutated in cancer and have unveiled specific signatures of the mutagenic mechanisms, including carcinogen exposures or DNA-repair defects, implicated in the development of different malignant tumors.[83,84,87,131] Furthermore, these cancer genome studies have also contributed to define clinically relevant subtypes of tumors for prognosis and therapeutic management, and in some cases have identified new targets and strategies for cancer treatment.[74–76] The rapid technological advances in DNA sequencing will likely drop the costs of sequencing cancer genomes to a small fraction of

the current price and will allow researchers to overcome some of the current limitations of these global sequencing efforts. Hopefully, worldwide coordination of cancer genome projects, including Pan-Cancer initiative, with those involving large-scale, functional analyses of genes in both cellular and animal models will likely provide us with the most comprehensive collection of information generated to date about the causes and molecular mechanisms of cancer.

## THE GENOMIC LANDSCAPE OF CANCERS

Examining the overall distribution of the identified mutations redefined the cancer genome landscapes whereby the *mountains* are the handful of commonly mutated genes and the *hills* represent the vast majority of genes that are infrequently mutated.

One of the most striking features of the tumor genomic landscape is that it involves different sets of cancer genes that are mutated in a tissue-specific fashion.[132,133] To continue with the analogy, the scenery is very different if we observe a colorectal, a lung, or a breast tumor. This indicates that mutations in specific genes cause tumors at specific sites, or are associated with specific stages of development, cell differentiation, or tumorigenesis, despite many of those genes being expressed in various fetal and adult tissues. Moreover, different types of tumors follow specific genetic pathways in terms of the combination of genetic alterations that it must acquire. For example, no cancer outside the bowel has been shown to follow the classic genetic pathway of colorectal tumorigenesis. Additionally, *KRAS* mutations are almost always present in pancreatic cancers but are very rare or absent in breast cancers. Similarly, *BRAF* mutations are present in 60% of melanomas, but are very infrequent in lung cancers.[1] Another intriguing feature is that alterations in ubiquitous housekeeping genes, such as those involved in DNA repair or energy production, occur only in particular types of tumors.

In addition to tissue specificity, the genomic landscape of tumors can also be associated with gender and hormonal status. For example, *HER2* amplification and *PIK3C2A* mutations, two genetic alterations associated with breast cancer development, are correlated with the estrogen-receptor hormonal status.[134] The molecular basis for the occurrence of cancer mutations in tissue- and gender-specific profiles is still largely unknown. Organ-specific expression profiles and cell-specific neoplastic transformation requirements are often mentioned as possible causes for this phenomenon. Identifying tissue and gender cancer mutations patterns is relevant because it may allow for the definition of individualized therapeutic avenues.

## INTEGRATIVE ANALYSIS OF CANCER GENOMICS

The implementation of novel high-throughput technologies is generating an extraordinary amount of information on cancer samples in many different ways other than those derived from whole-exome or whole-genome sequencing. Accordingly, there is a growing need to integrate genomic, epigenomic, transcriptomic, and proteomic landscapes from tumor samples, and then linking this integrated information with clinical outcomes of cancer patients. There are some examples of human malignancies in which this integrative approach has been already performed, such as for AML, glioblastoma, medulloblastoma, and renal cell, colorectal, ovarian, endometrial, prostate, and breast carcinomas.[135–142] In these cases, the integration of whole-exome and whole-genome sequencing with studies involving genomic DNA copy number arrays, DNA methylation, transcriptomic arrays, miRNA sequencing, and proteomic profiling has contributed to improving the molecular classification of complex and heterogeneous tumors. These integrative molecular analyses have also provided new insights into the mechanisms disrupted in each particular cancer type or subtype and have facilitated the association of genomic information with distinct clinical parameters of cancer patients and the discovery of novel therapeutic targets.[143] Also in this regard, there has been significant progress in the definition of the mechanisms by which the cancer genome and epigenome influence each other and cooperate to facilitate malignant transformation.[144,145] Thus, many tumor-suppressor genes are inactivated by either mutation or epigenetic silencing, and in some cases such as colorectal carcinomas, both mechanisms work coordinately to create a permissive environment for oncogenic transformation.[146] Moreover, mutations in epigenetic regulators such as DNA methyl transferases, chromatin remodelers, histones, and histone modifiers, are very frequent events in many tumors,

including hepatocellular carcinomas, renal carcinomas leukemias, lymphomas, glioblastomas, and medulloblastomas. These genetic alterations of epigenetic modulators cause widespread transcriptomic changes, thereby amplifying the initial effect of the mutational event at the cancer genome level.[145]

The recent availability of different platforms for integrative cancer genome analyses will be very helpful in enabling the classification, biologic characterization, and personalized clinical management of human cancers (Table 1.3).[144,147]

## THE CANCER GENOME AND THE NEW TAXONOMY OF TUMORS

Deciphering the cancer genome has already impacted clinical practice at multiple levels. On the one hand, it allowed for the identification of new cancer genes such as *IDH1*, a gene involved in glioma, which was discovered recently (see previous), and on the other hand, it is redesigning the taxonomy of tumors.

Until the genomic revolution, tumors had been classified based on two criteria: their localization (site of occurrence) and their appearance (histology). These criteria are also currently used as primary determinants of prognosis and to establish the best treatments. For many decades, it has been known that patients with histologically similar tumors have different clinical outcomes. Furthermore, tumors that cannot be distinguished based on an histologic analysis can respond very differently to identical therapies.[148]

It is becoming increasingly clear that the frequency and distribution of mutations affecting cancer genes can be used to redefine the histology-based taxonomy of a given tumor type. Lung and colorectal tumors represent paradigmatic examples. Genomic analyses led to the identification of activating mutations in the receptor tyrosine kinase *EGFR* in lung adenocarcinomas.[149] The occurrence of *EGFR* mutations molecularly defines a subtype of non–small-cell lung cancers (NSCLC) that occur mainly in nonsmoking women, that tend to have a distinctly enhanced prognosis, and that typically respond to epidermal growth factor receptor (EGFR)-targeted therapies.[150–152] Similarly, the recent discovery of the *EML4-ALK* fusion identifies yet another subset of NSCLC that is clearly distinct from those that harbor *EGFR* mutations, that have distinct epidemiologic and biologic features, and that respond to ALK inhibitors.[109,153]

The second example is colorectal cancers (CRC), the tumor type for which the genomic landscape has been refined with the highest accuracy. CRCs can be clearly categorized according to the mutational profile of the genes involved in the *KRAS* pathway (Fig. 1.10). It is now known that *KRAS* mutations occur in approximately 40% of CRCs. Another subtype of CRC (approximately 10%) harbors mutations in *BRAF*, the immediate downstream effectors of *KRAS*.[10]

In CRCs and other tumor types, *KRAS* and *BRAF* mutations are known to be mutually exclusive. The mutual exclusivity pattern indicates that these genes operate in the same signaling pathway. Large epidemiologic studies have shown that the prognosis of tumors harboring wild-type *KRAS/BRAF* genes is distinct, and typically more favorable, than that of the mutated ones.[154,155] Of note, *KRAS* and *BRAF* mutations have been recently shown to impair responsiveness to the anti-EGFR monoclonal antibodies therapies in CRC patients.[156–158] Clearly distinct subgroups can be genetically identified in both NSCLCs and CRCs with respect to prognosis and response to therapy. It is likely that as soon as the genomic landscapes of other tumor types are defined, molecular subgroups like those described previously will also become defined.

Genotyping tumor tissue in search of somatic genetic alterations for *actionable* information has become routine practice in clinical oncology. The genetic profile of solid tumors is currently obtained from surgical or biopsy specimens. As the techniques

## TABLE 1.3

### Useful Information for the Description and Management of Cancer

| Bioinformatic Tool or Webservices | Database Used | Webservice or Tool | Upload of Data Possible | Gene Search | Chromosomal Region Search | mRNA Expression | SNV | CNV | Methylation | miRNA Expression | Protein | Pathways |
|---|---|---|---|---|---|---|---|---|---|---|---|---|
| cBioPortal for Cancer Genomics | TCGA | Webservice | — | ✓ | — | ✓ | ✓ | ✓ | — | — | ✓ | ✓ |
| PARADIGM, Broad GDAC Firehose | TCGA | Webservice | ✓ | ✓ | ✓ | ✓ | ✓ | ✓ | ✓ | — | — | ✓ |
| WashU Epigenome Browser | ENCODE | Webservice | ✓ | ✓ | ✓ | ✓ | ✓ | ✓ | ✓ | — | — | ✓ |
| UCSC Cancer Genomics Browser | UCSC | Webservice | ✓ | ✓ | ✓ | ✓ | ✓ | ✓ | ✓ | ✓ | — | — |
| The Cancer Genome Workbench | TCGA | Webservice | — | ✓ | ✓ | ✓ | ✓ | ✓ | ✓ | — | — | — |
| EpiExplorer | ENCODE and ROADMAP | Webservice | ✓ | ✓ | ✓ | — | — | — | ✓ | — | — | — |
| EpiGRAPH | ENCODE | Webservice | ✓ | ✓ | ✓ | ✓ | ✓ | ✓ | ✓ | — | — | ✓ |
| Catalogue of Somatic Mutations in Cancer (COSMIC) | TCGA and ICGC | Webservice | — | ✓ | — | — | — | ✓ | — | — | — | — |
| PCmtl, MAGIA, miRvar, CoMeTa, etc.* | GEO and TCGA | Webservice | ✓ | ✓ | ✓ | ✓ | ✓ | ✓ | ✓ | ✓ | — | ✓ |
| ICGC | ICGC | Webservice | — | ✓ | — | ✓ | ✓ | ✓ | — | — | — | ✓ |
| Genomatix | User defined | Tool | — | ✓ | — | ✓ | ✓ | ✓ | — | — | — | ✓ |
| Caleydo | TCGA | Tool | — | ✓ | ✓ | ✓ | ✓ | ✓ | ✓ | — | — | ✓ |
| Integrative Genomics Viewer (IGV) | ENCODE | Tool | — | ✓ | ✓ | ✓ | — | ✓ | ✓ | ✓ | — | ✓ |
| iCluster and iCluster Plus | User defined | Tool | — | ✓ | — | ✓ | — | ✓ | — | — | — | — |

* Web Site with links for integrated analysis of microRNA and mRNA expression.

CNV, copy-number variation; ENCODE, Encyclopedia of DNA Elements; ICGC, the International Cancer Genome Consortium; GDAC, Genomic Data Analysis Center; GEO, Gene Expression Omnibus; miRNA, microRNA; SNV, single-nucleotide variation; TCGA, The Cancer Genome Atlas; USCS, University of California, Santa Cruz;
Based on Plass C, Pfister SM, Lindroth AM, et al. Mutations in regulators of the epigenome and their connections to global chromatin patterns in cancer. *Nat Rev Genet* 2013;14:765–780, Table 1.

**PRINCIPLES OF ONCOLOGY**

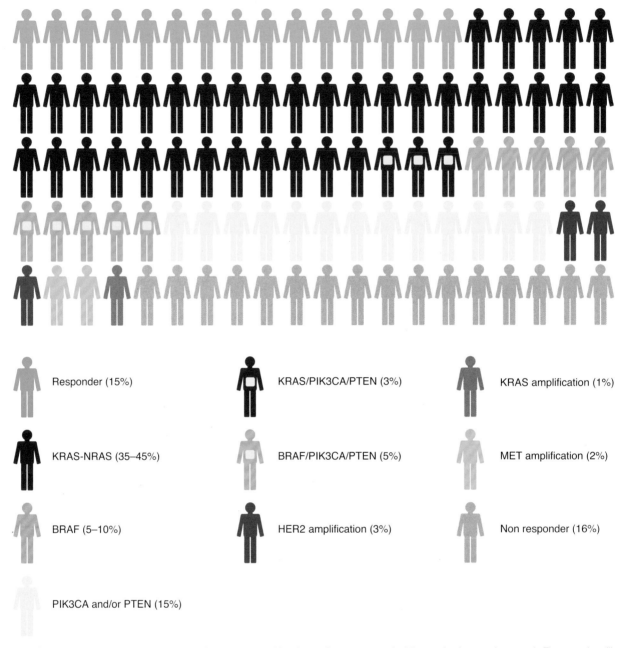

**Figure 1.10** Graphic representation of a cohort of 100 patients with colorectal cancer treated with cetuximab or panitumumab. The genetic milieu of individual tumors and their impacts on the clinical response are listed. *KRAS, BRAF,* and *PIK3CA* somatic mutations as well as loss of PTEN protein expression are indicated according to different color codes. Molecular alterations mutually exclusive or coexisting in individual tumors are indicated using different color variants. The relative frequencies at which the molecular alterations occur in colorectal cancers are described. (Redrawn from Bardelli A, Siena S. Molecular mechanisms of resistance to cetuximab and panitumumab in colorectal cancer. *J Clin Oncol* 2010;28:1254–1261.)

that have enabled us to analyze tumor tissues become ever more sophisticated, we have realized the limitations of this approach. As previously discussed, cancers are heterogeneous, with different areas of the same tumor showing different genetic profiles (i.e., intratumoral heterogeneity); likewise, heterogeneity exists between metastases within the same patient (i.e., intermetastatic heterogeneity).[159] A tissue section (or a biopsy) from one part of a solitary tumor will miss the molecular intratumoral as well as intermetastatic heterogeneity. To capture tumor heterogeneity, techniques that are capable of interrogating the genetic landscapes of the overall disease in a single patient are needed.

In 1948, the publication of a manuscript describing the presence of cell-free circulating DNA (cfDNA) in the blood of humans

offered—probably without realizing it—unprecedented opportunities in this area.[160] Only recently, the full potential of this seminal discovery has been appreciated. Several groups have reported that the analysis of circulating tumor DNA can, in principle, provide the same genetic information obtained from tumor tissue.[161] The levels of cfDNA are typically higher in cancer patients than healthy individuals, indicating that it is possible to screen for the presence of disease through a simple blood test. Furthermore, the specific detection of tumor-derived cfDNA has been shown to correlate with tumor burden, which changes in response to treatment or surgery.[162–164]

Although the detection of ctDNA has remarkable potential, it is also challenging for several reasons. The first is the need to discriminate DNA released from tumor cells (ctDNA) from circulating *normal* DNA. Discerning ctDNA from normal cfDNA is aided by the fact that tumor DNA is defined by the presence of mutations. These somatic mutations, commonly single base pair substitutions, are present only in the genomes of cancer cells or precancerous cells and are present in the DNA of normal cells of the same individual. Accordingly, ctDNA offers exquisite specificity as a biomarker. Unfortunately, cfDNA derived from tumor cells often represents a very small fraction (<1%) of the total cfDNA, thus limiting the applicability of the approach. The development and refinement of next-generation sequencing strategies as well as recently developed digital PCR techniques have made it possible to define rare mutant variants in complex mixtures of DNA. Using these approaches, it is possible to detect point mutations, rearrangements, and gene copy number changes in individual genes starting from a few milliliters of plasma.[165] Very recently, several groups have opened a new frontier by showing that exome analyses can also be performed from circulating DNA extracted from the blood of cancer patients.[166]

The detection of tumor-specific genetic alterations in patients' blood (often referred to as *liquid biopsies*) has several applications in the field of oncology, which are summarized as follows. Analyses of cfDNA can be used to genotype tumors when a tissue sample is not available or is difficult to obtain. Circulating tumor DNA fragments contain the identical genetic defects as the tumor themselves, thus the blood can reveal tumor point mutations (*EGFR, KRAS, BRAF, PIK3CA*), rearrangements (e.g., *EML4-ALK*), as well as tumor amplifications (*MET*).[167–169] *Liquid biopsies* may also be useful in monitoring tumor burden—a central aspect in the management of patients with cancer—that is typically assessed with imaging. In this regard, several investigational studies have shown that ctDNA can be a surrogate for tumor burden and that, much like viral load changes (e.g., HIV viral load), levels of ctDNA correspond with clinical course. Another application of ctDNA is the detection of minimal residual disease following surgery or therapy with curative intent.[163] Finally, *liquid biopsies* can be used to monitor the genomic drift (clonal evolution) of tumors upon treatment.[166] In this setting, the analysis of ctDNA in plasma samples obtained pretreatment, during, and posttreatment can lead to an understanding of the mechanisms of primary and, especially, acquired resistance to therapies.[170,171]

Importantly, the advances in sequencing technologies have made the idea of personalized treatment of cancer a reality, which is most evident in the field of adoptive cell therapy (ACT). Although already a treatment in use, the ability to use a patient's autologous tumor-infiltrating lymphocytes (TIL) is in position to benefit greatly from advances in sequencing technologies. A recent study demonstrated this when whole-exome data, along with a major histocompatibility complex (MHC)-binding algorithm, were utilized to identify candidate tumor epitopes that are recognized by the patients' TILs.[172] This study should allow for future work in which the information obtained from the direct sequencing of a patient's tumor can quickly be used to generate tumor-reactive T cells that can then be used for a personalized treatment.

In conclusion, the taxonomy of tumors is being rewritten using the presence of genetic lesions as major criteria. Genome-based information will improve the diagnosis and will be used to determine personalized therapeutic regimens based on the genetic landscape of individual tumors.

## CANCER GENOMICS AND DRUG RESISTANCE

Cancer genomics has dramatically impacted disease management, because its application is helping researchers determine which

patients are likely to benefit from which drug. As discussed in great detail in Chapter 22, good examples for such treatment include targeted therapy using imatinib for chronic myeloid leukemia (CML) patients and the use of gefitinib and erlotinib for NSCLC patients.

The key to the successful development and application of anticancer agents is a better understanding of the effect of the therapeutic regimens and of resistance mechanisms that may develop. In most tumor types, a fraction of patients' tumors are refractory to therapies (intrinsic resistance). Even if an initial response to therapies is obtained, the vast majority of tumors subsequently become refractory (i.e., acquired resistance), and patients eventually succumb to disease progression. Therefore, secondary resistance should be regarded as a key obstacle to treatment progress. The analysis of the cancer genome represents a powerful tool both for the identification of chemotherapeutic signatures as well as to understand resistance mechanisms to therapeutic agents. Examples for each of these are described as follows.

An important application of systematic sequencing experiments is the identification of the effects of chemotherapy on the cancer genome. For example, gliomas that recur after temozolomide treatment have been shown to harbor large numbers of mutations with a signature typical of a DNA alkylating agent.[173,174] Because these alterations were detected using Sanger sequencing, which as described previously has limited sensitivity, the data suggested that the detected alterations were clonal. The model that unfolds from this study indicates that although temozolomide has limited efficacy, almost all of the cells in a glioma respond to the drug. However, a single cell that was resistant to the chemotherapy proliferated and formed a cell clone. Later genomic analyses of the cell clone allowed for the identification of the underlying mutated resistance genes.[173,174]

Single-molecule–targeted therapy is almost always followed by acquired drug resistance.[175–177] Genomic analyses can be successfully exploited to decipher resistance mechanisms to such inhibitors. A few paradigmatic examples are presented as follows, which will be discussed extensively in other chapters. Despite the effectiveness of gefitinib and erlotinib in EGFR mutant cases of NSCLC,[178] drug resistance develops within 6 to 12 months after the initiation of therapy. The underlying reason for this resistance was identified as a secondary mutation in *EGFR* exon 20, T790M, which is detectable in 50% of patients who relapse.[179–181] Importantly, some studies have shown the mutation to be present before the patient was treated with the drug,[182,183] suggesting that exposure to the drug selected for these cells.[184] Because the drug-resistant *EGFR* mutation is structurally analogous to the mutated gatekeeper residue T315I in BCR-ABL, T670I in c-Kit, and L1196M in EML4-ALK, which have been shown previously to confer resistance to imatinib and other kinase inhibitors,[176,185,186] this mechanism of resistance represents a general problem that needs to be overcome.

A recent elegant study, which also represents the use of genomics in understanding drug-resistance mechanisms, focused on the inhibition of activating *BRAF* (V600E) mutations, which occur in 7% of human malignancies and in 60% of melanomas.[9] Clinical trials using PLX4032, a novel class I RAF-selective inhibitor, showed an 80% antitumor response rate in melanoma patients with *BRAF* (V600E) mutations; however, cases of drug resistance were observed.[187] The use of microarray and sequencing technologies showed that, in this case, the resistance was not due to secondary mutations in *BRAF*, but due rather to either upregulation of *PDGFRB* or *NRAS* mutations.[188]

It was, however, the introduction of two anti-EGFR monoclonal antibodies, cetuximab and panitumumab, for the treatment of metastatic colorectal cancer, that provided the largest body of knowledge on the relationship between tumors' genotypes and the response to targeted therapies. The initial clinical analysis pointed out that only a fraction of metastatic CRC patients benefited from this novel treatment. Different from the NSCLC paradigm, it was found that EGFR mutations do not play a major role in the response. On the contrary, from the initial retrospective analysis, it became clear that somatic *KRAS* mutations, thought to be present in 35% to 45% of metastatic colorectal cancers, are important negative predictors of efficacy in patients who are given panitumumab or cetuximab.[156–158] Among tumors carrying wild-type *KRAS*, mutations of *BRAF* or *PIK3CA*, or a loss of phosphatase and tensin homolog (PTEN) expression may also predict resistance to EGFR-targeted monoclonal antibodies, although the latter biomarkers require further validation before they can be incorporated into clinical practice. From these few examples, it is clear that a future, deeper genomic understanding of targeted drug resistance is crucial to the effective development of additional as well as alternative therapies to overcome this resistance.

## PERSPECTIVES OF CANCER GENOME ANALYSIS

The completion of the human genome project has marked a new beginning in biomedical sciences. Because human cancer is a genetic disease, the field of oncology has been one of the first to be impacted by this historic revolution. Knowledge of the sequence and organization of the human genome allows for the systematic analysis of the genetic alterations underlying the origin and evolution of tumors. High-throughput mutational profiling of common tumors, including lung, skin, breast, and colorectal cancers, and the application of next-generation sequencing to whole genome, whole exome, and whole transcriptome of cancer samples has allowed substantial advances in the understanding of this disease by facilitating the detection of all main types of somatic cancer genome alterations. These have also led to historical results, such as the identification of genetic alterations that are likely to be the major drivers of these diseases.

However, the genetic landscape of cancers is by no means complete, and what has been learned so far has raised new and exciting questions that must be addressed. There are still important technical challenges for the detection of somatic mutations.[60] Clinical tumor samples often contain large amounts of nonmalignant cells, which makes the identification of mutations in cancer genomes more challenging when compared with similar analyses of peripheral blood samples for germ-line genome studies. Moreover, the genomic instability inherent to cancer development and progression largely increases the complexity and diversity of genomic alterations of malignant tumors, making it necessary to distinguish between driver and passenger mutations. Likewise, the fact that malignant tumors are genetically heterogeneous and contain several clones simultaneously growing within the same tumor mass raises additional questions regarding the quality of the information currently derived from cancer genomes. Hopefully, in the near future, advances in third-generation sequencing technologies will make it feasible to obtain high-quality sequence data of a genome isolated from a single cell, an aspect of crucial relevance for cancer research.

One of the next imperatives is the definition of the oncogenomic profile of all tumor types. In particular, the less common—although not less lethal—ones are still largely mysterious to scientists and untreatable to clinicians. For some of these diseases, few new therapeutically amenable molecular targets have been discovered in the past years. For example, the identification of drugable genetic lesions associated with pancreatic and ovarian cancers could help define new therapeutic strategies for these aggressive diseases. To achieve this, detailed oncogenomic maps of the corresponding tumors must be drafted. The latter will hopefully be completed in the coming years, thanks to the systematic cancer genome projects that are presently being performed.

Even in the case of common cancers, a lot of genomic profiling efforts still lay ahead. For example, in a significant fraction of breast and lung tumors, the mutations that are likely to be drivers have not yet been found. This is not surprising considering that even in these tumor types only a limited number of samples have been systematically analyzed so far. Therefore, low incidence mutations that could represent potentially key therapeutic targets in a subset of tumors might have escaped detection. Consequently, the scaling up of the mutational profiling to large numbers of specimens for each tumor type is warranted.

Finally, understanding the cellular properties imparted by the hundreds of recently discovered cancer alleles is another area that must be developed. As a matter of fact, compared to the genomic discovery stage, the functional validation of putative novel cancer alleles, despite their potential clinical relevance, is substantially lagging behind. To achieve this, high-throughput functional studies in model systems that accurately recapitulate the genetic alterations found in human cancer must be developed.

To conclude, the eventual goal of profiling the cancer genome is not only to further understand the molecular basis of the disease, but also to discover novel diagnostic and drug targets. One might anticipate that the most immediate application of these new technologies will be noninvasive strategies for early cancer detection. Considering that oncogenic mutations are present only in cancer cells, screening for tumor-derived mutant DNA in patients' blood holds great potential and will progressively substitute current biomarkers, which have poor sensitivity and lack specificity.[171] Further improvements in next-generation sequencing technologies are likely to reduce their cost as well as make these analyses more facile in the future. Once this happens, most cancer patients will undergo in-depth genomic analyses as part of their initial evaluation and throughout their treatment. This will offer more precise diagnostic and prognostic information, which will affect treatment decisions. Although many challenges remain, the information gained from next-generation sequencing platforms is laying a foundation for personalized medicine, in which patients are managed with therapies that are tailored to the specific gene mutations found in their tumors. Ultimately, these should lead to therapeutic successes similar to the ones attained for CML patients with imatinib,[189,190] melanoma patients with PLX4032,[187] and NSCLC patients with gefitinib and erlotinib.[178] Clearly, this is the absolute goal for all of this work.

## ACKNOWLEDGMENTS

This work was supported by the Intramural Research Programs of the National Human Genome Research Institute, National Institutes of Health, USA, YS is supported by the Henry Chanoch Krenter Institute for Biomedical Imaging and Genomics, Louis and Fannie Tolz Collaborative Research Project, Dukler Fund for Cancer Research, De Benedetti Foundation-Cherasco 1547, Peter and Patricia Gruber Awards, Gideon Hamburger, Israel, Estate of Alice Schwarz-Gardos, Estate of John Hunter and the Knell Family. YS is supported by the Israel Science Foundation grant numbers 1604/13 and 877/13 and the ERC (StG-335377). A.B. is supported by the European Communityís Seventh Framework Programme under grant agreement no. 259015 COLTHERES, Associazione Italiana per la Ricerca sul Cancro (AIRC) IG grant no. 12812 and Fondazione Piemontese per la Ricerca sul Cancro–ONLUS. C.L-O. is an Investigator of the Botin Foundation supported by grants from Ministerio de Economía y Competitividad-Spain and Instituto de Salud Carlos III (RTICC), Spain.

1. Vogelstein B, Kinzler KW. Cancer genes and the pathways they control. *Nat Med* 2004;10:789–799.
2. Kinzler KW, Vogelstein B. Lessons from hereditary colon cancer. *Cell* 1996; 87:159–170.
3. International Human Genome Sequencing Consortium. Finishing the euchromatic sequence of the human genome. *Nature* 2004;431:931–945.
4. Stehelin D, Varmus HE, Bishop JM, et al. DNA related to the transforming gene(s) of avian sarcoma viruses is present in normal avian DNA. *Nature* 1976;260:170–173.
5. Rous P. Transmission of a malignant new growth by means of a cell-free filtrate. *J Am Med Assoc* 1911;56:198.
6. International HapMap Consortium. The International HapMap Project. *Nature* 2003;426:89–96.
7. International HapMap Consortium. A haplotype map of the human genome. *Nature* 2005;437:1299–1320.
8. Sanger F, Nicklen S, Coulson AR. DNA sequencing with chain-terminating inhibitors. *Proc Natl Acad Sci U S A* 1977;74:5463–5467.
9. Davies H, Bignell GR, Cox C, et al. Mutations of the BRAF gene in human cancer. *Nature* 2002;417:949–954.
10. Rajagopalan H, Bardelli A, Lengauer C, et al. Tumorigenesis: RAF/RAS oncogenes and mismatch-repair status. *Nature* 2002;418:934.
11. Moodie SA, Wolfman A. The 3Rs of life: Ras, Raf and growth regulation. *Trends Genet* 1994;10:44–48.
12. Hafen E, Dickson B, Brunner D, et al. Genetic dissection of signal transduction mediated by the sevenless receptor tyrosine kinase in Drosophila. *Prog Neurobiol* 1994;42:287–292.
13. Bardelli A, Parsons DW, Silliman N, et al. Mutational analysis of the tyrosine kinome in colorectal cancers. *Science* 2003;300:949.
14. Greenman C, Stephens P, Smith R, et al. Patterns of somatic mutation in human cancer genomes. *Nature* 2007;446:153–158.
15. Samuels Y, Wang Z, Bardelli A, et al. High frequency of mutations of the PIK3CA gene in human cancers. *Science* 2004;304:554.
16. Wang Z, Shen D, Parsons DW, et al. Mutational analysis of the tyrosine phosphatome in colorectal cancers. *Science* 2004;304:1164–1166.
17. Vivanco I, Sawyers CL. The phosphatidylinositol 3-Kinase AKT pathway in human cancer. *Nat Rev Cancer* 2002;2:489–501.
18. Broderick DK, Di C, Parrett TJ, et al. Mutations of PIK3CA in anaplastic oligodendrogliomas, high-grade astrocytomas, and medulloblastomas. *Cancer Res* 2004;64:5048–5050.
19. Lee JW, Soung YH, Kim SY, et al. PIK3CA gene is frequently mutated in breast carcinomas and hepatocellular carcinomas. *Oncogene* 2005;24:1477–1480.
20. Bachman KE, Argani P, Samuels Y, et al. The PIK3CA gene is mutated with high frequency in human breast cancers. *Cancer Biol Ther* 2004;3: 772–775.
21. Oda K, Stokoe D, Taketani Y, et al. High frequency of coexistent mutations of PIK3CA and PTEN genes in endometrial carcinoma. *Cancer Res* 2005;65:10669–10673.
22. Samuels Y, Waldman T. Oncogenic mutations of PIK3CA in human cancers. *Curr Top Microbiol Immunol* 2010;2:21–42.
23. Parsons DW, Wang TL, Samuels Y, et al. Colorectal cancer: mutations in a signalling pathway. *Nature* 2005;436:792.
24. Lopez-Otin C, Overall CM. Protease degradomics: a new challenge for proteomics. *Nat Rev Mol Cell Biol* 2002;3:509–519.
25. Liotta LA, Tryggvason K, Garbisa S, et al. Metastatic potential correlates with enzymatic degradation of basement membrane collagen. *Nature* 1980;284: 67–68.
26. Lopez-Otin C, Hunter T. The regulatory crosstalk between kinases and proteases in cancer. *Nat Rev Cancer* 2010;10:278–292.
27. Egeblad M, Werb Z. New functions for the matrix metalloproteinases in cancer progression. *Nat Rev Cancer* 2002;2:161–174.
28. Lopez-Otin C, Matrisian LM. Emerging roles of proteases in tumour suppression. *Nat Rev Cancer* 2007;7:800–808.
29. Wood LD, Parsons DW, Jones S, et al. The genomic landscapes of human breast and colorectal cancers. *Science* 2007;318:1108–1113.
30. Palavalli LH, Prickett TD, Wunderluch JR, et al. Analysis of the matrix metalloproteinase family reveals that MMP8 is often mutated in melanoma. *Nat Genet* 2009;41:518–520.
31. Lopez-Otin C, Palavalli LH, Samuels Y. Protective roles of matrix metalloproteinases: from mouse models to human cancer. *Cell Cycle* 2009;8:3657–3662.
32. Hanahan D, Weinberg RA. The hallmarks of cancer. *Cell* 2000;100:57–70.
33. Teitz T, Wei T, Valentine MB, et al. Caspase 8 is deleted or silenced preferentially in childhood neuroblastomas with amplification of MYCN. *Nat Med* 2000;6:529–535.
34. Mandruzzato S, Brasseur F, Andry G, et al. A CASP-8 mutation recognized by cytolytic T lymphocytes on a human head and neck carcinoma. *J Exp Med* 1997;186:785–793.
35. Soung YH, Lee JW, Kim SY, et al. CASPASE-8 gene is inactivated by somatic mutations in gastric carcinomas. *Cancer Res* 2005;65:815–821.
36. Fraile JM, Quesada V, Rodríguez D, et al. Deubiquitinases in cancer: new functions and therapeutic options. *Oncogene* 2012;31:2373–2388.
37. Bignell GR, Warren W, Seal S, et al. Identification of the familial cylindromatosis tumour-suppressor gene. *Nat Genet* 2000;25:160–165.
38. Schmitz R, Hansmann ML, Bohle V, et al. TNFAIP3 (A20) is a tumor suppressor gene in Hodgkin lymphoma and primary mediastinal B cell lymphoma. *J Exp Med* 2009;206:981–989.
39. Compagno M, Lim WK, Grunn A, et al. Mutations of multiple genes cause deregulation of NF-kappaB in diffuse large B-cell lymphoma. *Nature* 2009;459:717–721.
40. Kato M, Sanada M, Kato I, et al. Frequent inactivation of A20 in B-cell lymphomas. *Nature* 2009;459:712–716.
41. Novak U, Rinaldi A, Kwee I, et al. The NF-kappa B negative regulator TNFAIP3 (A20) is inactivated by somatic mutations and genomic deletions in marginal zone lymphomas. *Blood* 2009;113: 4918–4921.
42. Harbour JW, Onken MD, Roberson ED, et al. Frequent mutation of BAP1 in metastasizing uveal melanomas. *Science* 2010;330:1410–1413.
43. Carbone M, Yang H, Pass HI, et al. BAP1 and cancer. *Nat Rev Cancer* 2013; 13:153–159.
44. Sjöblom T, Jones S, Wood LD, et al. The consensus coding sequences of human breast and colorectal cancers. *Science* 2006;314:268–274.
45. Jones S, Zhang X, Parsons DW, et al. Core signaling pathways in human pancreatic cancers revealed by global genomic analyses. *Science* 2008;321:1801–1806.
46. Parsons DW, Jones S, Zhang X, et al. An integrated genomic analysis of human glioblastoma multiforme. *Science* 2008;321:1807–1812.
47. Jones S, Wang TL, Shih IeM, et al. Frequent mutations of chromatin remodeling gene ARID1A in ovarian clear cell carcinoma. *Science* 2010;330:228–231.
48. Parsons DW, Li M, Zhang X, et al. The genetic landscape of the childhood cancer medulloblastoma. *Science* 2011;331:435–439.
49. Yan H, Parsons DW, Jin G, et al. IDH1 and IDH2 mutations in gliomas. *N Engl J Med* 2009;360:765–773.
50. Bleeker FE, Lamba S, Leenstra S, et al. IDH1 mutations at residue p.R132 (IDH1(R132)) occur frequently in high-grade gliomas but not in other solid tumors. *Hum Mutat* 2009;30:7–11.
51. Hartmann C, Meyer J, Balss J, et al. Type and frequency of IDH1 and IDH2 mutations are related to astrocytic and oligodendroglial differentiation and age: a study of 1,010 diffuse gliomas. *Acta Neuropathol* 2009;118:469–474.
52. Hayden JT, Frühwald MC, Hasselblatt M, et al. Frequent IDH1 mutations in supratentorial primitive neuroectodermal tumors (sPNET) of adults but not children. *Cell Cycle* 2009;8:1806–1807.
53. Ichimura K, Pearson DM, Kocialkowski S, et al. IDH1 mutations are present in the majority of common adult gliomas but rare in primary glioblastomas. *Neuro Oncol* 2009;11:341–347.
54. Kang MR, Kim MS, Oh JE, et al. Mutational analysis of IDH1 codon 132 in glioblastomas and other common cancers. *Int J Cancer* 2009;125:353–355.
55. Watanabe T, Nobusawa S, Kleihues P, et al. IDH1 mutations are early events in the development of astrocytomas and oligodendrogliomas. *Am J Pathol* 2009;174:1149–1153.
56. Mardis ER, Ding L, Dooling DJ, et al. Recurring mutations found by sequencing an acute myeloid leukemia genome. *N Engl J Med* 2009;361:1058–1066.
57. Green A, Beer P. Somatic mutations of IDH1 and IDH2 in the leukemic transformation of myeloproliferative neoplasms. *N Engl J Med* 2010;362:369–370.
58. Gross S, Cairns RA, Minden Md, et al. Cancer-associated metabolite 2-hydroxyglutarate accumulates in acute myelogenous leukemia with isocitrate dehydrogenase 1 and 2 mutations. *J Exp Med* 2010;207:339–344.
59. Mardis ER, Wilson RK. Cancer genome sequencing: a review. *Hum Mol Genet* 2009;18:R163–R168.
60. Meyerson M, Gabriel S, Getz G. Advances in understanding cancer genomes through second-generation sequencing. *Nat Rev Genet* 2010;11:685–696.
61. Metzker ML. Sequencing technologies - the next generation. *Nat Rev Genet* 2010;11:31–46.
62. Bell DW. Our changing view of the genomic landscape of cancer. *J Pathol* 2010;220:231–243.
63. Campbell PJ, Pleasance ED, Stephens PJ, et al. Subclonal phylogenetic structures in cancer revealed by ultra-deep sequencing. *Proc Natl Acad Sci U S A* 2008;105:13081–13086.
64. Kidd JM, Cooper GM, Donahue WF, et al. Mapping and sequencing of structural variation from eight human genomes. *Nature* 2008;453:56–64.
65. Drmanac R, Sparks AB, Callow MJ, et al. Human genome sequencing using unchained base reads on self-assembling DNA nanoarrays. *Science* 2010; 327:78–81.
66. Clarke J, Wu HC, Jayasinghe L, et al. Continuous base identification for single-molecule nanopore DNA sequencing. *Nat Nanotechnol* 2009;4:265–270.
67. Schadt EE, Turner S, Kasarskis A. A window into third-generation sequencing. *Hum Mol Genet* 2010;19:R227–R240.
68. Dressman D, Yan H, Traverso G, et al. Transforming single DNA molecules into fluorescent magnetic particles for detection and enumeration of genetic variations. *Proc Natl Acad Sci U S A* 2003;100:8817–8822.
69. Fedurco M, Romieu A, Williams S, et al. BTA, a novel reagent for DNA attachment on glass and efficient generation of solid-phase amplified DNA colonies. *Nucleic Acids Res* 2006;34:e22.
70. Harris TD, Buzby PR, Babcock H, et al. Single-molecule DNA sequencing of a viral genome. *Science* 2008;320:106–109.
71. Morozova O, Hirst M, Marra MA. Applications of new sequencing technologies for transcriptome analysis. *Annu Rev Genomics Hum Genet* 2009;10: 135–151.

72. Pop M, Salzberg SL. Bioinformatics challenges of new sequencing technology. *Trends Genet* 2008;24:142–149.

73. Ley TJ, Mardis ER, Ding L, et al. DNA sequencing of a cytogenetically normal acute myeloid leukaemia genome. *Nature* 2008;456:66–72.

74. Garraway LA, Lander ES. Lessons from the cancer genome. *Cell* 2013;15:17–37.

75. Vogelstein B, Papadopoulos N, Velculescu VE, et al. Cancer genome landscapes. *Science* 2013;339:1546–1558.

76. Watson IR, Takahashi K, Futreal PA, et al. Emerging patterns of somatic mutations in cancer. *Nat Rev Genet* 2013;14:703–718.

77. Campbell PJ, Yachida S, Mudie LJ, et al. The patterns and dynamics of genomic instability in metastatic pancreatic cancer. *Nature* 2010;467:1109–1113.

78. Lee W, Jiang Z, Liu J, et al. The mutation spectrum revealed by paired genome sequences from a lung cancer patient. *Nature* 2010;465:473–477.

79. Marcucci G, Maharry K, Wu YZ, et al. IDH1 and IDH2 gene mutations identify novel molecular subsets within de novo cytogenetically normal acute myeloid leukemia: a Cancer and Leukemia Group B study. *J Clin Oncol* 2010;28:2348–2355.

80. Paschka P, Schlenk RF, Gaidzik VI, et al. IDH1 and IDH2 mutations are frequent genetic alterations in acute myeloid leukemia and confer adverse prognosis in cytogenetically normal acute myeloid leukemia with NPM1 mutation without FLT3 internal tandem duplication. *J Clin Oncol* 2010;28:3636–3643.

81. Shah SP, Morin Rd, Khattra J, et al. Mutational evolution in a lobular breast tumour profiled at single nucleotide resolution. *Nature* 2009;461:809–813.

82. Yachida S, Jones S, Bozic I, et al. Distant metastasis occurs late during the genetic evolution of pancreatic cancer. *Nature* 2010;467:1114–1117.

83. Pleasance ED, Cheetham RK, Stephens PJ, et al. A comprehensive catalogue of somatic mutations from a human cancer genome. *Nature* 2010;463:191–196.

84. Pleasance ED, Stephens PJ, O'Meara S, et al. A small-cell lung cancer genome with complex signatures of tobacco exposure. *Nature* 2010;463:184–190.

85. Ding L, Ellis MJ, Li S, et al. Genome remodelling in a basal-like breast cancer metastasis and xenograft. *Nature* 2010;464:999–1005.

86. Ley TJ, Ding L, Walter MJ, et al. DNMT3A mutations in acute myeloid leukemia. *N Engl J Med* 2010;363:2424–2433.

87. Alexandrov LB, Nik-Zainal S, Wedge DC, et al. Signatures of mutational processes in human cancer. *Nature* 2013;500:415–421.

88. Ward PS, Patel J, Wise DR, et al. The common feature of leukemia-associated IDH1 and IDH2 mutations is a neomorphic enzyme activity converting alpha-ketoglutarate to 2-hydroxyglutarate. *Cancer Cell* 2010;17:225–234.

89. Jones SJ, Laskin J, Lu YY, et al. Evolution of an adenocarcinoma in response to selection by targeted kinase inhibitors. *Genome Biol* 2010;11:R82.

90. Navin N, Kendall J, Troge J, et al. Tumour evolution inferred by single-cell sequencing. *Nature* 2011;472:90–94.

91. Vanharanta S, Massague J. Origins of metastatic traits. *Cancer Cell* 2013;24:410–421.

92. Huang FW, Hodis E, Xu MJ, et al. Highly recurrent TERT promoter mutations in human melanoma. *Science* 2013;339:957–959.

93. Horn S, Figl A, Rachakonda PS, et al. TERT promoter mutations in familial and sporadic melanoma. *Science* 2013;339:959–961.

94. Ying Z, Li Y, Wu J, et al. Loss of miR-204 expression enhances glioma migration and stem cell-like phenotype. *Cancer Res* 2013;73:990–999.

95. Liang YJ, Wang QY, Zhou CX, et al. MiR-124 targets Slug to regulate epithelial-mesenchymal transition and metastasis of breast cancer. *Carcinogenesis* 2013;34:713–722.

96. Cooper C, Guo J, Yan Y, et al. Increasing the relative expression of endogenous non-coding Steroid Receptor RNA Activator (SRA) in human breast cancer cells using modified oligonucleotides. *Nucleic Acids Res* 2009;37:4518–4531.

97. Stephens PJ, Greenman CD, Fu B, et al. Massive genomic rearrangement acquired in a single catastrophic event during cancer development. *Cell* 2011;144:27–40.

98. Korbel JO, Campbell PJ. Criteria for inference of chromothripsis in cancer genomes. *Cell* 2013;152:1226–1236.

99. Baca SC, Prandi D, Lawrence MS, et al. Punctuated evolution of prostate cancer genomes. *Cell* 2013;153:666–677.

100. Turner EH, Lee C, Ng SB, et al. Massively parallel exon capture and library-free resequencing across 16 genomes. *Nat Methods* 2009;6:315–316.

101. Gnirke A, Melnikov A, Maguire J, et al. Solution hybrid selection with ultra-long oligonucleotides for massively parallel targeted sequencing. *Nat Biotechnol* 2009;27:182–189.

102. Levin JZ, Berger MF, Adiconis X, et al. Targeted next-generation sequencing of a cancer transcriptome enhances detection of sequence variants and novel fusion transcripts. *Genome Biol* 2009;10:R115.

103. Lawrence MS, Stojanov P, Polak P, et al. Mutational heterogeneity in cancer and the search for new cancer-associated genes. *Nature* 2013;499:214–218.

104. Kandoth C, McLellan MD, Vandin F, et al. Mutational landscape and significance across 12 major cancer types. *Nature* 2013;502:333–339.

105. Gartner JJ, Parker SC, Prickett TD, et al. Whole-genome sequencing identifies a recurrent functional synonymous mutation in melanoma. *Proc Natl Acad Sci U S A* 2013;110:13481–13486.

106. Stegh AH, Brennan C, Mahoney JA, et al. Glioma oncoprotein Bcl2L12 inhibits the p53 tumor suppressor. *Genes Dev* 2010;24:2194–2204.

107. Mullaney JM, Mills RE, Pittard WS, et al. Small insertions and deletions (INDELs) in human genomes. *Hum Mol Genet* 2010;19:R131–R136.

108. Tomlins SA, Rhodes DR, Perner S, et al. Recurrent fusion of TMPRSS2 and ETS transcription factor genes in prostate cancer. *Science* 2005;310:644–648.

109. Soda M, Choi YL, Enomoto M, et al. Identification of the transforming EML4-ALK fusion gene in non-small-cell lung cancer. *Nature* 2007;448:561–566.

110. Palanisamy N, Ateeq B, Kalyana-Sundaram S, et al. Rearrangements of the RAF kinase pathway in prostate cancer, gastric cancer and melanoma. *Nat Med* 2010;16:793–798.

111. Leary RJ, Kinde I, Diehl F, et al. Development of personalized tumor biomarkers using massively parallel sequencing. *Sci Transl Med* 2010;2:20ra14.

112. Maher CA, Kumar-Sinha C, Cao X, et al. Transcriptome sequencing to detect gene fusions in cancer. *Nature* 2009;458:97–101.

113. Stephens PJ, McBride DJ, Lin ML, et al. Complex landscapes of somatic rearrangement in human breast cancer genomes. *Nature* 2009;462:1005–1010.

114. Feng H, Shuda M, Chang Y, et al. Clonal integration of a polyomavirus in human Merkel cell carcinoma. *Science* 2008;319:1096–1100.

115. Herner A, Sauliunaite D, Michalski CW, et al. Glutamate increases pancreatic cancer cell invasion and migration via AMPA receptor activation and Kras-MAPK signaling. *Int J Cancer* 2011;129:2349–2359.

116. Wei X, Walia V, Lin JC, et al. Exome sequencing identifies GRIN2A as frequently mutated in melanoma. *Nat Genet* 2011;43:442–446.

117. Prickett TD, Wei X, Cardenas-Navia I, et al. Exon capture analysis of G protein-coupled receptors identifies activating mutations in GRM3 in melanoma. *Nat Genet* 2011;43:1119–1126.

118. Krauthammer M, Kong Y, Ha BH, et al. Exome sequencing identifies recurrent somatic RAC1 mutations in melanoma. *Nat Genet* 2012;44:1006–1014.

119. Davies H, Hunter C, Smith R, et al. Somatic mutations of the protein kinase gene family in human lung cancer. *Cancer Res* 2005;65:7591–7595.

120. Bozic I, Antal T, Ohtsuki H, et al. Accumulation of driver and passenger mutations during tumor progression. *Proc Natl Acad Sci U S A* 2010;107:18545–18550.

121. Parmigiani G, Boca S, Lin J, et al. Design and analysis issues in genome-wide somatic mutation studies of cancer. *Genomics* 2009;93:17–21.

122. Kaminker JS, Zhang Y, Waugh A, et al. Distinguishing cancer-associated missense mutations from common polymorphisms. *Cancer Res* 2007;67:465–473.

123. Futreal PA. Backseat drivers take the wheel. *Cancer Cell* 2007;12:493–494.

124. Greenman C, Wooster R, Futreal PA, et al. Statistical analysis of pathogenicity of somatic mutations in cancer. *Genetics* 2006;173:2187–2198.

125. Baudot A, Real FX, Izarzugaza JM, et al. From cancer genomes to cancer models: bridging the gaps. *EMBO Rep* 2009;10:359–366.

126. Carter H, Chen S, Isik L, et al. Cancer-specific high-throughput annotation of somatic mutations: computational prediction of driver missense mutations. *Cancer Res* 2009;69:6660–6667.

127. Ng PC, Henikoff S. SIFT: Predicting amino acid changes that affect protein function. *Nucleic Acids Res* 2003;31:3812–3814.

128. Kohli M, Rago C, Lengauer C, et al. Facile methods for generating human somatic cell gene knockouts using recombinant adeno-associated viruses. *Nucleic Acids Res* 2004;32:e3.

129. Downing JR, Wilson RK, Zhang J, et al. The Pediatric Cancer Genome Project. *Nat Genet* 2012;44:619–622.

130. Hudson TJ, Anderson W, Artez A, et al. International network of cancer genome projects. *Nature* 2010;464:993–998.

131. Bignell GR, Greenman CD, Davies H, et al. Signatures of mutation and selection in the cancer genome. *Nature* 2010;463:893–898.

132. Sieber OM, Tomlinson SR, Tomlinson IP. Tissue, cell and stage specificity of (epi)mutations in cancers. *Nat Rev Cancer* 2005;5:649–655.

133. Benvenuti S, Frattini M, Arena S, et al. PIK3CA cancer mutations display gender and tissue specificity patterns. *Hum Mutat* 2008;29:284–288.

134. Karakas B, Bachman KE, Park BH. Mutation of the PIK3CA oncogene in human cancers. *Br J Cancer* 2006;94:455–459.

135. Brennan CW, Werhaak RG, McKenna A, et al. The somatic genomic landscape of glioblastoma. *Cell* 2013;155:462–477.

136. Cancer Genome Atlas Network. Comprehensive molecular characterization of human colon and rectal cancer. *Nature* 2012;487:330–337.

137. Cancer Genome Atlas Network. Comprehensive molecular portraits of human breast tumours. *Nature* 2012;490:61–70.

138. Cancer Genome Atlas Research Network. Integrated genomic analyses of ovarian carcinoma. *Nature* 2011;474:609–615.

139. Cancer Genome Atlas Research Network. Comprehensive molecular characterization of clear cell renal cell carcinoma. *Nature* 2013;499:43–49.

140. Cancer Genome Atlas Research Network. Integrated genomic characterization of endometrial carcinoma. *Nature* 2013;497:67–73.

141. Weischenfeldt J, Simon R, Feuerbach L, et al. Integrative genomic analyses reveal an androgen-driven somatic alteration landscape in early-onset prostate cancer. *Cancer Cell* 2013;23:159–170.

142. Cancer Genome Atlas Research Network. Genomic and epigenomic landscapes of adult de novo acute myeloid leukemia. *N Engl J Med* 2013;368:2059–2074.

143. Dawson SJ, Rueda OM, Aparicio S, et al. A new genome-driven integrated classification of breast cancer and its implications. *EMBO J* 2013;32:617–628.

144. Plass C, Pfister SM, Lindroth AM, et al. Mutations in regulators of the epigenome and their connections to global chromatin patterns in cancer. *Nat Rev Genet* 2013;14:765–780.

145. Shen H, Laird PW. Interplay between the cancer genome and epigenome. *Cell* 2013;153:38–55.

146. Yamamoto E, Suzuki H, Yamano HO, et al. Molecular dissection of premalignant colorectal lesions reveals early onset of the CpG island methylator phenotype. *Am J Pathol* 2012;181:1847–1861.

147. Gao J, Aksoy BA, Dogrusoz U, et al. Integrative analysis of complex cancer genomics and clinical profiles using the cBioPortal. *Sci Signal* 2013;6:pl1.

148. Bleeker FE, Bardelli A. Genomic landscapes of cancers: prospects for targeted therapies. *Pharmacogenomics* 2007;8:1629–1633.

149. Paez JG, Jänne PA, Lee JC, et al. EGFR mutations in lung cancer: correlation with clinical response to gefitinib therapy. *Science* 2004;304:1497–1500.

150. Ciardiello F, Tortora G. EGFR antagonists in cancer treatment. *N Engl J Med* 2008;358:1160–1174.

151. Janku F, Stewart DJ, Kurzrock R. Targeted therapy in non-small-cell lung cancer—is it becoming a reality? *Nat Rev Clin Oncol* 2010;7:401–414.

152. Pao W, Chmielecki J. Rational, biologically based treatment of EGFR-mutant non-small-cell lung cancer. *Nat Rev Cancer* 2010;10:760–774.

153. Gerber DE, Minna JD. ALK inhibition for non-small cell lung cancer: from discovery to therapy in record time. *Cancer Cell* 2010;18:548–551.

154. Andreyev HJ, Norman AR, Cunningham D, et al. Kirsten ras mutations in patients with colorectal cancer: the multicenter "RASCAL" study. *J Natl Cancer Inst* 1998;90:675–684.

155. Roth AD, Tejpar S, Delorenzi M, et al. Prognostic role of KRAS and BRAF in stage II and III resected colon cancer: results of the translational study on the PETACC-3, EORTC 40993, SAKK 60-00 trial. *J Clin Oncol* 2010;28:466–474.

156. Bardelli A, Siena S. Molecular mechanisms of resistance to cetuximab and panitumumab in colorectal cancer. *J Clin Oncol* 2010;28:1254–1261.

157. Siena S, Sartore-Bianchi A, Di Nicolantonio F, et al. Biomarkers predicting clinical outcome of epidermal growth factor receptor-targeted therapy in metastatic colorectal cancer. *J Natl Cancer Inst* 2009;101:1308–1324.

158. Tejpar S, Bertagnolli M, Bosman F, et al. Prognostic and predictive biomarkers in resected colon cancer: current status and future perspectives for integrating genomics into biomarker discovery. *Oncologist* 2010;15:390–404.

159. Gerlinger M, Rowan AJ, Horswell S, et al. Intratumor heterogeneity and branched evolution revealed by multiregion sequencing. *N Engl J Med* 2012;366:883–892.

160. Mandel P, Metais P. [Not Available]. *C R Seances Soc Biol Fil* 1948;142:241–243.

161. Crowley E, Di Nicolantonio F, Loupakis F, et al. Liquid biopsy: monitoring cancer-genetics in the blood. *Nat Rev Clin Oncol* 2013;10:472–484.

162. Diehl F, Li M, Dressman D, et al. Detection and quantification of mutations in the plasma of patients with colorectal tumors. *Proc Natl Acad Sci U S A* 2005;102:16368–16373.

163. Diehl F, Schmidt K, Choti MA, et al. Circulating mutant DNA to assess tumor dynamics. *Nat Med* 2008;14:985–990.

164. Frattini M, Gallino G, Signoroni S, et al. Quantitative and qualitative characterization of plasma DNA identifies primary and recurrent colorectal cancer. *Cancer Lett* 2008;263:170–181.

165. Chan KC, Jiang P, Zheng YW, et al. Cancer genome scanning in plasma: detection of tumor-associated copy number aberrations, single-nucleotide variants, and tumoral heterogeneity by massively parallel sequencing. *Clin Chem* 2013;59:211–224.

166. Murtaza M, Dawson SJ, Tsui DW, et al. Non-invasive analysis of acquired resistance to cancer therapy by sequencing of plasma DNA. *Nature* 2013;497:108–112.

167. Bardelli A, Corso S, Bertotti A, et al. Amplification of the MET receptor drives resistance to anti-EGFR therapies in colorectal cancer. *Cancer Discov* 2013;3:658–673.

168. Higgins MJ, Jelovac D, Barnathan E, et al. Detection of tumor PIK3CA status in metastatic breast cancer using peripheral blood. *Clin Cancer Res* 2012;18:3462–3469.

169. Leary RJ, Sausen M, Kinde I, et al. Detection of chromosomal alterations in the circulation of cancer patients with whole-genome sequencing. *Sci Transl Med* 2012;4:162ra154.

170. Misale S, Yaeger R, Hobor S, et al. Emergence of KRAS mutations and acquired resistance to anti-EGFR therapy in colorectal cancer. *Nature* 2012;486:532–536.

171. Diaz LA Jr, Williams RT, Wu J, et al. The molecular evolution of acquired resistance to targeted EGFR blockade in colorectal cancers. *Nature* 2012;486:537–540.

172. Robbins PF, Lu YC, El-Gamil M, et al. Mining exomic sequencing data to identify mutated antigens recognized by adoptively transferred tumor-reactive T cells. *Nat Med* 2013;19:747–752.

173. Hunter C, Smith R, Cahill DP, et al. A hypermutation phenotype and somatic MSH6 mutations in recurrent human malignant gliomas after alkylator chemotherapy. *Cancer Res* 2006;66:3987–3991.

174. Cahill DP, Levine KK, Betensky RA, et al. Loss of the mismatch repair protein MSH6 in human glioblastomas is associated with tumor progression during temozolomide treatment. *Clin Cancer Res* 2007;13:2038–2045.

175. Engelman JA, Zejnullahu K, Mitsudomi T, et al. MET amplification leads to gefitinib resistance in lung cancer by activating ERBB3 signaling. *Science* 2007;316:1039–1043.

176. Gorre ME, Mohmmed M, Ellwood K, et al. Clinical resistance to STI-571 cancer therapy caused by BCR-ABL gene mutation or amplification. *Science* 2001;293:876–880.

177. Heinrich MC, Corless CL, Blanke CD, et al. Molecular correlates of imatinib resistance in gastrointestinal stromal tumors. *J Clin Oncol* 2006;24:4764–4774.

178. Shepherd FA, Rodrigues Pereira J, Ciuleanu T, et al. Erlotinib in previously treated non-small-cell lung cancer. *N Engl J Med* 2005;353:123–132.

179. Kobayashi S, Boggon TJ, Dayaram T, et al. EGFR mutation and resistance of non-small-cell lung cancer to gefitinib. *N Engl J Med* 2005;352:786–792.

180. Kwak EL, Sordella R, Bell DW, et al. Irreversible inhibitors of the EGF receptor may circumvent acquired resistance to gefitinib. *Proc Natl Acad Sci U S A* 2005;102:7665–7670.

181. Pao W, Miller VA, Politi KA, et al. Acquired resistance of lung adenocarcinomas to gefitinib or erlotinib is associated with a second mutation in the EGFR kinase domain. *PLoS Med* 2005;2:e73.

182. Shih JY, Gow CH, Yang PC. EGFR mutation conferring primary resistance to gefitinib in non-small-cell lung cancer. *N Engl J Med* 2005;353:207–208.

183. Bell DW, Gore I, Okimoto Ra, et al. Inherited susceptibility to lung cancer may be associated with the T790M drug resistance mutation in EGFR. *Nat Genet* 2005;37:1315–1316.

184. Inukai M, Toyooka S, Ito S, et al. Presence of epidermal growth factor receptor gene T790M mutation as a minor clone in non-small cell lung cancer. *Cancer Res* 2006;66:7854–7858.

185. Daub H, Specht K, Ullrich A. Strategies to overcome resistance to targeted protein kinase inhibitors. *Nat Rev Drug Discov* 2004;3:1001–1010.

186. Choi YL, Soda M, Yamashita Y, et al. EML4-ALK mutations in lung cancer that confer resistance to ALK inhibitors. *N Engl J Med* 2010;363:1734–1739.

187. Flaherty KT, Puzanov I, Kim KB, et al. Inhibition of mutated, activated BRAF in metastatic melanoma. *N Engl J Med* 2010;363:809–819.

188. Nazarian R, Shi H, Wang Q, et al. Melanomas acquire resistance to B-RAF(V600E) inhibition by RTK or N-RAS upregulation. *Nature* 2010;468:973–977.

189. Pompetti F, Spadano A, Sau A, et al. Long-term remission in BCR/ABL-positive AML-M6 patient treated with Imatinib Mesylate. *Leuk Res* 2007;31:563–567.

190. Druker BJ, Builhot F, O'Brien SG, et al. Five-year follow-up of patients receiving imatinib for chronic myeloid leukemia. *N Engl J Med* 2006;355:2408–2417.

# 2 Hallmarks of Cancer: An Organizing Principle for Cancer Medicine

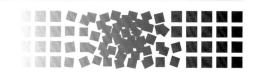

Douglas Hanahan and Robert A. Weinberg

## INTRODUCTION

The hallmarks of cancer comprise eight biologic capabilities acquired by incipient cancer cells during the multistep development of human tumors. The hallmarks constitute an organizing principle for rationalizing the complexities of neoplastic disease. They include sustaining proliferative signaling, evading growth suppressors, resisting cell death, enabling replicative immortality, inducing angiogenesis, activating invasion and metastasis, reprogramming energy metabolism, and evading immune destruction. Facilitating the acquisition of these hallmark capabilities are genome instability, which enables mutational alteration of hallmark-enabling genes, and immune inflammation, which fosters the acquisition of multiple hallmark functions. In addition to cancer cells, tumors exhibit another dimension of complexity: They contain a repertoire of recruited, ostensibly normal cells that contribute to the acquisition of hallmark traits by creating the *tumor microenvironment*. Recognition of the widespread applicability of these concepts will increasingly influence the development of new means to treat human cancer.

At the beginning of the new millennium, we proposed that six *hallmarks of cancer* embody an organizing principle that provides a logical framework for understanding the remarkable diversity of neoplastic diseases.[1] Implicit in our discussion was the notion that, as normal cells evolve progressively to a neoplastic state, they acquire a succession of these hallmark capabilities, and that the multistep process of human tumor pathogenesis can be rationalized by the need of incipient cancer cells to acquire the diverse traits that in aggregate enable them to become tumorigenic and, ultimately, malignant.

We noted as an ancillary proposition that tumors are more than insular masses of proliferating cancer cells. Instead, they are complex tissues composed of multiple distinct types of neoplastic and normal cells that participate in heterotypic interactions with one another. We depicted the recruited normal cells, which form tumor-associated stroma, as active participants in tumorigenesis rather than passive bystanders; as such, these stromal cells contribute to the development and expression of certain hallmark capabilities. This notion has been solidified and extended during the intervening period, and it is now clear that the biology of tumors can no longer be understood simply by enumerating the traits of the cancer cells, but instead must encompass the contributions of the *tumor microenvironment* to tumorigenesis. In 2011, we revisited the original hallmarks, adding two new ones to the roster, and expanded on the functional roles and contributions made by recruited stromal cells to tumor biology.[2] Herein we reiterate and further refine the hallmarks-of-cancer perspectives we presented in 2000 and 2011, with the goal of informing students of cancer medicine about the concept and its potential utility for understanding the pathogenesis of human cancer, and the potential relevance of this concept to the development of more effective treatments for this disease.

## HALLMARK CAPABILITIES, IN ESSENCE

The eight hallmarks of cancer—distinct and complementary capabilities that enable tumor growth and metastatic dissemination—continue to provide a solid foundation for understanding the biology of cancer (Fig. 2.1). The sections that follow summarize the essence of each hallmark, providing insights into their regulation and functional manifestations.

### Sustaining Proliferative Signaling

Arguably, the most fundamental trait of cancer cells involves their ability to sustain chronic proliferation. Normal tissues carefully control the production and release of growth-promoting signals that instruct entry of cells into and progression through the growth-and-division cycle, thereby ensuring proper control of cell number and thus maintenance of normal tissue architecture and function. Cancer cells, by deregulating these signals, become masters of their own destinies. The enabling signals are conveyed in large part by growth factors that bind cell-surface receptors, typically containing intracellular tyrosine kinase domains. The latter proceed to emit signals via branched intracellular signaling pathways that regulate progression through the cell cycle as well as cell growth (that is, increase in cell size); often, these signals influence yet other cell-biologic properties, such as cell survival and energy metabolism.

Remarkably, the precise identities and sources of the proliferative signals operating within normal tissues remain poorly understood. Moreover, we still know relatively little about the mechanisms controlling the release of these mitogenic signals. In part, the study of these mechanisms is complicated by the fact that the growth factor signals controlling cell number and position within normal tissues are thought to be transmitted in a temporally and spatially regulated fashion from one cell to its neighbors; such paracrine signaling is difficult to access experimentally. In addition, the bioavailability of growth factors is regulated by their sequestration in the pericellular space and associated extracellular matrix. Moreover, the actions of these extracellular mitogenic proteins is further controlled by a complex network of proteases, sulfatases, and possibly other enzymes that liberate and activate these factors, apparently in a highly specific and localized fashion.

The mitogenic signaling operating in cancer cells is, in contrast, far better understood.[3–6] Cancer cells can acquire the capability to sustain proliferative signaling in a number of alternative ways: They may produce growth factor ligands themselves, to which they can then respond via the coexpression of cognate receptors, resulting in autocrine proliferative stimulation. Alternatively, cancer cells may send signals to stimulate normal cells within the supporting tumor-associated stroma; the stromal cells then reciprocate by supplying the cancer cells with various growth factors.[7,8] Mitogenic signaling can also be deregulated by elevating the levels of receptor proteins displayed at the cancer cell

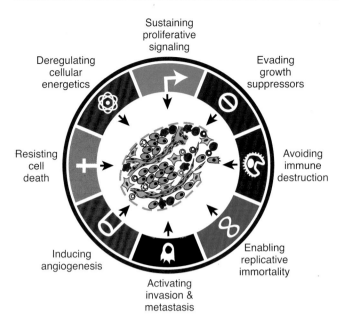

**Figure 2.1** The hallmarks of cancer. Eight functional capabilities—the hallmarks of cancer—are thought to be acquired by developing cancers in the course of the multistep carcinogenesis that leads to most forms of human cancer. The order in which these hallmark capabilities are acquired and the relative balance and importance of their contributions to malignant disease appears to vary across the spectrum of human cancers. (Adapted from Hanahan D, Weinberg R. The hallmarks of cancer. *Cell* 2000;100:57–70; Hanahan D, Weinberg RA. Hallmarks of cancer: the next generation. *Cell* 2011;144:646–674.)

surface, rendering such cells hyperresponsive to otherwise limiting amounts of growth factor ligands; the same outcome can result from structural alterations in the receptor molecules that facilitate ligand-independent firing.

Independence from externally supplied growth factors may also derive from the constitutive activation of components of intracellular signaling cascades operating downstream of these receptors within cancer cells. These intracellular alterations obviate the need to stimulate cell proliferation pathways by ligand-mediated activation of cell-surface receptors. Of note, because a number of distinct downstream signaling pathways radiate from ligand-stimulated receptors, the activation of one or another of these downstream branches (e.g., the pathway responding to the Ras signal transducer) may only provide a subset of the regulatory instructions transmitted by a ligand-activated receptor.

## Somatic Mutations Activate Additional Downstream Pathways

DNA sequencing analyses of cancer cell genomes have revealed somatic mutations in certain human tumors that predict constitutive activation of the signaling circuits, cited previously, that are normally triggered by activated growth factor receptors. The past 3 decades have witnessed the identification in tens of thousands of human tumors of mutant, oncogenic alleles of the *RAS* proto-oncogenes, most of which have sustained point mutations in the 12th codon, which results in RAS proteins that are constitutively active in downstream signaling. Thus, more than 90% of pancreatic adenocarcinomas carry mutant K-*RAS* alleles. More recently, the repertoire of frequently mutated genes has been expanded to include those encoding the downstream effectors of the RAS proteins. For example, we now know that ~40% of human melanomas contain activating mutations affecting the structure of the B-RAF protein, resulting in constitutive signaling through the RAF to the mitogen-activated protein (MAP)–kinase pathway.[9] Similarly, mutations in the catalytic subunit of phosphoinositide 3-kinase (PI3K)

isoforms are being detected in an array of tumor types; these mutations typically serve to hyperactivate the PI3K signaling pathway, causing in turn, excess signaling through the crucial Akt/PKB signal transducer.[10,11] The advantages to tumor cells of activating upstream (receptor) versus downstream (transducer) signaling remain obscure, as does the functional impact of cross-talk between the multiple branched pathways radiating from individual growth factor receptors.

## Disruptions of Negative-Feedback Mechanisms that Attenuate Proliferative Signaling

Recent observations have also highlighted the importance of negative-feedback loops that normally operate to dampen various types of signaling and thereby ensure homeostatic regulation of the flux of signals coursing through the intracellular circuitry.[12–15] Defects in these negative-feedback mechanisms are capable of enhancing proliferative signaling. The prototype of this type of regulation involves the RAS oncoprotein. The oncogenic effects of mutant RAS proteins do not result from a hyperactivation of its downstream signaling powers; instead, the oncogenic mutations affecting *RAS* genes impair the intrinsic GTPase activity of RAS that normally serves to turn its activity off, ensuring that active signal transmission (e.g., from upstream growth factor receptors) is transient; as such, oncogenic RAS mutations disrupt an autoregulatory negative-feedback mechanism, without which RAS generates chronic proliferative signals.

Analogous negative-feedback mechanisms operate at multiple nodes within the proliferative signaling circuitry. A prominent example involves phosphatase and tensin homolog (PTEN), which counteracts PI3K by degrading its product, phosphatidylinositol 3,4,5-phosphate (PIP$_3$). Loss-of-function mutations in PTEN amplify PI3K signaling and promote tumorigenesis in a variety of experimental models of cancer; in human tumors, PTEN expression is often lost by the methylation of DNA at specific sites associated with the promoter of the *PTEN* gene, resulting in the shutdown of its transcription.[10,11]

Yet another example involves the mammalian target of rapamycin (mTOR) kinase, a key coordinator of cell growth and metabolism that lies both upstream and downstream of the PI3K pathway. In the circuitry of some cancer cells, mTOR activation results, via negative feedback, in the inhibition of PI3K signaling. Accordingly, when mTOR is pharmacologically inhibited in such cancer cells (e.g., by the drug rapamycin), the associated loss of negative feedback results in increased activity of PI3K and its effector, the Akt/PKB kinase, thereby blunting the antiproliferative effects of mTOR inhibition.[16,17] It is likely that compromised negative feedback loops in this and other signaling pathways will prove to be widespread among human cancer cells, serving as important means by which cancer cells acquire the capability of signaling chronically through these pathways. Moreover, disruption of such normally self-attenuating signaling can contribute to the development of adaptive resistance toward therapeutic drugs targeting mitogenic signaling.

## Excessive Proliferative Signaling Can Trigger Cell Senescence

Early studies of oncogene action encouraged the notion that ever-increasing expression of such genes and the signals released by their protein products would result in proportionately increased cancer cell proliferation and, thus, tumor growth. More recent research has undermined this notion, in that it is now apparent that excessively elevated signaling by oncoproteins, such as RAS, MYC, and RAF, can provoke counteracting (protective) responses from cells, such as induction of cell death; alternatively, cancer cells expressing high levels of these oncoproteins may be forced to enter into the nonproliferative but viable state called senescence. These responses contrast with those seen in cells expressing lower levels of these proteins, which permit cells to avoid senescence or cell death and, thus, proliferate.[18–21]

Cells with morphologic features of senescence, including enlarged cytoplasm, the absence of proliferation markers, and the expression of the senescence-induced β-galactosidase enzyme, are abundant in the tissues of mice whose genomes have been reengineered to cause overexpression of certain oncogenes[19,20]; such senescent cells are also prevalent in some cases of human melanoma.[22]

These ostensibly paradoxical responses seem to reflect intrinsic cellular defense mechanisms designed to eliminate cells experiencing excessive levels of certain types of mitogenic signaling. Accordingly, the intensity of oncogenic signaling observed in naturally arising cancer cells may represent compromises between maximal mitogenic stimulation and avoidance of these anti-proliferative defenses. Alternatively, some cancer cells may adapt to high levels of oncogenic signaling by disabling their senescence- or apoptosis-inducing circuitry.

## Evading Growth Suppressors

In addition to the hallmark capability of inducing and sustaining positively acting growth-stimulatory signals, cancer cells must also circumvent powerful programs that negatively regulate cell proliferation; many of these programs depend on the actions of tumor suppressor genes. Dozens of tumor suppressors that operate in various ways to limit cell proliferation or survival have been discovered through their inactivation in one or another form of animal or human cancer; many of these genes have been validated as bona fide tumor suppressors through gain- or loss-of-function experiments in mice. The two prototypical tumor suppressor genes encode the retinoblastoma (RB)-associated and TP53 proteins; they operate as central control nodes within two key, complementary cellular regulatory circuits that govern the decisions of cells to proliferate, or alternatively, to activate growth arrest, senescence, or the cell-suicide program known as apoptosis.

The RB protein integrates signals from diverse extracellular and intracellular sources and, in response, decides whether or not a cell should proceed through its growth-and-division cycle.[23–25] Cancer cells with defects in the RB pathway function are thus missing the services of a critical gatekeeper of cell-cycle progression whose absence permits persistent cell proliferation. Whereas RB transduces growth-inhibitory signals that largely originate outside of the cell, TP53 receives inputs from stress and abnormality sensors that function within the cell's intracellular operating systems. For example, if the degree of damage to a cell's genome is excessive, or if the levels of nucleotide pools, growth-promoting signals, glucose, or oxygenation are insufficient, TP53 can call a halt to further cell-cycle progression until these conditions have been normalized. Alternatively, in the face of alarm signals indicating overwhelming or irreparable damage to such cellular systems, TP53 can trigger apoptosis. Of note, the alternative effects of activated TP53 are complex and highly context dependent, varying by cell type as well as by the severity and persistence of conditions of cell-physiologic stress and genomic damage.

Although the two canonical suppressors of proliferation—TP53 and RB—have preeminent importance in regulating cell proliferation, various lines of evidence indicate that each operates as part of a larger network that is wired for functional redundancy. For example, chimeric mice populated throughout their bodies with individual cells lacking a functional *Rb* gene are surprisingly free of proliferative abnormalities, despite the expectation that a loss of RB function should result in unimpeded advance through the cell division cycle by these cells and their lineal descendants; some of the resulting clusters of *Rb*-null cells should, by all rights, progress to neoplasia. Instead, the *Rb*-null cells in such chimeric mice have been found to participate in relatively normal tissue morphogenesis throughout the body; the only neoplasia observed is of pituitary tumors developing late in life.[26] Similarly, *TP53*-null mice develop

normally, show largely normal cell and tissue homeostasis, and again develop abnormalities only later in life in the form of leukemias and sarcomas.[27]

### Mechanisms of Contact Inhibition and Its Evasion

Four decades of research have demonstrated that the cell-to-cell contacts formed by dense populations of normal cells growing in 2-dimensional culture operate to suppress further cell proliferation, yielding confluent cell monolayers. Importantly, such *contact inhibition* is abolished in various types of cancer cells in culture, suggesting that contact inhibition is an in vitro surrogate of a mechanism that operates in vivo to ensure normal tissue homeostasis that is abrogated during the course of tumorigenesis. Until recently, the mechanistic basis for this mode of growth control remained obscure. Now, however, mechanisms of contact inhibition are beginning to emerge.[28]

One mechanism involves the product of the *NF2* gene, long implicated as a tumor suppressor because its loss triggers a form of human neurofibromatosis. Merlin, the cytoplasmic *NF2* gene product, orchestrates contact inhibition by coupling cell-surface adhesion molecules (e.g., E-cadherin) to transmembrane receptor tyrosine kinases (e.g., the EGF receptor). In so doing, Merlin strengthens the adhesiveness of cadherin-mediated cell-to-cell attachments. Additionally, by sequestering such growth factor receptors, Merlin limits their ability to efficiently emit mitogenic signals.[28–31]

### Corruption of the TGF-β Pathway Promotes Malignancy

Transforming growth factor beta (TGF-β is best known for its anti-proliferative effects on epithelial cells. The responses of carcinoma cells to TGF-β's proliferation–suppressive effects is now appreciated to be far more elaborate than a simple shutdown of its signaling circuitry.[32–35] In normal cells, exposure to TGF-β blocks their progression through the G1 phase of the cell cycle. In many late-stage tumors, however, TGF-β signaling is redirected away from suppressing cell proliferation and is found instead to activate a cellular program, termed the epithelial-to-mesenchymal transition (EMT), which confers on cancer cells multiple traits associated with high-grade malignancy, as will be discussed in further detail.

## Resisting Cell Death

The ability to activate the normally latent apoptotic cell-death program appears to be associated with most types of normal cells throughout the body. Its actions in many if not all multicellular organisms seems to reflect the need to eliminate aberrant cells whose continued presence would otherwise threaten organismic integrity. This rationale explains why cancer cells often, if not invariably, inactivate or attenuate this program during their development.[21,36–38]

Elucidation of the detailed design of the signaling circuitry governing the apoptotic program has revealed how apoptosis is triggered in response to various physiologic stresses that cancer cells experience either during the course of tumorigenesis or as a result of anticancer therapy. Notable among the apoptosis-inducing stresses are signaling imbalances resulting from elevated levels of oncogene signaling and from DNA damage. The regulators of the apoptotic response are divided into two major circuits, one receiving and processing extracellular death-inducing signals (the extrinsic apoptotic program, involving for example the Fas ligand/Fas receptor), and the other sensing and integrating a variety of signals of intracellular origin (the intrinsic program). Each of these circuits culminates in the activation of a normally latent protease (caspase 8 or 9, respectively), which proceeds to initiate a cascade of proteolysis involving effector caspases that are responsible for the execution phase of apoptosis. During this final phase, an apoptotic cell is progressively disassembled and then consumed, both by its neighbors and by professional phagocytic cells. Currently, the intrinsic apoptotic program is more widely implicated as a barrier to cancer pathogenesis.

The molecular machinery that conveys signals between the apoptotic regulators and effectors is controlled by counterbalancing pro- and antiapoptotic members of the Bcl-2 family of regulatory proteins.[36,37] The archetype, Bcl-2, along with its closest relatives (Bcl-XL, Bcl-W, Mcl-1, A1) are inhibitors of apoptosis, acting in large part by binding to and thereby suppressing two proapoptotic triggering proteins (Bax and Bak); the latter are embedded in the mitochondrial outer membrane. When relieved of inhibition by their antiapoptotic relatives, Bax and Bax disrupt the integrity of the outer mitochondrial membrane, causing the release into the cytosol of proapoptotic signaling proteins, the most important of which is cytochrome C. When the normally sequestered cytochrome C is released, it activates a cascade of cytosolic caspase proteases that proceed to fragment multiple cellular structures, thereby executing the apoptotic death program.[37,39]

Several abnormality sensors have been identified that play key roles in triggering apoptosis.[21,37] Most notable is a DNA damage sensor that acts through the TP53 tumor suppressor[40]; TP53 induces apoptosis by upregulating expression of the proapoptotic, Bcl-2-related Noxa and Puma proteins, doing so in response to substantial levels of DNA breaks and other chromosomal abnormalities. Alternatively, insufficient survival factor signaling (e.g., inadequate levels of interleukin (IL)-3 in lymphocytes or of insulinlike growth factors 1/2 [IGF1/2] in epithelial cells) can elicit apoptosis through another proapoptotic Bcl-2-related protein called Bim. Yet another condition triggering apoptosis involves hyperactive signaling by certain oncoproteins, such as Myc, which acts in part via Bim and other Bcl-2-related proteins.[18,21,40]

Tumor cells evolve a variety of strategies to limit or circumvent apoptosis. Most common is the loss of TP53 tumor suppressor function, which eliminates this critical damage sensor from the apoptosis-inducing circuitry. Alternatively, tumors may achieve similar ends by increasing the expression of antiapoptotic regulators (Bcl-2, Bcl-XL) or of survival signals (IGF1/2), by downregulating proapoptotic Bcl-2-related factors (Bax, Bim, Puma), or by short-circuiting the extrinsic ligand-induced death pathway. The multiplicity of apoptosis-avoiding mechanisms presumably reflects the diversity of apoptosis-inducing signals that cancer cell populations encounter during their evolution from the normal to the neoplastic state.

## Autophagy Mediates Both Tumor Cell Survival and Death

Autophagy represents an important cell-physiologic response that, like apoptosis, normally operates at low, basal levels in cells but can be strongly induced in certain states of cellular stress, the most obvious of which is nutrient deficiency.[41–43] The autophagic program enables cells to break down cellular organelles, such as ribosomes and mitochondria, allowing the resulting catabolites to be recycled and thus used for biosynthesis and energy metabolism. As part of this program, intracellular vesicles (termed autophagosomes) envelope the cellular organelles destined for degradation; the resulting vesicles then fuse with lysosomes in which degradation occurs. In this fashion, low-molecular-weight metabolites are generated that support survival in the stressed, nutrient-limited environments experienced by many cancer cells. When acting in this fashion, autophagy favors cancer cell survival.

However, the autophagy program intersects in more complex ways with the life and death of cancer cells. Like apoptosis, the autophagy machinery has both regulatory and effector components.[41–43] Among the latter are proteins that mediate autophagosome formation and delivery to lysosomes. Of note, recent research has revealed intersections between the regulatory circuits governing autophagy, apoptosis, and cellular homeostasis. For example, the signaling pathway involving PI3K, AKT, and mTOR, which is stimulated by survival signals to block apoptosis, similarly inhibits autophagy; when survival signals are insufficient, the PI3K signaling pathway is downregulated, with the result that autophagy and/or apoptosis may be induced.[41,42,44,45]

Another interconnection between these two programs resides in the Beclin-1 protein, which has been shown by genetic studies to be necessary for the induction of autophagy.[41–44] Beclin-1 is a member of the Bcl-2 family of apoptotic regulatory proteins, and its BH3 domain allows it to bind the Bcl-2/Bcl-XL proteins. Stress sensor–coupled BH3-containing proteins (e.g. Bim, Noxa) can displace Beclin-1 from its association with Bcl-2/Bcl-XL, enabling the liberated Beclin-1 to trigger autophagy, much as they can release proapoptotic Bax and Bak to trigger apoptosis. Hence, stress-transducing Bcl-2–related proteins can induce apoptosis and/or autophagy depending on the physiologic state of the cell.

Genetically altered mice bearing inactivated alleles of the *Beclin-1* gene or of certain other components of the autophagy machinery exhibit increased susceptibility to cancer.[42,46] These results suggest that the induction of autophagy can serve as a barrier to tumorigenesis that may operate independently of or in concert with apoptosis. For example, excessive activation of the autophagy program may cause cells to devour too many of their own critical organelles, such that cell growth and division are crippled. Accordingly, autophagy may represent yet another barrier that needs to be circumvented by incipient cancer cells during multistep tumor development.[41,46]

Perhaps paradoxically, nutrient starvation, radiotherapy, and certain cytotoxic drugs can induce elevated levels of autophagy that apparently protect cancer cells.[45–48] Moreover, severely stressed cancer cells have been shown to shrink via autophagy to a state of reversible dormancy.[46,49] This particular survival response may enable the persistence and eventual regrowth of some late-stage tumors following treatment with potent anticancer agents. Together, observations like these indicate that autophagy can have dichotomous effects on tumor cells and, thus, tumor progression.[46,47] An important agenda for future research will involve clarifying the genetic and cell-physiologic conditions that determine when and how autophagy enables cancer cells to survive or, alternatively, causes them to die.

## Necrosis Has Proinflammatory and Tumor-Promoting Potential

In contrast to apoptosis, in which a dying cell contracts into an almost invisible corpse that is soon consumed by its neighbors, necrotic cells become bloated and explode, releasing their contents into the local tissue microenvironment. A body of evidence has shown that cell death by necrosis, like apoptosis, is an organized process under genetic control, rather than being a random and undirected process.[50–52]

Importantly, necrotic cell death releases proinflammatory signals into the surrounding tissue microenvironment, in contrast to apoptosis, which does not. As a consequence, necrotic cells can recruit inflammatory cells of the immune system,[51,53,54] whose dedicated function is to survey the extent of tissue damage and remove associated necrotic debris. In the context of neoplasia, however, multiple lines of evidence indicate that immune inflammatory cells can be actively tumor-promoting by fostering angiogenesis, cancer cell proliferation, and invasiveness (discussed in subsequent sections). Additionally, necrotic cells can release bioactive regulatory factors, such as IL1α, which can directly stimulate neighboring viable cells to proliferate, with the potential, once again, to facilitate neoplastic progression.[53] Consequently, necrotic cell death, while seemingly beneficial in counterbalancing cancer-associated hyperproliferation, may ultimately do more damage to the patient than good.

## Enabling Replicative Immortality

Cancer cells require unlimited replicative potential in order to generate macroscopic tumors. This capability stands in marked contrast to the behavior of the cells in most normal cell lineages in the body, which are only able to pass through a limited number of successive cell growth-and-division cycles. This limitation has been associated with two distinct barriers to proliferation: *replicative senescence*, a typically irreversible entrance into a nonproliferative but viable state, and *crisis*, which involves cell death. Accordingly, when cells are propagated in culture, repeated cycles of cell division lead first to induction of replicative senescence and then, for those cells that succeed in circumventing this barrier, to the crisis phase, in which the great majority of cells in the population die. On rare occasion, cells emerge from a population in crisis and exhibit unlimited replicative potential. This transition has been termed immortalization, a trait that most established cell lines possess by virtue of their ability to proliferate in culture without evidence of either senescence or crisis.

Multiple lines of evidence indicate that telomeres protecting the ends of chromosomes are centrally involved in the capability for unlimited proliferation.[55–58] The telomere-associated DNA, composed of multiple tandem hexanucleotide repeats, shortens progressively in the chromosomes of nonimmortalized cells propagated in culture, eventually losing the ability to protect the ends of chromosomal DNA from end-to-end fusions; such aberrant fusions generate unstable dicentric chromosomes, whose resolution during the anaphase of mitosis results in a scrambling of karyotype and entrance into crisis that threatens cell viability. Accordingly, the length of telomeric DNA in a cell dictates how many successive cell generations its progeny can pass through before telomeres are largely eroded and have consequently lost their protective functions.

Telomerase, the specialized DNA polymerase that adds telomere repeat segments to the ends of telomeric DNA, is almost absent in nonimmortalized cells but is expressed at functionally significant levels in the great majority (~90%) of spontaneously immortalized cells, including human cancer cells. By extending telomeric DNA, telomerase is able to counter the progressive telomere erosion that would otherwise occur in its absence. The presence of telomerase activity, either in spontaneously immortalized cells or in the context of cells engineered to express the enzyme, is correlated with a resistance to induction of both senescence and crisis/apoptosis; conversely, the suppression of telomerase activity leads to telomere shortening and to activation of one or the other of these proliferative barriers.

The two barriers to proliferation—replicative senescence and crisis/apoptosis—have been rationalized as crucial anticancer defenses that are hardwired into our cells and are deployed to impede the outgrowth of clones of preneoplastic and, frankly, neoplastic cells. According to this thinking, most incipient neoplasias exhaust their endowment of replicative doublings and are stopped in their tracks by either of these barriers. The eventual immortalization of rare variant cells that proceed to form tumors has been attributed to their ability to maintain telomeric DNA at lengths sufficient to avoid triggering either senescence or apoptosis, which is achieved most commonly by upregulating the expression of telomerase or, less frequently, via an alternative recombination-based (ALT) telomere maintenance mechanism.[59] Hence, telomere shortening has come to be viewed as a clocking device that determines the limited replicative potential of normal cells and, thus, one that must be overcome by cancer cells.

### Reassessing Replicative Senescence

The senescent state induced by oncogenes, as described previously, is remarkably similar to that induced when cells are explanted from living tissue and introduced into culture, the latter being the replicative senescence just discussed. Importantly,

the concept of replication-induced senescence as a general barrier requires refinement and reformulation. Recent experiments have revealed that the induction of senescence in certain cultured cells can be delayed and possibly eliminated by the use of improved cell culture conditions, suggesting that recently explanted primary cells may be intrinsically able to proliferate unimpeded in culture up to the point of crisis and the associated induction of apoptosis triggered by critically shortened telomeres.[60–63] This result indicates that telomere shortening does not necessarily induce senescence prior to crisis. Additional insight comes from experiments in mice engineered to lack telomerase; this work has revealed that shortening telomeres can shunt premalignant cells into a senescent state that contributes (along with apoptosis) to attenuated tumorigenesis in mice genetically destined to develop particular forms of cancer.[58] Such telomerase-null mice with highly eroded telomeres exhibit multiorgan dysfunction and abnormalities that provide evidence of both senescence and apoptosis, perhaps similar to the senescence and apoptosis observed in cell culture.[58,64] Thus, depending on the cellular context, the proliferative barrier of telomere shortening can be manifested by the induction of senescence and/or apoptosis.

### Delayed Activation of Telomerase May Both Limit and Foster Neoplastic Progression

There is now evidence that clones of incipient cancer cells in spontaneously arising tumors experience telomere loss-induced crisis relatively early during the course of multistep tumor progression due to their inability to express significant levels of telomerase. Thus, extensively eroded telomeres have been documented in premalignant growths through the use of fluorescence in situ hybridization (FISH), which has also revealed the end-to-end chromosomal fusions that signal telomere failure and crisis.[65,66] These results suggest that such incipient cancer cells have passed through a substantial number of successive telomere-shortening cell divisions during their evolution from fully normal cells of origin. Accordingly, the development of some human neoplasias may be aborted by telomere-induced crisis long before they have progressed to become macroscopic, frankly neoplastic growths.

A quite different situation is observed in cells that have lost the TP53-mediated surveillance of genomic integrity and, thereafter, experience critically eroded telomeres. The loss of the TP53 DNA damage sensor can enable such cells to avoid apoptosis that would otherwise be triggered by the DNA damage resulting from dysfunctional telomeres. Instead, such cells lacking TP53 continue to divide, suffering repeated cycles of interchromosomal fusion and subsequent breakage at mitosis. Such breakage-fusion-bridge (BFB) cycles result in deletions and amplifications of chromosomal segments, evidently serving to mutagenize the genome, thereby facilitating the generation and subsequent clonal selection of cancer cells that have acquired mutant oncogenes and tumor suppressor genes.[58,67] One infers, however, that the clones of cancer cells that survive this telomere collapse must eventually acquire the ability to stabilize and thus protect their telomeres via the activation of telomerase or the ALT mechanism noted previously.

These considerations present an interesting dichotomy: Although dysfunctional telomeres are an evident barrier to chronic proliferation, they can also facilitate the genomic instability that generates hallmark-enabling mutations, as will be discussed further. Both mechanisms may be at play in certain forms of carcinogenesis in the form of transitory telomere deficiency prior to telomere stabilization. Circumstantial support for this concept of transient telomere deficiency in facilitating malignant progression has come from comparative analyses of premalignant and malignant lesions in the human breast.[68,69] The premalignant lesions did not express significant levels of telomerase and were marked by telomere shortening and chromosomal aberrations. In contrast, overt carcinomas exhibited telomerase expression concordantly with the reconstruction of longer telomeres and the fixation of the aberrant karyotypes that would seem to have been acquired after telomere failure but before the acquisition of telomerase activity. When portrayed in this way, the delayed acquisition of telomerase function serves to generate tumor-promoting mutations, whereas its subsequent expression stabilizes the mutant genome and confers the unlimited replicative capacity that cancer cells require in order to generate clinically apparent tumors.

## Inducing Angiogenesis

Like normal tissues, tumors require sustenance in the form of nutrients and oxygen as well as an ability to evacuate metabolic wastes and carbon dioxide. The tumor-associated neovasculature, generated by the process of angiogenesis, addresses these needs. During embryogenesis, the development of the vasculature involves the birth of new endothelial cells and their assembly into tubes (vasculogenesis) in addition to the sprouting (angiogenesis) of new vessels from existing ones. Following this morphogenesis, the normal vasculature becomes largely quiescent. In the adult, as part of physiologic processes such as wound healing and female reproductive cycling, angiogenesis is turned on, but only transiently. In contrast, during tumor progression, an *angiogenic switch* is almost always activated and remains on, causing normally quiescent vasculature to continually sprout new vessels that help sustain expanding neoplastic growths.[70]

A compelling body of evidence indicates that the angiogenic switch is governed by countervailing factors that either induce or oppose angiogenesis.[71,72] Some of these angiogenic regulators are signaling proteins that bind to stimulatory or inhibitory cell-surface receptors displayed by vascular endothelial cells. The well-known prototypes of angiogenesis inducers and inhibitors are vascular endothelial growth factor-A (VEGF-A) and thrombospondin-1 (Tsp-1), respectively.

The VEGF-A gene encodes ligands that are involved in orchestrating new blood vessel growth during embryonic and postnatal development, in the survival of endothelial cells in already-formed vessels, and in certain physiologic and pathologic situations in the adult. VEGF signaling via three receptor tyrosine kinases (VEGFR1–3) is regulated at multiple levels, reflecting this complexity of purpose. VEGF gene expression can be upregulated both by hypoxia and by oncogene signaling.[73–75] Additionally, VEGF ligands can be sequestered in the extracellular matrix in latent forms that are subject to release and activation by extracellular matrix-degrading proteases (e.g., matrix metallopeptidase 9 [MMP-9]).[76] In addition, other proangiogenic proteins, such as members of the fibroblast growth factor (FGF) family, have been implicated in sustaining tumor angiogenesis.[71] TSP-1, a key counterbalance in the angiogenic switch, also binds transmembrane receptors displayed by endothelial cells and thereby triggers suppressive signals that can counteract proangiogenic stimuli.[77]

The blood vessels produced within tumors by an unbalanced mix of proangiogenic signals are typically aberrant: Tumor neovasculature is marked by precocious capillary sprouting, convoluted and excessive vessel branching, distorted and enlarged vessels, erratic blood flow, microhemorrhaging, leaking of plasma into the tissue parenchyma, and abnormal levels of endothelial cell proliferation and apoptosis.[78,79]

Angiogenesis is induced surprisingly early during the multistage development of invasive cancers both in animal models and in humans. Histologic analyses of premalignant, noninvasive lesions, including dysplasias and in situ carcinomas arising in a variety of organs, have revealed the early tripping of the angiogenic switch.[70,80] Historically, angiogenesis was envisioned to be important only when rapidly growing macroscopic tumors had formed, but more recent data indicate that angiogenesis also contributes to the microscopic premalignant phase of neoplastic progression, further cementing its status as an integral hallmark of cancer.

## Gradations of the Angiogenic Switch

Once angiogenesis has been activated, tumors exhibit diverse patterns of neovascularization. Some tumors, including highly aggressive types such as pancreatic ductal adenocarcinomas, are hypovascularized and replete with stromal deserts that are largely avascular and indeed may even be actively antiangiogenic.[81] In contrast, many other tumors, including human renal and pancreatic neuroendocrine carcinomas, are highly angiogenic and, consequently, densely vascularized.[82,83]

Collectively, such observations suggest an initial tripping of the angiogenic switch during tumor development, which is followed by a variable intensity of ongoing neovascularization, the latter being controlled by a complex biologic rheostat that involves both the cancer cells and the associated stromal microenvironment.[71,72] Of note, the switching mechanisms can vary, even though the net result is a common inductive signal (e.g., VEGF). In some tumors, dominant oncogenes operating within tumor cells, such as *Ras* and *Myc*, can upregulate the expression of angiogenic factors, whereas in others, such inductive signals are produced indirectly by immune inflammatory cells, as will be discussed.

## Endogenous Angiogenesis Inhibitors Present Natural Barriers to Tumor Angiogenesis

A variety of secreted proteins have been reported to have the capability to help shut off normally transitory angiogenesis, including thrombospondin-1 (TSP-1), fragments of plasmin (angiostatin) and type 18 collagen (endostatin), along with another dozen candidate antiangiogenic proteins.[77,84–88] Most are proteins, and many are derived by proteolytic cleavage of structural proteins that are not themselves angiogenic regulators.

A number of these endogenous inhibitors of angiogenesis can be detected in the circulation of normal mice and humans. Genes that encode several endogenous angiogenesis inhibitors have been deleted from the mouse germ line without untoward developmental or physiologic effects; however, the growth of autochthonous and implanted tumors is enhanced as a consequence.[84,85,88] By contrast, if the circulating levels of an endogenous inhibitor are genetically increased (e.g., via overexpression in transgenic mice or in xenotransplanted tumors), tumor growth is impaired.[85,88] Interestingly, wound healing and fat deposition are impaired or accelerated by elevated or ablated expression of such genes.[89,90] The data suggest that, under normal conditions, endogenous angiogenesis inhibitors serve as physiologic regulators modulating the transitory angiogenesis that occurs during tissue remodeling and wound healing; they may also act as intrinsic barriers to the induction and/or persistence of angiogenesis by incipient neoplasias.

## Pericytes Are Important Components of the Tumor Neovasculature

Pericytes have long been known as supporting cells that are closely apposed to the outer surfaces of the endothelial tubes in normal tissue vasculature, where they provide important mechanical and physiologic support to the endothelial cells. Microscopic studies conducted in recent years have revealed that pericytes are associated, albeit loosely, with the neovasculature of most, if not all, tumors.[91–93] More importantly, mechanistic studies (discussed subsequently) have revealed that pericyte coverage is important for the maintenance of a functional tumor neovasculature.

## A Variety of Bone Marrow-Derived Cells Contribute to Tumor Angiogenesis

It is now clear that a repertoire of cell types originating in the bone marrow play crucial roles in pathologic angiogenesis.[94–97] These include cells of the innate immune system—notably, macrophages, neutrophils, mast cells, and myeloid progenitors—that assemble at the margins of such lesions or infiltrate deeply within them; the tumor-associated inflammatory cells can help to trip the angiogenic switch in quiescent tissue and sustain ongoing angiogenesis associated with tumor growth. In addition, they can help protect the vasculature from the effects of drugs targeting endothelial cell signaling.[98] Moreover, several types of bone marrow–derived *vascular progenitor cells* have been observed to have migrated into neoplastic lesions and become intercalated into the existing neovasculature, where they assumed the roles of either pericytes or endothelial cells.[92,99,100]

## Activating Invasion and Metastasis

The multistep process of invasion and metastasis has been schematized as a sequence of discrete steps, often termed the invasion–metastasis cascade.[101,102] This depiction portrays a succession of cell-biologic changes, beginning with local invasion, then intravasation by cancer cells into nearby blood and lymphatic vessels, transit of cancer cells through the lymphatic and hematogenous systems, followed by the escape of cancer cells from the lumina of such vessels into the parenchyma of distant tissues (extravasation), the formation of small nests of cancer cells (micrometastases), and finally, the growth of micrometastatic lesions into macroscopic tumors, this last step being termed *colonization*. These steps have largely been studied in the context of carcinoma pathogenesis. Indeed, when viewed through the prism of the invasion–metastasis cascade, the diverse tumors of this class appear to behave in similar ways.

During the malignant progression of carcinomas, the neoplastic cells typically develop alterations in their shape as well as their attachment to other cells and to the extracellular matrix (ECM). The best-characterized alteration involves the loss by carcinoma cells of E-cadherin, a key epithelial cell-to-cell adhesion molecule. By forming adherens junctions between adjacent epithelial cells, E-cadherin helps to assemble epithelial cell sheets and to maintain the quiescence of the cells within these sheets. Moreover, increased expression of E-cadherin has been well established as an antagonist of invasion and metastasis, whereas a reduction of its expression is known to potentiate these behaviors. The frequently observed downregulation and occasional mutational inactivation of the E-cadherin–encoding gene, *CDH1*, in human carcinomas provides strong support for its role as a key suppressor of the invasion–metastasis hallmark capability.[103,104]

Notably, the expression of genes encoding other cell-to-cell and cell-to-ECM adhesion molecules is also significantly altered in the cells of many highly aggressive carcinomas, with those favoring cytostasis typically being downregulated. Conversely, adhesion molecules normally associated with the cell migrations that occur during embryogenesis and inflammation are often upregulated. For example, N-cadherin, which is normally expressed in migrating neurons and mesenchymal cells during organogenesis, is upregulated in many invasive carcinoma cells, replacing the previously expressed E-cadherin.[104]

Research into the capability for invasion and metastasis has accelerated dramatically over the past decade as powerful new research tools, and refined experimental models have become available. Although still an emerging field replete with major unanswered questions, significant progress has been made in delineating important features of this complex hallmark capability. An admittedly incomplete representation of these advances is highlighted as follows.

### The Epithelial-to-Mesenchymal Transition Program Broadly Regulates Invasion and Metastasis

A developmental regulatory program, termed the EMT, has become implicated as a prominent means by which neoplastic epithelial cells can acquire the abilities to invade, resist apoptosis, and disseminate.[105–110] By co-opting a process involved in various steps of embryonic morphogenesis and wound healing, carcinoma cells can concomitantly acquire multiple attributes that enable invasion and metastasis. This multifaceted EMT program can be activated transiently or stably, and to differing degrees, by carcinoma cells during the course of invasion and metastasis.

A set of pleiotropically acting transcriptional factors (TF), including Snail, Slug, Twist, and Zeb1/2, orchestrate the EMT and related migratory processes during embryogenesis; most were initially identified by developmental genetics. These transcriptional regulators are expressed in various combinations in a number of malignant tumor types. Some of these EMT-TFs have been shown in experimental models of carcinoma formation to be causally important for programming invasion; others have been found to elicit metastasis when experimentally expressed in primary tumor cells.[105,111–114] Included among the cell-biologic traits evoked by these EMT-TFs are loss of adherens junctions and associated conversion from a polygonal/epithelial to a spindly/fibroblastic morphology, concomitant with expression of secreted matrix-degrading enzymes, increased motility, and heightened resistance to apoptosis, which are implicated in the processes of invasion and metastasis. Several of these transcription factors can directly repress E-cadherin gene expression, thereby releasing neoplastic epithelial cells from this key suppressor of motility and invasiveness.[115]

The available data suggest that EMT-TFs regulate one another as well as overlapping sets of target genes. Results from developmental genetics indicate that contextual signals received from neighboring cells in the embryo are involved in triggering expression of these transcription factors in cells that are destined to pass through an EMT[111]; in an analogous fashion, heterotypic interactions of cancer cells with adjacent tumor-associated stromal cells have been shown to induce expression of the malignant cell phenotypes that are known to be choreographed by one or more of these EMT-TFs.[116,117] Moreover, cancer cells at the invasive margins of certain carcinomas can be seen to have undergone an EMT, suggesting that these cancer cells are subject to microenvironmental stimuli distinct from those received by cancer cells located in the cores of these lesions.[118] Although the evidence is still incomplete, it would appear that EMT-TFs are able to orchestrate most steps of the invasion–metastasis cascade, except perhaps the final step of colonization, which involves adaptation of cells originating in one tissue to the microenvironment of a foreign, potentially inhospitable tissue.

We still know rather little about the various manifestations and temporal stability of the mesenchymal state produced by an EMT. Indeed, it seems increasingly likely that many human carcinoma cells only experience a *partial EMT*, in which they acquire mesenchymal markers while retaining many preexisting epithelial ones. Although the expression of EMT-TFs has been observed in certain nonepithelial tumor types, such as sarcomas and neuroectodermal tumors, their roles in programming malignant traits in these tumors are presently poorly documented. Additionally, it remains to be determined whether aggressive carcinoma cells invariably acquire their malignant capabilities through activation of components of the EMT program, or whether alternative regulatory programs can also enable expression of these traits.

### Heterotypic Contributions of Stromal Cells to Invasion and Metastasis

As mentioned previously, cross-talk between cancer cells and cell types of the neoplastic stroma is involved in the acquired capabilities of invasiveness and metastasis.[94,119–121] For example, mesenchymal stem cells (MSC) present in the tumor stroma have been found to secrete CCL5/RANTES in response to signals released by cancer cells; CCL5 then acts reciprocally on the cancer cells to stimulate invasive behavior.[122] In other work, carcinoma cells secreting IL-1 have been shown to induce MSCs to synthesize a spectrum of other cytokines that proceed thereafter to promote activation of the EMT program in the carcinoma cells; these effectors include IL-6, IL-8, growth-regulated oncogene alpha (GRO-α), and prostaglandin E2.[123]

Macrophages at the tumor periphery can foster local invasion by supplying matrix-degrading enzymes such as metalloproteinases and cysteine cathepsin proteases[76,120,124,125]; in one model system, the invasion-promoting macrophages are activated by IL-4 produced by the cancer cells.[126] And in an experimental model of metastatic breast cancer, tumor-associated macrophages (TAM) supply epidermal growth factor (EGF) to breast cancer cells, while the cancer cells reciprocally stimulate the macrophages with colony stimulating factor 1 (CSF-1). Their concerted interactions facilitate intravasation into the circulatory system and metastatic dissemination of the cancer cells.[94,127]

Observations like these indicate that the phenotypes of high-grade malignancy do not arise in a strictly cell-autonomous manner, and that their manifestation cannot be understood solely through analyses of signaling occurring within tumor cells. One important implication of the EMT model, still untested, is that the ability of carcinoma cells in primary tumors to negotiate most of the steps of the invasion–metastasis cascade may be acquired in certain tumors without the requirement that these cells undergo additional mutations beyond those that were needed for primary tumor formation.

## Plasticity in the Invasive Growth Program

The role of contextual signals in inducing an invasive growth capability (often via an EMT) implies the possibility of reversibility, in that cancer cells that have disseminated from a primary tumor to more distant tissue sites may no longer benefit from the activated stroma and the EMT-inducing signals that they experienced while residing in the primary tumor. In the absence of ongoing exposure to these signals, carcinoma cells may revert in their new tissue environment to a noninvasive state. Thus, carcinoma cells that underwent an EMT during initial invasion and metastatic dissemination may reverse this metamorphosis, doing so via a mesenchymal-to-epithelial transition (MET). This plasticity may result in the formation of new tumor colonies of carcinoma cells exhibiting an organization and histopathology similar to those created by carcinoma cells in the primary tumor that never experienced an EMT.[128]

## Distinct Forms of Invasion May Underlie Different Cancer Types

The EMT program regulates a particular type of invasiveness that has been termed *mesenchymal*. In addition, two other distinct modes of invasion have been identified and implicated in cancer cell invasion.[129,130] *Collective invasion* involves phalanxes of cancer cells advancing en masse into adjacent tissues and is characteristic of, for example, squamous cell carcinomas. Interestingly, such cancers are rarely metastatic, suggesting that this form of invasion lacks certain functional attributes that facilitate metastasis. Less clear is the prevalence of an *amoeboid* form of invasion,[131,132] in which individual cancer cells show morphologic plasticity, enabling them to slither through existing interstices in the ECM rather than clearing a path for themselves, as occurs in both the mesenchymal and collective forms of invasion. It is presently unresolved whether cancer cells participating in the collective and amoeboid forms of invasion employ components of the EMT program, or whether entirely different cell-biologic programs are responsible for choreographing these alternative invasion programs.

Another emerging concept, noted previously, involves the facilitation of cancer cell invasion by inflammatory cells that assemble at the boundaries of tumors, producing the ECM-degrading enzymes and other factors that enable invasive growth.[76,94,120,133] These functions may obviate the need of invading cancer cells to produce these proteins through activation of EMT programs. Thus, rather than synthesizing these proteases themselves, cancer cells may secrete chemoattractants that recruit proinvasive inflammatory cells; the latter then proceed to produce matrix-degrading enzymes that enable invasive growth.

## The Daunting Complexity of Metastatic Colonization

Metastasis can be broken down into two major phases: the physical dissemination of cancer cells from the primary tumor to distant tissues, and the adaptation of these cells to foreign tissue microenvironments that results in successful colonization (i.e., the growth of micrometastases into macroscopic tumors). The multiple steps of dissemination would seem to lie within the purview of the EMT and similarly acting migratory programs. Colonization, however, is not strictly coupled with physical dissemination, as evidenced by the presence in many patients of myriad micrometastases that have disseminated but never progress to form macroscopic metastatic tumors.[101,102,134–136]

In some types of cancer, the primary tumor may release systemic suppressor factors that render such micrometastases dormant, as revealed clinically by explosive metastatic growth soon after resection of the primary growth.[87,137] In others, however, such as breast cancer and melanoma, macroscopic metastases may erupt decades after a primary tumor has been surgically removed or pharmacologically destroyed. These metastatic tumor growths evidently reflect dormant micrometastases that have solved, after much trial and error, the complex problem of adaptation to foreign tissue microenvironments, allowing subsequent tissue colonization.[135,136,138] Implicit here is the notion that most disseminated cancer cells are likely to be poorly adapted, at least initially, to the microenvironment of the tissue in which they have landed. Accordingly, each type of disseminated cancer cell may need to develop its own set of ad hoc solutions to the problem of thriving in the microenvironment of one or another foreign tissue.[139]

One can infer from such natural histories that micrometastases may lack certain hallmark capabilities necessary for vigorous growth, such as the ability to activate angiogenesis. Indeed, the inability of certain experimentally generated dormant micrometastases to form macroscopic tumors has been ascribed to their failure to activate tumor angiogenesis.[135,140] Additionally, recent experiments have shown that nutrient starvation can induce intense autophagy that causes cancer cells to shrink and adopt a state of reversible dormancy. Such cells may exit this state and resume active growth and proliferation when permitted by changes in tissue microenvironment, such as increased availability of nutrients, inflammation from causes such as infection or wound healing, or other local abnormalities.[49,141] Other mechanisms of micrometastatic dormancy may involve antigrowth signals embedded in normal tissue ECM[138] and tumor-suppressing actions of the immune system.[135,142]

Metastatic dissemination has long been depicted as the last step in multistep primary tumor progression; indeed, for many tumors, that is likely the case, as illustrated by recent genome sequencing studies that provide genetic evidence for clonal evolution of pancreatic ductal adenocarcinoma to a metastatic stage.[143–145] Importantly, however, recent results have revealed that some cancer cells can disseminate remarkably early, dispersing from apparently noninvasive premalignant lesions in both mice and humans.[146,147] Additionally, micrometastases can be spawned from primary tumors that are not obviously invasive but possess a neovasculature lacking in luminal integrity.[148] Although cancer cells can clearly disseminate from such preneoplastic lesions and seed the bone marrow and other tissues, their capability to colonize these sites and develop into pathologically significant macrometastases remains unproven. At present, we view this early metastatic dissemination as a demonstrable phenomenon in mice and humans, the clinical significance of which is yet to be established.

Having developed such a tissue-specific colonizing ability, the cells in metastatic colonies may proceed to disseminate further, not only to new sites in the body, but also back to the primary tumors in which their ancestors arose. Accordingly, tissue-specific colonization programs that are evident among certain cells within a primary tumor may originate not from classical tumor progression occurring entirely within the primary lesion, but instead from immigrants that have returned home.[149] Such reseeding is consistent with the aforementioned studies of human pancreatic cancer metastasis.[143–145] Stated differently, the phenotypes and underlying gene expression programs in focal subpopulations of cancer cells within primary tumors may reflect, in part, the reverse migration of their distant metastatic progeny.

Implicit in this *self-seeding* process is another notion: The supportive stroma that arises in a primary tumor and contributes to its acquisition of malignant traits provides a hospitable site for reseeding and colonization by circulating cancer cells released from metastatic lesions.

Clarifying the regulatory programs that enable metastatic colonization represents an important agenda for future research. Substantial progress is being made, for example, in defining sets of genes (*metastatic signatures*) that correlate with and appear to facilitate the establishment of macroscopic metastases in specific tissues.[139,146,150–152] Importantly, metastatic colonization almost certainly requires the establishment of a permissive tumor microenvironment composed of critical stromal support cells. For these reasons, the process of colonization is likely to encompass a large number of cell-biologic programs that are, in aggregate, considerably more complex and diverse than the preceding steps of metastatic dissemination that allow carcinoma cells to depart from primary tumors to sites of lodging and extravasation throughout the body.

## Reprogramming Energy Metabolism

The chronic and often uncontrolled cell proliferation that represents the essence of neoplastic disease involves not only deregulated control of cell proliferation but also corresponding adjustments of energy metabolism in order to fuel cell growth and division. Under aerobic conditions, normal cells process glucose, first to pyruvate via glycolysis in the cytosol and thereafter via oxidative phosphorylation to carbon dioxide in the mitochondria. Under anaerobic conditions, glycolysis is favored and relatively little pyruvate is dispatched to the oxygen-consuming mitochondria. Otto Warburg first observed an anomalous characteristic of cancer cell energy metabolism[153–155]: Even in the presence of oxygen, cancer cells can reprogram their glucose metabolism, and thus their energy production, leading to a state that has been termed *aerobic glycolysis*.

The existence of this metabolic specialization operating in cancer cells has been substantiated in the ensuing decades. A key signature of aerobic glycolysis is upregulation of glucose transporters, notably GLUT1, which substantially increases glucose import into the cytoplasm.[156–158] Indeed, markedly increased uptake and utilization of glucose has been documented in many human tumor types, most readily by noninvasively visualizing glucose uptake using positron-emission tomography (PET) with a radiolabeled analog of glucose ([18]F-fluorodeoxyglucose [FDG]) as a reporter.

Glycolytic fueling has been shown to be associated with activated oncogenes (e.g., *RAS*, *MYC*) and mutant tumor suppressors (e.g., *TP53*),[18,156,157,159] whose alterations in tumor cells have been selected primarily for their benefits in conferring the hallmark capabilities of cell proliferation, subversion of cytostatic controls, and attenuation of apoptosis. This reliance on glycolysis can be further accentuated under the hypoxic conditions that operate within many tumors: The hypoxia response system acts pleiotropically to upregulate glucose transporters and multiple enzymes of the glycolytic pathway.[156,157,160] Thus, both the Ras oncoprotein and hypoxia can independently increase the levels of the HIF1α and HIF2α hypoxia-response transcription factors, which in turn upregulate glycolysis.[160–162]

The reprogramming of energy metabolism is seemingly counterintuitive, in that cancer cells must compensate for the ~18-fold lower efficiency of ATP production afforded by glycolysis relative to mitochondrial oxidative phosphorylation. According to one long-forgotten[163] and a recently revived and refined hypothesis,[164] increased glycolysis allows the diversion of glycolytic intermediates into various biosynthetic pathways, including those generating nucleosides and amino acids. In turn, this facilitates the biosynthesis of the macromolecules and organelles required for assembling new cells. Moreover, Warburg-like metabolism seems to be present in many rapidly dividing embryonic tissues, once again suggesting a role in supporting the large-scale biosynthetic programs that are required for active cell proliferation.

Interestingly, some tumors have been found to contain two subpopulations of cancer cells that differ in their energy-generating pathways. One subpopulation consists of glucose-dependent (Warburg-effect) cells that secrete lactate, whereas cells of the second subpopulation preferentially import and utilize the lactate produced by their neighbors as their main energy source, employing part of the citric acid cycle to do so.[165–168] These two populations evidently function symbiotically: The hypoxic cancer cells depend on glucose for fuel and secrete lactate as waste, which is imported and preferentially used as fuel by their better oxygenated brethren. Although this provocative mode of intratumoral symbiosis has yet to be generalized, the cooperation between lactate-secreting and lactate-utilizing cells to fuel tumor growth is in fact not an invention of tumors, but rather again reflects the co-opting of a normal physiologic mechanism, in this case one operative in muscle[165,167,168] and the brain.[169] Additionally, it is becoming apparent that oxygenation, ranging from normoxia to hypoxia, is not necessarily static in tumors, but instead fluctuates temporally and regionally,[170] likely as a result of the instability and chaotic organization of the tumor-associated neovasculature.

Finally, the notion of the Warburg effect needs to be refined for most if not all tumors exhibiting aerobic glycolysis. The effect does not involve a switching off oxidative phosphorylation concurrent with activation of glycolysis, the latter then serving as the sole source of energy. Rather, cancer cells become highly adaptive, utilizing both mitochondrial oxidative phosphorylation and glycolysis in varying proportions to generate fuel (ATP) and biosynthetic precursors needed for chronic cell proliferation. Finally, this capability for reprograming energy metabolism, dubbed to be an *emerging hallmark* in 2011,[2] is clearly intertwined with the hallmarks conveying deregulated proliferative signals and evasion of growth suppressors, as discussed earlier. As such, its status as a discrete, independently acquired hallmark remains unclear, despite growing appreciation of its importance as a crucial component of the neoplastic growth state.

## Evading Immune Destruction

The eighth hallmark reflects the role played by the immune system in antagonizing the formation and progression of tumors. A longstanding theory of immune surveillance posited that cells and tissues are constantly monitored by an ever alert immune system, and that such immune surveillance is responsible for recognizing and eliminating the vast majority of incipient cancer cells and, thus, nascent tumors.[171,172] According to this logic, clinical detectable cancers have somehow managed to avoid detection by the various arms of the immune system, or have been able to limit the extent of immunologic killing, thereby evading eradication.

The role of defective immunologic monitoring of tumors would seem to be validated by the striking increases of certain cancers in immune-compromised individuals.[173] However, the great majority of these are virus-induced cancers, suggesting that much of the control of this class of cancers normally depends on reducing viral burden in infected individuals, in part through eliminating virus-infected cells. These observations, therefore, shed little light on the possible role of the immune system in limiting formation of the >80% of tumors of nonviral etiology. In recent years, however, an increasing body of evidence, both from genetically engineered mice and from clinical epidemiology, suggests that the immune system operates as a significant barrier to tumor formation and progression, at least in some forms of non–virus-induced cancer.[174–177]

When mice genetically engineered to be deficient for various components of the immune system were assessed for the development of carcinogen-induced tumors, it was observed that tumors arose more frequently and/or grew more rapidly in the immunodeficient mice relative to immune-competent controls. In particular, deficiencies in the development or function of either CD8$^+$ cytotoxic T lymphocytes (CTL), CD4$^+$ T$_H$1 helper T cells, or natural killer (NK) cells, each led to demonstrable increases in tumor incidence. Moreover, mice with combined immunodeficiencies in both T cells and NK cells were even more susceptible to cancer development. The results indicated that, at least in certain experimental models, both the innate and adaptive cellular arms of the immune system are able to contribute significantly to immune surveillance and, thus, tumor eradication.[142,178]

In addition, transplantation experiments have shown that cancer cells that originally arose in immunodeficient mice are often inefficient at initiating secondary tumors in syngeneic immunocompetent hosts, whereas cancer cells from tumors arising in immunocompetent mice are equally efficient at initiating transplanted tumors in both types of hosts.[142,178] Such behavior has been interpreted as follows: Highly immunogenic cancer cell clones are routinely eliminated in immunocompetent hosts—a process that has been referred to as *immunoediting*—leaving behind only weakly immunogenic variants to grow and generate solid tumors. Such weakly immunogenic cells can thereafter successfully colonize both immunodeficient and immunocompetent hosts. Conversely, when arising in immunodeficient hosts, the immunogenic cancer cells are not selectively depleted and can, instead, prosper along with their weakly immunogenic counterparts. When cells from such nonedited tumors are serially transplanted into syngeneic recipients, the immunogenic cancer cells are rejected when they confront, for the first time, the competent immune systems of their secondary hosts.[179] (Unanswered in these particular experiments is the question of whether the chemical carcinogens used to induce such tumors are prone to generate cancer cells that are especially immunogenic.)

Clinical epidemiology also increasingly supports the existence of antitumoral immune responses in some forms of human cancer.[180–182] For example, patients with colon and ovarian tumors that are heavily infiltrated with CTLs and NK cells have a better prognosis than those who lack such abundant killer lymphocytes.[176,177,182,183] The case for other cancers is suggestive but less compelling and is the subject of ongoing investigation. Additionally, some immunosuppressed organ transplant recipients have been observed to develop donor-derived cancers, suggesting that in ostensibly tumor-free organ donors, the cancer cells were held in check in a dormant state by a functional immune system,[184] only to launch into proliferative expansion once these *passenger cells* in the transplanted organ found themselves in immunocompromised patients who lack the physiologically important capabilities to mount immune responses that would otherwise hold latent cancer cells in check or eradicate them.

Still, the epidemiology of chronically immunosuppressed patients does not indicate significantly increased incidences of the major forms of nonviral human cancers, as noted previously. This might be taken as an argument against the importance of immune surveillance as an effective barrier to tumorigenesis and tumor progression. We note, however, that HIV and pharmacologically immunosuppressed patients are predominantly immunodeficient in the T- and B-cell compartments and thus do not present with the multicomponent immunologic deficiencies that have been produced in the genetically engineered mutant mice lacking both NK cells and CTLs. This leaves open the possibility that such

patients still have residual capability for mounting an anticancer immunologic defense that is mediated by NK and other innate immune cells.

In truth, the previous discussions of cancer immunology simplify tumor–host immunologic interactions, because highly immunogenic cancer cells may well succeed in evading immune destruction by disabling components of the immune system that have been dispatched to eliminate them. For example, cancer cells may paralyze infiltrating CTLs and NK cells by secreting TGF-β or other immunosuppressive factors.[32,185,186] Alternatively, cancer cells may express immunosuppressive cell-surface ligands, such as PD-L1, that prevent activation of the cytotoxic mechanisms of the CTLs. These PD-L1 molecules serve as ligands for the PD-1 receptors displayed by the CTLs, together exemplifying a system of *checkpoint* ligands and receptors that serve to constrain immune responses in order to avoid autoimmunity.[187–189] Yet other localized immunosuppressive mechanisms operate through the recruitment of inflammatory cells that can actively suppress CTL activity, including regulatory T cells (Tregs) and myeloid-derived suppressor cells (MDSC).[174,190–193]

In summary, these eight hallmarks each contribute qualitatively distinct capabilities that seem integral to most lethal forms of human cancer. Certainly, the balance and relative importance of their respective contributions to disease pathogenesis will vary among cancer types, and some hallmarks may be absent or of minor importance in some cases. Still, there is reason to postulate their generality and, thus, their applicability to understanding the biology of human cancer. Next, we turn to the question of how these capabilities are acquired during the multistep pathways through which cancers develop, focusing on two facilitators that are commonly involved.

## TWO UBIQUITOUS CHARACTERISTICS FACILITATE THE ACQUISITION OF HALLMARK CAPABILITIES

We have defined the hallmarks of cancer as acquired functional capabilities that allow cancer cells to survive, proliferate, and disseminate. Their acquisition is made possible by two *enabling characteristics* (Fig. 2.2). Most prominent is the development of genomic instability in cancer cells, which generates random mutations, including chromosomal rearrangements, among which are rare genetic changes that can orchestrate individual hallmark capabilities. A second enabling characteristic involves the inflammatory state of premalignant and frankly malignant lesions. A variety of cells of the innate and adaptive immune system infiltrate neoplasias, some of which serve to promote tumor progression through various means.

### An Enabling Characteristic: Genome Instability and Mutation

Acquisition of the multiple hallmarks enumerated previously depends in large part on a succession of alterations in the genomes of neoplastic cells. Basically, certain mutant genotypes can confer selective advantage to particular subclones among proliferating nests of incipient cancer cells, enabling their outgrowth and eventual dominance in a local tissue environment. Accordingly, multistep tumor progression can be portrayed as a succession of clonal expansions, most of which are triggered by the chance acquisition of an enabling mutation.

Indeed, it is apparent that virtually every human cancer cell genome carries mutant alleles of one or several growth-regulating genes, underscoring the central importance of these genetic alterations in driving malignant progression.[194] Still, we note that many heritable phenotypes—including, notably, inactivation of tumor suppressor genes—can be acquired through epigenetic

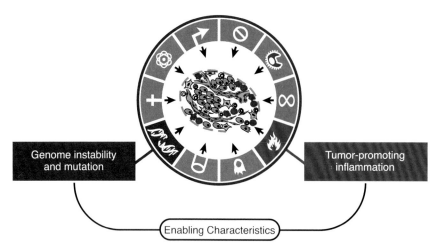

**Figure 2.2** Enabling characteristics. Two ostensibly generic characteristics of cancer cells and the neoplasias they create are involved in the acquisition of the hallmark capabilities. First and foremost, the impairment of genome maintenance systems in aberrantly proliferating cancer cells enables the generation of mutations in genes that contribute to multiple hallmarks. Secondarily, neoplasias invariably attract cells of the innate immune system that are programmed to heal wounds and fight infections; these cells, including macrophages, neutrophils, and partially differentiated myeloid cells, can contribute functionally to acquisition of many of the hallmark capabilities. (Adapted from Hanahan D, Weinberg RA. Hallmarks of cancer: the next generation. *Cell* 2011;144:646–674.)

mechanisms, such as DNA methylation and histone modifications.[195–198] Thus, many clonal expansions may also be triggered by heritable nonmutational changes affecting the regulation of gene expression. At present, the relative importance of genetic versus heritable epigenetic alterations to the various clonal expansions remains unclear, and, likely, varies broadly amongst the catalog of human cancer types.

The extraordinary ability of genome maintenance systems to detect and resolve defects in the DNA ensures that rates of spontaneous mutation in normal cells of the body are typically very low, both in quiescent cells and during cell division. The genomes of most cancer cells, by contrast, are replete with these alterations, reflecting loss of genomic integrity with concomitantly increased rates of mutation. This heightened mutability appears to accelerate the generation of variant cells, facilitating the selection of those cells whose advantageous phenotypes enable their clonal expansion.[199,200] This mutability is achieved through increased sensitivity to mutagenic agents, through a breakdown in one or several components of the genomic maintenance machinery, or both. In addition, the accumulation of mutations can be accelerated by aberrations that compromise the surveillance systems that normally monitor genomic integrity and force such genetically damaged cells into either quiescence, senescence, or apoptosis.[201–203] The role of TP53 is central here, leading to its being called the *guardian of the genome*.[204]

A diverse array of defects affecting various components of the DNA-maintenance machinery, referred to as the *caretakers* of the genome,[205] have been documented. The catalog of defects in these caretaker genes includes those whose products are involved in (1) detecting DNA damage and activating the repair machinery, (2) directly repairing damaged DNA, and (3) inactivating or intercepting mutagenic molecules before they have damaged the DNA.[199,201,202,206–208] From a genetic perspective, these caretaker genes behave much like tumor suppressor genes, in that their functions are often lost during the course of tumor progression, with such losses being achieved either through inactivating mutations or via epigenetic repression. Mutant copies of many of these caretaker genes have been introduced into the mouse germ line, resulting, not unexpectedly, in increased cancer incidence, thus supporting their involvement in human cancer development.[209]

In addition, research over the past decade has revealed another major source of tumor-associated genomic instability. As described earlier, the loss of telomeric DNA in many tumors generates karyotypic instability and associated amplification and deletion of chromosomal segments.[58] When viewed in this light, telomerase is more than an enabler of the hallmark capability for unlimited replicative potential. It must also be added to the list of critical caretakers responsible for maintaining genome integrity.

Advances in the molecular–genetic analysis of cancer cell genomes have provided the most compelling demonstrations of function-altering mutations and of ongoing genomic instability during tumor progression. One type of analysis—comparative genomic hybridization (CGH)—documents the gains and losses of gene copy number across the cell genome. In many tumors, the pervasive genomic aberrations revealed by CGH provide clear evidence for loss of control of genome integrity. Importantly, the recurrence of specific aberrations (both amplifications and deletions) at particular locations in the genome indicates that such sites are likely to harbor genes whose alteration favors neoplastic progression.[210]

More recently, with the advent of efficient and economical DNA sequencing technologies, higher resolution analyses of cancer cell genomes have become possible. Early studies are revealing distinctive patterns of DNA mutations in different tumor types (see: http://cancergenome.nih.gov/). In the not-too-distant future, the sequencing of entire cancer cell genomes promises to clarify the importance of ostensibly random mutations scattered across cancer cell genomes.[194] Thus, the use of whole genome resequencing offers the prospect of revealing recurrent genetic alterations (i.e., those found in multiple independently arising tumors) that in aggregate represent only minor proportions of the tumors of a given type. The recurrence of such mutations, despite their infrequency, may provide clues about the regulatory pathways playing causal roles in the pathogenesis of the tumors under study.

These surveys of cancer cell genomes have shown that the specifics of genome alteration vary dramatically between different tumor types. Nonetheless, the large number of already documented genome maintenance and repair defects, together with abundant evidence of widespread destabilization of gene copy number and nucleotide sequence, persuade us that instability of the genome is inherent to the cancer cells forming virtually all types of human tumors. This leads, in turn, to the conclusion that the defects in genome maintenance and repair are selectively advantageous and, therefore, instrumental for tumor progression, if only because they accelerate the rate at which evolving premalignant cells can accumulate favorable genotypes. As such, genome instability is clearly an *enabling characteristic* that is causally associated with the acquisition of hallmark capabilities.

## An Enabling Characteristic: Tumor-Promoting Inflammation

Among the cells recruited to the stroma of carcinomas are a variety of cell types of the immune system that mediate various inflammatory functions. Pathologists have long recognized that some (but not all) tumors are densely infiltrated by cells of both the innate and adaptive arms of the immune system, thereby mirroring inflammatory conditions arising in nonneoplastic tissues.[211] With the advent of better markers for accurately identifying the distinct cell types of the immune system, it is now clear that virtually every neoplastic lesion contains immune cells present at densities ranging from subtle infiltrations detectable only with cell type–specific antibodies to gross inflammations that are apparent even by standard histochemical staining techniques.[183] Historically, such immune responses were largely thought to reflect an attempt by the immune system to eradicate tumors, and indeed, there is increasing evidence for antitumoral responses to many tumor types with an attendant pressure on the tumor to evade immune destruction,[174,176,177,183] as discussed earlier.

By 2000, however, there were also clues that tumor-associated inflammatory responses can have the unanticipated effect of facilitating multiple steps of tumor progression, thereby helping incipient neoplasias to acquire hallmark capabilities. In the ensuing years, research on the intersections between inflammation and cancer pathogenesis has blossomed, producing abundant and compelling demonstrations of the functionally important tumor-promoting effects that immune cells—largely of the innate immune system—have on neoplastic progression.[19,53,94,174,212,213] Inflammatory cells can contribute to multiple hallmark capabilities by supplying signaling molecules to the tumor microenvironment, including growth factors that sustain proliferative signaling; survival factors that limit cell death; proangiogenic factors; extracellular matrix-modifying enzymes that facilitate angiogenesis, invasion, and metastasis; and inductive signals that lead to activation of EMT and other hallmark-promoting programs.[53,94,116,212,213]

Importantly, localized inflammation is often apparent at the earliest stages of neoplastic progression and is demonstrably capable of fostering the development of incipient neoplasias into full-blown cancers.[94,214] Additionally, inflammatory cells can release chemicals—notably, reactive oxygen species—that are actively mutagenic for nearby cancer cells, thus accelerating their genetic evolution toward states of heightened malignancy.[53] As such, inflammation by selective cell types of the immune system is demonstrably an *enabling characteristic* for its contributions to the acquisition of hallmark capabilities. The cells responsible for this enabling characteristic are described in the following section.

## THE CONSTITUENT CELL TYPES OF THE TUMOR MICROENVIRONMENT

Over the past 2 decades, tumors have increasingly been recognized as tissues whose complexity approaches and may even exceed that of normal healthy tissues. This realization contrasts starkly with the earlier, reductionist view of a tumor as nothing more than a collection of relatively homogeneous cancer cells, whose entire biology could be understood by elucidating the cell-autonomous properties of these cells (Fig. 2.3A). Rather, assemblages of diverse cell types associated with malignant lesions are increasingly documented to be functionally important for the manifestation of symptomatic disease (Fig. 2.3B). When viewed from this perspective, the biology of a tumor can only be fully understood by studying the individual specialized cell types within it. We enumerate as follows a set of accessory cell types recruited directly or indirectly by neoplastic cells into tumors, where they contribute in important ways to the biology of many tumors, and we discuss the regulatory mechanisms that control their individual and collective functions. Most of these observations stem from the study of carcinomas, in which the neoplastic epithelial cells constitute a compartment (the parenchyma) that is clearly distinct from the mesenchymal cells forming the tumor-associated stroma.

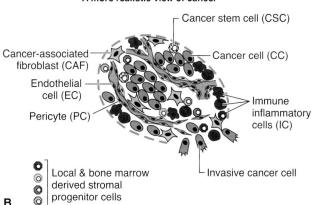

**A simple view of cancer**

Cancer cell (CC)

Invasive cancer cell

**A**

**A more realistic view of cancer**

Cancer stem cell (CSC)

Cancer-associated fibroblast (CAF)

Cancer cell (CC)

Endothelial cell (EC)

Pericyte (PC)

Immune inflammatory cells (IC)

Local & bone marrow derived stromal progenitor cells

Invasive cancer cell

**B**

**Figure 2.3** Tumors as outlaw organs. Research aimed at understanding the biology of tumors has historically focused on the cancer cells, which constitute the drivers of neoplastic disease. This view of tumors as nothing more than masses of cancer cells **(A)** ignores an important reality, that cancer cells recruit and corrupt a variety of normal cell types that form the tumor-associated stroma. Once formed, the stroma acts reciprocally on the cancer cells, affecting almost all of the traits that define the neoplastic behavior of the tumor as a whole **(B)**. The assemblage of heterogeneous populations of cancer cells and stromal cells is often referred to as the tumor microenvironment (TME). (Adapted from Hanahan D, Weinberg R. The hallmarks of cancer. *Cell* 2000;100:57–70; Hanahan D, Weinberg RA. Hallmarks of cancer: the next generation. *Cell* 2011;144:646–674.)

## Cancer-Associated Fibroblasts

Fibroblasts are found in various proportions across the spectrum of carcinomas, in many cases constituting the preponderant cell population of the tumor stroma. The term *cancer-associated fibroblasts* (CAFs) subsumes at least two distinct cell types: (1) cells with similarities to the fibroblasts that create the structural foundation supporting most normal epithelial tissues, and (2) myofibroblasts, whose biologic roles and properties differ markedly from those of the widely distributed tissue-derived fibroblasts. Myofibroblasts are identifiable by their expression of α-smooth muscle actin (αSMA). They are rare in most healthy epithelial tissues, although certain tissues, such as the liver and pancreas, contain appreciable numbers of αSMA-expressing cells. Myofibroblasts transiently increase in abundance in wounds and are also found in sites of chronic inflammation. Although beneficial to tissue repair, myofibroblasts are problematic in chronic inflammation, in that they contribute to the pathologic fibrosis observed in tissues such as the lung, kidney, and liver.

Recruited myofibroblasts and variants of normal tissue-derived fibroblastic cells have been demonstrated to enhance tumor phenotypes, notably cancer cell proliferation, angiogenesis, invasion, and metastasis. Their tumor-promoting activities have largely been defined by transplantation of cancer-associated fibroblasts admixed with cancer cells into mice, and more recently by genetic and pharmacologic perturbation of their functions in tumor-prone mice.[8,121,133,215–219] Because they secrete a variety of ECM components, cancer-associated fibroblasts are implicated in the formation of the desmoplastic stroma that characterizes many advanced carcinomas. The full spectrum of functions contributed by both subtypes of cancer-associated fibroblasts to tumor pathogenesis remains to be elucidated.

## Endothelial Cells

Prominent among the stromal constituents of the TME are the endothelial cells forming the tumor-associated vasculature. Quiescent tissue capillary endothelial cells are activated by *angiogenic* regulatory factors to produce a neovasculature that sustains tumor growth concomitant with continuing endothelial cell proliferation and vessel morphogenesis. A network of interconnected signaling pathways involving ligands of signal-transducing receptors (e.g., the Angiopoeitin-1/2, Notch ligands, Semaphorin, Neuropilin, Robo, and Ephrin-A/B) is now known to be involved in regulating quiescent versus activated angiogenic endothelial cells, in addition to the aforementioned counterbalancing VEGF and TSP signals. This network of signaling pathways has been functionally implicated in developmental and tumor-associated angiogenesis, further illustrating the complex regulation of endothelial cell phenotypes.[220–224]

Other avenues of research are revealing distinctive gene expression profiles of tumor-associated endothelial cells and identifying cell-surface markers displayed on the luminal surfaces of normal versus tumor endothelial cells.[78,225,226] Differences in signaling, in transcriptome profiles, and in vascular *ZIP codes* will likely prove to be important for understanding the conversion of normal endothelial cells into tumor-associated endothelial cells. Such knowledge may lead, in turn, to opportunities to develop novel therapies that exploit these differences in order to selectively target tumor-associated endothelial cells. Additionally, the activated (*angiogenic*) tumor vasculature has been revealed as a barrier to efficient intravasation and a functional suppressor of cytotoxic T cells,[227] and thus, tumor endothelial cells can contribute to the hallmark capability for evading immune destruction. As such, another emerging concept is to normalize rather than ablate them, so as to improve immunotherapy[190] as well as delivery of chemotherapy.[228]

Closely related to the endothelial cells of the circulatory system are those forming lymphatic vessels.[229] Their role in the tumor-associated stroma, specifically in supporting tumor growth, is poorly understood. Indeed, because of high interstitial pressure within solid tumors, intratumoral lymphatic vessels are typically collapsed and nonfunctional; in contrast, however, there are often functional, actively growing (*lymphangiogenic*) lymphatic vessels at the periphery of tumors and in the adjacent normal tissues that cancer cells invade. These associated lymphatics likely serve as channels for the seeding of metastatic cells in the draining lymph nodes that are commonly observed in a number of cancer types. Recent results that are yet to be generalized suggest an alternative role for the activated (i.e., lymphangiogenic) lymphatic endothelial cells associated with tumors, not in supporting tumor growth like the blood vessels, but in inducing (via VEGF-C–mediated signaling) a lymphatic tissue microenvironment that suppresses immune responses ordinarily marshaled from the draining lymph nodes.[230] As such, the real value to a tumor from activating the signaling circuit involving the ligand VEGF-C and its receptor VEGFR3 may be to facilitate the evasion of antitumor immunity by abrogating the otherwise immunostimulatory functions of draining lymphatic vessels and lymph nodes, with the collateral effect of inducing lymphatic endothelial cells to form the new lymphatic vessels that are commonly detected in association with tumors.

## Pericytes

Pericytes represent a specialized mesenchymal cell type that are closely related to smooth muscle cells, with fingerlike projections that wrap around the endothelial tubing of blood vessels. In normal tissues, pericytes are known to provide paracrine support signals to the quiescent endothelium. For example, Ang-1 secreted by pericytes conveys antiproliferative stabilizing signals that are received by the Tie2 receptors expressed on the surface of endothelial cells. Some pericytes also produce low levels of VEGF that serve a trophic function in endothelial homeostasis.[93,231] Pericytes also collaborate with the endothelial cells to synthesize the vascular basement membrane that anchors both pericytes and endothelial cells and helps vessel walls to withstand the hydrostatic pressure created by the blood.

Genetic and pharmacologic perturbation of the recruitment and association of pericytes has demonstrated the functional importance of these cells in supporting the tumor endothelium.[93,217,231] For example, the pharmacologic inhibition of signaling through the platelet-derived growth factor (PDGF) receptor expressed by tumor pericytes and bone marrow–derived pericyte progenitors results in reduced pericyte coverage of tumor vessels, which in turn destabilizes vascular integrity and function.[91,217,231] Interestingly, and in contrast, the pericytes of normal vessels are not prone to such pharmacologic disruption, providing another example of the differences in the regulation of normal quiescent and tumor vasculature. An intriguing hypothesis, still to be fully substantiated, is that tumors with poor pericyte coverage of their vasculature may be more prone to permit cancer cell intravasation into the circulatory system, thereby enabling subsequent hematogenous dissemination.[91,148]

## Immune Inflammatory Cells

Infiltrating cells of the immune system are increasingly accepted to be generic constituents of tumors. These inflammatory cells operate in conflicting ways: Both tumor-antagonizing and tumor-promoting leukocytes can be found in various proportions in most, if not all, neoplastic lesions. Evidence began to accumulate in the late 1990s that the infiltration of neoplastic tissues by cells of the immune system serves, perhaps counterintuitively, to promote tumor progression. Such work traced its conceptual roots back to the observed association of tumor formation with sites of chronic inflammation. Indeed, this led some to liken tumors to "wounds that do not heal."[211,232] In the course of normal wound healing and the resolution of infections, immune inflammatory cells appear transiently and then disappear, in contrast to their persistence in sites of chronic inflammation, where their presence has been associated with a variety of tissue pathologies, including fibrosis, aberrant angiogenesis, and as mentioned, neoplasia.[53,233]

We now know that immune cells play diverse and critical roles in fostering tumorigenesis. The roster of tumor-promoting inflammatory cells includes macrophage subtypes, mast cells, and neutrophils, as well as T and B lymphocytes.[96,97,119,133,212,234,235] Studies of these cells are yielding a growing list of tumor-promoting signaling molecules that they release, which include the tumor growth factor EGF, the angiogenic growth factors VEGF-A/-C, other proangiogenic factors such as FGF2, plus chemokines and cytokines that amplify the inflammatory state. In addition, these cells may produce proangiogenic and/or proinvasive matrix-degrading enzymes, including MMP-9 and other MMPs, cysteine cathepsin proteases, and heparanase.[94,96] Consistent with the expression of these diverse signals, tumor-infiltrating inflammatory cells have been shown to induce and help sustain tumor angiogenesis, to stimulate cancer cell proliferation, to facilitate tissue invasion, and to support the metastatic dissemination and seeding of cancer cells.[94,96,97,119,120,234–237]

In addition to fully differentiated immune cells present in tumor stroma, a variety of partially differentiated myeloid progenitors have been identified in tumors.[96] Such cells represent intermediaries between circulating cells of bone marrow origin and the differentiated immune cells typically found in normal and inflamed tissues. Importantly, these progenitors, like their more differentiated derivatives, have demonstrable tumor-promoting activity. Of particular interest, a class of tumor-infiltrating myeloid cells has been shown to suppress CTL and NK cell activity, having been identified as MDSCs that function to block the attack on tumors by the adaptive (i.e., CTL) and innate (i.e., NK) arms of the immune system.[94,133,193] Hence, recruitment of certain myeloid cells may be doubly beneficial for the developing tumor, by directly promoting angiogenesis and tumor progression, while at the same time affording a means of evading immune destruction.

These conflicting roles of the immune system in confronting tumors would seem to reflect similar situations that arise routinely in normal tissues. Thus, the immune system detects and targets infectious agents through cells of the adaptive immune response. Cells of the innate immune system, in contrast, are involved in wound healing and in clearing dead cells and cellular debris. The balance between the conflicting immune responses within particular tumor types (and indeed in individual patients' tumors) is likely to prove critical in determining the characteristics of tumor growth and the stepwise progression to stages of heightened aggressiveness (i.e., invasion and metastasis). Moreover, there is increasing evidence supporting the proposition that this balance can be modulated for therapeutic purposes in order to redirect or reprogram the immune response to focus its functional capabilities on destroying tumors.[133,238,239]

## Stem and Progenitor Cells of the Tumor Stroma

The various stromal cell types that constitute the tumor microenvironment may be recruited from adjacent normal tissue—the most obvious reservoir of such cell types. However, in recent years, bone marrow (BM) has increasingly been implicated as a key source of tumor-associated stromal cells.[99,100,240–243] Thus, mesenchymal stem and progenitor cells can be recruited into tumors from BM, where they may subsequently differentiate into the various well-characterized stromal cell types. Some of these recent arrivals may also persist in an undifferentiated or partially differentiated state, exhibiting functions that their more differentiated progeny lack.

The BM origins of stromal cell types have been demonstrated using tumor-bearing mice in which the BM cells (and thus their disseminated progeny) have been selectively labeled with reporters such as green fluorescent protein (GFP). Although immune inflammatory cells have been long known to derive from BM, more recently progenitors of endothelial cells, pericytes, and several subtypes of cancer-associated fibroblasts have also been shown to originate from BM in various mouse models of cancer.[100,240–243] The prevalence and functional importance of endothelial progenitors for tumor angiogenesis is, however, currently unresolved.[99,242] Taken together, these various lines of evidence indicate that tumor-associated stromal cells may be supplied to growing tumors by the proliferation of preexisting stromal cells or via recruitment of BM-derived stem/progenitor cells.

In summary, it is evident that virtually all cancers, including even the *liquid tumors* of hematopoietic malignancies, depend not only on neoplastic cells for their pathogenic effects, but also on diverse cell types recruited from local and distant tissue sources to assemble specialized, supporting tumor microenvironments. Importantly, the composition of stromal cell types supporting a particular cancer evidently varies considerably from one tumor type to another; even within a particular type, the patterns and abundance can be informative about malignant grade and prognosis. The inescapable conclusion is that cancer cells are not fully autonomous, and rather depend to various degrees on stromal cells of the tumor microenvironment, which can contribute functionally to seven of the eight hallmarks of cancer (Fig. 2.4).

## Heterotypic Signaling Orchestrates the Cells of the Tumor Microenvironment

Every cell in our bodies is governed by an elaborate intracellular signaling circuit—in effect, its own microcomputer. In cancer cells, key subcircuits in this integrated circuit are reprogrammed so as to activate and sustain hallmark capabilities. These changes are induced by mutations in the cells' genomes, by epigenetic alterations affecting gene expression, and by the receipt of a diverse array of signals from the tumor microenvironment. Figure 2.5A illustrates some of the circuits that are reprogrammed to enable cancer cells to proliferate chronically, to avoid proliferative brakes and cell death, and to become invasive and metastatic. Similarly, the intracellular integrated circuits that regulate the actions of stromal cells are also evidently reprogrammed. Current evidence suggests that stromal cell reprogramming is primarily affected by extracellular cues and epigenetic alterations in gene expression, rather than gene mutation.

Given the alterations in the signaling within both neoplastic cells and their stromal neighbors, a tumor can be depicted as a network of interconnected (cellular) microcomputers. This dictates that a complete elucidation of a particular tumor's biology will require far more than an elucidation of the aberrantly functioning integrated circuits within its neoplastic cells. Accordingly, the rapidly growing catalog of the function-enabling genetic mutations within cancer cell genomes[194] provides only one dimension to this problem. A reasonably complete, graphical depiction of the network of microenvironmental signaling interactions remains far beyond our reach, because the great majority of signaling molecules and their circuitry are still to be identified. Instead, we provide a hint of such interactions in Figure 2.5B. These few well-established examples are intended to exemplify a signaling network of remarkable complexity that is of critical importance to tumor pathogenesis.

## Coevolution of the Tumor Microenvironment During Carcinogenesis

The tumor microenvironment described previously is not static during multistage tumor development and progression, thus creating another dimension of complexity. Rather, the abundance and functional contributions of the stromal cells populating neoplastic lesions will likely vary during progression in two respects. First, as the neoplastic cells evolve, there will be a parallel coevolution occurring in the stroma, as indicated by the shifting composition of stroma-associated cell types. Second, as cancer cells enter into different locations, they encounter distinct stromal microenvironments. Thus, the microenvironment in the interior of a primary tumor will likely be distinct both from locally invasive breakout lesions and from the one encountered by disseminated cells in distant organs (Fig. 2.6A). This dictates that the observed histopathologic progression of a tumor reflects underlying changes in heterotypic signaling between tumor parenchyma and stroma.

We envision back-and-forth reciprocal interactions between the neoplastic cells and the supporting stromal cells that change during the course of multistep tumor development and progression, as depicted in Figure 2.6B. Thus, incipient neoplasias begin the interplay by recruiting and activating stromal cell types that assemble into an initial preneoplastic stroma, which in turn responds reciprocally by enhancing the neoplastic phenotypes of the nearby cancer cells. The cancer cells, in response, may then undergo further genetic evolution, causing them to feed signals back to the stroma. Ultimately, signals originating in the stroma of primary tumors enable cancer cells to invade normal adjacent tissues and disseminate, seeding distant tissues and, with low efficiency, metastatic colonies (see Fig. 2.6B).

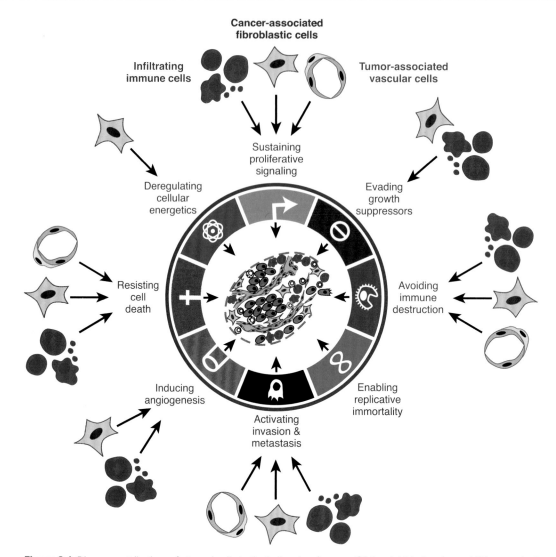

**Figure 2.4** Diverse contributions of stromal cells to the hallmarks of cancer. Of the eight hallmark capabilities acquired by cancer cells, seven depend on contributions by stromal cells forming the tumor microenvironment.[2,213] The stromal cells can be divided into three general classes: infiltrating immune cells, cancer-associated fibroblastic cells, and tumor-associated vascular cells. The association of these corrupted cell types with the acquisition of individual hallmark capabilities has been documented through a variety of experimental approaches that are often supported by descriptive studies in human cancers. The relative importance of each of these stromal cell classes to a particular hallmark varies according to tumor type and stage of progression. (Adapted from Hanahan D, Coussens LM. Accessories to the crime: functions of cells recruited to the tumor microenvironment. *Cancer Cell* 2012;21:309–322.)

The circulating cancer cells that are released from primary tumors leave a microenvironment supported by this coevolved stroma. Upon landing in a distant organ, however, disseminated cancer cells must find a means to grow in a quite different tissue microenvironment. In some cases, newly seeded cancer cells must survive and expand in naïve, fully normal tissue microenvironments. In other cases, the newly encountered tissue microenvironments may already be supportive of such disseminated cancer cells, having been preconditioned prior to their arrival. Such permissive sites have been referred to as *premetastatic niches*.[146,244,245] These supportive niches may already preexist in distant tissues for various physiologic reasons,[101] including the actions of circulating factors dispatched systemically by primary tumors.[245]

The fact that signaling interactions between cancer cells and their supporting stroma are likely to evolve during the course of multistage primary tumor development and metastatic colonization clearly complicates the goal of fully elucidating the mechanisms of cancer pathogenesis. For example, this complexity poses challenges to systems biologists seeking to chart the crucial regulatory networks that orchestrate malignant progression, because much of the critical signaling is not intrinsic to cancer cells and instead operates through the interactions that these cells establish with their neighbors.

## Cancer Cells, Cancer Stem Cells, and Intratumoral Heterogeneity

Cancer cells are the foundation of the disease. They initiate neoplastic development and drive tumor progression forward, having acquired the oncogenic and tumor suppressor mutations that define cancer as a genetic disease. Traditionally, the cancer cells within tumors have been portrayed as reasonably homogeneous cell populations until relatively late in the course of tumor progression, when hyperproliferation combined with increased genetic instability spawn genetically distinct clonal subpopulations. Reflecting such clonal heterogeneity, many human tumors are histopathologically diverse, containing regions demarcated by various

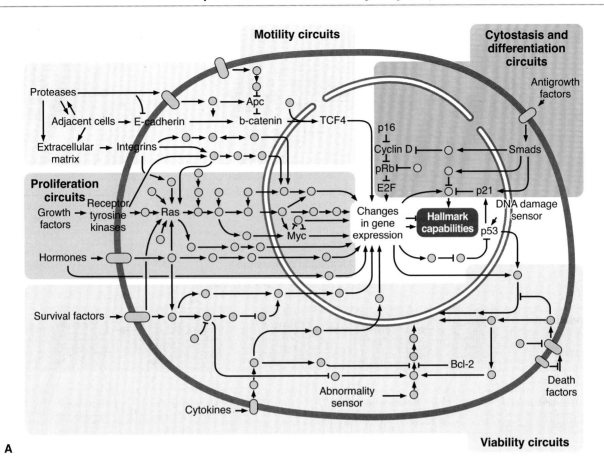

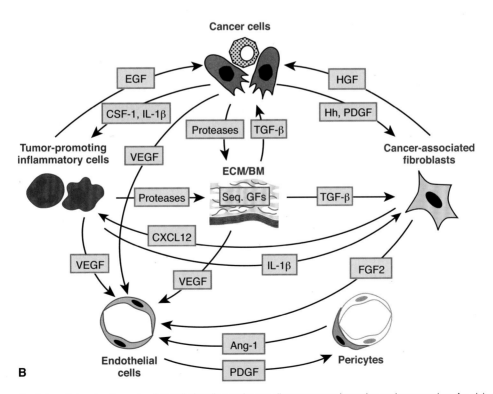

**Figure 2.5** Reprogramming intracellular circuits and cell-to-cell signaling pathways dictates tumor inception and progression. An elaborate integrated circuit operating within normal cells is reprogrammed to regulate the hallmark capabilities acquired by cancer cells **(A)** and by associated stromal cells. Separate subcircuits, depicted here in differently colored fields, are specialized to orchestrate distinct capabilities. At one level, this depiction is simplistic, because there is considerable cross-talk between such subcircuits. More broadly, the integrated circuits operating inside cancer cells and stromal cells are interconnected via a complex network of signals transmitted by the various cells in the tumor microenvironment (in some cases via the extracellular matrix *[ECM]* and basement membranes *[BM]* they synthesize), of which a few signals are exemplified **(B)**. HGF, hepatocyte growth factor for the cMet receptor; Hh, hedgehog ligand for the Patched (PTCH) receptor; Seq. GF, growth factors sequestered in the ECM/BM. (Adapted from Hanahan D, Weinberg RA. Hallmarks of cancer: the next generation. *Cell* 2011;144:646–674.)

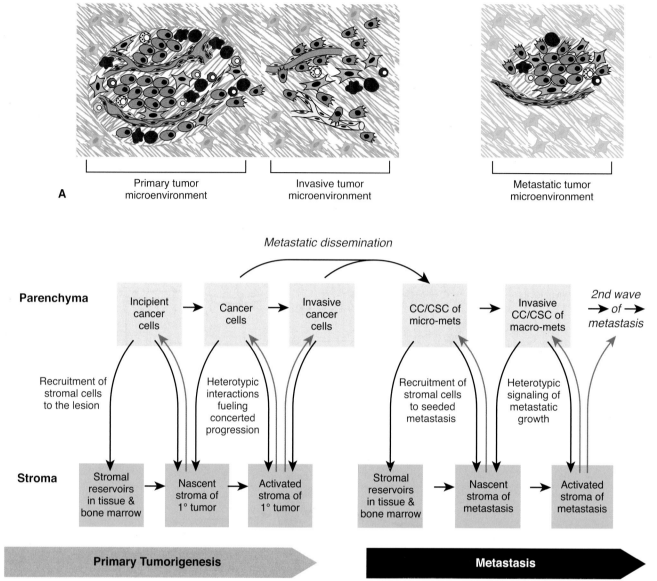

**Figure 2.6** The dynamic variation and coevolution of the tumor microenvironment during the lesional progression of cancer. **(A)** Interactions between multiple stromal cell types and heterogeneously evolving mutant cancer cells create a succession of tumor microenvironments that change dynamically as tumors are initiated, invade normal tissues, and thereafter seed and colonize distant tissues. The abundance, histologic organization, and characteristics of the stromal cell types and associated extracellular matrix *(hatched background)* evolves during progression, thereby enabling primary, invasive, and then metastatic growth. **(B)** Importantly, the signaling networks depicted in Figure 2.5 involving cancer cells and their stromal collaborators change during tumor progression as a result of reciprocal signaling interactions between these various cells. CC, cancer cell; CSC, cancer stem cell; mets, metastases. (Adapted from Hanahan D, Weinberg RA. Hallmarks of cancer: the next generation. *Cell* 2011;144:646–674.)

degrees of differentiation, proliferation, vascularity, and invasiveness. In recent years, however, evidence has accumulated pointing to the existence of a new dimension of intratumor heterogeneity and a hitherto unappreciated subclass of neoplastic cells within tumors, termed cancer stem cells (CSC).

CSCs were initially implicated in the pathogenesis of hematopoietic malignancies,[246,247] and years later, were identified in solid tumors, in particular breast carcinomas and neuroectodermal tumors.[248,249] The fractionation of cancer cells on the basis of cell-surface markers has yielded subpopulations of neoplastic cells with a greatly enhanced ability, relative to the corresponding majority populations of non-CSCs, to seed new tumors upon implantation in immunodeficient mice. These, often rare, tumor-initiating cells have proven to share transcriptional profiles with certain normal tissue stem cells, thus justifying their designation as stemlike.

Although the evidence is still fragmentary, CSCs may prove to be a constituent of many, if not most tumors, albeit being present with highly variable abundance. CSCs are defined operationally through their ability to efficiently seed new tumors upon implantation into recipient host mice.[250–253] This functional definition is often complemented by profiling the expression of certain CSC-associated markers that are typically expressed by the normal stem cells in the corresponding normal tissues of origin.[249] Importantly, recent in vivo lineage-tracing experiments have provided an additional functional test of CSCs by demonstrating their ability to spawn large numbers of progeny, including non-CSCs within tumors.[250] At the same time, these experiments have provided the most compelling evidence to date that CSCs exist, and that they can be defined functionally through tests that do not depend on the implantation of tumor cells into appropriate mouse hosts.

The origins of CSCs within a solid tumor have not been clarified and, indeed, may well vary from one tumor type to another.[250,251,254] In some tumors, normal tissue stem cells may serve as the cells of origin that undergo oncogenic transformation to yield CSCs; in others, partially differentiated transit-amplifying cells, also termed progenitor cells, may suffer the initial oncogenic transformation, thereafter assuming more stemlike characters. Once primary tumors have formed, the CSCs, like their normal counterparts, may self-renew as well as spawn more differentiated derivatives. In the case of neoplastic CSCs, these descendant cells form the great bulk of many tumors and thus are responsible for creating many tumor-associated phenotypes. It remains to be established whether multiple distinct classes of increasingly neoplastic stem cells form during the inception and subsequent multistep progression of tumors, ultimately yielding the CSCs that have been described in fully developed cancers.

Recent research has interrelated the acquisition of CSC traits with the EMT transdifferentiation program discussed previously.[250,255] The induction of this program in certain model systems can induce many of the defining features of stem cells, including self-renewal ability and the antigenic phenotypes associated with both normal and cancer stem cells. This concordance suggests that the EMT program may not only enable cancer cells to physically disseminate from primary tumors, but can also confer on such cells the self-renewal capability that is crucial to their subsequent role as founders of new neoplastic colonies at sites of dissemination.[256] If generalized, this connection raises an important corollary hypothesis: The heterotypic signals that trigger an EMT, such as those released by an activated, inflammatory stroma, may also be important in creating and maintaining CSCs.

An increasing number of human tumors are reported to contain subpopulations with the properties of CSCs, as defined operationally through their efficient tumor-initiating capabilities upon xenotransplantation into mice. Nevertheless, the importance of CSCs as a distinct phenotypic subclass of neoplastic cells remains a matter of debate, as does their oft cited rarity within tumors.[254,257–259] Indeed, it is plausible that the phenotypic plasticity operating within tumors may produce bidirectional interconversion between CSCs and non-CSCs, resulting in dynamic variation in the relative abundance of CSCs.[250,260] Such plasticity could complicate a definitive measurement of their characteristic abundance. Analogous plasticity is already implicated in the EMT program, which can be engaged reversibly.[261]

These complexities notwithstanding, it is already evident that this new dimension of tumor heterogeneity holds important implications for successful cancer therapies. Increasing evidence in a variety of tumor types suggests that cells exhibiting the properties of CSCs are more resistant to various commonly used chemotherapeutic treatments.[255,262,263] Their persistence following initial treatment may help to explain the almost inevitable disease recurrence occurring after apparently successful debulking of human solid tumors by radiation and various forms of chemotherapy. Moreover, CSCs may well prove to underlie certain forms of tumor dormancy, whereby latent cancer cells persist for years or even decades after initial surgical resection or radio/chemotherapy, only to suddenly erupt and generate life-threatening disease. Hence, CSCs represent a double threat in that they are more resistant to therapeutic killing, and at the same time, are endowed with the ability to regenerate a tumor once therapy has been halted.

This phenotypic plasticity implicit in the CSC state may also enable the formation of functionally distinct subpopulations within a tumor that support overall tumor growth in various ways. Thus, an EMT can convert epithelial carcinoma cells into mesenchymal, fibroblast-like cancer cells that may well assume the duties of CAFs in some tumors (e.g., pancreatic ductal adenocarcinoma).[264] Intriguingly, several recent reports that have yet to be thoroughly validated in terms of generality, functional importance, or prevalence have documented the ability of glioblastoma cells (or possibly their associated CSC subpopulations) to transdifferentiate into endothelial-like cells that can substitute for bona fide host-derived endothelial cells in forming a tumor-associated neovasculature.[265–267] These examples suggest that certain tumors may induce some of their own cancer cells to undergo various types of metamorphoses in order to generate stromal cell types needed to support tumor growth and progression, rather than relying on recruited host cells to provide the requisite hallmark-enabling functions.

Another form of phenotypic variability resides in the genetic heterogeneity of cancer cells within a tumor. Genomewide sequencing of cancer cells microdissected from different sectors of the same tumor[145] has revealed striking intratumoral genetic heterogeneity. Some of this genetic diversity may be reflected in the long recognized histologic heterogeneity within individual human tumors. Thus, genetic diversification may produce subpopulations of cancer cells that contribute distinct and complementary capabilities, which then accrue to the common benefit of overall tumor growth, progression, and resistance to therapy, as described earlier. Alternatively, such heterogeneity may simply reflect the genetic chaos that arises as tumor cell genomes become increasingly destabilized.

## THERAPEUTIC TARGETING OF THE HALLMARKS OF CANCER

We do not attempt here to enumerate the myriad therapies that are currently under development or have been introduced of late into the clinic. Instead, we consider how the description of hallmark principles is likely to inform therapeutic development at present and may increasingly do so in the future. Thus, the rapidly growing armamentarium of therapeutics directed against specific molecular targets can be categorized according to their respective effects on one or more hallmark capabilities, as illustrated in the examples presented in Figure 2.7. Indeed, the observed efficacy of these drugs represents, in each case, a validation of a particular capability: If a capability is truly critical to the biology of tumors, then its inhibition should impair tumor growth and progression.

Unfortunately, however, the clinical responses elicited by these targeted therapies have generally been transitory, being followed all too often by relapse. One interpretation, which is supported by growing experimental evidence, is that each of the core hallmark capabilities is regulated by a set of partially redundant signaling pathways. Consequently, a targeted therapeutic agent inhibiting one key pathway in a tumor may not completely eliminate a hallmark capability, allowing some cancer cells to survive with residual function until they or their progeny eventually adapt to the selective pressure imposed by the initially applied therapy. Such adaptation can reestablish the expression of the functional capability, permitting renewed tumor growth and clinical relapse. Because the number of parallel signaling pathways supporting a given hallmark must be limited, it may become possible to therapeutically cotarget all of these supporting pathways, thereby preventing the development of adaptive resistance.

Another dimension of the plasticity of tumors under therapeutic attack is illustrated by the unanticipated responses to antiangiogenic therapy, in which cancer cells reduce their dependence on this hallmark capability by increasing their dependence on another. Thus, many observers anticipated that potent inhibition of angiogenesis would starve tumors of vital nutrients and oxygen, forcing them into dormancy and possibly leading to their dissolution.[86,87,268] Instead, the clinical responses to antiangiogenic therapies have been found to be transitory, followed by relapse, implicating adaptive or evasive resistance mechanisms.[220,269–271] One such mechanism of evasive resistance, observed in certain preclinical models of antiangiogenic therapy, involves reduced dependence on continuing angiogenesis by increasing the activity of two other capabilities: invasiveness and metastasis.[269–271] By invading nearby and distant tissues, initially hypoxic cancer cells gain access to normal,

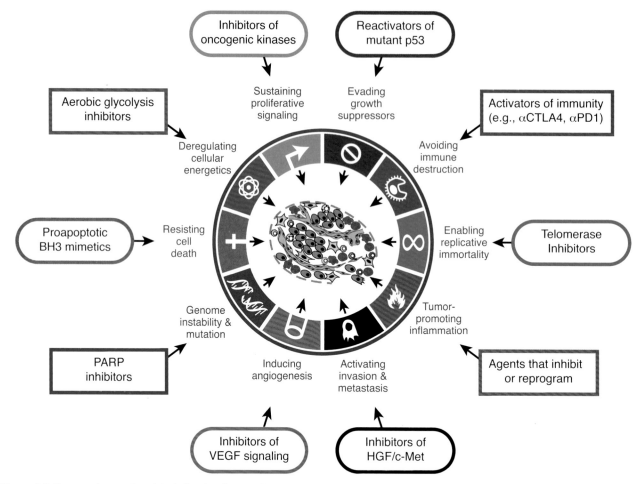

**Figure 2.7** Therapeutic targeting of the hallmarks of cancer. Drugs that interfere with each of the hallmark capabilities and hallmark-enabling processes have been developed and are in preclinical and/or clinical testing, and in some cases, approved for use in treating certain forms of human cancer. A focus on antagonizing specific hallmark capabilities is likely to yield insights into developing novel, highly effective therapeutic strategies. PARP, poly ADP ribose polymerase. (Adapted from Hanahan D, Weinberg RA. Hallmarks of cancer: the next generation. *Cell* 2011;144:646–674.)

preexisting tissue vasculature. The initial clinical validation of this adaptive/evasive resistance is apparent in the increased invasion and local metastasis seen when human glioblastomas are treated with antiangiogenic therapies.[272–274] The applicability of this lesson to other human cancers has yet to be established.

Analogous adaptive shifts in dependence on other hallmark traits may also limit the efficacy of analogous hallmark-targeting therapies. For example, the deployment of apoptosis-inducing drugs may induce cancer cells to hyperactivate mitogenic signaling, enabling them to compensate for the initial attrition triggered by such treatments. Such considerations suggest that drug development and the design of treatment protocols will benefit from incorporating the concepts of functionally discrete hallmark capabilities and of the multiple biochemical pathways involved in supporting each of them. For these reasons, we envisage that attacking multiple hallmark capabilities with hallmark-targeting drugs (see Fig. 2.7), in carefully considered combinations, sequences, and temporal regimens,[275] will result in increasingly effective therapies that produce more durable clinical responses.

## CONCLUSION AND A VISION FOR THE FUTURE

Looking ahead, we envision significant advances in our understanding of invasion and metastasis during the coming decade. Similarly, the role of altered energy metabolism in malignant growth will be

elucidated, including a resolution of whether this metabolic reprogramming is a discrete capability separable from the core hallmark of chronically sustained proliferation. We are excited about the new frontier of immunotherapy, which will be empowered to leverage detailed knowledge about the regulation of immune responses in order to develop pharmacologic tools that can modulate them therapeutically for the purpose of effectively and sustainably attacking tumors and, most importantly, their metastases.

Other areas are currently in rapid flux. In recent years, elaborate molecular mechanisms controlling transcription through chromatin modifications have been uncovered, and there are clues that specific shifts in chromatin configuration occur during the acquisition of certain hallmark capabilities.[195,196] Functionally significant epigenetic alterations seem likely to be factors not only in the cancer cells, but also in the altered cells of the tumor-associated stroma. At present, it is unclear whether an elucidation of these epigenetic mechanisms will materially change our overall understanding of the means by which hallmark capabilities are acquired, or simply add additional detail to the regulatory circuitry that is already known to govern them.

Similarly, the discovery of hundreds of distinct regulatory microRNAs has already led to profound changes in our understanding of the molecular control mechanisms that operate in health and disease. By now, dozens of microRNAs have been implicated in various tumor phenotypes.[276,277] Still, these only scratch the surface of the true complexity, because the functions of hundreds of microRNAs known to be present in our cells and to be altered in expression levels in different forms of cancer remain total mysteries. Here again, we are unclear whether future progress will cause fundamental shifts in our understanding of the pathogenic mechanisms of cancer, or only add detail to the elaborate regulatory circuits that have already been mapped out.

Finally, the existing diagrams of heterotypic interactions between the multiple distinct cell types that collaborate to produce malignant tumors are still rudimentary. We anticipate that, in another decade, the signaling pathways describing the intercommunication between these various cell types within tumors will be charted in far greater detail and clarity, eclipsing our current knowledge. And, as before,[1,2] we continue to foresee cancer research as an increasingly logical science, in which myriad phenotypic complexities are manifestations of an underlying organizing principle.

## ACKNOWLEDGMENT

This chapter is modified from Hanahan D, Weinberg RA. Hallmarks of cancer: the next generation. *Cell* 2011;144(5):646–674.

## REFERENCES

1. Hanahan D, Weinberg R. The hallmarks of cancer. *Cell* 2000;100:57–70.
2. Hanahan D, Weinberg RA. Hallmarks of cancer: the next generation. *Cell* 2011;144:646–674.
3. Lemmon MA, Schlessinger J. Cell signaling by receptor tyrosine kinases. *Cell* 2010;141:1117–1134.
4. Witsch E, Sela M, Yarden Y. Roles for growth factors in cancer progression. *Physiology* 2010;25:85–101.
5. Hynes NE, MacDonald G. ErbB receptors and signaling pathways in cancer. *Curr Opin Cell Biol* 2009;21:177–184.
6. Perona T. Cell signalling: growth factors and tyrosine kinase receptors. *Clin Transl Oncol* 2006;8:77–82.
7. Franco OE, Shaw AK, Strand DW, et al. Cancer associated fibroblasts in cancer pathogenesis. *Semin Cell Dev Biol* 2010;21:33–39.
8. Bhowmick NA, Neilson EG, Moses HL. Stromal fibroblasts in cancer initiation and progression. *Nature* 2004;432:332–337.
9. Davies MA, Samuels Y. Analysis of the genome to personalize therapy for melanoma. *Oncogene* 2010;29:5545–5555.
10. Jiang BH, Liu LZ. PI3K/PTEN signaling in angiogenesis and tumorigenesis. *Adv Cancer Res* 2009;102:19–65.
11. Yuan TL, Cantley LC. PI3K pathway alterations in cancer: variations on a theme. *Oncogene* 2008;27:5497–5510.
12. Wertz IE, Dixit VM. Regulation of death receptor signaling by the ubiquitin system. *Cell Death Differ* 2010;17:14–24.
13. Cabrita MA, Christofori G. Sprouty proteins, masterminds of receptor tyrosine kinase signaling. *Angiogenesis* 2008;11:53–62.
14. Amit I, Citri A, Shay T, et al. A module of negative feedback regulators defines growth factor signaling. *Nature Genet* 2007;39:503–512.
15. Mosesson Y, Mills GB, Yarden Y. Derailed endocytosis: an emerging feature of cancer. *Nat Rev Cancer* 2008;8:835–850.
16. Sudarsanam S, Johnson DE. Functional consequences of mTOR inhibition. *Curr Opin Drug Discov Devel* 2010;13:31–40.
17. O'Reilly KE, Rojo F, She QB, et al. mTOR inhibition induces upstream receptor tyrosine kinase signaling and activates Akt. *Cancer Res* 2006;66:1500–1508.
18. Dang CV. MYC on the path to cancer. *Cell* 2012;149:22–35.
19. Collado M, Serrano M. Senescence in tumours: evidence from mice and humans. *Nat Rev Cancer* 2010;10:51–57.
20. Evan GI, d'Adda di Fagagna F. Cellular senescence: hot or what? *Curr Opin Genet Dev* 2009;19:25–31.
21. Lowe SW, Cepero E, Evan G. Intrinsic tumour suppression. *Nature* 2004;432:307–315.
22. Mooi WJ, Peeper DS. Oncogene-induced cell senescence—halting on the road to cancer. *N Engl J Med* 2006;355:1037–1046.
23. Burkhart DL, Sage J. Cellular mechanisms of tumour suppression by the retinoblastoma gene. *Nat Rev Cancer* 2008;8:671–682.
24. Deshpande A, Sicinski P, Hinds PW. Cyclins and cdks in development and cancer: a perspective. *Oncogene* 2005;24:2909–2915.
25. Sherr CJ, McCormick F. The RB and p53 pathways in cancer. *Cancer Cell* 2002;2:103–112.
26. Lipinski MM, Jacks T. The retinoblastoma gene family in differentiation and development. *Oncogene* 1999;18:7873–7882.
27. Ghebranious N, Donehower LA. Mouse models in tumor suppression. *Oncogene* 1998;17:3385–3400.
28. McClatchey AI, Yap AS. Contact inhibition (of proliferation) redux. *Curr Opin Cell Biol* 2012;24:685–694.
29. Curto M, Cole BK, Lallemand D, et al. Contact-dependent inhibition of EGFR signaling by Nf2/Merlin. *J Cell Biol* 2007;177:893–903.
30. Okada T, Lopez-Lago M, Giancotti FG. Merlin/NF-2 mediates contact inhibition of growth by suppressing recruitment of Rac to the plasma membrane. *J Cell Biol* 2005;171:361–371.
31. Stamenkovic I, Yu Q. Merlin, a "magic" linker between the extracellular cues and intracellular signaling pathways that regulate cell motility, proliferation, and survival. *Curr Protein Pept Sci* 2010;11:471–484.
32. Pickup M, Novitskiy S, Moses HL. The roles of TGFβ in the tumour microenvironment. *Nat Rev Cancer* 2013;13:788–799.
33. Ikushima H, Miyazono K. TGFbeta signalling: a complex web in cancer progression. *Nat Rev Cancer* 2010;10:415–424.
34. Massagué J. TGF-beta in cancer. *Cell* 2008;134:215–230.
35. Bierie B, Moses HL. Tumour microenvironment: TGF-beta: the molecular Jekyll and Hyde of cancer. *Nat Rev Cancer* 2006;6:506–520.
36. Strasser A, Cory S, Adams JM. Deciphering the rules of programmed cell death to improve therapy of cancer and other diseases. *EMBO J* 2011;30:3667–3683.
37. Adams JM, Cory S. The Bcl-2 apoptotic switch in cancer development and therapy. *Oncogene* 2007;26:1324–1337.
38. Evan G, Littlewood T. A matter of life and cell death. *Science* 2004;281:1317–1322.
39. Willis SN, Adams JM. Life in the balance: how BH3-only proteins induce apoptosis. *Curr Opin Cell Biol* 2005;17:617–625.
40. Junttila MR, Evan GI. p53 — a jack of all trades but master of none. *Nat Rev Cancer* 2009;9:821–829.
41. White E. Deconvoluting the context-dependent role for autophagy in cancer. *Nat Rev Cancer* 2012;12:401–410.
42. Levine B, Kroemer G. Autophagy in the pathogenesis of disease. *Cell* 2008;132:27–42.
43. Mizushima N. Autophagy: process and function. *Genes Dev* 2007;21:2861–2873.
44. Sinha S, Levine B. The autophagy effector Beclin 1: a novel BH3-only protein. *Oncogene* 2008;27:S137–S148.
45. Mathew R, Karantza-Wadsworth V, White E. Role of autophagy in cancer. *Nat Rev Cancer* 2007;7:961–967.
46. White E, DiPaola RS. The double-edged sword of autophagy modulation in cancer. *Clin Cancer Res* 2009;15:5308–5316.
47. Apel A, Zentgraf H, Büchler MW, et al. Autophagy—A double-edged sword in oncology. *Int J Cancer* 2009;125:991–995.
48. Amaravadi RK, Thompson CB. The roles of therapy-induced autophagy and necrosis in cancer treatment. *Clin Cancer Res* 2007;13:7271–7279.
49. Lu Z, Luo RZ, Lu Y, et al. The tumor suppressor gene ARHI regulates autophagy and tumor dormancy in human ovarian cancer cells. *J Clin Invest* 2008;118:3917–3929.
50. Vanden Berghe T, Linkermann A, Jouan-Lanhouet S, et al. Regulated necrosis: the expanding network of non-apoptotic cell death pathways. *Nat Rev Mol Cell Biol* 2014;15:135–147.
51. Galluzzi L, Kroemer G. Necroptosis: a specialized pathway of programmed necrosis. *Cell* 2008;135:1161–1163.
52. Zong WX, Thompson CB. Necrotic death as a cell fate. *Genes Dev* 2006;20:1–15.
53. Grivennikov SI, Greten FR, Karin M. Immunity, inflammation, and cancer. *Cell* 2010;140:883–899.
54. White E, Karp C, Strohecker AM, et al. Role of autophagy in suppression of inflammation and cancer. *Curr Opin Cell Biol* 2010;22:212–217.
55. Blasco MA. Telomeres and human disease: ageing, cancer and beyond. *Nat Rev Genet* 2005;6:611–622.
56. Shay JW, Wright WE. Hayflick, his limit, and cellular ageing. *Nat Rev Mol Cell Biol* 2000;1:72–76.
57. Shay JW, Wright WE. Telomeres and telomerase in cancer. *Sem Cancer Biol* 2011;21:349–353.
58. Artandi SE, DePinho RA. Telomeres and telomerase in cancer. *Carcinogenesis* 2010;31:9–18.
59. Cesare AJ, Reddel RR. Alternative lengthening of telomeres: models, mechanisms and implications. *Nat Rev Genet* 2010;11:319–330.
60. Ince TA, Richardson AL, Bell GW, et al. Transformation of different human breast epithelial cell types leads to distinct tumor phenotypes. *Cancer Cell* 2007;12:160–170.
61. Passos JF, Saretzki G, von Zglinicki T. DNA damage in telomeres and mitochondria during cellular senescence: is there a connection? *Nucleic Acids Res* 2007;35:7505–7513.
62. Zhang H, Herbert BS, Pan KH, et al. Disparate effects of telomere attrition on gene expression during replicative senescence of human mammary epithelial cells cultured under different conditions. *Oncogene* 2004;23:6193–6198.
63. Sherr CJ, DePinho RA. Cellular senescence: mitotic clock or culture shock? *Cell* 2000;102:407–410.
64. Feldser DM, Greider CW. Short telomeres limit tumor progression in vivo by inducing senescence. *Cancer Cell* 2007;11:461–469.
65. Kawai T, Hiroi S, Nakanishi K, et al. Telomere length and telomerase expression in atypical adenomatous hyperplasia and small bronchioloalveolar carcinoma of the lung. *Am J Clin Pathol* 2007;127:254–262.

PRINCIPLES OF ONCOLOGY

66. Hansel DE, Meeker AK, Hicks J. Telomere length variation in biliary tract metaplasia, dysplasia, and carcinoma. *Mod Pathol* 2006;19:772–779.

67. Artandi SE, DePinho RA. Mice without telomerase: what can they teach us about human cancer? *Nature Med* 2000;6:852–855.

68. Raynaud CM, Hernandez J, Llorca FP, et al. DNA damage repair and telomere length in normal breast, preoplastic lesions, and invasive cancer. *Am J Clin Oncol* 2010;33:341–345.

69. Chin K, de Solorzano CO, Knowles D, et al. In situ analyses of genome instability in breast cancer. *Nature Genet* 2004;36:984–988.

70. Hanahan D, Folkman J. Patterns and emerging mechanisms of the angiogenic switch during tumorigenesis. *Cell* 1996;86:353–364.

71. Baeriswyl V, Christofori G. The angiogenic switch in carcinogenesis. *Semin Cancer Biol* 2009;19:329–337.

72. Bergers G, Benjamin LE. Tumorigenesis and the angiogenic switch. *Nat Rev Cancer* 2003;3:401–410.

73. Ferrara N. Vascular endothelial growth factor. *Arterioscler Thromb Vasc Biol* 2009;29:789–791.

74. Mac Gabhann F, Popel AS. Systems biology of vascular endothelial growth factors. *Microcirculation* 2008;15:715–738.

75. Carmeliet P. VEGF as a key mediator of angiogenesis in cancer. *Oncology* 2005;69:4–10.

76. Kessenbrock K, Plaks V, Werb Z. Matrix metalloproteinases: regulators of the tumor microenvironment. *Cell* 2010;141:52–67.

77. Kazerounian S, Yee KO, Lawler J. Thrombospondins in cancer. *Cell Mol Life Sci* 2008;65:700–712.

78. Nagy JA, Chang SH, Shih SC, et al. Heterogeneity of the tumor vasculature. *Semin Thromb Hemost* 2010;36:321–331.

79. Baluk P, Hashizume H, McDonald DM. Cellular abnormalities of blood vessels as targets in cancer. *Curr Opin Genet Dev* 2005;15:102–111.

80. Raica M, Cimpean AM, Ribatti D. Angiogenesis in pre-malignant conditions. *Eur J Cancer* 2009;45:1924–1934.

81. Olive KP, Jacobetz MA, Davidson CJ, et al. Inhibition of Hedgehog signaling enhances delivery of chemotherapy in a mouse model of pancreatic cancer. *Science* 2009;324:1457–1461.

82. Zee YK, O'Connor JP, Parker GJ, et al. Imaging angiogenesis of genitourinary tumors. *Nat Rev Urol* 2010;7:69–82.

83. Turner HE, Harris AL, Melmed S, et al. Angiogenesis in endocrine tumors. *Endocr Rev* 2003;24:600–632.

84. Xie L, Duncan MB, Pahler J, et al. Counterbalancing angiogenic regulatory factors control the rate of cancer progression and survival in a stage-specific manner. *Proc Natl Acad Sci U S A* 2011;108:9939–9944.

85. Ribatti D. Endogenous inhibitors of angiogenesis: a historical review. *Leuk Res* 2009;33:638–644.

86. Folkman J. Angiogenesis. *Annu Rev Med* 2006;57:1–18.

87. Folkman J. Role of angiogenesis in tumor growth and metastasis. *Semin Oncol* 2002;29:15–18.

88. Nyberg P, Xie L, Kalluri R. Endogenous inhibitors of angiogenesis. *Cancer Res* 2005;65:3967–3979.

89. Cao Y. Adipose tissue angiogenesis as a therapeutic target for obesity and metabolic diseases. *Nat Rev Drug Discov* 2010;9:107–115.

90. Seppinen L, Sormunen R, Soini Y, et al. Lack of collagen XVIII accelerates cutaneous wound healing, while overexpression of its endostatin domain leads to delayed healing. *Matrix Biol* 2008;27:535–546.

91. Raza A, Franklin MJ, Dudek AZ. Pericytes and vessel maturation during tumor angiogenesis and metastasis. *Am J Hematol* 2010;85:593–598.

92. Kovacic JC, Boehm M. Resident vascular progenitor cells: an emerging role for non-terminally differentiated vessel-resident cells in vascular biology. *Stem Cell Res* 2009;2:2–15.

93. Bergers G, Song S. The role of pericytes in blood-vessel formation and maintenance. *Neuro Oncol* 2005;7:452–464.

94. Qian BZ, Pollard JW. Macrophage diversity enhances tumor progression and metastasis. *Cell* 2010;141:39–51.

95. Zumsteg A, Christofori G. Corrupt policemen: inflammatory cells promote tumor angiogenesis. *Curr Opin Oncol* 2009;21:60–70.

96. Murdoch C, Muthana M, Coffelt SB, et al. The role of myeloid cells in the promotion of tumour angiogenesis. *Nat Rev Cancer* 2008;8:618–631.

97. De Palma M, Murdoch C, Venneri MA, et al. Tie2-expressing monocytes: regulation of tumor angiogenesis and therapeutic implications. *Trends Immunol* 2007;28:519–524.

98. Ferrara N. Pathways mediating VEGF-independent tumor angiogenesis. *Cytokine Growth Factor Rev* 2010;21:21–26.

99. Patenaude A, Parker J, Karsan A. Involvement of endothelial progenitor cells in tumor vascularization. *Microvasc Res* 2010;79:217–223.

100. Lamagna C, Bergers G. The bone marrow constitutes a reservoir of pericyte progenitors. *J Leukoc Biol* 2006;80:677–681.

101. Talmadge JE, Fidler IJ. AACR centennial series: the biology of cancer metastasis: historical perspective. *Cancer Res* 2010;70:5649–5669.

102. Fidler IJ. The pathogenesis of cancer metastasis: the "seed and soil" hypothesis revisited. *Nat Rev Cancer* 2003;3:453–458.

103. Berx G, van Roy F. Involvement of members of the cadherin superfamily in cancer. *Cold Spring Harb Perspect Biol* 2009;1:a003129.

104. Cavallaro U, Christofori G. Cell adhesion and signaling by cadherins and Ig-CAMs in cancer. *Nat Rev Cancer* 2004;4:118–132.

105. De Craene B, Berx G. Regulatory networks defining EMT during cancer initiation and progression. *Nat Rev Cancer* 2013;13:97–110.

106. Klymkowsky MW, Savagner P. Epithelial-mesenchymal transition: a cancer researcher's conceptual friend and foe. *Am J Pathol* 2009;174:1588–1592.

107. Polyak K, Weinberg RA. Transitions between epithelial and mesenchymal states: acquisition of malignant and stem cell traits. *Nat Rev Cancer* 2009;9:265–273.

108. Thiery JP, Acloque H, Huang RY, et al. Epithelial-mesenchymal transitions in development and disease. *Cell* 2009;139:871–890.

109. Yilmaz M, Christofori G. EMT, the cytoskeleton, and cancer cell invasion. *Cancer Metastasis Rev* 2009;28:15–33.

110. Barrallo-Gimeno A, Nieto MA. The Snail genes as inducers of cell movement and survival: implications in development and cancer. *Development* 2005;132:3151–3161.

111. Micalizzi DS, Farabaugh SM, Ford HL. Epithelial-mesenchymal transition in cancer: parallels between normal development and tumor progression. *J Mammary Gland Biol Neoplasia* 2010;15:117–134.

112. Taube JH, Herschkowitz JI, Komurov K, et al. Core epithelial-to-mesenchymal transition interactome gene-expression signature is associated with claudin-low and metaplastic breast cancer subtypes. *Proc Natl Acad Sci U S A* 2010;107:15449–15454.

113. Schmalhofer O, Brabletz S, Brabletz T. E-cadherin, beta-catenin, and ZEB1 in malignant progression of cancer. *Cancer Metastasis Rev* 2009;28:151–166.

114. Yang J, Weinberg RA. Epithelial-mesenchymal transition: at the crossroads of development and tumor metastasis. *Develop Cell* 2008;14:818–829.

115. Peinado H, Marin F, Cubillo E, et al. Snail and E47 repressors of E-cadherin induce distinct invasive and angiogenic properties in vivo. *J Cell Sci* 2004;117:2827–2839.

116. Karnoub AE, Weinberg RA. Chemokine networks and breast cancer metastasis. *Breast Dis* 2006;26:75–85.

117. Brabletz T, Jung A, Reu S, et al. Variable beta-catenin expression in colorectal cancers indicates tumor progression driven by the tumor environment. *Proc Natl Acad Sci U S A* 2001;98:10356–10361.

118. Hlubek F, Brabletz T, Budczies J, et al. Heterogeneous expression of Wnt/beta-catenin target genes within colorectal cancer. *Int J Cancer* 2007;121:1941–1948.

119. Egeblad M, Nakasone ES, Werb Z. Tumors as organs: complex tissues that interface with the entire organism. *Dev Cell* 2010;18:884–901.

120. Joyce JA, Pollard JW. Microenvironmental regulation of metastasis. *Nat Rev Cancer* 2009;9:239–252.

121. Kalluri R, Zeisberg M. Fibroblasts in cancer. *Nat Rev Cancer* 2006;6:392–401.

122. Karnoub AE, Dash AB, Vo AP, et al. Mesenchymal stem cells within tumour stroma promote breast cancer metastasis. *Nature* 2007;449:557–563.

123. Li HJ, Reinhart F, Herschman HR, et al. Cancer-stimulated mesenchymal stem cells create a carcinoma stem cell niche via prostaglandin E2 signaling. *Cancer Discov* 2012;2:840–855.

124. Palermo C, Joyce JA. Cysteine cathepsin proteases as pharmacological targets in cancer. *Trends Pharmacol Sci* 2008;29:22–28.

125. Mohamed MM, Sloane BF. Cysteine cathepsins: multifunctional enzymes in cancer. *Nat Rev Cancer* 2006;6:764–775.

126. Gocheva V, Wang HW, Gadea BB, et al. IL-4 induces cathepsin protease activity in tumor-associated macrophages to promote cancer growth and invasion. *Genes Dev* 2010;24:241–255.

127. Wyckoff JB, Wang Y, Lin EY, et al. Direct visualization of macrophage-assisted tumor cell intravasation in mammary tumors. *Cancer Res* 2007;67:2649–2656.

128. Hugo H, Ackland ML, Blick T, et al. Epithelial-mesenchymal and mesenchymal-epithelial transitions in carcinoma progression. *J Cell Physiol* 2007;213:374–383.

129. Friedl P, Wolf K. Plasticity of cell migration: a multiscale tuning model. *J Cell Biol* 2009;188:11–19.

130. Friedl P, Wolf K. Tube travel: the role of proteases in individual and collective cancer cell invasion. *Cancer Res* 2008;68:7247–7249.

131. Madsen CD, Sahai E. Cancer dissemination—lessons from leukocytes. *Dev Cell* 2010;19:13–26.

132. Sabeh F, Shimizu-Hirota R, Weiss SJ. Protease-dependent versus-independent cancer cell invasion programs: three-dimensional amoeboid movement revisited. *J Cell Biol* 2009;185:11–19.

133. Quail DF, Joyce JA. Microenvironmental regulation of tumor progression and metastasis. *Nat Med* 2013;19:1423–1437.

134. McGowan PM, Kirstein JM, Chambers AF. Micrometastatic disease and metastatic outgrowth: clinical issues and experimental approaches. *Future Oncol* 2009;5:1083–1098.

135. Aguirre-Ghiso JA. Models, mechanisms and clinical evidence for cancer dormancy. *Nat Rev Cancer* 2007;7:834–846.

136. Townson JL, Chambers AF. Dormancy of solitary metastatic cells. *Cell Cycle* 2006;5:1744–1750.

137. Demicheli R, Retsky MW, Hrushesky WJ, et al. The effects of surgery on tumor growth: a century of investigations. *Ann Oncol* 2008;19:1821–1828.

138. Barkan D, Green JE, Chambers AF. Extracellular matrix: a gatekeeper in the transition from dormancy to metastatic growth. *Eur J Cancer* 2010;46:1181–1188.

139. Gupta GP, Minn AJ, Kang,Y, et al. Identifying site-specific metastasis genes and functions. *Cold Spring Harb Symp Quant Biol* 2005;70:149–158.

140. Naumov GN, Folkman J, Straume O, et al. Tumor-vascular interactions and tumor dormancy. *APMIS* 2008;116:569–585.

141. Kenific CM, Thorburn A, Debnath J. Autophagy and metastasis: another double-edged sword. *Curr Opin Cell Biol* 2010;22:241–245.

142. Teng MW, Swann JB, Koebel CM, et al. Immune-mediated dormancy: an equilibrium with cancer. *J Leukoc Biol* 2008;84:988–993.

143. Campbell PJ, Yachida S, Mudie LJ, et al. The patterns and dynamics of genomic instability in metastatic pancreatic cancer. *Nature* 2010;467:1109–1113.

144. Luebeck EG. Cancer: genomic evolution of metastasis. *Nature* 2010;467:1053–1055.

145. Yachida S, Jones S, Bozic I, et al. Distant metastasis occurs late during the genetic evolution of pancreatic cancer. *Nature* 2010;467:1114–1117.

146. Coghlin C, Murray GI. Current and emerging concepts in tumour metastasis. *J Pathol* 2010;222:1–15.

147. Klein CA. Parallel progression of primary tumours and metastases. *Nat Rev Cancer* 2009;9:302–312.

148. Gerhardt H, Semb H. Pericytes: gatekeepers in tumour cell metastasis? *J Mol Med* 2008;86:135–144.

149. Kim MY, Oskarsson T, Acharyya S, et al. Tumor self-seeding by circulating cancer cells. *Cell* 2009;139:1315–1326.

150. Bos PD, Zhang XH, Nadal C, et al. Genes that mediate breast cancer metastasis to the brain. *Nature* 2009;459:1005–1009.

151. Olson P, Lu J, Zhang H, et al. MicroRNA dynamics in the stages of tumorigenesis correlate with hallmark capabilities of cancer. *Genes Dev* 2009;23:2152–2165.

152. Nguyen DX, Bos PD, Massagué J. Metastasis: from dissemination to organspecific colonization. *Nat Rev Cancer* 2009;9:274–284.

153. Warburg OH. *The Metabolism of Tumours: Investigations from the Kaiser Wilhelm Institute for Biology, Berlin-Dahlem.* London, UK: Arnold Constable; 1930.

154. Warburg O. On the origin of cancer cells. *Science* 1956;123:309–314.

155. Warburg O. On respiratory impairment in cancer cells. *Science* 1956;124:269–270.

156. Jones RG, Thompson CB. Tumor suppressors and cell metabolism: a recipe for cancer growth. *Genes Dev* 2009;23:537–548.

157. DeBerardinis RJ, Lum JJ, Hatzivassiliou G, et al. The biology of cancer: metabolic reprogramming fuels cell growth and proliferation. *Cell Metab* 2008;7:11–20.

158. Hsu PP, Sabatini DM. Cancer cell metabolism: Warburg and beyond. *Cell* 2008;134:703–707.

159. Ward PS, Thompson CB. Metabolic reprogramming: a cancer hallmark even warburg did not anticipate. *Cancer Cell* 2012;21:297–308.

160. Semenza GL. HIF-1: upstream and downstream of cancer metabolism. *Curr Opin Genet Dev* 2010;20:51–56.

161. Semenza GL. Defining the role of hypoxia-inducible factor 1 in cancer biology and therapeutics. *Oncogene* 2010;29:625–634.

162. Kroemer G, Pouyssegur J. Tumor cell metabolism: cancer's Achilles' heel. *Cancer Cell* 2008;13:472–482.

163. Potter V. The biochemical approach to the cancer problem. *Fed Proc* 1958;17:691–697.

164. Vander Heiden MG, Cantley LC, Thompson CB. Understanding the Warburg effect: the metabolic requirements of cell proliferation. *Science* 2009;324:1029–1033.

165. Semenza GL. Tumor metabolism: cancer cells give and take lactate. *J Clin Invest* 2008;118:3835–3837.

166. Nakajima EC, Van Houten B. Metabolic symbiosis in cancer: refocusing the Warburg lens. *Mol Carcinog* 2013;52:329–337.

167. Kennedy KM, Dewhirst MW. Tumor metabolism of lactate: the influence and therapeutic potential for MCT and CD147 regulation. *Future Oncol* 2010;6:127–148.

168. Feron O. Pyruvate into lactate and back: from the Warburg effect to symbiotic energy fuel exchange in cancer cells. *Radiother Oncol* 2009;92:329–333.

169. Magistretti PJ. Neuron-glia metabolic coupling and plasticity. *J Exp Biol* 2006;209:2304–2311.

170. Hardee ME, Dewhirst MW, Agarwal N, et al. Novel imaging provides new insights into mechanisms of oxygen transport in tumors. *Curr Mol Med* 2009;9:435–441.

171. Burnet FM. The concept of immunological surveillance. *Prog Exp Tumor Res* 1970;13:1–27.

172. Thomas L. On immuosurveillance in human cancer. *Yale J Biol Med* 1982;55:329–333.

173. Vajdic CM, van Leeuwen MT. Cancer incidence and risk factors after solid organ transplantation. *Int J Cancer* 2009;125:1747–1754.

174. Elinav E, Nowarski R, Thaiss CA, et al. Inflammation-induced cancer: crosstalk between tumours, immune cells and microorganisms. *Nat Rev Cancer* 2013;13:759–771.

175. Swann JB, Smyth MJ. Immune surveillance of tumors. *J Clin Invest* 2007;117:1137–1146.

176. Fridman WH, Mlecnik B, Bindea G, et al. Immunosurveillance in human non-viral cancers. *Curr Opin Immunol* 2011;23:272–278.

177. Galon J, Angell HK, Bedognetti D, et al. The continuum of cancer immunosurveillance: prognostic, predictive, and mechanistic signatures. *Immunity* 2013;39:11–26.

178. Kim R, Emi M, Tanabe K. Cancer immunoediting from immune surveillance to immune escape. *Immunology* 2007;121:1–14.

179. Smyth MJ, Dunn GP, Schreiber RD. Cancer immunosurveillance and immune-editing: the roles of immunity in suppressing tumor development and shaping tumor immunogenicity. *Adv Immunol* 2006;90:1–50.

180. Bindea G, Mlecnik B, Fridman WH, et al. Natural immunity to cancer in humans. *Curr Opin Immunol* 2010;22:215–222.

181. Ferrone C, Dranoff G. Dual roles for immunity in gastrointestinal cancers. *J Clin Oncol* 2010;28:4045–4051.

182. Nelson BH. The impact of T-cell immunity on ovarian cancer outcomes. *Immunol Rev* 2008;222:101–116.

183. Pagès F, Galon J, Dieu-Nosjean MC, et al. Immune infiltration in human tumors: a prognostic factor that should not be ignored. *Oncogene* 2010;29:1093–1102.

184. Strauss DC, Thomas JM. Transmission of donor melanoma by organ transplantation. *Lancet Oncol* 2010;11:790–796.

185. Yang L, Pang Y, Moses HL. TGF-beta and immune cells: an important regulatory axis in the tumor microenvironment and progression. *Trends Immunol* 2010;31:220–227.

186. Shields JD, Kourtis IC, Tomei AA, et al. Induction of lymphoidlike stroma and immune escape by tumors that express the chemokine CCL21. *Science* 2010;328:749–752.

187. Korman AJ, Peggs KS, Allison J. Checkpoint blockade in cancer immunotherapy. *Adv Immunol* 2006;90:297–339.

188. Fife BT, Pauken KE, Eagar TN, et al. Interactions between programmed death-1 and programmed death ligand-1 promote tolerance by blocking the T cell receptor-induced stop signal. *Nat Immunol* 2009;10:1185–1192.

189. Pardoll DM. The blockade of immune checkpoints in cancer immunotherapy. *Nat Rev Cancer* 2012;12:252–264.

190. Motz GT, Coukos G. Deciphering and reversing tumor immune suppression. *Immunity* 2013;39:61–73.

191. Gabrilovich DI, Nagaraj S. Myeloid-derived suppressor cells as regulators of the immune system. *Nat Rev Immunol* 2009;9:162–174.

192. Mougiakakos D, Choudhury A, Lladser A, et al. Regulatory T cells in cancer. *Adv Cancer Res* 2010;107:57–117.

193. Ostrand-Rosenberg S, Sinha P. Myeloid-derived suppressor cells: linking inflammation and cancer. *J Immunol* 2009;182:4499–4506.

194. Garraway LA, Lander ES. Lessons from the cancer genome. *Cell* 2013;153:17–37.

195. You JS, Jones PA. Cancer genetics and epigenetics: two sides of the same coin? *Cancer Cell* 2012;22:9–20.

196. Berdasco M, Esteller M. Aberrant epigenetic landscape in cancer: how cellular identity goes awry. *Dev Cell* 2010;19:698–711.

197. Esteller M. Cancer epigenomics: DNA methylomes and histone-modification maps. *Nat Rev Genet* 2007;8:286–298.

198. Jones PA, Baylin SB. The epigenomics of cancer. *Cell* 2007;128:683–692.

199. Negrini S, Gorgoulis VG, Halazonetis TD. Genomic instability—an evolving hallmark of cancer. *Nat Rev Mol Cell Bio* 2010;11:220–228.

200. Loeb LA. A mutator phenotype in cancer. *Cancer Res* 2001;61:3230–3239.

201. Jackson SP, Bartek J. The DNA-damage response in human biology and disease. *Nature* 2009;461:1071–1078.

202. Kastan MB. DNA damage responses: mechanisms and roles in human disease. *Mol Cancer Res* 2008;6:517–524.

203. Sigal A, Rotter V. Oncogenic mutations of the p53 tumor suppressor: the demons of the guardian of the genome. *Cancer Res* 2000;60:6788–6793.

204. Lane DP. Cancer. p53, guardian of the genome. *Nature* 1992;358:15–16.

205. Kinzler KW, Vogelstein B. Cancer-susceptibility genes. Gatekeepers and caretakers. *Nature* 1997;386:761–763.

206. Ciccia A, Elledge SJ. The DNA damage response: making it safe to play with knives. *Mol Cell* 2010;40:179–204.

207. Harper JW, Elledge SJ. The DNA damage response: ten years after. *Mol Cell* 2007;28:739–745.

208. Friedberg EC, Aguilera A, Gellert M, et al. DNA repair: from molecular mechanism to human disease. *DNA Repair (Amst)* 2006;5:986–996.

209. Barnes DE, Lindahl T. Repair and genetic consequences of endogenous DNA base damage in mammalian cells. *Annu Rev Genet* 2004;38:445–476.

210. Korkola J, Gray JW. Breast cancer genomes—form and function. *Curr Opin Genet Dev* 2010;20:4–14.

211. Dvorak HF. Tumors: wounds that do not heal. Similarities between tumor stroma generation and wound healing. *N Engl J Med* 1986;315:1650–1659.

212. De Nardo DG, Andreu P, Coussens LM. Interactions between lymphocytes and myeloid cells regulate pro- versus anti-tumor immunity. *Cancer Metastasis Rev* 2010;29:309–316.

213. Hanahan D, Coussens LM. Accessories to the crime: functions of cells recruited to the tumor microenvironment. *Cancer Cell* 2012;21:309–322.

214. de Visser KE, Eichten A, Coussens LM. Paradoxical roles of the immune system during cancer development. *Nat Rev Cancer* 2006;6:24–37.

215. Servais C, Erez N. From sentinel cells to inflammatory culprits: cancerassociated fibroblasts in tumour-related inflammation. *J Pathol* 2013;229:198–207.

216. Dirat B, Bochet L, Escourrou G, et al. Unraveling the obesity and breast cancer links: a role for cancer-associated adipocytes? *Endocr Dev* 2010;19:45–52.

217. Pietras K, Ostman A. Hallmarks of cancer: interactions with the tumor stroma. *Exp Cell Res* 2010;316:1324–1331.

218. Räsänen K, Vaheri A. Activation of fibroblasts in cancer stroma. *Exp Cell Res* 2010;316:2713–2722.

219. Shimoda M, Mellody KT, Orimo A. Carcinoma-associated fibroblasts are a ratelimiting determinant for tumour progression. *Sem Cell Dev Biol* 2010;21:19–25.

220. Welti J, Loges S, Dimmeler S, et al. Recent molecular discoveries in angiogenesis and antiangiogenic therapies in cancer. *J Clin Invest* 2013;123:3190–3200.

**PRINCIPLES OF ONCOLOGY**

221. Pasquale EB. Eph receptors and ephrins in cancer: bidirectional signalling and beyond. *Nat Rev Cancer* 2010;10:165–180.

222. Ahmed Z, Bicknell R. Angiogenic signalling pathways. *Methods Mol Biol* 2009;467:3–24.

223. Dejana E, Orsenigo F, Molendini C, et al. Organization and signaling of endothelial cell-to-cell junctions in various regions of the blood and lymphatic vascular trees. *Cell Tissue Res* 2009;335:17–25.

224. Carmeliet P, Jain RK. Angiogenesis in cancer and other diseases. *Nature* 2000;407:249–257.

225. Ruoslahti E, Bhatia SN, Sailor MJ. Targeting of drugs and nanoparticles to tumors. *J Cell Biol* 2010;188:759–768.

226. Ruoslahti E. Specialization of tumour vasculature. *Nat Rev Cancer* 2002;2: 83–90.

227. Motz GT, Coukos G. The parallel lives of angiogenesis and immunosuppression: cancer and other tales. *Nat Rev Immunol* 2011;11:702–711.

228. Carmeliet P, Jain RK. Principles and mechanisms of vessel normalization for cancer and other angiogenic diseases. *Nat Rev Drug Discov* 2011;10: 417–427.

229. Tammela T, Alitalo K. Lymphangiogenesis: Molecular mechanisms and future promise. *Cell* 2010;140:460–476.

230. Card CM, Yu SS, Swartz MA. Emerging roles of lymphatic endothelium in regulating adaptive immunity. *J Clin Invest* 2014;124:943–952.

231. Gaengel K, Genové G, Armulik A, et al. Endothelial-mural cell signaling in vascular development and angiogenesis. *Arterioscler Thromb Vasc Biol* 2009;29:630–638.

232. Schäfer M, Werner S. Cancer as an overhealing wound: an old hypothesis revisited. *Nat Rev Mol Cell Biol* 2008;9:628–638.

233. Karin M, Lawrence T, Nizet V. Innate immunity gone awry: linking microbial infections to chronic inflammation and cancer. *Cell* 2006;124:823–835.

234. Coffeldt SB, Lewis CE, Naldini L, et al. Elusive identities and overlapping phenotypes of proangiogenic myeloid cells in tumors. *Am J Pathol* 2010;176: 1564–1576.

235. Johansson M, Denardo DG, Coussens LM. Polarized immune responses differentially regulate cancer development. *Immunol Rev* 2008;222:145–154.

236. Mantovani A. Molecular pathways linking inflammation and cancer. *Curr Mol Med* 2010;10:369–373.

237. Mantovani A, Allavena P, Sica A, et al. Cancer-related inflammation. *Nature* 2008;454:436–444

238. DeNardo DG, Brennan DJ, Rexhepaj E, et al. Leukocyte complexity predicts breast cancer survival and functionally regulates response to chemotherapy. *Cancer Discov* 2011;1:54–67.

239. De Palma M, Coukos G, Hanahan D. A new twist on radiation oncology: low-dose irradiation elicits immunostimulatory macrophages that unlock barriers to tumor immunotherapy. *Cancer Cell* 2013;24:559–561.

240. Koh BI, Kang Y. The pro-metastatic role of bone marrow-derived cells: a focus on MSCs and regulatory T cells. *EMBO Rep* 2012;13:412–422.

241. Bergfeld SA, DeClerck YA. Bone marrow-derived mesenchymal stem cells and the tumor microenvironment. *Cancer Metastasis Rev* 2010;29:249–261.

242. Fang S, Salven P. Stem cells in tumor angiogenesis. *J Mol Cell Cardiol* 2011;50:290–295.

243. Giaccia AJ, Schipani E. Role of carcinoma-associated fibroblasts and hypoxia in tumor progression. *Curr Top Microbiol Immunol* 2010;345:31–45.

244. Labelle M, Hynes RO. The initial hours of metastasis: the importance of cooperative host-tumor cell interactions during hematogenous dissemination. *Cancer Discov* 2012;2:1091–1099.

245. Peinado H, Lavothskin S, Lyden D. The secreted factors responsible for pre-metastatic niche formation: old sayings and new thoughts. *Semin Cancer Biol* 2011;21:139–146.

246. Reya T, Morrison SJ, Clarke MF, et al. Stem cells, cancer, and cancer stem cells. *Nature* 2001;414:105–111.

247. Bonnet D, Dick JE. Human acute myeloid leukemia is organized as a hierarchy that originates from a primitive hematopoietic cell. *Nature Med* 1997;3: 730–737.

248. Gilbertson RJ, Rich JN. Making a tumour's bed: glioblastoma stem cells and the vascular niche. *Nat Rev Cancer* 2007;7:733–736.

249. al-Hajj M, Wicha M, Benito-Hernandez A, et al. Prospective identification of tumorigenic breast cancer cells. *Proc Natl Acad Sci U S A* 2003;100:3983–3988.

250. Beck B, Blanpain C. Unravelling cancer stem cell potential. *Nat Rev Cancer* 2013;13:727–738.

251. Magee JA, Piskounova E, Morrison SJ. Cancer stem cells: impact, heterogeneity, and uncertainty. *Cancer Cell* 2012;21:283–296.

252. Cho RW, Clarke MF. Recent advances in cancer stem cells. *Curr Opin Genet Devel* 2008;18:1–6.

253. Lobo NA, Shimono Y, Qian D, et al. The biology of cancer stem cells. *Annu Rev Cell Dev Biol* 2007;23:675–699.

254. Meacham CE, Morrison SJ. Tumour heterogeneity and cancer cell plasticity. *Nature* 2013;501:328–337.

255. Singh A, Settleman J. EMT, cancer stem cells and drug resistance: an emerging axis of evil in the war on cancer. *Oncogene* 2010;29:4741–4751.

256. Brabletz T, Jung A, Spaderna S, et al. Opinion: migrating cancer stem cells – an integrated concept of malignant tumor progression. *Nat Rev Cancer* 2005;5:744–749.

257. Boiko AD, Razorenova OV, van de Rijn M, et al. Human melanoma-initiating cells express neural crest nerve growth factor receptor CD271. *Nature* 2010;466:133–137.

258. Gupta P, Chaffer CL, Weinberg RA. Cancer stem cells: mirage or reality? *Nature Med* 2009;15:1010–1012.

259. Quintana E, Shackleton M, Sabel MS, et al. Efficient tumour formation by single human melanoma cells. *Nature* 2008;456:593–598.

260. Chaffer CL, Brueckmann I, Scheel C, et al. Normal and neoplastic nonstem cells can spontaneously convert to stem-like state. *Proc Natl Acad Sci U S A* 2011;108:7950–7955.

261. Thiery JP, Sleeman JR. Complex networks orchestrate epithelial-mesenchymal transitions. *Nat Rev Mol Cell Biol* 2006;7:131–142.

262. Creighton CJ, Li X, Landis M, et al. Residual breast cancers after conventional therapy display mesenchymal as well as tumor-initiating features. *Proc Natl Acad Sci U S A* 2009;106:13820–13825.

263. Buck E, Eyzaguirre A, Barr S, et al. Loss of homotypic cell adhesion by epithelial-mesenchymal transition or mutation limits sensitivity to epidermal growth factor receptor inhibition. *Mol Cancer Therap* 2007;6:532–541.

264. Rhim AD, Mirek ET, Aiello NM, et al. EMT and dissemination precede pancreatic tumor formation. *Cell* 2012;148:349–361.

265. Soda Y, Marumoto T, Friedmann-Morvinski D, et al. Transdifferentiation of glioblastoma cells into vascular endothelial cells. *Proc Natl Acad Sci U S A* 2011;108:4274–4280.

266. El Hallani S, Boisselier B, Peglion F, et al. A new alternative mechanism in glioblastoma vascularization: tubular vasculogenic mimicry. *Brain* 2010;133: 973–982.

267. Wang R, Chadalavada K, Wilshire J, et al. Glioblastoma stem-like cells give rise to tumour endothelium. *Nature* 2010;468:829–833.

268. Folkman J, Kalluri R. Cancer without disease. *Nature* 2004;427:787.

269. Azam F, Mehta S, Harris AL. Mechanisms of resistance to antiangiogenic therapy. *Eur J Cancer* 2010;46:1323–1332.

270. Ebos JM, Lee CR, Kerbel RS. Tumor and host-mediated pathways of resistance and disease progression in response to antiangiogenic therapy. *Clin Cancer Res* 2009;15:5020–5025.

271. Bergers G, Hanahan D. Modes of resistance to anti-angiogenic therapy. *Nat Rev Cancer* 2008;8:592–603.

272. Ellis LM, Reardon DA. Cancer: the nuances of therapy. *Nature* 2009;458: 290–292.

273. Norden AD, Drappatz J, Wen PY. Antiangiogenic therapies for high-grade glioma. *Nat Rev Neurol* 2009;5:610–620.

274. Verhoeff JJ, van Tellingen O, Claes A, et al. Concerns about anti-angiogenic treatment in patients with glioblastoma multiforme. *BMC Cancer* 2009; 9:444.

275. Hanahan D. Rethinking the war on cancer. *Lancet* 2014;383:558–563.

276. Pencheva N, Tavazoie SF. Control of metastatic progression by microRNA regulatory networks. *Nat Cell Biol* 2013;15:546–554.

277. Garzon R, Marcucci G, Croce CM. Targeting microRNAs in cancer: rationale, strategies and challenges. *Nat Rev Drug Discov* 2010;9:775–789.

# 3  Molecular Methods in Cancer

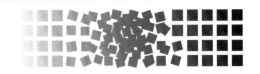

Larissa V. Furtado, Jay L. Hess, and Bryan L. Betz

## APPLICATIONS OF MOLECULAR DIAGNOSTICS IN ONCOLOGY

Molecular diagnostics is increasingly impacting a number of areas of cancer care delivery including diagnosis, prognosis, in predicting response to particular therapies, and in minimal residual disease monitoring. Each of these depends on detection or measurement of one or more disease-specific molecular biomarkers representing abnormalities in genetic or epigenetic pathways controlling cellular proliferation, differentiation, or cell death (Table 3.1). In addition, molecular diagnostics is beginning to play a role in predicting host metabolism of drugs—for example, in predicting fast versus slow thiopurine metabolizers using polymorphisms in the thiopurine methyltransferase (TPMT) allele and in use in dosing patients with thiopurine drugs.[1] Molecular diagnostics has also had a major impact on assessing an engraftment after bone marrow transplantation and in tissue typing for bone marrow and solid organ transplantation.

The ideal cancer biomarker is only associated with the disease and not the normal state. The utility of the biomarker largely depends on what the clinical effect the biomarker predicts for, how large the effect is, and how strong the evidence is for the effect. For clinical application, biomarkers need a high level of *analytic validity, clinical validity,* and *clinical utility.* Analytic validity refers to the ability of the overall testing process to accurately detect and, in many cases, measure the biomarker. Clinical validity is the ability of a biomarker to predict a particular disease behavior or response to therapy. Clinical utility, arguably the most difficult to assess, addresses whether the information available from the biomarker is actually beneficial for patient care.

Biomarkers can take many forms including *chromosomal translocations* and *other chromosomal rearrangements, gene amplification, copy number variation, point mutations, single nucleotide polymorphisms, changes in gene expression* (including micro RNAs), and *epigenetic alterations.* Most biomarkers in widespread use represent either gain of function or loss of function alterations in key signaling pathways. Those that occur early and at a high frequency in tumors tend to be *driver mutations,* whose function is important for the cancer cell's proliferation and/or survival. These are particularly useful as biomarkers because they often represent important therapeutic targets. However, cancer cells accumulate many genetic alterations, called *passenger mutations,* which tend to occur at a lower frequency overall and in a subset of a heterogeneous population of tumor cells that may contribute to the cancer phenotype but are not absolutely essential.[2] Distinguishing passenger from driver mutations using various functional assays has become a major focus of translational research in cancer. The same biomarker may have utility in a variety of settings. For example, the detection of the *BCR-ABL1* translocation, pathognomonic for chronic myelogenous leukemia (CML), is used for establishing the diagnosis, for the selection of therapy, and for monitoring for minimal residual disease during and after therapy.

Some of the most heavily used genetic biomarkers in cancer, particularly in hematologic malignancies, are *chromosomal translocations.* For certain diseases such as CML, detection of the *BCR-ABL1* translocation or in Burkitt lymphoma the immunoglobulin gene-*MYC* translocation is required, according to current World Health Organization (WHO) guidelines, to make the diagnosis. Identification of translocations is important in the diagnosis and subtyping of acute leukemias (e.g., detection of *PML-RARA* and variant translocations in acute promyelocytic leukemia) and is also extremely important for the diagnosis of sarcomas such as Ewing sarcoma. The discovery of chromosomal translocations, such as the *TMPRSS-ETS* in prostate cancer and *ALK* translocations in non–small-cell lung cancer, portends an importance of detecting translocations in solid tumors.[3] Chromosomal translocations, especially for hematologic malignancies, have been traditionally detected by classical karyotyping. This approach has limitations; in particular, it requires viable, dividing cells, which are often not readily available from solid tumor biopsies. In addition, a significant proportion of chromosomal translocations are not detectable by conventional karyotyping. For example, 5% to 10% of CML cases lack detectable t(9;22) by G banding. Such "cryptic" translocations require other approaches for detection, which are to be discussed, including *fluorescent in situ hybridization* (FISH), *polymerase chain reaction* (PCR), as well as *nucleic acid sequencing-based methods.*

In certain settings, it can be helpful to detect if a population of cells is clonal. For example, in some lymphoid infiltrates, the cells are well differentiated and it can be difficult to determine whether these represent a reactive or neoplastic infiltrate. If dispersed, cells are available and these could be analyzed by flow cytometer to detect whether a monotypic population expressing either immunoglobulin kappa or lambda light chains is present. In theory, immunohistochemical staining (IHC) for immunoglobulin light chains could be used to assess clonality; however, in practice this is done with more sensitivity using RNA in situ hybridization for immunoglobulin kappa and lambda light chain transcripts. The most sensitive way to detect clonality in a B-cell population is to analyze the size of the break point cluster region that arises as a result of VDJ recombination by *PCR.* Reactive B cells will show a distribution in the size of the VDJ recombination for the *IGH* or *IGK* or *IGL,* whereas clonal cells will show a predominant band that represents the size of the VDJ region of the dominant clone. Similarly, sometimes it can be difficult to distinguish neoplastic from reactive T-cell infiltrates. Given the large number of T-cell antigen receptors, it is not as simple to detect clonality by IHC or flow cytometry in T-cell proliferations. One approach is to use aberrant loss of T-cell antigen expression to aid in the diagnosis of T-cell neoplasms. Another is to detect clonal rearrangement of the VDJ region of the T-cell receptor gamma (*TCRγ*) gene, which can be done by PCR on both fresh and formalin-fixed paraffin-embedded (FFPE) tissue.

*Gene amplification* is another important mechanism in cancer that has been found to have high utility in a subset of cancers. *MYCN* amplification occurs in approximately 40% of undifferentiated or poorly differentiated neuroblastoma subtypes,[4,5] either appearing as double minute chromosomes or homogeneously

| TABLE 3.1 | | | | |
|---|---|---|---|---|
| **Genomic Alterations as Putative Predictive Biomarkers for Cancer Therapy** | | | | |
| **Genes** | **Pathways** | **Aberration Type** | **Disease Examples** | **Putative or Proven Drugs** |
| *PIK3CA*,[51,52] *PIK3R1*,[53] *PIK3R2*, *AKT1*, *AKT2*, and *AKT3*[54,55] | Phosphoinositide 3-kinase (PI3K) | Mutation or amplification | Breast, colorectal, and endometrial cancer | ■ PI3K inhibitors ■ AKT inhibitors |
| *PTEN*[56] | PI3K | Deletion | Numerous cancers | ■ PI3K inhibitors |
| *MTOR*,[57] *TSC1*,[58] and *TSC2*[59] | mTOR | Mutation | Tuberous sclerosis and bladder cancer | ■ mTOR inhibitors |
| RAS family (*HRAS*, *NRAS*, *KRAS*), *BRAF*,[60] and *MEK1* | RAS–MEK | Mutation, rearrangement, or amplification | Numerous cancers, including melanoma and prostate cancers | ■ RAF inhibitors ■ MEK inhibitors ■ PI3K inhibitors |
| Fibroblast growth factor receptor 1 (*FGFR1*), *FGFR2*, *FGFR3*, *FGFR4*[36] | FGFR | Mutation, amplification, or rearrangement | Myeloma, sarcoma, and bladder, breast, ovarian, lung, endometrial, and myeloid cancers | ■ FGFR inhibitors ■ FGFR antibodies |
| Epidermal growth factor receptor (*EGFR*) | EGFR | Mutation, deletion, or amplification | Lung and gastrointestinal cancer | ■ EGFR inhibitors ■ EGFR antibodies |
| *ERBB2*[61] | ERBB2 | Amplification or mutation | Breast, bladder, gastric, and lung cancers | ■ ERBB2 inhibitors ■ ERBB2 antibodies |
| *SMO*[62,63] and *PTCH1*[64] | Hedgehog | Mutation | Basal cell carcinoma | ■ Hedgehog inhibitor |
| *MET*[65] | MET | Amplification or mutation | Bladder, gastric, and renal cancers | ■ MET inhibitors ■ MET antibodies |
| *JAK1*, *JAK2*, *JAK3*,[66] *STAT1*, *STAT3* | JAK–STAT | Mutation or rearrangement | Leukemia and lymphoma | ■ JAK–STAT inhibitors ■ STAT decoys |
| Discoidin domain-containing receptor 2 (*DDR2*) | RTK | Mutation | Lung cancer | ■ Some tyrosine kinase inhibitors |
| Erythropoietin receptor (*EPOR*) | JAK–STAT | Rearrangement | Leukemia | ■ JAK–STAT inhibitors |
| Interleukin-7 receptor (*IL-7R*) | JAK–STAT | Mutation | Leukemia | ■ JAK–STAT inhibitors |
| Cyclin-dependent kinases (*CDKs*[67]; *CDK4*, *CDK6*, *CDK8*), *CDKN2A*, and cyclin D1 (*CCND1*) | CDK | Amplification, mutation, deletion, or rearrangement | Sarcoma, colorectal cancer, melanoma, and lymphoma | ■ CDK inhibitors |
| *ABL1* | ABL | Rearrangement | Leukemia | ■ ABL inhibitors |
| Retinoic acid receptor-α (*RARA*) | RARα | Rearrangement | Leukemia | ■ All-trans retinoic acid |
| Aurora kinase A (*AURKA*)[68] | Aurora kinases | Amplification | Prostate and breast cancers | ■ Aurora kinase inhibitors |
| Androgen receptor (*AR*)[69] | Androgen | Mutation, amplification, or splice variant | Prostate cancer | ■ Androgen synthesis inhibitors ■ Androgen receptor inhibitors |
| *FLT3*[70] | FLT3 | Mutation or deletion | Leukemia | ■ FLT3 inhibitors |
| *MET* | MET–HGF | Mutation or amplification | Lung and gastric cancers | ■ MET inhibitors |
| Myeloproliferative leukemia (*MPL*) | THPO, JAK–STAT | Mutation | Myeloproliferative neoplasms | ■ JAK–STAT inhibitors |
| *MDM2*[71] | MDM2 | Amplification | Sarcoma and adrenal carcinomas | ■ MDM2 antagonist |
| *KIT*[72] | KIT | Mutation | GIST, mastocytosis, and leukemia | ■ KIT inhibitors |
| *PDGFRA* and *PDGFRB* | PDGFR | Deletion, rearrangement, or amplification | Hematologic cancer, GIST, sarcoma, and brain cancer | ■ PDGFR inhibitors |
| Anaplastic lymphoma kinase (*ALK*)[9,37,73,74] | ALK | Rearrangement or mutation | Lung cancer and neuroblastoma | ■ ALK inhibitors |

*(continued)*

## TABLE 3.1

### Genomic Alterations as Putative Predictive Biomarkers for Cancer Therapy *(continued)*

| Genes | Pathways | Aberration Type | Disease Examples | Putative or Proven Drugs |
|---|---|---|---|---|
| *RET* | RET | Rearrangement or mutation | Lung and thyroid cancers | ▪ RET inhibitors |
| *ROS1*[75] | ROS1 | Rearrangement | Lung cancer and cholangiocarcinoma | ▪ ROS1 inhibitors |
| *NOTCH1* and *NOTCH2* | Notch | Rearrangement or mutation | Leukemia and breast cancer | ▪ Notch signalling pathway inhibitors |

*PIK3CA*, PI3K catalytic subunit-α; *PIK3R1*, PI3K regulatory subunit 1; *PI3K*, phosphoinositide 3-kinase; *AKT*, v-akt murine thymoma viral oncogene homolog; *PTEN*, phosphatase and tensin homolog; mTOR, mechanistic target of rapamycin; *TSC1*, tuberous sclerosis 1 protein; RAS–MEK, rat sarcoma; *MEK*, MAPK/ERK (mitogen-activated protein kinase/extracellular signal-regulated kinase) kinase; RAF, v-raf murine sarcoma viral oncogene homolog; *ERBB2*, also known as HER2; *SMO*, smoothened homolog; *PTCH1*, patched homolog; *MET*, hepatocyte growth factor receptor; *JAK*, Janus kinase; *THPO*, thrombopoietin; *STAT*, signal transducer and activator of transcription; RTK, receptor tyrosine kinase; *CDKN2A*, cyclin-dependent kinase inhibitor 2A; ABL, Abelson murine leukemia viral oncogene homolog 1; *FLT3*, FMS-like tyrosine kinase 3; *HGF*, hepatocyte growth factor; *MDM2*, mouse double minute 2; *KIT*, v-kit Hardy-Zuckerman 4 feline sarcoma viral oncogene homolog; GIST, gastrointestinal stromal tumor; PDGFR, platelet-derived growth factor receptor; *ROS1*, v-ros avian UR2 sarcoma virus oncogene homolog.
Reprinted by permission from Macmillan Publishers Limited: Nature Reviews Drug Discovery, Simon, R. and Rowchodhury, S. 12:358–369, 2013, ©2013.

staining regions. MYCN amplification is a very strong predictor of poor outcomes, particularly in patients with localized (stage 1 or stage 2) disease or in infants with stage 4S metastatic disease, where fewer than half of patients survive beyond 5 years.[6]

Use of *other chromosome abnormalities* has been largely limited to the diagnosis and prognostication of hematologic disorders. Roughly half of all myelodysplastic disorders show cytogenetically detectable chromosomal abnormalities, such as monosomy 5 or 7, partial chromosomal loss (5q-, 7q-), or complex chromosomal abnormalities. Certain abnormalities in isolation (e.g., 5q-) have a favorable prognosis, whereas many others (e.g., "complex" karyotypes with three or more abnormalities) carry a worse prognosis. Differences in ploidy have proven to be useful predictors in pediatric acute lymphocytic leukemia (ALL), with hyperdiploid cases (>50 chromosomes) showing a distinctly more favorable course compared with hypodiploid or near diploid cases.[7] Overall, DNA ploidy can be assessed by flow cytometry. Specific chromosomal

copy number alterations can be detected by *conventional karyotyping, array hybridization methods*, or *FISH*.

*Copy number variation (CNV)* represents the most common type of structural chromosomal alteration. Regions affected by CNVs range from approximately 1 kilobase to several megabases that are either amplified or deleted. It is estimated that about 0.4% of the genomes of healthy individuals differ in copy number.[8] CNVs resulting in deletion of genes such as *BRCA1, BRCA2, APC*, mismatch repair genes, and *TP53* have been implicated in a wide range of highly penetrant cancers.[9,10] CNVs can be detected by a variety of means including *FISH, comparative or array genomic hybridization*, or *virtual karyotyping* using *single nucleotide polymorphism (SNP) arrays*. Increasingly, CNV is detected using *next-generation sequencing*.

Large-scale sequencing of tumors has identified many *mutations* that are of potential prognostic and therapeutic significance. As will be discussed further, a wide range of strategies is available for the detection of point mutations (Fig. 3.1). It is important to

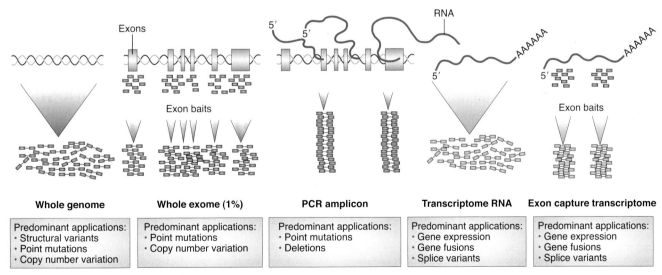

**Figure 3.1** Strategies for the detection of mutations, translocations, and other structural genomic abnormalities in cancer. Whole genome sequencing, which involves determining the entire sequence of both introns and exons, is not only the most comprehensive, but also the most laborious and expensive approach. Exome sequencing uses *baits* to capture either the entire exome (roughly 20,000 genes [about 1% of the genome]) or else a subset of genes of interest. Amplicon-based sequencing uses PCR or other amplification techniques to amplify targets of interest for sequencing. Transcriptome sequencing, also known as RNAseq, is based on sequencing expressed RNA and can be used to detect not only mutations, but also translocations, other structural abnormalities, as well as differences in expression levels. This can be combined methods exome capture techniques for a higher sensitivity analysis of genes of particular interest. (Reprinted by permission from Macmillan Publishers Limited: Nature Reviews Drug Discovery, Simon, R. and Rowchodhury, S. 12:358–369, 2013, ©2013.)

recognize that many nucleotide variations occur at any given allele in populations. Formally, the term *polymorphism* is used to describe genetic differences present in ≥1% of the human population, whereas *mutation* describes less frequent differences. However, in practice, *polymorphism* is often used to describe a nonpathogenic genetic change, and mutation a deleterious change, regardless of their frequencies.

Mutations can be classified according to their effect in the structure of a gene. The most common of these disease-associated alterations are single nucleotide substitutions (point mutations); however, many deletions, insertions, gene rearrangements, gene amplification, and copy number variations have been identified that have clinical significance. Point mutations may affect promoters, splicing sites, or coding regions. Coding region mutations can be classified into three kinds, depending on the impact on the codon: *missense mutation*, a nucleotide change leads to the substitution of an amino acid to another; *nonsense mutation*, a nucleotide substitution causes premature termination of codons with protein truncation; and *silent mutation*, a nucleotide change does not change the coded amino acid.

Loss of function mutations, either through point mutations or deletions in tumor suppression genes such as *APC* and *TP53*, are the most common mutations in cancers. Tumor suppression genes require two-hit (biallelic) mutations that inactivate both copies of the gene in order to allow tumorigenesis to occur. The first hit is usually an inherited or somatic point mutation, and the second hit is assumed to be an acquired deletion mutation that deletes the second copy of the tumor suppression gene. Promoter methylation of tumor suppressor genes is an alternative route to tumorigenesis that, to date, has not been commonly employed for molecular diagnostics.

Oncogenes originate from the deregulation of genes that normally encode for proteins associated with cell growth, differentiation, apoptosis, and signal transduction (proto-oncogenes, [e.g., *BRAF* and *KRAS*]). Proto-oncogenes generally require only one gain of function or activating mutation to become oncogenic. Common mutation types that result in proto-oncogene activation include point mutations, gene amplifications, and chromosomal translocations. One example is mutations in the epidermal growth factor receptor (*EGFR*) that occur in lung cancer, which are almost exclusively seen in nonmucinous bronchoalveolar carcinomas. Somatic mutations of *EGFR* constitutively activate the receptor tyrosine kinase (TK). Importantly, responsiveness of tumors harboring these mutations to the inhibitor gefitinib is highly coordinated with a mutation of the EGFR TK domain.[11,12]

One of the challenges with using mutations as biomarkers is that there can be many nucleotide alterations that affect a given gene. For example, there are over 100 known different point mutations in *EGFR* reported in non–small-cell lung cancer. Many of these mutations occur at low frequency and have an unknown clinical significance.[13,14] Another important concept is that the same driver oncogene may be mutated in a variety of different tumors. For example, lung cancers harbor a number of other different alterations that are common in other solid tumors, which generally occur at lower frequencies than *EGFR* mutations such as *KRAS*, *BRAF*, and *HER2*. Some lung cancers have translocations involving the *ALK* kinase gene. *ALK*, interestingly, is also activated by point mutations in a neuroblastoma as by translocation in anaplastic large cell lymphoma (Fig. 3.2). Hence, a therapy targeted to a genetic alteration in one cancer may demonstrate efficacy in other cancers.

The detection of mutations is also important in the evaluation of chemotherapy resistance. Roughly a third of CML patients are resistant to the frontline ABL1 kinase inhibitor imatinib, either at the time of initial treatment or, more commonly, secondarily. In cases of primary failure or secondary failure, over 100 different *ABL1* mutations have been identified, including particularly common ones such as T315I and P loop mutations. While some

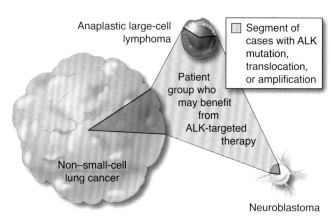

**Figure 3.2** Activating genomic alterations occur in a variety of tumor types. *ALK* translocations, mutations, and amplifications occur in non–small-cell lung cancer, neuroblastomas, and in anaplastic large cell lymphomas. Such recurrent alterations in cancer, together with effective inhibitors of these pathways, are transforming oncologic therapies from organ-specific to pathway-specific interventions and are driving the use of molecular diagnostics in a wider range of tumor types. (Modified from McDermott, U. and Settleman, J. *J Clin Oncol* 2009;27:5650–5659.)

mutations, such as Y253H, respond to second generation TK inhibitors (TKI), others, such as the T315I mutation, are noteworthy because they confer resistance not only to imatinib, but also to nilotinib and dasatinib.

Mutations are also used as important predictive biomarkers (Table 3.1). Two of the most notable examples are the use of the *BRCA1* and *BRCA2* mutation analysis for women with a strong family history of breast cancer. Over 200 mutations (loss of function point mutations, small deletions, or insertions) occur in *BRCA* genes, which are distributed across the genes necessitating full sequencing for their detection. The overall prevalence of these occur in about 0.1% of the general population.[15,16] The lifetime risk of breast cancer for women carrying *BRCA1* mutations is in the range of 47% to 66%, whereas for *BRCA2* mutations, it is in the range of 40% to 57%.[17,18] In addition, the risk of other tumors including ovarian, fallopian, and pancreatic cancer is also increased. Detection of *BRCA1* and *BRCA2* mutations is, therefore, important for cancer prevention and risk reduction.

## THE CLINICAL MOLECULAR DIAGNOSTICS LABORATORY: RULES AND REGULATIONS

Laboratories in the United States that perform molecular diagnostic testing are categorized as high-complexity laboratories under the Clinical Laboratory Improvement Amendments of 1988 (CLIA).[19] The CLIA program sets the minimum administrative and technical standards that must be met in order to ensure quality laboratory testing. Most laboratories in the United States that perform clinical testing in humans are regulated under CLIA. CLIA-certified laboratories must be accredited by professional organizations such as the Joint Commission, the College of American Pathologists, or another agency officially approved by the Centers for Medicare & Medicaid Services (CMS), and must comply with CLIA standards and guidelines for quality assurance. Although the regulation of laboratory services is in the U.S. Food and Drug Administration's (FDA) jurisdiction, the FDA has historically exercised enforcement discretion. Therefore, FDA approval is not currently required for clinical implementation of molecular tests as long as other regulations are met.[20,21]

# SPECIMEN REQUIREMENTS FOR MOLECULAR DIAGNOSTICS

Samples typically received for molecular oncology testing include blood, bone marrow aspirates and biopsies, fluids, organ-specific fresh tissues in saline or tissue culture media such as Roswell Park Memorial Institute (RPMI), FFPE tissues, and cytology cell blocks. Molecular tests can be ordered electronically or through written requisition forms, but never through verbal requests only. All samples submitted for molecular testing need to be appropriately identified. Sample type, quantity, and specimen handling and transport requirements should conform to the laboratory's stated requirements in order to ensure valid test results.

Blood and bone marrow samples should be drawn into anticoagulated tubes. The preferred anticoagulant for most molecular assays is ethylenediaminetetraacetic acid (EDTA; lavender). Other acceptable collection tubes include ACD (yellow) solutions A and B. Heparinized tubes are not preferred for most molecular tests because heparin inhibits the polymerase enzyme utilized in PCR, which may lead to assay failure. Blood and bone marrow samples can be transported at ambient temperature. Blood samples should never be frozen prior to separation of cellular elements because this causes hemolysis, which interferes with DNA amplification. Fluids should be transported on ice. Tissues should be frozen (preferred method) as soon as possible and sent on dry ice to minimize degradation. Fresh tissues in RPMI should be sent on ice or cold packs. Cells should be kept frozen and sent on dry ice; DNA samples can be sent at ambient temperature or on ice.

For FFPE tissue blocks, typical collection and handling procedures include cutting 4 to 6 microtome sections of 10-micron thickness each on uncoated slides, air-drying unstained sections at room temperature, and staining one of the slides with hematoxylin and eosin (H&E). A board-certified pathologist reviews the H&E slides to ensure the tissue block contains a sufficient quantity of neoplastic tumor cells, and circles an area on the H&E slide that will be used as a template to guide macrodissection or microdissection of the adjacent, unstained slides. The pathologist also provides an estimate of the percentage of neoplastic cells in the area that will be tested, which should exceed the established limit of detection (LOD) of the assay.

# MOLECULAR DIAGNOSTICS TESTING PROCESS

The workflow of a molecular test begins with receipt and accessioning of the specimen in the clinical molecular diagnostics laboratory followed by extraction of the nucleic acid (DNA or RNA), test setup, detection of analyte (e.g., PCR products), data analysis, and result reporting to the patient medical record (Fig. 3.3).

An extraction of intact, moderately high-quality DNA is essential for molecular assays. For DNA extraction, the preferred age for blood, bone marrow, and fluid samples is less than 5 days; for frozen or fixed tissue, it is indefinite; and for fresh tissue, it is overnight. Although there is no age limit for the use of a fixed and embedded tissue specimen for analysis, older specimens may yield a lower quantity and quality of DNA. Because RNA is significantly more labile than DNA, the preferred age for blood and bone marrow is less than 48 hours (from time of collection). Tissue samples intended for an RNA analysis should be promptly processed in fresh state, snap frozen, or preserved with RNA stabilizing agents for transport.

Dedicated areas, equipment, and materials are designated for various stages of DNA and RNA extraction procedures. DNA and RNA isolation can be done by manual or automated methods. Currently, most clinical laboratories employ commercial protocols based on liquid- or solid-phase extractions. Nucleated cells are isolated from biological samples prior to nucleic acid extraction.

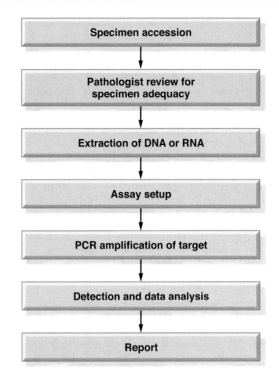

**Figure 3.3** Simplified workflow of clinical molecular diagnostic testing.

White blood cells (WBC) can be isolated from blood and bone marrow samples by different methods. One method involves lysing the red blood cells with an ammonium chloride solution, which yields the total WBC population and other nucleated cells present. Another method involves a gradient preparation with a Ficoll solution, which yields the mononuclear cell population only. Sections of FFPE tissue blocks are prepared for DNA extraction by first removing the paraffin and disrupting the cell membranes with proteinase K digestion. Fresh and frozen tissues also undergo proteinase K digestion prior to nucleic acid extraction. DNA isolation protocols consist of several steps, including cell lysis, DNA purification by salting out the proteins and other debris (nonorganic method), or by solvent extractions of the proteins with phenol and chloroform solutions (organic method). The DNA is then precipitated out of the solution with isopropanol or ethanol. The pellet is washed with 70% to 80% ethanol and then solubilized in buffer, such as Tris-EDTA solution. Proteinase K can be added to assist in the disruption and to prevent nonspecific degradation of the DNA. RNase is sometimes added to eliminate contaminating RNA. The DNA yield is quantitated spectrophotometrically, and the DNA sample integrity is visually checked, if necessary, on an agarose gel followed by ethidium bromide staining. Intact DNA appears as a high–molecular-weight single band, whereas degraded DNA is identified as a smear of variably sized fragments. After extraction, the DNA is stored at 4°C prior to use in a PCR assay, and is then stored at −70°C after completion of the assay. Because the DNA extracted from formalin-fixed tissue is degraded to a variable extent, an analysis of the extraction product by gel electrophoresis is not informative. Yield and integrity of the extracted DNA is best assessed by an amplification control to ensure that the quality and quantity of input DNA is adequate to yield a valid result.

RNA isolation steps are similar to the ones described previously for DNA extraction. However, RNA is inherently less stable than DNA due to its single-strand conformation and susceptibility to degradation by RNase, which is ubiquitous in the environment. To ensure preservation of target RNA, special precautions are required, including the use of diethylpyrocarbonate (DEPC) water in all reagents used in RNA procedures, and special decontamination of work area and pipettes to prevent RNase contamination. The extracted RNA is usually degraded to a variable extent so that the analysis of the extraction product by gel electrophoresis is not informative. The quality of the RNA and its suitability for use in a reverse transcriptase polymerase chain reaction (RT-PCR)–based assay is assessed most appropriately by the demonstration of a positive result in an assay designed to detect the RNA transcripts for a "housekeeping gene," such as *ABL1* or *GAPDH*. Any RNA sample in which the 260/280-nm absorption ratio is below 1.9 or greater than 2.0 may contain contaminants and must be cleaned prior to analysis.

Following nucleic acid extraction, the assay is set up according to written procedures established during validation/verification of the assay by qualified laboratory staff. Dedicated areas, equipment, and materials are designated for various stages of the test (e.g., extraction, pre-PCR and post-PCR for amplification-based assays). For each molecular oncology test, appropriated positive and negative control specimens are included to each run as a matter of routine quality assessment. A no template (blank) control, containing the complete reaction mixture except for nucleic acids, is also included in amplification-based assays to evaluate for amplicon contamination in the assay reagents that may lead to inaccurate results. The controls are processed in the same manner as patient samples to ensure that established performance characteristics are being met for each step of the assay (extraction, amplification, and detection). All assay controls and overall performance of the run must be examined prior to interpretation of sample results. Following acceptance of the controls, results are electronically entered into reports. The final report is reviewed and signed by the laboratory director or a qualified designee who meets the same qualifications as the director, as defined by CLIA (see previous).

## TECHNOLOGIES

Several traditional and emerging techniques are currently available for mutation detection in cancer (Table 3.2). In the era of personalized medicine, molecular oncology assays are rapidly moving from a mutational analysis of single genes toward a multigene panel analysis. As the number of "actionable" mutations such as *ALK, EGFR, BRAF,* and others increase, the use of next-generation sequencing platforms is expected to become much more widespread. Both traditional and emerging testing approaches have advantages and disadvantages that need to be balanced before a test platform is implemented into practice.

An important consideration when adding a new oncology test in the clinical laboratory menu is to define the intended use of the assay (e.g., diagnosis, prognosis, prediction of therapy response). The clinical utility of the assay, appropriate types of specimens, the spectrum of possible mutations that can be found in the genomic region of interest, and available methods for testing should also be determined. The laboratory director and ordering physicians should also discuss the estimated test volume, optimal reporting format, and required turnaround time for the proposed new test.[21–23]

### Polymerase Chain Reaction

Polymerase chain reaction (PCR)[24,25] is widely used in all molecular diagnostics laboratories for the rapid amplification of targeted DNA sequences. The reaction includes the specimen template DNA, forward and reverse primers (18 to 24 oligonucleotides long), Taq DNA polymerase, and each of the four nucleotides bases (dATP, dTTP, dCTP, dGTP). During PCR, selected genomic sequences undergo repetitive temperature cycling (sequential heat and cooling) that allows for *denaturation* of double-stranded DNA template, *annealing* of the primers to the targeted complementary sequences on the template, and *extension* of new strands of DNA by Taq polymerase from nucleotides, using the primers as the starting point. Each cycle doubles the copy number of PCR

templates for the next round of polymerase activity, resulting in an exponential amplification of the selected target sequence. The PCR products (amplicons) are detected by electrophoresis or in real-time systems simultaneously to the amplification reaction (see real-time PCR, which follows).

PCR is specifically designed to work on DNA templates because the Taq polymerase does not recognize RNA as a starting material. Nonetheless, PCR can be adapted to RNA testing by including a reverse transcription step to convert a RNA sequence into its cognate cDNA sequence before the PCR reaction is performed (see reverse-transcription PCR, which follows). Multiplex PCR reactions can also be designed with multiple primers for simultaneous amplification of multiple genomic targets. PCR is a highly sensitive and specific technique that can be employed in different capacities for the detection of point mutations, small deletions, insertions and duplications, as well as gene rearrangements and clonality assessment. Limits of detection can reach 0.1% mutant allele or lower, which is important for the detection of somatic mutations in oncology because tumor specimens are usually composed of a mixture of tumor and normal cells. Reverse transcription PCR can also be used for the relative quantification of target RNA in minimal residual disease testing, such as *BCR-ABL1* transcripts in CML. Another advantage of PCR is its ability to amplify small amounts of low quality FFPE-derived DNA. However, applications of PCR can be limited because it cannot amplify across large or highly repetitive genomic regions. Also, the PCR reaction can be inhibited by heparin or melanin if present in the extracted DNA, which may lead to assay failure. Finally, the risk of false positives due to specimen or amplicon contamination is an important issue when using PCR-based techniques; therefore, stringent laboratory procedures, as described previously, are used to minimize contamination. With the exception of hybridization assays, such as fluorescence in situ hybridization and genomic microarrays, PCR is the necessary initial step in all current molecular oncology assays.

### Targeted Mutation Analysis Methods

#### Real-Time PCR (q-PCR)

In real-time PCR (q-PCR), the polymerase chain reaction is performed with a PCR reporter that is usually a fluorescent double-stranded DNA binding dye or a fluorescent reporter probe. The intensity of the fluorescence produced at each amplification cycle is monitored in real time, and both quantification and detection of targeted sequences is accomplished in the reaction tube as the PCR amplification proceeds.

The intensity of the fluorescent signal for a given DNA fragment (wild type or mutant) is correlated with its quantity, based on the PCR cycle in which the fluorescence rises above the background (crossing threshold [Ct] or crossing point [Cp]).[26] The Ct value can be used for qualitative or quantitative analysis. Qualitative assays use the Ct as a cutoff for determining "presence" or "absence" of a given target in the reaction. A qualitative analysis by q-PCR is particularly useful for a targeted detection of point mutations that are located in mutational hotspots. Examples include the *JAK2* V617F mutation, which is located within exon 14, and is found in several myeloproliferative neoplasms (polycythemia vera, essential thrombocythemia, and primary myelofibrosis),[27] and the *BRAF* V600E,[28] which is located within exon 15, and is found in various cancer types including melanomas and thyroid and lung cancers.

For a quantitative analysis, the Ct of standards with known template concentration is used to generate a standard curve to which Ct values of unknown samples are compared. The concentration of the unknown samples is then extrapolated from values from the standard curve. The quantity of amplicons produced in a PCR reaction is proportional to the prevalence of the targeted sequence;

## TABLE 3.2

**Molecular Methods in Oncology**

| Method | Advantages | Disadvantages | Analytic Sensitivity | Examples of Applications in Oncology |
|---|---|---|---|---|
| Real-time PCR (q-PCR) Allele-specific PCR (AS-PCR) Reverse transcriptase PCR (RT-PCR) | Flexible platforms that permit detection of a variety of conserved hotspot mutations including nucleotide substitutions, small length mutations (deletions, insertions), and translocations High sensitivity is beneficial for residual disease testing and specimens with limited tumor content Adaptable to quantitative assays | Detects only specific targeted mutations/ chromosomal translocations Not suitable for variable mutations May not determine the exact change in nucleotide sequence | Very high | *KRAS, BRAF,* and *EGFR* mutations in solid tumors *JAK2* V617F and *MPL* mutations in myeloproliferative neoplasms *KIT* D816V mutation in systemic mastocytosis and AML Quantitation of *BCR-ABL1* and *PML-RARA* transcripts for residual disease monitoring in CML and APL, respectively |
| Fragment analysis | Detects small to medium insertions and deletions Detects variable insertions and deletions regardless of specific alteration Provides semiquantitative information regarding mutation level | Does not determine the exact change in nucleotide sequence Does not detect single nucleotide substitution mutations Limited multiplex capability | High | *NPM1* insertion mutations in AML *FLT3* internal tandem duplications in AML *JAK2* exon 12 insertions and deletions in PV *EGFR* exon 19 deletions in NSCLC |
| FISH | Detects chromosomal translocation, gene amplification, and deletion Morphology of tumor is preserved, allowing for a more accurate interpretation of heterogeneous samples | High cost Unable to detect small insertions and deletions Limited multiplex capability Does not determine the exact breakpoint and change in nucleotide sequence | High | *IGH/BCL2* translocation detection in follicular lymphoma and in a subset of diffuse large B-cell lymphoma *ALK* translocation in NSCLC *EWSR1* translocation in soft tissue tumors *HER2* amplification in breast cancer 1p/19q deletion in oligodendroglioma |
| High-resolution melting (HRM) curve analysis | Qualitative detection of variable single nucleotide substitutions and small insertions and deletions | Does not determine the exact mutation Result interpretation may require testing via an alternate technology Limited multiplex capability | Medium | *KRAS* and *BRAF* mutations in solid tumors *JAK2* exon 12 mutations in PV |
| Sanger sequencing | Detects variable single nucleotide substitutions and small insertions and deletions Provides semiquantitative information about mutation level Current gold standard for mutation detection | Low throughput Low analytic sensitivity limits application in specimens with low tumor burden Does not detect copy number changes or large (>500 bp) insertions and deletions | Low | *KIT* mutations in GIST and melanoma *CEBPA* mutations in AML *EGFR* mutations in NSCLC |
| Pyrosequencing | Higher analytical sensitivity than Sanger sequencing Detects variable single nucleotide substitutions and small insertions and deletions Provides quantitative information about mutation level | Short read lengths limit analysis to mutational hotspots Low throughput | Medium | *KRAS* and *BRAF* mutations in solid tumors |
| Single nucleotide extension assay (SNaPshot) | Simultaneous detection of targeted nucleotide substitution mutations Multiplex capability | Detects only targeted mutations | High | Small gene panels (3–10) for melanoma, NSCLC, breast cancer, and metastatic colorectal cancer |

*(continued)*

PRINCIPLES OF ONCOLOGY

**Molecular Methods in Oncology** *(continued)*

| Method | Advantages | Disadvantages | Analytic Sensitivity | Examples of Applications in Oncology |
|---|---|---|---|---|
| Next-generation sequencing (NGS) | Quantitative detection of variable single nucleotide substitutions, small insertions and deletions, chromosomal translocations, and gene copy number variations<br>Highly multiplexed<br>High throughput | Requires costly investment in instrumentation and bioinformatics<br>Technology is rapidly evolving<br>Higher error rates for insertion and deletion mutations<br>Limited ability to sequence GC-rich regions | High | Small to large gene panels (3–500) for solid tumor and hematologic malignancies |
| Genomic microarray | Simultaneous detection of copy number variation and LOH (SNP array) | Limited application to FFPE tissue<br>Does not detect balanced translocations<br>May not detect low-level mutant allele burden | Medium | Analysis of recurrent copy number variation and LOH in chronic lymphocytic leukemia and myeloproliferative neoplasms |

AML, acute myelogenous leukemia; CML, chronic myelogenous leukemia; APL, acute promyelocytic leukemia; PV, polycythemia vera; NSCLC, non–small-cell lung carcinoma; GIST, gastrointestinal stromal tumor; GC, guanine-cytosine; LOH, loss of heterozygosity; FFPE, formalin-fixed paraffin-embedded.

therefore, samples with a higher template concentration reaches the Ct at earlier PCR cycles than one with a low concentration of the amplified target. Quantitative q-PCR has high analytical sensitivity for the detection of low mutant allele burden. For that reason, this method has been widely utilized for monitoring minimal residual disease.

## Allele-Specific PCR

Allele-specific PCR (AS-PCR) is a variant of conventional PCR. The method is based on the principle that Taq polymerase is incapable of catalyzing chain elongation in the presence of a mismatch between the 3′ end of the primer and the template DNA. Selective amplification by AS-PCR is achieved by designing a forward primer that matches the mutant sequence at the 3′ end primer. A second mismatch within the primer can be introduced at the adjacent -1 or -2 position to decrease the efficiency of mismatched amplification products. This will minimize the chance of amplifying and, therefore, detecting the wild-type target. AS-PCR is usually performed as two PCR reactions: one employing a forward primer specific for the mutant sequence, the other using a forward primer specific for the correspondent wild-type sequence. In this case, a common reverse primer is used for both reactions. Following amplification, the PCR products are detected by electrophoresis (capillary or agarose gel) or in q-PCR systems. The detection of adequate PCR product in the wild-type amplification reaction is important to control for adequate specimen quality and quantity, particularly when the specimen is negative in the mutation-specific PCR reaction.

AS-PCR is particularly useful for the detection of targeted point mutations. Multiplex AS-PCR reactions can be designed for the simultaneous detection of multiple mutations by including several mutation-specific primers. The method has high analytical sensitivity and specificity and can be easily deployed in most clinical laboratories. However, an important limitation is that this approach will not detect mutations other than those for which specific primers are designed. Therefore, it is utilized for highly recurrent mutations that occur at specific locations within genes, rather than for the detection of variable mutations that may occur throughout a gene.

Examples of AS-PCR applications in oncology include the detection of *JAK2* V617F and *MPL* mutations in myeloprolifera-tive neoplasms (primary myelofibrosis, essential thrombocythemia, and/or polycythemia vera),[29] the *BRAF* V600E mutation,[30] and *KIT* D816V mutations in cases of systemic mastocytosis and in acute myelogenous leukemia (AML).

## Reverse Transcriptase PCR

RT-PCR is utilized for the detection and quantification of RNA transcripts. The first step for all amplification-based assays that use RNA as a starting material is reverse transcription of RNA into cDNA, because RNA is not a suitable substrate for Taq polymerase. In RT-PCR, RNA is isolated and reverse transcribed into cDNA by using a reverse transcriptase enzyme and one of the following: (1) random hexamer primers, which anneal randomly to RNA and reverse transcribe all RNA in the cell; (2) oligo dT primers, which anneal to the polyA tail of mRNA and reverse transcribe only mRNA; or (3) gene-specific primers that reverse transcribe only the target of interest. PCR is subsequently performed on the cDNA with forward and reverse primers specific to the gene(s) of interest. The RT-PCR products may then be analyzed by capillary electrophoresis or in real-time systems as in a standard PCR reaction.

RT-PCR is commonly used for detecting gene fusions during translocation analysis because breakpoints frequently occur within the intron of each partner gene and the precise intronic breakpoint locations may be variable. This variability complicates the design of primers used in DNA-based PCR assays. RT-PCR tests are advantageous because mature mRNA has intronic sequence spliced out, allowing for simplified primer design within the affected exon of each partner gene. In this setting, RT-PCR is useful in tests where both translocation partners are recurrent and only one or a few exons are involved in each partner gene. For instance, 95% of acute promyelocytic leukemia (APL) cases harbor the reciprocal t(15;17) chromosomal translocation and these breakpoints always occur within intron 2 of the *RARA* gene. By contrast, three distinct chromosome 15 breakpoints are involved, all occurring within the *PML* gene: intron 6, exon 6, and intron 3. Because the breakpoints in the two genes are recurrent, most of the reported *PML-RARA* fusions can be detected by targeting these three transcript isoforms.

RT-PCR is the method of choice when high sensitivity is required to detect gene translocations. For example, *PML-RARA*

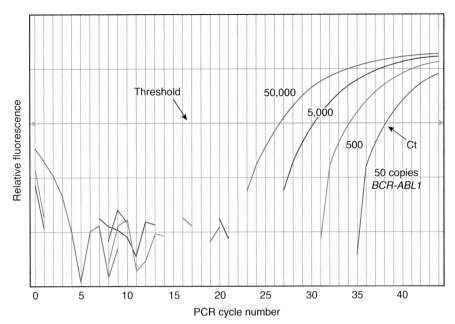

**Figure 3.4** Reverse transcriptase PCR (RT-PCR) is a sensitive means to detect *BCR-ABL1* fusion transcripts in CML. RT-PCR can be combined with real-time PCR (q-PCR) to quantitate *BCR-ABL1* transcripts across four to six log range levels. Amplification products are detected during each PCR cycle using a fluorescent probe specific to the PCR product. The accumulated fluorescence in log(10) value is plotted against the number of PCR cycles. For a given specimen, the PCR cycle number is measured when the increase in fluorescence is exponential and exceeds a threshold. This point is called the Ct, which is inversely proportional to the amount of PCR target in the specimen (i.e., lower Ct values indicate a greater amount of target). Calibration standards of known quantity are used in standard curves to calculate the amount of target in a tested specimen. These are shown in the chart as different colored plots. Note that PCR increases the amount of amplification product by a factor of two with each PCR cycle. Therefore, specimens that produce a Ct value that is one cycle lower are expected to have a twofold higher concentration of target. Specimens that differ in target concentration by a factor of 10 (as shown) are expected to have a Ct value 3.3 cycles apart ($2^{3.3} = 10$).

transcript detection by RT-PCR can detect this fusion transcript down to 1 tumor cell in the background of 100,000 normal cells. Detecting low levels of fusion transcript can reveal relapse after consolidation and guide further treatment.[31] RT-PCR can also be used to quantitate the amount of expression of a gene. One major application of RT-PCR in this setting includes quantitative detection of *BCR-ABL1* fusion transcript for prognostication and minimal residual disease testing in CML (Fig. 3.4). In this setting, a three log decrease in *BCR-ABL1* levels is associated with an improved outcome.[32,33]

## Fragment Analysis

A fragment analysis is a PCR amplicon-sizing technique that is relevant for the detection of small- to medium-length–affecting mutations (deletions, insertions, and duplications). This is typically performed by capillary electrophoresis, which is capable of resolving length mutations from approximately 1 to 500 base pairs in size.

Fragment analysis represents a practical strategy because it enables comprehensive detection of a wide variety of possible length mutations and has high analytic sensitivity. Further, it can provide semiquantitative information regarding the relative amount of mutated alleles. Limitations of this approach include the inability to objectively quantitate mutant allele burdens, the inability to determine the exact change in nucleotide sequence, and the inability to detect non–length-affecting mutations such as substitution mutations.

Examples of fragment analysis applications in oncology include the detection of *NPM1* insertion mutations (Fig. 3.5),[34] *EGFR* exon 19 deletions, *FLT3* internal tandem duplications, and *JAK2* exon 12 mutations.[35]

## High-Resolution Melting Curve Analysis

A high-resolution melting (HRM) curve analysis is a mutation screening method that allows for the detection of DNA sequence variations based on specific sequence-related melting profiles of PCR products.[36] Because the melting property of DNA duplexes is dependent on the biophysical and chemical properties of the nucleotide sequences, mutant and wild-type DNA sequences can be differentiated from one another based on their melting characteristics.

An HRM analysis is preceded by a PCR. The reaction employs a pair of gene-specific forward and reverse primers, template DNA, and a reporter that can either be a double-stranded DNA binding dye or a fluorescent reporter probe. Following the last cycle of the PCR, the amplification products undergo a cooling step that generates homoduplexes (double-stranded molecules with perfect complementarity between alleles) and heteroduplexes (double-stranded molecules with sequence mismatch between alleles) followed by a heating step that denatures (i.e., melts) the double-stranded products. Heteroduplexes (mutant DNA) produce a melting profile different from that of wild-type samples (homoduplexes). In most cases, the reaction is performed in a q-PCR system that allows for an analysis of amplification and

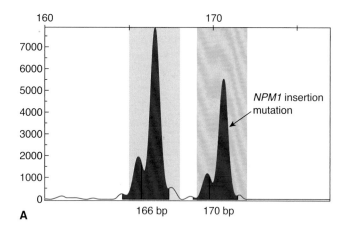

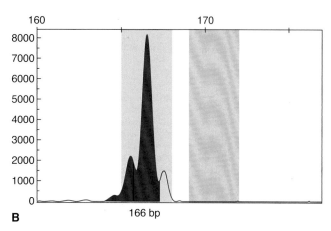

**Figure 3.5** Fragment analysis. *NPM1* mutations are important prognostic markers in acute myeloid leukemia. Virtually all *NPM1* mutations result in a four nucleotide insertion within exon 12. Detection of these mutations can be accomplished by PCR utilizing primers that flank the mutation region. The amplification products are sized using capillary electrophoresis. A mutation is indicated by a PCR fragment that is 4 bp larger than the wild-type fragment. Mutation positive **(A)** and negative **(B)** cases are shown.

melting data in a close-tube format, thereby minimizing the risk of amplicon contamination.

An HRM analysis is useful for the qualitative detection of variable point mutations and small length-affecting mutations that occur within mutational hotspot regions. This method has high analytical sensitivity and can detect mutations even in a small fraction of alleles in a background of wild-type DNA. However, this assay does not characterize the specific sequence alteration in the mutant allele and may be challenging to interpret, especially for cases with mutation levels that approach the detection limit of the assay. Samples with a lower abundance of mutant alleles, and consequently a decreased fraction of heteroduplexes that produced fluorescence decay during the melting analysis, usually produce a melting curve that may not differ significantly from that of wild-type samples. Likewise, the detection of duplication mutations may be hampered by the similarity between the mutant and the duplicated wild-type genome sequences, which may produce only subtle differences in the melting behavior of the DNA duplexes, especially for samples with low mutant allele burden. Therefore, both the mutant sequence and the allelic burden play in the ability of an HRM analysis to detect mutations.[37] Poor quality and impurity of genomic DNA may also lower the sensitivity of an HRM analysis.[38] In instances of patients with a low mutant allelic burden, equivocal mutations identified by this approach may not be confirmable by an alternate method such as Sanger sequencing.

Examples of HRM applications in oncology include a mutational analysis of *KRAS* codons 12, 13, and 61[39]; a mutation screening of *BRAF* codon 600[39]; and the detection of *JAK2* exon 12 mutations (Fig. 3.6).[40]

## Sanger Sequencing

Mutations in single gene assays are commonly analyzed by targeted nucleic acid sequencing, most commonly by Sanger sequencing.[41] This method, also known as dideoxy sequencing, is based on random incorporation of modified nucleotides (dideoxynucleotides [ddNTP]) into a DNA sequence during rounds of template extension that result in termination of the chain reaction at various fragment lengths. Because dideoxynucleotides lack a 3′ hydroxyl group on the DNA pentose ring, which is required for the addition of further nucleotides during extension of the new DNA strand, the chain reaction is terminated at different lengths with the random incorporation of ddNTPs to the sequence. In addition to the dideoxy modification, each ddNTP (ddATP, ddTTP, ddCTP, ddGTP) is labeled with fluorescent tags of different fluorescence wavelengths.

In this method, repetitive cycles of primer extension are performed using denatured PCR products (amplicons) as templates. Unlike PCR, in which both forward and reverse primers are added to the same reaction, in Sanger sequencing, the forward and reverse reactions are performed separately. Bidirectional sequencing is performed to ensure that the entire region of interest

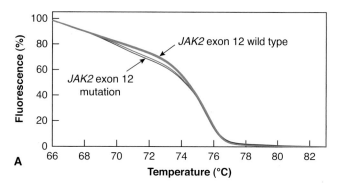

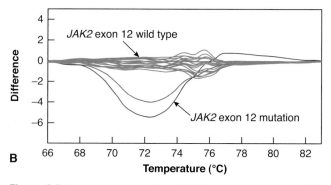

**Figure 3.6** High resolution melting (HRM) curve analysis. An HRM analysis can be an efficient screening method for detecting a variety of mutations that may cluster in one or more hotspot regions, such as occurs with *JAK2* exon 12 mutations in polycythemia vera. PCR is utilized to amplify the target region in the presence of a fluorescent double-stranded DNA-binding dye. Following PCR, the product is gradually melted, and the emitted fluorescence is measured. **(A)** Plotting fluorescence versus temperature generates a melt curve characteristic of each amplicon. The presence of a mutation alters the melt profile due to mismatched double-stranded heteroduplexes of mutant and wild-type fragments. **(B)** A difference plot in which sample curves are subtracted from a wild-type control can accentuate the different melt profiles.

for each analysis is visualized adequately to produce unequivocal sequence readout. The sequencing products of increasing size are resolved by capillary electrophoresis, and the DNA sequence is determined by detection of the fluorescently labeled nucleotide sequences.

Sanger sequencing has the ability to detect a wide variety of nucleotide alterations in the DNA, including point mutations, deletions, insertions, and duplications. This technique is especially useful when mutations are scattered across the entire gene, when genes have not been sufficiently studied to determine mutational hot spots, or when it is relevant to determine the exact change in DNA sequence. Sanger sequencing can also provide semiquantitative information about mutation levels in a sample based on the evaluation of average peak drop values from forward and reverse mutant peaks on sequence chromatograms. Limitations of this approach include low throughput and limited diagnostic sensitivity. In general, heterozygous mutations at allelic levels lower than 20% may be difficult to detect by Sanger sequencing. This may be particularly problematic when testing for somatic mutations in oncogenes, such as *JAK2* exon 12 in polycythemia vera, which may occur at low levels.[35]

Examples of Sanger sequencing applications in oncology include the detection of *KIT* mutations for gastrointestinal stromal tumors (GIST) and melanomas that arise from mucosal membranes and acral skin, *EGFR* mutations for non–small-cell lung cancers, and *KRAS* mutations for colorectal and lung carcinomas (Fig. 3.7).

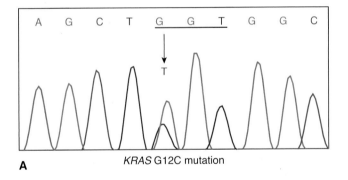

**A**    *KRAS* G12C mutation

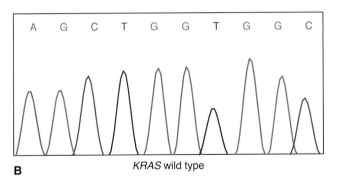

**B**    *KRAS* wild type

**Figure 3.7** Sanger sequencing. *KRAS* mutation testing requires a technology like Sanger sequencing, which can detect the diverse variety of mutations that span multiple nucleotide sites. Overlapping peaks in the DNA sequence chromatogram indicate the presence of a mutation. The top panel **(A)** displays a G to T nucleotide substitution in codon 12. This results in a GGT to TGT codon change, leading to a glycine to cysteine (G12C) amino acid substitution. Activating mutations in *KRAS* such as G12C are associated with resistance to epidermal growth factor receptor (EGFR) targeted therapies in colon cancer. The bottom panel **(B)** displays a wild-type *KRAS* sequence.

## Pyrosequencing

Pyrosequencing, also known as *sequencing by synthesis*, is based on the real-time detection of pyrophosphate release by nucleotide incorporation during DNA synthesis.[42] In the pyrosequencing reaction, as nucleotides are added to the nucleic acid chain by polymerase, pyrophosphate molecules are released and subsequently converted to ATP by ATP sulfurylase. Light is produced by an ATP-driven luciferase reaction via oxidation of a luciferin molecule. The amount of light produced is proportional to the number of incorporated nucleotides in the sequence. When a nucleotide is not incorporated into the reaction, no pyrophosphate is released and the unused nucleotide is degraded by apyrase. Light is converted into peaks in a charge-coupled device (CCD) camera. Individual dNTP nucleotides are sequentially added to the reaction, and the sequence of nucleotides that produce chemiluminescent signals allow the template sequence to be determined. Mutations appear as new peaks in the pyrogram sequence or variations of the expected peak heights.[43]

Pyrosequencing is particularly useful for the detection of point mutations and insertion/deletion mutations that occur at short stretches in mutational hotspots. This method has higher analytical sensitivity than Sanger sequencing and can provide quantitative information about mutation levels in a sample. Pyrosequencing can also be used for the detection and quantification of gene-specific DNA methylation and gene copy number assessments. A microfluidic pyrosequencing platform is available for massive parallel sequencing. However, this method is not well suited for detecting mutations that are scattered across the entire gene because pyrosequencing read lengths are limited to ~100 to 250 base pairs.[43]

Examples of pyrosequencing applications in oncology include the mutational analysis of *BRAF* (codon 600),[44,45] *KRAS* (codons 12, 13, 61),[45] *NRAS* (codon 61),[45] and the methylation analysis of *MGMT* in glioblastoma multiforme.[46,47]

## Single Nucleotide Extension Assay (SNaPshot®)

The single nucleotide extension assay is a variant of dideoxy sequencing. This method consists of a single base extension of an unlabeled primer that anneals one base upstream to the relevant mutation with fluorophore-labeled dideoxynucleotides (ddNTP). Multiplexed reactions can be designed with multiple primers of differing lengths for simultaneous amplification of multiple genomic targets.[48] Mutations are identified based on amplicon size and fluorophore color via capillary electrophoresis. When a mutation is present, an alternative dideoxynucleotide triphosphate is incorporated, resulting in a different colored peak with a different amplicon length than the expected wild-type one.

The single nucleotide extension assay is particularly useful for the simultaneous detection of recurrent point mutations. Clinically, it has been employed for analyses of mutational hotspots in multiple genes involved in melanomas, non–small-cell lung cancers, breast cancers, and metastatic colorectal cancers.[49] The assay has higher analytical sensitivity than Sanger sequencing and can detect low-level mutations in FFPE-derived DNA, making it advantageous for biopsy specimens with limited tumor involvement. This assay, however, can only detect mutations that are immediately adjacent to the 3′ to the end of the primer.

## Fluorescence In Situ Hybridization

FISH allows for the visualization of specific chromosome nucleic acid sequences within a cellular preparation. This method involves the annealing of a large single-stranded fluorophore-labeled oligonucleotide probe to complementary DNA target sequences within a tissue or cell preparation. The hybridization of the probe at the specific DNA region within a nucleus is visible by direct detection using fluorescence microscopy.

FISH can be used for the quantitative assessment of gene amplification or deletion and for the qualitative evaluation of gene rearrangements. Many oncologic FISH assays employ two probe types: *locus specific probes*, which are complementary to the gene of interest, and *centromeric probes*, which hybridize to the alpha-satellite regions near the centromere of a specific chromosome and help in the enumeration of the number of copies of that chromosome.

For the quantitative assessment of gene amplification, a locus-specific probe and a centromeric probe are labeled with two different fluorophores. The signals generated by each of these probes are counted and a ratio of the targeted gene to the chromosome copy number is calculated. The amount of signal produced by the locus-specific probe is proportional to the number of copies of the targeted gene in a cell. This type of gene amplification assay can be used for the detection of *HER2* gene amplification as an adjunct to existing clinical and pathologic information as an aid in the assessment of stage II, node-positive breast cancer patients for whom Herceptin treatment is being considered. It can also be used for an assessment of *MYCN* amplification in neuroblastoma.

For the detection of deletion mutations, dual-probe hybridization is usually performed using locus-specific probes. For instance, for the detection of 1p/19q codeletion in oligodendrogliomas, locus-specific probe sets for 1p36 and 19q13, and 1q25 and 19p13 (control) are used. The frequencies of signal patterns for each of these loci are evaluated. A signal pattern with 1p and 19q signals that are less than control signals is consistent with deletion of these loci.

Gene rearrangements/chromosomal translocations in hematologic or solid malignancies can be tested using locus-specific dual-fusion or break-apart probes. Dual-color, dual-fusion translocation assays employ two probes that are located in two separate genes involved in a specific rearrangement. Each gene probe is labeled in a different color. This design detects translocations by the juxtaposition of both probe signals. Dual-color, dual-fusion translocation assays are very specific for detecting a selected translocation. But, it can only be used for detecting translocations that involve consistent partners, where both partners are known. Alternate translocations with different fusion partners are not detected by this approach. Examples of application of dual-fusion probes in oncology include for the detection of the *IGH-BCL2* translocation that occurs in most follicular lymphomas and a subset of diffuse large B-cell lymphomas (Fig. 3.8) and for the detection of *IGH-CCND1* rearrangements in mantle cell lymphomas.

In break-apart FISH assays, both dual-colored probes flank the breakpoint region in a single gene that represents the constant partner in the translocation. By this approach, rearranged alleles show two split signals, whereas normal alleles show fusion signals. This design is particularly useful for genes that fuse with multiple translocation partners (e.g., *EWSR1* gene, which may undergo rearrangement with multiple partner genes, including *FLI1*, *ERG*, *ETV1*, *FEV*, and *E1AF* in Ewing sarcoma/primitive neuroectodermal tumor [PNET]; *WT1* in desmoplastic small round cell tumors; *CHN* in extraskeletal myxoid chondrosarcoma; and *ATF1* in clear cell sarcoma and angiomatoid fibrous histiocytoma).[50] The disadvantage of this approach is that break-apart FISH does not allow for the identification of the "unknown" partner in the translocation.

FISH has the advantage of being applicable to a variety of specimen types, including FFPE tissue. Because probes are hybridized to tissue in situ, the tumor morphology is preserved, which allows for an interpretation of the assay even in the context of heterogeneous samples. However, FISH is a targeted approach that will only detect specific alterations. Because most probes are large (e.g., >100 kb), small deletions or insertions will not be detected. In addition, poor tissue fixation, fixation artifacts, nuclear truncation on tissue slides, and nuclear overlaps are potential pitfalls of this technique that may hamper interpretation. Some intrachromosomal rearrangements (e.g., *RET-PTC* and *EML4-ALK*) may be challenging to interpret by FISH due to subtle rearrangements of the probe signals on the same chromosome arm.

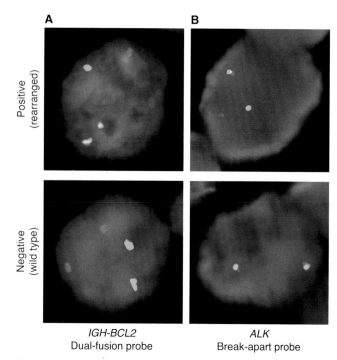

**Figure 3.8** Fluorescence in situ hybridization (FISH). **(A)** Recurrent chromosomal translocations such as *IGH-BCL2* (occurring in B-cell lymphomas) can be effectively detected with a dual-fusion probe strategy. This design utilizes a green probe specific to the *IGH* locus and a red probe specific to the *BCL2* gene, with each probe spanning their respective breakpoint region. Individual green and red probe signals indicate a lack of translocation. Colocalization of green and red probes is observed when an *IGH-BCL2* translocation is present. **(B)** *ALK* rearrangements in non–small-cell lung cancers may involve a variety of translocation partners, including *EML4*, *TFG*, and *KIF5B*. Therefore, a break-apart FISH probe strategy is utilized that will detect any *ALK* rearrangement, regardless of the partner gene. Fluorescently labeled red and green probes are designed on opposite sides of the *ALK* gene breakpoint region. With this design, a normal *ALK* gene is observed as overlapping or adjacent red and green fluorescent signals, whereas a rearranged *ALK* gene is indicated by split red and green signals. *ALK* testing in lung cancer has become widespread in use because of the significant therapeutic implications.

## Methylation Analysis

Changes in the methylation status of cytosine in DNA regions enriched for the sequence CpG (also known as CpG islands) are early events in many cancers and permanent changes found in many tumors. The detection of aberrant methylation of cancer-related genes may aid in the diagnosis, prognosis, and/or determination of the metastatic potential of tumors.

The most common approaches for the detection of methylation are based on the conversion of unmethylated cytosine bases into uracil after sodium bisulfite treatment, which is then converted to thymidine during PCR. By this approach, bisulfite-treated methylated alleles have different DNA sequences as compared with their corresponding unmethylated alleles. The differences between methylated and unmethylated DNA sequences can be evaluated by several methods, including methylation-sensitive restriction enzyme analysis, methylation-specific PCR, semiquantitative q-PCR, Sanger sequencing, pyrosequencing, and next-generation sequencing.

The methylation status of oncogenic genes can also be assessed by methylation-sensitive multiplex ligation-dependent probe amplification (MS-MLPA) assay.[51,52] MS-MLPA is a variant of multiplex PCR in which oligonucleotide probes hybridized to the targeted DNA samples are directly amplified using one pair of universal primers. This method is not based on bisulfite conversion of unmethylated cytosine bases into uracil. Instead, the target sequences detected by MS-MLPA probes contain a restriction site recognized by methylation-sensitive endonucleases. A probe amplification product will only be obtained if the CpG site is methylated because digested probes cannot be amplified during PCR. The level of methylation is determined by resolving PCR products by capillary electrophoresis and calculating the normalized ratio of each target probe peak area in both digested and undigested specimens. The ratio corresponds to the percentage of methylation present in the specimen.

Examples of applications of methylation analysis in oncology include an analysis of *MLH1* promoter hypermethylation in microsatellite unstable sporadic colorectal carcinomas, an analysis of *MGMT* promoter methylation status in glioblastoma multiforme patients treated with alkylating chemotherapy, and *SEPT9* promoter methylation in DNA derived from blood plasma in colorectal cancer patients.[53]

## Microsatellite Instability Analysis

Microsatellites are short, tandem-repeated DNA sequences with repeating units of one to six base pairs in length. Microsatellites are distributed throughout the human genome, and individual repeat loci often vary in length from one individual to another. Microsatellite instability (MSI) is the change in length of a microsatellite allele due to either insertion or deletion of repeating units and a failure of the DNA mismatch repair (MMR) system to repair these replication errors. This genomic instability arises in a variety of human neoplasms where tumor cells have a decreased ability to faithfully replicate DNA. MSI is particularly associated with colorectal cancer, where 15% to 20% of sporadic tumors show MSI, in contrast to the more common chromosomal instability (CIN) phenotype, with MSI status being an independent prognostic indicator. MSI analysis is also clinically useful in identifying patients at increased risk of hereditary nonpolyposis colorectal cancer (HNPCC)/Lynch syndrome, where a germline mutation of an MMR gene causes a familial predisposition to colorectal cancer. MSI analysis alone is not sufficient to make a diagnosis of a germline MMR mutation given the high rate of sporadic MSI-positive colorectal tumors, but a positive result is an indication for follow-up genetic testing and counseling.

In an MSI analysis, DNA is extracted from tumor tissue and the corresponding adjacent normal mucosa. The DNA is subjected to multiplex PCR using fluorescent-labeled primers for coamplification of five mononucleotide repeat markers for MSI determination and two pentanucleotide markers for confirming tumor/normal sample identity. The resulting PCR fragments are separated and detected using capillary electrophoresis. Allelic profiles of normal versus tumor tissues are compared, and MSI is scored as the presence of novel microsatellite lengths in tumor DNA compared to normal DNA. Instability in two or more out of five mononucleotide microsatellite markers in tumor DNA compared to normal DNA is defined as MSI-H (high). MSI-L (low) is defined as instability in one out of five mononucleotide markers in tumor DNA compared to normal DNA. Tumors with no instability (zero out of five altered mononucleotide markers) are defined as microsatellite stable (MSS).[54,55]

## Loss of Heterozygosity Analysis

Loss of heterozygosity (LOH) is a common event in cancer that usually occurs due to deletion of a chromosome segment and results in a loss of one copy of an allele. LOH is a common occurrence in tumor suppressor genes and may contribute to tumorigenesis when the second allele is subsequently inactivated by a second "hit" due to mutation or deletion.

LOH studies are used to identify genomic imbalance in tumors, indicating possible sites of tumor suppressor gene (TSG) deletion. LOH studies can be done by multiplex PCR analysis of microsatellites (short tandem repeats [STRs]), FISH, and genomic

microarrays). By PCR, microsatellites located in the vicinity of a tumor suppressor gene are used as surrogate markers for the presence of the gene of interest. DNA is extracted from tumor tissue and corresponding adjacent normal mucosa. The DNA is subjected to multiplex PCR using fluorescent-labeled STR primers. Peak height ratio of informative (nonhomozygous) alleles at each locus is calculated from both normal and tumor tissues. LOH is defined as the decrease in peak height of one of the two alleles, relative to the allele peak heights of the normal sample.

An example of applications of LOH studies in oncology include an analysis of 1p/19q loss in oligodendrogliomas, and an analysis of 1p loss in parathyroid carcinomas.

# Whole Genome Analysis Methods

## Next-Generation Sequencing

Next-generation sequencing (NGS), also known as massive parallel sequencing or deep sequencing, is an emerging technology that has revolutionized the speed, throughput, and cost of sequencing and has facilitated the discovery of clinically relevant genetic biomarkers for diagnosis, prognosis, and personalized therapeutics. By way of this technology, multiple genes or the entire exome or genome can be interrogated simultaneously in multiple parallel reactions instead of a single-gene basis as in Sanger sequencing or pyrosequencing. Currently, the most common NGS approach for cancer testing in the clinical setting employs targeted sequencing of specific genes and mutation hotspot regions. This targeted approach increases sensitivity for the detection of low-level mutations by increasing the depth of sequence coverage.

Presently, there are numerous NGS platforms that employ different sequencing technologies. A comprehensive review and comparison of NGS platforms is beyond the scope of this chapter and has been reviewed elsewhere.[56,57] A generalized clinical workflow is shown (Fig. 3.9). Frequently, multiple DNA samples are individually barcoded and pooled together to leverage platform throughput. Pooled libraries are prepared and enriched, and single DNA molecules are arrayed in solid surfaces, glass slides, or beads and sequenced in situ using reversible DNA chain terminators or iterative cycles of oligonucleotide ligation. NGS signal outputs are based on luminescence, fluorescence, or changes in ion concentration. Robust bioinformatics pipelines are required for an alignment of reads to a reference genome sequence, variant calling, variant annotation, and to assist with result reporting.[58]

NGS can be used for the detection of single nucleotide variants, small insertions and deletions, translocations, inversions, alternative splicing, and copy number variations given sufficient depth of genomic DNA sequence (Fig. 3.10). Technical limitations of this technique include difficulty in sequencing guanine-cytosine (GC)–rich genomic regions, and erroneous sequencing of homologous DNA regions (e.g., pseudogenes) that may confound interpretation.

Examples of applications of NGS in oncology include small targeted panels (3 to 50 genes) for non–small-cell lung cancers, melanomas, colon cancers, and acute myeloid leukemias.[57,59–62] Larger panels (50 to 500 genes) are increasingly being utilized, particularly in both clinical trials and research.

Massively parallel sequencing of RNA (RNA-Seq) can be used for determining sequence variants, alternative splicing, gene rearrangements, and allelic expression of mutant transcripts. To date, this technique has been used primarily for discovery rather than clinical applications, but it is likely to play an increasing role in clinical diagnostics as the technology improves. For transcriptome sequencing, the RNA must first be converted to cDNA, which is then fragmented and entered into library construction. After sequencing, reads are aligned to a reference genome, compared with known transcript sequences, or assembled de novo

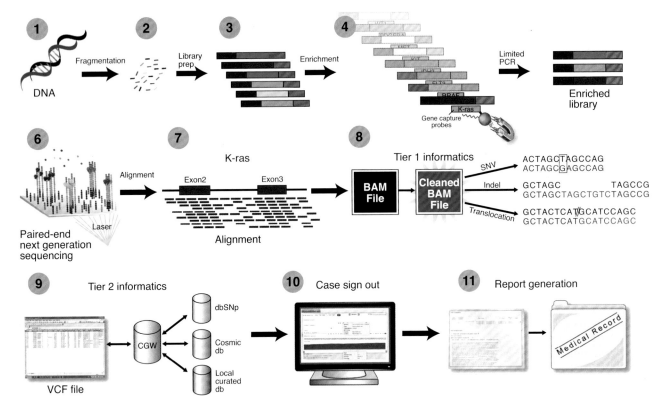

**Figure 3.9** Next-generation sequencing (NGS) workflow in a clinical laboratory. Targeted-panel sequencing offers tremendous promise for cancer diagnostics due to the massive improvement in throughput, speed, and cost. NGS is a complex, multiday process that requires significant infrastructure and expertise to deploy in a clinical setting. The process begins with genomic DNA extraction, which is fragmented and to which linkers are ligated. In this targeted gene panel–based example, the sequencing libraries are enriched for the target genes, which are subjected to a limited PCR prior to sequencing. Sequence reads are mapped to a reference genome and subjected to several bioinformatics tools to provide variant calling results and variant annotation. Clinical interpretation and case sign out is performed by a physician with expertise in molecular pathology. BAM, Binary Sequence Alignment/Map; SNV, Single Nucleotide Variant; VCF, Variant Call Format; CGW, Clinical Genomicist Workstation; dbSNP, The Single Nucleotide Polymorphism Database. (Used with permission from Shashikant Kulkarni PhD and Eric Duncavage MD.)

to construct a genome-scale transcription map. Expression levels are determined from the total number of sequence reads that map to the exons of a particular gene, normalized by the length of exons that can be uniquely mapped.[56] Compared with genomic microarrays, RNA-Seq has a greater ability to distinguish RNA isoforms, determine allelic expression, and reveal sequence variants.

Chromatin immunoprecipitation with sequencing (ChIP-Seq) can be used to determine the genome-wide location of chromatin-binding transcription factors or specific epigenetic modifications of histones. This has proved to be a very powerful research tool, which to date has not been used for clinical diagnostics. Proteins in contact with genomic DNA are chemically cross-linked (usually with formaldehyde treatment) to their binding sites, the DNA is fragmented, and the proteins cross-linked with DNA are then immunoprecipitated with antibodies specific for the proteins (or specific epigenetic histone modification) of interest. The DNA harvested from the immunoprecipitate is converted into a library for NGS. The obtained reads are mapped to the reference genome of interest to generate a genome-wide protein binding map.[63,64] ChIP-Seq is rapidly replacing chromatin immunoprecipitation and microarray hybridization (ChIP-on-chip) technology[65] because of its higher sensitivity and resolution.[66]

## Genomic Microarrays

High-density genomic microarrays are widely used for whole genome assessment of copy number changes, LOH, and geno-

typing. In array comparative genomic hybridization (aCGH), cloned genomic probes are arrayed onto glass slides and serves as targets for the competitive hybridization of normal and tumor DNA. In the aCGH reaction, tumor DNA and DNA from a normal control sample are labeled with different fluorophores. These samples are denatured and hybridized together to the arrayed single-strand probes. Digital imaging systems are used to quantify the relative fluorescence intensities of the labeled DNA probes that have hybridized to each target probe. The fluorescence ratio of the tumor and control hybridization signals is determined at different positions along the genome, which provides information on the relative copy number of sequences in the tumor genome as compared to the normal genome.[67] This method is able to detect copy number variation, such as deletions, duplications, and gene amplification, but it cannot detect polymorphic allele changes.

An SNP array has the ability to detect LOH profiles in addition to high-resolution detection of copy number aberrations, such as amplifications and deletions. This method employs thousands of unique fluorescent-labeled nucleotide probe sequences arrayed on a chip to which a fragmented single-stranded specimen DNA binds to their complementary partners. Each SNP site is interrogated by complementary sets of probes containing perfect matches and mismatches to each SNP site. Each probe is associated with one of the two alleles of an SNP (also known as A and B). Relative fluorescence intensity depends on both the amount of target DNA in the sample, as well as the affinity between target and probe. An analysis of the raw fluorescence intensity is done by computational

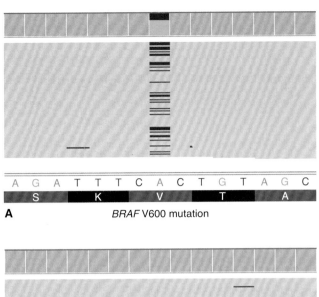

**A** *BRAF* V600 mutation

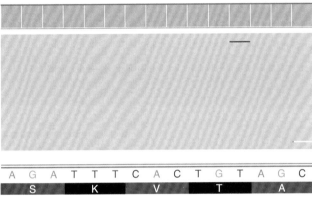

**B** *BRAF* wild type

**Figure 3.10** Next-generation sequencing (NGS). Hundreds to thousands of sequence reads are mapped and horizontally aligned to specific targeted regions in the reference genome (sequence shown on *bottom* of each panel). A software-assisted analysis assists in the detection of mutations, displayed as colored bars in each read above the mutation site. A wild-type sequence within each read is displayed in *gray*. Mutation frequency correlates to the number of times the mutant sequence is detected compared to the total number of reads at that nucleotide position. Shown are sequencing results from *BRAF* V600E mutation positive **(A)** and negative **(B)** melanomas. The A to T base substitution that leads to the V600E mutation is displayed in red. Patients with metastatic melanoma that harbors the *BRAF* V600E mutation are candidates for targeted therapy.

algorithms that convert the set of probe intensities into genotypes. Deleted genomic regions are identified as having an LOH associated with copy number reduction. A copy-neutral LOH is detected when SNPs expected to be heterozygous in the normal sample are detected as homozygous in the tumor sample without copy number variation. A copy neutral LOH may arise from somatic homologous recombination of a mutated tumor suppressor allele and its surrounding DNA that replaces the other allele (uniparental disomy [UPD]). SNP microarrays are the only genomic microarrays that are able to identify UPD. Array technologies cannot detect true balanced chromosome abnormalities and low-level mosaicism.

Examples of genomic microarrays applications in oncology include the detection of copy number variations and LOH in chronic lymphocytic leukemia[68] and recurrent cytogenetic abnormalities in MDS (e.g., 5q-, -7 or 7q-, +8, 20q-).[69]

## Expression Panels

Gene expression signatures of multiple cancer biomarkers are starting to be incorporated into clinical practice as an adjunct to clinical and pathologic information in diverse cancer management settings. An example of a multigene expression–based test in current use includes Oncotype DX, which is a quantitative RT-PCR–based assay that measures the expression of 21 genes in FFPE breast tumors. The test is designed to predict the potential benefit of chemotherapy and the likelihood of distant breast cancer recurrence in women with node negative or node positive, estrogen receptor (ER)-positive, and *HER2*-negative invasive breast cancer. This test has been in-corporated into current American Society of Clinical Oncology (ASCO) and National Comprehensive Cancer Network (NCCN) for breast cancer management.[70] Prospective trials are in progress to evaluate other multigene tests for early stage breast cancer.

With the rapid advances in molecular diagnostic technologies, it is likely that many mutation- and expression-based panels analyzing hundreds if not thousands of genes, or even the complete genome or transcriptome, will enter widespread use. Some of the many challenges to address will be to provide evidence-based, actionable reports that guide the oncologist to more effective therapies, to learn from the results of such testing to improve the algorithms guiding therapy, to handle the incidental findings in such testing in an ethically responsible way, and ultimately, with the drugs available, to provide sufficient improvements in outcomes so that society will be willing to bear the costs.

# REFERENCES

1. Lennard L, Cartwright CS, Wade R, et al. Thiopurine methyltransferase genotype-phenotype discordance and thiopurine active metabolite formation in childhood acute lymphoblastic leukaemia. *Br J Clin Pharmacol* 2013;76(1):125–136.
2. Haber DA, Settleman J. Cancer: drivers and passengers. *Nature* 2007; 446(7132):145–146.
3. Hayashi T, Sudo J. Relieving effect of saline on cephaloridine nephrotoxicity in rats. *Chem Pharm Bull (Tokyo)* 1989;37(3):785–790.
4. Brodeur GM, Seeger RC, Schwab M, et al. Amplification of N-myc in untreated human neuroblastomas correlates with advanced disease stage. *Science* 1984;224(4653):1121–1124.
5. Seeger RC, Brodeur GM, Sather H, et al. Association of multiple copies of the N-myc oncogene with rapid progression of neuroblastomas. *N Engl J Med* 1985;313(18):1111–1116.
6. Weinstein JL, Katzenstein HM, Cohn SL. Advances in the diagnosis and treatment of neuroblastoma. *Oncologist* 2003;8(3):278–292.
7. Pui CH, Crist WM, Look AT. Biology and clinical significance of cytogenetic abnormalities in childhood acute lymphoblastic leukemia. *Blood* 1990;76(8):1449–1463.
8. Lee JA, Lupski JR. Genomic rearrangements and gene copy-number alterations as a cause of nervous system disorders. *Neuron* 2006;52(1):103–121.
9. Kuiper RP, Ligtenberg MJ, Hoogerbrugge N, et al. Germline copy number variation and cancer risk. *Curr Opin Genet Dev* 2010;20(3):282–289.
10. Shlien A, Malkin D. Copy number variations and cancer. *Genome Med* 2009;1(6):62.
11. Lynch TJ, Bell DW, Sordella R, et al. Activating mutations in the epidermal growth factor receptor underlying responsiveness of non–small-cell lung cancer to gefitinib. *N Engl J Med* 2004;350(21):2129–2139.
12. Paez JG, Janne PA, Lee JC, et al. EGFR mutations in lung cancer: correlation with clinical response to gefitinib therapy. *Science* 2004;304(5676): 1497–1500.
13. Forbes SA, Bindal N, Bamford S, et al. COSMIC: mining complete cancer genomes in the Catalogue of Somatic Mutations in Cancer. *Nucleic Acids Res* 2011;39(Database issue):D945–950.
14. Van Allen EM, Wagle N, Levy MA. Clinical analysis and interpretation of cancer genome data. *J Clin Oncol* 2013;31(15):1825–1833.
15. Newman B, Mu H, Butler LM, et al. Frequency of breast cancer attributable to BRCA1 in a population-based series of American women. *JAMA* 1998;279(12):915–921.
16. Ford D, Easton DF, Stratton M, et al. Genetic heterogeneity and penetrance analysis of the BRCA1 and BRCA2 genes in breast cancer families. The Breast Cancer Linkage Consortium. *Am J Hum Genet* 1998;62(3): 676–689.
17. Antoniou A, Pharoah PD, Narod S, et al. Average risks of breast and ovarian cancer associated with BRCA1 or BRCA2 mutations detected in case series unselected for family history: a combined analysis of 22 studies. *Am J Hum Genet* 2003;72(5):1117–1130.
18. Chen S, Iversen ES, Friebel T, et al. Characterization of BRCA1 and BRCA2 mutations in a large United States sample. *J Clin Oncol* 2006;24(6):863–871.

19. Bachner P, Hamlin W. Federal regulation of clinical laboratories and the Clinical Laboratory Improvement Amendments of 1988—Part II. *Clin Lab Med* 1993;13(4):987–994.

20. Halling KC, Schrijver I, Persons DL. Test verification and validation for molecular diagnostic assays. *Arch Pathol Lab Med* 2012;136(1):11–13.

21. Jennings L, Van Deerlin VM, Gulley ML, College of American Pathologists Molecular Pathology Resource C. Recommended principles and practices for validating clinical molecular pathology tests. *Arch Pathol Lab Med* 2009;133(5):743–755.

22. Jennings LJ, Smith FA, Halling KC, et al. Design and analytic validation of BCR-ABL1 quantitative reverse transcription polymerase chain reaction assay for monitoring minimal residual disease. *Arch Pathol Lab Med* 2012;136(1): 33–40.

23. Pont-Kingdon G, Gedge F, Wooderchak-Donahue W, et al. Design and analytical validation of clinical DNA sequencing assays. *Arch Pathol Lab Med* 2012;136(1):41–46.

24. Saiki RK, Gelfand DH, Stoffel S, et al. Primer-directed enzymatic amplification of DNA with a thermostable DNA polymerase. *Science* 1988;239(4839): 487–491.

25. Mullis KB. The unusual origin of the polymerase chain reaction. *Sci Am* 1990;262(4):56–61, 64–65.

26. Bernard PS, Wittwer CT. Real-time PCR technology for cancer diagnostics. *Clin Chem* 2002;48(8):1178–1185.

27. Bench AJ, Baxter EJ, Green AR. Methods for detecting mutations in the human JAK2 gene. *Methods Mol Biol* 2013;967:115–131.

28. Halait H, Demartin K, Shah S, et al. Analytical performance of a real-time PCR-based assay for V600 mutations in the BRAF gene, used as the companion diagnostic test for the novel BRAF inhibitor vemurafenib in metastatic melanoma. *Diagn Mol Pathol* 2012;21(1):1–8.

29. Furtado LV, Weigelin HC, Elenitoba-Johnson KS, et al. Detection of MPL mutations by a novel allele-specific PCR-based strategy. *J Mol Diagn* 2013;15(6):810–818.

30. Lang AH, Drexel H, Geller-Rhomberg S, et al. Optimized allele-specific real-time PCR assays for the detection of common mutations in KRAS and BRAF. *J Mol Diagn* 2011;13(1):23–28.

31. Wang ZY, Chen Z. Acute promyelocytic leukemia: from highly fatal to highly curable. *Blood* 2008;111(5):2505–2515.

32. O'Brien SG, Guilhot F, Larson RA, et al. Imatinib compared with interferon and low-dose cytarabine for newly diagnosed chronic-phase chronic myeloid leukemia. *N Engl J Med* 2003;348(11):994–1004.

33. Hughes TP, Kaeda J, Branford S, et al. Frequency of major molecular responses to imatinib or interferon alfa plus cytarabine in newly diagnosed chronic myeloid leukemia. *N Engl J Med* 2003;349(15):1423–1432.

34. Szankasi P, Jama M, Bahler DW. A new DNA-based test for detection of nucleophosmin exon 12 mutations by capillary electrophoresis. *J Mol Diagn* 2008;10(3):236–241.

35. Furtado LV, Weigelin HC, Elenitoba-Johnson KS, et al. A multiplexed fragment analysis-based assay for detection of JAK2 exon 12 mutations. *J Mol Diagn* 2013;15(5):592–599.

36. Reed GH, Kent JO, Wittwer CT. High-resolution DNA melting analysis for simple and efficient molecular diagnostics. *Pharmacogenomics* 2007;8(6): 597–608.

37. Palais RA, Liew MA, Wittwer CT. Quantitative heteroduplex analysis for single nucleotide polymorphism genotyping. *Anal Biochem* 2005;346(1):167–175.

38. Carillo S, Henry L, Lippert E, et al. Nested high-resolution melting curve analysis a highly sensitive, reliable, and simple method for detection of JAK2 exon 12 mutations—clinical relevance in the monitoring of polycythemia. *J Mol Diagn* 2011;13(3):263–270.

39. Ney JT, Froehner S, Roesler A, et al. High-resolution melting analysis as a sensitive prescreening diagnostic tool to detect KRAS, BRAF, PIK3CA, and AKT1 mutations in formalin-fixed, paraffin-embedded tissues. *Arch Pathol Lab Med* 2012;136(9):983–992.

40. Jones AV, Cross NC, White HE, et al. Rapid identification of JAK2 exon 12 mutations using high resolution melting analysis. *Haematologica* Oct 2008;93(10):1560–1564.

41. Sanger F, Nicklen S, Coulson AR. DNA sequencing with chain-terminating inhibitors. *Proc Natl Acad Sci U S A* 1977;74(12):5463–5467.

42. Ronaghi M, Uhlén M, Nyrén P. A sequencing method based on real-time pyrophosphate. *Science* 1998;281(5375):363, 365.

43. Ronaghi M, Shokralla S, Gharizadeh B. Pyrosequencing for discovery and analysis of DNA sequence variations. *Pharmacogenomics* 2007;8(10): 1437–1441.

44. Shigaki H, Baba Y, Watanabe M, et al. KRAS and BRAF mutations in 203 esophageal squamous cell carcinomas: pyrosequencing technology and literature review. *Ann Surg Oncol* 2013;20:485–491.

45. Vaughn CP, Zobell SD, Furtado LV, et al. Frequency of KRAS, BRAF, and NRAS mutations in colorectal cancer. *Genes Chromosomes Cancer* 2011;50(5):307–312.

46. Everhard S, Tost J, El Abdalaoui H, et al. Identification of regions correlating MGMT promoter methylation and gene expression in glioblastomas. *Neuro Oncol* 2009;11(4):348–356.

47. Mikeska T, Bock C, El-Maarri O, et al. Optimization of quantitative MGMT promoter methylation analysis using pyrosequencing and combined bisulfite restriction analysis. *J Mol Diagn* 2007;9(3):368–381.

48. Dias-Santagata D, Akhavanfard S, David SS, et al. Rapid targeted mutational analysis of human tumours: a clinical platform to guide personalized cancer medicine. *EMBO Mol Med* 2010;2(5):146–158.

49. Su Z, Dias-Santagata D, Duke M, et al. A platform for rapid detection of multiple oncogenic mutations with relevance to targeted therapy in non–small-cell lung cancer. *J Mol Diagn* 2011;13(1):74–84.

50. Lazar A, Abruzzo LV, Pollock RE, et al. Molecular diagnosis of sarcomas: chromosomal translocations in sarcomas. *Arch Pathol Lab Med* 2006;130(8): 1199–1207.

51. Nygren AO, Ameziane N, Duarte HM, et al. Methylation-specific MLPA (MS-MLPA): simultaneous detection of CpG methylation and copy number changes of up to 40 sequences. *Nucleic Acids Res* 2005;33(14):e128.

52. Hömig-Hölzel C, Savola S. Multiplex ligation-dependent probe amplification (MLPA) in tumor diagnostics and prognostics. *Diagn Mol Pathol* 2012;21(4):189–206.

53. Warren JD, Xiong W, Bunker AM, et al. Septin 9 methylated DNA is a sensitive and specific blood test for colorectal cancer. *BMC Med* 2011;9:133.

54. Boland CR, Thibodeau SN, Hamilton SR, et al. A National Cancer Institute Workshop on Microsatellite Instability for cancer detection and familial predisposition: development of international criteria for the determination of microsatellite instability in colorectal cancer. *Cancer Res* 1998;58(22): 5248–5257.

55. Umar A, Boland CR, Terdiman JP, et al. Revised Bethesda Guidelines for hereditary nonpolyposis colorectal cancer (Lynch syndrome) and microsatellite instability. *J Natl Cancer Inst* 2004;96(4):261–268.

56. Voelkerding KV, Dames SA, Durtschi JD. Next-generation sequencing: from basic research to diagnostics. *Clin Chem* 2009;55(4):641–658.

57. Cronin M, Ross JS. Comprehensive next-generation cancer genome sequencing in the era of targeted therapy and personalized oncology. *Biomarker Med* 2011;5(3):293–305.

58. Coonrod EM, Durtschi JD, Margraf RL, et al. Developing genome and exome sequencing for candidate gene identification in inherited disorders: an integrated technical and bioinformatics approach. *Arch Pathol Lab Med* 2013;137(3):415–433.

59. Grossmann V, Kohlmann A, Klein HU, et al. Targeted next-generation sequencing detects point mutations, insertions, deletions and balanced chromosomal rearrangements as well as identifies novel leukemia-specific fusion genes in a single procedure. *Leukemia* 2011;25(4):671–680.

60. Marchetti A, Del Grammastro M, Filice G, et al. Complex mutations & subpopulations of deletions at exon 19 of EGFR in NSCLC revealed by next generation sequencing: potential clinical implications. *PloS One* 2012;7(7):e42164.

61. McCourt CM, McArt DG, Mills K, et al. Validation of next generation sequencing technologies in comparison to current diagnostic gold standards for BRAF, EGFR and KRAS mutational analysis. *PloS One* 2013;8(7):e69604.

62. Thol F, Kölking B, Damm F, et al. Next-generation sequencing for minimal residual disease monitoring in acute myeloid leukemia patients with FLT3-ITD or NPM1 mutations. *Genes Chromosomes Cancer* 2012;51(7):689–695.

63. Barski A, Cuddapah S, Cui K, et al. High-resolution profiling of histone methylations in the human genome. *Cell* 2007;129(4):823–837.

64. Schones DE, Zhao K. Genome-wide approaches to studying chromatin modifications. *Nat Rev Genet* 2008;9(3):179–191.

65. Ren B, Robert F, Wyrick JJ, et al. Genome-wide location and function of DNA binding proteins. *Science* 2000;290(5500):2306–2309.

66. Robertson G, Hirst M, Bainbridge M, et al. Genome-wide profiles of STAT1 DNA association using chromatin immunoprecipitation and massively parallel sequencing. *Nat Methods* 2007;4(8):651–657.

67. Shinawi M, Cheung SW. The array CGH and its clinical applications. *Drug Discov Today* 2008;13(17–18):760–770.

68. Iacobucci I, Lonetti A, Papayannidis C, Martinelli G. Use of single nucleotide polymorphism array technology to improve the identification of chromosomal lesions in leukemia. *Curr Cancer Drug Targets* 2013;13(7):791–810.

69. Ahmad A, Iqbal MA. Significance of genome-wide analysis of copy number alterations and UPD in myelodysplastic syndromes using combined CGH - SNP arrays. *Curr Med Chem* 2012;19(22):3739–3747.

70. Goncalves R, Bose R. Using multigene tests to select treatment for early-stage breast cancer. *J Natl Compr Canc Netw* 2013;11(2):174–182.

## PART II

# Etiology and Epidemiology of Cancer

# Section 1  Etiology of Cancer

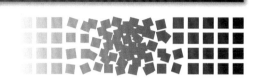

# 4  Tobacco

Richard J. O'Connor

## INTRODUCTION

Regrettably, tobacco use remains one of the leading causes of death worldwide. It is projected to leave over 1 billion dead in the 21st century, after killing nearly 100 million during the course of the 20th century.[1] Data from the Global Adult Tobacco Survey (GATS), which conducted representative household surveys in 14 low- and middle-income countries (Bangladesh, Brazil, China, Egypt, India, Mexico, Philippines, Poland, Russia, Thailand, Turkey, Ukraine, Uruguay, and Vietnam), suggest 41% of men and 5% of women across these countries currently smoke.[2] Compare this to approximately 24% of men and 16% of women in the United States.[3] A preponderance of the death and disease associated with tobacco use is associated with its combusted forms, particularly the cigarette. However, all forms of tobacco use have negative health consequences, the severity of which can vary among products. From the introduction of the mass-manufactured, mass-marketed cigarette (e.g., Camel in 1913), smoking rates grew, first among men then among women, and peaked in Western countries in the 1960s to 1970s, before beginning a steady decline.[4] The smoking rate among US adults has dropped from its peak in 1965 of 42% to 19% in 2011.[3] Per capita consumption has been dropping almost continuously since the 1960s, although the rate of decline has slowed since the early 2000s.[5] Among youth, smoking rates have been in decline since the 1990s,[6,7] although there is some evidence of growth in use of other forms of tobacco (e.g., cigars, water pipes, electronic cigarettes) in 2011 to 2012 that may be displacing cigarette use.[8]

Tobacco control policy interventions can impact both smoking prevalence and lung cancer incidence.[9] For example, a recent analysis suggests that implementation of graphic health warnings in Canada in 1999 resulted in a significant reduction (up to 4.5 percentage points) in smoking prevalence over a decade.[10] Increases in tobacco taxes have long been shown to reduce youth smoking initiation and to prompt more attempts to quit smoking.[11] Evidence from state comparisons in the United States suggests that comprehensive tobacco control measures effectively implemented (such as in California and Massachusetts) can reduce lung cancer incidence.[12] Indeed, Holford and colleagues[13] have shown that since the seminal 1964 Report of the Surgeon General, an estimated 157 million years of life (approximately 20 years per person) have been saved by tobacco control activities in the United States over 50 years. That is, tobacco control activities are estimated to have averted 8 million premature deaths and extended mean life span by 19 to 20 years.[13] However, the marketing of cigarettes has since shifted focus to the developing world, where smoking rates are on the increase. In an attempt to head off an epidemic of smoking and associated diseases, the World Health Organization initiated a public health treaty, the Framework Convention on Tobacco Control (FCTC), to coordinate international efforts to reduce tobacco use.[14] The FCTC binds parties to enact measures to control the labeling and marketing of tobacco products,

create a framework for testing and regulating product contents and emissions, combat smuggling and counterfeiting, and protect nonsmokers from secondhand smoke.[15] To date, the FCTC has been ratified by more than 150 countries. The FCTC provides governments the opportunity to regulate the marketing, labeling, and contents/emissions of tobacco products, as well as control the global trade in tobacco products. In the United States, which is currently not a party to FCTC, the U.S. Food and Drug Administration (FDA) has, since 2009, had authority to regulate tobacco products and their marketing along similar lines.[16]

## EPIDEMIOLOGY OF TOBACCO AND CANCER

Linkages between tobacco use and cancers at various sites had been noted for several decades. In the late 1800s, it was believed that excessive cigar use created irritation that led to oral cancers.[17] In the 1930s, German scientists began to establish links between cigarette smoking and lung cancers.[18] However, it was not until the Doll and Hill[19] and Wynder and Graham[20] studies were published that the association was demonstrated in large samples and well-designed studies. Table 4.1 lists the cancers currently recognized by the U.S. Surgeon General as caused by smoking, along with their corresponding estimated mortality statistics.[21–23] Of these, the most well-publicized link is between smoking and lung cancer. In a recent examination of National Health and Nutrition Examination Survey (NHANES) data, Jha[24] showed a hazard ratio for lung cancer in smokers versus nonsmokers of 17.8 in women and 14.6 in men. However, smoking contributes substantially to overall cancer burden across multiple sites, including the oropharynx, cervix, and pancreas. Hazard ratios of 1.7 for women and 2.2 for men are seen for cancers other than in the lung in smokers versus nonsmokers.[24] Emerging evidence also links smoking with breast cancer, although the data are as yet insufficient to make causal conclusions.[23,25] Cancer risks associated with smoking, as well as outcomes and survival, depend on a number of factors. A common index of cancer risk is pack-years, or the number of packs of cigarettes smoked per day multiplied by the number of years smoked in the lifetime. In general, the higher the number of pack-years, the greater the cancer risk. Risks for lung cancer decline with smoking cessation, and the longer a former smoker remains off of cigarettes, the more the risk declines.[26] However, excepting those smokers who quit with relatively few pack years accumulated (typically before age 40), cancer risk rarely approaches that of a never smoker.[24,27]

A recent study using several large cohort studies examined death rates and the relative risks associated with smoking and smoking cessation for 3 epochs (1959 to 1965, 1982 to 1988, and 2000 to 2010).[27] Of most interest here is death from lung cancer. For men, the age-adjusted death rate from lung cancer increased from 1959 through 1965 to 1982 through1988, but then fell for 2000

## TABLE 4.1

**Level of Evidence for Smoking-Attributable Cancers According to the United States Office of the Surgeon General by Cancer Site and Yearly Smoking-Attributable Mortality at Sites with Available Estimates, United States, 2004**

| | Cancer Site | Yearly Smoking-Attributable Mortality |
|---|---|---|
| **Evidence Sufficient to Infer Causal Relationship** | Bladder | 4,983 |
| | Cervix | 447 |
| | Colon and rectum | N/A |
| | Esophagus | 8,592 |
| | Kidney | 3,043 |
| | Larynx | 3,009 |
| | Leukemia (AML) | 1,192 |
| | Liver | N/A |
| | Lung | 125,522 |
| | Oral cavity and pharynx | 4,893 |
| | Pancreas | 6,683 |
| | Stomach | 2,484 |
| **Evidence Suggestive but Not Sufficient to Infer Causal Relationship** | Breast | |
| **Inadequate to Infer Presence or Absence of Causal Relationship** | Ovary | |
| **Evidence Sufficient to Infer No Causal Relationship** | Prostate | |

N/A, not available; AML, acute myeloid leukemia.

through 2010; for women, the age-adjusted death rate continued to rise over time, with the biggest increase between 1982 through 1988 to 2000 through 2010.[27] In relative risk terms, the likelihood of dying from lung cancer given current smoking has increased from 2.73 to 12.65 to 25.66 among women, and 12.22 to 23.81 to 24.97 for men. Equivalent risks for former smokers increased from 1.3 to 3.85 to 6.7 among women, versus 3.48 to 7.41 to 6.75 for men. These and other analyses suggest that the cancer risks from smoking may have increased with time.[27,28] The histologic subtypes of lung cancer seen in the US population have also shifted with time. Into the early 1980s, squamous cell carcinoma (SCC) were the most common manifestations of lung cancer. However, a rapid rise in adenocarcinomas has been noted, and by the 1990s, had overtaken SCC as the leading type of lung cancer.[23]

## Tobacco Use Behaviors

The level of tobacco exposure is ultimately driven by use behaviors, including the number of cigarettes smoked, the patterns of smoking on individual cigarettes, and the number of years smoked. The primary driver of smoking behavior is nicotine—the major addictive substance and primary reinforcer of continued smoking.[29–31] Over time, smokers learn an *acceptable* level of nicotine intake that attains the beneficial effects they seek while avoiding negative withdrawal symptoms. Smokers can affect the amount of nicotine (and accompanying toxicants) they draw from a cigarette by altering the number of puffs taken, puff size,

frequency, duration, and velocity (collectively referred to as smoking topography).[32] Smokers tend to consume a relatively stable number of cigarettes per day and to smoke those cigarettes in a relatively consistent manner in order to maintain an acceptable level of nicotine in their system across the day.[33] The number of cigarettes smoked per day and the smoking pattern of an individual may be influenced by the rate of nicotine metabolism.[30] Nicotine is metabolized primarily to cotinine, which is further metabolized to trans-3′-hydroxycotinine (3HC), catalyzed by the liver cytochrome P450 2A6 enzyme.[34] Functional polymorphisms in the genes coding for these enzymes allow for the identification of *fast* metabolizers, who have more rapid nicotine clearance and show greater cigarette intake and more intensive smoking topography profiles relative to *normal* or *slow* metabolizers.[35–37] The ratio of 3HC to cotinine in plasma or saliva can be used as a reliable noninvasive phenotypic marker for CYP2A6 activity.[38,39] CYP2A6 activity is known to vary across racial/ethnic groups, with those of African or Asian descent showing slower metabolism than those of Caucasian descent.[40–42] Clinical trial data clearly show that the metabolite ratio can be used to predict success in quitting, and that the likelihood of quitting decreases as the ratio increases, such that slower metabolizers are more successful at achieving abstinence.[37,41,43] Despite their addiction to nicotine, most smokers in Western countries report that they regret ever starting to smoke and want to quit smoking, and there is evidence for similar regret in developing countries as well.[44–46] However, most smokers are unsuccessful in their attempts to quit smoking; the most effective evidence-based treatments increase the odds of quitting by 3 times, with 12-month cessation rates of approximately 40% relative to placebo.[47]

## Evolution of Tobacco Products

Historically, tar was believed to be the main contributor to smoking-caused disease.[48] It is important to note that *tar* is not a specific substance, but simply the collected particulate matter from cigarette smoke, less water and nicotine (in technical reports, it is often referred to as nicotine-free dry particulate matter). Soon after the first studies were done showing that painting mice with cigarette tar caused cancerous tumors, it was theorized that reducing tar yields of cigarettes might also reduce the disease burden of smoking.[48] Concurrently, cigarette manufacturers were seeking to reassure their customers that their products were safe, that if hazardous compounds were identified they would be removed, and that product modifications could help to reduce risks.[4,49–51] Indeed, in the United States and United Kingdom, average tar levels of cigarettes dropped dramatically from the 1960s through the 1990s, and have since leveled off.[52,53] The European Union took the tar reduction mentality to heart in crafting maximum levels of tar in cigarettes that could be sold in member countries, beginning at 15 mg in 1992, then dropping to 12 mg in 1998, and 10 mg in 2005.[54] Unfortunately, these reductions in tar yields have not translated into changes in disease risks among smokers.[55] Despite initial optimism about these products, both laboratory-based and epidemiologic studies indicate neither an individual, nor a public health benefit from *low-tar* cigarettes as compared to *full-flavor* varieties.[56–58] The health consequences of mistakenly accepting the purported benefits of lower tar and nicotine products have been significant. The increases in adenocarcinoma of the lung observed in the United States over recent decades may reflect changes made to the cigarette, such as filters, filter ventilation, and tobacco-specific nitrosamines (TSNA) in smoke produced by the relatively high amount of burley tobacco used in the typical US cigarette blend.[23,59] Tobacco manufacturers engineered cigarettes be *elastic*; that is, cigarettes allow smokers to adjust their puffing patterns to regulate their intake of nicotine, regardless of how the cigarette might perform under the standard

ETIOLOGY AND EPIDEMIOLOGY OF CANCER

testing conditions that drove the labeling and advertising of the products.[55] Researchers have since come to determine that filter vents are the main design feature the industry relied on in creating elastic products.[54,55,60,61] Vents facilitate taking larger puffs and also contribute to sensory perceptions, because they dilute the smoke with air.[62] So, even with a larger puff, the same mass of toxins can seem less harsh and irritating because it is diluted by a proportionate amount of air, which may in turn underscore smokers' beliefs that they are smoking safer cigarettes.[62–64] Other smoke components (e.g., acetaldehyde, ammonia, minor tobacco alkaloids) and aspects of cigarette engineering (e.g., menthol, flavor additives) may further contribute to the addictiveness of cigarettes.[65]

Since the 1980s, manufacturers have introduced products that make more explicit claims about reduced health risks. Examples of modified cigarettelike products include Premier (RJ Reynolds), Eclipse (RJ Reynolds), Accord/Heatbar (Philip Morris), Omni (Vector Tobacco), and Advance (Brown and Williamson).[66] In the 2000s, as evidence of reduced lung cancer incidence and coincident increases in snus use in Sweden appeared,[67,68] manufacturers began to promote smokeless tobacco products as reduced harm alternatives. Most recently, electronic cigarettes, which vaporize a nicotine solution, have gained increasing popularity and generated concern among public health practitioners, particularly with regard to effects on youth.[8,69,70] In the United States, the FDA has authority to authorize marketing claims about reduced risk, which an Institute of Medicine panel concluded should be based on extensive testing of abuse liability, likely health effects, and effects on the whole population.[71]

## CARCINOGENS IN TOBACCO PRODUCTS AND PROCESSES OF CANCER DEVELOPMENT

Cigarette smoke has been identified as carcinogenic since the 1950s, and efforts have continued to identify specific carcinogens in smoke and smokeless tobacco products. The International Agency for Research on Cancer (IARC) has classified both cigarette smoke and smokeless tobacco as Group 1 carcinogens.[72,73] IARC has also identified 72 measurable carcinogens in cigarette smoke where evidence is sufficient to classify them as Group 1 (carcinogenic to humans), 2A (probably carcinogenic to humans), or 2B (possibly carcinogenic to humans).[72] The IARC list, in addition to data from the U.S. Environmental Protection Agency (EPA), the National Toxicology Program, and the National Institute for Occupational Safety and Health (NIOSH), informed the FDA's development of a list of Harmful and Potentially Harmful Constituents (HPHC) in tobacco and tobacco smoke, which manufacturers will be required to report.[74] Table 4.2 illustrates the carcinogens listed as HPHC alongside their carcinogenicity classifications by IARC or the EPA.

### Compounds of Particular Concern

Research groups have listed components of cigarette smoke theorized to impact health risk, often relying on carcinogenic potency indices and relative concentrations in smoke.[75,76] In these analyses, the N-nitrosamines, benzene, 1,3-butadiene, aromatic amines, and cadmium often rank highly. Polycyclic aromatic hydrocarbons (PAH), many of which are carcinogenic, consist of three or more fused aromatic rings resulting from incomplete combustion of organic (carbonaceous) materials, and are often found in coal tar, soot, broiled foods, and automobile engine exhaust.[77] A compound of particular concern in cigarette smoke historically has been benzo(a)pyrene (BaP), which has substantial carcinogenic activity and is considered carcinogenic to humans by the IARC.[77] In addition to PAH, other hydrocarbons found in significant quantities in cigarette smoke include benzene (a long-established cause

of leukemia), 1,3-butadiene (a potent multiorgan carcinogen), naphthalene, and styrene. Carbonyl compounds, such as formaldehyde and acetaldehyde, are found in copious amounts in cigarette smoke, primarily coming from the combustion of sugars and cellulose.[78] However, there are numerous other noncigarette exposures to these compounds, including endogenous formation during metabolism. Smoke contains a number of aromatic amines, such as known bladder carcinogens 2-aminonaphthalene and 4-aminobiphenyl, heterocyclic amines, and furans. Toxic metals, including beryllium, cadmium, lead, and polonium-210, are also present in cigarette smoke in measurable quantities,[79,80] levels of which may depend in part on the region of the world where the tobacco was grown.[81] Much attention has been focused on the N-nitrosamines, primarily because they are well-established carcinogens.[82–85] Nitrosamines form through reactions of nitrite with amino groups. In tobacco, two compounds of concern are 4-(methylnitrosamino)-1-(3-pyridyl)-1-butanone (NNK), which is derived from nitrosation of nicotine, and $N'$-nitrosonornicotine (NNN), which is derived from nitrosation of nornicotine. Both of these compounds are tobacco specific. NNN and NNK primarily form during the curing process for tobacco, where the leaves are dried through contact with combustion gases from heat (flue) curing or microbial activity in air curing.[78] NNK is known to be a potent lung carcinogen, but also shows tumor induction activity in the nasal cavity, the pancreas, and the liver, whereas NNN has been shown to induce tumors along the respiratory tract and esophagus in various animal models. Because they are produced in the curing process and transfer into smoke, rather than being formed by combustion, it is possible to reduce nitrosamines by changing curing and storage practices.[78,86,87]

Smokeless tobacco products, although they are not burned, nonetheless contain substantial levels of carcinogens, most prominently the N-nitrosamines.[73] Here, product type and composition has an enormous effect on nitrosamine levels. For example, US moist snuff has substantially higher levels than that sold in Sweden (snus), whereas smokeless products available in India are often far higher in nitrosamines.[88] US smokeless products also can contain PAH and carbonyl compounds, likely derived from fire curing the constituent tobacco.[89] Similar to cigarettes, smokeless products would also contain toxic metals.[79,80]

Although tobacco is an exceedingly complex mixture, it is possible to use animal model and epidemiologic evidence to postulate relationships between specific components and known tobacco-induced cancers.[90–92] There is strong evidence from multiple studies to suggest that PAH and N-nitrosamines are involved in lung carcinogenesis. For example, PAH–DNA adducts are observed in lung tissues, and p53 tumor suppressor mutations in lung tumors resemble the damage created by PAH diol epoxide metabolites in vitro.[93–96] NNK appears to preferentially induce lung tumors in the rat, regardless of the route of administration, and DNA–nitrosamine adducts are detectable in lung tissues.[97,98] Most importantly, nitrosamine metabolite levels measured in smokers were prospectively related to the risk of lung cancer in cohort studies, even adjusting for other indices of smoking exposure (e.g., cotinine, pack-years).[98–102] PAH and nitrosamines are also likely to be implicated in cancers along the respiratory tract and the cervix.[103,104] Considerable evidence exist that aromatic amines such as 4-aminobiphenyl and 2-naphthylamine are potent bladder carcinogens, and smokers are known to be at an elevated risk of bladder cancer, so these are presumed to be the primary causative agents.[105–107] Similarly, as benzene is a known cause of leukemia, it is presumed that this is the link to leukemia observed in smokers.

Important to examining the role of various smoke components in cancer is the ability to measure the exposure of smokers to these components. Biomarkers of exposure may also be crucial for examining products for their potential to reduce health risks associated with tobacco use.[71,108,109] Validation of tobacco exposure biomarkers is threefold: method validation, validation with respect to product use, and validation with respect to disease risk.[71]

TABLE 4.2

**Carcinogens in Tobacco and Tobacco Smoke Identified as Harmful and Potentially Harmful by the U.S. Food and Drug Administration, with International Agency for Research on Cancer Carcinogenecity (IARC) Classifications as of 2013**

| Compound | CAS No. | IARC Group | IARC Volume | Year |
|---|---|---|---|---|
| 1,3-Butadiene | 106-99-0 | 1 | 100F | 2012 |
| 2-Aminonaphthalene | 91-59-8 | 1 | 100F | 2012 |
| 4-(Methylnitrosamino)-1-(3-pyridyl)-1-butanone (NNK) | 64091-91-4 | 1 | 100E | 2012 |
| 4-Aminobiphenyl | 92-67-1 | 1 | 100F | 2012 |
| Aflatoxin B1 | 1162-65-8 | 1 | 100F | 2012 |
| Arsenic | 7440-38-2 | 1 | 100C | 2012 |
| Benzene | 71-43-2 | 1 | 100F | 2012 |
| Benzo[a]pyrene | 50-32-8 | 1 | 100F | 2012 |
| Beryllium | 7440-41-7 | 1 | 100C | 2012 |
| Cadmium | 7440-43-9 | 1 | 100C | 2012 |
| Chromium (Hexavalent compounds) | 18540-29-9 | 1 | 100C | 2012 |
| Ethylene oxide | 75-21-8 | 1 | 100F | 2012 |
| Formaldehyde | 50-00-0 | 1 | 100F | 2012 |
| N-Nitrosonornicotine (NNN) | 16543-55-8 | 1 | 100E | 2012 |
| Nickel (compounds) | | 1 | 100C | 2012 |
| o-Toluidine | 95-53-4 | 1 | 100F | 2012 |
| Polonium-210 | 7440-08-6 | 1 | 100D | 2012 |
| Uranium (235, 238 Isotopes) | 7440-61-1 | 1 | 100D | 2012 |
| Vinyl chloride | 75-01-4 | 1 | 100F | 2012 |
| Acrylamide | 79-06-1 | 2A | 60 | 1994 |
| Cyclopenta[c,d]pyrene | 27208-37-3 | 2A | 92 | 2010 |
| Dibenz[a,h]anthracene | 53-70-3 | 2A | 92 | 2010 |
| Dibenzo[a,l]pyrene | 191-30-0 | 2A | 92 | 2010 |
| Ethyl carbamate (urethane) | 51-79-6 | 2A | 96 | 2010 |
| IQ (2-Amino-3-methylimidazo[4,5-f]quinoline) | 76180-96-6 | 2A | 56 | 1993 |
| N-Nitrosodiethylamine | 55-18-5 | 2A | SUP 7 | 1987 |
| N-Nitrosodimethylamine (NDMA) | 62-75-9 | 2A | SUP 7 | 1987 |
| 2-Nitropropane | 79-46-9 | 2B | 71 | 1999 |
| 2,6-Dimethylaniline | 87-62-7 | 2B | 57 | 1993 |
| 5-Methylchrysene | 3697-24-3 | 2B | 92 | 2010 |
| A-α-C (2-Amino-9H-pyrido[2,3-b]indole) | 26148-68-5 | 2B | SUP 7 | 1987 |
| Acetaldehyde | 75-07-0 | 2B | 71 | 1999 |
| Acetamide | 60-35-5 | 2B | 71 | 1999 |
| Acrylonitrile | 107-13-1 | 2B | 71 | 1999 |
| Benz[a]anthracene | 56-55-3 | 2B | 92 | 2010 |
| Benz[j]aceanthrylene | 202-33-5 | 2B | 92 | 2012 |
| Benzo[b]fluoranthene | 205-99-2 | 2B | 92 | 2010 |
| Benzo[b]furan | 271-89-6 | 2B | 63 | 1995 |
| Benzo[c]phenanthrene | 195-19-7 | 2B | 92 | 2010 |
| Benzo[k]fluoranthene | 207-08-9 | 2B | 92 | 2010 |
| Caffeic acid | 331-39-5 | 2B | 56 | 1993 |
| Catechol | 120-80-9 | 2B | 71 | 1999 |
| Chrysene | 218-01-9 | 2B | 92 | 2010 |
| Cobalt | 7440-48-4 | 2B | 52 | 1991 |

*(continued)*

ETIOLOGY AND EPIDEMIOLOGY OF CANCER

TABLE 4.2

**Carcinogens in Tobacco and Tobacco Smoke Identified as Harmful and Potentially Harmful by the U.S. Food and Drug Administration, with International Agency for Research on Cancer Carcinogenecity (IARC) Classifications as of 2013 (continued)**

| Compound | CAS No. | IARC Group | IARC Volume | Year |
|---|---|---|---|---|
| Dibenzo[a,h]pyrene | 189-64-0 | 2B | 92 | 2010 |
| Dibenzo[a,i]pyrene | 189-55-9 | 2B | 92 | 2010 |
| Ethylbenzene | 100-41-4 | 2B | 77 | 2000 |
| Furan | 110-00-9 | 2B | 63 | 1995 |
| Glu-P-1 (2-Amino-6-methyldipyrido[1,2-a:3′,2′-d]imidazole) | 67730-11-4 | 2B | SUP 7 | 1987 |
| Glu-P-2 (2-Aminodipyrido[1,2-a:3′,2′-d]imidazole) | 67730-10-3 | 2B | SUP 7 | 1987 |
| Hydrazine | 302-01-2 | 2B | 71 | 1999 |
| Indeno[1,2,3-cd]pyrene | 193-39-5 | 2B | 92 | 2010 |
| Isoprene | 78-79-5 | 2B | 71 | 1999 |
| Lead | 7439-92-1 | 2B | SUP 7 | 1987 |
| MeA-α-C (2-Amino-3-methyl)-9H-pyrido[2,3-b]indole) | 68006-83-7 | 2B | SUP 7 | 1987 |
| N-Nitrosodiethanolamine (NDELA) | 1116-54-7 | 2B | 77 | 2000 |
| N-Nitrosomethylethylamine | 10595-95-6 | 2B | SUP 7 | 1987 |
| N-Nitrosomorpholine (NMOR) | 59-89-2 | 2B | SUP 7 | 1987 |
| N-Nitrosopiperidine (NPIP) | 100-75-4 | 2B | SUP 7 | 1987 |
| N-Nitrosopyrrolidine (NPYR) | 930-55-2 | 2B | SUP 7 | 1987 |
| N-Nitrososarcosine (NSAR) | 13256-22-9 | 2B | SUP 7 | 1987 |
| Naphthalene | 91-20-3 | 2B | 82 | 2002 |
| Nickel | 7440-02-0 | 2B | 49 | 1990 |
| Nitrobenzene | 98-95-3 | 2B | 65 | 1996 |
| Nitromethane | 75-52-5 | 2B | 77 | 2000 |
| o-Anisidine | 90-04-0 | 2B | 73 | 1999 |
| PhIP (2-Amino-1-methyl-6-phenylimidazo[4,5-b]pyridine) | 105650-23-5 | 2B | 56 | 1993 |
| Propylene oxide | 75-56-9 | 2B | 60 | 1994 |
| Styrene | 100-42-5 | 2B | 82 | 2002 |
| Trp-P-1 (3-Amino-1,4-dimethyl-5H-pyrido[4,3-b]indole) | 62450-06-0 | 2B | SUP 7 | 1987 |
| Trp-P-2 (3-Amino-1-Methyl-5H-pyrido[4,3-b]indole ) | 62450-07-1 | 2B | SUP 7 | 1987 |
| Vinyl acetate | 108-05-4 | 2B | 63 | 1995 |
| 1-Aminonaphthalene | 134-32-7 | 3 | SUP 7 | 1987 |
| Chromium | 7440-47-3 | 3 | 49 | 1990 |
| Crotonaldehyde | 4170-30-3 | 3 | 63 | 1995 |
| Dibenzo[a,e]pyrene | 192-65-4 | 3 | 92 | 2010 |
| Mercury | 7439-97-6 | 3 | 58 | 1993 |
| Quinoline | 91-22-5 | EPA Group B2 | | |
| Cresols (o-, m-, and p-cresol) | 1319-77-3 | EPA Group C | | |

Notes: Most recently published IARC monograph for each compound is listed.
Quinoline and cresols have not been evaluated by IARC, but have been evaluated by U.S. Environmental Protection Agency.
IARC Groups: 1, Carcinogenic to humans; 2A, Probably carcinogenic to humans; 2B, Possibly carcinogenic to humans; 3, Not classifiable as to its carcinogenicity to humans; http://monographs.iarc.fr/ENG/Classification/ClassificationsAlphaOrder.pdf
EPA Groups: B2, Likely to be carcinogenic in humans; C, Possible human carcinogen.
CAS No., Chemical Abstracts Service registry number. CAS Registry Number is a Registered Trademark of the American Chemical Society. EPA, Environmental Protection Agency.
Quinoline: http://www.epa.gov/iris/subst/1004.htm
Cresols: http://www.epa.gov/iris/subst/0300.htm; http://www.epa.gov/iris/subst/0301.htm; http://www.epa.gov/iris/subst/0302.htm

## TABLE 4.3

### Commonly Used Biomarkers of Exposure to Carcinogens in Tobacco Smoke

| Biomarker | Tobacco Smoke Source | Matrices |
|---|---|---|
| Monohydroxy-30butenyl mercapturic acid (MHBMA) | 1,3-butadiene | Urine |
| 4-Aminobiphenyl-globin | 4-aminobiphenyl | Blood |
| N-(2-hydroxypropyl)methacrylamide (HPMA) | Acrolein | Urine |
| Carbamoylethylvaline | Acrylamide | Blood |
| Cyanoethylvaline | Acrylonitrile | Blood |
| S-phenylmercapturic acid (SPMA) | Benzene | Urine |
| Cd | Cadmium | Urine |
| 3-hydroxypropyl mercapturic acid (HBMA) | Crotonaldehyde | Urine |
| 2-hydroxyethyl mercapturic acid (HEMA) | Ethylene oxide | Urine |
| Nicotine equivalents (nicotine, cotinine, trans-3'-hydroxycotinine, and their respective glucuronides) | Nicotine | Urine |
| Total 4-(methylnitrosamino)-1-(3-pyridyl)-1-butanol (NNAL) (NNAL + NNAL glucuronide) | NNK | Urine |
| Total NNN (NNN + NNN glucuronide) | NNN | Urine |
| 1-Hydroxypyrene | Pyrene (representative of other PAH) | Urine |

Adapted from Hecht SS, Yuan JM, Hatsukami D. Applying tobacco carcinogen and toxicant biomarkers in product regulation and cancer prevention. *Chem Res Toxicol* 2010;23:1001–1008.

Validation with respect to product use means that levels of a given biomarker differ substantially between users and nonusers, and that biomarker levels decrease substantially when product use is stopped. Validation with respect to disease risk implies that variation in biomarker levels in product users are predictive of variations in disease outcomes. Over the last decade, the development of modern high-throughput, high-resolution mass spectrometry has allowed for the measurement of multiple metabolites of tobacco carcinogens.[110–113] Commonly used biomarkers of tobacco exposure are listed in Table 4.3.

## How Tobacco Use Leads to Cancer

A recent U.S. Surgeon General's report provides extensive detail on the current state of knowledge of how smoking causes cancer.[65] Therefore, only a brief overview is provided here. Hecht[101,113–116] has argued for a major pathway by which tobacco use leads to cancer: carcinogen exposure leads to the formation of carcinogen–DNA adducts, which then cause mutations that, if not repaired or removed by apoptosis, will eventually give rise to cancer. It is important to keep perspective that, whereas each cigarette may contain seemingly low levels of a given carcinogen, smoking is, for most people, a long-term addiction. Thus, a mixture of numerous carcinogens is administered multiple times per day over the course of decades. Further, compounds taken in during smokers can be metabolically activated, thus increasing their activity. Cigarette smoke compounds appear to induce the cytochrome P450 system, which facilitates the metabolic activation of carcinogens to electrophilic entities that are able to covalently bind DNA.[117,118] DNA adducts appear to be crucial to the cancer process, and numerous studies show that smoker tissues contain higher levels of DNA adducts than nonsmokers, and that DNA adduct levels are associated with cancer risk.[119,120] At the same time, other systems are involved in the detoxification and deactivation of smoke constituents, typically catalyzed by UDP-glucuronosyltransferases and glutathione-S-transferases, resulting in excretion of inactive compounds.[121,122] An individual's balance of activation and deactivation of toxicants

may be an important predictor of cancer risk, although evidence for this is mixed in the literature.[123,124] Similarly, DNA repair capacity is an important consideration, because, even if adducts are formed, processes exist to remove such perturbations to normalize DNA structure. Enzymatic processes of DNA repair include alkytransferases, nucleotide excision, and mismatch repair. Polymorphisms in genes coding for these enzymes may relate to individual cancer susceptibility. Table 4.4 outlines the metabolic activation/detoxification, DNA-adduct formation, and repair processes believed to be involved for four tobacco carcinogens (nitrosamines, PAH, benzene, 4-aminobiphenyl).[65,120]

Those DNA adducts that persist can cause miscoding during DNA replication. Smoke carcinogens are known to cause G:A and G:T mutations, and mutations in the *KRAS* oncogene and the *P53* tumor suppressor gene are strongly associated with tobacco-caused cancers.[95,114,125–127] Inactivation of *P53*, together with the activation of *KRAS*, appear to reduce survival in non–small-cell lung cancer.[65] Gene mutations that do not result in apoptosis may go on to influence a number of downstream processes, which may lead to genomic instability, proliferation, and eventually, malignancy.[128–130] Some smoke constituents may also act in ways that indirectly support the development of cancer. Nicotine, although not a carcinogen in itself, is known to reduce apoptosis and increase angiogenesis and transformation processes via nuclear factor kappa B (NF-κB).[65,131] Activation of nicotinic acetylcholine receptors (nAChR) in lung epithelium by nicotine or NNK is associated with survival and proliferation of malignant cells.[65] Nitrosamines also appear to have similar activities via the activation of protein kinases A and B.[132] NNK may bind β-adrenergic receptors to stimulate the release of arachidonic acid, which is converted to prostaglandin E2 by cyclooxygenase (COX)-2. Smoke compounds appear to activate epidermal growth factor receptor (EGFR) and COX-2, both of which are found to be elevated in many cancers.[133] Ciliatoxic, inflammatory, and oxidizing compounds, such as acrolein and ethylene oxide in smoke, may also impact the likelihood of cancer development. Epigenetic changes such as hypermethylation, particularly at P16, may also play a role in lung cancer development.[65]

## TABLE 4.4

### Key Pathways and Processes Where Selected Smoke Constituents Are Activated and Detoxified

|  | NNN, NNK | PAH | Benzene | 4-ABP |
|---|---|---|---|---|
| **Metabolic Activation** | Alpha hydroxylation | Diol epoxide formation | Epoxide/oxepin formation | N-oxidation |
| **Cytochrome P450 Enzymes Involved** | 2A6, 2A13, 2E1 | 1A1, 1B1 | 2E1 | 1A2 |
| **Enzymes Involved in Detoxification/ Activation** | UGT | MEH, GST, UGT | MEH, GST | UGT, NAT |
| **DNA Adduct Formation Sites** |  |  |  |  |
| **Lung** | O6-POB-deoxyguanosine | BPDE-N2-deoxyguanosine |  |  |
| **Bladder** |  |  |  | C-8 deoxyguanosine |
| **DNA Repair Pathways** | AGT, BER | NER, MMR | BER, NER, NIR | NER |

UGT, uridine-5′-diphosphate-glucuronosyltransferases; MEH, microsomal epoxide hydrolases; NAT, N-Acetyltransferases; GST, glutathione-S-transferases; AGT, O6-alkylguanine–DNA alkyltransferase; BER, base excision repair; NER, nucleotide excision repair; MMR, mismatch repair; NIR, nucleotide incision repair.

## REFERENCES

1. World Health Organization, Research for International Tobacco Control. WHO *Report on the Global Tobacco Epidemic, 2008: the MPOWER Package.* Geneva: World Health Organization; 2008.
2. Giovino GA, Mirza SA, Samet JM, et al. Tobacco use in 3 billion individuals from 16 countries: an analysis of nationally representative cross-sectional household surveys. *Lancet* 2012;380:668–679.
3. Centers for Disease Control and Prevention (CDC). Current cigarette smoking among adults—United States, 2011. *MMWR Morb Mortal Wkly Rep* 2012;61:889–894.
4. Proctor R. *Golden Holocaust: Origins of the Cigarette Catastrophe and the Case for Abolition.* Berkeley: University of California Press; 2011.
5. Centers for Disease Control and Prevention (CDC). Consumption of cigarettes and combustible tobacco—United States, 2000-2011. *MMWR Morb Mortal Wkly Rep* 2012;61:565–569.
6. Centers for Disease Control and Prevention (CDC). Cigarette use among high school students—United States, 1991–2009. *MMWR Morb Mortal Wkly Rep* 2010;59:797–801.
7. Centers for Disease Control and Prevention (CDC). Tobacco use among middle and high school students—United States, 2000–2009. *MMWR Morb Mortal Wkly Rep* 2010;59:1063–1068.
8. Centers for Disease Control and Prevention (CDC). Tobacco product use among middle and high school students—United States, 2011 and 2012. *MMWR Morb Mortal Wkly Rep* 2013;62:893–897.
9. Cummings KM, Fong GT, Borland R. Environmental influences on tobacco use: evidence from societal and community influences on tobacco use and dependence. *Annu Rev Clin Psychol* 2009;5:433–458.
10. Huang J, Chaloupka FJ, Fong GT. Cigarette graphic warning labels and smoking prevalence in Canada: a critical examination and reformulation of the FDA regulatory impact analysis. *Tob Control* 2014;1:i7–i12.
11. Chaloupka FJ, Yurekli A, Fong GT. Tobacco taxes as a tobacco control strategy. *Tob Control* 2012;21:172–180.
12. Centers for Disease Control and Prevention (CDC). State-specific trends in lung cancer incidence and smoking—United States, 1999-2008. *MMWR Morb Mortal Wkly Rep* 2011;60:1243–1247.
13. Holford TR, Meza R, Warner KE, et al. Tobacco control and the reduction in smoking-related premature deaths in the United States, 1964–2012. *JAMA* 2014;311:164–171.
14. Slama K. The FCTC enters into effect in 2005. *Int J Tuberc Lung Dis* 2005;9:119.
15. Liberman J. Four COPs and counting: achievements, underachievements and looming challenges in the early life of the WHO FCTC Conference of the Parties. *Tob Control* 2012;21:215–220.
16. Deyton LR. FDA tobacco product regulations: a powerful tool for tobacco control. *Public Health Rep* 2011;126:167–169.
17. Patterson JT. *The Dread Disease: Cancer and Modern American Culture.* Cambridge, MA: Harvard University Press; 1987.
18. Proctor R. *The Nazi War on Cancer.* Princeton: Princeton University Press; 1999.
19. Doll R, Hill AB. Smoking and carcinoma of the lung: a preliminary report. *BMJ* 1950;2:739–748.
20. Wynder EL, Graham EA. Tobacco smoking as a possible etiologic factor in bronchiogenic carcinoma: a study of six hundred and eighty-four proved cases. *JAMA* 1950;143:329–336.
21. US Department of Health and Human Services. *The Health Consequences of Smoking: A Report of the Surgeon General.* Atlanta: Department of Health and Human Services, Centers for Disease Control and Prevention, National Center for Chronic Disease Prevention and Health Promotion, Office on Smoking and Health; 2004.
22. Centers for Disease Control and Prevention (CDC). Smoking-attributable mortality, years of potential life lost, and productivity losses—United States, 2000-2004. *MMWR Morb Mortal Wkly Rep* 2008;57:1226–1228.
23. US Department of Health and Human Services. *The Health Consequences of Smoking—50 Years of Progress. A Report of the Surgeon General.* Atlanta: U.S. Department of Health and Human Services, Centers for Disease Control and Prevention, National Center for Chronic Disease Prevention and Health Promotion, Office on Smoking and Health; 2014.
24. Jha P, Ramasundarahettige C, Landsman V, et al. 21st-century hazards of smoking and benefits of cessation in the United States. *N Engl J Med* 2013;368:341–350.
25. Gaudet MM, Gapstur SM, Sun J, et al. Active smoking and breast cancer risk: original cohort data and meta-analysis. *J Natl Cancer Inst* 2013;105:515–525.
26. Peto R, Darby S, Deo H, et al. Smoking, smoking cessation, and lung cancer in the UK since 1950: combination of national statistics with two case-control studies. *BMJ* 2000;321:323–329.
27. Thun MJ, Carter BD, Feskanich D, et al. 50-year trends in smoking-related mortality in the United States. *N Engl J Med* 2013;368:351–364.
28. Burns DM, Anderson CM, Gray N. Has the lung cancer risk from smoking increased over the last fifty years? *Cancer Causes Control* 2011;22:389–397.
29. Benowitz NL. Clinical pharmacology of nicotine: implications for understanding, preventing, and treating tobacco addiction. *Clin Pharmacol Ther* 2008;83:531–541.
30. Benowitz NL. Pharmacology of nicotine: addiction, smoking-induced disease, and therapeutics. *Annu Rev Pharmacol Toxicol* 2009;49:57–71.
31. Benowitz NL. Nicotine addiction. *N Engl J Med* 2010;362:2295–2303.
32. Scherer G. Smoking behaviour and compensation: a review of the literature. *Psychopharmacology (Berl)* 1999;145:1–20.
33. Hammond D, Fong GT, Cummings KM, et al. Smoking topography, brand switching, and nicotine delivery: results from an in vivo study. *Cancer Epidemiol Biomarkers Prev* 2005;14:1370–1375.
34. Benowitz NL, Hukkanen J, Jacob P. Nicotine chemistry, metabolism, kinetics and biomarkers. *Handb Exp Pharmacol* 2009:29–60.
35. Benowitz NL, Swan GE, Jacob P, et al. CYP2A6 genotype and the metabolism and disposition kinetics of nicotine. *Clin Pharmacol Ther* 2006;80:457–467.
36. Johnstone E, Benowitz N, Cargill A, et al. Determinants of the rate of nicotine metabolism and effects on smoking behavior. *Clin Pharmacol Ther* 2006;80:319–330.
37. Malaiyandi V, Lerman C, Benowitz NL, et al. Impact of CYP2A6 genotype on pretreatment smoking behaviour and nicotine levels from and usage of nicotine replacement therapy. *Mol Psychiatry* 2006;11:400–409.
38. Lea RA, Dickson S, Benowitz NL. Within-subject variation of the salivary 3HC/COT ratio in regular daily smokers: prospects for estimating CYP2A6 enzyme activity in large-scale surveys of nicotine metabolic rate. *J Anal Toxicol* 2006;30:386–389.
39. St Helen G, Novalen M, Heitjan DF, et al. Reproducibility of the nicotine metabolite ratio in cigarette smokers. *Cancer Epidemiol Biomarkers Prev* 2012;21:1105–1114.

40. Benowitz NL, Dains KM, Dempsey D, et al. Racial differences in the relationship between number of cigarettes smoked and nicotine and carcinogen exposure. *Nicotine Tob Res* 2011;13:772–783.

41. Dempsey DA, St Helen G, Jacob P, et al. Genetic and pharmacokinetic determinants of response to transdermal nicotine in white, black, and asian nonsmokers. *Clin Pharmacol Ther* 2013;94:687–694.

42. Zhu AZ, Renner CC, Hatsukami DK, et al. The ability of plasma cotinine to predict nicotine and carcinogen exposure is altered by differences in CYP2A6: the influence of genetics, race, and sex. *Cancer Epidemiol Biomarkers Prev* 2013;22:708–718.

43. Schnoll RA, Patterson F, Wileyto EP, et al. Nicotine metabolic rate predicts successful smoking cessation with transdermal nicotine: a validation study. *Pharmacol Biochem Behav* 2009;92:6–11.

44. Fong GT, Hammond D, Laux FL, et al. The near-universal experience of regret among smokers in four countries: findings from the International Tobacco Control Policy Evaluation Survey. *Nicotine Tob Res* 2004;6:S341–S351.

45. Lee WB, Fong GT, Zanna MP, et al. Regret and rationalization among smokers in Thailand and Malaysia: findings from the International Tobacco Control Southeast Asia Survey. *Health Psychol* 2009;28:457–464.

46. Sansone N, Fong GT, Lee WB, et al. Comparing the experience of regret and its predictors among smokers in four Asian countries: findings from the ITC surveys in Thailand, South Korea, Malaysia, and China. *Nicotine Tob Res* 2013;15:1663–1672.

47. Tobacco Use and Dependence Guideline Panel. *Treating Tobacco Use and Dependence: 2008 Update.* Rockville, MD: U.S. Department of Health and Human Services; 2008.

48. Wynder EL, Hoffmann D. *Tobacco and Tobacco Smoke.* New York: Academic Press; 1967.

49. Cummings KM, Morley CP, Hyland A. Failed promises of the cigarette industry and its effect on consumer misperceptions about the health risks of smoking. *Tob Control* 2002;11:I110–I117.

50. Pollay RW, Dewhirst T. The dark side of marketing seemingly "Light" cigarettes: successful images and failed fact. *Tob Control* 2002;11:I18–I31.

51. Fairchild A, Colgrove J. Out of the ashes: the life, death, and rebirth of the "safer" cigarette in the United States. *Am J Public Health* 2004;94:192–204.

52. Hoffmann D, Hoffmann I. The changing cigarette, 1950–1995. *J Toxicol Environ Health.* 1997;50:307–364.

53. Jarvis MJ. Trends in sales weighted tar, nicotine, and carbon monoxide yields of UK cigarettes. *Thorax* 2001;56:960–963.

54. O'Connor RJ, Cummings KM, Giovino GA, et al. How did UK cigarette makers reduce tar to 10 mg or less? *BMJ.* 2006;332:302.

55. National Cancer Institute. *Risks Associated with Smoking Cigarettes with Low Machine-Measured Yields of Tar and Nicotine.* Bethesda, MD: The Institute; 2001.

56. Harris JE, Thun MJ, Mondul AM, et al. Cigarette tar yields in relation to mortality from lung cancer in the cancer prevention study II prospective cohort, 1982-8. *BMJ* 2004;328:72.

57. Thun MJ, Burns DM. Health impact of "reduced yield" cigarettes: a critical assessment of the epidemiological evidence. *Tob Control* 2001;10:i4–i11.

58. Benowitz NL, Jacob P, Bernert JT, et al. Carcinogen exposure during short-term switching from regular to "light" cigarettes. *Cancer Epidemiol Biomarkers Prev* 2005;14:1376–1383.

59. Burns DM, Anderson CM, Gray N. Do changes in cigarette design influence the rise in adenocarcinoma of the lung? *Cancer Causes Control* 2011;22:13–22.

60. Kozlowski LT, Mehta NY, Sweeney CT, et al. Filter ventilation and nicotine content of tobacco in cigarettes from Canada, the United Kingdom, and the United States. *Tob Control* 1998;7:369–375.

61. Kozlowski LT, O'Connor RJ, Giovino GA, et al. Maximum yields might improve public health—if filter were banned: a lesson from the history of vented filters. *Tob Control* 2006;15:262–266.

62. Kozlowski LT, O'Connor RJ. Cigarette filter ventilation is a defective design because of misleading taste, bigger puffs, and blocked vents. *Tob Control* 2002;11:I40–I50.

63. Kozlowski LT, Goldberg ME, Yost BA, et al. Smokers are unaware of the filter vents now on most cigarettes: results of a national survey. *Tob Control* 1996;5:265–270.

64. O'Connor RJ, Caruso RV, Borland R, et al. Relationship of cigarette-related perceptions to cigarette design features: findings from the 2009 ITC U.S. Survey. *Nicotine Tob Res* 2013;15:1943–1947.

65. Centers for Disease Control and Prevention, National Center for Chronic Disease Prevention and Health Promotion, Office on Smoking and Health. *How Tobacco Smoke Causes Disease: The Biology and Behavioral Basis for Smoking-Attributable Disease: A Report of the Surgeon General.* Rockville, MD: Centers for Disease Control and Prevetion; 2010.

66. Stratton KR. *Clearing the Smoke: Assessing the Science Base for Tobacco Harm Reduction.* Washington, DC: Institute of Medicine, National Academy Press; 2001.

67. Foulds J, Ramstrom L, Burke M, et al. Effect of smokeless tobacco (snus) on smoking and public health in Sweden. *Tob Control* 2003;12:349–359.

68. Henningfield JE, Fagerstrom KO. Swedish Match Company, Swedish snus and public health: a harm reduction experiment in progress? *Tob Control* 2001;10:253–257.

69. Pepper JK, Brewer NT. Electronic nicotine delivery system (electronic cigarette) awareness, use, reactions and beliefs: a systematic review. *Tob Control* 2013 [Epub ahead of print].

70. Schaller K, Ruppert L, Kahnert S, et al. *Electronic Cigarettes—An Overview.* Heidelberg: German Cancer Research Center (DKFZ); 2013. http://www.dkfz.de/en/presse/download/RS-Vol19-E-Cigarettes-EN.pdf

71. Institute of Medicine. *Scientific Standards for Studies on Modified Risk Tobacco Products.* Washington, DC: National Academies Press; 2012.

72. International Agency for Research on Cancer. *Tobacco Smoke and Involuntary Smoking.* Vol 83. Lyon: International Agency for Research on Cancer, World Health Organization; 2004.

73. International Agency for Research on Cancer. *Smokeless Tobacco and Tobacco-Specific Nitrosamines.* Vol 89. Lyon: International Agency for Research on Cancer, World Health Organization; 2007.

74. Center for Tobacco Products. *Reporting Harmful and Potentially Harmful Constituents in Tobacco Products and Tobacco Smoke Under Section 904(a)(3) of the Federal Food, Drug, and Cosmetic Act.* Rockville, MD: Department of Health and Human Services; 2012.

75. Fowles J, Dybing E.. Application of toxicological risk assessment principles to the chemical constituents of cigarette smoke. *Tob Control* 2003;12:424–430.

76. Burns DM, Dybing E, Gray N, et al. Mandated lowering of toxicants in cigarette smoke: a description of the World Health Organization tobacco regulation proposal. *Tob Control* 2008;17:132–141.

77. Straif K, Baan R, Gosse Y, et al. Carcinogenicity of polycyclic aromatic hydrocarbons. *Lancet Oncol* 2005;6:931–932.

78. O'Connor RJ, Hurley PJ. Existing technologies to reduce specific toxicant emissions in cigarette smoke. *Tob Control* 2008;17:i39–i48.

79. Pappas RS. Toxic elements in tobacco and in cigarette smoke: inflammation and sensitization. *Metallomics* 2011;3:1181–1198.

80. Marano KM, Naufal ZS, Kathman SJ, et al. Cadmium exposure and tobacco consumption: biomarkers and risk assessment. *Regul Toxicol Pharmacol* 2012;64:243–252.

81. Stephens WE, Calder A, Newton J. Source and health implications of high toxic metal concentrations in illicit tobacco products. *Environ Sci Technol* 2005;39:479–488.

82. Hecht SS, Hoffmann D. Tobacco-specific nitrosamines, an important group of carcinogens in tobacco and tobacco smoke. *Carcinogenesis* 1988;9:875–884.

83. Hecht SS. Biochemistry, biology, and carcinogenicity of tobacco-specific N-nitrosamines. *Chem Res Toxicol* 1998;11:559–603.

84. Hoffmann D, Rivenson A, Hecht SS. The biological significance of tobacco-specific N-nitrosamines: smoking and adenocarcinoma of the lung. *Crit Rev Toxicol* 1996;26:199–211.

85. Nilsson R. The molecular basis for induction of human cancers by tobacco specific nitrosamines. *Regul Toxicol Pharmacol* 2011;60:268–280.

86. Hecht SS, Stepanov I, Hatsukami DK. Major tobacco companies have technology to reduce carcinogen levels but do not apply it to popular smokeless tobacco products. *Tob Control* 2011;20:443.

87. Stepanov I, Knezevich A, Zhang L, et al. Carcinogenic tobacco-specific N-nitrosamines in US cigarettes: three decades of remarkable neglect by the tobacco industry. *Tob Control* 2012;21:44–48.

88. Stanfill SB, Connolly GN, Zhang L, et al. Global surveillance of oral tobacco products: total nicotine, unionised nicotine and tobacco-specific N-nitrosamines. *Tob Control* 2011;20:e2.

89. Stepanov I, Villalta PW, Knezevich A, et al. Analysis of 23 polycyclic aromatic hydrocarbons in smokeless tobacco by gas chromatography-mass spectrometry. *Chem Res Toxicol* 2010;23:66–73.

90. Stanton MF, Miller E, Wrench C, et al. Experimental induction of epidermoid carcinoma in the lungs of rats by cigarette smoke condensate. *J Natl Cancer Inst* 1972;49:867–877.

91. Hoffmann D, Stepanov I, Hecht SS, et al. *Tobacco Carcinogenesis.* New York: Academic Press; 1978.

92. Deutsch-Wenzel R, Brune H, Grimmer G. Experimental studies in rat lungs on the carcinogenicity and dose-response relationships of eight frequently occurring environmental polycyclic aromatic hydrocarbons. *J Natl Cancer Inst* 1983;71:539–544.

93. Pfeifer GP, Denissenko MF, Olivier M, et al. Tobacco smoke carcinogens, DNA damage and p53 mutations in smoking-associated cancers. *Oncogene* 2002;21:7435–7451.

94. Boysen G, Hecht SS. Analysis of DNA and protein adducts of benzo[a]pyrene in human tissues using structure-specific methods. *Mutat Res* 2003;543:17–30.

95. Phillips DH. Smoking-related DNA and protein adducts in human tissues. *Carcinogenesis* 2002;23:1979–2004.

96. Liu Z, Muehlbauer KR, Schmeiser HH, et al. p53 Mutations in benzo[a]pyrene-exposed human p53 knock-in murine fibroblasts correlate with p53 mutations in human lung tumors. *Cancer Res* 2005;65:2583–2587.

97. Belinsky SA, Foley JF, White CM, et al. Dose-response relationship between O6-methylguanine formation in Clara cells and induction of pulmonary neoplasia in the rat by 4-(methylnitrosamino)-1-(3-pyridyl)-1-butanone. *Cancer Res* 1990;50:3772–3780.

98. Stepanov I, Sebero E, Wang R, et al. Tobacco-specific N-nitrosamine exposures and cancer risk in the Shanghai cohort study: remarkable coherence with rat tumor sites. *Int J Cancer* 2014;134:2278–2283.

99. Yuan JM, Koh WP, Murphy SE, et al. Urinary levels of tobacco-specific nitrosamine metabolites in relation to lung cancer development in two prospective cohorts of cigarette smokers. *Cancer Res* 2009;69:2990–2995.

ETIOLOGY AND EPIDEMIOLOGY OF CANCER

100. Church TR, Anderson SE, Caporaso NE, et al. A prospectively measured serum biomarker for a tobacco-specific carcinogen and lung cancer in smokers. *Cancer Epidemiol Biomarkers Prev* 2009;18:260–266.

101. Hecht SS, Murphy SE, Stepanov I, et al. Tobacco smoke biomarkers and cancer risk among male smokers in the Shanghai Cohort Study. *Cancer Lett* 2012 [Epub ahead of print].

102. Yuan JM, Butler LM, Gao YT, et al. Urinary metabolites of a polycyclic aromatic hydrocarbon and volatile organic compounds in relation to lung cancer development in lifelong never smokers in the Shanghai Cohort Study. *Carcinogenesis* 2014;35:339–345.

103. Melikian AA, Sun P, Prokopczyk B, et al. Identification of benzo[a]pyrene metabolites in cervical mucus and DNA adducts in cervical tissues in humans by gas chromatography-mass spectrometry. *Cancer Lett* 1999;146: 127–134.

104. Prokopczyk B, Trushin N, Leszczynska J, et al. Human cervical tissue metabolizes the tobacco-specific nitrosamine, 4-(methylnitrosamino)-1-(3-pyridyl)-1-butanone, via alpha-hydroxylation and carbonyl reduction pathways. *Carcinogenesis* 2001;22:107–114.

105. Castelao JE, Yuan JM, Skipper PL, et al. Gender- and smoking-related bladder cancer risk. *J Natl Cancer Inst* 2001;93:538–545.

106. Sugimura T. History, present and future, of heterocyclic amines, cooked food mutagens. *Princess Takamatsu Symp* 1995;23:214–231.

107. Turesky RJ. Heterocyclic aromatic amine metabolism, DNA adduct formation, mutagenesis, and carcinogenesis. *Drug Metab Rev* 2002; 34:625–650.

108. Ashley DL, O'Connor RJ, Bernert JT, et al. Effect of differing levels of tobacco-specific nitrosamines in cigarette smoke on the levels of biomarkers in smokers. *Cancer Epidemiol Biomarkers Prev* 2010;19:1389–1398.

109. Hatsukami DK, Benowitz NL, Rennard SI, et al. Biomarkers to assess the utility of potential reduced exposure tobacco products. *Nicotine Tob Res* 2008;8: 169–191.

110. Carmella SG, Chen M, Han S, et al. Effects of smoking cessation on eight urinary tobacco carcinogen and toxicant biomarkers. *Chem Res Toxicol* 2009;22:734–741.

111. Carmella SG, Ming X, Olvera N, et al. High throughput liquid and gas chromatography-tandem mass spectrometry assays for tobacco-specific nitrosamine and polycyclic aromatic hydrocarbon metabolites associated with lung cancer in smokers. *Chem Res Toxicol* 2013;26:1209–1217.

112. Church TR, Anderson KE, Le C, et al. Temporal stability of urinary and plasma biomarkers of tobacco smoke exposure among cigarette smokers. *Biomarkers* 2010;15:345–352.

113. Hecht SS, Yuan JM, Hatsukami D. Applying tobacco carcinogen and toxicant biomarkers in product regulation and cancer prevention. *Chem Res Toxicol* 2010;23:1001–1008.

114. Hecht SS. Tobacco smoke carcinogens and lung cancer. *J Natl Cancer Inst* 1999;91:1194–1210.

115. Hecht SS. Tobacco carcinogens, their biomarkers, and tobacco-induced cancer. *Nature Rev Cancer* 2003;3:733–744.

116. Hecht SS. Lung carcinogenesis by tobacco smoke. *Int J Cancer* 2012;131: 2724–2732.

117. Guengerich FP. Common and uncommon cytochrome P450 reactions related to metabolism and chemical toxicity. *Chem Res Toxicol* 2001; 14:611–650.

118. Jalas J, Hecht SS, Murphy SE. Cytochrome P450 2A enzymes as catalysts of metabolism of 4-(methylnitrosamino)-1-(3-pyridyl)-1-butanone (NNK), a tobacco-specific carcinogen. *Chem Res Toxicol* 2005;18:95–110.

119. Nebert DW, Dalton TP, Okey AB, et al. Role of aryl hydrocarbon receptor-mediated induction of the CYP1 enzymes in environmental toxicity and cancer. *J Biol Chem* 2004;279:23847–23850.

120. Hang B. Formation and repair of tobacco carcinogen-derived bulky DNA adducts. *J Nucleic Acids* 2010;2010:709521.

121. Burchell B, McGurk K, Brierley CH, et al. *UDP-Glucuronosyltransferases.* Vol 3. New York: Elsevier Science; 1997.

122. Armstrong RN. *Glutathione-S-Transferases.* Vol 3. New York: Elsevier Science; 1997.

123. Vineis P, Veglia F, Benhamou S, et al. CYP1A1 T3801 C polymorphism and lung cancer: a pooled analysis of 2451 cases and 3358 controls. *Int J Cancer* 2003;104:650–657.

124. Carlsten C, Sagoo GS, Frodsham AJ, et al. Glutathione S-transferase M1 (GSTM1) polymorphisms and lung cancer: a literature-based systematic HuGE review and meta-analysis. *Am J Epidemiol* 2008;167:759–774.

125. Ahrendt SA, Decker PA, Alawi EA, et al. Cigarette smoking is strongly associated with mutation of the K-ras gene in patients with primary adenocarcinoma of the lung. *Cancer* 2001;92:1525–1530.

126. Ding L, Getz G, Wheeler DA, et al. Somatic mutations affect key pathways in lung adenocarcinoma. *Nature* 2008;455:1069–1075.

127. Johnson L, Mercer K, Greenbaum D, et al. Somatic activation of the K-ras oncogene causes early onset lung cancer in mice. *Nature* 2001;410:1111–1116.

128. Sekido Y, Fong KW, Minna JD. Progress in understanding the molecular pathogenesis of human lung cancer. *Biochim Biophys Acta* 1998;1378:F21–F59.

129. Bode AM, Dong A. Signal transduction pathways in cancer development and as targets for cancer prevention. *Prog Nucleic Acid Res Mol Biol* 2005;79:237–297.

130. Schuller HM. Mechanisms of smoking-related lung and pancreatic adenocarcinoma development. *Nat Rev Cancer* 2002;2:455–463.

131. Heeschen C, Jang JJ, Weis M, et al. Nicotine stimulates angiogenesis and promotes tumor growth and atherosclerosis. *Nat Med* 2001;7:833–839.

132. West KA, Brognard J, Clark AS, et al. Rapid Akt activation by nicotine and a tobacco carcinogen modulates the phenotype of normal human airway epithelial cells. *J Clin Invest* 2003;111:81–90.

133. Moraitis D, Du B, De Lorenzo MS, et al. Levels of cyclooxygenase-2 are increased in the oral mucosa of smokers: evidence for the role of epidermal growth factor receptor and its ligands. *Cancer Res* 2005;65:664–670.

# 5 Oncogenic Viruses

Christopher B. Buck and Lee Ratner

## PRINCIPLES OF TUMOR VIROLOGY

Viral infections are estimated to play a causal role in at least 11% of all new cancer diagnoses worldwide.[1] A vast majority of cases (>85%) occur in developing countries, where poor sanitation, high rates of cocarcinogenic factors such as HIV/AIDS, and lack of access to vaccines and cancer screening all contribute to increased rates of virally induced cancers. Even in developed countries, where effective countermeasures are widely available, cancers attributable to viral infection account for at least 4% of new cases.[2,3]

Viruses thought to cause various forms of human cancer come from six distinct viral families with a range of physical characteristics (Table 5.1). All known human cancer viruses are capable of establishing durable, long-term infections and cause cancer only in a minority of persistently infected individuals. The low penetrance of cancer induction is consistent with the idea that a virus capable of establishing a durable productive infection would not benefit from inducing a disease that kills the host.[4] The slow course of cancer induction (typically over a course of many years after the initial infection) suggests that viral infection alone is rarely sufficient to cause human malignancy and that virally induced cancers arise only after additional oncogenic "hits" have had time to accumulate stochastically.

In broad terms, viruses can cause cancer through either (or both) of two broad mechanisms: direct or indirect. Direct mechanisms, in which the virus-infected cell ultimately becomes malignant, are typically driven by the effects of viral oncogene expression or through direct genotoxic effects of viral gene products. In most established examples of direct viral oncogenesis, the cancerous cell remains "addicted" to viral oncogene expression for ongoing growth and viability.

A common feature of DNA viruses that depend on host cell DNA polymerases for replication (e.g., papillomaviruses, herpesviruses, and polyomaviruses) is the expression of viral gene products that promote progression into the cell cycle. A typical mechanism of direct oncogenic effects is through the inactivation of tumor suppressor proteins, such as the guardian of the genome, p53, and retinoblastoma protein (pRB). This effectively primes the cell to express the host machinery necessary for replicating the viral DNA. The study of tumor viruses has been instrumental in uncovering the existence and function of key tumor suppressor proteins, as well as key cellular proto-oncogenes, such as Src and Myc.

In theory, viruses could cause cancer via direct hit-and-run effects. In this model, viral gene products may serve to preserve cellular viability and promote cell growth in the face of otherwise proapoptotic genetic damage during the early phases of tumor development. In principle, the precancerous cell might eventually accumulate enough additional genetic hits to allow for cell growth and survival independent of viral oncogene expression. This would allow for stochastic loss of viral nucleic acids from the nascent tumor, perhaps giving a growth advantage due to the loss of "foreign" viral antigens that might otherwise serve as targets for immune-mediated clearance of the nascent tumor. Although hit-and-run effects have been observed in animal models of virally

induced cancer,[5] these effects are extremely difficult to address in humans. Currently, there are no clearly established examples of hit-and-run effects in human cancer.

In indirect oncogenic mechanisms, the cells that give rise to the malignant tumor have never been infected by the virus. Instead, the viral infection is thought to lead to cancer by attracting inflammatory immune responses that, in turn, lead to accelerated cycles of tissue damage and regeneration of noninfected cells. In some instances, virally infected cells may secrete paracrine signals that drive the proliferation of uninfected cells. At a theoretical level, it may be difficult to distinguish between indirect carcinogenesis and hit-and-run direct carcinogenesis, because, in both cases, the metastatic tumor may not contain any viral nucleic acids.

A variety of hunting approaches have been used to uncover etiologic roles for viruses in human cancer. The first clues that high-risk human papillomaviruses (HPVs), Epstein-Barr virus (EBV), Kaposi's sarcoma–associated herpesvirus (KSHV), and Merkel cell polyomavirus (MCPyV) might be carcinogenic were based on the detection of virions, viral DNA, or viral RNA in the tumors these viruses cause. A common feature of known virally induced cancers is that they are more prevalent in immunosuppressed individuals, such as individuals suffering from HIV/AIDS or patients on immunosuppressive therapy after organ transplantation. This is thought to reflect the lack of immunologic control over the cancer-causing virus. Studies focused on AIDS-associated cancers provided the first evidence for the carcinogenic potential of KSHV and MCPyV. A theoretical limitation of this approach is that some virally induced cancers may not occur at dramatically elevated rates in all types of immunosuppressed subjects, particularly if the virus causes only a fraction of cases (e.g., HPV-induced head and neck cancers). Fortunately, the unbiased analysis of nucleic acid sequences found in tumors has become substantially more tractable as deep-sequencing methods have continued to fall in price. In the coming years, it should be increasingly possible to search for viral sequences without making the starting assumption that all virally induced tumors are associated with immunosuppression.[6]

One limitation of tumor sequencing approaches is that they might miss undiscovered divergent viral species within viral families known to have extensive sequence diversity[7] and could miss viral families that have not yet been discovered.[8] Tumor-sequencing approaches might also miss viruses that cause cancer by hit-and-run or indirect mechanisms. It is conceivable that this caveat could be addressed by focusing on sequencing early precancerous lesions thought to ultimately give rise to metastatic cancer.

An additional successful approach to hunting cancer viruses involves showing that individuals who are infected with a particular virus have an increased long-term risk of developing particular forms of cancer. This approach was successful for identifying and validating the carcinogenic roles of high-risk HPV types, hepatitis B virus (HBV), hepatitis C virus (HCV), KSHV, and human T-lymphotropic virus 1 (HTLV-1). Although viruses that are extremely prevalent, such as EBV and MCPyV, are not amenable to this approach per se, it may still be possible to draw connections

## TABLE 5.1
## Oncogenic Viruses

| Virus | Taxon | Viral Genome | Virion | Infection Rate | Site of Persistance | Diseases in Normal Hosts | Diseases in Immunocompromised Hosts | Associated Cancers |
|---|---|---|---|---|---|---|---|---|
| High-risk human papillomavirus types (e.g., HPV16) | Alphapapillomavirus | 8 kb circular dsDNA | Nonenveloped | >70% | Anogenital mucosa, oral mucosa | Carcinomas of the cervix, penis, anus, vagina, vulva, tonsils, base of tongue | Increased incidence of same diseases | 610,000 |
| Hepatitis B virus (HBV) | Hepadnaviridae | 3 kb ss/dsDNA | Enveloped | 2%–8% | Hepatocytes | Cirrhosis, hepatocellular carcinoma | Same diseases, increased incidence with AIDS | 380,000 |
| Hepatitis C virus (HCV) | Flaviviridae | 10 kb +RNA | Enveloped | ~3% | Hepatocytes | Cirrhosis, hepatocellular carcinoma, splenic marginal zone lymphoma | Same diseases, increased incidence with AIDS | 220,000 |
| Epstein-Barr virus (EBV, HHV-4) | Gammaherpesvirinae | 170 kb linear DNA | Enveloped | 90% | B cells, pharyngeal mucosa | Mononucleosis, Burkitt lymphoma, other non-Hodgkin lymphoma, nasopharyngeal carcinoma | Increased incidence of same diseases, lymphoproliferative disease, other lymphomas, oral hairy leukoplakia, leiomyosarcoma | 110,000 |
| Kaposi's sarcoma herpesvirus (KSHV, HHV-8) | Gammaherpesvirinae | 170 kb linear DNA | Enveloped | 2%–60% | Oral mucosa, endothelium, B cells | Kaposi's sarcoma (KS), multicentric Castleman disease (MCD) | Increased KS, MCD incidence, primary effusion lymphoma | 43,000 |
| Merkel cell polyomavirus (MCPyV, MCV) | Orthopolyomavirus | 5 kb circular dsDNA | Nonenveloped | 75% | Skin (lymphocytes?) | Merkel cell carcinoma (MCC) | Increased MCC incidence | 1,500 (US) |
| Human T-cell leukemia virus (HTLV-1) | Deltaretrovirus | 9 kb +RNA (RT) | Enveloped | 0.01%–6% | T and B cells | Adult T-cell leukemia/lymphoma, tropical spastic paraparesis, myelopathy, uveitis, dermatitis | Unknown | 2,100 |

*Note:* Ranges for infection rates imply major variations in prevalence among populations in different world regions. *Associated cancers* indicates the annual number of new cases clearly attributable to viral infection. An estimate for the worldwide incidence of Merkel cell carcinoma is not currently available and an estimate of the annual new cases in the United States alone is given instead.

ds, double-stranded; ss, single-stranded; HHV, human herpesvirus; RT, reverse transcriptase.

Adapted from de Martel C, Ferlay J, Franceschi S, et al. Global burden of cancers attributable to infections in 2008: a review and synthetic analysis. *Lancet Oncol* 2012;13(6):607–615; Schiller JT, Lowy DR. Virus infection and human cancer: an overview. *Recent Results Cancer Res* 2014;193:1–10; Chen CJ, Hsu WL, Yang HI, et al. Epidemiology of virus infection and human cancer. *Recent Results Cancer Res* 2014;193:11–32; and Virgin HW, Wherry EJ, Ahmed R. Redefining chronic viral infection. *Cell* 2009;138(1):30–50.

between cancer risk and either unusually high serum antibody titers against viral antigens or unusually high viral load. Relatively high serologic titers reflect either comparatively poor control of the viral infection in at-risk individuals or expression of viral antigens in tumors or tumor precursor cells.[9,10]

The finding that a virus causes cancer is good news, in the sense that it can suggest possible paths to clinical intervention. These can include the development of vaccines or antiviral agents that prevent, attenuate, or eradicate the viral infection and thereby prevent cancer; the development of methods for early detection or diagnosis of cancer based on assays for viral nucleic acids or gene products; or the development of drugs or immunotherapeutics that treat cancer by targeting viral gene products. Unfortunately, establishing the carcinogenicity of a given viral species is an arduous process that must inevitably integrate multiple lines of evidence.[11] The demonstration that the virus can transform cells in culture and/or cause cancer in animal models provides circumstantial evidence of the oncogenic potential of a virus. All known human cancer viruses meet this criterion. However, it is important to recognize that viruses can theoretically coevolve to be noncarcinogenic in their native host (e.g., humans) and cause cancer only in the dysregulated environment of a nonnative host animal. This caveat may apply to human adenoviruses.

Finding that viral DNA is clonally integrated in a primary tumor and its metastatic lesions helps address the caveat that the virus might merely be a hitchhiker that finds the tumor cell a conducive environment in which to replicate (as opposed to playing a causal carcinogenic role). This caveat is also addressed by the observation that, in most instances, viruses found in tumors have lost the ability to exit viral latency and are functionally unable to produce new progeny virions. An unfortunate consequence of this is that vaccines or antiviral agents that target virion proteins (e.g., vaccines against high-risk HPVs or HBV) or gene products expressed late in the viral life cycle (e.g., herpesvirus thymidine kinase, which is the target of drugs such as ganciclovir) are rarely effective for treating existing virally induced tumors.

Demonstrating that a vaccine or antiviral agent targeting the virus either prevents or treats human cancer is by far the strongest form of evidence that a given virus causes human cancer. This type of proof has fully validated the causal role of HBV in human liver cancer. Compelling clinical trial data also show that antiherpesvirus therapeutics can prevent KSHV- or EBV-associated lymphoproliferative disorders, and that vaccination against HPV can prevent the development of precancerous lesions on the uterine cervix.

# PAPILLOMAVIRUSES

## History

The idea that cancer of the uterine cervix might be linked to sexual behavior was first proposed in the mid 19th century by Dominico Rigoni-Stern, who observed that nuns rarely contracted cervical cancer, whereas prostitutes suffered from cervical cancer more often than the general populace.[12] Another major milestone in cervical cancer research was Georgios Papanikolaou's development of the so-called Pap smear for early cytologic diagnosis of precancerous cervical lesions.[13] This form of screening, which allows for surgical intervention to remove precancerous lesions, has saved many millions of lives in developed countries, where public health campaigns have made testing widely available.

Although observations in the early 1980s suggested the possibility of a hit-and-run carcinogenic role for herpes simplex viruses in cervical cancer,[14] this hypothesis was abandoned in light of studies led by Harald zur Hausen. Low-stringency hybridization approaches revealed the presence of two previously unknown papillomavirus types, HPV16 and HPV18, in various cervical cancer cell lines, including the famous HeLa cell line.[15,16] There is now

overwhelming evidence that a group of more than a dozen sexually transmitted HPV types, including HPV16 and HPV18, play a causal role in essentially all cases of cervical cancer. HPVs associated with a high risk of cancer also cause about half of all penile cancers, 88% of anal cancers, 43% of vulvar cancers, 70% of vaginal cancers,[2] and an increasing fraction of head and neck cancers (see the following). In 2008, zur Hausen was awarded the Nobel Prize for his groundbreaking work establishing the link between HPVs and human cancer.

The viral family *Papillomaviridae* is named for the benign skin warts (papillomas) that some members of the family cause. In the early 1930s, Richard Edwin Shope and colleagues demonstrated viral transmission of papillomas in a rabbit model system.[17] Using this system, Peyton Rous and others showed that cottontail rabbit papillomavirus-induced lesions can progress to malignant skin cancer.[18,19] This was the first demonstration of a cancer-causing virus in mammals, building on Rous' prior work demonstrating a virus capable of causing cancer in chickens (the Rous sarcoma retrovirus).

## Tissue Tropism and Gene Functions

Although papillomaviruses can achieve infectious entry into a wide variety of cell types in vitro and in vivo, the late phase of the viral life cycle, during which the viral genome undergoes vegetative replication and the L1 and L2 capsid proteins are expressed, is strictly dependent on host cell factors found only in differentiating keratinocytes near the surface of the skin or mucosa. Interestingly, a majority of HPV-induced cancers appear to arise primarily at zones of transition between stratified squamous epithelia and the single-layer (columnar) epithelia of the endocervix, the inner surface of the anus, and tonsillar crypts. It is thought that the mixed phenotypic milieu in cells at squamocolumnar transition zones may cause dysregulation of the normal coupling of the HPV life cycle to keratinocyte differentiation.

There are nearly 200 known HPV types.[20] In general, each papillomavirus type is a functionally distinct serotype, meaning that serum antibodies that neutralize one HPV type do not robustly neutralize other HPV types. Various HPV types preferentially infect different skin or mucosal surfaces. Different types tend to establish either transient infections that may be cleared over the course of months, or stable infections where virions are chronically shed from the infected skin surface for the lifetime of the host. HPV infections may or may not be associated with the formation of visible warts or other lesions. High-risk HPV types, with clearly established causal links to human cancer, are preferentially tropic for the anogenital mucosa and the oral mucosa, are usually transmitted by sexual contact, rarely cause visible warts, and usually establish only transient infections in a great majority of exposed individuals. The lifetime risk of sexual exposure to a high-risk HPV type has been estimated to be >70%. Individuals who fail to clear their infection with a high-risk HPV type and remain persistently infected are at much greater risk of developing cancer. Polymerase chain reaction (PCR)-based screening for the presence of high-risk HPV types thus serves as a useful adjunct to, or even a replacement for, the traditional Pap test.[21]

A consequence of the strict tissue-differentiation specificity of the papillomavirus life cycle is that HPVs do not replicate in standard monolayer cell cultures. Papillomaviruses also seem to be highly species restricted, and there are no known examples of an HPV type capable of infecting animals.[22] Thus, the investigation of key details of papillomavirus biology has relied almost entirely on modern recombinant DNA and molecular biologic analyses.

Papillomavirus genomes are roughly 8 kb, double-stranded, closed-circular DNA molecules (essentially reminiscent of a plasmid). During the normal viral life cycle, the genome does not adopt a linear form, does not integrate into the host cell chromosome, and remains as an extrachromosomal episome or minichromosome.

All the viral protein-coding sequences are arranged on one strand of the genome. The expression of various proteins is regulated by differential transcription and polyadenylation, as well as effects at the level of RNA splicing, export from the nucleus, and translation. In addition to the late half of the viral genome, which encodes the L1 and L2 capsid proteins, all papillomaviruses encode six key early region genes: E1, E2, E4, E5, E6, and E7.

The master transcriptional regulator E2 serves as a transcriptional repressor, and loss of E2 expression (typically through integration of the viral episome into the host cell DNA) results in the upregulation of early gene expression. The most extensively studied early region proteins are the E6 and E7 oncogenes of HPV16 and HPV18. The E6 protein of high-risk HPV types triggers the destruction of p53 by recruiting a host cell ubiquitin–protein ligase, E6AP.[23–25] Another important oncogenic function of E6 is the activation of cellular telomerase.[26] A wide variety of additional high-risk E6 activities that do not involve p53 have been identified.[27]

Most E7 proteins, including those of many low-risk HPV types, contain a conserved LXCXE motif that mediates interaction with pRB and the related "pocket" proteins p107 and p130.[28] Interestingly, the LXCXE motif is present in a wide variety of other oncogenes, most notably the T antigens of polyomaviruses and the E1A oncogenes of adenoviruses. The interaction of E7 with pRB disrupts the formation of a complex between pRB and E2F transcription factors, thereby blocking the ability of pRB to trigger cell cycle arrest.[29] The E7 proteins of high-risk HPVs can also contribute to chromosomal mis-segregation and aneuploidy, which may in turn contribute to malignant progression.[30] Like E6, E7 interacts with a wide variety of additional cellular targets, the spectrum of which seems to vary with different HPV types.[27]

Some papillomavirus types express an E5 oncogene, which functions as an agonist for cell surface growth factor receptors such as platelet-derived growth factor beta (PDGF-β) and epidermal growth factor (EGF) receptor.[31] Because E5 expression is uncommon in cervical tumors, it is uncertain whether the protein plays a key role in human cancer.

## Human Papilloma Virus Vaccines

Two preventive vaccines against cancer-causing HPVs, trade named Gardasil (Merck) and Cervarix (GSK), are currently marketed worldwide for the prevention of cervical cancer. Both vaccines contain recombinant L1 capsid proteins based on HPV16 and HPV18 that are assembled in vitro into virus-like particles (VLPs). Together, HPV16 and HPV18 cause about 70% of all cases of cervical cancer worldwide. Gardasil also includes VLPs based on HPV types 6 and 11, which rarely cause cervical cancer but together cause about 90% of all genital warts. The VLPs contained in the vaccines are highly immunogenic in humans, eliciting high-titer serum antibody responses against L1 that are capable of neutralizing the infectivity of the cognate HPV types represented in the vaccine. It appears that the current HPV vaccines may confer lifelong immunity against new infection with the HPV types represented in the vaccine.[32] The vaccines elicit lower titer cross-neutralizing responses against a subset of cancer-causing HPV types that are closely related to HPV16 and HPV18.[33] Although these cross-neutralizing responses can at least partially protect vaccinees against a new infection with additional high-risk types, such as HPV31 and HPV45, it remains unclear how durable the lower level cross-protection will be.[33]

Because L1 is not expressed in latently infected keratinocyte stem cells residing on the epithelial basement membrane, current HPV vaccines are very unlikely to eradicate existing infections.[34,35] Like keratinocyte stem cells, cervical cancers and precursor lesions rarely or never express L1. Thus, the existing L1-based vaccines seem unlikely to serve as therapeutic agents for treating cervical cancer.

Three types of next-generation HPV vaccines are currently in human clinical trials. Merck has recently announced that a newer version of Gardasil, which contains VLPs based on a total of nine different HPV types, remained highly effective against HPV16 and HPV18 and also prevented 97% of precancerous cervical lesions caused by a wider variety of high-risk HPV types.[36] Another class of second-generation vaccines targets the papillomavirus minor capsid protein L2. An N-terminal portion of L2 appears to represent a highly conserved "Achilles' heel", which contains conserved protein motifs required for key steps of the infectious entry process.[37] Anti-L2 antibodies can neutralize a broad range of different human and animal HPV types, and thus, L2 vaccines are hoped to offer protection against all HPVs that cause cervical cancer, all low-risk HPV types that cause abnormal Pap smear results, as well as the full range of HPV types that cause skin warts. Finally, a wide variety of vaccines that seek to elicit cell-mediated immune responses against the E6 and E7 oncoproteins are aimed at a therapeutic intervention for the treatment of cervical cancer.[38]

## Oropharyngeal Cancer

It is well established that tobacco products and alcohol cause head and neck cancer. In the late 1990s, Maura Gillison and colleagues noted a surprising number of new cases of tonsillar cancer in nonsmokers.[39] Many of the tumors found in nonsmokers were found to have wild-type p53 genes, raising the possibility that the tumor might be dependent on a p53-suppressing viral oncogene (as seen in cervical cancer). Gillison and colleagues went on to show that nearly half of all tonsillar cancers contain HPV DNA, most commonly HPV16. Interestingly, HPV-positive oropharyngeal cancers tend to be less lethal than tobacco-associated HPV-negative tumors. This finding has important implications for treatment of HPV-positive head and neck cancers.[40]

Although the incidence of tobacco-associated head and neck cancer has been declining in recent decades due to decreased tobacco use, recent studies suggest an ongoing increase in the incidence of HPV-associated cancers of the tonsils and the base of the tongue. By 2025, the number of new HPV-induced head and neck cancer cases in the United States is expected to roughly equal the number of new cervical cancer cases.[39] Based in part on these observations, the U.S. Centers for Disease Control and Prevention recommends that boys, in addition to girls, should be vaccinated against high-risk HPVs.

## Nonmelanoma Skin Cancer

Epidermodysplasia verruciformis (EV) is a rare immunodeficiency that is characterized by the appearance of numerous flat, wartlike lesions across wide areas of skin. The lesions typically contain genus betapapillomaviruses, such as HPV5 or HPV8. EV patients frequently develop squamous cell carcinomas (SCC) in sun-exposed skin areas (suggesting that ultraviolet [UV] light exposure is a cofactor). It is also well established that other immunosuppressed individuals, such as organ transplant recipients and HIV-infected individuals, are at increased risk of developing SCC.[41,42] Although the E6 and E7 proteins of betapapillomaviruses appear to exert a different spectrum of effects than the E6 and E7 proteins of HPV types associated with cervical cancer,[43–45] Betapapillomavirus oncogenes can transform cells in vitro.[46] Although these circumstantial lines of evidence suggest that infectious agents, such as Betapapillomaviruses, might play a causal role in SCC, recent deep sequencing studies have observed few or no viral sequences in SCC tumors.[47] Although the results argue against durable direct oncogenic effects of any known viral species in SCC, an animal model system using bovine papillomavirus type 4 strongly suggests that papillomaviruses can cause cancer by hit and run mechanisms.[5] Thus, the question of whether hit-and-run or indirect oncogenic effects of HPVs may be at play in human SCC remains open.

# POLYOMAVIRUSES

## History

In the early 1950s, Ludwik Gross showed that a filterable infectious agent could cause salivary gland cancer in laboratory mice.[48] Later work by Bernice Eddy and Sarah Stewart showed that the murine polyoma (Greek for "many tumors") virus caused many different types of cancer in experimentally infected mice.[49] The discovery that murine polyomavirus could be grown in cell culture helped rekindle research interest in tumor virology and interest in the question of whether viruses might cause human cancer.

Like papillomaviruses, polyomaviruses have a nonenveloped capsid assembled from 72 pentamers of a single major capsid protein (VP1). Both viral families also carry circular dsDNA genomes. These physical similarities initially led to the classification of both groups into a single family, *Papovaviridae*. When sequencing studies ultimately revealed that polyomaviruses have a unique genome organization (with early and late genes being arranged on opposing strands of the genome) and almost no sequence homology to papillomaviruses, the two groups of viruses were divided into separate families.

In the early 1960s, Bernice Eddy, Maurice Hilleman, and Benjamin Sweet reported the discovery of simian vacuolating virus 40 (SV40), a previously unknown polyomavirus that was found as a contaminant in vaccines against poliovirus.[50,51] SV40 was derived from the rhesus monkey kidney cells used to amplify poliovirus virions in culture.[52] SV40 rapidly became an important model polyomavirus, and studies of its major and minor tumor antigens (large T [LT] and small t [ST], respectively) have played an important role in understanding various aspects of carcinogenesis. Despite significant alarm about the possible risk SV40 might pose to exposed individuals, a comprehensive, decades long series of studies have failed to uncover compelling evidence that SV40 exposure is causally associated with human cancer.[53]

Two naturally human-tropic polyomaviruses, BK virus (BKV) and John Cunningham virus (JCV), were first reported in back-to-back publications in 1971.[54,55] BKV and JCV are known to cause kidney disease and a lethal brain disease called progressive multifocal leukoencephalopathy, respectively, in immunosuppressed individuals. Although both viruses can cause cancer in experimentally exposed animals, it remains unclear whether either virus plays a causal role in human cancer. Although BKV LT expression can frequently be observed in the inflammatory precursor lesions that

are thought to give rise to prostate cancer,[56] there is no evidence for the persistence of BKV DNA in malignant prostate tumors.[57] There have been case studies finding BKV T-antigen expression in bladder cancer,[58] and some reports have indicated the presence of JCV DNA in colorectal tumors. The long history of conflicting evidence concerning possible roles for BKV or JCV in human cancer is reviewed elsewhere.[59,60]

## Merkel Cell Polyomavirus

In 2008, Yuan Chang and Patrick Moore reported their lab's discovery of the fifth known human polyomavirus species, which they named Merkel cell polyomavirus (MCV or MCPyV) based on its presence in Merkel cell carcinoma (MCC).[61] The discovery used an RNA deep sequencing approach called digital transcriptome subtraction. Using classic Southern blotting, this report demonstrated the clonal integration of MCPyV in an MCC tumor and its distant metastases. Many other labs worldwide have independently confirmed the presence of MCPyV DNA in about 80% of MCC tumors.[11]

MCC is a rare but highly lethal form of cancer that typically presents as a fast-growing lesion on sun-exposed skin surfaces (Fig. 5.1).[62] The risk of MCC is dramatically higher in HIV/AIDS patients, offering an initial clue that MCC might be a virally induced cancer.[63] Although MCC tumors express neuroendocrine markers associated with sensory Merkel cells of the epidermis, one recent report has shown that some MCC tumors also express B-cell markers, including rearranged antibody loci.[64] Currently, there is no clear evidence for the involvement of MCPyV in other tumors with neuroendocrine features.

In 2012, the International Agency for Research on Cancer (IARC) concluded that MCPyV is a class 2A carcinogen (probably carcinogenic to humans).[10,53] It should be noted that IARC evaluations rely heavily on animal carcinogenicity studies, and the 2A designation was assigned prior to a recent report showing that MCV-positive MCC lines are tumorigenic in a mouse model system.[65]

A great majority of healthy adults have serum antibodies specific for the MCPyV major capsid protein VP1. A majority also shed MCPyV virions from apparently healthy skin surfaces, and there is a strong correlation between individual subjects' serologic titer against VP1 and the amount of MCPyV DNA they shed.[66–68] Interestingly, MCC patients tend to have exceptionally strong serologic titers against VP1.[69] MCC tumors do not express detectable amounts of VP1, so this is unlikely to reflect direct exposure to

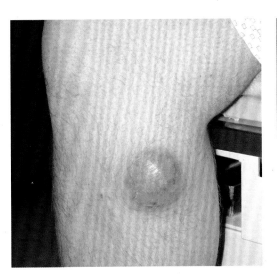
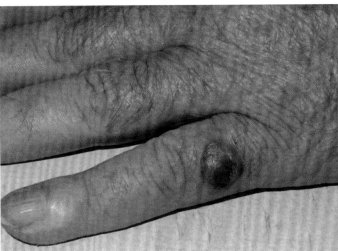

**Figure 5.1** Merkel cell carcinoma (MCC). The *left panel* shows an MCC tumor on the calf. The *right panel* shows an MCC tumor on the finger. Photographs provided with permission by Dr. Paul Nghiem (University of Washington, www.merkelcell.org).

the tumor and instead likely represents a history of a high MCPyV load in MCC patients. A recent study of archived serum samples shows that unusually high serologic titers against MCPyV VP1 often precede the development of MCC by many years.[70]

Like the LT protein of SV40 (and the E7 proteins of high-risk HPVs), an N-terminal portion of the MCPyV LT protein contains an LXCXE motif that mediates inactivation of pRB function. In contrast to SV40 LT, which carries a p53-inactivation domain that overlaps the C-terminal helicase domain, MCPyV LT does not appear to inactivate p53 function.[71] Instead, the MCPyV LT helicase domain activates DNA damage responses and induces cell cycle arrest in cultured cell lines.[72] This may explain why the LT genes found in MCC tumors essentially always carry mutations that truncate LT upstream of the helicase domain. siRNA experiments indicate that most (although possibly not all) MCC tumors are "addicted" to the expression of MCPyV T antigens.[73–75] Interestingly, patients with higher levels of MCPyV DNA in their tumors, stronger T-antigen expression, and tumors that have been infiltrated by CD8+ T cells appear to have better prognoses.[76] This is consistent with the idea that cell-mediated immunity can help clear MCC tumors that express MCPyV antigens.

Recent work has shown that the pRB interacting domain of LT mediates increased expression of the cellular gene survivin. The knockdown of survivin using siRNAs results in MCC tumor cell death and YM155, a small molecule inhibitor of survivin expression, protects mice from MCC tumors in a xenograft challenge system.[77,78]

In contrast to SV40, where LT appears to be the dominant oncogene, the MCPyV ST protein appears to play a key role in cell transformation. In addition to modifying the signaling functions of the cellular proto-oncogene PP2A, ST triggers the phosphorylation of eukaryotic translation initiation factor 4E binding protein 1.[79] This results in dysregulation of cap-dependent translation and cellular transformation.

Although there is an intriguing epidemiologic correlation between MCC and chronic lymphocytic leukemia (CLL),[80] there are conflicting reports concerning the presence of MCPyV in CLL and other lymphocytic cancers.[81–83]

## Other Human Polyomaviruses

In recent years, the number of known human polyomaviruses has expanded dramatically. Of the 12 currently known HPyV species, only MCPyV has been clearly linked to human cancer. One new HPyV, trichodysplasia spinulosa polyomavirus (TSV or TSPyV) has been found in association with abnormal spiny growths on the facial skin of a small number of immunocompromised individuals.

## EPSTEIN-BARR VIRUS

### History

In 1958, Denis Burkitt provided the first clear clinical description of an unusual B-cell–derived tumor that frequently affects the jawbones of children in equatorial Africa.[84] After hearing Burkitt give a 1961 lecture entitled "The Commonest Children's Cancer in Tropical Africa – A Hitherto Unrecognized Syndrome," Michael Epstein became interested in the idea that an insect vector-borne infection might account for the high incidence of Burkitt lymphoma in tropical Africa. Epstein, together with then PhD candidate Yvonne Barr, began examining tumor samples sent to them by Burkitt. Electron micrographs of lymphoid cells that grew out of the tumors in culture revealed viral particles with a morphology strikingly similar to herpes simplex viruses.[85] It was soon shown that Epstein-Barr herpesvirus (EBV, later designated human herpesvirus 4 [HHV-4]) can transform cultured B cells and is the agent responsible for infectious mononucleosis.[86–88]

Although the initial conjecture that tropically endemic Burkitt lymphoma depends on a geographically restricted infectious agent ultimately proved correct, it was quickly established that the EBV infection is not restricted to the tropics. It instead appears likely that the malaria parasite *Plasmodium falciparum* is a key geographically restricted cocarcinogen responsible for endemic Burkitt lymphoma.[53] In areas where children suffer repeated malaria infections, it appears that the parasite triggers abnormal B-cell responses, as well as weakened cell-mediated immune function, and these effects of recurring malaria infection in turn promote or allow the development of EBV-induced Burkitt tumors.[11]

### Epstein-Barr Virus Life Cycle

EBV chronically infects nearly all humans. In a great majority of individuals, the infection is initially established in early childhood and is never associated with any noticeable symptoms. The infection is typically transmitted when virions, shed in the saliva of a chronically infected individual, come in contact with the oropharyngeal epithelium of a naïve individual. Although infected epithelial cells, such as keratinocytes, might serve to amplify the virus in some circumstances,[89] the establishment of chronic infection is ultimately dependent on mature B cells, as subjects with X-linked agammaglobulinemia (who lack mature B cells) appear to be immune to stable EBV infection.[90] Individuals who escape infection during childhood and instead first become infected during adolescence or adulthood often develop mononucleosis, which is associated with fevers and extreme fatigue lasting for weeks or sometimes months. Interestingly, late-infected individuals who experience mononucleosis and high EBV viral load are at increased risk of developing EBV-positive Hodgkin lymphoma.[91]

EBV-infected B cells can either go on to produce new virions, which are typically associated with cell lysis, or the virus can enter a nonproductive state known as latency. Viral latency is defined as a condition in which the virus expresses few (or possibly no) gene products but can, under some conditions, "reawaken" to express the full range of viral gene products and produce new progeny virions. Latently infected cells are highly resistant to immune clearance.

There are three recognized forms of EBV latency. In latency I, EBV nuclear antigen-1 (EBNA1), which is required for the stable maintenance of the circularized viral DNA minichromosome, is the only viral protein expressed. EBV-derived microRNAs (miRs) may also be expressed. At the other end of the spectrum, latency III is characterized by the expression of EBNA1–6, several latent membrane proteins (LMP1, 2A, and 2B), two noncoding RNAs (EBER1 and 2), the BCL-2 homolog BHRF1, BARF0, and multiple miRs. Although the initial discovery of EBV involved the visualization of virions, indicating that the virus had exited latency and entered the productive lytic phase of the life cycle, viral gene expression in EBV-induced cancers generally follows one of the three latent patterns. The oncogenic activities of various EBV gene products have recently been reviewed.[87,88]

In a great majority of healthy individuals, EBV exists almost exclusively in a latent state, with the occasional asymptomatic shedding of virions in the saliva. The infection is controlled, at least in part, by CD8+ T cells specific for various latency proteins. EBV, like other herpesviruses, expresses a variety of proteins that interfere with cell-mediated immune responses. Intriguingly, results from mouse model systems suggest that the chronic immunostimulatory effects of persistent gammaherpesvirus emergence (or abortive emergence) from latency in healthy hosts can nonspecifically boost immunity to other infections.[92]

### Lymphomas

In addition to endemic Burkitt lymphoma, EBV is often present in sporadic cases of Burkitt lymphoma in individuals who have not been exposed to malaria. Although nearly all cases of endemic

Burkitt's lymphoma contain EBV DNA in the tumor (typically in a latency I–like state), only about 20% of sporadic cases arising in immunocompetent individuals contain EBV. Rates of Burkitt lymphoma are elevated in HIV-infected individuals, and HIV-associated Burkitt lymphomas contain EBV in about 30% of cases.

A common hallmark of all types of Burkitt's lymphomas is deregulation of the cellular Myc proto-oncogene. A classic mutation involves chromosomal translocation of the Myc gene to the antibody heavy chain locus. Burkitt's lymphoma tumors that lack detectable EBV DNA tend to carry multiple additional mutations in host cell genes, raising the possibility that an originally EBV-positive precursor cell ultimately accumulated mutations that rendered it independent of viral genes.[88,93]

In addition to Burkitt lymphoma, EBV is associated, to varying extents, with a histologically diverse range of other lymphoid cancers, including Hodgkin lymphoma, natural killer (NK)/T-cell lymphoma, primary central nervous system (CNS) lymphoma, and diffuse large B-cell lymphoma. The incidence of these various forms of lymphoma is significantly increased both in AIDS patients as well as in iatrogenically and congenitally immunosuppressed individuals.[88] In particular, the essentially universal presence of EBV in CNS lymphomas in AIDS patients makes it possible to diagnose the disease with a PCR test for EBV that, together with radiologic findings, can obviate the need for a brain biopsy.

EBV is almost invariably associated with lymphoproliferative disorders, such as plasmacytic hyperplasia and polymorphic B cell hyperplasia, which are often observed in organ transplant recipients. These polyclonal lymphoproliferative responses can, in some instances, progress to oligoclonal or monoclonal lymphomas of various types. The occurrence of EBV-associated lymphoproliferative disease in immunosuppressed patients is generally heralded by the increased detection of EBV DNA in the peripheral blood and the oral cavity. This presumably reflects the failure of cellular immune responses to drive the virus into full latency and perhaps also a failure of cell-mediated immune responses targeting latency-associated EBV gene products present in the nascent tumor.

## Carcinomas

In Southern China, NPC affects 25 out of 100,000 people, accounting for 18% of all cancers in China as a whole.[94] Most other world regions have a 25- to 100-fold lower rate of NPC. EBV is present in nearly all cases of NPC, both in endemic and nonendemic regions. Although there is support for the idea that dietary intake of salted fish and other preserved foods is a factor in endemic NPC, it remains possible that genetic traits or as yet unidentified environmental cocarcinogenic factors may play a role as well. Individuals with rising or relatively high IgA antibody responses to EBNA1, DNase, and/or EBV capsid antigens have a dramatically increased risk of developing NPC, offering an early detection method for at-risk individuals.[87]

EBV is also present in a small percentage (5% to 15%) of gastric adenocarcinomas and over 90% of gastric lymphoepithelioma-like carcinomas. In contrast to NPC, the prevalence of EBV-associated gastric cancer is similar in all world regions. As with NPC, elevated antibody responsiveness to EBV antigens may offer a method for identifying individuals at greater risk of gastric cancer.

## Prevention and Treatment

The reduction of immunosuppression in response to increasing EBV loads is a standard approach to preventing EBV diseases in T-cell immunosuppressed individuals. Another approach to the prevention of EBV disease relies on ganciclovir (or related antiherpesvirus drugs), which can trigger the death of cells that express the EBV thymidine kinase gene. Pretreating at-risk individuals, such as organ transplant recipients, with ganciclovir has been shown to effectively prevent the development of EBV-induced

lymphoproliferative disorders.[95] However, it is important to note that thymidine kinase is only expressed in the lytic phase of the viral life cycle, and drugs of this class are not generally effective for treating existing tumors, presumably due to the fact that EBV gene expression in tumors is typically of a latent type.

Although a recently developed vaccine targeting the EBV gp350 virion surface antigen did not provide sterilizing immunity to EBV infection, vaccinees did experience lower peak EBV viral loads upon infection.[96] Given the strong correlation between high EBV loads and the development of EBV diseases, it is hoped that the vaccine's ability to merely blunt the acute infection may offer significant protection against disease.

Most forms of EBV-associated lymphoid cancers express the B-cell marker CD20, making rituximab (an anti-CD20 mAb) a potentially effective adjunct therapy.[97,98] An emerging treatment approach that has recently entered clinical trials involves stimulating T cells ex vivo against peptides based on EBV antigens or against autologous EBV-transformed B cells.

# KAPOSI'S SARCOMA HERPESVIRUS

## History and Epidemiology

In the late 19th century, Hungarian dermatologist Moritz Kaposi's described a relatively rare type of indolent pigmented skin sarcoma affecting older men.[99] Kaposi's sarcoma (KS) was later found to be more prevalent in the Mediterranean region and in eastern portions of sub-Saharan Africa.[100] An early clue to the emergence of the HIV/AIDS pandemic in the early 1980s was a dramatic increase in the incidence of highly aggressive forms of KS, particularly in gay men who were much younger than typical KS patients. After the discovery of HIV, it was briefly hypothesized that HIV might be a direct cause of KS. However, this hypothesis failed to explain the existence of KS long prior to the HIV pandemic and the low incidence of KS in individuals who became infected with HIV via blood products. This latter observation was more easily explained by the existence of a sexually transmitted cofactor other than HIV.[101]

Using a subtractive DNA hybridization approach known as representational difference analysis, Yuan Chang, Patrick Moore, and colleagues discovered the presence of a previously unknown herpesvirus in KS tumors.[102] The newly founded field of research rapidly established key lines of evidence supporting the conclusion that KSHV (later designated human herpesvirus-8 [HHV-8]) is a causal factor in KS.[11]

It is now clear that the rate of KSHV infection varies greatly in different world regions.[11,103] In North America and Western Europe, KSHV seroprevalence in the general population ranges from 1% to 7%. Seroprevalence among gay men in these regions is substantially higher (25% to 60%), suggesting a possible link to sexual transmission. KSHV infection is much more prevalent in the general population in central and eastern Africa, where seroprevalence ranges from 23% to 70%. In endemic areas, up to 15% of children are seropositive, suggesting either vertical transmission or transmission via nonsexual casual contact (presumably via saliva). In endemic regions, KS is estimated to be the third most common cancer among adults.[104]

## Kaposi's Sarcoma-Associated Herpesvirus in Kaposi's Sarcoma

KS tumors are complex on a number of levels. In contrast to most other forms of cancer, where it is often clear that a single cell type has proliferated out of control, KS tumors are composed of cells from multiple lineages (Fig. 5.2). KSHV-infected cells in the tumor often have a spindle-shaped morphology. Interestingly,

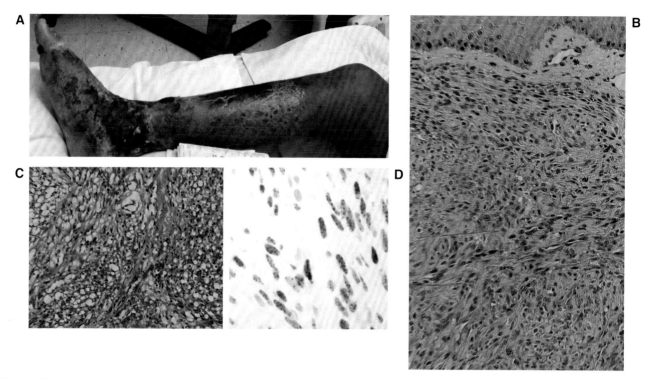

**Figure 5.2** Kaposi's sarcoma (KS). **(A)** Photograph of the lower leg of an individual with severe, diffuse KS involving the lower leg. **(B)** Histology of the skin. **(C)** Lung shows a mixture of spindle to epithelioid cells, with slitlike vascular spaces intermixed with red blood cells and red blood cell fragments. **(D)** Immunohistochemical detection of KSHV LANA in the cutaneous tumor. Photographs provided with permission by Drs. Odey Ukpo and Ethel Cesarman.

spindle cells do not exhibit a highly transformed phenotype and tend to show relatively little chromosomal instability. In a culture, the cells are highly dependent on exogenous cytokines and other factors present in the tumor microenvironment in vivo. Although spindle cells express a number of markers of the endothelial lineage, it is uncertain whether they are derived from mature endothelial cells, the early precursor cells that give rise to smooth muscle and vascular endothelial cells, or cells of the lymphatic endothelial lineage. KS tumors also contain infiltrating lymphocytes and monocytes, as well as aberrant neovascular spaces lined with infected and uninfected endothelial cells. The aberrant blood vessels in KS lesion vessels rupture easily and leak red blood cells, giving KS tumors their classic dark red, brown, or purple color.

The latency status of KSHV in KS tumors is also complex, with the expression of gene products typical of latency (e.g., LANA) as well as lytic-phase genes (e.g., RTA/ORF50). Some of these gene products, such as the viral interleukin (IL)-6 homolog (vIL-6), trigger proliferation and secondary cytokine signaling in noninfected cells within the tumor. The tumorigenic effects of individual KSHV gene products have recently been reviewed.[88,103] In contrast to EBV, where tumorigenesis is driven by latency gene expression, it appears that KS pathogenesis is often dependent on lytic phase gene expression. This may explain why ganciclovir, which is not a particularly effective treatment for EBV tumors, was found to prevent the formation of new KS lesions in HIV-positive patients.[105] However, it should be noted that this outcome has more recently proven difficult to reproduce.[106] At present, there are no recommended preventive therapies for individuals at risk of KS, but this is an area of active investigation.

There are a variety of possible explanations for the need for lytic-phase KSHV gene expression during tumor development. For example, infected spindle cells may lose the viral DNA during cell division and require reinfection for ongoing tumorigenicity. Alternatively, factors secreted by a small fraction of tumor cells that enter the lytic phase may be required for tumorigenesis. An important area of current research focus is the role of KSHV gene products in the regulation of angiogenesis in KS lesions[107] and several current trials are investigating inhibitors of angiogenic pathways for the treatment of KS.

## Lymphoproliferative Disorders

KSHV causes two forms of B-cell proliferative disorder: multicentric Castleman disease (MCD) and primary effusion lymphoma (PEL). Both diseases are most commonly found in association with HIV infection. In HIV-infected individuals, MCD tumors contain KSHV in nearly all cases, whereas in HIV-negative individuals, the tumor contains KSHV in only about 50% of cases.[108] KSHV in MCD exhibits periodic activation of lytic replication and the expression of lytic phase genes.[109] The expression of vIL-6 during disease flare-ups appears to play a role in MCD pathogenesis, raising the possibility that tocilizumab (a mAb therapeutic that targets the IL-6 receptor) may be of therapeutic benefit.

PEL comprises about 4% of all HIV-associated non-Hodgkin lymphomas.[110] Typically, PEL tumors express markers of both plasma cells (akin to multiple myeloma tumors) and immunoblasts (similar to some EBV-induced tumors). In AIDS patients, essentially all PEL tumors are infected with KSHV and a great majority are also coinfected with EBV.[88] Although PEL is rare in HIV-negative individuals, PEL tumors in such individuals contain KSHV in about 50% of cases.

A common approach to the treatment of all KSHV-associated diseases is the restoration of immune function, either through antiretroviral therapy of HIV/AIDS or through a reduction of immunosuppressive therapy. The general success of immune reconstitution in many KSHV-associated diseases presumably involves an immune-mediated attack of cells expressing KSHV gene products, particularly the many lytic-phase gene products the virus can produce in various disease states.

# ANIMAL AND HUMAN RETROVIRUSES

The first oncogenic retroviruses were discovered by Ellerman and Bang in 1908 and by Rous in 1911, but it was many years before the significance of these findings was appreciated.[111] One reason the field was stymied was the failure to identify RNA forms of the viral genome in infected cells. This led to the discovery of the reverse transcriptase independently by Baltimore and Temin in 1970. Another major development was the finding in 1976 of viral oncogenes derived from cellular genes, with the identification by Varmus and Bishop of the first dominant oncogene, *src*. With the discovery of IL-2 by Gallo in 1976, it became possible to culture the first human retrovirus, HTLV-1, from a form of adult T-cell leukemia/lymphoma (ATLL) that was first recognized by Takatsuki and coworkers.[112] These advances opened the door for Montagnier and colleagues' isolation of HIV-1 in 1983, a discovery confirmed independently by Gallo and Levy. This breakthrough led to the first licensed HIV test in 1985.

Retroviruses are positive single-strand RNA viruses that utilize transcription of their RNA genome into a DNA intermediate during virus replication.[111] This accounts for their name, retroviruses, because this is opposite to the normal flow of eukaryotic genetic information. They infect a wide range of vertebrate animal species and are distantly related to repetitive elements in the human genome, known as retrotransposons. Retroviruses are also related to hepadnaviruses, double-stranded DNA viruses, such as hepatitis B virus, which also undergo a reverse transcription step in their replication.

Retroviruses may be classified as *endogenous* or *exogenous* depending on whether they appear in the genome of the host species. There are approximately 100,000 endogenous retroviral elements in the human genome, making up nearly 8% of the genetic information, but their potential roles in disease are unclear.[113] Retroviruses may also be classified as *ecotropic, xenotropic*, or *polytropic* depending on whether they infect cells of the same animal species from which they are derived, infect cells of a different species, or both. *Amphotropic* retroviruses infect cells of the species of origin without producing disease, but infect cells of other species and may produce disease.

Retroviruses that produce disease after a long incubation period are termed *lentiviruses* and include human, simian, feline, ovine, caprine, and bovine immunodeficiency viruses. Another group of retroviruses that are not clearly associated with disease are known as *spumaviruses* and include human and simian foamy viruses. HTLV-1, which is classified in the genus Delta, is the only retrovirus known to be oncogenic in humans. A member of the retroviral genus Gamma identified in 2008, designated xenotropic murine leukemia virus-related virus (XMRV), was thought to be associated with human prostate cancer; however, more recent studies showed XMRV to be a lab-derived artifact.[114] A genus betaretrovirus related to the mouse mammary tumor virus has been suggested to be associated with biliary cirrhosis, but this finding requires independent validation.[115]

Retroviruses producing tumors in animals or birds are designated transforming viruses and may be classified as acute or chronic transforming retroviruses. Acute transforming retroviruses have acquired a mutated cellular gene, termed *oncogene*, and induce cancer in an animal within a few weeks. Many dominant acting proto-oncogenes in humans (e.g., *ras, myc*, and *erbB*), were first identified as retroviral oncogenes.

Chronic transforming retroviruses integrate almost randomly in the genome, but when integrated in the vicinity of specific genes disrupt their regulation and induce cell proliferation or resistance to apoptosis. Chronic transforming retroviruses induce malignancy only after many weeks to months of infection. The use of a murine leukemia virus vector for gene therapy in children with a form of severe combined immune deficiency syndrome characterized by defective expression of the common gamma chain of the IL-2 receptor resulted in T-cell acute lymphoblastic leukemia.

This was found to be the result of persistent expression of the LIM domain only 2 (LMO2) gene triggered by the nearby integration of the retroviral vector.[116]

In addition to acute or chronic transformation mechanisms, retroviruses can transform cells through direct effects on cell physiology mediated by structural or nonstructural viral proteins. Transforming genes of HTLV-1 are nonstructural viral proteins that activate host cell signaling pathways.[117] Because the oncogenic effects of HTLV-1 transforming genes generally take many years to cause cancer, the virus does not fit the precise definition of having either an acute or a chronic oncogenic mechanism.

HIV-1 infection is also associated with a variety of malignancies, but only by indirect effects of suppressing immunity to oncogenic virus infections, such as gammaherpesviruses, high-risk human papillomaviruses, and hepatitis viruses.

## Human T-Cell Leukemia Virus Epidemiology

Four species of human T-cell leukemia virus have been identified. HTLV-1 was identified in 1980 as the first human retrovirus associated with cancer, and it is the focus of the remainder of this section.[118] HTLV-2 was discovered in 1982 and shares 70% genomic homology with HTLV-1.[119] HTLV-3 and -4 were sporadically isolated from individuals who had contact with monkeys.[120] HTLV-2, -3, and -4 do not appear to be associated with disease in humans.

HTLV-1 is present in 15 to 20 million individuals worldwide, most commonly in the Caribbean Islands, South America, southern Japan, and parts of Australia, Melanesia, Africa, and Iran.[121] In the United States, Canada, and Europe, 0.01% to 0.03% of blood donors are infected with HTLV-1. It is most commonly found in individuals who emigrated from endemic regions or among African Americans. HTLV-1 is transmitted sexually, by contaminated cell-associated blood products, or by breast-feeding.[122] Only 2% to 5% of HTLV-1–infected individuals develop disease, and ATLL only occurs in individuals who acquired HTLV-1 by breast-feeding.

## Human T-Cell Leukemia Virus Molecular Biology

HTLV-1, like other retroviruses, encodes Gag, Protease, Pol, and Envelope proteins.[123] Gag proteins compose the inner nucleocapsid core of the virus. The Pol proteins include the reverse transcriptase and integrase. The reverse transcriptase copies the single-stranded viral RNA into double-stranded DNA, and it is inhibited by several nucleoside analogs, but not by the nonnucleoside reverse transcriptase inhibitors approved for HIV-1.[124] The integrase is responsible for inserting the linear double-stranded DNA product of reverse transcription into the host chromosomal DNA. At least one integrase inhibitor, raltegravir, now approved for HIV-1, is active against HTLV-1.[125] Integration occurs throughout the human genome, but there is preference for integration into transcriptionally active genomic regions.[126] The viral protease proteolytically processes Gag, Protease, and Pol precursor proteins to the mature individual proteins, but it is not affected by inhibitors of HIV-1 protease. The envelope proteins include the transmembrane protein, which anchors the surface envelope protein on the virion, which mediates binding to the viral receptor.[127]

The viral genome also encodes regulatory proteins, including Tax and HTLV-1 bZIP factor (HBZ).[117] Tax is a transcriptional transactivator protein that functions as a coactivator to induce members of the cAMP response element-binding protein/activating transcription factor (CREB/ATF) family, nuclear factor kappa B (NF-κB), and serum response factor (SRF) pathways. Tax activation of the CREB/ATF pathway is responsible for upregulation of the viral promoter. Tax induction of NF-κB promotes cell proliferation and resistance to apoptosis. Tax also binds and activates cyclin-dependent kinases and inhibits cell cycle checkpoint proteins. Tax is important for tumor initiation, whereas HBZ may be important in tumor maintenance.[128]

HTLV-1 preferentially immortalizes CD4+ T lymphocytes and induces tumors in mice.[129] Tax also promotes the leukemia-initiating activity of ATLL cells in mouse models.[130] In immunodeficient mice reconstituted with human hematopoietic cells, HTLV-1 causes CD4+ lymphomas.[131]

## Clinical Characteristics and Treatment of HTLV-Associated Malignancies

The diagnosis of HTLV-1 is based on serologic assays.[132] HTLV-1 is associated with various inflammatory disorders, including uveitis, polymyositits, pneumonitis, Sjögren syndrome, and myelopathy. Infected patients are susceptible to certain infectious disorders (e.g. staphylococcal dermatitis) and opportunistic infections such as pneumocystis pneumonia, disseminated cryptococcosis, strongyloidiasis, or toxoplasmosis.[133] Vaccines have not been developed for HTLV infections.

T-lymphocyte proliferative disorders develop in 1% to 5% of infected individuals and are generally CD2+, CD3+, CD4+, CD5+, CD25+, CD29+, CD45RO+, CD52+, HLA-DR+, T-cell receptor αβ+, and variably CD30+, and lack CD7, CD8, and CD26 expression. The virus is clonally integrated in the malignant cells. Complex karyotypes are often found, and cytogenetic analysis is rarely useful. The histologic features of lymph nodes in ATLL may be indistinguishable from those of other peripheral T-cell lymphomas.[134] Circulating tumor "flower cells" are helpful in the diagnosis (Fig. 5.3).

ATLL is categorized in four subtypes.[135] (1) Smoldering ATLL is defined as 5% or more abnormal T lymphocytes and lactate dehydrogenase (LDH) levels up to 1.5× the upper limit of normal, with normal lymphocyte count, calcium, and no lymph node or visceral disease other than skin or pulmonary disease. (2) Chronic ATLL is characterized by lymphocytosis, LDH up to 2× the upper limit of normal, no hypercalcemia, and no CNS, bone, pleural, peritoneal, or gastrointestinal involvement, although the lymph nodes, liver, spleen, skin, or lungs may be involved. The mean survival of these forms of ATLL is 2 to 5 years.[136] No intervention in these subtypes of ATLL has been defined that prevents progression to the more aggressive forms of ATLL. Although chronic or smoldering ATLL may respond to zidovudine and interferon, randomized studies have not been conducted.[137] (3) Lymphoma-type ATLL is characterized by ≤1% abnormal T lymphocytes and features of non-Hodgkin lymphoma. (4) Acute-type ATLL includes the remaining patients. Even with optimal therapy, the median survival of lymphoma and acute-type ATLL is less than 1 year.[138] Lymphoma and acute types of ATLL are the most common presenting subtypes. Other major prognostic factors include performance status, age, the presence of more than three involved lesions, and hypercalcemia.[139]

Combination chemotherapy for lymphoma or acute-type ATLL with the infusional etoposide, prednisone, vincristine, and doxorubicin (EPOCH) regimen or the LSG-15 regimen results in complete remission rates of 15% to 40%.[140,141] However, responses are short lived, with <10% of patients free of disease at 4 years. The addition of anti-CCR4 antibody, mogamulizumab, may improve response rates, but studies are still underway.[142]

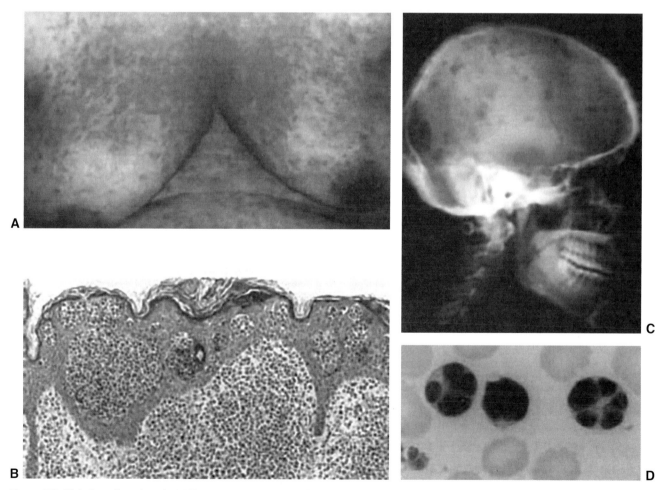

**Figure 5.3** Clinical manifestation of adult T-cell leukemia/lymphoma. **(A–B)** Infiltration of malignant T lymphocytes into the skin. **(C)** Lytic bone lesions seen on lateral skull x-ray. **(D)** "Flower cells" in the blood.

The combination of interferon and zidovudine with or without arsenic may result in the remission of acute, but not lymphoma subtypes.[143] Allogenic transplantation may result in long-term, disease-free survival for patients with complete or near complete remission of disease, although infectious complications have been notable in these studies.[144]

# HEPATITIS VIRUSES

The earliest record of an epidemic caused by a hepatitis virus was in 1885, occurring in individuals vaccinated for smallpox with lymph from other people.[145] The cause of the epidemic, HBV, was not identified until 1966, when Blumberg discovered the *Australian antigen* now known to be the hepatitis B surface antigen (HBsAg). This was followed by the discovery of the virus particle by Dane in 1970. In the early 1980s, the HBV genome was sequenced and the first vaccines were tested. In the mid 1970s, Alter described cases of hepatitis not due to hepatitis A or B viruses, and the suspected agent was designated non-A, non-B hepatitis virus, now known as HCV.[146] In 1987, Houghton used molecular cloning to identify the HCV genome and develop a diagnostic test, which was licensed in 1990.

Approximately 240 million people are chronically infected with HBV and 150 to 200 million people are infected with HCV worldwide, according to the World Health Organization (WHO). About 1 million deaths per year are attributed to the chronic diseases such as liver cirrhosis and hepatocellular carcinoma (HCC) that result from viral hepatitis infections. HBV and HCV are the leading cause of liver cancer in the world, accounting for almost 80% of the cases. In the United States, Europe, Egypt, and Japan, more than 60% of HCC cases are associated with HCV, and 20% are related to HBV and chronic alcoholism.[147] In Africa and Asia, 60% of HCC is associated with HBV, 20% related to HCV, and the remainder related to other risk factors, such as alcohol and aflatoxin. HCC is the sixth most common cancer worldwide and is the third most common cause of cancer death.[148]

In Asia and Africa, up to 70% of individuals have serologic evidence of current or prior HBV infection, and 8% to 15% of these subjects have a chronic active infection. Rates of HCV infection of >3.5% occur in Central and East Asia, North Africa, and the Middle East. In the United States, 0.8 to 1.4 million individuals are infected with HBV, and 3.2 million with HCV. The incidence of HCC in the United States tripled between 1975 and 2005, particularly in African American and Hispanic males.[149]

HBV is transmitted primarily through exposure to infected blood, semen, and other body fluids, whereas HCV is transmitted primarily by contact with contaminated blood. Acute HCV infection causes mild and vague symptoms in about 15% of individuals and resolves spontaneously in 10% to 50% of cases.[150] Liver enzymes are normal in 5% to 50% of individuals with chronic HCV infection.[151] After 20 years of an HCV infection, the likelihood of cirrhosis is 10% to 15% for men, and 1.5% for women.[152] Cofactors that increase the likelihood of cirrhosis are coinfection with both hepatitis viruses, persistently high levels of HBV or HCV viremia, HBeAg, certain viral genotypes, schistosoma, HIV, alcoholism, male gender, advanced age at the time of infection, diabetes, and obesity.[153,154]

## Hepatitis B Virus

HBV is an enveloped DNA virus that is a member of the *Hepadnaviridae* family.[155] HBV has a strong preference for infecting hepatocytes, but small amounts of viral DNA can also be found in kidney, pancreas, and mononuclear cells, although it is not linked to extrahepatic disease. The viral genome is a relaxed circular, partially double-stranded (ds) DNA of 3.2 kb. The genome exists as an episomal covalently closed circular dsDNA (cccDNA)

molecule in the nucleus of infected cells, although chromosomal integration of viral genomic sequences can occur during cycles of hepatocyte regeneration and proliferation. In addition to 40 to 42 nm virions, HBV-infected cells also produce noninfectious 20-nm spherical and filamentous particles. The viral genome encodes four open reading frames. The presurface–surface (preS-S) region encodes three proteins from different translational initiation sites; these include the S (HBsAg), M (or pre-S2), and L (or pre-S1) proteins. The L protein is responsible for receptor binding and virion assembly. The precore–core (preC-C) region encodes the HBcAg and HBeAg. The P region encodes the viral polymerase, and the X (HBx) protein modulates host-signal transduction.

After infection, the viral genome is transcribed by host RNA polymerase II, and viral proteins are translated. Nucleocapsids assemble in the cytosol, incorporating a molecule of pregenomic RNA into the viral core, where reverse transcription occurs to produce the dsDNA viral genome. Viral cores are enveloped with intracellular membranes and viral L, M, and S surface antigens, which are exported from the cells.

HBV replication is not cytotoxic. Instead, liver injury is due to the host immune response, primarily T-cell and proinflammatory cytokine responses. Chronic HBV carriers exhibit an attenuated virus-specific T-cells response, although a vigorous humoral response is still evident. About 5% of infections in adults and up to 90% of infections in neonates result in a persistent infection, which may or may not be associated with symptoms and elevated serum aminotransferase levels. About 20% of such individuals develop cirrhosis. Immunosuppressed individuals also have a higher likelihood of a persistent infection.

With acute infection, viral titers of $10^9$ to $10^{10}$ virions per milliliter are present, whereas levels of $10^7$ to $10^9$ virions per mililiter and HBsAg, and in some cases, HBeAg are present in the blood of individuals with a persistent infection. The resolution of infection, which is associated with declining viral DNA titers, is observed at a rate of 5% to 10% per year in persistently infected individuals. However, even subjects who have resolved the infection continue to have very low levels of viral DNA ($10^3$ to $10^5$ copies per mililiter) for most of their lives.

HBV infection can be managed with alpha interferon or nucleos(t)ide analogs that inhibit the viral polymerase, such as lamivudine, telbivudine, entecavir, adefovir, and tenofovir.[156] Entecavir and tenofovir are both effective at inducing viral suppression, and may be used in combination in patients with high HBV DNA load or multidrug resistance. Because these agents are all associated with some toxicity, current guidelines recommend therapy only when liver disease is clinically apparent, with continued treatment for 6 to 12 months after clearance of HBeAg or HBsAg. Although these drugs effectively control HBV, they typically fail to cure the infection due to the long-term persistence of the cccDNA form of the viral genome. Other nucleos(t)ide analogs are currently in clinical trials, as well as a novel form of interferon (IFN-λ) and an inhibitor of virus release.[157]

Hepatitis D virus (HDV) occurs only in individuals coinfected with HBV. HDV is composed a single-stranded circular viral RNA genome of 1,679 nucleotides, a central core of HDAg, and an outer coat with all three HBV envelope proteins. HDV infection results in more severe complications than infection with HBV alone, with a higher likelihood and more rapid progression to cirrhosis and HCC.

## Hepatits C Virus

HCV is an enveloped RNA virus associated with cancer, primarily HCC and, rarely, splenic marginal zone lymphoma.[158] HCV is a positive-sense, single-stranded RNA virus of the *Flaviviridae* family.[159] There are seven genotypes of HCV; in the United States, about 70% of infections are caused by genotype 1.[160] HCV replicates in the cytoplasm and does not integrate into the host cell genome. The viral RNA is 9.6 kb and encodes a single polyprotein of 3,010 amino acids that is proteolytically processed into structural and nonstructural proteins. In addition to the structural roles of the core (C) protein, it has also been reported to affect various host cell functions. The envelope glycoproteins E1 and E2 mediate infectious entry through tetraspanin CD81 and other receptors on hepatocytes and B lymphocytes.

HCV non structural proteins NS2, NS3, NS4A, NS4B, NS5A, NS5B, and p7 are required for virus replication and assembly. NS2 is a membrane-associated cysteine protease. NS3 is a helicase and NTPase that unwinds RNA and DNA substrates. The complex of NS3 with NS4A forms a serine protease. NS4B induces the formation of a membranous web associated with the viral RNA replicase. NS5A is an RNA-binding phosphoprotein, whereas NS5B is the RNA-dependent RNA polymerase. The p7 protein forms a cation channel in infected cells that has a role in particle maturation and release.

Treating an HCV infection typically utilizes 24 to 48 weeks of pegylated IFN-α and ribavirin.[161] Treatment with IFN and ribavirin alone produces sustained virologic responses in 70% to 80% of subjects with genotype 2 or 3 infections. Recently approved inhibitors of the NS3-4A protease (e.g., telaprevir, boceprevir, or simeprevir) may be included in IFN-based regimens, particularly if the patient has failed prior therapy. Protease inhibitors are currently approved for use in IFN/ribavirin combination therapy for HCV genotype 1 or 4 infection. Sofosbuvir, a nucleoside analog inhibitor of the viral NS5B polymerase, has recently been approved for use in combination with ribavirin alone for genotypes 2 or 3, or in triple therapy for genotypes 1 and 4. Recently, IFN-free regimens have also been approved. Additional protease and polymerase inhibitors are currently in development. A recent meta-analysis of eight randomized controlled trials comparing antiviral therapy with placebo suggested that antiviral therapy resulted in a 50% reduced risk of HCC.[162]

## Hepatitis Virus Pathogenesis

HBV and HCV depress innate immune responses by inhibiting Toll-like receptor signaling through effects of HBx and NS3-4A.[147] In addition, HCV C inhibits the Janus kinase (JAK)-signal transducer and activator of transcription (STAT) signaling, and NS5A and E2 inhibit IFN signaling. Through an undefined mechanism, HBV can inhibit JAK-STAT signaling as well.

HBV and HCV induce HCC by direct and indirect mechanisms.[147] Both HBV and HCV encode proteins that have pro- and antiapoptotic properties. High levels of HBx block activation of the NF-κB pathway, whereas HCV C and NS5A block apoptosis by the activation of AKT and NF-κB, respectively. The C and NS5A proteins may also induce epithelial–mesenchymal transition (EMT), which is important for liver fibrosis, through effects on transforming growth factor β and Src signaling. Mice transgenic for NS5A develop steatosis and HCC.

HBx and HCV C are associated with mitochondria, where they trigger oxidative stress that induces apoptosis. In addition, HBs and HBx and NS3-4A alter calcium signaling and increase reactive oxygen species, which trigger endoplasmic reticulum (ER) stress, an unfolded protein response, and the production of proinflammatory cytokines that induce collagen synthesis, which drives the development of fibrosis. Autophagy is triggered by both viruses to restore ER integrity, which promotes cell survival and viral persistence.

HBV and HCV also disrupt tumor suppressor proteins. HCV NS5B recruits an ubiquitin ligase protein to modify pRB and induce its degradation, whereas HBx and HCV C proteins both inhibit p16INK4a and p21 cell cycle inhibitors, which leads to the inactivating phosphorylation of pRB. The HBx and HCV C, NS3, and NS5A proteins deregulate p53 tumor suppressor activity, by compromising p53-mediated DNA repair. HBV and HCV also induce alterations in micro-RNAs that are partially responsible for cell cycle effects.

Although not part of the normal virus replication cycle, the tendency of HBV genomic DNA sequences to integrate within the host cell chromosomes also contributes to the pathogenesis of HBV-associated HCC. In most hepatoma cells, HBV replication is extinguished, and integration at certain sites provides a growth or survival advantage, leading to tumors that are clonal with respect to viral integration. Whole-genome sequencing studies have identified a number of cellular loci, including *TERT* and *MLL*, where HBV integration is associated with HCC.[163,164]

Both HBV and HCV promote characteristics of cancer stem cells. HBx promotes the expression of Nanog, Kruppel-like factor 4, octamer-binding transcription factor 4, and Myc. These markers are also induced by HBV and HCV-induced hypoxia and hypoxia-induced factors.

## Clinical Characteristics and Treatment of Hepatitis Virus-Associated Malignancies

HBV and HCV infections are diagnosed by serologic assays, and/or antigen assays in the case of HBV.[153] Quantitative HBV DNA and HCV RNA polymerase chain reactions are utilized to measure virus load. No vaccine has been identified that protects against HCV because infections consist of a genetically heterogenous "swarm" of virus particles, some of which escape neutralization. However, a vaccine, which now utilizes a recombinant HBsAg produced in yeast cells, has been available for HBV prevention for more than 30 years. The HBV vaccine reduces the risk of infection by more than 70%.[157] Factors associated with HBV vaccination failure in adults include increased age, obesity, smoking, diabetes, end-stage renal disease, HIV infection, alcoholism, or recipients of liver or kidney transplantation. There have been recent suggestions that emerging HBV strains may be evolving to escape neutralizing antibodies elicited by the current vaccine.[165] Novel vaccine adjuvants are currently in clinical trials, as well as studies of a therapeutic HBV vaccine.

Because an early diagnosis of HCC is key to a successful treatment, there has been extensive research on surveillance techniques in HBV- and HCV-infected individuals.[166] The U.S. Centers for Disease Control and Prevention has recently recommended that all individuals born between 1945 and 1965 be tested for HCV infection. The American Association for the Study of Liver Diseases, as well as the European and Asian Pacific Associations for the Study of the Liver, endorse surveillance in HCV-infected individuals with cirrhosis using ultrasound every 6 months. Viral eradication does not fully eliminate the risk of HCC, and thus, continued surveillance is still recommended in cirrhotic patients.

Therapeutic options for HCC are determined not only by the number and size of HCC nodules as well as the presence or absence of vascular invasion and metastases, but also by liver function and the presence or absence of portal hypertension.[167] HCC amenable to liver transplantation is usually defined as either one tumor measuring ≤50 mm in diameter or two to three tumors measuring ≤30 mm in diameter without vascular extension or metastasis (Milan criteria).[168] Up to 30% of all cases of HCC present with multiple nodules of HCC, suggesting a field carcinogenesis effect of HBV and HCV.[169] HBV- and HCV-infected patients may have a lower survival than noninfected patients after liver transplantation.[170] Hepatitis B immune globulin and nucleos(t)ide analogs are recommended for reinfection prophylaxis in the posttransplant period for HBV-infected individuals.[171] Studies are underway to examine the appropriate use of antiviral therapy for HCV-infected patients undergoing liver transplantation.

Reactivation of HCV can occur with chemotherapy or monoclonal antibody-based immunosuppressive therapies, but is less frequent as compared to HBV infection.[172] Individuals who appear to have cleared an HBV infection and who have an undetectable viral load can experience HBV reactivation on rituximab therapy. Monitoring hepatic function and virus load is indicated during chemoimmunotherapy of HBV- or HCV-positive patients.[173] Although there is controversy regarding the role of virus screening for patients undergoing chemotherapy, antiviral therapy is recommended for high-risk HBV-infected patients undergoing chemoimmunotherapy, such as rituximab-based chemotherapy regimens.[174]

An association between HCV and B-cell non-Hodgkin lymphoma (NHL) has also been demonstrated in highly endemic geographic areas.[175] Lymphoproliferation has been linked to type II mixed cryoglobulinemia in many of these individuals. In addition to diffuse large B-cell lymphoma, marginal zone lymphomas and lymphoplasmacytic lymphomas are the histologic subtypes most frequently associated with HCV infection. Antiviral treatment with IFNα with or without ribavirin has been effective in the treatment of HCV-infected patients with indolent lymphoma, but rarely in individuals with aggressive lymphomas.

## CONCLUSION

Oncogenic viruses are important causes of cancer, especially in less industrialized countries and in immunosuppressed individuals. They are common causes of anogenital cancers, lymphomas, oral and hepatocellular carcinomas and are associated with a variety of other malignancies. Vaccines and antiviral agents play an important role in the prevention of virus-induced cancers. Studies of virus pathogenesis will continue to establish paradigms that are critical to our understanding of cancer etiology in general.

## REFERENCES

1. de Martel C, Ferlay J, Franceschi S, et al. Global burden of cancers attributable to infections in 2008: a review and synthetic analysis. *Lancet Oncol* 2012;13(6):607–615.
2. Schiller JT, Lowy DR. Virus infection and human cancer: an overview. *Recent Results Cancer Res* 2014;193:1–10.
3. Chen CJ, Hsu WL, Yang HI, et al. Epidemiology of virus infection and human cancer. *Recent Results Cancer Res* 2014;193:11–32.
4. Virgin HW, Wherry EJ, Ahmed R. Redefining chronic viral infection. *Cell* 2009;138(1):30–50.
5. Campo MS, O'Neil BW, Barron RJ, et al. Experimental reproduction of the papilloma-carcinoma complex of the alimentary canal in cattle. *Carcinogenesis* 1994;15(8):1597–1601.
6. Khoury JD, Tannir NM, Williams MD, et al. Landscape of DNA virus associations across human malignant cancers: analysis of 3,775 cases using RNA-Seq. *J Virol* 2013;87(16):8916–8926.
7. zur Hausen H, de Villiers EM. TT viruses: oncogenic or tumor-suppressive properties? *Curr Top Microbiol Immunol* 2009;331:109–116.
8. Mizutani T, Sayama Y, Nakanishi A, et al. Novel DNA virus isolated from samples showing endothelial cell necrosis in the Japanese eel, Anguilla japonica. *Virology* 2011;412(1):179–187.
9. Paulson KG, Carter JJ, Johnson LG, et al. Antibodies to merkel cell polyomavirus T antigen oncoproteins reflect tumor burden in merkel cell carcinoma patients. *Cancer Res* 2010;70:8388–8397.
10. International Agency for Research on Cancer (IARC) Working Group. *IARC Monographs on the Evalation of Carcinogenic Risks to Humans. Malaria and Some Polyomaviruses (SV40, BK, JC, and Merkel Cell Viruses)*, Vol. 104. Lyon, France: IARC; 2013.
11. Moore PS, Chang Y. The conundrum of causality in tumor virology: the cases of KSHV and MCV. *Semin Cancer Biol* 2013;26C:4–12.
12. Rigoni-Stern E. Fatti statistici relativi alle malattie cancrose. *Giornale Service Progr Pathol Terap Ser* 1842;2:507–517.
13. Lowy DR. History of papillomavirus research. In: Garcea RL, DiMaio D, eds. *The Papillomaviruses*. New York, NY: Springer; 2007:13–28.
14. zur Hausen H. Herpes simplex virus in human genital cancer. *Int Rev Exp Pathol* 1983;25:307–326.
15. Durst M, Gissmann L, Ikenberg H, et al. A papillomavirus DNA from a cervical carcinoma and its prevalence in cancer biopsy samples from different geographic regions. *Proc Natl Acad Sci U S A* 1983;80(12):3812–3815.
16. Boshart M, Gissmann L, Ikenberg H, et al. A new type of papillomavirus DNA, its presence in genital cancer biopsies and in cell lines derived from cervical cancer. *Embo J* 1984;3(5):1151–1157.
17. Christensen ND. Cottontail rabbit papillomavirus (CRPV) model system to test antiviral and immunotherapeutic strategies. *Antivir Chem Chemother* 2005;16(6):355–362.
18. Rous P, Beard J. The progression to carcinoma of virus induced rabbit papillomas (Shope). *J Exp Med* 1935;62:523–545.
19. Syverton JT, Berry GP. Carcinoma in the cottontail rabbit following spontaneous virus papilloma (Shope). *Proc Soc Exp Biol Med* 1935;33:399–400.
20. de Villiers EM. Cross-roads in the classification of papillomaviruses. *Virology* 2013;445(1–2):2–10.
21. Bosch FX, Broker TR, Forman D, et al. Comprehensive control of human papillomavirus infections and related diseases. *Vaccine* 2013;31 Suppl 8:I1–I31.
22. Van Doorslaer K. Evolution of the papillomaviridae. *Virology* 2013;445(1–2):11–20.
23. Scheffner M, Werness BA, Huibregtse JM, et al. The E6 oncoprotein encoded by human papillomavirus types 16 and 18 promotes the degradation of p53. *Cell* 1990;63(6):1129–1136.
24. Scheffner M, Huibregtse JM, Vierstra RD, Howley PM. The HPV-16 E6 and E6-AP complex functions as a ubiquitin-protein ligase in the ubiquitination of p53. *Cell* 1993;75(3):495–505.
25. Huibregtse JM, Scheffner M, Howley PM. Cloning and expression of the cDNA for E6-AP, a protein that mediates the interaction of the human papillomavirus E6 oncoprotein with p53. *Mol Cell Biol* 1993;13(2):775–784.
26. Klingelhutz AJ, Foster SA, McDougall JK. Telomerase activation by the E6 gene product of human papillomavirus type 16. *Nature* 1996;380(6569):79–82.
27. White EA, Howley PM. Proteomic approaches to the study of papillomavirus-host interactions. *Virology* 2013;435(1):57–69.
28. Dyson N, Howley PM, Munger K, et al. The human papilloma virus-16 E7 oncoprotein is able to bind to the retinoblastoma gene product. *Science* 1989;243(4893):934–937.
29. Munger K, Howley PM. Human papillomavirus immortalization and transformation functions. *Virus Res* 2002;89(2):213–228.
30. Duensing S, Lee LY, Duensing A, et al. The human papillomavirus type 16 E6 and E7 oncoproteins cooperate to induce mitotic defects and genomic instability by uncoupling centrosome duplication from the cell division cycle. *Proc Natl Acad Sci U S A* 2000;97(18):10002–10007.
31. DiMaio D, Petti LM. The E5 proteins. *Virology* 2013;445(1–2):99–114.
32. Schiller JT, Lowy DR. Understanding and learning from the success of prophylactic human papillomavirus vaccines. *Nat Rev Microbiol* 2012;10(10):681–692.
33. Kemp TJ, Safaeian M, Hildesheim A, et al. Kinetic and HPV infection effects on cross-type neutralizing antibody and avidity responses induced by Cervarix((R)). *Vaccine* 2012;31(1):165–170.
34. Haupt RM, Wheeler CM, Brown DR, et al. Impact of an HPV6/11/16/18 L1 virus-like particle vaccine on progression to cervical intraepithelial neoplasia in seropositive women with HPV16/18 infection. *Int J Cancer* 2011;129(11):2632–2642.
35. Kreuter A, Wieland U. Lack of efficacy in treating condyloma acuminata and preventing recurrences with the recombinant quadrivalent human papillomavirus vaccine in a case series of immunocompetent patients. *J Am Acad Dermatol* 2013;68(1):179–180.
36. Joura E, Team V-S, eds. Abstract SS 8–4: Efficacy and immunogenicity of a novel 9-valent HPV L1 virus-like particle vaccine in 16- to 26-year-old women. Paper presented at: Eurogin 2013 International Multidisciplinary Congress; 2013; Florence, Italy.
37. Wang JW, Roden RB. L2, the minor capsid protein of papillomavirus. *Virology* 2013;445(1–2):175–186.
38. Ma B, Maraj B, Tran NP, et al. Emerging human papillomavirus vaccines. *Expert Opin Emerg Drugs* 2012;17(4):469–492.
39. Scudellari M. HPV: sex, cancer and a virus. *Nature* 2013;503(7476):330–332.
40. Gillison ML, Alemany L, Snijders PJ, et al. Human papillomavirus and diseases of the upper airway: head and neck cancer and respiratory papillomatosis. *Vaccine* 2012;30 Suppl 5:F34–54.
41. Silverberg MJ, Leyden W, Warton EM, et al. HIV infection status, immunodeficiency, and the incidence of non-melanoma skin cancer. *J Natl Cancer Inst* 2013;105(5):350–360.
42. Kempf W, Mertz KD, Hofbauer GF, et al. Skin cancer in organ transplant recipients. *Pathobiology* 2013;80(6):302–309.
43. Wallace NA, Gasior SL, Faber ZJ, et al. HPV 5 and 8 E6 expression reduces ATM protein levels and attenuates LINE-1 retrotposition. *Virology* 2013;443(1):69–79.
44. White EA, Kramer RE, Tan MJ, et al. Comprehensive analysis of host cellular interactions with human papillomavirus E6 proteins identifies new E6 binding partners and reflects viral diversity. *J Virol* 2012;86(24):13174–13186.
45. White EA, Sowa ME, Tan MJ, et al. Systematic identification of interactions between host cell proteins and E7 oncoproteins from diverse human papillomaviruses. *Proc Natl Acad Sci U S A* 2012;109(5):E260–267.
46. Caldeira S, Zehbe I, Accardi R, et al. The E6 and E7 proteins of the cutaneous human papillomavirus type 38 display transforming properties. *J Virol* 2003;77(3):2195–2206.
47. Arron ST, Ruby JG, Dybbro E, et al. Transcriptome sequencing demonstrates that human papillomavirus is not active in cutaneous squamous cell carcinoma. *J Invest Dermatol* 2011;131(8):1745–1753.
48. Gross L. A filterable agent, recovered from Ak leukemic extracts, causing salivary gland carcinomas in C3H mice. *Proc Soc Exp Biol Med* 1953;83(2):414–421.

49. Eddy BE, Stewart SE. Characteristics of the SE polyoma virus. *Am J Public Health Nations Health* 1959;49:1486–1492.

50. Sweet BH, Hilleman MR. The vacuolating virus, S.V. 40. *Proc Soc Exp Biol Med* 1960;105:420–427.

51. Eddy BE, Borman GS, Grubbs GE, et al. Identification of the oncogenic substance in rhesus monkey kidney cell culture as simian virus 40. *Virology* 1962;17:65–75.

52. Dang-Tan T, Mahmud SM, Puntoni R, et al. Polio vaccines, simian virus 40, and human cancer: the epidemiologic evidence for a causal association. *Oncogene* 2004;23(38):6535–6540.

53. Bouvard V, Baan RA, Grosse Y, et al. Carcinogenicity of malaria and of some polyomaviruses. *Lancet Oncol* 2012;13(4):339–340.

54. Gardner SD, Field AM, Coleman DV, et al. New human papovavirus (B.K.) isolated from urine after renal transplantation. *Lancet.*1971;1(7712): 1253–1257.

55. Padgett BL, Walker DL, ZuRhein GM, et al. Cultivation of papova-like virus from human brain with progressive multifocal leucoencephalopathy. *Lancet* 1971;1(7712):1257–1260.

56. Das D, Wojno K, Imperiale MJ. BK virus as a cofactor in the etiology of prostate cancer in its early stages. *J Virol* 2008;82(6):2705–2714.

57. Akgul B, Pfister D, Knuchel R, et al. No evidence for a role of xenotropic murine leukaemia virus-related virus and BK virus in prostate cancer of German patients. *Med Microbiol Immunol* 2012;201(2):245–248.

58. Alexiev BA, Randhawa P, Vazquez Martul E, et al. BK virus-associated urinary bladder carcinoma in transplant recipients: report of 2 cases, review of the literature, and proposed pathogenetic model. *Human Pathol* 2013;44(5):908–917.

59. Abend JR, Jiang M, Imperiale MJ. BK virus and human cancer: innocent until proven guilty. *Semin Cancer Biol* 2009;19(4):252–260.

60. Maginnis MS, Atwood WJ. JC virus: an oncogenic virus in animals and humans? *Semin Cancer Biol* 2009;19(4):261–269.

61. Feng H, Shuda M, Chang Y, et al. Clonal integration of a polyomavirus in human Merkel cell carcinoma. *Science* 2008;319(5866):1096–1100.

62. Hodgson NC. Merkel cell carcinoma: changing incidence trends. *J Surg Oncol* 2005;89(1):1–4.

63. Engels EA, Frisch M, Goedert JJ, et al. Merkel cell carcinoma and HIV infection. *Lancet* 2002;359(9305):497–498.

64. Zur Hausen A, Rennspiess D, Winnepenninckx V, et al. Early B-cell differentiation in Merkel cell carcinomas: clues to cellular ancestry. *Cancer Res* 2013;73(16):4982–4987.

65. Guastafierro A, Feng H, Thant M, et al. Characterization of an early passage Merkel cell polyomavirus-positive Merkel cell carcinoma cell line, MS-1, and its growth in NOD scid gamma mice. *J Virol Methods* 2013;187(1):6–14.

66. Schowalter RM, Pastrana DV, Pumphrey KA, et al. Merkel cell polyomavirus and two previously unknown polyomaviruses are chronically shed from human skin. *Cell Host Microbe* 2010;7(6):509–515.

67. Faust H, Pastrana DV, Buck CB, et al. Antibodies to Merkel cell polyomavirus correlate to presence of viral DNA in the skin. *J Infect Dis* 2011;203(8):1096–1100.

68. Pastrana DV, Wieland U, Silling S, et al. Positive correlation between Merkel cell polyomavirus viral load and capsid-specific antibody titer. *Med Microbiol Immunol* 2011;201(1):17–23.

69. Pastrana DV, Tolstov YL, Becker JC, et al. Quantitation of human seroresponsiveness to Merkel cell polyomavirus. *PLoS Pathog* 2009;5(9):e1000578.

70. Faust H, Andersson K, Ekstrom J, et al. Prospective study of Merkel cell polyomavirus and risk of Merkel cell carcinoma. *Int J Cancer* 2014;134(4):844–848.

71. Cheng J, Rozenblatt-Rosen O, Paulson KG, et al. Merkel cell polyomavirus large T antigen has growth-promoting and inhibitory activities. *J Virol* 2013;87(11):6118–6126.

72. Li J, Wang X, Diaz J, et al. Merkel cell polyomavirus large T antigen disrupts host genomic integrity and inhibits cellular proliferation. *J Virol* 2013;87(16):9173–9188.

73. Houben R, Shuda M, Weinkam R, et al. Merkel cell polyomavirus-infected Merkel cell carcinoma cells require expression of viral T antigens. *J Virol* 2010;84(14):7064–7072.

74. Houben R, Grimm J, Willmes C, et al. Merkel cell carcinoma and Merkel cell carcinoma polyomavirus: evidence for hit-and-run oncogenesis. *J Invest Dermatol* 2012;132(1):254–256.

75. Shuda M, Chang Y, Moore PS. Merkel cell polyomavirus positive Merkel cell carcinoma requires viral small T antigen for cell proliferation. *J Invest Dermatol* 2013 [Epub ahead of print].

76. Paulson KG, Iyer JG, Tegeder AR, et al. Transcriptome-wide studies of merkel cell carcinoma and validation of intratumoral CD8+ lymphocyte invasion as an independent predictor of survival. *J Clin Oncol* 2011;29(12):1539–1546.

77. Arora R, Shuda M, Guastafierro A, et al. Survivin is a therapeutic target in Merkel cell carcinoma. *Sci Transl Med* 2012;4(133):133ra56.

78. Dresang LR, Guastafierro A, Arora R, et al. Response of merkel cell polyomavirus-positive merkel cell carcinoma xenografts to a survivin inhibitor. *PloS One* 2013;8(11):e80543.

79. Shuda M, Kwun HJ, Feng H, et al. Human Merkel cell polyomavirus small T antigen is an oncoprotein targeting the 4E-BP1 translation regulator. *J Clin Invest* 2011;121(9):3623–3634.

80. Howard RA, Dores GM, Curtis RE, et al. Merkel cell carcinoma and multiple primary cancers. *Cancer Epidemiol Biomarkers Prev* 2006;15(8): 1545–1549.

81. Pantulu ND, Pallasch CP, Kurz AK, et al. Detection of a novel truncating Merkel cell polyomavirus large T antigen deletion in chronic lymphocytic leukemia cells. *Blood* 2010;116(24):5280–5284.

82. Tolstov YL, Arora R, Scudiere SC, et al. Lack of evidence for direct involvement of Merkel cell polyomavirus (MCV) in chronic lymphocytic leukemia (CLL). *Blood* 2010;115(23):4973–4974.

83. Cimino PJ, Jr., Bahler DW, Duncavage EJ. Detection of Merkel cell polyomavirus in chronic lymphocytic leukemia T-cells. *Exp Mol Pathol* 2013;94(1):40–44.

84. Burkitt D. A sarcoma involving the jaws in African children. *Br J Surg* 1958;46(197):218–223.

85. Epstein MA, Achong BG, Barr YM. Virus particles in cultured lymphoblasts from Burkitt's lymphoma. *Lancet* 1964;1(7335):702–703.

86. Henle G, Henle W, Diehl V. Relation of Burkitt's tumor-associated herpesytpe virus to infectious mononucleosis. *Proc Natl Acad Sci U S A* 1968;59(1): 94–101.

87. Longnecker RM, Kieff E, Cohen JI. Epstein-Barr virus. In: Knipe DM, Howley PM, eds. *Fields Virology*. 6th ed. Philadelphia, PA: Lippincott Williams & Wilkins; 2013.

88. Cesarman E. Gammaherpesviruses and lymphoproliferative disorders. *Annu Rev Pathol* 2014;9:349–372.

89. Shannon-Lowe C, Rowe M. Epstein-Barr virus infection of polarized epithelial cells via the basolateral surface by memory B cell-mediated transfer infection. *PLoS Pathog* 2011;7(5):e1001338.

90. Faulkner GC, Burrows SR, Khanna R, et al. X-Linked agammaglobulinemia patients are not infected with Epstein-Barr virus: implications for the biology of the virus. *J Virol* 1999;73(2):1555–1564.

91. Hjalgrim H, Smedby KE, Rostgaard K, et al. Infectious mononucleosis, childhood social environment, and risk of Hodgkin lymphoma. *Cancer Res* 2007;67(5):2382–2388.

92. Barton ES, White DW, Cathelyn JS, et al. Herpesvirus latency confers symbiotic protection from bacterial infection. *Nature* 2007;447(7142):326–329.

93. Giulino-Roth L, Cesarman E. Molecular biology of Burkitt lymphoma. In: Robertson E, ed. *Burkitt's Lymphoma*. New York, NY: Springer; 2013: 211–226.

94. Chang ET, Adami HO. The enigmatic epidemiology of nasopharyngeal carcinoma. *Cancer Epidemiol Biomarkers Prev* 2006;15(10):1765–1777.

95. Murukesan V, Mukherjee S. Managing post-transplant lymphoproliferative disorders in solid-organ transplant recipients: a review of immunosuppressant regimens. *Drugs* 2012;72(12):1631–1643.

96. Cohen JI, Mocarski ES, Raab-Traub N, et al. The need and challenges for development of an Epstein-Barr virus vaccine. *Vaccine* 2013;31(Suppl 2): B194–196.

97. Choquet S, Leblond V, Herbrecht R, et al. Efficacy and safety of rituximab in B-cell post-transplantation lymphoproliferative disorders: results of a prospective multicenter phase 2 study. *Blood* 2006;107(8):3053–3057.

98. Barnes JA, Lacasce AS, Feng Y, et al. Evaluation of the addition of rituximab to CODOX-M/IVAC for Burkitt's lymphoma: a retrospective analysis. *Ann Oncol* 2011;22(8):1859–1864.

99. Kaposi M. Idiopathisches multiples Pigmentsarkom der Haut. *Archiv für Dermatologie und Syphilis* 1872;4(2):265–273.

100. Antman K, Chang Y. Kaposi's sarcoma. *N Engl J Med* 2000;342(14):1027–1038.

101. Beral V, Peterman TA, Berkelman RL, et al. Kaposi's sarcoma among persons with AIDS: a sexually transmitted infection? *Lancet* 1990;335(8682):123–128.

102. Chang Y, Cesarman E, Pessin MS, et al. Identification of herpesvirus-like DNA sequences in AIDS-associated Kaposi's sarcoma. *Science* 1994;266(5192): 1865–1869.

103. Damania BA, Cesarman E. Kaposi's sarcoma-associated herpesvirus. In: Knipe DM, Howley PM, eds. *Fields Virology*. 6th ed. Philadelphia, PA: Lippincott Williams & Wilkins; 2013.

104. Cook-Mozaffari P, Newton R, Beral V, et al. The geographical distribution of Kaposi's sarcoma and of lymphomas in Africa before the AIDS epidemic. *Br J Cancer* 1998;78(11):1521–1528.

105. Martin DF, Kuppermann BD, Wolitz RA, et al. Oral ganciclovir for patients with cytomegalovirus retinitis treated with a ganciclovir implant. Roche Ganciclovir Study Group. *N Engl J Med* 1999;340(14):1063–1070.

106. Krown SE, Dittmer DP, Cesarman E. Pilot study of oral valganciclovir therapy in patients with classic Kaposi's sarcoma. *J Infect Dis* 2011;203(8):1082–1086.

107. Sakakibara S, Tosato G. Regulation of angiogenesis in malignancies associated with Epstein-Barr virus and Kaposi's sarcoma-associated herpes virus. *Future Microbiol* 2009;4(7):903–917.

108. Soulier J, Grollet L, Oksenhendler E, et al. Kaposi's sarcoma-associated herpesvirus-like DNA sequences in multicentric Castleman's disease. *Blood* 1995;86(4):1276–1280.

109. Polizzotto MN, Uldrick TS, Wang V, et al. Human and viral interleukin-6 and other cytokines in Kaposi sarcoma herpesvirus-associated multicentric Castleman disease. *Blood* 2013;122(26):4189–4198.

110. Simonelli C, Spina M, Cinelli R, et al. Clinical features and outcome of primary effusion lymphoma in HIV-infected patients: a single-institution study. *J Clin Oncol* 2003;21(21):3948–3954.

111. Coffin JM, Hughes SH, Varmus HE, eds. The interactions of retroviruses and their hosts. *Retroviruses*. Cold Spring Harbor, NY: Cold Spring Harbor Laboratory Press; 1997.

112. Gallo RC. History of the discovery of the first human retroviruses: HTLV-1 and HTLV-2. *Oncogene* 2005;24:5926–5930.

113. Smit AF, Riggs AD. Tiggers and DNA transposon fossils in the human genome. *Proc Natl Acad Sci U S A* 1996;93:1443–1448.

114. Delviks-Frankenberry K, Paprotka T, Cingöz O, et al. Generation of multiple replication-competent retroviruses through recombination between PreXMRV-1 and PreXMRV-2. *J Virol* 2013;87:11525–11537.

115. Mason AL, Zhang G. Linking human beta retrovirus infection with primary biliary cirrhosis. *Gastroenterol Clin Biol* 2010;34:359–366.

116. Hacein-Bey-Abina S, VonKalle C, Schmidt M, et al. LMO2-associated clonal T cell proliferation in two patients after gene therapy for SCID-X1. *Science* 2003;302:415–419.

117. Matsuoka M, Jeang K-T. Human T-cell leukaemia virus type 1 (HTLV-1) infectivity and cellular transformation. *Nat Rev Cancer* 2007;7:270–280.

118. Poiesz BJ, Ruscetti FW, Mier JW, et al. T-cell lines established from human T-lymphocytic neoplasias by direct response to T-cell growth factor. *Proc Natl Acad Sci U S A* 1980;77:6815–6819.

119. Kalyanaraman VS, Sarngadharan MG, Robert-Guroff M, et al. A new subtype of human T-cell leukemia virus (HTLV-II) associated with a T-cell variant of hairy cell leukemia. *Science* 1982;218:571–573.

120. Wolfe ND, Heneine W, Carr JK, et al. Emergence of unique primate T-lymphotropic viruses among central African bushmeat hunters. *Proc Natl Acad Sci U S A* 2005;102:7994–7999.

121. Goncalves DU, Proietti FA, Ribas JGR, et al. Epidemiology, treatment, and prevention of human T-cell leukemia virus type 1-associated diseases. *Clin Microbiol Rev* 2010;23:577–589.

122. Hino S, Sugiyama H, Doi H, et al. Breaking the cycle of HTLV-1 transmission via carrier mothers' milk. *Lancet Oncol* 1987;2:158–159.

123. Kannian P, Green PL. Human T lymphotropic virus type 1 (HTLV-1): molecular biology and oncogenesis. *Viruses* 2010;2:2037–2077.

124. Hill SA, Lloyd PA, McDonald S, et al. Susceptibility of human T cell leukemia virus type I to nucleoside reverse transcriptase inhibitors. *J Infec Dis* 2003;188:424–427.

125. Seegulam ME, Ratner L. Integrase inhibitors effective against human T-cell leukemia virus type 1. *Antimicrob Agents Chemother* 2011;55:2011–2017.

126. Derse D, Crise B, Li Y, et al. Human T-cell leukemia virus type 1 integration target sites in the human genome: comparison with those of other retroviruses. *J Virol* 2007;81:6731–6741.

127. Jones KS, Lambert S, Bouttier M, et al. Molecular aspects of HTLV-1 entry: functional domains of the HTLV-1 surface subunit (SU) and their relationships to the entry receptors. *Viruses* 2011;3:794–810.

128. Matsuoka M, Green PL. The HBZ gene, a key player in HTLV-1 pathogenesis. *Retrovirology* 2009;6:71.

129. Grossman WJ, Kimata JT, Wong FH, et al. Development of leukemia in mice transgenic for the tax gene of human T-cell leukemia virus type I. *Proc Natl Acad Sci U S A* 1995;92:1057–1061.

130. El Hajj H, El-Sabban M, Hasegawa H, et al. Therapy-induced selective loss of leukemia-initiating activity in murine adult T cell leukemia. *J Exp Med* 2010;207:2785–2792.

131. Villaudy J, Wencker M, Gadot N, et al. HTLV-1 propels thymic human T cell development in "human immune system" Rag2-/-IL-2Rgammac-/- mice. *PLoS Pathog* 2011;7:e1002231.

132. Costa EAS, Magri MC, Caterino-de-Arujo A. The best algorithm to confirm the diagnosis of HTLV-1 and HTLV-2 in at-risk individuals from Sao Paulo, Brazil. *J Virol Methods* 2011;173:280–286.

133. Barros N, Woll F, Watanabe L, et al. Are increased Foxp3+ regulatory T cells responsible for immunosuppression during HTLV-1 infection? Case reports and review of the literature. *BMJ Case Rep* 2012;bcr2012006574.

134. Cook LB, Rowan AG, Melamed A, et al. HTLV-1-infected T cells contain a single integrated provirus in natural infection. *Blood* 2012;120:3488–3490.

135. Shimoyama M. Diagnostic criteria and classification of clinical subtypes of adult T-cell leukemia-lymphoma: a report from the Lymphoma Study Group. *Br J Hematol* 1991;79:426–437.

136. Takasaki Y, Iwanaga M, Imaizumi Y, et al. Long-term study of indolent adult T-cell leukemia-lymphoma. *Blood* 2010;115:4337–4343.

137. Bazarbachi A, Plumelle Y, Ramos JC, et al. Meta-analysis on the use of zidovudine and interferon-alfa in adult T-cell leukemia/lymphoma showing improved survival in the leukemic subtypes. *J Clin Oncol* 2010;28:4177–4183.

138. Katsuya H, Yamanka T, Ishitsuka K, et al. Prognostic index for acute- and lymphoma-type adult T-cell leukemia/lymphoma. *J Clin Oncol* 2012;30:1635–1640.

139. Tsukasaki K, Hermine O, Bazarbachi A, et al. Definition, prognostic factors, treatment, and reponse criteria of adult T-cell leukemia-lymphoma: a proposal from an international consensus meeting. *J Clin Oncol* 2009;27:453–459.

140. Yamada Y, Tomonaga M, Fukuda H, et al. A new G-CSF supported combination chemotherapy, LSG15, for adult T-cell leukaemia-lymphoma: Japan Clinical Oncology Group Study 9303. *Br J Hematol* 2001;113:375–382.

141. Ratner L, Harrington W, Feng X, et al. Human T cell leukemia virus reactivation with progression of adult T-cell leukemia-lymphoma. *PLoS One* 2009;4:e4420.

142. Tatsuro J, Ishida T, Takemoto S, et al., eds. Randomized phase II study of mogamulizumab (KW-0761) plus VCAP-AMP-VECP (mLSG15) versus mLSG15 alone for newly diagnosed aggressive adult T-cell leukemia-lymphoma (ATL). Paper presented at: 2013 ASCO Annual Meeting; 2013; Chicago, IL.

143. Bazarbachi A, Suarez F, Fields P, et al. How I treat adult T-cell leukemia/lymphoma. *Blood* 2011;118:1736–1745.

144. Utsonomiya A, Miyazaki Y, Takasuka Y, et al. Improved outcome of adult T cell leukemia/lymphoma with allogeneic hematopoietic stem cell transplanation. *Bone Marrow Transplant* 2001;27:15–20.

145. Blumberg BS. The discovery of the hepatitis B virus and the intervention of the vaccine: a scientific memoir. *J Gastroenterol Hepatol* 2002;17(Supplement s4):S502–S503.

146. Houghton M. Discovery of the hepatitis C virus. *Liver Int* 2009;29(Supplement 1):82–88.

147. Arzumanyan A, Reis HM, Feitelson MA. Pathogenic mechanisms in HBV- and HCV-associated hepatocellular carcinoma. *Nat Rev Cancer* 2013;13:123–135.

148. Soerjomataram I, Lortet-Tieulent J, Parkin DM, et al. Global burden of cancer in 2008: a systematic analysis of disability-adjusted life-years in 12 world regions. *Lancet* 2012;380:1840–1850.

149. Altekruse SF, McGlynn KA, Reichman ME. Hepatocellular carcinoma incidence, mortality, and survival trends in the United States from 1975 to 2005. *J Clin Oncol* 2009;27:1485–1491.

150. Shiffman ML, ed. *Chronic Hepatitis C Virus: Advances in Treatment, Promise for the Future*. New York: Springer Verlag; 2011.

151. Nicot F, Nassim K, Lionel R, et al. Occult hepatitis C virus infection: Where are we now? *Liver Biopsy in Modern Med* 2004;307–334.

152. Freeman AJ, Dore GJ, Law MG, et al. Estimating progression to cirrhosis in chronic hepatitis C virus infection. *Hepatology* 2001;34:809–816.

153. Wilkins T, Malcom JK, Raina D, et al. Hepatitis C: diagnosis and treatment. *Am Fam Physician* 2010;81:1351–1357.

154. Fallot G, Neuveut C, Buendia M-A. Diverse roles of hepatitis B virus in liver cancer. *Curr Opin Virol* 2012;2:467–473.

155. Ganem D, Prince AM. Hepatitis B virus infection - natural history and clinical consequences. *N Engl J Med* 2004;350:1118–1129.

156. Tujios SR, Lee WM. Update in the management of chronic hepatitis B. *Curr Opin Gastroenterol* 2013;29:250–256.

157. Seto W-K, Fung J, Yuen M-F, et al. Future prevention and treatment of chronic hepatitis B infection. *J Clin Gastroenterol* 2012;46:725–734.

158. Wang WK, Levy S. Hepatitis C virus (HCV) and lymphomagenesis. *Leuk Lymphoma* 2003;44:1113–1120.

159. Fernandez-Garcia M-D, Mazzon M, Jacobs M, et al. Pathogenesis of flavivirus infections: using and abusing the host cell. *Cell Host Microbe* 2009;318:318–328.

160. Moradpour D, Penin F, Rice CM. Replication of hepatitis c virus. *Nat Rev Microbiol* 2007;5:453–463.

161. Liang TJ, Ghany MG. Current and future therapies for hepatitis C virus infection. *N Engl J Med* 2013;368:1907–1917.

162. Kimer N, Dahl EK, Gluud LL, et al. Antiviral therapy for prevention of hepatocellular carcinoma in chronic hepatitis C: systematic review and meta-analysis of randomised controlled trials. *BMJ Open* 2012;2:e001313.

163. Fujimoto A, Totoki Y, Abe T, et al. Whole-genome sequencing of liver cancers identifies etiological influences on mutation patterns and recurrent mutations in chromatin regulators. *Nat Genet* 2012;44:760–764.

164. Sung WK, Zheng H, Li S, et al. Genome-wide survey of recurrent HBV integration in hepatocellular carcinoma. *Nat Genet* 2012;44:765–769.

165. Devi U, Locarnini S. Hepatitis B antivirals and resistance. *Curr Opin Virol* 2013;3:495–500.

166. Aghemo A, Colombo M. Hepatocellular carcinoma in chronic hepatitis C: from bench to bedside. *Semin Immunopathol* 2013;35:111–120.

167. Bruix J, Sherman M. Management of hepatocellular carcinoma: an update. *Hepatology* 2011;53:1020–1022.

168. Mazzaferro V, Regalia E, Doci R, et al. Liver transplantation for the treatment of small hepatocellular carcinomas in patients with cirrhosis. *N Engl J Med* 1996;334:693–699.

169. Mino M, Lauwers GY. Pathologic spectrum and prognostic significance of underlying liver disease in hepatocellular carcinoma. *Surg Oncol Clin N Am* 2003;12:13–24.

170. Burton JR, Everson GT. Management of the transplant recipient with chronic hepatitis C. *Clin Liver Dis* 2013;17:73–91.

171. Beckebaum S, Kabar I, Cicinnati VR. Hepatitis B and C in liver transplantation: new strategies to combat the enemies. *Rev Med Virol* 2012;23:172–193.

172. Torres HA, Davila M. Reactivation of hepatitis B virus and hepatitis C virus in patients with cancer. *Nat Rev Clin Oncol* 2012;9:156–166.

173. Huang Y-H, Hsaio L-T, Hong Y-C, et al. Randomized controlled trial of entecavir prophylaxis for rituximab-associated hepatitis B virus reactivation in patients with lymhoma and resolved hepatitis. *J Clin Oncol* 2013;31:2765–2772.

174. Artz AS, Somerfield MR, Feld JJ, et al. American Society of Clinical Oncology provisional clinical opinion: chronic hepatitis B virus infection screening in patients receiving cytotoxic chemotherapy for treatment of malignant diseases. *J Clin Oncol* 2010;28:3199–3202.

175. Forghieri F, Luppi M, Barozzi P, et al. Pathogenetic mechanisms of hepatitits C virus-induced B-cell lymphomagenesis. *Clin Dev Immunol* 2012;2012:807351.

**ETIOLOGY AND EPIDEMIOLOGY OF CANCER**

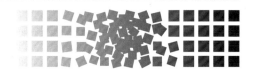

# 6 Inflammation

Sahdeo Prasad and Bharat B. Aggarwal

## INTRODUCTION

Extensive research over the last half a century indicates that inflammation plays an important role in cancer. Although acute inflammation can play a therapeutic role, low-level chronic inflammation can promote cancer. Different inflammatory cells, the various cell signaling pathways that lead to inflammation, and biomarkers of inflammation have now been well defined. These inflammatory pathways, which are primarily mediated through the transcription factors nuclear factor kappa B (NF-κB) and signal transducer and activator of transcription 3 (STAT3), have been linked to cellular transformation, tumor survival, proliferation, invasion, angiogenesis, and metastasis of cancer. These pathways have also now been linked with chemoresistance and radioresistance. This chapter considers the role of inflammation in cancer and its potential for cancer prevention and treatment.

Inflammation is the complex biologic responses of the body to irritation, injury, or infection. The recognition of inflammation dates back to antiquity. As documented by Aulus Cornelius Celsus, a Roman of the 1st century AD, inflammation is characterized by the tissue response to injury that results in *rubor* (redness, due to hyperemia), *tumor* (swelling, caused by increased permeability of the microvasculature and leakage of protein into the interstitial space), *calor* (heat, associated with increased blood flow and the metabolic activity of the cellular mediators of inflammation), and *dolor* (pain, in part due to changes in the perivasculature and associated nerve endings). Rudolf Virchow subsequently added *functio laesa* (dysfunction of the organs involved) in the 1850s. The process includes increased blood flow with an influx of white blood cells and other chemical substances that facilitate healing. Inflammation is also considered the body's self-protective attempt to remove harmful stimuli, including damaged cells, irritants, or pathogens, and to begin the healing process.

The word inflammation is derived from the Latin *inflammo* (meaning "I set alight, I ignite"). Because inflammation is a stereotyped response, it is considered a mechanism of innate immunity, as compared with adaptive immunity. On the basis of longevity, inflammation is classified as acute or chronic. When inflammation is short term, usually appearing within a few minutes or hours and ceasing upon the removal of the injurious stimulus, it is called acute. However, if it persists longer, it is called chronic inflammation, which leads to simultaneous destruction from the inflammatory process. Inflammation is beneficial when it is acute; however, chronic inflammation leads to several diseases, including cancer. Cancer is primarily a disease of lifestyle, with 30% of all cancers having been linked to smoking, 35% to diet, 14% to 20% to obesity, 18% to infection, and 7% to environmental pollution and radiation (Fig. 6.1).[1] Smoking, obesity, infections, pollution, and radiation are all known to activate proinflammatory pathways.[2] Therefore, understanding how inflammation contributes to cancer etiology is important for both cancer prevention and treatment.[3]

## MOLECULAR BASIS OF INFLAMMATION

Although it is clear that inflammation and cancer are closely related, the mechanisms underlying persistent and chronic inflammation in chronic diseases remain unclear. Numerous cytokines have been linked with inflammation, including tumor necrosis factor (TNF), interleukin (IL)-1, IL-6, IL-8, IL-17, and vascular endothelial growth factor (VEGF). Among various cytokines that have been linked with inflammation, TNF is a primary mediator of inflammation linked to cancer.[4] However, it has been shown that proinflammatory transcriptional factors (activator protein [AP]-1, STAT3, NF-κB, hypoxia-inducible factor [HIF]-1, and β-catenin/Wnt) are ubiquitously expressed and control numerous physiologic processes, including development, differentiation, immunity, and metabolism in chronic diseases. Although these transcription factors are regulated by completely different signaling mechanisms, they are activated in response to various stimuli, including stresses and cytokines, and are involved in inflammation-induced tumor development and its metastasis.[5] Interestingly, inflammation plays a role at all stages of tumor development: initiation, progression, and metastasis.[2] In initiation, inflammation induces the release of a variety of cytokines and chemokines that promote the release of inflammatory cells and associated factors. This further causes oxidative damage, DNA mutations, and other changes in the tissue microenvironment, making it more conducive to cell transformation, increased survival, and proliferation. Inflammation also contributes to tissue injury, remodeling of the extracellular matrix, angiogenesis, and fibrosis in diverse target tissues. Among all the inflammatory cell signaling pathways, NF-κB has been shown to play a major role in cancer,[6,7] and TNF is one of the most potent activators of NF-κB.[8,9]

## ROLE OF INFLAMMATION IN TRANSFORMATION

Transformation is the process by which the cellular and molecular makeup of a cell is altered as it becomes malignant. Numerous factors are involved in the process of cell transformation, including inflammation. A clinical study has shown that chronic inflammation due to heavy metal deposition in lymph nodes leads to malignant transformation and, finally, to patient death.[10] More recently, chronic exposure to cigarette smoke extract[11] and arsenite[12] has been shown to induce inflammation followed by epithelial–mesenchymal transition and transformation of human bronchial epithelial (HBE) cells. Furthermore, activation of NF-κB and HIF-2α increased the levels of the proinflammatory IL-6, IL-8, and IL-1β, which are essential for the malignant progression of transformed HBE cells. Sox2, another important molecular factor, cooperates with inflammation-mediated STAT3 activation, which precedes the malignant transformation of foregut basal progenitor cells.[13] A clinical study reported that the p53 mutation is a critical event for the malignant transformation of sinonasal inverted papilloma. This p53 mutation resulted in cyclooxygenase (COX)-2–mediated inflammatory signals that contribute to the proliferation

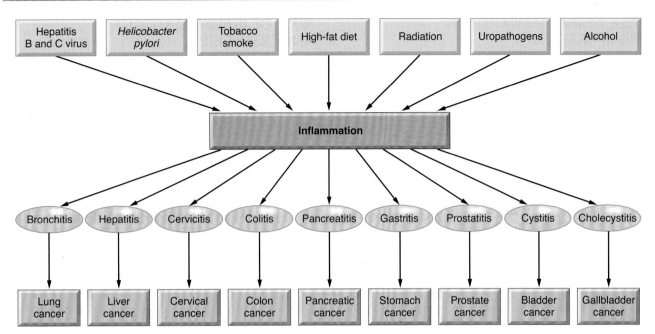

**Figure 6.1** Origin of inflammation and its role in various cancers.

of advanced sinonasal inverted papilloma.[14] In another study in patients, the YKL-40 protein was found to be involved in chronic inflammation and oncogenic transformation of human breast tissues.[15] Inflammation-mediated transformation was also found to be regulated by MyD88 in a mouse model through Ras signaling.[16] In addition, inflammation contributed to the activation of the epidermal growth factor receptor (EGFR) and its subsequent interaction with PKCδ, which leads to the transformation of normal esophageal epithelia to squamous cell carcinoma.[17] Activation of Src oncoprotein triggers an inflammatory response mediated by NF-κB that directly activates Lin28 transcription and rapidly reduces let-7 microRNA levels. The inflammatory cytokine IL-6 mediates the activation of STAT3 transcription factor, which results in the transformation of cells.[18]

## ROLE OF INFLAMMATION IN SURVIVAL

Numerous findings across different cancer populations have suggested that inflammation has an important role in carcinogenesis and disease progression.[19,20] The important markers of systemic inflammatory response in both in vitro findings and clinical outcomes include plasma C-reactive protein (CRP) concentration,[21,22] hypoalbuminemia,[23] and the Glasgow Prognostic Score (GPS), which combines CRP and albumin.[24,25] In addition to these, hematologic markers of systemic inflammatory response such as absolute white-cell count or its components (neutrophils, neutrophil-to-lymphocyte ratio [NLR]),[26–28] platelets, and a platelet-to-lymphocyte ratio[29,30] are also prognostic indicators for cancer clinical outcomes. Whether these inflammatory biomarkers influence the survival of cancer patients is discussed in this section.

In a study of 416 patients with renal cell carcinoma, with 362 patients included in the analysis, elevated neutrophil count, elevated platelet counts, and a high NLR were found. This inflammatory response was predictive for shorter overall patient survival.[31] Another study in unresectable malignant biliary obstruction (UMBO) found that patients with low GPS (0 and 1) had better postoperative survivals than did patients with a higher GPS. The 6-month and 1-year survival rates were 58.1% to 27.3%, respectively, for patients with low GPS and 25% to 6.2%, respectively, for patients with a higher GPS.[32] It has been also shown that prostate

cancer patients with aggressive, clinically significant disease and an elevated GPS[2] had a higher risk of death overall as well as high-grade disease.[33] Other than GPS, age and gastrectomy have also been shown to independently influence the disease-specific and progression-free survival of gastric cancer patients.[34] A biomarker of systemic inflammation, the blood NLR, predicted patient survival with hepatocellular carcinoma (HCC) after transarterial chemoembolization. Patients in whom the NLR remained stable or became normalized after transarterial chemoembolization showed improved overall survival compared with patients showing a persistently abnormal index of NLR.[35]

A further study found that inflammatory transcription factors and cytokines contribute to the overall survival of patients. One study found that 97% of patients with epithelial tumors of malignant pleural mesothelioma and 95% of patients with nonepithelial tumors expressed IL-4Rα protein, and this strong IL-4Rα expression was correlated with a worse survival. In response to IL-4, human malignant pleural mesothelioma cells showed increased STAT6 phosphorylation and increased production of IL-6, IL-8, and VEGF without any effect on proliferation or apoptosis. This finding indicates that high expression of STAT6 as well as STAT3 and cytokines is inversely correlated with survival in patients.[36,37] NF-κB, along with IL-6, contributes to the survival of mammospheres in culture, because NF-κB and IL-6 were hyperactive in breast cancer–derived mammospheres.[38] In addition, elevated CRP and serum amyloid A (SAA) were associated with reduced disease-free survival of breast cancer patients.[39] In gastroesophageal cancer, proinflammatory cytokines IL-1β, IL-6, IL-8, and TNF-α and acute phase protein concentrations (CRP) were found to be elevated, and these levels were associated with reduced survival of patients.[40] Additionally, the Bcl-2 family protein COX-2, which is regulated by inflammatory transcription factors, is also involved in the survival of cancer cells.[41,42] Thus, we conclude that inflammation in general contributes to poor survival of patients.

In contrast to these findings, an in vivo study of dogs with osteosarcoma showed that survival improvement was apparent with inflammation or lymphocyte-infiltration scores >1, as well as in dogs that had apoptosis scores in the top 50th percentile.[43] Also, in patients with epithelioid malignant pleural mesothelioma, a high degree of chronic inflammatory cell infiltration in the stromal component was associated with improved overall survival.[44]

# ROLE OF INFLAMMATION IN PROLIFERATION

Several studies have shown that cell proliferation is affected by inflammation.[45] More significantly, proliferation in the setting of chronic inflammation predisposes humans to carcinoma in the esophagus, stomach, colon, liver, and urinary bladder.[46] In postgastrectomy patients, *Helicobacter pylori* induced inflammation and was associated with increased epithelial cell proliferation.[47] Even in the mouse model, chronic infection with *Helicobacter hepaticus* induced hepatic inflammation, which further led to hepatic cell proliferation.[48] Other reports found an increased expression of the cell proliferative markers PCNA and Ki-67 in the linings of inflamed odontogenic keratocysts compared with noninflamed lesions.[49,50] These findings suggest the existence of greater proliferative activity in the cells with inflammation. Wang et al.[51] showed an increased expression of cell proliferative markers PCNA and Ki-67 in a sample of 45 patients with benign prostatic hyperplasia.

The inflammatory biomarker COX-2 was also associated with the proliferation of cells. The highest proliferation index was found in COX-2–positive epithelium.[51] The association of COX-2 and proliferation was also reported in a rat model. The carcinogen dimethylhydrazine (DMH) induces an increase in epithelial cell proliferation and in the expression of COX-2 in the colon of rats.[52] Erbb2, a kinase, regulates inflammation through the induction of NF-κB, Comp1, IL-1β, COX-2, and multiple chemokines in the skin by ultraviolet (UV) exposure. This inflammation has been shown to increase the proliferation of skin tissue after UV irradiation.[53]

# ROLE OF INFLAMMATION IN INVASION

A characteristic of invasive cancer cells is survival and growth under nonadhesive conditions. This invasion of cancer cells causes the disease to spread, which results in poor patient survival.[54] A strong relationship has been documented between inflammation and cancer cell invasion.[55,56] In a study of 150 patients with HCC, a high GPS score was associated with a high vascular invasion of cancer cells.[57] Another study of colorectal cancer also supports the links between inflammation and the invasion of cancer cells, with a finding that a high GPS increased the invasion of colorectal cancer cells.[58] In patients with esophageal squamous cell carcinoma, a high GPS score also showed a close relationship with lymphatic and venous invasion.[59]

At the molecular level, various proteins are known to be involved in tumor cell invasion. MMP-9, a gelatinase that degrades type IV collagen—the major structural protein component in the extracellular matrix and basement membrane—is thought to play an important role in facilitating tumor invasion, as it is highly expressed in various malignant tumors.[60,61] Additionally, the high expression of HIF-1α has been proposed as being associated with a greater incidence of vascular invasion of HCC. This expression of HIF-1α was further correlated with high expression of the inflammatory molecule COX-2.[62]

Breast cancer invasion has been linked to proteolytic activity at the tumor cell surface. In inflammatory breast cancer (IBC) cells, high expression of cathepsin B, a cell surface proteolytic enzyme, has been shown to be associated with invasiveness of IBC. In addition, a high coexpression of cathepsin B and caveolin-1 was found in IBC patient biopsies. Thus, proteolytic activity of cathepsin B and its coexpression with caveolin-1 contributes to the invasiveness of IBC.[63] In IBC, RhoC GTPase is also responsible for the invasive phenotype.[64] In addition, the PI3K/Akt signaling pathway is crucial in IBC invasion. The molecules involved in cell motility are specifically upregulated in IBC patients compared with stage-matched and cell-type-of-origin–matched non-IBCs patients. Distinctively, RhoC GTPase is a substrate for Akt1, and its phosphorylation is absolutely essential for IBC cell invasion.[65]

# ROLE OF INFLAMMATION IN ANGIOGENESIS

Angiogenesis—the formation of new blood vessels from existing vessels—is tightly linked to chronic inflammation and cancer. Angiogenesis is one of the molecular events that bridges the gap between inflammation and cancer. Angiogenesis results from multiple signals acting on endothelial cells. Mature vessels control exchanges of hematopoietic cells and solutes between blood and surrounding tissues by responding to microenvironmental cues, including inflammation. Although inflammation is essential to defend the body against pathogens, it has adverse effects on the surrounding tissue, and some of these effects induce angiogenesis. Inflammation and angiogenesis are thereby linked processes, but exactly how they are related has not been well understood. Both inflammation and angiogenesis are exacerbated by an increased production of chemokines/cytokines, growth factors, proteolytic enzymes, proteoglycans, lipid mediators, and prostaglandins.

A close relationship has been reported between inflammation and angiogenesis in breast cancer. Tissue section staining showed increased vascularity with the intensity of diffuse inflammation.[66] Offersen et al.[67] found that inflammation was significantly correlated in bladder carcinoma with microvessel density, which is a marker of angiogenesis. Leukocytes have been described as mediators of inflammation-associated angiogenesis. In addition, the stable expression of TNF-α in endothelial cells increased angiogenic sprout formation independently of angiogenic growth factors. Furthermore, in work using the Matrigel plug assay in vivo, increased angiogenesis was observed in endothelial TNF-α–expressing mice. Thus, chronic inflammatory changes mediated by TNF-α can induce angiogenesis in vitro and in vivo, suggesting a direct link between inflammation and angiogenesis.[68] TNF-α–induced inhibitor of nuclear factor kappa kinase (IKK)-β activation also activates the angiogenic process. IKK-β activates the mammalian target of rapamycin (mTOR) pathway and enhances angiogenesis through VEGF production.[66] In addition to TNF-α, proinflammatory cytokines IL-1 (mainly IL-1β) and IL-8 were also found to be major proangiogenic stimuli of both physiologic and pathologic angiogenesis.[69,70] Recently, another cytokine macrophage migration inhibitory factor (MIF) was found to play a role in neoangiogenesis/vasculogenesis by endothelial cell activation along with inflammation.[71]

Benest et al.[72] found that a well-known regulator of angiogenesis, angiopoietin-2 (Ang-2), can upregulate inflammatory responses, indicating a common signaling pathway for inflammation and angiogenesis. TGF-β induction was also reported in head and neck epithelia and human head and neck squamous cell carcinomas (HNSCC), with severe inflammation that leads to angiogenesis.[73] The tumor-derived cytokine endothelial monocyte-activating polypeptide II (EMAP-II) has been shown to have profound effects on inflammation as well as on the processes involved in angiogenesis.[74] NF-κB plays an important role in inflammation as well as in angiogenesis, because the suppression of NF-κB and IkB-2A blocks basic fibroblast growth factor–induced angiogenesis in vivo. NF-κB regulates the angiogenic protein VEGF promoted by α5β1 integrin, which coordinately regulates angiogenesis and inflammation.[75] It has been also reported that a coculture of cancer cells with macrophages synergistically increased the production of various angiogenesis-related factors when stimulated by the inflammatory cytokine. This inflammatory angiogenesis was mediated by the activation of NF-κB and activator protein 1 (Jun/Fos), because the administration of either NF-κB–targeting drugs or COX-2 inhibitors or the depletion of macrophages blocked inflammatory angiogenesis.[76]

In a mouse model, cigarette smoke induced the inflammatory protein 5-lipoxygenase (5-LOX), and this induction activated matrix metalloproteinase 2 (MMP-2) and VEGF to induce the angiogenic process.[77] A cellular enzyme, Tank-binding kinase 1

(TBK-1), has been proposed as a putative mediator in tumor angiogenesis. TBK-1 mediates angiogenesis through the upregulation of VEGF and exerts proinflammatory effects via the induction of inflammatory cytokines. Thus, these pathways, including TBK-1, are an important cross-link between angiogenesis and inflammation.[78]

## ROLE OF INFLAMMATION IN METASTASIS

Inflammation plays a regulatory role in cancer progression and metastasis. Chronic or tumor-derived inflammation and inflammation-related stimuli within the tumor microenvironment promote blood and lymphatic vessel formation and aid in invasion and metastasis.[79,80] The association of inflammation and metastasis has been observed in several cancer types. In an immunohistochemical analysis of lung cancer tissues, a remarkably high level of metastasis was observed with severe inflammation.[81] A mouse model of breast cancer found that mammary tumors increased the frequency of lung metastases, and this effect was associated with the recruitment of inflammatory cells to the lung as well as elevated levels of IL-6 in the lung airways.[82] In another murine model, implanting human ovarian tumor cells into the ovaries of severe combined immunodeficient mice resulted in peritoneal inflammation and tumor cell dissemination from the ovaries. In addition, enhancement of the inflammatory response with thioglycolate accelerated the development of ascites and metastases, and its suppression with acetylsalicylic acid delayed metastasis.[83] Thus, it can be concluded that inflammation facilitates ovarian tumor metastasis by a mechanism largely mediated by cytokines.

It has been shown that metastatic tumor cells entering a distant organ such as the liver trigger a proinflammatory response involving the Kupffer cell–mediated release of TNF-α and the upregulation of vascular endothelial cell adhesion receptors, such as E-selectin.[84] The physiologic expression of the selectins is tightly controlled to limit the inflammatory response, but dysregulated expression of selectins contributes to inflammatory and thrombotic disorders as well as tumor metastases.[85] Using P-selectin knockout mice, the importance of P-selectin–mediated cell adhesive interactions in the pathogenesis of inflammation and metastasis of cancers has been clearly demonstrated.[86]

Tumor-associated inflammatory monocytes and macrophages are essential promoters of tumor cell migration, invasion, and metastasis.[87] Macrophages and their mediators affect the multistep process of invasion and metastasis, from interaction with the extracellular matrix to the construction of a premetastatic niche. Monocytes are attracted by cytokines and chemokines (e.g., CSF-1, GM-CSF, and MCP-1), which are released by tumor cells or cells of the tumor microenvironment. These monocytes are then induced to express proangiogenic and metastatic factors, including VEGF, fibroblast growth factor (FGF)-2, platelet-derived growth factor (PDGF), intercellular adhesion molecule (ICAM)-1, vascular cell adhesion molecule (VCAM)-1, E-selectin, P- selectin, and MMP-9.[88] Versican, a large extracellular matrix proteoglycan, has been shown to activate tumor-infiltrating myeloid cells through Toll-like receptor (TLR) 2 and its coreceptors TLR6 and CD14 and to elicit the production of proinflammatory cytokines (including TNF-α), which enhance tumor metastasis. TLR2 increases the secretion of IL-8, which potentiates metastatic growth. Ligation of TLR2 by versican induces inflammatory cytokine secretion, providing a link between inflammation and cancer metastasis.[89]

IKK-α has been shown to be important in the inflammation-associated metastasis of cancer cells. Luo et al.[90] demonstrated that activation and nuclear localization of IKK-α by tumor-infiltrating immune cells in prostatic epithelial tumor cells leads to malignant prostatic epithelial cells with a metastatic fate. Src family kinases, when inappropriately activated, promote pathologic inflammatory processes and tumor metastasis, in part through their effects on the regulation of endothelial monolayer permeability.[91] Platelet-activating factor (PAF), an inflammatory biolipid, has also been shown to increase metastasis. In particular, Melnikova et al.[92] demonstrated that PAF receptor antagonists can effectively inhibit the metastatic potential of human melanoma cells in nude mice. Mesenchymal stem cells promote HCC metastasis under the influence of inflammation through TGF-β.[93]

## EPIGENETIC CHANGES AND INFLAMMATION

Epigenetics considers the heritable changes in the activity of gene expression without the alteration of DNA sequences, and such changes have been linked to many human diseases, including cancer.[94] DNA methylation and histone modification are well-known epigenetic changes that can lead to gene activation or inactivation.[94–96] DNA methylation occurs primarily at cytosine-phosphate-guanine (CpG) dinucleotides as well as at transcriptional regulatory sites on the gene promoter.[96–98] Epigenetic abnormalities result in dysregulated gene expression and function, which can further lead to cancer. Inflammation and epigenetic abnormalities in cancer are highly associated. Inflammation induces aberrant epigenetic alterations in a tissue early in the process of carcinogenesis, and accumulation of such alterations forms an epigenetic field for cancer. Yara et al.[99] have shown that increased inflammation, as evidenced by the activation of NF-κB, production of IL-6 and COX-2, as well as the decrease of IκB, leads to the promoter's methylation. However, preincubation of cells with a demethylating agent prevented inflammation.

Infectious agents also contribute to inflammation-induced epigenetic changes. Infectious agents such as H. pylori and hepatitis C virus as well as intrinsic mediators of inflammatory responses, including proinflammatory cytokines, induce genetic and epigenetic changes, including point mutations, deletions, duplications, recombinations, and methylation of various tumor-related genes. Interestingly, disturbances in cytokine and chemokine signals and the induction of cell proliferation are important ways that inflammation induces aberrant DNA methylation. A study has shown that infection of human gastric mucosae with H. pylori induces chronic inflammation and further gastric cancers.[100] This inflammation is associated with high methylation levels or high incidences of methylation.[101–103]

Furthermore, numerous reports have documented the fact that inflammation is linked with epigenetic changes in carcinogenesis. Recently, Achyut[104] reported that inflammation in stromal fibroblasts caused epigenetic silencing of p21 and further tumor progression. Chronic inflammation also led to epigenetic regulation of p16 and activation of DNA damage in a lung carcinogenesis model.[105]

A transient inflammatory signal has been shown to initiate an epigenetic switch from nontransformed cells to cancer cells via a positive feedback loop involving NF-κB, Lin28, let-7, and IL-6. This IL-6 induced STAT3, directly activated miR-21 and miR-181b-1, and further induced the epigenetic switch. Thus, STAT3 underlies the epigenetic switch of mir-21 and mir-181b-1 that links inflammation to cancer.[106] Another report also showed that transient activation of Src oncoprotein mediates an epigenetic switch from immortalized breast cells to a stably transformed line that contained cancer stem cells. Thus, inflammation activates a positive feedback loop that maintains the epigenetic transformed state for many generations in the absence of the inducing signal.[18]

DNA hypermethylation at promoter CpG islands is an important mechanism by which carcinogenesis occurs through the inactivation of tumor-suppressor genes. Aberrant CpG island hypermethylation is also frequently observed in chronic inflammation and precancerous lesions, which again suggests links between inflammation and epigenetic change.[107] In addition, inflammation induced the halogenation of cytosine nucleotide. Damage products of this inflammation-mediated halogenated cytosine interfere with normal epigenetic control by altering DNA-protein interactions that are critical for gene regulation and the heritable transmission of methylation patterns. These inflammation-mediated cytosine damage products also provide a mechanistic link between inflammation and cancer.[108]

## ROLE OF INFLAMMATION IN CANCER DIAGNOSIS

Chronic inflammation plays an important role in the etiology and progression of chronic diseases, including cancer. Hence, chronic inflammation may have an important diagnostic role in cancer. Inflammation induced by inflammatory cells such as infiltrating cells and mesothelial cells is mediated via the release of various mediators and proteins, including PDGF, IL-8, monocyte chemotactic peptide (MCP-1), nitric oxide (NO), collagen, antioxidant enzymes, and the plasminogen activation inhibitor (PAI). Furthermore, several inflammatory mediators have been shown to be detected at increased concentrations, thereby aiding in the disease diagnosis.[109]

In one study, numerous inflammatory disorders were detected based on inflammation measured in gastric biopsies of patients by Fourier transform infrared spectroscopy (FT-IR). Using endoscopic samples, gastritis and gastric cancer were diagnosed.[110] Furthermore, the degree of prostate inflammation has been used to determine the level of incidental prostatitis.[111] An assessment of the expression of cytokines and other immune stimulatory molecules that drive B-cell activation provides insight into the etiology of cancers. It has been shown that the dysregulation of cytokine production precedes the diagnosis of non-Hodgkin lymphoma.[112]

Inflammation parameters have been used to diagnose cancer in patients. Inflammation parameters, including CRP, were found to differ in patients with cancer and in those without. In clinical practice, however, such parameters are considered to have modest diagnostic value for cancer.[113] In a study with 1,275 patients, granulomatous inflammation was identified in 154 patients (12.1%), of whom 12 out of 154 (7.8%) had a concurrent diagnosis of cancer.[114] In another study with 173 patients, 52% had lung adenocarcinoma. Patients with high systemic inflammation were more likely to have more than two sites of metastatic disease and to have poor performance status and less likely to receive any chemotherapy. Systemic inflammation at diagnosis is considered to be

an independent marker of poor outcome in patients with advanced non-small cell lung cancer (NSCLC).[115]

## INFLAMMATION AND GENOMICS

Recently, the genomic landscape of the most common forms of human cancer have been examined.[116] Almost 140 genes and 12 cell signaling pathways have been linked with most cancers. Several of these genes and pathways are directly or indirectly linked with inflammation. A cytokine pattern in patients with cancer has been identified.[117]

## INFLAMMATION AND TARGETED THERAPIES

That inflammation can be used as a target for cancer prevention and treatment is indicated by the fact that several drugs approved by the U.S. Food and Drug Administration (FDA) actually modulate proinflammatory pathways. For instance, EGFR, HER2, VEGF, CXCR4, and proteasome have been shown to activate NF-κB–mediated proinflammatory pathways, and their inhibitors have been approved by the FDA for the treatment of various cancers. Similarly, steroids such as dexamethasone, nonsteroidal anti-inflammatory drugs (NSAIDs), and statins that are currently used for prevention or treatment have also been found to suppress the NF-κB pathway. Thus, these observations indicate that inflammatory pathways are excellent targets for cancer.

## CONCLUSIONS

According to Colditz et al.,[118] almost 50% of all cancers can be prevented based on what we know today. All the studies summarized previously suggest that inflammation is closely linked to cancer, and the incidence of most cancers can be reduced by controlling inflammation. Proinflammatory conditions such as colitis, bronchitis, hepatitis, and gastritis can all eventually lead to cancer. Thus, one must find ways to treat these conditions before the appearance of cancer. All these studies indicate that an anti-inflammatory lifestyle could play an important role in both the prevention and treatment of cancer.

## REFERENCES

1. Anand P, Kunnumakkara AB, Sundaram C, et al. Cancer is a preventable disease that requires major lifestyle changes. *Pharm Res* 2008;25:2097–2116.
2. Aggarwal BB, Gehlot P. Inflammation and cancer: how friendly is the relationship for cancer patients? *Curr Opin Pharmacol* 2009;9:351–369.
3. Coussens LM, Zitvogel L, Palucka AK. Neutralizing tumor-promoting chronic inflammation: a magic bullet? *Science* 2013;339:286–291.
4. Sethi G, Sung B, Aggarwal BB. TNF: a master switch for inflammation to cancer. *Front Biosci* 2008;13:5094–5107.
5. Karin M. Nuclear factor-kappaB in cancer development and progression. *Nature* 2006;441:431–436.
6. Aggarwal BB. Nuclear factor-kappaB: the enemy within. *Cancer Cell* 2004; 6:203–208.
7. Chaturvedi MM, Sung B, Yadav VR, et al. NF-kappaB addiction and its role in cancer: 'one size does not fit all'. *Oncogene* 2011;30:1615–1630.
8. Aggarwal BB. Signalling pathways of the TNF superfamily: a double-edged sword. *Nat Rev Immunol* 2003;3:745–756.
9. Aggarwal BB, Gupta SC, Kim JH. Historical perspectives on tumor necrosis factor and its superfamily: 25 years later, a golden journey. *Blood* 2012; 119:651–665.
10. Iannitti T, Capone S, Gatti A, et al. Intracellular heavy metal nanoparticle storage: progressive accumulation within lymph nodes with transformation from chronic inflammation to malignancy. *Int J Nanomed* 2010;5:955–960.
11. Zhao Y, Xu Y, Li Y, et al. NF-kappaB-mediated inflammation leading to EMT via miR-200c is involved in cell transformation induced by cigarette smoke extract. *Toxicol Sci* 2013;135:265–276.
12. Xu Y, Zhao Y, Xu W, et al. Involvement of HIF-2alpha-mediated inflammation in arsenite-induced transformation of human bronchial epithelial cells. *Toxicol Appl Pharmacol* 2013;272:542–550.

13. Liu K, Jiang M, Lu Y, et al. Sox2 cooperates with inflammation-mediated Stat3 activation in the malignant transformation of foregut basal progenitor cells. *Cell Stem Cell* 2013;12:304–315.
14. Yoon BN, Chon KM, Hong SL, et al. Inflammation and apoptosis in malignant transformation of sinonasal inverted papilloma: the role of the bridge molecules, cyclooxygenase-2, and nuclear factor kappaB. *Am J Otolaryngol* 2013;34:22–30.
15. Roslind A, Johansen JS. YKL-40: a novel marker shared by chronic inflammation and oncogenic transformation. *Methods Mol Biol* 2009;511:159–184.
16. Coste I, Le Corf K, Kfoury A, et al. Dual function of MyD88 in RAS signaling and inflammation, leading to mouse and human cell transformation. *J Clin Invest* 2010;120:3663–3667.
17. Parthasarathy S, Dhayaparan D, Jayanthi V, et al. Aberrant expression of epidermal growth factor receptor and its interaction with protein kinase C delta in inflammation associated neoplastic transformation of human esophageal epithelium in high risk populations. *J Gastroenterol Hepatol* 2011;26:382–390.
18. Iliopoulos D, Hirsch HA, Struhl K. An epigenetic switch involving NF-kappaB, Lin28, Let-7 MicroRNA, and IL6 links inflammation to cell transformation. *Cell* 2009;139:693–706.
19. Colotta F, Allavena P, Sica A, et al. Cancer-related inflammation, the seventh hallmark of cancer: links to genetic instability. *Carcinogenesis* 2009;30: 1073–1081.
20. Hanahan D, Weinberg RA. Hallmarks of cancer: the next generation. *Cell* 2011;144:646–674.
21. Canna K, McMillan DC, McKee RF, et al. Evaluation of a cumulative prognostic score based on the systemic inflammatory response in patients undergoing potentially curative surgery for colorectal cancer. *Br J Cancer* 2004;90: 1707–1709.

22. Hilmy M, Bartlett JM, Underwood MA, et al. The relationship between the systemic inflammatory response and survival in patients with transitional cell carcinoma of the urinary bladder. *Br J Cancer* 2005;92:625–627.

23. Forrest LM, McMillan DC, McArdle CS, et al. Evaluation of cumulative prognostic scores based on the systemic inflammatory response in patients with inoperable non-small-cell lung cancer. *Br J Cancer* 2003;89:1028–1030.

24. Ramsey S, Lamb GW, Aitchison M, et al. Evaluation of an inflammation-based prognostic score in patients with metastatic renal cancer. *Cancer* 2007;109:205–212.

25. Crumley AB, Stuart RC, McKernan M, et al. Comparison of an inflammation-based prognostic score (GPS) with performance status (ECOG-ps) in patients receiving palliative chemotherapy for gastroesophageal cancer. *J Gastroenterol Hepatol* 2008;23:e325–329.

26. Yamanaka T, Matsumoto S, Teramukai S, et al. The baseline ratio of neutrophils to lymphocytes is associated with patient prognosis in advanced gastric cancer. *Oncology* 2007;73:215–220.

27. Halazun KJ, Aldoori A, Malik HZ, et al. Elevated preoperative neutrophil to lymphocyte ratio predicts survival following hepatic resection for colorectal liver metastases. *Eur J Surg Oncol* 2008;34:55–60.

28. Huang ZL, Luo J, Chen MS, et al. Blood neutrophil-to-lymphocyte ratio predicts survival in patients with unresectable hepatocellular carcinoma undergoing transarterial chemoembolization. *J Vasc Interv Radiol* 2011;22:702–709.

29. Heng DY, Xie W, Regan MM, et al. Prognostic factors for overall survival in patients with metastatic renal cell carcinoma treated with vascular endothelial growth factor-targeted agents: results from a large, multicenter study. *J Clin Oncol* 2009;27:5794–5799.

30. Smith RA, Bosonnet L, Raraty M, et al. Preoperative platelet-lymphocyte ratio is an independent significant prognostic marker in resected pancreatic ductal adenocarcinoma. *Am J Surg* 2009;197:466–472.

31. Fox P, Hudson M, Brown C, et al. Markers of systemic inflammation predict survival in patients with advanced renal cell cancer. *Br J Cancer* 2013;109:147–153.

32. Iwasaki Y, Ishizuka M, Kato M, et al. Usefulness of an inflammation-based prognostic score (mGPS) for predicting survival in patients with unresectable malignant biliary obstruction. *World J Surg* 2013;37:2222–2228.

33. Shafique K, Proctor MJ, McMillan DC, et al. Systemic inflammation and survival of patients with prostate cancer: evidence from the Glasgow Inflammation Outcome Study. *Prostate Cancer Prostatic Dis* 2012;15:195–201.

34. Kunisaki C, Takahashi M, Ono HA, et al. Inflammation-based prognostic score predicts survival in patients with advanced gastric cancer receiving biweekly docetaxel and s-1 combination chemotherapy. *Oncology* 2012;83:183–191.

35. Pinato DJ, Sharma R. An inflammation-based prognostic index predicts survival advantage after transarterial chemoembolization in hepatocellular carcinoma. *Transl Res* 2012;160:146–152.

36. Burt BM, Bader A, Winter D, et al. Expression of interleukin-4 receptor alpha in human pleural mesothelioma is associated with poor survival and promotion of tumor inflammation. *Clin Cancer Res* 2012;18:1568–1577.

37. Sethi G, Shanmugam MK, Ramachandran L, et al. Multifaceted link between cancer and inflammation. *Biosci Rep* 2012;32:1–15.

38. Papi A, Guarnieri T, Storci G, et al. Nuclear receptors agonists exert opposing effects on the inflammation dependent survival of breast cancer stem cells. *Cell Death Differ* 2012;19:1208–1219.

39. Pierce BL, Ballard-Barbash R, Bernstein L, et al. Elevated biomarkers of inflammation are associated with reduced survival among breast cancer patients. *J Clin Oncol* 2009;27:3437–3444.

40. Deans DA, Wigmore SJ, Gilmour H, et al. Elevated tumour interleukin-1beta is associated with systemic inflammation: a marker of reduced survival in gastro-oesophageal cancer. *Br J Cancer* 2006;95:1568–1575.

41. Chen LS, Balakrishnan K, Gandhi V. Inflammation and survival pathways: chronic lymphocytic leukemia as a model system. *Biochem Pharmacol* 2010;80:1936–1945.

42. Sharma-Walia N, Paul AG, Bottero V, et al. Kaposi's sarcoma associated herpes virus (KSHV) induced COX-2: a key factor in latency, inflammation, angiogenesis, cell survival and invasion. *PLoS Pathog* 2010;6:e1000777.

43. Modiano JF, Bellgrau D, Cutter GR, et al. Inflammation, apoptosis, and necrosis induced by neoadjuvant fas ligand gene therapy improves survival of dogs with spontaneous bone cancer. *Mol Ther* 2012;20:2234–2243.

44. Suzuki K, Kadota K, Sima CS, et al. Chronic inflammation in tumor stroma is an independent predictor of prolonged survival in epithelioid malignant pleural mesothelioma patients. *Cancer Immunol Immunother* 2011;60:1721–1728.

45. Hu B, Elinav E, Flavell RA. Inflammasome-mediated suppression of inflammation-induced colorectal cancer progression is mediated by direct regulation of epithelial cell proliferation. *Cell Cycle* 2011;10:1936–1939.

46. Sugar LM. Inflammation and prostate cancer. *Can J Urol* 2006;13(Suppl 1):46–47.

47. Safatle-Ribeiro AV, Ribeiro U, Jr., Clarke MR, et al. Relationship between persistence of *Helicobacter pylori* and dysplasia, intestinal metaplasia, atrophy, inflammation, and cell proliferation following partial gastrectomy. *Dig Dis Sci* 1999;44:243–252.

48. Ihrig M, Schrenzel MD, Fox JG. Differential susceptibility to hepatic inflammation and proliferation in AXB recombinant inbred mice chronically infected with *Helicobacter hepaticus*. *Am J Pathol* 1999;155:571–582.

49. de Paula AM, Carvalhais JN, Domingues MG, et al. Cell proliferation markers in the odontogenic keratocyst: effect of inflammation. *J Oral Pathol Med* 2000;29:477–482.

50. Kaplan I, Hirshberg A. The correlation between epithelial cell proliferation and inflammation in odontogenic keratocyst. *Oral Oncol* 2004;40:985–991.

51. Wang W, Bergh A, Damber JE. Chronic inflammation in benign prostate hyperplasia is associated with focal upregulation of cyclooxygenase-2, Bcl-2, and cell proliferation in the glandular epithelium. *Prostate* 2004;61:60–72.

52. Demarzo MM, Martins LV, Fernandes CR, et al. Exercise reduces inflammation and cell proliferation in rat colon carcinogenesis. *Med Sci Sports Exerc* 2008;40:618–621.

53. Madson JG, Lynch DT, Tinkum KL, et al. Erbb2 regulates inflammation and proliferation in the skin after ultraviolet irradiation. *Am J Pathol* 2006;169:1402–1414.

54. Bondong S, Kiefel H, Hielscher T, et al. Prognostic significance of L1CAM in ovarian cancer and its role in constitutive NF-kappaB activation. *Ann Oncol* 2012;23:1795–1802.

55. Wu Y, Zhou BP. Inflammation: a driving force speeds cancer metastasis. *Cell Cycle* 2009;8:3267–3273.

56. Aggarwal BB, Vijayalekshmi RV, Sung B. Targeting inflammatory pathways for prevention and therapy of cancer: short-term friend, long-term foe. *Clin Cancer Res* 2009;15:425–430.

57. Kinoshita A, Onoda H, Imai N, et al. The Glasgow Prognostic Score, an inflammation based prognostic score, predicts survival in patients with hepatocellular carcinoma. *BMC Cancer* 2013;13:52.

58. Toiyama Y, Miki C, Inoue Y, et al. Evaluation of an inflammation-based prognostic score for the identification of patients requiring postoperative adjuvant chemotherapy for stage II colorectal cancer. *Exp Ther Med* 2011;2:95–101.

59. Kobayashi T, Teruya M, Kishiki T, et al. Inflammation-based prognostic score, prior to neoadjuvant chemoradiotherapy, predicts postoperative outcome in patients with esophageal squamous cell carcinoma. *Surgery* 2008;144:729–735.

60. Nelson AR, Fingleton B, Rothenberg ML, et al. Matrix metalloproteinases: biologic activity and clinical implications. *J Clin Oncol* 2000;18:1135–1149.

61. Clark ES, Weaver AM. A new role for cortactin in invadopodia: regulation of protease secretion. *Eur J Cell Biol* 2008;87:581–590.

62. Dai CX, Gao Q, Qiu SJ, et al. Hypoxia-inducible factor-1 alpha, in association with inflammation, angiogenesis and MYC, is a critical prognostic factor in patients with HCC after surgery. *BMC Cancer* 2009;9:418.

63. Victor BC, Anbalagan A, Mohamed MM, et al. Inhibition of cathepsin B activity attenuates extracellular matrix degradation and inflammatory breast cancer invasion. *Breast Cancer Res* 2011;13:R115.

64. van Golen KL, Bao LW, Pan Q, et al. Mitogen activated protein kinase pathway is involved in RhoC GTPase induced motility, invasion and angiogenesis in inflammatory breast cancer. *Clin Exp Metastasis* 2002;19:301–311.

65. Lehman HL, Van Laere SJ, van Golen CM, et al. Regulation of inflammatory breast cancer cell invasion through Akt1/PKBalpha phosphorylation of RhoC GTPase. *Mol Cancer Res* 2012;10:1306–1318.

66. Lee DF, Kuo HP, Chen CT, et al. IKK beta suppression of TSC1 links inflammation and tumor angiogenesis via the mTOR pathway. *Cell* 2007;130:440–455.

67. Offersen BV, Knap MM, Marcussen N, et al. Intense inflammation in bladder carcinoma is associated with angiogenesis and indicates good prognosis. *Br J Cancer* 2002;87:1422–1430.

68. Rajashekhar G, Willuweit A, Patterson CE, et al. Continuous endothelial cell activation increases angiogenesis: evidence for the direct role of endothelium linking angiogenesis and inflammation. *J Vasc Res* 2006;43:193–204.

69. Voronov E, Carmi Y, Apte RN. Role of IL-1-mediated inflammation in tumor angiogenesis. *Adv Exp Med Biol* 2007;601:265–270.

70. Qazi BS, Tang K, Qazi A. Recent advances in underlying pathologies provide insight into interleukin-8 expression-mediated inflammation and angiogenesis. *Int J Inflam* 2011;2011:908468.

71. Asare Y, Schmitt M, Bernhagen J. The vascular biology of macrophage migration inhibitory factor (MIF). Expression and effects in inflammation, atherogenesis and angiogenesis. *Thromb Haemost* 2013;109:391–398.

72. Benest AV, Kruse K, Savant S, et al. Angiopoietin-2 is critical for cytokine-induced vascular leakage. *PLoS One* 2013;8: e70459.

73. Lu SL, Reh D, Li AG, et al. Overexpression of transforming growth factor beta1 in head and neck epithelia results in inflammation, angiogenesis, and epithelial hyperproliferation. *Cancer Res* 2004;64:4405–4410.

74. Berger AC, Tang G, Alexander HR, et al. Endothelial monocyte-activating polypeptide II, a tumor-derived cytokine that plays an important role in inflammation, apoptosis, and angiogenesis. *J Immunother* 2000;23:519–527.

75. Klein S, de Fougerolles AR, Blaikie P, et al. Alpha 5 beta 1 integrin activates an NF-kappa B-dependent program of gene expression important for angiogenesis and inflammation. *Mol Cell Biol* 2002;22:5912–5922.

76. Ono M. Molecular links between tumor angiogenesis and inflammation: inflammatory stimuli of macrophages and cancer cells as targets for therapeutic strategy. *Cancer Sci* 2008;99:1501–1506.

77. Ye YN, Liu ES, Shin VY, et al. Contributory role of 5-lipoxygenase and its association with angiogenesis in the promotion of inflammation-associated colonic tumorigenesis by cigarette smoking. *Toxicology* 2004;203:179–188.

78. Czabanka M, Korherr C, Brinkmann U, et al. Influence of TBK-1 on tumor angiogenesis and microvascular inflammation. *Front Biosci* 2008;13:7243–7249.

79. Solinas G, Marchesi F, Garlanda C, et al. Inflammation-mediated promotion of invasion and metastasis. *Cancer Metastasis Rev* 2010;29:243–248.

80. Affara NI, Coussens LM. IKKalpha at the crossroads of inflammation and metastasis. *Cell* 2007;129:25–26.

81. Kayser K, Bulzebruck H, Ebert W, et al. Local tumor inflammation, lymph node metastasis, and survival of operated bronchus carcinoma patients. *J Natl Cancer Inst* 1986;77:77–81.

82. Hobson J, Gummadidala P, Silverstrim B, et al. Acute inflammation induced by the biopsy of mouse mammary tumors promotes the development of metastasis. *Breast Cancer Res Treat* 2013;139:391–401.

83. Robinson-Smith TM, Isaacsohn I, Mercer CA, et al. Macrophages mediate inflammation-enhanced metastasis of ovarian tumors in mice. *Cancer Res* 2007;67:5708–5716.

84. Khatib AM, Auguste P, Fallavollita L, et al. Characterization of the host proinflammatory response to tumor cells during the initial stages of liver metastasis. *Am J Pathol* 2005;167:749–759.

85. McEver RP. Selectin-carbohydrate interactions during inflammation and metastasis. *Glycoconj J* 1997;14:585–591.

86. Geng JG, Chen M, Chou KC. P-selectin cell adhesion molecule in inflammation, thrombosis, cancer growth and metastasis. *Curr Med Chem* 2004; 11:2153–2160.

87. Condeelis J, Pollard JW. Macrophages: obligate partners for tumor cell migration, invasion, and metastasis. *Cell* 2006;124:263–266.

88. Siegel G, Malmsten M. The role of the endothelium in inflammation and tumor metastasis. *Int J Microcirc Clin Exp* 1997;17:257–272.

89. Wang W, Xu GL, Jia WD, et al. Ligation of TLR2 by versican: a link between inflammation and metastasis. *Arch Med Res* 2009;40:321–323.

90. Luo JL, Tan W, Ricono JM, et al. Nuclear cytokine-activated IKKalpha controls prostate cancer metastasis by repressing Maspin. *Nature* 2007;446:690–694.

91. Kim MP, Park SI, Kopetz S, et al. Src family kinases as mediators of endothelial permeability: effects on inflammation and metastasis. *Cell Tissue Res* 2009;335:249–259.

92. Melnikova V, Bar-Eli M. Inflammation and melanoma growth and metastasis: the role of platelet-activating factor (PAF) and its receptor. *Cancer Metastasis Rev* 2007;26:359–371.

93. Jing Y, Han Z, Liu Y, et al. Mesenchymal stem cells in inflammation microenvironment accelerates hepatocellular carcinoma metastasis by inducing epithelial-mesenchymal transition. *PLoS One* 2012;7:e43272.

94. Jones PA, Baylin SB. The epigenomics of cancer. *Cell* 2007;128:683–692.

95. Esteller M. Aberrant DNA methylation as a cancer-inducing mechanism. *Annu Rev Pharmacol Toxicol* 2005;45:629–656.

96. Thiagalingam S, Cheng KH, Lee HJ, et al. Histone deacetylases: unique players in shaping the epigenetic histone code. *Ann N Y Acad Sci* 2003; 983:84–100.

97. Li E, Beard C, Jaenisch R. Role for DNA methylation in genomic imprinting. *Nature* 1993;366:362–365.

98. Antequera F, Bird A. Number of CpG islands and genes in human and mouse. *Proc Natl Acad Sci U S A* 1993;90:11995–11999.

99. Yara S, Lavoie JC, Beaulieu JF, et al. Iron-ascorbate-mediated lipid peroxidation causes epigenetic changes in the antioxidant defense in intestinal epithelial cells: impact on inflammation. *PLoS One* 2013;8:e63456.

100. Uemura N, Okamoto S, Yamamoto S, et al. Helicobacter pylori infection and the development of gastric cancer. *N Engl J Med* 2001;345:784–789.

101. Maekita T, Nakazawa K, Mihara M, et al. High levels of aberrant DNA methylation in Helicobacter pylori-infected gastric mucosae and its possible association with gastric cancer risk. *Clin Cancer Res* 2006;12:989–995.

102. Nakajima T, Maekita T, Oda I, et al. Higher methylation levels in gastric mucosae significantly correlate with higher risk of gastric cancers. *Cancer Epidemiol Biomarkers Prev* 2006;15:2317–2321.

103. Perri F, Cotugno R, Piepoli A, et al. Aberrant DNA methylation in non-neoplastic gastric mucosa of H. Pylori infected patients and effect of eradication. *Am J Gastroenterol* 2007;102:1361–1371.

104. Achyut BR, Bader DA, Robles AI, et al. Inflammation-mediated genetic and epigenetic alterations drive cancer development in the neighboring epithelium upon stromal abrogation of TGF-beta signaling. *PLoS Genet* 2013;9:e1003251.

105. Blanco D, Vicent S, Fraga MF, et al. Molecular analysis of a multistep lung cancer model induced by chronic inflammation reveals epigenetic regulation of p16 and activation of the DNA damage response pathway. *Neoplasia* 2007;9:840–852.

106. Iliopoulos D, Jaeger SA, Hirsch HA, et al. STAT3 activation of miR-21 and miR-181b-1 via PTEN and CYLD are part of the epigenetic switch linking inflammation to cancer. *Mol Cell* 2010;39:493–506.

107. Suzuki H, Toyota M, Kondo Y, et al. Inflammation-related aberrant patterns of DNA methylation: detection and role in epigenetic deregulation of cancer cell transcriptome. *Methods Mol Biol* 2009;512:55–69.

108. Valinluck V, Sowers LC. Inflammation-mediated cytosine damage: a mechanistic link between inflammation and the epigenetic alterations in human cancers. *Cancer Res* 2007;67:5583–5586.

109. Kroegel C, Antony VB. Immunobiology of pleural inflammation: potential implications for pathogenesis, diagnosis and therapy. *Eur Respir J* 1997; 10:2411–2418.

110. Li QB, Sun XJ, Xu YZ, et al. Use of Fourier-transform infrared spectroscopy to rapidly diagnose gastric endoscopic biopsies. *World J Gastroenterol* 2005;11:3842–3845.

111. Difuccia B, Keith I, Teunissen B, et al. Diagnosis of prostatic inflammation: efficacy of needle biopsies versus tissue blocks. *Urology* 2005;65:445–448.

112. Vendrame E, Martinez-Maza O. Assessment of pre-diagnosis biomarkers of immune activation and inflammation: insights on the etiology of lymphoma. *J Proteome Res* 2011;10:113–119.

113. Baicus C, Caraiola S, Rimbas M, et al. Utility of routine hematological and inflammation parameters for the diagnosis of cancer in involuntary weight loss. *J Investig Med* 2011;59:951–955.

114. DePew ZS, Gonsalves WI, Roden AC, et al. Granulomatous inflammation detected by endobronchial ultrasound-guided transbronchial needle aspiration in patients with a concurrent diagnosis of cancer: a clinical conundrum. *J Bronchology Interv Pulmonol* 2012;19:176–181.

115. Jafri SH, Shi R, Mills G. Advance lung cancer inflammation index (ALI) at diagnosis is a prognostic marker in patients with metastatic non-small cell lung cancer (NSCLC): a retrospective review. *BMC Cancer* 2013;13:158.

116. Vogelstein B, Papadopoulos N, Velculescu VE, et al. Cancer genome landscapes. *Science* 2013;339:1546–1558.

117. Lippitz BE. Cytokine patterns in patients with cancer: a systematic review. *Lancet Oncol* 2013;14:e218–228.

118. Colditz GA, Wolin KY, Gehlert S. Applying what we know to accelerate cancer prevention. *Sci Transl Med* 2012;4(127):127rv4.

# 7 Chemical Factors

Stuart H. Yuspa and Peter G. Shields

## INTRODUCTION

As early as the 1800s, initial observations of unusual cancer incidences in occupational groups provided the first indications that chemicals were a cause of human cancer, which was then confirmed in experimental animal studies during the early and mid 1900s. However, the extent to which chemical exposures contribute to cancer incidence was not fully appreciated until population-based studies documented differing organ-specific cancer rates in geographically distinct populations and in cohort studies such as those that linked smoking to lung cancer.[1] The most commonly occurring chemical exposures that increase cancer risk are tobacco, alcoholic beverages, diet, and reproductive factors (e.g., hormones). Today, it is recognized that cancer results not solely from chemical exposure (e.g., in the workplace or at home), but that a variety of biologic, social, and physical factors contribute to cancer pathogenesis.[2,3] For some common cancers, it also has been recognized that heritable factors also contribute to cancer risk from chemical exposure (e.g., genes involved in carcinogen metabolism, DNA repair, a variety of cancer pathways).[4] Twin studies show that for common cancers, nongenetic risk factors are dominant, and the best associations for genetic risks of sporadic cancers indicate that the risks for specific genetic traits are typically less than 1.5-fold.[5–7] The role of the tumor microenvironment, the cancer stem cells, and feedback signaling to and from the tumor also have been recently recognized as important contributors to carcinogenesis, although how chemicals affect these have yet been clearly demonstrated.[8–10]

The experimental induction of tumors in animals, the neoplastic transformation of cultured cells by chemicals, and the molecular analysis of human tumors have revealed important concepts regarding the pathogenesis of cancer and how laboratory studies can be used to better understand human cancer pathogenesis.[7,11,12] Chemical carcinogens usually affect specific organs, targeting the epithelial cells (or other susceptible cells within an organ) and causing genetic damage (genotoxic) or epigenetic effects regulating DNA transcription and translation. Chemically related DNA damage and consequent somatic mutations relevant to human cancer can occur either directly from exogenous exposures or indirectly by activation of endogenous mutagenic pathways (e.g., nitric oxide, oxyradicals).[13,14] The risk of developing a chemically induced tumor may be modified by nongenotoxic exogenous and endogenous exposures and factors (e.g., hormones, immunosuppression triggered by the tumor), and by accumulated exposure to the same or different genotoxic carcinogens.[7,15]

Analyses of how chemicals induce cancer in animal models and human populations has had a major impact on human health. Experimental studies have been instrumental in replicating hypotheses generated from human studies and identifying pathobiologic mechanisms. For example, animal experiments confirmed the carcinogenic and cocarcinogenic properties of cigarette smoke and identified bioactive chemical and gaseous components.[1] The transplacental carcinogenicity of diethylstilbestrol and the hazards of specific occupational carcinogens such as vinyl chloride, benzene, aromatic amines, and bis(chloromethyl)ether led to a reduction in allowable exposures of suspected human carcinogens from the workplace and a reduction in cancer rates. Dietary factors that enhance or inhibit cancer development and the contribution of obesity to specific organ sites have been identified in models of chemical carcinogenesis, and alterations in diet and obesity are expected to result in reduced cancer risk. Experimental animal studies are the mainstay of risk assessment as a screening tool to identify potential carcinogens in the workplace and the environment, although these studies do not prove specific chemical etiologies as a cause of human cancer because of interspecies differences and the use of maximally tolerated doses that do not replicate human exposure.

## THE NATURE OF CHEMICAL CARCINOGENS: CHEMISTRY AND METABOLISM

The National Toxicology Program, based mostly on experimental animal studies and supported by epidemiology studies when available, lists 45 chemical, physical, and infectious agents as known human carcinogens and about 175 that are reasonably anticipated to be human carcinogens (http://ntp.niehs. nih.gov/?objectid=035E57E7-BDD9-2D9B-AFB9D1CADC8 D09C1), whereas the International Agency for Research on Cancer (IARC) lists 113 agents as carcinogenic to humans and 66 that are probably carcinogenic to humans (http://monographs. iarc.fr/ENG/Classification/index.php). Table 7.1 provides a selected list of known human carcinogens, as indicated by the IARC, which are continuously updated.[16] Most chemical carcinogens first undergo metabolic activation by cytochrome P450s or other metabolic pathways so that they react with DNA and/or alter epigenetic mechanisms.[11,17] This process, evolutionarily presumed to have been developed to rid the body of foreign chemicals for excretion, inadvertently generates reactive carcinogenic intermediates that can bind cellular molecules, including DNA, and cause mutations or other alterations.[18] Recent data indicate that metabolizing enzymes also have the ability to cross-talk with transcription factors involved in the regulation of other metabolizing and antioxidant enzymes.[19] DNA is considered the ultimate target for most carcinogens to cause either mutations or gross chromosomal changes, but epigenetic effects, such as altered DNA methylation and gene transcription, also promote carcinogenesis.[20] The formation of DNA adducts, where chemicals bind directly to DNA to promote mutations, is likely necessary but not sufficient to cause cancer.

Genotoxic carcinogens may transfer simple alkyl or complexed (aryl) alkyl groups to specific sites on DNA bases.[18,21] These alkylating and aryl-alkylating agents include, but are not limited to, N-nitroso compounds, aliphatic epoxides, aflatoxins, mustards, polycyclic aromatic hydrocarbons, and other combustion products of fossil fuels and vegetable matter. Others transfer arylamine residues to DNA, as exemplified by aryl aromatic

95

| TABLE 7.1 |
| :-- |

**Known Chemical Carcinogens in Humans**[a]

| Target Organ | Agents | Industries | Tumor Type |
| :-- | :-- | :-- | :-- |
| Lung | Tobacco smoke, arsenic, asbestos, crystalline silica, benzo(a)pyrene, beryllium, bis(chloro)methyl ether, 1,3-butadiene, chromium VI compounds, coal tar and pitch, diesel exhaust, nickel compounds, soot, mustard gas, cobalt-tungsten carbide powders | Aluminum production, coal gasification, coke production, painting, hematite mining, painting, grinding in oil and gas | Squamous, large cell, and small cell cancer and adenocarcinoma |
| Pleura | Asbestos, erionite, painting | Insulation, mining | Mesothelioma |
| Oral cavity | Tobacco smoke, alcoholic beverages, nickel compounds, betel quid | – | Squamous cell cancer |
| Esophagus | Tobacco smoke, alcoholic beverages, betel quid | – | Squamous cell cancer |
| Gastric | Tobacco smoking | Rubber industry | Adenocarcinoma |
| Colon | Alcohol, tobacco smoking | – | Adenocarcinoma |
| Liver | Aflatoxin, vinyl chloride, tobacco smoke, alcoholic beverages | – | Hepatocellular carcinoma, hemangiosarcoma |
| Kidney | Tobacco smoke, trichloroethylene | – | Renal cell cancer |
| Bladder | Tobacco smoke, 4-aminobiphenyl, benzidine, 2-napthylamine, cyclophosphamide, phenacetin | Magenta manufacturing, auramine manufacturing, painting, rubber production | Transitional cell cancer |
| Prostate | Cadmium | – | Adenocarcinoma |
| Skin | Arsenic, benzo(a)pyrene, coal tar and pitch, mineral oils, soot, cyclosporin A, azathioprine, shale oils | – | Squamous cell cancer, basal cell cancer |
| Bone marrow | Benzene, tobacco smoke, ethylene oxide, antineoplastic agents, cyclosporin A, formaldehyde | Rubber workers | Leukemia, lymphoma |

[a] The carcinogen designations are determined by the International Agency for Research on Cancer (http://monographs.iarc.fr/index.php). They do not imply proof of carcinogenicity in individuals. This table is not all inclusive. For additional information, the reader is referred to agency documents and publications.

amines, aminoazo dyes, and heterocyclic aromatic amines. For genotoxic carcinogens, the interaction with DNA is not random, and each class of agents reacts selectively with purine and pyrimidine targets.[7,18,21] Furthermore, targeting carcinogens to particular sites in DNA is determined by nucleotide sequence, by host cell, and by selective DNA repair processes (see later discussion), making some genetic material at risk over others. As expected from this chemistry, genotoxic carcinogens can be potent mutagens and particularly adept at causing nucleotide base mispairing or small deletions, leading to missense or nonsense mutations. Others may cause macrogenetic damage, such as chromosome breaks and large deletions. In some cases, such genotoxic damage may result in changes in transcription and translation that affect protein levels or function, which in turn alter the behavior of the specific host cell type. For example, there may be effects on cell proliferation, programmed cell death, or DNA repair. This is best typified by the signature mutations detected in the p53 gene caused by ingested aflatoxin in human liver cancer[22] and by polycyclic aromatic hydrocarbons human lung cancer caused by the inhalation of cigarette smoke.[15,23,24] Similarly, a distinct pattern of mutations is detected in pancreatic cancers from smokers when compared with pancreatic cancers from nonsmokers.[25]

Some chemicals that cause cancers in laboratory rodents are not demonstrably genotoxic. In general, these agents are carcinogenic in laboratory animals at high doses and require prolonged exposure. Synthetic pesticides and herbicides fall within this group, as do a number of natural products that are ingested. The mechanism of action by nongenotoxic carcinogens is not well understood, and may be related in some cases to toxic cell death and regenerative hyperplasia. They may also induce endogenous mutagenic mechanisms through the production of free radicals, increasing

rates of depurination, and the deamination of 5-methylcytosine. In other cases, nongenotoxic carcinogens may have hormonal effects on hormone-dependent tissues. For example, some pesticides, herbicides, and fungicides have endocrine-disrupting properties in experimental models, although the relation to human cancer risk is unknown.

## ANIMAL MODEL SYSTEMS AND CHEMICAL CARCINOGENESIS

Most human chemical carcinogens can induce tumors in experimental animals; however, the tumors may not be in the same organ, the exposure pathways may differ from human exposure, and the causative mechanisms may not exist in humans. In many cases, however, the cell of origin, morphogenesis, phenotypic markers, and genetic alterations are qualitatively identical to corresponding human cancers. Furthermore, animal models have revealed the constancy of carcinogen–host interaction among mammalian species by reproducing organ-specific cancers in animals with chemicals identified as human carcinogens, such as coal tar and squamous cell carcinomas, vinyl chloride and hepatic angiosarcomas, aflatoxin and hepatocellular carcinoma, and aromatic amines and bladder cancer. The introduction of genetically modified mice designed to reproduce specific human cancer syndromes and precancer models has accelerated both the understanding of the contributions of chemicals to cancer causation and the identification of potential exogenous carcinogens.[26,27] Furthermore, construction of mouse strains genetically altered to express human drug–metabolizing enzymes has added both to the relevance of mouse studies for understanding human carcinogen metabolism and the prediction of genotoxicity from suspected human carcinogens and other chemical exposures.[28] Together, these studies have indicated that carcinogenic agents can directly activate oncogenes, inactivate tumor suppressor genes, and cause the genomic changes that are associated with autonomous growth, enhanced survival, and modified gene expression profiles that are required for the malignant phenotype.[29]

## Genetic Susceptibility to Chemical Carcinogenesis in Experimental Animal Models

The use of inbred strains of rodents and spontaneous or genetically modified mutant strains have led to the identification and characterization of genes that modify risks for cancer development.[30–32] For a variety of tissue sites, including the lungs, the liver, the breast, and the skin, pairs of inbred mice can differ by 100-fold in the risk for tumor development after carcinogen exposure. Genetically determined differences in the affinity for the aryl hydrocarbon hydroxylase (Ah) receptor or other differences in metabolic processing of carcinogens is one modifier that has a major impact on experimental and presumed human cancer risk.[33–35] The development of mice reconstituted with components of the human carcinogen–metabolizing genome should facilitate the extrapolation of metabolic activity by human enzymes and cancer risk.[27,28,36] Such mice also show that other loci regulate the growth of premalignant foci, the response to tumor promoters, the immune response to metastatic cells, and the basal proliferation rate of target cells.[30] In mice susceptible to colon cancer due to a carcinogen-induced constitutive mutation in the APC gene, a locus on mouse chromosome 4 confers resistance to colon cancer.[31] The identification of the phospholipase A2 gene at this locus and subsequent functional testing in transgenic mice revealed an interesting paracrine protective influence on tumor development.[31] This gene, and several other genes mapped for susceptibility to chemically induced mouse tumors (PTPRJ, a receptor type tyrosine phosphatase, and STK6/STK15, an aurora kinase), have now been shown to influence susceptibility to organ-specific cancer induction in humans.[30,31]

## MOLECULAR EPIDEMIOLOGY, CHEMICAL CARCINOGENESIS, AND CANCER RISK IN HUMAN POPULATIONS

Molecular epidemiology is the application of biologically based hypotheses using molecular and epidemiologic methods and measures. New technologies continue to allow epidemiologic studies to improve the testing of biologically based hypotheses and to develop large datasets for hypothesis generation, most notably the application of various –omics technologies via next-generation sequencing (e.g., genomics, epigenomics, transcriptomics), proteomics, and metabolomics. The greatest challenge now is to develop methods that allow for analysis cutting across various technologies.[37–43] Recent advances now include the role of microRNA and long noncoding RNAs in tumor development and progression because of their impact on the regulation of gene expression.[44,45] Chemical effects on microRNAs and the resultant gene expression is currently being identified.[46] Using such technologies, emerging evidence is noting the importance of the microbiome and associated infections as a risk of human cancer.[47–50] The complexity of environmental exposure and how it interacts with humans to affect numerous biologic pathways has been characterized as the exposome, also expressed as a multidimensional complex dataset.[51] Therefore, the important goal remains: to characterize cancer risk based on gene–environment interactions. However, we remain challenged because cancer is a complex disease of diverse etiologies by multiple exposures causing damage in different genes; for

example, gene$^n$–environment$^n$ interactions, for which the variable $n$ is not known.

Two fundamental principles underlie current studies of molecular epidemiology. First, carcinogenesis is a multistage process, and behind each stage are numerous genetic events that occur either due to an exogenous insult such as a chemical exposure or an endogenous insult, such as from free radicals generated via cellular processes or errors in DNA replication. Therefore, identifying a cancer risk factor can be challenging because of the multifactorial nature of carcinogenesis, given that any one risk factor occurs within a background of many risk factors. Second, wide interindividual variation in response to carcinogen exposure and other carcinogenic processes indicate that the human response is not homogeneous, so that experimental models and epidemiology (e.g., the use of a single cell clone to study a gene's effect experimentally or the assumption that the population responds similarly to the mean in epidemiology studies), might not be representative of susceptible and resistant groups within a population.

## Genetic Susceptibility

In humans, the determination of genetic susceptibility can be assessed by phenotyping or genotyping methods. Phenotypes generally represent complex genotypes. Examples of phenotypes include the assessment of DNA repair capacity in cultured blood cells, mammographic breast density, or the quantitation of carcinogen-DNA adducts in a target organ. Phenotypes now also include profiles of methylation that affect gene expression, a so-called epigenetic effect, for example, identified though next-generation sequencing or other methods.[52] The contribution of genetics to cancer risk from chemical carcinogens can range from small to large, depending on its penetrance.[4] Highly penetrant cancer-susceptibility genes cause familial cancers, but account for less than 5% of all cancers. Low-penetrant genes cause common sporadic cancers, which have large public health consequences.

A genetic polymorphism (e.g., single nucleotide polymorphisms) is defined as a genetic variant present in at least 1% of the population. Because of the advent of improved genotyping methods that have reduced cost and increased high throughput, haplotyping and whole genomewide association studies are ongoing. Although haplotyping studies, facilitated through the International HapMap Project (www.hapmap.org), have not proven useful for predicting human cancers; high-density, whole genomewide, single nucleotide polymorphism association studies have shown remarkable consistency for many gene loci, although the risk estimates are only 1.0 to 1.4, which are not useful in the clinic for individual risk assessment.[6] For example, the contribution of genetic polymorphisms to cancer risk, at least for breast cancer, appears to improve risk modeling by only a few percent; known breast cancer risk factors account for about 58% of risk, and adding 10 genetic variants increases the risk prediction only to 62%.[53] Genes under study are from pathways that affect behavior, activate and detoxify carcinogens, affect DNA repair, govern cell-cycle control, trigger apoptosis, effect cell signaling, and so forth.

## Biomarkers of Cancer Risk

The evaluation of dose and risk estimates in epidemiologic studies can include four components: namely, external exposure measurements, internal exposure measurements, biomarkers estimating the biologically effective dose, and biomarkers of effect or harm. The latter three measurements are biomarkers that improve on the first by quantifying exposure inside the individual and at the cellular level to characterize low-dose exposures in low-risk populations, providing a relative contribution of individual chemical carcinogens from complex mixtures, and/or estimating total burden of a particular exposure where there are many sources.[54]

Chemicals cause genetic damage in different ways, namely in the formation of carcinogen-DNA adducts leading to base mutations or gross chromosomal changes. Adducts are formed when a mutagen, or part of it, irreversibly binds to DNA so that it can cause a base substitution, insertion, or deletion during DNA replication. Gross chromosomal mutations are chromosome breaks, gaps, or translocations. The level of DNA damage is the biologically effective dose in a target organ, and reflects the net result of carcinogen exposure, activation, lack of detoxification, lack of effective DNA repair, and lack of programmed cell death. A variety of assays have been used for determining carcinogen-macromolecular adducts in human tissues; for example, for assessing risk from tobacco smoking for lung cancer and aflatoxin and liver cancer.[55,56] Important considerations for the assessment of biomarkers include sensitivity, specificity, reproducibility, accessibility for human use, and whether it represents a risk measured in a target organ or surrogate tissue. No single biomarker has been considered to be sufficiently validated for use as a cancer risk marker in an individual as it relates to chemical carcinogenesis.[57] However, there is some evidence that DNA adducts are cancer risk factors in both cohort and case-control studies.[58]

People are commonly exposed to N-nitrosamine and other N-nitroso compounds from dietary and tobacco exposures, which are associated with DNA adduct formation and cancer. Exposure can occur through endogenous formation of N-nitrosamines from nitrates in food or directly from dietary sources, cosmetics, drugs, household commodities, and tobacco smoke. Endogenous formation occurs in the stomach from the reaction of nitrosatable amines and nitrate (used as a preservative), which is converted to nitrites by bacteria. The N-nitrosamines undergo metabolic activation by cytochrome P450s (CYP2E1, CYP2A6, and CYP2D6) and form DNA adducts. Biomarkers are available to assess N-nitrosamine exposure from tobacco smoke (e.g., urinary tobacco-specific nitrosamine levels) or DNA, including in target organs such as the lungs. Recent data indicate that increasing levels of tobacco-specific nitrosamine metabolites are associated with increased lung cancer risk.[55]

Heterocyclic amines are formed from the overheating of food with creatine, such as meat, chicken, and fish.[59] Heterocyclic amines, estimated based on consumption of well-done meat, have been associated with breast and colon cancer, presumably through metabolic activation mechanisms and DNA damage.[59] Aflatoxins, another food contaminant, are considered to be a major contributor to liver cancer in China and parts of Africa, especially interacting with hepatitis viruses, and urinary aflatoxin adduct levels are predictors of liver cancer risk.[56]

Aromatic amines are another class of human carcinogens. Aryl aromatic amines have been implicated in bladder carcinogenesis, especially in occupationally exposed cohorts (e.g., dye workers) and tobacco smokers.[60] These compounds are activated by cytochrome P4501A2 and excreted via the N-acetyltransferase 2 gene. They are genotoxic, and the quantitative assessment using biomarkers has been more difficult, but some persons have studied DNA adducts as well.[61]

Polycyclic aromatic hydrocarbons (PAH) are large, aromatic (three or more fused benzene rings) compounds that are a class of more than 200 chemicals. These compounds are ubiquitous in the environment and present in the ambient air. They are formed from overcooking foods, fireplaces, charcoal barbeques, burning of coal and crude oil, tobacco smoke, and can be found in various occupational settings. In order for PAHs to exert their toxic effect, they must undergo metabolic activation via cytochromes P4501A1 and P4503A4 to form DNA adducts, or are excreted via pathways involving the glutathione-S-transferase genes. PAHs are associated with an increased risk of lung and skin cancer in the occupational setting, although risk varies by type of industry and the individual being exposed.[62,63] Benzo(a)pyrene (BaP), the most frequently studied PAH, serves as a model for chemical carcinogens. The bay region diol epoxide binds to DNA, mostly as the N2-deoxyguanosine adduct. The evidence linking BaP-deoxyguanosine adducts with a carcinogenic effect in lung cancer is very strong, including site-specific hotspot mutations in the p53 tumor suppressor gene.[64–68] Various biomarkers of exposure have been developed for assessing PAH exposure. These include measuring DNA adducts, protein adducts, and urinary 1-hydroxypyrene; only the latter is a validated biomarker of exposure and no adducts have been validated as biomarkers of cancer risk. However, recent data indicate that PAH metabolites might be risk factors for lung cancer.[58]

Air pollution has been recently classified by the IARC as a known human lung carcinogen.[69] Studies that support the conclusion include cohort studies that use biomarkers of exposure.[70] Such markers include measurements of 1-hydroxypyrene, DNA adducts, chromosomal aberrations, micronuclei, oxidative damage to nucleobases, and methylation changes.[71]

Epidemiologic and experimental studies have linked benzene to hematologic toxicity, including aplastic anemia, myelodysplastic syndrome, and acute myeloid leukemia.[72–74] Benzene is metabolized by hepatic P4502E1 (CYP2E1), yielding benzene oxide and hydroquinone, among other reactive metabolites. Circulating hydroquinones may be further metabolized to reactive benzoquinones by myeloperoxidase in bone marrow white blood cell precursors and stroma. Benzene metabolites are reported to have a variety of biologic consequences on bone marrow cells, including covalent binding to DNA and protein, alterations in gene expression, cytokine and chemokine abnormalities, and chromosomal aberrations.[75] There are well-established biomarkers of exposure to benzene, but to date, biomarkers of toxicity have not been validated (except for high-level exposure workplaces and effects of peripheral blood counts).

# ARISTOLOCHIC ACID AND UROTHELIAL CANCERS AS A MODEL FOR IDENTIFYING HUMAN CARCINOGENS

Aristolochic acids come from the Aristolochia genus of plants, which have been used for herbal remedies (e.g., birthwort, Dutchman's pipe). The case of the carcinogen aristolochic acid, which is identified as a Class 1 human carcinogen by the IARC (http://monographs.iarc.fr/ENG/Monographs/vol100A/mono100A-23.pdf), presents a powerful example of how the forces of epidemiology, classical chemical carcinogenesis, and genomics collaborate to unravel the pathogenesis and prevention of a specific human cancer.[76] In the 1990s, epidemiologists independently reported on three distinct unrelated population groups that developed nephrotoxicity (interstitial fibrosis) and an extraordinary high incidence of urothelial cancer of the upper urinary track after exposure for different reasons and in different parts of the world (Belgium, the Balkans, and China). In Belgian women ingesting an extract from plants of the Aristolochia species for weight reduction, which was provided to them in a weight loss clinic, nearly 50% developed this unusual syndrome. A similar clinical picture (so-called Balkan endemic nephropathy) was reported for residents farming around the Danube River and eating home-baked bread from wheat contaminated with seeds from Aristolochia weeds grown in the same fields. In China, the Aristolochia herbs have been used for centuries in Chinese medicine and are prominently prescribed in Taiwan, a nation with the highest incidence of urothelial cancer in the world, as remedies for ailments of the heart, liver, snake bites, arthritis, gout, childbirth, and others.

Common to all Aristolochia species are one of two major nitrophenanthrene carboxylic acid toxicants, namely, aristolochic acid I and II (http://monographs.iarc.fr/ENG/Monographs/vol100A/

mono100A-23.pdf).[77,78] The oral administration of aristolochic acid to rodents is highly carcinogenic, producing predominantly forestomach cancers and lymphomas, along with cancers of the lung, kidney, and urothelium (http://monographs.iarc.fr/ENG/Monographs/vol100A/mono100A-23.pdf). The major route of excretion of aristolochic acid is through the kidneys. These clinical and experimental observations inspired further analyses of the mechanism of action of these potent human carcinogens. Studies in intact mice and mice reconstituted with humanized P450 revealed that CYP1a and CYP2a were responsible for both the activation and the detoxification of aristolochic acid I and II, and that NAD(P)H:quinone oxidoreductase produced the ultimate reactive aristolactam I nitrenium species.[78] The molecular action of the ultimate carcinogen is remarkably specific, targeting purine nucleotides in DNA to form DNA adducts and binding at the exocyclic amino group of deoxyadenosine and deoxyguanosine with a far greater affinity for dA over dG (Fig. 7.1). DNA adducts from aristolochic acids have been found in both experimental animals and humans. Furthermore, unlike any other human carcinogen, the predominant mutagenic outcome is an A:T transversion with a marked preference for the nontranscribed strand of DNA, notably in the p53 gene.[77,79] The A:T to T:A transversions

are extremely uncommon among the mutation spectrum in all eukaryotes. These unique properties of aristolochic acid DNA adducts appear to elude DNA repair mechanisms that commonly focus on transcribing DNA, resulting in persistent carcinogen-DNA adducts in human tissues and surgical tumor specimens, thus confirming the association of exposure with a biologic effect.[80] In experimental models in mice where human p53 is substituted for the mouse gene, multiple sites on p53 are mutated, almost all of which are those unusual A:T transversions.[81] Modern genomic techniques have unraveled other selective properties of this unusual but potent human chemical carcinogen. Whole genome and exome sequencing of multiple aristolochic-associated kidney cancers from patients confirmed the high frequency of the unusual A:T to T:A transversion mutations. Furthermore, an unusual pattern emerges where there is selectivity for mutations at splice sites with a preferable consensus sequence of T/CAG. Among the many mutations detected, certain targets stand out, particularly in p53, MLL2, and other genes the products of which function in regulating gene expression through higher chromosome order.[82,83] This cancer story covers the gamut of all elements of chemical carcinogenesis, and its illumination has opened a door for cancer prevention.

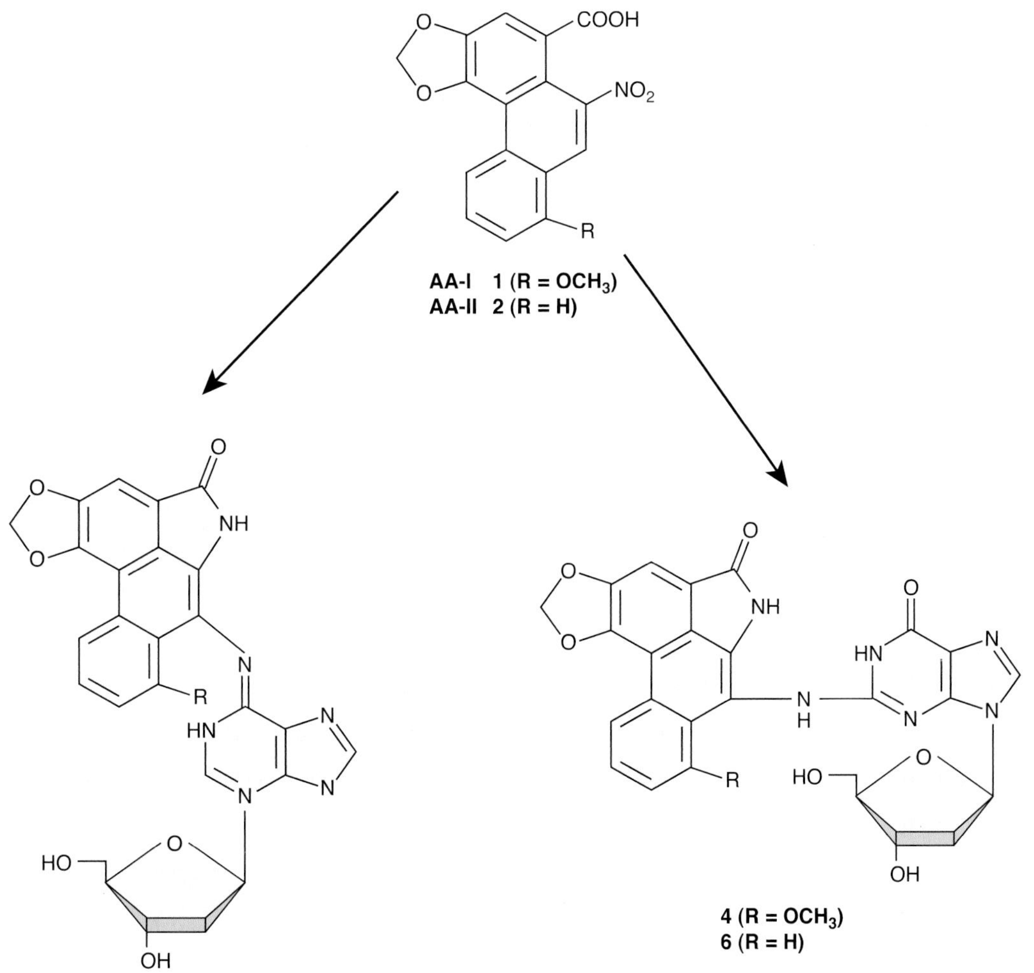

**Figure 7.1** Aristolochic acid I and II form DNA adducts through the exocyclic amino group of deoxyadenosine and deoxyguanosine. The deoxyadenosine adduct is highly favored. For more detailed analysis of the complete metabolic profile, see Attaluri et al.[79]

# REFERENCES

1. U.S. Department of Health and Human Services. *The Health Consequences of Smoking: 50 Years of Progress. A Report of the Surgeon General.* Atlanta: Author; 2014.
2. Colditz GA, Wei EK. Preventability of cancer: the relative contributions of biologic and social and physical environmental determinants of cancer mortality. *Annu Rev Public Health* 2012;33:137–156.
3. Lynch SM, Rebbeck TR. Bridging the gap between biologic, individual, and macroenvironmental factors in cancer: a multilevel approach. *Cancer Epidemiol Biomarkers Prev* 2013;22:485–495.
4. Rahman N. Realizing the promise of cancer predisposition genes. *Nature* 2014;505:302–308.
5. Lichtenstein P, Holm NV, Verkasalo PK, et al. Environmental and heritable factors in the causation of cancer—analyses of cohorts of twins from Sweden, Denmark, and Finland. *N Engl J Med* 2000;343:78–85.
6. Hunter DJ, Chanock SJ. Genome-wide association studies and "the art of the soluble." *J Natl Cancer Inst* 2010;102:836–837.
7. Luch A. Nature and nurture - lessons from chemical carcinogenesis. *Nat Rev Cancer* 2005;5:113–125.
8. Taddei ML, Giannoni E, Comito G, et al. Microenvironment and tumor cell plasticity: an easy way out. *Cancer Lett* 2013;341:80–96.
9. Fessler E, Dijkgraaf FE, De Sousa E Melo, et al. Cancer stem cell dynamics in tumor progression and metastasis: is the microenvironment to blame? *Cancer Lett* 2013;341:97–104.
10. Hanahan D, Coussens LM. Accessories to the crime: functions of cells recruited to the tumor microenvironment. *Cancer Cell* 2012;21:309–322.
11. Irigaray P, Belpomme D. Basic properties and molecular mechanisms of exogenous chemical carcinogens. *Carcinogenesis* 2010;31:135–148.
12. Xia HJ, Chen CS. Progress of non-human primate animal models of cancers. *Dongwuxue Yanjiu* 2011;32:70–80.
13. Yi C, He C. DNA repair by reversal of DNA damage. *Cold Spring Harb Perspect Biol* 2013;5:a012575.
14. Dizdaroglu M. Oxidatively induced DNA damage: mechanisms, repair and disease. *Cancer Lett* 2012;327:26–47.
15. Wogan GN, Hecht SS, Felton JS, et al. Environmental and chemical carcinogenesis. *Semin Cancer Biol* 2004;14:473–486.
16. Baan R, Grosse Y, Straif K, et al. A review of human carcinogens—Part F: chemical agents and related occupations. *Lancet Oncol* 2009;10:1143–1144.
17. Rendic S, Guengerich FP. Contributions of human enzymes in carcinogen metabolism. *Chem Res Toxicol* 2012;25:1316–1383.
18. Luch A. The mode of action of organic carcinogens on cellular structures. *EXS* 2006;65–95.
19. Anttila S, Raunio H, Hakkola J. Cytochrome P450-mediated pulmonary metabolism of carcinogens: regulation and cross-talk in lung carcinogenesis. *Am J Respir Cell Mol Biol* 2011;44:583–590.
20. Pogribny IP, Beland FA. DNA methylome alterations in chemical carcinogenesis. *Cancer Lett* 2012 [Epub ahead of print].
21. Shrivastav N, Li D, Essigmann JM. Chemical biology of mutagenesis and DNA repair: cellular responses to DNA alkylation. *Carcinogenesis* 2010;31:59–70.
22. Kew MC. Aflatoxins as a cause of hepatocellular carcinoma. *J Gastrointestin Liver Dis* 2013;22:305–310.
23. Feng Z, Hu W, Hu Y, et al. Acrolein is a major cigarette-related lung cancer agent: preferential binding at p53 mutational hotspots and inhibition of DNA repair. *Proc Natl Acad Sci U S A* 2006;103:15404–15409.
24. Porta M, Crous-Bou M, Wark PA, et al. Cigarette smoking and K-ras mutations in pancreas, lung and colorectal adenocarcinomas: etiopathogenic similarities, differences and paradoxes. *Mutat Res* 2009;682:83–93.
25. Blackford A, Parmigiani G, Kensler TW, et al. Genetic mutations associated with cigarette smoking in pancreatic cancer. *Cancer Res* 2009;69:3681–3688.
26. Eastmond DA, Vulimiri SV, French JE, et al. The use of genetically modified mice in cancer risk assessment: challenges and limitations. *Crit Rev Toxicol* 2013;43:611–631.
27. Boverhof DR, Chamberlain MP, Elcombe CR, et al. Transgenic animal models in toxicology: historical perspectives and future outlook. *Toxicol Sci* 2011;121:207–233.
28. Cheung C, Gonzalez FJ. Humanized mouse lines and their application for prediction of human drug metabolism and toxicological risk assessment. *J Pharmacol Exp Ther* 2008;327:288–299.
29. Hanahan D, Weinberg RA. Hallmarks of cancer: the next generation. *Cell* 2011;144:646–674.
30. Demant P. Cancer susceptibility in the mouse: genetics, biology and implications for human cancer. *Nat Rev Genet* 2003;4:721–734.
31. Klatt P, Serrano M. Engineering cancer resistance in mice. *Carcinogenesis* 2003;24:817–826.
32. Lynch D, Svoboda J, Putta S, et al. Mouse skin models for carcinogenic hazard identification: utilities and challenges. *Toxicol Pathol* 2007;35:853–864.
33. Lash LH, Hines RN, Gonzalez FJ, et al. Genetics and susceptibility to toxic chemicals: do you (or should you) know your genetic profile? *J Pharmacol Exp Ther* 2003;305:403–409.
34. Di PG, Magno LA, Rios-Santos F. Glutathione S-transferases: an overview in cancer research. *Expert Opin Drug Metab Toxicol* 2010;6:153–170.
35. Feng S, Cao Z, Wang X. Role of aryl hydrocarbon receptor in cancer. *Biochim Biophys Acta* 2013;1836:197–210.
36. Jiang XL, Gonzalez FJ, Yu AM. Drug-metabolizing enzyme, transporter, and nuclear receptor genetically modified mouse models. *Drug Metab Rev* 2011;43:27–40.
37. Tuna M, Amos CI. Genomic sequencing in cancer. *Cancer Lett* 2013;340:161–170.
38. MacConaill LE. Existing and emerging technologies for tumor genomic profiling. *J Clin Oncol* 2013;31:1815–1824.
39. Watson IR, Takahashi K, Futreal PA, et al. Emerging patterns of somatic mutations in cancer. *Nat Rev Genet* 2013;14:703–718.
40. Dumas ME. Metabolome 2.0: quantitative genetics and network biology of metabolic phenotypes. *Mol Biosyst* 2012;8:2494–2502.
41. Adamski J, Suhre K. Metabolomics platforms for genome wide association studies—linking the genome to the metabolome. *Curr Opin Biotechnol* 2013;24:39–47.
42. Verma M, Khoury MJ, Ioannidis JP. Opportunities and challenges for selected emerging technologies in cancer epidemiology: mitochondrial, epigenomic, metabolomic, and telomerase profiling. *Cancer Epidemiol Biomarkers Prev* 2013;22:189–200.
43. Edwards SL, Beesley J, French JD, et al. Beyond GWASs: illuminating the dark road from association to function. *Am J Hum Genet* 2013;93:779–797.
44. Di LG, Garofalo M, Croce CM. MicroRNAs in cancer. *Annu Rev Pathol* 2014;9:287–314.
45. Cheetham SW, Gruhl F, Mattick JS, et al. Long noncoding RNAs and the genetics of cancer. *Br J Cancer* 2013;108:2419–2425.
46. Izzotti A, Pulliero A. The effects of environmental chemical carcinogens on the microRNA machinery. *Int J Hyg Environ Health* 2014 [Epub ahead of print].
47. Kostic AD, Gevers D, Pedamallu CS, et al. Genomic analysis identifies association of Fusobacterium with colorectal carcinoma. *Genome Res* 2012;22:292–298.
48. Compare D, Nardone G. Contribution of gut microbiota to colonic and extracolonic cancer development. *Dig Dis* 2011;29:554–561.
49. Ahn J, Chen CY, Hayes RB. Oral microbiome and oral and gastrointestinal cancer risk. *Cancer Causes Control* 2012;23:399–404.
50. Schwabe RF, Jobin C. The microbiome and cancer. *Nat Rev Cancer* 2013;13:800–812.
51. Wild CP, Scalbert A, Herceg Z. Measuring the exposome: a powerful basis for evaluating environmental exposures and cancer risk. *Environ Mol Mutagen* 2013;54:480–499.
52. Brennan K, Flanagan JM. Epigenetic epidemiology for cancer risk: harnessing germline epigenetic variation. *Methods Mol Biol* 2012;863:439–465.
53. Wacholder S, Hartge P, Prentice R, et al. Performance of common genetic variants in breast-cancer risk models. *N Engl J Med* 2010;362:986–993.
54. Boffetta P, van der Hel O, Norppa H, et al. Chromosomal aberrations and cancer risk: results of a cohort study from Central Europe. *Am J Epidemiol* 2007;165:36–43.
55. Yuan JM, Gao YT, Wang R, et al. Urinary levels of volatile organic carcinogen and toxicant biomarkers in relation to lung cancer development in smokers. *Carcinogenesis* 2012;33:804–809.
56. Wogan GN, Kensler TW, Groopman JD. Present and future directions of translational research on aflatoxin and hepatocellular carcinoma. A review. *Food Addit Contam Part A Chem Anal Control Expo Risk Assess* 2012;29:249–257.
57. Hatsukami DK, Benowitz NL, Rennard SI, et al. Biomarkers to assess the utility of potential reduced exposure tobacco products. *Nicotine Tob Res* 2006;8:599–622.
58. Yuan JM, Gao YT, Murphy SE, et al. Urinary levels of cigarette smoke constituent metabolites do you (or should you) know your genetic profile? *Cancer Res* 2011;71:6749–6757.
59. Turesky RJ, Le ML. Metabolism and biomarkers of heterocyclic aromatic amines in molecular epidemiology studies: lessons learned from aromatic amines. *Chem Res Toxicol* 2011;24:1169–1214.
60. Burger M, Catto JW, Dalbagni G, et al. Epidemiology and risk factors of urothelial bladder cancer. *Eur Urol* 2013;63:234–241.
61. Besaratinia A, Tommasi S. Genotoxicity of tobacco smoke-derived aromatic amines and bladder cancer: current state of knowledge and future research directions. *FASEB J* 2013;27:2090–2100.
62. International Agency for Research on Cancer. *IARC Monographs on the Evaluation of Carcinogenic Risks to Humans: Some Non-Heterocyclic Polycyclic Aromatic Hydrocarbons and Some Related Exposures.* Volume 92. Lyon, France: World Health Organization; 2010.
63. Boffetta P, Autier P, Boniol M, et al. An estimate of cancers attributable to occupational exposures in France. *J Occup Environ Med* 2010;52:399–406.
64. Mordukhovich I, Rossner P Jr, Terry MB, et al. Associations between polycyclic aromatic hydrocarbon-related exposures and p53 mutations in breast tumors. *Environ Health Perspect* 2010;118:511–518.
65. Pfeifer GP, Denissenko MF, Olivier M, et al. Tobacco smoke carcinogens, DNA damage and p53 mutations in smoking-associated cancers. *Oncogene* 2002;21:7435–7451.
66. Pfeifer GP, Hainaut P. On the origin of G → T transversions in lung cancer. *Mutat Res* 2003;526:39–43.
67. Sjaastad AK, Jorgensen RB, Svendsen K. Exposure to polycyclic aromatic hydrocarbons (PAHs), mutagenic aldehydes and particulate matter during pan frying of beefsteak. *Occup Environ Med* 2010;67:228–232.

68. Hussain SP, Amstad P, Raja K, et al. Mutability of p53 hotspot codons to benzo(a)pyrene diol epoxide (BPDE) and the frequency of p53 mutations in nontumorous human lung. *Cancer Res* 2001;61:6350–6355.

69. Loomis D, Grosse Y, Lauby-Secretan B, et al. The carcinogenicity of outdoor air pollution. *Lancet Oncol* 2013;14:1262–1263.

70. Raaschou-Nielsen O, Andersen ZJ, Beelen R, et al. Air pollution and lung cancer incidence in 17 European cohorts: prospective analyses from the European Study of Cohorts for Air Pollution Effects (ESCAPE). *Lancet Oncol* 2013;14:813–822.

71. Demetriou CA, Raaschou-Nielsen O, Loft S, et al. Biomarkers of ambient air pollution and lung cancer: a systematic review. *Occup Environ Med* 2012;69:619–627.

72. Galbraith D, Gross SA, Paustenbach D. Benzene and human health: A historical review and appraisal of associations with various diseases. *Crit Rev Toxicol* 2010;40:1–46.

73. Vlaanderen J, Portengen L, Rothman N, et al. Flexible meta-regression to assess the shape of the benzene-leukemia exposure-response curve. *Environ Health Perspect* 2010;118:526–532.

74. Vlaanderen J, Lan Q, Kromhout H, et al. Occupational benzene exposure and the risk of chronic myeloid leukemia: a meta-analysis of cohort studies incorporating study quality dimensions. *Am J Ind Med* 2012;55:779–785.

75. Snyder R. Leukemia and benzene. *Int J Environ Res Public Health* 2012;9: 2875–2893.

76. Grollman AP. Aristolochic acid nephropathy: harbinger of a global iatrogenic disease. *Environ Mol Mutagen* 2013;54:1–7.

77. Hollstein M, Moriya M, Grollman AP, et al. Analysis of TP53 mutation spectra reveals the fingerprint of the potent environmental carcinogen, aristolochic acid. *Mutat Res* 2013;753:41–49.

78. Stiborova M, Martinek V, Frei E, et al. Enzymes metabolizing aristolochic acid and their contribution to the development of aristolochic acid nephropathy and urothelial cancer. *Curr Drug Metab* 2013;14:695–705.

79. Attaluri S, Bonala RR, Yang IY, et al. DNA adducts of aristolochic acid II: total synthesis and site-specific mutagenesis studies in mammalian cells. *Nucleic Acids Res* 2010;38:339–352.

80. Sidorenko VS, Yeo JE, Bonala RR, et al. Lack of recognition by global-genome nucleotide excision repair accounts for the high mutagenicity and persistence of aristolactam-DNA adducts. *Nucleic Acids Res* 2012;40:2494–2505.

81. Nedelko T, Arlt VM, Phillips DH, et al. TP53 mutation signature supports involvement of aristolochic acid in the aetiology of endemic nephropathy-associated tumours. *Int J Cancer* 2009;124:987–990.

82. Hoang ML, Chen CH, Sidorenko VS, et al. Mutational signature of aristolochic acid exposure as revealed by whole-exome sequencing. *Sci Transl Med* 2013;5:197ra102.

83. Poon SL, Pang ST, McPherson JR, et al. Genome-wide mutational signatures of aristolochic acid and its application as a screening tool. *Sci Transl Med* 2013;5:197ra101.

ETIOLOGY AND EPIDEMIOLOGY OF CANCER

# 8 Physical Factors

Mats Ljungman

## INTRODUCTION

Ionizing radiation (IR) and ultraviolet (UV) light have challenged the genetic integrity of all living organisms throughout time. By inducing DNA damage and subsequent mutations, these physical agents have promoted diversity through natural selection, and, as a result, organisms from all kingdoms of life carry genes that encode proteins that repair damaged DNA. In higher, multicellular organisms, many additional mechanisms of genome preservation have evolved, such as cell cycle checkpoints and apoptosis. Despite the many sophisticated mechanisms to safeguard the human genome from the mutagenic actions of DNA-damaging agents, not all exposed cells successfully restore the integrity of their DNA and some cells may subsequently progress into malignant cancer cells. Furthermore, through manmade activities, we are now exposed to many new physical agents, such as radiofrequency and microwave radiation, electromagnetic fields, asbestos, and nanoparticles, for which evolution has not yet had time to deliver genome-preserving response mechanisms. This chapter will highlight the molecular mechanisms by which these physical agents affect cells and how human exposure may lead to cancer.

## IONIZING RADIATION

IR is defined as radiation that has sufficient energy to ionize molecules by displacing electrons from atoms. IR can be electromagnetic, such as x-rays and gamma rays, or can consist of particles, such as electrons, protons, neutrons, alpha particles, or carbon ions. Natural sources of IR make up about 80% of human exposure and medical sources make up about 20%.[1] The increased medical use of diagnostic x-rays and computed tomography (CT) scanning procedures likely translates into higher incidences of cancer. Of the natural sources, radon exposure is the most significant exposure risk to humans. Importantly, with better and more comprehensive screening techniques, the human exposure to radon could be dramatically lowered.

### Mechanisms of Damage Induction

#### Linear Energy Transfer

The biologic effects of IR are unique in that the induced damage is clustered due to the local deposition of energy in radiation tracks. The distance between the depositions of energy is biologically very relevant and unique to the energy and the type of radiation. The term *linear energy transfer (LET)* denotes the energy transferred per unit length of a track of radiation. Electromagnetic radiation, such as x-rays or gamma rays, are sparsely ionizing and therefore classified as low LET radiation, whereas particulate radiation, such as neutrons, protons, and alpha particles, are examples of high LET radiation.[1]

#### Radiation Biochemistry

Radiation-induced damage to cellular target molecules, such as DNA, proteins, and lipids, can be either direct or indirect

(Fig. 8.1). The *direct action* of radiation, which is the dominant mode of action of high LET radiation, is due to the deposition of energy directly to the target molecule, resulting in one or more ionization events. The *indirect action* of radiation is due to the radiolysis of water molecules, which, after initial absorption of radiation energy, become excited and generate different types of radiolysis products where the reactive hydroxyl radical ($\bullet OH$), can damage both DNA and proteins. About two-thirds of the damage induced by low LET radiation is due to the indirect action of radiation. Since the hydroxyl radical is very reactive (half-life is $10^{-9}$ seconds), it does not diffuse more than a few nanometers after it is formed before it reacts with other molecules, and, thus, only radicals formed in close proximity to the target molecule will contribute to the damage of that target.[2] However, by chemical recombination of the primary radiolysis products, hydrogen peroxide ($H_2O_2$) is formed, which in turn can produce hydroxyl radicals at a later time through the Fenton reaction, involving free metals. Because $H_2O_2$ is not very reactive, it can diffuse long distances away from the initial site of energy deposition.

Radical scavengers normally present in cells, such as glutathione, can protect target molecules by reacting with the hydroxyl radical (see Fig. 8.1). Even after the target molecule has been hit and ionized, glutathione can contribute to cell protection by donating a hydrogen atom to the radical, allowing the unpaired electron present in the radical to pair up with the electron from the hydrogen atom. This is considered the simplest of all types of repair and is called *chemical repair*.[3] However, if oxygen molecules are present, they will compete with scavenger molecules for the ionized molecule, and if oxygen reacts with the ionized target molecule before the hydrogen donation occurs, the damage will be solidified as a peroxide, which is not amendable to chemical repair. Instead, this lesion will require enzymatic repair for the restoration of DNA. This augmenting biologic effect of oxygen is called the *oxygen effect* and is considered an important factor for the effectiveness of radiation therapy.[1]

### Damage to DNA

The direct and indirect effects of radiation induce more or less identical types of lesions in DNA. However, the density of lesions induced in a stretch of DNA is higher for high LET radiation, and this increased complexity is thought to complicate the repair of these lesions. Radiation-induced lesions consist of more than 100 chemically distinct base lesions, such as the mutagenic lesions thymine glycol and 8-hydroxyguanine.[2,4,5] Furthermore, damage to the sugar moiety in the backbone of DNA and some types of base damage can result in single-strand breaks (SSB). Because the energy deposition of radiation is clustered even for low LET radiation, it is possible that two individual strand breaks are formed in close proximity on opposite strands, resulting in the formation of a double-strand break (DSB). It has been estimated that 1 Gy of ionizing radiation gives rise to about 40 DSBs, 1,000 SSBs, 1,000 base lesions, and 150 DNA-protein cross-links per cell.[2] For a similarly lethal dose of UV light, about 400,000 lesions are required, demonstrating that the lesions induced by IR are much more toxic

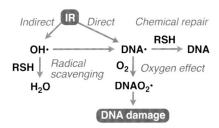

**Figure 8.1** Factors affecting the induction of DNA damage by ionizing radiation (IR). Ionizing radiation can ionize DNA either by direct action or by indirect action, in which radiation energy is absorbed by neighboring molecules, such as water, leading to the generation of hydroxyl radicals that attack DNA. Sulfur-containing cellular molecules (RSH), such as glutathione, can scavenge hydroxyl radicals by hydrogen atom donations and thereby protect the DNA from the indirect action of radiation. Glutathione can also donate hydrogen atoms to ionized DNA, thereby restoring the integrity of DNA in a process termed *chemical repair.* Oxygen can compete with chemical repair in a process termed the *oxygen effect,* resulting in the enhancement of the biologic effect of ionizing radiation by the fixation of the initial DNA damage into DNA peroxides (DNAO$_2$•).

than lesions induced by UV light. It is believed that DSBs are the critical lesions that lead to cell lethality following exposure to ionizing radiation.[6]

## Damage to Proteins

Although proteins and lipids are subject to damage following exposure to IR, the common belief is that DNA is the critical target for the biologic effects of radiation. Indeed, abrogation of DNA damage surveillance or repair processes in cells results in the enhanced induction of mutations and decreased cell survival following radiation.[5] However, studies of radiation-sensitive and radiation-resistant bacteria imply that mechanisms that suppress protein damage may also play important roles in radiation resistance.[7] *Deinococcus radiodurans* is a bacterium that can survive radiation exposures of up to 17,000 Gy, and its extreme radioresistance has been linked to high intracellular levels of manganese, which protect proteins from oxidation. The thought is that if a cell can limit protein oxidation, then its enzymes will remain active, and cellular functions such as DNA repair will be able to restore the integrity of DNA even after severe DNA damage.[8] It would be interesting to explore whether the concentration of manganese can be manipulated to sensitize tumor cells to radiation therapy. Furthermore, because protein damage due to reactive oxygen species (ROS) accumulate during the aging process, could supplements of manganese turn back the clock on aging?

## Cellular Responses

### DNA Repair

Ever since organisms started to utilize atmospheric oxygen for metabolic respiration many millions of years ago, they have been forced to deal with the cellular damage induced by ROS. Base excision repair (BER) evolved to remove many of the different types of oxidative base lesions and DNA SSBs induced by ROS. However, ROS seldom induce DSBs unless the generation of hydroxyl radicals is clustered near the DNA molecule. A more important source of intracellular generation of DSBs may instead be the process of DNA replication, and it is possible that homologous recombination (HR) repair primarily evolved to overcome DSBs sporadically induced during the replication process. The other major pathway of DSB repair is the nonhomologous end-joining (NHEJ) pathway, which is utilized by immune cells in the process of antibody generation. Although the HR pathway has high fidelity due to the utilization of homologous sister chromatids to ensure that correct DNA ends are joined, the NHEJ pathway lacks this

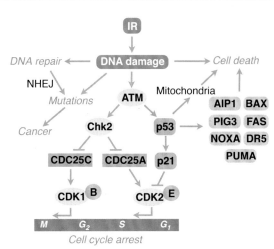

**Figure 8.2** Cellular responses to ionizing radiation. Ionizing radiation induces predominantly base lesions and single- and double-strand breaks. Base lesions and single-strand breaks are repaired by base excision repair (BER), whereas double-strand breaks are repaired by nonhomologous end joining (NHEJ) and homologous recombination (HR). If DNA lesions are misrepaired by NHEJ or not repaired at all before cells enter S phase or mitosis, genomic instability is manifested as mutations or chromosome aberrations that promote carcinogenesis. In order for cells to assist DNA repair and safeguard against genetic instability and cancer, cells can induce cell cycle arrest or apoptosis. The ATM kinase is an early responder to DNA damage induced by ionizing radiation that activates the cell cycle checkpoint kinase Chk2 and the tumor suppressor p53. Chk2 inactivates the CDC25A and CDC25C phosphatases that are critical in promoting cell cycle progression by activating the cyclin-dependent kinases CDK2 or CDK1 and thereby arresting the cells at the G$_1$/S or G$_2$/M checkpoints. In addition, p53 can arrest cells at the G$_1$/S checkpoint by inducing the CDK inhibitor p21. p53 also plays a role in promoting apoptosis by inducing a number of proapoptotic proteins as well as translocating to mitochondria where it inhibits the actions of antiapoptotic factors. AIP1, actin interacting protein 1; BAX, bcl-2-like protein; PIG3, p53-inducible gene 3.

control mechanism and therefore occasionally rejoins ends incorrectly. Thus, the NHEJ pathway may contribute to the generation of mutations following radiation (Fig. 8.2). However, NHEJ is the only mechanism available for DSB repair in postmitotic cells and cells in the G$_1$ phase of the cell cycle because no sister chromatids are available in these cells to support HR repair.

### Ataxia-Telangiectasia Mutated and Cell Cycle Checkpoints

Due to the enormous task of replicating the whole genome during the S phase and segregating the chromosomes during mitosis, proliferating cells are generally much more vulnerable to radiation than stationary cells. To prevent cells with damaged DNA from entering into these critical stages of the cell cycle, cells can activate cell cycle checkpoints (see Fig. 8.2). The major sensor of radiation-induced damage in cells is the ataxia-telangiectasia mutated (ATM) kinase, which, following activation, can phosphorylate more than 700 proteins in cells.[9] Two ATM substrates, p53 and Chk2, are critical for the activation of cell cycle arrests at multiple sites in the cell cycle.[10,11] The kinase p53 regulates the gene expression of specific genes such as *p21*, which inhibits cyclin-dependent kinase (CDK)2- and CDK4-mediated phosphorylation of the retinoblastoma protein, resulting in a block in the progression from the G$_1$ phase to the S phase of the cell cycle.[12,13] The Chk2 kinase promotes checkpoint activation in G$_1$ by targeting the cell division cycle 25 homolog A (CDC25A) phosphatase[14] and, in G$_2$/M, by targeting the CDC25C phosphatase.[15] The activation of a cell cycle arrest following DNA damage provides the cell with additional time to repair the DNA before entering critical cell cycle stages, which promotes genetic stability. Loss or defects in the *ATM* or *p53* genes result in abrogation of radiation-induced cell cycle checkpoints, which manifests itself as the highly cancer-prone human syndromes ataxia telangiectasia[16] or Li-Fraumeni,[17] respectively.

### Radiation-Induced Cell Death

Terminally differentiated and stationary cells, such as kidney, lung, brain, muscle, and liver cells, are generally more resistant to radiation-induced killing than are cells with a high turnover rate, such as different epithelial cells, spermatogonia, and hair follicles. However, the spleen and thymus, which consist of mostly nondividing cells, are among the most radiosensitive tissues, implying that the rate of cell proliferation is not the sole determiner of the radiation sensitivity of a tissue. An important factor regulating the induction of programmed cell death (apoptosis) in tissues is the tumor suppressor p53.[18] The p53 protein is activated in cells following exposure to IR by the ATM kinase (see Fig. 8.2). When activated, it regulates the expression of multiple genes that have roles in DNA repair, cell cycle arrest, and apoptosis. p53 can also localize to mitochondria following irradiation, where it triggers apoptosis through the inactivation of antiapoptotic regulatory proteins.[19] Not all tissues induce the p53 response to the same degree after similar doses of IR, nor do they activate downstream pathways, such as DNA repair, cell cycle arrest, and apoptosis, in a similar way. For example, thymocytes have an intrinsic setting that favors apoptosis over cell cycle arrest following IR, whereas fibroblasts rarely induce apoptosis, but instead activate a strong and lasting cell cycle arrest.[18]

IR can induce cell death in tissues by many different mechanisms. Apoptosis can occur rapidly in a p53-dependent manner or later in a p53-independent manner. This later wave of radiation-induced apoptosis is often initiated by mitotic catastrophe, which occurs as a result of complications during chromosome segregation. Cell death induced by IR may in some cases be associated with autophagy, also called autophagocytosis, in which cells degrade cellular components via the lysosomal machinery. Whether autophagy is a programmed cell death or occurs in parallel with cell death is not clear. Interestingly, for some cell types, autophagy has been shown to actually protect the cells from radiation-induced death. Finally, tissue can undergo necrotic cell death following exposure to IR. Necrosis is a clinical problem following radiation therapy that can occur in normal tissues many months after treatment and can contribute to the inflammatory response.

## Cancer Risks

It is clear from epidemiologic studies of radiation workers and atomic bomb and Chernobyl victims that IR can induce cancer.[20] Twenty years after the atomic bomb explosions in Japan during World War II, significant increases in the incidence of thyroid cancer and leukemia were observed. However, it took almost 50 years before solid tumors appeared in the population as a result of radiation exposure from the atomic bombs.[21] The incidences of solid tumors, such as breast, ovary, bladder, lung, and colon cancers, were estimated to have increased by a factor of 2 in the exposed group during this time period. The epidemiology studies following the nuclear power plant disaster in Chernobyl showed a clear increase in thyroid cancer as early as 4 years after the accident.[22] Young children were the most vulnerable to radiation exposure, with 1-year-old children being 237-fold more susceptible to thyroid cancer than the control group, while 10-year-old children were found to be sixfold more susceptible to thyroid cancer. Many of the thyroid cancers that developed following the Chernobyl disaster could have been prevented if the population had not consumed locally produced milk that was contaminated with radioactive iodine.

The molecular signatures of radiation-induced tumors are complex but involve point mutations that could lead to the activation of the *RAS* oncogene or inactivation of the tumor suppressor gene *p53*. Furthermore, IR induces DNA DSBs that may be unfaithfully repaired by the NHEJ pathway, leading to chromosome rearrangements. One such rearrangement found in 50% to 90% of the thyroid cancers examined following the Chernobyl accident involved the receptor tyrosine kinase c-RET, which promotes cell growth when activated.[22] Furthermore, a great majority of the thyroid cancers found in the exposed children harbored kinase fusion oncogenes affecting the mitogen-activated protein kinase (MAPK) signaling pathway.[23]

The correlation between high exposure to IR and cancer following the atomic bomb explosions and the Chernobyl accident is clear. What about the cancer risk following lower radiation exposures occurring in daily life? There are four theoretical risk models of radiation-induced cancer to consider. First, the *linear, no threshold* (LNT) *model* suggests that the induction of cancer is directly proportional to the dose of radiation, even at low doses of exposure. Second, the *sublinear* or *threshold model* suggests that below a certain threshold dose the risk of radiation-induced cancers is negligible. At these lower doses of radiation exposure, the DNA damage surveillance and repair mechanisms are thought to be fully capable of safeguarding the DNA to avoid the induction of mutations and cancer. Third, the *supralinear* or *stealth model* suggests that doses below a certain threshold or radiation with sufficiently low dose rates may not trigger the activation of DNA damage surveillance and repair mechanisms, resulting in suboptimal activation of cell cycle checkpoints and repair. This would be expected to lead to a higher rate of mutations and cancers than predicted by the LNT model, but may be balanced by a higher incident of cell death. Fourth, the *linear-quadratic model* suggest that radiation effects at low doses are due to a single track of radiation hitting multiple targets, resulting in a linear induction rate, whereas at higher doses, multiple radiation tracks hit multiple cellular targets, resulting in a quadratic induction rate.

The Biological Effects of Ionizing Radiation (BEIR) VII report, released by the Committee on Biological Effects of Ionizing Radiation of the National Academy of Sciences and commissioned by the US Environmental Protection Agency (EPA), is a review of published data regarding human health and cancer risks from exposure to low levels of IR. Although this topic is controversial and not fully settled, the BIER VII report favored the LNT model.[24] Thus, the "official" view is that no level of radiation is safe; therefore, a careful consideration of risks versus benefits is necessary to ensure that the general population only receives radiation doses as low as reasonably achievable. Furthermore, the BIER VII committee concluded that the heritable effects of radiation were not evident in the published data, indicating that an individual is not likely to develop cancer due to radiation exposure of his or her parents.

The largest source of radiation exposure to the population is radon, which is a natural radioactive gas formed as a decay product of radium in the decay chain of uranium. Radon gas can accumulate to high levels in poorly ventilated basements in houses built on rock containing uranium. The major risk with radon is that some of its radioactive decay products can attach to dust particles that accumulate in the lungs, leading to a continuous exposure of the lung tissues to high LET alpha particles. Due to this radiation exposure, the EPA claims that radon is the second leading cause of lung cancer in the United States. Another important source of human exposure to IR is medical x-ray devices, and there is a growing concern about the dramatically increased use of whole body CT scans for diagnostic purposes. For a typical CT scan, a patient will receive about 100-fold more radiation than from a typical mammogram.[24] It is recommended that the use of whole body CT scans for children be very restricted due to the elevated risk of developing radiation-induced cancer for this age group.

Cancer patients who receive radiation therapy are at risk of developing secondary tumors induced by the radiation therapy treatment.[1] This is particularly a concern for young patients since (1) children are more prone to radiation-induced cancer,

(2) children have a relatively good chance of surviving the primary cancer and would have long life expectancies so a secondary tumor would have plenty of time to develop, and (3) many childhood cancers are promoted by genetic defects in DNA damage response pathways, making these patients highly prone to the genotoxic effects of radiation and subsequent secondary cancers. The most sensitive tissues for the development of secondary cancer have been found to be bone marrow (leukemia), the thyroid, breast, and lung.[1]

## ULTRAVIOLET LIGHT

Depending on the wavelength, UV light is categorized into UVA (320 to 400 nm), UVB (290 to 320 nm), and UVC (240 to 290 nm) radiation. Most of the UVC light emitted from the sun is absorbed by the ozone layer in the atmosphere, and, thus, living organisms are mostly exposed to UVA and UVB irradiation.

### Mechanisms of Damage Induction

UVC light is more damaging to DNA than UVA and UVB because the absorption maximum of DNA is around 260 nm. UVB and UVC induce predominantly pyrimidine dimers and 6-4 photoproducts, which consist of covalent ring structures that link two adjacent pyrimidines on the same DNA strand.[5] The formation of these lesions results in the bending of the DNA helix, resulting in the interference with both DNA and RNA synthesis. UVA light does not induce pyrimidine dimers or 6-4 photoproducts but can induce ROS, which in turn can form SSBs and base lesions in DNA of exposed cells.

### Cellular Responses

#### DNA Repair

The nucleotide excision repair (NER) pathway removes pyrimidine dimers and 6-4 photoproducts from cellular DNA.[5] This pathway involves proteins that recognize the DNA lesions, nucleases that excise the DNA strand that contains the lesion, a DNA polymerase that synthesizes new DNA to fill the gap, and a DNA ligase that joins the backbone in the newly synthesized strand. Genetic defects in the NER pathway result in the human syndrome xeroderma pigmentosum, with individuals more than 1,000-fold more prone to sun-induced skin cancer than normal individuals. In addition, human polymorphisms in certain NER genes are thought to predispose individuals to cancers such as lung cancer, nonmelanoma skin cancer, head and neck cancer, and bladder cancer, indicating that NER is responsible for safeguarding the genome against many types of DNA adducts in addition to UV-induced lesions.[5]

UV-induced lesions formed in the transcribed strand of active genes block the elongation of RNA polymerase II, and if a cell does not restore transcription within a certain time frame, it may undergo apoptosis (Fig. 8.3).[25,26] To rapidly restore RNA synthesis and avoid cell death, NER enzymes are recruited to the sites of blocked RNA polymerase II and the lesions are removed in a process called transcription-coupled repair (TCR).[27] Individuals with Cockayne syndrome (CS), trichothiodystrophy, or the UV-sensitive syndrome, are unable to utilize the TCR pathway following UV irradiation.[5] Cells from these individuals do not recover RNA synthesis following UV irradiation and are therefore very prone to UV-induced apoptosis. Interestingly, despite a clear DNA repair defect, these individuals are not predisposed to UV-induced skin cancer. It is thought that the inability of CS cells to remove the toxic lesions that block transcription following UV irradiation results in the suppression of tumorigenesis by the elimination of damaged cells by apoptosis. However, while protecting against

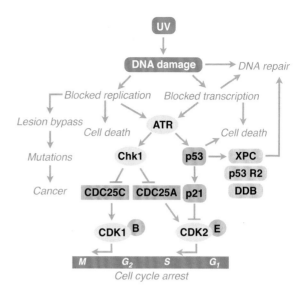

**Figure 8.3** Cellular responses to ultraviolet (UV) light–induced DNA damage. UV light predominantly induces bulky DNA lesions that interfere with the processes of DNA replication and transcription. These lesions are removed from the global genome by global genomic nucleotide excision repair (GG-NER) and from transcribed DNA strands by transcription-coupled NER (TC-NER). Lesions blocking replication can be bypassed by exchanging processive DNA polymerases with less processive translesion DNA polymerases. While these polymerases allow cells to continue DNA synthesis and progress through the cell cycle, they have low fidelity, resulting in the potential induction of mutations promoting UV-induced carcinogenesis. To suppress mutations and support DNA repair efforts, the ataxia-telangiectasia and Rad3-related (ATR) kinase is activated in response to blocked replication or transcription. ATR activates the cell cycle checkpoint kinase Chk1, which, similar to Chk2, arrests cells in the $G_1/S$ and $G_2/M$ checkpoints by inhibiting CDC25A and CDC25C. ATR also activates p53, promoting $G_1/S$ checkpoint activation via the induction of the Cdk-inhibitor p21. p53 also stimulates GG-NER by the transactivation of various NER genes and can promote apoptosis by the induction of proapoptotic factors and translocation to mitochondria. Finally, apoptosis is induced if cells do not recover transcription in a certain time frame, potentially due to the loss of survival factors or complications in the S phase when replication encounters stall the transcription complexes.

tumorigenesis, the elevated level of apoptosis in these cells leads to increased cell loss, which in turn may lead to neurologic degeneration.[25,28] Persistent transcription-blocking lesions in the genome have also been linked to aging.[29–31]

### Translesion DNA Synthesis

Proliferating skin cells are very vulnerable to UV light because UV lesions block DNA replication (see Fig. 8.3). Cells that have entered the S phase and have initiated DNA synthesis have no choice but to finish replicating the whole genome or they will die. If DNA repair enzymes are not able to remove the blocking lesions from the template, the processive DNA polymerases may be exchanged for other, less processive DNA polymerases that can bypass the lesions. This is part of a "tolerance" mechanism, which allows cells to complete replication and eventually divide.[5] However, the translesion DNA polymerases do not have the same fidelity as the processive DNA polymerases; thus, mutations may occur. This is thought to be a major pathway by which UV light induces mutagenesis and, subsequently, cancer (see Fig. 8.3).

### ATM and Rad3-Related Mediated Cell Cycle Checkpoints

In addition to utilizing the NER and BER pathways to repair UV-induced DNA damage, proliferating cells activate cell cycle checkpoints to allow more time for repair before entering critical parts of the cell cycle, such as the S phase and mitosis. The ATM and Rad3-related (ATR) kinase is activated following UV irradiation by blocked replication or transcription (see Fig. 8.3).[32] ATR phosphorylates a large number of proteins, many of which are the same as those phosphorylated by ATM after exposure to ionizing radiation.[9] Two important substrates of ATR are p53 and Chk1, which are critical in promoting cell cycle arrest. When induced by ATR, p53 transactivates the gene that encodes the cell cycle inhibitor p21, leading to the arrest of cells in the $G_1$ phase of the cell cycle, while Chk1 phosphorylates the CDK-activating phosphatases CDC25A and CDC25C, which targets them for degradation, resulting in an S-phase or $G_2$-phase arrest (see Fig. 8.3).[33]

### Activation of Cell Membrane Receptors

In addition to triggering cellular stress responses by inducing DNA damage, UV light can directly induce membrane receptor signaling by receptor phosphorylation. This is thought to be due to the direct UV-mediated inhibition of protein-tyrosine phosphatases that regulate the phosphorylation levels of various membrane receptors.[34] In addition, membrane receptors may physically aggregate following UV irradiation, leading to the activation of signal transduction pathways that regulate cell growth[35] or apoptosis.[36]

### Cell Death

UV light effectively induces apoptosis in skin cells. The mechanism by which UV light induces cell death is not fully understood, but failure to adequately resume RNA synthesis following UV light exposure is strongly linked to apoptosis (see Fig. 8.3).[25] Many potential mechanisms of how blocked transcription results in apoptosis have been suggested, such as a physical clash during the S phase between elongating replication machineries and transcription complexes stalled at UV lesions. Another possible mechanism involves the preferential loss of survival factors coded by highly unstable mRNAs.[37] The induction of p53 may also contribute to UV-induced apoptosis,[38] although p53 appears to protect human fibroblasts[39] and keratinocytes[40] from UV-induced apoptosis. Although complications induced by DNA damage may be the predominant mechanism by which cells die following UV irradiation, UV light may induce apoptosis in certain cell types by directly promoting the physical aggregation of the death receptor Fas/APO1.[36]

### Cancer Risks

The incidence of sun-induced skin cancer, especially melanoma, is on the increase due to higher rates of sun exposure in the general population. The link between UV light exposure and skin cancer is very strong, but the role of UV light in the etiology of nonmelanoma and melanoma skin cancer differs. Although the risk of nonmelanoma cancer relates to the cumulative lifetime exposure to UV light, the risk of contracting melanoma appears to be linked to high sunlight exposure during childhood.[41] What makes UV light such a potent carcinogen is that it can initiate carcinogenesis by inducing DNA lesions as well as suppressing the immune system, resulting in a greater probability that initiated cells will survive and grow into tumors.[42,43]

### Nonmelanoma Skin Cancer

Basal cell carcinoma (BCC) and squamous cell carcinoma (SCC) are the two most common skin cancer types. BCC and SCC occur predominantly in sun-exposed areas of the skin, but there are examples of these cancers forming in nonexposed areas as well. The tumor suppressor genes *p53* and *p16* are frequently inactivated in BCC and SCC, while the hedgehog-signaling pathway is activated primarily by mutations to the patched gene (percutaneous transhepatic cholangiography [*PTCH*]). This scenario promotes proliferation without the opposition of the cell cycle inhibitors p53 and p16.

### Melanoma

Melanoma arises from mutations in epidermal melanocytes and is the most dangerous form of skin cancer because it has the highest propensity to metastasize. It is formed in both sun-exposed and shielded areas of the skin; therefore, the role of UV light as the major carcinogen in melanoma has been controversial.[41] Defects in the NER pathway do not seem to predispose the development of melanoma, suggesting that pyrimidine dimers or 6-4 photoproducts induced by UVB are not the initiators of melanoma carcinogenesis. Instead, ROS induced by UVA may be responsible for the development of melanoma.[41] However, a study using next-generation sequencing techniques to catalog all mutations in a melanoma cell line found a mutational spectrum of the over 33,000 mutations detected that strongly indicated that pyrimidine dimers and 6-4 photoproducts are the major mutagenic lesions in melanoma, whereas a subset of mutations may be induced by ROS.[44] The incidence of mutations in the *p16* and *ARF* genes is high, whereas *p53* and *RAS* mutations are fairly uncommon in melanoma.

### Photoimmunosuppression

Studies of transplantation of mouse skin cancers into syngeneic mice revealed that prior UVB irradiation of recipient mice promoted tumor growth, whereas transplantation into naïve nonirradiated mice led to rejection.[43] These studies established that UV light has local immunosuppressing ability, and subsequent studies found that UV light preferentially depletes Langerhans cells from irradiated skin.[42] Langerhans cells play an important role in the immune response by presenting antigens to the immune cells, and, thus, depletion of these cells leads to local immunosuppression. In addition to local immunosuppression, UV light has been shown to promote systemic immunosuppression.[45] This response is complex, but it is known that UV-induced DNA lesions in skin cells contribute to the systemic immunosuppression response.[46] The secretion of the immunosuppressing cytokine interleukin (IL)-10 from irradiated keratinocytes as well as UV-induced structural alteration of the epidermal chromophore urocanic acid may mediate the long-range immunosuppressive effects of UV light.[42,45]

## RADIOFREQUENCY AND MICROWAVE RADIATION

Radiofrequency radiation (RFR) is electromagnetic radiation in the frequency range 3 kHz to 300 MHz, whereas microwave radiation (MR) is in the frequency range between 300 MHz to 300 GHz. RFR and MR do not have sufficient energies to cause ionizations in target tissues. Rather, the radiation energy is converted into heat as the radiation energy is absorbed. Sources of radiofrequency and microwave radiation include mobile phones, radio transmitters of wireless communication, radars, medical devices, and kitchen appliances.

### Mechanism of Damage Induction

Because human exposure to RFR has increased dramatically in recent years, it is important to know whether this type of radiation gives rise to genotoxic damage. Although there are many studies showing that RFR can induce ROS, leading to genetic damage in cell culture systems, other studies have generated conflicting results.[47] One confounding factor when assessing the genotoxic effect of RFR, and especially MR, is the heating effect that occurs in the tissue when the radiation energy is absorbed. A recent study controlling for the potential heating effect of exposure found that RFR induces ROS and DNA damage in human spermatozoa in vitro, which is an alarming finding considering the potential hereditary implications.[48] It has been suggested that MR may affect the folding of proteins in cells that promote new protein synthesis.[49] Furthermore, exposure of cells to MR has been shown to lead to the phosphorylation of numerous cellular proteins largely through the activation of the p38/MAPK stress response pathway.[50] However, the biologic consequences of these cellular changes are not clear. Epidemiology studies that monitored the genetic effects in individuals exposed to high levels of RF have revealed evidence of increased induction of chromosome aberrations in lymphocytes.[51] However, there is a level of uncertainty in these studies about exposure levels, making it difficult to come to meaningful conclusions.

## Cancer Risks

Because the population's exposure to RFR and MR has dramatically increased in recent years, it is of great importance to assess the potential cancer risks of these types of radiation so that appropriate exposure limits can be implemented. A number of studies have focused on the potential cancer risks from mobile phone usage, and some of these studies indicate that long-term mobile phone usage may be associated with increased risks of developing brain tumors (see the following). Other epidemiologic studies of cancer incidences in populations living near radio towers or mobile phone base stations are inconclusive. Some studies have shown a connection between proximity to mobile phone base stations and increased cancer incidence,[52] whereas another study found no association between exposure to RFR from mobile phone base stations and early childhood cancers.[53]

# ELECTROMAGNETIC FIELDS

An electromagnetic field (EMF) is a physical field produced by electrically charged objects that can affect other charged objects in the field. Typical sources of EMFs are electric power lines, electrical devices, and magnetic resonance imaging (MRI) machines.

## Mechanisms of Damage Induction

A low frequency EMF does not transmit energy high enough to break chemical bonds; therefore, it is not thought to directly damage DNA or proteins in cells. The data obtained from studies to assess the potential genotoxic effects of EMF do not provide a clear conclusion. Some of the results obtained in cell culture studies suggest a harmful effect of EMFs, but the concerns are that these effects may be related to heat production induced by EMFs rather than from the magnetic field itself. A recent in vitro study detected DNA strand breaks in cells exposed to EMFs, but this induction was thought to not be the result of ROS production, but rather due to indirect effects through interference with DNA replication and induction of apoptosis in a subset of cells.[54] A study using an MRI found no evidence of an induced formation of DNA DSBs in cell cultures.[55] EMFs have been shown to induce nongenotoxic effects in cells, such as interference with cellular signaling pathways,[56] which could contribute to neurodegeneration.[57]

## Cancer Risks

Studies with rodents have largely failed to detect an association between exposure to EMFs and cancer. This is also true for numerous epidemiology studies, with the only exception being the association between EMF exposure and childhood leukemia where children exposed to doses of 0.4 mcT or above may have about a twofold increased risk of developing leukemia.[58,59] There is no strong link between EMF exposure and increased risks of contracting adult leukemia, brain tumors, or breast cancer.[60,61] Furthermore, a study investigating whether EMF exposure was associated with heritable effects found no correlation between parental exposure and childhood cancer.[62]

## Potential Cancer Risks from Mobile Phone Usage

Mobile phones emit RFR and generate EMFs. The biggest health concern with mobile phone usage is its potential role in the development of brain tumors. During mobile phone use, the brain tissue is exposed to doses, giving peak specific absorption rates (SAR) of 4 to 8 W/kg. At these intensities, the induction of DNA damage has been detected in laboratory studies.[63] The current epidemiologic data are largely inconclusive on the association between mobile phone usage and brain tumor incidence. Meta-analysis studies of populations who had used mobile phones for more than 10 years concluded that mobile phone usage was associated with an elevated risk for brain tumors, such as acoustic neuroma and glioma cancer.[64–66] In contrast, other large prospective studies did not observe a correlation between mobile phone usage and incidences of glioma, meningioma, or non–central nervous system (CNS) cancers.[67,68] It is important to point out that, generally, it takes 30 to 40 years for brain tumors to develop, and because mobile phones have only been in general use for about 15 years, there has not been sufficient time to fully evaluate the brain cancer risks of mobile phone usage.

# ASBESTOS

Asbestos is a class of naturally occurring silicate minerals that have been widely used in building materials for its heat, sound, and electrical insulating qualities. Asbestos becomes a serious health hazard if the fibers are inhaled over a long period of time, and these health effects are increased dramatically if the exposed individual is a smoker. It was first reported in 1935 that asbestos might be an occupational health hazard that could induce cancer.[69,70] However, it was not until 1986 that the International Labor Organization recommended banning asbestos.[71] The use of asbestos products peaked in the 1970s, yet remains a major health hazard in many places around the world today.

## Mechanisms of Damage Induction

Asbestos fibers can enter cells and induce ROS, especially if they contain high levels of iron.[72] In addition, ROS can be generated by "frustrated" phagocytosis, and this in turn can lead to the release of proinflammatory cytokines with subsequent inflammation of the tissue. ROS have been implicated to originate from affected mitochondria leading to induction of SSBs and base damage, such as 8-hydroxyguanine in DNA.[73] Furthermore, if not successfully repaired, asbestos-induced DNA damage has been shown to result in chromosome aberrations, micronuclei formation, and increased rates of sister chromatid exchanges.[74]

## Cellular and Tissue Responses

Asbestos-induced ROS cause base lesions and DNA strand breaks, which require base excision repair for the restoration of DNA and for minimizing mutagenesis. In addition to DNA repair, a number of cellular signaling pathways are activated by asbestos. These include the epidermal growth factor receptor (EGFR) and the MAPK pathway, leading to the activation of nuclear factor kappa B

(NF-κB) and transcription factor AP-1.[72,74] Activation of the NF-κB pathway leads to the induction of proinflammatory genes such as tumor necrosis factor (TNF), *IL-6*, *IL-8*, and proliferation-promoting genes such as *c-Myc*, leading to inflammation and increased cell proliferation. Asbestos exposure also stimulates the expression of the transforming growth factor beta (TGF-β), which, in turn, stimulates fibrogenesis in exposed tissues.[74]

## Cancer Risks

### Lung Cancer

Epidemiologic studies have found a strong link between asbestos exposure and lung cancer.[74] It has been estimated that about 5% to 7% of all lung cancers are attributable to asbestos exposure, and asbestos and tobacco smoking act in synergy to induce lung cancer. Mutational spectra due to 8-hydroxyguanine lesions formed by ROS can be linked to asbestos exposure, and point mutations in the tumor suppressor genes *p53* and *p16/INK4A* and in the *KRAS* oncogene have been found in tumors from asbestos-exposed individuals.

### Mesothelioma

After being taken up by lung tissues, asbestos fibers can translocate into the pleura, the body cavity that surrounds the lungs. The pleura are covered with a protective lining, the mesothelium, which consists of squamouslike epithelial cells. Mesothelial cells can internalize asbestos fibers, resulting in the induction of ROS and inflammatory responses, subsequently leading to the initiation and progression of malignant mesothelioma.[75] Asbestos is considered one of the major causes of malignant mesothelioma, and frequent mutations are found in the *p16/INK4A* and *NF2* genes, whereas *p53* mutations are fairly rare.

## NANOPARTICLES

Nanoparticles are defined as ultrafine particles of the size range 1 to 100 nm in diameter. Nanoparticle chemistry of a certain compound is different from bulk chemistry of that compound because of the high percentage of atoms at the surface of the particle. The production of nanoparticles has increased dramatically in recent years, and they are found in many industrial and consumer products such as paint, cosmetics, and sunscreens. They also have many potential medical applications, such as delivery vehicles for specific drugs to specific target tissues or tumors.

## Mechanisms of DNA Damage Induction

Many of the cellular effects of nanoparticles are similar to the effects exerted by asbestos, such as the generation of ROS and inflammation.[72] Nanoparticles have been shown to induce oxidative DNA damage, such as DNA strand breaks and 8-hydroxyguanine lesions both in cell culture[76, 77] and in vivo.[78] Nanoparticle-induced DNA lesions are manifested as histone γ-H2AX nuclear foci, chromosome deletions, and micronuclei.

## Cellular Responses

Nanoparticles induce ROS either directly or indirectly, resulting in DNA lesions, such as 8-hydroxyguanine–base damage and DNA strand breaks. These lesions are repaired by the base excision repair. The phosphorylation of histone H2AX has been shown to occur following exposure of cells to nanoparticles, suggesting that the DNA lesions trigger the activation of ATM or ATR stress kinases.[79] Nanoparticles have also been found to affect the immune system[80] and can induce the release of the proinflammatory cytokine TNF-α from cells.

## Cancer Risks

Some nanoparticles, such as titanium dioxide, which is used as pigments in paint, have been classified by the International Agency for Research on Cancer (IARC) as a group 2B carcinogen, "possible carcinogenic to humans." However, rigorous epidemiologic data is lacking to fully evaluate the cancer-inducing potential of nanoparticles.[81]

## REFERENCES

1. Hall E, Giaccia A. *Radiobiology for the Radiologist*. Philadelphia: Lippincott Williams & Wilkins; 2012.
2. Ward JF. DNA damage produced by ionizing radiation in mammalian cells: identities, mechanisms of formation, and repairability. *Prog Nucleic Acid Res Mol Biol* 1988;35:95–125.
3. Prutz WA. 'Chemical repair' in irradiated DNA solutions containing thiols and/or disulphides. Further evidence for disulphide radical anions acting as electron donors. *Int J Radiat Biol* 1989;56:21–33.
4. Hutchinson F. Chemical changes induced in DNA by ionizing radiation. *Prog Nucleic Acid Res Mol Biol* 1985;32:115–154.
5. Friedberg E, Walker G, Siede W, et al. *DNA Repair and Mutagenesis*. 2nd ed. Washington, D.C.: ASM Press; 2006.
6. Radford IR. The level of induced DNA double-strand breakage correlates with cell killing after X-irradiation. *Int J Radiat Biol Relat Stud Phys Chem Med* 1985;48:45–54.
7. Daly MJ. A new perspective on radiation resistance based on *Deinococcus radiodurans*. *Nat Rev Microbiol* 2009;7:237–245.
8. Krisko A, Radman M. Biology of extreme radiation resistance: the way of *Deinococcus radiodurans*. *Cold Spring Harb Perspect Biol* 2013;5.
9. Matsuoka S, Ballif BA, Smogorzewska A, et al. ATM and ATR substrate analysis reveals extensive protein networks responsive to DNA damage. *Science* 2007;316:1160–1166.
10. Kastan M, Onyekwere O, Sidransky D, et al. Participation of p53 protein in the cellular response to DNA damage. *Cancer Res* 1991;51:6304–6311.
11. Matsuoka S, Huang M, Elledge SJ. Linkage of ATM to cell cycle regulation by the Chk2 protein kinase. *Science* 1998;282:1893–1897.
12. Harper J, Adami G, Wei N, et al. The p21 cdk-interacting protein Cip1 is a potent inhibitor of G1 cyclin-dependent kinases. *Cell* 1993;75:805–816.
13. El-Deiry W, Tokino T, Velculescu V, et al. WAF1, a potential mediater of p53 tumor suppression. *Cell* 1993;75:817–825.
14. Falck J, Mailand N, Syljuasen RG, et al. The ATM-Chk2-Cdc25A checkpoint pathway guards against radioresistant DNA synthesis. *Nature* 2001;410:842–847.
15. Bartek J, Falck J, Lukas J. Chk2 kinase—a busy messenger [Review]. *Nat Rev Mol Cell Biol* 2001;2:877–886.
16. Savitsky K, Bar-Shira A, Gilad S, et al. A single ataxia telangiectasia gene with a product similar to PI-3 kinase. *Science* 1995;268:1749–1753.
17. Srivastava S, Zou ZQ, Pirollo K, et al. Germ-line transmission of a mutated p53 gene in a cancer-prone family with Li-Fraumeni syndrome. *Nature* 1990;348:747–749.
18. Gudkov AV, Komarova EA. The role of p53 in determining sensitivity to radiotherapy. *Nat Rev Cancer* 2003;3:117–129.
19. Mihara M, Erster S, Zaika A, et al. p53 has a direct apoptogenic role at the mitochondria. *Mol Cell* 2003;11:577–590.
20. Williams D, Baverstock K. Chernobyl and the future: too soon for a final diagnosis. *Nature* 2006;440:993–994.
21. Thompson DE, Mabuchi K, Ron E, et al. Cancer incidence in atomic bomb survivors. Part II: Solid tumors, 1958–1987. *Radiat Res* 1994;137:S17–67.
22. Williams D. Cancer after nuclear fallout: lessons from the Chernobyl accident. *Nat Rev Cancer* 2002;2:543–549.
23. Ricarte-Filho JC, Li S, Garcia-Rendueles ME, et al. Identification of kinase fusion oncogenes in post-Chernobyl radiation-induced thyroid cancers. *J Clin Invest* 2013;123:4935–4944.
24. National Research Council. *Health Risks from Exposure to Low Levels of Ionizing Radiation: BEIR VII Phase 2*. Washington, D.C.: National Academy Press; 2006.
25. Ljungman M, Zhang F. Blockage of RNA polymerase as a possible trigger for u.v. light-induced apoptosis. *Oncogene* 1996;13:823–831.
26. Brash DE, Wikonkal NM, Remenyik E, et al. The DNA damage signal for Mdm2 regulation, Trp53 induction, and sunburn cell formation in vivo originates from actively transcribed genes. *J Invest Derm* 2001;117:1234–1240.

27. Hanawalt PC, Spivak G. Transcription-coupled DNA repair: two decades of progress and surprises. *Nat Rev Mol Cell Biol* 2008;9:958–970.
28. Lehmann AR. DNA repair-deficient diseases, xeroderma pigmentosum, Cockayne syndrome and trichothiodystrophy. *Biochimie* 2003;85:1101–1111.
29. Andressoo JO, Hoeijmakers JH. Transcription-coupled repair and premature ageing. *Mutat Res* 2005;577:179–194.
30. de Boer J, Andressoo JO, de Wit J, et al. Premature aging in mice deficient in DNA repair and transcription. *Science* 2002;296:1276–1279.
31. Garinis GA, Uittenboogaard LM, Stachelscheid H, et al. Persistent transcription-blocking DNA lesions trigger somatic growth attenuation associated with longevity. *Nat Cell Biol* 2009;11:604–615.
32. Derheimer FA, O'Hagan HM, Krueger HM, et al. RPA and ATR link transcriptional stress to p53. *Proc Natl Acad Sci U S A* 2007;104:12778–12783.
33. Kastan MB, Bartek J. Cell-cycle checkpoints and cancer. *Nature* 2004;432:316–323.
34. Gross S, Knebel A, Tenev T, et al. Inactivation of protein-tyrosine phosphatases as mechanism of UV-induced signal transduction. *J Biol Chem* 1999;274:26378–26386.
35. Sachsenmaier C, Radlerpohl A, Zinck R, et al. Involvement of growth factor receptors in the mammalian UVC response. *Cell* 1994;78:963–972.
36. Rehemtulla A, Hamilton CA, Chinnaiyan AM, et al. Ultraviolet radiation-induced apoptosis is mediated by activation of CD-95 (Fas/APO-1). *J Biol Chem* 1997;272:25783–25786.
37. Ljungman M, Lane DP. Transcription - guarding the genome by sensing DNA damage. *Nat Rev Cancer* 2004;4:727–737.
38. Ziegler A, Jonason AS, Leffell DJ, et al. Sunburn and p53 in the onset of skin cancer. *Nature* 1994;372:773–776.
39. McKay B, Ljungman M. Role for p53 in the recovery of transcription and protection against apoptosis induced by ultraviolet light. *Neoplasia* 1999;1:276–284.
40. Chaturvedi V, Sitailo LA, Qin JZ, et al. Knockdown of p53 levels in human keratinocytes accelerates Mcl-1 and Bcl-x(L) reduction thereby enhancing UV-light induced apoptosis. *Oncogene* 2005;24:5299–5312.
41. Maddodi N, Setaluri V. Role of UV in cutaneous melanoma. *Photochem Photobiol* 2008;84:528–536.
42. Murphy GM. Ultraviolet radiation and immunosuppression. *Br J Dermatol* 2009;161(Suppl 3):90–95.
43. Fisher MS, Kripke ML. Systemic alteration induced in mice by ultraviolet light irradiation and its relationship to ultraviolet carcinogenesis. *Proc Natl Acad Sci U S A* 1977;74:1688–1692.
44. Pleasance ED, Cheetham RK, Stephens PJ, et al. A comprehensive catalogue of somatic mutations from a human cancer genome. *Nature* 2010;463:191–196.
45. Schwarz T. Photoimmunosuppression. *Photodermatol Photoimmunol Photomed* 2002;18:141–145.
46. Kripke ML, Cox PA, Alas LG, et al. Pyrimidine dimers in DNA initiate systemic immunosuppression in UV-irradiated mice. *Proc Natl Acad Sci U S A* 1992;89:7516–7520.
47. Vijayalaxmi, Prihoda TJ. Genetic damage in mammalian somatic cells exposed to radiofrequency radiation: a meta-analysis of data from 63 publications (1990–2005). *Radiat Res* 2008;169:561–574.
48. De Iuliis GN, Newey RJ, King BV, et al. Mobile phone radiation induces reactive oxygen species production and DNA damage in human spermatozoa in vitro. *PLoS One* 2009;4:e6446.
49. Gerner C, Haudek V, Schandl U, et al. Increased protein synthesis by cells exposed to a 1,800-MHz radio-frequency mobile phone electromagnetic field, detected by proteome profiling. *Int Arch Occup Environ Health* 2010;83:691–702.
50. Leszczynski D, Joenvaara S, Reivinen J, et al. Non-thermal activation of the hsp27/p38MAPK stress pathway by mobile phone radiation in human endothelial cells: molecular mechanism for cancer- and blood-brain barrier-related effects. *Differentiation* 2002;70:120–129.
51. Verschaeve L. Genetic damage in subjects exposed to radiofrequency radiation. *Mutat Res* 2009;681:259–270.
52. Khurana VG, Hardell L, Everaert J, et al. Epidemiological evidence for a health risk from mobile phone base stations. *Int J Occup Environ Health* 2010;16:263–267.
53. Elliott P, Toledano MB, Bennett J, et al. Mobile phone base stations and early childhood cancers: case-control study. *BMJ* 2010;340:c3077.
54. Focke F, Schuermann D, Kuster N, et al. DNA fragmentation in human fibroblasts under extremely low frequency electromagnetic field exposure. *Mutat Res* 2010;683:74–83.
55. Schwenzer NF, Bantleon R, Maurer B, et al. Detection of DNA double-strand breaks using gammaH2AX after MRI exposure at 3 Tesla: an in vitro study. *J Magn Reson Imaging* 2007;26:1308–1314.
56. Girgert R, Hanf V, Emons G, et al. Signal transduction of the melatonin receptor MT1 is disrupted in breast cancer cells by electromagnetic fields. *Bioelectromagnetics* 2010;31:237–245.
57. Consales C, Merla C, Marino C, et al. Electromagnetic fields, oxidative stress, and neurodegeneration. *Int J Cell Biol* 2012;2012:683897.
58. Ahlbom A, Day N, Feychting M, et al. A pooled analysis of magnetic fields and childhood leukaemia. *Br J Cancer* 2000;83:692–698.
59. Malagoli C, Fabbi S, Teggi S, et al. Risk of hematological malignancies associated with magnetic fields exposure from power lines: a case-control study in two municipalities of northern Italy. *Environ Health* 2010;9:16.
60. Kheifets L, Monroe J, Vergara X, et al. Occupational electromagnetic fields and leukemia and brain cancer: an update to two meta-analyses. *J Occup Environ Med* 2008;50:677–688.
61. Chen C, Ma X, Zhong M, et al. Extremely low-frequency electromagnetic fields exposure and female breast cancer risk: a meta-analysis based on 24,338 cases and 60,628 controls. *Breast Cancer Res Treat* 2010;123:569–576.
62. Hug K, Grize L, Seidler A, et al. Parental occupational exposure to extremely low frequency magnetic fields and childhood cancer: a German case-control study. *Am J Epidemiol* 2010;171:27–35.
63. Hardell L, Sage C. Biological effects from electromagnetic field exposure and public exposure standards. *Biomed Pharmacother* 2008;62:104–109.
64. Hardell L, Carlberg M, Hansson Mild K. Mobile phone use and the risk for malignant brain tumors: a case-control study on deceased cases and controls. *Neuroepidemiology* 2010;35:109–114.
65. Hardell L, Carlberg M, Soderqvist F, et al. Meta-analysis of long-term mobile phone use and the association with brain tumours. *Int J Oncol* 2008;32:1097–1103.
66. Myung SK, Ju W, McDonnell DD, et al. Mobile phone use and risk of tumors: a meta-analysis. *J Clin Oncol* 2009;27:5565–5572.
67. Benson VS, Pirie K, Schuz J, et al. Mobile phone use and risk of brain neoplasms and other cancers: prospective study. *Int J Epidemiol* 2013;42:792–802.
68. Poulsen AH, Friis S, Johansen C, et al. Mobile phone use and the risk of skin cancer: a nationwide cohort study in Denmark. *Am J Epidemiol* 2013;178:190–197.
69. Lynch K, Smith W. Pulmonary asbestosis. III. Carcinoma of lung in asbestos-silicosis. *Am J Cancer* 1935;24:56–64.
70. Gloyne S. Two cases of squamous carcinoma of the lung occuring in asbestosis. *Tubercele* 1935;17:5–10.
71. LaDou J. The asbestos cancer epidemic. *Environ Health Perspect* 2004;112:285–290.
72. Pacurari M, Castranova V, Vallyathan V. Single- and multi-wall carbon nanotubes versus asbestos: are the carbon nanotubes a new health risk to humans? *J Toxicol Environ Health A* 2010;73:378–395.
73. Liu G, Cheresh P, Kamp DW. Molecular basis of asbestos-induced lung disease. *Annu Rev Pathol* 2013;8:161–187.
74. Nymark P, Wikman H, Hienonen-Kempas T, et al. Molecular and genetic changes in asbestos-related lung cancer. *Cancer Lett* 2008;265:1–15.
75. Jaurand MC, Renier A, Daubriac J. Mesothelioma: do asbestos and carbon nanotubes pose the same health risk? *Part Fibre Toxicol* 2009;6:16.
76. Shukla RK, Kumar A, Gurbani D, et al. TiO(2) nanoparticles induce oxidative DNA damage and apoptosis in human liver cells. *Nanotoxicology* 2013;7:48–60.
77. Horie M, Nishio K, Endoh S, et al. Chromium(III) oxide nanoparticles induced remarkable oxidative stress and apoptosis on culture cells. *Environ Toxicol* 2013;28:61–75.
78. Trouiller B, Reliene R, Westbrook A, et al. Titanium dioxide nanoparticles induce DNA damage and genetic instability in vivo in mice. *Cancer Res* 2009;69:8784–8789.
79. Prasad RY, Chastain PD, Nikolaishvili-Feinberg N, et al. Titanium dioxide nanoparticles activate the ATM-Chk2 DNA damage response in human dermal fibroblasts. *Nanotoxicology* 2013;7:1111–1119.
80. Zolnik BS, Gonzalez-Fernandez A, Sadrieh N, et al. Nanoparticles and the immune system. *Endocrinology* 2010;151:458–465.
81. Shi H, Magaye R, Castranova V, et al. Titanium dioxide nanoparticles: a review of current toxicological data. *Part Fibre Toxicol* 2013;10:15.

ETIOLOGY AND EPIDEMIOLOGY OF CANCER

# 9 Dietary Factors

Karin B. Michels and Walter C. Willett

## INTRODUCTION

Over two decades ago, Doll and Peto[1] speculated that 35% (range: 10% to 70%) of all cancer deaths in the United States may be preventable by alterations in diet. The magnitude of the estimate for dietary factors exceeded that for tobacco (30%) and infections (10%).

Studies of cancer incidence among populations migrating to countries with different lifestyle factors have indicated that most cancers have a large environmental etiology. Although the contribution of environmental influences differs by cancer type, the incidence of many cancers changes by as much as five- to tenfold among migrants over time, approaching that of the host country. The age at migration affects the degree of adaptation among first-generation migrants for some cancers, suggesting that the susceptibility to environmental carcinogenic influences varies with age by cancer type. Identifying the specific environmental and lifestyle factors most important to cancer etiology, however, has proven difficult.

Environmental factors such as diet may influence the incidence of cancer through many different mechanisms and at different stages in the cancer process. Simple mutagens in foods, such as those produced by the heating of proteins, can cause damage to DNA, but dietary factors can also influence this process by inducing enzymes that activate or inactivate these mutagens, or by blocking the action of the mutagen. Dietary factors can also affect every pathway hypothesized to mediate cancer risk–for example, the rate of cell cycling through hormonal or antihormonal effects, aiding or inhibiting DNA repair, promoting or inhibiting apoptosis, and DNA methylation. Because of the complexity of these mechanisms, knowledge of dietary influences on risk of cancer will require an empirical basis with human cancer as the outcome.

## METHODOLOGIC CHALLENGES

### Study Types and Biases

The association between diet and the risk of cancer has been the subject of a number of epidemiologic studies. The most prevalent designs are the case-control study, the cohort study, and the randomized clinical trial. When the results from epidemiologic studies are interpreted, the potential for confounding must be considered. Individuals who maintain a healthy diet are likely to exhibit other indicators of a healthy lifestyle, including regular physical activity, lower body weight, use of multivitamin supplements, lower smoking rates, and lower alcohol consumption. Even if the influence of these confounding variables is analytically controlled, residual confounding remains possible.

### Ecologic Studies

In ecologic studies or international correlation studies, variation in food disappearance data and the prevalence of a certain disease are correlated, generally across different countries. A linear association may provide preliminary data to inform future research but, due to the high probability of confounding, cannot provide strong evidence for a causal link. Food disappearance data also may not provide a good estimate for human consumption. The gross national product is correlated with many dietary factors such as fat intake.[2] Many other differences besides dietary fat exist between the countries with low fat consumption (less affluent) and high fat consumption (more affluent); reproductive behaviors, physical activity level, and body fatness are particularly notable and are strongly associated with specific cancers.

### Migrant Studies

Studies of populations migrating from areas with low incidence of disease to areas with high incidence of disease (or vice versa) can help sort out the role of environmental factors versus genetics in the etiology of a cancer, depending on whether the migrating group adopts the cancer rates of the new environment. Specific dietary components linked to disease are difficult to identify in a migrant study.

### Case-Control Studies

Case-control studies of diet may be affected by recall bias, control selection bias, and confounding. In a case-control study, participants affected by the disease under study (cases) and healthy controls are asked to recall their past dietary habits. Cases may overestimate their consumption of foods that are commonly considered "unhealthy" and underestimate their consumption of foods considered "healthy." Giovannucci et al.[3] have documented differential reporting of fat intake before and after disease occurrence. Thus, the possibility of recall bias in a case-control study poses a real threat to the validity of the observed associations. Even more importantly, in contemporary case-control studies using a population sample of controls, the participation rate of controls is usually far from complete, often 50% to 70%. Unfortunately, health-conscious individuals may be more likely to participate as controls and will thus be less overweight, will consume fruits and vegetables more frequently, and will consume less fat and red meat, which can substantially distort associations observed.

### Cohort Studies

Prospective cohort studies of the effects of diet are likely to have a much higher validity than retrospective case-control studies because diet is recorded by participants before disease occurrence. Cohort studies are still affected by measurement error because diet consists of a large number of foods eaten in complex combinations. Confounding by other unmeasured or imperfectly measured lifestyle factors can remain a problem in cohort studies.

Now that the results of a substantial number of cohort studies have become available, their findings can be compared with those of case-control studies that have examined the same relations. In many cases, the findings of the case-control studies have not been confirmed; for example, the consistent finding of lower risk of many cancers with higher intake of fruits and vegetables in case-control studies has generally not been seen in cohort studies.[4] These findings suggest that the concerns about biases in case-control studies of diet, and probably many other lifestyle factors, are justified, and findings from such studies must be interpreted cautiously.

## Randomized Clinical Trials

The gold standard in medical research is the randomized clinical trial (RCT). In an RCT on nutrition, participants are randomly assigned to one of two or more diets; hence, the association between diet and the cancer of interest should not be confounded by other factors. The problem with RCTs of diet is that maintaining the assigned diet strictly over many years, as would be necessary for diet to have an impact on cancer incidence, is difficult. For example, in the dietary fat reduction trial of the Women's Health Initiative (WHI), participants randomized to the intervention arm reduced their fat intake much less than planned.[5] The remaining limited contrast between the two groups left the lack of difference in disease outcomes difficult to interpret. Furthermore, the relevant time window for intervention and the necessary duration of intervention are unclear, especially with cancer outcomes. Hence, randomized trials are rarely used to examine the effect of diet on cancer but have better promise for the study of diet and outcomes that require a considerably shorter follow-up time (e.g., adenoma recurrence). Also, the randomized design may lend itself better to the study of the effects of dietary supplements such as multivitamin or fiber supplements, although the control group may adopt the intervention behavior because nutritional supplements are widely available. For example, in the WHI trial of calcium and vitamin D supplementation, two-thirds of the study population used vitamin D or calcium supplements that they obtained outside of the trial, again rendering the lack of effect in the trial uninterpretable.

## Diet Assessment Instruments

Observational studies depend on a reasonably valid assessment of dietary intake. Although, for some nutrients, biochemical measurements can be used to assess intake, for most dietary constituents, a useful biochemical indicator does not exist. In population-based studies, diet is generally assessed with a self-administered instrument. Since 1980, considerable effort has been directed at the development of standardized questionnaires for measuring diet, and numerous studies have been conducted to assess the validity of these methods. The most widely used diet assessment instruments are the food frequency questionnaire, the 7-day diet record, and the 24-hour recall. Although the 7-day diet record may provide the most accurate documentation of intake during the week the participant keeps a diet diary, the burden of computerizing the information and extracting foods and nutrients has prohibited the use of the 7-day diet record in most large-scale studies. The 24-hour recall provides only a snapshot of diet on one day, which may or may not be representative of the participant's usual diet and is thus affected by both personal variation and seasonal variation. The food frequency questionnaire, the most widely used instrument in large population-based studies, asks participants to report their average intake of a large number of foods during the previous year. Participants tend to substantially overreport their fruit and vegetable consumption on the food frequency questionnaire.[6] This tendency may reflect social desirability bias, which leads to overreporting healthy foods and underreporting less healthy foods. Studies of validity using biomarkers or detailed measurements of diet as comparisons have suggested that carefully designed questionnaires can have sufficient validity to detect moderate to strong associations. Validity can be enhanced by using the average of repeated assessments over time.[7]

# THE ROLE OF INDIVIDUAL FOOD AND NUTRIENTS IN CANCER ETIOLOGY

## Energy

The most important impact of diet on the risk of cancer is mediated through body weight. Overweight, obesity, and inactivity are major contributors to cancer risk. (A more detailed discussion is provided in Chapter 10.) In the large American Cancer Society Cohort, obese individuals had substantially higher mortality from all cancers and, in particular, from colorectal cancer, postmenopausal breast cancer, uterine cancer, cervical cancer, pancreatic cancer, and gallbladder cancer than their normal-weight counterparts.[8] Adiposity and, in particular, waist circumference are predictors of colon cancer incidence among women and men.[9,10] A weight gain of 10 kg or more is associated with a significant increase in postmenopausal breast cancer incidence among women who never used hormone replacement therapy, whereas a weight loss of comparable magnitude after menopause substantially decreases breast cancer risk.[11] Regular physical activity contributes to a lower prevalence of being overweight and obesity and consequently reduces the burden of cancer through this pathway.

The mechanisms whereby adiposity increases the risk of various cancers are probably multiple. Being overweight is strongly associated with endogenous estrogen levels, which likely contribute to the excess risks of endometrial and postmenopausal breast cancers. The reasons for the association with other cancers are less clear, but excess body fat is also related to higher circulating levels of insulin, insulin-like growth factor (IGF)-1, and C-peptide (a marker of insulin secretion), lower levels of binding proteins for sex hormones and IGF-1, and higher levels of various inflammatory factors, all of which have been hypothesized to be related to risks of various cancers.

Energy restriction is one of the most effective measures to prevent cancer in the animal model. While energy restriction is more difficult to study in humans, voluntary starvation among anorectics and situations of food rationing during famines provide related models. Breast cancer rates were substantially reduced among women with a history of severe anorexia.[12] Although breast cancer incidence was higher among women exposed to the Dutch famine during childhood or adolescence, such short-term involuntary food rationing for 9 months or less was often followed by overnutrition.[13] A more prolonged deficit in food availability during World War II in Norway was associated with a reduction in adult risk of breast cancer if it occurred during early adolescence.[14]

## Alcohol

Aside from body weight, alcohol consumption is the best established dietary risk factor for cancer. Alcohol is classified as a carcinogen by the International Agency for Research on Cancer. The consumption of alcohol increases the risk of numerous cancers, including those of the liver, esophagus, pharynx, oral cavity, larynx, breast, and colorectum in a dose-dependent fashion.[15] Evidence is convincing that excessive alcohol consumption increases the risk of primary liver cancer, probably through cirrhosis and alcoholic hepatitis. At least in the developed world, about 75% of cancers of the esophagus, pharynx, oral cavity, and larynx are attributable to alcohol and tobacco, with a marked increase in risk among drinkers who also smoke, suggesting a multiplicative effect. Mechanisms may include direct damage to the cells in the upper gastrointestinal tract; modulation of DNA methylation, which affects susceptibility to DNA mutations; and an increase in acetaldehyde, the main metabolite of alcohol, which enhances the proliferation of epithelial cells, forms DNA adducts, and is a recognized carcinogen. The association between alcohol consumption and breast cancer is notable because a small but significant risk has been found even with one drink per day. Mechanisms may include an interaction with folate, an increase in endogenous estrogen levels, and an elevation of acetaldehyde. Some evidence suggests that the excess risk is mitigated by adequate folate intake possibly through an effect on DNA methylation.[16] Notably, for most cancer sites, no important difference in associations was found with the type of alcoholic beverage, suggesting a critical role of ethanol in carcinogenesis.

## Dietary Fat

In recent years, reducing dietary fat has been at the center of cancer prevention efforts. In the landmark 1982 National Academy of Sciences review of diet, nutrition, and cancer, a reduction in fat intake to 30% of calories was the primary recommendation.

Interest in dietary fat as a cause of cancer began in the first half of the 20th century, when studies by Tannenbaum[17] indicated that diets high in fat could promote tumor growth in animal models. Dietary fat has a clear effect on tumor incidence in many models, although not in all; however, a central issue has been whether this is independent of the effect of energy intake. In the 1970s, the possible relation of dietary fat intake to cancer incidence gained greater attention as the large international differences in rates of many cancers were noted to be strongly correlated with apparent per capita fat consumption in ecologic studies.[2] Particularly strong associations were seen with cancers of the breast, colon, prostate, and endometrium, which include the most important cancers not due to smoking in affluent countries. These correlations were observed to be limited to animal, not vegetable, fat.

### Dietary Fat and Breast Cancer

Breast cancer is the most common malignancy among women, and incidence has been increasing for decades, although a decline has been noted starting with the new millennium. Rates in most parts of Asia, South America, and Africa have been only approximately one-fifth that of the United States, but in almost all these areas rates of breast cancer are also increasing. Populations that migrate from low- to high-incidence countries develop breast cancer rates that approximate those of the new host country. However, rates do not approach those of the general US population until the second or third generation.[18] This slower rate of change for immigrants may indicate delayed acculturation; although because a similar delay in rate increase is not observed for colon cancer, it may suggest an origin of breast cancer earlier in the life course.

The results from 12 smaller case-control studies that included 4,312 cases and 5,978 controls have been summarized in a meta-analysis.[19] The pooled relative risk (RR) was 1.35 ($P$ <.0001) for a 100-g increase in daily total fat intake, although the risk was somewhat stronger for postmenopausal women (RR, 1.48; $P$ <.001). This magnitude of association, however, could be compatible with biases due to recall of diet or the selection of controls.

Because of the prospective design of cohort studies, most of the methodologic biases of case-control studies are avoided. In an analysis of the Nurses' Health Study that included 121,700 US female registered nurses, no association with total fat intake was observed, and there was no suggestion of any reduction in risk at intakes below 25% of energy.[20] Because repeated assessments of diet were obtained at 2- to 4-year intervals, this analysis provided a particularly detailed evaluation of fat intake over an extended period in relation to breast cancer risk. Similar observations were made in the National Institutes of Health (NIH)–American Association of Retired Persons (AARP) Diet and Health Study including 188,736 postmenopausal women[21] and in the European Prospective Investigation into Cancer and Nutrition (EPIC), which included 7,119 incident cases.[22] In a pooled analysis of seven prospective studies, which included 337,000 women who developed 4,980 incident cases of breast cancer, no overall association was seen for fat intake over the range of less than 20% to more than 45% energy (reflecting the current range observed

internationally).[23] A similar lack of association was seen for specific types of fat. This lack of association with total fat intake was confirmed in a subsequent analysis of the pooled prospective studies of diet and breast cancer, which included over 7,000 cases.[24] Therefore, these cohort findings do not support the hypothesis that dietary fat is an important contributor to breast cancer incidence.

Endogenous estrogen levels have now been established as a risk factor for breast cancer. Thus, the effects of fat and other dietary factors on estrogen levels are of potential interest. Vegetarian women, who consume higher amounts of fiber and lower amounts of fat, have lower blood levels and reduced urinary excretion of estrogens, apparently due to increased fecal excretion. A meta-analysis has suggested that a reduction in dietary fat reduces plasma estrogen levels,[25] but the studies included were plagued by the lack of concurrent controls, the short duration, and the negative energy balance. In a large, randomized trial among postmenopausal women with a previous diagnosis of breast cancer, a reduction in dietary fat did not affect estradiol levels when the data were appropriately analyzed.[26]

The WHI Randomized Controlled Dietary Modification Trial similarly suggested no association between fat intake and breast cancer incidence,[5] but these results are difficult to interpret.[27] The data on biomarkers that reflect fat intake suggest little if any difference in fat intake between the intervention and control groups.[28] Even if dietary fat does truly have an effect on cancer incidence and other outcomes, this lack of adherence to the dietary intervention could explain the absence of an observed effect on total cancer incidence and total mortality. In another randomized trial in Canada that tested an intervention target of 15% of calories from fat, a small but significant difference in high-density lipoprotein (HDL) levels was observed after 8 to 9 years of follow-up suggesting a difference in fat intake in the two groups.[29] The incidence of breast cancer in the intervention and the control group did not differ significantly.

Some prospective cohort studies suggest an inverse association between monounsaturated fat and breast cancer. This is an intriguing observation because of the relatively low rates of breast cancer in southern European countries with high intakes of monounsaturated fats due to the use of olive oil as the primary fat. In case-control studies in Spain, Greece, and Italy, women who used more olive oil had reduced risks of breast cancer.

In a report of findings from the Nurses' Health Study II cohort of premenopausal women, a higher intake of animal fat was associated with an approximately 50% greater risk of breast cancer, but no association was seen with intake of vegetable fat.[30] This suggests that factors in foods containing animal fats, rather than fat per se, may account for the findings. In the same cohort, an intake of red meat and total fat during adolescence was also associated with the risk of premenopausal breast cancer.[31,32]

### Dietary Fat and Colon Cancer

In comparisons among countries, rates of colon cancer are strongly correlated with a national per capita disappearance of animal fat and meat, with correlation coefficients ranging between 0.8 and 0.9.[2] Rates of colon cancer rose sharply in Japan after World War II, paralleling a 2.5-fold increase in fat intake. Based on these epidemiologic investigations and on animal studies, a hypothesis has developed that higher dietary fat increases the excretion of bile acids, which can be converted to carcinogens or act as promoters. However, evidence from many studies on obesity and low levels of physical activity increasing the risk of colon cancer suggests that at least part of the high rates in affluent countries previously attributed to fat intake is probably due to a sedentary lifestyle.

The Nurses' Health Study suggested an approximately twofold higher risk of colon cancer among women in the highest quintile of animal fat intake than in those in the lowest quintile.[33] In a multivariate analysis of these data, which included red meat intake and animal fat intake in the same model, red meat intake remained significantly predictive of colon cancer risk, whereas the association with animal fat was eliminated. Other cohort studies have supported associations of colon cancer and the consumption of red meat and processed meats but not other sources of fat or total fat.[34–36] Similar associations were also observed for colorectal adenomas. In a meta-analysis of prospective studies, red meat consumption was associated with a risk of colon cancer (RR = 1.24; 95% confidence interval [CI], 1.09 to 1.41 for an increment of 120 g per day).[37] The association with the consumption of processed meats was particularly strong (RR = 1.36; 95% CI, 1.15 to 1.61 for an increment of 30 g per day).

The apparently stronger association with red meat consumption than with fat intake in most large cohort studies needs further confirmation, but such an association could result if the fatty acids or nonfat components of meat (e.g., the heme iron or carcinogens created by cooking) were the primary etiologic factors. This issue has major practical implications because current dietary recommendations support the daily consumption of red meat as long as it is lean.[38]

## Dietary Fat and Prostate Cancer

Although further data are desirable, the evidence from international correlations, case-control[39] and cohort studies[40–44] provides some support for an association between the consumption of fat-containing animal products and prostate cancer incidence. This evidence does not generally support a relation with intake of vegetable fat, which suggests that either the type of fat or other components of animal products are responsible. Some evidence also indicates that animal fat consumption may be most strongly associated with the incidence of aggressive prostate cancer, which suggests an influence on the transition from the widespread indolent form to the more lethal form of this malignancy. Data are limited on the relation of fat intake to the probability of survival after the diagnosis of prostate cancer.

## Dietary Fat and Other Cancers

Rates of other cancers that are common in affluent countries, including those of the endometrium and ovary, are also correlated with fat intake internationally. In prospective studies between Iowa and Canadian women, no evidence of a relation between fat intake and risk of endometrial cancer was found. Positive associations between dietary fat and lung cancer have been observed in many case-control studies. However, in a pooled analysis of large prospective studies that included over 3,000 incident cases, no association was observed.[45] These findings provide further evidence that the results of case-control studies of diet and cancer are likely to be misleading.

## Summary

Largely on the basis of the results of animal studies, international correlations, and a few case-control studies, great enthusiasm developed in the 1980s that modest reductions in total fat intake would have a major impact on breast cancer incidence. As the findings from large prospective studies have become available, however, support for this relation has greatly weakened. Although evidence suggests that a high intake of animal fat early in adult life may increase the risk of premenopausal breast cancer, this is not likely to be due to fat per se because vegetable fat intake was not related to risk. For colon cancer, the associations seen with animal fat intake internationally have been supported in numerous case-control and cohort studies, but this also appears to be explained by factors in red meat other than simply its fat content. Further, the importance of physical activity and leanness as protective factors against colon cancer indicates that international correlations probably overstate the contribution of diet to differences in colon cancer incidence. At present, the available evidence most strongly suggests an association between animal fat consumption and risk of prostate cancer, particularly the aggressive form of this disease.

As with colon cancer, the possibility remains that other factors in animal products contribute to risk.

Despite the large body of data on dietary fat and cancer that has accumulated since 1985, any conclusions should be regarded as tentative, because these are disease processes that are poorly understood and are likely to take many decades to develop. Because most of the reported literature from prospective studies is based on fewer than 20 years' follow-up, further evaluations of the effects of diet earlier in life and at longer intervals of observation are needed to fully understand these complex relations. Nevertheless, persons interested in reducing their risk of cancer could be advised, as a prudent measure, to minimize their intake of foods high in animal fat, particularly red meat. Such a dietary pattern is also likely to be beneficial for the risk of cardiovascular disease. On the other hand, unsaturated fats (with the exception of *transfatty* acids) reduce blood low-density lipoprotein cholesterol levels and the risk of cardiovascular disease, and little evidence suggests that they adversely affect cancer risk. Thus, efforts to reduce unsaturated fat intake are not warranted at this time and are likely to have adverse effects on cardiovascular disease risk. Because excess adiposity increases the risk of several cancers and cardiovascular disease, balancing calories from any source with adequate physical activity is extremely important.

# Fruits and Vegetables

## General Properties

Fruits and vegetables have been hypothesized to be major dietary contributors to cancer prevention because they are rich in potential anticarcinogenic substances. Fruits and vegetables contain antioxidants and minerals and are good sources of fiber, potassium, carotenoids, vitamin C, folate, and other vitamins. Although fruits and vegetables supply less than 5% of total energy intake in most countries worldwide on a population basis, the concentration of micronutrients in these foods is greater than in most others.

The comprehensive report of the World Cancer Research Fund and the American Institute for Cancer Research, published in 2007 and titled *Food, Nutrition, Physical Activity, and the Prevention of Cancer: A Global Perspective*, reached the consensus based on the available evidence: "findings from cohort studies conducted since the mid-1990s have made the overall evidence, that vegetables or fruits protect against cancers, somewhat less impressive. In no case now is the evidence of protection judged to be convincing."[15]

## Fruit and Vegetable Consumption and Colorectal Cancer

The association between fruit and vegetable consumption and the incidence of colon or rectal cancer has been examined prospectively in at least six studies. In some of these prospective cohorts, inverse associations were observed for individual foods or particular subgroups of fruits or vegetables, but no consistent pattern emerged and many comparisons revealed no such links. The results from the largest studies, the Nurses' Health Study and the Health Professionals' Follow-Up Study, suggested no important association between the consumption of fruits and vegetables and the incidence of cancers of the colon or rectum during 1,743,645 person-years of follow-up.[46] In these two large cohorts, diet was assessed repeatedly during follow-up with a detailed food frequency questionnaire. Similarly, in the Pooling Project of Prospective Studies of Diet and Cancer, including 14 studies, 756,217 participants, and 5,838 cases of colon cancer, no association with overall colon cancer risk was found.[47]

## Fruit and Vegetable Consumption and Stomach Cancer

At least 12 prospective cohort studies have examined the consumption of some fruits and vegetables and the incidence of stomach cancer.[15] Seven of these studies considered total vegetable intake. Three found significant protection from stomach cancer, whereas three did not. All other comparisons were made for subgroups of vegetables and produced inconsistent results. Nine prospective cohort studies investigated the association between fruit consumption and stomach cancer risk. Four studies found an inverse association of borderline statistical significance.

## Fruit and Vegetable Consumption and Breast Cancer

The most comprehensive evaluation of fruit and vegetable consumption and the incidence of breast cancer was provided by a pooled analysis of all cohort studies.[48] Data were pooled from eight prospective studies that included 351,825 women, 7,377 of whom developed incident invasive breast cancer during follow-up. The pooled relative risk adjusted for potential confounding variables was 0.93 (95% CI, 0.86 to 1.0; P for trend, .08) for the highest versus the lowest quartile of fruit consumption, 0.96 (95% CI, 0.89 to 1.04; P for trend, .54) for vegetable intake, and 0.93 (95% CI, 0.86 to 1.0; P for trend, .12) for total consumption of fruits and vegetables combined. The EPIC study confirmed this lack of association.[49] In a recent analysis within the Nurses' Health Study, an inverse association was seen between vegetable intake and the risk of estrogen receptor–negative breast cancer.[50] This observation was confirmed in the pooling project of prospective studies: The pooled relative risk for the highest vs. the lowest quintile of total vegetable consumption was 0.82 (95% CI 0.74 to 0.90) for estrogen-receptor negative breast cancer.[51]

## Fruit and Vegetable Consumption and Lung Cancer

The relation between fruit and vegetable consumption and the incidence of lung cancer was examined in the pooled analysis of cohort studies.[52] Overall, no association was observed, although a modest increase in lung cancer incidence was evident among participants with the lowest fruit and vegetable consumption.

## Fruit and Vegetable Consumption and Total Cancer

An analysis of the Nurses' Health Study and the Health Professionals' Follow-Up Study, including over 9,000 incident cases of cancer, did not reveal a benefit of fruit and vegetable consumption for total cancer incidence.[53] Observations from the EPIC cohort were essentially consistent with these findings.[54] Although there may be no or only a very weak protection conferred for cancer from consuming an abundance of fruits and vegetables, there is a substantial benefit for protection from cardiovascular disease.

## Summary

The consumption of fruits and vegetables and some of their main micronutrients appear to be less important in cancer prevention than previously assumed. With an accumulation of data from prospective cohort studies and randomized trials, a lack of association of these foods and nutrients with cancer outcomes has become apparent. A modest association cannot be excluded because of an imperfect measurement of diet, and it remains possible that a high consumption of fruits and vegetables during childhood and adolescence is more effective at reducing cancer risk than consumption in adult life due to the long latency of cancer manifestation.

Conversely, it is possible that, with the fortification of breakfast cereal, flour, and other staple foods, the frequent consumption of fruits and vegetables has become less essential for cancer prevention. Nevertheless, an abundance of fruits and vegetables as part of a healthy diet is recommended, because evidence consistently suggests that it lowers the incidence of hypertension, heart disease, and stroke.

## Fiber

### General Properties

Dietary fiber was defined in 1976 as "all plant polysaccharides and lignin which are resistant to hydrolysis by the digestive enzymes of men."[55] Fiber, both soluble and insoluble, is fermented by the luminal bacteria of the colon. Among the properties of fiber that make it a candidate for cancer prevention are its "bulking" effect, which reduces colonic transit time, and the binding of potentially carcinogenic luminal chemicals. Fiber may also aid in producing short-chain fatty acids that may be directly anticarcinogenic. Fiber may also induce apoptosis.

### Dietary Fiber and Colorectal Cancer

In 1969, Dennis Burkitt hypothesized that dietary fiber is involved in colon carcinogenesis.[56] While working as a physician in Africa, Burkitt noticed the low incidence of colon cancer among African populations whose diets were high in fiber. Burkitt concluded that a link might exist between the fiber-rich diet and the low incidence of colon cancer. Burkitt's observations were followed by numerous case-control studies that seemed to confirm his theories. A combined analysis of 13 case-control studies[57] as well as a meta-analysis of 16 case-control studies[58] suggested an inverse association between fiber intake and the risk of colorectal cancer. The inclusion of studies was selective, however, and effect estimates unadjusted for potential confounders were used for most studies. Moreover, recall bias is a severe threat to the validity of retrospective case-control studies of fiber intake and any disease outcome.

Data from prospective cohort studies have largely failed to support an inverse association between dietary fiber and colorectal cancer incidence. Initial analyses from the Nurses' Health Study and the Health Professionals' Follow-Up Study[36] found no important association between dietary fiber and colorectal cancer. A significant inverse association between fiber intake and incidence of colorectal cancer was reported from the EPIC study. The analysis presented on dietary fiber and colorectal cancer encompassed 434,209 women and men from eight European countries.[59] The analytic model used by the EPIC investigators included adjustments for age, height, weight, total caloric intake, sex, and center assessed at baseline and identified[60] a significant inverse association between fiber intake and colorectal cancer. Applying the same analytic model used in EPIC to data from the Nurses' Health Study and the Health Professionals' Follow-Up Study encompassing 1.8 million person-years of follow-up and 1,572 cases of colorectal cancer revealed associations similar to those found in the EPIC study.[61] After a more complete adjustment for confounding variables, however, the association vanished.[61] Results from the pooled analysis of 13 prospective cohort studies, including 8,081 colorectal cancer cases diagnosed during over 7 million person-years of follow-up, suggested an inverse relation between dietary fiber and colorectal cancer incidence in age-adjusted analyses, but this association disappeared after appropriate adjustment for confounding variables, particularly other dietary factors.[62] The NIH–AARP study, which included 2,974 cases of colorectal cancer, confirmed the lack of association between total dietary fiber and colorectal cancer risk.[63]

The association between dietary fiber and colorectal cancer appears to be confounded by a number of other dietary and nondietary factors. These methodologic considerations must be taken into account when interpreting the evidence. It is possible that other dietary factors such as folate intake are more important for colorectal cancer pathogenesis than dietary fiber.

### Dietary Fiber and Colorectal Adenomas

In a few prospective cohort studies, the primary occurrence of colorectal polyps was investigated, but no consistent relation was found.

The study of fiber intake and colorectal adenoma recurrence lends itself to a randomized clinical trial design because of the relatively short follow-up necessary and because fiber can be provided as a supplement. A number of RCTs have explored the effect of fiber supplementation on colorectal adenoma recurrence. Evidence has fairly consistently indicated no effect of fiber intake.[64–68] In one RCT, an increase in adenoma recurrence was observed among participants randomly assigned to use a fiber supplement, which was stronger among those with high dietary calcium.[69]

### Dietary Fiber and Breast Cancer

Investigators have speculated that dietary fiber may reduce the risk of breast cancer through a reduction in intestinal absorption of estrogens excreted via the biliary system.

Relatively few epidemiologic studies have examined the association between fiber intake and breast cancer. In a meta-analysis of 10 case-control studies, a significant inverse association was observed. However, these retrospective studies were likely affected by the aforementioned biases—selection and recall bias, in particular. Results from at least six prospective cohort studies consistently suggested no association between fiber intake and breast cancer incidence.[70–75]

### Dietary Fiber and Stomach Cancer

The results from retrospective case-control studies of fiber intake and gastric cancer risk are inconsistent. In the Netherlands Cohort Study, dietary fiber was not associated with an incidence of gastric carcinoma.[76] Further investigations through prospective cohort studies must be completed before conclusions about the relation between fiber intake and stomach cancer incidence can be drawn.

### Summary

The observational data presently available do not indicate an important role for dietary fiber in the prevention of cancer, although small effects cannot be excluded. The long-held perception that a high intake of fiber conveys protection originated largely from retrospectively conducted studies, which are affected by a number of biases, in particular, the potential for differential recall of diet, and from studies that were not well controlled for potential confounding variables.

## OTHER FOODS AND NUTRIENTS

### Red Meat

The regular consumption of red meat has been associated with an increased risk of colorectal cancer. In a recent meta-analysis, the increase in risk associated with an increase in intake of 120 g per day was 24% (95% CI, 9% to 41%).[37] The association was strongest for processed meat; the relative risk of colorectal cancer was 1.36 (95% CI, 1.15 to 1.61) for a consumption of 30 g per day.[37] No overall association has been observed between red meat consumption and breast cancer in a pooled analysis of prospective cohorts.[77] However, among premenopausal women in the Nurses' Health Study II, the risk for estrogen-receptor–positive and progesterone-receptor–positive breast cancer doubled with 1.5 servings of red meat per day compared to three or fewer servings per week.[78] No associations have been found in studies on poultry or fish.[15] Mechanisms through which red meat may increase cancer risk include anabolic hormones routinely used in meat production in the United States, heterocyclic amines, and polycyclic aromatic hydrocarbons formed during cooking at high temperatures, the high amounts of heme iron, and nitrates and related compounds in smoked, salted, and some processed meats that can convert to carcinogenic nitrosamines in the colon.

## Milk, Dairy Products, and Calcium

Regular milk consumption has been associated with a modest reduction in colorectal cancer in both a pooling project[79] and a meta-analysis of cohort studies,[80] possibly due to its calcium content. In the pooling project of prospective studies of diet and cancer, a modest inverse association was also seen for calcium intake.[79] This finding is consistent with the results of a randomized trial in which calcium supplements reduced the risk of colorectal adenomas.[81] Associations with cheese and other dairy products have been less consistent.[79,80]

Conversely, in multiple studies, a high intake of calcium or dairy products has been associated with an increased risk of prostate cancer,[80,82–86] specifically fatal prostate cancer.[87,88] Similar observations were made in the NIH–AARP study, although the increase in risk there did not reach statistical significance.[89] While the Multiethnic Cohort[90] and the Prostate, Lung, Colorectal, and Ovarian Cancer Screening Trial[91] did not find an important association between dairy consumption and prostate cancer, these cohort studies did not specifically include fatal prostate cancer cases. A meta-analysis of prospective studies generated an overall relative risk of advanced prostate cancer of 1.33 (95% CI, 1.00 to 1.78) for the highest versus the lowest intake categories of dairy products.[92] In another meta-analysis, no significant association was found for cohort studies on dairy or milk consumption, but relative risk estimates suggested a positive association.[93] Thus, although the findings are not entirely consistent and are complicated by the widespread use of prostate-specific antigen (PSA) screening in the United States, the global evidence suggests a positive association between the regular consumption of dairy products and the risk of fatal prostate cancer. Consuming three or more servings of dairy products per day has been associated with endometrial cancer among postmenopausal women not using hormonal therapy.[94] A high intake of lactose from dairy products has also been associated with a modestly higher risk of ovarian cancer.[95]

These observations are particularly important in the context of national dietary recommendations to drink three glasses of milk per day.[38] Possible mechanisms include an increase in endogenous IGF-1 levels[96] and steroid hormones contained in cows' milk.[97]

## Vitamin D

In 1980, Garland and Garland[98] hypothesized that sunlight and vitamin D may reduce the risk of colon cancer. Since then, substantial research has been conducted in this area supporting an inverse association between circulating 25-hydroxyvitamin D (25[OH]D) levels and colorectal cancer risk.[99–103] A meta-analysis, including five nested case-control studies with prediagnostic serum, suggested a reduction of colorectal cancer risk by about half among individuals with serum 25(OH)D levels of more than 82 nmol/L compared to individuals with less than 30 nmol/L.[104] A subsequent meta-analysis including eight studies confirmed these associations.[105] These observations are supported by similar findings for colorectal adenomas.[106] Vitamin D levels may particularly affect colorectal cancer prognosis; colorectal cancer mortality was 72% lower among individuals with 25(OH)D concentrations of 80 nmol/L or higher.[107]

The evidence for other cancers has been less consistent. High plasma levels of vitamin D have been associated with a decreased risk of several other cancers, including cancer of the breast[108–111]; prostate, especially fatal prostate cancer[112]; and ovary.[113,114] Whether vitamin D plays a role in pancreatic cancerogenesis remains to be determined with one pooling project, suggesting a positive association,[115] whereas other prospective studies[116] and a pooling project of cohort studies found inverse associations.[117]

The activation of vitamin D receptors by $1,25(OH)^2D$ induces cell differentiation and inhibits proliferation and angiogenesis.[118] Solar ultraviolet B radiation is the major source of plasma vitamin D, and dietary vitamin D without supplementation has a minor effect on plasma vitamin D. To achieve sufficient plasma levels through sun exposure, at least 15 minutes of full-body exposure to bright sunlight is necessary. Physical activity has to be considered as possible confounder of studies on plasma levels of vitamin D and cancer. Sunscreen effectively blocks vitamin D production. Populations who live in geographic areas with limited or seasonal sun exposure may benefit from a vitamin D supplementation of 1,000 IU per day.

## Folate

Folate is a micronutrient commonly found in fruits and vegetables, particularly oranges, orange juice, asparagus, beets, and peas. Folate may affect carcinogenesis through various mechanisms: DNA methylation, DNA synthesis, and DNA repair. In the animal model, folate deficiency enhances intestinal carcinogenesis.[119] Folate deficiency is related to the incorporation of uracil into human DNA and to an increased frequency of chromosomal breaks. A number of epidemiologic studies suggest that a diet rich in folate lowers the risk of colorectal adenomas and colorectal cancer.[15] Because the folate content in foods is generally relatively low, is susceptible to oxidative destruction by cooking and food processing, and is not well absorbed, folic acid from supplements and fortification plays an important role. Pooled results from 13 prospective studies suggests that intake of 400 to 500 μg per day is required to minimize risk.[120]

Potential interactions among alcohol consumption, folic acid intake, and methionine intake have been described. Although alcohol consumption has been fairly consistently related to an increase in breast cancer incidence, the potential detrimental effect of alcohol seems to be eliminated in women with high folic acid intake.[16] A similar folic acid or methionine–alcohol interaction has been observed for colorectal cancer risk.[119]

Genetic susceptibility may also modify the relation between folate intake and cancer risk. A polymorphism of the *methylenetetrahydrofolate reductase* (MTHFR) gene (cytosine to thymine transition at position 677) may result in a relative deficiency of methionine. Individuals with the common C677T mutation appear to experience the greatest protection from high folic acid or methionine intake and low alcohol consumption.[121] Although the interaction between this polymorphism and dietary factors needs to be investigated further, the consistently observed association between this polymorphism and the risk of colorectal cancer supports a role of folate in the etiology of colorectal cancer.

Folate levels also affect the availability of methyl groups via S-adenosylmethionine in the one-carbon metabolism.[122] Low red blood cell folate levels are associated with low DNA methylation status among homozygous MTHFR 677T/T mutation carriers, whereas at high red blood cell folate levels, the amount of methylated cytosine in DNA is similar to that of the heterozygote MTHFR C677T genotype.[123]

Conversely, evidence from animal and human studies suggests that a high folate status may promote the progression of existing neoplasias.[122,124,125] The randomization of folic acid supplements among individuals with a history of colorectal adenoma resulted in either no effect on recurrent adenoma recurrence[126] or an increase in recurrence with over 6 to 8 years of follow-up.[127] The high proliferation rate of neoplastic cells requiring increased DNA synthesis is likely supported by folate, which is necessary for thymidine synthesis.[122,125] The effects of folate on de novo methylation and subsequent gene silencing have been insufficiently studied. An increase in colorectal cancer rates has been observed in the United States and Canada concurrent with the introduction of the folic acid fortification program, but this could be an artifact due to increased use of colonoscopies.[128] The lack of increase in mortality, but an acceleration in a long-term downward trend suggests the latter explanation (http://progressreport.cancer.gov/).

## Carotenoids

Carotenoids, antioxidants prevalent in fruits and vegetables, enhance cell-to-cell communication, promote cell differentiation, and modulate immune response. In 1981, Doll and Peto[1] speculated that beta-carotene may be a major player in cancer prevention and encouraged testing its anticarcinogenic properties. Indeed, subsequent observational studies, mostly case-control investigations, suggested a reduced cancer risk—especially of lung cancer—with a high intake of carotenoids. In contrast, clinical trials randomizing the intake of beta-carotene supplements have not revealed the evidence of a protective effect of beta-carotene. In fact, beta-carotene was found to increase the risk of lung cancer and total mortality among smokers in the Finnish Alpha-Tocopherol, Beta-Carotene Cancer Prevention Study.[129] However, these adverse affects disappeared during longer periods of follow-up.[130] In a detailed analysis of prospective studies, no association was seen between the intake of beta-carotene and the risk of lung cancer.[131]

The pooled analysis of 18 cohort studies including more than 33,000 breast cancer cases suggested inverse associations between the intake of several carotenoids (beta-carotene, alpha-carotene, luteine/zeaxanthin) and estrogen-receptor–negative breast cancer incidence, whereas no association was found for estrogen-receptor–positive tumors.[132] Similarly, in a pooled analysis of data from eight prospective studies including about 3,055 breast cancer cases, blood levels of carotenoids were inversely related to estrogen-receptor–negative mammary tumor incidence.[133] Women in the highest quintile of beta-carotene levels had about half the risk of developing estrogen-receptor–negative breast cancer than women in the lowest quintile (hazard ratio [HR] = 0.52; 95% CI, 0.36 to 0.77).

The particularly pronounced antioxidant properties of lycopene, a carotenoid mainly found in tomatoes, may explain the inverse associations with some cancers. The frequent consumption of tomato-based products has been associated with a decreased risk of prostate, lung, and stomach cancers.[134] The bioavailability of lycopene from cooked tomatoes is higher than from fresh tomatoes, making tomato soup and sauce excellent sources of the carotenoid.

## Selenium

Selenium has long been of interest in cancer prevention due to its antioxidative properties. Its intake is difficult to estimate because food content depends on the selenium content of the soil it is grown in. Selenium enriches in toenails, which provide an integrative measure of intake during the previous year and therefore are popular biomarkers in epidemiologic studies. Inverse associations with toenail selenium levels have been found in several prospective studies, especially for fatal prostate cancer.[135–137] In a recent meta-analysis, plasma/serum selenium was also inversely correlated with prostate cancer.[138] In the Selenium and Vitamin E Cancer Prevention Trial (SELECT), no protective effect of selenium was found for prostate cancer. However, the trial was terminated prematurely after 4 years, which is a short period in which to expect a reduction in cancer.[139]

## Soy Products

The role of soy products has been considered for breast carcinogenesis. In Asian countries, which traditionally have a high consumption of soy foods, breast cancer rates have been low until recently. In Western countries, soy consumption is generally low, and between-person variation may be insufficient to allow meaningful comparisons. Soybeans contain isoflavones, which are phytoestrogens that compete with estrogen for the estrogen receptor. Hence, soy consumption may affect estrogen concentrations differently depending on the endogenous baseline level. This mechanism may also contribute to the equivocal results of studies on soy foods and breast cancer risk. In a recent meta-analysis of 18 epidemiologic studies, including over 9,000 breast cancer cases, frequent soy intake was associated with a modest decrease in risk (odds ratio = 0.86; 95% CI, 0.75 to 0.99).[140] Wu et al.[141] observed that childhood intake of soy was more relevant to breast cancer prevention than adult consumption.

## Carbohydrates

The Warburg hypothesis postulated in 1924 that tumor cells mainly generate energy by the nonoxidative breakdown of glucose (glucolysis) instead of pyrovate.[142] Carbohydrates with a high glycemic load increase blood glucose levels after consumption, which results in insulin spikes increasing the risk for type 2 diabetes. Several cancers, including colorectal cancer[143] and breast cancer,[144] have been associated with type 2 diabetes. The evidence on the consumption of sucrose and refined, processed flour and cancer incidence is heterogeneous.[145] Whereas in some prospective cohort studies an increase in colon cancer incidence was observed,[146] this was not found in other studies.[147] In large cohort studies, associations have been observed for pancreatic[148] and endometrial[145] cancer risk, but not for postmenopausal breast cancer.[149] Especially in obese, sedentary individuals, abnormal glucose and insulin metabolism may contribute to tumorigenesis.

## DIETARY PATTERNS

Foods and nutrients are not consumed in isolation, and, when evaluating the role of diet in disease prevention and causation, it is sensible to consider the entire dietary pattern of individuals. Public health messages may be better framed in the context of a global diet than individual constituents.

The role of vegetarian diets for cancer incidence has been examined in a few studies. In the Adventist Health Study-2, vegetarians had an 8% lower incidence of cancer than nonvegetarians (95% CI, 1 to 15%).[150] The protective association was strongest for cancers of the gastrointestinal tract with 24% (95% CI, 10 to 37%). Vegans had a 16% (95%, 1 to 28%) lower incidence of cancer, with a particular protection conferred to female cancers of 34% (95% CI, 8 to 53%). A combined analysis of data from the Oxford Vegetarian Study and EPIC similarly suggest a 12% (95% CI, 4 to 19%) reduction in cancer incidence among vegetarians compared to meat eaters.[151]

During the past decade, dietary pattern analyses have gained popularity in observational studies. The most commonly employed methods are factor analyses and cluster analyses, which are largely data-driven methods, and investigator-determined methods such as dietary indices and scores. The search for associations between distinct patterns such as the "Western pattern," which is characterized by a high consumption of red and processed meats; high fat dairy products, including butter and eggs; and refined carbohydrates, such as sweets, desserts, and refined grains, and the "prudent pattern," which is defined by the frequent consumption of a variety of fruits and vegetables, whole grains, legumes, fish, and poultry, and the risk of cancer has been largely disappointing. Notable exceptions were the link between a Western dietary pattern and colon cancer incidence and an inverse relation between a prudent diet[152] and estrogen-receptor–negative breast cancer.[153] These findings were subsequently in the California Teachers Study.[154] The general lack of association between global dietary patterns and cancer supports a more modest role of nutrition during adult life in carcinogenesis than previously assumed.

## DIET DURING THE EARLY PHASES OF LIFE

Some cancers may originate early in the course of life. A high birth weight is associated with an increase in the risk of childhood leukemia,[155] premenopausal breast cancer,[156] and testicular cancer.[157] Tall height is an indicator of the risk of many cancers and is in part determined by nutrition during childhood.[15] Until recently, most studies focused on the role of diet during adult life. However, the critical exposure period for nutrition to affect cancer risk may be earlier, and because the latent period for cancer may span several decades, diet during childhood and adolescence may be important. However, relating dietary information during early life and cancer outcomes prospectively is difficult because nutrition records from the remote past are not available. Studies in which recalled diet during youth is used have to be interpreted cautiously due to misclassification, although recall has been found reasonably reproducible and consistent with recalls provided by participants' mothers.[158,159] The role of early life diet has been explored in only a few studies in relation to breast cancer risk. In a study nested in the Nurses' Health Study cohorts that used data recalled by mothers, frequent consumption of french fries was associated with an increased risk of breast cancer, whereas whole milk consumption was inversely related to risk.[160] Similarly, an inverse association with milk consumption during childhood was found among younger women (30 to 39 years), but not among older premenopausal women (40 to 49 years) in a Norwegian cohort.[161] Dietary habits during high school recalled by adult participants of the Nurses' Health Study II (but before the diagnosis of breast cancer) suggested a positive association of total fat and red meat consumption.[31,32] More data are needed in this promising area of research.[162]

## DIET AFTER A DIAGNOSIS OF CANCER

The role of diet in the secondary prevention of cancer recurrence and survival is generally of great interest to cancer patients because they are highly motivated to make lifestyle changes to optimize their prognosis. The compliance of cancer patients makes the RCTs a more feasible design to evaluate the role of diet than among healthy individuals. However, concurrent cancer treatments may make any effect of diet more difficult to isolate.

Most evidence is available for breast cancer, colorectal, and prostate cancer. Observational data suggest a limited role of diet in the prevention of breast cancer recurrence and survival. The Life After Cancer Epidemiology (LACE) Cohort supported a beneficial role for vitamin C and E supplement use but the effect of other health-seeking behaviors is difficult to exclude.[163] In a pooled analysis, alcohol consumption after a diagnosis did not affect survival.[164] Several randomized trials have addressed the role of diet in breast cancer prognosis. In the Women's Intervention Nutrition Study (WINS), 2,437 women with early stage breast cancer were randomized to a dietary goal of 15% of calories from fat or maintenance of their usual dietary habits.[165] The intervention group received dietary counseling by registered dieticians and, according to self-reports, a difference of 19 g in daily fat intake was maintained between the intervention and the control group after 60 months of follow-up. However, at that time, women in the intervention group were also 6 pounds lighter, making it difficult to separate an effect of dietary fat from a nonspecific effect of intensive dietary intervention, which quite consistently produces weight loss. Breast cancer recurrence was 29% lower in the intervention group (95% CI, 6% to 47%), whereas overall survival was not affected. In the Women's Healthy Eating and Living (WHEL) RCT, 3,088 early stage breast cancer patients were randomly assigned to a target of five vegetable servings, three fruit servings, 30 g fiber per day, and 15% to 20% of calories from fat.[166] After 72 months, the intervention versus control group reports were 5.8 versus 3.6 servings of vegetables, 3.4 versus 2.6 servings of fruit, 24.2 versus 18.9 g fiber per day, and 28.9% versus 32.4% of calories from fat. The total plasma carotenoid concentration, a biomarker of vegetable and fruit intake, was 43% higher in the intervention group than the comparison group after 4 years (p<0.001). Neither recurrence rates nor mortality were affected by the intervention after the 7.3-year follow-up. Overall, diet is unlikely a major factor influencing breast cancer prognosis. However, because the prognosis for breast cancer is relatively good, women diagnosed with breast cancer remain at risk for cardiovascular disease and other causes of death that affect those without breast cancer. Thus, among women in the Nurses' Health Study diagnosed with breast cancer, a higher diet quality, which was assessed by the Alternative Healthy Eating Index, was not associated with mortality due to breast cancer but was associated with substantially lower mortality due to other causes.[167] Similarly, among over 4,000 women with breast cancer, intakes of saturated and trans fat, but not of total fat, were associated with significantly greater total mortality but not specifically breast cancer mortality. Thus, there is good reason for women with breast cancer to adopt a healthy diet even if it does not affect the prognosis of breast cancer.

In a systematic review, no consistent association between individual dietary components and colorectal cancer prognosis outcome was found.[168] However, in an observational study including 1,009 patients with stage III colon cancer, a Western dietary pattern was associated with lower rates of disease-free survival, recurrence-free survival, and overall survivals.[169] In the same patient population, higher dietary glycemic load and total carbohydrate intake were significantly associated with an increased risk of recurrence and mortality.[170] These findings support a possible role of glycemic load in colon cancer progression.

In the Physician's Health Study, whole milk consumption among men with incident prostate cancer was associated with double the risk of progression to fatal disease.[171] Among men with nonmetastatic prostate cancer in the Health Professionals' Follow-up Study, replacing 10% of energy intake from carbohydrates with vegetable fat was associated with a lower risk of lethal prostate cancer.[172] A marginally increased risk of progression of localized to lethal prostate cancer among these men was also associated with postdiagnostic poultry and processed red meat consumption,[173] whereas postdiagnostic consumption of fish and tomato sauce were inversely related with a risk of progression.[174] In an intervention study, 93 patients with early stage prostate cancer (PSA = 4 to 10 ng per mililiter and Gleason score <7) were randomized to comprehensive lifestyle changes, including a vegan diet based on 10% of calories from fat and consisting predominantly of vegetables, fruit, whole grains, legumes, and soy protein.[175] Other interventions included moderate exercise, stress management, and relaxation. After 1 year, PSA values decreased 4% in the intervention group, but increased 6% in the control group. Six patients in the control group, but none in the experimental group, underwent conventional prostate cancer treatment. Although the impact of the different intervention components are difficult to separate in this study, further data on diet and the prognosis for patients with localized prostate cancer are needed.

## SUMMARY

A considerable proportion of cancers are potentially preventable through lifestyle changes. Besides a curtailment of smoking, the most important strategies are maintaining a healthy body weight and regular physical activity, which contribute to a lower prevalence of being overweight and obesity. The avoidance of a positive energy balance and becoming overweight are the most important nutritional factors in cancer prevention.

Although dietary patterns, including frequent fruit and vegetable consumption, appear to play a modest role in cancer prevention, knowledge gained about some specific foods and nutrients might inform a targeted approach. Vitamin D is a strong candidate to counter carcinogenesis, thus supplementation could be a feasible and safe route to avoid several types of cancer. Although the data on vitamin D and cancer incidence are not conclusive, the

prevention of bone fractures is a sufficient reason to maintain good vitamin D status.

Limiting or avoiding red meat, processed meat, and alcohol reduces the risk of breast, colorectal, stomach, esophageal, and other cancers. Although the role of dairy products and milk remains to be more fully elucidated, current evidence suggests a probable increase in the risk of prostate cancer with frequent milk consumption, and possibly endometrial cancer, which raises concern regarding current dietary recommendations of three glasses of milk per day. The relation of calcium and dairy intake to cancer is complex, as the evidence for a reduction in the risk of colorectal cancer is strong, but high intakes appear likely to increase the risk of fatal prostate cancer. The consumption of tomato-based products may contribute to the prevention of prostate cancer. Finally, diet may influence the prognosis of colorectal and prostate cancer, but more data are needed in this area. Because most people with cancer remain at risk of cardiovascular disease and other common conditions related to unhealthy diets, an overall healthy diet can be recommended while further research on diet and cancer survival is ongoing.

## LIMITATIONS

Studying the role of diet in health and disease requires overcoming a number of hurdles. Because biomarkers reflecting nutrient intake with sufficient accuracy are largely lacking, assessing nutrition in a population-based study has to rely on self-reports by individuals, which inevitably leads to imprecision or error in the diet assessment. Such misclassification may produce spurious associations in case-control studies or may lead to an underestimation of true associations in prospective cohort studies. Ideally, hypotheses relating dietary factors to cancer risks would be tested in large randomized trials. Besides being extremely expensive, maintaining adherence to assigned diets has been challenging; for example, in the WHI trial that focused on dietary fat reduction, there were no differences between intervention and control groups in blood lipid fractions that are known to change with a reduction in fat intake, indicating a failure to test the hypothesis.[28]

Most observational studies are conducted within populations or countries. Although reasonable variations in nutritional habits exist within populations, allowing for the detection of substantial dietary risk factors for cardiovascular disease and diabetes, these contrasts may be too limited to detect small relative risks as they may exist for cancer. The pooled analysis of large prospective cohort studies across countries and continents attempts to overcome this limitation. Studies taking advantage of the large between-population variation in diets across developed and developing countries would appear to be advantageous, but would be plagued by confounding by other differences in lifestyle factors that might be difficult to assess and control adequately.

Few epidemiologic studies repeatedly capture dietary habits over time and thus account for potential changes in diet over time. Furthermore, the length of follow-up in prospective studies may not be sufficient to capture the impact of diets assessed at baseline. In case-control studies, a recall of dietary habits prior to the disease onset may be influenced by current disease status; moreover, the relevant time for nutrition to act may be decades earlier, which is more difficult to remember.

Most epidemiologic studies of diet and cancer have assessed intake among adults. Due to greater susceptibility to genotoxic influences earlier in life, it is possible that data on diet during childhood or early adolescence are more relevant for carcinogenesis and cancer prevention. Studies that have collected dietary data during childhood and followed the subjects for cancer incidence would be most informative but are virtually nonexistent and will be challenging to conduct.

Finally, data on special diets including organic foods, whole foods, raw foods, and a vegan diet are limited.

# FUTURE DIRECTIONS

Some of the most promising research at present is in the areas of vitamin D, milk consumption, and the effect of diet early in life on cancer incidence. Recent nutrition changes in countries previously maintaining a more traditional diet such as Japan and some developing countries have already been followed by increased rates of some cancers (but declines in stomach cancer), providing a setting to study the effect of change over time. Additional insight may come from studies on gene–nutrient interaction and epigenetic changes induced by the diet. To improve observational research methods, refined dietary assessment methods, including the identification of new biomarkers, will be advantageous.

# RECOMMENDATIONS

A wealth of data are available from observational studies on diet and cancer, and the current evidence supports suggestions made by Doll and Peto[1] that approximately 30% to 40% of cancers may be avoidable with changes in nutrition; however, much of this risk of cancer is related to being overweight and to inactivity. Excessive energy intake and lack of physical activity, marked by rapid growth in childhood and being overweight, have become growing threats to population health and are important contributors to risks of many cancers. Nevertheless, the cumulative incidence for many cancers has decreased over the past decade, in part due to the decreasing prevalence of smoking and use of hormone therapy.

Dietary recommendations must integrate the goal of overall avoidance of disease and maintenance of health and, thus, should not focus singularly on cancer prevention. The strength of the evidence and magnitude of the expected benefit should also be considered in recommendations. With these considerations in mind, the following recommendations are outlined, which are largely in agreement with the guidelines put forth by the American Cancer Society in 2012:[176]

1. *Engage in regular physical activity.* Physical activity is a primary method of weight control and it also reduces risk of several cancers, especially colon cancer, through independent mechanisms. Moderate to vigorous exercise for at least 30 minutes on most days is a minimum and more will provide additional benefits.

2. *Avoid being overweight and weight gain in adulthood.* A positive energy balance that results in excess body fat is one of the most important contributors to cancer risk. Staying within 10 pounds of body weight at age 20 may be a simple guide, assuming no adolescent obesity.

3. *Limit alcohol consumption.* Alcohol consumption contributes to the risk of many cancers and increases the risk of accidents and addiction, but low to moderate consumption has benefits for coronary heart disease risk. The individual family history of disease as well as personal preferences should be considered.

4. *Consume lots of fruits and vegetables.* Frequent consumption of fruits and vegetables during adult life is not likely to have a major effect on cancer incidence, but will reduce the risk of cardiovascular disease.

5. *Consume whole grains and avoid refined carbohydrates and sugars.* A regular consumption of whole grain products instead of refined flour and a low consumption of refined sugars lower the risk of cardiovascular disease and diabetes. The effect on cancer risk is less clear.

6. *Replace red meat and dairy products with fish, nuts, and legumes.* Red meat consumption increases the risk of colorectal cancer, diabetes, and coronary heart disease and should be largely avoided. Frequent dairy consumption may increase the risk of prostate cancer. Fish, nuts, and legumes are excellent sources of valuable mono- and polyunsaturated fats and vegetable proteins and may contribute to lower rates of cardiovascular disease and diabetes.

7. *Consider taking a vitamin D supplement.* A substantial proportion of the population, especially those living at higher latitudes, are vitamin D deficient. Most adults may benefit from taking 1,000 IU of vitamin D[3] per day during months of low sunlight intensity. Vitamin D supplementation will, at a minimum, reduce bone fracture rates, probably colorectal cancer incidence, and possibly other cancers.

ETIOLOGY AND EPIDEMIOLOGY OF CANCER

# REFERENCES

1. Doll R, Peto R. The causes of cancer: quantitative estimates of avoidable risks of cancer in the United States today. *J Natl Cancer Inst* 1981;66:1191–1308.
2. Armstrong B, Doll R. Environmental factors and cancer incidence and mortality in different countries, with special reference to dietary practices. *Int J Cancer* 1975;15:617–631.
3. Giovannucci E, Stampfer MJ, Colditz GA, et al. A comparison of prospective and retrospective assessments of diet in the study of breast cancer. *Am J Epidemiol* 1993;137:502–511.
4. Riboli E, Norat T. Epidemiologic evidence of the protective effect of fruit and vegetables on cancer risk. *Am J Clin Nutr* 2003;78:559S–569S.
5. Prentice RL, Caan B, Chlebowski RT, et al. Low-fat dietary pattern and risk of invasive breast cancer: the Women's Health Initiative Randomized Controlled Dietary Modification Trial. *JAMA* 2006;295:629–642.
6. Michels KB, Bingham SA, Luben R, et al. The effect of correlated measurement error in multivariate models of diet. *Am J Epidemiol* 2004;160:59–67.
7. Willett W. *Nutritional Epidemiology*. 3rd ed. New York: Oxford University Press; 2013.
8. Calle EE, Rodriguez C, Walker-Thurmond K, et al. Overweight, obesity, and mortality from cancer in a prospectively studied cohort of U.S. adults. *N Engl J Med* 2003;348:1625–1638.
9. Giovannucci E, Ascherio A, Rimm EB, et al. Physical activity, obesity, and risk for colon cancer and adenoma in men. *Ann Intern Med* 1995;122:327–334.
10. Martinez ME, Giovannucci E, Spiegelman D, et al. Leisure-time physical activity, body size, and colon cancer in women. Nurses' Health Study Research Group. *J Natl Cancer Inst* 1997;89:948–955.
11. Eliassen AH, Colditz GA, Rosner B, et al. Adult weight change and risk of postmenopausal breast cancer. *JAMA* 2006;296:193–201.
12. Michels KB, Ekbom A. Caloric restriction and incidence of breast cancer. *JAMA* 2004;291:1226–1230.
13. Elias SG, Peeters PH, Grobbee DE, et al. Breast cancer risk after caloric restriction during the 1944–1945 Dutch famine. *J Natl Cancer Inst* 2004;96:539–546.
14. Tretli S, Gaard M. Lifestyle changes during adolescence and risk of breast cancer: an ecologic study of the effect of World War II in Norway. *Cancer Causes Control* 1996;7:507–512.
15. World Cancer Research Fund/American Institute for Cancer Research. *Food, Nutrition, Physical Activity, and the Prevention of Cancer: A Global Perspective*. Washington, D.C.: AICR; 2007.
16. Zhang S, Hunter DJ, Hankinson SE, et al. A prospective study of folate intake and the risk of breast cancer. *JAMA* 1999;281:1632–1637.
17. Tannenbaum A. The genesis and growth of tumors. III. Effects of a high-fat diet. *Cancer Res* 1942;2:468–475.
18. Kolonel L, Hinds M, Hankin J. *Cancer Patterns Among Migrant and Native-Born Japanese in Hawaii in Relation to Smoking, Drinking, and Dietary Habits*. Tokyo: Japan Scientific Societies Press; 1980.
19. Howe GR, Hirohata T, Hislop TG, et al. Dietary factors and risk of breast cancer: combined analysis of 12 case-control studies. *J Natl Cancer Inst* 1990;82:561–569.
20. Kim EH, Willett WC, Colditz GA, et al. Dietary fat and risk of postmenopausal breast cancer in a 20-year follow-up. *Am J Epidemiol* 2006;164:990–997.
21. Thiebaut AC, Kipnis V, Chang SC, et al. Dietary fat and postmenopausal invasive breast cancer in the National Institutes of Health-AARP Diet and Health Study cohort. *J Natl Cancer Inst* 2007;99:451–462.
22. Sieri S, Krogh V, Ferrari P, et al. Dietary fat and breast cancer risk in the European Prospective Investigation into Cancer and Nutrition. *Am J Clin Nutr* 2008;88:1304–1312.
23. Hunter DJ, Spiegelman D, Adami HO, et al. Cohort studies of fat intake and the risk of breast cancer—a pooled analysis. *N Engl J Med* 1996;334:356–361.
24. Smith-Warner SA, Spiegelman D, Adami HO, et al. Types of dietary fat and breast cancer: a pooled analysis of cohort studies. *Int J Cancer* 2001;92:767–774.
25. Wu AH, Pike MC, Stram DO. Meta-analysis: dietary fat intake, serum estrogen levels, and the risk of breast cancer. *J Natl Cancer Inst* 1999;91:529–534.

26. Rose DP, Connolly JM, Chlebowski RT, et al. The effects of a low-fat dietary intervention and tamoxifen adjuvant therapy on the serum estrogen and sex hormone-binding globulin concentrations of postmenopausal breast cancer patients. *Breast Cancer Res Treat* 1993;27:253–262.

27. Michels KB. The women's health initiative—curse or blessing? *Int J Epidemiol* 2006;35:814–816.

28. Michels KB, Willett WC. The Women's Health Initiative Randomized Controlled Dietary Modification Trial: a post-mortem. *Breast Cancer Res Treat* 2009;114:1–6.

29. Martin LJ, Li Q, Melnichouk O, et al. A randomized trial of dietary intervention for breast cancer prevention. *Cancer Res* 2011;71:123–133.

30. Cho E, Spiegelman D, Hunter DJ, et al. Premenopausal fat intake and risk of breast cancer. *J Natl Cancer Inst* 2003;95:1079–1085.

31. Linos E, Willett WC, Cho E, et al. Red meat consumption during adolescence among premenopausal women and risk of breast cancer. *Cancer Epidemiol Biomarkers Prev* 2008;17:2146–2151.

32. Linos E, Willett WC, Cho E, et al. Adolescent diet in relation to breast cancer risk among premenopausal women. *Cancer Epidemiol Biomarkers Prev* 2010;19:689–696.

33. Willett WC, Stampfer MJ, Colditz GA, et al. Relation of meat, fat, and fiber intake to the risk of colon cancer in a prospective study among women. *N Engl J Med* 1990;323:1664–1672.

34. Bostick RM, Potter JD, Kushi LH, et al. Sugar, meat, and fat intake, and non-dietary risk factors for colon cancer incidence in Iowa women (United States). *Cancer Causes Control* 1994;5:38–52.

35. Goldbohm RA, van den Brandt PA, van't Veer P, et al. A prospective cohort study on the relation between meat consumption and the risk of colon cancer. *Cancer Res* 1994;54:718–723.

36. Giovannucci E, Rimm EB, Stampfer MJ, et al. Intake of fat, meat, and fiber in relation to risk of colon cancer in men. *Cancer Res* 1994;54:2390–2397.

37. Norat T, Lukanova A, Ferrari P, et al. Meat consumption and colorectal cancer risk: dose-response meta-analysis of epidemiological studies. *Int J Cancer* 2002;98:241–256.

38. Dietary Guidelines for Americans. DietaryGuidelines.gov Web site. http://www.health.gov/dietaryguidelines/.

39. Whittemore AS, Kolonel LN, Wu AH, et al. Prostate cancer in relation to diet, physical activity, and body size in blacks, whites, and Asians in the United States and Canada. *J Natl Cancer Inst* 1995;87:652–661.

40. Crowe FL, Key TJ, Appleby PN, et al. Dietary fat intake and risk of prostate cancer in the European Prospective Investigation into Cancer and Nutrition. *Am J Clin Nutr* 2008;87:1405–1413.

41. Giovannucci E, Rimm EB, Colditz GA, et al. A prospective study of dietary fat and risk of prostate cancer. *J Natl Cancer Inst* 1993;85:1571–1579.

42. Mills PK, Beeson WL, Phillips RL, et al. Cohort study of diet, lifestyle, and prostate cancer in Adventist men. *Cancer* 1989;64:598–604.

43. Park S-Y, Murphy SP, Wilkens LR, et al. Fat and meat intake and prostate cancer risk: The multiethnic cohort study. *Int J Cancer* 2007;121:1339–1345.

44. Schuurman AG, van den Brandt PA, Dorant E, et al. Association of energy and fat intake with prostate carcinoma risk: results from The Netherlands Cohort Study. *Cancer* 1999;86:1019–1027.

45. Smith-Warner SA, Ritz J, Hunter DJ, et al. Dietary fat and risk of lung cancer in a pooled analysis of prospective studies. *Cancer Epidemiol Biomarkers Prev* 2002;11:987–992.

46. Michels KB, Edward G, Joshipura KJ, et al. Prospective study of fruit and vegetable consumption and incidence of colon and rectal cancers. *J Natl Cancer Inst* 2000;92:1740–1752.

47. Koushik A, Hunter DJ, Spiegelman D, et al. Fruits, vegetables, and colon cancer risk in a pooled analysis of 14 cohort studies. *J Natl Cancer Inst* 2007;99:1471–1483.

48. Smith-Warner SA, Spiegelman D, Yaun SS, et al. Intake of fruits and vegetables and risk of breast cancer: a pooled analysis of cohort studies. *JAMA* 2001;285:769–776.

49. van Gils CH, Peeters PH, Bueno-de-Mesquita HB, et al. Consumption of vegetables and fruits and risk of breast cancer. *JAMA* 2005;293:183–193.

50. Fung TT, Hu FB, McCullough ML, et al. Diet quality is associated with the risk of estrogen receptor-negative breast cancer in postmenopausal women. *J Nutr* 2006;136:466–472.

51. Jung S, Spiegelman D, Baglietto L, et al. Fruit and vegetable intake and risk of breast cancer by hormone receptor status. *J Natl Cancer Inst* 2013;105:219–236.

52. Smith-Warner SA, Spiegelman D, Yaun SS, et al. Fruits, vegetables and lung cancer: a pooled analysis of cohort studies. *Int J Cancer* 2003;107:1001–1011.

53. Hung HC, Joshipura KJ, Jiang R, et al. Fruit and vegetable intake and risk of major chronic disease. *J Natl Cancer Inst* 2004;96:1577–1584.

54. Boffetta P, Couto E, Wichmann J, et al. Fruit and vegetable intake and overall cancer risk in the European Prospective Investigation into Cancer and Nutrition (EPIC). *J Natl Cancer Inst* 2010;102:529–537.

55. Trowell H, Southgate DA, Woolever TM, et al. Letter: Dietary fibre redefined. *Lancet* 1976;1:967.

56. Burkitt DP. Related disease—related cause? *Lancet* 1969;2:1229–1231.

57. Howe GR, Benito E, Castelleto R, et al. Dietary intake of fiber and decreased risk of cancers of the colon and rectum: evidence from the combined analysis of 13 case-control studies. *J Natl Cancer Inst* 1992;84:1887–1896.

58. Trock B, Lanza E, Greenwald P. Dietary fiber, vegetables, and colon cancer: critical review and meta-analyses of the epidemiologic evidence. *J Natl Cancer Inst* 1990;82:650–661.

59. Bingham SA, Day NE, Luben R, et al. Dietary fibre in food and protection against colorectal cancer in the European Prospective Investigation into Cancer and Nutrition (EPIC): an observational study. *Lancet* 2003;361: 1496–1501.

60. Fuchs CS, Giovannucci EL, Colditz GA, et al. Dietary fiber and the risk of colorectal cancer and adenoma in women. *N Engl J Med* 1999;340:169–176.

61. Michels KB, Fuchs CS, Giovannucci E, et al. Fiber intake and incidence of colorectal cancer among 76,947 women and 47,279 men. *Cancer Epidemiol Biomarkers Prev* 2005;14:842–849.

62. Park Y, Hunter DJ, Spiegelman D, et al. Dietary fiber intake and risk of colorectal cancer: a pooled analysis of prospective cohort studies. *JAMA* 2005;294:2849–2857.

63. Schatzkin A, Mouw T, Park Y, et al. Dietary fiber and whole-grain consumption in relation to colorectal cancer in the NIH-AARP Diet and Health Study. *Am J Clin Nutr* 2007;85:1353–1360.

64. Alberts DS, Martinez ME, Roe DJ, et al. Lack of effect of a high-fiber cereal supplement on the recurrence of colorectal adenomas. Phoenix Colon Cancer Prevention Physicians' Network. *N Engl J Med* 2000;342: 1156–1162.

65. Jacobs ET, Giuliano AR, Roe DJ, et al. Intake of supplemental and total fiber and risk of colorectal adenoma recurrence in the wheat bran fiber trial. *Cancer Epidemiol Biomarkers Prev* 2002;11:906–914.

66. MacLennan R, Macrae F, Bain C, et al. Randomized trial of intake of fat, fiber, and beta carotene to prevent colorectal adenomas. The Australian Polyp Prevention Project. *J Natl Cancer Inst* 1995;87:1760–1766.

67. McKeown-Eyssen GE, Bright-See E, Bruce WR, et al. A randomized trial of a low fat high fibre diet in the recurrence of colorectal polyps. Toronto Polyp Prevention Group. *J Clin Epidemiol* 1994;47:525–536.

68. Schatzkin A, Lanza E, Corle D, et al. Lack of effect of a low-fat, high-fiber diet on the recurrence of colorectal adenomas. Polyp Prevention Trial Study Group. *N Engl J Med* 2000;342:1149–1155.

69. Bonithon-Kopp C, Kronborg O, Giacosa A, et al. Calcium and fibre supplementation in prevention of colorectal adenoma recurrence: a randomised intervention trial. European Cancer Prevention Organisation Study Group. *Lancet* 2000;356:1300–1306.

70. Graham S, Zielezny M, Marshall J, et al. Diet in the epidemiology of postmenopausal breast cancer in the New York State Cohort. *Am J Epidemiol* 1992;136:1327–1337.

71. Horn-Ross PL, Hoggatt KJ, West DW, et al. Recent diet and breast cancer risk: the California Teachers Study (USA). *Cancer Causes Control* 2002;13: 407–415.

72. Jarvinen R, Knekt P, Seppanen R, et al. Diet and breast cancer risk in a cohort of Finnish women. *Cancer Lett* 1997;114:251–253.

73. Terry P, Jain M, Miller AB, et al. No association among total dietary fiber, fiber fractions, and risk of breast cancer. *Cancer Epidemiol Biomarkers Prev* 2002;11:1507–1508.

74. Verhoeven DT, Assen N, Goldbohm RA, et al. Vitamins C and E, retinol, beta-carotene and dietary fibre in relation to breast cancer risk: a prospective cohort study. *Br J Cancer* 1997;75:149–155.

75. Willett WC, Hunter DJ, Stampfer MJ, et al. Dietary fat and fiber in relation to risk of breast cancer. An 8-year follow-up. *JAMA* 1992;268:2037–2044.

76. Botterweck AA, van den Brandt PA, Goldbohm RA. Vitamins, carotenoids, dietary fiber, and the risk of gastric carcinoma: results from a prospective study after 6.3 years of follow-up. *Cancer* 2000;88:737–748.

77. Missmer SA, Smith-Warner SA, Spiegelman D, et al. Meat and dairy food consumption and breast cancer: a pooled analysis of cohort studies. *Int J Epidemiol* 2002;31:78–85.

78. Cho E, Chen WY, Hunter DJ, et al. Red meat intake and risk of breast cancer among premenopausal women. *Arch Intern Med* 2006;166:2253–2259.

79. Cho E, Smith-Warner SA, Spiegelman D, et al. Dairy foods, calcium, and colorectal cancer: a pooled analysis of 10 cohort studies. *J Natl Cancer Inst* 2004;96:1015–1022.

80. Aune D, Lau R, Chan DS, et al. Dairy products and colorectal cancer risk: a systematic review and meta-analysis of cohort studies. *Ann Oncol* 2012; 23:37–45.

81. Baron JA, Beach M, Mandel JS, et al. Calcium supplements for the prevention of colorectal adenomas. Calcium Polyp Prevention Study Group. *N Engl J Med* 1999;340:101–107.

82. Allen NE, Key TJ, Appleby PN, et al. Animal foods, protein, calcium and prostate cancer risk: the European Prospective Investigation into Cancer and Nutrition. *Br J Cancer* 2008;98:1574–1581.

83. Kurahashi N, Inoue M, Iwasaki M, et al. Dairy product, saturated fatty acid, and calcium intake and prostate cancer in a prospective cohort of Japanese men. *Cancer Epidemiol Biomarkers Prev* 2008;17:930–937.

84. Chan JM, Stampfer MJ, Ma J, et al. Dairy products, calcium, and prostate cancer risk in the Physicians' Health Study. *Am J Clin Nut* 2001;74:549–554.

85. Mitrou PN, Albanes D, Weinstein SJ, et al. A prospective study of dietary calcium, dairy products and prostate cancer risk (Finland). *Int J Cancer* 2007;120:2466–2473.

86. Tseng M, Breslow RA, Graubard BI, et al. Dairy, calcium, and vitamin D intakes and prostate cancer risk in the National Health and Nutrition Examination Epidemiologic Follow-up Study cohort. *Am J Clin Nutr* 2005; 81:1147–1154.

87. Giovannucci E, Liu Y, Stampfer MJ, et al. A prospective study of calcium intake and incident and fatal prostate cancer. *Cancer Epidemiol Biomarkers Prev* 2006;15:203–210.

88. Snowdon DA, Phillips RL, Choi W. Diet, obesity, and risk of fatal prostate cancer. *Am J Epidemiol* 1984;120:244–250.

89. Park Y, Mitrou PN, Kipnis V, et al. Calcium, dairy foods, and risk of incident and fatal prostate cancer: the NIH-AARP Diet and Health Study. *Am J Epidemiol* 2007;166:1270–1279.

90. Park SY, Murphy SP, Wilkens LR, et al. Calcium, vitamin D, and dairy product intake and prostate cancer risk: the Multiethnic Cohort Study. *Am J Epidemiol* 2007;166:1259–1269.

91. Ahn J, Albanes D, Peters U, et al. Dairy products, calcium intake, and risk of prostate cancer in the prostate, lung, colorectal, and ovarian cancer screening trial. *Cancer Epidemiol Biomarkers Prev* 2007;16:2623–2630.

92. Gao X, LaValley MP, Tucker KL. Prospective studies of dairy product and calcium intakes and prostate cancer risk: a meta-analysis. *J Natl Cancer Inst* 2005;97:1768–1777.

93. Huncharek M, Muscat J, Kupelnick B. Dairy products, dietary calcium and vitamin D intake as risk factors for prostate cancer: a meta-analysis of 26,769 cases from 45 observational studies. *Nutr Cancer* 2008;60:421–441.

94. Ganmaa D, Cui X, Feskanich D, et al. Milk, dairy intake and risk of endometrial cancer: a 26-year follow-up. *Int J Cancer* 2012;130:2664–2671.

95. Genkinger JM, Hunter DJ, Spiegelman D, et al. Dairy products and ovarian cancer: a pooled analysis of 12 cohort studies. *Cancer Epidemiol Biomarkers Prev* 2006;15:364–372.

96. Hoppe C, Molgaard C, Juul A, et al. High intakes of skimmed milk, but not meat, increase serum IGF-I and IGFBP-3 in eight-year-old boys. *Eur J Clin Nutr* 2004;58:1211–1216.

97. Ganmaa D, Wang PY, Qin LQ, et al. Is milk responsible for male reproductive disorders? *Med Hypotheses* 2001;57:510–514.

98. Garland CF, Garland FC. Do sunlight and vitamin D reduce the likelihood of colon cancer? *Int J Epidemiol* 1980;9:227–231.

99. Feskanich D, Ma J, Fuchs CS, et al. Plasma vitamin D metabolites and risk of colorectal cancer in women. *Cancer Epidemiol Biomarkers Prev* 2004;13:1502–1508.

100. Woolcott CG, Wilkens LR, Nomura AM, et al. Plasma 25-hydroxyvitamin D levels and the risk of colorectal cancer: the multiethnic cohort study. *Cancer Epidemiol Biomarkers Prev* 2010;19:130–134.

101. Jenab M, Bueno-de-Mesquita HB, Ferrari P, et al. Association between pre-diagnostic circulating vitamin D concentration and risk of colorectal cancer in European populations: a nested case-control study. *BMJ* 2010;340:b5500.

102. Wactawski-Wende J, Kotchen JM, Anderson GL, et al. Calcium plus vitamin D supplementation and the risk of colorectal cancer. *N Engl J Med* 2006;354:684–696.

103. Park SY, Murphy SP, Wilkens LR, et al. Calcium and vitamin D intake and risk of colorectal cancer: the Multiethnic Cohort Study. *Am J Epidemiol* 2007;165:784–793.

104. Gorham ED, Garland CF, Garland FC, et al. Optimal vitamin D status for colorectal cancer prevention: a quantitative meta analysis. *Am J Prev Med* 2007;32:210–216.

105. Yin L, Grandi N, Raum E, et al. Meta-analysis: longitudinal studies of serum vitamin D and colorectal cancer risk. *Aliment Pharmacol Ther* 2009;30:113–125.

106. Wei MY, Garland CF, Gorham ED, et al. Vitamin D and prevention of colorectal adenoma: a meta-analysis. *Cancer Epidemiol Biomarkers Prev* 2008;17:2958–2969.

107. Freedman DM, Looker AC, Chang SC, et al. Prospective study of serum vitamin D and cancer mortality in the United States. *J Natl Cancer Inst* 2007;99:1594–1602.

108. Bertone-Johnson ER, Chen WY, Holick MF, et al. Plasma 25-hydroxyvitamin D and 1,25-dihydroxyvitamin D and risk of breast cancer. *Cancer Epidemiol Biomarkers Prev* 2005;14:1991–1997.

109. McCullough ML, Rodriguez C, Diver WR, et al. Dairy, calcium, and vitamin D intake and postmenopausal breast cancer risk in the Cancer Prevention Study II Nutrition Cohort. *Cancer Epidemiol Biomarkers Prev* 2005;14:2898–2904.

110. Chen P, Hu P, Xie D, et al. Meta-analysis of vitamin D, calcium and the prevention of breast cancer. *Breast Cancer Res Treat* 2010;121:469–477.

111. Platz EA, Leitzmann MF, Hollis BW, et al. Plasma 1,25-dihydroxy- and 25-hydroxyvitamin D and subsequent risk of prostate cancer. *Cancer Causes Control* 2004;15:255–265.

112. Shui IM, Mucci LA, Kraft P, et al. Vitamin D-related genetic variation, plasma vitamin D, and risk of lethal prostate cancer: a prospective nested case-control study. *J Natl Cancer Inst* 2012;104:690–699.

113. Tworoger SS, Lee IM, Buring JE, et al. Plasma 25-hydroxyvitamin D and 1,25-dihydroxyvitamin D and risk of incident ovarian cancer. *Cancer Epidemiol Biomarkers Prev* 2007;16:783–788.

114. Toriola AT, Surcel HM, Agborsangaya C, et al. Serum 25-hydroxyvitamin D and the risk of ovarian cancer. *Eur J Cancer* 2010;46:364–369.

115. Stolzenberg-Solomon RZ, Jacobs EJ, Arslan AA, et al. Circulating 25-hydroxyvitamin D and risk of pancreatic cancer: Cohort Consortium Vitamin D Pooling Project of Rarer Cancers. *Am J Epidemiol* 2010;172:81–93.

116. Skinner HG, Michaud DS, Giovannucci E, et al. Vitamin D intake and the risk for pancreatic cancer in two cohort studies. *Cancer Epidemiol Biomarkers Prev* 2006;15:1688–1695.

117. Wolpin BM, Ng K, Bao Y, et al. Plasma 25-hydroxyvitamin D and risk of pancreatic cancer. *Cancer Epidemiol Biomarkers Prev* 2012;21:82–91.

118. Giovannucci E. Epidemiology of vitamin D and colorectal cancer: casual or causal link? *J Steroid Biochem Mol Biol* 2010;121(1–2):349–354.

119. Giovannucci E. Epidemiologic studies of folate and colorectal neoplasia: a review. *J Nutr* 2002;132:2350S–2355S.

120. Kim D, Smith-Warner S, Spiegelman D, et al. Pooled analysis of 13 prospective cohort studies on folate and colon cancer. *Cancer Causes Control* 2010;21:1919-1930.

121. Chen J, Giovannucci E, Kelsey K, et al. A methylenetetrahydrofolate reductase polymorphism and the risk of colorectal cancer. *Cancer Res* 1996;56:4862–4864.

122. Osterhues A, Holzgreve W, Michels KB. Shall we put the world on folate? *Lancet* 2009;374:959–961.

123. Friso S, Choi SW, Girelli D, et al. A common mutation in the 5,10-methylene-tetrahydrofolate reductase gene affects genomic DNA methylation through an interaction with folate status. *Proc Natl Acad Sci U S A* 2002;99:5606–5611.

124. Kim YI. Folate: a magic bullet or a double edged sword for colorectal cancer prevention? *Gut* 2006;55:1387–1389.

125. Mason JB. Folate, cancer risk, and the Greek god, Proteus: a tale of two chameleons. *Nutr Rev* 2009;67:206–212.

126. Wu K, Platz EA, Willett W, et al. A randomized trial on folic acid supplementation and risk of recurrent colorectal adenoma. *Am J Clin Nutr* 2009;90:1623–1631.

127. Cole BF, Baron JA, Sandler RS, et al. Folic acid for the prevention of colorectal adenomas: a randomized clinical trial. *JAMA* 2007;297:2351–2359.

128. Mason JB, Dickstein A, Jacques PF, et al. A temporal association between folic acid fortification and an increase in colorectal cancer rates may be illuminating important biological principles: a hypothesis. *Cancer Epidemiol Biomarkers Prev* 2007;16:1325–1329.

129. The effect of vitamin E and beta carotene on the incidence of lung cancer and other cancers in male smokers. The Alpha-Tocopherol, Beta Carotene Cancer Prevention Study Group. *N Engl J Med* 1994;330:1029–1035.

130. Virtamo J, Pietinen P, Huttunen JK, et al. Incidence of cancer and mortality following alpha-tocopherol and beta-carotene supplementation: a postintervention follow-up. *JAMA* 2003;290:476–485.

131. Mannisto S, Smith-Warner SA, Spiegelman D, et al. Dietary carotenoids and risk of lung cancer in a pooled analysis of seven cohort studies. *Cancer Epidemiol Biomarkers Prev* 2004;13:40–48.

132. Zhang X, Spiegelman D, Baglietto L, et al. Carotenoid intakes and risk of breast cancer defined by estrogen receptor and progesterone receptor status: a pooled analysis of 18 prospective cohort studies. *Am J Clin Nutr* 2012;95:713–725.

133. Eliassen AH, Hendrickson SJ, Brinton LA, et al. Circulating carotenoids and risk of breast cancer: pooled analysis of eight prospective studies. *J Natl Cancer Inst* 2012;104:1905–1916.

134. Giovannucci E. Tomatoes, tomato-based products, lycopene, and cancer: review of the epidemiologic literature. *J Natl Cancer Inst* 1999;91:317–331.

135. Yoshizawa K, Willett WC, Morris SJ, et al. Study of prediagnostic selenium level in toenails and the risk of advanced prostate cancer. *J Natl Cancer Inst* 1998;90:1219–1224.

136. Amaral AF, Cantor KP, Silverman DT, et al. Selenium and bladder cancer risk: a meta-analysis. *Cancer Epidemiol Biomarkers Prev* 2010;19:2407–2415.

137. Geybels MS, Verhage BA, van Schooten FJ, et al. Advanced prostate cancer risk in relation to toenail selenium levels. *J Natl Cancer Inst* 2013;105:1394–1401.

138. Hurst R, Hooper L, Norat T, et al. Selenium and prostate cancer: systematic review and meta-analysis. *Am J Clinical Nutr* 2012;96:111–122.

139. Lippman SM, Klein EA, Goodman PJ, et al. Effect of selenium and vitamin E on risk of prostate cancer and other cancers: the Selenium and Vitamin E Cancer Prevention Trial (SELECT). *JAMA* 2009;301:39–51.

140. Trock BJ, Hilakivi-Clarke L, Clarke R. Meta-analysis of soy intake and breast cancer risk. *J Natl Cancer Inst* 2006;98:459–471.

141. Wu AH, Wan P, Hankin J, et al. Adolescent and adult soy intake and risk of breast cancer in Asian-Americans. *Carcinogenesis* 2002;23:1491–1496.

142. Warburg O, Posener K, Negelein E. Ueber den Stoffwechsel der Tumoren. *Biochemische Zeitschrift* 1924;152:319.

143. Hu FB, Manson JE, Liu S, et al. Prospective study of adult onset diabetes mellitus (type 2) and risk of colorectal cancer in women. *J Natl Cancer Inst* 1999;91:542–547.

144. Michels KB, Solomon CG, Hu FB, et al. Type 2 diabetes and subsequent incidence of breast cancer in the Nurses' Health Study. *Diabetes Care* 2003;26:1752–1758.

145. Gnagnarella P, Gandini S, La Vecchia C, et al. Glycemic index, glycemic load, and cancer risk: a meta-analysis. *Am J Clinical Nutr* 2008;87:1793–1801.

146. Slattery ML, Benson J, Berry TD, et al. Dietary sugar and colon cancer. *Cancer Epidemiol Biomarkers Prev* 1997;6:677–685.

147. Terry PD, Jain M, Miller AB, et al. Glycemic load, carbohydrate intake, and risk of colorectal cancer in women: a prospective cohort study. *J Natl Cancer Inst* 2003;95:914–916.

148. Michaud DS, Liu S, Giovannucci E, et al. Dietary sugar, glycemic load, and pancreatic cancer risk in a prospective study. *J Natl Cancer Inst* 2002;94:1293–1300.

149. Jonas CR, McCullough ML, Teras LR, et al. Dietary glycemic index, glycemic load, and risk of incident breast cancer in postmenopausal women. *Cancer Epidemiol Biomarkers Prev* 2003;12:573–577.

150. Tantamango-Bartley Y, Jaceldo-Siegl K, Fan J, et al. Vegetarian diets and the incidence of cancer in a low-risk population. *Cancer Epidemiol Biomarkers Prev* 2013;22:286–294.

151. Key TJ, Appleby PN, Spencer EA, et al. Cancer incidence in British vegetarians. *Br J Cancer* 2009;101:192–197.

**ETIOLOGY AND EPIDEMIOLOGY OF CANCER**

152. Fung T, Hu FB, Fuchs C, et al. Major dietary patterns and the risk of colorectal cancer in women. *Arch Intern Med* 2003;163:309–314.

153. Fung TT, Hu FB, Holmes MD, et al. Dietary patterns and the risk of postmenopausal breast cancer. *Int J Cancer* 2005;116:116–121.

154. Link LB, Canchola AJ, Bernstein L, et al. Dietary patterns and breast cancer risk in the California Teachers Study cohort. *Am J Clin Nutr* 2013;98:1524–1532.

155. Caughey RW, Michels KB. Birth weight and childhood leukemia: a meta-analysis and review of the current evidence. *Int J Cancer* 2009;124:2658–2670.

156. Michels KB, Xue F. Role of birthweight in the etiology of breast cancer. *Int J Cancer* 2006;119:2007–2025.

157. Michos A, Xue F, Michels KB. Birth weight and the risk of testicular cancer: a meta-analysis. *Int J Cancer* 2007;121:1123–1131.

158. Chavarro JE, Rosner BA, Sampson L, et al. Validity of adolescent diet recall 48 years later. *Am J Epidemiol* 2009;170:1563–1570.

159. Maruti SS, Feskanich D, Colditz GA, et al. Adult recall of adolescent diet: reproducibility and comparison with maternal reporting. *Am J Epidemiol* 2005;161:89–97.

160. Michels KB, Rosner BA, Chumlea WC, et al. Preschool diet and adult risk of breast cancer. *Int J Cancer* 2006;118:749–754.

161. Hjartaker A, Laake P, Lund E. Childhood and adult milk consumption and risk of premenopausal breast cancer in a cohort of 48,844 women - the Norwegian women and cancer study. *Int J Cancer* 2001;93:888–893.

162. Michels KB, Mohllajee AP, Roset-Bahmanyar E, et al. Diet and breast cancer: a review of the prospective observational studies. *Cancer* 2007;109:2712–2749.

163. Greenlee H, Kwan ML, Kushi LH, et al. Antioxidant supplement use after breast cancer diagnosis and mortality in the Life After Cancer Epidemiology (LACE) cohort. *Cancer* 2012;118:2048–2058.

164. Kwan ML, Chen WY, Flatt SW, et al. Postdiagnosis alcohol consumption and breast cancer prognosis in the after breast cancer pooling project. *Cancer Epidemiol Biomarkers Prev* 2013;22:32–41.

165. Chlebowski RT, Blackburn GL, Thomson CA, et al. Dietary fat reduction and breast cancer outcome: interim efficacy results from the Women's Intervention Nutrition Study. *J Natl Cancer Inst* 2006;98:1767–1776.

166. Pierce JP, Natarajan L, Caan BJ, et al. Influence of a diet very high in vegetables, fruit, and fiber and low in fat on prognosis following treatment for breast cancer: the Women's Healthy Eating and Living (WHEL) randomized trial. *JAMA* 2007;298:289–298.

167. Izano MA, Fung TT, Chiuve SS, et al. Are diet quality scores after breast cancer diagnosis associated with improved breast cancer survival? *Nutr Cancer* 2013;65:820–826.

168. van Meer S, Leufkens AM, Bueno-de-Mesquita HB, et al. Role of dietary factors in survival and mortality in colorectal cancer: a systematic review. *Nutrition Rev* 2013;71:631–641.

169. Meyerhardt JA, Niedzwiecki D, Hollis D, et al. Association of dietary patterns with cancer recurrence and survival in patients with stage III colon cancer. *JAMA* 2007;298:754–764.

170. Meyerhardt JA, Sato K, Niedzwiecki D, et al. Dietary glycemic load and cancer recurrence and survival in patients with stage III colon cancer: findings from CALGB 89803. *J Natl Cancer Inst* 2012;104:1702–1711.

171. Song Y, Chavarro JE, Cao Y, et al. Whole milk intake is associated with prostate cancer-specific mortality among U.S. male physicians. *J Nutr* 2013;143:189–196.

172. Richman EL, Kenfield SA, Chavarro JE, et al. Fat intake after diagnosis and risk of lethal prostate cancer and all-cause mortality. *JAMA Intern Med* 2013;173:1318–1326.

173. Richman EL, Kenfield SA, Stampfer MJ, et al. Egg, red meat, and poultry intake and risk of lethal prostate cancer in the prostate-specific antigen-era: incidence and survival. *Cancer Prev Res (Phila)* 2011;4:2110–2121.

174. Chan JM, Holick CN, Leitzmann MF, et al. Diet after diagnosis and the risk of prostate cancer progression, recurrence, and death (United States). *Cancer Causes Control* 2006;17:199–208.

175. Ornish D, Weidner G, Fair WR, et al. Intensive lifestyle changes may affect the progression of prostate cancer. *J Urol* 2005;174:1065–1070.

176. Kushi LH, Doyle C, McCullough M, et al. American Cancer Society Guidelines on nutrition and physical activity for cancer prevention: reducing the risk of cancer with healthy food choices and physical activity. *CA Cancer J Clin* 2012;62:30–67.

# 10 Obesity and Physical Activity

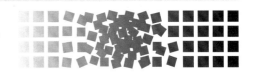

Yani Lu, Jessica Clague, and Leslie Bernstein

## INTRODUCTION

Evidence showing that physical activity is associated with decreased cancer risk and that obesity is associated with increased cancer risk at certain sites is rapidly accumulating. It is not yet known whether these two factors are interrelated or independent. Physical activity may act to decrease cancer risk primarily by preventing weight gain and obesity. However, physical activity may also have independent effects on cancer risk. In this chapter, we present a summary of the current epidemiologic literature on the possible associations between physical activity and obesity and risk of cancer at several organ sites.

Physical activity is defined as any movement of the body that results in energy expenditure. In this chapter, we focus on recreational physical activity, also called leisure-time physical activity or exercise, and occupational physical activity, including household activity.[1] Occupational physical activity typically occurs over a longer period of time and generally requires less energy expenditure per hour than bouts of strenuous or moderate recreational physical activity. The distinction between recreational and occupational activity is important because increasing mechanization and technologic advances have led to decreased occupational physical activity in developed areas of the world, perhaps contributing to a decrease in overall physical activity.

Obesity is defined as the condition of being extremely overweight. In epidemiologic studies, the usual, but not necessarily the best, measure of body mass in adults is Quetelet's Index, or body mass index (BMI), which is measured as weight in kilograms (kg) divided by the square of height in meters (m²). In the year spanning 2009 to 2010, the prevalence of obesity, defined by having a BMI of 30 kg/m² or greater, in the US population was 35.5% for adult men and 35.8% for adult women.[2] Physical inactivity has likely contributed to the high prevalence of obesity in the United States; data from the 2003 to 2004 National Health and Nutritional Examination Survey, a cross-sectional study of a sample of the civilian, noninstitutionalized population of the United States, has indicated that less than 5% of US adults achieve 30 minutes per day of physical activity, and that men are more physically active than women.[3]

Epidemiologic evidence on the associations of physical activity and obesity with cancer come from observational studies, including cohort studies, which follow populations forward in time after collecting exposure information, and case-control studies, which optimally identify a population-based series of newly diagnosed cases and healthy control subjects, collecting information retrospectively on exposures. In both study designs, physical activity information is usually self-reported and measures vary substantially with respect to timing and level of detail. Studies have measured lifetime or long-term physical activity, activity at defined ages or time points in life, and/or current or recent activity. Ideally, a study would capture activity by type (recreational, occupational, or other, such as an activity related to transportation), duration (minutes per session), frequency (sessions per day), and intensity (low, moderate, or strenuous as defined by examples of activity types) across the lifetime. These studies have often measured height and weight by self-report at one time point, such as at the time of study entry. Some studies have collected other or more detailed anthropometric information, such as waist circumference, hip circumference, or weight at an additional time point like at age 18. Anthropometrics are directly measured by trained study personnel in only a few studies.

Epidemiologic evidence for a role of physical activity or obesity in relation to cancer risk exists for cancers of the breast, colon, endometrium, esophagus, kidney, and pancreatic cancer. Evidence is accumulating to link at least one of these "exposures" to the incidence of gallbladder cancer, non-Hodgkin lymphoma (NHL), and advanced prostate cancer. The evidence for an association between either physical activity or obesity and lung and ovarian cancer is inconclusive.

In addition to specific biologic mechanisms pertinent to physical activity or to obesity at each specific organ site, several global mechanisms have been implicated in both relationships across a number of these organ sites. The steroid hormone and insulin/insulinlike growth factor (IGF) pathways are two such global mechanisms hypothesized to be involved in the links between physical activity or obesity and cancer.[4] The role of steroid hormones as a mediator in these relationships is perhaps best understood in the context of breast cancer and endometrial cancer, and will be discussed in those sections. The roles of the insulin and IGF pathways have been discussed in depth with respect to colon cancer and, thus, will be presented in that context. Other global mechanisms have been proposed that have more generalized anticancer impacts and may explain associations between physical activity and several cancer sites; these include heightening immune surveillance, reducing inflammation, increasing insulin sensitivity, controlling growth factor production and activation, decreasing obesity and central adiposity, optimizing DNA repair capacity, and reducing oxidative stress.[5,6] Further, obesity has been shown to produce a proinflammatory state and, thus, inflammation may mediate the relationship between obesity and cancer risk.[7] It is highly plausible that several of these mechanisms act simultaneously and that they interact synergistically to mediate the associations between physical activity, obesity, and cancer.

## BREAST CANCER

Low level of physical activity is an established breast cancer risk factor among postmenopausal women and, to a lesser extent, premenopausal women.[4,8,9] The evidence for an association between physical activity and breast cancer has been classified as convincing, with a 20% to 40% reduced risk among physically active women.[10] Obesity appears to have a paradoxical relationship with breast cancer risk in that it is an established breast cancer risk factor among postmenopausal women, but may offer some protection for breast cancer among premenopausal women.[4]

The epidemiologic literature has shown with relative consistency that breast cancer risk is reduced by increasing one's amount of physical activity.[4,8,9,11–13] One of the earliest studies, a case-control study of women age 40 years or younger, showed a dramatic reduction in risk of approximately 50% among women who averaged about 4 hours of activity per week during their reproductive years.[14] Similarly, among postmenopausal women, those with higher levels of recreational physical activity during their lifetimes have been shown to have lower breast cancer risk.[15] A meta-analysis of 29 case-control studies and 19 cohort studies published between 1994 and 2006 provided strong evidence for an inverse association between physical activity and risk of breast cancer, citing that the evidence for an association between physical activity and premenopausal breast cancer was not as strong as that for postmenopausal breast cancer.[8] The conclusion of the meta-analysis was that each additional hour of physical activity per week decreases breast cancer by approximately 6%.

Epidemiologists require that a risk factor demonstrate consistency across populations before considering it as accepted. Recently, studies have been published on the association between physical activity and breast cancer risk among Japanese,[16] Chinese,[17] Mexican,[18] Tunisian,[19] and African American women.[20] All studies showed a decreased risk of breast cancer with increasing physical activity. Interestingly, both Suzuki et al.[17] and Pronk et al.[21] observed the strongest associations among "heavier" women (BMI $\geq$25 kg/m$^2$ and 23.73 kg/m$^2$, respectively). In the California Teachers Study (CTS), a prospective cohort study of over 133,000 female public school professionals, a variable combining strenuous and moderate long-term recreational physical activity was associated with a reduced risk of estrogen receptor (ER)-negative but not ER-positive invasive breast cancer.[11] On the contrary, the Women's Health Initiative (WHI) observed decreases in breast cancer risk associated with recreational physical activity among postmenopausal women with ER-positive breast cancer and triple negative breast cancer, with only results for ER-positive breast cancer demonstrating a 15% statistically significant reduced risk (when comparing the highest versus lowest tertile of moderate-intensity physical activity).[22] Similar but not statistically significant results were observed for strenuous recreational physical activity.[22] A major limitation to this and previous studies stratifying by hormone receptor status is the inability to comprehensively classify triple negative breast cancer due to missing HER2 status (unknown in 40% of cases in the WHI study). The use of hormone therapy did not alter the inverse association between recreational physical activity and invasive breast cancer in the Women's Contraceptive and Reproductive Experiences (CARE) Study.[23] Most recently, in the American Cancer Society Cancer Prevention Study II Nutrition Cohort, it was observed that postmenopausal women who engage in at least 7 hours of walking over the course of a week had a modest decreased risk of breast cancer, even in the absence of more vigorous exercise.[24] Further, this association did not differ by ER status, BMI, adult weight gain, postmenopausal hormone therapy use, or time spent sitting.[24]

Lastly, whether physical activity reduces breast cancer risk by impacting preinvasive disease has been studied by assessing the associations with in situ breast cancer and benign breast disease. In the CTS cohort, increasing levels of long-term strenuous recreational physical activity were associated with a decreasing risk of in situ breast cancer.[11] Furthermore, a report from the Nurses' Health Study II cohort showed that lifetime recreational physical activity was associated with a decreased risk of benign breast disease and columnar cell lesions, which may be precursors to breast cancer.[25]

In summary, epidemiologic studies investigating the association between physical activity and breast cancer risk have produced relatively consistent results showing a reduction in breast cancer risk with increasing level of physical activity. Results to date suggest that moderate-to-strenuous activity may be required for the effect between physical activity and breast cancer risk to be clear; however, clarification of other key details, such as the importance of timing and intensity of activity or variation in effects by tumor characteristics, is pending.

Adult obesity and adult weight gain have both been associated with increased breast cancer risk among postmenopausal women, especially among women who were not current users of menopausal hormone therapy.[4,26,27] Most studies among postmenopausal women show a 1.5- to 2-fold increase in risk of invasive breast cancer when comparing the most obese women or those with the largest weight gain to normal-weight women (BMI: 18.5 to 24.9 kg/m$^2$) or those with the least weight gain.[4] Paradoxically, overweight or obese premenopausal women have a slightly decreased risk of breast cancer compared with normal-weight or thinner women. Whether larger waist circumference is more important than BMI has been studied in order to separate overall weight gain from abdominal obesity (i.e., visceral fat, which is one element of metabolic syndrome); however, most studies have reported a null association between waist circumference, used as a surrogate for visceral fat, and risk of postmenopausal breast cancer after adjustment for BMI.[26] In contrast to the results for postmenopausal women, waist circumference and a positive association with premenopausal breast cancer was found after adjustment for BMI.[26] A recent analysis of the Nurses' Health Study suggests that self-rated body fatness during youth and BMI at age 18 years are both inversely associated with breast cancer risk, with similar results for premenopausal and postmenopausal breast cancer.[28]

Hormones are central to the discussion of biologic mechanisms linking both physical activity and obesity with breast cancer risk. Physical activity can alter menstrual cycle patterns in premenopausal women, and hormone profiles in both premenopausal and postmenopausal women. Physical activity may lower body fat among children,[29] which in turn may delay age at menarche.[30] Later age at menarche has been associated with reduced breast cancer risk.[31] Physical activity may reduce the frequency of ovulatory cycles.[32] Having less frequent and therefore fewer cumulative ovulatory cycles is likely to reduce the lifetime exposure of the breast to endogenous ovarian hormones,[31] which are proven proliferative agents.[33] Physical activity also can have a direct impact on circulating estrogen levels among postmenopausal women.[34]

In the postmenopausal period, adipose tissue is the primary source of endogenous hormones via aromatization of androstenedione to estrone.[35] Thus, heavier postmenopausal women have higher levels of circulating estrogen than women with less adipose tissue. The involvement of estrogen in the relationship between obesity and breast cancer risk is supported by the observation that obesity does not independently increase breast cancer risk among menopausal hormone therapy users[27]; the obesity-related increase in estrogen over that provided by exogenous estrogens is negligible. The breast tissue of overweight or obese perimenopausal and postmenopausal women with relatively high risk of breast cancer has been shown to have cytologic abnormalities and higher epithelial cell counts than that of normal-weight women.[36] In contrast, obese premenopausal women experience menstrual cycle disturbances, including anovulatory cycles and secondary amenorrhea, thereby lowering their cumulative exposure to estradiol and progesterone.[31] A possible explanation for the inverse association between youth body fatness and breast cancer risk is that youth body size is inversely associated with adult IGF-1 levels.[28]

Other likely mechanisms that may link physical activity[37,38] and obesity[39,40] with breast cancer risk include aspects of immune function, inflammatory mechanisms, oxidative stress and DNA repair capability, metabolic hormones, and growth factors.

## COLON AND RECTAL CANCER

An inverse association between physical activity and colon cancer risk has been consistently observed among epidemiologic studies; however, the evidence for rectal cancer remains inconclusive. Historically, comprehensive reviews have estimated that physical activity may reduce colon cancer risk by 20% to 25% when comparing individuals with the highest levels to those with the lowest levels of activity.[41] Risk reductions are greater for case-control studies (24%) than for cohort studies (17%), and risk reductions for occupational activity (22%) and recreational activity (23%) are similar.[41] In cohort studies, colon cancer risk reduction associated with physical activity is greater for men than for women, which may be due to the influence of hormone therapy on colon cancer risk,[42] although case-control studies suggest similar benefits for men and women.[43]

Whether physical activity preferentially protects against proximal or distal colon cancer is of interest. A meta-analysis including 21 cohort and case-control studies that examined associations between physical activity and the risks of proximal colon and distal colon cancers produced results suggesting that physical activity is associated with a reduced risk of both proximal colon and distal colon cancers, and that the magnitude of the association does not differ by subsite.[44]

Although the majority of previous studies have not found an association between physical activity and rectal cancer,[41] the National Institutes of Health (NIH)–AARP Diet and Health Study observed a modest reduction in rectal cancer risk for men but not for women after 6.9 years of follow-up.[45] Further, in a case-control study conducted in Australia, rectal cancer risk was reduced among men but not among women who participated in vigorous recreational physical activity averaging at least 6 metabolic equivalent task (MET)-hours per week during their adult years.[46]

An emphasis has been made on trying to identify risk factors for colon adenomas, which are considered precursor lesions for colon cancer; these are detected and removed during colonoscopy or sigmoidoscopy. Wolin et al. conducted a meta-analysis of 20 studies published through April 2010 that investigated the association between recreational physical activity and colon adenomas.[47] Adenoma risk was reduced by 19% among men and by 13% among women and, when combining men and women, the inverse association with physical activity was strongest for large/advanced polyps.

Obesity is an established risk factor for colon cancer in both men and women, although the relative risks for men have been higher than those for women.[4,26] The adverse impact of being overweight or obese on colon cancer risk is stronger for distal than for proximal colon cancers. In addition, visceral adiposity appears to confer greater risk than general adiposity.[26] In the European Prospective Investigation into Cancer and Nutrition (EPIC) study, abdominal obesity as well as adult weight gain were strongly associated with colon cancer risk in both men and women.[48,49] No association between these adiposity measures and colon cancer risk was evident among postmenopausal women who had used menopausal hormone therapy, and no association was observed between any measure of adiposity and rectal cancer risk.[48] The positive association between obesity and risk of colon cancer was further supported by the findings that both general obesity and abdominal obesity increase the risk of colon adenomas[47] with one study of women indicating that the distal colon is the main target site.[50]

Given that a higher BMI and lack of physical activity are both risk factors for colon cancer, several statistical approaches have been employed to tease apart their joint and independent effects on colon cancer risk. In the Netherlands Cohort Study,[51] colorectal cancer risk was increased at each subsite among larger women in the lowest recreational activity category (<30 minutes per day) than in smaller women in the highest recreational activity category (>90 minutes per day); however, the interaction between physical activity and body size was statistically significant only for proximal tumors. Using different fatness measures for men, the only similar finding was that men with low levels of physical activity whose trouser size was below the median of that for the cohort had an increased risk of distal colon cancer; no differences in risk were noted for other subsites or for men with larger trouser sizes.[51]

The mechanisms explaining the relationship between physical activity and colon cancer are not clearly established, but include the impact on insulin sensitivity and IGF profiles, and inflammation, as well as some colon-specific mechanisms. Physical activity may stimulate stool transit in the colon, thereby decreasing the exposure of colonic mucosa to carcinogens in the stool.[6] Alternatively, physical activity–induced decreases in prostaglandin $E_2$ may decrease colonic cell proliferation rates and increase colonic motility.[6] In addition to steroid hormones, which have been clearly implicated as biologic modifiers of the effect of physical activity and obesity on colon cancer risk, the insulin and IGF pathways may mediate the associations between these exposures and colon cancer risk. For obesity in particular, the link can be inferred because obesity can lead to insulin resistance,[52] a syndrome characterized by high circulating insulin levels. High insulin levels appear to promote cell proliferation and tumor growth in the colon[7] and may also suppress the expression of IGF-binding proteins 1 and 2, leading to increased bioavailable IGF-1 levels.[53] Another possible mechanism is obesity-enhanced inflammation in which increases in adipose tissue macrophages lead to the secretion of inflammatory cytokines associated with colon cancer risk (e.g., tumor necrosis factor [TNF]-α, monocyte chemoattractant protein [MCP]-1, and interleukin [IL]-6).

## ENDOMETRIAL CANCER

The evidence for an association between physical activity and endometrial cancer risk is accumulating[4,54–58] but is not definitive. A meta-analysis of prospective cohort studies results published through 2009 indicates that recreational physical activity lowers endometrial cancer risk by 27%, and occupational activity lowers risk by 21%.[59] Adjustments for BMI minimally change relative risk estimates, suggesting that physical activity is independently associated with endometrial cancer. Although physical activity is associated with a decreased risk of endometrial cancer in both normal-weight and obese women, two recent studies have suggested that this association is more pronounced for obese women.[54,58]

Two meta-analyses of the association between physical activity and endometrial cancer have identified some inconsistencies in dose-response relationships, indicating the importance of differences in activity type and intensity.[55,56] Little evidence exists on how long-term or lifetime physical activity and activity patterns during different life periods might influence endometrial cancer risk; it has been suggested that recent or long-term activity might be more important than activity at early ages.[56] In the CTS, higher levels of recent (at cohort formation) strenuous recreational physical activity was associated with lower levels of endometrial cancer risk; among women exercising >3 hours per week per year, risk was approximately 25% lower than that of women exercising <0.5 hour per week per year.[60] This inverse association was limited to overweight and obese women (BMI ≥25 kg/m²). Finally, sitting time has been independently associated with increased endometrial cancer risk.[59]

Epidemiologic studies have established a strong association between obesity and endometrial cancer risk.[26] Recent studies have suggested a linear trend between increasing body weight or BMI and increasing endometrial cancer risk among postmenopausal women, whereas among premenopausal women, no trend is observed, but rather, only obese women have an increased risk.[26] Furthermore, the strong association among postmenopausal women is only observed among those who are not using hormone therapy.[26] Finally, BMI appears to exert an effect on the risk of endometrial cancer that is independent of physical activity.[55]

Physical activity and obesity are likely to influence endometrial cancer risk by altering endogenous hormone profiles.[31,53] Heavier postmenopausal women have higher circulating levels of estrogen than do lighter postmenopausal women because of the aromatization of androstenedione to estrone in adipose tissue. This is pertinent to endometrial cancer risk because this aromatization occurs in the absence of progesterone, which opposes the proliferative effects of estrogen on endometrial tissue. Physical activity may counter the proliferative effects of estrogen either directly or by restricting weight gain. Some evidence also links elevated insulin levels and diabetes to endometrial cancer risk.[61] Physical inactivity and obesity play a role in the development of insulin insensitivity and diabetes, providing another mechanism by which they may influence endometrial cancer risk.

# ADENOCARCINOMA OF THE ESOPHAGUS

Several case-control studies[62–64] and one cohort study[65] have examined the association between physical activity and risk of adenocarcinoma of the esophagus. Zhang et al.[62] reported a modest association between participation in recreational physical activity more than once per week and a decreased risk of all esophageal cancer (adenocarcinomas and squamous cell tumors), although the result was not statistically significant. Lagergren et al.[63] reported no association between total, usual recreational and occupational physical activity and esophageal adenocarcinoma. Vigen et al.[64] showed that lifetime occupational physical activity was modestly associated with a lower risk of adenocarcinoma of the esophagus: the average annual level of occupational physical activity before age 65 years was associated with an approximately 40% reduction in risk of esophageal adenocarcinoma when the highest was compared with the lowest occupational physical activity category. Results from the NIH–AARP Diet and Health Study also support the hypothesis that physical activity lowers the risk of esophageal adenocarcinoma, but no association between physical activity and the risk of squamous cell esophageal cancer was found.[65]

Obesity is strongly associated with an increased risk of esophageal adenocarcinoma.[66,67] A pooled analysis of existing data showed that individuals with severe obesity (BMI $\geq$40 kg/m$^2$) had a 4.8-fold greater risk than individuals who were not overweight (BMI <25 kg/m$^2$), with similar risk estimates for men and women.[68] Several studies have examined the effect of abdominal adiposity, which have suggested that the risk associated with obesity is driven primarily by abdominal fatness.[26]

It is likely that obesity impacts esophageal adenocarcinoma risk because it is associated with the risk of gastroesophageal reflux disease (GERD). GERD may cause changes in the esophageal epithelium, leading to Barrett esophagus, a well-established precancerous condition for esophageal adenocarcinoma. On the other hand, obesity is associated with a systemic inflammatory state, which includes the exposure to adipocytokines and procoagulant factors released by adipocytes in central fat, which may also contribute to the development of esophageal adenocarcinoma.[67] Physical activity may influence the risk of esophageal adenocarcinoma by increasing digestive track transit time, thus reducing exposure of the esophagus to putative cancer-causing agents.

# KIDNEY/RENAL CELL CANCER

Physical activity has been studied in relation to renal cell carcinoma in part because of the known deleterious effects of high BMI and hypertension on the risk of renal cell cancer; however, no association has been firmly established. A review of physical activity and risk of genitourinary cancers noted significant protective effects in 8 of 15 studies of physical activity in relation to renal cell carcinoma, with an average 8% reduction in risk when comparing individuals with the highest level of physical activity to those with the lowest level of activity.[69] Reductions in risk were greater for recreational than for other forms of activity and for activity performed later in life.

Obesity, in addition to high blood pressure and diabetes, is an established risk factor for kidney cancer.[26] It is still uncertain whether a gender difference exists, however. A meta-analysis has suggested a similar impact of BMI on kidney cancer risk among women and men, with an approximate 7% increase in risk per unit increase in BMI.[26] The effect of obesity may differ by histology; a recent study reported an increased risk observed for clear cell and chromophobe cancers, but not papillary renal cell cancer.[70]

# PANCREATIC CANCER

Pancreatic cancer is generally diagnosed at an advanced stage and is associated with high mortality rates. A meta-analysis of 28 stud-

ies of pancreatic cancer showed that higher total lifetime physical activity and occupational activity were associated with a lower risk.[71] Nonsignificant reductions in risk were observed for recreational physical activity and transportation (walking and cycling as a form of commuting). Significant heterogeneity was present across the studies, making it difficult to find a definitive answer.

Evidence indicating that obesity is a risk factor for pancreatic cancer is convincing. Three large pooled analyses and three of four meta-analyses that encompass a range of well-designed, independent observational epidemiologic studies have demonstrated a positive association between obesity and pancreatic cancer risk.[72,73] Effects were relatively consistent across studies, with an approximate 10% or greater increase in risk for every 5 kg/m$^2$ increase in BMI. Two of the pooled analyses and one of the meta-analyses assessed measures of adiposity such as waist circumference or waist-to-hip ratio (WHR); each of the results suggested positive associations with pancreatic cancer risk.[72,74,75] The pooled analyses reported at least a 35% greater risk when the fourth quartile of WHR was compared to the first quartile. The meta-analysis study reported an 11% increase in risk associated with each 10-cm increase in waist circumference and a 19% increase in risk for each 0.1-unit increment in WHR.

# GALLBLADDER CANCER

Gallbladder cancer occurs more frequently in women than in men, and the major risk factor is a history of gallstones,[10] which has been associated with the use of exogenous estrogens.[76] To date, we have found no epidemiologic literature investigating the possible association of physical activity and gallbladder cancer, although several studies have suggested a positive association between obesity and gallbladder cancer. In a meta-analysis comprised of 3,288 cases derived from eight cohort studies and three case-control studies, obesity was associated with a 66% increased risk of gallbladder cancer, and the increase in risk was larger for women than for men.[77] Further, two studies found that WHR was positively associated with gallbladder cancer risk among men and women with and without a history of gallstones, suggesting that abdominal obesity may be important in the etiology of this disease.[78,79]

# NON-HODGKIN LYMPHOMA

Studies addressing physical inactivity and obesity as potential risk factors for NHL have been mixed, in part because they have not had a sufficient number of cases to assess risk by NHL subtype. Generally, studies have shown no overall association between physical activity and NHL risk.[4] The results of four cohort studies, the CTS,[80] WHI,[81] EPIC,[82] and the American Cancer Society Prevention Study-II[83] have been unconvincing, with WHI showing a nonstatistically significant positive association, whereas the other studies showed no association.

In 2008, the International Lymphoma Epidemiology Consortium (InterLymph) published a pooled analysis of 18 case-control studies with more than 10,000 cases reporting no association between BMI around the time of diagnosis and NHL risk overall, but an increased risk of diffuse NHL for severe obesity (BMI $\geq$40 kg/m$^2$).[84] The results from meta-analyses of cohort studies suggested a weak positive association overall and for diffuse NHL.[85,86] An analysis of two cohort studies has suggested that body size in early adulthood may be more predictive of NHL risk than that later in life for all NHL and for the diffuse and follicular subtypes.[87]

# PROSTATE CANCER

More than 20 studies have assessed the potential association between physical activity and prostate cancer.[4,88,89] Regardless of the different approaches used, the populations studied, or the sample sizes of the studies, the majority of studies have suggested a modest reduction in risk with an increased level of physical activity.[4] In a review of the literature, Friedenreich and Orenstein[88] concluded that prostate cancer risk is reduced 10% to 30% when comparing the most active with the least active men and suggested that it may be high levels of physical activity earlier in life that are most relevant to this disease. An update to this review, based on 22 additional studies, indicates that the majority of recent research studies observed protective effects.[90] Leitzmann and Rohrmann[91] added that the associations with reduced risk may be most apparent for fatal prostate cancer. A current systematic review and meta-analysis, including 19 cohort and 24 case-control studies, agrees.[92] A pooled 19% reduction in risk was observed for occupational physical activity, and a 5% reduction was observed for recreational physical activity comparing the most physically active men to the least active.[92] An issue that somewhat reduces our confidence in these estimates is that considerable heterogeneity between studies was observed. Further, it is not yet clear whether these results reflect a true causal association or whether they are due to confounding by prostate-specific antigen testing, which may be more common among physically active men.

The early epidemiologic literature on the potential association between obesity and prostate cancer provided no consistent evidence of any relationship.[4] Recent studies have suggested that obesity may have a dual effect on prostate cancer risk. One meta-analysis reported that the risk of early-stage prostate cancer decreased by 6%, whereas the risk of advanced prostate cancer increased 9% per 5-kg/m$^2$ increase in BMI.[93] Another possibility is that obesity may decrease the likelihood of diagnosis of less aggressive prostate cancer. Proposed mechanisms include the paradoxical effects of testosterone on low-grade versus more advanced prostate cancer and alterations in insulin and circulating IGF-1.[94]

## LUNG CANCER

Physical activity may reduce lung cancer risk by 30% to 40%,[88] but no definitive conclusion can be drawn because one cannot ignore potential residual confounding or effect modification due to smoking as an explanation for any observed association. Recent studies have attempted to address this issue by estimating risk within subgroups defined by smoking status. A recent review suggests an inverse relationship between heavy lifetime physical activity and lung cancer in former and current smokers that is consistent across all histologies, but is not observed among never smokers.[5] A small case-control study of current and former smokers enrolled in the Cologne Smoking Study came to a similar conclusion, observing a lower risk of lung cancer among participants who were physically active compared to those who were not.[95] In the large NIH–AARP Diet and Health Study, no associations were observed between occupational or recreation physical activity and lung cancer risk among those who never smoked.[96]

Due to sex differences in lung cancer pathology, risk factors, and prognosis, current research has also begun to investigate the association for men and women separately.[97] The recent literature consists of small case-control studies,[98] which lack statistical power to examine risks in subgroups defined by histology, smoking status, or sex, and which may be affected by survival bias in that rapidly fatal cases or those who are too ill to be interviewed are excluded from the study population.

Several studies have suggested the existence of an inverse association between increasing BMI and lung cancer risk.[99–102] Nevertheless, this inverse effect may have been due to residual confounding by smoking because the inverse association was restricted to ever smokers. One meta-analysis showed an inverse association between BMI and lung cancer in nonsmokers[103]; however, caution should be exercised when interpreting the results due to concerns about heterogeneity of risk estimates across studies, the quality of the original studies, and confounding by smoking.[104]

## OVARIAN CANCER

The literature on ovarian cancer risk in relation to physical activity and obesity has been inconclusive. More than 18 studies have assessed the impact of physical activity on ovarian cancer risk. A meta-analysis of 12 studies found an approximate 20% decrease in ovarian cancer risk associated with physical activity when the highest category of exercise was compared to the lowest.[105] Four[106–109] of five[110] additional studies found no association; the fifth study found a nonsignificant 10% to 20% reduction in ovarian cancer risk for women who participated in at least 1 hour per week of recreational aerobic activity.

The evidence for an association between obesity and increased ovarian cancer risk is weak, with few studies showing a statistically significant result.[4,111] A meta-analysis of 16 studies indicated that adult obesity increases the risk for ovarian cancer; the overall pooled effect estimate was a 30% increase in ovarian cancer risk associated with adult obesity with a possible dose-response effect, but no variation in risk estimates across histologic subtypes.[111] In contrast, the results from the Ovarian Cancer Association Consortium, based on original data from 15 case-control studies, suggest that obesity only increases the risk of the less common histologic subtypes of ovarian cancer; obesity does not increase risk of high-grade invasive serous cancers, the most common subtype.[112] A pooled analysis of 12 cohort studies reported that BMI was not associated with ovarian cancer risk in postmenopausal women, but was positively associated with risk in premenopausal women.[113] Another meta-analysis, using 47 studies, showed that the positive association between BMI and ovarian cancer was restricted to women who had never used hormone therapy; among these women, risk increased by 10% with every 5 kg/m$^2$ increase in BMI.[114]

## CONCLUSIONS

Table 10.1 illustrates the strength of evidence regarding increased physical activity as a protective factor and obesity as a risk factor

**TABLE 10.1**

**Summary of the Strength of the Observational Epidemiologic Evidence for Physical Activity as a Protective Factor and Obesity as a Risk Factor for Cancer, By Type of Cancer**

|  | Physical Activity | Overweight/ Obesity |
|---|---|---|
| Breast, postmenopausal | +++ | +++ |
| Breast, premenopausal | ++ | ++ (protection) |
| Colon | +++ | +++ |
| Endometrium | + | +++ |
| Esophagus, adenocarcinoma | ? | +++ |
| Kidney/renal cell | ? | +++ |
| Gallbladder | ? | ++ |
| Pancreas | ? | +++ |
| Non-Hodgkin lymphoma | ? | + |
| Prostate, aggressive | + | + |
| Lung | + | ? |
| Ovary | ? | ? |

+++, evidence is convincing; ++, evidence is probable; +, evidence is possible; ?, evidence remains insufficient/inconclusive.

ETIOLOGY AND EPIDEMIOLOGY OF CANCER

for cancer. The strength of evidence for each exposure is classified as convincing (+++), probable (++), possible (+), or insufficient and inconclusive (?). Overall, for physical activity, convincing evidence exists for an association with postmenopausal breast cancer and colon cancer; for obesity, the evidence is convincing for breast, colon, endometrial, esophageal, and kidney/renal cell cancer. Evidence for associations between these exposures and several other cancer sites is accumulating. Despite some convincing evidence of the effects of physical activity and obesity on the risk of certain cancers, it is difficult to make recommendations as to appropriate changes in lifestyle that will reduce a person's chances of developing cancer. We have no physical activity prescriptions to give at this time. Many questions remain to be answered: What are

the ages at which physical activity will provide the most benefit? What types of activity should one do and at what intensity, frequency (times per week), and duration (hours per week)? Similarly, for BMI, is there some threshold below which the individual will not have excess cancer risk? Does purposeful weight loss during the adult years lower the risk associated with being overweight or obese? Finally, necessary research is ongoing to identify the biologic mechanisms that account for these effects and to determine whether all persons are affected equally. For instance, it is possible that genetically defined subgroups of the population respond to physical activity or obesity differently. Understanding mechanisms and population variation in these effects will illuminate appropriate prescriptions for lifestyle change.

# REFERENCES

1. Caspersen CJ, Powell KE, Christenson GM. Physical activity, exercise, and physical fitness: definitions and distinctions for health-related research. *Public Health Rep* 1985;100(2):126–131.
2. Flegal KM, Carroll MD, Kit BK, et al. Prevalence of obesity and trends in the distribution of body mass index among US adults, 1999-2010. *JAMA* 2012;307(5):491–497.
3. Troiano RP, Berrigan D, Dodd KW, et al. Physical activity in the United States measured by accelerometer. *Med Sci Sports Exerc* 2008;40(1):181–188.
4. Vainio H, Bianchini F, eds. *IARC Handbooks of Cancer Prevention Volume 6: Weight Control and Physical Activity.* Lyon, France: IARC Press; 2000.
5. Anzuini F, Battistella A, Izzotti A. Physical activity and cancer prevention: a review of current evidence and biological mechanisms. *J Prev Med Hyg* 2011;52(4):174–180.
6. Hardman AE. Physical activity and cancer risk. *Proc Nutr Soc* 2001;60(1):107–113.
7. Gunter MJ, Leitzmann MF. Obesity and colorectal cancer: epidemiology, mechanisms and candidate genes. *J Nutr Biochem* 2006;17(3):145–156.
8. Monninkhof EM, Elias SG, Vlems FA, et al. Physical activity and breast cancer: a systematic review. *Epidemiol* 2007;18(1):137–157.
9. World Cancer Research Fund/American Institute for Cancer Research. *Food, Nutrition, Physical Activity, and the Prevention of Cancer: A Global Perspective.* Washington, D.C.: World Cancer Research Fund/American Institute for Cancer Research; 2007.
10. Ishiguro S, Inoue M, Kurahashi N, et al. Risk factors of biliary tract cancer in a large-scale population-based cohort study in Japan (JPHC study); with special focus on cholelithiasis, body mass index, and their effect modification. *Cancer Causes Control* 2008;19(1):33–41.
11. Dallal CM, Sullivan-Halley J, Ross RK, et al. Long-term recreational physical activity and risk of invasive and in situ breast cancer: The California Teachers Study. *Arch Intern Med* 2007;167(4):408–415.
12. Lahmann P, Friedenreich C, Schuit A, et al. Physical activity and breast cancer risk: The European Prospective Investigation into Cancer and Nutrition. *Cancer Epidemiol Biomarkers Prev* 2007;16(1):36–42.
13. Maruti SS, Willett WC, Feskanich D, et al. A prospective study of age-specific physical activity and premenopausal breast cancer. *J Natl Cancer Inst* 2008;100(10):728–737.
14. Bernstein L, Henderson BE, Hanisch R, et al. Physical exercise and reduced risk of breast cancer in young women. *J Natl Cancer Inst* 1994;86(18):1403–1408.
15. Carpenter CL, Ross RK, Paganini-Hill A, et al. Effect of family history, obesity and exercise on breast cancer risk among postmenopausal women. *Int J Cancer* 2003;106(1):96–102.
16. Iwasaki M, Tsugane S. Risk factors for breast cancer: epidemiological evidence from Japanese studies. *Cancer Sci* 2011;102(9):1607–1614.
17. Pronk A, Ji BT, Shu XO, et al. Physical activity and breast cancer risk in Chinese women. *Br J Cancer* 2011;105(9):1443–1450.
18. Sanchez-Zamorano LM, Flores-Luna L, Angeles-Llerenas A, et al. Healthy lifestyle on the risk of breast cancer. *Cancer Epidemiol Biomarkers Prev* 2011;20(5):912–922.
19. Awatef M, Olfa G, Rim C, et al. Physical activity reduces breast cancer risk: a case-control study in Tunisia. *Cancer Epidemiol* 2011;35(6):540–544.
20. Sheppard VB, Makambi K, Taylor T, et al. Physical activity reduces breast cancer risk in African American women. *Ethn Dis* 2011;21(4):406–411.
21. Suzuki R, Iwasaki M, Yamamoto S, et al. Leisure-time physical activity and breast cancer risk defined by estrogen and progesterone receptor status—the Japan Public Health Center-based Prospective Study. *Prev Med* 2011;52(3-4):227–233.
22. Phipps AI, Chlebowski RT, Prentice R, et al. Body size, physical activity, and risk of triple-negative and estrogen receptor-positive breast cancer. *Cancer Epidemiol Biomarkers Prev* 2011;20(3):454–463.
23. Dieli-Conwright CM, Sullivan-Halley J, Patel A, et al. Does hormone therapy counter the beneficial effects of physical activity on breast cancer risk in postmenopausal women? *Cancer Causes Control* 2011;22(3):515–522.
24. Hildebrand JS, Gapstur SM, Campbell PT, et al. Recreational physical activity and leisure-time sitting in relation to postmenopausal breast cancer risk. *Cancer Epidemiol Biomarkers Prev* 2013;22(10):1906–1912.
25. Jung MM, Colditz GA, Collins LC, et al. Lifetime physical activity and the incidence of proliferative benign breast disease. *Cancer Causes Control* 2011;22(9):1297–1305.
26. Boeing H. Obesity and cancer—the update 2013. *Best Pract Res Clin Endocrinol Metab* 2013;27(2):219–227.
27. Lahmann PH, Schulz M, Hoffmann K, et al. Long-term weight change and breast cancer risk: The European Prospective Investigation into Cancer and Nutrition (EPIC). *Br J Cancer* 2005;93(5):582–589.
28. Harris HR, Tamimi RM, Willett WC, et al. Body size across the life course, mammographic density, and risk of breast cancer. *Am J Epidemiol* 2011;174(8):909–918.
29. Goran MI. Energy metabolism and obesity. *Med Clin North Am* 2000;84(2):347–362.
30. Frisch R, McArthur J. Menstrual cycles: fatness as a determinant of minimum weight for height necessary for their maintenance or onset. *Science* 1974;185:949–951.
31. Bernstein L. Epidemiology of endocrine-related risk factors for breast cancer. *J Mammary Gland Biol Neoplasia* 2002;7(1):3–15.
32. Bernstein L, Ross RK, Lobo RA, et al. The effects of moderate physical activity on menstrual cycle patterns in adolescence: implications for breast cancer prevention. *Br J Cancer* 1987;55(6):681–685.
33. Anderson E, Clarke RB, Howell A. Estrogen responsiveness and control of normal human breast proliferation. *J Mammary Gland Biol Neoplasia* 1998;3(1):23–35.
34. Cauley JA, Gutai JP, Kuller LH, et al. The epidemiology of serum sex hormones in postmenopausal women. *Am J Epidemiol* 1989;129(6):1120–1131.
35. MacDonald PC, Edman CD, Hemsell DL, et al. Effect of obesity on conversion of plasma androstenedione to estrone in postmenopausal women with and without endometrial cancer. *Am J Obstet Gynecol* 1978;130(4):448–455.
36. Seewaldt FL, Goldenberg V, Jones LW, et al. Overweight and obese perimenopausal and postmenopausal women exhibit increased abnormal mammary epithelial cytology. *Cancer Epidemiol Biomarkers Prev* 2007;16:613–616.
37. Bernstein L. Exercise and breast cancer prevention. *Curr Oncol Reports* 2009;11(6):490–496.
38. Neilson HK, Friedenreich CM, Brockton NT, et al. Physical activity and postmenopausal breast cancer: proposed biologic mechanisms and areas for future research. *Cancer Epidemiol Biomarkers Prev* 2009;18(1):11–27.
39. Cleary MP, Grossmann ME. Obesity and breast cancer: the estrogen connection. *Endocrinol* 2009;150(6):2537–2542.
40. Brown KA, Simpson ER. Obesity and breast cancer: progress to understanding the relationship. *Cancer Res* 2010;70(1):4–7.
41. Friedenreich CM, Neilson HK, Lynch BM. State of the epidemiological evidence on physical activity and cancer prevention. *Eur J Cancer* 2010;46(14):2593–2604.
42. Mai PL, Sullivan-Halley J, Ursin G, et al. Physical activity and colon cancer risk among women in the California Teachers Study. *Cancer Epidemiol Biomarkers Prev* 2007;16(3):517–525.
43. Wolin KY, Yan Y, Colditz GA, et al. Physical activity and colon cancer prevention: a meta-analysis. *Br J Cancer* 2009;100(4):611–616.
44. Boyle T, Keegel T, Bull F, et al. Physical activity and risks of proximal and distal colon cancers: a systematic review and meta-analysis. *J Natl Cancer Inst* 2012;104(20):1548–1561.
45. Howard RA, Freedman DM, Park Y, et al. Physical activity, sedentary behavior, and the risk of colon and rectal cancer in the NIH-AARP Diet and Health Study. *Cancer Causes Control* 2008;19(9):939–953.
46. Boyle T, Heyworth J, Bull F, et al. Timing and intensity of recreational physical activity and the risk of subsite-specific colorectal cancer. *Cancer Causes Control* 2011;22(12):1647–1658.
47. Wolin KY, Yan Y, Colditz GA. Physical activity and risk of colon adenoma: a meta-analysis. *Br J Cancer* 2011;104(5):882–885.
48. Pischon T, Lahmann PH, Boeing H, et al. Body size and risk of colon and rectal cancer in the European Prospective Investigation Into Cancer and Nutrition (EPIC). *J Natl Cancer Inst* 2006;98(13):920–931.
49. Aleksandrova K, Pischon T, Buijsse B, et al. Adult weight change and risk of colorectal cancer in the European Prospective Investigation into Cancer and Nutrition. *Eur J Cancer* 2013;49(16):3526–3536.
50. Nimptsch K, Giovannucci E, Willett WC, et al. Body fatness during childhood and adolescence, adult height, and risk of colorectal adenoma in women. *Cancer Prev Res* 2011;4(10):1710–1718.

51. Hughes LA, Simons CC, van den Brandt PA, et al. Body size and colorectal cancer risk after 16.3 years of follow-up: an analysis from the Netherlands Cohort Study. *Am J Epidemiol* 2011;174(10):1127–1139.

52. Abate N. Insulin resistance and obesity. The role of fat distribution pattern. *Diabetes Care* 1996;19(3):292–294.

53. Calle EE, Kaaks R. Overweight, obesity and cancer: epidemiological evidence and proposed mechanisms. *Nat Rev Cancer* 2004;4(8):579–591.

54. Gierach GL, Chang SC, Brinton LA, et al. Physical activity, sedentary behavior, and endometrial cancer risk in the NIH-AARP Diet and Health Study. *Int J Cancer* 2009;124(9):2139–2147.

55. Voskuil DW, Monninkhof EM, Elias SG, et al. Physical activity and endometrial cancer risk, a systematic review of current evidence. *Cancer Epidemiol Biomarkers Prev* 2007;16(4):639–648.

56. Cust AE, Armstrong BK, Friedenreich CM, et al. Physical activity and endometrial cancer risk: a review of the current evidence, biologic mechanisms and the quality of physical activity assessment methods. *Cancer Causes Control* 2007;18(3):243–258.

57. Friedenreich C, Cust A, Lahmann PH, et al. Physical activity and risk of endometrial cancer: The European Prospective Investigation into Cancer and Nutrition. *Int J Cancer* 2007;121(2):347–355.

58. Patel AV, Feigelson HS, Talbot JT, et al. The role of body weight in the relationship between physical activity and endometrial cancer: results from a large cohort of US women. *Int J Cancer* 2008;123(8):1877–1882.

59. Moore SC, Gierach GL, Schatzkin A, et al. Physical activity, sedentary behaviours, and the prevention of endometrial cancer. *Br J Cancer* 2010;103(7):933–938.

60. Dieli-Conwright CM, Ma H, Lacey JV, Jr., et al. Long-term and baseline recreational physical activity and risk of endometrial cancer: The California Teachers Study. *Br J Cancer* 2013;109(3):761–768.

61. Kaaks R, Lukanova A, Kurzer MS. Obesity, endogenous hormones, and endometrial cancer risk: a synthetic review. *Cancer Epidemiol Biomarkers Prev* 2002;11(12):1531–1543.

62. Zhang ZF, Kurtz RC, Sun M, et al. Adenocarcinomas of the esophagus and gastric cardia: medical conditions, tobacco, alcohol, and socioeconomic factors. *Cancer Epidemiol Biomarkers Prev* 1996;5(10):761–768.

63. Lagergren J, Bergstrom R, Nyren O. Association between body mass and adenocarcinoma of the esophagus and gastric cardia. *Ann Intern Med* 1999;130(11):883–890.

64. Vigen C, Bernstein L, Wu AH. Occupational physical activity and risk of adenocarcinomas of the esophagus and stomach. *Int J Cancer* 2006;118(4):1004–1009.

65. Leitzmann MF, Koebnick S, Freedman ND, et al. Physical activity and esophageal and gastric carcinoma in a large prospective study. *Am J Prev Med* 2009;36(2):112–119.

66. Lepage C, Drouillard A, Jouve JL, et al. Epidemiology and risk factors for oesophageal adenocarcinoma. *Dig Liver Dis* 2013;45(8):625–629.

67. Ryan AM, Duong M, Healy L, et al. Obesity, metabolic syndrome and esophageal adenocarcinoma: epidemiology, etiology and new targets. *Cancer Epidemiol* 2011;35(4):309–319.

68. Hoyo C, Cook MB, Kamangar F, et al. Body mass index in relation to oesophageal and oesophagogastric junction adenocarcinomas: a pooled analysis from the International BEACON Consortium. *Int J Epidemiol* 2012;41(6):1706–1718.

69. Leitzmann MF. Physical activity and genitourinary cancer prevention. *Recent Results Cancer Res* 2011;186:43–71.

70. Purdue MP, Moore LE, Merino MJ, et al. An investigation of risk factors for renal cell carcinoma by histologic subtype in two case-control studies. *Int J Cancer* 2013;132(11):2640–2647.

71. O'Rorke MA, Cantwell MM, Cardwell CR, et al. Can physical activity modulate pancreatic cancer risk? A systematic review and meta-analysis. *Int J Cancer* 2010;126(12):2957–2968.

72. Aune D, Greenwood DC, Chan DS, et al. Body mass index, abdominal fatness and pancreatic cancer risk: a systematic review and non-linear dose-response meta-analysis of prospective studies. *Ann Oncol* 2012;23(4):843–852.

73. Bracci PM. Obesity and pancreatic cancer: overview of epidemiologic evidence and biologic mechanisms. *Mol Carcinog* 2012;51(1):53–63.

74. Arslan AA, Helzlsouer KJ, Kooperberg C, et al. Anthropometric measures, body mass index, and pancreatic cancer: a pooled analysis from the Pancreatic Cancer Cohort Consortium (PanScan). *Arch Intern Med* 2010;170(9):791–802.

75. Genkinger JM, Spiegelman D, Anderson KE, et al. A pooled analysis of 14 cohort studies of anthropometric factors and pancreatic cancer risk. *Int J Cancer* 2010;129(7):1708–1717.

76. Uhler ML, Marks JW, Judd HL. Estrogen replacement therapy and gallbladder disease in postmenopausal women. *Menopause* 2000;7(3):162–167.

77. Larsson SC, Wolk A. Obesity and the risk of gallbladder cancer: a meta-analysis. *Br J Cancer* 2007;96(9):1457–1461.

78. Hsing AW, Sakoda LC, Rashid A, et al. Body size and the risk of biliary tract cancer: a population-based study in China. *Br J Cancer* 2008;99(5):811–815.

79. Schlesinger S, Aleksandrova K, Pischon T, et al. Abdominal obesity, weight gain during adulthood and risk of liver and biliary tract cancer in a European cohort. *Int J Cancer* 2013;132(3):645–657.

80. Lu Y, Prescott J, Sullivan-Halley J, et al. Body size, recreational physical activity, and B-cell non-Hodgkin lymphoma risk among women in the California Teachers Study. *Am J Epidemiol* 2009;170(10):1231–1240.

81. Kabat GC, Kim MY, Jean Wactawski W, et al. Anthropometric factors, physical activity, and risk of non-Hodgkin's lymphoma in the Women's Health Initiative. *Cancer Epidemiol* 2012;36(1):52–59.

82. van Veldhoven CM, Khan AE, Teucher B, et al. Physical activity and lymphoid neoplasms in the European Prospective Investigation into Cancer and Nutrition (EPIC). *Eur J Cancer* 2011;47(5):748–760.

83. Teras LR, Gapstur SM, Diver WR, et al. Recreational physical activity, leisure sitting time and risk of non-Hodgkin lymphoid neoplasms in the American Cancer Society Cancer Prevention Study II Cohort. *Int J Cancer* 2012;131(8):1912–1920.

84. Willett EV, Morton LM, Hartge P, et al. Non-Hodgkin lymphoma and obesity: a pooled analysis from the InterLymph Consortium. *Int J Cancer* 2008;122(9):2062–2070.

85. Larsson SC, Wolk A. Body mass index and risk of non-Hodgkin's and Hodgkin's lymphoma: a meta-analysis of prospective studies. *Eur J Cancer* 2011;47(16):2422–2430.

86. Larsson SC, Wolk A. Obesity and risk of non-Hodgkin's lymphoma: a meta-analysis. *Int J Cancer* 2007;121(7):1564–1570.

87. Bertrand KA, Giovannucci E, Zhang SM, et al. A prospective analysis of body size during childhood, adolescence, and adulthood and risk of non-Hodgkin lymphoma. *Cancer Prev Res* 2013;6(8):864–873.

88. Friedenreich CM, Orenstein MR. Physical activity and cancer prevention: Etiologic evidence and biological mechanisms. *J Nutr* 2002;132(11 Suppl):3456S–3464S.

89. Friedenreich CM, McGregor SE, Courneya KS, et al. Case-control study of lifetime total physical activity and prostate cancer risk. *Am J Epidemiol* 2004;159(8):740–749.

90. Young-McCaughan S. Potential for prostate cancer prevention through physical activity. *World J Urol* 2012;30(2):167–179.

91. Leitzmann MF, Rohrmann S. Risk factors for the onset of prostatic cancer: age, location, and behavioral correlates. *Clin Epidemiol* 2012;4:1–11.

92. Liu Y, Hu F, Li D, et al. Does physical activity reduce the risk of prostate cancer? A systematic review and meta-analysis. *Eur Urol* 2011;60(5):1029–1044.

93. Discacciati A, Orsini N, Wolk A. Body mass index and incidence of localized and advanced prostate cancer—a dose-response meta-analysis of prospective studies. *Ann Oncol* 2012;23(7):1665–1671.

94. Rodriguez C, Freedland SJ, Deka A, et al. Body mass index, weight change, and risk of prostate cancer in the Cancer Prevention Study II Nutrition Cohort. *Cancer Epidemiol Biomarkers Prev* 2007;16(1):63–69.

95. Schmidt A, Jung J, Ernstmann N, et al. The association between active participation in a sports club, physical activity and social network on the development of lung cancer in smokers: A case-control study. *BMC Res Notes* 2012;5:2.

96. Lam TK, Moore SC, Brinton LA, et al. Anthropometric measures and physical activity and the risk of lung cancer in never-smokers: a prospective cohort study. *PLoS One* 2013;8(8):e70672.

97. Tardon A, Lee WJ, Delgado-Rodriguez M, et al. Leisure-time physical activity and lung cancer: a meta-analysis. *Cancer Causes Control* 2005;16(4):389–397.

98. Lin Y, Cai L. Environmental and dietary factors and lung cancer risk among Chinese women: a case-control study in Southeast China. *Nutr Cancer* 2012;64(4):508–514.

99. Bethea TN, Rosenberg L, Charlot M, et al. Obesity in relation to lung cancer incidence in African American women. *Cancer Causes Control* 2013;24(9):1695–1703.

100. Smith L, Brinton LA, Spitz MR, et al. Body mass index and risk of lung cancer among never, former, and current smokers. *J Natl Cancer Inst* 2012;104(10):778–789.

101. Andreotti G, Hou L, Beane Freeman LE, et al. Body mass index, agricultural pesticide use, and cancer incidence in the Agricultural Health Study cohort. *Cancer Causes Control* 2010;21(11):1759–1775.

102. Tarnaud C, Guida F, Papadopoulos A, et al. Body mass index and lung cancer risk: results from the ICARE Study, a large, population-based case-control study. *Cancer Causes Control* 2012;23(7):1113–1126.

103. Yang Y, Dong J, Sun K, et al. Obesity and incidence of lung cancer: a meta-analysis. *Int J Cancer* 2013;132(5):1162–1169.

104. El-Zein M, Parent ME, Rousseau MC. Comments on a recent meta-analysis: obesity and lung cancer. *Int J Cancer* 2012;132(8):1962–1963.

105. Olsen CM, Bain CJ, Jordan SJ, et al. Recreational physical activity and epithelial ovarian cancer. A case-control study, systematic review, and meta-analysis. *Cancer Epidemiol Biomarkers Prev* 2007;16(11):2321–2330.

106. Weiderpass E, Margolis KL, Sandin S, et al. Prospective study of physical activity in different periods of life and the risk of ovarian cancer. *Int J Cancer* 2006;118(12):3153–3160.

107. Lahmann PH, Friedenreich C, Schulz M, et al. Physical activity and ovarian cancer risk: The European Prospective Investigation into Cancer and Nutrition. *Cancer Epidemiol Biomarkers Prev* 2009;18(1):351–354.

108. Leitzmann MF, Koebnick C, Moore SC, et al. Prospective study of physical activity and risk of ovarian cancer. *Cancer Causes Control* 2009;20(5):765–773.

109. Xiao Q, Yang HP, Wentzensen N, et al. Physical activity in different periods of life, sedentary behavior, and the risk of ovarian cancer in the NIH-AARP Diet and Health Study. *Cancer Epidemiol Biomarkers Prev* 2013;22(11):2000–2008.

110. Moorman PG, Jones LW, Akushevich L, et al. Recreational physical activity and ovarian cancer risk and survival. *Ann Epidemiol* 2011;21(3):178–187.

111. Olsen CM, Green AC, Whiteman DC, et al. Obesity and the risk of epithelial ovarian cancer: a systematic review and meta-analysis. *Eur J Cancer* 2007;43(4):690–709.

112. Olsen CM, Nagle CM, Whiteman DC, et al. Obesity and risk of ovarian cancer subtypes: evidence from the Ovarian Cancer Association Consortium. *Endocr Relat Cancer* 2013;20(2):251–262.

113. Schouten LJ, Rivera C, Hunter DJ, et al. Height, body mass index, and ovarian cancer: a pooled analysis of 12 cohort studies. *Cancer Epidemiol Biomarkers Prev* 2008;17(4):902–912.

114. Collaborative Group on Epidemiological Studies of Ovarian Cancer. Ovarian cancer and body size: individual participant meta-analysis including 25,157 women with ovarian cancer from 47 epidemiological studies. *PLoS Med* 2012;9(4):e1001200.

**ETIOLOGY AND EPIDEMIOLOGY OF CANCER**

# 11 Epidemiologic Methods

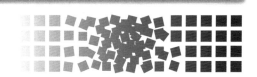

Xiaomei Ma and Herbert Yu

## INTRODUCTION

Epidemiology is the study of the distribution and determinants of health-related states or events in specified populations and the application of this study to control health problems.[1] Epidemiologic principles and methods have long been applied to cancer research, with the assumptions that cancer does not occur at random and the nonrandomness of carcinogenesis can be elucidated through systematic research. An example of such applications is the lung cancer study conducted by Doll and Hill in the early 1950s, which linked tobacco smoking to an increased mortality of lung cancer in over 40,000 medical professionals in the United Kingdom.[2] The observation from this study and many other studies, in conjunction with laboratory findings regarding the underlying biologic mechanisms for the effect of tobacco smoking, helped establish the role of tobacco smoking in the etiology of lung cancer. Epidemiologic methods are also used in clinical settings, where trials are conducted to evaluate the efficacy of new treatment protocols or preventive measures and where observational studies of prognostic factors are done.

Epidemiologic studies can take different forms, but generally they can be classified into two broad categories, observational studies and experimental studies (Fig. 11.1). In experimental studies, an investigator allocates different study regimens to the subjects, usually with randomization (experimental studies without randomization are sometimes referred to as "quasi-experiments").[3] Experimental studies can be individual based or community based. An experimental study most closely resembles laboratory experiments in that the investigator has control over the study condition. Experimental studies can be used to evaluate the efficacy of a treatment protocol (e.g., low-dose compared with standard-dose chemotherapy for non-Hodgkin's lymphoma)[4] or preventive measures (e.g., tamoxifen for women at an increased risk of breast cancer).[5] Although experimental studies are often considered the "gold standard" because of well-controlled study situations, they are only suitable for the evaluation of effects that are beneficial or at least not harmful due to ethical concerns. Experimental studies are discussed in detail in other chapters of this book. This section will focus on observational studies.

Observational studies do not involve the artificial manipulation of study regimens. In an observational study, an investigator stands by to observe what happens or happened to the subjects, in terms of exposure and outcome. Observational studies can be further divided into descriptive and analytical studies (see Fig. 11.1). Descriptive studies focus on the *distribution* of diseases with respect to person, place, and time (i.e., who, where, and when), whereas analytical studies focus on the *determinants* of diseases. Descriptive studies are often used to *generate* hypotheses, whereas analytical studies are often used to *test* hypotheses. However, the two types of studies should not be considered mutually exclusive entities; rather, they are the opposite ends of a continuum. Descriptive studies are discussed in detail in other chapters of this book.

## ANALYTICAL STUDIES

### Ecologic Studies

As in experimental studies, the unit of analysis can be individuals or groups of people in observational studies. Studies that use groups of people as the unit of analysis are called ecologic studies, which are relatively easy to carry out when group level measures are available. However, a relationship observed between variables on a group level does not necessarily reflect the relationship that exists at an individual level. For example, the fraction of energy supply from animal products was found to be positively correlated with breast cancer mortality in a recent ecologic study, which used preexisting data on both dietary supply and breast cancer mortality rates from 35 countries.[6] Because the data were country based, no reliable inference can be made at an individual level. Within each country, it could be that the people who had a low fraction of energy supply from animal products were actually dying from breast cancer. Results from ecologic studies are useful for inference at an individual level only when the within-group variability of the exposure is low so that a group-level measure can reasonably reflect exposure at an individual level. Alternatively, if the implications for prevention or intervention are at a group level (e.g., taxation of cigarettes to reduce smoking), results from ecologic studies are very useful.

### Cross-Sectional Studies

There are three main types of analytical studies in which the unit of analysis is individuals: cross-sectional, cohort, and case-control studies. In a cross-sectional study, the information on various factors is collected from the study population at a given point in time. From a public health perspective, data collected in cross-sectional studies can be of great value in assessing the general health status of a population and allocating resources. For example, the National Health and Nutrition Examination Survey has provided valuable national estimates of health and nutritional status of the US civilian, noninstitutionalized population.[7] Findings from cross-sectional studies can also help generate hypotheses that may be tested later in other types of studies. However, it should be noted that cross-sectional studies have serious methodologic limitations if the research purpose is etiologic inference. Because exposures and disease status are evaluated simultaneously, it is usually not possible to know the temporality of events unless the exposure cannot change over time (e.g., blood type, skin color, race, country of birth). If one observes that more brain cancer patients are depressed than people without brain cancer in a cross-sectional study, the correlation does not necessarily mean that depression causes brain cancer. Depression may simply have resulted from the pathogenesis and diagnosis of brain cancer, or depression may

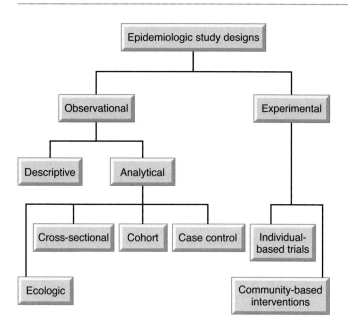

**Figure 11.1** Classification of epidemiologic study designs.

have caused brain cancer in some patients and resulted from brain cancer in other patients. Without additional information on the timing of events, no conclusions can be made. Another concern in cross-sectional studies is the enrollment of prevalent cases, who survived different lengths of time after the incidence of disease. Factors that affect survival may also influence incidence. Prevalent cases may not be representative of incident cases, which makes etiologic inferences based on cross-sectional studies suspect at best.

## Cohort Studies

In a cohort study, a study population free of a specific disease (or any other health-related condition) is grouped based on their exposure status and followed up for a certain period of time. Then the exposed and unexposed subjects are compared with respect to disease status at the end of the follow-up. The objective of a cohort study is usually to evaluate whether the incidence of a disease is associated with an exposure. The cohort design is fundamental in observational epidemiology and is considered "ideal" in that, if unbiased, cohort data reflect the real-life cause/effect sequence of disease.[8] Subjects in cohort studies may be a sample of the general population in a geographic area, a group of workers who are exposed to certain occupational hazards in a specific industry, or people who are considered at a high risk for a specific disease. A cohort study is considered prospective or concurrent if the investigator starts following up the cohort from the present time into the future, and retrospective or historical if the cohort is established in the past based on existing records (e.g., an occupational cohort based on employment records) and the follow-up ends before or at the time of the study. Alternatively, a cohort study can be ambidirectional in that data collection goes both directions.[9] Whether a cohort study is prospective, retrospective, or ambidirectional, the key feature is that all the subjects were free of the disease at the beginning of the follow-up and the study tracks the subjects from exposure to disease. Follow-up time, ranging from days to decades, is an essential element in cohort studies.

In a cohort study, the incidence of disease in the exposed group and the unexposed group is compared. The incidence measure can be cumulative incidence or incidence density, depending on the availability of data. When comparing the incidence in the two groups, both relative differences and absolute differences can be assessed. In cohort studies, the relative risk of developing

the disease is expressed as the ratio of the cumulative incidence in the exposed group to that in the unexposed group, which is also called cumulative incidence ratio or risk ratio. If we have data on the exact person-time of follow-up for every subject, we can also calculate an incidence density ratio (also called rate ratio) in a similar way. The numeric value of the risk or rate ratio reflects the magnitude of the association between an exposure and a disease. For example, a risk ratio of 2 would be interpreted as exposed individuals have a doubled risk of developing a disease than unexposed individuals, whereas a risk ratio of 5 indicates that exposed individuals have 5 times the risk of developing a disease compared with unexposed individuals. To put in another way, a factor with a risk ratio of 5 has a stronger effect than another factor with a risk ratio of 2. In addition to risk ratio and rate ratio, another relative measure called probability odds ratio can be calculated in cohort studies. The probability odds of disease is the number of subjects who developed a disease divided by the number of subjects who did not develop the disease, and the probability odds ratio is the probability odds in the exposed group divided by the probability odds in the unexposed group. Many investigators prefer risk ratio or rate ratio to probability odds ratio in cohort studies, because the ability to directly measure the risk of developing a disease is one of the most significant advantages in cohort studies. In practice, however, a probability odds ratio is often used as an approximation for risk or rate ratio, especially when multivariate logistic regression models are employed to adjust for the effect of other factors that may influence the relationship between an exposure and a disease.

As for absolute differences, a commonly used measure is called attributable risk in the exposed, which is the incidence in the exposed group minus the incidence in the unexposed group. Attributable risk reflects the disease incidence that could be attributed to the exposure in exposed individuals and the reduction in incidence that we would expect if the exposure can be removed from the exposed individuals, provided that there is a causal relationship between the exposure and the disease. Another absolute measure called population attributable risk extends this concept to the general population; it estimates the disease incidence that could be attributed to an exposure in the general population. Because both relative and absolute differences can be assessed in cohort studies, a natural question to ask is what measures to choose. In general, the relative differences are used more often if the main research objective is etiologic inference, and they can be used for the judgment of causality. Once causality is established, or at least assumed, measures of absolute differences are more important from a public health perspective. This point can be illustrated using the following hypothetical example. Assume the following: toxin X in the environment triples the risk of bladder cancer and toxin Y doubles the risk of bladder cancer, the effects of X and Y are entirely independent of each other, the prevalence of exposure to toxin Y in the general population is 20 times higher than the prevalence of exposure to toxin X, and there are only resources available to reduce the exposure to one toxin. It would be more effective to use the resources to reduce the exposure to toxin Y instead of toxin X. This is because the population attributable risk due to Y is higher than that due to X, although the risk ratio associated with toxin Y is smaller than that associated with toxin X.

Cohort studies have many advantages. A cohort design is the best way to study the natural history of a disease.[9] There is usually a clear temporal relationship between an exposure and a disease because all the subjects are free of the disease at the beginning of the follow-up (it can be a problem if a subject has a subclinical disease such as undetected prostate cancer). Furthermore, multiple diseases can be studied with respect to the same exposure. On the other hand, cohort studies, especially prospective cohort studies, are costly in terms of both time and money. A cohort design requires the follow-up of a large number of study participants over a sometimes extremely lengthy period of time and usually extensive data collection through questionnaires, physical measurements, and/or biologic specimens at regular intervals. Participants may be "lost" during the follow-up because they became tired of the study, moved away from the study area, or died from some causes other than the disease under study. If the subjects who were lost during the follow-up are different from those who remained under observation with respect to exposure, disease, or other factors that may influence the relationship between the exposure and the disease, results from the study may be biased. To date, cohort studies have been used to study the etiology of a wide spectrum of diseases, including different types of cancer. If a cohort study is conducted to evaluate the etiology of cancer, usually the study sample size would need to be very large (such as the National Institutes of Health-AARP Diet and Health Study, which included more than half million subjects[10]) and the follow-up time would need to be long, unless the cohort selected is a high-risk population.

For simplicity, we have discussed cohort studies in which the outcome of interest is the incidence of a specific disease and there are only two exposure groups. In practice, any health-related event can be the outcome of interest, and multiple exposure groups can be compared.

## Case-Control Studies

Case-control design is an alternative to cohort design for the evaluation of the relationship between an exposure and a disease (or any other health condition). A case-control approach compares the odds of past exposure between cases and noncases (controls) and uses the exposure odds ratio as an estimate for relative risk. A primary goal in a case-control study is to reach the same conclusions as what would have been obtained from a cohort study, if one had been done.[11] If appropriately designed and conducted, a case-control study can optimize speed and efficiency as the need for follow-up is avoided.[8] The starting point of a case-control study is a source population from which the cases arise. Instead of obtaining the denominators for the calculation of risks or rates in a cohort study, a control group is sampled from the entire source population. After selecting control subjects, who ideally would have become cases had they developed the disease, an investigator collects data on past exposures from both the cases and the controls and then calculates an odds ratio, which is the odds of exposure in the cases divided by the odds of exposure in the controls.

There are two main types of case-control studies: case-based case-control studies and case-control studies within defined cohorts.[8] Some variations of the case-control design also exist. For instance, if the effect of an exposure is transient, sometimes a case can be used as his/her own control (case cross-over design). In case-based case-control studies, cases and controls are selected at a given point in time from a hypothetical cohort (e.g., at the end of follow-up). A cross-sectional ascertainment of cases will result in a case group that mostly contains prevalent cases who may have survived for different lengths of time after disease incidence. Cases who died before an investigator began subject ascertainment would not be eligible to be included in the study. As a result, the cases finally included in the study may not be representative of all the cases from the entire hypothetical cohort. Another disadvantage of enrolling prevalent cases is that cases that were diagnosed a long time ago will likely have difficulties recalling exposures that occurred before the disease incidence. In case-control studies, it is preferable to ascertain incident cases as soon as they are diagnosed and to select controls as soon as cases are identified. Case-control studies that enroll only incident cases are sometimes called *prospective* case-control studies because the investigators need to wait for the incident cases to develop and get diagnosed. For cancer studies, the cases can be ascertained from population-based cancer registries or hospitals. A major advantage of using a cancer registry is the completeness of case ascertainment; however, the reporting of cancer cases to registries is usually not instantaneous. There could be a lag time of several months or even over a year, and some cases could have died during the lag time. If the cancer

under study has a poor survival rate and/or clinical specimens need to be obtained in a timely manner, it may be preferable to identify cases directly from hospitals using a rapid ascertainment protocol. As for the selection of controls, the key issue is that controls should be representative of the source population from which the cases arise and, theoretically, the controls would have been ascertained as cases had they developed the disease. The most common types of controls include population-based controls (often selected through random digit dialing in case-control studies of cancer etiology), hospital controls, and friend controls. The advantages and disadvantages of different types of controls have been nicely summarized by Wacholder et al.[12] Because no follow-up is involved in case-based case-control studies, the incidence risk or rate cannot be calculated directly for case and control groups. The odds ratio will be a good estimate of relative risk if the disease is uncommon.

In addition to case-based case-control studies, there are also case-control studies within defined cohorts (also known as hybrid or ambidirectional designs), including case-cohort studies and nested case-control studies. In case-cohort studies, cases are identified from a well-defined cohort after some follow-up time, and controls are selected from the baseline cohort. In nested case-control studies, cases are also identified from a cohort, but controls are selected from the individuals at risk at the time each case occurs (i.e., incidence density sampling).[8] In these types of designs, controls are a sample of the cohort and the controls selected can theoretically become cases at some point. The possibility of selection bias in case-control studies within defined cohorts is lower than that in case-based case-control studies because the cases and the controls are selected from the same source population. Because of an increased awareness of the methodological issues inherent in the design of case-based case-control studies and the availability of a growing number of large cohorts, case-control studies within defined cohorts have become more common in recent years. The advantage of case-control studies within cohorts over traditional cohort studies is mainly the efficiency in additional data collection. For instance, a recent nested case-control study evaluated the relationship between endogenous sex hormones and prostate cancer risk.[13] Instead of measuring the serum hormones levels of the entire cohort (over 12,000 subjects), investigators chose to measure 300 cases and 300 controls selected from the cohort. Doing so not only significantly reduced the cost of measurements and the time it took to address the research question, but also helped preserve valuable serum samples for possible analyses in the future. In a case-cohort design, an odds ratio estimates risk ratio; in a nested case-control design, an odds ratio estimates rate ratio. In both designs, the disease under study does not have to be rare for the odds ratio to be a good estimate of the risk ratio or rate ratio.[8,14]

The biggest advantage of a case-control design is the speed and efficiency of obtaining data. It is claimed that investigators implement case-control studies more frequently than any other analytical epidemiologic study.[15] Because most types of cancer are uncommon and take a long time to develop, to date, most epidemiologic studies of cancer have been case-control instead of cohort in design. A case-control study can be conducted to evaluate the relationship between many different exposures and a specific disease, but the study will have limited statistical power if the exposure is rare. In general, a case-control design tends to be more susceptible to biases than a cohort design. Such biases include, but are not limited to, selection bias when choosing and enrolling subjects (especially controls) and recall bias when obtaining data from the subjects. The status of the subjects—that is, case or control—may affect how they recall and report previous exposures, some of which occurred years or even decades ago. It is important for investigators to explicitly define the diagnostic and eligibility criteria for cases, to select controls from the same population as the cases independent of the exposures of interest, to blind data collection staff to the case or control status of subjects and/or the main hypotheses of the study, to ascertain exposure in a similar manner from cases and controls, and to take into account other factors that may influence the relationship between an exposure and a disease.[15]

## INTERPRETATION OF EPIDEMIOLOGIC FINDINGS

We have discussed measures of effects in various study designs. However, a risk ratio of 3 from a cohort study or an odds ratio of 2.5 from a case-control study does not necessarily mean that there is an association between an exposure and a disease. Several alternative explanations need to be assessed, including chance (random error), bias (systematic error), and confounding. Potential interaction also needs be evaluated.

Statistical methods are required to evaluate the role of chance. A usual way is to calculate the upper and lower limits of a 95% confidence interval around a point estimate for relative risk (risk ratio, rate ratio, or odds ratio). If the confidence interval does not include one, one would say that the observed association is statistically significant; if the confidence interval includes one, one would say that the observed relationship is not statistically significant. The width of a confidence interval is directly related to the number of participants in a study, which is called sample size. A larger sample size leads to less variability in the data, a tighter confidence interval, and a higher possibility in finding a statistically significant association if one truly exists. A 95% confidence interval means that if the data collection and analysis could be replicated many times, the confidence interval should include the correct value of the measure 95% of the time.[16] It is better to consider a confidence interval to be a general guide to the amount of random error in the data but not necessarily a literal measure of statistical variability.[16]

Bias can be defined as any systematic error in an epidemiologic study that results in an incorrect estimate of the association between exposure and disease, and it can occur in every type of epidemiologic study design. There are two main types of bias: selection bias and information bias. Selection bias is present when individuals included in a study are systematically different from the target population. For example, a selection bias would occur if a study aimed to generate a sample representing all women in the United States, but of the women contacted, more with a family history of breast cancer agreed to participate. This sample would be at a higher risk for breast cancer than the target population. Refusal to participate poses a constant challenge in epidemiologic studies. As individuals have become more concerned about privacy issues and as studies have become more demanding of time, biologic specimens, and other impositions, participation rates have dropped substantially in recent years. If nonparticipants are different from the participants with respect to study-related characteristics, the validity of the study is threatened. Information bias occurs when the data collected from the study subjects are erroneous. Information bias is also known as misclassification if the variable is measured on a categorical scale and the error causes a subject to be placed in a wrong category. Misclassification can happen to both exposure and disease. For example, in a case-control study of previous reproductive history and ovarian cancer, a woman who had an extremely early pregnancy loss might not even realize that she was ever pregnant and would mistakenly report no pregnancy, and another woman who has only subclinical presentations of ovarian cancer might be mistakenly selected as a control. Misclassification can be differential or nondifferential. An exposure misclassification is considered differential if it is related to disease status and nondifferential if not related to disease status. Similarly, a disease misclassification is considered differential if it is related to exposure status and nondifferential if not related to exposure status. If a binary exposure variable and a binary disease variable are analyzed, a nondifferential misclassification will result in an underestimate of the true association. Differential misclassification can either exaggerate or underestimate a true effect. Usually not much can be done to control or correct bias at the data analysis stage; therefore,

it is important to establish research protocols that are not prone to bias. The evaluation of potential bias is critical to the interpretation of study results. An invalid estimate is worse than no estimate.

Confounding refers to a situation in which the association between an exposure and a disease (or any health-related condition) is influenced by a third variable. This third variable is considered a confounding variable or confounder. A confounder must fulfill three criteria: (1) be associated with the exposure, (2) be associated with the disease independent of the exposure, and (3) not be an intermediate step between the exposure and the disease (i.e., not on the causal pathway). Unlike bias, which is primarily introduced by the investigator or study participants, confounding is a function of the complex interrelationship between various exposures and disease.[17] In a hypothetical case-control study of the effect of alcohol drinking on lung cancer, we may observe an odds ratio of 2.5 (usually called a "crude" odds ratio in the sense that no other variables were taken into account), which indicates that alcohol drinking increases the risk of lung cancer by 1.5-fold. However, if we classify all study subjects into two strata based on a history of cigarette smoking and then calculate the odds ratio in the two strata (smokers and nonsmokers) separately, we may have two stratum-specific odds ratios both equal to one, indicating that alcohol drinking is not associated with lung cancer risk. In this example, the crude odds ratio calculated to estimate the association between alcohol drinking and lung cancer without considering smoking is simply misleading. Being associated with both the exposure (i.e., alcohol drinking) and the disease (i.e., lung cancer), smoking acted as a confounder in this example. A stratified analysis is needed to evaluate the potential confounding effect of a third variable, whether it is done with pencil and paper or statistical modeling. Usually data are stratified based on the level of a third variable. If the stratum-specific effect measures are similar to each other but different from the crude effect measure, confounding is said to be present. In this section, we have illustrated basic epidemiologic principles using an overly simplified scenario and only considered a single exposure. In practice, most if not all diseases, cancer included, have a multifactorial etiology. Consequently, it is usually necessary to assess the potential confounding effect of a group of variables simultaneously using multivariate statistical models. The effect measure derived from a multivariate model will then be called an "adjusted" one in the sense that the effect of other factors was also adjusted for. Without controlling for the potential effect of other variables, an investigator cannot really judge whether an observed association between a given exposure and a specific disease is spurious.

If the effect of an exposure on the risk of a disease is not homogeneous in strata formed by a third variable, the third variable is considered an effect modifier, and the situation is called interaction or effect modification. Put in other words, interaction exists when the stratum-specific effect measures are different from each other. In the lung cancer example given previously, if the odds ratio for alcohol drinking is 1 in smokers but 3 in nonsmokers, then there is interaction and smoking is an effect modifier. The evaluation of interaction is essentially a stratified analysis, which is similar to the evaluation of confounding. Confounding and interaction can be both present in a given study. However, when interaction occurs, the stratum-specific effect measures should be reported. It is no longer appropriate to report a summary measure in the presence of interaction. Unlike confounding, which is a nuisance that an investigator hopes to remove, interaction is a more detailed description of the true relationship between an exposure and a disease.

## CANCER OUTCOMES RESEARCH

The discussion of epidemiologic methods in this section focuses primarily on etiological research, which aims at identifying the risk factors of cancer. However, similar principles and methods are applicable to cancer outcomes research, which aims at studying a variety of factors related to the early identification, treatment, prognosis, health related quality of life, and cost of care. Cancer outcomes research can be experimental or observational in nature. For example, randomized clinical trials have been conducted to assess the impact of screening on prostate cancer mortality[18] and to compare the effect of radical prostatectomy versus observation in patients with localized prostate cancer.[19] Observational studies of cancer outcomes, especially those that build upon preexisting resources,[20,21] can be carried out in a large group of patients with relatively little cost to capture the patterns and cost of care and to address many other research questions that have important clinical implications. Although the findings of such observation studies are subject to bias and confounding inherent in an observational design, these studies are complementary to experimental studies and have their unique value. Given an increasing interest in improving the effectiveness and value of cancer care, more cancer outcomes research is to be expected in the future.

## MOLECULAR EPIDEMIOLOGY

Molecular epidemiology involves multidisciplinary and transdisciplinary research that entails not only traditional epidemiology and biostatistics, but also genetics, molecular biology, biochemistry, cellular biology, analytical chemistry, toxicology, pharmacology, and laboratory medicine. Unlike traditional epidemiology research of cancer, which focuses on exposures or risk factors ascertained through questionnaire-based interviews or surveys, molecular epidemiology studies expand the assessment of exposure to a much broader scope that includes an analysis of biomarkers underlying internal exposure of exogenous and endogenous carcinogenic agents or risk factors, molecular alterations in response to exposure, and genetic susceptibility to cancer. The biomarkers often measured in molecular epidemiology research include DNA, RNA, proteins, chromosomes, compound molecules (e.g., DNA and protein adducts), and various metabolites as well as other endogenous and exogenous substances (e.g., steroids, nutrients, chemical or biologic toxins, and phytochemicals). Molecular markers can reflect different aspects of the tumorigenic process, which include biomarkers of internal exposure, biomarkers of molecular or cellular changes in response to exposure, and biomarkers of precursor lesions or early diseases.[22,23] Depending on the source of molecules and location of diseases, surrogates are often used in epidemiologic studies. When using a surrogate marker or tissue, the relevance of a proxy to its underlying target needs to be established or justified.[23] This justification is especially important when conducting population-based epidemiologic studies that focus on organ-specific cancers, because assessing biomarkers in target tissue is difficult for controls; molecular markers from blood samples are often used as substitutes. If a biomarker in the blood does not travel to or act on the tissue or organ of interest, an association between the circulating marker and the cancer may not be relevant. Thus, establishing a close link between a surrogate and its target is crucial in molecular epidemiology research.

Gene-environment interaction plays an essential role in cancer development.[24] Common genetic variations are considered an important determinant of host susceptibility and are a major focus of molecular epidemiology research. Depending on the biologic mechanism involved, genetic variations can influence every aspect of the carcinogenic process, ranging from external and internal exposure to carcinogens or risk factors to molecular and cellular damage, alteration, and response.[22,23] Currently, single nucleotide polymorphisms (SNPs) are the most studied genetic variations. It is believed that even if SNPs confer a small risk, they may still be important at the population level because these variations are common in the general population. It is also important that the impacts of SNPs on cancer are considered under the context of gene–gene and gene–environment interactions. As genotyping technology has advanced substantially with respect to its analytic

quality, capacity, and cost, research of genetic polymorphisms has evolved rapidly from investigations of a single SNP to studies of haplotypes and tag SNPs, and from a pathway-based candidate gene approach to genome-wide association studies (GWAS).[25] A GWAS analyzes hundreds of thousands of SNPs simultaneously for hundreds or even thousands of study subjects. When these data are further combined with questionnaire information such as environmental exposures, lifestyle factors, dietary habits, and medical history, enormous information is generated, which requires a huge sample size to allow for a reliable and complete assessment of these variables individually and jointly. A single epidemiologic study can no longer provide sufficient power for this type of investigation. Multicenter investigations or study consortia that pool study information and specimens together are developed to address the sample size issue.[26] False-positive findings resulting from multiple comparisons constitute a major challenge in epidemiologic studies of genetic associations with cancer.[27] A meta-analysis or pooled analysis can be used to address this problem if sufficient studies are already published and available for evaluation. To address this issue at the time of study design, one may adopt a two- or multiphase study design in which study subjects are divided into two or multiple groups for genotyping and data analysis. Selected or genomewide SNPs are first screened in one group of the study subjects (discovery phase), and then the significant findings determined by stringent statistical criteria (usually p values less than $1 \times 10^{-5}$ or $1 \times 10^{-7}$) are reanalyzed in one or several other groups of subjects for verification (validation phase). This study design also lowers the cost of genotyping. False-positive findings can also be addressed with various statistical methods, such as bootstrap, permutation test, estimate of false positive report probability, prediction of false discovery rate, and the use of a much more stringent p value to accommodate multiple comparisons. For epidemiologic studies that are not population based or not conducted strictly following epidemiology principles, population stratification is a potential source of bias that may distort genetic associations.[28]

A large number of GWAS have been completed in search for SNPs that influence host susceptibility to cancer. Considering that more than 5 million SNPs are present in the human genome, the numbers of SNPs that are found to be associated with cancer risk after rigorous validation are much fewer than what one would have anticipated. In addition, the risk associations detected are quite weak, with most of the odds ratios ranging from 1.1 to 1.5, and the functional relevance or biologic implications are unclear for most of the SNPs. Furthermore, not many SNPs associated with cancer risk are located in protein-coding regions, and even fewer are in the loci of candidate genes suspected to be involved in tumorigenesis, such as oncogenes, tumor suppressor genes, DNA repair genes, and xenobiotic metabolizing or detoxification genes. Genes where SNPs are found to be linked to cancer by GWAS include *FGFR2, MAP3K1, MRPS30, LSP1, TNRC9, TOX3, STXBP1,* and *RAD51L1* for breast cancer[29–31]; *JAZF1, HNF1B, MSMB, CTBP2,* and *KLK2/KLK3* for prostate cancer[29,32]; *SMAD7, CRAC1, EIF3H, BMP4, CDH1,* and *RHPN2* for colorectal cancer[29,33]; *CHRNA3* and *CHRNA5* for lung cancer[34,35]; *ABO* for pancreatic cancer[36]; *TACC3* and *PSCA* for bladder cancer[37,38]; and *KRT5* for basal cell carcinoma.[39] Among these genes identified by GWAS, two findings are considered especially interesting. One is the association of lung cancer with *CHRNA3* and *CHRNA5*, which encode neuronal nicotinic acetylcholine receptor subunits. Different genotypes of these receptor subunits appear to influence individual's addiction to tobacco, which further leads to different smoking exposure and lung cancer risk.[40,41] Another is the link of the *ABO* gene to pancreatic cancer. The association between pancreatic cancer risk and ABO blood type was observed 50 years ago. The GWAS finding not only confirms the relationship, but also provides new clues for understanding the underlying biologic mechanism.

Besides intragenic SNPs, GWAS also found many intergenic SNPs in association to cancer risk, which include those in the regions of 8q24, 5p15, 1p11, 1p36, 1q42, 2p15, 2q35, 3p12, 3p24,

3q28, 6p21, 6q25, 7q21, 7q32, 9p21, 9p22, 9p24, 9q22, 10p14, 11q13, 11q23, 14q13, 18q23, and 20p12.[29–31,33,39,42–48] Of these loci, SNPs in 8q24 are associated with several cancer sites, including prostate, breast, colon, and bladder.[29,31–33,47–49] Further analysis of 8q24 indicates that there are nine SNPs in five regions and each region is independently related to different types of cancer, with SNPs in regions 1, 4, and 5 associated exclusively with prostate cancer, a SNP in region 2 related to breast cancer, and SNPs in region 3 linked to prostate, colon, and ovarian cancers.[50] No known genes are located within the region of 8q24, but an oncogene c-MYC resides about 330 kb downstream of the region.[51] An initial investigation found no evidence of the SNPs' influence on c-MYC expression,[47] but a later study suggests that the SNPs in 8q24 may be distal enhancers of c-MYC, interacting with its promoter through a chromatin loop.[52] Another genomic region that is associated with the risk of multiple cancer sites is 5p15, a region involving telomerase reverse transcriptase (TERT) cleft lip and palate transmembrane protein 1–like protein (CLPTM1L). Five types of cancer are found to be linked to this region, including basal cell carcinoma, lung, bladder, prostate, and cervical cancers.[53] TERT extends the length of telomere and is associated with cell proliferation and abnormal telomere maintenance.[54] The risk alleles of TERT are associated with shorter telomere length among the elderly and with higher DNA adduct in the lungs.[53,55]

GWAS has demonstrated its value in identifying disease-related SNPs in unknown regions of the genome, which provides new clues for investigators to interrogate and understand different regions of the human genome, especially in the gene-desert areas. Despite the strength, the low yield of significant findings from the GWAS has raised concerns in several areas, including the SNP coverage in the genome (rare SNPs and SNP representativeness in unknown regions), associations with low statistical significance (p value between 0.01 and $1 \times 10^{-5}$, the GWAS cutoff), other forms of genetic variations (copy number variation and other structural variations), cancer subtypes, and genetic interplay with environmental factors (gene–environment interaction).[56,57] To address these issues, investigators propose to perform fine-mapping and resequencing to examine genetic regions more specifically and meticulously. Epidemiologists suggest that detailed environmental exposure and lifestyle factors should be included in the next wave of GWAS. Furthermore, to make the study more reliable and compelling, DNA specimens, instead of convenient samples, should come from well-designed and well-executed epidemiologic studies that pay close attention to the selection of study subjects and the measurement of environmental and lifestyle factors to eliminate or minimize selection bias and measurement errors.

As described earlier, analytical epidemiology has two major study designs: the case-control study and the cohort study. It is important that investigators choose an appropriate study design to investigate molecular markers in epidemiologic studies. Two types of molecular markers, genotypic and phenotypic markers, can be considered. Genotypic markers refer to nucleotide sequences of genomic DNA, and all other molecules are considered phenotypic markers, including most of the chemical modifications on DNA, such as cytosine methylation. The distinction between the two is a marker's status in relation to an outcome variable, usually a disease. Genotypic markers generally do not change over time and are not affected by the development of a disease, whereas phenotypic markers are likely to change over time or be influenced by the presence of a disease, either itself or the treatment associated with it. If measurements of a phenotypic marker are made from the specimens that are collected after or at the time of cancer diagnosis, investigators will have difficulties determining the status of the phenotypic marker before the cancer was diagnosed. A disease condition, however, does not affect genotypic markers such as SNPs; therefore, a temporal relationship can be easily established even if the samples are collected after the disease is diagnosed. Based on this distinction, one can evaluate genotypic markers either in case-control or cohort studies, but a case-control study would be

the design of choice because of efficiency and cost-effectiveness. A prospective cohort study design is ideal for phenotypic markers. Investigators, however, may use other study designs if they can demonstrate that the disease status does not influence the phenotypic markers of interest. To reduce study cost, investigators usually use nested case-control or case-cohort designs to avoid analyzing specimens from the entire cohort. The main purpose in choosing a cohort study design for a molecular epidemiology investigation is to ensure that biospecimens are collected before the development of a disease so that a temporal relationship between a marker and disease development can be established.

The differences between molecular epidemiology and genetic epidemiology are the scope of the molecular analysis and the emphasis on heredity. Sometimes molecular and genetic epidemiology both investigate genetic factors in association with cancer risk, but each has its own emphasis. The former assesses genetic involvement, but not necessarily inheritance, whereas the latter focuses mainly on heredity. Because of the difference in focus, study populations are different between the two types of investigation. Molecular epidemiology studies unrelated individuals, whereas genetic epidemiology investigates family members in the format of pedigrees, parent–child trios, or sibling pairs. Given the different research focus between genetic and molecular epidemiology, these investigations evaluate different genetic markers. Genetic epidemiology research is designed to identify genetic markers with high penetrance (strong association with an underlying disease) but low prevalence in the general populations, whereas a molecular epidemiology investigation targets low penetrance markers that are commonly present in the general population. Given the difference in study design, the analysis of genetic marker's link to cancer is also different between the studies. Relative risks or odds ratios are calculated in molecular epidemiology studies because study participants are unrelated individuals, whereas linkage analysis is used in genetic epidemiology because individuals in the study are genetically related family members. Recently, both genetic and molecular epidemiology study designs have been considered in GWAS to improve study validity and to minimize false positive findings. Another difference between genetic and molecular epidemiology research is that molecular epidemiology also studies nongenetic molecules. Thus, the scope of molecular analysis is much broader in molecular epidemiology research than in genetic epidemiology studies.

A laboratory analysis of molecular markers is another integral part of molecular epidemiology research, which has unique features that are different from basic science research. Collecting biologic specimens is difficult and expensive in population-based epidemiologic studies. It not only increases the study cost, but also imposes constraints to multiple areas of epidemiology research. Specimen collection may adversely influence the response rate of study participants, potentially compromising study validity. For organ-specific cancer research, investigating molecular markers in target tissue is difficult. Blood is the most common and versatile specimen used in molecular epidemiology research; other specimens used include urine, stool, nail, hair, sputum, buccal cells, and saliva. Tissue samples, either fresh frozen or chemically fixed, are also used, but the availability of these samples is highly limited to patients or selected subgroups of a general study population. Comparability and generalizability are always problems in epidemiologic studies involving tissue specimens, except for those investigations that focus on cancer prognosis or treatment in which only cancer patients are involved. Attempts have been made to use special body fluids for epidemiologic research, such as nipple aspirate and breast or pulmonary lavage, but the difficulty in specimen collection and preparation makes these samples impractical in large population-based studies.

Given the research value of biologic specimens and the difficulty in collecting them for population-based studies, technical issues related to specimen collection, processing, and storage become especially important in molecular epidemiology research.

These include time and conditions for specimen transportation and processing, a sample aliquot and labeling system, a sample special treatment for storage and analysis, a sample storage and tracking system, as well as backup plans and equipment for unexpected adverse events during long-term storage (e.g., power failure, earthquake, flooding). Laboratory methods used to analyze biomarkers are also important in molecular epidemiology. Because large numbers of specimens are involved, laboratory methods are required to be robust, reproducible, high throughput, low cost, and easy to use. These requirements are often met in the analysis of nucleotide sequences that serve as genotypic markers. However, for phenotypic markers, many methods do not readily meet these requirements. Moreover, many phenotypic markers, such as proteins, require both qualitative and quantitative assessments. An ideal laboratory method should be quantitative (able to measure a wide range of values), sensitive (able to detect a small amount of analyte), specific (able to detect only the molecule of interest, no other molecules), reproducible (high precision and low variation), and versatile (easy to use). In addition, investigators need to implement appropriate quality assurance procedures during sample processing and testing as well as include appropriate quality control samples in specimen analysis.

Host–environment interaction is believed to play a key role in the etiology of most types of cancer. Genetic factors, including mutations and polymorphisms, are initially considered important host factors, but recent developments in cancer research has indicated that epigenetic factors may also play a critical role in cancer as a host factor involved in host–environment interaction. Epigenetic factors, which regulate the function of human genome without altering the physical sequences of nucleotides, include pretranscription regulation through nucleotide modification (e.g., cytosine methylation at CpG sites), chromosome modification (e.g., histone acetylation), and posttranscription regulation by noncoding small RNA (e.g., microRNAs). These epigenetic factors have two unique features that have captured the attention of cancer researchers, especially cancer epidemiologists who are interested in the gene–environment interaction. It is known that epigenetic factors are heritable, but these inherited features are readily modifiable by environmental and lifestyle factors. Monozygotic twins have an identical genome as well as epigenome at birth, but the latter undergoes substantial changes over time, resulting in distinct epigenetic profiles that depend heavily on their environmental exposures.[58] Animal studies also indicated that the maternal intake of dietary nutrients involving one-carbon metabolism could influence offsprings' growth phenotypes, which are regulated by DNA methylation.[59] As evidence mounts on epigenetic involvement in cancer, molecular epidemiologists will start to look for clues in human populations that can link epigenetic factors to both lifestyle factors and cancer risk. Given that epigenetic regulation is tissue specific and time dependent, investigators face challenges in accurately assessing these phenotypic markers in etiologic studies. However, progress in the analysis of circulating methylation markers and microRNAs may provide an alternative to study epigenetic regulation in human cancer. Furthermore, methods for a genome-wide analysis of DNA methylation have been developed and applied in epidemiologic studies, which can substantially accelerate the search for cancer-related DNA methylation. Together with the high-throughput, high-dimensional analysis of DNA methylation, two other evolving fields that will have significant impacts on molecular epidemiology of cancer research are metagenomics and metabolomics. The former focuses on environmental genomics of the microbiome that resides in our body and influences one's biologic functions and health status. The latter refers to the analysis of hundreds or thousands of metabolites in a biologic specimen, including tissue, blood, urine, body fluids, and fecal samples. These new analyses will add tremendous value to epidemiologic studies.

# REFERENCES

1. Last J. A *Dictionary of Epidemiology*. 3rd ed. New York: Oxford University Press; 1995.
2. Doll R, Hill AB. Lung cancer and other causes of death in relation to smoking: a second report on the mortality of British doctors. *Br Med J* 1956;12:1071–1081.
3. Kleinbaum D, Kupper L, Morgenstern H. *Epidemiologic Research*. New York: Van Nostrand Reinhold; 1982.
4. Kaplan LD, Straus DJ, Testa MA, et al. Low-dose compared with standard-dose m-BACOD chemotherapy for non-Hodgkin's lymphoma associated with human immunodeficiency virus infection. National Institute of Allergy and Infectious Diseases AIDS Clinical Trials Group. *N Engl J Med* 1997;336:1641–1648.
5. Dunn BK, Kramer BS, Ford LG. Phase III, large-scale chemoprevention trials. Approach to chemoprevention clinical trials and phase III clinical trial of tamoxifen as a chemopreventive for breast cancer—the US National Cancer Institute experience. *Hematol Oncol Clin North Am* 1998;12:1019–1036, vii.
6. Grant WB. An ecologic study of dietary and solar ultraviolet-B links to breast carcinoma mortality rates. *Cancer* 2002;94:272–281.
7. National Center for Health Statistics. Third National Health and Nutrition Examination Survey, 1988–1994, Plan and Operations Procedures Manuals (CD-ROM). Hyattsville, MD: U.S. Department of Health and Human Services (DHHS), Centers for Disease Control and Prevention; 1996.
8. Szklo M, Nieto F. *Epidemiology: Beyond the Basics*. Gaithersburg, MD: Aspen Publishers; 2000.
9. Grimes DA, Schulz KF. Cohort studies: marching towards outcomes. *Lancet* 2002;359:341–345.
10. Schatzkin A, Subar AF, Thompson FE, et al. Design and serendipity in establishing a large cohort with wide dietary intake distributions: the National Institutes of Health-American Association of Retired Persons Diet and Health Study. *Am J Epidemiol* 2001;154:1119–1125.
11. Mantel N, Haenszel W. Statistical aspects of the analysis of data from retrospective studies of disease. *J Natl Cancer Inst* 1959;22:719–748.
12. Wacholder S, Silverman DT, McLaughlin JK, et al. Selection of controls in case-control studies. II. Types of controls. *Am J Epidemiol* 1992;135:1029–1041.
13. Chen C, Weiss NS, Stanczyk FZ, et al. Endogenous sex hormones and prostate cancer risk: a case-control study nested within the Carotene and Retinol Efficacy Trial. *Cancer Epidemiol Biomarkers Prev* 2003;12:1410–1416.
14. Pearce N. What does the odds ratio estimate in a case-control study? *Int J Epidemiol* 1993;22:1189–1192.
15. Schulz KF, Grimes DA. Case-control studies: research in reverse. *Lancet* 2002;359:431–434.
16. Rothman K. *Epidemiology: An Introduction*. New York: Oxford University Press; 2002.
17. Hennekens C, Buring J. *Epidemiology in Medicine*. Boston: Little, Brown and Company; 1987.
18. Andriole GL, Crawford ED, Grubb RL 3rd, et al. Mortality results from a randomized prostate-cancer screening trial. *N Engl J Med* 2009;360:1310–1319.
19. Wilt TJ, Brawer MK, Jones KM, et al. Radical prostatectomy versus observation for localized prostate cancer. *N Engl J Med* 2012;367:203–213.
20. Yu JB, Soulos PR, Herrin J, et al. Proton versus intensity-modulated radiotherapy for prostate cancer: patterns of care and early toxicity. *J Natl Cancer Inst* 2013;105:25–32.
21. Ma X, Wang R, Long JB, et al. The cost implications of prostate cancer screening in the Medicare population. *Cancer* 2014;120(1):96–102.
22. Rundle A, Schwartz S. Issues in the epidemiological analysis and interpretation of intermediate biomarkers. *Cancer Epidemiol Biomarkers Prev* 2003;12:491–496.
23. Shields PG. Tobacco smoking, harm reduction, and biomarkers. *J Natl Cancer Inst* 2002;94:1435–1444.
24. Hunter DJ. Gene-environment interactions in human diseases. *Nat Rev Genet* 2005;6:287–298.
25. Hirschhorn JN, Daly MJ. Genome-wide association studies for common diseases and complex traits. *Nat Rev Genet* 2005;6:95–108.
26. Breast Cancer Association Consortium. Commonly studied single-nucleotide polymorphisms and breast cancer: results from the Breast Cancer Association Consortium. *J Natl Cancer Inst* 2006;98:1382–1396.
27. Wacholder S, Chanock S, Garcia-Closas M, et al. Assessing the probability that a positive report is false: an approach for molecular epidemiology studies. *J Natl Cancer Inst* 2004;96:434–442.
28. Clayton DG, Walker NM, Smyth DJ, et al. Population structure, differential bias and genomic control in a large-scale, case-control association study. *Nat Genet* 2005;37:1243–1246.
29. Easton DF, Eeles RA. Genome-wide association studies in cancer. *Hum Mol Genet* 2008;17:R109–115.
30. Ahmed S, Thomas G, Ghoussaini M, et al. Newly discovered breast cancer susceptibility loci on 3p24 and 17q23.2. *Nat Genet* 2009;41:585–590.
31. Thomas G, Jacobs KB, Kraft P, et al. A multistage genome-wide association study in breast cancer identifies two new risk alleles at 1p11.2 and 14q24.1 (RAD51L1). *Nat Genet* 2009;41:579–584.
32. Thomas G, Jacobs KB, Yeager M, et al. Multiple loci identified in a genome-wide association study of prostate cancer. *Nat Genet* 2008;40:310–315.

33. Le Marchand L. Genome-wide association studies and colorectal cancer. *Surg Oncol Clin N Am* 2009;18:663–668.
34. Hung RJ, McKay JD, Gaborieau V, et al. A susceptibility locus for lung cancer maps to nicotinic acetylcholine receptor subunit genes on 15q25. *Nature* 2008;452:633–637.
35. Amos CI, Wu X, Broderick P, et al. Genome-wide association scan of tag SNPs identifies a susceptibility locus for lung cancer at 15q25.1. *Nat Genet* 2008;40:616–622.
36. Amundadottir L, Kraft P, Stolzenberg-Solomon RZ, et al. Genome-wide association study identifies variants in the ABO locus associated with susceptibility to pancreatic cancer. *Nat Genet* 2009;41:986–990.
37. Kiemeney LA, Sulem P, Besenbacher S, et al. A sequence variant at 4p16.3 confers susceptibility to urinary bladder cancer. *Nat Genet* 2010;42(5):415–419.
38. Wu X, Ye Y, Kiemeney LA, et al. Genetic variation in the prostate stem cell antigen gene PSCA confers susceptibility to urinary bladder cancer. *Nat Genet* 2009;41:991–995.
39. Stacey SN, Sulem P, Masson G, et al. New common variants affecting susceptibility to basal cell carcinoma. *Nat Genet* 2009;41:909–914.
40. Thorgeirsson TE, Geller F, Sulem P, et al. A variant associated with nicotine dependence, lung cancer and peripheral arterial disease. *Nature* 2008;452:638–642.
41. Spitz MR, Amos CI, Dong Q, et al. The CHRNA5-A3 region on chromosome 15q24-25.1 is a risk factor both for nicotine dependence and for lung cancer. *J Natl Cancer Inst* 2008;100:1552–1556.
42. Zheng W, Long J, Gao YT, et al. Genome-wide association study identifies a new breast cancer susceptibility locus at 6q25.1. *Nat Genet* 2009;41:324–328.
43. Gudmundsson J, Sulem P, Gudbjartsson DF, et al. Common variants on 9q22.33 and 14q13.3 predispose to thyroid cancer in European populations. *Nat Genet* 2009;41:460–464.
44. Gudmundsson J, Sulem P, Gudbjartsson DF, et al. Genome-wide association and replication studies identify four variants associated with prostate cancer susceptibility. *Nat Genet* 2009;41:1122–1126.
45. Song H, Ramus SJ, Tyrer J, et al. A genome-wide association study identifies a new ovarian cancer susceptibility locus on 9p22.2. *Nat Genet* 2009;41:996–1000.
46. Stacey SN, Gudbjartsson DF, Sulem P, et al. Common variants on 1p36 and 1q42 are associated with cutaneous basal cell carcinoma but not with melanoma or pigmentation traits. *Nat Genet* 2008;40:1313–1318.
47. Zanke BW, Greenwood CM, Rangrej J, et al. Genome-wide association scan identifies a colorectal cancer susceptibility locus on chromosome 8q24. *Nat Genet* 2007;39:989–994.
48. Haiman CA, Patterson N, Freedman ML, et al. Multiple regions within 8q24 independently affect risk for prostate cancer. *Nat Genet* 2007;39:638–644.
49. Kiemeney LA, Thorlacius S, Sulem P, et al. Sequence variant on 8q24 confers susceptibility to urinary bladder cancer. *Nat Genet* 2008;40:1307–1312.
50. Ghoussaini M, Song H, Koessler T, et al. Multiple loci with different cancer specificities within the 8q24 gene desert. *J Natl Cancer Inst* 2008;100:962–966.
51. Harismendy O, Frazer KA. Elucidating the role of 8q24 in colorectal cancer. *Nat Genet* 2009;41:868–869.
52. Wright JB, Brown SJ, Cole MD. Upregulation of c-MYC in cis through a large chromatin loop linked to a cancer risk-associated single-nucleotide polymorphism in colorectal cancer cells. *Mol Cell Biol* 2010;30:1411–1420.
53. Rafnar T, Sulem P, Stacey SN, et al. Sequence variants at the TERT-CLPTM1L locus associate with many cancer types. *Nat Genet* 2009;41:221–227.
54. Fernandez-Garcia I, Ortiz-de-Solorzano C, Montuenga LM. Telomeres and telomerase in lung cancer. *J Thorac Oncol* 2008;3:1085–1088.
55. Zienolddiny S, Skaug V, Landvik NE, et al. The TERT-CLPTM1L lung cancer susceptibility variant associates with higher DNA adduct formation in the lung. *Carcinogenesis* 2009;30:1368–1371.
56. Ioannidis JP, Thomas G, Daly MJ. Validating, augmenting and refining genome-wide association signals. *Nat Rev Genet* 2009;10:318–329.
57. Chung CC, Magalhaes WC, Gonzalez-Bosquet J, et al. Genome-wide association studies in cancer—current and future directions. *Carcinogenesis* 2010;31:111–120.
58. Fraga MF, Ballestar E, Paz MF, et al. Epigenetic differences arise during the lifetime of monozygotic twins. *Proc Natl Acad Sci U S A* 2005;102:10604–10609.
59. Dolinoy DC, Weidman JR, Waterland RA, et al. Maternal genistein alters coat color and protects Avy mouse offspring from obesity by modifying the fetal epigenome. *Environ Health Perspect* 2006;114:567–572.

ETIOLOGY AND EPIDEMIOLOGY OF CANCER

# 12 Trends in United States Cancer Mortality

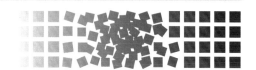

Tim E. Byers

## INTRODUCTION

Cancer incidence registries now cover nearly all of the US population. State-based vital records systems and aggregate national systems regularly report trends in both cancer incidence and mortality, and national surveys routinely monitor cancer-related risk factors in the population. These surveillance systems have documented substantial changes in both risk factors for cancer and in cancer incidence and mortality rates in the United States over the past 3 decades. In 1996, the American Cancer Society (ACS) set an ambitious challenge for the United States: to reduce cancer mortality rates from their apparent peak in 1990 by 50% in the 25-year period ending in 2015.[1] In 1998, the ACS then challenged the United States to also reduce cancer incidence rates from their peak in 1992 by 25% by the year 2015.[2] In this chapter, we will examine trends in cancer risk factors as well as trends in cancer incidence and mortality rates in the United States over the 25-year period between 1990 and 2015.

## CANCER SURVEILLANCE SYSTEMS

Collecting cancer incidence rates is largely a state-based activity in the United States, because cancer is a reportable disease in all states. The Centers for Disease Control and Prevention (CDC) organizes all state-based cancer registries within the National Program of Cancer Registries, which now reports collective data on cancer incidence from over 40 different state-based registries, providing data that meets strict quality standards.[3] The National Cancer Institute has supported high-quality cancer incidence and outcomes registration in selected states and cities since 1973 within the Surveillance, Epidemiology, and End Results (SEER) Program.[4] The most precise measures of long-term trends in cancer incidence come from SEER-9, a set of nine SEER registries that together include about 10% of the US population. The populations included in the SEER-9 registries document the most detailed history of cancer trends beginning in the 1970s based on highly standardized cancer case ascertainment, staging, treatment, and outcomes. Deaths from cancer are well ascertained in all states via state-based vital records, which are aggregated into annual national mortality reports by the CDC's National Center for Health Statistics.[5] Each year, the ACS, the National Cancer Institute, and the CDC publish a *Report to the Nation* on trends in cancer incidence and mortality in the United States.[6] Trends in the prevalence of behavioral factors that affect cancer risk are tracked by the Health Interview Survey, an ongoing, in-person interview of a nationally representative sample of adults, and in annual reports by the Behavioral Risk Factor Surveillance System, a continuously operating telephone-based survey operated by state departments of health and organized by the CDC.[7]

## MAKING SENSE OF CANCER TRENDS

Understanding the reasons for cancer trends requires understanding trends in cancer-related risk factors. For factors like tobacco,

relating trends in exposure to trends in rates is easy, because those effects are large and single. However, for many other cancer risk factors, because effects are much smaller and multifactorial, simple correlations over time are less apparent. In most situations, all that maybe possible are crude qualitative relationships between temporal trends in cancer risk factors and subsequent trends in cancer rates. Statistical methods such as linear regression joinpoint analysis can tell us when inflections in cancer trends occur, but accounting for the precise reasons for changing rates is often impaired by our incomplete knowledge about the interacting impacts of variations in cancer screening, diagnosis, and treatment, and by uncertainties about latencies between interventions and outcomes.[8]

## TRENDS IN CANCER RISK FACTORS AND SCREENING

Trends in major cancer risk factors have been mixed (Table 12.1). Although the downward trends in tobacco smoking among adults that began in the 1960s slowed after 1990, there has been a continuing downward trend in the number of cigarettes smoked per day by continuing smokers.[9] Obesity trends have been adverse among both men and women since the 1970s, with more than a doubling of the prevalence of obesity between 1990 and 2010. Long-term trends in the use of hormone replacement therapy (HRT) are not routinely monitored in the Behavioral Risk Factor Surveillance System (BRFSS), but HRT use increased substantially in the last 2 decades of the 20th century. Then, following the 2002 publication of the Women's Health Initiative trial, which showed clear adverse effects of HRT, there was a rapid and substantial drop in HRT use.[10,11] The use of endoscopic screening for colorectal cancer (sigmoidoscopy or colonoscopy) has increased substantially in recent years, approximately doubling since the mid 1990s, so that, as of 2010, about two-thirds of Americans age 50 and older reported ever having had an endoscopic examination. Mammography use increased progressively through the 1990s, but mammogram rates then leveled off after 2000.[12] Widespread prostate-specific antigen (PSA) testing began in the mid to late 1980s, then increased substantially during the 1990s. By 2002, a majority of US men age 50 and older reported having been tested.

## CANCER INCIDENCE AND MORTALITY

In this chapter, we describe and discuss cancer trends for the time period 1990 through 2010 using cancer incidence data from the SEER-9 registry (Table 12.2 and Fig. 12.1) and US cancer mortality data from the National Center for Health Statistics (Table 12.3).[4,5] All rates were age-adjusted to the US 2000 standard population by the direct method, using 10-year age intervals.

### Lung Cancer

The lung is the second leading site for cancer incidence and the leading site for cancer death among both men and women in the

TABLE 12.1

**Trends in Risk Factors and Cancer Screening Practices in the United States, 1990–2010**[a]

| | Men | | Women | | Both Genders | |
|---|---|---|---|---|---|---|
| | Smoking | PSA Screening | Smoking | Mammography | Obesity | CRC Screening |
| 1990 | 24.9 | — | 21.3 | 58.3 | 11.6 | — |
| 1991 | 25.1 | — | 21.3 | 62.2 | 12.6 | — |
| 1992 | 24.2 | — | 21.0 | 63.1 | 12.6 | — |
| 1993 | 24.0 | — | 21.1 | 66.5 | 13.7 | — |
| 1994 | 23.9 | — | 21.6 | 66.6 | 14.4 | — |
| 1995 | 24.8 | — | 20.9 | 68.6 | 15.8 | 29.4 |
| 1996 | 25.5 | — | 21.9 | 69.2 | 16.8 | — |
| 1997 | 25.4 | — | 21.1 | 70.3 | 16.6 | 32.4 |
| 1998 | 25.3 | — | 20.9 | 72.3 | 18.3 | — |
| 1999 | 24.2 | — | 20.8 | 72.8 | 19.7 | 43.7 |
| 2000 | 24.4 | — | 21.2 | 76.1 | 20.1 | — |
| 2001 | 25.4 | — | 21.2 | — | 21.0 | — |
| 2002 | 25.7 | 53.9 | 20.8 | 75.9 | 22.1 | 48.1 |
| 2003 | 24.8 | — | 20.2 | — | — | — |
| 2004 | 23.0 | 52.1 | 19.0 | 74.7 | 23.2 | 53.0 |
| 2005 | 22.1 | — | 19.2 | — | 24.4 | — |
| 2006 | 22.2 | 53.8 | 18.4 | 76.5 | 25.1 | 57.1 |
| 2007 | 21.2 | — | 18.4 | — | 26.3 | — |
| 2008 | 20.3 | 54.8 | 16.7 | 76.0 | 26.6 | 61.8 |
| 2009 | 19.5 | — | 16.7 | — | 27.1 | — |
| 2010 | 18.5 | 53.2 | 15.8 | 75.2 | 27.5 | 65.2 |

CRC, colorectal cancer; PSA, prostate-specific antigen.

[a] Median percent of the population across all states in the Behavioral Risk Factor Surveillance System. The survey covered such areas as body mass index and was based on self-reported height and weight. Questions included: Are you a regular cigarette smoker? Have you ever had a sigmoidoscopy or proctoscopic examination? For women age 40 and older, the following question was included: Have you had a mammogram in the past 2 years? For men aged 50 and older, the following question was included: Have you had a PSA test in the last 2 years? (From Centers for Disease Control and Prevention. Behavioral Risk Factor Surveillance System Web site. http://cdc.gov/brfss.)

ETIOLOGY AND EPIDEMIOLOGY OF CANCER

United States.[6] There are now more deaths from lung cancer in the United States than from the sum of colorectal, breast, and prostate cancers. Trends in lung cancer incidence and mortality have been nearly identical because there are few effective treatments for lung cancer, and survival time remains short. Lung cancer trends follow historic declines in tobacco use, lagged by about 20 years.[13] Between 1965 and 1985, tobacco use among US adults dropped substantially, and more in men than in women. Lung cancer mortality rates began to decline among men in 1990, but rates increased among women throughout the 1990s. The stabilization of lung cancer incidence trends among women from 2000 to 2005 and the beginning of a decline in the period 2005 to 2010 foretells a coming persistent decline in lung cancer mortality among women in the United States.

The effectiveness of annual examinations by use of chest radiographs in reducing lung cancer mortality was studied as part of the Prostate, Lung, Colorectal, Ovary (PLCO) trial, and the effectiveness of annual screening by low-dose computed tomography (LDCT) of the lung fields was studied in the National Lung Screening Trial (NLST).[14,15] In brief, screening with standard chest radiography finds more cancers earlier but does not affect mortality, whereas screening with LDCT reduces the risk of death from lung cancer by at least 20%.[14,15] Therefore, both the ACS and the US Preventive Services Task Force have issued recommendations that favor informed decision making for lung cancer screening using LDCT.[16,17]

The major factor that will determine lung cancer incidence in the coming decade is the past history of tobacco use, but future screening will also reduce future mortality rates. Considering all factors, it is likely that over the coming decade the downward trends in mortality from lung cancer will continue at about the same rate among men, and soon will become more apparent among women.

## Colorectal Cancer

The colorectum is the third leading site for cancer incidence and the second leading site for cancer death in the United States.[6] Colorectal cancer incidence rates increased until 1985, when they began to decline. The reasons for this decline are not clear, but could be related to downward trends in cigarette smoking and the increasing use of both nonsteroidal anti-inflammatory drugs (NSAIDs) and HRT.[18] The rapid decline in HRT use following the publication of the Women's Health Initiative trial results in 2002 may adversely affect colorectal trends among women in the coming years, because HRT reduces the risk for colorectal cancer among women.[11] Recent trials have demonstrated the potential for NSAIDs to reduce colorectal neoplasia, but adverse effects from these agents will limit their widespread use for that explicit purpose. Nonetheless, even the common sporadic use of NSAIDs for other indications will contribute to continuing declines in colorectal cancer incidence in the coming years.

Screening with either sigmoidoscopy or colonoscopy leads to the identification and removal of adenomas, thus preventing the development of colorectal cancer.[19,20] Medicare included

## TABLE 12.2

**Trends in Age-Adjusted Cancer Incidence Rates in the United States by Cancer Site, 1990–2010[a]**

| | Men | | Women | | Both Genders | |
|---|---|---|---|---|---|---|
| | Lung | Prostate | Lung | Breast | Colorectal | All Sites |
| 1990 | 96.9 | 171.0 | 47.8 | 131.8 | 60.7 | 482.0 |
| 1991 | 97.2 | 214.8 | 49.6 | 133.9 | 59.5 | 503.0 |
| 1992 | 97.2 | 237.4 | 49.9 | 132.1 | 58.0 | 510.6 |
| 1993 | 94.0 | 209.5 | 49.2 | 129.2 | 56.8 | 493.4 |
| 1994 | 90.9 | 180.3 | 50.5 | 131.0 | 55.6 | 483.5 |
| 1995 | 89.8 | 169.3 | 50.4 | 132.6 | 54.0 | 476.9 |
| 1996 | 88.0 | 169.5 | 50.2 | 133.7 | 54.8 | 479.1 |
| 1997 | 86.3 | 173.5 | 52.6 | 138.0 | 56.4 | 486.4 |
| 1998 | 88.0 | 171.0 | 53.0 | 141.4 | 56.8 | 488.2 |
| 1999 | 84.6 | 183.4 | 52.4 | 141.5 | 55.5 | 490.4 |
| 2000 | 82.1 | 183.0 | 51.2 | 136.4 | 54.1 | 486.0 |
| 2001 | 81.4 | 184.8 | 51.7 | 138.7 | 53.6 | 489.7 |
| 2002 | 80.4 | 182.2 | 52.5 | 135.6 | 53.1 | 487.5 |
| 2003 | 81.0 | 169.6 | 53.0 | 126.8 | 50.8 | 475.2 |
| 2004 | 76.2 | 165.7 | 52.0 | 128.0 | 50.0 | 476.1 |
| 2005 | 75.8 | 156.5 | 53.7 | 126.4 | 47.8 | 471.9 |
| 2006 | 74.2 | 171.5 | 53.4 | 126.0 | 46.8 | 475.0 |
| 2007 | 73.5 | 174.3 | 53.4 | 127.9 | 46.3 | 480.5 |
| 2008 | 72.0 | 157.0 | 51.6 | 128.0 | 45.2 | 473.4 |
| 2009 | 70.2 | 153.7 | 51.8 | 130.3 | 43.0 | 470.5 |
| 2010 | 66.8 | 145.1 | 49.2 | 126.0 | 40.6 | 457.5 |
| Average annual % change 1990–2010 | −1.8 | −0.5 | +0.2 | −0.2 | −2.0 | −0.2 |

[a] Data source is the Surveillance, Epidemiology, and End Results-9 populations for cancer incidence. Rates are age-adjusted to the year 2000 population standard. The annual percent change is the mean percent change per year across the 20-year period, 1990 to 2010. (From National Cancer Institute. Surveillance, Epidemiology, and End Results Program Web site. http://seer.cancer.gov.)

coverage for all recommended colorectal screening methods in 2001, and national publicity has substantially increased public interest in screening.[21] Colorectal screening rates have increased over time, now with about two-thirds of adults over age 50 reporting having ever been screened by lower gastrointestinal endoscopy (see Table 12.1).

Decreasing rates of colorectal cancer incidence are occurring in spite of the obesity epidemic, which is an adverse force on colorectal cancer risk, because obesity may account for as much as 20% of colorectal cancer in the United States.[22] Recently, however, obesity trends have stabilized in the United States.[23] As a result of the increased use of lower gastrointestinal endoscopy for colorectal screening and this stabilization of obesity trends, the incidence of colorectal cancer may exceed the ACS goal for 2015 of a 25% reduction, and there is a high likelihood that the rate of decline in deaths from colorectal cancer will be steep enough to reach the 2015 ACS mortality reduction goal of 50%.

## Breast Cancer

The breast is the leading site of cancer incidence and the second leading site for cancer death among women in the United States.[6] Over the period 1990 to 2001, no substantial changes in incidence rates were observed, but after 2000, breast cancer incidence began to decline. The decline in breast cancer incidence observed after 2002 seems to have been the result of the sudden decline in the use of HRT following the 2002 publication of the Women's Health Initiative results.[10,11] It is likely that persisting lower rates of HRT use will cause a continued decline in breast cancer incidence in the coming years. Countering this favorable trend, however, are the adverse effects of the obesity epidemic. Obesity, a major risk factor for postmenopausal breast cancer, increased substantially between 1990 and 2005, now with over 25% of US women being obese. However, the slowing of the obesity epidemic since 2005 may have substantial beneficial effects on the future trends in breast cancer incidence.

After persistent increases in the use of mammography over a 20-year period, mammography rates declined modestly between 2000 and 2004, and then leveled off. The downgrading of the evidence recommendations by the US Preventive Services Task Force for mammography for women age 40 to 49 and recommendations for every other year mammographies for women age 50 and older have resulted in lower mammogram utilization, which is likely to continue into the coming decade.[17] This trend will have an adverse effect on breast cancer mortality, but will tend to reduce breast cancer incidence somewhat because of a lack of detection of very early stage cancers.

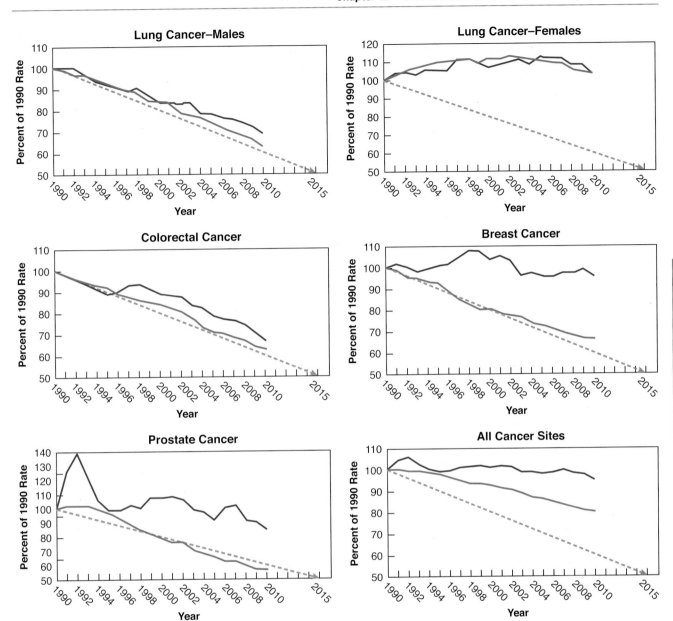

**Figure 12.1 (A–F)** Trends in cancer incidence and mortality between 1990 and 2010. Incidence rates are for the populations in the Surveillance, Epidemiology, and End Results Program; registries and mortality rates are for the entire United States. Rates are age-adjusted to the year 2000 standard. The y-axis rates are expressed as a percentage of the 1990 incidence and mortality rates. The *red lines* represent incidence rates, and the *blue lines* represent mortality rates. The *straight dotted green lines* represent the linear trend that would need to be followed to achieve a 50% mortality reduction between 1990 and 2015. (Data from National Cancer Institute. Surveillance, Epidemiology, and End Results Program Web site. http://seer.cancer.gov, and Centers for Disease Control and Prevention. U.S. mortality data. http://wonder.cdc.gov/ucd-icd10.html)

The antiestrogens tamoxifen and raloxifene have both been shown to reduce the risk of incident breast cancer.[24] The safety profile for tamoxifen discourages its widespread use, but there is a more favorable risk/benefit balance of raloxifene. Nonetheless, neither of these drugs is commonly used for breast cancer prevention among postmenopausal women in the United States.

The average decline in breast cancer death rates of 2% per year since 1990 is the combined result of earlier diagnosis and better treatment.[25] Progress in breast cancer treatment is continuing, especially in the development and application of hormone-targeted therapies. Aromatase inhibitors have largely replaced tamoxifen therapy for breast cancer treatment for postmenopausal women. Because all antiestrogens substantially reduce the incidence of second primary cancers in the contralateral breast, they impact both therapy and prevention. In the coming decade, the longer term effects of decreased HRT use, increased antiestrogen use, reversal of the obesity trends, and continued improvements in therapies will likely lead to continued decreases in both the incidence and mortality rates from breast cancer.

## Prostate Cancer

The prostate is the leading site for cancer incidence and the second leading site for cancer death among men in the United States.[6] The incidence of prostate cancer has been extremely variable over the period 1990 to 2010. The incidence spike observed in the early 1990s actually began in the late 1980s, coincident with the advent of PSA testing. The reasons for the 2.8% annual downward trend in prostate cancer mortality since 1990 are uncertain, however, because the ongoing PSA screening trials have not yet demonstrated a mortality benefit from screening anywhere as large as the downward mortality

**ETIOLOGY AND EPIDEMIOLOGY OF CANCER**

## TABLE 12.3

**Trends in Age-Adjusted Cancer Mortality Rates in the United States by Cancer Site, 1990–2010**[a]

| | Men | | Women | | Both Genders | |
|---|---|---|---|---|---|---|
| | Lung | Prostate | Lung | Breast | Colorectal | All Sites |
| 1990 | 90.6 | 38.6 | 36.8 | 33.1 | 24.6 | 214.9 |
| 1991 | 89.9 | 39.3 | 37.6 | 32.7 | 24.0 | 215.1 |
| 1992 | 88.0 | 39.2 | 38.7 | 31.6 | 23.6 | 213.5 |
| 1993 | 87.6 | 39.3 | 39.3 | 31.4 | 23.3 | 213.4 |
| 1994 | 85.7 | 38.5 | 39.6 | 30.9 | 22.9 | 211.7 |
| 1995 | 84.4 | 37.3 | 40.3 | 30.6 | 22.6 | 210.0 |
| 1996 | 82.8 | 36.0 | 40.4 | 29.5 | 21.9 | 207.0 |
| 1997 | 81.3 | 34.2 | 40.8 | 28.2 | 21.5 | 203.6 |
| 1998 | 79.9 | 32.6 | 41.0 | 27.5 | 21.2 | 200.8 |
| 1999 | 77.0 | 31.6 | 40.2 | 26.6 | 20.9 | 200.7 |
| 2000 | 76.5 | 30.4 | 41.1 | 26.6 | 20.7 | 198.8 |
| 2001 | 75.3 | 29.5 | 41.0 | 26.0 | 20.2 | 196.3 |
| 2002 | 73.7 | 28.7 | 41.6 | 25.6 | 19.8 | 194.4 |
| 2003 | 72.0 | 27.2 | 41.3 | 25.3 | 19.1 | 190.9 |
| 2004 | 70.4 | 26.2 | 41.0 | 24.5 | 18.1 | 186.8 |
| 2005 | 69.5 | 25.4 | 40.7 | 24.1 | 17.6 | 185.2 |
| 2006 | 67.4 | 24.2 | 40.3 | 23.6 | 17.3 | 182.0 |
| 2007 | 65.2 | 24.2 | 40.1 | 23.0 | 16.9 | 179.3 |
| 2008 | 63.7 | 23.0 | 39.1 | 22.6 | 16.5 | 176.3 |
| 2009 | 61.5 | 22.1 | 38.6 | 22.2 | 15.8 | 173.4 |
| 2010 | 60.1 | 21.8 | 38.0 | 22.0 | 15.5 | 171.8 |
| Average annual % change 1990–2010 | −2.0 | −2.8 | +0.2 | −2.0 | −2.3 | −1.1 |

[a] Data source is the National Center for Health Statistics national mortality data set. Rates are age-adjusted to the year 2000 population standard. The average percentage change per year is the mean percent change per year across the 20-year period, 1990 to 2010. (From Centers for Disease Control and Prevention. U.S. mortality data. http://wonder.cdc.gov/ucd-icd10.html)

decline observed since 1990.[26,27] In fact, the US trial findings suggest that there was virtually no mortality benefit within the first decade following the initiation of screening.[28] Therefore, it is not possible to know how much of this favorable trend was related to early diagnosis, how much was related to improvements in treatment, or how much might have been related to other factors, such as changes in the way cause of death has been listed on death certificates.

The Prostate Cancer Prevention Trial provided an important proof of principle that antiandrogen therapies can reduce prostate cancer risk.[29] Although the net benefits of finasteride for prevention are not clearly demonstrated from this trial, other agents that interfere with androgen effects on prostate cancer growth could prove to be useful for prostate cancer chemoprevention in the future. Prostate cancer incidence trends will likely continue to be largely driven by rates of PSA screening in the coming decade. Longer term results of a clearer benefit to mortality from either the PLCO trial in the United States or the European PSA trial would help to better specify screening recommendations.

## Other Cancers

Even though mortality rates have been declining by about 2% per year from the four most common causes of cancer death (lung, colorectal, breast, and prostate), very little progress has been made in reducing death rates from the other half of all adult cancers in the United States. Continuing progress in tobacco control will have beneficial effects on many other types of cancer linked to tobacco, and stopping the obesity epidemic will have favorable effects on many obesity-related cancers that have been increasing in recent years, such as adenocarcinoma of the esophagus and renal cancer.[30] Melanoma incidence rates have been increasing substantially in recent years, likely the result of the combined effects of previous sun exposure and increased awareness and surveillance for pigmented skin lesions, but recent advances in therapy for metastatic melanoma may foretell future declines in melanoma morality. Declining rates of stomach cancer incidence and mortality over several decades may be related to the combined effects of historic improvements in nutrition and the declining prevalence of chronic infection with *Helicobacter pylori*. Liver cancer incidence has been substantially increasing in recent years, likely resulting from historic trends in chronic infection with hepatitis B and C viruses. As a result, liver cancer will likely continue to rise in the United States over the coming decade.

The incidence of thyroid cancer has been increasing in the United States for the past several decades, but thyroid cancer mortality rates have been stable, a pattern most likely due to increased detection from improved diagnostic techniques. Invasive cervical cancer is uncommon in the United States because of widespread screening using Pap smears. Although the vaccination for human papillomavirus (HPV) has been shown to be highly effective in protecting against the serotypes that together account for 70% of cervical cancer cases, so far, HPV vaccine coverage has been low among young women in the United States.[6] For many of the other cancers, such as cancers of the pancreas, brain, ovary, and the hematopoietic malignancies, risk factors are poorly understood, and there are no effective early detection methods. For these cancers, the current hope for improvement resides in the development of better methods for early cancer detection and treatment.

## PREDICTING FUTURE CANCER TRENDS

In the United States, cancer is now the leading cause of death under age 85 years. Over the first half of the ACS 25-year challenge period, overall cancer incidence rates have declined by about 0.2% per year, and mortality rates have declined by about 1% per year. The trends in both incidence and mortality from the four leading cancer sites are summarized in Figure 12.1. Using simple linear extrapolation, it therefore seems that the ACS challenge goals of reducing cancer incidence by 25% and mortality by 50% over 25 years may be only half achieved.[31,32] Clearly, though, estimating future trends only by linear extrapolation is a crude way to foretell future events. Projecting cancer trends into the more distant future using complex modeling is possible, however, as knowledge about changes in major cancer risk factors can lead to reasonable predictions about the direction and approximate slope of future trends. One method to incorporate knowledge about trends in risk factors into estimates of future cancer trends is to estimate the impact of changes in the attributable risk (also called the *preventable fraction*) in the population for each risk factor. By making assumptions about latency period, then tying changes in factors to changes in cancer incidence and mortality, cancer trends resulting from risk factor changes can be predicted. For example, if there were a factor that explained 30% of a particular cancer, then cutting that exposure in half would eventually lead to a projected 15% reduction in rates (50% of 30%). This method was used to project cancer mortality trends to 2015 and seems to have projected trends that are quite similar to those observed in recent years.[33]

Progress in cancer prevention, early detection, and treatment since 1990 has been persistent, and there are many reasons to be optimistic about the future. Just how much steeper the future downward slope in cancer death rates can be driven will depend on the extent to which we can discover new factors causing cancer, and effectively deploy ways to better act on our current knowledge about how to prevent and control cancer. Especially important will be progress in reversing the epidemics of tobacco use and obesity, and ensuring that the coming improvements to health care access will lead to access to state-of-the-art cancer screening and therapy for all.

## REFERENCES

1. American Cancer Society Board of Directors. ACS Challenge goals for U.S. Cancer Mortality for the Year 2015. *Proceedings of the Board of Directors.* Atlanta, GA: American Cancer Society, 1996.
2. American Cancer Society Board of Directors. ACS Challenge goals for U.S. Cancer Incidence for the Year 2015. *Proceedings of the Board of Directors.* Atlanta, GA: American Cancer Society, 1998.
3. Centers for Disease Control and Prevention. National Program of Cancer Registries (NPCR) Web site. http://cdc.gov/cancer/npcr.
4. National Cancer Institute. Surveillance, Epidemiology, and End Results Program Web site. http://seer.cancer.gov.
5. Centers for Disease Control and Prevention. U.S. mortality data. http://wonder.cdc.gov/ucd-icd10.html
6. Jemal A, Simard E, Dorell C, et al. Annual report to the nation on the status of cancer, 1975–2009, featuring the burden and trends in human papillomavirus (HPV)–associated cancers and HPV vaccination coverage levels. *J Natl Cancer Inst* 2013;105:175–201.
7. Centers for Disease Control and Prevention. Behavioral Risk Factor Surveillance System Web site. http://cdc.gov/brfss.
8. Ward E, Thun M, Hannan L, et al. Interpreting cancer trends. *Ann N Y Acad Sci* 2006;1076:29–53.
9. Centers for Disease Control and Prevention. Smoking & Tobacco Use Web site. http://cdc.gov/tobacco.
10. Rossouw JE, Anderson GL, Prentice RL, et al. Risks and benefits of estrogen plus progestin in healthy postmenopausal women: principal results from the Women's Health Initiative randomized controlled trial. *JAMA* 2002; 288:321–333.
11. Hersh A, Stefanick M, Stafford R. National use of postmenopausal hormone therapy: annual trends and response to recent evidence. *JAMA* 2004;291:47–53.
12. Ryerson AB, Miller J, Eheman CR, et al. Use of mammograms among women aged ≥40 years—United States, 2000–2005. *MMWR* 2007;56:49–51.
13. Giovino GA. Epidemiology of tobacco use in the United States. *Oncogene* 2002;21:7326–7340.
14. Oken M, Hocking W, Kvale P, et al. Screening by chest radiograph and lung cancer mortality. *JAMA* 2011;306:1865–1873.
15. The National Lung Screening Trial Research Team. Reduced lung-cancer mortality with low-dose computed tomographic screening. *N Engl J Med* 2011; 365:395–409.
16. Smith R, Brooks D, Cokkinides V, et al. Cancer screening in the United States, 2013: a review of current American Cancer Society guidelines, current issues in cancer screening, and new guidance on cervical cancer screening and lung cancer screening. *CA Cancer J Clin* 2013;63:88–105.
17. U.S. Preventive Services Task Force. U.S. Preventive Services Task Force Web site. http://uspreventiveservicestaskforce.org.
18. Martinez ME. Primary prevention of colorectal cancer: lifestyle, nutrition, exercise. *Recent Results Cancer Res* 2005;166:177–211.
19. Atkin W, Edwards R, Kralj-Hans I, et al. Once-only flexible sigmoidoscopy screening in prevention of colorectal cancer: a multicentre randomized controlled trial. *Lancet* 2010;375:1624–1633.
20. Schoen RE, Pinsky PF, Weissfeld JL, et al. Colorectal-cancer incidence and mortality with screening flexible sigmoidoscopy. *N Engl J Med* 2012; 366:2345–2357.
21. Cram P, Fendrick A, Inadomi J, et al. The impact of celebrity promotional campaign on the use of colon cancer screening: the Katie Couric effect. *Arch Intern Med* 2003;163(13):1601–1605.
22. World Cancer Research Fund/American Institute for Cancer Prevention. *Policy and Action for Cancer Prevention. Food, Nutrition, and Physical Activity: A Global Perspective.* Washington, DC: AICR; 2009.
23. Ogden CL, Carroll MD, Curtin LR, et al. Prevalence of overweight and obesity in the United States, 1999–2004. *JAMA* 2006;295:1549–1555.
24. Vogel V, Constantino J, Wickerham D, et al. Effects of tamoxifen vs raloxifene on the risks of developing invasive breast cancer and other disease outcomes: the NSABP Study of Tamoxifen and Raloxifene (STAR) P-2 trial. *JAMA* 2006;295:2727–2741.
25. Berry D, Cronin K, Plevritis S, et al. Effect of screening and adjuvant therapy on mortality from breast cancer. *N Engl J Med* 2005;353:1784–1792.
26. Andriole GL, Crawford ED, Grubb RL 3rd, et al. Mortality results from a randomized prostate-cancer screening trial. *N Engl J Med* 2009;360(13):1310–1319.
27. Schröder FH, Hugosson J, Roobol MJ, et al. Screening and prostate-cancer mortality in a randomized European study. *N Engl J Med* 2009;360(13):1320–1328.
28. Andriole G, Crawford D, Grubb R, et al. Prostate cancer screening in the randomized Prostate, Lung, Colorectal, and Ovarian Cancer Screening Trial: mortality results after 13 years of follow-up. *J Natl Cancer Inst* 2012;104: 125–132.
29. Thompson I, Goodman P, Tangen C, et al. Long-term survival of participants in the prostate cancer prevention trial. *N Engl J Med* 2013;369:603–610.
30. International Agency for Cancer Research. *Weight Control and Physical Activity. Handbook 6.* Lyon, France: IARC Press; 2002.
31. Sedjo R, Byers T, Barrera E, et al. A midpoint assessment of the American Cancer Society challenge goal to decrease cancer incidence by 25% between 1992 and 2015. *CA Cancer J Clin* 2007;57:326–340.
32. Byers T, Barrera E, Fontham E, et al. A midpoint assessment of the American Cancer Society challenge goal to halve the U.S. cancer mortality rates between the years 1990 and 2015. *Cancer* 2006;107:396–405.
33. Byers T, Mouchawar J, Marks J, et al. The American Cancer Society challenge goals. How far can cancer rates decline in the U.S. by the year 2015? *Cancer* 1999;86:715–727.

ETIOLOGY AND EPIDEMIOLOGY OF CANCER

## PART III

# Cancer Therapeutics

# 13 Essentials of Radiation Therapy

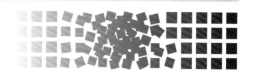

Meredith A. Morgan, Randall K. Ten Haken, and Theodore S. Lawrence

## INTRODUCTION

The beneficial use of radiation was launched by the experiments of Wilhelm Roentgen, who, in 1895, found that x-rays could pass through materials that were impenetrable to light. Emil Grubbe provided one of the early examples of the therapeutic use of radiation by treating an advanced ulcerated breast cancer with x-rays in January 1896. We have made great progress since these early days, which has been strongly influenced by research in radiation chemistry, biology, and physics.

## BIOLOGIC ASPECTS OF RADIATION ONCOLOGY

### Radiation-Induced DNA Damage

Radiation is administered to cells either in the form of photons (x-rays and gamma rays) or particles (protons, neutrons, and electrons). When photons or particles interact with biologic material, they cause ionizations that can either directly interact with subcellular structures or they can interact with water, the major constituent of cells, and generate free radicals that can then interact with subcellular structures (Fig. 13.1).

The direct effects of radiation are the consequence of the DNA in chromosomes absorbing energy that leads to ionizations. This is the major mechanism of DNA damage induced by charged nuclei (such as a carbon nucleus) and neutrons and is termed *high linear energy transfer* (Fig. 13.2). In contrast, the interaction of photons with other molecules, such as water, results in the production of free radicals, some of which possess a lifetime long enough to be able to diffuse to the nucleus and interact with DNA in the chromosomes. This is the major mechanism of DNA damage induced by x-rays and has been termed *low linear energy transfer*.[1]

A free radical generated through the interaction of photons with other molecules that possess an unpaired electron in their outermost shell (e.g., hydroxyl radicals) can abstract a hydrogen molecule from a macromolecule such as DNA to generate damage. Cells that have increased levels of free radical scavengers, such as glutathione, would have less DNA damage induced by x-rays, but would have similar levels of DNA damage induced by a carbon nucleus that is directly absorbed by chromosomal DNA. Furthermore, a low oxygen environment would also protect cells from x-ray–induced damage because there would be fewer radicals available to induce DNA damage in the absence of oxygen, but this environment would have little impact on DNA damage induced by carbon nuclei.[2]

### Cellular Responses to Radiation-Induced DNA Damage

#### Checkpoint Pathways

The cell cycle must progress in a specific order; checkpoint genes ensure that the initiation of late events is delayed until earlier events are complete. There are three principal places in the cell cycle at which checkpoints induced by DNA damage function: the border between G1 phase and S phase, intra-S phase, and the border between G2 phase and mitosis (Fig. 13.3). Cells with an intact checkpoint function that have sustained DNA damage stop progressing through the cycle and become arrested at the next checkpoint in the cell cycle. For example, cells with damaged DNA in G1 phase avoid replicating that damage by arresting at the G1/S interface. If irradiated cells have already passed the restriction point, a position in G1 phase that is regulated by the phosphorylation of the retinoblastoma tumor suppressor gene (*Rb*) and its dissociation from the E2F family of transcription factors, they will transiently arrest in S phase. The G1/S and intra-S phase checkpoints inhibit the replication of damaged DNA and work in a coordinated manner with the DNA repair machinery to permit the restitution of DNA integrity, thereby increasing cell survival.

The earliest response to radiation is the activation of ataxia-telangiectasia mutated (ATM), which involves a conformational change that results in the activation of its kinase domain and phosphorylation of serine 1981 (see Fig. 13.3).[3] This phosphorylation causes the ATM homodimer to dissociate into active monomers that phosphorylate a wide range of proteins such as 53BP1, the histone variant H2AX, Nbs1 (Nijmegen breakage syndrome; a member of the *MRN complex*, composed of Mre11, Rad50, and Nbs1), BRCA1, and SMC1 (structural maintenance of chromosomes), and these proteins coordinate repair with the cell cycle.[4] In response to DNA damage, H2AX is rapidly phosphorylated by ATM and localizes to sites of DNA double-strand breaks in multiprotein complexes described as foci (Fig. 13.4). Phosphorylation of H2AX by ATM results in the direct recruitment of Mdc1 and forms a complex with H2AX to recruit additional ATM molecules, forming a positive feedback loop.

The G1/S phase checkpoint is the best understood. In response to DNA damage, activated ATM can directly phosphorylate p53 and mdm2, the ubiquitin ligase that targets p53 for degradation. These phosphorylations are important for increasing the stability of the p53 protein. In addition to ATM, checkpoint kinase 2 (Chk2) also phosphorylates p53 and can enhance p53 stability. Activated p53 transcriptionally increases the expression of the *p21*[WAF1/CIP1] gene, which results in a sustained inhibition of G1 cyclin/Cdk, and prevents phosphorylation of pRb and progression from G1 into S.[5] Mutations in p53 that are commonly found in solid tumors result in loss of transcriptional activity and compromised checkpoint function.

Control of the S-phase checkpoint is mediated in part by the Cdc25A phosphatase inhibiting Cdk2 activity and the loading of Cdc45 onto chromatin. If Cdc45 fails to bind to chromatin, DNA polymerase α is not recruited to replication origins and replicon initiation fails to occur.[6] A more prominent mechanism for S-phase arrest is signaled through the MRN complex and the cohesin protein SMC1 by ATM.[7] Loss of ATM, MRN components, or SMC1 leads to the loss of the intra-S phase checkpoint function and increased radiosensitivity. Both the CDC45 and ATM pathways represent parallel, but seemingly independent, pathways to protect replication forks from trying to replicate through DNA strand

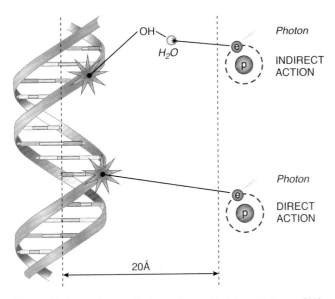

**Figure 13.1** The direct and indirect effects of ionizing radiation on DNA. Incident photons transfer part of their energy to free electrons (Compton scattering). These electrons can directly interact with DNA to induce DNA damage, or they can first interact with water to produce hydroxyl radicals that can then induce damage.

breaks. Although ATM has received the lion's share of attention in signaling checkpoint activation in response to ionizing radiation, its family member ATR (ataxia telangiectasia and rad3-related) also plays a role in S-phase checkpoint responses.[8] ATM kinase activity is inducible by radiation, whereas ATR kinase activity is constitutive and does not significantly change with irradiation. (ATR is described in more detail in Chapter 19.) In contrast to Cdc45 and ATM, ATR is probably more important in monitoring

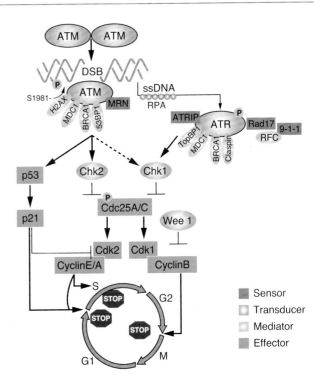

**Figure 13.3** In response to DNA damage, the MRN complex—composed of MRE11, Rad50, and NBS1—together with ataxia-telangiectasia mutation (ATM) and H2AX are the earliest proteins recruited to the site of the break. ATM is released from its homodimer complex, activated by transautophosphorylation and, in turn, phosphorylates H2AX. Other members are recruited to the complex such as BRCA1 and 53BP1. As the DNA at the double-strand break (DSB) is resected, single-stranded DNA is formed and bound by replication protein A (RPA), resulting in the activation of the ataxia-telangiectasia and Rad3-related (ATR) pathway. The net result of ATM/ATR activation is the downstream activation of p53, leading to the transcription of the Cdk inhibitor, p21, and the activation of Chk1/Chk2, resulting in the degradation of Cdc25 phosphatases, Cdk-cyclin complex inactivation, and cell cycle arrest at phase G1, intra S, or G2. Note that ATM is also partially activated by changes in chromatin structure induced by DNA double-strand breaks.

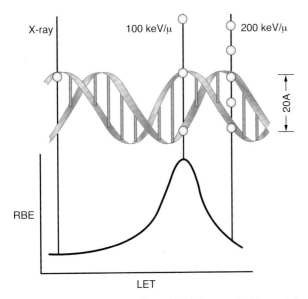

**Figure 13.2** Linear energy transfer and DNA damage. Ionizing radiation deposits energy along the track (linear energy transfer [LET]), which causes DNA damage and cell killing. The most biologically potent (highest relative biologic effectiveness [RBE]) LET is 100 keV per μm because the separation between ionizing events is the same as the diameter of the DNA double helix (2 nm). (From Hall EJ, Giaccia AJ. *Radiobiology for the Radiologist.* Philadelphia: Lippincott Williams & Williams; 2012, with permission.)

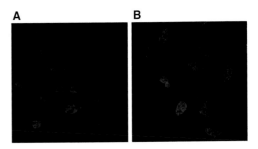

**Figure 13.4** Phosphorylated histone variant H2AX as a marker of DNA damage. Phosphorylated histone variant H2AX (also called gamma H2AX) localizes to sites of DNA double-strand breaks, so that its appearance and disappearance correspond with induction and repair of breaks. The cells in panels **A** and **B** have been stained with DAPI (4′,6-diamidino-2-phenylindole) (*blue*) in order to visualize cell nuclei and stained with an antibody, which recognizes *gamma* H2AX (*red*). The cells in **A** are untreated and exhibit little to no gamma H2AX staining, whereas the cells in **B** are treated with 7.5 Gy radiation and exhibit strong gamma H2AX staining at punctate foci in the nuclei, which are thought to correlate with sites of DNA double-strand breaks. (Image provided by Dr. Leslie Parsels, University of Michigan.)

perturbations in replication that are the result of stalled replication forks to prevent the formation of DNA double-strand breaks.

The arrest of cells in the G2 phase following DNA damage is one of the most conserved evolutionary responses to ionizing radiation. It makes sense to have a final checkpoint in the G2 phase to prevent cells from entering into mitosis with damaged DNA that could be transmitted to their progeny. It follows that cells lacking the G2 checkpoint are radiosensitive because they try to divide with damaged chromosomes that cannot be aligned at metaphase to be properly apportioned to daughter cells. At the biochemical level, the regulation of the mitosis-promoting factor cyclin B/Cdk1 is the critical step in the activation of this checkpoint. At the molecular level, ATM and Chk1/2 are activated by DNA damage in the G2 phase and inhibit the activation of Cdc25A and C phosphatases, which are essential for the activation of cyclin B/Cdk1.[9,10] The pololike kinase family (Plk1 and Plk3) also responds to DNA damage and can inhibit Cdc25C activation.[11] A great deal of effort has been focused on the development of small molecules to inhibit checkpoint response proteins, such as Chk1, with the idea that they would inhibit radiation-induced G2 arrest and perhaps repair and thus be used as radiation sensitizers.[12]

## DNA Repair

Ionizing radiation causes base damage, single-strand breaks, double-strand breaks, and sugar damage, as well as DNA–DNA, and DNA–protein cross-links. The critical target for ionizing radiation-induced cell inactivation and cell killing is the DNA double-strand break.[13,14] In eukaryotic cells, DNA double-strand breaks can be repaired by two processes: homologous recombination repair (HRR), which requires an undamaged DNA strand as a participant in the repair, and nonhomologous end joining (NHEJ), which mediates end-to-end joining.[15] In lower eukaryotes, such as yeast, HRR is the predominant pathway used for repairing DNA double-strand breaks, whereas mammalian cells use both HHR and non-HHR to repair their DNA. In mammalian cells, the choice of repair is biased by the phase of the cell cycle and by the abundance of repetitive DNA. HRR is used primarily in the late S phase/G2 phases of the cell-cycle, and NHEJ predominates in the G1-phase of the cell cycle (Fig. 13.5). NHEJ and HRR are not mutually exclusive, and both have been found to be active in the late S/G2 phase of the cell cycle, indicating that factors in addition to the cell-cycle phase are important in determining which mechanism will be used to repair DNA strand breaks.

**Nonhomologous End Joining.** In the G1-phase of the cell cycle, the ligation of DNA double-strand breaks is primarily through NHEJ because a sister chromatid does not exist to provide a template for HRR. The damaged ends of DNA double-strand breaks must first be modified before rejoining. The process of NHEJ can be divided into at least four steps: synapsis, end processing, fill-in synthesis, and ligation (Fig. 13.6).[16] Synapsis is the critical initial step where the Ku heterodimer and the DNA-dependent protein kinase catalytic subunit (DNA-PKcs) bind to the ends of the DNA double-strand break. Ku recruits not only DNA-PKcs to

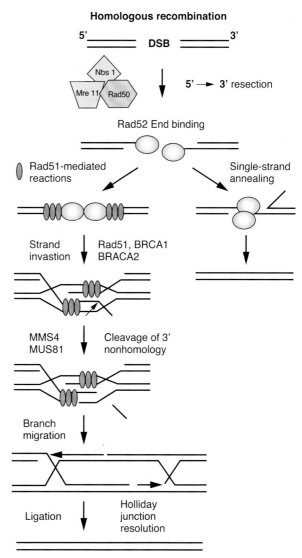

**Figure 13.6** Schematic of the critical steps and proteins involved in homologous recombination repair (HRR). The process of HRR can be divided into the following steps: double-strand break (DSB) targeting by H2AX and the MRN complex, recruitment of the ataxia-telangiectasia mutation (ATM) kinase, end processing and protection, strand exchange, single-strand gap filling, and resolution into unique double-stranded molecules.

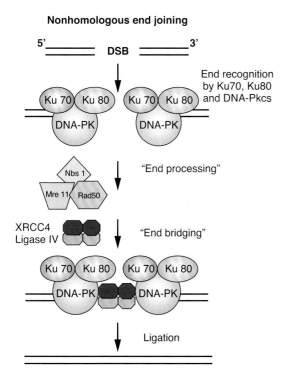

**Figure 13.5** Schematic of the critical steps and proteins involved in nonhomologous end joining (NHEJ). The process of NHEJ can be divided into at least four steps: synapsis, end processing, fill-in synthesis, and ligation. DSB, double-strand break.

the DNA ends, but also artemis, a protein that possesses endonuclease activity for 5′ and 3′ overhangs as well as hairpins.[17] DNA-PKcs that is bound to the broken DNA ends phosphorylates artemis and activates its endonuclease activity for end processing. This role of artemis' endonuclease activity in NHEJ may not necessarily be required for the ligation of blunt ends or ends with compatible termini. DNA polymerase μ is associated with the Ku/DNA/XRCC4/DNA ligase IV complex, and is probably the polymerase that is used in the fill-in reaction. The actual rejoining of DNA ends is mediated by a XRCC4/DNA ligase IV complex, which is also probably recruited by the Ku heterodimer.[18,19] Although NHEJ is effective at rejoining DNA double-strand breaks, it is highly error prone. In fact, the main physiologic role of NHEJ is to generate antibodies through V(D)J rejoining, and the error-prone nature of NHEJ is essential for generating antibody diversity.

*Homologous Recombination.* HRR provides the mammalian genome a high-fidelity pathway of repairing DNA double-strand breaks. In contrast to NHEJ, HRR requires physical contact with an undamaged DNA template, such as a sister chromatid, for repair to occur. In response to a double-strand break, ATM as well as the complex of Mre11, Rad50, and Nbs1 proteins (MRN complex), are recruited to sites of DNA double-strand breaks (Fig. 13.6).[20] The MRN complex is also involved in the recruitment of the breast cancer tumor suppressor gene, *BRCA1*, to the site of the break.[21] In addition to recruiting *BRCA1* to the site of the DNA strand break, Mre11 and as yet unidentified endonucleases resect the DNA, resulting in a 3′ single-strand DNA that serves as a binding site for Rad51. *BRCA2*, which is recruited to the double-strand break by BRCA1, facilitates the loading of the Rad51 protein onto replication protein A (RPA)-coated single-strand overhangs that are produced by endonuclease resection.[22] The Rad51 protein is a homolog of the *Escherichia coli* recombinase RecA, and possesses the ability to form nucleofilaments and catalyze strand exchange with the complementary strand of the undamaged chromatid, an essential step in HRR. Five additional paralogs of Rad51 also bind to the RPA-coated single-stranded region and recruit Rad52, which binds DNA and protects against exonucleolytic degradation.[23] To facilitate repair, the Rad54 protein uses its ATPase activity to unwind the double-stranded molecule. The two invading ends serve as primers for DNA synthesis, resulting in structures known as Holliday junctions. These Holliday junctions are resolved either by noncrossing over, in which case the Holliday junctions disengage and the DNA strands align followed by gap filling, or by crossing over of the Holliday junctions and gap filling. Because inactivation of most of the HRR genes discussed previously results in radiosensitivity and genomic instability, these genes provide a critical link between HRR and chromosome stability.

## Chromosome Aberrations Result from Faulty DNA Double-Strand Break Repair

Unfaithful restitution of DNA strand breaks can lead to chromosome aberrations such as acentric fragments (no centromeres) or terminal deletions (uncapped chromosome ends). Radiation-induced DNA double-strand breaks also induce exchange-type aberrations that are the consequence of symmetric translocations between two DNA double-strand breaks in two different chromosomes (Fig. 13.7). Symmetrical chromosome translocations often do not lead to lethality, because genetic information is not lost in subsequent cell divisions. In contrast, when two DNA double-strand breaks in two different chromosomes recombine to form one chromosome with two centromeres and two fragments of chromosomes without centromeres or telomeres, cell death is inevitable. These types of chromosome aberrations are the consequence of asymmetrical chromosome translocations where the genetic material is recombined in what has been termed an *illegitimate* manner (e.g., a chromosome containing an extra centromere).

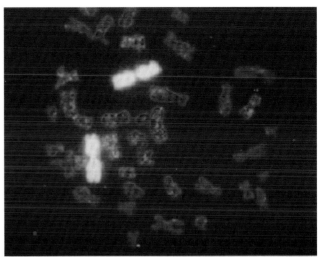
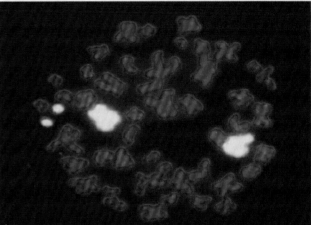

**Figure 13.7** Fluorescent in situ hybridization of DNA probes that specifically recognize chromosome 4. In unirradiated cells **(top)**, two chromosome 4s are visualized. In irradiated cells **(bottom)**, one chromosome 4 illegitimately recombined with another chromosome to produce an asymmetrical chromosome aberration, with resulting acentric fragments that will be lost in subsequent cell divisions.

During mitosis, when a cell divides, aberrant chromosomes that have two centromeres, lack a centromere, or are in the shape of a ring have difficulty in separating, resulting in daughter cells with unequal or asymmetric distribution of the parental genetic material. The quantification of asymmetric chromosome aberrations induced by radiation is difficult and has to be performed by the first cell division because these aberrations will be lost during subsequent cell divisions. For this reason, symmetrical chromosome aberrations have been used to assess radiation-induced damage many generations after exposure because they are not lost from the population of exposed cells. In fact, symmetrical chromosome aberrations can be detected in the descendants of survivors of Hiroshima and Nagasaki, indicating that they are stable biomarkers of radiation exposure.[24]

## Membrane Signaling

Apart from the direct of effects on DNA, radiation also affects cellular membranes. As part of the cellular stress response, radiation activates membrane receptor signaling pathways such those initiated via epidermal growth factor receptor (EGFR) and transforming growth factor β (TGF-β).[25,26] Activation of these pathways promotes overall survival in response to radiation by promoting DNA damage repair and/or cellular proliferation. In addition,

## Cellular Response to Genotoxic Stress

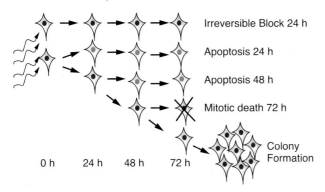

**Figure 13.8** Consequences of exposure to ionizing radiation at the cellular level. Cells exposed to ionizing radiation can enter a state of senescence where they are unable to divide, but are still able to secrete growth factors. Alternatively, cells can die through apoptosis, mitotic linked cell death, or they can repair their DNA damage and produce viable progeny.

radiation also induces ceramide production at the membrane via activation of sphingomyelinases, which hydrolyze sphingomyelin to form ceramide. Ceramide production is linked to radiation-induced apoptosis.[27]

## The Effect of Radiation on Cell Survival

The major potential consequences of cells exposed to ionizing radiation are normal cell division, DNA damage–induced senescence (reproductively inactive but metabolically active), apoptosis, or mitotic-linked cell death (Fig. 13.8). These manifestations of DNA damage can occur within one or two cell divisions or can manifest at later times after many cell divisions.[28] Effects that occur

at later times have been termed *delayed reproductive cell death* and may also be influenced by secreted factors that are induced in response to radiation.[29]

The ability to culture cells derived from both normal and tumor tissues has allowed us to gain insight into how radiosensitivity varies between tissues by analyzing the shape of survival curves. Survival curves of tumor cells often possess a shouldered region at low doses that becomes shallower as the dose increases and eventually becomes exponential. A shoulder on a survival means that these low doses of radiation are less efficient in cell killing, presumably because cells are efficient at repairing DNA strand breaks.[13,14] Killing at low doses of radiation can be described in the form of a linear quadratic equation: $S = e^{-\alpha D - \beta D^2}$ (Fig. 13.9).[30] In this equation, S is the fraction of cells that survive a dose (D) of radiation, whereas $\alpha$ and $\beta$ are constants. Cell killing by the linear and quadratic components are equal when $\alpha D = \beta D^2$ or $D = \alpha/\beta$. Over a larger dose range, the relationship between cell killing and dose is more complex and is described by three different components: an initial slope ($D_1$), a final slope ($D_0$), and the width of the shoulder (n, the extrapolation number) or Dq, the quasi-threshold dose (Fig. 13.10). The extrapolation number, n, defines the place where the shoulder intersects the ordinate when the dose is extrapolated to zero, and the quasithreshold dose, Dq, defines the width of the shoulder by cutting the dose axis when there is a survival fraction of unity. In contrast to photons, the shoulder on the survival curve disappears when cells are exposed to densely ionizing radiation from particles, indicating that this form of radiation is highly effective at killing cells at both low and high doses.

### In Vivo Survival Determination of Normal Tissue Response to Radiation

Although much of our knowledge on the effects of radiation on cell survival has come from cell culture studies, investigators have also devised experimental approaches to assess the clonogenic survival of normal tissues. The earliest example came from McCulloch and Till,[31] who developed an assay to measure the

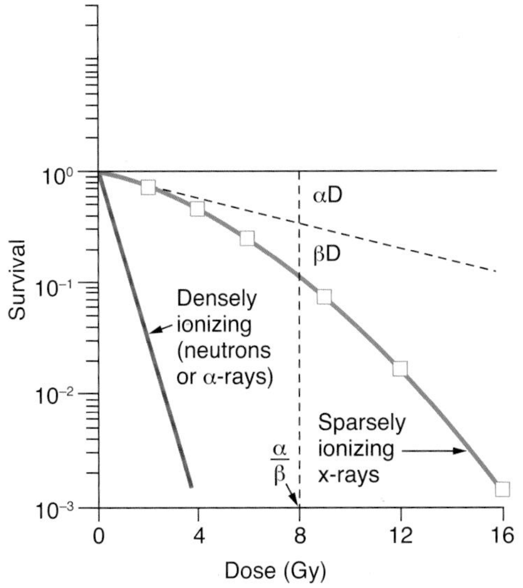

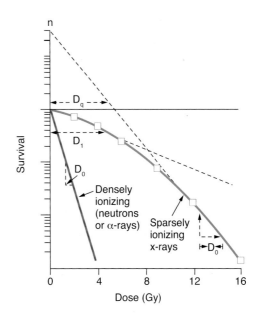

**Figure 13.9** An analysis of survival curves for mammalian cells exposed to radiation by the linear quadratic model. The probability of hitting a critical target is proportional to dose (aD): the alpha component. The probability of hitting two critical targets will be the product of those probabilities; therefore, it will be proportional to dose² ($\beta D^2$): the beta component. The dose at which killing by both the alpha and beta components is equal is defined as $D = \alpha/\beta$. (From Hall EJ, Giaccia AJ. *Radiobiology for the Radiologist.* Philadelphia: Lippincott Williams & Williams; 2012, with permission.)

**Figure 13.10** An analysis of survival curves for mammalian cells exposed to radiation by the multitarget model. This survival is described by an initial slope ($D_1$; dose to decreased survival to 37% on initial portion of the curve), a final slope ($D_0$; dose to decrease survival from starting point to 37% of that point on straight line portion of the curve), an extrapolation number (n; an estimate of the width of the shoulder), and a quasithreshold ($D_q$; a type of threshold dose below which radiation has no effect). (From Hall EJ, Giaccia AJ. *Radiobiology for the Radiologist.* Philadelphia: Lippincott Williams & Williams; 2012, with permission.)

clonogenic survival of bone marrow–derived cells in response to radiation by injecting them into a recipient mouse and quantifying the number of colonies that developed in the spleen. An analysis of these in vivo spleen assays indicated that bone marrow cells are highly radiosensitive (perhaps the most radiosensitive of all mammalian cells) in that their cell survival curve lacked a shoulder. These experiments represent two important firsts in the radiation sciences: They described the first development of an in vivo assay to assess normal tissue survival to radiation, and they demonstrated the first existence of normal tissue stem cells. Soon after, Withers and colleagues[32] developed an assay to assess the survival of skin stem cells, and Withers and Elkind[33] developed an assay to quantify the viability of small intestinal clonogens.

Because these ingenious approaches cannot be applied to all normal tissues, loss of tissue function instead of clonogenic survival has been used as an end point to assess radiation effects. Effects on tissue function can be grouped into the acute or late variety. Desquamation of skin by radiation is an example of an acute loss of function, whereas loss of spinal cord function is an example of a late functional effect. Acutely sensitive tissues such as skin, bone marrow, and intestinal mucosa possess a significant component of tissue cell division, whereas delayed sensitive tissues, such as spinal cord, breast, and bone, do not possess a significant amount of cell division or turnover and manifest radiation effects at later times.

### In Vivo Determination of Tumor Response to Radiation

Assays have also been developed to assess the clonogenic survival of tumor cells in animals. Perhaps the most relevant of these assays is the tumor control dose 50% ($TCD_{50}$) assay,[34] in which the dose of radiation needed to control the growth of 50% of the tumors is determined in large cohorts of tumor-bearing animals. The $TCD_{50}$ assay in animals most closely approximates the clinical situation because tumors are irradiated in animals and the ability to kill all viable tumor cells is assessed. Unlike assays in which tumor cells are irradiated ex vivo, the $TCD_{50}$ assay takes into account the effects of the tumor microenvironment on tumor response. In contrast to the $TCD_{50}$ assay, the tumor growth delay assay reflects the time after irradiation that a transplanted tumor reaches a fixed multiple of the pretreatment volume compared to an unirradiated control. This end point can be achieved by measuring tumor volume through the use of calipers or by a noninvasive measurement of tumor volume using bioluminescent molecules such as luciferase or fluorescent proteins. In the latter approach, all the tumor cells are stably transfected with a bioluminescent marker before implantation, and tumor growth is measured by bioluminescent activity.[35] The advantage of this approach is that tumor cells can be assessed even if they are orthotopically transplanted into their tissue of origin. In another approach, tumors or cells are first irradiated in vivo, the tumor is excised and made into a single-cell suspension, and these cells are then injected into a non–tumor-bearing animal. If the cells are injected subcutaneously under the skin, the end point is tumor formation.[36] If the tumor cells are injected in the tail vein of the mouse, the end point is colony formation in the lungs.[37] The major advantage of these assays is that the actual number of viable cells can be determined.

## FACTORS THAT AFFECT RADIATION RESPONSE

### The Fundamental Principles of Radiobiology

Studies on split-dose repair (SDR) by Elkind et al.[38] uncovered three of what we now recognize as the most fundamental principles of fractionated radiotherapy: repair, reassortment, and repopulation (Fig. 13.11). (Reoxygenation, described in the following paragraphs, is the fourth). SDR describes the increased survival

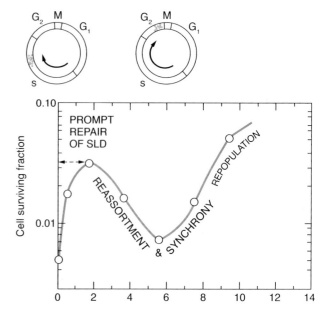

**Figure 13.11** Idealized survival curve of rodent cells exposed to two fractions of x-rays. This figure illustrates how the time interval between doses alters the sensitivity of cells when exposed to multiple fractions. In this case, cells move from a resistant phase of the cell cycle (late S phase) to a sensitive phase of the cell cycle (G2 phase). This is known as *reassortment*. If longer periods of time occur between fractions of radiation, cells will undergo division. This latter process is called *repopulation*. SLD, sublethal damage. (From Hall EJ, Giaccia AJ. *Radiobiology for the Radiologist*. Philadelphia: Lippincott Williams & Williams; 2012, with permission.)

or tumor growth delay found if a dose of radiation is split into two fractions compared to the same dose administered in one fraction. This repair is likely due to DNA double-strand break rejoining. Elkind et al. found that the survival of cells increased with an increase in time between doses for up to a maximum of about 6 hours. This finding is consistent with the clinical observation that a separation of radiation treatments by 6 hours produces similar normal tissue injury as a 24-hour separation. The shoulder of a survival curve is strongly influenced by SDR: The broader the shoulder, the more SDR and the smaller $\alpha/\beta$ ratio.

Similar to repair, reassortment and repopulation are also dependent on the interval of time between radiation fractions. If cells are given short time intervals between doses, they can progress from a resistant portion of the cell cycle (e.g., S phase) to a sensitive portion of the cell cycle (e.g., G2 phase). This transit between resistant and sensitive phases of the cell cycle is termed *reassortment*. If irradiated cells are provided even longer intervals of time between doses, the survival of the population of irradiated cells will increase. This increase in split-dose survival after longer periods of time is the result of cell division and has been termed *repopulation*. Reassortment and repopulation appear to have more protracted kinetics in normal tissues than rapidly proliferating tumor cells, and thereby enhance the tumor response to fractionated radiotherapy compared to normal tissues.

### Dose-Rate Effects

For sparsely ionizing radiation, dose rate plays a critical factor in cell killing. Lowering the dose rate, and thereby increasing exposure time, reduces the effectiveness of killing by x-rays because of increased SDR. A further reduction in dose rate results in more SDR and reduces the shoulder of the survival curve. Thus, if one plots the survival for individual doses in a multifraction experiment so that there is sufficient time for SDR to occur, the resulting survival curve would have little shoulder and appear almost linear.[39]

In some cell types, there is a threshold to the lowering of dose rate, and in fact, one paradoxically finds an increase, instead of a decrease, in cell killing. This increase in cell killing under these conditions of protracted dose rate is due to the accumulation of cells in a radiosensitive portion of the cell cycle. In summary, the magnitude of the dose rate effect varies between cell types because of SDR, the redistribution of cells through the cell cycle, and the time for cell division to occur.

## Cell Cycle

The phase of the cell cycle at the time of radiation influences the cell's inherent sensitivity to radiation. Cells synchronized in late G1/early S and G2/M phases are most sensitive, whereas cells in G1 and mid to late S phase are more resistant to radiation.[1] These differences in sensitivity during the cell cycle are exploited by the concept of reassortment during fractioned radiotherapy as well by the use of chemotherapeutic agents, which reassort cells into more sensitive phases of the cell cycle in combination with radiation.

## Tumor Oxygenation

The major microenvironmental influence on tumor response to radiation is molecular oxygen.[40] Decreased levels of oxygen (hypoxia) in tissue culture result in decreased killing after radiation, which can be expressed as an *oxygen enhancement ratio* (OER). Operationally, OER is defined as the ratio of doses to give the same killing under hypoxic and normoxic conditions. At high doses of radiation, the OER is approximately 3, whereas at low doses, it is closer to 2.[41] Oxygen must be present within 10 $\mu$s of irradiation to achieve its radiosensitizing effect. Under hypoxic conditions, damage to DNA can be repaired more readily than under oxic conditions, where damage to DNA is "fixed" because of the interaction of oxygen with free radicals generated by radiation. These changes in radiation sensitivity are detectable at oxygen ranges below 30 mm Hg. Most tumor cells exhibit a survival difference halfway between fully aerobic and fully anoxic cells when exposed to a partial pressure of oxygen between 3 and 10 mm Hg.[1] The presence of hypoxia has greater significance for single-dose fractions used in the treatment of certain primary tumors and metastases and is less important for fractionated radiotherapy, where reoxygenation occurs between fractions. Furthermore, most hypoxic cells are not actively undergoing cell division, thus impeding the efficacy of conventional chemotherapeutic agents that are targeted to actively dividing cells.

Although normal tissue and tumors vary in their oxygen concentrations, only tumors possess levels of oxygen low enough to influence the effectiveness of radiation killing. Although the variations in normal tissue oxygenation are in large part due to physiology governing acute changes in oxygen consumption, the variations in tumor oxygen can be directly attributed to abnormal vasculature that results in a more chronic condition. Thomlinson and Gray[42] observed that variations in tumor oxygen occur because there is insufficient vasculature to provide oxygen to all tumor cells. They hypothesized that oxygen is unable to reach tumor cells beyond 10 to 12 cell diameters from the lumen of a tumor blood vessel because of metabolic consumption by respiring tumor cells. This form of hypoxia caused by metabolic consumption of oxygen has been termed *chronic* or *diffusion-mediated hypoxia*. In contrast, changes in blood flow due either to interstitial pressure changes in tumor blood vessels that lack a smooth muscle component or red blood cell fluxes can cause transient occlusion of blood vessels resulting in *acute* or *transient hypoxia*. Chronically, hypoxic cells will only become reoxygenated when their distance from the lumen of a blood vessel decreases, such as during fractionated radiotherapy when tumor cords shrink. In contrast, tumor cells that are acutely hypoxic because of changes in blood flow or interstitial pressure often cycle in an unpredictable manner between oxic and hypoxic states as blood flow changes.

Based on studies demonstrating that hypoxia can alter radiation sensitivity and decrease tumor control by radiotherapy, strategies have been developed to increase tumor oxygenation. Most importantly, it appears that tumor oxygen levels increase during a course of fractionated radiation. This may be one of the most important benefits of fractionated radiation and is termed *reoxygenation* (the fourth of the four Rs of radiobiology). Tumor reoxygenation during a course of fractionated radiation may also offer an explanation for the general lack of clinical efficacy of hypoxic cell sensitizers despite the clear evidence that hypoxia causes radioresistance.

Aside from using fractionated radiation, the most direct approach to increasing tumor oxygenation is to expose patients receiving radiotherapy to hyperbaric oxygen therapy. The underlying concept is that increasing the amount of oxygen in the bloodstream should result in more oxygen being available for diffusion to the hypoxic regions of tumors. Experimentally, hyperbaric oxygen therapy increases the sensitivity of transplanted tumors to radiation. The results of clinical studies with hyperbaric oxygen therapy, when combined with radiotherapy, showed improvement for two sites—head and neck cancers, and cervix cancers—but failed to show an improvement with other sites, thus calling into question its general usefulness in radiotherapy.[43] In a related approach, erythropoietin (EPO), a hormone released by the kidney that increases red blood cell production, should also increase tumor oxygenation by increasing the delivery of hemoglobin-bound oxygen molecules. EPO has been effective at correcting anemia, but has not been successful in combination with radiation to control head and neck cancer and may, in fact, stimulate tumor growth.[44, 45]

Another strategy to increase tumor oxygenation has been the combined use of nicotinamide, which increases tissue perfusion and carbogen (95% $O_2$ and 5% $CO_2$) breathing (accelerated radiotherapy with carbogen and nicotinamide [ARCON] therapy). Recently, a randomized phase III clinical trial demonstrated improved regional but not local tumor control in larynx cancer patients treated with nicotinamide, carbogen, and radiation versus radiation alone.[46] Biologics such as antivascular endothelial growth factor (anti-VEGF) therapy have also been demonstrated to increase tumor oxygenation.[47] Anti-VEGF therapy may increase tumor oxygenation by eliminating abnormal vessels that are inadequate in perfusing tumor cells—the so-called *vascular normalization hypothesis*. Although there is solid experimental evidence to support this hypothesis, there appears to be only a short window of time in which it could be effectively combined with radiotherapy.

Because the presence of hypoxia has both prognostic and potential therapeutic implications, a substantial effort has been invested in trying to image hypoxia.[48] The goal of using imaging to "paint" radiation doses to different regions of tumors, although technically possible (as described in the next section, Radiation Physics), faces the problem that changes in oxygenation are dynamic.[49] In the future, hypoxia-directed treatment may evolve from the use of hypoxic cell cytotoxins to targeted drugs that exploit cellular signaling changes induced by hypoxia such as hypoxia-inducible factor 1$\alpha$ (HIF-1$\alpha$). However, despite the strong rationale supporting their use, at this time, there are no agents used in the clinic that target hypoxia.

## Immune Response

The abscopal effects of radiation (i.e., tumor cell killing outside of the radiation field) have been attributed to the activation of antigen and cytokine release by radiation, which subsequently activates a systemic immune response against tumor cells.[50,51] This response begins with the transfer of tumor cell antigens to dendritic cells and, subsequently, the activation of tumor-specific T cells and *immunogenic tumor cell death*. It is likely that radiation dose and fractionation influence the optimal immune response with higher doses and fewer fractions of radiation than those used in conventional fractionation schemes appearing superior in experimental models. Unfortunately, abscopal effects are uncommon because immune system evasion is an inherent characteristic of cancer cells that often dominates, even in the presence of a radiation-induced immune response. Strategies to amplify radiation-induced immune responses, and thus to overcome tumor cell evasion of the immune system, are under investigation. The combination of radiation with immune *checkpoint* modulators such as ipilimumab, an antibody against cytotoxic T-lymphocyte antigen 4 (CTLA-4), have shown promising, albeit anecdotal, clinical effects.

# DRUGS THAT AFFECT RADIATION SENSITIVITY

For over 30 years now, chemotherapy and radiotherapy have been administered concurrently. In order to maximize the efficacy of radiochemotherapy, it is necessary to understand the biologic mechanisms underlying radiosensitization by chemotherapeutic agents. The several classes of standard chemotherapeutic agents as well as novel molecularly targeted agents that possess radiosensitizing properties will be discussed in this section.

## Antimetabolites

5-fluorouracil is among the most commonly used chemotherapeutic radiation sensitizers. Given in combination with radiation, it has led to clinical improvements in a variety of cancers, including those of the head and neck, the esophagus, the stomach, the pancreas, the rectum, the anus, and the cervix. The combination of 5-fluorouracil with radiation is now a standard therapy for cancers of the stomach (adjuvant), the pancreas (unresectable), and the rectum. For other cancers such as head and neck, esophagus, or anal, 5-fluorouracil and radiation are combined with cisplatin or mitomycin C, respectively. Being an analog of uracil, 5-flourouracil is misincorporated into RNA and DNA. However, the ability of 5-fluorouracil to radiosensitize is related to its ability to inhibit thymidylate synthase, which leads to the depletion of thymidine triphosphate (dTTP) and the inhibition of DNA synthesis. This slowed, inappropriate progression through S phase in response to 5-fluorouracil is thought to be the mechanism underlying radiosensitization.[52] Similar to 5-fluorouracil, the oral thymidylate synthase inhibitor, capecitabine, is also being increasingly used in combination with radiation.

Gemcitabine (2′, 2′-deoxyfluorocytidine [dFdCyd]) is another potent antimetabolite radiosensitizer. Preclinical studies have demonstrated that radiosensitization by gemcitabine involves the depletion of deoxyadenosine triphosphate (dATP) (related to the ability of gemcitabine diphosphate (dFdCDP) to inhibit ribonucleotide reductase) as well as the redistribution of cells into the early S phase of the cell cycle.[53] The combination of gemcitabine with radiation in clinical trials has suggested improved clinical outcomes for patients with cancers of the lung, pancreas, and bladder. Gemcitabine-based chemoradiation has developed into a standard therapy for locally advanced pancreatic cancer. However, in some clinical trials, such as those in lung and head and neck cancers, the combination of gemcitabine with radiation has led to increased mucositis and esophagitis.[54] Thus, it should be emphasized that in the presence of gemcitabine, radiation fields must be defined with great caution. Such is the case with pancreatic cancer, where the combination of full-dose gemcitabine with radiation to the gross tumor can be safely administered if clinically uninvolved lymph nodes are excluded.[55] Conversely, the inclusion of the regional lymphatics in the treatment field in combination with full-dose gemcitabine produces unacceptable toxicities.[56]

## Platinums and Temozolomide

Cisplatin is likely the most commonly used chemotherapeutic agent in combination with radiation. Although cisplatin was the prototype for several other platinum analogs, carboplatin was also frequently used in combination with radiation. Cisplatin, in combination with radiation, and sometimes in conjunction with a second chemotherapeutic agent, is indicated for cancers of the head and neck, esophagus (with 5-fluorouracil), the lung, the cervix, and the anus. Radiosensitization by cisplatin is related to its ability to cause inter- and intra-strand DNA cross-links. Removal of these cross-links during the repair process results in DNA strand breaks. Although there are multiple theories to explain the mechanism(s) of radiosensitization by cisplatin, two plausible explanations are that cisplatin inhibits the repair (both homologous and nonhomologous) of radiation-induced DNA double-strand breaks and/or increases the number of lethal radiation-induced double-strand breaks.[57]

Temozolomide in combination with radiation is standard therapy for glioblastoma. Temozolomide is an alkylating agent, which forms methyl adducts at the $O^6$ position of guanine (as well as at $N^7$ and $N^3$-guanine) that are subsequently improperly repaired by the mismatch repair pathway. Radiosensitization by temozolomide involves the inhibition of DNA repair and/or an increase in radiation-induced DNA double-strand breaks due to radiation-induced single-strand breaks in proximity to $O^6$ methyl adducts. Like cisplatin, temozolomide-mediated radiosensitization does not seem to require cell cycle redistribution.

## Taxanes

The taxanes, paclitaxel and docetaxel, act to stabilize microtubules resulting in the accumulation of cells in G2/M, the most radiation-sensitive phase of the cell cycle. The radiosensitizing properties of the taxanes are thought to be attributable to the redistribution of cells into G2/M. Paclitaxel, in combination with radiation (and carboplatin), has demonstrated a clinical benefit in the treatment of resectable lung carcinoma.[58]

## Molecularly Targeted Agents

Molecularly targeted agents are especially appealing in the context of radiosensitization because they are generally less toxic than standard chemotherapeutic agents and need to be given in multimodality regimens (given their often inadequate efficacy as single agents). The EGFR has been intensely pursued as a target; both antibody and small molecule EGFR inhibitors, such as cetuximab and erlotinib, respectively, have been developed. The head and neck seem to be the most promising tumor sites for the combination of EGFR inhibitors with radiation therapy. Preclinical data have demonstrated that the schedule of administration of EGFR inhibitors with radiation is important; EGFR inhibition before chemoradiation may produce antagonism.[59] In a randomized phase III trial, cetuximab plus radiation produced a significant survival advantage over radiation alone in patients with locally advanced head and neck cancer.[60] In a subsequent trial, however, cetuximab in combination with concurrent, cisplatin-based chemoradiation failed to produce a survival benefit in head and neck cancer patients.[61] The combination of EGFR inhibitor with cisplatin-radiation requires further preclinical investigation.

Although EGFR inhibition, concurrent with radiation, is by far the best established combination of a molecularly targeted agent with radiation, other exciting molecularly targeted agents are being developed as radiation sensitizers. Targeting DNA damage response pathways is one approach to radiosensitization. Recently, agents that abrogate radiation-induced cell cycle checkpoints, such as Wee1 and Chk1 inhibitors, have been shown to radiosensitize tumor cells and are currently in clinical development in combination with chemotherapy, with clinical trials planned in combination with radiation.[62,63] In addition, poly(ADP-ribose) polymerase (PARP) inhibitors have been demonstrated to preclinically induce radiosensitization, and several clinical trials combining PARP inhibitors with radiation therapy are underway.[64]

## Other Agents

Although the most common clinically used agents in combination with radiation have been shown to produce significant clinical benefit, as described previously, other agents with different mechanisms of action have been used as radiation sensitizers as well as radiation protectors. The vinca alkaloids, such as vincristine, possess radiosensitizing properties due to their ability to block mitotic spindle assembly and, thus, arrest cells in M phase. Although vincristine is used in combination with radiation to treat medulloblastoma, rhabdomyosarcoma, and brain stem glioma, its use is principally based on its lack of myelosuppressive side effects, which are dose limiting for radiation in these types of tumors, rather than its potential radiosensitizing properties.

Also worth mention in a discussion of modulators of radiation sensitivity are agents designed to radioprotect normal tissues. One such type of drug, amifostine, is a free radical scavenger with some selectivity toward normal tissues that express more alkaline phosphatase than tumor cells, the enzyme of which converts amifostine to a free thiol metabolite. Clinical trials in head and neck as well as lung cancers have shown a reduction in radiation-related toxicities such as xerostomia, mucositis, esophagitis, and pneumonitis, respectively.[65,66] However, further clinical investigations are necessary to conclusively demonstrate a lack of tumor protection and safety in combination with chemoradiotherapy regimens.

## RADIATION PHYSICS

### Physics of Photon Interactions

Tumors requiring radiation can be found at depths ranging from zero to 10s of centimeters below the skin. The goal of treatment is to deliver sufficient ionizing radiation to the tumor site, which can result in an absorbed dose. This involves both the availability of treatment beams and delivery techniques, and the methods to plan the treatments and ensure their safe delivery. This section will establish the general physical basis for the use of ionizing radiation in the treatment of tumors, briefly describe some of the treatment equipment, indicate physical qualities of the treatment beams themselves, and summarize the treatment planning process. Those who desire more in-depth details are referred to textbooks and other resources dedicated to medical physics and the technologic aspects of radiation oncology.[67] Most patients who are treated with radiation receive high-energy, external-beam photon therapy. Here, *external* indicates that the treatment beam is generated and delivered from outside of the body. High-energy (6 to 20 MV) photon beams (electromagnetic radiation) penetrate tissue, enabling the treatment of deep-seated tumors. Modern equipment generates these beams with sufficient fluence to ensure delivery of therapeutic fractions of dose in short treatment sessions. Other types of particles and beams also exist for use in treating tumors both externally and internally. They are mentioned briefly later. However, as external photon beams dominate the practice (and as common basic physics principles related to delivered dose exist among the modalities), the focus here will be on photon beam generation and interactions in tissue.

As mentioned earlier, ionizing radiation kills cells via both direct and indirect mechanisms. Radiation therapy aims to instigate those ionizations and events in the tumor cells. Photons are massless, uncharged packets of energy that primarily interact with matter via electromagnetic processes. As a consequence of those interactions, an incident photon can become either entirely absorbed (giving up its energy to the ejection of an atomic electron [photoelectric effect]), or create an energetic electron-positron pair (pair production), or scatter off an electron with a reduction in energy and a change in direction and subsequent transfer of parts of its energy to the free electron (Compton scattering). The secondary electrons generated as a consequence of these interactions have residual energy, mass, and, most importantly, electric charge. They slow down in matter through multiple interactions with (primarily) the electrons of atoms, leading to excitation and ionization of those atoms. These ionizations (hence the term *ionizing radiation*) lead to a local absorption of energy (i.e., dose = energy absorbed per unit mass) and the direct and indirect cell killing effects necessary to treat tumors.

Thus, the use of external photon beams for cancer therapy involves a two-step process: interaction (scattering) of the photons, with subsequent dose deposition via the secondary electrons. The probability of photon interactions is energy dependent. Photoelectric interactions dominate at lower photon energies. Whereas these beams are ideal for diagnostic procedures (for their preferential absorption by tissues of differing atomic number, leading to good subject contrast), they are attenuated too quickly in tissues to supply enough interactions to be useful for therapy for any but the most superficial tumors. Pair production interactions dominate at higher photon energies; however, the probability of interacting in tissues for those high-energy photons is so low as to preclude them from general use as well. In the 10s to 100s of kiloelectron volt (keV) to the few megaelectron volt (MeV) photon energy range, Compton scattering dominates. As will be shown, these beams have sufficient penetration and can be generated with sufficient intensity to be useful for tumor treatments, especially when combined in treatment plans that comprise multiple beams entering the patient from different directions but overlapping at the tumor.

It is useful to point out physical scales of reference for external photon beam therapy. A typical megavoltage photon beam may have an average photon energy near 2 MeV. Those photons primarily undergo Compton scattering with a mean free path in tissue of approximately 20 cm. An average Compton interaction results in a secondary electron with a mean energy near 0.5 MeV (and a Compton scattered photon near 1.5 MeV, which likely escapes or scatters elsewhere in the patient). A typical secondary electron of approximately 0.5 MeV will cause excitations and ionizations of atoms as it dissipates its energy over a path length of approximately 2 mm. This could be expected to lead to approximately 10,000 ionizations, or about 5 ionizations per micron of tissue. As can be seen, therapeutic damage to the DNA of cancer cells (2 nm; see Fig. 13.2) will require very many Compton scatterings with statistical interaction among the ionizations resulting from the slowing down of the secondary electrons.

### Photon Beam Generation and Treatment Delivery

As previously mentioned, effective external-beam photon treatments require higher energy beams capable of reaching deep-seated tumors with sufficient fluence to make it likely that the dose deposition will kill the tumor cells. To spare normal tissues and maximize targeting, beams are arranged to enter the patient from several directions and to intersect at the center of the tumor (treatment isocenter). Although machines containing collimated beams from high-intensity radioactive sources (primarily cobalt 60 [$^{60}$Co]) are still in use, today's modern treatment machine accelerates electrons to high (MeV) energy and impinges them onto an x-ray production target, leading to the generation of intense beams of Bremsstrahlung x-rays. A typical photon beam treatment machine[68,69] (Fig. 13.12) consists of a high-energy (6 to 20 MeV) linear electron accelerator, electromagnetic beam steering and

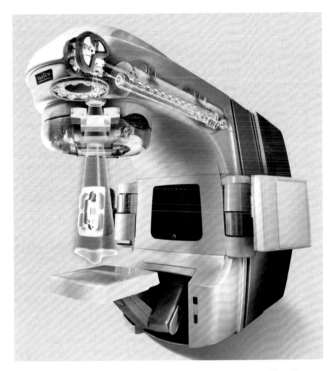

**Figure 13.12** A shadow view of a C-arm linear accelerator. The electron beam (originating at upper right) is accelerated through a linear accelerator wave guide, selected for correct energy in a bending magnet, and then impinges on an x-ray production target. The x-ray beam (originating at target upper left) is flattened and collimated before leaving the treatment head. Also illustrated (downstream from the beam) is an electric portal imager that is used to measure (image) the beam exiting a patient. (From Varian Medical Systems, Palo Alto, CA, with permission.)

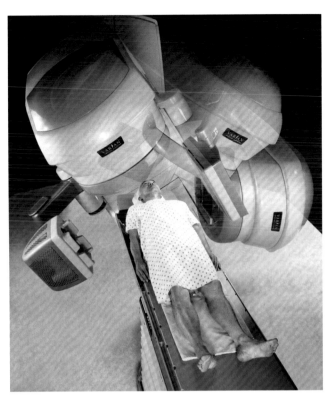

**Figure 13.13** Model in treatment position on the patient support table. The treatment delivery head on the gantry's C-arm rotates about the patient, enabling the delivery of beams throughout 360 degrees of rotation. (From Varian Medical Systems, Palo Alto, CA, with permission.)

monitoring systems, x-ray generation targets, high-density treatment field-shaping devices (collimators), and up to a ton of radiation shielding on a mechanical C-arm gantry that can rotate precisely around a treatment couch (Fig. 13.13). These treatment-delivery machines routinely maintain mechanical isocenters for patient treatments to within a sphere of 1 mm radius. The development of *stereotactic radiotherapy*, which will be described in the section titled Clinical Application of Types of Radiation, depends on this level of machine precision.

X-ray production by monoenergetic high-energy electrons results in an x-ray (photon) beam that contains a continuous spectrum of energies with maximum photon energy near that of the incident electron beam. Lower energy photons appear with a much greater probability than do the highest energy ones, but they also become preferentially filtered out of the beam through the absorption in the target and the attenuation in the flattening filter. This generally results in a treatment beam energy spectrum with a mean photon energy of approximately one-third of the initial electron beam energy. In this energy range, the resulting photon beam exits the production target with a narrow angular spread focused primarily in the forward direction. These forward-peaked intensity distributions generally need to be modulated (flattened) to produce a large (up to 40 cm diameter at the patient) photon beam with uniform intensity across the beam. All modern treatment units take advantage of extensive computer control, monitoring, and feedback to produce highly stable and reproducible treatment beams.

The resulting photon beam requires beam shaping for conformal dose delivery. Some combination of primary, high-density field blocks (collimators) together with additional edge blocks generally provide the required shaping and shielding. Modern machines use computer-controlled multileaf collimators (Fig. 13.14)

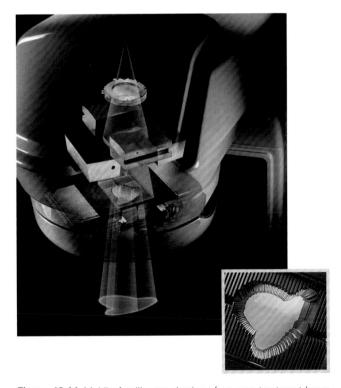

**Figure 13.14** Multileaf collimator shaping of an x-ray treatment beam from a linear accelerator. *Inset* shows a view of the multileaf collimator. (From Varian Medical Systems, Palo Alto, CA, with permission.)

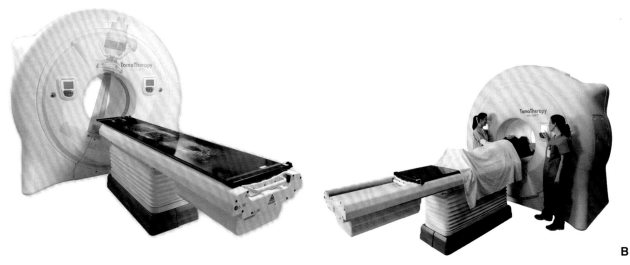

**A**                                                                                          **B**

**Figure 13.15** **(A)** A shadow view of linear accelerator, x-ray beam production system, and x-ray fan beam for helical tomotherapy treatment delivery. The beam production system rotates within its enclosed gantry. **(B)** The model patient on treatment table slides into the treatment unit. During treatment, the table moves as the collimated fan beam rotates about the patient, creating a modulated helical dose delivery pattern. (From TomoTherapy, Inc., Madison, WI, with permission.)

for the edge sculpting subsequent to setting the primary collimators for maximal shielding. This computer control provides high precision and reproducibility in the definition of field edges. Additionally, automation allows for a precise reshaping of the treatment beam for each angle of incidence, allowing not only conformation of irradiation to target volumes, but also modulation of the beam intensity patterns across the field (intensity-modulated radiation therapy [IMRT]).

Variations on the standard linear accelerator (linac) plus C-arm scenario that are being used for external-beam radiation treatments throughout the body include helical tomotherapy and nonisocentric miniature linac robotic delivery systems.[70] In helical tomotherapy, the accelerator, photon-production target, and collimation system are mounted on a ring gantry (similar to those found on diagnostic computed tomography [CT] scanners) (Fig. 13.15). It produces a fan beam of photons, and the intensity of each part of the fan being modulated by a binary collimator. As the gantry rotates, the patient simultaneously slides through the bore of the machine (again analogous to modern x-ray/CT imagers), which allows for the continuous delivery of intensity-modulated radiation in a helical pattern from all angles around a patient. Another delivery system uses an industrial robot to hold a miniature accelerator plus photon beam-production system (Fig. 13.16). The bulk of the system is reduced by keeping the field sizes small (spotlike). However, computer control of the robot provides flexibility in irradiating tumors from nearly any position external to the patient. The same control allows for the selection and use of many differing beam angles to build up the dose at the tumor location.

To take advantage of the precision of modern beam delivery, it is crucial to localize the patient's tumor and normal tissue.[71] This process can be divided into patient immobilization (i.e., limiting the motion of the patient) and localization (i.e., knowing the tumor and normal tissue location precisely in space). Although these concepts of immobilization and localization are related, they are not identical. Patients can be held reasonably comfortable in their treatment pose with the aid of foam molds and meshes (i.e., immobilization devices). Traditionally, localization has been achieved by indexing the immobilization device to the computer-controlled treatment couch and by using low-power laser beams aligned to skin marks. These techniques make it possible to reproducibly couple the surface of each patient with the treatment machine isocenter.

However, what is truly needed is to localize the tumor and normal tissues. The development of in-room, online x-ray, ultrasound, and infrared imaging equipment can now be used to ensure that the intended portions of each patient's internal anatomy are correctly positioned at the time of treatment. In particular, the development of rugged, low-profile, active matrix, flat-panel imaging devices, either attached to the treatment gantry or placed in the vicinity of the treatment couch, together with diagnostic x-ray generators or the patient treatment beam (see Fig. 13.13), allows the digital capture of projection x-ray images of patient anatomy with respect to the isocenter and treatment field borders. These digitized electronic images are immediately available for analysis. Software tools allow for a comparison to reference images and the generation of correction coordinates, which are in turn available for downloading to the treatment couch for automated fine adjustment of the patient's treatment position. Other precise localization systems rely on the identification of the positions of small, implanted radiopaque markers or other types of *smart* position-reporting devices. Careful use of these image-guided radiation

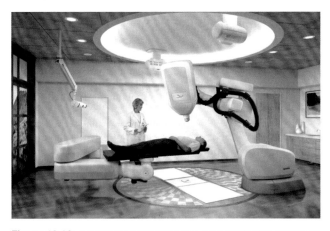

**Figure 13.16** A miniature accelerator plus x-ray production system on a robotic delivery arm. Both the treatment table and the treatment head is set by a computer for multiple arbitrary angles of incidence. (From Accuray, Sunnyvale, CA, with permission.)

therapy (IGRT) systems[71, 72] can result in the repeated reducibility of patient position to within a few millimeters over a 5- to 8-week course of treatment.

The final part of external-beam patient treatment is dose delivery. All modern treatment units have computer monitoring (and often control) of all mechanical and dose-delivery components. Treatment-planning information (treatment machine parameters, treatment field configurations, dose per treatment field segment) is downloaded to a work station at the treatment unit that first assists with and then records treatment. This information, together with the readbacks from the treatment machine, are used to reproducibly set up and then verify each patient's treatment parameters, which prevents many of the variations that used to occur when all treatment was performed simply by following instructions written in a treatment chart.

## Treatment Beam Characteristics and Dose-Calculation Algorithms

Beyond a basic understanding of the interactions of ionizing radiation with matter lies the requirement of being able to characterize the treatment beams for purposes of planning and verifying treatments. By virtue of a few underlying principles, this generally can be accomplished via a two-step process of absolute calibration of the dose at some reference point in a phantom (i.e., measurement media representative of a patient's tissues), with relative scaling of dose values in other parts of the beam or phantom with respect to that point.

As mentioned earlier, the predominant mode of interaction for therapeutic energy photon beams in tissuelike materials is through Compton scattering. The probability of Compton scattering events is primarily proportional to the relative electron density of the media with which they interact. Because many body tissues are waterlike in composition, it has been possible to make photon beam dosimetric measurements in phantoms consisting mostly of water (water tanks) or tissue-equivalent plastic and to then scale the interactions via relative electron density values (for example, as can be derived from computed x-ray/CT) to other waterlike materials. Thus, the relative fluence of photons in a therapeutic treatment beam is attenuated as it passes through a phantom, primarily via Compton scattering.

It was stated earlier that the photon beam is generated at a small region in the head of the machine. That fluence of photons spreads out through the collimating system before reaching the patient. Thus, without any interactions (e.g., if the beam were in a vacuum), the number of photons crossing any plane perpendicular to the beam direction would remain constant. However, the cross-sectional area of the plane gets larger the farther it is located from the source point. In fact, both the width and length of the cross-sectional area increase in proportion to the distance from the source, and thus the area increases in proportion to the square of the distance. This means that the primary photon fluence per unit area in a plane perpendicular to the beam direction of a pointlike source also decreases as one over the square of the distance, the so-called $1/r^2$ reduction in fluence as a function of distance, r, from the source.

Thus, we have two processes, attenuation and $1/r^2$ reduction, which reduce the photon fluence from an external therapeutic beam as a function of depth in a patient. There is also a process that can increase the photon fluence at a point downstream. Recall that Compton scattering interactions lead not only to secondary electrons (which are responsible for deposition of dose), but also to Compton scattered photons. These photons are scattered from the interaction sites in multiple, predominantly forward-looking directions. Thus, Compton-scattered photons originating from many other places can add to the photon fluence at another point. As the irradiated area (field size) increases, the amount of scattered radiation also increases.

As mentioned earlier, dose *deposition* is a two-step process of photon interaction (proportional to the local fluence of photons) and energy transfer to the medium via the slowing down of secondary electrons. Thus, the point where a photon interacts is not the place where the dose is actually deposited, which happens over the track of the secondary electron. Dose has a very strict definition of energy *absorbed* per unit mass (i.e., due to the slowing down charged particles) and should be distinguished from the energy released at a point, defined as kerma (e.g., energy transfer from the scattering incident photon). Thus, although the photon beam fluence will always be greatest at the entrance to a patient or phantom, the actual *absorbed dose* for a megavoltage photon beam builds up over the first couple of centimeters, reaching a maximum (d-max) at a depth corresponding to the range of the higher energy Compton electrons set in motion. This turns out to be a second desirable characteristic of these beams (beyond their ability to treat deep-seated lesions), because the dose to the skin (a primary dose-limiting structure in earlier times) is greatly reduced.

The relative distributions of dose, normalized to an absolute dose measurement (using a small thimblelike air ionization chamber at a standard depth and for a standard field size according to nationally and internationally accepted protocols), are the major inputs into treatment-planning systems. The major features of these distributions are (1) the initial dose buildup up to a depth of d-max, with a more gradual drop off in dose as a function of depth into the phantom due to the attenuation and $1/r^2$ factors at deeper depths (relative depth dose), and (2) the shape of the dose in the plane perpendicular to the direction of the beams; both as a function of field size. Central axis depth dose curves for typical external photon beams are shown in Figure 13.17 for two beam energies and for both a large and smaller field size. Notice both the expected increase in penetration with increasing beam energy and the increase in dose at a particular depth with increasing field size; the latter effect due to increased numbers of secondary Compton-scattered photons for larger irradiated areas. The change in dose perpendicular to the central axis is less remarkable, because the beams are designed to be uniform across a field as a function of depth.

It is useful to also point out the depth dose characteristics of clinical external treatment beams produced using ionizing

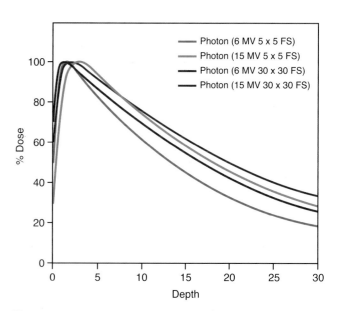

**Figure 13.17** Sample depth-dose curves (change in delivered dose as a function of depth) along the central axis of some typical photon treatment beams for low (6 MV) and intermediate (15 MV) energy beams, and large (30 × 30 cm²) and smaller (5 × 5 cm²) field sizes (FS).

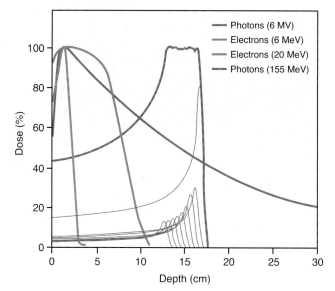

**Figure 13.18** Sample depth-dose curves along the central axis of some typical charged particle treatment beams compared with that of a 6-MV proton beam. The spread out Bragg peak at the end of the 155-MeV proton beam (*thick pink curve*) is a composite dose deposition pattern from the addition of the multiple range-shifted proton curves (*thinner pink curves*).

radiations other than photons, primarily through the direct use of charged particles. Those beams (Fig. 13.18) illustrate interesting characteristics, which, when added to the options available for treatment planning (or used by themselves), can produce advantageous results. Relative to the photon beam, the direct use of electron beams leads to deposition of dose over a more localized range, but at the expense of a relative lack of penetration. Thus, electron beams are most widely used for treating, or boosting the treatment of, more superficial tumors and regions (see the section titled Clinical Application of Types of Radiation). The heavier charged particle beams (protons and carbon ions) appear to exhibit even more interesting *depth-dose* characteristics, with the advantage of both (when necessary) being highly penetrating and also lacking a significant dose beyond a certain depth (a depth that can be controlled and purposefully placed, for example, at the distal edge of a target volume).

The results of measurements such as these have been modeled so as to develop dose-calculation algorithms used in treatment-planning systems. These models all use measured beam data to set or adjust parameters used by those algorithms in their dose-distribution computations. Because most of the input data used for beam fitting come from measurements in water phantoms (or waterlike plastic phantoms), patient-specific adjustments are needed for the water phantom data to account for both geometry and tissue properties. It is the task of the dose-calculation algorithms to take those changes into account. The accuracy and precision actually realized for all dose-calculation algorithms generally need to be traded off against the time required to complete the calculation. Although the availability of ever more powerful computers has made calculation time less of a concern for broad, open-beam treatment planning, issues still remain for more specialized planning exercises that use many small beams or parts of beams such as IMRT (discussed later). Typically, relative dose distributions can be computed within patients on the scale of a few millimeters with a precision of better than a few percentage points.

An important area of research is the development of treatment-planning systems that calculate dose based on the principles of how radiation interacts with tissues, rather than simply by fitting data. These approaches use Monte Carlo techniques,[71,73] which

build a dose distribution by summing the calculated paths of thousands of photons and scattered electrons. This approach is more accurate than beam-fitting algorithms in regions of differing tissue densities, such as the lung, and therefore, will ultimately replace the current generation of treatment-planning systems, particularly for complex conditions. However, the time to perform these calculations is still prohibitive for a clinic, and it is anticipated that Monte Carlo calculations will be introduced over a period of years by balancing the need for accuracy in a particular clinical situation with the need to initiate patient treatment.

## TREATMENT PLANNING

As discussed in the previous section, single-treatment beams usually deposit more of the dose closer to where they enter the patient than they do at depths corresponding to where a deep-seated tumor might be located. The use of multiple beams entering the patient from different directions that overlap at the target produces more dose per unit volume throughout the tumor volume than is received by normal tissues. In fact, as noted earlier, the treatment-delivery machines are designed to make this easy to accomplish. Planning patient treatments under these circumstances should be a somewhat trivial matter of first selecting a sufficient number of beam angles to realize the desired buildup of the dose in the overlap region relative to the doses in the upstream parts of each beam, and then second, designing beam apertures that shape the edges of the beams to match the target. However, dose-limiting normal tissues often also lie in the paths of one or more of the beams. These normal tissues are often more sensitive to radiation damage than the tumor, and regardless, it is best practice to minimize the dose in any case as a general principle. Computerized treatment-planning systems function to develop patient-specific anatomic or geometric models and then use these models together with the beam-specific dose deposition properties (derived from phantom measurements, as previously described) to select beam angles, shapes, and intensities that meet an overall prescribed objective. That is, modern radiation oncology dose prescriptions contain both tumor and normal tissue objectives, and the modern computerized treatment-planning systems make it possible to design treatments that meet these objectives.

The development and use of three-dimensional (3D) models of each patient's anatomy, treatment geometry, and dose distribution led to a paradigm shift in radiation therapy treatment planning. Computerized radiation treatment planning began in the 1980s as a mainly x-ray/CT–based reconstruction of 3D geometries from information manually contoured on multiple two-dimensional (2D) transverse CT images. Today, these models often incorporate imaging data from multiple sources. Geometrically accurate anatomic information from an x-ray/CT scan still anchors these studies (as well as provides tissue density information necessary for dose calculations). However, it is now quite common to also register the CT data set with other studies such as magnetic resonance imaging (MRI), which may add anatomic detail for soft tissues, or functional MRI or positron emission tomography (PET) studies,[74,75] which provide physiologic or molecular information about tumors and normal tissues. Once registered with each other, the unique or complementary information from each data set can be fused for inspection and incorporated into the design of each patient's target and normal tissue volumes (Fig. 13.19). Beyond the ability to more fully define the extent of the primary target volume (for instance, as the encompassing envelope of disease appreciated on all the imaging studies) lies the ability to define subvolumes of the tumor volume that might be appropriate for simultaneous treatment to higher dose. For example, it should soon become possible to define different biologic components of the tumor that could potentially be targeted and then monitored for response using these same imaging techniques.[76]

Current treatment planning makes the tacit assumption that the planning image yields "the truth" about the location and condition

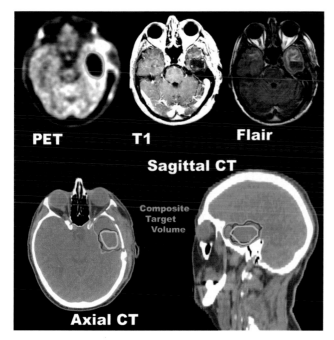

**Figure 13.19** An illustration of the brain tumor target volume delineated on coregistered nuclear medicine and magnetic resonance imaging studies fused with computed tomography (CT) data for treatment planning. PET, positron emission tomography.

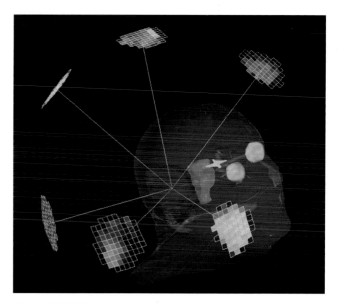

**Figure 13.20** Six intensity-modulated treatment ports planned for treatment of a brain tumor (*large object in red*). Differing intensities of the 5 × 5 mm *beamlets* in each port illustrated by gray scale (brighter beamlet = higher intensity). The computer optimization of the beamlet intensities is designed to generate a delivered dose distribution that will conform to the tumor region, yet avoid critical normal tissues such as the brain stem (*dark pink*), optic chiasm (*green*), and optic nerves (*red tubular structures*).

of tumors and normal tissues throughout the course of treatment. However, this ignores the complexity inherent in attempting to build accurate 3D models from multimodality imaging for purposes of planning patient treatments. First, patients breathe and undergo other physiologic processes during a single treatment, changes that require dynamic modeling or other methods of accounting for the changes. Furthermore, the patient's condition may change over time (and hence their model). Thus, a complete design and assessment of a patient undergoing high-precision treatment requires the construction of four-dimensional (4D) patient models. Indeed, the recent ready availability of multidetector CT scanners with subsecond gantry rotations, and even more recently, the availability of cone-beam CT capabilities on the radiation therapy treatment simulators and treatment machines themselves, now makes it possible to construct 4D patient models. A very active area of physics research[72,75] deals with IGRT, including the formation of 4D patient models (including distortions and changes in anatomy) of the motion over time and the determination of the accumulated dose received by a moving tumor as well as the surrounding normal tissues such as uninvolved lung.

Complementary to the availability of these patient and dose models has come a much better understanding of the doses safely tolerated by normal tissues adjacent to a tumor volume (e.g., spinal cord) or surrounding it (e.g., brain, lung, liver).[77] Indeed, not only has knowledge of whole organ tolerances to irradiation been obtained, but it has also become possible to characterize in some detail the complex dependence of the probability of incurring a complication with respect to the highly (intentionally) inhomogeneous dose distributions these normal tissues receive as part of the planning process designed to avoid treating them. Modeling partial organ tolerances to irradiation is of great use in planning patient treatments because it enables[78] integration and manipulation of variable dose and volume distributions with respect to possible clinical outcomes.

Making the vast amount of tumor and normal tissue information useful for planning treatments requires equally sophisticated new ways of planning and delivering dose, potentially preferentially targeting subvolumes of the tumor regions or specifically

avoiding selected portions of adjacent organs at risk. As mentioned earlier, modern treatment machines are capable of either varying the intensity of the radiation across each treatment port or projecting many small beams at a targeted region. This modulation of beam intensities (IMRT) from a given beam direction, together with the use of multiple beams (or parts of beams) from different directions, gives many degrees of freedom to create highly sculpted dose distributions, given that a system for designing the intensity modulation is available. Much computer programming and computational analysis has gone into the design of treatment-planning optimization systems to perform these functions.[79,80]

In IMRT, as most often applied, each treatment beam portal is broken down into simple basic components called beamlets, typically 0.5 to 1 cm × 1 cm in size, evenly distributed on a grid over the cross-section of each beam. Optimization begins with precomputation of the relative dose contribution that each of these beamlets gives to every subportion of tumor and normal tissue that the beamlet traverses as it goes through the patient model. Sophisticated optimization engines and search routines then iteratively alter the relative intensities of each beamlet in all the beams to minimize a cost function associated with target and normal tissue treatment goals. These, often hundreds of beamlets (each with its own intensity) (Fig. 13.20), provide the necessary flexibility and degrees of freedom to create dose distributions that can preferentially irradiate subportions of targets and also produce sharp dose gradients to avoid nearby organs at risk (Fig. 13.21). The cost-function approach also facilitates the ability to include factors such as the normal tissue and tumor-response models, mentioned previously in the optimization process, thus integrating the overall effects of the complex dose distributions across whole organ systems or target volumes within the planning process.

## OTHER TREATMENT MODALITIES

Other types of external-beam radiation treatments use atomic or nuclear particles rather than photons. Beams of fast neutrons have been used for some cancers,[81] primarily because of the

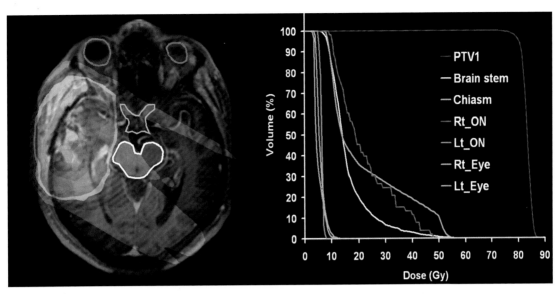

**Figure 13.21** Resulting isodose distribution for an optimized intensity-modulated brain treatment. Dose-intensity pattern in the *left panel* is overlaid on the patient's magnetic resonance images used in planning. Also contoured are the optic chiasm (*green*), the brain stem (*white*), and the eyes (*orange*). In the *right panel*, the dose distribution throughout all slices of the patient's anatomy is summarized via cumulative dose-volume histograms for the various tissues and volumes that have been previously segmented. Each location on each curve represents the fraction of the volume of that tissue (%) that receives greater than or the same as the corresponding dose level.

dense ionization patterns they produce as they slow down in tissue (making cell killing less dependent on the indirect effect previously discussed). Being uncharged particles, neutron beams of therapeutic energy penetrate in tissue (have depth-dose characteristics) similar to photon beams, but with denser dose deposition in the cellular scale. Most other external-beam treatments use charged particles, primarily either electrons[82] (produced on the same machines used for photon beam treatments) or protons or heavier particles such as carbon ions.[83,84] The latter beams have desirable dose-deposition properties (see Fig. 13.18), because they can spare tissues downstream from the target volume and generally give less overall dose to normal tissue. There can also be some radiobiologic advantage to the heavier charged particle beams, similar to neutrons. The generation and delivery of proton beams and heavier charged particle beams generally requires an accelerator (in its own vault) plus a beam transport system and some sort of treatment nozzle, often located on an isocentric gantry. The cost of the accelerator is generally leveraged by having it supply beams to multiple treatment rooms, but these units still cost many times that of a standard linear accelerator.

Brachytherapy[85] is a form of treatment that uses direct placement of radioactive sources or materials within tumors (interstitial brachytherapy) or within body or surgical cavities (intracavitary brachytherapy), either permanently (allowing for full decay of short-lived radioactive materials) or temporarily (either in one extended application or over several shorter term applications). The ability to irradiate tumors from close range (even from the inside out) can lead to conformal treatments with low normal tissue doses. The radioactive isotopes most generally used for these treatments are contained within small tubelike or seedlike sealed source enclosures (which prevents direct contamination). They emit photons (gamma and x-rays) during their decay, which penetrate the source cover and interact with tissue via the same physical processes as described for external-beam treatments. The treatments have the advantage of providing a high fluence (and dose) very near each source that drops in intensity as 1 over the square of the distance from the source ($1/r^2$). Radioactive sources decay in an exponential fashion characterized by their individual half-lives. After each half-life ($T_{1/2}$) the strength of each source decreases by half. Brachytherapy treatments are further generally classified into the two broad categories of low–dose-rate and

high–dose-rate treatments. Low–dose-rate treatments attempt to deliver tumoricidal doses via continuous irradiation from implanted sources over a period of several days. High–dose-rate treatments use one or more higher activity sources (stored external to the patient) together with a remote applicator or source transfer system to give one or more higher dose treatments on time scales and schedules more like external-beam treatments.

Isotopes for brachytherapy treatments are selected on the basis of a combination of specific activity (i.e., how much activity can be achieved per unit mass [i.e., to keep the source sizes small]), the penetrating ability of the decay photons (together with the $1/r^2$ fall off determines how many sources or source location will be required for treatment), and the half-life of the radioactive material (which must be accounted for in computation of dose, but also determines how often reusable sources will need to be replaced). Table 13.1 lists those isotopes most commonly used, along with some of their primary applications.

The dose-deposition patterns surrounding each type of source can be measured or computed. These data (or the parameterization

### TABLE 13.1

### Common Isotopes for Brachytherapy Treatment

| Isotope | Form | Primary Applications |
|---------|------|----------------------|
| $^{125}$I | Implantable sealed seed | LDR: Permanent prostate implants, brain implants, tumor bed implants, eye plaques |
| $^{192}$Ir | Implantable sealed seed | LDR: Interstitial solid tumor treatments |
| $^{192}$Ir | High activity sealed source on a remote transfer wire | HDR: Intracavitary GYN treatments, intraluminal irradiations |
| $^{137}$Cs | Sealed source tubes | LDR: Intracavitary GYN treatments |

LDR, low-dose rate; HDR, high-dose rate; GYN, gynecologic; $^{137}$Cs, caesium-137.

of same) can be stored within a computerized treatment-planning system. Planning a brachytherapy treatment-delivery scheme (desirable source strengths and arrangements) proceeds within the planning system by distributing the sources throughout the treatment area and having the computer add up the contributions of each source to designated tumor and normal tissue locations (e.g., obtained from a CT scan). Source strengths or spacing can be adjusted until an acceptable result is obtained. Indeed, optimization systems are now routinely used to fine tune this process.

Other types of therapeutic treatments with internal sources of ionizing radiation, generally classified as systemic targeted radionuclide therapy (STaRT), use antibodies or other conjugates or carriers such as microspheres to selectively deliver radionuclides to cancer cells.[86] Computing the effective dose to tumors and normal tissues via these techniques requires information on how much of the injected activity reaches the targets (biodistribution) as well as the energy and decay properties of the radionuclide being delivered. Imaging techniques and computer models are aiding in these computations.

# CLINICAL APPLICATIONS OF RADIATION THERAPY

In contrast to surgical oncology and medical oncology, which focus on early- or late-stage disease, respectively, the field of radiation oncology encompasses the1p8.49 entire spectrum of oncology. Board certification requires 5 years of postdoctoral training, typically beginning with an internship in internal medicine or surgery, followed by 4 years of radiation oncology residency. Education, as defined by leaders in the field,[87] begins with a thorough knowledge of the biology, physics, and clinical applications of radiation. It also includes training in the theoretical and practical aspects of the administration of radiation protectors and anticancer agents used as radiation sensitizers and the management of toxicities resulting from those treatments. In addition, residents receive education in palliative care, supportive care, and symptom and pain management. This training is in preparation for a practice that, in a given week, might include patients with a 2-mm vocal cord lesion or a 20-cm soft tissue sarcoma, both of whom can be treated with curative intent, as well as a patient with widely metastatic disease who needs palliative radiation, medical care for pain and depression, and discussion of end-of-life issues. More than 50% of (nonskin) cancer patients receive radiation therapy during the course of their illness.[88]

## Clinical Application of Types of Radiation

Electrons are now the most widely used form of radiation for superficial treatments. Because the depth of penetration can be well controlled by the energy of the beam, it is possible to treat, for instance, skin cancer, a small part of the breast while sparing the underlying lung, or the cervical lymph nodes but not the spinal cord, which lies several centimeters more deeply. Superficial tumors, such as of skin cancers, can also be treated very effectively with low-energy (kilovoltage) photons, but their use has decreased because a separate machine is required for their production.

The main form of treatment for deep tumors is photons. As described in the Radiation Physics section, photons spare the skin and deposit dose along their entire path until the beam leaves the body. The use of multiple beams that intersect on the tumor permit high doses to be delivered to the tumor with a relative sparing of normal tissue. The pinnacle of this concept is IMRT, which uses hundreds of beams and can treat concave shapes with relative sparing of the central region (see Figs. 13.20 and 13.21). However, as each beam continues on its path beyond the tumor, this use of multiple beams means that a significant volume of normal tissue receives a low dose. There has been considerable debate concerning the magnitude of the risk of second cancers produced by radiating large volumes with low doses of radiation.[89] Charged particle beams (proton and carbon, in this discussion) differ from photons in that they interact only modestly with tissue until they reach the end of their path, where they then deposit the majority of their energy and stop (the Bragg peak; see Fig. 13.18). This ability to stop at a chosen depth decreases the region of low dose. The chief form of charged particle used today is the proton. In the decade from 1980 to 1990, proton therapy could deliver higher doses of radiation to the target than photon therapy because protons could produce a more rapid fall off of dose between the target and the critical normal tissue (e.g., tumor and brain stem). Therefore, initially, their main application was in the treatment uveal melanomas, base-of-skull chondrosarcomas, and chordomas. In contrast, today's IMRT photons are more conformal in the high-dose region than protons due to the range uncertainty of the latter.[90] Thus, it seems unlikely that protons will permit a higher target dose to be delivered than photons. In contrast, protons have the potential to decrease regions of low dose. This would be of particular advantage in the treatment of pediatric malignancies, where low doses of radiation would tend to increase the chance of second cancers and could affect neurocognitive function in the treatment of brain tumors.

A carbon ion beam has an additional potential biologic advantage over protons. As discussed in the section Biologic Aspects of Radiation Oncology, hypoxic cells, which are found in many tumors, are up to 3 times more resistant to photon or proton radiation than well-oxygenated cells. In contrast, hypoxia does not cause resistance to a carbon beam. Whether hypoxia is a cause of clinical resistance to fractionated radiation is still debated.[91] A carbon beam is available at a few sites in Europe and Japan.

Two major issues have affected the widespread acceptance of protons. The most widely recognized is cost. Proton (approximately $120 million) and carbon beam facilities (in excess of $200 million) are substantially more expensive than a similar-sized photon facility (approximately $25 million). The operating costs appear to be significantly higher as well. Although the majority of patients who have received proton therapy have prostate cancer, there is no evidence that protons produce superior results to those obtained with IMRT planned photons.[92,93] The lack of solid evidence that protons are superior to photons for any disease site and the magnitude of these costs are of societal importance.[94] Although less expensive single gantry proton units are under construction, there are no functioning units at the time of this writing. A second, less well-appreciated issue concerns the need to develop full integration of charged particle beams with IGRT, as has already been accomplished with photons, although this feature is being incorporated into second-generation proton units.

Neutron therapy attracted significant interest in the 1980s, based on the principle that it would be more effective than photons against hypoxic cells that some have thought are responsible for radiation resistance of tumors. The effectiveness of neutron therapy has been limited by initial difficulties with collimation and targeting, although there is evidence that they have a role in the treatment of refractory parotid gland tumors.[95]

Brachytherapy refers to the placement of radioactive sources next to or inside the tumor. The chief sites where brachytherapy plays a role are in prostate and cervical cancer, although it has applications in head and neck cancers, soft tissue sarcomas, and other sites. In the case of prostate cancer, most experience is with low–dose-rate permanent implants using iodine-125 ($^{125}$I) or, more recently, palladium-103 ($^{103}$Pd). Over the last 5 years, there has been an increasing emphasis on improving the accuracy of seed placement, guided by ultrasound and confirmed by CT or MRI, and in skilled hands, outstanding results can be achieved.[96] In the case of cervical cancer, high–dose-rate treatment, which can be performed in an outpatient setting, has essentially replaced low–dose-rate treatment, which typically requires general anesthesia and a 2-day hospital stay. The results from both techniques appear to be approximately equivalent.

Yttrium microspheres represent a distinct form of brachytherapy. These spheres carry yttrium-90 ($^{90}$Y), a pure beta emitter with a range of about 1 cm. These have been used to treat both primary hepatocellular cancer and colorectal cancer metastatic to the liver (hepatic arterial or systemic chemotherapy) by administration through the hepatic artery.

## TREATMENT INTENT

Radiation doses are chosen so as to maximize the chance of tumor control without producing unacceptable toxicity. The dose of radiation required depends on the tumor type, the volume of disease (number of tumor cells), and the use of radiation-modifying agents (such as chemotherapeutic drugs used as radiation sensitizers). Except for a subset of tumors that are exquisitely sensitive to radiation (e.g., seminoma, lymphoma), doses that are required are often close to the tolerance of the normal tissue. A key fact driving the choice of dose is that a 1-cm$^3$ tumor contains approximately 1 billion cells. It follows that the reduction of a tumor that is 3 cm in diameter to 3 mm, which would be called a complete response by CT scan, would still leave 1 million tumor cells. Because each radiation fraction appears to kill a fixed fraction of the tumor, the dose to cure occult disease needs to be more similar to the dose for gross disease than one might otherwise expect. Thus, radiation doses (using the standard fractionation) of 45 to 54 Gy are typically used in the adjuvant setting when there is moderate suspicion for occult disease, 60 to 65 Gy for positive margins or when there is a high suspicion for occult disease, and 70 Gy or more for gross disease.

It is common during the course of radiation to give higher doses of radiation to regions that have a higher tumor burden. For example, regions that are suspected of harboring occult disease may be targeted to receive (in once daily 2-Gy fractions) 54 Gy, whereas, to control the gross tumor, the goal may be to administer a total dose of 70 Gy. Because the gross tumor will invariably reside within the region at risk for occult disease, it has become standard practice to deliver 50 Gy to the entire region, and then an additional *boost* dose of 20 Gy to the tumor. This sequence is called the *shrinking field technique*. With the development of IMRT, it has become possible to treat both regions with a different dose each day and achieve both goals simultaneously. For example, on each of the 35 days of treatment, the gross tumor might receive 2 Gy, and the region of occult disease 1.7 Gy, for a total dose of 59.5 Gy, which is of approximately equal biologic effectiveness to 54 Gy in 1.8-Gy fractions because of the lower dose per fraction (see the section Biologic Aspects of Radiation Oncology).

Radiation therapy alone is often used with curative intent for localized tumors. The decision to use surgery or radiation therapy involves factors determined by the tumor (e.g., is it resectable without a serious compromise in function?) and the patient (e.g., is the patient a good operative candidate?). The most common tumor in this group is prostate cancer, but patients with early-stage larynx cancer often receive radiation for voice preservation, and there are many patients with early-stage lung cancer who are not operative candidates. Control rates for these early-stage lesions are in excess of 70% (and as high as 90% for early-stage larynx cancer) and are usually a function of tumor size.

Stereotactic body radiation therapy (SBRT; sometimes called *stereotactic ablative radiation*) uses many (typically more than eight) cross-firing beams and provides an improved method of curing early-stage lung cancer[97] and liver metastases.[98] This approach uses precise localization and image guidance to deliver a small number (less than five) of high doses of radiation, with the concept of ablating the tumor, rather than using fractionation to achieve a therapeutic index (see the section title Fractionation). SBRT can provide long-term, local control rates of >90% for tumors less than 4 to 5 cm with minimal side effects.

Locally advanced or aggressive cancers can be cured with radiation alone or with a combination of radiation and chemotherapy or a molecularly targeted therapy. The most common examples here are locally advanced lung cancer, head and neck, esophageal, and cervix cancers, with cure rates in the 15% to 40% range, and are discussed in detail in their own chapters. A general principle that has emerged during the last decade is that combination chemoradiation has increased the cure rates of locally advanced cancers by 5% to 10% at the cost of increased toxicity.

An important consideration in the use of radiation (with or without chemotherapy) with curative intent is the concept of organ preservation. Perhaps the best example of achieving organ preservation in the face of gross disease involves the use of chemotherapy and radiation to replace laryngectomy in the treatment of advanced larynx cancer. Combined radiation and chemotherapy does not improve overall survival compared with radical surgery; however, the organ-conservation approach permits voice preservation in approximately two-thirds of patients with advanced larynx cancer.[99] The treatment of anal cancer with chemoradiation can also be viewed in this light, with chemoradiotherapy producing organ conservation and cure rates superior to radical surgery used decades ago.[100] Multiple randomized trials have demonstrated that lumpectomy plus radiation for breast cancer produces survival rates equal to that of modified radical mastectomy, while allowing for the preservation of the breast.

In the last decade, it has become clear that some patients with metastatic disease can be cured with radiation (with or without chemotherapy). The concept underlying this approach was established by the surgical practice of resecting a limited number of liver or lung metastases. A significant fraction of patients have a limited number of liver metastases that cannot be resected because of location, but are able to undergo high-dose radiation (often combined with chemotherapy). This radical approach to *oligometastases*[101] can produce 5-year survivals in the range of 20% in selected patients.[102] Patients with a limited number of lung metastases from colorectal cancer or soft tissue sarcomas are now being approached with stereotactic body radiation with a similar concept as has been used to justify surgical resection.[102] In addition to the direct effect of radiation on metastatic tumor, there is now anecdotal but provocative evidence that radiation can stimulate the immune system so that tumors distant from the irradiated tumor can respond. Distant (abscopal) responses have been reported in patients who receive immune checkpoint inhibitors such as ipilimumab.[103]

Radiation therapy can also contribute to the cure of patients when used in an adjuvant setting. If the risk of recurrence after surgery is low or if a recurrence could be easily addressed by a second resection, adjuvant radiation therapy is not usually given. However, when a gross total resection of the tumor is still associated with a high risk of residual occult disease or if local recurrence is morbid, adjuvant treatment is often recommended. A general finding across many disease sites is that adjuvant radiation can reduce local failure rates to below 10%, even in high-risk patients, if a gross total resection is achieved. If gross disease or positive margins remain, higher doses and/or larger volumes may be required, which may be less well tolerated and are less successful in achieving tumor control.

Adjuvant therapy can be delivered before or after definitive surgery. There are some advantages to giving radiation therapy after surgery. The details of the tumor location are known and, with the surgeon's cooperation, clips can be placed in the tumor bed, permitting increased treatment accuracy. In addition, compared with preoperative therapy, postoperative therapy is associated with fewer wound complications. However, in some cases, it is preferable to deliver preoperative radiation. Radiation can shrink the tumor, diminishing the extent of the resection, or making an unresectable tumor resectable. In the case of rectal cancer, the response to treatment may carry more prognostic information than the initial TNM staging.[104] In patients who will undergo significant surgeries (particularly a Whipple procedure or an esophageal resection), preoperative (sometimes called neoadjuvant) therapy can be more reliably administered than postoperative therapy. Most importantly, after resection of abdominal or pelvic tumors (such as rectal cancers or retroperitoneal sarcomas), the small bowel may become fixed by adhesions in the region requiring treatment, thus increasing the morbidity of postoperative treatment. A randomized trial has shown that preoperative therapy produces fewer gastrointestinal side effects and has at least as good efficacy as postoperative adjuvant therapy for locally advanced rectal cancer.[105] Taken together, there appears to be a trend toward preoperative or neoadjuvant therapy in cancers of the gastrointestinal track (esophagus, stomach, pancreas, rectum), postoperative radiation seems to be favored in head and neck, lung, and breast cancer, and soft tissue sarcoma seems equally split.

The effectiveness of adjuvant therapy in decreasing local recurrence has been demonstrated in randomized trials in lung, rectal, and breast cancers. More recently, randomized trials have shown that postmastectomy radiation improved the survival for women with breast cancer and four or more positive lymph nodes, all of whom also received adjuvant chemotherapy. A fascinating analysis has revealed that, across many treatment conditions, each 4% increase in 5-year local control is associated with a 1% increase in 5-year survival.[106] It has been proposed that the long-term survival benefit of radiation in these more recent studies was revealed by the introduction of effective chemotherapy, which prevented such a high fraction of women from dying early with metastatic disease.[107] This concept has been developed into a hypothesis that the effect of adjuvant radiation on survival will depend on the effectiveness of adjuvant chemotherapy. If chemotherapy is either ineffective or very effective, adjuvant radiation may have little influence on the survival in a disease in which systemic relapse dominates survival. Radiation will have its greatest impact on survival when chemotherapy is moderately effective.[108]

In addition to these curative roles, radiation plays an important part in palliative treatment. Perhaps most importantly, emergency irradiation can begin to reverse the devastating effects of spinal cord compression and of superior vena cava syndrome. A single 8-Gy fraction is highly effective for many patients with bone pain from a metastatic lesion. There is increasing evidence of the effectiveness of body stereotactic radiation to treat vertebral body metastases in patients who have a long projected survival or who need retreatment after previous radiation.[109] Stereotactic treatment can relieve symptoms from a small number of brain metastasis, and fractionated whole-brain radiation can mitigate the effects of multiple metastases. Bronchial obstruction can often be relieved by a brief course of treatment as can duodenal obstruction from pancreatic cancer. Palliative treatment is usually delivered in a smaller number of larger radiation fractions (see the section titled Fractionation) because the desire to simplify the treatment for a patient with limited life expectancy outweighs the somewhat increased potential for late side effects.

## FRACTIONATION

Two crucial features that influence the effectiveness of a physical dose of radiation are the dose given in each radiation treatment (i.e., the fraction) and the total amount of time required to complete the course of radiation. Standard fractionation for radiation therapy is defined as the delivery of one treatment of 1.8 to 2.25 Gy per day. This approach produces a fairly well-understood chance of tumor control and risk of normal tissue damage (as a function of volume). By altering the fractionation schemes, one may be able to improve the outcome for patients undergoing curative treatment or to simplify the treatment for patients receiving palliative therapy.

Two forms of altered fractionation have been tested for patients undergoing curative treatment: accelerated fractionation and hyperfractionation. Accelerated fractionation emerged from analyses of the control of head and neck cancer as a function of dose administered and total treatment time. It was found that with an increasing dose there was increasing local control, but that protraction of treatment was associated with a loss of local control that

was equivalent to about 0.75 Gy per day.[110] The data were best modeled by assuming that, approximately 2 weeks into treatment, tumor cells began to proliferate more rapidly than they were proliferating early in treatment (called *accelerated repopulation*).[111] In accelerated fractionation, the goal is to complete radiation before the accelerated tumor cell proliferation occurs. The most common method of achieving accelerated fractionation is to give a standard fraction to the entire field in the morning and to give a second treatment to the boost field in the afternoon (called *concomitant boost*). As in standard radiation, the boost would be given by extending the length of the treatment course; this concomitant boost approach can shorten treatment from 7 weeks to 5 weeks in head and neck cancer.

The second approach to altering fractionation is called *hyperfractionation*. Hyperfractionation is defined as the use of more than one fraction per day separated by more than 6 hours (see the section titled Biologic Aspects of Radiation Oncology), with a dose per fraction that is less than standard. Hyperfractionation is expected to produce fewer late complications for the same acute effects against both rapidly dividing normal tissues and tumors. Pure hyperfractionation might give 1 Gy twice a day, so that the total dose per day would be 2 Gy, and thus be equal to standard fractionation. In practice, hyperfractionated treatments are usually in the range of 1.2 Gy, which means that, compared with a standard fractionation, a somewhat higher dose is administered during the same period of time (so that most hyperfractionation also includes modest acceleration). The overall effect is to increase the acute toxicity (which resolves) and tumor response, while not increasing the (dose-limiting) late toxicity, which can improve cure rate. Both accelerated fractionation and hyperfractionation have been demonstrated in a meta-analysis to be superior to standard fractionation in the treatment of head and neck cancer with radiation alone.[112] However, a recent randomized trial has shown that there is no increase in control or survival, but there is an increase toxicity using chemotherapy with hyperfractionation compared to standard chemoradiation; therefore, the use of altered fractionation schemes has decreased dramatically during the last few years.[113]

*Hypofractionation* refers to the administration of a smaller number of larger fractions than is standard. Hypofractionation might be expected to cause more late toxicity for the same antitumor effect than standard or hyperfractionation. In the past, this approach was reserved for palliative cases, with the sense that a modest potential for increased late toxicity was not a major concern in patients with limited life expectancy. However, more recently, it has been proposed that the ability to better exclude normal tissue by using IGRT may permit hypofractionation to be used safely and that, in the specific case of prostate cancer, hypofractionation may have beneficial effects.[114]

## ADVERSE EFFECTS

Radiation produces adverse effects in normal tissues. Although these are discussed in detail in later chapters as part of comprehensive discussions of organ toxicity, it is worth making some general comments here from the perspective of how radiation biology relates to the clinical toxicities. The term *radiation toxicity* is used to describe the adverse effects caused by radiation alone and radiation plus chemotherapy. Although this latter toxicity would be better labeled as *combined modality toxicity*, the pattern typically resembles a more severe form of the toxicity produced by radiation alone. Adverse effects from radiation can be divided into acute, subacute, and chronic (or late) effects. Acute effects are common, rarely serious, and usually self-limiting. Acute effects tend to occur in organs that depend on rapid self-renewal, most commonly the skin or mucosal surfaces (oropharynx, esophagus, small intestine, rectum, and bladder). This is due to radiation-induced cell death that occurs during mitosis, so that cells that divide rapidly show the most rapid cell loss. In the treatment of head and neck cancer, mucositis becomes worse during the first 3 to 4 weeks of therapy, but then will often stabilize as the normal mucosa cell proliferation increases in response to mucosal cell loss. It seems likely that normal tissue stem cells are relatively resistant to radiation compared with the more differentiated cells, because these stem cells survive to permit the normal mucosa to reepithelialize. Acute side effects typically resolve within 1 to 2 weeks of treatment completion, although occasionally these effects are so severe that they lead to consequential late effects, as described later.

Because lymphocytes are exquisitely sensitive to radiation, there has been considerable investigation into the effects of radiation on immune function. In contrast to mucosal cell killing, which requires mitosis, radiation kills lymphocytes in all phases of the cell cycle by apoptosis, so that lymphocyte counts decrease within days of initiating treatment. These effects do not tend to put patients at risk for infection, because granulocytes, which are chiefly responsible for combating infections, are relatively unaffected.

Two acute side effects of radiation do not fit neatly into these models relating to cell kill: nausea[115,116] and fatigue.[117,118] The origin of radiation-induced nausea is not related to acute cell loss, because it can occur within hours of the first treatment. Nausea is usually associated with radiation of the stomach, but it can sometimes occur during brain irradiation or from large-volume irradiation that involves neither the brain nor the stomach. Irradiation typically produces fatigue, even if relatively small volumes are irradiated. It seems likely that the origins of both of these *abscopal* effects of radiation (i.e., effects that occur systemically or at a distance for the site of irradiation) are related to the release of cytokines, but little is known.

Radiation can also produce subacute toxicities in the form of radiation pneumonitis and radiation-induced liver disease. These typically occur 2 weeks to 3 months after radiation is completed. The risk of radiation pneumonitis and radiation-induced liver disease is proportional to the mean dose delivered.[119,120] Thus, the 3D tools that permit the calculation of dose-volume histograms (described in the physics section) are currently used to determine the maximum safe treatment that can be delivered in terms of dose

and volume. These toxicities appear to be initiated subclinically during the course of radiation as a cascade of cytokines in which TGF-β, tumor necrosis factor α, interleukin 6, and other cytokines play a role.[121] High TGF-β plasma levels during a course of treatment have been found to be associated with a greater risk of radiation pneumonitis.[122] Thus, in the future, we might look toward a combination of physical dose delivery, measured by the dose-volume histogram, the functional imaging of normal tissue damage, and the detection of biomarkers of toxicity, such as TGF-β, to improve the ability to individualize therapy. Attempts to determine the genomic basis of radiation sensitivity, beyond the known rare genetic defects such as ataxia telangiectasia, have not yet been successful.[123]

Late effects, which are typically seen 6 or more months after a course of radiation, include fibrosis, fistula formation, or long-term organ damage. Two theories for the origin of late effects have been put forth: late damage to the microvasculature and direct damage to the parenchyma. Although the vascular damage theory is attractive, it does not account for the differing sensitivities of organs to radiation. Perhaps the microvasculature is unique in each organ.[124] Regardless of the mechanism of toxicity, the tolerance of whole-organ radiation is now fairly well established (Table 13.2). Late complications can also be divided into two categories: consequential and true late effects. The best example of a consequential late effect is fibrosis and dysphagia after high-dose chemoradiation for head and neck cancer. Here, late fibrosis or ulceration appears to be the result of the mucosa becoming denuded for a prolonged time period. Late consequential effects are distinct from true late effects, which can follow a normal treatment course of self-limited toxicity and a 6-month or more symptom-free period. Examples of true late effects are radiation myelitis, radiation brain necrosis, and radiation-induced bowel obstruction. In the past, radiation fibrosis was thought to be an irreversible condition. Therefore, an exciting recent development is that severe radiation-induced breast fibrosis is an active process that can be reversed by drug therapy (pentoxifylline and vitamin E).[125]

**CANCER THERAPEUTICS**

## TABLE 13.2

**Radiation Tolerance Doses for Normal Tissues**

| Site | TD 5/5 (Gy)[a] Portion of Organ Irradiated | | | TD 50/5 (Gy)[b] Portion of Organ Irradiated | | | Complication End Point(s) |
|---|---|---|---|---|---|---|---|
| | $1/3$ | $2/3$ | $3/3$ | $1/3$ | $2/3$ | $3/3$ | |
| Kidney | 50 | 30 | 23 | — | 40 | 28 | Nephritis |
| Rain | 60 | 50 | 45 | 75 | 65 | 60 | Necrosis, infarct |
| Brain stem | 60 | 53 | 50 | — | — | 65 | Necrosis, infarct |
| Spinal cord | 50 (5–10 cm) | — | 47 (20 cm) | 70 (5–10 cm) | — | — | Myelitis, necrosis |
| Lung | 45 | 30 | 17.5 | 65 | 40 | 24.5 | Radiation pneumonitis |
| Heart | 60 | 45 | 40 | 70 | 55 | 50 | Pericarditis |
| Esophagus | 60 | 58 | 55 | 72 | 70 | 68 | Stricture, perforation |
| Stomach | 60 | 55 | 50 | 70 | 67 | 65 | Ulceration, perforation |
| Small intestine | 50 | — | 40 | 60 | — | 55 | Obstruction, perforation, fistula |
| Colon | 55 | — | 45 | 65 | — | 55 | Obstruction, perforation, fistula, ulceration |
| Rectum | (100 cm³ volume) | | 60 | (100 cm³ volume) | | 80 | Severe proctitis, necrosis, fistula |
| Liver | 50 | 35 | 30 | 55 | 45 | 40 | Liver failure |

[a] TD 5/5, the average dose that results in a 5% complication risk within 5 years.
[b] TD 50/5, the average dose that results in a 50% complication risk within 5 years.
Adapted from Emami B, Lyman J, Brown A, et al. Tolerance of normal tissue to therapeutic irradiation. *Int J Radiat Oncol Biol Phys* 1991;21:109–122.

# PRINCIPLES OF COMBINING ANTICANCER AGENTS WITH RADIATION THERAPY

Combining chemotherapy with radiation therapy has produced important improvements in treatment outcome. Randomized clinical trials show improved local control and survival through the use of concurrent chemotherapy and radiation therapy for patients with high-grade gliomas and locally advanced cancers of the head and neck, lung, esophagus, stomach, rectum, prostate, and anus. There are least two proposed reasons why chemoradiotherapy might be successful. The first is radiosensitization. In the laboratory, radiosensitization is defined as a synergistic relationship, using mathematical approaches such as isobologram or median effect analysis.[126,127] The underlying concept is that the observed effect of using chemotherapy and radiation concurrently is greater than simply adding the two together. A second proposed reason to combine radiation and chemotherapy is to realize the benefit of improved local control radiation along with the systemic effect of chemotherapy, a concept called *spatial additivity*.[128]

Clinical results show that both radiosensitization and spatial additivity contribute to varying extents in different clinical settings. In the case of head and neck cancer, radiosensitization predominates. This conclusion is supported by the meta-analysis of head and neck cancer: sequential chemotherapy and radiotherapy produces little if any improvement in survival, whereas concurrent chemoradiation produces a significant increase in survival.[129] Furthermore, in the early positive studies using concurrent chemoradiation, systemic metastases were unaffected even though survival was improved. Radiosensitization may also predominate in the success of chemoradiotherapy for locally advanced lung cancer. For instance, although initial studies indicated that sequential chemotherapy and radiation had some benefit for lung cancer,[130] more recent work indicates that concurrent therapy is superior, and it is now the standard treatment.[131] However, there are also examples of spatial additivity. For example, both radiosensitization and spatial additivity is provided by the use of chemoradiation for locally advanced cervical cancer in that both local and systemic relapses are decreased by combined therapy.[132]

By targeting the aberrant growth factor or proangiogenic pathways that are specific to cancer cells rather than all rapidly proliferating cells, molecularly targeted therapies offer the potential to improve outcome without increasing toxicity. Even a selective cytostatic effect against the tumor would be predicted to act synergistically with radiation (Fig. 13.22). Although preclinical studies (summarized in the previous biology section) have highlighted the potential therapeutic gains that could be achieved by adding EGFR inhibitors to radiation, the best validation of this combination has been from the results of clinical trials in head and neck cancer. A phase III clinical trial demonstrated that, in a cohort of 424 patients with local–regionally advanced squamous cell carcinoma of the head and neck, the addition of cetuximab nearly doubled the median survival of patients (compared to radiotherapy alone), from 28 to 54 months. This study represents the first major success

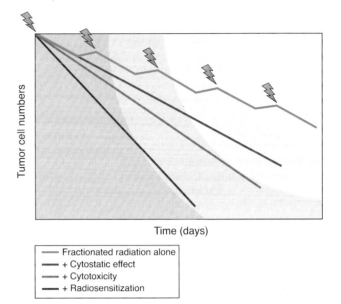

Time (days)

— Fractionated radiation alone
— + Cytostatic effect
— + Cytotoxicity
— + Radiosensitization

**Figure 13.22** Potential mechanisms of synergy between epidermal growth factor receptor (EGFR) inhibitors and radiation. Although each daily radiation treatment kills a fraction of the cells, some cells grow back by the next day, which attenuates the effectiveness of radiation. If an EGFR inhibitor has only a selective cytostatic effect and blocks regrowth between fractions, the result would be a dramatic increase in radiation efficacy. The benefit of the inhibitor would be even greater if it caused tumor cell cytotoxicity or radiosensitization.

achieved by the addition of an EGFR antagonist to radiotherapy. This improvement was achieved without enhanced toxicity. Notably, the rates of pharyngitis and weight loss were identical in the two arms.[60] Local control was improved rather than the development of metastases, suggesting synergy rather than spatial additivity. Thus, the principle that can be derived from this study is that in tumors expressing high EGFR levels and that are likely to depend on aberrant EGF signaling, combining a true cytotoxic agent such as radiation with a cytostatic agent such as cetuximab has considerable promise.

Because of the success of chemoradiotherapy, the natural tendency has not been to substitute molecularly targeted agents such as cetuximab for chemotherapy, but to add cetuximab to chemoradiotherapy. Thus, the combination of cisplatin, cetuximab, and radiation was recently found to have the same control rate as cisplatin and radiation for patients with locally advanced head and neck cancer, but the cetuximab arm had greater toxicity. Unfortunately, the triple therapy was never evaluated preclinically, and it has been shown preclinically that when EGFR inhibitors are given prior to chemotherapy, they can produce antagonism.[133] The principles of adding molecularly targeted therapy to chemoradiation are still evolving.[63]

## REFERENCES

1. Hall EJ, Giaccia AJ. *Radiobiology for the Radiologist.* Philadelphia: Lippincott Williams & Williams; 2012.
2. Fowler JF. Developing aspects of radiation oncology. *Med Phys* 1981;8:427–434.
3. Lavin MF. Ataxia-telangiectasia: from a rare disorder to a paradigm for cell signalling and cancer. *Nat Rev Mol Cell Biol* 2008;9:759–769.
4. Thompson LH. Recognition, signaling, and repair of DNA double-strand breaks produced by ionizing radiation in mammalian cells: the molecular choreography. *Mutat Res* 2012;751:158–246.
5. Sherr CJ, McCormick F. The RB and p53 pathways in cancer. *Cancer Cell* 2002;2:103–112.
6. Bartek J, Lukas J. Chk1 and Chk2 kinases in checkpoint control and cancer. *Cancer Cell* 2003;3:421–429.

7. Kitagawa R, Bakkenist CJ, McKinnon PJ, et al. Phosphorylation of SMC1 is a critical downstream event in the ATM-NBS1-BRCA1 pathway. *Genes Dev* 2004;18:1423–1438.
8. Abraham RT. Cell cycle checkpoint signaling through the ATM and ATR kinases. *Genes Dev* 2001;15:2177–2196.
9. Mailand N, Podtelejnikov AV, Groth A, et al. Regulation of G(2)/M events by Cdc25A through phosphorylation-dependent modulation of its stability. *EMBO J* 2002;21:5911–5920.
10. Donzelli M, Draetta GF. Regulating mammalian checkpoints through Cdc25 inactivation. *EMBO Rep* 2003;4:671–677.
11. Tsvetkov L. Polo-like kinases and Chk2 at the interface of DNA damage checkpoint pathways and mitotic regulation. *IUBMB Life* 2004;56:449–456.

12. Dai Y, Grant S. New insights into checkpoint kinase 1 in the DNA damage response signaling network. *Clin Cancer Res* 2010;16:376–383.
13. Giaccia A, Weinstein R, Hu J, et al. Cell cycle-dependent repair of double-strand DNA breaks in a gamma-ray-sensitive Chinese hamster cell. *Somat Cell Mol Genet* 1985;11:485–491.
14. Kemp LM, Sedgwick SG, Jeggo PA. X-ray sensitive mutants of Chinese hamster ovary cells defective in double-strand break rejoining. *Mutat Res* 1984;132:189–196.
15. Helleday T, Lo J, van Gent DC, et al. DNA double-strand break repair: from mechanistic understanding to cancer treatment. *DNA Repair (Amst)* 2007;6:923–935.
16. Hefferin ML, Tomkinson AE. Mechanism of DNA double-strand break repair by non-homologous end joining. *DNA Repair (Amst)* 2005;4:639–648.
17. Ma Y, Pannicke U, Schwarz K, et al. Hairpin opening and overhang processing by an Artemis/DNA-dependent protein kinase complex in nonhomologous end joining and V(D)J recombination. *Cell* 2002;108:781–794.
18. Grawunder U, Wilm M, Wu X, et al. Activity of DNA ligase IV stimulated by complex formation with XRCC4 protein in mammalian cells. *Nature* 1997;388:492–495.
19. Chen L, Trujillo K, Sung P, et al. Interactions of the DNA ligase IV-XRCC4 complex with DNA ends and the DNA-dependent protein kinase. *J Biol Chem* 2000;275:26196–26205.
20. Tsukuda T, Fleming AB, Nickoloff JA, et al. Chromatin remodelling at a DNA double-strand break site in Saccharomyces cerevisiae. *Nature* 2005;438:379–383.
21. Yang YG, Saidi A, Frappart PO, et al. Conditional deletion of Nbs1 in murine cells reveals its role in branching repair pathways of DNA double-strand breaks. *EMBO J* 2006;25:5527–5538.
22. Esashi F, Galkin VE, Yu X, et al. Stabilization of RAD51 nucleoprotein filaments by the C-terminal region of BRCA2. *Nat Struct Mol Biol* 2007;14:468–474.
23. Sleeth KM, Sorensen CS, Issaeva N, et al. RPA mediates recombination repair during replication stress and is displaced from DNA by checkpoint signalling in human cells. *J Mol Biol* 2007;373:38–47.
24. Littlefield LG, Kleinerman RA, Sayer AM, et al. Chromosome aberrations in lymphocytes—biomonitors of radiation exposure. *Prog Clin Biol Res* 1991;372:387–397.
25. Toulany M, Rodemann HP. Membrane receptor signaling and control of DNA repair after exposure to ionizing radiation. *Nuklearmedizin* 2010;49:S26–S30.
26. Barcellos-Hoff MH, Akhurst RJ. Transforming growth factor-beta in breast cancer: too much, too late. *Breast Cancer Res* 2009;11:202.
27. Deng X, Yin X, Allan R, et al. Ceramide biogenesis is required for radiation-induced apoptosis in the germ line of C. elegans. *Science* 2008;322:110–115.
28. Thompson LH, Suit HD. Proliferation kinetics of x-irradiated mouse L cells studied WITH TIME-lapse photography. II. *Int J Radiat Biol Relat Stud Phys Chem Med* 1969;15:347–362.
29. Sowa Resat MB, Morgan WF. Radiation-induced genomic instability: a role for secreted soluble factors in communicating the radiation response to non-irradiated cells. *J Cell Biochem* 2004;92:1013–1019.
30. Elkind MM. The initial part of the survival curve: does it predict the outcome of fractionated radiotherapy? *Radiat Res* 1988;114:425–436.
31. McCulloch EA, Till JE. The sensitivity of cells from normal mouse bone marrow to gamma radiation in vitro and in vivo. *Radiat Res* 1962;16:822–832.
32. Withers HR. Recovery and repopulation in vivo by mouse skin epithelial cells during fractionated irradiation. *Radiat Res* 1967;32:227–239.
33. Withers HR, Elkind MM. Microcolony survival assay for cells of mouse intestinal mucosa exposed to radiation. *Int J Radiat Biol Relat Stud Phys Chem Med* 1970;17:261–267.
34. Suit H, Wette R. Radiation dose fractionation and tumor control probability. *Radiat Res* 1966;29:267–281.
35. O'Neill K, Lyons SK, Gallagher WM, et al. Bioluminescent imaging: a critical tool in pre-clinical oncology research. *J Pathol* 2010;220:317–327.
36. Hewitt HB, Wilson CW. Survival curves for tumor cells irradiated in vivo. *Ann N Y Acad Sci* 1961;95:818–827.
37. Hill RP, Bush RS. A lung-colony assay to determine the radiosensitivity of cells of a solid tumour. *Int J Radiat Biol Relat Stud Phys Chem Med* 1969;15:435–444.
38. Elkind MM, Sutton-Gilbert H, Moses WB, et al. Radiation response of mammalian cells grown in culture. V. Temperature dependence of the repair of x-ray damage in surviving cells (aerobic and hypoxic). *Radiat Res* 1965;25:359–376.
39. Elkind MM, Whitmore GF. *Radiobiology of Cultured Mammalian Cells*. New York: Gordon and Breach; 1967.
40. Mottram JC. Factors of importance in radiosensitivity of tumors. *Br J Radiol* 1936;9:606.
41. Palcic B, Skarsgard LD. Reduced oxygen enhancement ratio at low doses of ionizing radiation. *Radiat Res* 1984;100:328–339.
42. Thomlinson RH, Gray LH. The histological structure of some human lung cancers and the possible implications for radiotherapy. *Br J Cancer* 1955;9:539–549.
43. Overgaard J, Horsman MR. Modification of hypoxia-induced radioresistance in tumors by the use of oxygen and sensitizers. *Semin Radiat Oncol* 1996;6:10–21.
44. Machtay M, Pajak TF, Suntharalingam M, et al. Radiotherapy with or without erythropoietin for anemic patients with head and neck cancer: a randomized trial of the Radiation Therapy Oncology Group (RTOG 99-03). *Int J Radiat Oncol Biol Phys* 2007;69:1008–1017.
45. Henke M, Laszig R, Rube C, et al. Erythropoietin to treat head and neck cancer patients with anaemia undergoing radiotherapy: randomised, double-blind, placebo-controlled trial. *Lancet* 2003;362:1255–1260.
46. Janssens GO, Rademakers SE, Terhaard CH, et al. Accelerated radiotherapy with carbogen and nicotinamide for laryngeal cancer: results of a phase III randomized trial. *J Clin Oncol* 2012;30:1777–1783.
47. Willett CG, Boucher Y, di Tomaso E, et al. Direct evidence that the VEGF-specific antibody bevacizumab has antivascular effects in human rectal cancer. *Nat Med* 2004;10:145–147.
48. Lapi SE, Voller TF, Welch MJ. Positron emission tomography imaging of hypoxia. *PET Clin* 2009;4:39–47.
49. Lee NY, Mechalakos JG, Nehmeh S, et al. Fluorine-18-labeled fluoromisonidazole positron emission and computed tomography-guided intensity-modulated radiotherapy for head and neck cancer: a feasibility study. *Int J Radiat Oncol Biol Phys* 2008;70:2–13.
50. Schaue D, Xie MW, Ratikan JA, et al. Regulatory T cells in radiotherapeutic responses. *Front Oncol* 2012;2:90.
51. Formenti SC, Demaria S. Combining radiotherapy and cancer immunotherapy: a paradigm shift. *J Natl Cancer Inst* 2013;105:256–265.
52. Lawrence TS, Davis MA, Tang HY, et al. Fluorodeoxyuridine-mediated cytotoxicity and radiosensitization require S phase progression. *Int J Radiat Biol* 1996;70:273–280.
53. Lawrence TS, Chang EY, Hahn TM, et al. Radiosensitization of pancreatic cancer cells by 2′,2′-difluoro-2′-deoxycytidine. *Int J Radiat Oncol Biol Phys* 1996;34:867–872.
54. Eisbruch A, Shewach DS, Bradford CR, et al. Radiation concurrent with gemcitabine for locally advanced head and neck cancer: a phase I trial and intracellular drug incorporation study. *J Clin Oncol* 2001;19:792–799.
55. Ben-Josef E, Schipper M, Francis IR, et al. A phase I/II trial of intensity modulated radiation (IMRT) dose escalation with concurrent fixed-dose rate gemcitabine (FDR-G) in patients with unresectable pancreatic cancer. *Int J Radiat Oncol Biol Phys* 2012;84:1166–1171.
56. Wolff RA, Evans DB, Gravel DM, et al. Phase I trial of gemcitabine combined with radiation for the treatment of locally advanced pancreatic adenocarcinoma. *Clin Cancer Res* 2001;7:2246–2253.
57. Wilson GD, Bentzen SM, Harari PM. Biologic basis for combining drugs with radiation. *Semin Radiat Oncol* 2006;16:2–9.
58. Bradley JD, Paulus R, Graham MV, et al. Phase II trial of postoperative adjuvant paclitaxel/carboplatin and thoracic radiotherapy in resected stage II and IIIA non-small-cell lung cancer: promising long-term results of the Radiation Therapy Oncology Group—RTOG 9705. *J Clin Oncol* 2005;23:3480–3487.
59. Nyati MK, Morgan MA, Feng FY, et al. Integration of EGFR inhibitors with radiochemotherapy. *Nat Rev Cancer* 2006;6:876–885.
60. Bonner JA, Harari PM, Giralt J, et al. Radiotherapy plus cetuximab for locoregionally advanced head and neck cancer: 5-year survival data from a phase 3 randomised trial, and relation between cetuximab-induced rash and survival. *Lancet Oncol* 2010;11:21–28.
61. Ang KK, Zhang QE, Rosenthal DI, et al. A randomized phase III trial (RTOG 0522) of concurrent accelerated radiation plus cisplatin with or without cetuximab for stage III-IV head and neck squamous cell carcinomas (HNC). *J Clin Oncol* 2011;29.
62. Engelke CG, Parsels LA, Qian Y, et al. Sensitization of pancreatic cancer to chemoradiation by the Chk1 inhibitor MK8776. *Clin Cancer Res* 2013;19:4412–4421.
63. Morgan MA, Parsels LA, Maybaum J, et al. Improving the efficacy of chemoradiation with targeted agents. *Cancer Discov* 2014;4:280–291.
64. Chalmers AJ, Lakshman M, Chan N, et al. Poly(ADP-ribose) polymerase inhibition as a model for synthetic lethality in developing radiation oncology targets. *Semin Radiat Oncol* 2010;20:274–281.
65. Brizel DM, Wasserman TH, Henke M, et al. Phase III randomized trial of amifostine as a radioprotector in head and neck cancer. *J Clin Oncol* 2000;18:3339–3345.
66. Winczura P, Jassem J. Combined treatment with cytoprotective agents and radiotherapy. *Cancer Treat Rev* 2010;36:268–275.
67. Van Dyk J, ed. Radiation oncology medical physics resources for working, teaching, and learning. In: *The Modern Technology of Radiation Oncology*. Volume 3. Medical Physics Publishing Web site. http://www.medicalphysics.org/vandykch16.pdf. Madison, WI: Medical Physics Publishing; 2013.
68. Karzmark C, Nunan C, Tanabe E. *Medical Electron Accelerators*. New York: McGraw-Hill Ryerson; 1993.
69. Greene D, Williams P. *Linear Accelerators for Radiation Therapy*. 2nd ed. New York: Taylor and Francis Group; 1997.
70. Fenwick JD, Tome WA, Soisson ET, et al. Tomotherapy and other innovative IMRT delivery systems. *Semin Radiat Oncol* 2006;16:199–208.
71. Curran B, Balter J, Chetty I, eds. *Integrating New Technologies into the Clinic: Monte Carlo and Image-Guided Radiation Therapy*. Madison, WI: Medical Physics Publishing; 2006.
72. Bourland J, ed. *Image-Guided Radiation Therapy*. Boca Raton, FL: Taylor & Francis; 2012.
73. Seco J, Verhaegen F, eds. *Monte Carlo Techniques in Radiation Therapy*. Boca Raton, FL: Taylor & Francis; 2013.
74. Kessler ML. Image registration and data fusion in radiation therapy. *Br J Radiol* 2006;79:S99–S108.
75. Brock K, ed. *Image Processing in Radiation Therapy*. Boca Raton, FL: Taylor & Francis Group; 2014.
76. Sovik A, Malinen E, Olsen DR. Strategies for biologic image-guided dose escalation: a review. *Int J Radiat Oncol Biol Phys* 2009;73:650–658.
77. Marks LB, Ten Haken RK, Martel MK. Guest editor's introduction to QUANTEC: a users guide. *Int J Radiat Oncol Biol Phys* 2010;76:S1–S2.

**CANCER THERAPEUTICS**

78. Li A, Alber M, Deasy JO, et al. The use and QA of biologically related models for treatment planning: short report of the TG-166 of the therapy physics committee of the AAPM. *Med Phys* 2012;39:1386–1409.
79. Bortfeld T. IMRT: a review and preview. *Phys Med Biol* 2006;51:R363–R379.
80. Webb S. *Contemporary IMRT Developing Physics and Clinical Implementation.* London: IOP Publishing; 2005.
81. Maughan R, Yudelev M. Neutron therapy. In: Van Dyk J, ed. *The Modern Technology of Radiation Oncology.* Madison, WI: Medical Physics Publishing; 1999.
82. Hogstrom KR, Almond PR. Review of electron beam therapy physics. *Phys Med Biol* 2006;51:R455–R489.
83. Schlegel W, Bortfeld T, Grosu A, eds. *New Technologies in Radiation Oncology.* Heidelberg: Springer-Verlag; 2006.
84. Ma C-MC, Lomax T, eds. *Proton and Carbon Ion Therapy.* Boca Raton, FL: Taylor & Francis Group; 2012.
85. Venselaar J, Meigooni A, Baltas D, et al., eds. *Comprehensive Brachytherapy: Physical and Clinical Aspects.* Boca Raton, FL: Taylor & Francis Group; 2012.
86. Meredith RF. Systemic targeted radionuclide therapy symposium introduction. *Int J Radiat Oncol Biol Phys* 2006;66:S7.
87. Tripuraneni P, Watson RL, Ang KK, et al. Intersociety Radiation Oncology Summit-SCOPE II. *Int J Radiat Oncol Biol Phys* 2008;72:323–326.
88. Delaney G, Jacob S, Featherstone C, et al. The role of radiotherapy in cancer treatment: estimating optimal utilization from a review of evidence-based clinical guidelines. *Cancer* 2005;104:1129–1137.
89. Zelefsky MJ, Housman DM, Pei X, et al. Incidence of secondary cancer development after high-dose intensity-modulated radiotherapy and image-guided brachytherapy for the treatment of localized prostate cancer. *Int J Radiat Oncol Biol Phys* 2012;83:953–959.
90. Combs SE, Laperriere N, Brada M. Clinical controversies: proton radiation therapy for brain and skull base tumors. *Semin Radiat Oncol* 2013;23:120–126.
91. Overgaard J. Hypoxic radiosensitization: adored and ignored. *J Clin Oncol* 2007;25:4066–4074.
92. Mouw KW, Trofimov A, Zietman AL, et al. Clinical controversies: proton therapy for prostate cancer. *Semin Radiat Oncol* 2013;23:109–114.
93. Yu JB, Soulos PR, Herrin J, et al. Proton versus intensity-modulated radiotherapy for prostate cancer: patterns of care and early toxicity. *J Natl Cancer Inst* 2013;105:25–32.
94. Brada M, Pijls-Johannesma M, De Ruysscher D. Proton therapy in clinical practice: current clinical evidence. *J Clin Oncol* 2007;25:965–970.
95. Douglas JG, Koh WJ, Austin-Seymour M, et al. Treatment of salivary gland neoplasms with fast neutron radiotherapy. *Arch Otolaryngol Head Neck Surg* 2003;129:944–948.
96. Shilkrut M, Merrick GS, McLaughlin PW, et al. The addition of low-dose-rate brachytherapy and androgen-deprivation therapy decreases biochemical failure and prostate cancer death compared with dose-escalated external-beam radiation therapy for high-risk prostate cancer. *Cancer* 2013;119:681–690.
97. Iyengar P, Timmerman R. Stereotactic ablative radiotherapy for non-small cell lung cancer: rationale and outcomes. *J Natl Compr Canc Netw* 2012;10:1514–1520.
98. Lo SS, Moffatt-Bruce SD, Dawson LA, et al. The role of local therapy in the management of lung and liver oligometastases. *Nat Rev Clin Oncol* 2011;8:405–416.
99. Forastiere AA, Zhang Q, Weber RS, et al. Long-term results of RTOG 91-11: a comparison of three nonsurgical treatment strategies to preserve the larynx in patients with locally advanced larynx cancer. *J Clin Oncol* 2013;31:845–852.
100. Gunderson LL, Winter KA, Ajani JA, et al. Long-term update of US GI intergroup RTOG 98-11 phase III trial for anal carcinoma: survival, relapse, and colostomy failure with concurrent chemoradiation involving fluorouracil/mitomycin versus fluorouracil/cisplatin. *J Clin Oncol* 2012;30:4344–4351.
101. Hellman S, Weichselbaum RR. Oligometastases. *J Clin Oncol* 1995;13:8–10.
102. Hortobagyi GN. Can we cure limited metastatic breast cancer? *J Clin Oncol* 2002;20:620–623.
103. Stamell EF, Wolchok JD, Gnjatic S, et al. The abscopal effect associated with a systemic anti-melanoma immune response. *Int J Radiat Oncol Biol Phys* 2013;85:293–295.
104. Nagtegaal ID, Gosens MJ, Marijnen CA, et al. Combinations of tumor and treatment parameters are more discriminative for prognosis than the present TNM system in rectal cancer. *J Clin Oncol* 2007;25:1647–1650.
105. Sauer R, Becker H, Hohenberger W, et al. Preoperative versus postoperative chemoradiotherapy for rectal cancer. *N Engl J Med* 2004;351:1731–1740.
106. Clarke M, Collins R, Darby S, et al. Effects of radiotherapy and of differences in the extent of surgery for early breast cancer on local recurrence and 15-year survival: an overview of the randomised trials. *Lancet* 2005;366:2087–2106.
107. Hellman S. Stopping metastases at their source. *N Engl J Med* 1997;337:996–997.
108. Marks LB, Prosnitz LR. Postoperative radiotherapy for lung cancer: the breast cancer story all over again? *Int J Radiat Oncol Biol Phys* 2000;48:625–627.
109. Wang XS, Rhines LD, Shiu AS, et al. Stereotactic body radiation therapy for management of spinal metastases in patients without spinal cord compression: a phase 1-2 trial. *Lancet Oncol* 2012;13:395–402.
110. Tarnawski R, Fowler J, Skladowski K, et al. How fast is repopulation of tumor cells during the treatment gap? *Int J Radiat Oncol Biol Phys* 2002;54:229–236.
111. Peters LJ, Withers HR. Applying radiobiological principles to combined modality treatment of head and neck cancer—the time factor. *Int J Radiat Oncol Biol Phys* 1997;39:831–836.
112. Bourhis J, Overgaard J, Audry H, et al. Hyperfractionated or accelerated radiotherapy in head and neck cancer: a meta-analysis. *Lancet* 2006;368:843–854.
113. Bourhis J, Sire C, Graff P, et al. Concomitant chemoradiotherapy versus acceleration of radiotherapy with or without concomitant chemotherapy in locally advanced head and neck carcinoma (GORTEC 99-02): an open-label phase 3 randomised trial. *Lancet Oncol* 2012;13:145–153.
114. Adkison JB, McHaffie DR, Bentzen SM, et al. Phase I trial of pelvic nodal dose escalation with hypofractionated IMRT for high-risk prostate cancer. *Int J Radiat Oncol Biol Phys* 2012;82:184–190.
115. Feyer P, Maranzano E, Molassiotis A, et al. Radiotherapy-induced nausea and vomiting (RINV): antiemetic guidelines. *Support Care Cancer* 2005;13:122–128.
116. Horiot JC. Prophylaxis versus treatment: is there a better way to manage radiotherapy-induced nausea and vomiting? *Int J Radiat Oncol Biol Phys* 2004;60:1018–1025.
117. Hickok JT, Roscoe JA, Morrow GR, et al. Frequency, severity, clinical course, and correlates of fatigue in 372 patients during 5 weeks of radiotherapy for cancer. *Cancer* 2005;104:1772–1778.
118. Schwartz AL, Nail LM, Chen S, et al. Fatigue patterns observed in patients receiving chemotherapy and radiotherapy. *Cancer Invest* 2000;18:11–19.
119. Dawson LA, Ten Haken RK. Partial volume tolerance of the liver to radiation. *Semin Radiat Oncol* 2005;15:279–283.
120. Kong FM, Hayman JA, Griffith KA, et al. Final toxicity results of a radiation-dose escalation study in patients with non-small-cell lung cancer (NSCLC): predictors for radiation pneumonitis and fibrosis. *Int J Radiat Oncol Biol Phys* 2006;65:1075–1086.
121. Fleckenstein K, Gauter-Fleckenstein B, Jackson IL, et al. Using biological markers to predict risk of radiation injury. *Semin Radiat Oncol* 2007;17:89–98.
122. Hart JP, Broadwater G, Rabbani Z, et al. Cytokine profiling for prediction of symptomatic radiation-induced lung injury. *Int J Radiat Oncol Biol Phys* 2005;63:1448–1454.
123. Barnett GC, Coles CE, Elliott RM, et al. Independent validation of genes and polymorphisms reported to be associated with radiation toxicity: a prospective analysis study. *Lancet Oncol* 2012;13:65–77.
124. Fajardo LF. Is the pathology of radiation injury different in small vs large blood vessels? *Cardiovasc Radiat Med* 1999;1:108–110.
125. Delanian S, Porcher R, Rudant J, et al. Kinetics of response to long-term treatment combining pentoxifylline and tocopherol in patients with superficial radiation-induced fibrosis. *J Clin Oncol* 2005;23:8570–8579.
126. Chou TC, Talalay P. Quantitative analysis of dose-effect relationships: the combined effects of multiple drugs or enzyme inhibitors. *Adv Enzyme Regul* 1984;22:27–55.
127. Steel GG, Peckham MJ. Exploitable mechanisms in combined radiotherapy-chemotherapy: the concept of additivity. *Int J Radiat Oncol Biol Phys* 1979;5:85–91.
128. Tannock IF. Treatment of cancer with radiation and drugs. *J Clin Oncol* 1996;14:3156–3174.
129. Blanchard P, Baujat B, Holostenco V, et al. Meta-analysis of chemotherapy in head and neck cancer (MACH-NC): a comprehensive analysis by tumour site. *Radiother Oncol* 2011;100:33–40.
130. Dillman RO, Herndon J, Seagren SL, et al. Improved survival in stage III non-small-cell lung cancer: seven-year follow-up of cancer and leukemia group B (CALGB) 8433 trial. *J Natl Cancer Inst* 1996;88:1210–1215.
131. De Ruysscher D, Belderbos J, Reymen B, et al. State of the art radiation therapy for lung cancer 2012: a glimpse of the future. *Clin Lung Cancer* 2013;14:89–95.
132. Klopp AH, Eifel PJ. Chemoradiotherapy for cervical cancer in 2010. *Curr Oncol Rep* 2011;13:77–85.
133. Chun PY, Feng FY, Scheurer AM, et al. Synergistic effects of gemcitabine and gefitinib in the treatment of head and neck carcinoma. *Cancer Res* 2006;66:981–988.

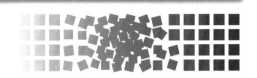

# 14 Cancer Immunotherapy

Steven A. Rosenberg, Paul F. Robbins, Giao Q. Phan,
Steven A. Feldman, and James N. Kochenderfer

## INTRODUCTION

Progress in understanding basic aspects of cellular immunology and tumor–host immune interactions have led to the development of immune-based therapies capable of mediating the rejection of metastatic cancer in humans. Early studies of allografts and transplanted syngeneic tumors in mice demonstrated that it was the cellular arm of the immune response rather than the action of antibodies (humoral immunity) that was responsible for tissue rejection. Thus, studies of immunotherapy have focused on enhancing antitumor immune responses of T cells that recognize cancer antigens. Antibodies that recognize growth factors on the surface of tumors can contribute to tumor regression, primarily by interfering with growth signals rather than by the direct destruction of tumor cells. The use of monoclonal antibodies in cancer treatment will be considered in Chapter 29.

Evidence for specific tumor recognition by cells of the immune system was obtained in experiments first conducted in the 1940s using murine tumors generated or induced by the mutagen methylcholanthrene (MCA). Mice that received a surgical resection of previously inoculated tumors could be protected against a subsequent tumor challenge with the immunizing tumor but not generally protected against challenge with additional MCA tumors. The observation that CD8+ cytotoxic T cells were primarily responsible for mediating the rejection of MCA-induced tumors in mice led to the identification of genes that encoded tumor rejection antigens expressed on murine tumors as well as the subsequent identification of antigens recognized by human tumor-reactive T cells. The identification of widely shared nonmutated tumor antigens led to the expectation that effective vaccine therapies could be developed for the treatment of cancer patients; however, the response rates in clinical cancer vaccine trials targeting these antigens have, to this point, been disappointingly low. Vaccination with viruslike particles expressing human papilloma virus (HPV) proteins are successful in preventing the establishment of cervical cancer and immunization with peptides derived from the oncogenic HPV E6 and E7 proteins can mediate tumor regression in woman with high vulvar neoplasia.[1] Immune-based therapies have, however, been identified that mediate the regression of large, established tumor metastases. Nonspecific immune stimulation with interleukin-2 (IL-2) administration can lead to objective clinical responses in patients with melanoma and renal cancer,[2] and inhibition of regulatory pathways mediated by CTLA-4[3] or PD-1[4] can lead to tumor regression in patients with metastatic melanoma and lung cancer. The adoptive transfer of melanoma reactive T cells can mediate objective clinical responses in 50% to 70% of patients with melanoma,[5] and the ability to genetically modify antitumor lymphocytes is expanding this cell transfer therapy approach to the treatment of patients with other cancer histologies.[6] Studies aimed at identifying potent tumor rejection antigens, as well as mechanisms that regulate immune responses to cancer, are being actively pursued.

## HUMAN TUMOR ANTIGENS

To be recognized by immune lymphocytes, intracellular proteins must be digested and the resulting peptides transported to the cell surface and bound to Class I or II main histocompatibility molecules (Fig. 14.1). A variety of approaches have been used to identify the antigens that are naturally processed and presented on tumor cells. These include evaluating the ability of cells transfected with tumor cDNA library pools along with genes encoding autologous major histocompatibility complex (MHC) molecules, as well as the ability of target cells pulsed with peptides eluted from tumor cell surface MHC molecules for their ability to stimulate tumor reactive T cells. Reverse immunology approaches that involve either repeated in vitro T cell sensitization or in vivo immunization with candidate peptides or proteins have also lead to the identification of tumor antigens. Candidate epitopes identified on the basis of their ability to bind to a particular MHC molecule, however, may not necessarily be naturally processed and presented on the tumor cell surface, and there are conflicting reports on the ability of T cells generated using some candidate epitopes to recognize unmanipulated tumor targets, as discussed further.

Additional tumor antigens have been identified using antisera from cancer patients to screen tumor cell cDNA libraries, a method that has been termed serological analysis of recombinant cDNA expression (SEREX).[7] Although some of the proteins identified using this technique are expressed in a tumor-specific manner, many of these antigens are simply expressed at higher levels in tumor cells than in normal cells. This may occur due to the release of normal self-proteins from necrotic and apoptotic tumor cells leading to the generation of antibodies against intracellular proteins that are normally sequestered from the immune system.

Finally, the use of recently described approaches involving whole exomic sequencing of tumor cells has led to the identification of mutated tumor antigens. These studies will be discussed further in the section devoted to mutated tumor antigens

### Cancer/Germ-Line Antigens

The first antigen identified as a target of human tumor reactive T cells was isolated by screening a melanoma genomic DNA library with an autologous cytotoxic T lymphocyte (CTL) clone.[8] The gene that was isolated, termed *MAGE-1*, was found to be a nonmutated gene that was a member of a large, previously unidentified gene family, many of whose members encode antigens recognized by tumor reactive T cells.[9] Members of this family of antigens are expressed in the testes and placenta, both of which lack an expression of MHC molecules, but often not in other normal tissues, which has led to their designation as cancer germ-line (CG) antigens. Members of the MAGE gene family are expressed in a variety of tumor types, including melanoma, breast, prostate, and esophageal cancers. The expression patterns of three

CANCER THERAPEUTICS

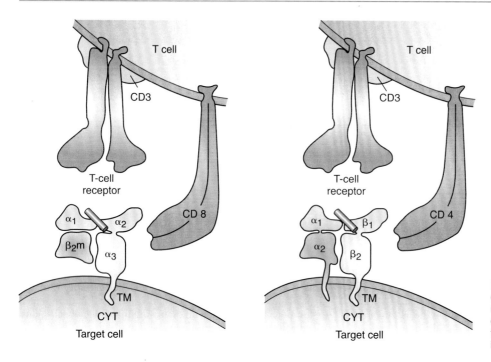

**Figure 14.1** CD8 and CD4 cells use different molecules that interact with major histocompatibility complex (MHC) class I and II molecules respectively on the cell surface and serve to potentiate immune reactions.

different cancer/testes antigens in multiple tumor types is shown in Figure 14.2. The NY-ESO-1 antigen—a CG antigen that is unrelated to the MAGE family of genes—is expressed in approximately 30% of breast, prostate, and melanoma tumors, as well as between 70% and 80% of synovial cell sarcomas.[10]

Clinical adoptive immunotherapy trials targeting CG antigens have now been conducted in patients with melanoma as well as other tumor types. In a recent trial, objective clinical responses were seen in approximately 50% of patients with melanoma and 80% of patients with synovial cell sarcoma receiving autologous peripheral blood mononuclear cell (PBMC) transduced with a T-cell receptor directed against an HLA-A*02:01 restricted NY-ESO-1 epitope.[6] A trial targeting a MAGEA3

epitopes was recently carried out using a T-cell receptor (TCR) isolated from an HLA-A*02:01+ transgenic mouse immunized with the MAGEA3:112–120 peptide.[11] Objective clinical responses were observed in five of nine melanoma patients receiving the adoptively transferred PBMC that were transduced with the MAGEA3-reactive TCR.[12] Unexpectedly, neural toxicity was observed in three of the patients treated in this trial, two of whom lapsed into a coma and subsequently died. Autopsy samples of patients' brains revealed that *MAGEA12*, which encodes a crossreactive epitope recognized by the MAGEA3 TCR, was expressed at low levels in patients' brains, which may have been responsible for the observed neurologic toxicities. In a recent trial carried out using an affinity-enhanced human TCR directed against the

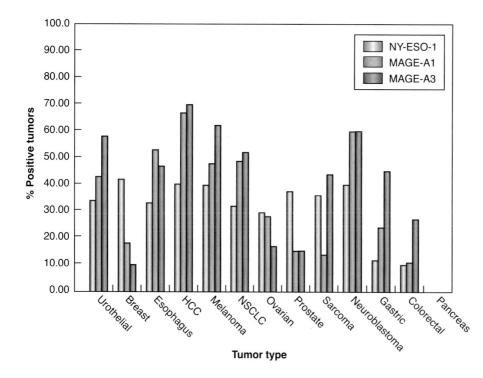

**Figure 14.2** Expression of three different cancer/testes antigens in many different tumor types is shown. These data reflect reverse transcription–polymerase chain reaction measurements and is more sensitive than results obtained by immunohistochemistry. NSCLC, non–small-cell lung cancer. (Data compiled by Dr. J. Wargo. Massachusetts General Hospital.)

HLA-A*01:01-restricted, MAGEA3:168-176 epitope, the first two patients receiving TCR-transduced autologous PBMC died of cardiac arrest 4 to 5 days following infusion, which was attributed to cross-reactivity with titin, a protein expressed at high levels in cardimyocytes.[13] Taken together, these findings demonstrate the need for caution in evaluating cross-reactivity of high affinity TCRs recognizing tumor antigens.

## Melanocyte Differentiation Antigens

Melanoma-reactive T cells have been frequently found to recognize gene products, termed melanocyte differentiation antigens (MDA), that are expressed in melanomas as well as in normal melanocytes present in the skin, eye, and ear but not in other normal tissues or tumor types. These include epitopes derived from gp100,[14,15] tyrosinase,[16] TRP-1,[17] and TRP-2,[18] proteins that had previously been found to play important roles in melanin synthesis. The screening of melanoma cDNA libraries with an HLA-A2–restricted tumor reactive T cells lead to the isolation of a previously unidentified gene, termed MART-1[19] or Melan-A.[20] The MART-1 antigen, which is expressed in 80% to 90% of fresh melanomas and cultured melanoma cell lines as well as normal melanocytes, represents an MDA of unknown function. The majority of melanoma reactive, HLA-A2–restricted tumor-infiltrating lymphocytes (TIL) recognize a single MART-1 epitope.[21] Studies carried out using a variety of approaches have also resulted in the identification of human leukocyte antigen (HLA) class II restricted epitopes of tyrosinase, TRP-1, TRP-2, and gp100.[9]

## Overexpressed Gene Products

Gene products that are expressed at low levels in a variety of normal tissues but are overexpressed in a variety of tumor types have also been shown to be recognized by T cells. Screening of an autologous renal carcinoma cDNA library with a tumor reactive, HLA-A3–restricted T-cell clone resulted in the isolation of FGF5,[22] a protein that was expressed only at low levels in normal tissues but upregulated in multiple renal carcinomas as well as prostate and breast carcinomas. The peptide epitope recognized by FGF5-reactive T cells was generated by protein splicing, a process in which distant protein regions are joined together in the proteasome that had previously only been described in plants[23] and unicellular organisms.[24] Subsequent studies have led to the identification of multiple epitopes that result from protein splicing, suggesting that this represents a general mechanism for generating T-cell epitopes.[25–28] Screening of an autologous cDNA library led to the identification of a previously unknown gene that was termed PRAME.[29] This gene product was expressed in relatively high levels in melanomas as well as in additional tumor types but was also expressed at lower levels in a variety of normal tissues that included the testis, endometrium, ovary, and adrenals. The HLA-A24–restricted PRAME reactive T-cell clone, however, expressed the natural killer (NK) inhibitory receptor p58.2, and tumor cell recognition was dependent on the loss of expression of the HLA C*07 allele that represented the ligand for the inhibitory receptor, which may explain the lack of recognition of normal tissues that express relatively high levels of this HLA gene product.

Attempts have also been made to generate T cells directed against overexpressed candidate antigens by repeatedly stimulating PBMC in vitro with peptides that were identified as high binders for particular MHC molecules either using direct binding assays or in silico analysis carried out using peptide/MHC binding algorithms.[30,31] Using this approach, candidate epitopes have been identified from a variety of proteins that include prostate-specific antigen (PSA)[32] and prostate-specific membrane antigen (PSMA),[33] as well as Her-2/neu, a protein that is frequently overexpressed in a variety of tumor types, including breast carcinomas. Initial studies indicated that T cells derived by in vitro stimulation

with a peptide that was predicted to bind with high affinity to HLA-A*02:01, Her-2/neu:369–377, recognized the appropriate natural tumor targets.[34] In one study, T cells generated following two in vitro stimulations of postvaccination PBMC from three of the four patients who were tested efficiently recognized peptide-pulsed targets but failed to recognize appropriate tumor targets.[35] Similarly, although stimulation with a peptide corresponding to amino acids 540 through 548 of the human telomerase reverse transcriptase (hTERT) catalytic subunit was initially reported to generate tumor-reactive T cells,[36] additional observations indicated that T cells generated using this peptide failed to recognize tumor targets.[37] These factors responsible for these discrepancies remain unresolved, although the in vitro stimulation of T cells with target cells pulsed with relatively high peptide concentrations could have led to the generation of low-avidity T cells that were incapable of recognizing naturally processed antigens.

Alternative screening approaches employed for tumor antigen discovery that may help to address these issues include the use of tandem mass spectrometry to sequence peptides that have been eluted from tumor cell surface MHC molecules. Use of this technique, coupled with microarray gene expression profiling, resulted in the identification of peptides derived from proteins that appeared to be overexpressed in tumor cells.[38] Peptides identified using this approach may, in many cases, not be immunogenic due to the fact that their expression in normal tissues, although lower than in tumor cells, may be high enough to lead to central or peripheral tolerance. Nevertheless, one of the peptides that were identified in this study also appeared to be recognized by human tumor reactive T cells. Recently, a similar approach was used to identify candidate peptides presented on cell surface MHC molecules that appeared to be derived from proteins that were overexpressed on glioblastomas.[39] In a clinical trial involving vaccination of patients with pools of the identified peptides, overall survival was associated with the number of peptides in the vaccine pool that elicited immune response[40]; however, this may simply reflect the fact that T cells from healthier patients can more readily generate peptide-specific responses.

Transgenic mice that express human HLA molecules have also been immunized with candidate antigens in an attempt to identify high avidity tumor-reactive T cells. Immunization of transgenic mice expressing HLA-A*0201 with the native human p53:264–272 peptide that differed from the corresponding murine p53 sequence at a single position lead to the generation of T cells that recognized tumor cells expressing high levels of p53.[41] Human T cells transduced with a murine p53 TCR isolated from an immunized mouse recognized a variety of human tumor cells; however, transduced T cells also recognized normal cells expressing lower p53 levels, indicating the dangers of targeting a normal self-protein whose expression is not strictly limited to tumor cells.[42] Similarly, a TCR that was highly reactive with HLA-A*02:01+ tumor cells expressing the human carcinoembryonic antigen (CEA), a protein that is overexpressed in colon and breast carcinomas, was isolated by immunizing HLA-A*02:01+ transgenic mice with the CEA:691–699 peptide.[43] The adoptive transfer of human PBMC transduced with the CEA-reactive TCR lead to an objective clinical response in one of the three treated patients; however, severe colitis was observed in all three of the treated patients.[44] In general, immunotherapies that target antigens present even in small amounts on normal tissues have led to normal tissue destruction and must be applied with caution.

## Mutated Gene Products Recognized by CD8+ and CD4+ T Cells

A variety of mutated antigens have also been identified as targets of tumor reactive T cells. The majority of mutated antigens identified using these approaches appear to be unique or only expressed in a relatively small percentage of cancers, and so do not represent targets that are broadly applicable to the treatment of multiple patients. Nevertheless, these studies have in some cases provided insights into mechanisms involved with tumor development, as the mutations may represent drivers of the transformed phenotype. The CDK4 gene product that was cloned using a CTL clone contained a point mutation that enhanced the binding to the HLA-A2 restriction element.[45] This mutation, which was identified in 1 of an additional 28 melanomas that were analyzed, led to the inhibition of binding to the cell cycle inhibitory protein p16[INK4a] and may have played a role in the loss of growth control in this tumor cell. A point-mutated product of the β-catenin gene, containing a substitution of phenylalanine for serine at position 37, was isolated by screening a cDNA library with an HLA-24–restricted, melanoma reactive TIL.[46] This mutation was found to stabilize the β-catenin gene product by altering a critical serine phosphorylation site, and 2 of 24 additional melanoma cell lines were found to express transcripts with identical mutations.[47]

The observation that immunization against individual murine tumors did not generally cross-protect against challenge with additional syngeneic murine tumors has provided support for the hypothesis that mutant T-cell epitopes represent the predominant antigens responsible for tumor rejection.[48] Mutated epitopes also represent a foreign antigen, which may render them more immunogenic than the majority of normal self-antigens. Although many of the mutations are specific for individual tumors, T cells have been generated by carrying out in vitro sensitization with peptides encoded at mutational hot spots present in *driver* genes.[49]

Recently, novel approaches have been developed that involve the sequencing of tumor cell DNA to identify potential mutated epitopes. In one study, whole exome sequencing of the murine B16 melanoma led to the identification of mutated epitopes that elicited a T cell that appeared to specifically recognize the mutated but not the corresponding wild-type peptides.[50] In a second study, a mutated antigen was identified by screening candidate epitopes that were expressed by tumors derived from immunodeficient mice that regressed in immune-competent mice.[51] More recently, melanomas from three patients who responded to adoptive immunotherapy were subjected to whole exome sequencing, followed by *in silico* analysis using peptide/MHC binding algorithms to identify candidate epitopes that were predicted to bind to the patients' MHC molecules.[52] Using this approach, a total of seven peptides were identified as targets of the TIL that were administered to these patients. Two mutated epitopes were recently identified by whole exome sequencing of a melanoma from a patient who demonstrated a partial response to treatment with the anti–CTLA-4 antibody ipilimumab, followed by a screening of a panel of mutated candidate peptide/MHC tetramers that were predicted to bind to the patient's HLA-A and B alleles.[53] In addition, a mutated epitope expressed by a bile duct cancer was identified by screening tandem minigenes encoding all mutated epitopes that were identified by whole exome sequencing.[54] The adoptive transfer of T cells directed against this mutation-mediated regression of the patient's cancer. Mutations unique to each cancer represent ideal targets for immunotherapy and can potentially lead to the development of personalized therapies directed against these unique targets.

## Antigens Identified in Viral-Associated Cancers

Viruses do not appear to play a role in the development of the majority of human cancers; however, an infection with HPV, a group of double-stranded DNA viruses that infect squamous epithelium, is highly associated with the development of a variety of genital lesions that range from warts to carcinomas, as well as the majority of oropharyngeal carcinomas. Recombinant vaccines have been produced by the generation of viruslike particles (VLP),

self-assembling particles that form following the expression of the HPV L1 protein in recombinant viral and yeast systems that were initially found to be protective in animal models. The results of a phase II trial in which 2,392 women between 16 and 23 years of age were immunized with HPV-16 VLPs indicated that 100% of those who were vaccinated were protected against infection with HPV-16.[55,56] Although vaccination with VLP does not lead to the regression of established disease, some success has been seen in therapeutic vaccination trials that target the oncogenic viral proteins E6 and E7. In a trial involving the vaccination of women with HPV-16–positive high-grade vulvar intraepithelial neoplasia with synthetic long peptides that encompass both HLA class I and class II restricted epitopes from the oncogenic HPV proteins E6 and E, clinical responses were observed in 15 of the 19 vaccinated patients, and complete regression of all lesions were seen in 9 of the 19 patients in this trial.[1]

Targeting foreign antigens thus may represent a strategy that can lead to more effective immunotherapies. These include viral epitopes as well as mutated epitopes that are also foreign to the host and therefore may represent more effective targets for these therapies than normal self-antigen.

## HUMAN CANCER IMMUNOTHERAPIES

A wide variety of therapies have been evaluated in model systems and are now being developed for the treatment of patients with cancer. These include nonspecific approaches, those that involve direct immunization of patients with a variety of immunogens and approaches that involve the adoptive transfer of activated effector cells (Table 14.1). Much confusion related to the effectiveness of cancer immunotherapy has resulted from the lack of proper evaluation of the results of therapy using standard, accepted oncologic criteria such as the World Health Organization or the Response Evaluation Criteria in Solid Tumors (RECIST). Many clinical trials reported a positive use of *soft* criteria such as lymphoid infiltration or tumor necrosis that can occur in the natural course of cancer growth. Because of the delayed responses seen with some immunotherapy approaches, including tumor regression after initial tumor growth, guidelines have been published suggesting the use of an alternate set of immune-related response criteria for the evaluation of immune-based cancer treatments.[57,58] Other confusion has arisen from the use of inappropriate animal models. Although animal model systems have provided important clues that may lead to improved therapies, model systems that employ artificially introduced foreign antigens or that evaluate protection from tumor challenge do not appear to be relevant to the treatment of patients with bulky metastases. Short-term lung metastasis models involve the treatment of relatively small, nonvascularized tumors and also may not be directly relevant to the majority of tumors that are the targets of current clinical trials.

---

### TABLE 14.1

#### Three Main Approaches to Cancer Immunotherapy

1. Nonspecific stimulation of immune reactions
   a) Stimulate effector cells
      IL-2 (melanoma and renal cancer)
   b) Inhibit regulatory factors
      Anti-CTLA4 (melanoma)
      Anti–PD-1 (melanoma, lung cancer)
2. Active immunization to enhance antitumor reactions (cancer vaccines)
3. Passively transfer activated immune cells with antitumor activity (adoptive immunotherapy)

# Nonspecific Approaches to Cancer Immunotherapy

Progress has surged in the past 10 years in the understanding and utilization of nonspecific immune stimulation for the treatment of metastatic cancers. These agents aim to activate quiescent tumor-reactive immune cells or to remove inhibitory mechanisms to allow immunosuppressed cells to function to their full capacity. Although IL-2 and ipilimumab are currently the only immune stimulants approved by the U.S. Food and Drug Administration (FDA) for the treatment of metastatic renal cell carcinoma (IL-2) and melanoma (IL-2 and ipilimumab), new immune checkpoint inhibitors such as anti–programmed cell death 1 (anti–PD-1) have shown impressive results in recent clinical trials for patients with melanoma, renal cell cancer, and also non–small-cell lung cancer (NSCLC), and will likely be approved in the near future. As expected with nonspecific immunostimulation, systemic and bystander immune-related adverse events such as colitis has been reported with all agents in varying degrees, although most side effects are controllable and reversible if addressed aggressively and promptly by experienced clinicians. Importantly, antitumor responses seen with these immune-based modalities appear to be durable for some patients and may even be potentially curative. As with many therapies for metastatic solid tumors, preliminary trials using combination therapies have suggested better than expected response rates and survival, and confirmatory trials are in process to validate and ensure that toxicities from combining agents would not be prohibitive. Overall, patients with metastatic solid tumors may soon have wider armamentarium of off-the-shelf immunotherapy options.

## Interleukin-2

Morgan et al.[59] showed that a *factor* produced in the medium from stimulated normal human blood lymphocytes can allow ex vivo growth and expansion of human T lymphocytes. The identification of this soluble T-cell growth factor (IL-2)[60,61] allowed the ability to culture T cells in vitro. IL-2 is a 15-kd glycoprotein produced in minute amounts by activated peripheral blood lymphocytes, and even with using T-cell hybridomas, minimal quantities could be purified; thus, research using IL-2 was impeded by the limited amounts of purified IL-2 available. The isolation of the cDNA clone in 1983[62] enabled the development in 1984 of recombinant IL-2,[63] which permitted the ability to mass manufacture IL-2. Although murine studies demonstrated the ability of IL-2 to mediate tumor regression,[64] early phase I clinical trials did not show any antitumor response,[65] but was instructive in showing pharmacokinetics and toxicities, which led to more effective regimens. Subsequently, IL-2 was given in higher doses (up to 720,000 IU/kg intravenously every 8 hours) in a landmark trial involving 25 patients, along with nonspecific lymphokine-activated natural killer (LAK) cells, which are non-T and non-B lymphocytes.[66] This report was the first to document the regression of advanced solid cancers (melanoma, renal cell, lung, and colon) using immunotherapy in humans.[66] A follow-up trial randomizing 181 patients to either high-dose IL-2 alone (720,000 IU/kg intravenously every 8 hours) or high-dose IL-2 and LAK cells showed that the tumor response was due to IL-2 alone and not to the nonspecific LAK cells.[67] This study also narrowed the IL-2–sensitive histologies to melanoma and renal cell cancer, which had more consistent responses.

## IL-2 Therapy for Metastatic Renal Cell Cancer

Subsequent to the studies discussed previously, high-dose IL-2 was tested by additional centers and in combination with other agents for renal cell cancer. A randomized phase II trial involving 99 kidney cancer patients showed no increase in antitumor responses with the addition of interferon alfa-2b (IFNα-2b). Responses were seen for 12 (17%) of 71 patients who received high-dose IL-2 alone, with 4 complete regressions.[68] A summary report of 227 patients with metastatic renal cell cancer treated with high-dose IL-2 (defined as 600,000 IU/kg or 720,000 IU/kg given intravenously every 8 hours as tolerated up to 15 doses) from 1985 to 1996 at the Surgery Branch of the National Cancer Institute (NCI) documented a total response rate of 19%, with 10% partial and 9% complete; the longest duration of a complete response was over 10 years ongoing (134+ months).[69] Another summary report from seven phase II clinical trials from multiple institutions involving 255 patients with metastatic renal cell cancer receiving high-dose IL-2 showed the overall response rate was 14%, with 9% partial and 5% complete, and responses occurred in all sites of disease, including primary kidney tumors, bone metastases, and bulking visceral tumor burdens.[70] Although the response rates were modest, the durability of the responses was remarkable, with many responses lasting over 5 years ongoing (see Fig. 14.2). Because of the striking durability of the antitumor responses, IL-2 received FDA approval for the treatment of metastatic renal cell cancer in 1992. A follow-up report in 2000 showing the response rates of the 255 renal cell patients in the seven phase II studies to be the same, with complete responses lasting over 10 years ongoing (131+ months for the longest responder), suggesting a potential cure.[71]

To ascertain whether lower doses and/or different administration routes, which would decrease toxicity and obviate the need for inpatient hospitalization for IL-2 therapy, a trial randomizing 400 patients with metastatic renal cell cancer to either standard high-dose intravenous IL-2, low-dose intravenous IL-2 (at 72,000 IU/kg), or low-dose subcutaneous IL-2 (250,000 U/kg per dose daily Monday through Friday in the first week and then 125,000 U/kg per dose daily during the next 5 weeks).[72] Although responses were seen with all three regimens, including complete responses in the low-dose subcutaneous regimen, standard high-dose IL-2 had higher overall response rates (21%) versus low-dose intravenous IL-2 (13%; p = 0.048) and low-dose subcutaneous IL-2 (10%; p = 0.033), suggesting the superiority of the high-dose intravenous regimen.[72]

The administration of IL-2 represents the only known curative treatment for patients with metastatic renal cell cancer and should be considered as front-line therapy for suitable patients.

## IL-2 Therapy for Metastatic Melanoma

Between 1985 and 1993, 270 patients with metastatic melanoma enrolled into eight clinical trials in multiple centers using high-dose IL-2 (defined as 600,000 IU/kg or 720,000 IU/kg given intravenously every 8 hours as tolerated up to 15 doses). Atkins et al.[73] reported overall response rates of 16% (43 patients), with 10% partial and 6% complete; responses occurred at all tumor sites and regardless of initial tumor burden. With median follow-up at that time of 62 months, 20 responders (47%) were still alive, with 15 surviving over 5 years.[73] A follow-up report on those patients in 2000 showed that the response rates were unchanged; with the longest response duration of >12 years ongoing, disease progression was not observed in any patient responding greater than 30 months.[74] As with renal cell cancer, the flat *tail* of the Kaplan-Meier response duration and overall survival curves (Fig. 14.3), showing the potential curative nature of the antitumor responses, was the main compelling reason the FDA approved IL-2 for the treatment of metastatic melanoma in 1998.

Research in subsequent years aimed to increase the response rates of IL-2, led by increasing interests in tumor vaccinations as melanoma-associated antigens were being characterized.[75] Pilot studies suggested that vaccinations using modified melanoma differentiation antigens such as gp100:209–217(210M) could elicit immunologic responses in nearly all patients, and when combined with high-dose IL-2, could elicit potentially higher than expected clinical antitumor responses.[75] A follow-up phase III study[76] randomized 185 patients with HLA*A0201 from 21 centers to either high-dose IL-2 or high-dose IL-2 plus gp100:209–217(210M) concurrent immunization. Although the response rates for the

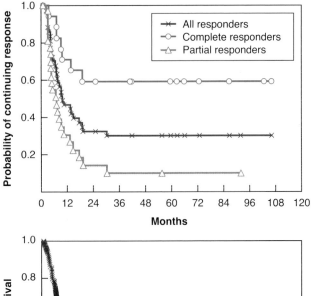

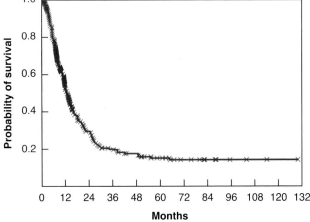

**Figure 14.3** Kaplain-Meier plots of response duration (*top*) and overall survival (*bottom*) for 270 patients with metastatic melanoma who were treated with high-dose bolus IL-2 from 1985 to 1993 in eight clinical trials.[73]

IL-2 plus vaccine arm was statistically improved compared to IL-2 alone (16% versus 6%; p = 0.03), the IL-2 alone arm was notable for being much lower than in all prior studies.[76] In addition, a pilot trial of 36 melanoma patients treated high-dose IL-2 concurrently with ipilimumab (an antibody against cytotoxic T lymphocyte–associated antigen 4 discussed in the following section) gave a 25% OR rate, with 17% achieving complete response[77]; however, these data have not been further tested.

Correlative studies suggest that the total doses of IL-2 received during the first treatment course was significantly higher in patients achieving a complete response[69]; however, when limited to patients who were able to complete both cycles of the course, there was no statistical significance, suggesting that patients whose tumors progressed significantly after one cycle (and was not able to complete the second cycle of the course) accounted for some of the difference seen.[78] Responders did have a higher maximal lymphocyte count[69,78] immediately posttherapy and were more likely to develop vitiligo and thyroid dysfunction.[78] There has not been a consistent pretherapy factor that is predictive of response, although one retrospective correlative study involving 374 patients showed that patients with M1a (subcutaneous- and/or cutaneous-only disease) have a response rate of 54% compared with 12% for those with visceral M1b/c ($P_2$ <0.0001).[78]

## Toxicities and Safe Administration of IL-2

High-dose IL-2 has been shown to be associated with adverse events that impact multiple organ systems.[73,79,80] The main component of

the toxicities is due to an inflammatory response mediated by the release of cytokines such as IFN$\gamma$ and tumor necrosis factor alpha (TNF-$\alpha$)[81] resulting in a capillary-leak syndrome[82] and decreased systemic vascular resistance, which can lead to fever, hypotension, cardiac arrhythmia, lethargy, renal insufficiency, hepatic dysfunction, body edema, pulmonary edema, and confusion; other side effects can also include nausea, diarrhea, rash, anemia, thrombocytopenia, lymphocytosis, and neutrophil chemotactic defect[83] that predispose patients to gram-positive line infections. Since the first clinical trials with IL-2 in 1984, however, much has been learned to permit its safe dosing for appropriately screened patients[82,84,85]; importantly, if patients are appropriately supported, side effects are quickly reversible once IL-2 dosing ceases.[85] Kammula et al.[86] compared the incidences of grade 3/4 toxicities between the 155 patients treated from 1985 to 1986 to 156 patients treated from 1993 through 1997 at the NCI Surgery Branch: grade 3/4 hypotension decreased from 81% to 31%, intubations from 12% to 3%, neuropsychiatric toxicities from 19% to 8%, diarrhea from 92% to 12%, line sepsis from 18% to 4%, cardiac ischemia from 3% to 0%, and mortality from 3% to 0%. In fact, no fatality occurred strictly due to IL-2 therapy since 1989.[86] Overall strategies for the safe administration of high-dose IL-2 include careful screening for appropriately selected patients with adequate cardiopulmonary reserve, having an experienced team of physicians and nurses who are cognizant of the expected toxicities of IL-2, having routine preemptive measures such as prophylactic antibiotics to prevent line infections, and aggressive and prompt management of toxicities.

## Checkpoint Modulators

### Anti–Cytotoxic T Lymphocyte Antigen 4

CTLA-4 is an immunosuppressive *costimulatory* receptor found on newly activated T cells (and on regulatory T cells) that binds with costimulatory ligands B7-1 and B7-2 on antigen-presenting cells.[87,88] When CTLA-4 is engaged by B7-1 or B7-2, the T cells becomes inhibited,[89,90] suggesting that CTLA-4 likely evolved as a self-protective mechanism to prevent autoimmunity (Fig. 14.4). Thus, overcoming this *checkpoint* molecule was an aim of cancer immunotherapy. After CTLA-4 blockade in murine models led to antitumor immunity,[91,92] anti–CTLA-4 antibodies were tested in clinical trials starting in 2002.

The combination of anti–CTLA-4 blocking antibodies and vaccination worked well in murine models and led to one of the early phase II studies using ipilimumab (a fully human immunoglobulin [IgG$_1$] monoclonal antibody previously called MDX-010) with two gp100 vaccines, gp100:209–217(210M) and gp100:280–288(288V), in patients with metastatic melanoma.[93] Antitumor regressions were seen (from 11% to 22% overall response rates, with up to 8% complete response rates), along with severe autoimmune toxicities such as colitis, dermatitis, and even hypophysitis,[93–95] as would be expected based on the mechanism of CTLA-4 blockade. In fact, autoimmunity adverse events appeared to correlate with response to ipilimumab.[3] The experience with these early studies led to management strategies to screen aggressively for immune-related adverse events (IRAE), such as routine screening of endocrinopathies, and to treat IRAEs promptly, including high-dose steroids if needed for severe colitis.[96,97] Overall, ipilimumab was in some ways easier to manage for the patients than IL-2 because it was an outpatient infusion given every 3 weeks; IRAEs were unpredictable, however, and can appear suddenly many weeks after receiving a dose.

In 2010, results from a landmark phase III randomized trial comparing three treatment strategies (ipilimumab alone, gp100 peptide vaccine alone, or ipilimumab plus gp100 peptide vaccine) in 676 patients with metastatic melanoma were published showing improvement in median survival in the two arms that received ipilimumab (10 months) compared to the gp100 alone arm (6 months, p <0.001), despite showing a low response rate of 7% (among 540 patients who received ipilimumab).[98] Another

## "Second Signal"

### Additional signal(s) via costimulatory molecules

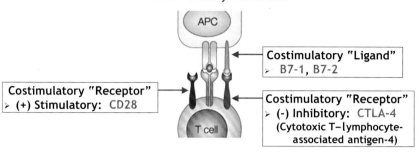

**Figure 14.4** Mechanism of action of cytotoxic T-lymphocyte–associated antigen 4 (CTLA-4). When CD28 is engaged on the T cell, reactivity of the T cell is enhanced. When CTLA-4 is engaged on the T cell, reactivity of the T cell is inhibited. Blocking of CTLA-4 with a monoclonal antibody can elicit antitumor immunity but also autoimmunity.

phase III randomized trial comparing dacarbazine plus ipilimumab versus dacarbazine alone again showed improved survival in that arm containing dacarbazine (11.2 months versus 9.1 months; p <0.001).[99] These studies showing survival benefit led to FDA approval of ipilimumab for advanced melanoma in 2011.

The responses seen with ipilimumab appear to be durable.[100] A follow-up study of 177 patients with metastatic melanoma treated on the earliest trials at the NCI Surgery Branch using ipilimumab showed that response duration could last 99+ months ongoing.[77] In fact, 14 out of the 15 complete responders remain disease free 54+ to 99+ months ongoing, suggesting a potential cure for some patients. Interestingly, several patients who were deemed partial responders converted to complete responders several years later, because it took an average of 30 months to have all visible tumor marks on imaging scans to disappear.[77]

Ipilimumab was also tested on other solid tumors, and renal cell cancer again appears to be the only other type beside melanoma that had significant responses. Sixty-one patients with metastatic renal cell cancer were treated, and six developed a response (10%); however, 33% developed grade 3/4 IRAEs.[101] Subsequently, the availability of agents with lower toxicity profiles such as sunitinib and sorafenib prevented further enthusiasm to pursue this drug for renal cell cancer.

Another anti–CTLA-4 antibody, tremelimumab (previously called CP-675,206), has also demonstrated durable responses in melanoma patients.[102,103] A phase III randomized trial randomizing 655 patients with metastatic melanoma to either tremelimumab or physician's choice chemotherapy, however, failed to show a survival difference (despite a significantly different response duration favoring tremelimumab, 35.8 months versus 13.7 months; p = 0.0011), possibly due to crossover of chemotherapy patients enrolling into ipilimumab trials and expanded access programs.[103]

### Anti–Programmed Death 1 and Anti–Programmed Death Ligand 1

PD-1 is another checkpoint modulator expressed on activated T cells. Although CTLA-4 appears to be involved in the early activation of T cells, PD-1 is involved in the later effector phase of T-cell activation and can function to prevent excessive damage to self by activated T cells in the periphery.[104,105] Interaction with its corresponding ligand, PD-L1 (B7-H1) and PD-L2 (B7-H2) leads to suppressed T-effector function. PD-L1 is expressed on hematopoietic and epithelial cells and is upregulated by cytokines such as IFNγ,[106] whereas PD-L1 is mainly on antigen-presenting cells. Given the clinical results with inhibiting the CTLA-4 checkpoint, recent efforts have focused on inhibiting the PD-1/PD-L1 and PD-1/PD-L2 interactions.

Nivolumab (previously known as BMS-936558, MDX-1106, and ONO-4538) is a fully human anti–PD-1 IgG4 monoclonal antibody that was initially tested in a phase I trial published in 2010

in which 39 patients with advanced solid cancers were treated in escalating doses.[107] Responses were seen in one patient with colon cancer, one with melanoma, and one with renal cell cancer; one patient developed colitis.[108] These hopeful results lead to a larger study in which 236 patients with either NSCLC (74 patients), melanoma (94 patients), or renal cell cancer (33 patients).[4] Objective responses were seen in 18% of patients with NSCLC, 28% with melanoma, and 27% with renal cell cancer.[4] Grade 3/4 adverse events occurred in 14% of patients, including those previously seen with ipilimumab (dermatitis, colitis, hepatitis, thyroiditis, hypophysitis, and pneumonitis). Nine patients developed pneumonitis, six of whom was reversible, and three (1%) with grade 3/4 died despite steroids and infliximab therapy.[4] An update on the status of 107 melanoma patients treated from 2008 to 2012 shows a 31% tumor response rate, with a median response duration of 2 years and a median overall survival of 16.8 months.[109]

Nivolumab was also tested in combination with ipilimumab in melanoma in either concurrent (53 patients) or sequenced (33 patients) regimens. The concurrent group experienced an overall response rate of 40%, whereas the sequenced group had a 20% response rate.[110] The concurrent group also experienced a higher rate of grade 3/4 adverse events (53%), compared to 18% in the sequenced group. Interestingly, 16 of 21 responders in the concurrent group experienced tumor reduction of 80% or greater by 12 weeks,[110] a tempo that is faster than was seen with ipilimumab.

Another anti–PD-1 developed independently, lambrolizumab (previously known as MK-3475, a humanized IgG4κ monoclonal antibody), was tested on 135 patients with metastatic melanoma.[111] The response rate was found to be 38% and was similar between those who had received ipilimumab and those who were ipilimumab naïve,[111] confirming that the antitumor response from lambrolizumab occurs via a different mechanism. Similar to nivolumab, 13% of patients developed grade 3/4 adverse events, with 4% developing pneumonitis, although none developed grade 3/4 pneumonitis.[111]

BMS-936559 is a fully human IgG4 monoclonal antibody that blocks PD-L1 ligation to both PD-1 and CD80. A phase I study was tested in 207 patients (75 with NSCLC, 55 with melanoma, 18 with colon cancer, and 17 with renal cell cancer, 17 with ovarian cancer, 14 with pancreatic cancer, 7 with gastric cancer, and 4 with breast cancer).[112] Among patients who were evaluated for response, objective responses were seen in 16% of melanoma patients, 17% of renal cell cancer patients, 10% of NSCLC patients, and 1 out of 17 ovarian cancer patients. Grade 3/4 toxicities were seen in 9% of patients.[112]

The advent of these checkpoint inhibitors brings additional treatment options to patients with selected advanced cancers, particularly those with histologies deemed previously to be outside the realm of immunotherapy such as NSCLC.[108,113] In addition, a new anti–PD-L1 (MPDL3280A) in clinical trials has also shown some efficacy in melanoma, renal cell cancer, and NSCLC in early reports.

## Active Immunization Approaches to Cancer Therapy (Cancer Vaccines)

The molecular characterization of multiple cancer antigens led to a large number of clinical trials that attempted to actively immunize against these antigens with the expectation that cellular immune reactions would be generated capable of inhibiting the growth of established cancers. The results of these efforts have yet to produce significant vaccine efforts of value in the treatment of human cancer. There is a paucity of murine tumor models that suggests that active vaccine approaches can mediate the regression of established vascularized tumors; therefore, it is not surprising that these approaches have, with a few exceptions, shown little efficacy in humans. Enthusiasm about the effectiveness of cancer vaccines has often been grounded in surrogate and subjective end points, rather than reliable objective cancer regressions using standard oncologic criteria. In a review of the world literature, including 107 published cancer vaccine trials involving 2,242 patients, a 3.4% overall objective response rate was observed (Table 14.2).[114,115] In many cases, relatively soft criteria such as stable disease or the regression of individual metastases in the presence of progressive disease at other sites have been reported. A variety of immunizing vectors have been used, including tumor-derived peptides, proteins, whole tumor cells, recombinant viruses, dendritic cells, and heat-shock proteins.[116–122] Although many of these approaches can lead to the development of circulating T cells that can recognize the immunizing tumor antigen, these T cells rarely cause the inhibition of established tumors, a point that has led to much confusion in the field of tumor immunology. The generation of antitumor T cells in vivo is likely a necessary, but certainly not a sufficient criteria for the development of a clinically active immunotherapy. Often, T cells with weak avidity for tumor recognition are generated, and the tolerizing and inhibitory influences that exist in vivo must be overcome for an effective immune response to cause tumor destruction.

A prospective randomized trial of immunization with antigen-presenting cells was carried out by the Dendreon Corporation (Seattle, Washington). This trial used an antigen-presenting cell vaccine loaded with prostatic acid phosphatase linked to GM-CSF compared to placebo in men with hormone-refractory prostate cancer.[123] Of 330 patients who received the vaccine treatment,

**TABLE 14.2**

### Experience with Therapeutic Cancer Vaccines

| | Number of Trials | Number of Patients | Objective Responses |
|---|---|---|---|
| Surgery Branch, National Cancer Institute | 25 | 541 | 14 (2.6%) |
| Published before 2005[114] | 33 | 765 | 29 (4.0%) |
| Published 2005–2010[115] | 49 | 936 | 34 (3.7%) |
| Total | 107 | 2,242 | 77 (3.4%) |

*Note*: Vaccines include: peptide, protein, dendritic cell, virus, plasmid DNA, and whole tumor cells.

1 objective partial response was seen. Only 8 patients experienced a PSA drop of at least 50%. There was no difference in the time to disease progression; however, the vaccine group had a median survival of 25.8 months compared to 21.7 months in the placebo group, and based on this statistically significant survival improvement, this treatment was approved by the FDA (Fig. 14.5).

## Adoptive Cell Transfer Immunotherapy

Adoptive cellular immunotherapy refers to the transfer to the tumor-bearing host of immune lymphocytes with anticancer activity. The first successful administration of adoptive cell therapy (ACT) involving TIL, in combination with high-dose IL-2 was carried out at the National Cancer Institute Surgery Branch in 1988.[124] Studies that used cell transfer therapy in patients with metastatic melanoma have provided the clearest evidence of the power of the immune system to mediate the regression of advanced metastatic cancers in humans. Adoptive cell therapy has several theoretical as well as practical advantages.[125] Lymphocytes with antitumor activity can be expanded to very large numbers ex vivo for infusion into cancer patients. These cells can be tested in vitro for antitumor activity, and cells with appropriate properties such as high avidity for tumor recognition and a high proliferative potential

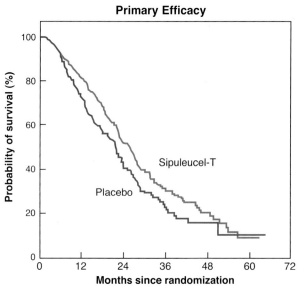

**Primary Efficacy**

Number at risk

| | | | | | | |
|---|---|---|---|---|---|---|
| Sipuleucel-T | 341 | 274 | 129 | 49 | 14 | 1 |
| Placebo | 171 | 123 | 55 | 19 | 4 | 1 |

**Figure 14.5** Kaplan-Meier estimate of the overall survival in patients with metastatic castration-resistant prostate cancer treated with Sipuleucel-T antigen–presenting cell immunotherapy. A modest but statistically significant improvement in survival was seen ($P = 0.03$).

## Adoptive Transfer of Tumor Infiltrating Lymphocytes (TIL)

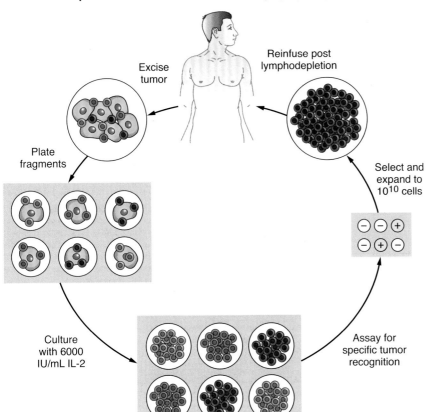

**Figure 14.6** Diagram of the adoptive cell therapy of patients with metastatic melanoma. Tumors are resected and individual cultures are grown and tested for antitumor reactivity. Optimal cultures are expanded in vitro and reinfused into the autologous patient who had received a preparative lymphodepleting chemotherapy.

can be identified and selectively expanded for treatment. These cells can be activated in vitro and thus are not subjected to the tolerizing influences that exist in vivo. Perhaps, most important, the host can be manipulated prior to the transfer of the anticancer cells to provide an optimal tumor microenvironment free of in vivo suppressive factors.[125] Studies have shown that the transfer of cultured lymphocytes with antiviral activity can prevent Epstein-Barr virus (EBV) infections as well as the subsequent development of posttransplant lymphoproliferative diseases. Cultured lymphocytes have been used for the treatment of patients with established EBV-induced lymphomas.[126]

The best evidence for the ability of adoptive cell transfer to successfully treat patients with solid tumors comes from the treatment of patients with metastatic melanoma. A diagram that describes the nature of this treatment is shown in Figure 14.6. In patients with metastatic melanoma, TILs can be obtained from resected tumor deposits and individual cultures tested to identify those with optimal anticancer activity.[124,127] These cells are then expanded ex vivo and reinfused along with IL-2, which is the requisite growth factor required for the survival and persistence of these cells. The administration of a preparative lymphodepleting chemotherapy regimen, consisting of cyclophosphamide and fludarabine with or without 2 or 12 Gy total body irradiation, could substantially enhance the survival and persistence of the transferred cells and increase their in vivo antitumor effectiveness.[128,129] In a series of three pilot trials with 93 patients, objective responses were seen in 49% to 72% of patients.[5,130] Of the 93 patients, 20 (22%) experienced a complete regression of all metastatic melanoma. Only 1 of these 20 patients has recurred, and the remaining patients have ongoing complete regressions from 80 to over 104 months (Table 14.3, Fig. 14.7).

| TABLE 14.3 | | | | |
|---|---|---|---|---|
| **Cell Transfer Therapy** | | | | |
| **Treatment** | **Total** | **PR** | **CR** | **OR** |
| | | *Number of Patients (Percentage) (Duration in Months)* | | |
| No TBI | 43 | 16 (37%)<br>(84, 36, 29, 28, 14, 12, 11, 7, 7, 7, 7, 4, 4, 2, 2, 2) | 5 (12%)<br>(114+, 112+, 111+, 97+, 86+) | 21 (49%) |
| 200 TBI | 25 | 8 (32%)<br>(14, 9, 6, 6, 5, 4, 3, 3) | 5 (20%)<br>(101+, 98+, 93+, 90+, 70+) | 13 (52%) |
| 1,200 TBI | 25 | 8 (32%)<br>(21, 13, 7, 6, 6, 5, 3, 2) | 10 (40%)<br>(81+, 78+, 77+, 72+, 72+, 71+, 71+, 70+, 70+, 19) | 18 (72%) |

*Note*: 20 complete responses: 19 ongoing at 70 to 114 months.

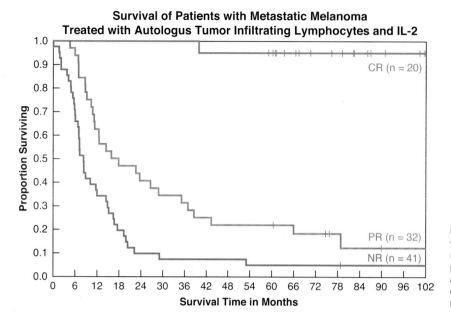

**Figure 14.7** Survival curves of 93 patients treated with adoptive cell transfer using autologous TIL. The results of three consecutive trials using different preparative regimens have been combined in this analysis. Of 20 patients who achieved a complete cancer regression, only one has recurred with a median follow-up of over 8 years.[5]

The 5-year survival of these 93 patients was 29% and was similar regardless of the prior treatments that these patients had received.

Extensive genomic studies have shown that TILs that mediate complete cancer regressions recognize mutated epitopes presented by the cancer.[52] The use of exomic sequencing combined with in vitro tests of antitumor activity can be used to select for T-cell populations reactive against the cancer. This approach has now been utilized to identify T cells used to successfully treat a patient with chemotherapy-refractory cholangiocarcinoma and provides a blueprint for the application of cell transfer therapy for a variety of common epithelial cancers.[54]

The difficulty in obtaining TILs with antitumor activity from cancers other than melanoma has also led to the development of approaches using lymphocytes genetically modified using retroviral transduction to insert antitumor T-cell receptors into the normal lymphocytes of patients.[131]

## Genetic Modification of Lymphocytes for Use in Adoptive Cell Therapy: Basic Principles and Applications to Solid Tumors

Efforts are in progress to genetically engineer autologous PBMCs through the introduction of exogenous high avidity receptors that specifically recognize tumor antigens (Fig. 14.8). These cells can then be expanded to large numbers in vitro and be readministered back to the patient similar to TILs in order to mediate tumor regression. The use of gene-modified cells for ACT has resulted in objective clinical responses for a variety of cancer histologies including melanoma, synovial sarcoma, and CD19-positive B-cell malignancies.[6,131–133]

There are two key requirements necessary for the use of gene-modified cells for the treatment of solid cancer. The first is the selection of an appropriate gene transfer method in order to achieve high receptor expression levels in the transferred T cells. For this discussion, we will consider both nonviral and viral-based gene delivery platforms. Generally speaking, there are two categories of nonviral gene transfer, chemical and physical. Chemical gene transfer involves the use of positively charged delivery vehicle such as calcium phosphate, cationic lipids, or polymers to form DNA complexes capable of entering a cell through endocytosis.[134] These reagents benefit from their ease of manufacture and ability to form complexes with large DNA sequences; however, low transfection efficiency of human T cells continues to be an issue.

Physical methods for gene delivery may involve direct delivery of DNA into a cell via microinjection or indirect DNA uptake via electroporation.[135] Electroporation of messenger RNA (mRNA) can achieve high levels of protein expression in cells, comparable to many of the viral-mediated gene delivery systems (gammaretroviral or lentiviral).[135,136] High-throughput electroporators should allow one to gene modify large numbers of T cells ex vivo.[137] mRNA electroporation appears to be most suited for this application, because there is significant loss of cell viability following electroporation of large amounts of DNA.[136] The electroporation of mRNA, although gaining traction as a means of redirecting T cell specificity,[137] provides for transient receptor expression because the mRNA will degrade over time. Currently, it is not clear if stable long-term receptor expression is required to mediate tumor regression. However, the main criticism of the non-viral methods described is the lack of stable gene transfer. To overcome this problem, many investigators are now using transposons such as *sleeping beauty* or *piggybac*.[138] Transposons are mobile DNA gene delivery elements encoding a gene of interest (i.e., TCR or chimeric antigen receptors [CAR]) that can randomly integrate into the genome in the presence of the transposase enzyme, thereby allowing for stable gene expression. This technology is currently being used for the ACT of CAR-modified cells targeting B-cell malignancies (see Fig. 14.8B).[139]

Viral-mediated gene delivery is currently the most common method for the genetic modification of immune cells for cancer ACT. Retroviridae is a family of RNA viruses that, upon entry into cells, undergo a process called reverse transcription whereby the viral RNA is converted into DNA as it stably integrates into the host genome. The two most common retroviral vector systems are based on the gammaretrovirus, Moloney murine leukemia virus (MLV), and the lentivirus, HIV type 1 (see Fig. 14.8B). Gammaretroviral vectors have been used in human clinical applications for over 20 years. The only reported toxicity associated with gammaretroviral engineering of human cells involved the retroviral transduction of hematopoietic stem cells for the treatment of children with severe combined immunodeficiency syndrome (X-SCID).[140] There have been no reports of clonal outgrowth following the retroviral transduction of mature T lymphocytes in adults. Highly active vectors have been generated from a variety of murine retroviruses including spleen focus forming virus (SFFV), myeloproliferative sarcoma virus (MPSV), and the murine stem cell virus (MSCV).[141–147] In most cases, these vectors are replication incompetent, but non–self-inactivating in

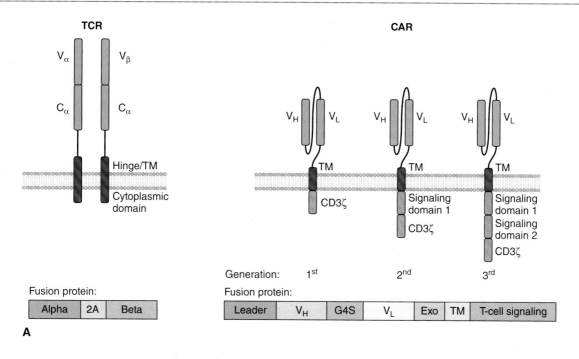

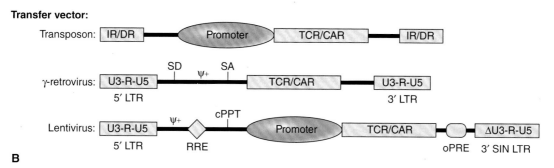

**Figure 14.8** Genetic modification of T cells for the treatment of solid cancers. **(A)** In order to gene-modify T cells to confer stable tumor-specific reactivity, one can transduce T cells with an exogenous TCR derived from a naturally occurring or murine T-cell clone or a CAR derived from a tumor-specific monoclonal antibody. The TCR or CAR is synthesized as fusion proteins and inserted into the appropriate gene transfer vector. **(B)** Depending on the transfer vector selected, the T cells are then electroporated (transposon) or transduced (viral vector) to confer tumor specificity. $V_\alpha$, $V_\beta$, and $C_\alpha$, $C_\beta$, TCR alpha and beta chain variable and constant regions, respectively; TM, transmembrane domain; $V_H$ and $V_L$, immunoglobulin variable regions; 2A and G4S, linker sequences; Exo, extracellular spacer domain; SD, splice donor; SA, splice acceptor; $\Psi$, packaging signal; LTR, long terminal repeat; U3, unique 3′ region; R, repeat region; U5, unique 5′ region; RRE, rev response element; cPPT, central polypurine tract; wPRE, woodchuck hepatitis virus posttranscriptional regulatory element; $\Delta$U3, truncated unique 3′ region; SIN, self-inactivating.

that the promoter for transgene expression is derived from the viral long terminal repeat (LTR). Self-inactivating (SIN) gammaretroviral vectors have been developed that require an internal promoter to drive transgene expression. The advantage of non-SIN vectors is the ability to use a variety of retroviral packaging cell lines (PG13, Phoenix) engineered to constitutively express gag (capsid protein), pol (reverse transcriptase, integrase, and RNase H enzymes) and env (envelope protein). Transduction of these packaging lines with a non-SIN retroviral vector encoding a transgene allows for the generation of a stable packaging cell line that constitutively releases vector into the medium. This platform is easily scaled up to support large-scale vector production efforts. An alternative to the gammaretroviral vector platform is the lentiviral vector platform. There are some advantages to selecting a lentiviral vector for T-cell engineering in that one can transduce large numbers of minimally stimulated T cells,[148] transfer more complex and larger gene expression cassettes, and yield a potentially safer chromosomal integration profile as compared to gammaretroviruses. However, there has been at least one instance of clonal outgrowth

following lentiviral vector transduction of CD34+ stem cells.[149] Therefore, more data will be needed to better understand the risk of insertional mutagenesis associated with the use of lentiviral vectors. The major disadvantage with using lentiviral vectors for ACT is the lack of a robust packaging cell line, which requires transient vector production and is difficult to scale up.

The first successful application ACT involved the use of autologous T cells genetically modified with a conventional $\alpha\beta$ TCR targeting MART-1 for the treatment of patients with melanoma.[131] The success of this approach relies on the ability to identify naturally occurring TCRs with sufficiently high avidity for the tumor antigen. For this clinical trial, a tumor-specific TCR was cloned directly from melanoma TIL. Exogenous TCR can also be generated from human PBMC following a variety of in vitro sensitization techniques or immunization of transgenic mice expressing HLA molecules. A T-cell clone expressing a low avidity TCR recognizing MART-1 was isolated and the $\alpha$ and $\beta$ chains cloned into a gammaretroviral vector. The objective response rate from this trial was 13% (2/15).[131] In a follow-up trial with a higher avidity TCR that was cloned from the same melanoma TIL, the objective response rate increased to 30% (6/20).[150] However, patients in this trial experienced significant on-target, off-tumor toxicity with the destruction of normal melanocytes in the skin, eye, and ear. These trials showed the potential to use ACT for the treatment of solid cancers, but also highlight the importance of selecting appropriate tumor antigens to target in order to minimize normal tissue toxicities. Perhaps a better class of antigen to target for ACT would be the cancer testes antigens (CTA) that are expressed only on germ cells during fetal development and then reexpressed on cancers but not other normal tissues with the exception of the testes (see Table 14.1). Because the testes do not express class I MHC molecules, they are protected from any adverse immune response.[151] NY-ESO-1 is a CTA overexpressed on melanoma, as well as a variety of solid epithelial cancers.[152–154] A high-avidity TCR was developed targeting NY-ESO-1 and patients with metastatic melanoma or synovial cell sarcoma were treated following adoptive cell transfer using autologous lymphocytes transduced with a gammaretrovirus encoding this receptor.[6] In updated results from this trial, 8 of 17 patients (47%) with melanoma showed objective tumor responses, two of which were complete responses and ongoing at 51 and 48 months after treatment. Nine of 19 patients (47%) with synovial cell sarcoma showed objective tumor response, only one of which is complete and ongoing at 12 months. Of note, no toxicities were observed in any of these trials. Thus, targeting NY-ESO-1 and other CTAs is an attractive strategy for the application of ACT for the treatment of solid cancers (see Table 14.4 for other trials conducted at the National Cancer Institute, Surgery Branch).

Redirection of T-cell specificity using conventional TCR is constrained by HLA restriction, which limits treatment only to patients expressing a particular MHC haplotype. An alternate approach is to use CAR comprised of an monoclonal antibody single chain variable fragment (scFv) fused in frame to T-cell intracellular signaling domains capable of T-cell activation following antigen-specific binding (see Fig. 14.8A).[155] CARs, unlike conventional TCRs, are not MHC restricted but are limited by the requirement for the tumor antigen to be expressed on the cell surface. CARs can also recognize carbohydrate and lipid moieties further expanding their application. To date, there has been limited success using

CAR-based ACT for the treatment of solid cancers. In 2008, the first successful CAR trial targeting the disialoganglioside, GD2, for the treatment of neuroblastoma was reported.[156] In this trial, 4 out of 8 patients (50%) with evaluable tumor experienced tumor regression or necrosis with one complete responder. In that same year, a second CAR trial targeting CD20 on non-Hodgkin and mantle cell lymphomas was reported.[157] Of the 7 patients treated, one achieved a partial response. Much greater success has now been achieved using a CAR targeting CD19, a molecule expressed on normal B cells and virtually all B-cell lymphomas. In a trial conducted at the National Cancer Institute, Surgery Branch, Kochenderfer et al.[132] first reported that autologous T cells expressing a CAR targeting CD19 was able to mediate tumor regression in a patient with B-cell lymphoma (hematologic malignancies will be discussed in more detail elsewhere). Successfully expanding CAR-based ACT to other cancer histologies has been limited by the inability to identify suitable tumor antigens to target. At the National Cancer Institute, Surgery Branch, there are active clinical programs with CAR targeting the mutated epidermal growth factor receptor, EGFRvIII, expressed on approximately 40% of glioblastomas as well as head and neck cancers[158]; the vascular endothelial growth factor-2 receptor, VEGFR-2, expressed on tumor vasculature[159]; and mesothelin, expressed on the mesothelial lining of the pleura, peritoneum, and pericardium, but overexpressed on mesothelioma, pancreatic, and ovarian cancers.[160] These trials are currently accruing patients; however, no objective clinical responses have been observed to date. A summary of clinical trials at the National Cancer Institute, Surgery Branch using gene-modified autologous T cells for ACT are shown in Table 14.4. ACT can mediate the regression of large, established tumors in humans. Efforts to identify and specifically target novel tumor antigens are currently underway with the hope that ACT using gene-modified T cells will develop into an effective treatment for patients with a variety of solid cancers.

## Genetic Modification of Lymphocytes to Treat Hematologic Malignancies

Immunologic therapies can be useful treatments for some hematologic malignancies as demonstrated by the effectiveness of mono-

## TABLE 14.4

**Surgery Branch, National Cancer Institute Program for the Application of Cell Transfer Therapy to a Wide Variety of Human Cancers**

| Receptor | Type | Cancers | Status |
| --- | --- | --- | --- |
| MART-1 | TCR | Melanoma | Closed |
| gp100 | TCR | Melanoma | Closed |
| NY-ESO-1 | TCR | Epithelial & sarcomas | Accruing |
| CEA | TCR | Colorectal | Closed |
| CD19 | CAR | Lymphomas | Accruing |
| VEGFR2 | CAR | All cancers | Accruing |
| 2G-1 | TCR | Kidney | Accruing |
| IL-12 | Cytokine | Adjuvant for all receptors | Accruing |
| MAGE-A3[a] | TCR | Epithelial | In development |
| EGFRvIII | CAR | Glioblastoma | Accruing |
| SSX-2 | TCR | Epithelial | In development |
| Mesothelin | CAR | Pancreas & mesothelioma | Accruing |
| HPV16 (E6&7) | TCR | Cervical, oropharyngeal | In development |

[a] MAGE-A3 TCRs; restricted by HLA-A2, A1, Cw7, DP4—covers 80% of patients.
EGFR, epidermal growth factor receptor; VEGFR2, vascular endothelial growth factor 2.

clonal antibodies in treating B-cell malignancies and the fact that allogeneic hematopoietic stem cell transplantation (alloHSCT) can cure a variety of hematologic malignancies.[161–167] The results with monoclonal antibodies and alloHSCT clearly prove that immunologic therapies have significant activity against hematologic malignancies, but monoclonal antibodies are not curative as single agents,[162,166] and alloHSCT has a substantial transplant-related mortality rate due to infections and an immunologic attack against normal tissues known as graft versus host disease (GVHD).[163,165] The proven curative potential of alloHSCT and the effectiveness of autologous T-cell transfer therapies for melanoma have encouraged the development of autologous T-cell therapies for hematologic malignancies.[125,129,163,165] Genetically engineering T cells to specifically recognize antigens expressed by malignant cells has emerged as a very promising strategy for cancer immunotherapy.[125,129,168]

T cells can be genetically engineered to express either of two types of receptors, CARs[168–171] or natural TCRs.[6,131,172] T cells expressing either a CAR or TCR gain the ability to specifically recognize an antigen.[171,172] CARs are artificial fusion proteins that incorporate antigen recognition domains and T-cell activation domains.[168,170,172] The antigen recognition domains are most often derived from monoclonal antibodies.[168,170,172] Antigen recognition by TCRs is major histocompatibility complex restricted.[125,128] In contrast to TCRs, recognition of antigens by CARs is not dependent on MHC molecules. An advantage of TCRs over CARs is that TCRs can recognize intracellular antigens, whereas CARs can only recognize cell-surface antigens.

## Chimeric Antigen Receptors

CARs targeting hematopoietic antigens have been extensively studied in preclinical experiments and early-stage clinical trials.[168,170,172,173] For a protein to be a promising target for CAR-expressing T cells, it should be uniformly expressed on the malignant cells being targeted but not expressed on essential normal cells. Many cell-surface proteins with restricted normal tissue expression patterns have been identified on malignant hematologic cells, and CARs targeting many of these proteins are under development (Table 14.5).

Many factors can affect CAR T-cell therapies. The types of gene-therapy vectors encoding the DNA of the CAR could be an important factor. The types of vectors currently being used in clinical trials of CAR T cells are gammaretroviruses, lentiviruses, and transposon-based systems.[132,133,174–181] The design of the CAR fusion protein is another important factor. CAR fusion proteins include an antigen-recognition domain that is most often derived from an antibody, costimulatory domains such as CD28 and 4-1BB, and T-cell activation domains that are usually derived from the CD3z molecule.[168,170,171,182] Other factors that could impact the effectiveness of CAR T-cell therapies include the cell culture method used to prepare the cells and administration of chemotherapy or radiation therapy prior to the CAR T-cell infusions.[170,178,179] In mouse models, a profound enhancement of the antimalignancy activity of infused T cells occurs when the T-cell infusions are preceded by lymphocyte-depleting chemotherapy or radiation therapy.[183–185] Because chemotherapy can have a direct antimalignancy effect against hematologic malignancies, the administration of chemotherapy prior to infusions of T cells is a confounding factor that must always be kept in mind when interpreting the results of clinical trials of T-cell therapies.

### Anti-CD19 Chimeric Antigen Receptors

CD19 is an appealing target antigen for CARs because CD19 is expressed on almost all malignant B cells, but CD19 is not expressed on normal cells except B cells.[186] The first preclinical studies of anti-CD19 CARs utilized either gammaretrovirus vectors[174] or plasmid electroporation[176] to insert genes encoding anti-CD19 CARs into human T cells. These studies and subsequent preclinical work by other groups showed that T cells expressing anti-CD19

## TABLE 14.5

### Hematologic Antigens Targeted by Genetically-Modified T-Cells

| Antigen | Malignancy Expressing Antigen | Targeted by CAR or TCR | References |
|---|---|---|---|
| CD19 | B-cell malignancies | CAR | 17, 19, 21, 22, 23, 24, 25, 26, 34, 35, 55, 56 |
| CD20 | B-cell malignancies | CAR | 36, 37, 38 |
| CD22 | B-cell malignancies | CAR | 39, 40 |
| CD23 | B-cell malignancies | CAR | 41 |
| ROR1 | B-cell malignancies | CAR | 42 |
| Kappa light chain | B-cell malignancies | CAR | 43 |
| B-cell maturation antigen (BCMA) | Multiple myeloma | CAR | 44 |
| Lewis Y antigen | Multiple myeloma and acute myeloid leukemia (AML) | CAR | 45, 46 |
| CD123 | AML | CAR | 47 |
| CD30 | Hodgkin lymphoma | CAR | 48, 49 |
| CD70 | Hodgkin lymphoma | CAR | 50 |
| Wilms tumor-1 (WT1) | AML and acute lymphoid leukemia (ALL) | TCR | 51 |
| Aurora kinase-A | AML and chronic myeloid leukemia (CML) | TCR | 52 |
| Hyaluronan-mediated motility receptor (HMMR) | AML and ALL | TCR | 53 |

CARs could specifically recognize and kill CD19-expressing malignant B cells in vitro and in vivo.[174–176,187] These preclinical studies compared many different CAR signaling moieties, which led most groups to utilize CARs with T-cell activation domains from the CD3z molecule and costimulatory molecules from either CD28 or 4-1BB (CD137).[165,180,182,187,188] Preclinical studies showed that lymphocyte-depleting radiation therapy administered before anti-CD19 CAR T-cell infusions was critical to the antimalignancy activity of CAR T cells.[183] The addition of lymphocyte-depleting radiation therapy prior to infusions of anti-CD19 CAR T cells increased the percentage of mice cured of lymphoma by the CAR T cells from 0% to 100%.[183] Preclinical experiments with anti-CD19 CARs have led to several early-phase clinical trials.

The first clinical trial to demonstrate in vivo activity of anti-CD19 CAR T cells in humans was conducted in the Surgery Branch of the National Cancer Institute.[132] The gammaretroviral vector used in this trial encoded a CAR with a CD28 costimulatory domain. Patients treated on this clinical trial received cyclophosphamide and fludarabine chemotherapy followed by an infusion of anti-CD19 CAR T cells and a short course of intravenous IL-2.[132,181] Clear antigen-specific activity of the anti-CD19 CAR T cells was demonstrated because blood B cells were selectively eliminated from four of the seven evaluable patients for several months.[181] The duration of B-cell depletion in these patients was much longer than the duration of B-cell depletion caused by the chemotherapy that the patients received.[132,181] This study also generated evidence of an antimalignancy effect by the anti-CD19 CAR T cells because six of seven evaluable patients with advanced B-cell malignancies obtained either complete remissions or partial remissions (Fig. 14.9).[181] One of these remissions is ongoing 45 months after treatment, and another remission is ongoing 31 months after treatment. Significant toxicity, including hypotension and neurologic toxicity, occurred during this clinical trial.[181] The severity of these toxicities correlated with the levels of serum inflammatory cytokines.[181] Except for one patient who died with influenza pneumonia, the toxicities were transient, with all toxicities resolving within 3 weeks of the anti-CD19 CAR T-cell infusions.[181]

Investigators at the Memorial Sloan Kettering Cancer Center treated nine patients with chronic lymphocytic leukemia (CLL) or acute lymphocytic leukemia (ALL) by infusing T cells that expressed a CAR with a CD28 costimulatory domain.[179] The gene therapy vector used in this work was a gammaretrovirus.[179] None of three patients treated with CAR T cells alone experienced a regression of leukemia, and CLL regressed in one of four evaluable patients treated with cyclophosphamide followed by an infusion of CAR T cells. Using the same CAR, the same group went on to treat five patients with ALL.[173] Patients received chemotherapy followed by an infusion of anti-CD19 CAR T cells. Four patients had detectable leukemia prior to their CAR T-cell infusions, and all of these patients became minimal residual disease negative after infusion of CAR T cells. Four of five patients on this trial rapidly underwent allogeneic stem cell transplantation after their CAR T-cell infusions.[173]

Investigators at the Baylor College of Medicine conducted clinical trials of anti-CD19 CAR T cells in which each patient simultaneously received infusions of two types of anti-CD19 CAR T cells.[189] One type of T cell expressed a CAR expressing a CD28 costimulatory domain. The other type of T cell was identical except that the CAR it expressed lacked a CD28 domain. Compared to the T cells lacking a CD28 moiety, the T cells expressing a CAR with a CD28 moiety had higher peak blood levels and longer in vivo persistence.[189] Patients on this trial did not receive chemotherapy, and there were no remissions of malignancy or long-term B-cell depletion.[189]

Investigators at the University of Pennsylvania reported results from three patients with CLL who were treated with chemotherapy followed by infusions of anti-CD19 CAR-expressing T cells.[133,180] The CAR used in this study was encoded by a lentiviral vector and contained a costimulatory domain from the 4-1BB molecule. Two

**Before treatment**

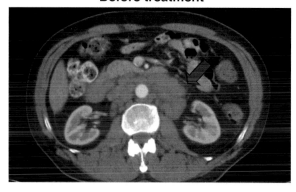

**32 days after infusion**

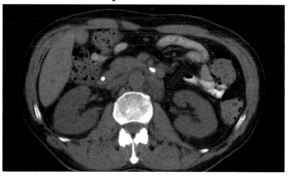

**132 days after infusion**

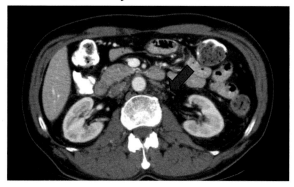

**645 days after infusion**

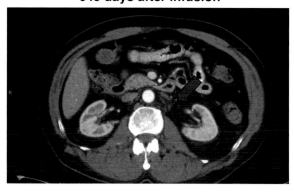

**Figure 14.9** Computed tomography (CT) scans show regression of adenopathy in a patient with chronic lymphocytic leukemia (CLL) after treatment with chemotherapy followed by an infusion of autologous anti-CD19 CAR T cells. The time after the cell infusion of each CT scan is indicated. The *arrow* points to a large lymph node mass that resolved completely over time. (Reproduced from Kochenderfer JN, Rosenberg SA. Treating B-Cell cancer with T cells expressing anti-CD19 chimeric antigen receptors. *Nature Rev Clin Oncology* 2013;10:267-276, with permission.)

of the three reported patients obtained prolonged complete remissions.[180] This same CAR design was subsequently evaluated in a clinical trial enrolling patients with ALL.[190] One ALL patient obtained a prolonged complete remission but also experienced significant toxicity that was associated with elevated levels of serum cytokines.[190]

Overall, the early results with anti-CD19 CAR T cells show that this strategy holds great promise to improve the treatment of B-cell malignancies, but anti-CD19 CAR T-cell infusions are also associated with significant toxicity that is usually of short duration. Future progress will require decreasing the toxicity of anti-CD19 CAR T cells while maintaining or enhancing their antimalignancy activity. Parameters that are being studied in an effort to improve anti-CD19 CAR therapy include vector selection, CAR design, cell culture methods, and clinical application.

## Chimeric Antigen Receptors and T-Cell Receptors Targeting Hematologic Antigens Other than CD19

CARs and TCRs targeting several hematologic antigens other than CD19 have been evaluated in preclinical or clinical studies. Except for CD19, the B-cell antigen CD20 has been the hematologic antigen most extensively studied as a target of CAR T cells.[191–193] Plasmid electroporation, which is not an optimal method of T-cell genetic modification, was used to transfer the anti-CD20 CAR gene to T cells in these studies. In one trial of anti-CD20 CAR T cells, patients received chemotherapy followed by infusions of T cells expressing a CAR without costimulatory domains.[192] One of seven patients obtained a partial remission that lasted 3 months. In a second trial, patients received chemotherapy followed by anti-CD20 CAR T cells expressing a CAR with both CD28 and 4-1BB costimulatory domains; in this trial, the only evaluable patient obtained a partial remission.[193]

CARs targeting other B-cell antigens including CD22,[157,194] CD23,[195] receptor tyrosine kinase–like orphan receptor-1 (ROR1),[196] and the immunoglobulin kappa light chain[197] have been evaluated in preclinical studies. CARs for treating multiple myeloma are currently being developed. B-cell maturation antigen (BCMA) is expressed on normal and malignant plasma cells, but it is not known to be expressed on other normal cells except for a small subset of mature B cells.[198] CARs targeting BCMA have undergone preclinical testing, and a clinical trial of an anti-BCMA CAR will open soon.[198] Preclinical studies have been performed on CARs targeting the Lewis Y antigen as a treatment for multiple myeloma and acute myeloid leukemia (AML),[199] and activity against AML was recently demonstrated in a phase I clinical trial of a CAR targeting the Lewis Y antigen.[200] CARs targeting the

CD123 protein are undergoing preclinical testing for potential use against AML.[201] For Hodgkin lymphoma, CARs have been developed that target the CD30 protein and the CD70 protein, and anti-CD30 CARs are entering early-phase clinical trials.[202–204]

MHC-restricted TCRs targeting some antigens expressed on hematologic malignancies have undergone preclinical testing, but TCRs for treating hematologic malignancies are at a much earlier stage of development than CARs (see Table 14.1). TCRs targeting the Wilms tumor antigen-1 (WT1) are under development to treat ALL and AML.[205] Aurora kinase-A–specific TCRs and hyaluronan-mediated motility receptor (HMMR)-specific TCRs are under preclinical development as leukemia treatments.[206,207]

## T-Cell Gene Therapy in the Setting of Allogeneic Hematopoietic Stem Cell Transplantation

A leading cause of death among patients undergoing alloHSCT is relapse of malignancy, and alloHSCT is often complicated by GVHD.[164,165,208] Therefore, a central goal in the field of alloHSCT is to increase the antimalignancy activity of allogeneic T cells without worsening GVHD. One way to accomplish this goal might be to genetically modify T cells to give them the ability to specifically recognize antigens expressed by malignant cells. CARs are well-suited for this task.

Two groups have recently reported promising early results treating B-cell malignancies after alloHSCT with allogeneic donor-derived T cells expressing anti-CD19 CARs.[209,210] Investigators at the National Cancer Institute treated 10 patients with B-cell malignancies that persisted despite alloHSCT and standard donor lymphocyte infusions.[209] Although patients on this trial did not receive chemotherapy before their T-cell infusions, 3 of 10 patients had objective regressions of their malignancies, and 1 patient with CLL remains in CR more than 1 year after treatment.[209] No patient developed GVHD after receiving allogeneic anti-CD19 CAR T cells on this trial.[209] Investigators at the Baylor College of Medicine reported objective antimalignancy responses in two of six patients with relapsed malignancy after infusion of donor-derived allogeneic anti-CD19 CAR T cells that were also specific for viral antigens.[210]

In an effort to improve the safety of infusions of allogeneic lymphocytes by limiting GVHD, investigators have genetically modified T cells to express *suicide genes* that cause death of the T cells containing the suicide gene when certain drugs are administered.[211–214] Suicide gene–expressing T cells are infused to treat malignancy after alloHSCT. This approach has been tested in clinical trials, and rapid abrogation of GVHD has been demonstrated.[211,213,214]

## REFERENCES

1. Kenter GG, Welters MJ, Valentijn AR, et al. Vaccination against HPV-16 oncoproteins for vulvar intraepithelial neoplasia. *N Engl J Med* 2009;361:1838–1847.
2. Gaffen SL, Liu KD. Overview of interleukin-2 function, production and clinical applications. *Cytokine* 2004;28:109–123.
3. Attia P, Phan GQ, Maker AV, et al. Autoimmunity correlates with tumor regression in patients with metastatic melanoma treated with anti-cytotoxic T-lymphocyte antigen-4. *J Clin Oncol* 2005;23:6043–6053.
4. Topalian SL, Hodi FS, Brahmer JR, et al. Safety, activity, and immune correlates of anti-PD-1 antibody in cancer. *N Engl J Med* 2012;366:2443–2454.
5. Rosenberg SA, Yang JC, Sherry RM, et al. Durable complete responses in heavily pretreated patients with metastatic melanoma using T-cell transfer immunotherapy. *Clin Cancer Res* 2011;17:4550–4557.
6. Robbins PF, Morgan RA, Feldman SA, et al. Tumor regression in patients with metastatic synovial sarcoma and melanoma using genetically engineered lymphocytes reactive with NY-ESO-1. *J Clin Oncol* 2011;29:917–924.
7. Chen YT, Scanlan MJ, Sahin U, et al. A testicular antigen aberrantly expressed in human cancers detected by autologous antibody screening. *Proc Natl Acad Sci U S A* 1997;94:1914–1918.

8. Van der Bruggen P, Traversari C, Chomez P, et al. A gene encoding an antigen recognized by cytolytic T lymphocytes on a human melanoma. *Science* 1991;254:1643–1647.
9. van der Bruggen P, Stroobant V, Vigneron N, et al. Peptide database: T cell-defined tumor antigens. *Cancer Immun* 2013. https://www.cancerimmunity.org/peptide/
10. Gnjatic S, Nishikawa H, Jungbluth AA, et al. NY-ESO-1: review of an immunogenic tumor antigen. *Adv Cancer Res* 2006;95:1–30.
11. Chinnasamy N, Wargo JA, Yu Z, et al. A TCR targeting the HLA-A*0201-restricted epitope of MAGE-A3 recognizes multiple epitopes of the MAGE-A antigen superfamily in several types of cancer. *J Immunol* 2011;186:685–696.
12. Morgan RA, Chinnasamy N, Abate-Daga D, et al. Cancer regression and neurological toxicity following anti-MAGE-A3 TCR gene therapy. *J Immunother* 2013;36:133–151.
13. Linette GP, Stadtmauer EA, Maus MV, et al. Cardiovascular toxicity and titin cross-reactivity of affinity-enhanced T cells in myeloma and melanoma. *Blood* 2013;122:863–871.
14. Cox AL, Skipper J, Chen Y, et al. Identification of a peptide recognized by five melanoma-specific human cytotoxic T cell lines. *Science* 1994;264:716–719.

15. Kawakami Y, Eliyahu S, Jennings C, et al. Recognition of multiple epitopes in the human melanoma antigen gp100 by tumor infiltrating T-lymphocytes associated with in vivo tumor regression. *J Immunol* 1995;154:3961–3968.

16. Brichard V, Van Pel A, Wolfel T, et al. The tyrosinase gene codes for an antigen recognized by autologous cytolytic T lymphocytes on HLA-A2 melanomas. *J Exp Med* 1993;178:489–495.

17. Wang RF, Robbins PF, Kawakami Y, et al. Identification of a gene encoding a melanoma tumor antigen recognized by HLA-A31-restricted tumor-infiltrating lymphocytes. *J Exp Med* 1995;181:799–804.

18. Wang R-F, Appella E, Kawakami Y, et al. Identification of TRP-2 as a human tumor antigen recognized by cytotoxic T lymphocytes. *J Exp Med* 1996;184:2207–2216.

19. Kawakami Y, Eliyahu S, Delgado CH, et al. Cloning of the gene coding for a shared human melanoma antigen recognized by autologous T cells infiltrating into tumor. *Proc Natl Acad Sci U S A* 1994;91:3515–3519.

20. Coulie PG, Brichard V, Van Pel A, et al. A new gene coding for a differentiation antigen recognized by autologous cytolytic T lymphocytes on HLA-A2 melanomas. *J Exp Med* 1994;180:35–42.

21. Kawakami Y, Eliyahu S, Sakaguchi K, et al. Identification of the immunodominant peptides of the MART-1 human melanoma antigen recognized by the majority of HLA-A2-restricted tumor infiltrating lymphocytes. *J Exp Med* 1994;180:347–352.

22. Hanada K, Yewdell JW, Yang JC. Immune recognition of a human renal cancer antigen through post-translational protein splicing. *Nature* 2004;427:252–256.

23. Carrington DM, Auffret A, Hanke DE. Polypeptide ligation occurs during post-translational modification of concanavalin A. *Nature* 1985;313:64–67.

24. Paulus H. Protein splicing and related forms of protein autoprocessing. *Annu Rev Biochem* 2000;69:447–496.

25. Vigneron N, Stroobant V, Chapiro J, et al. An antigenic peptide produced by peptide splicing in the proteasome. *Science* 2004;304:587–590.

26. Warren EH, Vigneron NJ, Gavin MA, et al. An antigen produced by splicing of noncontiguous peptides in the reverse order. *Science* 2006;313:1444–1447.

27. Dalet A, Robbins PF, Stroobant V, et al. An antigenic peptide produced by reverse splicing and double asparagine deamidation. *Proc Natl Acad Sci U S A* 2011;108:E323–E331.

28. Michaux A, Larrieu P, Stroobant V, et al. A spliced antigenic peptide comprising a single spliced amino acid is produced in the proteasome by reverse splicing of a longer peptide fragment followed by trimming. *J Immunol* 2014;192:1962–1971.

29. Ikeda H, Lethe B, Lehmann F. Characterization of an antigen that is recognized on a melanoma showing partial HLA loss by CTL expressing an NK inhibitory receptor. *Immunity* 1999;6:199–208.

30. Lundegaard C, Lamberth K, Harndahl M, et al. NetMHC-3.0: accurate web accessible predictions of human, mouse and monkey MHC class I affinities for peptides of length 8-11. *Nucleic Acids Res* 2008;36:W509–W512.

31. Peters B, Sette A. Generating quantitative models describing the sequence specificity of biological processes with the stabilized matrix method. *BMC Bioinformatics* 2005;6:132.

32. Xue BH, Zhang Y, Sosman JA, et al. Induction of human cytotoxic T lymphocytes specific for prostate-specific antigen. *Prostate* 1997;30:73–78.

33. Horiguchi Y, Nukaya I, Okazawa K, et al. Screening of HLA-A24-restricted epitope peptides from prostate-specific membrane antigen that induce specific antitumor cytotoxic T lymphocytes. *Clin Cancer Res* 2002;8:3885–3892.

34. Peoples GE, Goedegebuure PS, Smith R. Breast and ovarian cancer-specific cytotoxic T lymphocytes recognize the same HER2/neu-derived peptide. *Proc Natl Acad U S A* 1995;92:432–436.

35. Zaks TZ, Rosenberg SA. Immunization with a peptide epitope (p369-377) from HER-2/neu leads to peptide-specific cytotoxic T lymphocytes that fail to recognize HER-2/neu+ tumors. *Cancer Res* 1998;58:4902–4908.

36. Vonderheide RH, Hahn WC, Schultze JL, et al. The telomerase catalytic subunit is a widely expressed tumor-associated antigen recognized by cytotoxic T lymphocytes. *Immunity* 1999;10:673–679.

37. Parkhurst MR, Riley JP, Igarashi T, et al. Immunization of patients with the hTERT:540-548 peptide induces peptide-reactive T lymphocytes that do not recognize tumors endogenously expressing telomerase. *Clin Cancer Res* 2004;10:4688–4698.

38. Weinschenk T, Gouttefangeas C, Schirle M, et al. Integrated functional genomics approach for the design of patient-individual antitumor vaccines. *Cancer Res* 2002;62: 5818–5827.

39. Dutoit V, Herold-Mende C, Hilf N, et al. Exploiting the glioblastoma peptidome to discover novel tumour-associated antigens for immunotherapy. *Brain* 2012;135:1042–1054.

40. Walter S, Weinschenk T, Stenzl A, et al. Multipeptide immune response to cancer vaccine IMA901 after single-dose cyclophosphamide associates with longer patient survival. *Nat Med* 2012;18:1254–1261.

41. Theobald M, Biggs J, Dittmer D, et al. Targeting p53 as a general tumor antigen. *Proc Natl Acad Sci U S A* 1995;92:11993–11997.

42. Theoret MR, Cohen CJ, Nahvi AV, et al. Relationship of p53 overexpression on cancers and recognition by anti-p53 T cell receptor-transduced T cells. *Hum Gene Ther* 2008;19:1219–1231.

43. Parkhurst M, Joo J, Riley JP, et al. Characterization of genetically modified T cell receptors that recognize the CEA:691-699 peptide in the context of HLA-A2.1 on human colorectal cancer cells. *Clin Cancer Res* 2009;15:169–180.

44. Parkhurst MR, Yang JC, Langan RC, et al. T cells targeting carcinoembryonic antigen can mediate regression of metastatic colorectal cancer but induce severe transient colitis. *Mol Ther* 2011;19:620–626.

45. Wolfel T, Hauer M, Schneider J, et al. A p16INK4A-insensitive CDK4 mutant targeted by cytolytic T lymphocytes in a human melanoma. *Science* 1995;269:1281–1284.

46. Robbins PF, El-Gamil M, Li YF, et al. A mutated B-catenin gene encodes a melanoma-specific antigen recognized by tumor infiltrating lymphocytes. *J Exp Med* 1996;183:1185–1192.

47. Rubinfeld B, Robbins P, El-Gamil M. Stabilization of beta-catenin by genetic defects in melanoma cell lines. *Science* 1997;275:1790–1792.

48. Mumberg D, Wick M, Schreiber H. Unique tumor antigens redefined as mutant tumor-specific antigens. *Semin Immunol* 1996;8:289–293.

49. Cheever MA, Chen W, Disis ML, et al. T-cell immunity to oncogenic proteins including mutated ras and chimeric bcr-abl. *Ann N Y Acad Sci* 1993;690: 101–112.

50. Castle JC, Kreiter S, Diekmann J, et al. Exploiting the mutanome for tumor vaccination. *Cancer Res* 2012;72:1081–1091.

51. Matsushita H, Vesely MD, Koboldt DC, et al. Cancer exome analysis reveals a T-cell-dependent mechanism of cancer immunoediting. *Nature* 2012;482: 400–404.

52. Robbins PF, Lu YC, El-Gamil M, et al. Mining exomic sequencing data to identify mutated antigens recognized by adoptively transferred tumor-reactive T cells. *Nat Med* 2013;19:747–752.

53. van Rooij N, van Buuren MM, Philips D, et al. Tumor exome analysis reveals neoantigen-specific T-cell reactivity in an ipilimumab-responsive melanoma. *J Clin Oncol* 2013;31:e439–e442.

54. Tran E, Turcotte S, Gros A, et al. Cancer immunotherapy based on mutation-specific CD4+ T cells in a patient with epithelial cancer. *Science* 2014;344:641–645.

55. Koutsky LA, Ault KA, Wheeler CM, et al. A controlled trial of a human papillomavirus type 16 vaccine. *N Engl J Med* 2002;347:1645–1651.

56. Villa LL, Costa RL, Petta CA, et al. Prophylactic quadrivalent human papillomavirus (types 6, 11, 16, and 18) L1 virus-like particle vaccine in young women: a randomised double-blind placebo-controlled multicentre phase II efficacy trial. *Lancet Oncol* 2005;6:271–278.

57. Wolchok JD, Hoos A, O'Day S, et al. Guidelines for the evaluation of immune therapy activity in solid tumors: immune-related response criteria. *Clin Cancer Res* 2009;15:7412–7420.

58. Hoos A, Eggermont AM, Janetzki S, et al. Improved endpoints for cancer immunotherapy trials. *J Natl Cancer Inst* 2010;102:1388–1397.

59. Morgan DA, Ruscetti FW, Gallo R. Selective in vitro growth of T lymphocytes from normal human bone marrows. *Science* 1976;193:1007–1008.

60. Smith KA, Gilbride KJ, Favata MF. Lymphocyte activating factor promotes T-cell growth factor production by cloned murine lymphoma cells. *Nature* 1980;287:853–855.

61. Smith KA, Lachman LB, Oppenheim JJ, et al. The functional relationship of the interleukins. *J Exp Med* 1980;151:1551–1556.

62. Taniguchi T, Matsui H, Fujita T. Structure and expression of a cloned cDNA for human interleukin-2. *Nature* 1983;302:305–307.

63. Rosenberg SA, Grimm EA, McGrogan M, et al. Biological activity of recombinant human interleukin-2 produced in *Escherichia coli*. *Science* 1984;223:1412–1414.

64. Rosenberg SA, Mule JJ, Spiess PJ, et al. Regression of established pulmonary metastases and subcutaneous tumor mediated by the systemic administration of high dose recombinant IL-2. *J Exp Med* 1985;161:1169–1188.

65. Lotze MT, Matory YL, Ettinghausen SE, et al. In vivo administration of purified human interleukin-2. II. Half life, immunologic effects and expansion of peripheral lymphoid cells in vivo with recombinant IL-2. *J Immunol* 1985;135:2865–2875.

66. Rosenberg SA, Lotze MT, Muul LM, et al. Observations on the systemic administration of autologous lymphokine-activated killer cells and recombinant interleukin-2 to patients with metastatic cancer. *N Engl J Med* 1985;313: 1485–1492.

67. Rosenberg SA, Lotze MT, Yang JC, et al. Prospective randomized trial of high-dose interleukin-2 alone or in conjunction with lymphokine-activated killer cells for the treatment of patients with advanced cancer. *J Natl Cancer Inst* 1993;85:622–632.

68. Atkins MB, Sparano J, Fisher RI, et al. Randomized phase II trial of high-dose interleukin-2 either alone or in combination with interferon alfa-2b in advanced renal cell carcinoma. *J Clin Oncol* 1993;11:661–670.

69. Rosenberg SA, Yang JC, White DE, et al. Durability of complete responses in patients with metastatic cancer treated with high-dose interleukin-2: identification of the antigens mediating response. *Ann Surg* 1998;228:307–319.

70. Fyfe G, Fisher R, Sznol M, et al. Results of treatment of 255 patients with metastatic renal cell carcinoma who received high dose proleukin interleukin-2 therapy. *J Clin Oncol* 1995;13:688–696.

71. Fisher RI, Rosenberg SA, Fyfe G. Long-term survival update for high-dose recombinant interleukin-2 in patients with renal cell carcinoma. *Cancer J Sci Am* 2000;6:S55–S57.

72. Yang JC, Sherry RM, Steinberg SM, et al. Randomized study of high-dose and low-dose interleukin-2 in patients with metastatic renal cancer. *J Clin Oncol* 2003;21:3127–3132.

73. Atkins MB, Lotze MT, Dutcher JP, et al. High-dose recombinant interleukin 2 therapy for patients with metastatic melanoma: analysis of 270 patients treated between 1985 and 1993. *J Clin Oncol* 1999;17:2105–2116.

74. Atkins MB, Kunkel L, Sznol M, et al. High-dose recombinant interleukin-2 therapy in patients with metastatic melanoma: long-term survival update. *Cancer J Sci Am* 2000;6:S11–S14.

75. Rosenberg SA, Yang JC, Schwartzentruber DJ, et al. Immunologic and therapeutic evaluation of a synthetic peptide vaccine for the treatment of patients with metastatic melanoma. *Nat Med* 1998;4:321–327.

76. Schwartzentruber DJ, Lawson DH, Richards JM, et al. gp100 peptide vaccine and interleukin-2 in patients with advanced melanoma. *N Engl J Med* 2011;364:2119–2127.

77. Prieto PA, Yang JC, Sherry RM, et al. CTLA-4 blockade with ipilimumab: long-term follow-up of 177 patients with metastatic melanoma. *Clin Cancer Res* 2012;18:2039–2047.

78. Phan GQ, Attia P, Steinberg SM, et al. Factors associated with response to high-dose interleukin-2 in patients with metastatic melanoma. *J Clin Oncol* 2001;19:3477–3482.

79. Rosenberg SA, Yang JC, Topalian SL, et al. Treatment of 283 consecutive patients with metastatic melanoma or renal cell cancer using high-dose bolus interleukin 2. *JAMA* 1994;271:907–913.

80. Rosenberg SA, Lotze MT, Yang JC, et al. Experience with the use of high-dose interleukin-2 in the treatment of 652 cancer patients. *Ann Surg* 1989;210:474–484.

81. Gemlo BT, Palladino Jr MA, Jaffe HS, et al. Circulating cytokines in patients with metastatic cancer treated with recombinant interleukin 2 and lymphokine-activated killer cells. *Cancer Res* 1988;48:5864–5867.

82. Pockaj BA, Yang JC, Lotze MT, et al. A prospective randomized trial evaluating colloid versus crystalloid resuscitation in the treatment of the vascular leak syndrome associated with interleukin-2 therapy. *J Immunother Emphasis Tumor Immunol* 1994;15:22–28.

83. Klempner MS, Noring R, Mier JW, et al. An acquired chemotactic defect in neutrophils from patients receiving interleukin-2 immunotherapy. *N Engl J Med* 1990;322:959–965.

84. Lee RE, Lotze MT, Skibber JM, et al. Cardiorespiratory effects of immunotherapy with interleukin-2. *J Clin Oncol* 1989;7:7–20.

85. Schwartzentruber DJ. Guidelines for the safe administration of high-dose interleukin-2. *J Immunother* 2001;24:287–293.

86. Kammula US, White DE, Rosenberg SA. Trends in the safety of high dose bolus interleukin-2 administration in patients with metastatic cancer. *Cancer* 1998;83:797–805.

87. Brunet JF, Denizot F, Luciani MF, et al. A new member of the immunoglobulin superfamily—CTLA-4. *Nature* 1987;328:267–270.

88. Linsley PS, Brady W, Urnes M, et al. CTLA-4 is a second receptor for the B cell activation antigen B7. *J Exp Med* 1991;174:561–569.

89. Walunas TL, Lenschow DJ, Bakker CY, et al. CTLA-4 can function as a negative regulator of T cell activation. *Immunity* 1994;1:405–413.

90. Walunas TL, Bakker CY, Bluestone JA. CTLA-4 ligation blocks CD28-dependent T cell activation. *J Exp Med* 1996;183:2541–2550.

91. van Elsas A, Hurwitz AA, Allison JP. Combination immunotherapy of B16 melanoma using anti-cytotoxic T lymphocyte-associated antigen 4 (CTLA-4) and granulocyte/macrophage colony-stimulating factor (GM-CSF)-producing vaccines induces rejection of subcutaneous and metastatic tumors accompanied by autoimmune depigmentation. *J Exp Med* 1999;190:355–366.

92. Hurwitz AA, Yu TF, Leach DR, et al. CTLA-4 blockade synergizes with tumor-derived granulocyte-macrophage colony-stimulating factor for treatment of an experimental mammary carcinoma. *Proc Natl Acad Sci U S A* 1998;95:10067–10071.

93. Phan GQ, Yang JC, Sherry RM, et al. Cancer regression and autoimmunity induced by cytotoxic T lymphocyte-associated antigen 4 blockade in patients with metastatic melanoma. *Proc Natl Acad Sci U S A* 2003;100:8372–8377.

94. Maker AV, Phan GQ, Attia P, et al. Tumor regression and autoimmunity in patients treated with cytotoxic T lymphocyte-associated antigen 4 blockade and interleukin 2: a phase I/II study. *Ann Surg Oncol* 2005;12:1005–1016.

95. Maker AV, Yang JC, Sherry RM, et al. Intrapatient dose escalation of anti-CTLA-4 antibody in patients with metastatic melanoma. *J Immunother* 2006;29:455–463.

96. Beck KE, Blansfield JA, Tran KQ, et al. Enterocolitis in patients with cancer after antibody blockade of cytotoxic T-lymphocyte-associated antigen 4. *J Clin Oncol* 2006;24:2283–2289.

97. Robinson MR, Chan CC, Yang JC, et al. Cytotoxic T lymphocyte-associated antigen 4 blockade in patients with metastatic melanoma: a new cause of uveitis. *J Immunother* 2004;27:478–479.

98. Hodi FS, O'Day SJ, McDermott DF, et al. Improved survival with ipilimumab in patients with metastatic melanoma. *N Engl J Med* 2010;363:711–723.

99. Robert C, Thomas L, Bondarenko I, et al. Ipilimumab plus dacarbazine for previously untreated metastatic melanoma. *N Engl J Med* 2011;364:2517–2526.

100. Wolchok JD, Weber JS, Maio M, et al. Four-year survival rates for patients with metastatic melanoma who received ipilimumab in phase II clinical trials. *Ann Oncol* 2013;24:2174–2180.

101. Yang JC, Hughes M, Kammula U, et al. Ipilimumab (anti-CTLA4 antibody) causes regression of metastatic renal cell cancer associated with enteritis and hypophysitis. *J Immunother* 2007;30:825–830.

102. Kirkwood JM, Lorigan P, Hersey P, et al. Phase II trial of tremelimumab (CP-675,206) in patients with advanced refractory or relapsed melanoma. *Clin Cancer Res* 2010;16:1042–1048.

103. Ribas A, Kefford R, Marshall MA, et al. Phase III randomized clinical trial comparing tremelimumab with standard-of-care chemotherapy in patients with advanced melanoma. *J Clin Oncol* 2013;31:616–622.

104. Ott PA, Hodi FS, Robert C. CTLA-4 and PD-1/PD-L1 blockade: new immunotherapeutic modalities with durable clinical benefit in melanoma patients. *Clin Cancer Res* 2013;19:5300–5309.

105. Keir ME, Butte MJ, Freeman GJ, et al. PD-1 and its ligands in tolerance and immunity. *Annu Rev Immunol* 2008;26:677–704.

106. Dong H, Strome SE, Salomao DR, et al. Tumor-associated B7-H1 promotes T-cell apoptosis: a potential mechanism of immune evasion. *Nat Med* 2002;8:793–800.

107. Brahmer JR, Drake CG, Wollner I, et al. Phase I study of single-agent anti-programmed death-1 (MDX-1106) in refractory solid tumors: safety, clinical activity, pharmacodynamics, and immunologic correlates. *J Clin Oncol* 2010;28:3167–3175.

108. Brahmer JR. Immune checkpoint blockade: the hope for immunotherapy as a treatment of lung cancer? *Semin Oncol* 2014;41:126–132.

109. Topalian SL, Sznol M, McDermott DF, et al. Survival, durable tumor remission, and long-term safety in patients with advanced melanoma receiving nivolumab. *J Clin Oncol* 2014;32:1020–1030.

110. Wolchok JD, Kluger H, Callahan MK, et al. Nivolumab plus ipilimumab in advanced melanoma. *N Engl J Med* 2013;369:122–133.

111. Hamid O, Robert C, Daud A, et al. Safety and tumor responses with lambrolizumab (anti-PD-1) in melanoma. *N Engl J Med* 2013;369:134–144.

112. Brahmer JR, Tykodi SS, Chow LQ, et al. Safety and activity of anti-PD-L1 antibody in patients with advanced cancer. *N Engl J Med* 2012;366:2455–2465.

113. Drake CG, Lipson EJ, Brahmer JR. Breathing new life into immunotherapy: review of melanoma, lung and kidney cancer. *Nat Rev Clin Oncol* 2014;11:24–37.

114. Rosenberg SA, Yang JC, Restifo NP. Cancer immunotherapy: moving beyond current vaccines. *Nat Med* 2004;10:909–915.

115. Klebanoff CA, Acquavella N, Yu Z, et al. Therapeutic cancer vaccines: are we there yet? *Immunol Rev* 2011;239:27–44.

116. Slingluff CL, Yamshchikov G, Neese P, et al. Phase I trial of a melanoma vaccine with gp100 $_{280-288}$ peptide and tetanus helper peptide in adjuvant: immunologic and clinical outcomes. *Clin Cancer Res* 2001;7:3012–3024.

117. Schaed SG, Klimek VM, Panageas KS, et al. T-cell responses against tyrosinase 368-376(370D) peptide in HLA*A0201$^+$ melanoma patients: randomized trial comparing incomplete Freund's adjuvant, granulocyte macrophage colony-stimulating factor, and QS-21 as immunological adjuvants. *Clin Cancer Res* 2004;8:967–972.

118. Marshall JL, Hoyer RJ, Toomey MA, et al. Phase I study in advanced cancer patients of a diversified prime-and-boost vaccination protocol using recombinant vaccinia virus and recombinant nonreplicating avipox virus to elicit anti-carcinoembryonic antigen immune responses. *J Clin Oncol* 2000;18:3964–3973.

119. Eder JP, Kantoff PW, Roper K, et al. A phase I trial of a recombinant vaccinia virus expressing prostate-specific antigen in advanced prostate cancer. *Clin Cancer Res* 2003;6:1632–1638.

120. Lurquin C, Lethe B, De Plaen E, et al. Contrasting frequencies of antitumor and anti-vaccine T cells in metastases of a melanoma patient vaccinated with a MAGE tumor antigen. *J Exp Med* 2005;201:249–257.

121. Marincola FM, Rivoltini L, Salgaller ML, et al. Differential anti-MART-1/MelanA CTL activity in peripheral blood of HLA-A2 melanoma patients in comparison to healthy donors: evidence of in vivo priming by tumor cells. *J Immunother Emphasis Tumor Immunol* 1996;19:266–277.

122. Cormier JN, Salgaller ML, Prevette T, et al. Enhancement of cellular immunity in melanoma patients immunized with a peptide from MART-1/Melan A. *Cancer J Sci Am* 1997;3:37–44.

123. Kantoff PW, Higano CS, Shore ND, et al. Sipuleucel-T immunotherapy for castration-resistant prostate cancer. *N Engl J Med* 2010;363:422.

124. Rosenberg SA, Packard BS, Aebersold PM, et al. Use of tumor infiltrating lymphocytes and interleukin-2 in the immunotherapy of patients with metastatic melanoma. Preliminary report. *N Engl J Med* 1988;319:1676–1680.

125. Restifo NP, Dudley ME, Rosenberg SA. Adoptive immunotherapy for cancer: harnessing the T cell response. *Nat Rev Immunol* 2012;12:269–281.

126. Rooney CM, Smith CA, Ng CY, et al. Infusion of cytotoxic T cells for the prevention and treatment of Epstein-Barr virus-induced lymphoma in allogeneic transplant recipients. *Blood* 1998;92:1549–1555.

127. Rosenberg SA, Yannelli JR, Yang JC, et al. Treatment of patients with metastatic melanoma using autologous tumor-infiltrating lymphocytes and interleukin-2. *J Natl Cancer Inst* 1994;86:1159–1166.

128. Dudley ME, Wunderlich JR, Robbins PF, et al. Cancer regression and autoimmunity in patients after clonal repopulation with anti-tumor lymphocytes. *Science* 2002;298:850–854.

129. Dudley ME, Yang JC, Sherry R, et al. Adoptive cell therapy for patients with metastatic melanoma: Evaluation of intensive myeloablative chemoradiation preparative regimens. *J Clin Oncol* 2008;26:5233–5239.

130. Rosenberg SA. Cell transfer immunotherapy for metastatic solid cancer—what clinicians need to know. *Nat Rev Clin Oncol* 2011;8:577–585.

131. Morgan RA, Dudley ME, Wunderlich JR, et al. Cancer regression in patients after transfer of genetically engineered lymphocytes. *Science* 2006;314:126–129.

132. Kochenderfer JN, Wilson WH, Janik E, et al. Eradication of B-lineage cells and regression of lymphoma in a patient treated with autologous T cells genetically engineered to recognize CD19. *Blood* 2010;116:4099–4102.

133. Porter DL, Levine BL, Kalos M, et al. Chimeric antigen receptor-modified T cells in chronic lymphoid leukemia. *N Engl J Med* 2011;365:725–733.

134. Tiera MJ, Winnik FO, Fernandes JC. Synthetic and natural polycations for gene therapy: state of the art and new perspectives. *Curr Gene Ther* 2006;6:59–71.

135. Birkholz K, Hombach A, Krug C, et al. Transfer of mRNA encoding recombinant immunoreceptors reprograms CD4+ and CD8+ T cells for use in the adoptive immunotherapy of cancer. *Gene Ther* 2009;16:596–604.

136. Zhao Y, Zheng Z, Cohen CJ, et al. High-efficiency transfection of primary human and mouse T lymphocytes using RNA electroporation. *Mol Ther* 2006;13:151–159.

137. Li L, Liu LC, Feller S, et al. Expression of chimeric antigen receptors in natural killer cells with a regulatory-compliant non-viral method. *Cancer Gene Ther* 2010;17:147–154.

138. Zhao Y, Moon E, Carpenito C, et al. Multiple injections of electroporated autologous T cells expressing a chimeric antigen receptor mediate regression of human disseminated tumor. *Cancer Res* 2010;70:9053–9061.

139. Ivics Z, Izsvak Z. Transposons for gene therapy! *Curr Gene Ther* 2006;6:593–607.

140. Singh H, Huls H, Kebriaei P, et al. A new approach to gene therapy using Sleeping Beauty to genetically modify clinical-grade T cells to target CD19. *Immunol Rev* 2014;257:181–190.

141. Hacein-Bey-Abina S, von Kalle C, Schmidt M, et al. A serious adverse event after successful gene therapy for X-linked severe combined immunodeficiency. *N Engl J Med* 2003;348:255–256.

142. Riviere I, Brose K, Mulligan RC. Effects of retroviral vector design on expression of human adenosine deaminase in murine bone marrow transplant recipients engrafted with genetically modified cells. *Proc Natl Acad Sci U S A* 1995;92:6733–6737.

143. Maetzig T, Galla M, Baum C, et al. Gammaretroviral vectors: biology, technology and application. *Viruses* 2011;3:677–713.

144. Schambach A, Swaney WP, van der Loo JC. Design and production of retro- and lentiviral vectors for gene expression in hematopoietic cells. *Methods Mol Biol* 2009;506:191–205.

145. Hughes MS, Yu YYL, Dudley ME, et al. Transfer of a TCR gene derived from a patient with a marked antitumor response conveys highly active T-cell effector functions. *Hum Gene Ther* 2005;16:457–472.

146. Zhang X, Godbey WT. Viral vectors for gene delivery in tissue engineering. *Adv Drug Deliv Rev* 2006;58:515–534.

147. Yu SS, Han E, Hong Y, et al. Construction of a retroviral vector production system with the minimum possibility of a homologous recombination. *Gene Ther* 2003;10:706–711.

148. Cavalieri S, Cazzaniga S, Geuna M, et al. Human T lymphocytes transduced by lentiviral vectors in the absence of TCR activation maintain an intact immune competence. *Blood* 2003;102:497–505.

149. Cavazzana-Calvo M, Payen E, Negre O, et al. Transfusion independence and HMGA2 activation after gene therapy of human beta-thalassaemia. *Nature* 2010;467:318–322.

150. Johnson LA, Morgan RA, Dudley ME, et al. Gene therapy with human and mouse T-cell receptors mediates cancer regression and targets normal tissues expressing cognate antigen. *Blood* 2009;114:535–546.

151. Simpson AJ, Caballero OL, Jungbluth A, et al. Cancer/testis antigens, gametogenesis and cancer. *Nat Rev Cancer* 2005;5:625.

152. Hofmann O, Caballero OL, Stevenson BJ, et al. Genome-wide analysis of cancer/testis gene expression. *Proc Natl Acad Sci U S A* 2008;105: 20422–20427.

153. Zhang Y, Wang Z, Liu H, et al. Pattern of gene expression and immune responses to Semenogelin 1 in chronic hematologic malignancies. *J Immunother* 2003;26:461–467.

154. Jungbluth AA, Antonescu CR, Busam KJ, et al. Monophasic and biphasic synovial sarcomas abundantly express cancer/testis antigen NY-ESO-1 but not MAGE-A1 or CT7. *Int J Cancer* 2001;94:252–256.

155. Gross G, Waks T, Eshhar Z. Expression of immunoglobulin-T-cell receptor chimeric molecules as functional receptors with antibody-type specificity. *Proc Natl Acad Sci U S A* 1989;86:10024–10028.

156. Pule MA, Savoldo B, Myers GD, et al. Virus-specific T cells engineered to coexpress tumor-specific receptors: persistence and antitumor activity in individuals with neuroblastoma. *Nat Med* 2008;14:1264–1270.

157. James SE, Greenberg PD, Jensen MC, et al. Antigen sensitivity of CD22-specific chimeric TCR is modulated by target epitope distance from the cell membrane. *J Immunol* 2008;180:7028–7038.

158. Morgan RA, Johnson LA, Davis JL, et al. Recognition of glioma stem cells by genetically modified T cells targeting EGFRvIII and development of adoptive cell therapy for glioma. *Hum Gene Ther* 2012;23:1043–1053.

159. Chinnasamy D, Yu Z, Theoret MR, et al. Gene therapy using genetically modified lymphocytes targeting VEGFR-2 inhibits the growth of vascularized syngenic tumors in mice. *J Clin Invest* 2010;120:3953–3968.

160. Carpenito C, Milone MC, Hassan R, et al. Control of large, established tumor xenografts with genetically retargeted human T cells containing CD28 and CD137 domains. *Proc Natl Acad Sci U S A* 2009;106:3360–3365.

161. Feugier P, Van HA, Sebban C, et al. Long-term results of the R-CHOP study in the treatment of elderly patients with diffuse large B-cell lymphoma: a study by the Groupe d'Etude des Lymphomes de l'Adulte. *J Clin Oncol* 2005;23:4117–4126.

162. Gribben JG, O'Brien S. Update on therapy of chronic lymphocytic leukemia. *J Clin Oncol* 2011;29:544–550.

163. Sorror ML, Sandmaier BM, Storer BE, et al. Long-term outcomes among older patients following nonmyeloablative conditioning and allogeneic hematopoietic cell transplantation for advanced hematologic malignancies. *JAMA* 2011;306:1874–1883.

164. Van BK. Current status of allogeneic transplantation for aggressive non-Hodgkin lymphoma. *Curr Opin Oncol* 2011;23:681–691.

165. Van BK. Stem cell transplantation for indolent lymphoma: a reappraisal. *Blood Rev* 2011;25:223–228.

166. McLaughlin P, Grillo-Lopez AJ, Link BK, et al. Rituximab chimeric anti-CD20 monoclonal antibody therapy for relapsed indolent lymphoma: half of patients respond to a four-dose treatment program. *J Clin Oncol* 1998;16:2825–2833.

167. Bacher U, Klyuchnikov E, Le-Rademacher J, et al. Conditioning regimens for allotransplants for diffuse large B-cell lymphoma: myeloablative or reduced intensity? *Blood* 2012;120:4256–4262.

168. Dotti G, Gottschalk S, Savoldo B, et al. Design and development of therapies using chimeric antigen receptor-expressing T cells. *Immunol Rev* 2014;257:107–126.

169. Eshhar Z, Waks T, Gross G, et al. Specific activation and targeting of cytotoxic lymphocytes through chimeric single chains consisting of antibody-binding domains and the gamma or zeta subunits of the immunoglobulin and T-cell receptors. *Proc Natl Acad Sci U S A* 1993;90:720–724.

170. Kochenderfer JN, Rosenberg SA. Treating B-cell cancer with T cells expressing anti-CD19 chimeric antigen receptors. *Nat Rev Clin Oncol* 2013;10:267–276.

171. Sadelain M, Brentjens R, Riviere I. The basic principles of chimeric antigen receptor design. *Cancer Discov* 2013;3:388–398.

172. Kershaw MH, Westwood JA, Darcy PK. Gene-engineered T cells for cancer therapy. *Nat Rev Cancer* 2013;13:525–541.

173. Brentjens RJ, Davila ML, Riviere I, et al. CD19-targeted T cells rapidly induce molecular remissions in adults with chemotherapy-refractory acute lymphoblastic leukemia. *Sci Transl Med* 2013;5:177ra38.

174. Brentjens RJ, Latouche JB, Santos E, et al. Eradication of systemic B-cell tumors by genetically targeted human T lymphocytes co-stimulated by CD80 and interleukin-15. *Nat Med* 2003;9:279–286.

175. Milone MC, Fish JD, Carpenito C, et al. Chimeric receptors containing CD137 signal transduction domains mediate enhanced survival of T cells and increased antileukemic efficacy in vivo. *Mol Ther* 2009;17:1453–1464.

176. Cooper LJ, Topp MS, Serrano LM, et al. T-cell clones can be rendered specific for CD19: toward the selective augmentation of the graft-versus-B lineage leukemia effect. *Blood* 2003;101:1637–1644.

177. Kebriaei P, Huls H, Jena B, et al. Infusing CD19-directed T cells to augment disease control in patients undergoing autologous hematopoietic stem-cell transplantation for advanced B-lymphoid malignancies. *Hum Gene Ther* 2012;23:444–450.

178. Wang X, Naranjo A, Brown CE, et al. Phenotypic and functional attributes of lentivirus-modified CD19-specific human CD8+ central memory T cells manufactured at clinical scale. *J Immunother* 2012;35:689–701.

179. Brentjens RJ, Rivière I, Park JH, et al. Safety and persistence of adoptively transferred autologous CD19-targeted T cells in patients with relapsed or chemotherapy refractory B-cell leukemias. *Blood* 2011;118:4817–4828.

180. Kalos M, Levine BL, Porter DL, et al. T cells with chimeric antigen receptors have potent antitumor effects and can establish memory in patients with advanced leukemia. *Sci Transl Med* 2011;3:95ra73.

181. Kochenderfer JN, Dudley ME, Feldman SA, et al. B-cell depletion and remissions of malignancy along with cytokine-associated toxicity in a clinical trial of anti-CD19 chimeric-antigen-receptor-transduced T cells. *Blood* 2011;119:2709–2720.

182. Imai C, Mihara K, Andreansky M, et al. Chimeric receptors with 4-1BB signaling capacity provoke potent cytotoxicity against acute lymphoblastic leukemia. *Leukemia* 2004;18:678–684.

183. Kochenderfer JN, Yu Z, Frasheri D, et al. Adoptive transfer of syngeneic T cells transduced with a chimeric antigen receptor that recognizes murine CD19 can eradicate lymphoma and normal B cells. *Blood* 2010;116:3875–3886.

184. North RJ. Cyclophosphamide-facilitated adoptive immunotherapy of an established tumor depends on elimination of tumor-induced suppressor T cells. *J Exp Med* 1982;155:1063–1074.

185. Gattinoni L, Finkelstein SE, Klebanoff CA, et al. Removal of homeostatic cytokine sinks by lymphodepletion enhances the efficacy of adoptively transferred tumor-specific CD8+ T cells. *J Exp Med* 2005;202:907–912.

186. Uckun FM, Jaszcz W, Ambrus JL, et al. Detailed studies on expression and function of CD19 surface determinant by using B43 monoclonal antibody and the clinical potential of anti-CD19 immunotoxins. *Blood* 1988;71:13–29.

187. Kochenderfer JN, Feldman SA, Zhao Y, et al. Construction and preclinical evaluation of an anti-CD19 chimeric antigen receptor. *J Immunother* 2009;32:689–702.

188. Brentjens RJ, Santos E, Nikhamin Y, et al. Genetically targeted T cells eradicate systemic acute lymphoblastic leukemia xenografts. *Clin Cancer Res* 2007;13:5426–5435.

189. Savoldo B, Ramos CA, Liu E, et al. CD28 costimulation improves expansion and persistence of chimeric antigen receptor-modified T cells in lymphoma patients. *J Clin Invest* 2011;121:1822–1826.

190. Grupp SA, Kalos M, Barrett D, et al. Chimeric antigen receptor-modified T cells for acute lymphoid leukemia. *N Engl J Med* 2013;368:1509–1518.

191. Jensen MC, Popplewell L, Cooper LJ, et al. Antitransgene rejection responses contribute to attenuated persistence of adoptively transferred CD20/CD19-specific chimeric antigen receptor redirected T cells in humans. *Biol Blood Marrow Transplant* 2010;16:1245–1356.

192. Till BG, Jensen MC, Wang J, et al. Adoptive immunotherapy for indolent non-Hodgkin lymphoma and mantle cell lymphoma using genetically modified autologous CD20-specific T cells. *Blood* 2008;112:2261–2271.

193. Till BG, Jensen MC, Wang J, et al. CD20-specific adoptive immunotherapy for lymphoma using a chimeric antigen receptor with both CD28 and 4-1BB domains: pilot clinical trial results. *Blood* 2012;119:3940–3950.

194. Haso W, Lee DW, Shah NN, et al. Anti-CD22-chimeric antigen receptors targeting B-cell precursor acute lymphoblastic leukemia. *Blood* 2013;121:1165–1174.

195. Giordano Attianese GM, Marin V, Hoyos V, et al. In vitro and in vivo model of a novel immunotherapy approach for chronic lymphocytic leukemia by anti-CD23 chimeric antigen receptor. *Blood* 2011;117:4736–4745.

196. Hudecek M, Schmitt TM, Baskar S, et al. The B-cell tumor-associated antigen ROR1 can be targeted with T cells modified to express a ROR1-specific chimeric antigen receptor. *Blood* 2010;116: 4532–4541.

197. Vera J, Savoldo B, Vigouroux S, et al. T lymphocytes redirected against the kappa light chain of human immunoglobulin efficiently kill mature B lymphocyte-derived malignant cells. *Blood* 2006;108:3890–3897.

198. Carpenter RO, Evbuomwan MO, Pittaluga S, et al. B-cell maturation antigen is a promising target for adoptive T-cell therapy of multiple myeloma. *Clin Cancer Res* 2013;19:2048–2060.

199. Peinert S, Prince HM, Guru PM, et al. Gene-modified T cells as immunotherapy for multiple myeloma and acute myeloid leukemia expressing the Lewis Y antigen. *Gene Ther* 2010;17:678–686.

200. Ritchie DS, Neeson PJ, Khot A, et al. Persistence and efficacy of second generation CAR T cell against the LeY antigen in acute myeloid leukemia. *Mol Ther* 2013;21:2122–2129.

201. Mardiros A, Dos SC, McDonald T, et al. T cells expressing CD123-specific chimeric antigen receptors exhibit specific cytolytic effector functions and antitumor effects against human acute myeloid leukemia. *Blood* 2013;122:3138–3148.

202. Savoldo B, Rooney CM, Di SA, et al. Epstein Barr virus specific cytotoxic T lymphocytes expressing the anti-CD30zeta artificial chimeric T-cell receptor for immunotherapy of Hodgkin disease. *Blood* 2007;110:2620–2630.

203. Hombach A, Heuser C, Sircar R, et al. An anti-CD30 chimeric receptor that mediates CD3-zeta-independent T-cell activation against Hodgkin's lymphoma cells in the presence of soluble CD30. *Cancer Res* 1998;58:1116–1119.

204. Shaffer DR, Savoldo B, Yi Z, et al. T cells redirected against CD70 for the immunotherapy of CD70-positive malignancies. *Blood* 2011;117:4304–4314.

205. Xue SA, Gao L, Hart D, et al. Elimination of human leukemia cells in NOD/SCID mice by WT1-TCR gene-transduced human T cells. *Blood* 2005;106:3062–3067.

206. Nagai K, Ochi T, Fujiwara H, et al. Aurora kinase A-specific T-cell receptor gene transfer redirects T lymphocytes to display effective antileukemia reactivity. *Blood* 2012;119:368–376.

207. Spranger S, Jeremias I, Wilde S, et al. TCR-transgenic lymphocytes specific for HMMR/Rhamm limit tumor outgrowth in vivo. *Blood* 2012;119:3440–3449.

208. Hale GA, Shrestha S, Le-Rademacher J, et al. Alternate donor hematopoietic cell transplantation (HCT) in non-Hodgkin lymphoma using lower intensity conditioning: a report from the CIBMTR. *Biol Blood Marrow Transplant* 2012;18:1036–1043.

209. Kochenderfer JN, Dudley ME, Carpenter RO, et al. Donor-derived CD19-targeted T cells cause regression of malignancy persisting after allogeneic hematopoietic stem cell transplantation. *Blood* 2013;122:4129–4139.

210. Cruz CR, Micklethwaite KP, Savoldo B, et al. Infusion of donor-derived CD19-redirected virus-specific T cells for B-cell malignancies relapsed after allogeneic stem cell transplant: a phase 1 study. *Blood* 2013;122:2965–2973.

211. Traversari C, Marktel S, Magnani Z, et al. The potential immunogenicity of the TK suicide gene does not prevent full clinical benefit associated with the use of TK-transduced donor lymphocytes in HSCT for hematologic malignancies. *Blood* 2007;109:4708–4715.

212. Tey S, Dotti G, Rooney CM, et al. Inducible caspase 9 suicide gene to improve the safety of allodepleted T cells after haploidentical stem cell transplantation. *Biol Blood Marrow Transplant* 2007;13:924.

213. Ciceri F, Bonini C, Stanghellini MT, et al. Infusion of suicide-gene-engineered donor lymphocytes after family haploidentical haemopoietic stem-cell transplantation for leukaemia (the TK007 trial): a non-randomised phase I-II study. *Lancet Oncol* 2009;10:489–500.

214. Di Stasi A, Tey SK, Dotti G, et al. Inducible apoptosis as a safety switch for adoptive cell therapy. *N Engl J Med* 2011;365:1673–1683.

**CANCER THERAPEUTICS**

# Pharmacokinetics and Pharmacodynamics of Anticancer Drugs

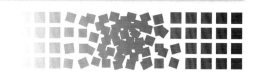

Alex Sparreboom and Sharyn D. Baker

## INTRODUCTION

Drug selection and therapy considerations in oncology were originally solely based on observations of the effects produced.[1] To overcome some of the limitations of this empirical approach and to answer questions related to considerations of dose, frequency, and duration of drug treatment, it is necessary to understand the events that follow drug administration. Preclinical in vitro and in vivo studies have shown that the magnitude of antitumor response is a function of the concentration of drug,[2] and this has led to the suggestion that the therapeutic objective can be achieved by maintaining an adequate concentration at the site of action for the duration of therapy.[3] However, drugs are rarely directly administered at their sites of action. Indeed, most anticancer drugs are given intravenously or orally, and yet are expected to act in the brain, lungs, or elsewhere. Drugs must, therefore, move from the site of administration to the site of action and, moreover, distribute to all other tissues including organs that eliminate them from the body, such as the kidneys and liver. To administer drugs optimally, knowledge is needed not only of the mechanisms of drug absorption, distribution, and elimination, but also of the kinetics of these processes.[4]

The treatment of human malignancies involving drugs can be divided into two pharmacologic phases, a *pharmacokinetic* phase in which the dose, dosage form, frequency, and route of administration are related to drug level–time relationships in the body, and a *pharmacodynamic* phase in which the concentration of drug at the site(s) of action is related to the magnitude of the effect(s) produced. Once both of these phases have been defined, a dosage regimen can be designed to achieve the therapeutic objective, although additional factors need to be taken into consideration (Fig. 15.1). The clinical application of this approach allows distinctions between pharmacokinetic and pharmacodynamic causes of an unusual drug response. A basic tenet of pharmacokinetics is that the magnitude of both the desired response and toxicity are functions of the drug concentration at the site(s) of action. Accordingly, therapeutic failure results when either the concentration is too low, resulting in ineffective therapy, or is too high, producing unacceptable toxicity. Between these limits of concentrations lies a region associated with therapeutic success, the so-called *therapeutic window*.[5] Because the concentration of a drug at the site of action can rarely be measured directly, with the exception of certain hematologic malignancies, plasma or blood is commonly measured instead as a more accessible alternative.

## PHARMACOKINETIC CONCEPTS

A drug's pharmacokinetic properties can be defined by two fundamental processes affecting drug behavior over time, *absorption* and *disposition*.

## Absorption

Historically, most anticancer drugs have been administered intravenously; however, the use of orally administered agents is growing with the development of small-molecule targeted cancer therapeutics, such as tyrosine kinase inhibitors.[6] Moreover, drugs may also be administered regionally, for example into the pleural or peritoneal cavities,[7] the cerebrospinal fluid, or intra-arterially into a vessel leading to a cancerous tissue.[8] The process by which the unchanged drug moves from the site of administration to the site of measurement within the body is referred to as *absorption*. Loss at any site prior to the site of measurement contributes to a decrease in the apparent absorption of a drug. For an orally administered agent, this complex series of events involves disintegration of the pharmaceutical dosage form, dissolution, diffusion through gastrointestinal fluids, permeation of the gut membrane, portal circulation uptake, passage through the liver, and, finally, entry into the systemic circulation. The loss of drug as it passes for the first time through organs of elimination, such as the gastrointestinal membranes and the liver, during the absorption process is known as the *first-pass effect*.[9]

The pharmacokinetic parameter most closely associated with absorption is availability or bioavailability (F), defined as the fraction (or percent) of the administered dose that is absorbed intact. Bioavailability can be estimated by dividing the area under the plasma concentration–time curve (AUC) achieved following extravascular administration by the AUC observed after intravenous administration, and can range from 0 to 1.0 (or 0% to 100%).

## Disposition

Disposition is defined as all the processes that occur subsequent to absorption of a drug; by definition, the components of disposition are *distribution* and *elimination*. Distribution is the process of reversible transfer of a drug to and from the site of measurement. Any drug that leaves the site of measurement and does not return has undergone elimination, which occurs by two processes, *excretion* and *metabolism*. Excretion is the irreversible loss of the chemically unchanged drug, whereas metabolism is the conversion of drug to another chemical species.

The extent of drug distribution can be determined by relating the concentration obtained with a known amount of drug in the body and is, in essence, a dilution space. The apparent volume into which a drug distributes in the body at equilibrium in called the volume of distribution ($V_d$), and may or may not correspond to an actual physiologic compartment.

The rate and extent to which a drug distributes into various tissues depend on a number of factors, including hydrophobicity, tissue permeability, tissue-binding constants, binding to serum proteins, and local organ blood flow.[10] Large apparent volumes of distribution are common for agents with high tissue binding or high lipid solubility,

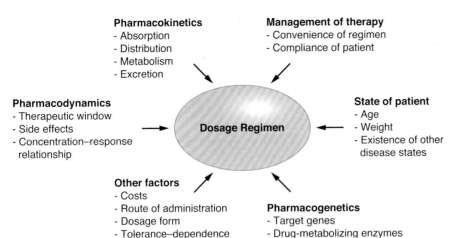

**Figure 15.1** Principal determinants of dosage regimen selection for an anticancer drug

although distribution into specific body compartments may be limited by physiologic processes, such as the blood–brain barrier protecting the central nervous system[11,12] or the blood–testes barrier.[13]

Just as $V_d$ is needed as a parameter to relate the concentration to the amount of drug in the body, there is also a need to have a parameter to relate the concentration to the rate of drug elimination, which is known as *clearance* (CL). Of all pharmacokinetic parameters, CL has the most clinical relevance because it defines the key relationship between drug dose and systemic drug exposure (AUC). Derived from $V_d$ and CL is the parameter *elimination rate constant*, which can be regarded as the fractional rate of drug removal. It is, however, more common to refer to the half-life than to the elimination rate constant of a drug. The half-life of a drug is a useful parameter to estimate the time required to reach steady state on a multidose schedule or during a continuous intravenous drug infusion.

## Dose Proportionality

When drug concentrations change in strict proportionality to the dose of drug administered, then the condition of dose proportionality (or linear pharmacokinetics) holds. If doubling the dose exactly doubles the plasma concentration or AUC, then pharmacokinetic parameters such $V_d$, and CL are constant and remain independent of dose and concentration.[14] By strict definition, drugs with linear pharmacokinetics are dose proportional. Dose proportionality is clinically important because it means that dose adjustments will generate predictable changes in systemic drug exposure. For drugs that lack dose proportionality, $V_d$ and CL will demonstrate concentration or time dependence, or both, making it difficult to predict the effect of dose adjustments on drug concentration (Fig. 15.2). Factors that can contribute to a lack of dose proportional pharmacokinetics include saturable oral absorption,[15] capacity-limited distribution or protein binding,[16] and/or saturable metabolism.[17] Dose proportionality of anticancer agents is typically assessed in Phase 1 dose-escalation trials in which small groups of patients are treated at a single dose level using a parallel study design, although the statistical power of such studies to detect deviations from dose proportionality is poor. An alternative, more robust study design is a crossover study in which each patient receives a low dose, an intermediate dose, and a high dose over consecutive cycles of treatment.[18] However, such studies are relatively rare in oncology because of the required use of low, potentially ineffective doses, which may raise ethical concerns for patients.

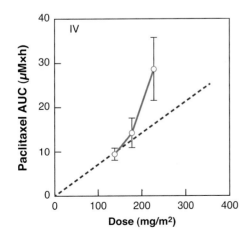

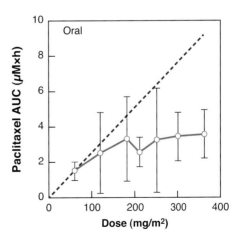

**Figure 15.2** Effect of drug dose on systemic exposure to paclitaxel following intravenous (IV) or oral administration in patients with cancer. Data are expressed as mean values (symbols) and standard deviation (error bars). The *dashed line* indicates the hypothetical dose-proportional increase in the area under the plasma concentration time curve (AUC). (Data derived from van Zuylen L, Karlsson MO, Verweij J, et al. Pharmacokinetic modeling of paclitaxel encapsulation in Cremophor EL micelles. *Cancer Chemother Pharmacol* 2001;47:309–318, and Malingre MM, Terwogt JM, Beijnen JH, et al. Phase I and pharmacokinetic study of oral paclitaxel. *J Clin Oncol* 2000;18:2468–2475, respectively.)

## TABLE 15.1

### Examples of Systemic Exposure as a Pharmacodynamic Marker of Anticancer Drug Effects

| Drug | Side Effect | Response/Survival |
| --- | --- | --- |
| Carboplatin | Thrombocytopenia | Ovarian cancer |
| Cisplatin | Nephrotoxicity | Head and neck cancer |
| Cyclophosphamide | Cardiotoxicity | |
| Docetaxel | Neutropenia | Non–small-cell lung cancer |
| Doxorubicin | Neutropenia | |
| Epirubicin | Neutropenia | |
| Erlotinib | Skin rash | Non–small-cell lung and head and neck cancer |
| Etoposide | | Non–small-cell lung cancer |
| 5-Fluorouracil | Diarrhea, mucositis | Head and neck cancer |
| Imatinib | | Chronic myeloid leukemia |
| Irinotecan | Diarrhea, neutropenia | |
| 6-Mercaptopurine | | Acute lymphoblastic leukemia |
| Methotrexate | Mucositis | Acute lymphoblastic leukemia |
| Nilotinib | Anemia, QT-interval prolongation | |
| Paclitaxel | Neutropenia | |
| Sorafenib | Hypertension, hand-foot skin reaction | Renal cell cancer |
| Sunitinib | Neutropenia | Renal cell cancer |
| Teniposide | | Lymphoma |

## PHARMACODYNAMIC CONCEPTS

Pharmacodynamic models relate clinical drug effects with drug dose, concentration, or other pharmacokinetic parameters indicative of drug exposures (Table 15.1). In oncology, pharmacodynamic variability may account for substantial differences in clinical outcomes, even when systemic exposures are uniform. Variability in pharmacodynamic response may be heavily influenced by clinical covariates such as age, gender, prior chemotherapy, prior radiotherapy, concomitant medications, or other variables.[19] The pharmacokinetic parameters that are most often correlated with drug effects are markers of drug exposure, such as AUC. In general, the specific parameter used as the independent variable in a pharmacodynamic analysis depends on the particular characteristics of the study drug.

In oncology, pharmacodynamic studies of drug effects have most often focused on toxicity endpoints.[20] Continuous response variables, such as the percentage fall in the absolute blood count from baseline, are easily analyzed using nonlinear regression methods. Dose-limiting neutropenia has been frequently analyzed using a sigmoid maximum effect model described by the modified Hill equation. The pharmacodynamic analysis of subjectively graded clinical endpoints, such as common toxicity criteria scores on a 4-point scale, may require more sophisticated statistical methods.[21,22] Logistical regression methods have been used to model these types of categorical (ordinal) response or outcome variables.

Physiologic pharmacodynamic models describing the severity and time course of drug-related myelosuppression have been derived using population mixed-effect methods for several agents, including paclitaxel[23,24] and pemetrexed.[25] The ability of these models to predict both the severity and duration of drug-induced neutropenia substantially enhances their clinical usefulness.[26] In contrast to small-molecule therapeutics, large-molecule therapeutics such as monoclonal antibodies may not demonstrate toxicities directly related to dose levels. For these agents, a thorough understanding of the pharmacokinetic/pharmacodynamic relationships using modeling approaches may be critical for optimal dose selection.[27]

The antitumor activity of certain chemotherapeutic agents is highly schedule dependent. For such drugs, the dose fractionated over several days can produce a different antitumor response or toxicity profile compared with the same dose given over a shorter period. For example, the efficacy of etoposide in the treatment of small-cell lung cancer is markedly increased when an identical total dose of etoposide is administered by a 5-day divided-dose schedule rather than a 24-hour infusion.[28] Pharmacokinetic analysis in that study showed that both schedules produced very similar overall drug exposure (as measured by AUC), but that the divided-dose schedule produced twice the duration of exposure to an etoposide plasma concentration of $>1$ $\mu$g/mL. This finding has led to the use of prolonged oral administration of etoposide to treat patients with cancer.[29] Similar schedule dependence has been demonstrated for a number of other anticancer agents, notably paclitaxel[30,31] and topotecan.[32] For these agents, the variability in clinically tested treatment schedules is enormous, ranging from short intravenous infusions of less than 30 minutes to 21-day or even 7-week continuous infusion administrations, with large differences in experienced toxicity profiles.

## VARIABILITY IN PHARMACOKINETICS/ PHARMACODYNAMICS

There is often a marked variation in drug handling between individual patients, resulting in variability in pharmacokinetic parameters (Fig. 15.3), which will often lead to variability in the pharmacodynamic effects of a given dose of a drug.[33] That is, an identical dose of drug may result in acceptable toxicity in one patient, and unacceptable and possibly life-threatening toxicity in another, or a clinical response in one individual and cancer progression in another. The principal underlying sources of this interindividual pharmacokinetic/pharmacodynamic variability are discussed in the following paragraphs.

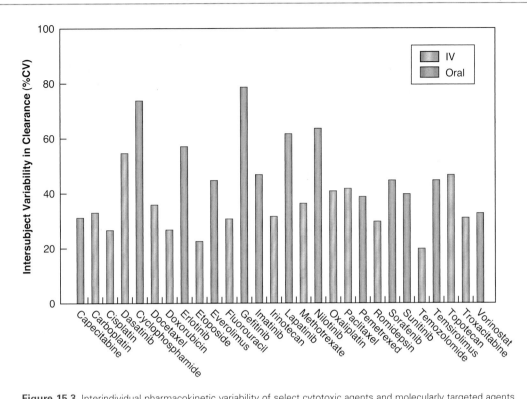

**Figure 15.3** Interindividual pharmacokinetic variability of select cytotoxic agents and molecularly targeted agents expressed as a percent coefficient of variation (%CV) in apparent (oral) clearance. IV, intravenous. (Data derived from Mathijssen RH, de Jong FA, Loos WJ, et al. Flat-fixed dosing versus body surface area based dosing of anticancer drugs in adults: does it make a difference? *Oncologist* 2007;12:913–923, and publicly available prescribing information.)

## Body Size and Body Composition

The traditional method of individualizing anticancer drug dosage is by using body surface area (BSA).[34] However, the usefulness of normalizing an anticancer drug dose to BSA in adults has been questioned, because, for many drugs, there is no relationship between BSA and CL.[35] Likewise, attempts to replace BSA as a size metric in dose calculation with alternate descriptors such as lean body weight, either in an average population or in individuals at the outer extremes of weight (i.e., frail, severely obese patients) have failed for many anticancer agents.[36,37] It should be pointed out that BSA is a much more important consideration in drug dose calculation for pediatric patients as compared to adults, because of the larger size range in the former population.[38] Based in part on the failure to reduce interindividual pharmacokinetic variability with the use of BSA normalization to obtain a starting dose, many of the more recently developed molecularly targeted agents are currently administered using a flat-fixed dose irrespective of an individual's BSA.[37]

## Age

Changes in body composition and organ function at the extremes of age can affect both drug disposition and drug effect.[39] For example, maturational processes in infancy may alter the absorption and distribution of drugs as well as change the capacity for drug metabolism and excretion.[4] The importance of understanding the influence of age on the pharmacokinetics and pharmacodynamics of individual anticancer agents has increased steadily as treatment for the malignancies of infants,[40] adolescents,[41] and the elderly[42] has advanced. Although pediatric cancers remain rare compared with cancers in adults and the elderly population, in particular, optimizing treatment in a patient group with a high cure rate and a long expected survival becomes critical to minimize the incidence of preventable late complications while maintaining efficacy.

## Pathophysiologic Changes

### Effects of Disease

Pathophysiologic changes associated with particular malignancies may cause dramatic alterations in drug disposition. For example, increases in the clearance of both antipyrine and lorazepam were noted after remission induction compared with the time of diagnosis in children with acute lymphoblastic leukemia (ALL).[43] The clearance of unbound teniposide is lower in children with ALL in relapse than during first remission.[44] Because leukemic infiltration of the liver at the time of diagnosis is common, drugs metabolized by the liver may have a reduced clearance, as has been documented in preclinical models.[45]

Furthermore, in mouse models, certain tumors elicited an acute phase response that coincided with downregulation of human CYP3A4 in the liver as well as the mouse ortholog Cyp3a11.[46] The reduction of murine hepatic Cyp3a gene expression in tumor-bearing mice resulted in decreased Cyp3a protein expression and, consequently, a significant reduction in Cyp3a-mediated metabolism of midazolam. These findings support the possibility that tumor-derived inflammation may alter the pharmacokinetic and pharmacodynamic properties of CYP3A4 substrates, leading to reduced metabolism of drugs in humans.[47] This supports a possible need for disease-specific design of early clinical trials with anticancer drugs,[48] as has been recommended for docetaxel.[49]

### Effects of Renal Impairment

The potential impact of pathophysiologic status on interindividual pharmacokinetic variability can be due to either the disease itself or to a dysfunction of specific organs involved in drug elimination. For example, if urinary excretion is an important elimination route for a given drug, any decrement in renal function could lead to decreased drug clearance, which may result in drug accumulation and toxicity.[50] Therefore, it would be logical to decrease the drug dose relative to the degree of impaired renal function in order to maintain plasma concentrations within a target therapeutic window. The best known example of this a priori dose adjustment of an anticancer agent remains carboplatin, which is excreted renally almost entirely by glomerular filtration. Various strategies have been developed to estimate carboplatin doses based on renal function among patients, either using creatinine clearance[51] or glomerular filtration rates as measured by a radioisotope method.[52] The application of these procedures has led to a substantial reduction in pharmacokinetic variability, such that carboplatin is currently one of the few drugs routinely administered to achieve a target exposure rather than on a milligram per square meter or milligram per kilogram basis.

The U.S. Food and Drug Administration (FDA) has developed a guidance on the impact of renal impairment on the pharmacokinetics, dosing, and labeling of drugs.[53] The impact of this guidance has been assessed following a survey of 94 new drug applications for small-molecule new molecular entities approved over the years 2003 to 2007. The survey results indicated that 41% of the applications that included renal impairment study data resulted in a recommendation of dose adjustment in renal impairment.[54] Interestingly, the survey results provided evidence that renal impairment can affect the pharmacokinetics of drugs that are predominantly eliminated by nonrenal processes such as metabolism and/or active transport. The latter finding supports the FDA recommendation to evaluate pharmacokinetic/pharmacodynamic alterations in renal impairment for those drugs that are predominantly eliminated by nonrenal processes, in addition to those that are mainly excreted unchanged by the kidneys. A striking example of a drug in the former category is imatinib, an agent that is predominantly eliminated by hepatic pathways but where predialysis renal impairment is associated with dramatically reduced drug clearance,[55] presumably due to a transporter-mediated process.[56]

### Effects of Hepatic Impairment

In contrast to the predictable decline in renal clearance of drugs when glomerular filtration is impaired, it is difficult to make general predictions on the effect of impaired liver function on drug clearance. The major problem is that commonly applied criteria to establish hepatic impairment are typically not good indicators of drug-metabolizing enzyme activity and that several alternative hepatic function tests, such as indocyanine green and antipyrine, have relatively limited value in predicting anticancer drug pharmacokinetics. An alternative dynamic measure of liver function has been proposed, which is based on totaled values (scored to the World Health Organization [WHO] grading system) of serum bilirubin, alkaline phosphatase, and either alanine aminotransferase or aspartate aminotransferase to give a hepatic dysfunction score.[57] Based on pharmacokinetic studies in patients with normal and impaired hepatic function, guidelines have been proposed for dose adjustments of several agents when administered to patients with severe liver dysfunction.[58] It should be emphasized that no uniform criteria have been used in the conduct of these studies and that, ultimately, substantial advances could be made through an a priori determination of the hepatic activity of enzymes of pertinent relevance to the chemotherapeutic drug(s) of interest, as has been done for docetaxel.[59]

### Effects of Serum Proteins

The binding of drugs to serum proteins, particularly those that are highly bound, may also have significant clinical implications for a therapeutic outcome.[60] Although protein binding is a major determinant of drug action, it is clearly only one of a myriad of factors that influence the disposition of anticancer drugs.[16] The extent of protein binding is a function of drug and protein concentrations, the affinity constants for the drug–protein interaction, and the number of protein-binding sites per class of binding site. Because only the unbound (or free) drug in plasma water is available for distribution, the therapeutic response will correlate with free drug concentration rather than total drug concentration. Several clinical situations, including liver and renal disease, can significantly decrease the extent of serum binding and may lead to higher free drug concentrations and a possible risk of unexpected toxicity, although the total (free plus bound forms) plasma drug concentrations are unaltered.[61] It is important to realize, however, that after therapeutic doses of most anticancer drugs, binding to serum proteins is independent of drug concentration, suggesting that the total plasma concentration is reflective of the unbound concentration. For some anticancer agents, including etoposide[62] and paclitaxel,[63] however, protein binding is highly dependent on dose and schedule.

## Sex Dependence

A number of pharmacokinetic analyses have suggested that male gender is positively correlated with the maximum elimination capacity of various anticancer drugs (e.g., paclitaxel)[8] or with increased clearance (e.g., imatinib)[64] compared with female gender. These observations have added to a growing body of evidence that the pharmacokinetic profile of various anticancer drugs exhibits significant sexual dimorphism, which is rarely considered in the design of clinical trials during oncology drug development.

## Drug Interactions

### Coadministration of Other Chemotherapeutic Drugs

Favorable and unfavorable interactions between drugs must be considered in developing combination regimens. These interactions may influence the effectiveness of each of the components of the combination, and typically occur when the pharmacokinetic profile of one drug is altered by the other. Such interactions are important in the design of trials evaluating drug combinations because, occasionally, the outcome of concurrent drug administration is diminished therapeutic efficacy or increased toxicity of one or more of the administered agents. Although a recent survey indicated that clinically significant pharmacokinetic interactions are relatively rare in Phase I trials of oncology drug combinations,[65] interactions appear to be more common for combinations of tyrosine kinase inhibitors with cytotoxic chemotherapeutics.[66]

### Coadministration of Nonchemotherapeutic Drugs

Many prescription and over-the-counter medications have the potential to cause interactions with anticancer agents by altering their pharmacokinetic characteristics and leading to clinically significant phenotypes. Most clinically relevant drug interactions in this category are due to changes in metabolic routes related to an altered expression or function of cytochrome P450 (CYP) isozymes. This class of enzymes, particularly the CYP3A4 isoform, is responsible for the oxidation of a large proportion of currently approved anticancer drugs. Elevated CYP activity (induction), translated into a more rapid metabolic rate, may result in a decrease in plasma concentrations and to a loss of therapeutic effect. For example, anticonvulsant drugs such as phenytoin, phenobarbital, and carbamazepine can induce drug-metabolizing enzymes and thereby increase the clearance of various anticancer agents.[33]

Conversely, the suppression (inhibition) of CYP activity, for example with ketoconazole,[13,67] may trigger a rise in plasma concentrations and can lead to exaggerated toxicity commensurate with overdose. It should be borne in mind that several pharmacokinetic parameters could be altered simultaneously. Especially in the development of anticancer agents given by the oral route,

**TABLE 15.2**

**Effect of Food on Exposure to Select Oral Anticancer Agents**

| Drug | Food | Effect on Drug Exposure | Manufacturer's Recommendations |
|---|---|---|---|
| Abiraterone | High-fat meal | ↑ AUC 1,000% | Without food |
| Dasatinib | High-fat meal | ↑ AUC 14% | With or without food |
| Erlotinib | High-fat, high-calorie breakfast | Single dose, ↑ AUC 200% Multiple dose, ↑ AUC 37%–66% | Without food[a] |
| Gefitinib | High-fat breakfast | ↓ AUC 14%, ↓ Cmax 35% | With or without food |
| | High-fat breakfast | ↑ AUC 32%, ↑ Cmax 35% | |
| Imatinib | High-fat meal | No change Variability (% CV) ↓ 37% | With food and a large glass of water[b] |
| Lapatinib | Low-fat meal (5% fat, 500 calories) | ↑ AUC 167%, ↑ Cmax 142% | Without food[c] |
| | High-fat meal (50% fat, 1,000 calories) | ↑ AUC 325%, ↑ Cmax 203% | |
| Nilotinib | High-fat meal | ↑ AUC 82% | Without food |
| Sorafenib | Moderate-fat meal (30% fat, 700 calories) | No change in bioavailability | Without food |
| | High-fat meal (50% fat, 900 calories) | ↓ Bioavailability 29% | |
| Sunitinib | High-fat, high-calorie meal | ↑ AUC 18% | With or without food |
| Everolimus | High-fat meal | ↓ AUC 16%, ↓ Cmax 60% | With or without food |
| Vismodegib | High-fat meal | ↑ AUC 74% for single dose; no effect at steady state | With or without food |
| Vorinostat | High-fat meal | ↑ AUC 37% | With food[d] |

[a] Recommended without food because the approved dose is the maximum tolerated dose.
[b] Recommended with food to reduce nausea.
[c] Recommended without food to achieve consistent drug exposure; was taken without food in clinical trials.
[d] Was taken with food in clinical trials.
AUC, area under the plasma concentration time curve; Cmax, maximum plasma concentration; CV, coefficient of variation.

oral bioavailability plays a crucial role[9]; this parameter is contingent on adequate absorption and the circumvention of intestinal and, subsequently, hepatic metabolism of the drug. It has been suggested that the prevalence of drug–drug interactions is particularly high in cancer patients receiving oral chemotherapy,[68] especially for agents that are weak bases that exhibit pH-dependent solubility.[69]

An additional consideration is related to a possible influence of food intake on the extent of drug absorption after oral administration, which can increase, decrease, or remain unchanged depending on specific physicochemical properties of the drug in question (Table 15.2). The relatively narrow therapeutic index of most of these agents means that significant inter- and intrapatient variability would predispose some individuals to excessive toxicity or, conversely, inadequate efficacy.[12]

## Coadministration of Complementary and Alternative Medicine

Surveys within the past decade estimate the prevalence of complementary and alternative medicine (CAM) use in oncology patients to be as high as 87%, and in many cases the treating physician is not aware of the patients' CAM use.[70] With a larger number of participants to phase I clinical trials[71] using herbal treatments combined with allopathic therapies, the risk for herb–drug interactions is a growing concern, and there is an increasing need to understand possible adverse drug interactions in oncology at the early stages of drug development.

A number of clinically important pharmacokinetic interactions involving CAM and cancer drugs have now been recognized, although causal relationships have not always been established.[72] Most of the observed interactions point to the herbs

affecting several isoforms of the CYP family, either through inhibition or induction. In the context of chemotherapeutic drugs, St. John's wort,[73] garlic,[74] milk thistle,[75] and Echinacea[11] have been formally evaluated for their pharmacokinetic drug–interaction potential in cancer patients. However, various other herbs have the potential to significantly modulate the expression and/or activity of drug-metabolizing enzymes and drug transporters (Table 15.3), including ginkgo, ginseng, and kava.[70] Because of the high prevalence of herbal medicine use, physicians should include herb usage in their routine drug histories in order to have an opportunity to outline to individual patients which potential hazards should be taken into consideration prior to participation in a clinical trial.

## Inherited Genetic Factors

The discipline of pharmacogenetics describes differences in the pharmacokinetics and pharmacodynamics of drugs as a result of inherited variation in drug metabolizing enzymes, drug transporters, and drug targets between patients.[76] These inherited variations are occasionally responsible for extensive interpatient variability in drug exposure or effects. Severe toxicity might occur in the absence of a typical metabolism of active compounds, while the therapeutic effect of a drug could be diminished in the case of an absence of activation of a prodrug, such as irinotecan.[77] The importance and detectability of polymorphisms for a given enzyme or transporter depends on the contribution of the variant gene product to pharmacologic response, the availability of alternative pathways of elimination, and the frequency of occurrence of the variant allele. Although many substrates have been identified for the known polymorphic drug metabolizing enzymes

| TABLE 15.3 |
|---|

**Effects of Common Herbal Products on Exposure to Anticancer Agents**

| Botanical | Concurrent Chemotherapy/Condition (Suspected Effect) |
|---|---|
| Ephedra | Avoid with all cardiovascular chemotherapy (synergistic increase in blood pressure) |
| Ginkgo | Caution with camptothecins, cyclophosphamide, TK inhibitors, epipodophyllotoxins, taxanes, and vinca alkaloids (CYP3A4 and CYP2C19 inhibition); discourage with alkylating agents, antitumor antibiotics, and platinum analogs (free-radical scavenging) |
| Ginseng | Discourage in patients with estrogen-receptor–positive breast cancer and endometrial cancer (stimulation of tumor growth) |
| Green tea | Discourage with erlotinib and pazopanib (CYP1A2 induction) |
| Japanese arrowroot | Avoid with methotrexate (ABC and OAT transporter inhibition) |
| St. John's wort | Avoid with all concurrent chemotherapy (CYP2B6, CYP2C9, CYP2C19, CYP2E1, CYP3A4, and ABCB1 induction) |
| Valerian | Caution with tamoxifen (CYP2C9 inhibition), cyclophosphamide, and teniposide (CYP2C19 inhibition) |
| Kava-kava | Avoid in all patients with preexisting liver disease, with evidence of hepatic injury (herb-induced hepatotoxicity), and/or in combination with hepatotoxic chemotherapy; caution with camptothecins, cyclophosphamide, TK inhibitors, epipodophyllotoxins, taxanes, and Vinca alkaloids (CYP3A4 induction) |

TK, tyrosine kinase; CYP, cytochrome P450; ABC, ATP-binding cassette; OAT, organic anion transporter.

and transporters, the contribution of a genetically determined source of interindividual pharmacokinetic variability has been established for only a few cancer chemotherapeutic agents. Most of these cases involve agents for which elimination is critically dependent on a rate-limiting breakdown by a polymorphic enzyme (e.g., 6-mercaptopurine by thiopurine-S-methyltransferase; 5-fluorouracil by dihydropyrimidine dehydrogenase) or when a polymorphic enzyme is involved in the formation of a toxic metabolite (e.g., tamoxifen by CYP2D6).[78]

In addition to drug metabolism, pharmacokinetic processes are highly dependent on the interplay with drug transport in organs such as the intestines, kidneys, and liver. Genetically determined variation in drug transporter function or expression is now increasingly recognized to have a significant role as a determinant of intersubject variability in response to various commonly prescribed drugs.[79] The most extensively studied class of drug transporters are those encoded by the family of ATP-binding cassette (ABC) genes, some of which also play a role in the resistance of malignant cells to anticancer agents. Among the 48 known ABC gene products, ABCB1 (P-glycoprotein), ABCC1 (multidrug-resistance associated protein-1 [MRP1]) and its homologue ABCC2 (MRP2; cMOAT), and ABCG2 (breast cancer resistance protein [BCRP]) are known to influence the oral absorption and disposition of a wide variety of drugs.[80] As a result, the expression levels of these proteins in humans have important consequences for an individual's susceptibility to certain anticancer drug–induced side effects, interactions, and treatment efficacy, for example, in the case of genetic variation in ABCG2 in relation to gefitinib-induced diarrhea.[81]

Similar to the discoveries of functional genetic variations in drug efflux transporters of the ABC family, there have been considerable advances in the identification of inherited variants in transporters that facilitate cellular drug uptake in tissues that play an important role in drug elimination, such as the liver (Fig. 15.4). Among these, members of the organic anion-transporting polypeptides (OATP), organic anion transporters (OAT), and organic cation transporters (OCT) can mediate the cellular uptake of a large number of structurally divergent compounds.[82,83] Accordingly, functionally relevant polymorphisms in these influx transporters may contribute to interindividual and interethnic variability in drug disposition and response,[84] for example, in the case of the impact of polymorphic variants in the OCT1 gene SLC22A1 on the survival of patients with chronic myeloid leukemia receiving treatment with imatinib.[85]

## DOSE-ADAPTATION USING PHARMACOKINETIC/PHARMACODYNAMIC PRINCIPLES

### Therapeutic Drug Monitoring

Prolonged infusion schedules of anticancer drugs offer a very convenient setting for dose adaptation in individual patients. At the time required to achieve steady-state concentration, it is possible to modify the infusion rate for the remainder of the treatment course if a relationship is known between this steady-state concentration and a desired pharmacodynamic endpoint. This method has been successfully used to adapt the dose during continuous infusions of 5-fluorouracil and etoposide, and for repeated oral administration of etoposide or repeated intravenous administration of cisplatin.[86] Methotrexate plasma concentrations are routinely monitored to identify patients at high risk of toxicity and to adjust leucovorin rescue in patients with delayed drug excretion. This monitoring has significantly reduced the incidence of serious toxicity, including toxic death, and in fact, has improved outcome by eliminating unacceptably low systemic exposure levels.[87] Therapeutic drug monitoring has also been applied to or is currently under investigation for several more recently developed anticancer drugs, including imatinib[88–90] and sorafenib.[91]

### Feedback-Controlled Dosing

It remains to be determined how information on interindividual pharmacokinetic variability can eventually be used to devise an optimal dosage regimen of a drug for the treatment of a given disease in an individual patient. Obviously, the desired objective would be most efficiently achieved if the individual's dosage requirements could be calculated prior to administering the drug. While this ideal cannot be met completely in clinical practice, with the notable exception of carboplatin, some success may be achieved by adopting feedback-controlled dosing. In the adaptive dosage with feedback control, population-based predictive models are used initially, but allow the possibility of dosage alteration based on feedback revision. In this approach, patients are first treated with standard dose and, during treatment, pharmacokinetic information is estimated by a limited-sampling strategy and compared with that predicted from the population model with which treatment was initiated. On the basis of the comparison,

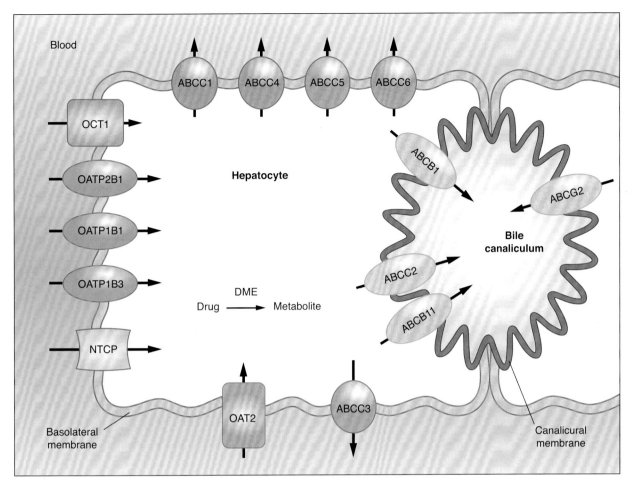

**Figure 15.4** Common mechanisms for possible interactions between xenobiotics and anticancer drugs in the liver. DME, drug-metabolizing enzyme(s).

more patient-specific pharmacokinetic parameters are calculated, and dosage is adjusted accordingly to maintain the target exposure measure producing the desired pharmacodynamic effect. Despite its mathematical complexity, this approach may be the only way to deliver the desired and precise exposure of an anticancer agent.

The study of population pharmacokinetics seeks to identify the measurable factors that cause changes in the dose-concentration relationship and the extent of these alterations so that, if these are associated with clinically significant shifts in the therapeutic index, dosage can be appropriately modified in the individual patient. It is obvious that a careful collection of data during the development of drugs and subsequent analyses could be helpful to collect some essential information on the drug. Unfortunately, important information is often lost by failing to analyze this data or due to the fact that the relevant samples or data were never collected. Historically, this has resulted in the notion that tools for the identification of patient population subgroups are inadequate for most of the currently approved anticancer drugs.

However, the use of population pharmacokinetic models is increasingly studied in an attempt to accommodate as much of the pharmacokinetic variability as possible in terms of measurable characteristics. This type of analysis has been conducted for a number of clinically important anticancer drugs, including carboplatin,[92] docetaxel,[93] topotecan,[94] gefitinib,[95] and erlotinib,[96] and provided mathematical equations based on morphometric, demographic, phenotypic enzyme activity, and/or physiologic characteristics of patients, in order to predict drug clearance with an acceptable degree of precision and bias.[97]

## REFERENCES

1. DeVita VT, Chu E. A history of cancer chemotherapy. *Cancer Res* 2008; 68:8643–8653.
2. Lieu CH, Tan AC, Leong S, et al. From bench to bedside: lessons learned in translating preclinical studies in cancer drug development. *J Natl Cancer Inst* 2013;105:1441–1456.
3. Sparreboom A, Verweij J. Advances in cancer therapeutics. *Clin Pharmacol Ther* 2009;85:113–117.
4. Fujita KI, Sasaki Y. Optimization of cancer chemotherapy on the basis of pharmacokinetics and pharmacodynamics: from patients enrolled in 'clinical trials' to those in the 'real world'. *Drug Metab Pharmacokin* 2014;29(1):20–28.
5. Liliemark J, Peterson C. Pharmacokinetic optimisation of anticancer therapy. *Clin Pharmacokinet* 1991;21:213–231.
6. Stuurman FE, Nuijen B, Beijnen JH, et al. Oral anticancer drugs: mechanisms of low bioavailability and strategies for improvement. *Clin Pharmacokinet* 2013;52:399–414.

7. Hasovits C, Clarke S. Pharmacokinetics and pharmacodynamics of intraperitoneal cancer chemotherapeutics. *Clin Pharmacokinet* 2012;51:203–224.
8. Cai S, Bagby TR, Forrest ML. Development of regional chemotherapies: feasibility, safety and efficacy in clinical use and preclinical studies. *Ther Deliv* 2011;2:1467–1484.
9. DeMario MD, Ratain MJ. Oral chemotherapy: rationale and future directions. *J Clin Oncol* 1998;16:2557–2567.
10. Zou P, Zheng N, Yang Y, et al. Prediction of volume of distribution at steady state in humans: comparison of different approaches. *Exp Opin Drug Metab Toxicol* 2012;8:855–872.
11. Deeken JF, Loscher W. The blood-brain barrier and cancer: transporters, treatment, and Trojan horses. *Clin Cancer Res* 2007;13:1663–1674.
12. Pitz MW, Desai A, Grossman SA, et al. Tissue concentration of systemically administered antineoplastic agents in human brain tumors. *J Neurooncol* 2011;104:629–638.

CANCER THERAPEUTICS

13. Mruk DD, Su L, Cheng CY. Emerging role for drug transporters at the blood-testis barrier. *Trends Pharmacol Sci* 2011;32:99–106.

14. Smith BP, Vandenhende FR, DeSante KA, et al. Confidence interval criteria for assessment of dose proportionality. *Pharm Res* 2000;17:1278–1283.

15. Malingre MM, Terwogt JM, Beijnen JH, et al. Phase I and pharmacokinetic study of oral paclitaxel. *J Clin Oncol* 2000;18:2468–2475.

16. Sparreboom A, Chen H, Acharya MR, et al. Effects of alpha1-acid glycoprotein on the clinical pharmacokinetics of 7-hydroxystaurosporine. *Clin Cancer Res* 2004;10:6840–6846.

17. Yamaoka K, Takakura Y. Analysis methods and recent advances in nonlinear pharmacokinetics from in vitro through in loci to in vivo. *Drug Metab Dispos* 2004;19:397–406.

18. van Zuylen L, Karlsson MO, Verweij J, et al. Pharmacokinetic modeling of paclitaxel encapsulation in Cremophor EL micelles. *Cancer Chemother Pharmacol* 2001;47:309–318.

19. Karlsson MO, Molnar V, Bergh J, et al. A general model for time-dissociated pharmacokinetic-pharmacodynamic relationship exemplified by paclitaxel myelosuppression. *Clin Pharmacol Ther* 1998;63:11–25.

20. Zhou Q, Gallo JM. The pharmacokinetic/pharmacodynamic pipeline: translating anticancer drug pharmacology to the clinic. *AAPS J* 2011;13:111–120.

21. Xie R, Mathijssen RH, Sparreboom A, et al. Clinical pharmacokinetics of irinotecan and its metabolites in relation with diarrhea. *Clin Pharmacol Ther* 2002;72:265–275.

22. Xie R, Mathijssen RH, Sparreboom A, et al. Clinical pharmacokinetics of irinotecan and its metabolites: a population analysis. *J Clin Oncol* 2002;20:3293–3301.

23. Kearns CM, Gianni L, Egorin MJ. Paclitaxel pharmacokinetics and pharmacodynamics. *Sem Oncol* 1995;22:16–23.

24. Minami H, Sasaki Y, Saijo N, et al. Indirect-response model for the time course of leukopenia with anticancer drugs. *Clin Pharmacol Ther* 1998;64:511–521.

25. Latz JE, Schneck KL, Nakagawa K, et al. Population pharmacokinetic/pharmacodynamic analyses of pemetrexed and neutropenia: effect of vitamin supplementation and differences between Japanese and Western patients. *Clin Cancer Res* 2009;15:346–354.

26. Karlsson MO, Anehall T, Friberg LE, et al. Pharmacokinetic/pharmacodynamic modelling in oncological drug development. *Basic Clin Pharmacol Toxicol* 2005;96:206–211.

27. Keizer RJ, Huitema AD, Schellens JH, et al. Clinical pharmacokinetics of therapeutic monoclonal antibodies. *Clin Pharmacokinet* 2010;49:493–507.

28. Slevin ML, Clark PI, Joel SP, et al. A randomized trial to evaluate the effect of schedule on the activity of etoposide in small-cell lung cancer. *J Clin Oncol* 1989;7:1333–1340.

29. Hainsworth JD. Extended-schedule oral etoposide in selected neoplasms and overview of administration and scheduling issues. *Drugs* 1999;58 Suppl 3:51–56.

30. Gelderblom H, Mross K, ten Tije AJ, et al. Comparative pharmacokinetics of unbound paclitaxel during 1- and 3-hour infusions. *J Clin Oncol* 2002;20:574–581.

31. Woodward EJ, Twelves C. Scheduling of taxanes: a review. *Curr Clin Pharmacol* 2010;5:226–231.

32. Soepenberg O, Sparreboom A, Verweij J. Clinical studies of camptothecin and derivatives. *Alkaloid Chem Biol* 2003;60:1–50.

33. Undevia SD, Gomez-Abuin G, Ratain MJ. Pharmacokinetic variability of anticancer agents. *Nat Rev Cancer* 2005;5:447–458.

34. Gurney H. Dose calculation of anticancer drugs: a review of the current practice and introduction of an alternative. *J Clin Oncol* 1996;14:2590–2611.

35. Baker SD, Verweij J, Rowinsky EK, et al. Role of body surface area in dosing of investigational anticancer agents in adults, 1991–2001. *J Natl Cancer Inst* 2002;94:1883–1888.

36. Mathijssen RH, Sparreboom A. Influence of lean body weight on anticancer drug clearance. *Clin Pharmacol Ther* 2009;85:23.

37. Sparreboom A, Wolff AC, Mathijssen RH, et al. Evaluation of alternate size descriptors for dose calculation of anticancer drugs in the obese. *J Clin Oncol* 2007;25:4707–4713.

38. Bartelink IH, Rademaker CM, Schobben AF, et al. Guidelines on paediatric dosing on the basis of developmental physiology and pharmacokinetic considerations. *Clin Pharmacokinet* 2006;45:1077–1097.

39. McLeod HL, Relling MV, Crom WR, et al. Disposition of antineoplastic agents in the very young child. *Br J Cancer* 1992;18:S23–S29.

40. Hutson JR, Weitzman S, Schechter T, et al. Pharmacokinetic and pharmacogenetic determinants and considerations in chemotherapy selection and dosing in infants. *Exp Opin Drug Metab Toxicol* 2012;8:709–722.

41. Veal GJ, Hartford CM, Stewart CF. Clinical pharmacology in the adolescent oncology patient. *J Clin Oncol* 2010;28:4790–4799.

42. Lichtman SM. Pharmacology of aging and cancer: how useful are pharmacokinetic tests? *Interdiscip Top Gerontol* 2013;38:104–123.

43. Relling MV, Crom WR, Pieper JA, et al. Hepatic drug clearance in children with leukemia: changes in clearance of model substrates during remission-induction therapy. *Clin Pharmacol Ther* 1987;41:651–660.

44. Evans WE, Rodman JH, Relling MV, et al. Differences in teniposide disposition and pharmacodynamics in patients with newly diagnosed and relapsed acute lymphocytic leukemia. *J Pharmacol Exp Ther* 1992;260:71–77.

45. Powis G, Harris RN, Basseches PJ, et al. Effects of advanced leukemia on hepatic drug-metabolizing activity in the mouse. *Cancer Chemother Pharmacol* 1986;16:43–49.

46. Charles KA, Rivory LP, Brown SL, et al. Transcriptional repression of hepatic cytochrome P450 3A4 gene in the presence of cancer. *Clin Cancer Res* 2006;12:7492–7497.

47. Moore MM, Chua W, Charles KA, et al. Inflammation and cancer: causes and consequences. *Clin Pharmacol Ther* 2010;87:504–508.

48. Albekairy A, Alkatheri A, Fujita S, et al. Cytochrome P450 3A4FNx011B as pharmacogenomic predictor of tacrolimus pharmacokinetics and clinical outcome in the liver transplant recipients. *Saudi J Gastroenterol* 2013;19:89–95.

49. Franke RM, Carducci MA, Rudek MA, et al. Castration-dependent pharmacokinetics of docetaxel in patients with prostate cancer. *J Clin Oncol* 2010;28:4562–4567.

50. Rahman A, White RM. Cytotoxic anticancer agents and renal impairment study: the challenge remains. *J Clin Oncol* 2006;24:533–536.

51. Egorin MJ, Van Echo DA, Olman EA, et al. Prospective validation of a pharmacologically based dosing scheme for the cis-diamminedichloroplatinum(II) analogue diamminecyclobutanedicarboxylatoplatinum. *Cancer Res* 1985;45:6502–6506.

52. Calvert AH, Newell DR, Gumbrell LA, et al. Carboplatin dosage: prospective evaluation of a simple formula based on renal function. *J Clin Oncol* 1989;7:1748–1756.

53. Huang SM, Temple R, Xiao S, et al. When to conduct a renal impairment study during drug development: US Food and Drug Administration perspective. *Clin Pharmacol Ther* 2009;86:475–479.

54. Zhang Y, Zhang L, Abraham S, et al. Assessment of the impact of renal impairment on systemic exposure of new molecular entities: evaluation of recent new drug applications. *Clin Pharmacol Ther* 2009;85:305–311.

55. Gibbons J, Egorin MJ, Ramanathan RK, et al. Phase I and pharmacokinetic study of imatinib mesylate in patients with advanced malignancies and varying degrees of renal dysfunction: a study by the National Cancer Institute Organ Dysfunction Working Group. *J Clin Oncol* 2008;26:570–576.

56. Franke RM, Sparreboom A. Inhibition of imatinib transport by uremic toxins during renal failure. *J Clin Oncol* 2008;26:4226–4227.

57. Twelves C, Glynne-Jones R, Cassidy J, et al. Effect of hepatic dysfunction due to liver metastases on the pharmacokinetics of capecitabine and its metabolites. *Clin Cancer Res* 1999;5:1696–1702.

58. Eklund JW, Trifilio S, Mulcahy MF. Chemotherapy dosing in the setting of liver dysfunction. *Oncology (Williston Park)* 2005;19:1057–1063.

59. Hooker AC, Ten Tije AJ, Carducci MA, et al. Population pharmacokinetic model for docetaxel in patients with varying degrees of liver function: incorporating cytochrome P4503A activity measurements. *Clin Pharmacol Ther* 2008;84:111–118.

60. Grandison MK, Boudinot FD. Age-related changes in protein binding of drugs: implications for therapy. *Clin Pharmacokinet* 2000;38:271–290.

61. Sparreboom A, Nooter K, Loos WJ, et al. The (ir)relevance of plasma protein binding of anticancer drugs. *Neth J Med* 2001;59:196–207.

62. Perdaems N, Bachaud JM, Rouzaud P, et al. Relation between unbound plasma concentrations and toxicity in a prolonged oral etoposide schedule. *Eur J Clin Pharmacol* 1998;54:677–683.

63. Sparreboom A, van ZL, Brouwer E, et al. Cremophor EL-mediated alteration of paclitaxel distribution in human blood: clinical pharmacokinetic implications. *Cancer Res* 1999;59:1454–1457.

64. Gardner ER, Burger H, van Schaik RH, et al. Association of enzyme and transporter genotypes with the pharmacokinetics of imatinib. *Clin Pharmacol Ther* 2006;80:192–201.

65. Wu K, House L, Ramirez J, et al. Evaluation of utility of pharmacokinetic studies in phase I trials of two oncology drugs. *Clin Cancer Res* 2013;19:6039–6043.

66. Hu S, Mathijssen RH, de Bruijn P, et al. Inhibition of OATP1B1 by tyrosine kinase inhibitors: in vitro-in vivo correlations. *Br J Cancer* 2014;110(4):894–898.

67. Kehrer DF, Mathijssen RH, Verweij J, et al. Modulation of irinotecan metabolism by ketoconazole. *J Clin Oncol* 2002;20:3122–3129.

68. van Leeuwen RW, Brundel DH, Neef C, et al. Prevalence of potential drug-drug interactions in cancer patients treated with oral anticancer drugs. *Br J Cancer* 2013;108:1071–1078.

69. Budha NR, Frymoyer A, Smelick GS, et al. Drug absorption interactions between oral targeted anticancer agents and PPIs: is pH-dependent solubility the Achilles heel of targeted therapy? *Clin Pharmacol Ther* 2012;92:203–213.

70. Sparreboom A, Cox MC, Acharya MR, et al. Herbal remedies in the United States: potential adverse interactions with anticancer agents. *J Clin Oncol* 2004;22:2489–2503.

71. Dy GK, Bekele L, Hanson LJ, et al. Complementary and alternative medicine use by patients enrolled onto phase I clinical trials. *J Clin Oncol* 2004;22:4810–4815.

72. Goey AK, Mooiman KD, Beijnen JH, et al. Relevance of in vitro and clinical data for predicting CYP3A4-mediated herb-drug interactions in cancer patients. *Cancer Treat Rev* 2013;39:773–783.

73. Mathijssen RH, Verweij J, De Bruijn P, et al. Effects of St. John's wort on irinotecan metabolism. *J Natl Cancer Inst* 2002;94:1247–1249.

74. Cox MC, Low J, Lee J, et al. Influence of garlic (Allium sativum) on the pharmacokinetics of docetaxel. *Clin Cancer Res* 2006;12:4636–4640.

75. van Erp NP, Baker SD, Zhao M, et al. Effect of milk thistle (Silybum marianum) on the pharmacokinetics of irinotecan. *Clin Cancer Res* 2005;11:7800–7806.

76. Wheeler HE, Maitland ML, Dolan ME, et al. Cancer pharmacogenomics: strategies and challenges. *Nat Rev Genet* 2013;14:23–34.

77. Fujita K, Sparreboom A. Pharmacogenetics of irinotecan disposition and toxicity: a review. *Curr Clin Pharmacol* 2010;5:209–217.

78. Huang RS, Ratain MJ. Pharmacogenetics and pharmacogenomics of anticancer agents. *CA Cancer J Clin* 2009;59:42–55.

79. Evans WE, McLeod HL. Pharmacogenomics—drug disposition, drug targets, and side effects. *N Engl J Med* 2003;348:538–549.

80. Sparreboom A, Danesi R, Ando Y, et al. Pharmacogenomics of ABC transporters and its role in cancer chemotherapy. *Drug Resist Updat* 2003;6:71–84.

81. Cusatis G, Gregorc V, Li J, et al. Pharmacogenetics of ABCG2 and adverse reactions to gefitinib. *J Natl Cancer Inst* 2006;98:1739–1742.

82. Kim RB. Organic anion-transporting polypeptide (OATP) transporter family and drug disposition. *Eur J Clin Invest* 2003;33 Suppl 2:1–5.

83. Smith NF, Figg WD, Sparreboom A. Role of the liver-specific transporters OATP1B1 and OATP1B3 in governing drug elimination. *Exp Opin Drug Metab Toxicol* 2005;1:429–445.

84. Sprowl JA, Mikkelsen TS, Giovinazzo H, et al. Contribution of tumoral and host solute carriers to clinical drug response. *Drug Resist Updat* 2012;15:5–20.

85. Kim DH, Sriharsha L, Xu W, et al. Clinical relevance of a pharmacogenetic approach using multiple candidate genes to predict response and resistance to imatinib therapy in chronic myeloid leukemia. *Clin Cancer Res* 2009;15:4750–4758.

86. Canal P, Chatelut E, Guichard S. Practical treatment guide for dose individualisation in cancer chemotherapy. *Drugs* 1998;56:1019–1038.

87. Evans WE, Relling MV, Rodman JH, et al. Conventional compared with individualized chemotherapy for childhood acute lymphoblastic leukemia. *N Engl J Med* 1998;338:499–505.

88. Blasdel C, Egorin MJ, Lagattuta TF, et al. Therapeutic drug monitoring in CML patients on imatinib. *Blood* 2007;110:1699–1701.

89. Larson RA, Druker BJ, Guilhot F, et al. Imatinib pharmacokinetics and its correlation with response and safety in chronic-phase chronic myeloid leukemia: a subanalysis of the IRIS study. *Blood* 2008;111:4022–4028.

90. Picard S, Titier K, Etienne G, et al. Trough imatinib plasma levels are associated with both cytogenetic and molecular responses to standard-dose imatinib in chronic myeloid leukemia. *Blood* 2007;109:3496–3499.

91. Blanchet B, Billemont B, Cramard J, et al. Validation of an HPLC-UV method for sorafenib determination in human plasma and application to cancer patients in routine clinical practice. *J Pharm Biomed Anal* 2009;49:1109–1114.

92. Chatelut E, Canal P, Brunner V, et al. Prediction of carboplatin clearance from standard morphological and biological patient characteristics. *J Natl Cancer Inst* 1995;87:573–580.

93. Bruno R, Hille D, Riva A, et al. Population pharmacokinetics/pharmacodynamics of docetaxel in phase II studies in patients with cancer. *J Clin Oncol* 1998;16:187–196.

94. Gallo JM, Laub PB, Rowinsky EK, et al. Population pharmacokinetic model for topotecan derived from phase I clinical trials. *J Clin Oncol* 2000;18:2459–2467.

95. Li J, Karlsson MO, Brahmer J, et al. CYP3A phenotyping approach to predict systemic exposure to EGFR tyrosine kinase inhibitors. *J Natl Cancer Inst* 2006;98:1714–1723.

96. Lu JF, Eppler SM, Wolf J, et al. Clinical pharmacokinetics of erlotinib in patients with solid tumors and exposure-safety relationship in patients with non-small cell lung cancer. *Clin Pharmacol Ther* 2006;80:136–145.

97. Mathijssen RH, de Jong FA, Loos WJ, et al. Flat-fixed dosing versus body surface area based dosing of anticancer drugs in adults: does it make a difference? *Oncologist* 2007;12:913–923.

CANCER THERAPEUTICS

# 16 Pharmacogenomics

Christine M. Walko and Howard L. McLeod

## INTRODUCTION

The evolution of understanding cancer biology has yielded many advances that have been translated into cancer treatment. Application of this knowledge has allowed for a shift in chemotherapeutics from traditional cytotoxic agents that worked by killing both healthy and malignant fast growing cells to chemical and biologic therapies aimed at targeting a specific gene or pathway critical to the particular cancer being treated.[1] This age of pathway-directed therapy has been made possible by the increased availability and feasibility of high throughput technology able to provide comprehensive and clinically useful molecular characterization of tumors. Translation of these efforts have resulted in improved degree to disease control for many common cancers including breast, colorectal, lung, and melanoma as well as long-term survival benefits for chronic myelogenous leukemia (CML), gastrointestinal stromal tumors (GIST), and childhood acute lymphoblastic leukemia (ALL).[2]

Pharmacogenomic-guided therapy aims the use information on DNA and RNA integrity to optimize not only the treatment choice for an individual patient, but also the dose and schedule of that treatment. The assessment of both somatic and germ-line mutations contribute to the overall individualization of cancer treatment. Somatic mutations are genetic variations found within the tumor DNA, but not DNA from the normal (germ-line) tissues, which also have functional consequences that influence disease outcomes and/or response to certain therapies. These types of mutations or biomarkers can be classified as either prognostic or predictive. Prognostic biomarkers identify subpopulations of patients with different disease courses or outcomes, independent of treatment. Predictive biomarkers identify subpopulations of patients most likely to have a response to a given therapy.[3] Germ-line mutations are heritable variations found within the individual and, in practical terms, are focused on DNA markers predictive for toxicity or therapeutic outcomes of a particular therapy as well as inheritable risk of certain cancers.[4] Pharmacogenomic mutations in the germ line provide some explanation for the interindividual and interracial variability in drug response and toxicity. For cancer chemotherapy, where cytotoxic agents are administered at doses close to their maximal tolerable dose, and therapeutic windows are relatively narrow, minor differences in individual drug handling may lead to severe toxicities. Therefore, an understanding of the sources of this variability would lead to the possibility of individualizing dosages or influencing clinical decisions that can improve patient care. Pharmacogenomics has putative utility in therapy selection, clinical study design, and as a tool to improve understanding of the pharmacology of a medication.

The term *pharmacogenetics* was initially used to define inherited differences in drug effects and typically focused on individual candidate genes. The field of pharmacogenomics now includes genomewide association studies and is used to describe genetic variations in all aspects of drug absorption, distribution, metabolism, and excretion in addition to drug targets and their downstream pathways.[5] Table 16.1 illustrates some current clinical examples of genotype-guided cancer chemotherapy. Variations in the DNA sequences encoding these proteins may take the form of deletions, insertions, repeats, frameshift mutations, nonsense mutations, and missense mutations, resulting in an inactive, truncated, unstable, or otherwise dysfunctional protein. The most common change involves single nucleotide substitutions, called single-nucleotide polymorphisms (SNP), which occur at approximately 1 per 1,000 base pairs on the human genome. Variability in toxicity or activity can also be mediated by postgenomic events, at the level of RNA, protein, or functional activity.

## PHARMACOGENOMICS OF TUMOR RESPONSE

Tumor response to chemotherapy is regulated by a complex, multigenic network of genes that encompasses inherent characteristics of the tumor, differentially activated pathways of cell signaling, proliferation and DNA repair, factors that control drug delivery to the tumor cells (e.g., metabolism, transport), and cell death. These may in turn be modulated by previously administered treatment or drug exposure, which may upregulate target proteins or activate alternative pathways of drug resistance. The polygenic nature of drug response implies that a better understanding of genotype–phenotype associations would require more than the usual single-gene pharmacogenetic strategies employed to date. However, there are instances where the genomic context of a single gene within a cancer will be of high impact for specific therapeutic agents (see Table 16.1).

### Pathway Directed Anticancer Therapy

One of the earliest success stories illustrating pathway-driven therapeutics is with CML. The hallmark chromosomal abnormality of this disease is the translocation of chromosomes 9 and 22 that ultimately produces the fusion gene *BCR-ABL*. This discovery in 1960 eventually led to the development of the targeted tyrosine-kinase inhibitor (TKI) imatinib and its subsequent Food and Drug Administration (FDA) approval for treatment of CML in 2001.[6] The International Randomized Study of Interferon and STI571 (IRIS) trial began enrollment in 2000 and compared imatinib with interferon and low-dose cytarabine, which was the previous standard of care for newly diagnosed patients with chronic-phase CML. All efficacy endpoints favored imatinib, including complete cytogenetic response of 76.2% with imatinib compared with 14.5% with interferon (p <0.001).[7] Overall survival (OS) after 60 months of follow-up was 89% with imatinib.[8] This example is just one of many where a once fatal disease can now be considered more akin to a chronic disease, requiring a daily medication and regular physician follow-up, similar to hypertension or diabetes. Drug development has also kept pace with these advances and now several other agents, including dasatinib, nilotinib, bosutinib, and ponatinib, have joined imatinib as treatment options for CML.

The idea of changing treatment focus from a disease-based model to a pathway-driven model is also evolving. Human epidermal

### TABLE 16.1

**Clinical Examples of Genotype-Guided Cancer Chemotherapy**

| Somatic Mutation Examples | | |
| --- | --- | --- |
| **Drug Target** | **Drug(s)** | **Malignancy** |
| EML4-ALK | Crizotinib | Non–small-cell lung cancer |
| BCR-ABL | Dasatinib, imatinib, nilotinib, bosutinib, ponatinib | Chronic myelogenous leukemia |
| BRAF | Vemurafenib, dabrafenib | Melanoma |
| Epidermal growth factor receptor (EGFR) | Erlotinib, afatinib | Non–small-cell lung cancer |
| HER2 | Trastuzumab, lapatinib, pertuzumab, Ado-trastuzumab emtansine | Breast cancer, gastric cancer |
| Janus kinase 2 (JAK2) | Ruxolitinib | Myelofibrosis |
| Kirsten rat sarcoma viral oncogene (KRAS) | Cetuximab, panitumumab | Colorectal cancer |
| Rearranged during transfection (RET) | Vandetanib | Medullary thyroid cancer |
| Germ-Line Mutation Examples | | |
| **Gene Mutation** | **Drug** | **Effect** |
| Cytochrome P450 (CYP) 2C19 | Voriconazole | Decreased serum levels of active drug and potential decreased efficacy in patients with high enzyme levels (ultrarapid metabolizers) |
| CYP2D6 | Tamoxifen, codeine, ondansetron | Decreased production of active metabolite and potential decreased efficacy in patients with low enzyme levels |
| Dihydropyrimidine dehydrogenase (DPYD) | 5-Fluorouracil | Decreased elimination and increased risk of myelosuppression, diarrhea, and mucositis in patients with low enzyme levels |
| Glucose-6-phosphate dehydrogenase (G6PD) | Rasburicase | Risk of severe hemolysis in patients with G6PD deficiency |
| Thiopurine methyltransferase (TPMT) | Mercaptopurine, thioguanine, azathioprine | Decreased methylation of the active metabolite resulting decreased elimination and increased risk of neutropenia in patients with low enzyme levels |
| UDP-glucuronosyltransferase (UGT) 1A1 | Irinotecan | Decreased glucuronidation of the active metabolite resulting decreased elimination and increased risk of neutropenia and diarrhea in patients with low enzyme levels |

**CANCER THERAPEUTICS**

growth factor receptor 2 (HER2) is a transmembrane receptor tyrosine kinase that is overexpressed or amplified in up to 25% of breast cancers. Trastuzumab is a humanized monoclonal antibody directed against HER2 and demonstrated improved response rates (RR) and time to disease progression in patients with metastatic HER2 positive breast cancer and improved disease-free survival (DFS) and OS in HER2-positive breast cancer patients treated with adjuvant trastuzumab.[9] Several additional agents are now available to target the HER2 pathway and vary in their pharmacology and mechanism of action. Lapatinib is an oral TKI directed against HER2 and the epidermal growth factor receptor (EGFR), pertuzumab is a humanized monoclonal antibody that binds at a different location than trastuzumab and inhibits the dimerization and subsequent activation of HER2 signaling, and ado-trastuzumab emtansine is an antibody-drug conjugate that targets HER2-positive cells and then releases the cytotoxic antimitotic agent emtansine through liposomal degradation of the linking compound. All of these agents illustrate the progress and pharmacologic diversity of pathway-directed therapy and remain as standard of care options for HER2-positive breast cancer in either the adjuvant and/or metastatic settings.[10] HER2 expression is not limited to breast cancer, however. Though less common, HER2 expression is seen in numerous solid tumors including bladder, gastric, prostate and non–small-cell lung cancer with varying

degrees of incidence depending on the method of detection. Based on results from a large, open-label phase III randomized, international trial of 594 patients with gastric or gastroesophageal junction cancer expressing HER2 by either immunohistochemistry or gene amplification by fluorescence in situ hybridization, trastuzumab is also approved for treatment of metastatic gastric or gastroesophageal junction adenocarcinoma that expresses HER2. Patients randomized to chemotherapy in combination with trastuzumab had a median OS of 13.8 months compared with 11.1 months in the patients receiving chemotherapy alone (hazard ratio [HR], 0.74; 0.60 to 0.91, p = 0.0046).[11] Numerous examples also support that pathway-directed therapy will cross the boundaries of disease sites and that tumor genetics will become one of the biggest determining factors for treatment.

Simple expression of the drug target does not always translate into desired clinical outcomes though. Cetuximab and panitumumab are monoclonal antibodies directed against EGFR; however, it was found that colorectal cancer (CRC) patients who did not have detectable EGFR still experienced responses to these agents similar in extent to EGFR-positive patients. Kirsten rat sarcoma viral oncogene (KRAS) is a downstream effector of the EGFR pathway. Ligand binding to EGFR on the cell surface activates pathway signaling through the KRAS-RAF-mitogen-activated protein kinase (MAPK) pathway, which is thought to control cell growth, differentiation, and apoptosis.[12] Eventually it was found that CRC patients with a KRAS mutation did not derive benefit from cetuximab or panitumumab. The RR in CRC receiving either cetuximab or panitumumab who were KRAS wild type was 10% to 40% compared with near zero percent in those with KRAS mutations.[13] This finding was the result of a retrospective analysis of small group of patients and was confirmed in large, prospective trials. Additionally, it underscores the importance of tissue collection for biomarker assessment in trials with novel therapeutics. A recent clinical trial genomic analysis suggests that mutations in *NRAS* may also have value in predicting the utility of EGFR antibody therapy in colorectal cancer. Although the predictive value of KRAS mutation status in colorectal cancer has been well established in clinical trials, the role of KRAS in lung cancer and other malignancies is less well elucidated. Lung cancers harboring KRAS mutations have been shown to have less clinical benefit from the EGFR-targeted erlotinib in some trials, although this has not consistently been the case across all trials. Additionally, lung cancer KRAS mutation status does not appear to reproducibly predict clinical benefit from the EGFR-targeted monoclonal antibodies, as is the case in colorectal cancer.[14] Unlike the HER2 example discussed previously, the clinical application of some genetic mutations will differ between tissue of origin.

Deeper investigations and understandings of mutations driving oncogenic pathways can also elucidate mechanisms of resistance and practical therapeutic strategies for treatment and prevention. Approximately half of all cutaneous melanomas carry mutations in *BRAF*, with the most common being the V600E mutation. Vemurafenib is a TKI directed against mutated BRAF that demonstrated improvements in both progression-free survival (PFS) and OS when compared with the cytotoxic agent dacarbazine in previously untreated patients with metastatic melanoma carrying the BRAF V600E mutation. Vemurafenib demonstrated a 63% relative reduction in the risk of death compared with dacarbazine (p <0.001) along with a higher response rate (48% compared with 5% for dacarbazine).[15] Based on these results, vemurafenib was the first BRAF targeted TKI approved by the FDA and was soon joined by dabrafenib. Although dramatic responses to these agents have been observed, relapse almost universally occurs after a median of 6 to 8 months. Activating BRAF mutations, like V600E, result in uncontrolled activity of the MAPK pathway through activation of the downstream kinase MEK, which when phosphorylated, subsequently activates extracellular signal-regulated kinase (ERK), which ultimately translocates to the cell nucleus, resulting in cell proliferation and survival (Fig. 16.1).[16] An assessment of serial biopsies from patients treated with vemurafenib suggested numerous mechanisms for acquired resistance, including the appearance of secondary mutations in MEK.[17] This finding supports the clinical rationale for using combination therapy with a BRAF and a MEK inhibitor. The combination of dabrafenib (BRAF inhibitor) and trametinib (MEK inhibitor) was assessed in 247 metastatic melanoma patients with BRAF V600 mutations compared with dabrafenib alone. Median PFS was 9.4 months in the combination group compared with 5.8 months in the patients who received single-agent therapy (HR, 0.39; 0.25 to 0.62, p <0.001). A complete or partial response was also higher in the combination therapy group (76% compared with 54%, p = 0.03). The occurrence of cutaneous squamous cell carcinoma, a known side effect of single-agent BRAF inhibitor therapy due to paradoxical activation of RAF in nonmutated cells, was also decreased in the combination therapy group (7% compared with 19%, p = 0.09), further supporting the evidence of downstream inhibition.[18] Although combination therapy does prolong the time to disease progression, resistance still occurs in patients through a variety of mechanisms. Utilization of sequential biopsies and a genetic assessment will help to inform rationale combination and sequential pathway-driven therapy trials that will ultimately aid in better understanding and mitigation of common mechanism of resistance.

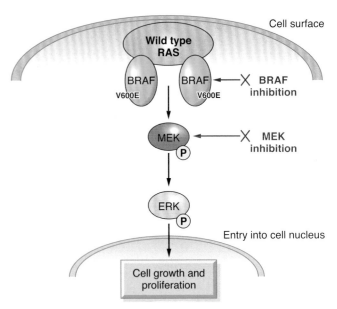

**Figure 16.1** MAPK pathway in BRAF mutated melanoma. The BRAF V600E mutation results in activation of the MAPK pathway independent of growth factor binding, initially by phosphorylation (P) of MEK. MEK subsequently phosphorylates ERK. ERK then translocates to the cell nucleus and causes transcription of cellular factors, resulting in cell proliferation and survival. Because one mechanism of resistance to BRAF inhibition is through mutations in MEK, inhibition at both the upstream target of BRAF and the downstream site of MEK can prolong the clinical benefit of the BRAF inhibitor.

Although advances in basic science and drug development have translated many oncogenic driver mutations across tumor types into pathway-directed therapy, this is not the case for the majority. There are numerous examples of functionally relevant recurrent driver mutations that affect protein targets that are not currently druggable. Regardless of malignancy, one of the most commonly mutated tumor suppressors is the protein p53. Mutations can result in p53 acquiring oncogenic functions that enable proliferation, invasion, metastasis, and cell survival as well as coordinating with different proteins, such as EGFR, to enhance or inhibit its effects. However, a clinical application of p53 mutation data or directly targeting p53 has been limited, to date.[19] *PIK3CA* encodes a catalytic subunit of phophoinositol-3 kinase (PI3K), which includes four distinct subfamily kinases involved in regulating cell growth, motility, proliferation, and survival. Direct inhibitors of the kinase, as well as downstream targets, including AKT (protein kinase B [PKB]) and mammalian target of rapamycin (mTOR), are being assessed to target these mutations. Therapeutic challenges include understanding the complex signaling network germane to each cancer and the role of kinases in each subfamily.[20] Both the examples of p53 and PI3K illustrate the challenge of translating the multitude of somatic mutations into applications of available therapeutic agents.

## Application of Genomewide Gene Expression Profiling to Guide Therapy

Single gene approaches may not reflect the overall complexity of genetic regulation of chemotherapy responses. Genomic strategies using global gene expression data are able to provide a more complete picture of the tumor through disease classification.[21] These strategies may identify subgroups of patients with early disease that need adjuvant chemotherapy, those who will not benefit from standard therapy, or help with the selection of chemotherapy from a menu of potentially active agents. Oncotype Dx is a 21-gene assay with 16 tumor-associated genes and 5 reference genes used to predict the risk of distant local recurrence in estrogen receptor (ER)-positive, HER2-negative patients with node-negative or select node-positive breast cancer. Additionally, the test also provides predictive information on which patients may benefit from the addition of chemotherapy to hormonal therapy alone. The test ultimately reports a recurrence score (RS) on a continuous scale from zero to 100. Patients with an RS <18 are considered low risk, with a 10-year distant recurrence rate (DRR) of 6.8% (95% confidence interval [CI], 4 to 9.6); RS scores of 18 to 30 are at intermediate risk, with a 10-year DRR of 14.3% (CI, 8.3 to 20.3); and RS scores ≥31 are at high risk, with a 10-year DRR of 30.5% (CI, 23.6 to 37.4).[22] Additionally, high-risk patients have the largest benefit from the addition of chemotherapy to hormonal therapy (HR, 0.26; 0.13 to 0.53), whereas low-risk patients have little benefit from the addition of chemotherapy and could consider hormonal treatment alone (HR, 1.31; 0.46 to 3.78). Intermediate risk patients are harder to classify, and clinical trials are underway to further address treatment recommendations for this group of patients.[23] These type of assays are also in development and in clinical trials for a variety of other solid tumor and hematologic malignancies.

## Genetic-Guided Therapy Practical Issues in Somatic Analysis

Currently, targeted DNA capture is the most common type of somatic genetic screening and involves focusing on a few relevant candidate genes followed by deeper sequencing. These types of techniques can reveal common genes associated with a particular malignancy but also may uncover a signaling pathway that would not be obviously associated with a particular histology or tumor site. Application of a next-generation sequencing assay in 40 CRC and 24 non–small-cell lung cancer (NSCLC) tissue samples that assessed 145 cancer-relevant genes demonstrated that somatic mutations were seen in 98% of the CRC tumors and 83% of the NSCLCs (Fig. 16.2).[24] The evolution of sequencing strategies and decreasing costs has made whole genome sequencing more available in the clinical setting, and several companies offer commercially available tumor profiling services. Several limitations exist that currently restrict the broad clinical implementation of these assays, however. Although germ-line genetic assessments can be done on a peripheral blood sample or buccal swab, somatic assessments typically require biopsy tissue, which is often in limited supply and of varying quality or may not be feasible depending on the site of the cancer. Ongoing studies are assessing the

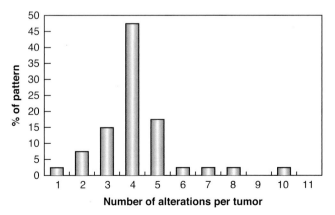

**Figure 16.2** Number of alterations per tumor. Deep sequencing of 145 genes in 40 colorectal cancers found a spectrum of incidence of somatic mutations, with more than half occurring in genes that are *druggable* with medication that is either FDA approved or in late stage clinical development.

value of liquid biopsies of circulating tumor DNA.[25] Optimizing and creating uniformity in quality control of gene panel or whole-genome assessment is also needed to decrease the reporting of uncertain or erroneous identification of mutations. Once sequencing is completed, a predictive analysis is needed for the 25% to 80% of instances where variants of unknown significance are identified in genes of interest. Translation of genomic sequencing into clinical practice will require a diverse team, including pathologists, medical oncologists, surgical oncologists, information technologists, geneticists, and pharmacologists.

# PHARMACOGENOMICS OF CHEMOTHERAPY DRUG TOXICITY

A drug's disposition and pharmacodynamic effects can be influenced by a number of variables, including patient age, diet, concomitant medications, and underlying disease processes. However, an individual's genetic constitution is an important regulator of variability in drug effect. Differences in drug effects are more pronounced between individuals compared to within an individual. Indeed, studies in monozygotic and dizygotic twins identified that 20% to 80% of the variation in drug disposition is mediated by inheritance.[26] Drug-metabolizing enzymes, cellular transporters, and tissue receptors are governed by genetic variation.

Advances in the treatment of most common malignancies have resulted in the availability of multiple distinct combination chemotherapy regimens with similar or equal anticancer efficacy. Therefore, differences in systemic toxicity have become a major determinant in the selection of therapy. The majority of pharmacogenomic examples affecting adverse events or efficacy from cytotoxic drugs involve hepatic metabolizing enzymes that detoxify or biotransform xenobiotics.[27,28]

## Thiopurine Methyltransferase

One of the best-studied pharmacogenetic syndrome involves the metabolism of the thiopurine drugs—6-mercaptopurine (6MP), 6-thioguanine, and azathioprine—which have wide applications, including maintenance therapy for childhood ALL and adult leukemias. These prodrugs must be activated to thioguanine nucleotides in order to have antiproliferative effects. However, most of the variability in the formation of active metabolites is mediated by methylation via thiopurine methyltransferase (TPMT).[29] TPMT is a cytosolic enzyme that catalyzes S-methylation of thiopurine agents, resulting in an inactive metabolite. Erythrocyte TPMT activity has a trimodal distribution, with 90% of patients having high activity, 10% intermediate activity, and 0.3% with very low or no detectable activity. TPMT deficiency results in higher intracellular activation of 6MP to form thioguanine nucleotides, resulting in severe or fatal hematologic toxicity from standard doses of therapy.[30] The variable activity results from polymorphism in the TPMT gene, located on chromosome locus 6p22.3. Genetic variants at codon 238 (TPMT*2), codon 719 (TPMT*3C), or both codons 460 and 719 (TPMT*3A) are the most clinically significant, accounting for 95% of the patients with reduced TPMT activity.[31] Heterozygotes (one wild type and one variant allele) are common (10% of patients), and have elevated levels of active metabolites (twofold more than homozygous wild type), and required more cumulative dose reductions of 6MP for maintenance ALL chemotherapy compared to homozygous wild-type patients (Fig. 16.3).[32] Patients with a homozygous variant TPMT genotype are at a fourfold risk of severe toxicity, compared with wild-type patients.[31] TPMT genotype tests are now available commercially in a Clinical Laboratory Improvement Amendments (CLIA)-certified environment. To date, patients homozygous for TPMT variant alleles appear to tolerate 10%, and heterozygotes appear to tolerate 65% of the recommended doses of 6MP, with no apparent

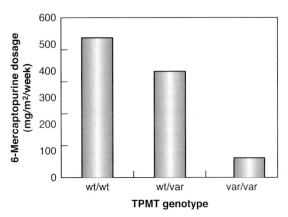

**Figure 16.3** Relationship between TPMT genotype and required 6MP dose. Compared with homozygous wild-type patients, those heterozygous for a thiopurine methyltransferase (TPMT) variant allele generally require at least a 30% dose reduction in 6MP, whereas homozygous variant patients require substantial dose reductions of approximately 90% that of wild-type patients.

decrease in clinical efficacy (Fig. 16.3).[32] This has formed the basis for prospective, TPMT genotype-guided dosing of 6MP to avoid severe toxicity. Clinical Pharmacogenomics Implementation Consortium (CPIC) Guidelines recommend that homozygous wild-type patients be started at the full standard dose. Heterozygous patients should start with reduced doses at 30% to 70% of the full dose with adjustments made after 2 to 4 weeks based on myelosuppression and disease-specific guidelines. Homozygous variant patients should start with 10% of the full dose due to the extremely high levels of the active metabolite and potential for fatal toxicity at standard doses. Adjustments should be made after 4 to 6 weeks based on myelosuppression and disease-specific guidelines.[33]

## Dihydropyrimidine Dehydrogenase (DPD)

Although 5-fluorouracil (5FU) has been available for over 40 years, it remains the cornerstone of colorectal cancer chemotherapy, both in the adjuvant and metastatic settings. Additionally, the oral prodrug capecitabine ultimately undergoes activation to 5FU and is commonly used in gastrointestinal and breast malignancies. 5FU is a prodrug that is activated intracellularly to 5-fluoro-2'-deoxyuridine monophosphate (5FdUMP), which inhibits thymidylate synthase (TS), among other mechanisms of action. TS inhibition results in impaired de novo pyrimidine synthesis and suppression of DNA synthesis. Approximately 85% of a 5FU dose is catabolized by dihydropyrimidine dehydrogenase (DPD) to inactive metabolites. Therefore, DPD is a primary regulator of 5FU activity. DPD deficiency has been described, resulting in higher 5FU blood levels, greater formation of active metabolites, and severe or fatal clinical toxicity, predominately myelosuppression, mucositis, and cerebellar toxicity.[34] In theory, this toxicity could be reduced or avoided by screening for DPD activity in surrogate tissues, such as peripheral mononuclear cells. However, the technical requirements for preparation of these samples make it impractical for many practice sites. Understanding the molecular basis for DPD deficiency will provide an approach for prospective identification of patients at high risk for severe 5FU toxicity. The gene encoding DPD is composed of 23 exons, and at least 23 SNPs have been found.[35] Studies in DPD-deficient patients have identified several distinct molecular variants associated with low enzyme activity. Many of these are rare, and base substitutions, splicing defects, and frame shift mutations, have been described. The prevalent variation is the splice recognition site in intron 14 (DPYD*2A), where a G to A substitution results in the skipping of exon 14, resulting in an inactive enzyme.[36–38] This polymorphism

has been associated with severe DPD deficiency in heterozygous patients, with a homozygous genotype associated with a mental retardation syndrome. Patients with severe 5FU toxicity may harbor one or more variant alleles of DPD, and a recent study showed that 61% of cancer patients experiencing severe 5FU toxicities had decreased DPD activity in peripheral mononuclear cells, and DPYD*2A was commonly found.[39] In the patients with grade 4 neutropenia, 50% harbored at least one DPYD*2A. It is estimated that in the Caucasian population, homozygotes for the variant alleles have an incidence of 0.1% and heterozygotes occur at an incidence of 0.5% to 2%. There are additional DPD mutations that have been associated with impaired enzyme activity, including DPYD *3 and DPYD*13. CPIC guidelines recommend standard dosing for homozygous wild-type patients. Reducing the dose by at least 50% in heterozygous patients (*1/*2A) is recommended, followed by dose adjustment based on toxicity and/or pharmacokinetic testing. The use of an alternative agent is recommended in homozygous-variant patients (*2A/*2A).[34] There are many patients with severe 5FU toxicity that have normal DPD activity. This highlights that many factors, including multiple genes, are potential causes of 5FU toxicity, and there will not be one simple test to avoid this important clinical problem.

## Cytochrome P450 2D6

Tamoxifen is a selective estrogen-receptor modulator used in ER-positive breast cancer in both the localized and metastatic settings. It is the drug of choice for premenopausal women and is a treatment option, along with aromatase inhibitors, for postmenopausal women. The low cost of tamoxifen also makes it a preferred therapy regardless of menopausal status in numerous countries. Tamoxifen metabolism is complex, with extensive metabolism through numerous phase I and II enzymes that produce several primary and secondary metabolites and their corresponding isomers, each possessing different antiestrogen effects.[40] The primary active metabolite is believed to be endoxifen, which is produced by the CYP3A4/5 mediated-conversion of tamoxifen to N-desmethyltamoxifen, which is then further converted to endoxifen (4-hydroxy-N-desmethyltamoxifen) via cytochrome P450 2D6 (CYP2D6). A direct relationship between endoxifen concentration and its antiestrogen effects has been demonstrated, potentially suggesting that a threshold concentration may be needed for optimal clinical effect.[41] CYP2D6 is highly polymorphic, with more than 80 allelic CYP2D6 variants described. These alleles vary in enzyme activity and prevalence with respect to race and ethnicity.[42] Based on genotype, patients can be classified by phenotype into ultrarapid metabolizers (UM; approximately 1% to 2% of patients [common alleles include *1xN, *2xN]) who carry more than two functional allele copies, extensive metabolizers (EM; 77% to 92% [e.g., *1, *2]), intermediate metabolizers (IM; 2% to 11% [e.g., *10, *17, *41]), or poor metabolizers (PM; 5% to 10% [*3, *4, *5]).[43] UM patients have the highest concentrations of endoxifen, followed by EM patients, then IM patients, and finally, PM patients have the lowest concentration. Up to a sixfold variation in endoxifen levels may be seen between homozygous PM and homozygous EM patients.[40]

The relationship between CYP2D6 genotype, endoxifen concentrations, and disease outcomes has been investigated in numerous clinical trials. One of the largest retrospective trials assessed this relationship in 1,325 women treated with adjuvant tamoxifen 20 mg daily. Approximately 46% of the patients were classified as EM, 48% were IM, and 5.9% were PM. A statistically significant increased risk of disease recurrence was seen in the IM and PM patients compared with the EM patients (HR, 1.40; 95% CI, 1.04 to 1.90 for IM; and HR 1.90, 95% CI, 1.10 to 3.28 for PM).[44] A large meta-analysis of 4,973 tamoxifen-treated patients across 12 international studies conducted by the International Tamoxifen Pharmacogenomics Consortium also supported this relationship.

CYP2D6 PM phenotypes were associated with decreased DFS (HR 1.25, 95% CI, 1.06 to 1.47, p = 0.009) when only considering the data from trials with postmenopausal women with ER-positive breast cancer who received tamoxifen 20 mg daily for 5 years.[45]

Not all trial results have been consistent, however, and dosing guidelines for genotype-guided therapy do not yet exist. Clinical trials do support the potential for genotype-guided therapy. IM patients who received an increased dose of 40 mg daily instead of the standard 20 mg were shown to have endoxifen concentrations similar to that of EM patients (p = 0.25).[46] This suggests that genotype-guided therapy with increased dose recommendations may be feasible, but additional prospective trials are needed to determine the clinical efficacy of this intervention.

## CONCLUSIONS AND FUTURE DIRECTIONS

Genomic-driven cancer medicine is being translated into clinical practice through increased understanding of somatic mutations in a specific tumor that can be translated to pathway-directed therapeutics as well as germ-line mutations that affect the pharmacokinetics and pharmacodynamics of individual medications. For the practicing oncologist, knowledge of pharmacogenomics is necessary because therapeutic decisions of drug selection and dosage are being based on more molecularly and genetically defined variables than the current phenotypic information of tumor type,

immunohistochemistry, and body surface area. Health-care policy changes preferring the bundling of care and reimbursement based on diagnosis coding may further drive individualized therapy where the goal is to optimize both treatment responses while minimizing toxicity. However, with advances always come challenges. Reimbursement for multiplex genomic testing is not universal, so deciding who and when to initiate testing is a consideration. Optimizing turnaround time, especially for referral patients who have had biopsies performed elsewhere, will require requesting this archived tissue prior to or during the initial patient visit to facilitate minimizing treatment delays. Although some variants have strong evidence supporting treatment recommendations, many currently do not yet. Multidisciplinary committees charged with reviewing the level of evidence for each genetic result and providing clinically actionable recommendations will be essential for translating these multigene tumor assay results into routine clinical practice. Decision tools and development of treatment guidelines will further assist with routine integration of this technology, especially for oncologists at smaller practice sites. Oncology fellowship training programs will also need to be expanded to ensure competence of new practitioners in the area of genomic-guided therapies.

Regardless of these challenges, the treatment paradigm of genomic-driven medicine and individualizing therapy has permitted the field of oncology to move beyond the limitations of nonselective cytotoxic therapy and toward the more optimal selection and dosing of oncology agents.

## REFERENCES

1. McLeod HL. Cancer pharmacogenomics: early promise, but concerted effort needed. *Science* 2013;339:1563–1566.
2. Garraway LA. Genomics-driven oncology: framework for an emerging paradigm. *J Clin Oncol* 2013;31:1806–1814.
3. Mandrekar SJ, Sargent DJ. Predictive biomarker validation in practice: lessons from real trials. *Clin Trials* 2010;7:567–573.
4. Evans WE, Relling MV. Pharmacogenomics: translating functional genomics into rational therapeutics. *Science* 1999;286:487–491.
5. Wang L, McLeod HL, Weinshilboum RM. Genomics and drug response. *N Engl J Med* 2011;364:1144–1153.
6. Druker BJ. Translation of the Philadelphia chromosome into therapy for CML. *Blood* 2008;112:4808–4817.
7. O'Brien SG, Guilhot F, Larson RA, et al. Imatinib compared with interferon and low-dose cytarabine for newly diagnosed chronic-phase chronic myeloid leukemia. *N Engl J Med* 2003;348:994–1004.
8. Druker BJ, Guilhot F, O'Brien SG, et al. Five-year follow-up of patients receiving imatinib for chronic myeloid leukemia. *N Engl J Med* 2006;355:2408–2417.
9. Hudis CA. Trastuzumab—mechanism of action and use in clinical practice. *N Engl J Med* 2007;357:39–51.
10. Figueroa-Magalhaes MC, Jelovac D, Connolly RM, et al. Treatment of HER2-positive breast cancer. *Breast* 2014;23:128–136.
11. Bang YJ, Van Cutsem E, Feyereislova A, et al. Trastuzumab in combination with chemotherapy versus chemotherapy alone for treatment of HER2-positive advanced gastric or gastro-oesophageal junction cancer (ToGA): a phase 3, open-label, randomised controlled trial. *Lancet* 2010;76:687–697.
12. Bardelli A, Siena S. Molecular mechanisms of resistance to cetuximab and panitumumab in colorectal cancer. *J Clin Oncol* 2010;28:1254–1261.
13. Jimeno A, Messersmith WA, Hirsch FR, et al. KRAS mutations and sensitivity to epidermal growth factor receptor inhibitors in colorectal cancer: practical application of patient selection. *J Clin Oncol* 2009;27:1130–1136.
14. Roberts PJ, Stinchcombe TE, Der CJ, et al. Personalized medicine in non-small-cell lung cancer: is KRAS a useful marker in selecting patients for epidermal growth factor receptor-targeted therapy? *J Clin Oncol* 2010;28:4769–4777.
15. Chapman PB, Hauschild A, Robert C, et al. Improved survival with vemurafenib in melanoma with BRAF V600E mutation. *N Engl J Med* 2011;364:2507–2516.
16. Dhillon AS, Hagan S, Rath O, et al. MAP kinase signalling pathways in cancer. *Oncogene* 2007;26:3279–3290.
17. Trunzer K, Pavlick AC, Schuchter L, et al. Pharmacodynamic effects and mechanisms of resistance to vemurafenib in patients with metastatic melanoma. *J Clin Oncol* 2013;31:1767–1774.
18. Flaherty KT, Infante JR, Daud A, et al. Combined BRAF and MEK inhibition in melanoma with BRAF V600 mutations. *N Engl J Med* 2012;367:1694–1703.
19. Muller PA, Vousden KH. p53 mutations in cancer. *Nat Cell Biol* 2013;15:2–8.
20. Clarke PA, Workman P. Phosphatidylinositide-3-kinase inhibitors: addressing questions of isoform selectivity and pharmacodynamic/predictive biomarkers in early clinical trials. *J Clin Oncol* 2012;30:331–333.
21. Ramaswamy S, Golub T. DNA microarrays in clinical oncology. *J Clin Oncol* 2002;20:1932–1941.
22. Paik S, Shak S, Tang G, et al. A multigene assay to predict recurrence of tamoxifen-treated, node-negative breast cancer. *N Engl J Med* 2004;351:2817–2826.
23. Paik S, Tang G, Shak S, et al. Gene expression and benefit of chemotherapy in women with node-negative, estrogen receptor-positive breast cancer. *J Clin Oncol* 2006;24:3726–3734.
24. Lipson D, Capelletti M, Yelensky R, et al. Identification of new ALK and RET gene fusions from colorectal and lung cancer biopsies. *Nat Med* 2012;18:382–384.
25. Diaz LA Jr, Bardelli A. Liquid biopsies: genotyping circulating tumor DNA. *J Clin Oncol* 2014;32:579–586.
26. Watters J, McLeod H. Cancer pharmacogenomics: current and future applications. *Biochim Biophys Acta* 2003;1603:99–111.
27. Evans W, Relling M. Pharmacogenomics: translating functional genomics into rational therapeutics. *Science* 1999;286:487–491.
28. Deenen MJ, Cats A, Beijnen H, et al. Part 2: pharmacogenetic variability in drug transport and phase I anticancer drug metabolism. *Oncologist* 2011;16:820–834.
29. Krynetski E, Evans W. Drug methylation in cancer therapy: lessons from the TPMT polymorphism. *Oncogene* 2003;22:7403–7413.
30. McLeod H, Krynetski EY, Relling MV, et al. Genetic polymorphism of thiopurine methyltransferase and its clinical relevance for childhood acute lymphoblastic leukemia. *Leukemia* 2000;14:567–572.
31. Evans W, Hon YY, Bomgaars L, et al. Preponderance of thiopurine S-methyltransferase deficiency and heterozygosity among patients intolerant to mercaptopurine or azathioprine. *J Clin Oncol* 2001;19:2293–2301.
32. Relling M, Hancock ML, Rivera GK, et al. Mercaptopurine therapy intolerance and heterozygosity at the thiopurine S-methyltransferase gene locus. *J Natl Cancer Inst* 1999;91:2001–2008.
33. Relling MV, Gardner EE, Sandborn WJ, et al. Clinical pharmacogenetics implementation consortium guidelines for thiopurine methyltransferase genotype and thiopurine dosing: 2013 update. *Clin Pharmacol Ther* 2013;93:324–325.
34. Caudle KE, Thorn CF, Klein TE, et al. Clinical Pharmacogenetics Implementation Consortium guidelines for dihydropyrimidine dehydrogenase genotype and fluoropyrimidine dosing. *Clin Pharmacol Ther* 2013;94:640–645.
35. McLeod H, Collie-Duguid ES, Vreken P, et al. Nomenclature for human DPYD alleles. *Pharmacogenetics* 1998;8:455–459.
36. Wei X, Elizondo G, Sapone A, et al. Characterization of the human dihydropyrimidine dehydrogenase gene. *Genomics* 1998;51:391–400.
37. Ridge S, Sludden J, Wei X, et al. Dihydropyrimidine dehydrogenase pharmacogenetics in patients with colorectal cancer. *Br J Cancer* 1998;77:497–500.
38. Johnson M, Wang K, Diasio R. Profound dihydropyrimidine dehydrogenase deficiency resulting from a novel compound heterozygote genotype. *Clin Cancer Res* 2002;8:768–774.
39. Van Kuilenburg A, Meinsma R, Zoetekouw L, et al. Increased risk of grade IV neutropenia after administration of 5-fluorouracil due to a dihydropyrimidine dehydrogenase deficiency: high prevalence of the IVS14+1g>a mutation. *Int J Cancer* 2002;101:253–258.

40. Mürdter TE, Schroth W, Bacchus-Gerybadze L, et al. Activity levels of tamoxifen metabolites at the estrogen receptor and the impact of genetic polymorphisms of phase I and II enzymes on their concentration levels in plasma. *Clin Pharmacol Ther* 2011;89:708–717.

41. Desta Z, Ward BA, Soukhova NV, et al. Comprehensive evaluation of tamoxifen sequential biotransformation by the human cytochrome P450 system in vitro: prominent roles for CYP3A and CYP2D6. *J Pharmacol Exp Ther* 2004;310:1062–1075.

42. Bradford LD. CYP2D6 allele frequency in European Caucasians, Asians, Africans and their descendants. *Pharmacogenomics* 2002;3:229–243.

43. Crews KR, Gaedigk A, Dunnenberger HM, et al. Clinical Pharmacogenetics Implementation Consortium (CPIC) guidelines for codeine therapy in the context of cytochrome P450 2D6 (CYP2D6) genotype. *Clin Pharmacol Ther* 2012;91:321–326.

44. Schroth W, Goetz MP, Hamann U, et al. Association between CYP2D6 polymorphisms and outcomes among women with early stage breast cancer treated with tamoxifen. *JAMA* 2009;302:1429–1436.

45. Province MA, Goetz MP, Brauch H, et al. CYP2D6 genotype and adjuvant tamoxifen: meta-analysis of heterogeneous study populations. *Clin Pharmacol Ther* 2014;95:216–227.

46. Irvin WJ Jr, Walko CM, Weck KE, et al. Genotype-guided tamoxifen dosing increases active metabolite exposure in women with reduced CYP2D6 metabolism: a multicenter study. *J Clin Oncol* 2011;29:3232–3239.

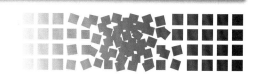

# 17 Alkylating Agents

Kenneth D. Tew

## PERSPECTIVES

Alkylating agents were the first anticancer molecules developed, and they are still used today. After more than 50 years of use, the basic chemistry and pharmacology of this drug family is well understood and has not changed substantially. The family contains six major classes: nitrogen mustards, aziridines, alkyl sulfonates, epoxides, nitrosoureas, and triazene compounds, although a few nonstandard agents have recently been developed. Most epoxides tend to be quite nonspecific with respect to their reactivity and, as such, few have useful clinical characteristics. This chapter provides perspective on how the limited varieties of alkylating agents continue to be useful in the therapeutic management of cancer patients.

The alkylating agents are a diverse group of anticancer agents with the commonality that they react in a manner such that an electrophilic alkyl group or a substituted alkyl group can covalently bind to cellular nucleophilic sites. Electrophilicity is achieved through the formation of carbonium ion intermediates and can result in transition complexes with target molecules. Ultimately, reactions result in the formation of covalent linkages by alkylation with a broad range of nucleophilic groups, including bases in DNA, and these are believed responsible for ultimate cytotoxicity and therapeutic effect. Although the alkylating agents react with cells in all phases of the cell cycle, their efficacy and toxicity result from interference with rapidly proliferating tissues. From a historical perspective, the vesicant properties of mustard gas used during World War I were shown to be accompanied by the suppression of lymphoid and hematologic functions in experimental animals[1] and led to the development of mechlorethamine as the first alkylating agent used in the management of human cancer.[2] Subsequently, a number of related drugs have been developed, and these have roles in the treatment of a range of leukemias, lymphomas, and solid tumors. Most of the alkylating agents cause dose-limiting toxicities to the bone marrow and, to a lesser degree, the intestinal mucosa, with other organ systems also affected contingent on the individual drug, dosage, and duration of therapy. Despite the present trend toward targeted therapies, this class of "nonspecific" drugs maintains an essential role in cancer chemotherapy.

Because of the classic nature of the drug family, there have been relatively few advances in either their use or utility since publication of the previous edition of this book.

## CHEMISTRY

Alkylating reactions are generally classified through their kinetic properties as $S_N1$ (nucleophilic substitution, first order) or $S_N2$ (nucleophilic substitution, second order) (Fig. 17.1). The first-order kinetics of the $S_N1$ reactions depend on the concentration of the original alkylating agent. The rate-limiting step is the initial formation of the reactive intermediate, and the rate is essentially independent of the concentration of the substrate. The $S_N2$ alkylation reaction is a bimolecular nucleophilic displacement with second-order kinetics, where the rate depends on the concentration of both alkylating agent and target nucleophile. Reactivity of electrophiles[3] suggests that the rates of alkylation of cellular nucleophiles (including thiols, phosphates, amino and imidazole groups of amino acids, and various reactive sites in nucleic acid bases) are most dependent on their potential energy states, which can be defined as "hard" or "soft," based on the polarizability of their reactive centers.[4] Although the metabolism and metabolites of nitrogen mustards and nitrosoureas differ, the active alkylating species of each is the alkyl carbonium ion (see Fig. 17.1), a highly polarized hard electrophile as a consequence of its highly positive charge density at the electrophilic center. Alkyl carbonium ions will react most readily with hard nucleophiles (possessing a highly polarized negative charge density), where the high-energy transition state (a potential energy barrier to the reaction) is most favorable. In specific terms, an active alkylating species from a nitrogen mustard will demonstrate selectivity for cellular nucleophiles in the following order: (1) oxygen in phosphate groups of RNA and DNA, (2) oxygens of purines and pyrimidines, (3) amino groups of purine bases, (4) primary and secondary amino groups of proteins, (5) sulfur atoms of methionine, and (6) thiol groups of cysteinyl residues of protein and glutathione.[3] The least favored reactions will still occur, but at much slower rates unless they are catalyzed.

Alkylation through highly reactive intermediates (e.g., mechlorethamine) would be expected to be less selective in their targets than the less reactive $S_N2$ reagents (e.g., busulfan). However, the therapeutic and toxic effects of alkylating agents do not correlate directly with their chemical reactivity. Clinically useful agents include drugs with $S_N1$ or $S_N2$ characteristics, and some with both.[5] These differ in their toxicity profiles and antitumor activity, but more as a consequence of differences in pharmacokinetics, lipid solubility, penetration of the central nervous system (CNS), membrane transport, metabolism and detoxification, and specific enzymatic reactions capable of repairing alkylation sites on DNA.

## CLASSIFICATION

The major classes of clinically useful alkylating agents are illustrated in Table 17.1 and summarized in the following sections. Doses and schedules of the various agents are shown in Table 17.2.

### Alkyl Sulfonates

Busulfan is used for the treatment of chronic myelogenous leukemia. It exhibits $S_N2$ alkylation kinetics and shows nucleophilic selectivity for thiol groups, suggesting that it may exert cytotoxicity through protein alkylation rather than through DNA. In contrast to the nitrogen mustards and nitrosoureas, busulfan has a greater effect on myeloid cells than lymphoid cells, thus the reason for its use against chronic myelogenous leukemia.[6]

### Aziridines

Aziridines are analogs of ring-closed intermediates of nitrogen mustards and are less chemically reactive, but they have

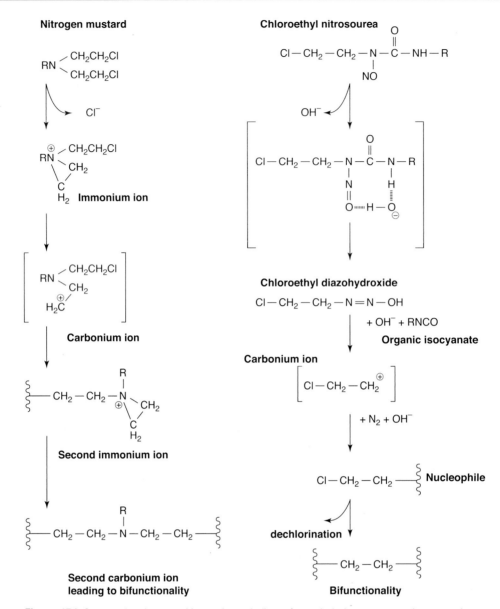

**Figure 17.1** Comparative decomposition and metabolism of a typical nitrogen mustard compared to a nitrosourea. Although intermediate metabolites are distinct, the active alkylating species is a carbonium ion in each case. This electrophilic moiety reacts with target cellular nucleophiles.

equivalent therapeutic properties. Thiotepa has been used in the treatment of carcinoma of the breast, ovary, for a variety of CNS diseases, and with increasing frequency as a component of high-dose chemotherapy regimens.[7] Thiotepa and its primary desulfurated metabolite triethylenethiophosphoramide (TEPA) alkylate through aziridine ring openings, a mechanism similar to the nitrogen mustards.

## Triazines

Perhaps the newest clinical development in the alkylating agent field is the emergence of temozolomide (TMZ). This agent acts as a prodrug and is an imidazotetrazine analog that undergoes spontaneous activation in solution to produce 5-(3-methyltriazen-1-yl)imidazole-4-carboxamide (MTIC), a triazine derivative. It crosses the blood–brain barrier with concentrations in the CNS approximating 30% of plasma concentrations.[8] Resistance to the methylating agent occurs quite frequently and has adversely affected the rate and durability of the clinical responses of patients. However, because of its favorable toxicity and pharmacokinetics, TMZ is

being combined with numerous other classes of anticancer drugs in an effort to improve response rates in diseases such as malignant melanomas, gliomas, brain metastasis from solid tumors, and refractory leukemias. Many of these trials are currently underway.[9]

## Nitrogen Mustards

Bischloroethylamines or nitrogen mustards are extensively administered in the clinic. As an initial step in alkylation, chlorine acts as a leaving group and the β-carbon reacts with the nucleophilic nitrogen atom to form the cyclic, positively charged, reactive aziridinium moiety. Reaction of the aziridinium ring with an electron-rich nucleophile creates an initial alkylation product. The remaining chloroethyl group achieves bifunctionality through the formation of a second aziridinium. Melphalan (L-phenylalanine mustard), chlorambucil, cyclophosphamide, and ifosfamide (see Table 17.1) replaced mechlorethamine as primary therapeutic agents. These derivatives have electron-withdrawing groups substituted on the nitrogen atom, reducing the nucleophilicity of the nitrogen and rendering them less reactive, but enhancing their antitumor efficacy.

**TABLE 17.1**

**Major Classes of Clinically Useful Alkylating Agents**

| Drug | Main Therapeutic Uses | Clinical Pharmacology | Major Toxicities | Notes |
|---|---|---|---|---|
| **ALKYL SULFONATES** | | | | |
| Busulfan | Bone marrow transplantation, especially in chronic myelogenous leukemia | Bioavailability, 80%; protein bound, 33%; $t_{1/2}$, 2.5 h | Pulmonary fibrosis, hyperpigmentation thrombocytopenia, lowered blood platelet count and activity | Oral or parenteral; high dose causes hepatic veno-occlusive disease |
| **ETHYLENEIMINES/METHYLMELAMINES** | | | | |
| Altretamine | | Protein bound, 94%; $t_{1/2}$, 5–10 h | Nausea, vomiting, diarrhea, and neurotoxicity | Not widely used |
| Thio TEPA | Breast, ovarian, and bladder cancer; also bone marrow transplant | $t_{1/2}$, 2.5 h; urinary excretion at 24 h, 25%; substrate for CYP2B6 and CYP2C11 | Myelosuppression | Nadirs of leukopenia, occur 2 wk; thrombocytopenia, 3 wk (correlates with AUC of parent drug) |
| **NITROGEN MUSTARDS** | | | | |
| Mechlorethamine | Hodgkin lymphoma | | Nausea, vomiting, myelosuppression | Precursor for other clinical mustards |
| Melphalan (L-phenylalanine mustard) | Multiple myeloma and ovarian cancer, and occasionally malignant melanoma | Bioavailability 25%–90%; $t_{1/2}$, 1.5 h; urinary excretion at 24 h, 13%; clearance, 9 mL/min/kg | Nausea, vomiting, myelosuppression | Causes less mucosal damage than others in class |
| Chlorambucil | Chronic lymphocytic leukemia | $t_{1/2}$, 1.5 h; urinary excretion at 24 h, 50% | Myelosuppression, gastrointestinal distress, CNS, skin reactions, hepatotoxicity | Oral |
| Cyclophosphamide | Variety of lymphomas, leukemias, and solid tumors | Bioavailability, >75%; protein bound, >60%; $t_{1/2}$, 3–12 h; urinary excretion at 24 h, <15% | Nausea and vomiting, bone marrow suppression, diarrhea, darkening of the skin/nails, alopecia (hair loss), lethargy, hemorrhagic cystitis | IV; primary excretion route is urine |
| Ifosfamide | Testicular, breast cancer; lymphoma (non-Hodgkin); soft tissue sarcoma; osteogenic sarcoma; lung, cervical, ovarian, bone cancer | $t_{1/2}$, 15 h; urinary excretion at 24 h, 15% | As for cyclophosphamide | Ifosfamide is often used in conjunction with mesna to avoid cystinuria |
| **NITROSOUREAS** | | | | |
| Carmustine | Glioma, glioblastoma multiforme, medulloblastoma and astrocytoma, multiple myeloma and lymphoma (Hodgkin and non-Hodgkin) | Bioavailability, 25%; protein bound, 80%; $t_{1/2}$, 30 min | Bone marrow and pulmonary toxicities are a function of lifetime cumulative dose | Clinically, nitrosoureas do not share cross-resistance with nitrogen mustards in lymphoma treatment |
| Streptozotocin | Cancers of the islets of Langerhans | $t_{1/2}$, 35 min; excreted in the urine (15%), feces (<1%), and in the expired air | Nausea and vomiting; nephrotoxicity can range from transient protein urea and azotemia to permanent tubular damage; can also cause aberrations of glucose metabolism | A natural product from *Streptomyces achromogenes* |
| **TRIAZENES** | | | | |
| Dacarbazine | Malignant melanoma and Hodgkin lymphoma | $t_{1/2}$, 5 h; protein bound, 5% hepatic metabolism | Nausea, vomiting, myelosuppression | IV or IM |
| Temozolomide | Glioblastoma; astrocytoma; metastatic melanoma | Protein bound, 15%; $t_{1/2}$, 1.8 h; clearance, 5.5 l/h/m² | Nausea, vomiting, myelosuppression | Oral; derivative of imidazotetrazine, prodrug of dacarbazine; rapidly absorbed |

$t_{1/2}$, half-life; TEPA, triethylenethiophosphoramide; AUC, area under curve; CNS, central nervous system; IV, intravenous; IM, intramuscular.

| TABLE 17.2 | | |
| --- | --- | --- |
| **Dose and Schedules of Clinically Useful Alkylating Agents** | | |
| **Alkylating Agent** | **Disease Sites and Dose Ranges Used Clinically** | **Notes** |
| BCNU (Carmustine) | General antineoplastic<br>150–200 mg/m$^2$ (IV, every 6 wks)<br>Cutaneous T-cell lymphoma 200–600 mg<br>  (topical solution)<br>Adjunct to surgical resection of brain tumor<br>  61.6 mg (implant) | Infusion 1–2 h; in combination, dose usually reduced by<br>  25%–50%<br>Side effects include irritant dermatitis, telangiectasia,<br>  erythema, and bone marrow suppression<br>Up to 8 wafers (7.7 mg of carmustine) implanted |
| Busulfan | Chronic myelogenous leukemia and<br>  myeloproliferative disorders<br>4–8 mg (daily PO)<br>1.8 mg/m$^2$ (daily PO)<br>Bone marrow transplant<br>640 mg/m$^2$ (daily PO) | Dispensed over 3–4 d, with cyclophosphamide |
| Carboplatin | Advanced ovarian cancer—monotherapy<br>360 mg/m$^2$ (IV, every 4 wks)<br>Ovarian cancer—combination<br>300 mg/m$^2$ (IV, every 4 wks for 6 cycles)<br>Ovarian cancer—IP<br>200–500 mg/m$^2$ (IP, 2 L dialysis fluid)<br>Ovarian and other sites phase 1/2 setting—<br>  high-dose therapy<br>800–1,600 mg/m$^2$ (IV) | With cyclophosphamide<br>Patients usually receive marrow transplantation or<br>  peripheral stem cell support |
| Cisplatin | Metastatic testicular cancer:<br>20 mg/m$^2$/d for 5 d of each cycle (IV)<br>Metastatic ovarian cancer:<br>75–100 mg/m$^2$ (IV, once every 4 wks)<br>Head and neck cancer:<br>100 mg/m$^2$ (IV)<br>Bladder cancer:<br>(combination prior to cystectomy)<br>50–70; initiate dosing at 50<br>mg/m$^2$ (IV, once every 3–4 wks)<br>Metastatic breast cancer:<br>20 mg/m$^2$ (IV, days 1–5 every 3 wks)<br>Cervical cancer:<br>70 mg/m$^2$ (IV, dosing cycled every 4 wks)<br>Non–small-cell lung cancer:<br>75 mg/m$^2$ (IV, every 3 wks)<br>Esophageal cancer:<br>75 mg/m$^2$ on day 1 of wks 1, 5, 8, and 11 (IV) | With other antineoplastic agents<br>With cyclophosphamide (600 mg/m$^2$ once every 4 wks)<br>With vincristine, bleomycin, and fluorouracil<br>With methotrexate and fluorouracil<br>MVAC regimen (methotrexate, vinblastine, doxorubicin,<br>  and cisplatin) used for cervical cancer<br>Administration preceded by paclitaxel 135 mg/m$^2$<br>  every 3 wks<br>With radiation therapy |
| Cyclophosphamide | General antineoplastic<br>1–5 mg/kg (daily PO)<br>40–50 mg/kg (IV, in divided doses over 2–5 d)<br>40–50 mg/kg (IV, in divided doses over 2–5 d)<br>10–15 mg/kg (IV, every 7–10 d)<br>10–15 mg/kg (IV, every 7–10 d)<br>3–5 mg/kg (IV twice per wk)<br>High-dose regimen in bone marrow transplantation<br>  and for other autoimmune disorders<br>200 mg/kg (IV)<br>1–2.5 mg/kg (daily PO 7–14 d/mo) | Dose used as monotherapy for patients with no<br>  hematologic toxicity |
| Dacarbazine | General antineoplastic<br>2–4.5 mg/kg/d (IV)<br>150 mg/m$^2$/d (IV) | Administered for 10 d, may be repeated at 4-week intervals<br>With other anticancer agents; treatment lasts 5 d,<br>  may be repeated every 4 wks |
| Etoposide | Testicular cancer<br>50–100 mg/m$^2$/day (IV, slow infusion over<br>  30–60+ min for 5 d)<br>Small cell lung cancer<br>35–50 mg/m$^2$/day (IV, slow infusion over<br>  30–60+ min for 4–5 d) | Alternatively, 100 mg/m$^2$/d on days 1, 3, and 5 may<br>  be used; doses for combination therapy and are<br>  repeated at 3- to 4-wk intervals after recovery from<br>  hematologic toxicity<br>Doses are for combination therapy and repeated at 3- to<br>  4-wk intervals after recovery from hematologic toxicity;<br>  oral dose is twice the IV, rounded to the nearest 50 mg |

*(continued)*

| TABLE 17.2 | | |
|---|---|---|
| **Dose and Schedules of Clinically Useful Alkylating Agents** *(continued)* | | |
| Ifosfamide | General antineoplastic<br>1.2 g/m$^2$/d (IV, for 5 consecutive days) | Repeat every 3 wks |
| Melphalan | Multiple myeloma:<br>16 mg/m$^2$ (IV, infusion over 15–20 min)<br>6 mg (daily PO)<br>Epithelial ovarian cancer:<br>0.2 mg/kg (daily PO) | 2-week intervals for 4 doses, 4-wk intervals thereafter<br>After 2–3 wks treatment, should be discontinued for up<br>to 4 wks, then reinstituted at 2–4 mg/d<br>Daily dose for a 5-d course, repeated every 4–5 wks |
| Streptozotocin | Pancreatic tumors<br>500 mg/m$^2$/d; 1,000 mg/m$^2$/d (IV; IV) | 500 mg for 5 consecutive days every 6 wks, 1,000 mg<br>is for 2 wks, followed by an increase in weekly dose<br>not to exceed 1,500 mg/m$^2$/wk |
| Temozolomide | Brain tumors<br>150 mg/m$^2$ (daily PO) | Dose adjusted on the basis of blood counts |
| Thiotepa | General antineoplastic:<br>0.3–0.4 mg/kg (IV)<br>Papillary carcinoma of the bladder:<br>60 mg/wk for 4 wks (bladder catheter)<br>Control of serous effusions:<br>0.6–0.8 mg/kg (intracavitary) | Rapid administration given at 1- to 4-wk intervals<br>30 or 60 mL should be retained for 2 h, so the patient is<br>usually dehydrated prior to administration of the drug |

IV, intravenously; PO, by mouth; IP, intraperitoneal.

One distinguishing feature of melphalan is that an amino acid transporter responsible for uptake influences its efficacy across cell membranes.[10] Although a number of glutathione (GSH) conjugates of alkylating agents are effluxed through adenosine triphosphate–dependent membrane transporters,[11] specific uptake mechanisms are generally rare for cancer drugs. Cyclophosphamide and ifosfamide are prodrugs that require cytochrome P-450 metabolism to release active alkylating species. Cyclophosphamide continues to be the most widely used alkylating agent and has activity against a variety of tumors.[12] A cost saving with equivalent therapeutic activity was recently shown in a modified regimen of high-dose cyclophosphamide plus cyclosporine in patients with severe or very severe aplastic anemia.[13]

## Nitrosoureas

The nitrosoureas form a diverse class of alkylating agents that have a distinct metabolism and pharmacology that separates them from others.[14] Under physiologic conditions, proton abstraction by a hydroxyl ion initiates spontaneous decomposition of the molecule to yield a diazonium hydroxide and an isocyanate (see Fig. 17.1). The chloroethyl carbonium ion generated is the active alkylating species. Through a subsequent dehalogenation step, a second electrophilic site imparts bifunctionality.[15] Thus, while cross-linking may occur similar to those lesions caused by nitrogen mustards, the chemistry leading to the endpoint is distinct. The isocyanate species generated are also electrophilic, showing nucleophilic selectivity toward sulfhydryl and amino groups that can inhibit a number of enzymes involved in nucleic acid synthesis and thiol balance.[16] Because carbamoylation is considered of minor importance to the therapeutic efficacy of clinically used nitrosoureas, chlorozotocin and streptozotocin were designed to undergo internal carbamoylation at the 1- or 3-OH group of the glucose ring, with the consequence that no carbamoylating species are produced.[17,18] Streptozotocin is also unusual in that most methylnitrosoureas have only modest therapeutic value. However, its lack of bone marrow toxicity and strong diabetogenic effect in animals led to its use in cancer of the pancreas (see Table 17.1).[19] The dose-limiting toxicities in humans are gastrointestinal and renal, but the drug has considerably less hematopoietic toxicity than the other nitrosoureas. Because of their lipophilicity and capacity to cross the blood–brain barrier, the chloroethylnitrosoureas

were found to be effective against intracranially inoculated murine tumors. Indeed, early preclinical studies showed that many mouse tumors were quite responsive to nitrosoureas. The same extent of efficacy was not found in humans. Subsequent analyses demonstrated that an enzyme responsible for repair of O-6-alkyl guanine (O$^6$-methylguanine-DNA methyltransferase [MGMT], or the Mer/Mex phenotype)[20] was expressed at low levels in mice, but at high levels in humans, a contributory factor in the reduced clinical efficacy of nitrosoureas in humans. In the 1980s, in particular, a number of new nitrosoureas were tested in patients in Europe and Japan, but none established a regular role in standard cancer treatment regimens.

MGMT promoter methylation is crucial in MGMT gene silencing and can predict a favorable outcome in glioblastoma patients receiving alkylating agents.[21] This biomarker is on the verge of entering clinical decision making and is currently used to stratify or even select glioblastoma patients for clinical trials. In other subtypes of glioma, such as anaplastic gliomas, the relevance of MGMT promoter methylation might extend beyond the prediction of chemosensitivity, and could reflect a distinct molecular profile. At this time, the standardization of MGMT assays will be critical in establishing prospective prognostic or predictive effects. In addition, eventual clinical trials will need to determine, for each subtype of glioma, the extent to which methylation patterns are predictive or prognostic and whether such assays could be incorporated into an individualized approach to clinical practice.[21]

## CLINICAL PHARMACOKINETICS/ PHARMACODYNAMICS

The pharmacokinetics of the alkylating agents are highly variable depending on the individual agent. Nevertheless, they are generally characterized by high reactivity and short half-lives. Although detailed studies on clinical pharmacology are available,[22] Table 17.1 summarizes some of the primary kinetic characteristics of the major clinically useful drugs. Mechlorethamine is unstable and is administered rapidly in a running intravenous infusion to avoid its rapid breakdown to inactive metabolites. In contrast, chlorambucil and cyclophosphamide are sufficiently stable to be given orally, and are rapidly and completely absorbed from the gastrointestinal tract, whereas others like melphalan have poor and variable

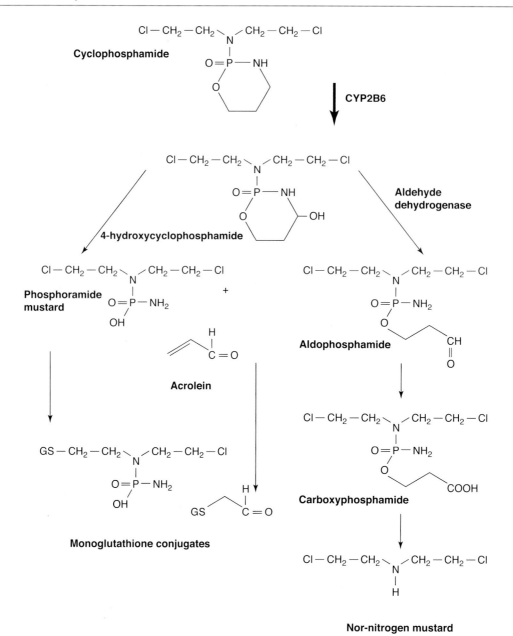

**Figure 17.2** Activation and detoxification routes of metabolism for cyclophosphamide.

oral absorption. Cyclophosphamide,[23] ifosfamide, and dacarbazine are unusual in that they require activation by cytochrome P-450 in the liver before they can alkylate cellular constituents. The nitrosoureas also require activation, albeit nonenzymatic. The major route of metabolism of most alkylating agents is spontaneous hydrolysis, although many can also undergo some degree of enzymatic metabolism. This is particularly pertinent for phase II metabolic conversions where reactivity with nucleophilic thiols precedes conversion to mercapturates, with the result that most of the alkylating agents are excreted in the urine. One example of complex multistep metabolism is provided by cyclophosphamide (see Fig. 17.2). Activation by CYP2B6 is followed by the conversion of aldehyde dehydrogenase to reactive alkylating species or possible detoxification through GSH conjugation reactions. The latter is particularly important for acrolein because it is believed to contribute to the bladder toxicities associated with the drug.

The alkylating agents form covalent bonds with a number of nucleophilic groups present in proteins, RNA, and DNA (e.g., amino, carboxyl, sulfhydryl, imidazole, phosphate). Under physiologic conditions, the chloroethyl group of the nitrogen mustards undergoes cyclization, with the chloride acting as a leaving group forming an intermediate carbonium ion that attacks nucleophilic sites (see Fig. 17.1). Bifunctional alkylating agents (with two chloroethyl side chains) can undergo a subsequent cyclization to form a covalent bond with an adjacent nucleophilic group, resulting in DNA–DNA or DNA–protein cross-links. The N7 or O6 positions of guanine are particularly susceptible and may represent primary targets that determine both the cytotoxic and mutagenic consequences of therapy.[24] The nitrosoureas have a similar, but distinct, mechanism of action, spontaneously forming both alkylating and carbamoylating agents in aqueous media (see Fig. 17.1). The carbamoylating moieties are generally believed to be inconsequential to the therapeutic properties of the nitrosoureas.

## THERAPEUTIC USES

The alkylating agents are frequently used in combination therapy to treat a variety of types of cancer. Perhaps the most versatile is cyclophosphamide, whereas the other alkylating agents are of more restricted clinical use. Because of early successes, many disease states are managed with drug combinations that contain several alkylating agents. Cyclophosphamide is employed to treat a variety of immune-related diseases and to purge bone marrow in autologous marrow transplant situations.[25] A general summary of the clinical uses of the primary alkylating agents is shown in Table 17.1.

# TOXICITIES

The alkylating agents show significant qualitative and quantitative variability in the sites and severities of their toxicities. The primary dose-limiting toxicity is suppression of bone marrow function, with secondary limiting effects on the proliferating cells of the intestinal mucosa.

Contraindications to the use of alkylating agents would identify patients with severely depressed bone marrow function and patients with hypersensitivity to these drugs. Other listed precautions to these drugs include carcinogenic and mutagenic effects and impairment of fertility. Precaution is also advised in patients with (1) leukopenia or thrombocytopenia, (2) previous exposure to chemotherapy or radiotherapy, (3) tumor cell infiltration of the bone marrow, and (4) impaired renal or hepatic function. These drugs can also increase toxicity in adrenalectomized patients and interfere with wound healing. A brief summary of dose-limiting toxicities is shown in Table 17.1, and a narrative of each follows here.

## Nausea and Vomiting

Nausea and vomiting are frequent side effects of alkylating agent therapy and are not well controlled by conventional antiemetics.[24] They are a major source of patient discomfort and a significant cause of lack of drug compliance and even discontinuation of therapy. Frequency and extent are highly variable among patients. The overall frequency of nausea and vomiting is directly proportional to the dose of alkylating agent. The onset of nausea may occur within a few minutes of the administration of the drug or may be delayed for several hours.

## Bone Marrow Toxicity

Bone marrow toxicity can involve all of the blood elements, leukocytes, platelets, and red cells.[26] The extent and time course of suppression show marked interindividual fluctuation. Relative platelet sparing is a characteristic of cyclophosphamide treatment. Even at the very high doses (<200 mg/kg) of cyclophosphamide (used in preparation for bone marrow transplantation), some recovery of hematopoietic elements occurs within 21 to 28 days. This stem cell–sparing property is further reflected by the fact that cumulative damage to the bone marrow is rarely seen when cyclophosphamide is given as a single agent, and repeated high doses can be given without progressive lowering of leukocyte and platelet counts. The biochemical basis for the stem cell–sparing effect of cyclophosphamide is related to the presence of high levels of aldehyde dehydrogenase in early bone marrow progenitor cells (see Fig. 17.2). Busulfan is particularly toxic to bone marrow stem cells,[26] and treatment can lead to prolonged hypoplasia. The hematopoietic depression produced by the nitrosoureas is characteristically delayed. The onset of leukocyte and platelet depression occurs 3 to 4 weeks after drug administration and may last an additional 2 to 3 weeks.[22,26] Thrombocytopenia appears earlier and usually is more severe than leukopenia. Even if the nitrosourea is given at 6-week intervals, hematopoietic recovery may not occur between courses, and the drug dose often must be decreased when repeated courses are used.

## Renal and Bladder Toxicity

Hemorrhagic cystitis is unique to the oxazaphosphorines (cyclophosphamide and ifosfamide) and may range from a mild cystitis to severe bladder damage with massive hemorrhage.[27] This toxicity is caused by the excretion of toxic metabolites (particularly acrolein) (see Fig. 17.2) in the urine, with subsequent direct irritation of the bladder mucosa. The incidence and severity can be lessened by adequate hydration and continuous irrigation of the bladder with a solution containing 2-mercaptoethane sulfonate (MESNA) and frequent bladder emptying.[26] MESNA is given in divided doses every 4 hours in dosages of 60% of those of the alkylating agent.

At high cumulative doses, all commonly used nitrosoureas can produce a dose-related renal toxicity that can result in renal failure and death.[29] In patients developing clinical evidence of toxicity, increases in serum creatinine usually appear after the completion of therapy and may be first detected up to 2 years after treatment.

## Interstitial Pneumonitis and Pulmonary Fibrosis

Long-term busulfan therapy can lead to the gradual onset of fever, a nonproductive cough, and dyspnea, followed by tachypnea and cyanosis, and progressing to severe pulmonary insufficiency and death.[30] If busulfan is stopped before the onset of clinical symptoms, pulmonary function may stabilize, but if clinical symptoms are manifest, the condition may be rapidly fatal. Cyclophosphamide, bischloroethylnitrosourea, and methyl-1-(2-chloroethyl)-3-cyclohexyl-1-nitrosourea in cumulative doses exceeding 1,000 mg/$m^2$ may also lead to similar side effects.[31] Other alkylating agents, including melphalan, chlorambucil, and mitomycin C, can lead to pulmonary fibrosis after therapy.[32] This effect is probably caused by a direct cytotoxicity of the alkylating agent to pulmonary epithelium, resulting in alveolitis and fibrosis.

## Gonadal Toxicity, Teratogenesis, and Carcinogenesis

Alkylating agents can have profound toxic effects on reproductive tissue.[33] A depletion of testicular germ (but not Sertoli) cells is accompanied by aspermia. In patients with a total absence of germ cells, an increase in plasma levels of follicle-stimulating hormone occurs. However, patients in remission and off alkylating agents for 2 to 7 years show complete spermatogenesis, indicating that testicular damage is reversible.

In women, a high incidence of amenorrhea and ovarian atrophy is associated with cyclophosphamide or melphalan therapy.[34] This seems to be age related because it developed after lower doses in older compared with younger patients, and was less likely to be reversible in the older cohort. A pathologic analysis reveals the absence of mature or primordial follicles, and endocrinology studies demonstrate decreased estrogen and progesterone levels and elevated serum follicle-stimulating hormone and luteinizing hormone levels typical of menopause.

The DNA-damaging properties of alkylating agents ensure that they are all teratogenic and carcinogenic to some degree. The administration of alkylating agents during the first trimester of pregnancy presents a definitive risk of a malformed fetus, but the administration of such drugs during the second and third trimesters does not increase the risk of fetal malformation above normal.[35]

Development of second cancer as a consequence of alkylating agent therapy has been documented. For example, a fulminant acute myeloid leukemia characterized by a preceding phase of myelodysplasia is found in some patients treated with melphalan, cyclophosphamide (which is much less leukemogenic than melphalan), chlorambucil, and the nitrosoureas.[33] This circumstance probably reflects the fact that these have been the most

CANCER THERAPEUTICS

widely used of the alkylating agents. Also, the preponderance of patients with multiple myeloma, Hodgkin lymphoma, and carcinoma of the ovary in the reports of leukemogenesis is probably because patients with these diseases may have good responses and are often treated with alkylating agents for a number of years. The rate of occurrence of acute leukemia in patients with ovarian cancer who survive for 10 years after treatment with alkylating agents might be as high as 10%. Acute leukemia has been the most frequently described second malignancy, and it usually develops 1 to 4 years after drug exposure.[36] Other malignancies, including solid tumors, also have been reported to develop in patients treated with alkylating agents.[37]

The last four decades have yielded a significant improvement in the survival of children diagnosed with cancer (5-year survival is approximately 80%). As many as two-thirds of the survivors of childhood malignancies can experience delayed drug toxicities that may be severe or even life threatening. Such complications include impairment in growth and development, neurocognitive dysfunction, cardiopulmonary compromise, endocrine dysfunction, renal impairment, gastrointestinal dysfunction, musculoskeletal sequelae, and second cancers.[38]

## Alopecia

The degree of alopecia after cyclophosphamide administration may be quite severe, especially when this drug is used in combination with vincristine sulfate or doxorubicin hydrochloride.[39] Regrowth of hair inevitably occurs after the cessation of therapy, but may be associated with a change in the color and greater curl. Use of a tourniquet or ice pack applied to the scalp during and for a short period after cyclophosphamide administration reduces the impact.

## Allergic Reactions

Alkylating agents covalently bind to proteins, and these conjugates can act as haptens and produce allergic reactions.[40] An increasing number of reports of skin eruption, angioneurotic edema, urticaria, and anaphylactic reactions after the systemic administration of alkylating agents have appeared.

## Immunosuppression

Alkylating agents suppress both humoral and cellular immunity in a variety of experimental systems.[41] The most immunosuppressive is cyclophosphamide, reported to cause (1) selective suppression of B-lymphocyte function, (2) depletion of B-lymphocytes, and (3) suppression of lymphocyte functions that are mediated by T cells, such as the graft-versus-host response and delayed hypersensitivity. Most intermittent antitumor regimens do not uniformly produce profound immunosuppression, and recovery is usually prompt. Sustained drug treatments can lead to severe lymphocyte depletion and profound immunosuppression and may be accompanied by an increase of viral, fungal, and protozoal infections.[41]

## COMPLICATIONS WITH HIGH-DOSE ALKYLATING AGENT THERAPY

At standard doses, alkylating agents produce myelosuppression as their dose-limiting toxicity. Less severe effects on the gastrointestinal epithelium, lungs, bladder, and kidneys may become problems with long-term treatment, but rarely limit initial therapy. For this reason, and because of their steep dose response to tumor-killing curves, the alkylating agents have become a logical tool, either alone or in combination, for high-dose chemotherapy

regimens in which bone marrow toxicity is expected, and is accommodated by bone marrow transplantation, stem cell reconstitution from peripheral blood monocytes, and growth factor rescue. In this high-dose setting, toxicities that affect the gut, lungs, liver, and CNS become dose limiting and life threatening.[42] The highly lipid-soluble alkylators, especially ifosfamide, busulfan, the nitrosoureas, and thiotepa, cause CNS dysfunction, including seizures, altered mental status, cerebellar dysfunction, cranial nerve palsies, and coma.[43] High-dose ifosfamide is most frequently the cause of neurotoxicity.[44] Clinical manifestations of grade 4 neurotoxicities were reported in approximately one-fourth of those patients receiving ifosfamide. The side-chain N-linked chloroethyl moiety of ifosfamide (see Table 17.1) is more likely than the bischloroethyl group of cyclophosphamide to undergo oxidation and subsequent N-deethylation and lead to the formation of chloroacetaldehyde. High-dose busulfan is also frequently used in a variety of conditioning regimens for hematopoietic cell transplantation. In this setting, busulfan causes neurotoxicity manifesting in seizures that generally are tonic–clonic in character. Phenytoin has been the preferred drug to treat busulfan-induced seizures, although some emerging clinical data support the use of benzodiazepines, most notably clonazepam and lorazepam, to prevent busulfan-induced seizures. Moreover, the second-generation antiepileptic drug levetiracetam possesses the characteristics of optimal prophylaxis for busulfan-induced seizures.[45] At least one recent study has suggested that a polymorphism in the glutathione S-transferase A2 family may be predictive of transplant-related mortality after allogeneic stem cell transplantation,[46] perhaps indicating that a pharmacogenetic approach might be possible in this disease setting. Moreover, in a preclinical setting, a proteomic analysis identified thioredoxin as a potentially important adjuvant therapy in enhancing donor cell graft enhancement in bone marrow transplantation.[47] The possibility that this approach may benefit patients following alkylating agent–based ablation remains to be tested in a clinical setting.

Cyclophosphamide at doses exceeding 100 mg/kg during a 48-hour period (preparatory to bone marrow transplantation) can cause cardiac toxicity.[48] No evidence exists for cumulative damage to the heart after repeated moderate or low doses of the drug. Cardiac toxicity occurs with greatest frequency in patients older than 50 years or in those previously treated with anthracyclines.[48]

## ALKYLATING AGENT–STEROID CONJUGATES

Adapting the rationale that steroid receptors may function to localize and concentrate attached drug species intracellularly in hormone-responsive cancers, a number of synthetic conjugates of nitrogen mustards and steroids have been developed. Of these, two made the transition into clinical use.

Prednimustine is an ester-linked conjugate of chlorambucil and prednisolone designed to function as a prodrug for chlorambucil. Release of the alkylating agent occurs after cleavage by serum esterases,[49] which can release the ester link of prednimustine, producing the hormone and active alkylating drug. The elimination phase of chlorambucil in patient plasma is significantly longer after the administration of prednimustine than after chlorambucil. Estramustine is a carbamate ester–linked conjugate of nor-nitrogen mustard and estradiol. Unlike prednimustine, the pharmacology of estramustine is governed by the presence of the carbamate group in the steroid–mustard linkage. The relative resistance of the carbamate bond to enzymatic cleavage eliminates the alkylating activity of the molecule and conveys an entirely new pharmacology.[50] The crystal structural and mechanism of action studies showed that estramustine has antimitotic activity, an activity shared by some other steroids.[51] Estramustine has found a clinical niche used in combination with other antimitotic drugs in the management of hormone refractory prostate cancer.[52]

# DRUG RESISTANCE AND MODULATION

As with all drugs, intrinsic or acquired resistance to alkylating agents occurs and limits the therapeutic utility of this class of anticancer drugs.[53] A plethora of preclinical studies have characterized mechanisms by which cells develop resistance and, to a lesser degree, these have been shown to occur clinically. Because alkylating agents have a narrow therapeutic index, the emergence of resistance can have a significant impact on clinical success. Some of the factors that can contribute to the expression of resistance to alkylating agents include (1) alterations in drug uptake or transport, (2) increased repair of drug-induced nucleic acid damage, (3) failure to activate alkylating agent prodrugs, (4) increased scavenging of drug species by nonessential cellular nucleophiles, (5) increased enzymatic detoxification of drug species, and (6) altered expression of genes coding for cellular commitment to apoptosis.

# RECENT DEVELOPMENTS

In the era of directed targeted therapies, the lack of specificity of alkylating agents would seem to limit the likelihood that novel drugs will be forthcoming. High toxicities, narrow therapeutic indices, and chemical instabilities are all properties that consign this drug class to the lower echelons of popularity in drug-discovery platforms. Although covalent bonding to specific target sites is one approach to direct targeting, the random electrophilic attraction toward nucleic acids and proteins is not an optimal property by today's standards. Nevertheless, the relative success of the alkylating agents in gaining therapeutic responses to diseases that are difficult to treat continues to serve as an impetus to use alkylating moieties as a means to kill cells. Some novel agents are presently in development. Cyclophosphamide and ifosfamide were prodrugs synthesized in the hope that high levels of phosphoamidase in epithelial tumors would selectively activate the drugs.[27] Other efforts to improve selectivity have centered on the synthesis of antibody–enzyme conjugates that bind to tumor-specific surface antigens. Enzymes frequently associated with the cell surface include peptidases, nitroreductases, and γ-glutamyl transpeptidase; to some degree, each has been targeted to cleave circulating alkylating prodrugs, thereby in a localized fashion releasing active alkylating species. Antibody-directed enzyme prodrug therapy is exemplified by the use of an antibody linked to the peptidase carboxypeptidase G-2, which releases an active alkylator from an inactive γ-glutamyl conjugate.[54] Linkage of the peptidase to any antibody that localizes selectively to a tumor cell membrane is a viable option. Expression of the peptidase on the cell surface then leads to prodrug activation and cell kill. Such approaches have had limited clinical impact to this time; however, their development does continue.

A further rationale for enhancing tumor-specific delivery takes advantage of the observation that glutathione-S-transferase *pi* (GSTP1-1) is preferentially expressed in a number of solid tumors and some lymphomas. In this case, the prodrug consists of an unusual alkylating agent conjugated to a substituted glutathione peptidomimetic. GSTP initiates the cleavage, thereby creating a cytotoxic alkylating species.[55] The initial canfosfamide design strategy relied on the principle that proton-abstracting sites at the active site of GST could initiate a cleavage reaction that would convert an inactive prodrug into a cytotoxic species. The presence of a histidine residue in proximity to the G binding site was integral to the removal of the sulfhydryl proton from the GSH cosubstrate, resulting in the generation of a nucleophilic sulfide anion. This moiety would be more reactive with electrophiles in the absence of GSH. Unlike other standard nitrogen mustard drugs, canfosfamide contains a tetrakis (chloroethyl) phosphorodiamidate moiety. Other compounds bearing this structure have been shown to be more cytotoxic than a similar structure with a single bis-(chloroethyl) amine group.[56]

As in other nitrogen mustards, the chlorines can act as leaving groups, thus creating aziridinium ions with electrophilic characteristics. Although the exact temporal or sequential formation of the four possible chlorine leaving events is not known, the assumption is that these species possess cytotoxic properties through their capacity to alkylate target nucleophiles, such as DNA bases. Tetrafunctionality could result in the formation of cross-links with bonding distances greater than for bifunctional agents. However, a number of caveats apply to this interpretation. For example, alkylating agents, whether mono-, bi-, or putatively tetrafunctional, generally lead to some form of myelosuppression. A number of clinical trials with canfosfamide have now been completed. These include, phase 1,[57] phase 1/2a,[58] phase 2,[59] and phase 3.[60] The phase 3 study was in platinum refractory ovarian cancer patients and proved negative for enhanced survival. Nevertheless, additional trials are still in progress.

Another targeting approach delivers the gene for a cytochrome P-450 isoenzyme to tumors by viral vector, thereby enhancing specific tumor cell activation of cyclophosphamide.[61] Because this therapy has its base in gene delivery technologies, successful development in humans will await further advances in this arena.

Laromustine is in the sulfonylhydrazine class of alkylating agents. It is presently in clinical development for the treatment of malignancies such as acute myelogenous leukemia (AML).[62] Similar to nitrosoureas, laromustine is a prodrug that yields a chloroethylating and a carbamoylating (methyl isocyanate) species. As with nitrosoureas, the cytotoxicity of laromustine is attributed primarily to the chloroethylating-mediated alkylation of DNA and subsequent interstrand cross-links.[63] The carbamoylating species can inhibit DNA repair and other cellular enzyme systems. Phase 1 trials in patients with solid tumors indicated the expected myelosuppression, although few extramedullary toxicities were observed, indicating potential efficacy in the treatment of hematologic malignancies. Phase 2 trials have been completed in patients with untreated AML, high-risk myelodysplastic syndrome, and relapsed AML. The most encouraging results have been found in patients older than 60 years with poor-risk, de novo AML for which no standard treatment exists. Laromustine is currently in phase 2/3 trials for AML and phase 2 trials for myelodysplastic syndrome and solid tumors.[64] Laromustine appears to be a promising agent in elderly patients who do not respond to or are not fit for intensive chemotherapy.

Although not a new drug, bendamustine is a unique cytotoxic agent with structural similarities to alkylating agents and antimetabolites, but it lacks cross-resistance with other established alkylating agents both in vitro and in the clinic.[65] Its mechanism of action is similar to other mustards in causing DNA intra- and interstrand cross-links. In comparison with other more commonly used alkylating agents, such as cyclophosphamide or phenylalanine mustard, more DNA double-strand breaks are formed at equitoxic dosages. Treatment with bendamustine induces a concentration-dependent apoptosis as evidenced by changes in Bcl-2 and Bax expression profiles in chronic B-cell lymphocytic leukemia.[66] DNA damage produced by bendamustine is repaired via base-excision repair mechanisms, implicating an unusual mode of action, which was recently confirmed through gene expression profiling analyses. This also provided an explanation for the lack of cross-resistance with other alkylating agents, as observed in vitro with anthracycline-resistant breast cancer and cisplatin-resistant ovarian cancer.[66,67]

Clinical studies conducted in Germany more than 30 years ago suggested activity in indolent non-Hodgkin lymphoma. Subsequent American trials showed responses in more than 70% of patients with drug refractory disease, with the implication that bendamustine may be the most effective drug in this patient population. Combinations of bendamustine and rituximab elicited response rates of 90% to 92%, with complete remission in 55% to 60% in follicular and mantle cell lymphoma. Superiority over chlorambucil in previously untreated patients with chronic lymphocytic leukemia (CLL) led to its recent approval for this disease in the United States. Bendamustine is approved in Germany for the treatment of patients with indolent non-Hodgkin lymphoma, CLL, and multiple myeloma. Activity has also been noted in patients with breast cancer and non–small-cell lung cancer.

Bendamustine has been used both as a single agent and in combination with other agents, including etoposide, fludarabine, mitoxantrone, methotrexate, prednisone, rituximab, and vincristine. A multicenter phase 2 trial in lymphomas had an overall response rate of 89%; (35% complete response and 54% partial response). In previously treated patients. the overall response rate was 76% (38% complete response and 38% partial response). The estimated median progression-free survival was 19 months.[67] In CLL patients, the drug is administered at 100 mg/m$^2$ intravenously over 30 minutes on days 1 and 2 of a 28-day cycle, for up to six cycles. Efficacy relative to first-line therapies other than chlorambucil has not been established. It is also indicated for the treatment of patients with indolent B-cell non-Hodgkin lymphoma that has progressed during, or within, 6 months of treatment with rituximab or rituximab-containing regimens. As with most alkylating agents, the primary dose-limiting toxicity is myelosuppression; nonhematologic toxicities were mild and included fatigue, nausea, loss of appetite, and vomiting. The optimization of dose and schedule, particularly relative to other drugs, and the management of toxicities has allowed its use in combination with a range of other chemotherapeutic agents, including prednisone, methotrexate, fludarabine, etoposide, mitoxantrone, vinca alkaloids, and rituximab. The availability of bendamustine provides another effective treatment option for patients with lymphoid malignancies, frequently reducing the side effects of the more standard cyclophosphamide, hydroxy doxorubicin, Oncovin, and prednisone (CHOP) regimen.[68] Recent approval by the U.S. Food and Drug Administration has allowed Cephalon, Inc. to market bendamustine under the trade name Treanda and, in combination with mitoxantrone and rituximab, it is now standard of care in indolent lymphomas. Trial results released in 2013 indicated that this combination more than doubled the progression-free survival in this disease[69] and there is early evidence that there may be utility in relapsed or refractory multiple myeloma.[70]

# REFERENCES

1. Adair FE, Bagg HJ. Experimental and clinical studies on the treatment of cancer by dichlorethylsulphide (mustard gas). *Ann Surg* 1931;93(1):190–199.
2. Rhoads C. Nitrogen mustards in treatment of neoplastic disease. *JAMA* 1946;131:656–658.
3. Coles B. Effects of modifying structure on electrophilic reactions with biological nucleophiles. *Drug Metab Rev* 1985;15:1307–1334.
4. Pearson R, Songstad J. Application of the principle of hard and soft acids and bases to organic chemistry. *J Am Chem Soc* 1967;89:1827.
5. Ross W. Alkylating agents. In: *Biological Alkylating Agents*. London: Butterworth; 1962.
6. Elson LA. Hematological effects of the alkylating agents. *Ann N Y Acad Sci* 1958;68(3):826–833.
7. Kushner BH, Kramer K, Modak S, et al. Topotecan, thiotepa, and carboplatin for neuroblastoma: failure to prevent relapse in the central nervous system. *Bone Marrow Transplant* 2006;37(3):271–276.
8. Agarwala SS, Kirkwood JM. Temozolomide, a novel alkylating agent with activity in the central nervous system, may improve the treatment of advanced metastatic melanoma. *Oncologist* 2000;5(2):144–151.
9. Tentori L, Graziani G. Recent approaches to improve the antitumor efficacy of temozolomide. *Curr Med Chem* 2009;16(2):245–257.
10. Vistica DT. Cytotoxicity as an indicator for transport mechanism: evidence that murine bone marrow progenitor cells lack a high-affinity leucine carrier that transports melphalan in murine L1210 leukemia cells. *Blood* 1980;56(3):427–429.
11. Dean M, Rzhetsky A, Allikmets R. The human ATP-binding cassette (ABC) transporter superfamily. *Genome Res* 2001;11(7):1156–1166.
12. Sensenbrenner LL, Marini JJ, Colvin M. Comparative effects of cyclophosphamide, isophosphamide, 4-methylcyclophosphamide, and phosphoramide mustard on murine hematopoietic and immunocompetent cells. *J Natl Cancer Inst* 1979;62(4):975–981.
13. Zhang F, Zhang L, Jing L, et al. (2013) High-dose cyclophosphamide compared with antithymocyte globulin for treatment of acquired severe aplastic anemia. *Exp Hematol* 2013;41:328–334.
14. Montgomery JA, James R, McCaleb GS, et al. The modes of decomposition of 1,3-bis(2-chloroethyl)-1-nitrosourea and related compounds. *J Med Chem* 1967;10(4):668–674.
15. Brundrett RB, Cowens JW, Colvin M. Chemistry of nitrosoureas: decomposition of Deuterated 1,3-bis(2-chloroethyl)-1-nitrosourea. *J Med Chem* 1976;19(7):958–961.
16. Tew KD, Kyle G, Johnson A, et al. Carbamoylation of glutathione reductase and changes in cellular and chromosome morphology in a rat cell line resistant to nitrogen mustards but collaterally sensitive to nitrosoureas. *Cancer Res* 1985;45(5):2326–2333.
17. Anderson T, Schein PS, McMenamin MG, et al. Streptozotocin diabetes: correlation with extent of depression of pancreatic islet nicotinamide adenine dinucleotide. *J Clin Invest* 1974;54(3):672–677.
18. Anderson T, McMenamin MG, Schein PS. Chlorozotocin, 2-(3-(2-chloroethyl)-3-nitrosoureido)-D-glucopyranose, an antitumor agent with modified bone marrow toxicity. *Cancer Res* 1975;35(3):761–765.
19. Schein PS, O'Connell MJ, Blom J, et al. Clinical antitumor activity and toxicity of streptozotocin (NSC-85998). *Cancer* 1974;34(4):993–1000.
20. Pieper RO. Understanding and manipulating O6-methylguanine-DNA methyltransferase expression. *Pharmacol Ther* 1997;74(3):285–297.
21. Weller M, Stupp R, Reifenberger G, et al. MGMT promoter methylation in malignant gliomas: ready for personalized medicine? *Nat Rev Neurol* 2010;6(1):39–51.
22. Tew K, Colvin OM, Jones RB. Clinical and high dose alkylating agents. In: Chabner BA, Longo DL, eds. *Cancer: Chemotherapy and Biotherapy: Principles and Practice*. Philadelphia: Lippincott-Raven; 2005: 283.

23. Brookes P, Lawley PD. The reaction of mono- and di-functional alkylating agents with nucleic acids. *Biochem J* 1961;80(3):496–503.
24. Penta JS, Poster DS, Bruno S, et al. Clinical trials with antiemetic agents in cancer patients receiving chemotherapy. *J Clin Pharmacol* 1981;21(8–9 Suppl):11S–22S.
25. Colvin M, Hilton J. Pharmacology of cyclophosphamide and metabolites. *Cancer Treat Rep* 1981;65(Suppl 3):89–95.
26. Elson L. Hematological effects of the alkylating agents. *Ann N Y Acad Sci* 1958;68:826–833.
27. Cox PJ. Cyclophosphamide cystitis—identification of acrolein as the causative agent. *Biochem Pharmacol* 1979;28(13):2045–2049.
28. Andriole GL, Sandlund JT, Miser JS, et al. The efficacy of mesna (2-mercaptoethane sodium sulfonate) as a uroprotectant in patients with hemorrhagic cystitis receiving further oxazaphosphorine chemotherapy. *J Clin Oncol* 1987;5(5):799–803.
29. Schacht RG, Feiner HD, Gallo GR, et al. Nephrotoxicity of nitrosoureas. *Cancer* 1981;48(6):1328–1334.
30. Littler WA, Ogilvie C. Lung function in patients receiving busulphan. *Br Med J* 1970;4(5734):530–532.
31. Mark GJ, Lehimgar-Zadeh A, Ragsdale BD. Cyclophosphamide pneumonitis. *Thorax* 1978;33(1):89–93.
32. Kreisman H, Wolkove N. Pulmonary toxicity of antineoplastic therapy. *Semin Oncol* 1992;19(5):508–520.
33. Kumar R, Biggart JD, McEvoy J, et al. Cyclophosphamide and reproductive function. *Lancet* 1972;1(7762):1212–1214.
34. Miller JJ 3rd, Williams GF, Leissring JC. Multiple late complications of therapy with cyclophosphamide, including ovarian destruction. *Am J Med* 1971;50(4):530–535.
35. Nicholson HO. Cytotoxic drugs in pregnancy: review of reported cases. *J Obstet Gynaecol Br Commonw* 1968;75(3):307–312.
36. Reimer RR, Hoover R, Fraumeni JF Jr, et al. Acute leukemia after alkylating-agent therapy of ovarian cancer. *N Engl J Med* 1977;297(4):177–181.
37. Penn I. Second malignant neoplasms associated with immunosuppressive medications. *Cancer* 1976;37(2 Suppl):1024–1032.
38. Bhatia S, Constine LS. Late morbidity after successful treatment of children with cancer. *Cancer J* 2009;15(3):174–180.
39. Calvert W. Alopecia and cytotoxic drugs. *Br Med J* 1966;2(5517):831.
40. Weiss RB, Bruno S. Hypersensitivity reactions to cancer chemotherapeutic agents. *Ann Intern Med* 1981;94(1):66–72.
41. Santos GW, Sensenbrenner LL, Burke PJ, et al. Marrow transplantation in man following cyclophosphamide. *Transplant Proc* 1971;3(1):400–404.
42. de Jonge ME, Huitema AD, Beijnen JH, et al. High exposures to bioactivated cyclophosphamide are related to the occurrence of veno-occlusive disease of the liver following high-dose chemotherapy. *Br J Cancer* 2006;94(9):1226–1230.
43. Baruchel S, Diezi M, Hargrave D, et al. Safety and pharmacokinetics of temozolomide using a dose-escalation, metronomic schedule in recurrent paediatric brain tumours. *Eur J Cancer* 2006;42(14):2335–2342.
44. Pratt CB, Goren MP, Meyer WH, et al. Ifosfamide neurotoxicity is related to previous cisplatin treatment for pediatric solid tumors. *J Clin Oncol* 1990;8(8):1399–1401.
45. Eberly AL, Anderson GD, Bubalo JS, et al. Optimal prevention of seizures induced by high-dose busulfan. *Pharmacotherapy* 2008;28(12):1502–1510.
46. Bonifazi F, Storci G, Bandini G, et al. Glutathione transferase-A2 S112T polymorphism predicts survival, transplant-related mortality, busulfan and bilirubin blood levels after allogeneic stem cell transplantation. *Haematologica* 2014;99(1):172–179.

47. An N, Janech MG, Bland AM, et al. Proteomic analysis of murine bone marrow niche microenvironment identifies thioredoxin as a novel agent for radioprotection and for enhancing donor cell reconstitution. *Exp Hematol* 2013;41:944–956.

48. Steinherz LJ, Steinherz PG, Mangiacasale D, et al. Cardiac changes with cyclophosphamide. *Med Pediatr Oncol* 1981;9(5):417–422.

49. Bastholt L, Johansson CJ, Pfeiffer P, et al. A pharmacokinetic study of prednimustine as compared with prednisolone plus chlorambucil in cancer patients. *Cancer Chemother Pharmacol* 1991;28(3):205–210.

50. Tew KD, Glusker JP, Hartley-Asp B, et al. Preclinical and clinical perspectives on the use of estramustine as an antimitotic drug. *Pharmacol Ther* 1992;56(3):323–339.

51. Punzi JS, Duax WL, Strong P, et al. Molecular conformation of estramustine and two analogues. *Mol Pharmacol* 1992;41(3):569–576.

52. Hudes GR, Greenberg R, Krigel RL, et al. Phase II study of estramustine and vinblastine, two microtubule inhibitors, in hormone-refractory prostate cancer. *J Clin Oncol* 1992;10(11):1754–1761.

53. Tew K, Houghton JA, Houghton PJ. *Preclinical and Clinical Modulation of Anticancer Drugs.* Boca Raton, FL: CRC Press; 1993.

54. Friedlos F, Davies L, Scanlon I, et al. Three new prodrugs for suicide gene therapy using carboxypeptidase G2 elicit bystander efficacy in two xenograft models. *Cancer Res* 2002;62(6):1724–1729.

55. Tew KD. TLK-286: a novel glutathione S-transferase-activated prodrug. *Expert Opin Investig Drugs* 2005;14(8):1047–1054.

56. Borch RF, Valente RR. Synthesis, activation, and cytotoxicity of aldophosphamide analogues. *J Med Chem* 1991;34(10):3052–3058.

57. Rosen LS, Laxa B, Boulos L, et al. Phase 1 study of TLK286 (Telcyta) administered weekly in advanced malignancies. *Clin Cancer Res* 2004;10(11):3689–3698.

58. Sequist LV, Fidias PM, Temel JS, et al. Phase 1–2a multicenter dose-ranging study of canfosfamide in combination with carboplatin and paclitaxel as first-line therapy for patients with advanced non-small cell lung cancer. *J Thorac Oncol* 2009;4(11):1389–1396.

59. Kavanagh JJ, Gershenson DM, Choi H, et al. Multi-institutional phase 2 study of TLK286 (TELCYTA, a glutathione S-transferase P1-1 activated glutathione analog prodrug) in patients with platinum and paclitaxel refractory or resistant ovarian cancer. *Int J Gynecol Cancer* 2005;15(4):593–600.

60. Vergote I, Finkler N, del Campo J, et al. Phase 3 randomised study of canfosfamide (Telcyta, TLK286) versus pegylated liposomal doxorubicin or topotecan as third-line therapy in patients with platinum-refractory or -resistant ovarian cancer. *Eur J Cancer* 2009;45(13):2324–2332.

61. Chase M, Chung RY, Chiocca EA. An oncolytic viral mutant that delivers the CYP2B1 transgene and augments cyclophosphamide chemotherapy. *Nat Biotechnol* 1998;16(5):444–448.

62. Vey N, Giles F. Laromustine (cloretazine). *Expert Opin Pharmacother* 2010;11(4):657–667.

63. Pigneux A. Laromustine, a sulfonyl hydrolyzing alkylating prodrug for cancer therapy. *IDrugs* 2009;12(1):39–53.

64. Schiller GJ, O'Brien SM, Pigneux A, et al. Single-agent laromustine, a novel alkylating agent, has significant activity in older patients with previously untreated poor-risk acute myeloid leukemia. *J Clin Oncol* 2010;28(5):815–821.

65. Eichbaum M, Bischofs E, Nehls K, et al. Bendamustine hydrochloride—a renaissance of alkylating strategies in anticancer medicine. *Drugs Today (Barc)* 2009;45(6):431–444.

66. Rasschaert M, Schrijvers D, Van den Brande J, et al. A phase I study of bendamustine hydrochloride administered day 1+2 every 3 weeks in patients with solid tumours. *Br J Cancer* 2007;96(11):1692–1698.

67. Weide R, Hess G, Köppler H, et al. High anti-lymphoma activity of bendamustine/mitoxantrone/rituximab in rituximab pretreated relapsed or refractory indolent lymphomas and mantle cell lymphomas: a multicenter phase II study of the German Low Grade Lymphoma Study Group (GLSG). *Leuk Lymphoma* 2007;48(7):1299–1306.

68. Cheson BD, Rummel MJ. Bendamustine: rebirth of an old drug. *J Clin Oncol* 2009;27(9):1492–1501.

69. van der Jagt R. Bendamustine for indolent non-Hodgkin lymphoma in the front-line or relapsed setting: a review of pharmacokinetics and clinical trial outcomes. *Expert Rev Hematol* 2013;6:525–537.

70. Ponisch W, Heyn S, Beck J, et al. Lenalidomide, bendamustine and prednisolone exhibits a favourable safety and efficacy profile in relapsed or refractory multiple myeloma: final results of a phase 1 clinical trial OSHO - #077. *Br J Haematol* 2013;162:202–209.

# 18  Platinum Analogs

Peter J. O'Dwyer and A. Hilary Calvert

## INTRODUCTION

The platinum drugs represent a unique and important class of antitumor compounds. Alone or in combination with other chemotherapeutic agents, *cis*-diamminedichloroplatinum (II) (cisplatin) and its analogs have made a significant impact on the treatment of a variety of solid tumors for nearly 40 years. The unique activity and toxicity profile observed with cisplatin in early clinical trials fueled the development of platinum analogs that are less toxic and more active against a variety of tumor types, including those that have developed resistance to cisplatin. In addition to cisplatin, two other platinum complexes are currently approved for use in the United States: *cis*-diamminecyclobutanedicarboxylate platinum (II) (carboplatin) and 1,2-diaminocyclohexaneoxalato platinum (II) (oxaliplatin). Several other analogs with unique activities are in various stages of clinical development, and nedaplatin (Japan) and lobaplatin (China) are locally registered. Progress in the development of superior analogs requires a thorough understanding of the chemical, biologic, pharmacokinetic, and pharmacodynamic properties of this important class of drugs.

## HISTORY

The realization that platinum complexes exhibited antitumor activity began serendipitously in a series of experiments to investigate the effect of electromagnetic radiation on the growth of bacteria, carried out by Dr. Barnett Rosenberg and colleagues beginning in 1961.[1,2] Exposure of the bacteria to an electric field resulted in a profound change in their morphology; this effect was found not to be from the electric field, but from electrolysis products produced by the platinum electrodes. An analysis of these products resulted in the identification of the cis-isomer of a platinum coordination complex as the active compound. Tests of *cis*-diamminedichloroplatinum (II) in mice bearing several model tumor types indicated that cisplatin exhibited a broad spectrum of antitumor activity. Although early clinical trials demonstrated responses in several tumor types, particularly testicular cancers, the severe renal and gastrointestinal toxicity caused by the drug nearly led to its abandonment. Work at Memorial Sloan-Kettering[3,4] showed that these effects could be ameliorated, in part, by aggressive prehydration, which rekindled interest in its clinical use. Currently, cisplatin is curative in testicular cancer and significantly prolongs survival in combination regimens for ovarian, lung, head and neck, bladder, and upper gastrointestinal (GI) cancers. Its role is being reexamined in other tumors, too, and especially breast cancer.

## PLATINUM CHEMISTRY

Platinum exists primarily in either a 2+ or 4+ oxidation state. These oxidation states dictate the stereochemistry of the ligands surrounding the platinum atom. Platinum (II) compounds exhibit a square planar geometry, in which the ammine ligands (also called carrier groups) are relatively stable, whereas the opposite, more polar ligands (leaving groups) are more easily displaced and

so confer reactivity toward charged macromolecules, including DNA.[5] The stereochemistry of platinum complexes is critical to their antitumor activity as evidenced by the significantly reduced efficacy observed with *trans*-diamminedichloroplatinum (II).

In an aqueous solution, the chloride leaving groups of cisplatin are subject to mono- and diaqua substitution, particularly at chloride concentrations below 100 mmol, which characterize the intracellular environment. The administration of cisplatin in high chloride solutions (normal saline usually), therefore, contributes to stability. Intracellular formation of partially and fully aquated complexes creates the chloroaqua and hydroxoaqua cisplatin species that bind DNA.[6]

## PLATINUM COMPLEXES AFTER CISPLATIN

Early in the clinical development of cisplatin, it became clear that its toxicity was a limitation to its therapeutic effectiveness, and that its activity, although striking in certain diseases, did not extend to all cancers. These observations then motivated a search for structural analogs with less toxicity and a different profile of antitumor activity. In addition, the side effects of cisplatin stimulated the development of antiemetics and other supportive care measures for use with chemotherapy. Progress in understanding the chemistry and pharmacokinetics of cisplatin has guided the development of new analogs. In general, modification of the chloride leaving groups of cisplatin results in compounds with different pharmacokinetics and reactivity towards DNA, whereas modification of the carrier ligands alters the activity of the resulting complex. The features of the more important platinum analogs that have been developed are shown in Figure 18.1.

### Carboplatin

The carboplatin molecule has the same ammine carrier ligands as cisplatin. Using a murine screen for nephrotoxicity, Harrap and Calvert discovered that substituting a cyclobutanedicarboxylate moiety for the two chloride ligands of cisplatin resulted in a complex with reduced renal toxicity. This observation was translated to the clinic in the form of carboplatin, a more stable and pharmacokinetically predictable analog.[7,8] The results in humans were accurately predicted by the animal models, and marrow toxicity rather than nephrotoxicity was the principal side effect. At effective doses, carboplatin produced less nausea, vomiting, nephrotoxicity, and neurotoxicity than cisplatin. Furthermore, the myelosuppression was closely associated with the pharmacokinetics. The work of Calvert et al.[9] and Egorin and colleagues[10] showed that toxicity can be made more predictable and dose intensity less variable by dosing strategies based on the exposure. Carboplatin was shown to be indistinguishable from cisplatin in its clinical activity in all but a handful of tumor types and is the most frequently used form of platinum in current use. Cisplatin and carboplatin have almost superimposable profiles of activity in the NCI60 cell line screen, which further emphasizes the dependence of spectrum of activity on the carrier ligand.

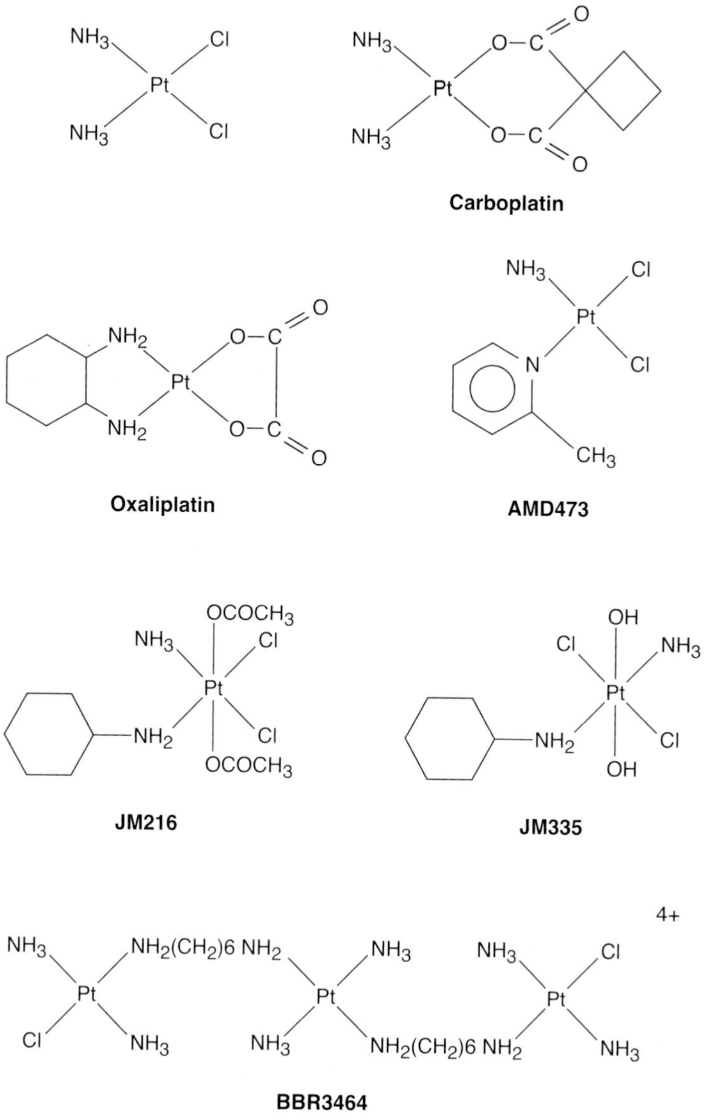

**Carboplatin**

**Nedaplatin**

**Oxaliplatin**

**AMD473**

**Lobaplatin**

**JM216**

**JM335**

4+

**BBR3464**

**Figure 18.1** Structures of cisplatin, analogs, lobaplatin, and nedaplatin.

## Oxaliplatin

Compounds with activity in cisplatin-resistant models emerged from modifications to the carrier group (see left side of the analogs in Fig. 18.1). Connors, in the late 1960s, synthesized platinum coordination compounds with varying physicochemical characteristics and found that the series that possessed a diaminocyclohexane (DACH) carrier group was active in models of cancer in vitro[11] and in vivo.[12] Subsequent studies supported the idea that DACH-based platinum complexes were non–cross-resistant with cisplatin, and DACH derivatives exhibited a unique cytotoxicity profile compared to cisplatin and carboplatin in the National Cancer Institute 60 cell line screen.[13–15] After a number of delays, a DACH analog that had been synthesized by Kidani and colleagues in the early 1970s, was developed in the clinic.[13] Oxaliplatin, a coordination compound of a DACH carrier group and an oxalato leaving group, was active in cisplatin-resistant tumor models. Like cisplatin, oxaliplatin preferentially forms adducts at the N7 position of guanine and, to a lesser extent, adenine. However, there is evidence that the three-dimensional structure of the DNA adducts and biologic response(s) they elicit are different from those of cisplatin. Oxaliplatin demonstrated activity in combination with 5-fluorouracil and leucovorin in colon cancer, a disease that is unresponsive to cisplatin. This finding validated the focus on cisplatin-resistant

preclinical models to identify new active molecules. Oxaliplatin is approved for the treatment of advanced colorectal cancer, and enhances cure rates in the adjuvant setting. The therapeutic role of oxaliplatin has been found to extend to pancreatic, gastric, and esophageal cancers, in all of which it is the more active platinum derivative.

## Nedaplatin and Lobaplatin

Nedaplatin is cis-diammineglycolatoplatinum, developed as a less nephrotoxic second-generation platinum analog, has been shown to be active in a range of tumors similar to that of cisplatin and carboplatin.[16] As a diammine structure, nedaplatin would fall among the cisplatin analogs analyzed in the NCI60 cell line screen,[17] and this activity is therefore anticipated. Lobaplatin is a platinum (II) complex in which the leaving group is lactic acid and the stable ammine ligand is 1,2-bis(aminomethyl)cyclobutane. In a similar way to oxaliplatin the stable ammine ligand may convey some non–cross-resistance compared to cisplatin or carboplatin. It is licensed in China for the breast cancer, small-cell lung cancer, and chronic myelogenous leukemia. It is unique among the platinum drugs for its approval for breast cancer, but there are few published clinical data and no randomized trials. It has not achieved approval in the United States or Europe.

## Newer Platinum Structures

The octahedral stereochemistry adopted by platinum (IV) compounds has led investigators to speculate that they may exhibit a different spectrum of activity than that of platinum (II) drugs. Two compounds that were tested clinically without much success are ormaplatin and iproplatin. Two other platinum (IV) compounds that exhibit novel structural features, satraplatin (previously JM216) and JM335 (*trans*-ammine[cyclohexylamine]dichlorodihydroxo platinum [IV]), underwent more limited development. Satraplatin was the first orally active platinum compound, and showed some activity in lung and ovarian cancers, but despite promising activity in prostate cancer, a phase III trial was not successful.[18,19]

An approach based on the chemistry of the platinum-DNA interaction led to design and synthesis by Farrell et al.[20] of a novel class of compounds containing multiple platinum atoms (see Fig. 18.1). These bi- and trinuclear structures form adducts that span greater distances across the minor groove of DNA and have a profile of cell kill that differs from that of the small molecules. These compounds are unique in that their interaction with DNA is considerably different from that of cisplatin, particularly in the abundance of interstrand cross-links formed. Clinical development of candidate compounds is at a preliminary stage.

Efforts have been made to design novel platinum analogs that can circumvent putative cisplatin resistance mechanisms. An example is *cis*-amminedichloro(2-methylpyridine) platinum (II) (also known as AMD473 and ZD0473). This compound is a sterically hindered platinum complex that was designed to have minimal reactivity with thiols and thus avoid inactivation by molecules such as glutathione.[21,22] Responses were identified with its use in the clinic, but development was curtailed based on low levels of activity. The recent description of a monofunctional platinum (II) analog, phenanthriplatin, from the lab of Lippard is potentially of great interest, based on both potency in vitro and a mechanistic profile different from existing analogs.[23] A renewed appreciation that chemotherapeutic drugs have a continuing role in managing cancer is likely to prompt additional clinical development of novel platinum structures.

## MECHANISM OF ACTION

### DNA Adduct Formation

DNA has long been thought to be the major therapeutic target for platinum compounds. The cytotoxic effects are determined, in part, by the structure and relative amount of DNA adducts formed. Cisplatin and its analogs react preferentially at the N7 position of guanine and adenine residues to form a variety of monofunctional and bifunctional adducts.[24] The monoadducts may form intrastrand or interstrand cross-links. The predominant lesions that are formed when platinum compounds bind DNA are d(GpG)Pt intrastrand cross-links. Cisplatin also forms interstrand cross-links between guanine residues located on opposite strands, and these account for less than 5% of the total DNA-bound platinum. The formation of adducts and cross-links has been associated with therapeutic efficacy.[25,26] These adducts may contribute to the drug's cytotoxicity because they impede certain cellular processes that require the separation of both DNA strands, such as replication and transcription. The adducts formed in the reaction between carboplatin and DNA in cultured cells are essentially the same as those of cisplatin; however, higher concentrations of carboplatin are required (20- to 40-fold for cells) to obtain equivalent total platinum-DNA adduct levels due to its slower rate of aquation.[27] Oxaliplatin intrastrand adducts form even more slowly due to a slower rate of conversion from monoadducts; however, they are formed at similar DNA sequences and regions as cisplatin adducts. At equitoxic doses, oxaliplatin forms fewer DNA adducts than

does cisplatin. This has been interpreted to mean that oxaliplatin lesions are more cytotoxic than those formed by cisplatin.

The differences observed in cytotoxicity between the diammine (e.g., cisplatin, carboplatin) and DACH platinum compounds may not depend on the type and relative amounts of the adducts formed, but on the overall three-dimensional structure of the adduct and its recognition by various cellular proteins. The major difference between them is the protrusion of the DACH moiety of oxaliplatin into the major groove of DNA, which thus produces a bulkier adduct than that of cisplatin. This bulkier, more hydrophobic adduct seems to be recognized differently by cellular proteins involved in sensing DNA damage.[28] The functional consequences are twofold: Proteins such as polymerases that recognize and participate in reactions on DNA under normal circumstances may be perturbed, whereas processes that are controlled by proteins that recognize damaged DNA may become activated (the DNA damage response). The latter group of proteins function both in the DNA repair process and in cellular signaling toward cell survival/death decisions.

### DNA Interstrand Cross-Links

Although the DNA adducts are well-recognized to result in G-G interstrand cross-links, like classical alkylating agents, platinum drugs have the capacity to form intrastrand cross-links, albeit to a lesser degree. By blocking essential aspects of DNA metabolism, such as replication and transcription, intrastrand cross-links are highly cytotoxic. Recent studies have drawn attention both to the cytotoxicity of these lesions, and their differing mechanisms of repair, both replication dependent and independent.[29,30] These studies may have clinical implications in selecting patients for therapy based on the repair competence of tumors.

## CELLULAR RESPONSES TO PLATINUM-INDUCED DNA DAMAGE

Multiple cellular outcomes may follow the formation of platinum-DNA adducts, including cell death by apoptosis, necrosis, or mitotic catastrophe, or cell survival by activation of various protective mechanisms including DNA repair, DNA damage signaling pathways, cell cycle arrest, and autophagy (the last may have a dual role, possibly context dependent).

### Cell Fate

The cellular effects following DNA binding by platinum drugs have been analyzed. The studies of Sorenson and Eastman,[31] using DNA repair-deficient Chinese hamster ovary (CHO) cells, indicated that passage through the S phase is necessary for G2 arrest and cell death, which suggests that DNA replication on a damaged template may result in the accumulation of further damage. An aberrant mitosis was observed before apoptosis in this model.

### DNA Damage Recognition

Among the initiation events that ultimately result in platinum drug–induced cell death are the binding of platinum-DNA damage recognition proteins, which then seed the accumulation of a large protein complex capable both of DNA damage signaling (as to cell cycle proteins to halt replication) and repair of the damaged DNA. Among the DNA-binding proteins are the high-mobility group proteins HMG1 and HMG2.[32–34] These proteins are capable of bending DNA as well as recognizing bent DNA structures, such as that produced by cisplatin, and different specificities for cisplatin and for oxaliplatin adducts are observed in structural studies.[35,36] Other candidate platinum-DNA damage recognition proteins include histone H1, RNA polymerase I transcription upstream binding factor (hUBF), the TATA binding protein (TBP), and proteins involved in mismatch repair (MMR). The MMR complex has been implicated in cisplatin sensitivity.[37] Studies have shown that the MSH2 and MLH1 proteins participate in the recognition of DNA adducts formed by cisplatin, but not oxaliplatin, which could contribute to differences in the cytotoxicity profiles observed between these two platinum complexes.

## DNA Damage Signaling

A number of signaling events have been shown to occur after treatment of cells with platinum drugs.[38] For example, the ATM- and Rad3-related (ATR) proteins that are involved in cell-cycle checkpoint activation are activated by cisplatin. These kinases phosphorylate and activate several downstream effectors that regulate cell cycle, DNA repair, cell survival, and apoptosis, including p53, CHK2, and members of the mitogen-activated protein kinase (MAPK) pathway (extracellular signal-related kinase [ERK], c-Jun amino-terminal kinase [JNK], and p38 kinase). Recent data especially implicate signaling through the JNK pathway, and inhibition at the level of JNK seems especially relevant to platinum drug cytotoxicity in vitro and in vivo.[39,40] The pleiotropic nature of this stress response only grows, because each of these molecules subsequently controls the activity and expression of many more proteins. As a result of this complexity, acting in the context of variable genomic tumor aberrations, therapeutic strategies directed to these pathways have been slow to emerge. However, clinical trials to investigate specific inhibitors of DNA damage responses are underway and hold promise. It is also relevant to point out that these signaling pathways affect not just the tumor cell, but also may communicate to cells in the microenvironment, the responses of which may also determine the effectiveness of therapy.

## IS DNA THE ONLY TARGET?

Early analyses of the action of cytotoxic drugs included a probe of whether effects on DNA were sufficient to explain drug effects. A pioneer in this field was Tritton,[41] who proposed that effects of DNA-intercalating agents on the plasma membrane could underlie the cytotoxicity of the drug. More recently, enucleated cells were shown to be susceptible to cisplatin, and a seminal paper from Voest and colleagues showed that platinum sensitivity was determined not solely by the accumulation of DNA damage in the tumor cell.[42] In analyzing the contribution of cells in the microenvironment of tumors, he showed that tumor infiltration with mesenchymal stem cells could confer drug resistance. A search for secreted factors defined platinum-induced fatty acids, metabolic products in the thromboxane synthetase, and cyclooxygenase-1 pathways as determining the effectiveness of drug therapy. A proteomic study in cisplatin-sensitive and -resistant cells confirmed the substantial effects of drug exposure on lipid metabolites and their relation to susceptibility. A current focus on therapies

directed to the microenvironment, including immunologic and anti-inflammatory interventions,[43] has the potential to expand our ability to apply platinum drugs in the clinic.

## MECHANISMS OF RESISTANCE

The major limitation to the successful treatment of solid tumors with platinum-based chemotherapy is the emergence of drug-resistant tumor cells.[44] Developments in tumor biology have advanced our thinking with regard to how and when these cells emerge; heterogeneity within a tumor even at its earliest diagnosis reflects the emergence of treatment-resistant clones even in advance of selection pressure and the realization that resistance may not be specific to the DNA-damaging drug. Indeed, this may be reflected clinically in the finding that after progression on initial chemotherapy, the use of second-line therapy is usually associated with a shorter duration of response.

Currently described mechanisms of platinum drug resistance (Fig. 18.2) include reduced cellular accumulation, intracellular detoxification, repair of Pt-DNA lesions, increased damage tolerance, and the activation of cellular defense mechanisms such as autophagy. In addition, we have already alluded to exogenous influences on mechanism, as may be mediated by other cells, metabolites, of physicochemical conditions (such as hypoxia) in the tumor microenvironment. It must be acknowledged, however, that our insights are very limited as to why some tumors respond and others do not to platinum chemotherapy. As genome sequencing yields increasing and often surprising revelations about the genes that drive cancers and the complexity inherent in cancers of a single histologic type, it is likely that when associated with outcomes in large patient populations, patterns will emerge to guide selection of therapies.

### Reduced Accumulation

Platinum uptake in cells occurs by simple diffusion and by carrier-mediated mechanisms. Inhibition of transport mechanisms has a marked effect on intracellular platinum accumulation, and Howell's group has shown the importance of the copper transporters CTR-1 and CTR-2 in regulating the influx of various platinum analogs in eukaryotic cells.[45,46] The contribution of these mechanisms to clinical platinum drug resistance is being explored.[47] Accumulation may also be influenced by enhanced efflux, and various transport proteins are upregulated in cell lines selected for acquired resistance, and in platinum-resistant ovarian cancers.

### Inactivation

Platinum complexes are highly reactive molecules and bind rapidly to multiple cellular macromolecules. Protection from such chemicals in the environment is afforded by cellular thiols, including

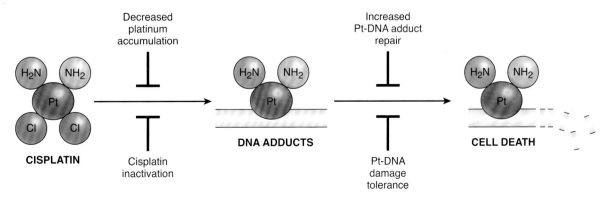

**Figure 18.2** Cellular mechanisms of cisplatin resistance.

small peptides such as glutathione (GSH) and larger proteins as exemplified by metallothionein (MT). There are many reports of an association between platinum drug sensitivity and glutathione levels[48–50]; however, reducing intracellular glutathione levels with drugs such as buthionine sulfoximine has resulted in only low to modest potentiation of cisplatin sensitivity.[51] Buthionine sulfoximine was developed for clinical use, and some impact on GSH content of tumors and normal tissues was demonstrated. However, the depletion of GSH was not consistent, and ultimately, the cost of producing the active stereoisomer of the drug was judged prohibitive. Inactivation of the platinum drugs may also occur through binding to the MTs, a family of sulfhydryl-rich, low–molecular-weight proteins that participate in heavy metal binding and detoxification; however, the contribution of MT to clinical platinum drug resistance is unclear, and a therapeutic role has not emerged.

## Increased DNA Repair

Once platinum-DNA adducts are formed, cells must either repair or tolerate the damage to survive. In general, the capacity to repair DNA damage seems to play a role in determining a tumor cell's sensitivity to platinum drugs and other DNA-damaging agents. For example, tumors that are unusually sensitive to cisplatin, such as testicular nonseminomatous germ cell tumors, may be deficient in their ability to repair platinum-DNA adducts.[52] The increased repair of platinum-DNA lesions in cisplatin-resistant cell lines as compared to their sensitive counterparts has been shown in several human cancer cell lines, but translation of these observations to the clinic has been difficult. The repair of platinum-DNA adducts appears to occur predominantly by nucleotide excision repair (NER), with a role for MMR under certain circumstances.[53] The molecular basis for the increased repair activity observed in cisplatin-resistant cells is not known precisely, but formation of the ERCC1/XPF protein complex may be a key step. Selvakumaran et al.[54] showed that the downregulation of ERCC-1 using an antisense approach sensitized a platinum-resistant cell line to cisplatin both in vitro and in vivo. There is substantial clinical evidence that implicates *ERCC1* expression in increased NER and cisplatin resistance, and high expression of ERCC1 has been demonstrated to confer a worse outcome after cisplatin treatment in several resistant tumors. The most extensive study of this as a marker has been in non–small-cell lung cancer, results in which were summarized and analyzed by Hubner et al.[55] In gastric cancer also, high levels of ERCC1 are associated with resistance to cisplatin treatment.[56–58] However, a recent reevaluation of discrepant results questioned the reliability of the assays of ERCC1 and their relationship to function.[59] These data suggest that there is a relationship between ERCC1 expression and treatment, but that the lag in marker development precludes implementation of a predictive assay until additional studies have been performed.

Perhaps the most striking evidence that DNA repair is a determinant of platinum drug responses is that breast and ovarian cancers occurring in BRCA1 or BRCA2 mutation carriers are particularly responsive to cisplatin or carboplatin. These cancers are also sensitive to inhibitors of poly(ADP-ribose)polymerase (PARPi), several of which are currently in clinical development. The mechanism of the sensitivity to PARPi has been elucidated. Both the BRCA1 and 2 proteins for part of the homologous recombination repair (HR) system that achieves error-free repair of double strand breaks. Carriers are heterozygous and, therefore, have normal repair function, but loss of the second allele leads to the use of error-prone backup systems and is therefore oncogenic. The cancers that arise are unable to perform HR and, therefore, are sensitive to drugs that induce single strand breaks, such as PARPi.[60,61] A mechanism of resistance to PARPi has been described, which is due to reactivation of the function of the BRCA2 leading to restoration of HR and sensitivity to PARPi.[62] This reactivation is accomplished by an intragenic deletion and the restoration of an open reading frame.

It has further been shown that such revertant cells are resistant to cisplatin as well as PARPi. Finally, recurrent cancers in BRCA2 mutation carriers, which have acquired platinum resistance, have been shown to have undergone reversion of the BRCA2 mutation.[63] This clearly shows that the HR system can be one cause of cisplatin resistance. However, not all cisplatin-resistant patients are also resistant to PARPi,[64] showing that there are multiple other causes of cis/carboplatin resistance.

Combinations of platinum drugs with PARPi are being actively pursued in patients with BRCA-related tumors and also in patients whose tumors are likely to have acquired loss of HR function (poorly differentiated serous ovarian cancer and triple negative breast cancer).

## Autophagy

After platinum-DNA adduct formation, the cell detects the DNA damage and initiates signaling through multiple pathways, the effects of which include mobilization of repair proteins; arrest of the cell cycle; altered transcriptional programs; redirection of energy production and consumption; activation of cell death pathways and, simultaneously, of pathways that would counter a cell death decision, and so to permit survival. A process recently characterized to perform the last function is autophagy. Initially described as a mechanism of cell death, autophagy represents a regulated dissolution of cellular elements into a characteristic set of subcellular organelles detectable by electron microscopy and linked by a particular profile of gene expression changes.[65] Multiple stimuli precipitate these changes and have in common scarcity of nutrients that are required for survival, from oxygen and glucose withdrawal to less specific calorie deprivation, and inhibition of metabolic pathways. Autophagy is also a consequence of cytotoxic drug treatment and, more recently, has been appreciated as a means by which cells might survive the stress of cellular insults, and so become resistant to treatment.[66] Amaravadi and colleagues[67] demonstrated that autophagy reversal can sensitize tumors to cytotoxic drugs and several trials of platinum compounds along with the autophagy inhibitor hydroxychloroquine are in progress.

## Increased DNA Damage Tolerance

The net result of DNA damage signaling in a sensitive tumor cell is engagement of cell death pathways, including apoptosis, and therapeutic benefit. In a resistant tumor cell, the cell survives as a consequence of one or many of these mechanisms, and this can result in platinum-DNA damage tolerance or multidrug resistance phenotype, or both. Contributors to the tolerance might include deficient DNA MMR (which could excise the adduct if NER failed), enhanced replicative bypass (which essentially ignores the adduct, allowing the cell to survive, but could contribute to the increase in mutation frequency observed in chemotherapy-treated cancers), and altered signaling through stress-related kinases such as JNK, which can both alter transcriptional programs and activate autophagy. Indeed JNK, by phosphorylating Bcl-2 or Bcl-XL, and releasing beclin-1 from inhibition, acts as a key switch to turn on autophagy. The enhanced DNA damage tolerance, in addition to permitting persistence of the cancer cell, may have an additional deleterious effect by fostering further mutagenesis within the tumor, facilitating its evolution to a more malignant phenotype.

# CLINICAL PHARMACOLOGY

## Pharmacokinetics

The pharmacokinetic differences observed between platinum drugs may be attributed to the structure of their leaving groups. Platinum complexes containing leaving groups that are less easily displaced exhibit reduced plasma protein binding, longer plasma half-lives, and higher rates of renal clearance. These features are

**TABLE 18.1**

**Comparative Parmacokinetics of Platinum Analogs After Bolus or Short Intravenous Infusion**

| | Cisplatin | Carboplatin | Oxaliplatin |
|---|---|---|---|
| $T_{1/2}\alpha$ | | | |
|   Total platinum | 14–49 min | 12–98 min | 26 min |
|   Ultrafiltrate | 9–30 min | 8–87 min | 21 min |
| $T_{1/2}\beta$ | | | |
|   Total platinum | 0.7–4.6 h | 1.3–1.7 h | — |
|   Ultrafiltrate | 0.7–0.8 h | 1.7–5.9 h | — |
| $T_{1/2}\gamma$ | | | |
|   Total platinum | 24–127 h | 8.2–40.0 h | 38–47 h |
|   Ultrafiltrate | — | — | 24–27 h |
| Protein binding | >90% | 24%–50% | 85% |
| Urinary excretion | 23%–50% | 54%–82% | >50% |

$T_{1/2}\alpha$, half-life of first phase; $T_{1/2}\beta$, half-life of second phase; $T_{1/2}\gamma$, half-life of terminal phase.

evident in the pharmacokinetic properties of cisplatin, carboplatin, and oxaliplatin, which are summarized in Table 18.1. Platinum drug pharmacokinetics have been reviewed.[68]

## Cisplatin

After intravenous infusion, cisplatin rapidly diffuses into tissues and is covalently bound to plasma protein. More than 90% of platinum is bound to plasma protein at 4 hours after infusion. The disappearance of ultrafilterable platinum is rapid and occurs in a biphasic fashion. Half-lives of 10 to 30 minutes and 0.7 to 0.8 hours have been reported for the initial and terminal phases, respectively. Cisplatin excretion is dependent on renal function, which accounts for the majority of its elimination. The percentage of platinum excreted in the urine has been reported to be between 23% and 40% at 24 hours after infusion. Only a small percentage of the total platinum is excreted in the bile.

## Carboplatin

The differences in pharmacokinetics observed between cisplatin and carboplatin depend primarily on the slower rate of conversion of carboplatin to a reactive species. Thus, the stability of carboplatin results in a low incidence of nephrotoxicity. Carboplatin diffuses rapidly into tissues after infusion; however, it is considerably more stable in plasma. Only 24% of a dose was bound to plasma protein at 4 hours after infusion. The disappearance of platinum from plasma after short intravenous infusions of carboplatin has been reported to occur in a biphasic or triphasic manner. The initial half-lives for total platinum, which vary considerably among several studies, are listed in Table 18.1. The half-lives for total platinum range from 12 to 98 minutes during the first phase ($T_{1/2}\alpha$) and from 1.3 to 1.7 hours during the second phase ($T_{1/2}\beta$). Half-lives reported for the terminal phase range from 8.2 to 40 hours. The disappearance of ultrafilterable platinum is biphasic with $T_{1/2}\alpha$ and $T_{1/2}\beta$ values ranging from 7.6 to 87 minutes and 1.7 to 5.9 hours, respectively. Carboplatin is excreted predominantly by the kidneys, and cumulative urinary excretion of platinum is 54% to 82%, most as unmodified carboplatin. The renal clearance of carboplatin is closely correlated with the glomerular filtration rate (GFR).[69] This observation enabled Calvert et al.[9] to design a carboplatin-dosing formula based on the individual patient's GFR.

## Oxaliplatin

After oxaliplatin infusion, platinum accumulates into three compartments: plasma-bound platinum, ultrafilterable platinum, and platinum associated with erythrocytes. When specific and sensitive mass spectrometric techniques are used, oxaliplatin itself is undetectable in plasma, even at end infusion.[70] The active forms of the drug have not been extensively characterized. Approximately 85% of the total platinum is bound to plasma protein at 2 to 5 hours after infusion.[71] Plasma elimination of total platinum and ultrafilterates is biphasic. The half-lives for the initial and terminal phases are 26 minutes and 38.7 hours, respectively, for total platinum and 21 minutes and 24.2 hours, respectively, for ultrafilterable platinum (see Table 18.1).[72] Thus, as with carboplatin, substantial differences between total and free platinum kinetics are not observed. As with cisplatin, a prolonged retention of oxaliplatin is observed in red blood cells. However, unlike cisplatin, oxaliplatin does not accumulate to any significant level after multiple courses of treatment.[71] This may explain why neurotoxicity associated with oxaliplatin is reversible. Oxaliplatin is eliminated predominantly by the kidneys, with more than 50% of the platinum being excreted in the urine at 48 hours.

## Pharmacodynamics

Pharmacodynamics relates pharmacokinetic indices of drug exposure to biologic measures of drug effect, usually toxicity to normal tissues or tumor cell kill. Two issues to be addressed in such studies are whether the effectiveness of the drug can be enhanced and whether the toxicity can be attenuated by knowledge of the platinum pharmacokinetics in an individual. These questions are appropriate to the use of cytotoxic agents with relatively narrow therapeutic indices. Toxicity to normal tissues can be quantitated as a continuous variable when the drug causes myelosuppression. Thus, the early studies of carboplatin demonstrated a close relationship of changes in platelet counts to the area under the concentration-time curve (AUC) in the individual. The AUC was itself closely related to renal function, which was determined as creatinine clearance. Based on these observations, Egorin et al.,[10] Calvert et al.,[9] and Chatelut and colleagues[73] derived formulas based on creatinine clearance to predict either the percentage change in platelet count or a target AUC. Application of pharmacodynamically guided dosing algorithms for carboplatin has been widely adopted as a means of avoiding overdosage (by producing acceptable nadir platelet counts) and of maximizing dose intensity in the individual. There is good evidence that this approach can decrease the risk of unacceptable toxicity. Accordingly, a dosing strategy based on renal function is recommended for the use of carboplatin.

A key question is whether maximizing carboplatin exposure in an individual can measurably increase the probability of tumor regression or survival. In an analysis by Jodrell et al.,[74] carboplatin AUC was a predictor of response, thrombocytopenia, and leukopenia. The likelihood of a tumor response increased with increasing AUC up to a level of 5 to 7 mg × hour per milliliter, after which a plateau was reached. Similar results were obtained with carboplatin in combination with cyclophosphamide, and neither response rate nor survival was determined by the carboplatin AUC in a cohort of ovarian cancer patients.[75] As a result, most carboplatin recommended doses are based on an AUC in this range (for every 3 to 4 week schedules), and modifications of these are used for more frequent administration (as in combined chemoradiotherapy regimens).

The relationship of pharmacokinetics to response has been sought by investigating the cellular pharmacology of these agents.[76] The formation and repair of the platinum-DNA adducts in human cells are not easily measured. Schellens and colleagues[77,78] analyzed the pharmacokinetic and pharmacodynamic interactions of cisplatin administered as a single agent. In a series of patients with head and neck cancer, they found that cisplatin exposure (measured as the AUC) closely correlated with both the peak DNA adduct content in leukocytes and the area under the DNA-adduct time curve. These measures were important predictors of response, both individually and in logistic regression analysis. However, as an approach to determine who should or should not be treated with platinum drugs, it seems more likely that genomic analyses will provide guidance in the near future.

## Pharmacogenomics

Variability in pharmacokinetics and pharmacodynamics of cytotoxic drugs is an important determinant of therapeutic index. This interindividual variation may be attributed in part to genetic differences among patients. Targeted analyses of germ-line DNA and, increasingly, Genome-wide association studies (GWAS) approaches, have yielded genotypic features associated with results of therapy. Detoxification pathways and DNA repair have emerged as having markers attributable to response of lack of it in response to platinum drugs. Single nucleotide polymorphisms (SNP) in genes related to glutathione metabolism and in several DNA repair genes have been identified in lung cancer, breast cancer, and various GI cancers. A concern is that larger trials have not always confirmed early findings. As yet, informative SNPs that could be used to define therapeutic strategies for individual patients have not yet been defined.

## FORMULATION AND ADMINISTRATION

### Cisplatin (Platinol)

Cisplatin is administered in a chloride-containing solution intravenously over 0.5 to 2.0 hours. To minimize the risk of nephrotoxicity, patients are prehydrated with at least 500 mL of salt-containing fluid. Immediately before cisplatin administration, mannitol (12.5 to 25.0 g) is given parenterally to maximize urine flow. A diuretic such as furosemide may be used also, along with parenteral antiemetics. These currently include dexamethasone together with a 5-hydroxytryptamine (5-HT$_3$) antagonist. A minimum of 1 L of posthydration fluid is usually given. The intensity of hydration varies somewhat with the dose of cisplatin. High-dose cisplatin (up to 200 mg/m$^2$ per course) may be administered in a formulation containing 3% sodium chloride, but this method is no longer widely used. Cisplatin may also be administered regionally to increase local drug exposure and diminish side effects. Its intraperitoneal use was defined by Ozols et al.[79] and by Howell and colleagues.[80] Measured drug exposure in the peritoneal cavity is some 50-fold higher compared to levels achieved with intravenous administration. At standard dosages in ovarian cancer patients with low-volume disease, a randomized intergroup trial suggested that intraperitoneal administration is superior to intravenous cisplatin in combination with intravenous cyclophosphamide.[81] The development of combinations of carboplatin and paclitaxel has, however, superseded this technique in the treatment of ovarian cancer, and the intraperitoneal route is now infrequently used. Regional uses also include intra-arterial delivery (as for hepatic tumors, melanoma, and glioblastoma), but none have been adopted as a standard method of treatment. There is growing interest in chemoembolization for the treatment of tumors confined to the liver, and cisplatin is a component of many popular regimens.[82]

### Carboplatin (Paraplatin)

Cisplatin treatment over 3 to 6 hours is burdensome for clinical resources and tiring for cancer patients. Previously given as an in-hospital treatment, it is now usually administered in the outpatient setting. The exigencies of the modern health-care environment have contributed to the expanding use of carboplatin as an alternative to cisplatin except in circumstances in which cisplatin is clearly the superior agent. Carboplatin is substantially easier to administer. Extensive hydration is not required because of the lack of nephrotoxicity at standard dosages. Carboplatin is reconstituted

in chloride-free solutions (unlike cisplatin, because chloride can displace the leaving groups) and administered over 30 minutes as a rapid intravenous infusion.

### Oxaliplatin (Eloxatin)

Oxaliplatin is also uncomplicated in its clinical administration. For bolus infusion, the required dose is administered in 500 mL of chloride-free diluent over a period of 2 hours. Oxaliplatin is most frequently given as a single dose every 2 weeks (85 mg/m$^2$) or every 3 weeks (130 mg/m$^2$), alone or with other active agents. It is common to pretreat patients with active antiemetics, such as a 5-HT$_3$ antagonist, but the nausea is not as severe as with cisplatin. No prehydration is required. Besides a relatively low incidence of myelosuppression, the predominant toxicity of oxaliplatin is cumulative neurotoxicity. The development of an oropharyngeal dysesthesia, often precipitated by exposure to cold, may require prolonging the duration of administration to 6 hours. On occasion, the occurrence of hypersensitivity also requires slowing the infusion.

## TOXICITY

A substantial body of literature documents the side effects of platinum compounds. As noted in the section titled History, earlier in this chapter, the toxicity of cisplatin was a driving force both in the search for less toxic analogs and for more effective treatments for its side effects, especially nausea and vomiting. The toxicities associated with cisplatin, carboplatin, and oxaliplatin are described in detail in the following sections and summarized in Table 18.2. Please review the package inserts for these drugs for full prescribing information and delineation of toxic effects.

### Cisplatin

The side effects associated with cisplatin (at single doses of more than 50 mg/m$^2$) include nausea and vomiting, nephrotoxicity, ototoxicity, neuropathy, and myelosuppression. Rare effects include visual impairment, seizures, arrhythmias, acute ischemic vascular events, glucose intolerance, and pancreatitis. The nausea and vomiting stimulated a search for new antiemetics. These effects are currently best managed with 5-HT$_3$ antagonists, usually given with a glucocorticoid, although other combinations of agents are still widely used. In the weeks after treatment, continuous antiemetic therapy may be required. Nephrotoxicity is ameliorated but not completely prevented by hydration. The renal damage to both glomeruli and tubules is cumulative, and after cisplatin treatment, serum creatinine levels are no longer a reliable guide to GFR. An acute elevation of serum creatinine level may follow a cisplatin dose, but this index returns to normal with time. Tubule damage may be reflected in a salt-losing syndrome that also resolves with time.

Ototoxicity is a cumulative and irreversible side effect of cisplatin treatment that results from damage to the inner ear. The initial audiographic manifestation is loss of high-frequency acuity (4,000 to 8,000 Hz). When acuity is affected in the range of speech, cisplatin

| **TABLE 18.2** | | | |
|---|---|---|---|
| **Toxicity Profiles of Platinum Analogs in Clinical Use** | | | |
| **Toxicity** | **Cisplatin** | **Carboplatin** | **Oxaliplatin** |
| Myelosuppression | | X | |
| Nephrotoxicity | X | | |
| Neurotoxicity | X | | X |
| Ototoxicity | X | | |
| Nausea and vomiting | X | X | X |

should be discontinued under most circumstances and carboplatin substituted where appropriate. Peripheral neuropathy is also cumulative, although less common than with agents such as vinca alkaloids. This neuropathy is usually reversible, although recovery is often slow. A number of agents with the potential for protection from neuropathy have been developed, but none is yet used widely.

## Carboplatin

Myelosuppression, which is not usually severe with cisplatin, is the dose-limiting toxicity of carboplatin. The drug is most toxic to the platelet precursors, but neutropenia and anemia are frequently observed. The lowest platelet counts after a single dose of carboplatin are observed 17 to 21 days later, and recovery usually occurs by day 28. The effect is dose dependent, but individuals vary widely in their susceptibility. As shown by Egorin et al.[10] and Calvert et al.,[9] the severity of platelet toxicity is best accounted for by a measure of the drug exposure in an individual, the AUC. Both groups derived pharmacologically based formulas to predict toxicity and guide carboplatin dosing. That of Calvert and colleagues targets a particular exposure to carboplatin:

$$\text{Dose (mg)} = \text{target AUC (mg} \cdot \text{min/mL)} \times \text{(GFR mL/min} + 25)$$

This formula has been widely used to individualize carboplatin dosing and permits targeting an acceptable level of toxicity. Patients who are elderly, have a poor performance status, or have a history of extensive pretreatment have a higher risk of toxicity even when dosage is calculated with these methods, but the safety of drug administration has been enhanced. In the combination of carboplatin and paclitaxel, AUC-based dosing has helped to maximize the dose intensity of carboplatin. Dosages some 30% higher than those using a dosing strategy based solely on body surface area may safely be used. A determination of whether this approach to dosing improves outcomes will require a randomized trial.

The other toxicities of carboplatin are generally milder and better tolerated than those of cisplatin. Nausea and vomiting, although frequent, are less severe, shorter in duration, and more easily controlled with standard antiemetics (i.e., prochlorperazine [Compazine]), dexamethasone, lorazepam) than that after cisplatin treatment. Renal impairment is infrequent, although alopecia is common, especially with the paclitaxel-containing combinations. Neurotoxicity is also less common than with cisplatin, although it

is observed more frequently with the increasing use of high-dose regimens. Ototoxicity is also less common.

## Oxaliplatin

The dose-limiting toxicity of oxaliplatin is sensory neuropathy, a characteristic of all DACH-containing platinum derivatives. This side effect takes two forms. First, a tingling of the extremities, which may also involve the perioral region, that occurs early and usually resolves within a few days. With repeated dosing, symptoms may last longer between cycles, but do not appear to be cumulative or of long duration. Laryngopharyngeal spasms and cold dysesthesias have also been reported but are not associated with significant respiratory symptoms and can be prevented by prolonging the duration of infusion. A second neuropathy, more typical of that seen with cisplatin, affects the extremities and increases with repeated doses. Definitive physiologic characterization of oxaliplatin-induced neuropathy has proven difficult in large studies. Electromyograms performed in six patients treated by Extra et al.[83] revealed an axonal sensory neuropathy, but nerve conduction velocities were unchanged. Specimens from peripheral nerve biopsies performed in this study showed decreased myelination and replacement with collagen pockets. The neurologic effects of oxaliplatin appear to be cumulative in that they become more pronounced and of greater duration with successive cycles; however, unlike those of cisplatin, they are reversible with drug cessation. In a review of 682 patient experiences, Brienza et al.[84] reported that 82% of patients who experienced grade 2 neurotoxicity or higher had their symptoms regress within 4 to 6 months. In a larger adjuvant trial, de Gramont et al.[85] reported that 12% of patients had grade 3 toxicity at the end of a 6-month treatment period and that the majority of these patients had relief, but not always complete resolution of the symptoms, by 1 year later. The persistence of the neurotoxicity has led to approaches to ameliorate it, including the use of protective agents. The use of calcium and magnesium salts intravenously before and after each infusion has been shown to be ineffective. Ototoxicity is not observed with oxaliplatin. Nausea and vomiting do occur and generally respond to 5-HT$_3$ antagonists. Myelosuppression is uncommon and is not severe with oxaliplatin as a single agent, but it is a feature of combinations including this drug. Oxaliplatin therapy is not associated with nephrotoxicity.

## REFERENCES

1. Rosenberg B, VanCamp L, Trosko J, et al. Platinum compounds: a new class of potent antitumor agents. *Nature* 1969;222:385–386.
2. Rosenberg B. Fundamental studies with cisplatin. *Cancer* 1985;55:2303–2316.
3. Cvitkovic E, Spaulding J, Bethune V, et al. Improvement of cis-dichlorodiammineplatinum (NSC 119875): therapeutic index in an animal model. *Cancer* 1977;39:1357–1361.
4. Hayes D, Cvitkovic E, Golbey R, et al. High dose cis-platinum diamine dichloride: amelioration of renal toxicity by mannitol diuresis. *Cancer* 1977;39:1372–1381.
5. Roberts J, Thomson A. The mechanism of action of antitumor platinum compounds. *Nucleic Acids Res* 1979;22:71–133.
6. Martin R. Platinum complexes: hydrolysis and binding to N(7) and N(1) of purines. In: Lippert B, ed. *Cisplatin: Chemistry and Biochemistry of a Leading Anticancer Drug.* Zurich: Verlag Helvetica Chimica Acta; 1999:183.
7. Harrap K. Preclinical studies identifying carboplatin as a viable cisplatin alternative. *Cancer Treat Rev* 1985;12:A21–A33.
8. Harrap K. Initiatives with platinum- and quinazoline-based antitumor molecules—Fourteenth Bruce F. Cain Memorial Award Lecture. *Cancer Res* 1995;55:2761–2768.
9. Calvert A, Newell D, Gumbrell L, et al. Carboplatin dosage: prospective evaluation of a simple formula based on renal function. *J Clin Oncol* 1989;7:1748–1756.
10. Egorin M, Echo DV, Olman E, et al. Prospective validation of a pharmacologically based dosing scheme for the cis-diamminedichloroplatinum(II) analogue diamminecyclobutanedicarboxylatoplatinum. *Cancer Res* 1985;45:6502–6506.
11. Connors T, Jones M, Ross W, et al. New platinum complexes with anti-tumour activity. *Chem Biol Interact* 1972;5:415–424.
12. Burchenal J, Kalaker K, Dew K, et al. Rationale for development of platinum analogs. *Cancer Treat Rep* 1979;63:1493–1498.
13. Kidani Y, Inagaki K, Tsukagoshi S. Examination of antitumor activities of platinum complexes of 1,2-diaminocyclohexane isomers and their related complexes. *Gann* 1976;67:921–922.
14. Burchenal J, Irani G, Kern K, et al. 1,2-Diaminocyclohexane platinum derivatives of potential clinical value. *Rec Res Cancer Res* 1980;74:146–155.
15. Rixe O, Ortuzar W, Alvarez M, et al. Oxaliplatin, tetraplatin, cisplatin, and carboplatin: spectrum of activity in drug-resistant cell lines and in the cell lines of the National Cancer Institute's anticancer drug screen panel. *Biochem Pharmacol* 1996;52:1855–1865.
16. Shimada M, Itamochi H, Kigawa J. Nedaplatin: a cisplatin derivative in cancer therapy. *Cancer Manag Res* 2013;5:67–76.
17. Fojo T, Farrell N, Ortuzar W, et al. Identification of non-cross-resistant platinum compounds with novel cytotoxicity profiles using the NCI anticancer drug screen and clustered image map visualizations. *Crit Rev Oncol Hematol* 2005;53:25–34.
18. Bates SE, Amiri-Kordestani L, Giaccone G. Drug development: portals of discovery. *Clin Cancer Res* 2012;18:23–32.
19. Kelland L. The development of orally active platinum drugs. In: Lippert B, ed. *Cisplatin: Chemistry and Biochemistry of a Leading Anticancer Drug.* Zurich: Verlag Helvetica Chimica Acta; 1999:497.
20. Farrell N, Qu Y, Bierbach U, et al. Structure-activity relationships within di- and trinuclear platinum phase-I clinical anticancer agents. In: Lippert B, ed. *Cisplatin: Chemistry and Biochemistry of a Leading Anticancer Drug.* Zurich: Verlag Helvetica Chimica Acta; 1999:477–496.
21. Holford J, Sharp S, Murrer B, et al. In vitro circumvention of cisplatin resistance by the novel sterically hindered platinum complex AMD473. *Br J Cancer* 1998;77:366–373.
22. Flaherty KT, Stevenson JP, Redlinger M, et al. A phase I, dose escalation trial of ZD0473, a novel platinum analogue, in combination with gemcitabine. *Cancer Chemother Pharmacol* 2004;53:404–408.
23. Park GY, Wilson JJ, Song Y, et al. Phenanthriplatin, a monofunctional DNA-binding platinum anticancer drug candidate with unusual potency and cellular activity profile. *Proc Natl Acad Sci U S A* 2012;109:11987–11992.

24. Eastman A. The formation, isolation and characterization of DNA adducts produced by anticancer platinum complexes. *Pharmacol Ther* 1987;34:155–166.

25. Zhu G, Song L, Lippard SJ. Visualizing inhibition of nucleosome mobility and transcription by cisplatin-DNA interstrand crosslinks in live mammalian cells. *Cancer Res* 2013;73:4451–4460.

26. Martens-de Kemp SR, Dalm SU, Wijnolts FM, et al. DNA-bound platinum is the major determinant of cisplatin sensitivity in head and neck squamous carcinoma cells. *PLoS One* 2013;8:e61555.

27. Blommaert F, van Kijk-Knijnenburg H, Dijt F, et al. Formation of DNA adducts by the anticancer drug carboplatin: different nucleotide sequence preferences in vitro and in cells. *Biochemistry* 1995;34:8474–8480.

28. Scheef E, Briggs J, Howell S. Molecular modeling of the intrastrand guanine-guanine DNA adducts produced by cisplatin and oxaliplatin. *Mol Pharmacol* 1999;56:633–643.

29. Enoiu M, Jiricny J, Schärer OD. Repair of cisplatin-induced DNA interstrand crosslinks by a replication-independent pathway involving transcription-coupled repair and translesion synthesis. *Nucleic Acids Res* 2012;40:8953–8964.

30. Zhu G, Song L, Lippard SJ. Visualizing inhibition of nucleosome mobility and transcription by cisplatin-DNA interstrand crosslinks in live mammalian cells. *Cancer Res* 2013;73:4451–4460.

31. Sorenson C, Eastman A. Mechanism of cis-diamminedichloroplatinum (II)-induced cytotoxicity: role of G2 arrest and DNA double-strand breaks. *Cancer Res* 1988;48:4484–4488.

32. Toney J, Donahue B, Kellett P, et al. Isolation of cDNAs encoding a human protein that binds selectively to DNA modified by the anticancer drug cis-diamminedichloroplatinum. *Proc Natl Acad Sci U S A* 1989;86:8328–8332.

33. Bruhn S, Pil P, Essigmann J, et al. Isolation and characterization of human cDNA clones encoding a high mobility group box protein that recognizes structural distortions to DNA caused by binding of the anticancer agent cisplatin. *Proc Natl Acad Sci U S A* 1989;89:2307–2311.

34. Hughes EN, Engelsberg BN, Billings PC. Purification of nuclear proteins that bind to cisplatin-damaged DNA. Identity with high mobility group proteins 1 and 2. *J Biol Chem* 1992;267:13520–13527.

35. Ramachandran S, Temple BR, Chaney SG, et al. Structural basis for the sequence-dependent effects of platinum-DNA adducts. *Nucleic Acids Res* 2009;37:2434–2448.

36. Ramachandran S, Temple B, Alexandrova AN, et al. Recognition of platinum-DNA adducts by HMGB1a. *Biochemistry* 2012;51:7608–7617.

37. Fink D, Zheng H, Nebel S, et al. In vitro and in vivo resistance to cisplatin in cells that have lost DNA mismatch repair. *Cancer Res* 1997;57:1841–1845.

38. Kelland L. The resurgence of platinum-based cancer chemotherapy. *Nat Rev Cancer* 2007;7:573–584.

39. Vasilevskaya IA, Rakitina TV, O'Dwyer PJ. Quantitative effects on c-Jun N-terminal protein kinase signaling determine synergistic interaction of cisplatin and 17-allylamino-17-demethoxygeldanamycin in colon cancer cell lines. *Mol Pharmacol* 2004;65:235–243.

40. Vasilevskaya IA, Selvakumaran M, O'Dwyer PJ. Disruption of signaling through SEK1 and MKK7 yields differential responses in hypoxic colon cancer cells treated with oxaliplatin. *Mol Pharmacol* 2008;74:246–254.

41. Maestre N, Tritton TR, Laurent G, et al. Cell surface-directed interaction of anthracyclines leads to cytotoxicity and nuclear factor kappaB activation but not apoptosis signaling. *Cancer Res* 2001;61:2558–2561.

42. Roodhart JM, Daenen LG, Stigter EC, et al. Mesenchymal stem cells induce resistance to chemotherapy through the release of platinum-induced fatty acids. *Cancer Cell* 2011;20:370–383.

43. Beatty GL, Chiorean EG, Fishman MP, et al. CD40 regulates cancer inflammation and induces regression of pancreatic carcinoma in mice and humans. *Science* 2011;331:1612–1616.

44. Galluzzi L, Senovilla L, Vitale I, et al. Molecular mechanisms of cisplatin resistance. *Oncogene* 2012;31:1869–1883.

45. Lin X, Okuda T, Holzer A, et al. The copper transporter CTR1 regulates cisplatin uptake in Saccharomyces cerevisiae. *Mol Pharmacol* 2002;62:1154–1159.

46. Blair BG, Larson CA, Safaei R, et al. Copper transporter 2 regulates the cellular accumulation and cytotoxicity of cisplatin and carboplatin. *Clin Cancer Res* 2009;15:4312–4321.

47. Samimi G, Varki NM, Wilczynski S, et al. Increase in the expression of the copper transporter ATP7A during platinum drug-based treatment is associated with poor survival in ovarian cancer patients. *Clin Cancer Res* 2003;9:5853–5859.

48. Britten RA, Green JA, Broughton C, et al. The relationship between nuclear glutathione levels and resistance to melphalan in human ovarian tumour cells. *Biochem Pharmacol* 1991;41:647–649.

49. Mistry P, Kelland L, Abel G, et al. The relationships between glutathione, glutathione-S-transferase and cytotoxicity of platinum drugs and melphalan in eight human ovarian carcinoma cell lines. *Br J Cancer* 1991;64:215–220.

50. Godwin A, Meister A, O'Dwyer P, et al. High resistance to cisplatin in human ovarian cancer cell lines is associated with marked increase in glutathione synthesis. *Proc Natl Acad Sci U S A* 1992;89:3070–3074.

51. Hamilton T, Winker M, Louie K, et al. Augmentation of adriamycin, melphalan and cisplatin cytotoxicity in drug-resistant and -sensitive human ovarian cancer cell lines by buthionine sulfoximine mediated glutathione depletion. *Biochem Pharmacol* 1985;34:2583–2586.

52. Koberle B, Grimaldi K, Sunters A, et al. DNA repair capacity and cisplatin sensitivity of human testis tumour cells. *Int J Cancer* 1997;70:551–555.

53. Martin LP, Hamilton TC, Schilder RJ. Platinum resistance: the role of DNA repair pathways. *Clin Cancer Res* 2008;14:1291–1295.

54. Selvakumaran M, Piscarcik DA, Bao R, et al. Enhanced cisplatin cytotoxicity by disturbing the nucleotide excision repair pathway in ovarian cancer cell lines. *Cancer Res* 2003;63:1311–1316.

55. Hubner RA, Riley RD, Billingham LJ, et al. Excision repair cross-complementation group 1 (ERCC1) status and lung cancer outcomes: a meta-analysis of published studies and recommendations. *PLoS One* 2011;6:e25164.

56. De Dosso S, Zanellato E, Nucifora M, et al. ERCC1 predicts outcome in patients with gastric cancer treated with adjuvant cisplatin-based chemotherapy. *Cancer Chemother Pharmacol* 2013;72:159–165.

57. Squires MH 3rd, Fisher SB, Fisher KE, et al. Differential expression and prognostic value of ERCC1 and thymidylate synthase in resected gastric adenocarcinoma. *Cancer* 2013;119:3242–3250.

58. Yamada Y, Boku N, Nishina T, et al. Impact of excision repair cross-complementing gene 1 (ERCC1) on the outcomes of patients with advanced gastric cancer: correlative study in Japan Clinical Oncology Group Trial JCOG9912. *Ann Oncol* 2013;24:2560–2565.

59. Friboulet L, Olaussen KA, Pignon JP, et al. ERCC1 isoform expression and DNA repair in non–small-cell lung cancer. *N Engl J Med* 2013;368:1101–1110.

60. Bryant HE, Schultz N, Thomas HD, et al. Specific killing of BRCA2-deficient tumours with inhibitors of poly(ADP-ribose) polymerase. *Nature* 2005;434:913–917.

61. Farmer H, McCabe1 N, Lord C, et al. Targeting the DNA repair defect in BRCA mutant cells as a therapeutic strategy. *Nature* 2005;434:917–921.

62. Edwards SL, Brough R, Lord CJ, et al. Resistance to therapy caused by intragenic deletion in BRCA2. *Nature* 2008;451:1111–1116.

63. Sakai W, Swisher EM, Karlan BM, et al. Secondary mutations as a mechanism of cisplatin resistance in BRCA2-mutated cancers. *Nature* 2008;451:1116–1121.

64. Gelmon KA, Tischkowitz M, Mackay H, et al. Olaparib in patients with recurrent high-grade serous or poorly differentiated ovarian carcinoma or triple-negative breast cancer: a phase 2, multicentre, open-label, non-randomised study. *Lancet Oncology* 2011;12:852–861.

65. Levine B, Kroemer G. Autophagy in the pathogenesis of disease. *Cell* 2008;132:27–42.

66. Matthew R, Karantza-Wadsworth V, White E. Role of autophagy in cancer. *Nat Rev Cancer* 2007;7:961–967.

67. Amaravadi RK, Yu D, Lum JJ, et al. Autophagy inhibition enhances therapy-induced apoptosis in a Myc-induced model of lymphoma. *J Clin Invest* 2007;117:326–336.

68. Duffull S, Robinson B. Clinical pharmacokinetics and dose optimization of carboplatin. *Clin Pharmacokinet* 1997;33:161–183.

69. Harland S, Newell D, Siddik Z, et al. Pharmacokinetics of cis-diammine-1,1-cyclobutane dicarboxylate platinum(II) in patients with normal and impaired renal function. *Cancer Res* 1984;44:1693–1697.

70. Graham MA, Lockwood GF, Greenslade D, et al. Clinical pharmacokinetics of oxaliplatin: a critical review. *Clin Cancer Res* 2000;6:1205–1218.

71. Gamelin E, Bouil A, Boisdron-Celle M, et al. Cumulative pharmacokinetic study of oxaliplatin, administered every three weeks, combined with 5-fluorouracil in colorectal cancer patients. *Clin Cancer Res* 1997;3:891–899.

72. Extra JM, Marty M, Brienza S, et al. Pharmacokinetics and safety profile of oxaliplatin. *Semin Oncol* 1998;25:13–22.

73. Chatelut E, Canal P, Brunner V, et al. Prediction of carboplatin clearance from standard morphological and biological patient characteristics. *J Natl Cancer Inst* 1995;87:573–580.

74. Jodrell D, Egorin M, Canetta R, et al. Relationships between carboplatin exposure and tumor response and toxicity in patients with ovarian cancer. *J Clin Oncol* 1992;10:520–528.

75. Reyno L, Egorin M, Canetta R, et al. Impact of cyclophosphamide on relationships between carboplatin exposure and response or toxicity when used in the treatment of advanced ovarian cancer. *J Clin Oncol* 1993;11:1156–1164.

76. Shen DW, Pouliot LM, Hall MD, et al. Cisplatin resistance: a cellular self-defense mechanism resulting from multiple epigenetic and genetic changes. *Pharmacol Rev* 2012;64:706–721.

77. Ma J, Verweij J, Planting A, et al. Current sample handling methods for measurement of platinum-DNA adducts in leucocytes in man lead to discrepant results in DNA adduct levels and DNA repair. *Br J Cancer* 1995;71:512–517.

78. Schellens J, Ma J, Planting A, et al. Relationship between the exposure to cisplatin, DNA-adduct formation in leucocytes and tumour response in patients with solid tumours. *Br J Cancer* 1996;73:1569–1575.

79. Ozols R, Corden B, Jacob J, et al. High-dose cisplatin in hypertonic saline. *Ann Intern Med* 1984;100:19–24.

80. Howell S, Pfeifle C, Wung W, et al. Intraperitoneal cis-diamminedichloroplatinum with systemic thiosulfate protection. *Cancer Res* 1983;43:1426–1431.

81. Alberts D, Liu P, Hannigan E, et al. Intraperitoneal cisplatin plus intravenous cyclophosphamide versus intravenous cisplatin plus intravenous cyclophosphamide for stage III ovarian cancer. *N Engl J Med* 1996;335:1950–1955.

82. Solomon B, Soulen M, Baum R, et al. Chemoembolization of hepatocellular carcinoma with cisplatin, doxorubicin, mitomycin-C, Ethiodol, and polyvinyl alcohol: prospective evaluation of response and survival in a US population. *J Vasc Interv Radiol* 1999;10:793–798.

83. Extra J, Marty M, Brienza S, et al. Pharmacokinetics and safety profile of oxaliplatin. *Semin Oncol* 1998;25:13–22.

84. Brienza S, Vignoud J, Itzhaki M, et al. Oxaliplatin (L-OHP): global safety in 682 patients. *Proc Am Soc Clin Oncol* 1995;14:209.

85. André T, Boni C, Mounedji-Boudiaf L, et al. Oxaliplatin, fluorouracil, and leucovorin as adjuvant treatment for colon cancer. *N Engl J Med* 2004;350:2343–2351.

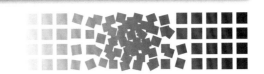

# 19 Antimetabolites

M. Wasif Saif and Edward Chu

CANCER THERAPEUTICS

## ANTIFOLATES

Reduced folates play a key role in one-carbon metabolism, and they are essential for the biosynthesis of purines, thymidylate, and protein biosynthesis. Aminopterin was the first antimetabolite with documented clinical activity in the treatment of children with acute leukemia in the 1940s. This antifolate analog was subsequently replaced by methotrexate (MTX), the 4-amino, 10-methyl analog of folic acid, which remains the most widely used antifolate analog, with activity against a wide range of cancers (Table 19.1), including hematologic malignancies (acute lymphoblastic leukemia and non-Hodgkin's lymphoma) and many solid tumors (breast cancer, head and neck cancer, osteogenic sarcoma, bladder cancer, and gestational trophoblastic cancer).

Pemetrexed is a pyrrolopyrimidine, multitargeted antifolate analog that targets multiple enzymes involved in folate metabolism, including thymidylate synthase (TS), dihydrofolate reductase (DHFR), glycinamide ribonucleotide (GAR) formyltransferase, and aminoimidazole carboxamide (AICAR) formyltransferase.[1,2] This agent has broad-spectrum activity against solid tumors, including malignant mesothelioma and breast, pancreatic, head and neck, non–small-cell lung, colon, gastric, cervical, and bladder cancers.[3–5]

The third antifolate compound to have entered clinical practice is pralatrexate (10-propargyl-10-deazaaminopterin), a 10-deazaaminopterin antifolate that was rationally designed to bind with higher affinity to the reduced folate carrier (RFC)-1 transport protein, when compared with MTX, leading to enhanced membrane transport into tumor cells. It is also an improved substrate for the enzyme folylpolyglutamyl synthetase (FPGS), resulting in enhanced formation of cytotoxic polyglutamate metabolites.[6,7] When compared with MTX, this analog is a more potent inhibitor of multiple enzymes involved in folate metabolism, including TS, DHFR, and GAR and AICAR formyltransferases. This agent is presently approved for the treatment of relapsed or refractory peripheral T-cell lymphomas.[8]

### Mechanism of Action

The antifolate compounds are tight-binding inhibitors of DHFR, a key enzyme in folate metabolism.[1] DHFR plays a pivotal role in maintaining the intracellular folate pools in their fully reduced form as tetrahydrofolates, and these compounds serve as one-carbon carriers required for the synthesis of thymidylate, purine nucleotides, and certain amino acids.

The cytotoxic effects of MTX, pemetrexed, and pralatrexate are mediated by their respective polyglutamate metabolites, with up to 5 to 7 glutamyl groups in a γ-peptide linkage. These polyglutamate metabolites exhibit prolonged intracellular half-lives, thereby allowing for prolonged drug action in tumor cells. Moreover, these polyglutamate metabolites are potent, direct inhibitors of several folate-dependent enzymes, including DHFR, TS, AICAR formyltransferase, and GAR formyltransferase.[1]

### Mechanisms of Resistance

The development of cellular resistance to antifolates remains a major obstacle to its clinical efficacy.[9,10] In experimental systems, resistance to antifolates arises from several mechanisms, including an alteration in antifolate transport because of either a defect in the reduced folate carrier or folate receptor systems, decreased capacity to polyglutamate the antifolate parent compound through either decreased expression of FPGS or increased expression of the catabolic enzyme γ-glutamyl hydrolase, and alterations in the target enzymes DHFR and/or TS through increased expression of wild-type protein or overexpression of a mutant protein with reduced binding affinity for the antifolate. Gene amplification is a common resistance mechanism observed in various experimental systems, including tumor samples from patients. In in vitro and in vivo experimental model systems, the levels of DHFR and/or TS protein acutely increase after exposure to MTX and other antifolate compounds. This acute induction of target protein in response to drug exposure is mediated, in part, by a translational regulatory mechanism, which may represent a clinically relevant mechanism for the acute development of cellular drug resistance.

### Clinical Pharmacology

The oral bioavailability of MTX is saturable and erratic at doses greater than 25 mg/m$^2$. MTX is completely absorbed from parenteral routes of administration, and peak serum levels are achieved within 30 to 60 minutes of administration.

The distribution of MTX into third-space fluid collections, such as pleural effusions and ascitic fluid, can substantially alter MTX pharmacokinetics. The slow release of accumulated MTX from these third spaces over time prolongs the terminal half-life of the drug, leading to potentially increased clinical toxicity. It is advisable to evacuate these fluid collections before treatment and monitor plasma drug concentrations closely.

Renal excretion is the main route of drug elimination, and this process is mediated by glomerular filtration and tubular secretion. About 80% to 90% of an administered dose is eliminated unchanged in the urine. Doses of MTX, therefore, should be reduced in proportion to reductions in creatinine clearance. Renal excretion of MTX is inhibited by probenecid, penicillins, cephalosporins, aspirin, and nonsteroidal anti-inflammatory drugs.

Pemetrexed enters the cell via the RFC system and, to a lesser extent, by the folate receptor protein. As with MTX, it undergoes polyglutamation within the cell to the pentaglutamate form, which is at least 60-fold more potent than the parent compound. This agent is mainly cleared by renal excretion, and in the setting of renal dysfunction, the terminal drug half-life is significantly prolonged to up to 20 hours. Pemetrexed, therefore, should be used with caution in patients with renal dysfunction. In addition, renal excretion is inhibited in the presence of other agents including probenecid, penicillins, cephalosporins, aspirin, and nonsteroidal anti-inflammatory drugs.

**223**

**TABLE 19.1**

**Antimetabolites: Indications, Doses and Schedules, and Toxicities**

| Drug | Main Therapeutic Uses | Main Doses and Schedule | Major Toxicities |
|---|---|---|---|
| Methotrexate | Non-Hodgkin's lymphoma<br>Primary CNS lymphoma<br>Acute lymphoblastic leukemia<br>Breast cancer<br>Bladder cancer<br>Osteogenic sarcoma<br>Gestational trophoblastic cancer | Low dose: 10–50 mg/m² IV every 3–4 weeks<br>Low dose weekly: 25 mg/m² IV weekly<br>Moderate dose: 100–500 m/m² IV every 2–3 weeks<br>High dose: 1–12 gm/m² IV over a 3- to 24-hour period every 1–3 weeks<br>Intrathecal (IT): 10–15 mg IT 2 times weekly until CSF is clear, then weekly dose for 2–6 weeks, followed by monthly dose | Mucositis, diarrhea, myelosuppression, acute renal failure, transient elevations in serum transaminases and bilirubin, pneumonitis, neurologic toxicity |
| Pemetrexed | Mesothelioma<br>Non–small-cell lung cancer | 500 mg/m² IV, every 3 weeks | Myelosuppression, skin rash, mucositis, diarrhea, fatigue |
| Pralatrexate | Peripheral T-cell lymphoma | 30 mg/m² IV, weekly for 6 weeks; cycles repeated every 7 weeks | Myelosuppression, skin rash, mucositis, diarrhea, elevation of serum transaminases and bilirubin, mild nausea/vomiting |
| 5-Fluorouracil | Breast cancer<br>Colorectal cancer<br>Anal cancer<br>Gastroesophageal cancer<br>Hepatocellular cancer<br>Pancreatic cancer<br>Head and neck cancer | Bolus monthly schedule: 425–450 mg/m² IV on days 1–5 every 28 days<br>Bolus weekly schedule: 500–600 mg/m² IV every week for 6 weeks every 8 weeks<br>Infusion schedule: 2,400–3,000 mg/m² IV over 46 hours every 2 weeks<br>120-hour infusion: 1,000 mg/m²/d IV on days 1–5 every 21–28 d<br>Protracted continuous infusion: 200–400 mg/m²/d IV | Nausea/vomiting, diarrhea, mucositis, myelosuppression, neurotoxicity, coronary artery vasospasm, conjunctivitis |
| Capecitabine | Breast cancer<br>Colorectal cancer<br>Gastroesophageal cancer<br>Hepatocellular cancer<br>Pancreatic cancer | Recommended dose for monotherapy is 1,250 mg/m² PO bid for 2 weeks with 1 wk rest<br>May decrease dose of capecitabine to 850–1,000 mg/m² bid on days 1–14 to reduce risk of toxicity without compromising efficacy<br>An alternative dosing schedule for monotherapy is 1,250–1,500 mg/m² PO bid for 1 week on and 1 week off; this schedule appears to be well tolerated, with no compromise in clinical efficacy<br>Capecitabine should be used at lower doses (850–1,000 mg/m² bid on days 1–14) when used in combination with other cytotoxic agents, such as oxaliplatin and lapatinib | Diarrhea, hand-foot syndrome, myelosuppression, mucositis, nausea/vomiting, neurologic toxicity, coronary artery vasospasm |
| Cytarabine | Hodgkin's lymphoma<br>Non-Hodgkin's lymphoma<br>Acute myelogenous leukemia<br>Acute lymphoblastic leukemia | Standard dose: 100 mg/m²/day IV on days 1–7 as a continuous IV infusion, in combination with an anthracycline as induction chemotherapy for acute myelogenous leukemia<br>High-dose: 1.5–3.0 gm/m² IV q 12 hours for 3 days as a high dose, intensification regimen for acute myelogenous leukemia<br>SC: 20 mg/m² SC for 10 days per month for 6 months, associated with IFN-α for treatment of chronic myelogenous leukemia<br>IT: 10–30 mg IT up to 3 times weekly in the treatment of leptomeningeal carcinomatosis secondary to leukemia or lymphoma. | Nausea/vomiting, myelosuppression, cerebellar ataxia, lethargy, confusion, acute pancreatitis, drug infusion reaction, hand-foot syndrome<br>High-dose therapy: noncardiogenic pulmonary edema, acute respiratory distress and *Streptococcus viridans* pneumonia, conjunctivitis, and keratitis |
| Gemcitabine | Pancreatic cancer<br>Non–small-cell lung cancer<br>Breast cancer<br>Bladder cancer<br>Hodgkin's lymphoma<br>Ovarian cancer<br>Soft tissue sarcoma | Pancreatic cancer: 1,000 mg/m² IV every week for 7 weeks with 1 week rest Treatment then continues weekly for 3 weeks followed by 1 week off<br>Bladder cancer: 1,000 mg/m² IV on days 1, 8, and 15 every 28 days<br>Non–small-cell lung cancer: 1,000-1,200 mg/m² IV on days 1 and 8 every 21 days | Nausea/vomiting, myelosuppression, flulike syndrome, elevation of serum transaminases and bilirubin, pneumonitis, infusion reaction, mild proteinuria, and rarely, hemolytic-uremic syndrome and thrombotic thrombocytopenic purpura |

*(continued)*

| TABLE 19.1 | | | |
|---|---|---|---|
| **Antimetabolites: Indications, Doses and Schedules, and Toxicities** *(continued)* | | | |
| **Drug** | **Main Therapeutic Uses** | **Main Doses and Schedule** | **Major Toxicities** |
| 6-Mercaptopurine | Acute lymphoblastic leukemia | Induction therapy: 2.5 mg/kg PO daily<br>Maintenance therapy: 1.5–2.5 mg/kg PO daily | Myelosuppression, nausea/vomiting, mucositis and diarrhea, hepatotoxicity, immunosuppression |
| 6-Thioguanine | Acute myelogenous leukemia<br>Acute lymphoblastic leukemia | Induction: 100 mg/m$^2$ PO every 12 hours on days 1–5, usually in combination with cytarabine<br>Maintenance: 100 mg/m$^2$ PO every 12 hours on days 1–5, every 4 weeks, usually in combination with other agents<br>Single agent: 1–3 mg/kg PO daily | Myelosuppression, nausea/vomiting, mucositis and diarrhea, hepatotoxicity, immunosuppression |
| Fludarabine | Chronic lymphocytic leukemia<br>Non-Hodgkin's lymphoma | 25 mg/m$^2$ IV on days 1–5 every 28 days For oral usage, the recommended dose is 40 mg/m$^2$ PO on days 1–5 every 28 days | Myelosuppression, immunosuppression with increased risk of opportunistic infections, mild nausea/vomiting, hypersensitivity reaction |
| Cladribine | Hairy cell leukemia<br>Chronic lymphocytic leukemia<br>Non-Hodgkin's lymphoma | Usual dose is 0.09 mg/kg/d IV via continuous infusion for 7 days; one course is usually administered | Myelosuppression, immunosuppression, mild nausea/vomiting, fever |
| Clofarabine | Acute lymphoblastic leukemia | 52 mg/m$^2$ IV daily for 5 days every 2–6 weeks | Myelosuppression nausea/vomiting, diarrhea, systemic inflammatory response syndrome, increased risk of opportunistic infections, renal toxicity |

CNS, central nervous system; IV, intravenously; CSF, cerebrospinal fluid; PO, by mouth; bid, twice daily; SC, subcutaneously; IFN-α, interferon alpha.

As with other antifolate analogs, pralatrexate is transported into the cell by the RFC carrier protein and then metabolized by FPGS to form longer chain polyglutamates, with up to four additional glutamate residues attached to the parent molecule. About 34% of the parent drug is cleared in the urine during the first 24 hours after drug administration. As such, caution is advised when using pralatrexate in patients with renal dysfunction. As with MTX and pemetrexed, the concomitant administration of other agents such as probenecid, penicillins, cephalosporins, aspirin, and nonsteroidal anti-inflammatory drugs, may inhibit renal clearance.

## Toxicity

The main side effects of MTX are myelosuppression and gastrointestinal (GI) toxicity, which are usually completely reversed within 14 days, unless drug-elimination mechanisms are impaired. In patients with compromised renal function, even small doses of MTX may result in serious toxicity. MTX-induced nephrotoxicity is thought to result from the intratubular precipitation of MTX and its metabolites in acidic urine. Antifolates may also exert a direct toxic effect on the renal tubules. Vigorous hydration and urinary alkalinization have greatly reduced the incidence of renal failure in patients on high-dose regimens. Acute elevations in hepatic enzyme levels and hyperbilirubinemia are often observed during high-dose therapy, but these levels usually return to normal within 10 days. Methotrexate given concomitantly with radiotherapy may increase the risk of soft tissue necrosis and osteonecrosis.

The original rationale for high-dose MTX therapy was based on the concept of selective rescue of normal tissues by the reduced folate leucovorin (LV). However, recent data suggest that high-dose MTX may also overcome resistance mechanisms caused by impaired active transport, decreased affinity of DHFR for MTX,

increased levels of DHFR resulting from gene amplification, and/or decreased polyglutamation of MTX.

The main toxicities of pemetrexed and pralatrexate include dose-limiting myelosuppression, mucositis, and skin rash, usually in the form of the hand-foot syndrome (HFS). Other toxicities include reversible transaminasemia, anorexia and fatigue syndrome, and GI toxicity. These side effects are reduced by supplementation with folic acid (350 μg orally daily) and vitamin B$_{12}$ (1,000 mg subcutaneously given at least 1 week before starting therapy, and then repeated every three cycles). To date, there is no evidence to suggest that vitamin supplementation adversely affects the clinical efficacy of pemetrexed or pralatrexate.

## 5-FLUOROPYRIMIDINES

The fluoropyrimidine, 5-fluorouracil (5-FU) was synthesized by Charles Heidelberger in the mid 1950s. Uracil is a normal component of RNA; as such, the rationale leading to the development of the drug was that cancer cells might be more sensitive to *decoy* molecules that mimic the natural compound than normal cells. 5-FU and its derivatives are an integral part of treatment for a broad range of solid tumors (see Table 19.1), including GI malignancies (esophageal, gastric, pancreatic, colorectal, anal, and hepatocellular cancers), breast, head and neck, and skin cancers.[11] It continues to serve as the main backbone for combination regimens used to treat metastatic colorectal cancer (mCRC) and as adjuvant therapy of early-stage colon cancer.

### Mechanism of Action

5-FU enters cells via the facilitated uracil base transport mechanism and is then anabolized to various cytotoxic nucleotide forms

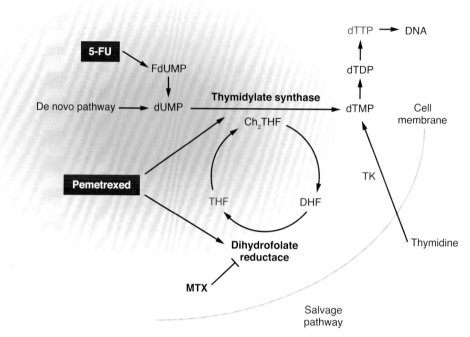

**Figure 19.1** Antifolates and 5-fluorouracil (5-FU) sites of action. FdUMP, fluorodeoxyuridine monophosphate; dUMP, deoxyuridine monophosphate; dTTP, deoxythymidine triphosphate; dTDP, deoxyuridine diphosphate; dTMP, deoxythymidine monophosphate; TK, thymidine kinase; CH$_2$THF, 5,10-methylenetetrahydrofolate; THF, tetrahydrofolate; DHF, dihydrofolate.

by several biochemical pathways. It is thought that 5-FU exerts its cytotoxic effects through various mechanisms, including (1) the inhibition of TS, (2) incorporation into RNA, and (3) incorporation into DNA (Fig. 19.1). In addition to these mechanisms, the genotoxic stress resulting from TS inhibition may also activate programmed cell-death pathways in susceptible cells, which leads to the induction of parental DNA fragmentation.

## Mechanisms of Resistance

Several resistance mechanisms to 5-FU have been identified in experimental and clinical settings. Alterations in the target enzyme TS represent the most commonly described mechanism of resistance. In vitro, in vivo, and clinical studies have documented a strong correlation between the levels of TS enzyme activity/TS protein and chemosensitivity to 5-FU. In this regard, cell lines and tumors with higher levels of TS are relatively more resistant to 5-FU. Mutations in the TS protein have been identified that lead to reduced binding affinity of the 5-FU metabolite fluorodeoxyuridine monophosphate (FdUMP) to the TS protein. Reduced expression and/or diminished activity of key activating enzymes may interfere with the formation of cytotoxic 5-FU metabolites. Decreased expression of mismatch repair enzymes, such as human mutL homolog 1 (hMLH1) and human mutS homolog 2 (hMSH2), and increased expression of the catabolic enzyme dihydropyrimidine dehydrogenase (DPD) are associated with fluoropyrimidine resistance. At this time, the relative contribution of each of these mechanisms in the development of cellular resistance to 5-FU in the actual clinical setting remains unclear.

## Clinical Pharmacology

5-FU is not orally administered, given its erratic bioavailability resulting from high levels of the catabolic enzyme DPD present

in the gut mucosa. After intravenous bolus doses, metabolic elimination is rapid, with a half-life of 8 to 14 minutes. More than 85% of an administered dose of 5-FU is enzymatically inactivated by DPD, the rate-limiting enzyme in the catabolism of 5-FU.

A pharmacogenetic syndrome has been identified in which partial or compete deficiency in the DPD enzyme is present in 3% to 5% and 0.1% of the general population, respectively. As DPD catalyzes the rate-limiting step in the catabolic pathway of 5-FU, a deficiency of DPD can result in a clinically dangerous increase in the anabolic products of 5-FU. Unfortunately, patients with DPD deficiency do not manifest a phenotype only until they are treated with 5-FU, and in that setting, they can develop severe GI toxicity in the form of mucositis and/or diarrhea, myelosuppression, neurologic toxicity, and in rare cases, death. In patients being treated with 5-FU or any other fluoropyrimidine, it is important to consider DPD deficiency in patients who present with excessive, severe toxicity.[12] It is now increasingly appreciated that DPD mutations are unable to account for all of the observed cases of excessive 5-FU toxicity, because up to 50% of patients who experience 5-FU toxicity will have no documented alterations in the *DPD* gene. Moreover, individuals with normal DPD enzyme activity may be diagnosed with high plasma levels of 5-FU, resulting in increased toxicity. Although DPD enzyme activity can be assayed from peripheral blood mononuclear cells in a specialized laboratory, routine phenotypic and genotypic screenings for DPD deficiency prior to 5-FU therapy are not yet available.

## Biomodulation of 5-FU

Significant efforts have focused on enhancing the antitumor activity of 5-FU through biochemical modulation in which 5-FU is combined with various agents, including leucovorin, MTX, N-phosphonacetyl-L-aspartic acid, interferon-α, interferon-γ, and

## TABLE 19.2

### Toxicities of Different Forms of 5-FU

| Route | Schedule | Dose | DLT |
|-------|----------|------|-----|
| IV | Daily × 5, bolus | 400–500 (mg/m²/d) | ⇓ BM<br>D<br>M |
| IV | Weekly bolus | 450–500 (mg/m²/d) | ⇓ BM |
| IV | Daily × 5, CI | 750–1,000 (mg/m²/d) | M<br>D |
| IV | PCI | 200–400 (mg/m²/d) | M<br>HFS |
| HAI | Daily × 14–21, CI | 750–1,000 (mg/m²/d) | M<br>D |
| IP | 32–120 hr | 5 nM | M<br>D |
| Oral (Xeloda) | 14–21 d | 2,000–2,500 (mg/m²/d) | HFS |

DLT, dose limiting toxicity; IV, intravenous; BM, bone marrow; D, diarrhea; M, mucositis; CI, continuous infusion; PCI, protracted continuous infusion; HFS, hand-foot syndrome; HAI, hepatic artery infusion; IP, intraperitoneal.

a whole host of other agents.[13] For the past 20 to 25 years, the reduced folate LV has been the main biochemical modulator of 5-FU. An alternative approach has been to alter the schedule of 5-FU administration. Given the S-phase specificity of this agent, prolonged exposure of tumor cells to 5-FU would increase the fraction of cells being exposed to the drug. Overall response rates are significantly higher in patients treated with infusional schedules of 5-FU than in those treated with bolus 5-FU, and this improvement in response rate has translated into an improved progression-free survival. Moreover, the overall safety profile is improved with infusional regimens. A hybrid schedule of bolus and infusional 5-FU was originally developed in France, and this regimen has shown superior clinical activity compared with bolus 5-FU schedules. This hybrid schedule has now been simplified by using only the 46-hour infusion of 5-FU and completely eliminating the 5-FU bolus doses.

## Toxicity

The spectrum of 5-FU toxicity is dose- and schedule-dependent (Table 19.2). The main side effects are diarrhea, mucositis, and myelosuppression. The dermatologic HFS is more commonly observed with infusional 5-FU therapy. Acute neurologic symptoms have also been reported, and they include somnolence, cerebellar ataxia, and upper motor signs. Treatment with 5-FU can, on rare occasions, cause coronary vasospasm, resulting in a syndrome of chest pain, cardiac enzyme elevations, and electrocardiographic changes. Cardiac toxicity seems to be related more to infusional 5-FU than bolus administration.[14]

# CAPECITABINE

Capecitabine is an oral fluoropyrimidine carbamate that was rationally designed to allow for selective 5-FU activation in tumor tissue.[15] This oral agent was initially approved in anthracycline- and taxane-resistant breast cancer and subsequently approved for use in combination with docetaxel as second-line therapy in metastatic breast cancer and in combination with lapatinib, a tyrosine-kinase inhibitor of human epidermal growth factor receptor type 2 (HER2) and epidermal growth factor receptor (EGFR) in women with HER2-positive metastatic breast cancer following progression on trastuzumab-based therapy.[16] This agent is also approved by the

U.S. Food and Drug Administration (FDA) for the first-line treatment of mCRC and as adjuvant therapy for stage III colon cancer when fluoropyrimidine therapy alone is preferred.[17] In Europe and throughout much of the world, the combination of capecitabine plus oxaliplatin (XELOX) is approved for the treatment of mCRC as well as for the adjuvant therapy of stage III colon cancer.[18] In addition, recent studies have documented the noninferiority of capecitabine to 5-FU when combined with cisplatin in the treatment of metastatic gastric cancer.

## Clinical Pharmacology

Capecitabine is rapidly and extensively absorbed by the gut mucosa, with nearly 80% oral bioavailability. It is inactive in its parent form and undergoes enzymatic conversion via three successive steps. Of note, the third and final step occurs in tumor tissue and involves the conversion of 5′-deoxy-5-fluorouridine to 5-FU by the enzyme thymidine phosphorylase (TP), which is expressed at much higher levels in tumors when compared with corresponding normal tissue. Capecitabine and capecitabine metabolites are primarily excreted by the kidneys, and in contrast to 5-FU, caution must be taken in the presence of renal dysfunction, with appropriate dose modification. The use of capecitabine is absolutely contraindicated in patients whose creatinine clearance is less than 30 mL per minute. The FDA and Roche have added a black box warning and strengthened the precautions section on the capecitabine label about the drug–drug interaction between warfarin and capecitabine-based chemotherapy. It is generally recommended to do weekly monitoring of the coagulation parameters (prothrombin time/international normalized ratio [PT/INR]) for all patients receiving concomitant warfarin and capecitabine, with an appropriate adjustment of warfarin dose.

## Toxicity

Similar to what is observed with infusional 5-FU, the main side effects of capecitabine include diarrhea and HFS. Of note, the incidence of myelosuppression, neutropenic fever, mucositis, alopecia, and nausea/vomiting is lower with capecitabine when compared with 5-FU. Elevations in indirect serum bilirubin can be observed, but are usually transient and clinically asymptomatic. Patients in the United States appear to be unable to tolerate as high doses of capecitabine as European patients, either as monotherapy or in combination with other cytotoxic chemotherapy.[19] Although the underlying reasons for this discrepancy are not known, it may in part be related to the increased fortification of the US diet with folate and the increased focus on vitamin and folic acid supplementation.

## S-1

S-1 is an oral fluoropyrimidine that consists of tegafur (FT), a prodrug of 5-FU, combined with two 5-FU biochemical modulators: 5-chloro-2,4-dihydroxypyridine (gimeracil or CDHP), a competitive inhibitor of DPD, and oteracil potassium, which inhibits phosphorylation of 5-flurouracil in the GI tract, thereby decreasing serious GI toxicities such as nausea/vomiting, mucositis, and diarrhea.[20] As with other oral agents, S-1 offers several advantages over 5-FU, including ease of administration, no risks associated with use of central venous access such as infection, thrombosis, etc., and reduced toxicities, especially neurotoxicity. Although S-1 has yet to be approved by the FDA, it has been approved for the treatment of gastric cancer, head and neck, colorectal cancer (CRC), non–small-cell lung, breast, pancreatic, and biliary tract cancers in several countries in Asia and for the treatment of advanced gastric cancer in combination with cisplatin in a large number of European countries.

## Clinical Pharmacology

S-1 was designed to provide continuous 5-FU plasma exposure comparable to the intravenous (IV) infusion. FT, the 5-FU prodrug, is absorbed in the small intestine and converted to 5-FU through the liver microsomal P-450 metabolizing enzyme system (CYP2A6). Most of the 5-FU is degraded (85%) by DPD, leading to the formation of fluoro-beta-alanine (FBAL).[21] CDHP inhibits DPD, thus allowing higher concentrations of 5-FU to enter the anabolic pathway and enhance its therapeutic effect. Additionally, the inhibition of DPD leads to a decreased amount of FBAL formation, which presumably leads to reduced neurotoxicity. Oteracil is the final component of the S-1 formulation, and it inhibits orotate phosphoribosyltransferase in the GI mucosa, which prevents the formation of fluorouridine monophosphate (FUMP), thereby decreasing GI toxicity.

The maximum tolerated dose was established at 80 mg/m² in two divided doses for a Japanese population and 25 mg/m² twice a day for a Caucasian population. This interethnic variability of S-1 pharmacokinetics and pharmacodynamics has been attributed to differences in the CYP2A6 genotypes.[22] Studies have demonstrated a high frequency of allelic variants CYP2A6*4, *7, and *9 in East Asians than in Caucasians, which might be associated with reduced enzymatic activity and decreased activation of FT. On the other hand, higher FT metabolism is seen in Caucasian patients due to higher CYP2A6 activity. However, investigators have established similar 5-FU exposure between these two ethnic groups. These findings were explained by higher CDHP exposure in Asians, resulting in increased DPD inhibition and slower catabolism of 5-FU, despite having low CYP2A6 activity, whereas Caucasians had higher CYP2A6 activity but faster 5-FU clearance.

## Clinical Toxicity

Clinical studies have shown that the GI toxicities associated with S-1, such as diarrhea, nausea, vomiting, and hyperbilirubinemia, are more prominent in Western patients, whereas hematologic toxicities are more prevalent in Japanese patients. The difference in safety profile cannot be explained by differences in 5-FU exposure, because pharmacokinetic studies have shown that overall drug exposures are similar. A potential explanation might involve interethnic variations in TS promoter enhancer region polymorphisms, which are more frequently seen in Asians or in Caucasians on a higher folate diet.

# CYTARABINE

Cytarabine (ara-C) is a deoxycytidine nucleoside analog isolated from the sponge *Cryptotethya crypta*, and it differs from its physiologic counterpart by virtue of a stereotypic inversion of the 2′-hydroxyl group of the sugar moiety.[23] A regimen of ara-C, combined with an anthracycline and given as a 5- or 7-day continuous infusion, is considered the standard induction treatment for acute myeloid leukemia (AML). Ara-C is active against other hematologic malignancies, such as non-Hodgkin's lymphoma, chronic myelogenous leukemia, and acute lymphocytic leukemia (see Table 19.1). However, this agent has absolutely no activity against solid tumors.

## Mechanism of Action

Ara-C enters cells via nucleoside transport proteins, the most important one being the equilibrative inhibitor-sensitive (ES) receptor. Once inside the cell, ara-C requires activation for its cytotoxic effects.[23,24] The first metabolic step is the conversion of ara-C to the monophosphate form ara-cytidine monophosphate (ara-CMP) by the enzyme deoxycytidine kinase (dCK) with subsequent phosphorylation to the di- and triphosphate metabolites, respectively. Ara-cytidine triphosphate (ara-CTP) is a potent inhibitor of DNA polymerases α, β, and γ, which in turn interferes with DNA chain elongation, DNA synthesis, and DNA repair. Ara-CTP is also incorporated directly into DNA and functions as a DNA chain terminator, interfering with chain elongation. Catabolism of ara-C involves two key enzymes, cytidine deaminase and deoxycytidylate deaminase. These breakdown enzymes convert ara-C and ara-CMP into the inactive metabolites, ara-uridine (ara-U) and ara-uridine monophosphate (ara-UMP), respectively. The balance between intracellular activation and degradation is critical in determining the amount of drug that is ultimately converted to ara-CTP and, thus, its subsequent cytotoxic and antitumor activity.

## Mechanisms of Resistance

Several resistance mechanisms to ara-C have been described. An impaired transmembrane transport, a decreased rate of anabolism, and an increased rate of catabolism may result in the development of ara-C resistance.[23,25,26] The level of cytidine deaminase enzyme activity has been shown to correlate with clinical response in patients with AML undergoing induction chemotherapy with ara-C–containing regimens.

## Clinical Pharmacology

Ara-C has poor oral bioavailability given its extensive deamination within the GI tract. Thus, ara-C is administered intravenously via continuous infusion. After administration, ara-C undergoes extensive metabolism in the liver, plasma, and peripheral tissues. Within 24 hours, up to 80% of drug is recovered in the urine as the ara-U metabolite. Ara-C crosses the blood–brain barrier when used at high doses, with cerebrospinal fluid levels between 7% and 14% of plasma levels and reaching peak levels of up to 10 μM.

## Toxicity

The toxicity profile of ara-C is highly dependent on the dose and schedule of administration. Myelosuppression is dose-limiting with a standard 7-day regimen. Leukopenia and thrombocytopenia are observed most frequently, with nadirs occurring between days 7 and 14 after drug administration. GI toxicity commonly manifests as a mild-to-moderate degree of anorexia, nausea, and vomiting along with mucositis, diarrhea, and abdominal pain. In rare cases, acute pancreatitis has been observed. The ara-C syndrome has been described in pediatric patients with hematologic malignancies, usually begins within 12 hours after the start of drug infusion, and is characterized by fever, myalgia, bone pain, maculopapular rash, conjunctivitis, malaise, and occasional chest pain.

The administration of ara-C at high doses (2 to 3 g/m² with each dose) is associated with profound myelosuppression.[27] Severe GI toxicity in the form of mucositis and/or diarrhea is also observed. Neurologic toxicity is significantly more common with high-dose ara-C than with standard doses, and presents with seizures, cerebral and cerebellar dysfunction, and peripheral neuropathy. Clinical signs of cerebellar dysfunction occur in up to 15% of patients and include dysarthria, dysmetria, and ataxia. Change in alertness and cognitive ability, memory loss, and frontal lobe release signs reflect cerebral toxicity. Despite discontinuation of therapy, clinical recovery is incomplete in up to 30% of affected patients. Pulmonary complications may include noncardiogenic pulmonary edema, acute respiratory distress, and pneumonia, resulting from *Streptococcus viridans* infection. Other side effects associated with high-dose ara-C include conjunctivitis (often responsive to topical corticosteroids), a painful HFS, and rarely, anaphylactic reactions.

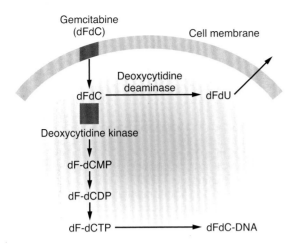

**Figure 19.2** Transport and metabolism of gemcitabine. dFdC, gemcitabine; dFdU, 2′,2′-difluorodeoxyuridine; dF-dCMP, gemcitabine monophosphate; dF-dCDP, gemcitabine diphosphate; dF-dCTP, gemcitabine triphosphate.

# GEMCITABINE

Gemcitabine (2′,2′-difluorodeoxycytidine) is a difluorinated deoxycytidine analog. Despite its similarity in structure, metabolism, and mechanism of action to ara-C, the spectrum of antitumor activity of gemcitabine is much broader.[23,28] This compound has significant clinical activity against several human solid tumors, including pancreatic, bile duct, gall bladder, small cell and non–small-cell lung, bladder, ovary, and breast cancers as well as hematologic malignancies, namely Hodgkin's and non-Hodgkin's lymphoma (see Table 19.1).

## Mechanism of Action

The transport of gemcitabine into cells requires the nucleoside transporter system. Gemcitabine is inactive in its parent form and requires intracellular activation for its cytotoxic effects. The steps involved in the metabolic activation of gemcitabine are similar to those observed with ara-C, with both drugs being activated by the same enzymatic machinery to the active triphosphate metabolite (see Fig. 19.2). Gemcitabine triphosphate is then incorporated into DNA, resulting in chain termination and the inhibition of DNA synthesis and function, or the triphosphate form can directly inhibit DNA polymerases α, β, and γ, which in turn, interferes with DNA chain elongation, DNA synthesis, and DNA repair. The triphosphate metabolite is also a potent inhibitor of ribonucleotide reductase, which further mediates inhibition of DNA biosynthesis by reducing the levels of key deoxynucleotide pools.[29]

## Mechanisms of Resistance

Several mechanisms of resistance to gemcitabine have been described in various preclinical experimental models.[30] Gemcitabine is a polar nucleoside analog that requires the activity of human equilibrative nucleoside transporter 1 (hENT1) to enter cells and exert its cytotoxic effects. Preclinical data in human pancreatic cancer cell lines showed that gemcitabine resistance is negatively correlated with hENT1 expression and can be induced by specific inhibitors of hENT1.[31] Clinical data also support the concept that a lack of hENT1 may be predictive of resistance to gemcitabine. CO-101, a lipid-drug conjugate of gemcitabine, was rationally designed to enter cells independently of hENT1. Unfortunately, two studies in pancreatic cancer failed to show any benefit of CO-101.

Additionally, several enzymes involved in the intracellular metabolism of gemcitabine have been implicated in the development of cellular drug resistance, including reduced expression and/or deficiency in dCK enzyme activity as well as increased expression and/or activity of the catabolic enzymes cytidine deaminase and dCMP deaminase. Recent studies have also identified a subset of CD44-positive cancer stem cells within pancreatic tumors that sustain tumor formation and growth, and are resistant to gemcitabine therapy.[33]

## Clinical Pharmacology

Gemcitabine is administered via the intravenous route, typically over a 30-minute intravenous infusion, and it undergoes extensive metabolism by deamination to the catabolic metabolite, difluorodeoxyuridine (dFdU), with more than 90% of the metabolized drug being recovered in urine. Plasma clearance is about 30% lower in women and in elderly patients, and this pharmacokinetic difference may result in an increased risk of toxicity in these respective patient populations. The initial findings from pilot pharmacokinetic studies suggested that gemcitabine, when given at a fixed dose rate (FDR) intravenous infusion of 10 mg/m² per minute, produced the highest accumulation of active dFdCTP metabolites in peripheral blood mononuclear cells, which led to a randomized phase II trial that compared gemcitabine 1,500 mg/m² by FDR or 2,200 mg/m² of gemcitabine over 30 minutes. Although this phase II study suggested an improved overall survival with FDR, a subsequent phase III trial failed to confirm the survival advantage of gemcitabine by FDR over its conventional administration schedule.[34]

## Toxicity

Gemcitabine is a relatively well-tolerated drug when used as a single agent. The main dose-limiting toxicity is myelosuppression, with neutropenia more commonly experienced than thrombocytopenia. Toxicity is schedule dependent, with longer infusions producing greater hematologic toxicity. Transient flulike symptoms, including fever, headache, arthralgias, and myalgias, occur in 45% of patients. Asthenia and transient transaminasemia may occur. Renal microangiopathy syndromes, including hemolytic-uremic syndrome and thrombotic thrombocytopenic purpura, have been reported rarely.

# 6-THIOPURINES

The development of the purine analogs in cancer chemotherapy began in the early 1950s with the synthesis of the thiopurines, 6-mercaptopurine (6-MP) and 6-thioguanine (6-TG). 6-MP has an important role in maintenance therapy for acute lymphoblastic leukemia, whereas 6-TG is active in remission induction and in maintenance therapy for AML (see Table 19.1).

## Mechanism of Action

The thiopurines, 6-MP and 6-TG, act similarly with respect to their cellular biochemistry.[34] In their respective monophosphate nucleotide forms, they inhibit enzymes involved in de novo purine synthesis and purine interconversion reactions. The triphosphate nucleotide forms can get directly incorporated into either cellular RNA or DNA, leading to the inhibition of RNA and DNA synthesis and function, respectively.

## Mechanisms of Resistance

The development of cellular resistance to 6-thiopurines results from a decreased level of key cytotoxic nucleotide metabolites, either through decreased formation or increased breakdown. Resistant cells have been identified that express either complete or partial deficiency of the activating enzyme hypoxanthine-guanine phosphoribosyltransferase (HGPRT). In clinical samples derived from patients with AML, drug resistance has been associated with increased concentrations of a membrane-bound alkaline phosphatase or a conjugating enzyme, 6-thiopurine methyltransferase (TPMT), the end-result being reduced formation of cytotoxic thiopurine nucleotides. Finally, the decreased expression of mismatch repair enzymes, including hMLH1 and hMSH2, has been associated with cellular drug resistance.

## Clinical Pharmacology

Oral absorption of 6-MP is highly erratic, and the relatively poor oral bioavailability is mainly related to rapid first-pass metabolism in the liver. The major route of drug elimination is via metabolism by several enzymatic pathways. 6-MP is oxidized to the inactive metabolite 6-thiouric acid by xanthine oxidase. Enhanced 6-MP toxicity may result from the concomitant administration of 6-MP and the xanthine oxidase inhibitor allopurinol. In patients receiving both 6-MP and allopurinol, the 6-MP dose must be reduced by at least 50% to 75%. 6-MP also undergoes S-methylation by the enzyme TPMT to yield 6-methylmercaptopurine.[35]

6-TG is administered orally in the treatment of AML. Its oral bioavailability is erratic, with peak plasma levels occurring 2 to 4 hours after ingestion. The catabolism of 6-TG differs from 6-MP in that it is not a direct substrate for xanthine oxidase.

TPMT enzyme activity may vary considerably among patients as a result of point mutations or loss of alleles of TPMT.[36] Approximately 0.3% of the Caucasian population expresses either a homozygous deletion or a mutation of both alleles of the *TPMT* gene. In these patients, grossly elevated thiopurine nucleotides concentrations, profound myelosuppression with pancytopenia, and extensive GI symptoms are observed after only a brief course of thiopurine treatment. An estimated 10% of patients may be at increased risk for toxicity because of heterozygous loss of the gene or a mutant allele coding for a less enzymatically active TPMT.

## Toxicity

The major dose-related toxicities of the thiopurines are myelosuppression and GI toxicity in the form of nausea/vomiting, anorexia, diarrhea, and stomatitis.[37] In TPMT-deficient patients, dosage reduction to 5% to 25% of the standard dosage is necessary to prevent severe excessive toxicity. Thiopurine hepatotoxicity occurs in up to 30% of adult patients and presents mainly as cholestatic jaundice, although elevations of hepatic transaminases may also be seen. Combinations of thiopurines with other known hepatotoxic agents should be avoided, and liver function should be closely monitored. The thiopurines are also potent suppressors of cell-mediated immunity, and prolonged therapy results in an increased predisposition to bacterial and parasitic infections.

## FLUDARABINE

Fludarabine (9-β-D-arabinosyl-2-fluoroadenine monophosphate, F-ara-AMP) is an active agent in the treatment of chronic lymphocytic leukemia (CLL) (see Table 19.1).[38,39] It is also active against indolent non-Hodgkin's lymphoma, prolymphocytic leukemia, cutaneous T-cell lymphoma, and Waldenström macroglobulinemia. This agent has also shown promising activity in mantle cell lymphoma. In contrast to its activity in hematologic malignancies, this compound has virtually no activity against solid tumors.

## Mechanism of Action

The active cytotoxic metabolite is the triphosphate metabolite F-ara-ATP, which competes with deoxyadenosine triphosphate (dATP) for incorporation into DNA and serves as a highly effective chain terminator. In addition, F-ara-ATP directly inhibits enzymes involved in DNA replication, including DNA polymerases, DNA primase, DNA ligase I, and ribonucleotide reductase.[37] F-ara-ATP is also incorporated into RNA, causing the inhibition of RNA function, processing, and mRNA translation. In contrast to other antimetabolites, fludarabine is active against nondividing cells. In fact, the primary effect of fludarabine may result from activation of apoptosis, through an as yet ill-defined mechanisms.[39] This finding may explain the activity of fludarabine in indolent lymphoproliferative diseases with relatively low growth fractions.

## Mechanisms of Resistance

The decreased expression of the activating enzyme dCK resulting in diminished intracellular formation of F-ara-AMP is one of the main resistance mechanisms identified in preclinical models.[38] A high degree of cross-resistance develops to multiple nucleoside analogs, requiring activation by dCK, including cytarabine, gemcitabine, cladribine, and clofarabine. Reduced cellular transport of drug has also been identified as a resistance mechanism.

## Clinical Pharmacology

Peak concentrations of F-ara-A are reached 3 to 4 hours after intravenous administration.[40] The main route of elimination is via the kidneys, with about 25% of a given dose of drug being excreted unchanged in the urine.

## Toxicity

Myelosuppression and immunosuppression are the major side effects of fludarabine as highlighted by dose-limiting and possibly cumulative lymphopenia and thrombocytopenia. Suppression of the immune system affects T-cell function more than B-cell function. Fevers, often in the setting of neutropenia, occur in 20% to 30% of patients. Lymphocyte counts, specifically CD4-positive cells, decrease rapidly after the initiation of therapy, and recovery of CD4-positive cells to normal levels may take longer than 1 year. Common opportunistic pathogens include the varicella-zoster virus, *Candida*, and *Pneumocystis carinii*. In general, patients are empirically placed on sulfamethoxazole trimethoprim prophylaxis to prevent the development of *P. carinii* infection.

## CLADRIBINE

Cladribine (2-CdA) is a purine deoxyadenosine analog, and it is the drug of choice for hairy cell leukemia with activity in low-grade lymphoproliferative disorders (see Table 19.1).[41,42] Salvage treatment of patients previously treated with interferon-α or splenectomy is as effective as first-line treatment. Retreatment with cladribine results in a complete response in up to 60% of relapsing patients. In addition, this agent has promising activity in patients with CLL and non-Hodgkin's lymphoma.

## Mechanism of Action

Upon entry into the cell, 2-CdA undergoes an initial conversion to cladribine-monophosphate (Cd-AMP) via the reaction catalyzed by dCK, and Cd-AMP is subsequently metabolized to the active metabolite, cladribine-triphosphate. The triphosphate metabolite competitively inhibits incorporation of the normal dATP nucleotide into DNA, a process that results in the termination of chain elongation.[43] Progressive accumulation of the triphosphate metabolite leads to an imbalance in deoxyribonucleotide pools, thereby inhibiting further DNA synthesis and repair. Finally, the triphosphate metabolite is a potent inhibitor of ribonucleotide reductase, which further facilitates the inhibition of DNA biosynthesis.

## Mechanisms of Resistance

Resistance to 2-CdA has been attributed to altered intracellular drug metabolism. A reduction in the activity of dCK, the enzyme responsible for generating cytotoxic nucleotide metabolites, is a major determinant of acquired resistance. The monophosphate and triphosphate metabolites are dephosphorylated by the cytoplasmic enzyme 5′-nucleotidase. Interestingly, resistant cells derived from a patient with CLL exhibited both low levels of dCK expression and high levels of 5′-nucleotidase.

## Clinical Pharmacology

2-CdA is orally bioavailable, with 50% of an administered dose orally absorbed. Approximately 50% of an administered dose of drug is cleared by the kidneys, and 20% to 35% of the drug is excreted unchanged in the urine. Of note, this nucleoside can cross the blood–brain barrier with penetration into the cerebrospinal fluid.

## Toxicity

At conventional doses, myelosuppression is dose limiting. After a single course of drug, recovery from thrombocytopenia usually occurs within 2 to 4 weeks, whereas recovery from neutropenia takes place in 3 to 5 weeks. GI toxicities are generally mild, with nausea/vomiting and diarrhea. Mild-to-moderate neurotoxicity occurs in 15% of patients and is at least partly reversible with discontinuation of the drug. Immunosuppression accounts for the late morbidity observed in 2-CdA–treated patients. Lymphocyte counts, particularly CD4-positive cells, decrease within 1 to 4 weeks of drug administration and may remain depressed for several years.[44] After discontinuation of 2-CdA, a median time of up to 40 months may be required for complete recovery of normal CD4-positive counts. Although opportunistic infections occur, they do so less frequently than with fludarabine therapy. Infectious complications correlate with decreases in the CD4-positive count, and they include herpes zoster, *Candida*, *Pneumocystis*, *Pseudomonas aeruginosa*, *Listeria monocytogenes*, *Cryptococcus neoformans*, *Aspergillus*, *P. carinii*, and cytomegalovirus.

# CLOFARABINE

Clofarabine is a purine deoxyadenosine nucleoside analog, and it is approved for the treatment of pediatric patients with relapsed or refractory acute lymphoblastic leukemia (see Table 19.1).[45]

Ongoing studies are exploring the benefit of clofarabine alone and in combination with other agents in less heavily pretreated patients and in the use of different dose schedules for other hematologic malignancies.[46]

## Mechanism of Action

Clofarabine is inactive in its parent form and, like other purine analogs, it requires intracellular activation by dCK to form the monophosphate nucleotide, which undergoes further metabolism to the cytotoxic triphosphate metabolite. Clofarabine triphosphate is then incorporated into DNA, resulting in chain termination, and inhibition of DNA synthesis and function or the triphosphate form can directly inhibit DNA polymerases $\alpha$, $\beta$, and $\gamma$, which in turn, interferes with DNA chain elongation, DNA synthesis, and DNA repair. The triphosphate metabolite is also a potent inhibitor of ribonucleotide reductase, further mediating the inhibition of DNA biosynthesis by reducing the levels of key deoxyribonucleotide pools.

## Mechanisms of Resistance

Several resistance mechanisms have been identified in various preclinical systems, and they include decreased activation of the drug through the reduced expression of the anabolic enzyme deoxycytidine kinase, the decreased transport of drug into cells via the nucleoside transporter protein, and the increased expression of CTP synthetase activity resulting in increased concentrations of competing physiologic nucleotide substrate dCTP. To date, the precise resistance mechanism(s) that are relevant in the clinical setting remain to be determined.

## Clinical Pharmacology

Approximately 50% to 60% of an administered dose of drug is excreted unchanged in the urine, and the terminal half-life is on the order of 5 hours. To date, the pathways for nonrenal elimination have not been well defined. Caution should be exercised in patients with abnormal renal function, and concomitant use of medications known to cause renal toxicity should be avoided during drug treatment.

## Toxicity

Myelosuppression is dose limiting with neutropenia, anemia, and thrombocytopenia. The capillary leak syndrome (systemic inflammatory response syndrome) presents with tachypnea, tachycardia, pulmonary edema, and hypotension.[47] In essence, this adverse event is part of the tumor lysis syndrome and results from rapid cytoreduction of peripheral leukemic cells following treatment.[47] Other side effects may include nausea/vomiting, reversible liver dysfunction (hyperbilirubinemia and elevated serum transaminases), renal dysfunction (approximately 10%), and cardiac toxicity in the form of tachycardia and acute pump dysfunction.

# REFERENCES

1. Wright DL, Anderson AC. Antifolate agents: a patent review (2006–2010). *Expert Opin Ther Pat* 2011;21:1293–1308.
2. Chattopadhyay S, Moran RG, Goldman ID. Pemetrexed: biochemical and cellular pharmacology, mechanisms, and clinical applications. *Mol Cancer Ther* 2007;6:404–417.
3. Vogelzang NJ, Rusthoven JJ, Symanowski J, et al. Phase III study of pemetrexed in combination with cisplatin versus cisplatin alone in patients with malignant pleural mesothelioma. *J Clin Oncol* 2003;21:2636–2644.
4. Kindler HL. Systemic treatments for mesothelioma: standard and novel. *Curr Treat Options Oncol* 2008;9:171–179.
5. Joerger M, Omlin A, Cerny T, et al. The role of pemetrexed in advanced non small-cell lung cancer: special focus on pharmacology and mechanism of action. *Curr Drug Targets* 2010;11:37–47.
6. Zain J, O'Connor O. Pralatrexate: basic understanding and clinical development. *Expert Opin Pharmacother* 2010;11:1705–1714.
7. Sirotnak FM, DeGraw JI, Moccio DM, et al. New folate analogs of the 10-deaza-aminopterin series. Basis for structural design and biochemical and pharmacologic properties. *Cancer Chemother Pharmacol* 1984;12:18–25.
8. O'Connor OA. Pralatrexate: an emerging new agent with activity in T-cell lymphomas. *Curr Opin Oncol* 2006;18:591–597.

9. Bertino JR, Göker E, Gorlick R, et al. Resistance mechanisms to methotrexate in tumors. *Oncologist* 1996;1:223–226.

10. Zhao R, Goldman ID. Resistance to antifolates. *Oncogene* 2003;22:7431–7457.

11. Grem JL. 5-Fluorouracil: forty-plus and still ticking. A review of its preclinical and clinical development. *Invest New Drugs* 2000;18:299–313.

12. Saif MW, Ezzeldin H, Vance K, et al. DPYD*2A mutation: the most common mutation associated with DPD deficiency. *Cancer Chemother Pharmacol* 2007;60:503–507.

13. Grem JL. Biochemical modulation of 5-FU in systemic treatment of advanced colorectal cancer. *Oncology (Williston Park)* 2001;15:13–19.

14. Saif MW, Shah MM, Shah AR. Fluoropyrimidine-associated cardiotoxicity: revisited. *Expert Opin Drug Saf* 2009;8:191–202.

15. Saif MW, Eloubeidi MA, Russo S, et al. Phase I study of capecitabine with concomitant radiotherapy for patients with locally advanced pancreatic cancer: expression analysis of genes related to outcome. *J Clin Oncol* 2005;23:8679–8687.

16. Geyer CE, Forster J, Lindquist D, et al. Lapatinib plus capecitabine for HER2-positive advanced breast cancer. *N Engl J Med* 2006;355:2733–2743.

17. Saif MW, Katirtzoglou NA, Syrigos KN. Capecitabine: an overview of the side effects and their management. *Anticancer Drugs* 2008;19:447–464.

18. Van Custem E, Verslype C, Tejpar S. Oral capecitabine: bridging the Atlantic divide in colon cancer treatment. *Semin Oncol* 2005;32:43–51.

19. Haller DG, Cassidy J, Clarke SJ, et al. Potential regional differences for the tolerability profiles of fluoropyrimidines. *J Clin Oncol* 2008;26:2118–2123.

20. Saif MW, Syrigos KN, Katirtzoglou NA. S-1: a promising new oral fluoropyrimidine derivative. *Expert Opin Investig Drugs* 2009;18:335–348.

21. Saif MW, Rosen LS, Saito K, et al. A phase I study evaluating the effect of CDHP as a component of S-1 on the pharmacokinetics of 5-fluorouracil. *Anticancer Res* 2011;31:625–632.

22. Daigo S, Takahashi Y, Fujieda M, et al. A novel mutant allele of the CYP2A6 gene (CYP2A6*11) found in a cancer patient who showed poor metabolic phenotype towards tegafur. *Pharmacogenetics* 2002;12:299–306.

23. Reiter A, Hochhaus A, Berger U, et al. AraC-based pharmacotherapy of chronic myeloid leukaemia. *Expert Opin Pharmacother* 2001;2:1129–1135.

24. Braess J, Wegendt C, Feuring-Buske M, et al. Leukemic blasts differ from normal bone marrow mononuclear cells and CD34+ hematopoietic stem cells in their metabolism of cytosine arabinoside. *Br J Haematol* 1999;105:388–393.

25. Momparler RL, Laliberte J, Eliopoulos N, et al. Transfection of murine fibroblast cells with human cytidine deaminase cDNA confers resistance to cytosine arabinoside. *Anticancer Drugs* 1996;7:266–274.

26. Cai J, Damaraju VL, Groulx N, et al. Two distinct molecular mechanisms underlying cytarabine resistance in human leukemic cells. *Cancer Res* 2008;68:2349–2357.

27. Kern W, Estey EH. High-dose cytosine arabinoside in the treatment of acute myeloid leukemia: review of three randomized trials. *Cancer* 2006;107:116–124.

28. Mini E, Nobili S, Caciagli B, et al. Cellular pharmacology of gemcitabine. *Ann Oncol* 2006;17:v7–v12.

29. Saif MW, Sellers S, Li M, et al. A phase I study of bi-weekly administration of 24-h gemcitabine followed by 24-h irinotecan in patients with solid tumors. *Cancer Chemother Pharmacol* 2007;60:871–882.

30. Bergman AM, Pinedo HM, Peters GJ. Determinants of resistance to 2′,2′-difluorodeoxycytidine (gemcitabine). *Drug Resist Update* 2002;5:19–33.

31. Saif MW, Lee Y, Kim R. Harnessing gemcitabine metabolism: a step towards personalized medicine for pancreatic cancer. *Ther Adv Med Oncol* 2012;4:341–346.

32. Hong SP, Wen J, Bang S, et al. CD44-positive cells are responsible for gemcitabine resistance in pancreatic cancer cells. *Int J Cancer* 2009;125:2323–2331.

33. Poplin E, Feng Y, Berlin J, et al. Phase III, randomized study of gemcitabine and oxaliplatin versus gemcitabine (fixed-dose rate infusion) compared with gemcitabine (30-minute infusion) in patients with pancreatic carcinoma E6201: a trial of the Eastern Cooperative Oncology Group. *J Clin Oncol* 2009;27:3778–3785.

34. Hande KR. Purine antimetabolites. In: Chabner BA, Longo DL, eds. *Cancer Chemotherapy and Biotherapy: Principles and Practice*, 4th ed. Philadelphia: Lippincott–Raven; 2006: 212.

35. Evans WE. Pharmacogenetics of thiopurine S-methyltransferase and thiopurine therapy. *Ther Drug Monitor* 2004;26:186–191.

36. Wang L, Weinshilboum R. Thiopurine S-methyltransferase pharmacogenetics: insights, challenges, and future directions. *Oncogene* 2006;25:1629–1638.

37. Vora A, Mitchell CD, Lennard L, et al. Toxicity and efficacy of 6-thioguanine versus 6-mercaptopurine in childhood lymphoblastic leukaemia: a randomised trial. *Lancet* 2006;368:1339–1348.

38. Montillo M, Ricci F, Tedeschi A. Role of fludarabine in hematological malignancies. *Expert Rev Anticancer Ther* 2006;6:1141–1161.

39. Gandhi V, Plunkett W. Cellular and clinical pharmacology of fludarabine. *Clin Pharmacokinet* 2002;41:93–103.

40. van den Neste E, Cardoen S, Offner F, et al. Old and new insights into the mechanism of action of two nucleoside analogs active in lymphoid malignancies: flludarabine and cladribine. *Int J Oncol* 2005;27:1113–1124.

41. Gidron A, Tallman MS. 2-CdA in the treatment of hairy cell leukemia: a review of long-term follow-up. *Leuk Lymphoma* 2006;47:2301–2307.

42. Huang P, Robertson LE, Wright S, et al. High molecular weight DNA fragmentation: a critical event in nucleoside analog-induced apoptosis in leukemia cells. *Clin Cancer Res* 1995;1:1005–1013.

43. Grevz N, Saven A. Cladribine: from the bench to the bedside: focus on hairy cell leukemia. *Expert Rev Anticancer Ther* 2004;4:745–757.

44. Seto S, Carrera CJ, Kubota M, et al. Mechanism of deoxyadenosine and 2-chlorodeoxyadenosine toxicity to nondividing human lymphocytes. *J Clin Invest* 1985;75:377–383.

45. Bonate PL, Arthaud L, Cantrell WR Jr, et al. Discovery and development of clofarabine: a nucleoside analogue for treating cancer. *Nat Rev Drug Discov* 2006;5:855–863.

46. Faderi S, Gandhi V, Keating MJ, et al. The role of clofarabine in hematologic and solid malignancies: development of a next generation nucleoside analog. *Cancer* 2005;102:1985–1995.

47. Baytan B, Ozdemir O, Gunes AM, et al. Clofarabine-induced capillary leak syndrome in a child with refractory acute lymphoblastic leukemia. *J Pediatr Hematol Oncol* 2010;32:144–146.

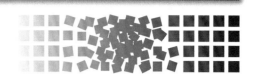

# 20 Topoisomerase Interactive Agents

Khanh T. Do, Shivaani Kummar, James H. Doroshow, and Yves Pommier

## CLASSIFICATION, BIOCHEMICAL, AND BIOLOGIC FUNCTIONS OF TOPOISOMERASES

Nucleic acids (DNA and RNA) being long polymers, topoisomerases fulfill the need for cellular DNA to be densely packaged in the cell nucleus, transcribed, replicated, and evenly distributed between daughter cells following replication without tangles. Topoisomerases are ubiquitous and essential for all organisms as they prevent and resolve DNA and RNA entanglements and resolve DNA supercoiling during transcription and replication. This chapter first summarizes the basic elements necessary to understand the mechanism of action of topoisomerases and their inhibitors. More detailed information can be found in recent reviews[1–7] and two recent books.[8,9] The second part of the chapter summarizes the use of topoisomerase inhibitors as anticancer drugs.

### Classification of Topoisomerases

Human cells contain six topoisomerase genes (Table 20.1), which have been numbered historically. The commonly used abbreviations are Top1 for topoisomerases I (Top1mt being the mitochondrial topoisomerase whose gene is encoded in the cell nucleus),[10] Top2 for topoisomerases II, and Top3 for topoisomerases III. Top1 was the first eukaryotic topoisomerase discovered by Champoux and Dulbecco.[11] Topoisomerases solve DNA topologic problems by cutting the DNA backbone and religating without the assistance of any additional ligase. Top1 and Top3 act by cleaving/religating a single strand of the DNA duplex, whereas Top2 enzymes cleave and religate both strands, making a four–base pair reversible staggered cut (Fig. 20.1). It is convenient to remember that odd-numbered topoisomerases (Top1 and Top3) cleave and religate one strand, whereas the even numbered topoisomerases (Top2s) cleave and religate both strands.

### Biochemical Characteristics and Cleavage Complexes of the Different Topoisomerases

The DNA cutting/relegation mechanism is common to all topoisomerases and utilizes an enzyme catalytic tyrosine residue acting as a nucleophile and becoming covalently attached to the end of the broken DNA. These catalytic intermediates are referred to as cleavage complexes (see Fig. 20.1B, E). The reverse religation reaction is carried out by the attack of the ribose hydroxyl ends toward the tyrosyl-DNA bond.

Top1 (and Top1mt) attaches to the 3′-end of the break, whereas the other topoisomerases (Top2 and Top3) have opposite polarity and covalently attach to the 5′-end of the breaks (see Table 20.1 [second column] and Fig. 20.1B, E). Topoisomerases have distinct biochemical requirements. Top1 and Top1mt are the simplest, nicking/closing, and relaxing DNA as monomers in the absence of cofactor, and even at ice temperature. Top2 enzymes, on the other hand, are the most complex topoisomerases working as dimers, requiring

ATP binding and hydrolysis, and a divalent metal ($Mg^{2+}$) for catalysis. Top3 enzymes also require $Mg^{2+}$ for catalysis but function as monomers without ATP requirement. Notably, the DNA substrates differ for Top3 enzymes. Whereas both Top1 and Top2 process double-stranded DNA, the Top3 substrates need to be single-stranded nucleic acids (DNA for Top3α and DNA or RNA for Top3β).[10,12,13]

### Differential Topoisomerization Mechanisms: Swiveling Versus Strand Passage, DNA Versus RNA Topoisomerases

Topoisomerases use two main mechanisms to change nucleic topology. The first is by "untwisting" the DNA duplex. This mechanism is unique to Top1, which, by an enzyme-associated single-strand break, allows the broken strand to rotate around the intact strand (see Fig. 20.1B) until DNA supercoiling is dissipated. At this point, the stacking energy of adjacent DNA bases realigns the broken ends, and the 5′-hydroxyl end attacks the 3′-phosphotyrosyl end, thereby relegating the DNA. A remarkable feature of this Top1 untwisting mechanism is its extreme efficiency with a rotation speed around 6,000 rpm and relative independence from torque, thereby allowing full relaxation of DNA supercoiling.[14]

The second topologic mechanism is by "strand passage." This mechanism allows the passage of a double- or a single-stranded DNA (or RNA) through the cleavage complexes. Top2α and Top2β both act by allowing the passage of an intact DNA duplex through the DNA double-strand break generated by the enzymes. After which, Top2 religates the broken duplex. Such reactions permit DNA decatenation, unknotting, and relaxation of supercoils.[3] Top3 enzymes also act by strand passage but only pass one nucleic acid strand through the single-strand break generated by the enzymes. In the case of Top3α, the substrate is a single-stranded DNA segment (such as a double-Holliday junction), whereas in the case of Top3β, the substrate can be a single-stranded RNA segment, with Top3β acting as a RNA topoisomerase.[13,15]

## TOPOISOMERASE INHIBITORS AS INTERFACIAL POISONS

### Topoisomerase Inhibitors Act as Interfacial Inhibitors by Binding at the Topoisomerase–DNA Interface and Trapping Topoisomerase Cleavage Complexes

Relegation of the cleavage complexes is dependent on the structure of the ends of the broken DNA (i.e., the realignment of the broken ends). Binding the drugs at the enzyme–DNA interface misaligns the ends of the DNA and precludes relegation, resulting in the stabilization of the topoisomerase cleavage complexes (Top1cc and Top2cc). Crystal structures of drug-bound cleavage complexes have firmly established this mechanism for both Top1- and Top2-targeted drugs.[16]

**TABLE 20.1**

**Classification of Human Topoisomerases and Topoisomerase Inhibitors**

| Type | Polarity | Mechanism | Genes | Proteins | Main Functions | Drugs |
|------|----------|-----------|-------|----------|----------------|-------|
| IB | 3'-PY | Rotation/swiveling | TOP1 | Top1 | DNA supercoiling relaxation, replication, and transcription | Camptothecins, noncamptothecins |
| | | | TOP1MT | Top1mt | | |
| IIA | 5'-PY | Strand passage ATPase | TOP2A | Top2α | Decatenation/replication | Anthracyclines, anthracenediones, epipodophyllotoxins |
| | | | TOP2B | Top2β | Transcription | |
| IA | 5'-PY | Strand passage | TOP3A | Top3α | DNA replication with BLM | None |
| | | | TOP3B | Top3β | RNA topoisomerase | |

Top1mt, mitochondrial DNA topoisomerase; BLM, Bloom's syndrome helicare.

It is critical to understand that the cytotoxic mechanism of topoisomerase inhibitors requires the drugs to trap the topoisomerase cleavage complexes rather than block catalytic activity. This sets apart topoisomerase inhibitors from classical enzyme inhibitors such as antifolates. Indeed, knocking out Top1 renders yeast cells totally immune to camptothecin,[17,18] and reducing enzyme levels in cancer cells confers drug resistance. Conversely, in breast cancers, amplification of TOP2A, which is on the same locus as HER2, contributes to the efficacy of doxorubicin.[19] Also, cellular mutations of Top1 and Top2 that renders cells insensitive to the trapping of topoisomerase cleavage complexes produce high resistance to Top1 or Top2 inhibitors. Based on this trapping of cleavage complexes mechanism, we refer to topoisomerase inhibitors as topoisomerase cleavage complex-targeted drugs.

## Top1cc-Targeted Drugs (Camptothecin and Noncamptothecin Derivatives) Kill Cancer Cells by Replication Collisions

Top1cc are cytotoxic by their conversion into DNA damage by replication and transcription fork collisions. This explains why cytotoxicity is directly related to drug exposure and why arresting DNA replication protects cells from camptothecin.[20,21] The collisions arise from the fact that the drugs, by slowing down the nicking/closing activity of Top1, uncouple the kinetics of Top1 with the polymerases and helicases, which lead polymerases to collide into Top1cc (Fig. 20.2A). Such collisions have two consequences. They generate double-strand breaks (replication and transcription runoff) and irreversible Top1–DNA adducts (see Fig. 20.2B). The replication double-strand breaks are repaired by homologous recombination, which explains the hypersensitivity of BRCA-deficient cancer cells to Top1cc-targeted drugs.[22] The Top1-covalent complexes can be removed by two pathways, the excision pathway centered around tyrosyl-DNA-phosphodiesterase 1 (TDP1)[23] and the endonuclease pathway involving 3'-flap endonucleases such as XPF-ERCC1.[24] It is also possible that drug-trapped Top1cc directly generate DNA double-strand breaks when they are within 10 base pairs on opposite strands of the DNA duplex or when they occur next to a preexisting single-strand break on the opposite strand. Finally, it is not excluded that topologic defects contribute to the cytotoxicity of Top1cc-targeted drugs (the accumulation of supercoils[25] and the formation of alternative structures such as R-loops) (see Fig. 20.2D).[26]

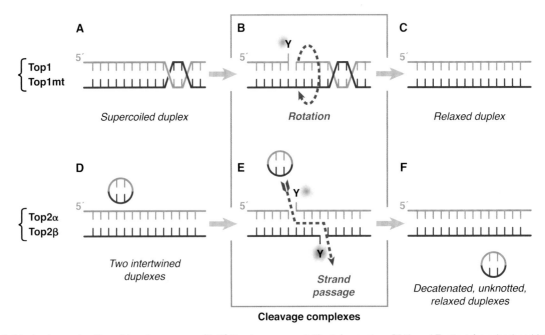

**Figure 20.1** Mechanisms of action of topoisomerases. **(A–C)** Topoisomerases I (Top1 for nuclear DNA and Top1mt for mitochondrial DNA) relax supercoiled DNA **(A)** by reversibly cleaving one DNA strand, forming a covalent bond between the enzyme catalytic tyrosine and the 3' end of the nicked DNA (the Top1 cleavage complex [Top1cc]) **(B)**. This reaction allows the swiveling of the broken strand around the intact strand. Rapid religation allows the dissociation of Top1. **(D–F)** Topoisomerases II (Top2α and Top2β) act on two DNA duplexes **(A)**. They act as homodimers, cleaving both strands and forming a covalent bond between their catalytic tyrosine and the 5' end of the DNA break (Top2cc) **(E)**. This reaction allows the passage of the intact duplex through the Top2 homodimer *(red dotted arrow)* **(E)**. Top2 inhibitors trap the Top2cc and prevent the normal religation **(F)**.

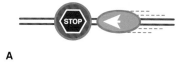

Collisions of polymerases and helicases *(green ellipse)* with trapped Top cleavage complexes *(Stop sign)*

=> Protein-DNA complexes blocking DNA metabolism

**A**

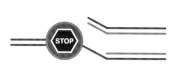

Conversion of Top1cc into DSB by replication "runoff"

=> Top1 needs to be removed by TDP1
        and /or 3'-flap endonucleases (XPF-ERCC1)

=> DSB repaired by homologous recombination

Top1cc also form DSB when on opposite strands or opposite to a preexisting single-strand break

**B**

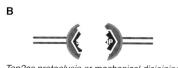

Top2cc readily form DSB when concerted cleavage on both strands and disjunction of the homodimer

*Top2cc proteolysis or mechanical disjoining*

**C**

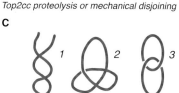

Topologic defects resulting from Top sequestration in the cleavage complexes: accumulation of

=> Supercoils (Top1 and Top2) *(1)*

=> Knots (Top2) *(2)*

=> Catenanes (Top2) *(3)*

**D**

**Figure 20.2** Mechanisms of action of topoisomerase inhibitors beyond the trapping of topoisomerase cleavage complexes. **(A)** Stalled or slow cleavage complexes lead to collisions with replication and transcription complexes. **(B)** Collisions of replication complexes with Top1cc on the leading strand for DNA synthesis generate DNA double-strand breaks by replication runoff. Top1cc can also form DNA double-strand breaks (DSBs) when they occur opposite to another Top1cc or preexisting nick. **(C)** Top2cc, which are normally held together by Top2 homodimers, can be converted to free DSBs upon Top2cc proteolysis or dimer disjunction. **(D)** Topologic defects resulting from functional topoisomerase deficiencies play a minor role in the anticancer activity of topoisomerase cleavage complex targeted drugs.

## Cytotoxic Mechanisms of Top2cc-Targeted Drugs (Intercalators and Demethyl Epipodophyllotoxins)

Contrary to camptothecins, Top2 inhibitors kill cancer cells without requiring DNA replication fork collisions. Indeed, even after a 30-minute exposure, doxorubicin and other Top2cc-targeted drugs can kill over 99% of the cells, which is in vast excess of the fraction of S-phase cells in tissue culture (generally less than 50%).[27,28] The collision mechanism in the case of Top2cc-targeted drugs (see Fig. 20.2A) appears to involve transcription and proteolysis of both Top2 and RNA polymerase II.[29] Such situation would then lead to DNA double-strand breaks by disruption of the Top2 dimer interface (see Fig. 20.2C). Alternatively, the Top2 homodimer interface could be disjoined by mechanical tension (see Fig. 20.2C). Yet, it is important to bear in mind that 90% of Top2cc trapped by etoposide are not concerted and, therefore, consist in single-strand breaks,[3,30,31] which is different from doxorubicin, which traps both Top2 monomers and produces a majority of DNA double-strand breaks.[32] Finally, it is not excluded that topologic defects resulting from Top2 sequestration by the drug-induced cleavage complexes could contribute to the cytotoxicity of Top2cc-targeted drugs (see Fig. 20.2D). Such topologic defects would include persistent DNA knots and catenanes, potentially leading to chromosome breaks during mitosis.

## TOPOISOMERASE I INHIBITORS: CAMPTOTHECINS AND BEYOND

Camptothecin is an alkaloid identified in the 1960s by Wall and Wani[33] in a screen of plant extracts for antineoplastic drugs. The two water-soluble derivatives of camptothecin containing the active lactone form are topotecan and irinotecan, which are approved by the U.S. Food and Drug Administration (FDA) for the treatment of several cancers. In addition, several Top1cc-targeting drugs are in clinical development, including camptothecin derivatives and formulations (including high–molecular-weight conjugates or liposomal formulations), as well as noncamptothecin compounds that exhibit greater potency or noncross resistance to irinotecan and topotecan in preclinical cancer models.[31,34–36]

## Irinotecan

Irinotecan, a prodrug containing a bulky dipiperidine side chain at C-10 (Fig. 20.3), is cleaved by a carboxylesterase-converting enzyme in the liver and other tissues to generate the active metabolite, SN-38. Irinotecan is FDA approved for the treatment of colorectal cancer in the metastatic setting as first-line treatment in combination with 5-fluorouracil/leucovorin (5-FU/LV) and as a single agent in the second-line treatment of progressive colorectal cancer after 5-FU–based therapy (see Table 20.1).[37,38] Newer therapeutic uses of irinotecan include a combination with oxaliplatin and 5-FU as first-line treatment in pancreatic cancer.[39] Irinotecan is additionally used in combination with cisplatin or carboplatin in extensive-stage small-cell lung cancer[40,41] as well as refractory esophageal and gastroesophageal junction (GEJ) cancers, gastric cancer, cervical cancer, anaplastic gliomas and glioblastomas, and non–small-cell lung cancer (Table 20.2). Irinotecan is usually administered intravenously at a dose of 125 mg/m² for 4 weeks with a 2-week rest period in combination with bolus 5-FU/LV, 180 mg/m² every 2 weeks in combination with an infusion of 5-FU/LV, or 350 mg/m² every 3 weeks as a single agent.

Diarrhea and myelosuppression are the most common toxicities associated with irinotecan administration. Two mechanisms explain irinotecan-induced diarrhea. Acute cholinergic effects resulting in abdominal cramping and diarrhea occur within 24 hours of drug administration are the result of acetylcholinesterase inhibition by the prodrug, and can be treated with the administration of atropine. Direct mucosal cytotoxicity with diarrhea is typically observed after 24 hours and can result in significant morbidity. Symptoms are managed with loperamide. Hepatic metabolism and biliary excretion accounts for >70% of the elimination of the administered dose, with renal excretion accounting for the remainder of the dose. SN-38 is glucuronidated in the liver by UGT1A1, and deficiencies in this pathway increase the risk of diarrhea and myelosuppression. Dose reductions are recommended for patients who are homozygous for the UGT1A1*28 allele, for which an FDA-approved test for detection of the UGT1A1*28 allele in patients is available.[42,43] Additionally, dose reductions of irinotecan are recommended for patients with hepatic dysfunction, with bilirubin greater than 1.5 mg/mL.[44]

CANCER THERAPEUTICS

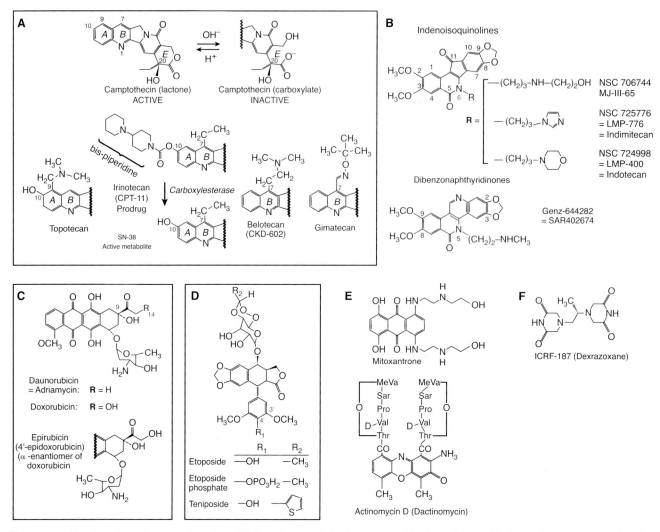

**Figure 20.3** Structure of topoisomerase inhibitors. **(A)** Camptothecin derivatives are instable at physiologic pH with the formation of a carboxylate derivative within minutes. Irinotecan is a prodrug and needs to be converted to SN-38 to trap Top1cc. **(B)** Non-camptothecin derivatives in clinical trials. **(C)** Anthracycline derivatives. **(D)** Demethyl epipodophyllotoxin derivatives. **(E)** Other intercalating Top2 inhibitors acting by trapping Top2cc. **(F)** Structure of dexrazoxane, which acts as a catalytic inhibitor of Top2.

## Topotecan

Topotecan contains a basic side chain at position C-9 that enhances its water solubility (see Fig. 20.3). Topotecan is approved for the treatment of ovarian cancer,[45] small-cell lung cancer,[46] and as a single agent and in combination with cisplatin for cervical cancer.[47] Additionally, it is active in acute myeloid leukemia (AML) and myelodysplastic syndrome (see Table 20.2). Topotecan is administered intravenously as a single agent at a dose of 1.5 mg/$m^2$ as a 30-minute infusion daily for 5 days, followed by a 2-week period of rest for the treatment of solid tumors or at a dose of 0.75 mg/$m^2$ as a 30-minute infusion daily for 3 days in combination with cisplatin on day 1, every 3 weeks, for the treatment of cervical cancer.

Myelosuppression is the most common dose-limiting toxicity. Extensive prior radiation or previous bone marrow–suppressive chemotherapy increases the risk of topotecan-induced myelosuppression. Other toxicities include nausea, vomiting, diarrhea, fatigue, alopecia, and transient hepatic transaminitis.

Topotecan and its metabolites are primarily cleared by the kidneys, requiring dose reduction in patients with renal dysfunction. A 50% dose reduction is recommended for patients with moderate renal impairment (creatinine clearance 20 to 39 mL per minute).

There are no formal guidelines for dose reductions in patients with hepatic dysfunction (defined as serum bilirubin >1.5 mg/dL to <10 mg/dL). Topotecan additionally penetrates the blood-brain barrier, achieving concentrations in cerebrospinal fluid that are approximately 30% that of plasma levels.[48]

## Camptothecin Conjugates and Analogs

New formulations of camptothecin conjugates and analogs are currently in clinical development in an effort to improve the therapeutic index (Table 20.3). The development of camptothecin conjugates is based on the notion that the addition of a bulky conjugate would allow for a more consistent delivery system and extend the half-life of the molecule.

CRLX101, formerly IT-101, a covalent cyclodextrin-polyethylene glycol copolymer camptothecin conjugate, has plasma concentrations and area under the curve (AUC) that are approximately 100-fold higher than camptothecin, with a half-life in the range of 17 to 20 hours compared to 1.3 hours for camptothecin.[49] It has demonstrated antitumor activity in preclinical studies in irinotecan-resistant tumors with complete tumor regression in human non–small-cell lung cancer, Ewing sarcoma, and

## TABLE 20.2

### U.S. Food and Drug Administration–Approved Camptothecin Analogs

| | | | |
|---|---|---|---|
| **Irinotecan (Camptosar)** | FDA approved for: Metastatic colorectal cancer | First-line therapy in combination with 5-FU/LV | Diarrhea (dose reductions are recommended for patients who are homozygous for the UGT1A1*28 allele) |
| | | Second-line therapy as a single agent | Myelosuppression |
| | Category 2A[a] recommendations: Pancreatic cancer | First-line therapy in combination with oxaliplatin, 5-FU/LV | |
| | Extensive-stage small-cell lung cancer | First-line therapy in combination with cisplatin or carboplatin | |
| | Category 2B[b] recommendations: Esophageal and GEJ cancers, gastric cancer, cervical cancer, anaplastic gliomas and glioblastomas, non–small-cell lung cancer, ovarian cancer | | |
| **Topotecan (Hycamtin)** | FDA approved for: Cervical cancer | Stage IVB, recurrent, or persistent carcinoma of the cervix not amenable to curative treatment with surgery and/or radiation therapy | Myelosuppression |
| | Ovarian cancer | After failure of initial therapy | |
| | Small-cell lung cancer | After failure of initial therapy | |
| | Class 2B recommendations: AML, MDS | | |

[a] Category 2A: Recommendations are based upon lower-level evidence, there is uniform National Comprehensive Cancer Network consensus that the intervention is appropriate.
[b] Category 2B: Recommendations are based upon lower-level evidence, there is National Comprehensive Cancer Network consensus that the intervention is appropriate.
MDS, myelodysplastic syndrome.

lymphoma xenograft models.[50] Preliminary data from Phase 1 studies indicate that CRLX101 is well tolerated at a dose of 15 mg/m$^2$ administered in a biweekly administration schedule.[51] It is currently being studied in Phase 2 studies as a single agent and in combination with chemotherapeutic agents in lung, renal cell cancer, and gynecologic malignancies.[52–54]

Etirinotecan pegol (NKTR-102), an irinotecan polymer conjugate, has a longer plasma circulation time with a lower maximum concentration of SN-38 compared with irinotecan. It was evaluated in a Phase 2 study in platinum-resistant refractory epithelial ovarian cancer at a dose of 145 mg/m$^2$ administered on a schedule of every 21 days; a median progression-free survival of 5.3 months and median overall survival of 11.7 months was observed.[55] Two schedules of administration, 145 mg/m$^2$ administered every 14 days versus every 21 days, have been tested in a Phase 2 study of NKTR-102 in patients with previously treated metastatic breast cancer.[56] Of the 70 patients evaluated in this study, 20 patients achieved an objective response (29%; 95% confidence interval [CI] 18.4 to 40.6). For both these studies, the most common adverse events on the 21-day administration schedule were dehydration and diarrhea. Etirinotecan pegol is currently being evaluated in several phase 2 studies in lung cancer, colorectal cancer, and high-grade gliomas,[57–60] with evidence of clinical activity in refractory solid tumors. A Phase 3 trial (The BEACON Study) is underway evaluating NKTR-102 against the physicians' choice in refractory breast cancer.[61]

As an alternative to macromolecular conjugates, attempts have also been made to alter the camptothecin pentacyclic ring structure with modifications of the A and B ring (see Fig. 20.3A) in an effort to improve solubility and enhance antitumor activity. Structure–activity relationship studies have shown that substitutions at the 7, 9, and 10 positions serve to enhance the antitumor activity of camptothecin.[62] Belotecan, a novel camptothecin analog, has a water-solubilizing group at the 7 position of the B ring of camptothecin (see Fig. 20.3A). Several Phase 2 studies have evaluated belotecan in combination with carboplatin in recurrent ovarian cancer[63] and in combination with cisplatin in extensive-stage small-cell lung cancer,[64] demonstrating activity in these cancers; however, these combinations were associated with prominent hematologic toxicities. Phase 2 studies evaluating belotecan as a single agent in patients with recurrent or progressive carcinoma of the uterine cervix failed to show activity.[65] Gimatecan is a lipophilic oral camptothecin analog (see Fig. 20.3A). Pharmacokinetic studies demonstrate that gimatecan is primarily present in plasma as the lactone form (>85%), and has a long half-life of 77.1 +/− 29.6 hours, with an increase in maximum concentration (Cmax) and AUC of three- to six-fold after multiple dosing.[66] Phase 2 studies show that gimatecan has demonstrated activity in previously treated ovarian cancer, with myelosuppression as the main toxicity.[67]

Newer development of analogs have attempted to modify the E-ring through introduction of an electron-withdrawing group at

## TABLE 20.3

### Topoisomerase I Inhibitors in Development

| Camptothecin Conjugates | Camptothecin Analogs | Noncamptothecin Agents |
|---|---|---|
| CRLX101 | Belotecan | Indenoisoquinoline |
| NKTR-102 | Gimatecan | Indotecan (LMP-400) |
| MM-398 | Homocamptothecin | Indimitecan (LMP-776) |
| | Elomotecan | Dibenzo naphthyridine |
| | Diflomotecan | Genz-644282 |

the α position in an effort to overcome the instability of the E-ring while maintaining the binding capability of the camptothecin analog to the Top1-DNA cleavage complex. Collectively called homocamptothecin analogs,[68] two have been tested in clinical trials and include diflomotecan[68] and elomotecan.[69] The dose-limiting toxicity in the Phase I study of elomotecan was neutropenia. A five-member E-ring derivative has also been developed and has reached a Phase 1 clinical trial.[70,71]

## Noncamptothecin Topoisomerase I Inhibitors

Noncamptothecin Top1 inhibitors are in clinical development, and include indenoisoquinolines and dibenzonaphthyridines (see Fig. 20.3B). Two indenoisoquinoline derivatives are currently in clinical development, indotecan (LMP400) and indimitecan (LMP776).[72,73] Early in vitro studies show enhanced potency compared with camptothecins, and persistence of Top1 cleavage complexes.[74] Genz-644282, a dibenzonaphthyridine derivative, demonstrated enhanced antitumor activity in preclinical studies[75] and is currently being evaluated in Phase 1 clinical trials.[76]

# TOPOISOMERASE II INHIBITORS: INTERCALATORS AND NONINTERCALATORS

Topoisomerase II inhibitors can be classified in two main classes: DNA intercalators, which encompass different chemical classes (Fig. 20.3C, E), and nonintercalators represented by the epipodophyllotoxin derivatives (see Fig. 20.3D). Although both act by trapping Top2 cleavage complexes (Top2cc), DNA intercalators exhibit a second effect as drug concentrations increase above low micromolar values: they block the formation of Top2cc by intercalating into DNA and destabilizing the binding of Top2 to DNA. This explains why Top2α and Top2β are trapped over a relatively narrow concentration range by anthracyclines, and why intercalators have additional effects besides trapping Top2cc, namely inhibition of a broad range of DNA processing enzymes including helicases, polymerase, and even nucleosome destabilization.

## Doxorubicin

Doxorubicin and daunorubicin were the first anthracyclines discovered in the 1960s and remain among the most widely used anticancer agents over a broad spectrum of malignancies. Although doxorubicin only differs by one hydroxyl substitution on position 14 (see Fig. 20.3C), doxorubicin has a much broader anticancer activity than daunorubicin. Anthracyclines are natural products derived from *Streptomyces peucetius* variation *caesius*. They were found to target Top2 well after their clinical approval.[77] Subsequent searches for less toxic drugs and formulations led to the approval of liposomal doxorubicin, idarubicin, and epirubicin.

Anthracyclines are flat, planar molecules that are relatively hydrophobic. The quinone structure of anthracyclines (see Fig. 20.3C) enhances the catalysis of oxidation-reduction reactions, thereby promoting the generation of oxygen free radicals, which may be involved in antitumor effects as well as the cardiotoxicity associated with these drugs.[78,79] Anthracyclines are also substrates for P-glycoprotein and Mrp-1, and drug efflux is thought to be a major drug resistance determinant.[80,81]

Doxorubicin is available in a standard salt form and as a liposomal formulation. FDA-labeled indications for standard doxorubicin include acute lymphocytic leukemia (ALL), AML, chronic lymphoid leukemia, Hodgkin lymphoma, non-Hodgkin lymphoma, mantle cell lymphoma, multiple myeloma, mycosis fungoides, Kaposi sarcoma, breast cancer (adjuvant therapy and advanced), advanced prostate cancer, advanced gastric cancer, Ewing sarcoma, thyroid cancer, advanced nephroblastoma,

advanced neuroblastoma, advanced non–small-cell lung cancer, advanced ovarian cancer, advanced transitional cell bladder cancer, cervical cancer, and Langerhans cell tumors. Doxorubicin has activity in other malignancies as well, including soft tissue sarcoma, osteosarcoma, carcinoid, and liver cancer (Table 20.4). Doxorubicin is typically administered at a recommended dose of 30 to 75 mg/m$^2$ every 3 weeks intravenously.

Major acute toxicities of doxorubicin include myelosuppression, mucositis, alopecia, nausea, and vomiting. Myelosuppression is the acute dose-limiting toxicity. Other toxicities, including diarrhea, nausea, vomiting, mucositis, and alopecia, are dose and schedule related. Prophylactic antiemetics are routinely given with bolus doses of doxorubicin, and longer infusions are associated with less nausea and less cardiotoxicity. Patients should also be warned to expect their urine to redden after drug administration. Doxorubicin is a potent vesicant, and extravasation can lead to severe necrosis of skin and local tissues, requiring surgical debridement and skin grafts. Infusions via a central venous catheter are recommended. Other toxicities of doxorubicin include *radiation recall* and the risk of developing secondary leukemia. *Radiation recall* is an inflammatory reaction at sites of previous radiation and can lead to pericarditis, pleural effusion, and skin rash. Secondary leukemias are thought to be a result of balanced translocations that result from Top2 poisoning by the anthracyclines, albeit to lesser degree than other Top2 poisons, such as the epipodophyllotoxins (see the following).[82]

Anthracyclines are cleared mainly by metabolism to less active forms and by biliary excretion. Less than 10% of the administered dose is cleared by the kidneys. Dose reductions should be made in patients with elevated plasma bilirubin. Doxorubicin should be dose reduced by 50% for plasma bilirubin concentrations ranging from 1.2 to 3.0 mg/dL, by 75% for values of 3.1 to 5.0 mg/dL, and withheld for values greater than 5 mg/dL.

## Liposomal Doxorubicin

Doxorubicin is also available in a polyethylene glycol (PEG)ylated liposomal form, which allows for enhancement of drug delivery. Use of liposomal doxorubicin has been associated with less cardiotoxicity even at doses exceeding 500 mg/m$^2$.[83] Additionally, liposomal doxorubicin produces less nausea and vomiting and relatively mild myelosuppression compared to doxorubicin. Unique to the liposomal formulation is the risk of hand–foot syndrome and an acute infusion reaction manifested by flushing, dyspnea, edema, fever, chills, rash, bronchospasm, and hypertension. These infusion reactions are related to the rate of infusion; therefore, the recommended administration schedule is set at an initial rate of 1 mg per minute for the first 10 to 15 minutes. The rate may be slowly increased to complete infusion over 60 minutes if no reaction occurs. Typical dosing schedules include 50 mg/m$^2$ intravenous infusion every 4 weeks for four courses in ovarian cancer, 20 mg/m$^2$ intravenous infusion every 3 weeks in AIDS-related Kaposi sarcoma, and 30 mg/m$^2$ intravenous infusion in combination with bortezomib to be given on days 1, 4, 8, and 11 every 3 weeks in multiple myeloma.

## Daunorubicin

Despite its chemical similarity (see Fig. 20.3C), daunorubicin is considerably less active in solid tumors compared to doxorubicin. It is FDA approved for the treatment of ALL and AML. Daunorubicin is typically administered via intravenous push over 3 to 5 minutes at a dose of 30 to 45 mg/m$^2$ per day on 3 consecutive days in combination chemotherapy. For induction therapy for pediatric acute lymphoblastic leukemia, daunorubicin is dosed at 25 mg/m$^2$ intravenously in combination with vincristine and prednisone. In children less than 2 years of age or in those who have a body surface area less than 0.5 m$^2$, current recommendations are based on

## TABLE 20.4

### U.S. Food And Drug Administration–Approved Topoisomerase II Inhibitors in Clinical Use

| Compound | Tumor Type | Clinical Indication | Major Toxicities |
|---|---|---|---|
| **I. Anthracyclines** | | | |
| Doxorubicin (Adriamycin) | Breast carcinoma | Adjuvant setting with axillary LN involvement following resection of primary breast cancer | Dose-dependent cardiotoxicity Myelosuppression |
| | ALL AML Wilms' tumor Neuroblastoma Sarcomas Ovarian cancer Transitional cell bladder cancer Thyroid cancer Gastric cancer Hodgkin lymphoma Non-Hodgkin lymphoma | In combination with other cytotoxic agents | |
| Pegylated liposomal doxorubicin (Doxil) | Ovarian cancer | After failure of platinum-based chemotherapy | Myelosuppression Stomatitis Hand-foot syndrome Dosage reduction recommended with hepatic dysfunction |
| | AIDS-related Kaposi sarcoma | After failure of prior systemic chemotherapy | |
| | Multiple myeloma | In combination with bortezomib | |
| Daunorubicin (Cerubidine) | ALL AML | Induction therapy | Dose-dependent cardiotoxicity Myelosuppression |
| Epirubicin (Ellence) | Breast cancer | Adjuvant therapy in patients with evidence of axillary node tumor involvement following primary resection | Dose-dependent cardiotoxicity Myelosuppression |
| Idarubicin (Idamycin) | AML | Induction therapy | Dose-dependent cardiotoxicity Myelosuppression |
| **II. Anthracenediones** | | | |
| Mitoxantrone (Novantrone) | Prostate cancer AML | Hormone-refractory prostate cancer | Myelosuppression |
| Dactinomycin (Cosmegen) | Wilms' tumor Rhabdomyosarcoma Ewing sarcoma Nonseminomatous testicular cancer Gestational trophoblastic neoplasia | | Myelosuppression |
| **III. Epipodophyllotoxins** | | | |
| Etoposide (VePesid) | Small-cell lung cancer Testicular cancer | First-line in combination First-line in combination | Myelosuppression |
| Teniposide (Vumon) | Pediatric lymphoblastic leukemia | Refractory setting | Myelosuppression |

LN, lymph node.

body mass index (1 mg/kg) rather than body surface area. A higher dose of daunorubicin at 60 mg/m$^2$ per day to 90 mg/m$^2$ per day intravenously for 3 consecutive days is currently recommended as part of the induction combination regimen for the treatment of acute myeloblastic leukemia. Daunorubicin has similar toxicities to doxorubicin, including myelosuppression, cardiac toxicity, nausea, vomiting, alopecia, and is also a vesicant. Daunorubicin is metabolized by the liver and undergoes substantial elimination by the kidneys, requiring dose reductions for both renal and hepatic dysfunction. A 50% dose reduction is recommended for either serum creatinine or bilirubin greater than 3 mg/dL, and a 25% reduction in dose for bilirubin concentrations ranging from 1.2 to 3.0 mg/dL.

## Epirubicin

Epirubicin is an epimer of doxorubicin (see Fig. 20.3C) with increased lipophilicity. It is FDA approved for adjuvant therapy of breast cancer but is also used in combination for the treatment of a variety of malignancies. Epirubicin is administered intravenously at doses ranging from 60 to 120 mg/m$^2$ every 3 to 4 weeks. Epirubicin has a similar toxicity profile to doxorubicin but is overall better tolerated.

In addition to being converted to an enol by an aldose reductase, epirubicin has a unique steric orientation of the C-4 hydroxyl group that allows it to serve as a substrate for conjugation reactions mediated by liver glucuronosyltransferases and sulfatases. As such, dose adjustments are recommended in the setting of hepatic dysfunction. For patients with serum bilirubin of 1.2 to 3 mg/dL or aspartate aminotransferase of 2 to 4 times the upper limit of normal, a 50% dose reduction is recommended. For patients with bilirubin greater than 3 mg/dL or aspartate aminotransferase greater than 4 times the upper limit of normal, a dose reduction of 75% is recommended. Due to limited data, no specific dose recommendations are currently available for patients with renal impairment, although current recommendations are for consideration of dose adjustments in patients with serum creatinine greater than 5 mg/dL.

## Idarubicin

Idarubicin is a synthetic derivative of daunorubicin, but lacks the 4-methoxy group (see Fig. 20.3C). It is FDA approved as part of combination chemotherapy regimen for AML and is also active in ALL. It is given intravenously at a dose of 12 mg/m$^2$ for 3 consecutive days, typically in combination with cytarabine. Idarubicin has similar toxicities as daunorubicin. Its primary active metabolite is idarubicinol, and elimination is mainly through the biliary system and, to a lesser extent, through renal excretion. A 50% dose reduction is recommended for serum bilirubin of 2.6 to 5 mg/dL and idarubicin should not be given if the bilirubin is greater than 5 mg/dL. Additionally, dose reductions in renal impairment are advised, but specific guidelines are not available.

## Cardiac Toxicity of Anthracyclines

Anthracyclines are responsible for cardiac toxicities, and special considerations are necessary to minimize this severe side effect. Acute doxorubicin cardiotoxicity is reversible, and clinical signs include tachycardia, hypotension, electrocardiogram changes, and arrhythmias. It develops during or within days of anthracycline infusion, and its incidence can be significantly reduced by slowing doxorubicin infusion rates.

Chronic and delayed cardiotoxicity is more common and more severe because it is irreversible. Chronic cardiotoxicity with congestive heart failure peaks at 1 to 3 months but can occur even years after therapy. Myocardial damage has been shown to occur by several mechanisms. The classical mechanism is by the direct generation of reactive oxygen species (ROS) during the electron transfer from the semiquinone to quinone moieties of the anthracycline,[84] which leads to myocardial damage. ROS can also be generated by mitochondrial damage resulting from drug-mediated inactivation of the oxidative phosphorylation chain because doxorubicin accumulates not only in chromatin, but also in mitochondria.[78,79] A recent study has also related doxorubicin cardiotoxicity to the poisoning of Top2β cleavage complexes in myocardiocytes.[85] Endomyocardial biopsy is characterized by a predominant finding of multifocal areas of patchy and interstitial fibrosis (stellate scars) and occasional vacuolated myocardial cells (Adria cells). Myocyte hypertrophy and degeneration, loss of cross-striations, and the absence of myocarditis are also characteristic of this diagnosis.[86] The incidence of cardiomyopathy is related to both the cumulative dose and the schedule of administration, and predisposition to cardiac damage includes a previous history of heart disease, hypertension, radiation to the mediastinum, age greater than 65 years or younger than 4 years, prior use of anthracyclines or other cardiac toxins, and coadministration of other chemotherapy agents (e.g., paclitaxel, cyclophosphamide, or trastuzumab).[87,88] Sequential administration of paclitaxel followed by doxorubicin in breast cancer patients is associated with cardiomyopathy at total doxorubicin doses above 340 to 380 mg/m$^2$, whereas the reverse sequence of drug administration did not yield the same systemic toxicities at these doses.[89] When doxorubicin is given in a low-dose weekly regimen (10 to 20 mg/m$^2$ per week) or by slow continuous infusion over 96 hours, cumulative doses of more than 500 mg/m$^2$ can be given. Doses of epirubicin less than 1,000 mg/m$^2$ and daunorubicin

less than 550 mg/m$^2$ are considered safe. Additionally, liposomal doxorubicin is associated with less cardiac toxicity.

Cardiac function can be monitored during treatment with anthracyclines by electrocardiography, echocardiography, or radionuclide scans. Numerous studies have established the danger of embarking on anthracycline therapy in patients with underlying cardiac disease (e.g., a baseline left ventricular ejection fraction of less than 50%) and of continuing therapy after a documented decrease in the ejection fraction by more than 10% (if this decrease falls below the lower limit of normal). Because anthracycline-induced cardiotoxicity has been related to the generation of free radicals, efforts have been aimed at attenuating this effect through the targeting of redox response and reduction in oxidative stress. Dexrazoxane is a metal chelator that decreases the myocardial toxicity of doxorubicin in breast cancer patients. In two multicenter, double-blind studies, advanced breast cancer patients were randomized to chemotherapy with dexrazoxane or a placebo; dexrazoxane was shown to have a cardioprotective effect based on serial, noninvasive cardiac testing during the course of the trial and is approved for that use by the FDA.[90] Dexrazoxane chelates iron and copper, thereby interfering with the redox reactions that generate free radicals and damage myocardial lipids. Notably, dexrazoxane is also a Top2 catalytic inhibitor (see Fig. 20.3F), which potentially might minimize the therapeutic activity of anthracyclines by interfering with the trapping of Top2 cleavage complexes by anthracyclines.[2,3,91] Other agents currently in use include β-blockers and statins. A recent meta-analysis of 12 randomized controlled trials and 2 observational studies involving the use of agents to prevent the cardiotoxicity associated with anthracyclines demonstrated relatively similar efficacy regardless of which prophylactic treatment was used.[92]

## Anthracenediones

Mitoxantrone (see Fig. 20.3E) is currently the only clinically approved anthracenedione. Compared to anthracyclines, mitoxantrone is less cardiotoxic owing to a decreased ability to undergo oxidation-reduction reactions and form free radicals.

Mitoxantrone is FDA approved for the treatment of advanced hormone-refractory prostate cancer[93] and AML.[94] It is typically administered intravenously at a dose of 12 to 14 mg/m$^2$ every 3 weeks in the treatment of prostate cancer, and at a dose of 12 mg/m$^2$ in combination with cytosine arabinoside for 3 days in the treatment of AML.

Toxicities are generally less severe compared to doxorubicin and include myelosuppression, nausea, vomiting, alopecia, and mucositis. Cardiac toxicity can be seen at cumulative doses greater than 160 mg/m$^2$.[95] Mitoxantrone is rapidly cleared from the plasma and is highly concentrated in tissues. The majority of the drug is eliminated in the feces, with a small amount undergoing renal excretion. Dose adjustments for hepatic dysfunction are recommended, but formal guidelines are currently not available.

## Dactinomycin

Dactinomycin was the first antibiotic shown to have antitumor activity[96] and consists of a planar phenoxazone ring attached to two peptide side chains. This unique structure allows for tight intercalation into DNA between adjacent guanine–cytosine bases, leading to Top2 and Top1 poisoning and transcription inhibition.[97] Dactinomycin was one of the first drugs shown to be transported by P-glycoprotein, and represents the major mechanism of resistance.[98]

Dactinomycin is FDA approved for Ewing sarcoma,[99] gestational trophoblastic neoplasm,[100] metastatic nonseminomatous testicular cancer,[101] nephroblastoma,[102] and rhabdomyosarcoma.[103] Typically, it is administered intravenously at doses of 15 μg/kg for 5 days in combination with other chemotherapeutic agents for the treatment of nephroblastoma, rhabdomyosarcoma, and Ewing sarcoma; at does of 12 µg/kg intravenously as a single agent in the treatment of gestational trophoblastic neoplasias; and at doses of 1,000 µg/m² intravenously on day 1 as part of a combination regimen with cyclophosphamide, bleomycin, vinblastine, and cisplatin in the treatment of metastatic nonseminomatous testicular cancer. Toxicities include myelosuppression, veno-occlusive disease of the liver, nausea, vomiting, alopecia, erythema, and acne. Additionally, similar to doxorubicin, dactinomycin can cause radiation recall and severe tissue necrosis in cases of extravasation. Dactinomycin is largely excreted unchanged in the feces and urine. Guidelines for dosing in patients with impaired renal or liver function are currently not available.

## Epipodophyllotoxins

Epipodophyllotoxins are glycoside derivatives of podophyllotoxin, an antimicrotubule agent extracted from the mandrake plant. Two derivatives, demethylated on the pendant ring (see R1 in Fig. 20.3D), etoposide and teniposide were shown to primarily function as Top2 poisons rather than through antimicrotubule mechanisms.[104,105] Epipodophyllotoxins poison Top2 through a mechanism distinct from that of anthracyclines and other DNA intercalators[106] without intercalating into normal DNA in the absence of Top2. Therefore, they are "cleaner" Top2 inhibitors than the anthracyclines, anthracenediones, and dactinomycin. However, etoposide and teniposide trap Top2 cleavage complexes by base stacking in a ternary complex at the interface of the DNA and the Top2 homodimer. Mechanisms that have been implicated in resistance to etoposide include drug efflux, because epipodophyllotoxins are substrates for P-glycoprotein[107]; altered localization of Top2α; decreased cellular expression of Top2α[108]; and impaired phosphorylation of Top2.[109]

## Etoposide

Etoposide (see Fig. 20.3D) is available in intravenous and oral forms. It is FDA approved for the treatment of small-cell lung cancer[110] and refractory testicular cancer.[111] It also has activity in hematologic malignancies and various solid tumors. The intravenous form is generally administered at doses of 35 to 50 mg/m² for 4 to 5 days every 3 to 4 weeks in combination therapy for small-cell lung cancer, and 50 to 100 mg/m² for 5 days every 3 to 4 weeks in combination therapy for refractory testicular cancer. The dose of oral etoposide is usually twice the intravenous dose. Oral bioavailability is highly variable due to dependence on intestinal P-glycoprotein.[112]

The dose-limiting toxicity for etoposide is myelosuppression, with white blood cell count nadirs typically occurring on days 10 to 14. Thrombocytopenia is less common than leukopenia. Additionally, mild to moderate nausea, vomiting, diarrhea, mucositis, and alopecia are associated with etoposide. Among topoisomerase inhibitors, epipodophyllotoxins have the greatest association with secondary malignancies, with etoposide having the highest risk, with an estimated 4% 6-year cumulative risk.[113] The majority of etoposide is cleared unchanged by the kidneys, and a 25% dose reduction is recommended in patients with a creatinine clearance of 15 to 50 mL per minute. A 50% dose reduction is recommended in patients with a creatinine clearance less than 15 mL per minute. Because the unbound fraction of etoposide is dependent on albumin and bilirubin concentrations, dose adjustments for hepatic dysfunction are advised, but consensus guidelines are currently not available.

## Teniposide

Teniposide contains a thiophene group in place of the methyl group on the glucose moiety of etoposide (Fig. 20.3D). Teniposide

is FDA approved for refractory pediatric ALL.[114,115] In pediatric ALL studies, doses ranged from 165 mg/m² intravenously in combination with cytarabine to 250 mg/m² intravenously weekly in combination with vincristine and prednisone. Similar to etoposide, the dose-limiting toxicity of teniposide is myelosuppression. Additional toxicities include mild-to-moderate nausea, vomiting, diarrhea, alopecia, and secondary leukemia. Teniposide is associated with greater frequency of hypersensitivity reactions compared to etoposide.

Teniposide is 99% bound to albumin and, as compared to etoposide, undergoes hepatic metabolism more extensively and renal clearance less extensively. No specific guidelines are currently available on dose adjustments for renal or hepatic dysfunction.

## THERAPY-RELATED SECONDARY ACUTE LEUKEMIA

One of the major complications of Top2 inhibitor therapies, especially for etoposide and mitoxantrone, is acute secondary leukemia, which occurs in approximately 5% of patients. Therapy-related AMLs (t-AML) are characterized by their relatively rapid onset (they can occur only a few months after therapy) and the presence of recurrent balanced translocations involving the mixed lineage leukemia (MLL) locus on 11q23 and over 50 partner genes.[116] The molecular mechanism is likely from the disjoining of two drug-trapped Top2 cleavage complexes on different chromosomes (see Fig. 20.2C) in relationship with transcription collisions and illegitimate relegation.[117] Top2β, rather than Top2α, has been implicated in the generation of these disjoined cleavage complexes.[117,118]

## FUTURE DIRECTIONS

Current challenges in the development of topoisomerase inhibitors lie in the inherent chemical instability of current and established agents. In addition to recent developments designed to enhance the stability with semisynthetic analogs and the development of novel delivery systems in an effort to achieve higher intratumoral concentrations, attention is also being focused on targeting other topoisomerase isoenzymes. Driving this trend has been the recent elucidation of the role of Top2β inhibition in the development of treatment-related cardiotoxicity and secondary AML.[86,117,118] In addition to combination chemotherapy regimens already in use, attempts have also been made for the sequential inhibition of Top1 and Top2. Based on early preclinical models suggesting synergy with sequential inhibition of Top1 and Top2,[120] phase 1 studies have evaluated the sequential administration of topotecan and etoposide in extensive-stage small-cell lung cancer and ovarian cancer, with significant myelosuppression as the dose-limiting toxicity.[121,122] Future rational drug combinations include targeting DNA repair pathways in combination with Top1 inhibition, although further characterization is needed of the specific DNA repair and stress response pathways invoked in response to DNA damage as a result of Top1 inhibition. However, one such attempt of combining topotecan with veliparib, a small molecule inhibitor of poly (ADP-ribose) polymerase, was poorly tolerated due to significant myelosuppression, thus limiting the doses of topotecan that could be safely administered.[123]

Molecular characterization of tumors to better define patient selection and the development of pharmacodynamic biomarkers to monitor the response to treatment and to optimize the combination dose and schedules is needed for the further clinical development of topoisomerase inhibitors. Validated assays have been developed to evaluate topoisomerase 1 levels and levels of plosphorylated histone H2AX (gamma-H2AX) as a marker of DNA damage response to topoisomerase inhibition,[124,125] and are being incorporated in current phase I studies of indenoisoquinolines.[72,73]

# REFERENCES

1. Nitiss JL. DNA topoisomerase II and its growing repertoire of biological functions. *Nat Rev Cancer* 2009;9(5):327–337.
2. Nitiss JL. Targeting DNA topoisomerase II in cancer chemotherapy. *Nat Rev Cancer* 2009;9(5):338–350.
3. Pommier Y, Leo E, Zhang H, et al. DNA topoisomerases and their poisoning by anticancer and antibacterial drugs. *Chem Biol* 2010;17(5):421–433.
4. Fortune JM, Osheroff N. Topoisomerase II as a target for anticancer drugs: when enzymes stop being nice. *Prog Nucleic Acid Res Mol Biol* 2000;64:221–253.
5. Wang JC. A journey in the world of DNA rings and beyond. *Annu Rev Biochem* 2009;78:31–54.
6. Wang JC. Cellular roles of DNA topoisomerases: a molecular perspective. *Nat Rev Mol Cell Biol* 2002;3(6):430–440.
7. Champoux JJ. DNA topoisomerases: structure, function, and mechanism. *Annu Rev Biochem* 2001;70:369–413.
8. Wang JC. *Untangling the Double Helix: DNA Entanglements and the Action of DNA Topoisomerases.* Cold Spring Harbor, NY: Cold Spring Harbor Laboratory Press; 2009.
9. Pommier Y. DNA Topoisomerases and cancer. In: Teicher BA, ed. *Cancer Discovery and Development.* New York: Springer & Humana Press; 2012.
10. Zhang H, Barceló JM, Lee B, et al. Human mitochondrial topoisomerase I. *Proc Natl Acad Sci U S A* 2001;98(10):10608–10613.
11. Champoux JJ, Dulbecco R. An activity from mammalian cells that untwists superhelical DNA—a possible swivel for DNA replication (polyoma-ethidium bromide-mouse-embryo cells-dye binding assay). *Proc Natl Acad Sci U S A* 1972;69(1):143–146.
12. Chen SH, Wu CH, Plank JL, et al. Essential functions of C terminus of Drosophila Topoisomerase IIIα in double Holliday junction dissolution. *J Biol Chem* 2012;287(23):19346–19353.
13. Xu D, Shen W, Guo R, et al. Top3β is an RNA topoisomerase that works with fragile X syndrome protein to promote synapse formation. *Nat Neurosci* 2013;16(9):1238–1247.
14. Seol Y, Gentry AC, Osheroff N, et al. Chiral discrimination and writhe-dependent relaxation mechanism of human topoisomerase IIα. *J Biol Chem* 2013;288(19):13695–13703.
15. Stoll G, Pietiläinen OP, Linder B, et al. Deletion of TOP3b, a component of FMRP-containing mRNPs, contributes to neurodevelopmental disorders. *Nat Neurosci* 2013;16(9):1228–1237.
16. Pommier Y, Marchand C. Interfacial inhibitors: targeting macromolecular complexes. *Nat Rev Drug Discov* 2011;11(1):25–36.
17. Nitiss J, Wang JC. DNA topoisomerase-targeting antitumor drugs can be studied in yeast. *Proc Natl Acad Sci U S A* 1988;85(20):7501–7505.
18. Bjornsti MA, Benedetti P, Viglianti GA, et al. Expression of human DNA topoisomerase I in yeast cells lacking yeast DNA topoisomerase I: restoration of sensitivity of the cells to the antitumor drug camptothecin. *Cancer Res* 1989;49(22):6318–6323.
19. Dressler LG, Berry DA, Broadwater G, et al. Comparison of HER2 status by fluorescence in situ hybridization and immunohistochemistry to predict benefit from dose escalation of adjuvant doxorubicin-based therapy in node-positive breast cancer patients. *J Clin Oncol* 2005;23(19):4287–4297.
20. Holm C, Covey JM, Kerrigan D, et al. Differential requirement of DNA replication for the cytotoxicity of DNA topoisomerase I and II inhibitors in Chinese hamster DC3F cell. *Cancer Res* 1989;49(22):6365–6368.
21. Hsiang YH, Lihou MG, Liu LF. Arrest of DNA replication by drug-stabilized topoisomerase I-DNA cleavable complexes as a mechanism of cell killing by camptothecin. *Cancer Res* 1989;49(18):5077–5082.
22. Maede Y, Shimizu H, Fukushima T, et al. Differential and common DNA repair pathways for topoisomerase I- and II-targeted drug in a genetic DT40 repair screen panel. *Mol Cancer Ther* 2014;13(1):214–220.
23. Huang SN, Pommier Y, Marchand C. Tyrosyl-DNA Phosphodiesterase 1(Tdp1) inhibitors. *Expert Opinion Ther Pat* 2011;21(9):1285–1292.
24. Zhang YW, Regairaz M, Seiler JA, et al. Poly(ADP-ribose) polymerase and XPF-ERCC1 participate in distinct pathways for the repair of topoisomerase I-induced DNA damage in mammalian cells. *Nucleic Acids Res* 2011;39(9):3607–3620.
25. Koster DA, Palle K, Bot ES, et al. Antitumor drugs impede DNA uncoiling by topoisomerase I. *Nature* 2007;448(7150):213–217.
26. Sordet O, Redon CE, Guirouilh-Barbat J, et al. Ataxia telangiectasia mutated activation by transcription- and topoisomerase I-induced DNA double-strand breaks. *EMBO Rep* 2009;10(8):887–893.
27. Pommier Y, Zwelling LA, Mattern MR, et al. Effects of dimethyl sulfoxide and thiourea upon intercalator-induced DNA single-strand breaks in mouse leukemia (L1210) cells. *Cancer Res* 1983;43(12 Pt 1):5718–5724.
28. Long BH, Musial ST, Brattain MG. Comparison of cytotoxicity and DNA breakage activity of congeners of podophyllotoxin including VP16-213 and VM26: a quantitative structure-activity relationship. *Biochemistry* 1984;23(6):1183–1188.
29. Ban Y, Ho CW, Lin RK, et al. Activation of a novel ubiquitin-independent proteasome pathway when RNA polymerase II encounters a protein roadblock. *Mol Cell Biol* 2013;33(20):4008–4016.
30. Long BH, Musial ST, Brattain MG. Single- and double-strand DNA breakage and repair in human lung adenocarcinoma cells exposed to etoposide and teniposide. *Cancer Res* 1985;45(7):3106–3112.
31. Pommier Y. Drugging topoisomerases: lessons and challenges. *ACS Chem Biol* 2013;8(1):82–95.
32. Zwelling LA, Michaels S, Erickson LC, et al. Protein-associated deoxyribonucleic acid strand breaks in L1210 cells treated with the deoxyribonucleic acid intercalating agents 4'-(9-acridinylamino) methanesulfon-m-anisidide and adriamycin. *Biochemistry* 1981;20(23):6553–6563.
33. Wall ME, Wani MC. Camptothecin and taxol: discovery to clinic—thirteenth Bruce F. Cain Memorial Award Lecture. *Cancer Res* 1995;55:753–760.
34. Pommier Y. Topoisomerase I inhibitors: camptothecins and beyond. *Nat Rev Cancer* 2006;6(10):789–802.
35. Teicher BA. Next generation topoisomerase I inhibitors: rationale and biomarker strategies. *Biochem Pharmacol* 2008;75(6):1262–1271.
36. Pommier Y, Cushman M. The indenoisoquinoline noncamptothecin topoisomerase I inhibitors: update and perspectives. *Mol Cancer Ther* 2009;8(5):1008–1014.
37. Douillard JY, Cunningham D, Roth AD, et al. Irinotecan combined with fluorouracil compared with fluorouracil alone as first-line treatment for metastatic colorectal cancer: a multicentre randomised trial. *Lancet* 2000;355:1041–1047.
38. Saltz LB, Cox JV, Blanke C, et al. Irinotecan plus fluorouracil and leucovorin for metastatic colorectal cancer. Irinotecan Study Group. *N Engl J Med* 2000;343:905–914.
39. Conroy T, Desseigne F, Tchou M, et al. FOLFIRINOX versus gemcitabine for metastatic pancreatic cancer. *N Engl J Med* 2011;364:1817–1825.
40. Hanna N, Bunn PA Jr, Langer C, et al. Randomized phase III trial comparing irinotecan/cisplatin with etoposide/cisplatin in patients with previously untreated extensive-stage disease small-cell lung cancer. *J Clin Oncol* 2006;24:2038–2043.
41. Schmittel A, Fischer von Weikersthal L, Sebastian M, et al. A randomized phase II trial of irinotecan plus carboplatin versus carboplatin treatment in patients with extended disease small-cell lung cancer. *Ann Oncol* 2006;17:663–667.
42. Iyer L, King CD, Whitington PF, et al. Genetic predisposition to the metabolism of irinotecan (CPT-11). Role of uridine diphosphate glucuronosyltransferase isoform 1A1 in the glucuronidation of its active metabolite (SN-38) in human liver microsomes. *J Clin Invest* 1998;101:847–854.
43. Innocenti F, Undevia SD, Iyer L, et al. Genetic variants in the UDP-glucuronosyltransferase 1A1 gene predict the risk of severe neutropenia of irinotecan. *J Clin Oncol* 2004;22:1382–1388.
44. Schaaf LJ, Hammond LA, Tipping SJ, et al. Phase 1 and pharmacokinetic study of intravenous irinotecan in refractory solid tumor patients with hepatic dysfunction. *Clin Cancer Res* 2006;12:3782–3791.
45. ten Bokkel Huinink W, Gore M, Carmichael J, et al. Topotecan versus paclitaxel for the treatment of recurrent epithelial ovarian cancer. *J Clin Oncol* 1997;15:2183–2193.
46. Ardizzoni A, Hansen H, Dombernowsky P, et al. Topotecan, a new active drug in the second-line treatment of small-cell lung cancer: a phase II study in patients with refractory and sensitive disease. The European Organization for Research and Treatment of Cancer Early Clinical Studies Group and New Drug Development Office, and the Lung Cancer Cooperative Group. *J Clin Oncol* 1997;15:2090–2096.
47. Long HJ 3rd, Bundy BN, Grendys EC Jr, et al. Randomized phase III trial of cisplatin with or without topotecan in carcinoma of the uterine cervix: a Gynecologic Oncology Group Study. *J Clin Oncol* 2005;23:4626–4633.
48. Baker SD, Heideman RL, Crom WR, et al. Cerebrospinal fluid pharmacokinetics and penetration of continuous infusion topotecan in children with central nervous system tumors. *Cancer Chemother Pharmacol* 1996;37:195–202.
49. Schluep T, Cheng J, Khin KT, et al. Pharmacokinetics and biodistribution of the camptothecin-polymer conjugate IT-101 in rats and tumor-bearing mice. *Cancer Chemother Pharmacol* 2006;57:654–662.
50. Young C, Schluep T, Hwang J, et al. CRLX101 (formerly IT-101)-A novel nanopharmaceutical of camptothecin in clinical development. *Curr Bioact Compd* 2011;7:8–14.
51. Weiss GJ, Chao J, Neidhart JD, et al. First-in-human phase 1/2a trial of CRLX101, a cyclodextrin-containing polymer-camptothecin nanopharmaceutical in patients with advanced solid tumor malignancies. *Invest New Drugs* 2013;31:986–1000.
52. University of Chicago. A randomized phase II study of IV Topotecan versus CRLX101 in the second line treatment of recurrent small cell lung cancer. ClinicalTrials.gov Identifier: NCT01803269.
53. Cerulean Pharma Inc. A randomized, phase 2, study to assess the safety and activity of CRLX101, a nanoparticle formulation of camptothecin, in patients with advanced non-small cell lung cancer who have failed one or two previous regimens of chemotherapy. ClinicalTrials Identifier: NCT01380769.
54. Massachusetts General Hospital. A Phase II, 2-stage Trial of CRLX101-202 in recurrent ovarian, tubal and peritoneal cancer. ClinicalTrials.gov Identifier: NCT01652079.
55. Vergote IB, Garcia A, Micha J et al. Randomized multicentre phase II trial comparing two schedules of etirinotecan pegol (NKTR-102) in women with recurrent platinum-resistant/refractory epithelial ovarian cancer. *J Clin Oncol* 2013;31(32):4060–4066.
56. Awada A, Garcia AA, Chan S et al. Two schedules of etirinotecan pegol (NKTR-102) in patients with previously treated metastatic breast cancer: a randomized phase 2 study. *Lancet Oncol* 2013;14(12):1216–1225.
57. Roswell Park Cancer Institute. A phase II study of single agent topoisomerase-I inhibitor polymer conjugate, Etirinotecan Pegol (NKTR-102), in patients with relapsed small cell lung cancer. ClinicalTrials Identifier: NCT01876446.
58. Abramson Cancer Center of the University of Pennsylvania. Phase 2 study of Etirinotecan Pegol (NKTR-102) in the treatment of patients with metastatic and recurrent non-small cell lung cancer (NSCLC) after failure of 2nd line treatment. ClinicalTrials Identifier: NCT01773109.

59. Nektar Therapeutics. A multicentre, open-label, randomized, phase 2 study to evaluate the efficacy and safety of NKTR-102 versus irinotecan in patients with second-line, irinotecan-naive, KRAS-mutant, metastatic colorectal cancer (mCRC). ClinicalTrials Identifier: NCT00856375.

60. Lawrence Recht. A phase II, single arm, open label study of NKTR-102 in bevacizumab-resistant high-grade glioma. ClinicalTrials Identifier: NCT01663012.

61. Nektar Therapeutics. The BEACON study (breast cancer outcomes with NKTR-102): a phase 3 open-label, randomized, multicenter study of NKTR-102 versus treatment of physician's choice (TPC) in patients with locally recurrent or metastatic breast cancer previously treated with an anthracycline, a taxane and capecitabine. ClinicalTrials Identifier: NCT01492101.

62. Basili S, Moro S. Novel camptothecin derivatives as topoisomerase I inhibitors. *Expert Opin Ther Pat* 2009;19:555–574.

63. Choi CH, Lee YY, Song TJ, et al. Phase II study of belotecan, a camptothecin analogue, in combination with carboplatin for the treatment of recurrent ovarian cancer. *Cancer* 2011;117:2104–2111.

64. Rhee CK, Lee SH, Kim JS, et al. A multicentre phase II study of belotecan, a new camptothecin analogue, as a second-line therapy in patients with small cell lung cancer. *Lung Cancer* 2011;72(1):64–67.

65. Hwang JH, Lim MC, Seo SS, et al. Phase II study of belotecan (CKD 602) as a single agent in patients with recurrent or progressive carcinoma of the uterine cervix. *Jpn J Clin Oncol* 2011;41:624–629.

66. Frapolli R, Zucchetti M, Sessa C, et al. Clinical pharmacokinetics of the new oral camptothecin gimatecan: the inter-patient variability is related to alpha1-acid glycoprotein plasma levels. *Eur J Cancer* 2010;46:505–516.

67. Pecorelli S, Ray-Coquard I, Tredan O, et al. Phase II of oral gimatecan in patients with recurrent epithelial ovarian, fallopian tube or peritoneal cancer, previously treated with platinum and taxanes. *Ann Oncol* 2010;21:759–765.

68. Graham JS, Falk S, Samuel LM et al. A multi-centre dose escalation and pharmacokinetic study of diflomotecan in patients with advanced malignancy. *Cancer Chemother Pharmacol* 2009;63:945–952.

69. Trocóniz IF, Cendrós JM, Soto E, et al. Population pharmacokinetic/pharmacodynamics modeling of drug-induced adverse effects of a novel homocamptothecin analog, elomotecan (BN80927), in a Phase I dose finding study in patients with advanced solid tumors. *Cancer Chemother Pharmacol* 2012;70:239–250.

70. Takagi K, Dexheimer TS, Redon C, et al. Novel E-ring camptothecin keto analogues (S38809 and S39625) are stable, potent, and selective topoisomerase I inhibitors without being substrates of drug efflux transporters. *Mol Cancer Ther* 2007;6(12 Pt 1):3229–3238.

71. Lansiaux A, Léonce S, Kraus-Berthier L, et al. Novel stable camptothecin derivatives replacing the E-ring lactone by a ketone function are potent inhibitors of topoisomerase I and promising antitumor drugs. *Mol Pharmacol* 2007;72(2):311–319.

72. National Cancer Institute. A Phase I Study of Indenoisoquinolines LMP400 and LMP776 in Adults With Relapsed Solid Tumors and Lymphomas. ClinicalTrials Identifier: NCT01051635.

73. National Cancer Institute. A phase I trial of weekly Indenoisoquinolines LMP400 in adults with relapsed solid tumors and lymphomas. ClinicalTrials Identifier: NCT01794104.

74. Antony S, Agama KK, Miao ZH, et al. Novel indenoisoquinolines NSC 725776 and NSC 724998 produce persistent topoisomerase I cleavage complexes and overcome multidrug resistance. *Cancer Res* 2007;67:10397–10405.

75. Kurtzberg LS, Roth S, Krumbholz R, et al. Genz-644282, a novel non-camptothecin topoisomerase I inhibitor for cancer treatment. *Clin Cancer Res* 2011;17:2777–2787.

76. Genzyme, a Sanofi Company. Dose Escalation Study to Assess the Safety and Tolerability of Genz-644282 in Patients With Solid Tumors. ClinicalTrials Identifier: NCT00942799.

77. Capranico G, Zunino F, Kohn KW, et al. Sequence-selective topoisomerase II inhibition by anthracycline derivatives in SV40 DNA: relationship with DNA binding affinity and cytotoxicity. *Biochemistry* 1990;29(2):562–569.

78. Davies KJ, Doroshow JH. Redox cycling of anthracyclines by cardiac mitochondria. I. Anthracycline radical formation by NADH dehydrogenase. *J Biol Chem* 1986;261(7):3060–3067.

79. Doroshow JH, Davies KJ. Redox cycling of anthracyclines by cardiac mitochondria. II. Formation of superoxide anion, hydrogen peroxide, and hydroxyl radical. *J Biol Chem* 1986;261:3068–3074.

80. Schneider E, Cowan KH. Multiple drug resistance in cancer therapy. *Med J Aust* 1994;160(6):371–373.

81. Alvarez M, Paull K, Monks A, et al. Generation of a drug resistance profile by quantitation of mdr-1/P-glycoprotein in the cell lines of the National Cancer Institute Anticancer Drug Screen. *J Clin Invest* 1995;95(5):2205–2214.

82. Felix CA, Kolaris CP, Osheroff N. Topoisomerase II and the etiology of chromosomal translocations. *DNA Repair* 2006;5:1093–1108.

83. O'Brien ME, Wigler N, Inbar M, et al. Reduced cardiotoxicity and comparable efficacy in a phase III trial of pegylated liposomal doxorubicin HCl (CAELYX/Doxil) versus conventional doxorubicin for first-line treatment of metastatic breast cancer. *Ann Oncol* 2004;15(3):440–449.

84. Doroshow JH. Effect of anthracycline antibiotics on oxygen radical formation in rat heart. *Cancer Res* 1983;43(2):460–472.

85. Zhang S, Liu X, Bawa-Khalfe T, et al. Identification of the molecular basis of doxorubicin-induced cardiotoxicity. *Nat Med* 2012;18:1639–1642.

86. Speyer J, Wasserheit C. Strategies for reduction of anthracycline cardiac toxicity. *Sem Oncol* 1998;25:525–537.

87. Chanan-Khan A, Srinivasan S, Czuczman MS. Prevention and management of cardiotoxicity from antineoplastic therapy. *J Support Oncol* 2004;2:251–256.

88. Von Hoff DD, Layard MW, Basa P, et al. Risk factors for doxorubicin-induced congestive heart failure. *Ann Intern Med* 1979;91:710–717.

89. Shan K, Lincoff AM, Young JB. Anthracycline-induced cardiotoxicity. *Ann Intern Med* 1996;125:47–58.

90. Swain SM, Whaley FS, Gerber MC, et al. Cardioprotection with dexrazoxane for doxorubicin-containing therapy in advanced breast cancer. *J Clin Oncol* 15(4):1318–1332.

91. Andoh T, Ishida R. Catalytic inhibitors of DNA topoisomerase II. *Biochim Biophys Acta* 1998;1400(1–3):155–171.

92. Kalam K, Marwick TH. Role of cardioprotective therapy for prevention of cardiotoxicity with chemotherapy: a systematic review and meta-analysis. *Eur J Cancer* 2013;49:2900–2909.

93. Tannock IF, Osoba D, Stockler MR, et al. Chemotherapy with mitoxantrone plus prednisone or prednisone alone for symptomatic hormone-resistant prostate cancer: a Canadian randomized trial with palliative end points. *J Clin Oncol* 1996;14:1756–1764.

94. Reece DE, Elmongy MB, Barnett MJ, et al. Chemotherapy with high-dose cytosine arabinoside and mitoxantrone for poor-prognosis myeloid leukemias. *Cancer Invest* 1993;11:509–516.

95. Shenkenberg TD, Von Hoff DD. Mitoxantrone: a new anticancer drug with significant clinical activity. *Ann Intern Med* 1986;105:67–81.

96. Hollstein U. Actinomycin. Chemistry and mechanism of action. *Chem Rev* 1974;74(6):625–652.

97. Wassermann K, Markovits J, Jaxel C, et al. Effects of morpholinyl doxorubicins, doxorubicin, and actinomycin D on mammalian DNA topoisomerases I and II. *Mol Pharmacol* 1990;38(1):38–45.

98. Biedler JL, Riehm H. Cellular resistance to actinomycin D in Chinese hamster cells in vitro: cross-resistance, radioautographic, and cytogenetic studies. *Cancer Res* 1970;30:1174–1184.

99. Jaffe N, Paed D, Traggis D, et al. Improved outlook for Ewing's sarcoma with combination chemotherapy (vincristine, actinomycin D and cyclophosphamide) and radiation therapy. *Cancer* 1976;38(5):1925–1930.

100. Turan T, Karacay O, Tulunay G, et al. Results of EMA/CO (etoposide, methotrexate, actinomycin D, cyclophosphamide, vincristine) chemotherapy in gestational trophoblastic neoplasia. *Int J Gynecol Cancer* 2006;16(3):1432–1438.

101. Early KS, Albert DJ. Single agent chemotherapy (actinomycin D) in the treatment of metastatic testicular carcinoma. *South Med J* 1976;69(8):1017–1021.

102. Fernbach DJ, Martyn DT. Role of dactinomycin in the improved survival of children with Wilm's tumor. *JAMA* 1966;195(1222):1005–1009.

103. Maurer HM, Moon T, Donaldson M, et al. The intergroup rhabdomyosarcoma study: a preliminary report. *Cancer* 1977;40(5):2015–2026.

104. Chen GL, Yang L, Rowe TC, et al. Nonintercalative antitumor drugs interfere with the breakage-reunion reaction of mammalian DNA topoisomerase. *J Biol Chem* 1984;259(21):13560–13566.

105. Long BH, Musial ST, Brattain MG. Comparison of cytotoxicity and DNA breakage activity of cogeners of podophyllotoxin including VP16-213 and VM26: a quantitative structure-activity relationship. *Biochemistry* 1984;23(6):1183–1188.

106. Ross W, Rowe T, Glisson B, et al. Role of topoisomerase II in mediating epipodophyllotoxin-induced DNA cleavage. *Cancer Res* 1984;44:5857–5860.

107. Meresse P, Dechaux E, Monneret C, et al. Etoposide: discovery and medicinal chemistry. *Curr Med Chem* 2004;11:2443–2466.

108. Valkov NI, Gump JL, Engel R, et al. Cell density-dependent VP-16 sensitivity of leukaemic cells is accompanied by the translocation of topoisomerase IIalpha from the nucleus to the cytoplasm. *Br J Haematol* 2000;108:331–345.

109. Takano H, Kohno K, Ono M, et al. Increased phosphorylation of DNA topoisomerase II in etoposide-resistant mutants of human cancer KB cells. *Cancer Res* 1991;51:3951–3957.

110. Sundstrøm S, Bremnes RM, Kaasa S, et al. Cisplatin and etoposide regimen is superior to cyclophosphamide, epirubicin, and vincristine regimen in small-cell lung cancer: results from a randomized phase III trial with 5 years' follow-up. *J Clin Oncol* 2002;20:4665–4672.

111. Nichols CR, Catalano PJ, Crawford ED, et al. Randomized comparison of cisplatin and etoposide and either bleomycin or ifosfamide in treatment of advanced disseminated germ cell tumors: an Eastern Cooperative Oncology Group, Southwest Oncology Group, and Cancer and Leukemia Group B Study. *J Clin Oncol* 1998;16:1287–1293.

112. Leu BL, Huang JD. Inhibition of intestinal P-glycoprotein and effects on etoposide absorption. *Cancer Chemother Pharmacol* 1995;35:432–436.

113. Smith MA, Rubinstein L, Anderson JR, et al. Secondary leukemia or myelodysplastic syndrome after treatment with epipodophyllotoxins. *J Clin Oncol* 1999;17:569–577.

114. Maluf PT, Odone Filho V, Cristofani LM, et al. Teniposide plus cytarabine as intensification therapy and in continuation therapy for advanced nonlymphoblastic lymphomas of childhood. *J Clin Oncol* 1994;12:1963–1968.

115. Rivera G, Bowman WP, Murphy SB, et al. VM-26 with prednisone and vincristine for treatment of refractory acute lymphocytic leukemia. *Med Pediatr Oncol* 1982;10:439–446.

116. Lovett BD, Lo Nigro L, Rappaport EF, et al. Near-precise interchromosomal recombination and functional DNA topoisomerase II cleavage sites at MLL and AF-4 genomic breakpoints in treatment-related acute lymphoblastic leukemia with t(4;11) translocation. *Proc Natl Acad Sci U S A* 2001;98(17):9802–9807.

117. Cowell IG, Sondka Z, Smith K, et al. Model for MLL translocations in therapy-related leukemia involving topoisomerase IIb-mediated DNA strand breaks and gene proximity. *Proc Natl Acad Sci U S A* 2012;109(23):8989–8994.

**CANCER THERAPEUTICS**

118. Azarova AM, Lyu YL, Lin CP, et al. Roles of DNA topoisomerases II isozymes in chemotherapy and secondary malignancies. *Proc Natl Acad Sci U S A* 2007;104:11014–11019.

119. Changela A, DiGate RJ, Mondragón A. Structural studies of E. Coli topoisomerase III-DNA complexes reveal a novel type IA topoisomerase-DNA conformational intermediate. *J Mol Biol* 2007;368:105–118.

120. Bertrand R, O'Connor PM, Kerrigan D, et al. Sequential administration of camptothecin and etoposide circumvents the antagonistic cytotoxicity of simultaneous drug administration in slowly growing human colon carcinoma HT-29 cells. *Eur J Cancer* 1992;28A(4–5):743–748.

121. Miller AA, Al Omari A, Murry DJ, et al. Phase I and pharmacologic study of sequential topotecan-carboplatin-etoposide in patients with extensive stage small cell lung cancer. *Lung Cancer* 2006;54:379–385.

122. Rose PG, Markham M, Bell JG, et al. Sequential prolonged oral topotecan and prolonged oral etoposide as second-line therapy in ovarian or peritoneal carcinoma: a phase I Gynecologic Oncology Study Group study. *Gynecol Oncol* 2006;102:236–239.

123. Kummar S, Chen A, Ji J, et al. Phase I study of PARP inhibitor ABT-888 in combination with topotecan in adults with refractory solid tumors and lymphomas. *Cancer Res* 2011;71(17):5626–5634.

124. Pfister TD, Hollingshead M, Kinders RJ, et al. Development and validation of an immunoassay for quantification of topoisomerase I in solid tumor tissues. *PLoS One* 2012;7:e50494.

125. Kinders RJ, Hollingshead M, Lawrence S, et al. Development of a validated immunofluorescence assay for gH2AX as a pharmacodynamics marker of topoisomerase I inhibitor activity. *Clin Cancer Res* 2010;16:5447–5457.

# 21 Antimicrotubule Agents

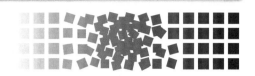

Christopher J. Hoimes and Lyndsay N. Harris

## MICROTUBULES

Microtubules are vital and dynamic cytoskeletal polymers that play a critical role in cell division, signaling, vesicle transport, shape, and polarity, which make them attractive targets in anticancer regimens and drug design.[1] Microtubules are composed of 13 linear protofilaments of polymerized α/β-tubulin heterodimers arranged in parallel around a cylindrical axis and associated with regulatory proteins such as microtubule-associated proteins, tau, and motor proteins kinesin and dynein.[2] The specific biologic functions of microtubules are due to their unique polymerization dynamics. Tubulin polymerization is mediated by a nucleation-elongation mechanism. One end of the microtubules, termed the *plus end*, is kinetically more dynamic than the other end, termed the *minus end* (Fig. 21.1). Microtubule dynamics are governed by two principal processes driven by guanosine 5′-triphosphate (GTP) hydrolysis: *treadmilling* or *poleward flux* is the net growth at one end of the microtubule and the net shortening at the opposite end, and *dynamic instability*, which is a process in which the microtubule ends switch spontaneously between states of slow sustained growth and rapid depolymerization.[2] Antimicrotubule agents are tubulin-binding drugs that directly bind tubules, inhibitors of tubulin-associated scaffold kinases, or inhibitors of their associated mitotic motor proteins to, ultimately, disrupt microtubule dynamics. They are broadly classified as microtubule stabilizing or microtubule destabilizing agents according to their effects on tubulin polymerization.

## TAXANES

Taxanes were the first-in-class microtubule stabilizing drugs. Ancient medicinal attempts at cardiac pharmacotherapy using material from the toxic coniferous yew tree, *Taxus* spp., were likely related to the plant's alkaloid *taxine* effect on sodium and calcium channels. Taxane compounds are the result of a drug screening of 35,000 plant extracts in 1963 that led to the identification of activity from the bark extract of the Pacific yew tree, *Taxus brevifolia*. Paclitaxel was identified as the active constituent with a report of its activity in carcinoma cell lines in 1971.[3] Motivation to identify taxanes derived from the more abundant and available needles of *Taxus baccata* led to the development of docetaxel, which is synthesized by the addition of a side chain to 10-deacetylbaccatin III, an inactive taxane precursor.[4] The taxane rings of paclitaxel and docetaxel are linked to an ester side chain attached to the C13 position of the ring, which is essential for antimicrotubule and antitumor activity. Nanoparticle albumin-bound paclitaxel (nab-paclitaxel) is a formulation that avoids the solvent related side effects of non–water-soluble paclitaxel and docetaxel. Overcoming docetaxel and paclitaxel's susceptibility to the P-glycoprotein efflux pump led to the development of cabazitaxel.[5] Cabazitaxel is synthesized by adding two methoxy groups to the 10-deacetylbaccatin III, which results in

the inhibition of the 5′-triphosphate–dependent efflux pump of P-glycoprotein.

Paclitaxel initially received regulatory approval in the United States in 1992 for the treatment of patients with ovarian cancer after failure of first-line or subsequent chemotherapy (Table 21.1).[1,4] Subsequently, it has been approved for several other indications, including advanced breast cancer after anthracycline-based regimens[6]; combination chemotherapy of lymph node–positive breast cancer in the adjuvant setting[7]; advanced ovarian cancer in combination with a platinum compound; second-line treatment of AIDS-related Kaposi sarcoma; and first-line treatment of non–small-cell lung cancer (NSCLC) in combination with cisplatin[8] (see Table 21.1). In addition to the U.S. Food and Drug Administration (FDA) on-label indications, paclitaxel is widely used for several other tumor types, such as cancers of unknown origin, bladder, esophagus, gastric, head and neck, and cervical cancers. The U.S. patent for paclitaxel expired in 2002, and a generic form of paclitaxel is now available.

Docetaxel was first approved for use in the United States in 1996 for patients with metastatic breast cancer that progressed or relapsed after anthracycline-based chemotherapy, which was later broadened to a general second-line indication (see Table 21.1).[4,6] Subsequently, it received regulatory approval in adjuvant chemotherapy of stage II breast cancer in combination with Adriamycin and cyclophosphamide (TAC)[9], and first-line treatment for locally advanced or metastatic breast cancer.[10] In addition, docetaxel has indications in nonresectable, locally advanced, or metastatic NSCLC after failure of or in combination with cisplatin therapy; metastatic castration-resistant prostate cancer in combination with prednisone[11]; first-line treatment of gastric adenocarcinoma, including gastroesophageal junction adenocarcinoma in combination with cisplatin and 5-fluorouracil (5-FU)[12]; and inoperable locally advanced squamous cell cancer of the head and neck in combination with cisplatin and 5-FU (see Table 21.1). Docetaxel came off patent in 2010 and a generic form is available.

### Mechanism of Action

The unique mechanism of action for paclitaxel was initially defined by Schiff et al.[13] in 1979, who showed that it bound to the interior surface of the microtubule lumen at binding sites completely distinct from those of exchangeable GTP, colchicine, podophyllotoxin, and the vinca alkaloids.[14] The taxanes profoundly alter the tubulin dissociation rate constants at both ends of the microtubule, suppressing treadmilling and dynamic instability. Dose-dependent taxane β-tubular binding induces mitotic arrest at the G2/M transition and induces cell death. By stabilizing microtubules, they also can stall ligand-dependent intracellular trafficking, as shown in sequestration of the androgen receptor to the cytosol in metastatic prostate cancer patients treated with docetaxel, and is associated with decreased androgen-regulated gene expression, such as prostate-specific antigen (PSA).[15,16] Peripheral neuropathy is a common dose-limiting toxicity across the antimicrotubule agents and likely is a result of their direct effect on microtubules. Studies

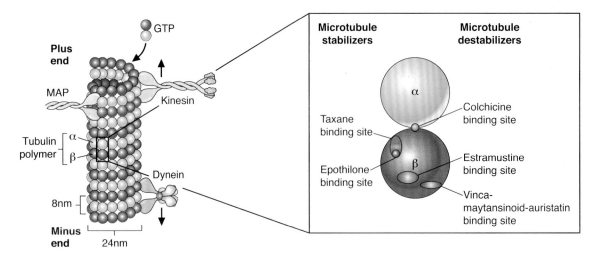

**Figure 21.1** Antimicrotubule agents bind tubulin directly or inhibit its associated proteins. Taxanes and epothilones have distinct binding pockets within the same site on the interior surface of the tubule. Estramustine has a distinct site on β-tubulin, although it also directly binds microtubule-associated proteins (MAP). (Adapted from Lieberman M, Marks A. *Mark's Basic Medical Biochemistry: A Clinical Approach.* 3rd ed. Philadelphia: Lippincott Williams & Wilkins; 2009.)

have shown that they inhibit anterograde and/or retrograde fast axonal transport and can explain the demyelinating "dying back" pattern seen and the vulnerability of sensory neurons with the longest axonal projections.[17]

Recent evidence suggests that microtubule inhibitors have collateral effects during interphase that lead to cell death. For instance, paclitaxel-stabilized microtubules serve as a scaffold for the binding of the death-effector domain of pro-caspase-8, and thereby enabling a caspase-8 downstream proteolytic cascade.[18,19] This caspase-8–dependent mechanism also serves as an important basis for the understanding of the loss of function and/or low expression of the breast cancer 1, early onset gene (*BRCA1*) association with resistance to taxane therapy.[20]

Another mechanism of the anticancer effect of taxanes is currently being elaborated and is tied to the B-cell lymphoma-2 (Bcl-2) antiapoptosis family of proteins. Paclitaxel has been shown to cause the phosphorylation of Bcl-2 and the sequestration of Bak and Bim; however, this seemingly cancer-protective phosphorylation needs to be reconciled and likely correlates with Bcl-2–expression levels.[21–23] Interestingly, neutralizing Bcl-2 homology 3 (BH3) domains with compounds such as ABT-737 is synergistic with docetaxel.[24]

## Clinical Pharmacology

### Paclitaxel

With prolonged infusion schedules (6 and 24 hours), drug disposition is a biphasic process with values for alpha and beta half-lives averaging approximately 20 minutes and 6 hours, respectively.[4] When administered as a 3-hour infusion, the pharmacokinetics are nonlinear and may lead to unexpected toxicity with a small dose escalation, or a disproportionate decrease in drug exposure and loss of tumor response with a dose reduction. Approximately 71% of an administered dose of paclitaxel is excreted in the stool via the enterohepatic circulation over 5 days as either the parent compound or metabolites in humans. Renal clearance of paclitaxel and metabolites is minimal, accounting for 14% of the administered dose. In humans, the bulk of drug disposition is metabolized by cytochrome P-450 mixed-function oxidases—specifically, the isoenzymes CYP2C8 and CYP3A4, which metabolize paclitaxel to hydroxylated 3′p-hydroxypaclitaxel (minor) and 6α-hydroxypaclitaxel (major), as well as dihydroxylated metabolites.

### Nanoparticle Albumin-Bound Paclitaxel

Nab-paclitaxel is a solvent-free colloidal suspension made by homogenizing paclitaxel with 3% to 4% albumin under high pressure to form nanoparticles of ~130 nm that disperse in plasma to ~10 nm (see Table 21.1).[25] It received regulatory approval in the United States in 2005 based on results in patients with metastatic breast cancer, and is now also approved in combination with carboplatin for first-line treatment of locally advanced or metastatic NSCLC, and in combination with gemcitabine for first-line treatment of metastatic pancreatic adenocarcinoma.[26–28] The improved responses seen with nab-paclitaxel, when compared to solvent-based paclitaxel, are not fully understood. Nab-paclitaxel likely capitalizes on several mechanisms, which include an improved pharmacokinetic profile with a larger volume of distribution and a higher maximal concentration of circulating, unbound, free drug; improved tumor accumulation by the enhanced permeability and retention (EPR) effect; and receptor-mediated transcytosis via an albumin-specific receptor (gp60) for endothelial transcytosis and binding of secreted protein acidic and rich in cysteine (SPARC) in the tumor interstitium.[29,30] In contrast to cremophor/ethanol (CrEL) solvent-based paclitaxel, nab-paclitaxel exhibits an extensive extravascular volume of distribution exceeding that of water, indicating extensive tissue and extravascular protein distribution. Some studies show that nab-paclitaxel achieves 33% higher drug concentration over CrEL-paclitaxel.[31] Additionally, the maximum concentration (Cmax), the mean plasma half-life of 15 to 18 hours, the area under curve (AUC), and the dose-independent plasma clearance correspond to linear pharmacokinetics over 80 to 300 mg/m[2].[29,32] The improved deposition of a nanoparticle, such as nab-paclitaxel in a tumor tissue, can occur passively through an EPR effect in areas of leaky vasculature, sufficient vascular pore size, and decreased lymphatic flow.[25,33] Once in the tissue, the nab-paclitaxel nanovehicle can deliver the drug locally or benefit from further receptor-mediated targeting to SPARC, which has been shown to be overexpressed, and correlates with disease progression in many tumor types.[34–38] Although preclinical models, as well as one clinical trial, have shown how nanoparticle therapy can benefit from this targeted approach,[39,40] correlative data for nab-paclitaxel is limited. The high stromal SPARC level was associated with longer survival in patients treated with nab-paclitaxel in the phase I/II study of patients with pancreatic cancer; however, this correlative analysis was not included in the phase III trial report and requires validation.[28,41]

## TABLE 21.1

**Antimicrotubule Agents: Dosages and Toxicities**

| Chemotherapeutic Agent | Dosage | Indications | Common Toxicities |
|---|---|---|---|
| Paclitaxel | 135–200 mg/m$^2$ IV over 3 h or 135 mg/m$^2$ IV over 24 h every 3 wk; or 80 mg/m$^2$ IV over 1 h weekly | Adjuvant therapy of node-positive breast cancer; metastatic breast, ovarian, non–small-cell lung, bladder, esophagus, cervical, gastric, and head and neck cancer; AIDS-related Kaposi sarcoma; cancer of unknown origin | Myelosuppression, hypersensitivity, nausea and vomiting, alopecia, arthralgia, myalgia, peripheral neuropathy |
| Docetaxel | 60–100 mg/m$^2$ IV over 1 h every 3 wk | Adjuvant therapy of node-positive breast cancer; metastatic breast, gastric, head and neck, prostate, non–small-cell lung, and ovarian cancer | Myelosuppression, hypersensitivity, edema, alopecia, nail damage, rash, diarrhea, nausea, vomiting, asthenia, neuropathy |
| Cabazitaxel | 25 mg/m$^2$ IV every 3 wk over 1 h | Docetaxel-refractory metastatic castration resistant prostate cancer | Neutropenia, infections, myelosuppression, diarrhea, nausea, vomiting, constipation, abdominal pain, asthenia |
| Nab-paclitaxel | 260 mg/m$^2$ IV over 30 min every 3 wk; or 125 mg/m$^2$ IV weekly on days 1, 8, and 15 every 28 d | Metastatic breast cancer, non–small-cell lung cancer, pancreatic cancer | Myelosuppression, nausea, vomiting, alopecia, myalgia, peripheral neuropathy |
| Ixabepilone | 40 mg/m$^2$ IV over 3 h every 3 wk | Metastatic and locally advanced breast cancer | Myelosuppression, fatigue/asthenia, myalgia/arthralgia, alopecia, nausea, vomiting, stomatitis/mucositis, diarrhea, musculoskeletal pain |
| Vincristine | 0.5–1.4 mg/m$^2$/wk IV (maximum 2 mg per dose); or 0.4 mg/d continuous infusion for 4 d | Lymphoma, acute leukemia, neuroblastoma, rhabdomyosarcoma, AIDS-related Kaposi sarcoma, multiple myeloma, testicular cancer | Constipation, nausea, vomiting, alopecia, diplopia, myelosuppression |
| Vinblastine | 6 mg/m$^2$ IV on days 1 and 15 as part of the ABVD regimen; 0.15 mg/kg IV on days 1 and 2 as part of the PVB regimen; 3 mg/m$^2$ IV as part of days 2, 15, 22 MVAC regimen | Hodgkin and non-Hodgkin lymphoma; Kaposi sarcoma; breast, testicular, bladder, prostate, and renal cell cancer | Myelosuppression, constipation, alopecia, malaise, bone pain |
| Vinorelbine | 25–30 mg/m$^2$ IV weekly | Non–small-cell lung, breast, cervical, and ovarian cancer | Alopecia, diarrhea, nausea, vomiting, asthenia, neuromyopathy |
| Estramustine | 14 mg/kg PO daily in 3 or 4 divided doses | Metastatic prostate cancer | Nausea, vomiting, gynecomastia, fluid retention |
| Ado-trastuzumab emtansine | 3.6 mg/kg IV every 3 wk | Metastatic breast cancer | Thrombocytopenia, nausea, constipation or diarrhea, peripheral neuropathy, fatigue, increased AST/ALT |
| Brentuximab vedotin | 1.8 mg/kg every 3 wk, maximum dose 180 mg | Refractory Hodgkin lymphoma, refractory systemic anaplastic large cell lymphoma | Neutropenia, anemia, thrombocytopenia, fatigue, fever, peripheral neuropathy |

ABVD, doxorubicin (Adriamycin), bleomycin, vinblastine, dacarbazine; PVB, cisplatin, vinblastine, bleomycin; MVAC, methotrexate, vinblastine, doxorubicin (Adriamycin), cisplatin; IV, intravenous; PO, by mouth; AST/ALT, aspartate amniotransferase–alanine amniotransferase.

## Docetaxel

The pharmacokinetics of docetaxel on a 1-hour schedule is triexponential and linear at doses of 115 mg/m$^2$ or less.[4] Terminal half-lives ranging from 11.1 to 18.5 hours has been reported. The most important determinants of docetaxel clearance were the body surface area (BSA), hepatic function, and plasma $\alpha_1$-acid glycoprotein concentration. Plasma protein binding is high (greater than 80%), and binding is primarily to $\alpha_1$-acid glycoprotein, albumin, and lipoproteins. The hepatic cytochrome P-450 mixed-function oxidases, particularly isoforms CYP3A4 and CYP3A5, are principally involved in biotransformation. The principal pharmacokinetic determinants of toxicity, particularly neutropenia, are drug exposure and the time that plasma concentrations exceed biologically relevant concentrations. The baseline level of $\alpha_1$-acid glycoprotein may be elevated as an acute phase reactant in advanced disease and is an independent predictor of response and a major objective prognostic factor of survival in patients with non–small-cell lung cancer treated with docetaxel chemotherapy.

**CANCER THERAPEUTICS**

## Cabazitaxel

Cabazitaxel is a semisynthetic derivative of the natural taxoid 10-deacetylbaccatin III. It binds to and stabilizes the β-tubulin subunit, resulting in the inhibition of microtubule depolymerization and cell division, cell cycle arrest in the $G_2$/M phase, and the inhibition of tumor cell proliferation.[5] It is active against diverse cancer cell lines and tumor models that are sensitive and resistant to docetaxel, including prostate, mammary, melanoma, kidney, colon, pancreas, lung, gastric, and head and neck.[5] Cabazitaxel is a poor substrate for the membrane-associated, multidrug resistance P-glycoprotein efflux pump; therefore, is useful for treating docetaxel-refractory prostate cancer for which it gained FDA approval in 2010.[5] In addition, it penetrates the blood–brain barrier.[42] Pharmacokinetics of cabazitaxel is similar to docetaxel; however, cabazitaxel has a larger volume of distribution and a longer terminal half-life (mean 77.3 hours versus 11.2 hours for docetaxel).[43,44]

## Tesetaxel

Tesetaxel (DJ-927, XRP6258) is a semisynthetic, orally bioavailable taxane currently in clinical trials in breast, gastric, and prostate cancer. Administration in phase I and II trials has been once per week or every 3 weeks and not associated with hypersensitivity and possibly less neurotoxicity compared to other taxanes. Dose-limiting toxicity has been neutropenia. Overall responses in phase II studies have been 50% and 38% in patients treated for first- and second-line breast cancer, respectively. A phase I/II study in advanced NSCLC showed an overall response rate of 5.6%. Tesetaxel activity is independent of P-glycoprotein expression.[45] Pharmacokinetics on a schedule of every 3 weeks have an AUC of ~1,750 ng/mL per hour, a half life of ~170 hours, and no drug interactions that have been noted.[46]

# Drug Interactions

Sequence-dependent pharmacokinetic and toxicologic interactions between paclitaxel and several other chemotherapy agents have been noted. The sequence of cisplatin followed by paclitaxel (on a 24-hour schedule) induces more profound neutropenia than the reverse sequence, which is explained by a 33% reduction in the clearance of paclitaxel after cisplatin.[47] Treatment with paclitaxel on either a 3- or 24-hour schedule followed by carboplatin has been demonstrated to produce equivalent neutropenia and less thrombocytopenia as compared to carboplatin as a single agent, which is not explained by pharmacokinetic interactions. Neutropenia and mucositis are more severe when paclitaxel is administered on a 24-hour schedule before doxorubicin, compared to the reverse sequence, which is most likely due to an approximately 32% reduction in the clearance rates of doxorubicin and doxorubicinol when doxorubicin is administered after paclitaxel. Several agents that inhibit cytochrome P-450 mixed-function oxidases interfere with the metabolism of paclitaxel and docetaxel in human microsomes in vitro; however, the clinical relevance of these findings is not known.[47]

# Toxicity

## Paclitaxel

The micelle-forming CrEL vehicle, which is required for suspension and intravenous delivery of paclitaxel, causes its nonlinear pharmacokinetics and thereby impacts its therapeutic index. CrEL causes hypersensitivity reactions, with major reactions usually occurring within the first 10 minutes after the first treatment and resolving completely after stopping the treatment. All patients should be premedicated with steroids, diphenhydramine, and an H2 antagonist, although up to 3% will still have reactions. Those who have major reactions have been rechallenged successfully after receiving high doses of corticosteroids.

Neuropathy is the principal toxicity of paclitaxel. Paclitaxel induces a peripheral neuropathy that presents in a symmetric stocking glove distribution, at first transient and then persistent.[48] A neurologic examination reveals sensory loss, and neurophysiologic studies reveal axonal degeneration and demyelination.[48] Compared with cisplatin, a loss of deep tendon reflexes occurs less commonly; however, autonomic and motor changes can occur. Severe neurotoxicity is uncommon when paclitaxel is given alone at doses below 200 mg/m$^2$ on a 3- or 24-hour schedule every 3 weeks, or below 100 mg/m$^2$ on a continuous weekly schedule. There is no convincing evidence that any specific measure is effective at ameliorating existing manifestations or preventing the development or worsening of neurotoxicity.[48]

Neutropenia is also frequent with paclitaxel. The onset is usually on days 8 to 11, and recovery is generally complete by days 15 to 21 with an every 3 weeks dosing regimen. Neutropenia is noncumulative, and the duration of severe neutropenia—even in heavily pretreated patients—is usually brief. Severity of neutropenia is related to the duration of exposure above the biologically relevant levels of 0.05 to 0.10 μM/L, and paclitaxel's nonlinear pharmacokinetics should be considered whenever adjusting dose.[49]

The most common cardiac rhythm disturbance, a transient sinus bradycardia, can be observed in up to 30% of patients. Routine cardiac monitoring during paclitaxel therapy is not necessary but is advisable for patients who may not be able to tolerate bradyarrhythmias. Drug-related gastrointestinal effects, such as vomiting and diarrhea, are uncommon. Severe hepatotoxicity and pancreatitis have also been noted rarely. Pulmonary toxicities, including acute bilateral pneumonitis, have been reported. Extravasation of large volumes can cause moderate soft tissue injury. Paclitaxel also induces reversible alopecia of the scalp in a dose-related fashion. Nail disorders have also been reported with paclitaxel use and include ridging, nail bed pigmentation, onychorrhexis, and onycholysis. These side effects have been reported more commonly with dose-intensified paclitaxel regimens.

Recent studies have suggested a role for the adenosine triphosphatase (ATP)-binding cassette (ABC) transporter polymorphisms in the development of neuropathy and neutropenia. Sissung et al.[50] reported that patients carrying two reference alleles for the *ABCB1* (P-glycoprotein, MDR1) 3435C greater than T polymorphism had a reduced risk to develop neuropathy as compared to patients carrying at least one variant allele ($P = .09$). Data from a large controlled trial to evaluate these and other candidate polymorphisms failed to detect a significant association between genotype and outcome or toxicity for any of the genes analyzed, although the correlative studies were retrospective and the sample size was inadequate to rule out smaller differences.[51] A large randomized trial of the CALGB 40101 using an integrated genomewide associate study found two polymorphisms associated with paclitaxel-induced polyneuropathy.[52] Both are involved in nerve development and maintenance, including the hereditary peripheral neuropathy Charcot-Marie-Tooth disease gene, *FGD4*. Further studies are required to adequately assess the role of these variants in predicting toxicity from taxane therapy.

## Nab-paclitaxel

Hypersensitivity reactions have not been observed during the infusion period and, therefore, steroid premedications are not necessary. The main dose-limiting toxicities are neutropenia and sensory neuropathy. In a trial comparing weekly paclitaxel 90 mg/m$^2$ to nab-paclitaxel 150 mg/m$^2$ to ixabepilone in patients with metastatic breast cancer, there was more hematologic toxicity and peripheral neuropathy in the nab-paclitaxel arm compared to the paclitaxel arm, although median progression-free survival was not significantly different at the 12-month follow-up.[53] This led to dose reductions in 45% of patients in the nab-paclitaxel arm compared with 15% for the paclitaxel arm.[53] Other toxicities include alopecia, diarrhea, nausea and vomiting, elevations in liver enzymes, arthralgia, myalgia, and asthenia.

## Docetaxel

Neutropenia is the main toxicity of docetaxel.[4] When docetaxel is administered on an every 3 weeks schedule, the onset of neutropenia is usually noted on day 8, with complete resolution by days 15 to 21. Neutropenia is significantly less when low doses are administered weekly. FDA black box warnings include increased toxicity in patients with abnormal liver function and, in select NSCLC patients that received prior platinum, severe hypersensitivity reactions and severe fluid retention despite dexamethasone at-home premedication.

Hypersensitivity reactions were noted in approximately 31% of patients who received the drug without premedications in early studies.[4] Symptoms include flushing, rash, chest tightness, back pain, dyspnea, and fever or chills. Severe hypotension, bronchospasm, generalized rash, and erythema may also occur.[54] Major reactions usually occur during the first two courses and within minutes after the start of treatment. Signs and symptoms generally resolve within 15 minutes after cessation of treatment, and docetaxel can usually be reinstituted without sequelae after treatment with diphenhydramine and an H2-receptor antagonist. Docetaxel induces a unique fluid retention syndrome characterized by edema, weight gain, and third-space fluid collection. Fluid retention is cumulative and is due to increased capillary permeability. Prophylactic treatment with corticosteroids has been demonstrated to reduce the incidence of fluid retention. Aggressive and early treatment with diuretics has been successfully used to manage fluid retention. Skin toxicity may occur in as many as 50% to 75% of patients; however, premedication may reduce the overall incidence of this effect.[4] Other cutaneous effects include palmar–plantar erythrodysesthesia and onychodystrophy. Docetaxel produces neurotoxicity, which is qualitatively similar to that of paclitaxel; however, neurosensory and neuromuscular effects are generally less frequent and less severe than with paclitaxel. Mild-to-moderate peripheral neurotoxicity occurs in approximately 40% of untreated patients.[55] Asthenia has been a prominent complaint in patients who have been treated with large cumulative doses. Stomatitis appears to occur more frequently with docetaxel than with paclitaxel. Other reported toxicities of note include necrotizing enterocolitis, interstitial pneumonitis, and organizing pneumonia.[56,57]

## Cabazitaxel

A phase III multi-institutional study of men with metastatic castration-resistant prostate cancer who had failed docetaxel improved overall median survival on cabazitaxel compared to mitoxantrone.[58] Cabazitaxel was approved by the FDA in June 2010 to treat metastatic castration-resistant prostate cancer in those who had received prior chemotherapy. This was despite a higher rate of adverse deaths (4.9%), a third of which were due to neutropenic sepsis. Cabazitaxel was associated with more grade 3 or 4 neutropenia (82%) than mitoxantrone (58%). Side effects reported in more than 20% of patients treated with cabazitaxel included myelosuppression, diarrhea, nausea, vomiting, constipation, abdominal pain, or asthenia. FDA black box warnings are similar to those for docetaxel.

## VINCA ALKALOIDS

The vinca alkaloids have been some of the most active agents in cancer chemotherapy since their introduction 40 years ago. The naturally occurring members of the family, vinblastine (VBL) and vincristine (VCR), were isolated from the leaves of the periwinkle plant *Catharanthus roseus G. Don.* In the late 1950s, their antimitotic and, therefore, cancer chemotherapeutic potential was discovered by groups both at Eli Lilly Research Laboratories and at the University of Western Ontario, and they came into widespread use for the single-agent treatment of childhood hematologic and solid malignancies and, shortly after, for adult hematologic

malignancies (see Table 21.1).[1] Their clinical efficacy in several combination therapies has led to the development of various novel semisynthetic analogs, including vinorelbine (VRL), vindesine (VDS), and vinflunine (VFL).

## Mechanism of Action

In contrast to the taxanes, the vinca alkaloids depolymerize microtubules and destroy mitotic spindles.[1] At low but clinically relevant concentrations, VBL does not depolymerize spindle microtubules, yet it powerfully blocks mitosis. This has been suggested to occur as a result of the suppression of microtubule dynamics rather than microtubule depolymerization. This group of compounds binds to the β subunit of tubulin dimers at a distinct region called the vinca-binding domain. Importantly, VBL binding induces a conformational change in tubulin in connection with tubulin self-association. In mitotic spindles, the slowing of the growth and shortening or treadmilling dynamics of the microtubules block mitotic progression. Disruption of the normal mitotic spindle assembly leads to delayed cell cycle progress with chromosomes stuck at the spindle poles and unable to pass from metaphase into anaphase, which eventually induces to apoptosis. The naturally occurring vinca alkaloids VCR and VBL, the semisynthetic analog VRL, and a novel bifluorinated analog VFL have similar mechanisms of action.

Tissue and tumor sensitivities to the vinca alkaloids, which, in part, relate to differences in drug transport and accumulation, also vary. Intracellular or extracellular concentration ratios range from five- to 500-fold depending on the individual cell type, lipophilicity, tissue-specific factors such as tubulin isotype composition, and tissue-specific microtubule-associated proteins (MAP).[59–61] Although the vinca alkaloids are retained in cells for long periods of time and thus may have prolonged cellular effects, intracellular retention is markedly different among the various vinca alkaloids. For instance, VBL appears to be retained in lipophilic tissue much more than either VCR or VDS.[59] Newer theories of antimicrotubule agents' mechanism of action have emerged, suggesting that the more important target of these drugs may be the tumor vasculature, as reviewed in the next section.

## Clinical Pharmacology

The vinca alkaloids are usually administered intravenously as a brief infusion, and their pharmacokinetic behavior in plasma has generally been explained by a three-compartment model. The vinca alkaloids share many pharmacokinetic properties, including large volumes of distribution, high clearance rates, and long terminal half-lives that reflect the high magnitude and avidity of drug binding in peripheral tissues. VCR has the longest terminal half-life and the lowest clearance rate; VBL has the shortest terminal half-life and the highest clearance rate; and VDS has intermediate characteristics. Although prolonged infusion schedules may avoid excessively toxic peak concentrations and increase the duration of drug exposure in plasma above biologically relevant threshold concentrations, there is little evidence to support the notion that prolonged infusions are more effective than bolus schedules. The longest half-life and lowest clearance rate of VCR may account for its greater propensity to induce neurotoxicity, but there are many other nonpharmacokinetic determinants of tissue sensitivity, as discussed in the previous section.

## Vincristine

After conventional doses of VCR (1.4 mg/m²) given as brief infusions, peak plasma levels approach 0.4 μmol. Plasma clearance is slow, and terminal half-lives that range from 23 to 85 hours have been reported. VCR is metabolized and excreted primarily by the hepatobiliary system. The nature of the VCR metabolites identified to date, as well as the results of metabolic studies in vitro, indicate that VCR metabolism is mediated principally by hepatic cytochrome P-450 CYP3A5.

## Vinblastine

The clinical pharmacology of VBL is similar to that of VCR. VBL binding to plasma proteins and formed elements of blood is extensive.[62,63] Peak plasma drug concentrations are approximately 0.4 $\mu$m after rapid intravenous injections of VBL at standard doses. Distribution is rapid, and terminal half-lives range from 20 to 24 hours. Like VCR, VBL disposition is principally through the hepatobiliary system with excretion in feces (approximately 95%); however, fecal excretion of the parent compound is low, indicating that hepatic metabolism is extensive.[59]

## Vinorelbine

The pharmacologic behavior of VRL is similar to that of the other vinca alkaloids, and plasma concentrations after rapid intravenous administration have been reported to decline in either a biexponential or triexponential manner.[64] After intravenous administration, there is a rapid decay of VRL concentrations followed by a much slower elimination phase (terminal half-life, 18 to 49 hours). Plasma protein binding, principally to $\alpha_1$-acid glycoprotein, albumin, and lipoproteins, has been reported to range from 80% to 91%, and drug binding to platelets is extensive.[64] VRL is widely distributed, and high concentrations are found in virtually all tissues, except the central nervous system.[64] The wide distribution of VRL reflects its lipophilicity, which is among the highest of the vinca alkaloids. As with other vinca alkaloids, the liver is the principal excretory organ, and up to 80% of VRL is excreted in the feces, whereas urinary excretion represents only 16% to 30% of total drug disposition, the bulk of which is unmetabolized VRL. Studies in humans indicate that 4-O-deacetyl-VRL and 3,6-epoxy-VRL are the principal metabolites, and several minor hydroxy-VRL isomer metabolites have been identified. Although most metabolites are inactive, the deacetyl-VRL metabolite may be as active as VRL. The cytochrome P-450 CYP3A isoenzyme appears to be principally involved in biotransformation.

## Vinflunine

VFL is a novel semisynthetic microtubule inhibitor with a fluorinated catharanthine moiety, which translates into lower affinity for the vinca binding site on tubulin and, therefore, different quantitative effects on microtubule dynamics.[65] The low affinity for tubulin may be responsible for its reduced clinical neurotoxicity. Despite this lower affinity, it is more active in vivo than other vinca alkaloids, and resistance develops more slowly. VFL is a new vinca and still under clinical development. Its volume of distribution is large, and has a terminal half-life of nearly 40 hours.[65] The only active metabolite is 4-O-deacetylvinflunine, which has a terminal half-life approximately 5 days longer than that of the parent compound.[65]

## Drug Interactions

Methotrexate accumulation in tumor cells is enhanced in vitro by the presence of VCR or VBL, an effect mediated by a vinca alkaloid–induced blockade of drug efflux; however, the minimal concentrations of VCR required to achieve this effect occur only transiently in vivo.[66] The vinca alkaloids also inhibit the cellular influx of the epipodophyllotoxins in vitro, resulting in less cytotoxicity. However, the clinical implications of this potential interaction are unknown. L-asparaginase may reduce the hepatic clearance of the vinca alkaloids, which may result in increased vinca-related toxicity. To minimize the possibility of this interaction, the vinca alkaloids should be given 12 to 24 hours before L-asparaginase. The combined use of mitomycin C and the vinca alkaloids has been associated with acute dyspnea and bronchospasm. The onset of these pulmonary toxicities has ranged from within minutes to hours after treatment with the vinca alkaloids, or up to 2 weeks after mitomycin C.

Treatment with the vinca alkaloids has precipitated seizures associated with subtherapeutic plasma phenytoin concentrations.[66] Reduced plasma phenytoin levels have been noted from 24 hours to 10 days after treatment with VCR and VBL. Because of the importance of the cytochrome P-450 CYP3A isoenzyme in vinca alkaloid metabolism, administration of the vinca alkaloids with erythromycin and other inhibitors of CYP3A may lead to severe toxicity.[67] Concomitantly administered drugs, such as pentobarbital and H$_2$-receptor antagonists, may also influence VCR clearance by modulating hepatic cytochrome P-450 metabolic processes.[66]

## Toxicity

Despite close similarities in structure, the vinca alkaloids differ in their safety profiles. Neutropenia is the principal dose-limiting toxicity of VBL and VRL. Thrombocytopenia and anemia occur less commonly. The onset of neutropenia is usually day 7 to 11, with recovery by day 14 to 21, and can be potentiated by hepatic dysfunction. Gastrointestinal autonomic dysfunction, as manifested by bloating, constipation, ileus, and abdominal pain, occur most commonly with VCR or high doses of the other vinca alkaloids. Mucositis occurs more frequently with VBL than with VRL and is least common with VCR. Nausea, vomiting, diarrhea,[31,43,45] and pancreatitis[53,54] also occur to a lesser extent.

VCR principally induces neurotoxicity characterized by a peripheral, symmetric mixed sensory motor and autonomic polyneuropathy.[68,69] Toxic manifestations include constipation, abdominal cramps, paralytic ileus, urinary retention, orthostatic hypotension, and hypertension. Its primary neuropathologic effects are due to interference with axonal microtubule function. Early symmetric sensory impairment and paresthesias can progress to neuritic pain and loss of deep tendon reflexes with continued treatment, which may be followed by foot drop, wrist drop, motor dysfunction, ataxia, and paralysis. Cranial nerves are rarely affected because the uptake of VCR into the central nervous system is low. Severe neurotoxicity occurs infrequently with VBL and VDS. VRL has been shown to have a lower affinity for axonal microtubules than either VCR or VBL, which seems to be confirmed by clinical observations.[70] Mild-to-moderate peripheral neuropathy, principally characterized by sensory effects, occurs in 7% to 31% of patients, and constipation and other autonomic effects are noted in 30% of patients, whereas severe toxicity occurs in 2% to 3%.

In adults, neurotoxicity may occur after treatment with cumulative doses as little as 5 to 6 mg, and manifestations may be profound after cumulative doses of 15 to 20 mg. Patients with delayed biliary excretion or hepatic dysfunction, and those with antecedent neurologic disorders, such as Charcot-Marie-Tooth disease, hereditary and sensory neuropathy type 1, and Guillain-Barré syndrome, are predisposed to neurotoxicity.

The vinca alkaloids are potent vesicants. To decrease the risk of phlebitis, the vein should be adequately flushed after treatment. If extravasation is suspected, treatment should be discontinued, aspiration of any residual drug remaining in the tissues should be attempted, and prompt application of heat (*not* ice) for 1 hour four times daily for 3 to 5 days can limit tissue damage.[71] Hyaluronidase, 150 to 1,500 U (15 U/mL in 6 mL 0.9% sodium chloride solution) subcutaneously, through six clockwise injections in a circumferential manner using a 25-gauge needle (changing the needle with each new injection) into the surrounding tissues may minimize discomfort and latent cellulitis. A surgical consultation to consider early debridement is also recommended. Mild and reversible alopecia occurs in approximately 10% and 20% of patients treated with VLR and VCR, respectively. Acute cardiac ischemia, chest pains without evidence of ischemia, fever, Raynaud syndrome, hand–foot syndrome, and pulmonary and liver toxicity (transaminitis and hyperbilirubinemia) have also been reported with use of the vinca alkaloids. All of the vinca alkaloids can cause a syndrome of inappropriate secretion of antidiuretic hormone (SIADH), and patients who are receiving intensive hydration are particularly prone to severe hyponatremia secondary to SIADH.

## MICROTUBULE ANTAGONISTS

### Estramustine Phosphate

Estramustine is a conjugate of nor-nitrogen mustard linked to 17β-estradiol by a carbamate ester bridge. Estramustine phosphate received regulatory approval in the United States in 1981 for treating patients with castration-resistant prostate cancer (CRPC). Although the recommended daily dose of estramustine phosphate is 14 mg/kg per day, patients are usually treated in the daily dosing range of 10 to 16 mg/kg in three to four divided daily doses (see Table 21.1). Estramustine has significant activity in CRPC and had been used in combination with VBL or docetaxel. However, phase III trials in patients with CRPC showed that when combined with docetaxel, there is no added benefit to overall survival compared to docetaxel alone.[72,73]

Estramustine binds to β-tubulin at a site distinct from the colchicine and vinca alkaloid binding sites. This agent depolymerizes microtubules and microfilaments, binds to and disrupts MAPs, and inhibits cell growth at high concentrations, resulting in mitotic arrest and apoptosis in tumor cells. The selective accumulation and actions of estramustine phosphate and its metabolite, *estromustine*, in specific tissues appear to be dependent on the expression of the estramustine-binding protein (EMBP). The disposition of estramustine is principally by rapid oxidative metabolism of the parent compound to estromustine. Estromustine concentrations in plasma are maximal within 2 to 4 hours after oral administration, and the mean elimination half-life of estromustine is 14 hours. Estromustine and estramustine are principally excreted in the feces, with only small amounts of conjugated estrone and estradiol detected in the urine (less than 1%).

In general, this agent has a manageable safety profile. Nausea and vomiting are the principal toxicities encountered. In contrast to the taxanes and the vinca alkaloids, myelosuppression is rarely clinically relevant. Common estrogenic side effects include gynecomastia, nipple tenderness, and fluid retention. Thromboembolic complications may occur in up to 10% of patients.

### Epothilones

The epothilones are macrolide compounds that were initially isolated from the mycobacterium *Sorangium cellulosum*. They exert their cytotoxic effects by promoting tubulin polymerization and inducing mitotic arrest.[74] In general, the epothilones are more potent than the taxanes. In contrast to the taxanes and vinca alkaloids, overexpression of the efflux protein P-glycoprotein minimally affects the cytotoxicity of epothilones. Epothilones include the natural epothilone B (patupilone; EPO906) and several semisynthetic epothilone compounds such as aza-epothilone B (ixabepilone; BMS-247550), epothilone D (deoxyepothilone B, KOS-862), and a fully synthetic analog, sagopilone (ZK-EPO).[75]

Ixabepilone has been evaluated in several schedules using a cremophor-based formulation and is FDA approved for the treatment of patients with breast cancer.[75] It is active in breast cancer previously treated with paclitaxel or docetaxel. The principal toxicities observed include neutropenia and peripheral neuropathy,

in addition to fatigue, nausea, emesis, and diarrhea.[55,74] It also has been evaluated in other solid tumors such as ovarian, prostate, and renal cell carcinomas.[75] Epothilones are still undergoing evaluations in several clinical trials. Pharmacokinetic studies based on patupilone have shown large volume of distribution (41-fold the total body water) and low body clearance (13% of hepatic blood flow).[76] There do not appear to be active metabolites once the parent drug is hydrolyzed, which is the main elimination pathway.[76]

## Maytansinoids and Auristatins: DM1, MMAE

Antibody drug conjugates (ADC) were first attempted with delivery of doxorubicin. Although tissue localization seemed promising, it became clear that the delivery of more potent chemotherapeutics was necessary.[77,78] One of the major advances for the promise of ADC came with the discovery and development of highly potent anticancer compounds such as calicheamicins, maytansinoids, and auristatins.[78] The next necessary advance was a linker that released the drug only when intended, and avoiding, or in some cases capitalizing on, in vivo proteases, oxidizing, or reducing environments. Gemtuzumab ozogamicin was the first ADC using calicheamicin, a potent DNA minor groove binder (and not a microtubule agent), approved in 2000 although withdrawn from the market in 2013 due to failed confirmatory studies. Maytansinoids and auristatins are unrelated, although are both tubulin-binding agents of the vinca binding site and inhibit tubulin polymerization.[78] They are 100- to 1,000-fold more cytotoxic that most cancer chemotherapeutics.[79]

Drug maytansinoid-1 (DM1) is the chemotherapeutic delivered using a thioether linker in the ADC ado-trastuzumab emtansine (T-DM1) that was FDA approved for patients with HER2- positive metastatic breast cancer previously treated with trastuzumab and taxane chemotherapy.[80,81] In the international phase III study, there was a 3.2-month improved progression-free survival among patients that received T-DM1 compared to those receiving standard treatment with capecitabine and lapatinib.[81] Despite a potent chemotherapeutic, the tolerability was much better in the experimental arm, which was dosed at 3.6 mg/kg intravenously every 21 days. The most common side effects in the trial were thrombocytopenia (12.8%), transient transaminitis (4.3%), as well as nausea, fatigue, myalgias, and arthralgias.[81]

Monomethyl auristatin E (MMAE) is linked to a monoclonal antibody against CD30 as an ADC (brentuximab vedotin, SGN35) and approved for refractory Hodgkin lymphoma or anaplastic large cell lymphoma. The linker is a peptide-based substrate for cathepsin-B and thereby designed to detect the lysosome/endosome compartment for drug release.[82,83] Dose-limiting toxicities include thrombocytopenia, hyperglycemia, diarrhea, and vomiting, and the most common side effects in this heavily pretreated population (including autologous stem cell transplant) includes peripheral neuropathy (42%), nausea (35%), and fatigue (34%).[84] The FDA black box warning includes contraindicated use with bleomycin due to increased pulmonary toxicity and the risk of John Cunningham (JC) virus–induced progressive multifocal leukoencephalopathy. Reports of severe pancreatitis are also emerging.[85]

## MITOTIC MOTOR PROTEIN INHIBITORS

### Aurora Kinase and Pololike Kinase Inhibitors

Aurora kinases are serine/threonine kinases crucial for mitosis in their recruitment of mitotic motor proteins for spindle formation. They are particularly overexpressed in high growth rate tumors. Aurora A and B kinases are expressed globally throughout all tissues, and Aurora C kinase is expressed in testes and participates in meiosis. Aurora A kinase is expressed and frequently amplified in many epithelial tumors and implicated in the microtubule-targeted agent-resistant phenotype.[86] Aurora A kinase interacts with p53, and there is evidence that p53 wild-type tumors are more sensitive to aurora A kinase inhibitors than p53 mutant tumors.[87] MLN-8237 has an $IC_{50}$ of 1 nm for aurora A kinase and >200 nm for aurora B kinase and is in clinical development for treatment-related neuroendocrine prostate cancer.[86,88] The main dose-limiting toxicity of these agents is neutropenia. Pololike kinases (PLKs) are serine or threonine kinases crucial for cell cycle process. Overexpression of PLKs has been shown to be related to histologic grading and poor prognosis in several types of cancer. BI-2536 and ON01910 are PLK inhibitors in early clinical development.[89]

## Kinesin Spindle Protein Inhibitor

### Ispinesib

Kinesin spindle protein (KSP; also known as EG5) is a kinesin motor protein required to establish mitotic-spindle bipolarity.[90] Several KSP inhibitors have been evaluated in early phase clinical trials. SB-715992 (ispinesib) is a small-molecule inhibitor of KSP ATPase and has been evaluated in two different schedules.[89] The dose-limiting toxicity is neutropenia. Ispinesib was found to be inactive in phase 2 studies evaluating efficacy in patients with castration-resistant and largely docetaxel-resistant prostate cancer, advanced renal cancer, and head and neck cancer.[90–92]

## MECHANISMS OF RESISTANCE TO MICROTUBULE INHIBITORS

Drug resistance is often complex and multifaceted and can involve diverse mechanisms such as (1) factors that reduce the ability of drugs to reach their cellular target (e.g., activation of detoxification pathways and decreased drug accumulation); (2) modifications in the drug target; and (3) events downstream of the target (e.g., decreased sensitivity to, or defective, apoptotic signals). Many tubulin binding agents are substrates for multidrug transporters such as P-glycoprotein and the multidrug resistance gene (MDR1).[93,94]

The MDR1-encoded gene product MDR1 (ABC subfamily B1; ABCB1) and MDR2 (ABC subfamily ABCB4) are the best-characterized ABC transporters thought to confer drug resistance to taxanes.[94,95] MDR-related taxane resistance can be reversed by many classes of drugs, including the calcium channel blockers, cyclosporin A, and antiarrhythmic agents.[94,95] However, the clinical utility of this approach has never been proven, despite several clinical trials. The role of ABC transporters in resistance to microtubule inhibitors remains to be determined.[96]

An increasing number of studies suggest that the expression of individual tubulin isotypes are altered in cells resistant to antimicrotubule drugs and may confer drug resistance.[93,97] Inherent differences in microtubule dynamics and drug interactions have been observed with some isotypes in vitro and in vivo.[98] Several taxane-resistant mutant cell lines that have structurally altered α- and β-tubulin proteins and an impaired ability to polymerize into microtubules have also been identified.[99] Mutations of tubulin isotype genes, gene amplifications, and isotype switching have also been reported in taxane-resistant cell lines.[99] In patients, levels of class III β-tubulin have been shown to correlate with response—those with high RNA levels have poor response—and immunohistochemical stains can correlate and may be predictive.[96,100,101] As opposed to taxanes, resistance to vinca alkaloids has been associated with decreased class II β-tubulin expression.[97,98]

MAPs are important structural and regulatory components of microtubules that act in concert to remodel the microtubule network by stabilizing or destabilizing microtubules during mitosis or cytokinesis. Alterations in the activity and/or balance of stabilizing or destabilizing MAPs can profoundly affect microtubule function.[99,102] The overexpression of stathmin, a destabilizing protein, has been reported to decrease sensitivity to paclitaxel and vinblastine.[1] An analysis of predictive or prognostic factors in a large phase 3 study (National Surgical Adjuvant Breast and Bowel Project NSABP-B 28) in patients with node-positive breast cancer showed that MAP-tau, a stabilizing protein, was a prognostic factor; however, it was not predictive for benefit from paclitaxel-based chemotherapy.[1,93] In a separate randomized controlled trial in breast cancer (TAX 307), where the only variable was docetaxel, MAP-tau was also shown to be prognostic, but not predictive of taxane benefit.[103]

Additional studies have shown a correlation with BRCA1 loss measured by gene or protein expression, or gene signatures, with resistance to taxane and sensitivity to DNA-damaging agents (such as cisplatin and anthracyclines).[104–107] BRCA1 is a tumor-suppressor gene with DNA damage response and repair, as well as cell cycle checkpoint activation, which explains why its loss leads to enhanced cisplatin sensitivity.[20] BRCA1 also indirectly regulates microtubule dynamics and stability and can favorably control how microtubules respond to paclitaxel treatment via their association with pro-caspase-8. The loss of BRCA1 can lead to impaired taxane-induced activation of apoptosis due to microtubules that are more dynamic and less susceptible to taxane-induced stabilization and proximity-induced activation of caspase-8 signaling.[20]

In addition to resistance, certain tumor subtypes may be sensitive to the taxane dosing schedule. In two randomized trials of low-dose, weekly paclitaxel, the luminal breast cancer subtype was found to have a better outcome compared with the control arm. This suggests that not only the drug, but also the schedule may influence the response to therapy and that genomic approaches may reveal these insights.[108]

## REFERENCES

1. Kavallaris M. Microtubules and resistance to tubulin-binding agents. *Nat Rev Cancer* 2010;10:194–204.
2. Nogales E. Structural insights into microtubule function. *Ann Rev Biophys Biomol Struct* 2001;30:397–420.
3. Wani MC, Taylor HL, Wall ME, et al. Plant antitumor agents. VI. Isolation and structure of taxol, a novel antileukemic and antitumor agent from Taxus brevifolia. *J Am Chem Soc* 1971;93:2325–2327.
4. Rowinsky E, Donehower R. Antimicrotubule agents. In: DeVita VT, Hellmann S, Rosenberg SA, eds. *Cancer: Principles and Practice of Oncology*. 5th ed. Philadelphia: Lippincott-Raven;1997.
5. Vrignaud P, Sémiond D, Lejeune P, et al. Preclinical antitumor activity of cabazitaxel, a semisynthetic taxane active in taxane-resistant tumors. *Clin Cancer Res* 2013;19:2973–2983.
6. Sparano JA. Taxanes for breast cancer: an evidence-based review of randomized phase II and phase III trials. *Clin Breast Cancer* 2000;1:32–40.
7. Mamounas E, Leinbersky B, Bryant J, et al. Paclitaxel after doxorubicin plus cyclophosphamide as adjuvant chemotherapy for node-positive breast cancer: results from NSABP B-28. *J Clin Oncol* 2005;23:3686–3696.
8. Bonomi P, Kim KM, Fairclough D, et al. Comparison of survival and quality of life in advanced non-small-cell lung cancer patients treated with two dose levels of paclitaxel combined with cisplatin versus etoposide with cisplatin: results of an Eastern Cooperative Oncology Group trial. *J Clin Oncol* 2000;18:623–631.
9. Martin M, Pienkowski T, Mackey J, et al. Adjuvant docetaxel for node-positive breast cancer. *N Engl J Med* 2005;352:2302–2313.
10. Jones SE, Erban J, Overmoyer B, et al. Randomized phase III study of docetaxel compared with paclitaxel in metastatic breast cancer. *J Clin Oncol* 2005;23:5542–5551.
11. Tannock IF, de Wit R, Berry WR, et al. Docetaxel plus prednisone or mitoxantrone plus prednisone for advanced prostate cancer. *N Engl J Med* 2004;351:1502–1512.
12. Van Cutsem E, Moiseyenko V, Tjulandin S, et al. Phase III study of docetaxel and cisplatin plus fluorouracil compared with cisplatin and fluorouracil as first-line therapy for advanced gastric cancer: a report of the V325 Study Group. *J Clin Oncol* 2006;24:4991–4997.
13. Schiff PB, Fant J, Horwitz SB. Promotion of microtubule assembly in vitro by taxol. *Nature* 1979;277:665–667.

14. Nogales E. Structural insight into microtubule function. *Annu Rev Biophys Biomol Struct* 2001;30:397–420.
15. Darshan MS, Loftus MS, Thadani-Mulero M, et al. Taxane-induced blockade to nuclear accumulation of the androgen receptor predicts clinical responses in metastatic prostate cancer. *Cancer Res* 2011;71:6019–6029.
16. Hoimes CJ, Kelly WK. Redefining hormone resistance in prostate cancer. *Ther Adv Med Oncol* 2010;2:107–123.
17. LaPointe NE, Morfini G, Brady ST, et al. Effects of eribulin, vincristine, paclitaxel and ixabepilone on fast axonal transport and kinesin-1 driven microtubule gliding: Implications for chemotherapy-induced peripheral neuropathy. *Neurotoxicology* 2013;37:231–239.
18. Mielgo A, Torres VA, Clair K, et al. Paclitaxel promotes a caspase 8-mediated apoptosis through death effector domain association with microtubules. *Oncogene* 2009;28:3551–3562.
19. Komlodi-Pasztor E, Sackett D, Wilkerson J, et al. Mitosis is not a key target of microtubule agents in patient tumors. *Nat Rev Clin Oncol* 2011;8:244–250.
20. Sung M, Giannakakou P. BRCA1 regulates microtubule dynamics and taxane-induced apoptotic cell signaling. *Oncogene* 2014;33(11):1418–1428.
21. Strobel T, Kraeft SK, Chen LB, et al. BAX expression is associated with enhanced intracellular accumulation of paclitaxel: a novel role for BAX during chemotherapy-induced cell death. *Cancer Res* 1998;58:4776–4781.
22. Srivastava RK, Mi QS, Hardwick JM, et al. Deletion of the loop region of Bcl-2 completely blocks paclitaxel-induced apoptosis. *Proc Natl Acad Sci U S A* 1999;96:3775–3780.
23. Dai H, Ding H, Meng XW, et al. Contribution of Bcl-2 phosphorylation to Bak binding and drug resistance. *Cancer Res* 2013;73(23)6998–7008.
24. Oakes SR, Vaillant F, Lim E, et al. Sensitization of BCL-2–expressing breast tumors to chemotherapy by the BH3 mimetic ABT-737. *Proc Natl Acad Sci* 2012;109:2766–2771.
25. Chauhan VP, Stylianopoulos T, Martin JD, et al. Normalization of tumour blood vessels improves the delivery of nanomedicines in a size-dependent manner. *Nat Nanotechnol* 2012;7:383–388.
26. Gradishar W, Tjulandin S, Davidson N, et al. Phase III trial of nanoparticle albumin-bound paclitaxel compared with polyethylated castor oil-based paclitaxel in women with breast cancer. *J Clin Oncol* 2005;23:7794–7803.
27. Socinski MA, Bondarenko I, Karaseva NA, et al. Weekly nab-paclitaxel in combination with carboplatin versus solvent-based paclitaxel plus carboplatin as first-line therapy in patients with advanced non–small-cell lung cancer: final results of a Phase III trial. *J Clin Oncol* 2012;30:2055–2062.
28. Von Hoff DD, Ervin T, Arena FP, et al. Increased survival in pancreatic cancer with nab-paclitaxel plus gemcitabine. *N Engl J Med* 2013;369:1691–1703.
29. Sparreboom A, Scripture CD, Trieu V, et al. Comparative preclinical and clinical pharmacokinetics of a cremophor-free, nanoparticle albumin-bound paclitaxel (ABI-007) and paclitaxel formulated in cremophor (Taxol). *Clin Cancer Res* 2005;11:4136–4143.
30. Yardley DA. nab-Paclitaxel mechanisms of action and delivery. *J Control Release* 2013;170:365–372.
31. Desai N, Trieu V, Yao Z, et al. Increased antitumor activity, intratumor paclitaxel concentrations, and endothelial cell transport of cremophor-free, albumin-bound paclitaxel, ABI-007, compared with cremophor-based paclitaxel. *Clin Cancer Res* 2006;12:1317–1324.
32. Nyman DW, Campbell KJ, Hersh E, et al. Phase I and pharmacokinetics trial of ABI-007, a novel nanoparticle formulation of paclitaxel in patients with advanced nonhematologic malignancies. *J Clin Oncol* 2005;23:7785–7793.
33. Cheng CJ, Saltzman WM. Nanomedicine: downsizing tumour therapeutics. *Nat Nanotechnol* 2012;7:346–347.
34. Infante JR, Matsubayashi H, Sato N, et al. Peritumoral fibroblast SPARC expression and patient outcome with resectable pancreatic adenocarcinoma. *J Clin Oncol* 2007;25:319–325.
35. Kato Y, Nagashima Y, Baba Y, et al. Expression of SPARC in tongue carcinoma of stage II is associated with poor prognosis: an immunohistochemical study of 86 cases. *Int J Mol Med* 2005;16:263–268.
36. Lau CPY, Poon RTP, Cheung ST, et al. SPARC and Hevin expression correlate with tumour angiogenesis in hepatocellular carcinoma. *J Pathol* 2006;210:459–468.
37. Thomas R, True LD, Bassuk JA, et al. Differential expression of osteonectin/SPARC during human prostate cancer progression. *Clin Cancer Res* 2000;6:1140–1149.
38. Watkins G, Douglas-Jones A, Bryce R, et al. Increased levels of SPARC (osteonectin) in human breast cancer tissues and its association with clinical outcomes. *Prostaglandins Leukot Essent Fatty Acids* 2005;72:267–272.
39. Cheng CJ, Saltzman WM. Enhanced siRNA delivery into cells by exploiting the synergy between targeting ligands and cell-penetrating peptides. *Biomaterials* 2011;32:6194–6203.
40. Davis ME, Zuckerman JE, Choi CH, et al. Evidence of RNAi in humans from systemically administered siRNA via targeted nanoparticles. *Nature* 2010;464:1067–1070.
41. Von Hoff DD, Ramanathan RK, Borad MJ, et al. Gemcitabine Plus nab-paclitaxel is an active regimen in patients with advanced pancreatic cancer: a Phase I/II trial. *J Clin Oncol* 2011;29:4548–4554.
42. Mita A, Denis L, Rowinsky E, et al. Phase I and pharmacokinetic study of XRP6258 (RPR 116258A), a novel taxane, administered as a 1-hour infusion every 3 weeks in patients with advanced solid tumors. *Clin Cancer Res* 2009;15:723–730.
43. Diéras V, Lortholary A, Laurence V, et al. Cabazitaxel in patients with advanced solid tumours: results of a Phase I and pharmacokinetic study. *Eur J Cancer* 2013;49:25–34.
44. Mita AC, Denis LJ, Rowinsky EK, et al. Phase I and pharmacokinetic study of XRP6258 (RPR 116258A), a novel taxane, administered as a 1-hour infusion every 3 weeks in patients with advanced solid tumors. *Clin Cancer Res* 2009;15:723–730.
45. Yared JA, Tkaczuk KH. Update on taxane development: new analogs and new formulations. *Drug Des Devel Ther* 2012;6:371–384.
46. Baas P, Szczesna A, Albert I, et al. Phase I/II study of a 3 weekly oral taxane (DJ-927) in patients with recurrent, advanced non-small cell lung cancer. *J Thorac Oncol* 2008;3:745–750.
47. Vigano L, Locatelli A, Grasselli G, et al. Drug interactions of paclitaxel and docetaxel and their relevance for the design of combination therapy. *Invest New Drugs* 2001;19:179–196.
48. Kudlowitz D, Muggia F. Defining risks of taxane neuropathy: insights from randomized clinical trials. *Clin Cancer Res* 2013;19:4570–4577.
49. Henningsson A, Karlsson MO, Viganò L, et al. Mechanism-based pharmacokinetic model for paclitaxel. *J Clin Oncol* 2001;19:4065–4073.
50. Sissung T, Mross K, Steinberg S, et al. Association of ABCB1 genotypes with paclitaxel-mediated peripheral neuropathy and neutropenia. *Eur J Cancer* 2006;42:2893–2896.
51. Marsh S, Paul J, King C, et al. Pharmacogenetic assessment of toxicity and outcome after platinum plus taxane chemotherapy in ovarian cancer: the Scottish Randomised Trial in Ovarian Cancer. *J Clin Oncol* 2007;25:4528–4535.
52. Baldwin RM, Owzar K, Zembutsu H, et al. A genome-wide association study identifies novel loci for paclitaxel-induced sensory peripheral neuropathy in CALGB 40101. *Clin Cancer Res* 2012;18:5099–5109.
53. Rugo H, Barry W, Moreno Aspitia A, et al. CALGB 40502/NCCTG N063H: Randomized phase III trial of weekly paclitaxel (P) compared to weekly nanoparticle albumin bound nab-paclitaxel (NP) or ixabepilone (Ix) with or without bevacizumab (B) as first-line therapy for locally recurrent or metastatic breast cancer (MBC). *J Clin Oncol* 2012;30.
54. Baker J, Ajani J, Scotté F, et al. Docetaxel-related side effects and their management. *Eur J Oncol Nurs* 2009;13:49–59.
55. Lee J, Swain S. Peripheral neuropathy induced by microtubule-stabilizing agents. *J Clin Oncol* 2006;24:1633–1642.
56. Alsamarai S, Charpidou AG, Matthay RA, et al. Pneumonitis related to docetaxel: case report and review of the literature. *In Vivo* 2009;23:635–637.
57. Dumitra S, Sideris L, Leclerc Y, et al. Neutropenic enterocolitis and docetaxel neoadjuvant chemotherapy. *Ann Oncol* 2009;20:795–796.
58. de Bono JS, Oudard S, Ozguroglu M, et al. Prednisone plus cabazitaxel or mitoxantrone for metastatic castration-resistant prostate cancer progressing after docetaxel treatment: a randomised open-label trial. *Lancet* 2010;376:1147–1154.
59. Zhou XJ, Placidi M, Rahmani R. Uptake and metabolism of vinca alkaloids by freshly isolated human hepatocytes in suspension. *Anticancer Res* 1994;14:1017–1022.
60. Zhou J, Giannakakou P. Targeting microtubules for cancer chemotherapy. *Curr Med Chem Anticancer Agents* 2005;5:65–71.
61. Jordan MA, Wilson L. Microtubules as a target for anticancer drugs. *Nat Rev Cancer* 2004;4:253–265.
62. Bender RA, Castle MC, Margileth DA, et al. The pharmacokinetics of [3H]-vincristine in man. *Clin Pharmacol Ther* 1977;22:430–435.
63. Zhou XJ, Martin M, Placidi M, et al. In-vivo and in-vitro pharmacokinetics and metabolism of vinca alkaloids in rat. II. Vinblastine and vincristine. *Eur J Drug Metab Pharmacokinet* 1990;15:323–332.
64. Rowinsky EK, Noe DA, Trump DL, et al. Pharmacokinetic, bioavailability, and feasibility study of oral vinorelbine in patients with solid tumors. *J Clin Oncol* 1994;12:1754–1763.
65. Fumoleau P, Guiu S. New vinca alkaloids in clinical development. *Curr Breast Cancer Rep* 2013;5:69–72.
66. Chan JD. Pharmacokinetic drug interactions of vinca alkaloids: summary of case reports. *Pharmacotherapy* 1998;18:1304–1307.
67. Tobe SW, Siu LL, Jamal SA, et al. Vinblastine and erythromycin: an unrecognized serious drug interaction. *Cancer Chemother Pharmacol* 1995;35:188–190.
68. Peltier A, Russell J. Recent advances in drug-induced neuropathies. *Curr Opin Neurol* 2002;15:633–638.
69. Quasthoff S, Hartung H. Chemotherapy-induced peripheral neuropathy. *J Neurol* 2002;249:9–17.
70. Lobert S, Vulevic B, Correia JJ. Interaction of vinca alkaloids with tubulin: a comparison of vinblastine, vincristine, and vinorelbine. *Biochemistry* 1996;35:6806–6814.
71. Schrijvers DL. Extravasation: a dreaded complication of chemotherapy. *Ann Oncol* 2003;14:iii26–iii30.
72. Petrylak D, Hussain MHA, Tangen C, et al. Docetaxel and estramustine compared with mitoxantrone and prednisone for advanced refractory prostate cancer. *N Engl J Med* 2004;351:1513–1520.
73. Tannock IF, de Wit R, Berry WR, et al. Docetaxel plus prednisone or mitoxantrone plus prednisone for advanced prostate cancer. *N Engl J Med* 2004;351:1502–1512.
74. Lee JJ, Kelly WK. Epothilones: tubulin polymerization as a novel target for prostate cancer therapy. *Nat Clin Pract Oncol* 2009;6:85–92.
75. Kelly WK. Epothilones in prostate cancer. *Urol Oncol* 2011;29:358–365.
76. Kelly K, Zollinger M, Lozac'h F, et al. Metabolism of patupilone in patients with advanced solid tumor malignancies. *Invest New Drugs* 2013;31:605–615.
77. Trail PA, Willner D, Lasch SJ, et al. Cure of xenografted human carcinomas by BR96-doxorubicin immunoconjugates. *Science* 1993;261:212–215.

78. Carter PJ, Senter PD. Antibody-drug conjugates for cancer therapy. *Cancer J* 2008;14:154–169.
79. Doronina SO, Toki BE, Torgov MY, et al. Development of potent monoclonal antibody auristatin conjugates for cancer therapy. *Nat Biotechnol* 2003;21: 778–784.
80. Lewis Phillips GD, Li G, Dugger DL, et al. Targeting HER2-positive breast cancer with trastuzumab-DM1, an antibody–cytotoxic drug conjugate. *Cancer Res* 2008;68:9280–9290.
81. Verma S, Miles D, Gianni L, et al. Trastuzumab emtansine for HER2-positive advanced breast cancer. *N Engl J Med* 2012;367:1783–1791.
82. Okeley NM, Miyamoto JB, Zhang X, et al. Intracellular activation of SGN-35, a potent anti-CD30 antibody-drug conjugate. *Clin Cancer Res* 2010;16:888–897.
83. Younes A, Bartlett NL, Leonard JP, et al. Brentuximab vedotin (SGN-35) for relapsed CD30-positive lymphomas. *N Engl J Med* 2010;363:1812–1821.
84. Younes A. Brentuximab vedotin for the treatment of patients with Hodgkin lymphoma. *Hematol Oncol Clin North Am* 2014;28:27–32.
85. Gandhi M, Evens AM, Fenske TS, et al. Pancreatitis in patients treated with brentuximab vedotin: a previously unrecognized serious adverse event. *Blood* 2013;122:4380.
86. Mosquera JM, Beltran H, Park K, et al. Concurrent AURKA and MYCN gene amplifications are harbingers of lethal treatment-related neuroendocrine prostate cancer. *Neoplasia* 2013;15:1–10.
87. Ujhazy P, Stewart D. DNA Repair. *J Thorac Oncol* 2009;4:S1068–S1070.
88. Green MR, Woolery JE, Mahadevan D. Update on aurora kinase targeted therapeutics in oncology. *Expert Opin Drug Discov* 2011;6:291–307.
89. Jackson JR, Patrick DR, Dar MM, et al. Targeted anti-mitotic therapies: can we improve on tubulin agents? *Nat Rev Cancer* 2007;7:107–117.
90. Tang PA, Siu LL, Chen EX, et al. Phase II study of ispinesib in recurrent or metastatic squamous cell carcinoma of the head and neck. *Invest New Drugs* 2008;26:257–264.
91. Beer TM, Goldman B, Synold TW, et al. Southwest oncology group phase II study of ispinesib in androgen-independent prostate cancer previously treated with taxanes. *Clin Genitourin Cancer* 2008;6:103–109.
92. Lee RT, Beekman KE, Hussain M, et al. A university of chicago consortium phase II trial of SB-715992 in advanced renal cell cancer. *Clin Genitourin Cancer* 2008;6:21–24.
93. Perez EA. Microtubule inhibitors: differentiating tubulin-inhibiting agents based on mechanisms of action, clinical activity, and resistance. *Mol Cancer Ther* 2009;8:2086–2095.
94. Gottesman MM, Fojo T, Bates SE. Multidrug resistance in cancer: role of ATP-dependent transporters. *Nat Rev Cancer* 2002;2:48–58.
95. Fojo AT, Menefee M. Microtubule targeting agents: basic mechanisms of multidrug resistance (MDR). *Semin Oncol* 2005;32:S3–S8.
96. Mozzetti S, Ferlini C, Concolino P, et al. Class III beta-tubulin overexpression is a prominent mechanism of paclitaxel resistance in ovarian cancer patients. *Clin Cancer Res* 2005;11:298–305.
97. Drukman S, Kavallaris M. Microtubule alterations and resistance to tubulin-binding agents (review). *Int J Oncol* 2002;21:621–628.
98. Verrills NM, Kavallaris M. Improving the targeting of tubulin-binding agents: lessons from drug resistance studies. *Curr Pharm Des* 2005;11:1719–1733.
99. Orr GA, Verdier-Pinard P, McDaid H, et al. Mechanisms of Taxol resistance related to microtubules. *Oncogene* 2003;22:7280–7295.
100. Monzó M, Rosell R, Sánchez JJ, et al. Paclitaxel resistance in non-small-cell lung cancer associated with beta-tubulin gene mutations. *J Clin Oncol* 1999;17:1786–1793.
101. Seve P, Mackey J, Isaac S, et al. Class III beta-tubulin expression in tumor cells predicts response and outcome in patients with non-small cell lung cancer receiving paclitaxel. *Mol Cancer Ther* 2005;4:2001–2007.
102. Baquero MT, Hanna JA, Neumeister V, et al. Stathmin expression and its relationship to microtubule-associated protein tau and outcome in breast cancer. *Cancer* 2012;118:4660–4669.
103. Baquero MT, Lostritto K, Gustavson MD, et al. Evaluation of prognostic and predictive value of microtubule associated protein tau in two independent cohorts. *Breast Cancer Res* 2011;13(5):R85.
104. Quinn JE, James CR, Stewart GE, et al. BRCA1 mRNA expression levels predict for overall survival in ovarian cancer after chemotherapy. *Clin Cancer Res* 2007;13:7413–7420.
105. Byrski T, Gronwald J, Huzarski T, et al. Response to neo-adjuvant chemotherapy in women with BRCA1-positive breast cancers. *Breast Cancer Res Treat* 2008;108:289–296.
106. Font A, Taron M, Gago JL, et al. BRCA1 mRNA expression and outcome to neoadjuvant cisplatin-based chemotherapy in bladder cancer. *Ann Oncol* 2011;22:139–144.
107. Reguart N, Cardona AF, Carrasco E, et al. BRCA1: a new genomic marker for non-small-cell lung cancer. *Clin Lung Cancer* 2008;9:331–339.
108. Martin M, Prat A, Rodriguez-Lescure A, et al. PAM50 proliferation score as a predictor of weekly paclitaxel benefit in breast cancer. *Breast Cancer Res Treat* 2013;138:457–466.

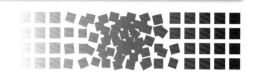

# 22 Kinase Inhibitors as Anticancer Drugs

Charles L. Sawyers

CANCER THERAPEUTICS

## INTRODUCTION

In 2001, the first tyrosine-kinase inhibitor imatinib was approved for clinical use in chronic myeloid leukemia. The spectacular success of this first-in-class agent ushered in a transformation in cancer drug discovery from efforts that were largely based on novel cytotoxic chemotherapy agents to an almost exclusive focus on molecularly targeted agents across the pharmaceutical and biotechnology industry and academia. This chapter summarizes this remarkable progress in this field over ~15 years, with the focus on the concepts underlying this paradigm shift as well as the considerable challenges that remain (Table 22.1). Readers in search of more specific details on individual drugs and their indications should consult the relevant disease-specific chapters elsewhere in this volume as well as references cited within this chapter. Readers should also note that the epidermal growth factor receptor (EGFR) and human epidermal growth factor receptor 2 (HER2) receptor tyrosine kinases covered here have also been successfully targeted by monoclonal antibodies that engage these proteins at the cell surface. These drugs, referred to as biologics rather than small molecule inhibitors, are covered in other chapters. The chapter is organized around kinase targets rather than diseases and, intentionally, has a historical flow to make certain thematic points and to illustrate the broad lessons that have been and continue to be learned through the clinical development of these exciting agents.

Perhaps the most stunning discovery from the clinical trials of the Abelson murine leukemia (ABL) kinase inhibitor imatinib was the recognition that tumor cells acquire exquisite dependence on the breakpoint cluster region protein BCR-ABL fusion oncogene, created by the Philadelphia chromosome translocation.[1] Although this may seem intuitive at first glance, consider the fact that the translocation arises in an otherwise normal hematopoietic stem cell, the survival of which is regulated by a complex array of growth factors and interactions with the bone marrow microenvironment. Although BCR-ABL clearly gives this cell a growth advantage that, over years, results in the clinical phenotype of chronic myeloid leukemia, there was no reason to expect that these cells would depend on BCR-ABL for their survival when confronted with an inhibitor. In the absence of BCR-ABL, these tumor cells could presumably rely on the marrow microenvironment, just like their normal, nontransformed neighbors. Thus, it seemed more likely that, by shutting down the driver oncogene, BCR-ABL inhibitors might halt the progression of chronic myeloid leukemia but not eliminate the preexisting tumor cells. In fact, chronic myeloid leukemia (CML) progenitors are eliminated after just a few months of anti–BCR-ABL therapy, indicating they are dependent on the driver oncogene for their survival and have "forgotten" how to return to normal. This phenomenon, subsequently documented in a variety of human malignancies, is colloquially termed *oncogene addiction*.[2] Although the molecular basis for this addiction still remains to be defined, the notion of finding an Achilles' heel for each cancer continues to captivate the cancer research community and has spawned a broad array of efforts to elucidate the molecular identity of these targets and discover relevant inhibitors.

## EARLY SUCCESSES: TARGETING CANCERS WITH WELL-KNOWN KINASE MUTATIONS (BCR-ABL, KIT, HER2)

From the beginning, clinical trials of imatinib were restricted to patients with Philadelphia chromosome–positive chronic myeloid leukemia. For what seem like obvious reasons, there was never any serious discussion about treating patients with Philadelphia chromosome–negative leukemia because the assumption was that only patients with the BCR-ABL fusion gene would have a chance of responding. This was clearly a wise decision because hematologic response rates approached 90% and cytogenetic remissions were seen in nearly half of the patients in the early phase studies.[3] It was obvious that the drug worked, and imatinib was approved in record time. Unwittingly, the power of genome-based patient selection was demonstrated in the clinical development of the very first kinase inhibitor. As we will see, it took nearly a decade for this lesson to be fully learned. Today, the much larger clinical experience, with an array of different kinase inhibitors across many tumor types, has led to a much better understanding of the principles that dictate oncogene addiction that, in retrospect, were staring us in the face. Foremost among them is the notion that tumors with a somatic mutation or amplification of a kinase drug target are much more likely to be dependent on that target for survival. Hence, a patient whose tumor has such a mutation is much more likely to respond to treatment with the appropriate inhibitor. This has also led to a new paradigm at the regulatory level of drug approval requiring codevelopment of a *companion diagnostic* (a molecularly based diagnostic test that reliably identifies patients with the mutation) with the new drug.

After chronic myeloid leukemia, the next example to illustrate this principle was gastrointestinal stromal tumor (GIST), which is associated with mutations in the KIT tyrosine-kinase receptor or, more rarely, in the platelet-derived growth factor (PDGF) receptor.[4,5] Serendipitously, imatinib inhibits both KIT and the PDGF receptor; therefore, the clinical test of KIT inhibition in GIST followed quickly on the heels of the success in CML.[6] In retrospect, the rapid progress made in these two diseases was based, in part, on the fact that the driver molecular lesion (BCR-ABL or KIT mutation, respectively) is present in nearly all patients who are diagnosed with these two diseases. The molecular analysis merely confirmed the diagnosis that was made using standard clinical and histologic criteria. Consequently, clinicians could identify the patients most likely to respond based on clinical criteria rather than rely on an elaborate molecular profiling infrastructure to prescreen patients. Consequently, clinical trials evaluating kinase inhibitors in CML and GIST accrued quickly, and the therapeutic benefit became clear almost immediately.

The notion that molecular alteration of a driver kinase determines sensitivity to a cognate kinase inhibitor was further validated during the development of the dual EGFR/HER2 kinase inhibitor lapatinib. Clinical trials of this kinase inhibitor were conducted in women with advanced HER2-positive breast cancer based on earlier success in these same patients with the monoclonal antibody trastuzumab, which targets the extracellular domain of the HER2

**TABLE 22.1**

## Kinase Inhibitors: Approved or Anticipated Approval In 2014

| Target | Drug | Approved Indications | Anticipated Future Indications |
|---|---|---|---|
| ALK | Crizotinib<br>Ceritinib | ALK mutant lung cancer | ALK mutant neuroblastoma,<br>anaplastic lymphoma |
| BCR-ABL | Imatinib<br>Dasatinib<br>Nilotinib<br>Bosutinib<br>Ponatinib | Chronic myeloid leukemia<br>Philadelphia chromosome–positive acute lymphoid leukemia<br>T315 mutation only (ponatinib) | |
| BRAF | Vemurafenib<br>Dabrafenib | BRAF mutant melanoma | Other BRAF mutant tumors |
| BTK | Ibrutinib | Chronic lymphocytic leukemia<br>Mantle cell lymphoma | |
| EGFR | Gefitinib<br>Erlotinib<br>Afatinib | Lung adenocarcinoma with EGFR mutation | |
| HER2 | Lapatinib | Her2$^+$ breast cancer | |
| JAK2 | Ruxolitinib | JAK2 mutant myelofibrosis | |
| KIT | Imatinib<br>Sunitinib | Gastrointestinal stromal tumor | |
| MEK | Trametinib | BRAF mutant melanoma | |
| PI3K delta[a] | Idelalisib | Chronic lymphocytic leukemia<br>Indolent non-Hodgkin lymphoma | |
| PDGFR- α/β | Imatinib | Chronic myelomonocytic leukemia (with TEL-PDGFR-β fusion)<br>    hypereosinophilic syndrome (with PDGFR-β fusion)<br>Dermatofibrosarcoma protuberans | |
| RET | Vandetanib<br>Sorafenib<br>Cabozantinib | Medullary thyroid cancer | |
| TORC1 | Sirolimus (rapamycin) | Kidney cancer | |
| (mTOR) | Everolimus<br>Temsirolimus | Breast cancer<br>Tuberous sclerosis | |
| VEGF<br>Receptor | Sorafenib<br>Sunitinib<br>Axitinib<br>Pazopanib | Kidney cancer<br>Hepatocellular carcinoma (sorafenib only)<br>Pancreatic neuroendocrine tumors (sunitinib) | |

[a] Approval is anticipated based on positive phase 3 data and announcement of accepted Food and Drug Administration submission by the sponsor.

kinase. Lapatinib was initially approved in combination with the cytotoxic agent capecitabine for women with resistance to trastuzumab,[7] and then was subsequently approved for frontline use in metastatic breast cancer in combination with chemotherapy or hormonal therapy, depending on estrogen receptor status. A key ingredient that enabled the clinical development of lapatinib was the routine use of HER2 gene amplification testing in the diagnosis of breast cancer, pioneered during the development of trastuzumab several years earlier. This widespread clinical practice allowed for the rapid identification of those patients most likely to benefit. If lapatinib trials had been conducted in unselected patients, the clinical signal in breast cancer would likely have been missed.

## The Serendipity of Unexpected Clinical Responses: EGFR in Lung Cancer

In contrast to the logical development of imatinib and lapatinib in molecularly defined patient populations, the EGFR kinase inhibitors gefitinib and erlotinib entered the clinic without the benefit

of such a focused clinical development plan. Although considerable preclinical data implicated EGFR as a cancer drug target, there was little insight into which patients were most likely to benefit. The first clue that EGFR inhibitors would have a role in lung cancer came from the recognition by several astute clinicians of remarkable responses in a small fraction of patients with lung adenocarcinoma.[8] Further studies revealed the curious clinical circumstance that those patients most likely to benefit tended to be those who never smoked, women, and those of Asian ethnicity.[9] Clearly, there was a strong clinical signal in a subgroup of patients, who could perhaps be enriched based on these clinical features, but it seemed that a unifying molecular lesion must be present. Three academic groups simultaneously converged on the answer. Mutations in the EGFR gene were detected in the 10% to 15% of patients with lung adenocarcinoma who had radiographic responses.[10–12] It may seem surprising that mutations in a gene as highly visible as EGFR and in such a prevalent cancer had not been detected earlier. But the motivation to search aggressively for EGFR mutations was not there until the clinical responses were seen. Perhaps even more surprising was the failure of the pharmaceutical company sponsors of the two most advanced compounds, gefitinib and erlotinib, to embrace this important discovery and refocus future clinical development plans on patients with EGFR mutant lung adenocarcinoma.

But that was 2004, when the prevailing approach to cancer drug development was an empiric one originally developed (with great success) for cytotoxic agents. Typically, small numbers of patients with different cancers were treated in *all comer* phase I studies (no enrichment for subgroups) with the goal of eliciting a clinical signal in at least one tumor type. A single-agent response rate of 20% to 30% in a disease-specific phase II trial would justify a randomized phase III registration trial, where the typical endpoint for drug approval is time to progression or survival. Cytotoxics were also typically evaluated in combination with existing standard of care treatment (typically approved chemotherapy agents) with the goal of increasing the response rate or enhancing the duration of response. (Note: The use of the past tense here is intentional. As we will see later in this chapter, nearly all cancer drug development today is based on selecting patients with a certain molecular profile.)

The clinical development of gefitinib and erlotinib followed the cytotoxic model. Both drugs had similarly low but convincing single-agent response rates (10% to 15%) in chemotherapy-refractory, advanced lung cancer. Indeed, gefitinib was originally granted accelerated approval by the U.S. Food and Drug Administration (FDA) in 2003 based on the impressive nature of these responses, contingent on the completion of formal phase III studies with survival endpoints.[13] The sponsors of both drugs, therefore, conducted phase III registration studies in patients with chemotherapy-refractory, advanced stage lung cancer but without prescreening patients for EGFR mutation status. (In fairness, these trials were initiated prior to the discovery of EGFR mutations in lung cancer but study amendments could have been considered.) Erlotinib was approved in 2004 on the basis of a modest survival advantage over placebo (the BR.21 trial); however, gefitinib failed to demonstrate a survival advantage in essentially the same patient population.[14,15] This difference in outcome was surprising because the two drugs have highly similar chemical structures and biologic properties. Perhaps the most important difference was drug dose. Erlotinib was given at the maximum tolerated dose, which produces a high frequency of rash and diarrhea. Both side effects are presumed *on target* consequences of EGFR inhibition because EGFR is highly expressed in skin and gastrointestinal epithelial cells. In contrast, gefitinib was dosed slightly lower to mitigate these toxicities, with the rationale that responses were clearly documented at lower doses.

In parallel with the single-agent phase III trials in chemotherapy-refractory patients, both gefitinib and erlotinib were studied as an upfront therapy for advanced lung cancer to determine if either would improve the efficacy of standard *doublet* (carboplatin/paclitaxel or gemcitabine/cisplatin) chemotherapy when all three drugs were given in combination. These trials, termed INTACT-1 and INTACT-2 (gefitinib with either gemcitabine/cisplatin or with carboplatin/paclitaxel) and TRIBUTE (erlotinib with carboplatin/paclitaxel), collectively enrolled over 3,000 patients.[16–18] Excitement in the oncology community was high based on the clear single-agent activity of both EGFR inhibitors. But, both trials were spectacular failures; neither drug showed any benefit over chemotherapy alone. The fact that EGFR mutations are present in only 10% to 15% of patients (i.e., those likely to benefit) provided a logical explanation. The clinical signal from those whose tumors had EGFR mutations was likely diluted out by all the patients whose tumors had no EGFR alterations, many of whom benefited from chemotherapy.

The convergence of the EGFR mutation discovery with these clinical trial results will be remembered as a remarkable time in the history of targeted cancer therapies, not just for the important role of these agents as lung cancer therapies, but also for missteps in deciding that the EGFR genotype should drive treatment selection. Perhaps the most egregious error came from a retrospective

analysis of tumors from patients treated on the BR.21 trial, which concluded that EGFR mutations did *not* predict for a survival advantage.[19] (EGFR gene amplification *was* associated with survival, but only in a univariate analysis.) This conclusion was concerning because less than 30% of patients on the trial had tissue available for EGFR mutation analysis, raising questions about the adequacy of the sample size. Furthermore, the EGFR mutation assay used by the authors was subsequently criticized because a significant number of the EGFR mutations reported in these patients were in residues not previously found by others, who had sequenced thousands of tumors. Many of these mutations were suspected to be an artifact of working from formalin-fixed biopsies. Fortunately, recent advances in DNA mutation detection, using massively parallel next-generation sequencing technology, have largely eliminated this concern. These new platforms are now being used in the clinical setting.

Clinical investigators in Asia, where a greater fraction of lung cancers (roughly 30%) are positive for EGFR mutations, addressed the question of whether mutations predict for clinical benefit in a prospective trial. In this study known as IPASS, gefitinib was clearly superior to standard doublet chemotherapy as frontline therapy for patients with advanced EGFR mutation–positive lung adenocarcinoma.[20] Conversely, EGFR mutation–negative patients fared much worse with gefitinib and benefited from chemotherapy. In addition, EGFR mutation–positive patients had a more favorable overall prognosis regardless of treatment, indicating that EGFR mutation is also a prognostic biomarker. The IPASS trial serves as a compelling example of a properly designed (and executed) biomarker-driven clinical trial. Although the rationale for this clinical development strategy had been demonstrated years earlier with BCR-ABL in leukemia, KIT in GIST, and HER2 in breast cancer, it was difficult to derail the empiric approach that had been used for decades in developing cytotoxic agents.

## A Mix of Science and Serendipity: PDGF Receptor–Driven Leukemias and Sarcoma

The discovery of EGFR mutations in lung cancer (motivated by dramatic clinical responses in a subset of patients treated with EGFR kinase inhibitors) is the most visible example of the power of bedside-to-bench science, but it is not the only (or the first) such example from the kinase inhibitor era. Shortly after the approval of imatinib for CML in 2001, two case reports documented dramatic remissions in patients with hypereosinophilic syndrome (HES), a blood disorder characterized by prolonged elevation of eosinophil counts and subsequent organ dysfunction from eosinophil infiltration, when treated with imatinib.[21,22] Although HES resembles myeloproliferative diseases such as CML, the molecular pathogenesis of HES was completely unknown at the time. Reasoning that these clinical responses must be explained by inhibition of a driver kinase, a team of laboratory-based physician/scientists quickly searched for mutations in the three kinases known to be inhibited by imatinib (ABL, KIT, and PDGF receptor). ABL and KIT were quickly excluded, but the PDGF receptor α (PDGFR-α) gene was targeted by an interstitial deletion that fused the upstream FIP1L1 gene to PDGFR-α[23] FIP1L1-PDGFR-α is a constitutively active tyrosine kinase, analogous to BCR-ABL, and is also inhibited by imatinib. As with EGFR-mutant lung cancer, the molecular pathophysiology of HES was discovered by dissecting the mechanism of response to the drug used to treat it.

The HES/FIP1L1-PDGFR-α story serves as a nice bookend to an earlier discovery that the t(5,12) chromosome translocation, found rarely in patients with chronic myelomonocytic leukemia, creates the TEL-PDGFR-β fusion tyrosine kinase.[24] Similar to HES, treatment of patients with t(5,12) translocation-positive leukemias with imatinib has also proven successful.[25] A third example comes from dermatofibrosarcoma protuberans, a sarcoma characterized by a t(17,22) translocation that fuses the COL1A gene to the PDGFB *ligand* (not the receptor). COL1A-PDGFB is oncogenic through autocrine stimulation of the normal PDGF receptor in these tumor cells. Patients with dermatofibrosarcoma protuberans respond to imatinib therapy because it targets the PDGF receptor, just one step downstream from the oncogenic lesion.[26]

## Exploiting the New Paradigm: Searching for Other Kinase-Driven Cancers

The benefits of serendipity notwithstanding, the growing number of examples of successful kinase inhibitor therapy in tumors with a mutation or amplification of the drug target begged for a more rational approach to drug discovery and development. In 2002, the list of human tumors known to have mutations in kinases was quite small. Due to advances in automated gene sequencing, it became possible to ask whether a much larger fraction of human cancers might also have such mutations through a brute force approach. To address this question comprehensively, one would have to sequence all of the kinases in the genome in hundreds of samples of each tumor type. Several early pilot studies demonstrated the potential of this approach by revealing important new targets for drug development. Perhaps the most spectacular was the discovery of mutations in the BRAF kinase in over half of patients with melanoma, as well as in a smaller fraction of colon and thyroid cancers.[27] Another was the discovery of mutations in the JAK2 kinase in nearly all patients with polycythemia vera, as well as a significant fraction of patients with myelofibrosis and essential thrombocytosis.[28–30] A third example was the identification of PIK3CA mutations in a variety of tumors, with the greatest frequencies in breast, endometrial, and colorectal cancers.[31] PIK3CA encodes a lipid kinase that generates the second messenger phosphatidyl inositol 3-phosphate (PIP3). PIP3 activates growth and survival signaling through the AKT family of kinases as well as other downstream effectors. Coupled with the well-established role of the phosphatase and tensin homolog (PTEN) lipid phosphatase in dephosphorylating PIP3, the discovery of PIK3CA mutations focused tremendous attention on developing inhibitors at multiple levels of this pathway, as discussed further in the follow paragraphs.

Each of these important discoveries—BRAF, JAK2, and PIK3CA—came from relatively small efforts (less than 100 tumors) and generally focused on resequencing only those exons that coded for regions of kinases where mutations had been found in other kinases (typically, the juxtamembrane and kinase domains). These restricted searches were largely driven by the high cost of DNA sequencing using the Sanger method. In 2006, a comprehensive effort to sequence all of the exons in all kinases in 100 tumors could easily exceed several million dollars. Financial support for such projects could not be obtained easily through traditional funding agencies because the risk/reward was considered too high. Furthermore, substantial infrastructure for sample acquisition, microdissection of the tumors from normal tissue, nucleic acid preparation, high throughput automated sequencing, and computational analysis of the resulting data was essential. Few institutions were equipped to address these challenges. In response, the National Cancer Institute in the United States (in partnership with the National Human Genome Research Institute) and an international group known as the International Cancer Genome Consortium (ICGC) launched large-scale efforts to sequence the complete genomes of thousands of cancers. In parallel, next-generation sequencing technologies resulted in massive reductions in cost, allowing a more comprehensive analysis of much larger numbers of tumors. At the time of this writing, the US effort (called The Cancer Genome Atlas [TCGA]) had reported data on 29 different tumor types (https://tcga-data.nci.nih.gov/tcga/). The international consortium has committed to sequencing 25,000 tumors representing 50 different cancer subtypes.[32] Both groups have enforced immediate release of all sequence information to the research community free of charge so that the entire scientific community can learn from the data. This policy enabled *pan cancer* mutational analyses that give an overall view of the genomic landscape of cancer, serving as a blueprint for the community of cancer researchers and drug developers.[33,34]

## Rounding Out the Treatment of Myeloproliferative Disorders: JAK2 and Myelofibrosis

Taken together with the BCR-ABL translocation in CML and FIP1L1-PDGFR-α in HES, the discovery of JAK2 mutations in polycythemia, essential thrombocytosis, and myelofibrosis provided a unifying understanding of myeloproliferative disorders as diseases of abnormal kinase activation. The JAK family kinases are the primary effectors of signaling through inflammatory cytokine receptors and, therefore, had been considered compelling targets for anti-inflammatory drugs. But the JAK2 mutation discovery immediately shifted these efforts toward developing JAK2 inhibitors for myeloproliferative disorders. Because most patients have a common JAK2 V617F mutation, these efforts could rapidly focus on screening for activity against a single genotype. Progress has been rapid. Myelofibrosis was selected as the initial indication (instead of essential thrombocytosis or polycythemia vera) because the time to registration is expected to be the shortest. Currently, ruxolitinib is approved for myelofibrosis based on shrinkage in spleen size as the primary endpoint. Clinical trials in essential thrombocytosis and polycythemia vera (versus hydroxyurea) are ongoing. Other JAK2 inhibitors are also in clinical development.

## BRAF Mutant Melanoma: Several Missteps Before Finding the Right Inhibitor

As with JAK2 mutations in myeloproliferative disorders, the discovery of BRAF mutations in patients with melanoma launched widespread efforts to find potent BRAF inhibitors. One early candidate was the drug sorafenib, which had been optimized during drug discovery to inhibit RAF kinases. (Sorafenib also inhibits vascular endothelial growth factor (VEGF) receptors, which led to its approval in kidney cancer, as discussed later in this chapter.) Despite the compelling molecular rationale for targeting BRAF, clinical results of sorafenib in melanoma were extremely disappointing and reduced enthusiasm for pursuing BRAF as a drug target.[35] In hindsight, this concern was completely misguided. Sorafenib dosing is limited by toxicities that preclude achieving serum levels in patients that potently inhibit RAF, but are sufficient to inhibit VEGF receptors. In addition, patients were enrolled without screening for BRAF mutations in their tumors. Although the frequency of BRAF mutations in melanoma is high, the inclusion of patients without the BRAF mutation diluted the chance of seeing any clinical signal. In short, the clinical evaluation of sorafenib in melanoma was poorly designed to test the hypothesis that BRAF is a therapeutic target. The danger is that negative data from such clinical experiments can slow subsequent progress. It is critical to know the pharmacodynamic properties of the drug and the molecular phenotype of the patients being studied when interpreting the results of a negative study.

The fact that RAF kinases are intermediate components of the well-characterized RAS/ mitogen-activated protein (MAP) kinase pathway (transducing signals from RAS to RAF to MEK to ERK) raised the possibility that tumors with BRAF mutations might respond to inhibitors of one of these downstream kinases (Fig. 22.1). Preclinical studies revealed that tumor cell lines with BRAF mutation were exquisitely sensitive to inhibitors of the downstream kinase MEK.[36] (Sorafenib, in contrast, does not show this profile of activity.[37] Thus, proper preclinical screening would have revealed the shortcomings of sorafenib as a BRAF inhibitor.) Curiously, cell lines with a mutation or amplification of EGFR or HER2, which

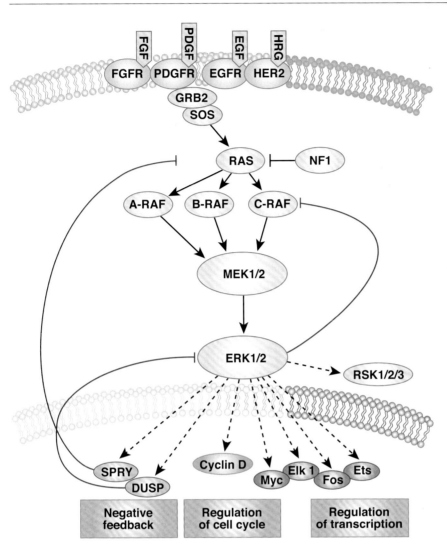

**Figure 22.1** The RAS–RAF–MEK–ERK signaling pathway. The classical mitogen-activated protein kinase (MAPK) pathway is activated in human tumors by several mechanisms, including the binding of ligand to receptor tyrosine kinases (RTK), the mutational activation of an RTK, by loss of the tumor suppressor NF1, or by mutations in RAS, BRAF, and MEK1. Phosphorylation and, thus, activation of ERK regulates the transcription of target genes that promote cell cycle progression and tumor survival. The ERK pathway contains a classical feedback loop in which the expression of feedback elements such as SPRY and DUSP family proteins are regulated by the level of ERK activity. Loss of expression of SPRY and DUSP family members due to promoter methylation or deletion is thus permissive for persistently elevated pathway output. In the case of tumors with mutant BRAF, pathway output is enhanced by impaired upstream feedback regulation. FGF, fibroblast growth factor; HRG, heregulin; NF1, neurofibromatosis 1. (From Bernt KM, Zhu N, Sinha AU, et al. MLL-rearranged leukemia is dependent on aberrant H3K79 methylation by DOT1L. *Cancer Cell* 2011;20(1):66–78, with permission.)

CANCER THERAPEUTICS

function upstream in the pathway, were insensitive to MEK inhibition. Even tumor lines with RAS mutations were variably sensitive. In short, the preclinical data made a strong case that MEK inhibitors should be effective in BRAF mutant melanoma, but not in other subtypes. The reason that HER2, EGFR, and RAS mutant tumors were not sensitive to MEK inhibitors is explained, at least in part, by the existence of negative feedback loops that modulate the flux of signal transduction through MEK.[38]

In parallel with the generation of these preclinical findings, clinical trials of several MEK inhibitors were initiated. Patients with various cancers were enrolled in the early studies, but there was a strong bias to include melanoma patients. Significant efforts were made to demonstrate MEK inhibition in tumor cells by measuring the phosphorylation status of the direct downstream substrate ERK using an immunohistochemical analysis of biopsies from patients with metastatic disease. Phase I studies of the two earliest compounds in clinical development (PD325901 and AZD6244) documented reduced phospho-ERK staining at multiple dose levels in several patients for whom baseline and treatment biopsies were obtained.[39,40] (In the following, we will learn that these pharmacodynamic studies, while well intentioned, were not quantitative enough to document the magnitude of MEK inhibition in these patients.) Furthermore, clinical responses were observed in a few patients with BRAF mutant melanoma. Armed with this confidence, a randomized phase II clinical trial of AZD6244 was conducted in advanced melanoma, with the chemotherapeutic agent temozolomide (which is approved for glioblastoma) as the comparator arm. (The clinical development

of PD325901 was discontinued because of safety concerns about ocular and neurologic toxicity.) Disappointingly, patients receiving AZD6244 had no benefit in progression-free survival when compared to temozolomide-treated patients, raising further concerns about the viability of BRAF as a drug target.[41] A closer examination of the data revealed that clinical responses were, indeed, seen in patients receiving AZD6244. The fact that BRAF mutation status was not required for study entry likely diminished the clinical signal in the AZD6244 arm, a lesson learned from the EGFR inhibitor trials in lung cancer. Indeed, a different MEK inhibitor, trametinib, received FDA approval in 2013 based on activity in melanoma patients with the BRAF mutation.[42]

All doubts about BRAF as a target vanished in 2009 to 2010 when dramatic clinical responses were observed with a novel BRAF inhibitor vemurafenib (PLX4032). Like sorafenib, this compound was optimized to inhibit RAF, but with an additional focus on mutant BRAF. Vemurafenib differs dramatically from sorafenib because it potently inhibits BRAF without the additional broad range of activities that sorafenib has against other kinases like the VEGF receptor.[43] The greater selectivity of vemurafenib relative to sorafenib resulted in a much greater tolerability, such that it could be given at high doses while avoiding significant toxicity. The early days of vemurafenib clinical development were plagued by challenges in maximizing the oral bioavailability of the drug.[44] Consequently, the initial phase I clinical trial was temporarily halted to develop a novel formulation (i.e., the coingredients in the drug capsule or tablet that improve solubility and absorption through the gastrointestinal tract). Much higher serum levels were obtained in patients who received the new vemurafenib formation and, shortly thereafter, complete and partial responses were observed in about 80% of the melanoma patients with B-RAF mutant tumors. Strikingly, no activity was observed in patients whose tumors were wild type for BRAF.[45,46] The data were so compelling that vemurafenib was immediately advanced to a phase III registration trial. Similarly impressive responses in BRAF mutant melanoma patients were observed with a second potent RAF inhibitor dabrafenib,[47] providing further proof that BRAF is a important cancer target.

The vemurafenib and dabrafenib data also provide insight into why sorafenib and the early MEK inhibitor trials failed to demonstrate activity. One lesson is the critical importance of achieving adequate target inhibition. Clinical responses with vemurafenib were observed only after the drug was reformulated to achieve substantially higher serum levels. Reductions in phospho-ERK staining (as documented by immunohistochemistry) were documented in the earlier trials but, in retrospect, the assays were not sensitive enough to distinguish between modest (~50%) kinase inhibition versus more complete BRAF or MEK inhibition. Efficacy in preclinical models is significantly improved using doses that give >80% inhibition, and the human trial data suggest that this degree of pathway blockade is also required for a high clinical response rate.[46] Collectively, these experiences illustrate the critical need for quantitative pharmacodynamic assays to measure target inhibition early in clinical development. A second lesson is the importance of genotyping all patients for mutation or amplification of the relevant drug target. Not only does this ensure that a sufficient number of patients with the biomarker of interest are included in the study, but also that the results provide compelling evidence early in clinical development in support (or not) of the preclinical hypothesis.

## Getting It Right: ALK and Lung Cancer

The development of the ALK inhibitor crizotinib (PF-02341066) illustrates how an unexpected signal obtained in a small number of patients can quickly shift a program in an entirely new direction with a high probability of success. The key ingredient in this story is a familiar one—a strong molecular hypothesis backed up by clinical response data in a small number of carefully selected patients. Crizotinib emerged from a drug discovery program at Pfizer that was focused on finding inhibitors of the MET receptor tyrosine kinase and entered the clinic with this target as its lead indication.[48] As we previously learned with imatinib, essentially all kinase inhibitors have activity against other targets (so called off-target activities), which can sometimes prove to be advantageous. Off-target activities are typically discovered by screening compounds against a large panel of kinases to establish profiles of relative selectivity against the intended target. Off-target activity, potency, and pharmaceutical properties (bioavailability, half-life) are all factors that influence the decision of which compound to advance to clinical development. The primary off-target activity of crizotinib is against the ALK tyrosine kinase.

ALK was first identified as a candidate driver oncogene in 1994 through the cloning of the t(2,5) chromosomal translocation associated with anaplastic large cell lymphoma, which creates the nucleophosmin/anaplastic lymphoma kinase (NPM-ALK) fusion gene.[49] This discovery, together with the demonstration that NPM-ALK causes lymphoma in mice, made a compelling case for ALK as a drug target in this disease. But there was limited interest in developing ALK inhibitors because this particular lymphoma subtype is rare and most commonly found in children. (Companies are generally reluctant to develop drugs solely for pediatric indications because of complexities related to dose selection and additional regulatory guidelines. Efforts to streamline this development process are underway, such as the Creating Hope Act, which provides new incentives for companies to pursue pediatric indications.) In

2007, a different ALK fusion gene called EML4-ALK was discovered in a small fraction of patients with lung adenocarcinoma, with an estimated frequency of 1% to 5%.[50] This discovery did not immediately capture the attention of drug developers, but several academic groups who had already begun testing lung cancer patients seen at their institutions for EGFR mutations simply added an EML4-ALK fusion test to the screening panel. Astute clinical investigators participating in the phase I trial of crizotinib, which was designed to include patients with a broad array of advanced cancers, were aware of the off-target ALK activity and enrolled several lung cancer patients with EML4-ALK fusions in the study. These patients had remarkably dramatic responses.[51] This serendipitous finding in a few ALK-positive patients was confirmed in a larger cohort, resulting in a strongly positive pivotal phase III study in ALK-positive lung cancer, just 2 years after the discovery of the EML4-ALK fusion.[52] Crizotinib is also being evaluated in other diseases associated with genomic alterations in ALK, including large-cell anaplastic lymphoma, neuroblastoma,[53] and inflammatory myofibroblastic sarcoma.[54]

## Extending the Model to RET Mutations in Thyroid Cancer: Clinical Responses, But Why?

Subsets of patients with papillary or medullary thyroid cancer have activating mutations or translocations targeting the RET tyrosine-kinase receptor, raising the question of whether RET inhibitors might have a role in this disease.[55] Although no drugs specifically designed to inhibit RET have entered the clinic, four compounds with off-target activity against RET (vandetanib, sorafenib, motesanib, and cabozantinib) have all shown single-agent activity in thyroid cancer studies.[56–60] Vandetanib and cabozantinib are currently approved in medullary thyroid cancer based on improved progression-free survival in phase III registration trials.[61,62] Because all four compounds also inhibit VEGF receptor, it is unclear whether the clinical benefit observed in these studies is explained by inhibition of RET, VEGF receptor, or both. Unlike the crizotinib trials in ALK-positive lung cancer, enrollment in these registration studies was not restricted to patients with RET mutations. In addition to the fact that thyroid cancer patients are not routinely screened for these mutations, the primary reason for including all comers in these studies is that clinical responses are observed in a larger fraction of patients than can be accounted for based on the suspected frequency of an RET mutation. Responses in patients without RET mutation (if they occur) might be explained by mutations in other genes in the RAS-MAP kinase pathway such as BRAF or HRAS, which are found in a substantial fraction of patients and typically do not overlap with RET alterations.[55] Clearly, detailed genotype/response correlations, as demonstrated in lung cancer and melanoma, will clarify the role of these mutations in predicting the response to these drugs. Thyroid cancer is also a compelling indication for the BRAF and MEK inhibitors discussed previously in melanoma.

## FLT3 Inhibitors in Acute Myeloid Leukemia: Did the Genomics Mislead Us?

Shortly after the success of imatinib, the receptor tyrosine–kinase FLT3 emerged as a compelling drug candidate based on the presence of activating mutations in about one-third of patients with acute myeloid leukemia.[63] Laboratory studies documented that FLT3 alleles bearing these mutations, which occur as internal tandem duplications (ITD) of the juxtamembrane domain or a point mutation in the kinase domain, function as driver oncogenes in mouse models, giving phenotypes analogous to BCR-ABL.[64] As with RET in thyroid cancer, no compounds had been specifically optimized to target FLT3, but several drugs with off-target FLT3 activity were redirected to acute myeloid leukemia (AML).

Disappointingly, the first three of the compounds tested (midostaurin, lestaurtinib, and sunitinib) showed only marginal single-agent activity in relapsed AML patients, even in those with FLT3 mutations.[65–67] Despite the strong molecular rationale for FLT3 as a driver lesion, questions were raised about the viability of FLT3 as a drug target. Pharmacodynamic studies showed evidence of FLT3 kinase inhibition in tumor cells, but the magnitude and duration of these effects were difficult to quantify, raising the possibility of inadequate target inhibition.[65] Indeed, the dose of all three compounds was limited by toxicities believed to be independent of FLT3. A more pessimistic interpretation was that FLT3, although presumably important for the initiation of AML, was no longer required for tumor maintenance due to the accumulation of additional driver genomic alterations. If true, even a complete FLT3 blockade with a highly selective inhibitor would be expected to fail. But this view was not supported by the fact that clinical responses were observed in the somewhat analogous situation of single-agent ABL kinase inhibitor treatment of CML in blast crisis, where BCR-ABL is just one of many additional genomic alterations that contribute to disease progression, yet complete remissions are observed in many patients.

Despite this pessimism about FLT3 as a viable drug target, several drugs are now advancing toward drug registration trials. Midostaurin, one of the early compounds that showed disappointing single-agent activity in relapsed AML, is being evaluated in a randomized phase III trial in newly diagnosed AML combined with standard induction chemotherapy. A single-arm phase II study showed higher and more durable remission rates in FLT3 mutant patients when compared to historical controls.[68] The second compound, quizartinib (AC220), is a next-generation FLT3 inhibitor with greater potency and specificity and with single-agent activity in FLT3 mutant relapsed AML—precisely the population where midostaurin and others failed.[69,70] The fact that some responder patients have relapsed with drug-resistant gatekeeper mutations in the FLT3 kinase domain provides formal proof that FLT3 is the relevant target.[71] Assuming these compounds prove successful in AML, it will be important to examine their activity in the rare cases of pediatric acute lymphoid leukemia associated with FLT3 mutation. Although the jury is still out on FLT3 inhibitors, the failure of early compounds in AML is reminiscent of the failures of early RAF and MEK inhibitors in melanoma. Collectively, these examples emphasize the importance of using optimized compounds to test a molecularly based hypothesis in patients and to focus enrollment on those patients with the relevant molecular lesion.

## Kidney Cancer: Targeting the Tumor and the Host With Mammalian Target of Rapamycin and VEGF Receptor Inhibitors

A recurring theme in this chapter is the critical role of driver kinase mutations in guiding the development of kinase inhibitors. Ironically, several kinase inhibitors have been approved for kidney cancer over the past 5 years in a tumor type with no known kinase mutations. The most common molecular alteration in kidney cancer is a loss of function in the Von Hippel-Lindau (VHL) tumor suppressor gene, resulting in the activation of the hypoxia inducible factor[68] pathway.[72] As a consequence of VHL loss, which normally targets hypoxia-inducible factor (HIF) proteins for proteasomal degradation, HIF-1α and HIF-2α are constitutively active transcription factors that function as oncogenes through activation of an array of downstream target genes. Among these is the angiogenesis factor VEGF, which is secreted by HIF-expressing cells and promotes the development and maintenance of tumor neovasculature. HIF-mediated secretion of VEGF by tumor cells likely explains the highly vascular histopathology of clear cell renal carcinoma. All three currently approved angiogenesis inhibitors (the monoclonal antibody bevacizumab targeting VEGF and the kinase inhibitors sorafenib and sunitinib targeting or its receptor

VEGF receptor) have single-agent clinical activity in clear cell carcinoma.[73–75] The high specificity of bevacizumab for VEGF leaves little doubt that the activity of this drug is explained by antiangiogenic effects. In contrast, the off-target activities of sorafenib and sunitinib include several kinases expressed in kidney tumor cells, stroma, and inflammatory cells (PDGFR, RAF, RET, FLT3, and others). Interestingly, the primary effect of bevacizumab in kidney cancer is disease stabilization, whereas sorafenib and sunitinib have substantial partial response rates. This raises the question of whether the superior antitumor activity of the VEGF receptor kinase inhibitors is due to the concurrent inhibition of other kinases. However, partial responses rates with next-generation VEGF receptor inhibitors (axitinib, pazopanib, and tivozanib), all of which have greater potency and selectivity for the VEGF receptor, are similarly high, and reinforce the importance of the VEGF receptor as the critical target in kidney cancer.[76–78] Pazopanib is approved for advanced kidney cancer, whereas axitinib is approved as second-line therapy.

Two inhibitors of the mammalian target of rapamycin (mTOR) kinase (temsirolimus and everolimus) are also approved for advanced renal cell carcinoma.[79,80] Both temsirolimus and everolimus are known as rapalogs because both are chemical derivatives of the natural product sirolimus (rapamycin). Sirolimus was approved more than 10 years ago to prevent graft rejection in transplant recipients based on its immunosuppressive properties against T cells. Sirolimus also has potent antiproliferative effects against vascular endothelial cells and, on that basis, is incorporated into drug-eluting cardiac stents to prevent coronary artery restenosis following angioplasty.[81] Rapalogs differ from all the other kinase inhibitors discussed in this chapter in that they inhibit the kinase through an allosteric mechanism rather than by targeting the mTOR kinase domain. Because rapalogs also inhibit the growth of cancer cell lines from different tissues of origin, clinical trials were initiated to study their potential role as anticancer agents in a broad range of tumor types. Based on responses in a few phase I patients with different tumor types (including kidney cancer), exploratory phase II studies were conducted in several diseases. Single-agent activity of temsirolimus was observed in a phase II kidney cancer study,[82] then confirmed in a phase III registration trial.[79] The phase III everolimus trial, which was initiated after temsirolimus, was noteworthy because clinical benefit was demonstrated in patients who had progressed on the VEGF receptor inhibitors sorafenib or sunitinib.[80]

In parallel with the empirical clinical development of rapalogs, various laboratories explored the molecular basis for mTOR dependence in cancer cells. mTOR functions at the center of a complex network that integrates signals from growth factor receptors and nutrient sensors to regulate cell growth and size (Fig. 22.2). It does so, in part, by controlling the translation of various mRNAs with complex 5′ untranslated regions into protein. mTOR exists in two distinct complexes known as TOR complex 1 (TORC1) and TORC2. Rapalogs only inhibit the TORC1 complex, which is largely responsible for downstream phosphorylation of targets such as S6K1/2 and 4EBP1/2 that regulate protein translation.[83] The TORC2 complex contributes to the activation of AKT by phosphorylating the important regulatory serine residue S473 and is unaffected by rapalogs.

Two hypotheses have emerged to explain the clinical activity of rapalogs in kidney cancer. The antiproliferative activity of these compounds against endothelial cells suggests an antiangiogenic mechanism, which is consistent with the clinical activity of the VEGF receptor inhibitors. But rapalogs also inhibit the growth of kidney cancer cell lines in laboratory models where the effects on tumor angiogenesis have been eliminated. Interestingly, mRNAs for HIF1/2 are among those whose translation is impaired by rapalogs, and this effect has been implicated as the primary mechanism of rapalog activity in kidney cancer xenograft models.[84] As with the VEGF receptor inhibitors, a detailed molecular annotation of tumors from responders and nonresponders will shed light on these issues.

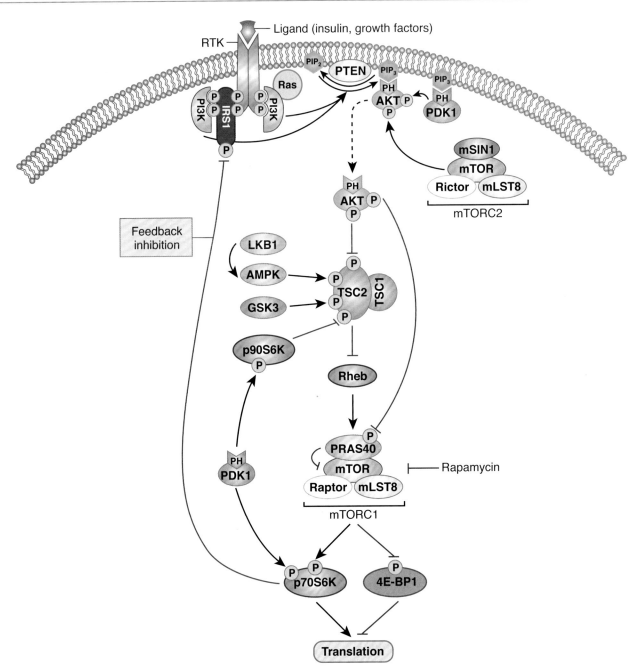

**Figure 22.2** Feedback inhibition of the phosphatidylinositol 3-kinase (PI3K) pathway. Activated AKT regulates cellular growth through mammalian target of rapamycin (mTOR), a key player in protein synthesis and translation. mTOR forms part of two distinct complexes known as mTORC1, which contains mTOR, Raptor, mLST8, and PRAS40, and mTORC2, which contains mTOR, Rictor, mLST8, and mSIN1. mTORC1 is sensitive to rapamycin and controls protein synthesis and translation, at least in part, through p70S6K and eukaryotic translation initiation factor 4E–binding protein 1 (4E-BP1). AKT phosphorylates and inhibits tuberous sclerosis complex 2 (TSC2), resulting in increased mTORC1 activity. AKT also phosphorylates PRAS40, thus relieving the PRAS40 inhibitory effect on mTOR and the mTORC1 complex. mTORC2 and 3-phosphoinositide–dependent kinase (PDK1) phosphorylate AKT on Ser473 and Thr308, respectively, rendering it fully active. mTORC1-activated p70S6K can phosphorylate insulin receptor substrate 1 (IRS1), resulting in inhibition of PI3K activity. In addition, PDK1 phosphorylates and activates p70S6K and p90S6K. The latter has been shown to inhibit TSC2 activity through direct phosphorylation. Conversely, LKB1-activated AMP-activated protein kinase (AMPK) and glycogen synthase kinase 3 (GSK3) activate the TSC1/TSC2 complex through direct phosphorylation of TSC2. Thus, signals through PI3K as well as through LKB1 and AMPK converge on mTORC1. Inhibition of mTORC1 can lead to increased insulin receptor–mediated signaling, and inhibition of PDK1 may lead to activation of mTORC1 and may, paradoxically, promote tumor growth. (From Daigle SR, Olhava EJ, Therkelsen CA, et al. Selective killing of mixed lineage leukemia cells by a potent small-molecule DOT1L inhibitor. *Cancer Cell* 2011;20(1):53–65, with permission.)

## Other Indications for mTOR Inhibitors: Breast Cancer and Tuberous Sclerosis Complex Mutant Cancers

Two other indications for mTOR have emerged, both based on fundamental insights from laboratory studies but from quite different angles. Preclinical studies of estrogen receptor (ER) therapy in breast cancer suggested that phosphatidylinositol 3-kinase (PI3K) pathway activation may be a mechanism of resistance and that this resistance could be prevented or overcome by combined treatment with ER-based drugs and rapalogs such as everolimus. Based on evidence that some women with progressive disease while receiving the aromatase inhibitor letrozole have clinical benefit from the addition of everolimus, randomized trials were initiated comparing everolimus + exemestane to exemestane alone (called BO-LERO-2), or everolimus + tamoxifen to tamoxifen alone (called TAMRAD). Both studies demonstrated substantial improvements in time to progression in women with metastatic breast cancer who had already failed one aromatase inhibitor,[85,86] resulting in FDA approval of the everolimus/exemestane combination. Evidence of cross-talk between the PI3K pathway and hormone receptor signaling (ER in breast cancer, androgen receptor in prostate cancer) provides a molecular rationale for the clinical benefit of combination therapy and is currently under investigation in metastatic prostate cancer.[87]

Yet another indication for rapalog therapy emerged from the genetics of children with tuberous sclerosis caused by a loss of function mutations in tuberous sclerosis complex 1 (TSC1) or TSC2, which encode the proteins hamartin and tuberin that function in the PI3K signaling pathway just upstream of mTOR. Based on laboratory studies showing that TSC1- or TSC2-deficient cells are exquisitely sensitive to rapalogs, a clinical trial was conducted in tuberous sclerosis patients with benign subependymal giant-cell astrocytomas (SEGA) that showed tumor shrinkage in 21 of 28 patients.[88] This genetic dependence on mTOR in tumors with tuberous sclerosis complex (TSC) loss has also been observed in bladder cancer. In a remarkable example of the power of comprehensive DNA sequencing to provide insight into rare clinical phenotypes, investigators examined the tumor genome of the single complete responder patient on a phase II trial of everolimus in bladder cancer and discovered somatic mutations in TSC2 as well as a second gene, NF2, that also controls mTOR activity.[89] This plus other examples of how a retrospective genomic analysis of *extraordinary responders* has led to a national effort to capture these cases, as well as prospective clinical trials of patients with the relevant tumor genotype regardless of histology (called *basket* trials).

It is unclear why rapalogs have failed in other tumor types. One explanation is the concurrence of PI3K pathway mutations with alterations in other pathways that mitigate sensitivity to rapalogs. Another possibility is the disruption of negative feedback loops regulated by mTOR that inhibit signaling from upstream receptor tyrosine kinases. Rapalogs paradoxically *increase* signaling through PI3K due to loss of this negative feedback. A primary consequence is *increased* AKT activation, which signals to an array of downstream substrates that can enhance cell proliferation and survival (other than TORC1, which remains inhibited by rapalog) (see Fig. 22.2). This problem might be overcome by combining rapalogs with an inhibitor of an upstream kinase in the feedback loop, such as HER kinases or the insulinlike growth factor receptor (IGFR), to block this undesired effect of rapalogs on PI3K activation.[90]

## DIRECTLY TARGETING THE PI3K PATHWAY

Mutations or copy number alterations (e.g., amplification or deletion of oncogenes or tumor suppressor genes) in PI3K pathway genes (PIK3CA, PIK3R1, PTEN, AKT1, and others) are among the most common abnormalities in cancer. Consequently, intensive efforts at many pharmaceutical companies have been devoted to the discovery of small-molecule inhibitors targeting kinases in the PI3K pathway. Inhibitors of PI3K, AKT, and ATP-competitive (rather than allosteric) inhibitors of mTOR that target both the TORC1 and TORC2 complex are all in clinical development. Phase I clinical trials have, in general, established that the pathway can be efficiently targeted without serious toxicity other than easily manageable effects on glucose metabolism (which is anticipated based on the importance of PI3K signaling in insulin signaling). Unfortunately, there has been no evidence to date of dramatic single-agent clinical activity with any of these agents, although early results with PI3K alpha selective inhibitor BYL719 in PIK3CA mutant breast cancer appear promising.[91]

However, the first approval of a direct PI3K inhibitor in cancer is likely to come in chronic lymphocytic leukemia and in lymphoma, but not on the basis of tumor genomics. Normal and malignant B cells are dependent on PI3K delta as well as Bruton tyrosine kinase (BTK) for proliferation and survival, raising the possibility that inhibitors of these kinases might be broadly active in B-cell malignancies. Concerns about toxicity to normal B cells were alleviated, in part, by the earlier clinical success of the CD20 antibody rituximab in lymphoma, which also eliminates normal circulating B cells, but without significant clinical sequelae. The first such PI3K delta inhibitor, idelalisib, has shown impressive activity in indolent non-Hodgkin lymphoma as a single agent and in relapsed chronic lymphocytic leukemia when given in combination with rituximab. The BTK inhibitor ibrutinib, following a similar clinical development path, was recently approved as second-line therapy for chronic lymphocytic leukemia and for mantle cell lymphoma.[92,93]

## COMBINATIONS OF KINASE INHIBITORS TO INDUCT RESPONSE AND PREVENT RESISTANCE

Preclinical studies indicate that combinations of kinase inhibitors are required to realize their full potential as anticancer agents. The most common rationale is to address the problem of concurrent mutations in different pathways that alleviate dependence on a single-driver oncogene. The best examples are cancers with mutations in both the RAS/MAP kinase pathway (RAS or BRAF) and the PI3K pathway (PIK3CA or PTEN). In mouse models, such doubly mutant tumors fail to respond to single-agent treatment with either an AKT inhibitor or a MEK inhibitor. However, combination treatment can give dramatic regressions.[94] Similarly, genetically engineered mice that develop KRAS-driven lung cancer respond only to combination therapy with a PI3K inhibitor and a MEK inhibitor.[95] To date, clinical trials combining different PI3K pathway and RAS/MAP kinase pathway inhibitors have been challenging due to toxicities associated with continuous, concurrent PI3K and RAS/MAP kinase pathway inhibition.

Many of the tumor types discussed in this chapter *do* respond to treatment with a single-agent kinase, but relapse despite continued inhibitor therapy. Research into the causes of "acquired" kinase inhibitor resistance has revealed two primary mechanisms: (1) novel mutations in the kinase domain of the drug target that preclude inhibition, or (2) *bypass* of the driver kinase signal by activation of a parallel kinase pathway. In both cases, the solution is combination therapy to prevent the emergence of resistance. An elegant demonstration of this approach comes from CML where resistance to imatinib is primarily caused by mutations in the BCR-ABL kinase domain.[96,97] The second-generation ABL inhibitors dasatinib and nilotinib are effective against most imatinib-resistant BCR-ABL mutants and were initially approved as single-agent therapy for imatinib-resistant CML.[98,99] Very recently, both drugs have proven superior to imatinib in the upfront treatment of CML due to increased potency and fewer mechanisms of acquired resistance.[100–102] However, one BCR-ABL mutation called T315I is resistant to all three drugs. The third-generation ABL kinase inhibitor ponatinib blocks T315I and showed activity in a phase II clinical trial that included CML patients with the T315I mutation,[103] resulting in FDA approval. However, subsequent reports of severe vascular occlusive events, such as stroke and heart failure, led to withdrawal from the market, followed by approval for restricted use in T315I-mutant patients. Analogous approaches are ongoing in other diseases such as EGFR-mutant lung cancer, where acquired resistance to the frontline kinase inhibitor is also associated with mutations in the target kinase.[104,105] Promising clinical results have been reported with irreversible EGFR inhibitors such as CO-1686 and AZD9291.

The clinical development of kinase inhibitor combinations to prevent acquired resistance is relatively straightforward. Because the frontline drug is already approved, success would be determined by an improvement in response duration using the combination. The situation is more complex when two experimental compounds (e.g., a PI3K pathway inhibitor and a MEK inhibitor) are combined, neither of which shows significant single-agent activity. Older regulatory guidelines required a four-arm study that compared each single agent to the combination and to a control group in order to obtain approval of the combination. Recognizing that this design could discourage drug developers as well as patients from moving forward because it requires a large sample size, the FDA has issued new guidelines for the development of novel combinations that require a two-arm registration study comparing the combination to standard of care http://www.fda.gov/downloads/Drugs/GuidanceComplianceRegulatory Information/Guidances/UCM236669.pdf. A more challenging issue may be dose optimization and dose schedule that is needed to safely combine two investigational drugs. Much like the development of combination chemotherapy several decades ago, it may be important to select compounds with nonoverlapping toxicities to allow for sufficient doses of each drug to be achieved.

## SPECULATIONS ON THE FUTURE ROLE OF KINASE INHIBITORS IN CANCER MEDICINE

The role of genomics in predicting a response to kinase inhibitor therapy is now irrefutable. As the number of kinase driver mutations continues to grow, the field is likely to move away from the current strategy of a *companion diagnostic* for each drug. Rather, comprehensive mutational profiling platforms that query each tumor for hundreds of potential cancer mutations are more likely to emerge as the diagnostic platform. The number of directly *actionable* mutations (meaning the presence of a mutation defines a treatment decision supported by clinical trial data) remains low, but this number will undoubtedly grow. In addition, it is becoming apparent that many patients have rare mutations (defined as rare in that histologic tumor type) but are, in theory, actionable. Because these examples are unlikely to be formally evaluated in clinical trials, many centers have opened *basket* studies (with eligibility based solely on mutation profile) to capture these cases with some reports of remarkable success.

More effort must be devoted to manipulating the dose and schedule of kinase inhibitor therapy to maximize efficacy and minimize toxicity. To date, all kinase inhibitors have been developed based on the assumption that a 24/7 coverage of the target is required for efficacy. Consequently, most compounds are optimized to have a long serum half-life (12 to 24 hours). Phase II doses are then selected based on the maximum tolerated dose determined with daily administration. But a recent clinical of the ABL inhibitor dasatinib in CML indicates that equivalent antitumor activity can be achieved with intermittent therapy.[106] By giving larger doses intermittently, higher peak drug concentrations were achieved that resulted in equivalent and possibly superior efficacy.[107] Similar results were observed in laboratory studies of EGFR inhibitors in EGFR-mutant lung cancer. Clinically robust, quantitative assays of target inhibition are needed to hasten progress in this area.

Although the focus of this chapter is kinase inhibitors, the themes developed here should apply broadly to inhibitors of other cancer targets. Inhibitors of the G-protein coupled receptor smoothened (SMO) in patients with metastatic basal cell carcinoma or medulloblastoma establish that the driver mutation hypothesis extends beyond kinase inhibitors. SMO is a component in the Hedgehog pathway, which is constitutively activated in subsets of patients with basal cell carcinoma and medulloblastoma due to mutations in the Hedgehog ligand-binding receptor Patched-1. Treatment with the SMO inhibitor vismodegib led to impressive responses in basal cell carcinoma and medulloblastoma patients whose tumors had Patched-1 mutations,[108,109] resulting in FDA approval. Other novel cancer targets are emerging from cancer genome sequencing projects. Somatic mutations in the Krebs cycle enzyme isocitrate dehydrogenase (IDH1/2) were found in subsets of patients with glioblastoma, AML, chondrosarcoma, and cholangiocarcinoma,[110–112] and the first IDH2 inhibitor has entered clinical trials in leukemia. Mutations in enzymes involved in chromatin remodeling, such as the histone methyltransferase EZH2, have been reported in lymphoma and have spurred the ongoing development of EZH2 inhibitors.[113,114] Inhibitors of another histone methyltransferase DOT1L, which is required for the maintenance of mixed lineage leukemia (MLL) fusion leukemias, are also in clinical development.[115,116] Kinase inhibitors are just the first wave of molecularly targeted drugs ushered in by our understanding of the molecular underpinnings of cancer cells. There is much more to follow.

## REFERENCES

1. Sawyers CL. Shifting paradigms: the seeds of oncogene addiction. *Nat Med* 2009;15(10):1158–1161.
2. Weinstein IB. Cancer. Addiction to oncogenes—the Achilles heal of cancer. *Science* 2002;297(5578):63–64.
3. Druker BJ, Talpaz M, Resta DJ, et al., Efficacy and safety of a specific inhibitor of the BCR-ABL tyrosine kinase in chronic myeloid leukemia. *N Engl J Med* 2001;344(14):1031–1037.
4. Hirota S, Isozaki K, Moriyama Y, et al. Gain-of-function mutations of c-kit in human gastrointestinal stromal tumors. *Science* 1998;279(5350):577–580.
5. Heinrich MC, Corless CL, Duensing A, et al. PDGFRA activating mutations in gastrointestinal stromal tumors. *Science* 2003;299(5607):708–710.
6. Demetri GD, von Mehren M, Blanke CD, et al. Efficacy and safety of imatinib mesylate in advanced gastrointestinal stromal tumors. *N Engl J Med* 2002;347(7):472–480.
7. Geyer CE, Forster J, Lindquist D, et al. Lapatinib plus capecitabine for HER2-positive advanced breast cancer. *N Engl J Med* 2006;355(26):2733–2743.
8. Kris MG, Natale RB, Herbst RS, et al. Efficacy of gefitinib, an inhibitor of the epidermal growth factor receptor tyrosine kinase, in symptomatic patients with non-small cell lung cancer: a randomized trial. *JAMA* 2003;290(16): 2149–2158.
9. Miller VA, Kris MG, Shah N, et al. Bronchioloalveolar pathologic subtype and smoking history predict sensitivity to gefitinib in advanced non-small-cell lung cancer. *J Clin Oncol* 2004;22(6):1103–1109.
10. Paez JG, Jänne PA, Lee JC, et al. EGFR mutations in lung cancer: correlation with clinical response to gefitinib therapy. *Science* 2004;304(5676):1497–1500.
11. Lynch TJ, Bell DW, Sordella R, et al. Activating mutations in the epidermal growth factor receptor underlying responsiveness of non-small-cell lung cancer to gefitinib. *N Engl J Med* 2004;350(21):2129–2139.
12. Pao W, Miller V, Zakowski M, et al. EGF receptor gene mutations are common in lung cancers from "never smokers" and are associated with sensitivity of tumors to gefitinib and erlotinib. *Proc Natl Acad Sci U S A* 2004;101(36): 13306–13311.
13. Cohen MH, Wlilliams GA, Sridhara R, et al. FDA drug approval summary: gefitinib (ZD1839) (Iressa) tablets. *Oncologist* 2003;8(4):303–306.
14. Shepherd FA, Rodrigues Pereira J, Ciuleanu T, et al. Erlotinib in previously treated non-small-cell lung cancer. *N Engl J Med* 2005;353(2):123–132.

15. Thatcher N, Chang A, Parikh P, et al. Gefitinib plus best supportive care in previously treated patients with refractory advanced non-small-cell lung cancer: results from a randomised, placebo-controlled, multicentre study (Iressa Survival Evaluation in Lung Cancer). *Lancet* 2005;366(9496):1527–1537.

16. Herbst RS, Giaccone G, Schiller JH, et al. Gefitinib in combination with paclitaxel and carboplatin in advanced non-small cell lung cancer: a phase III trial—INTACT 2. *J Clin Oncol* 2004;22(5):785–794.

17. Giaccone G, Herbst RS, Manegold C, et al. Gefitinib in combination with gemcitabine and cisplatin in advanced non-small-cell lung cancer: a phase III trial—INTACT 1. *J Clin Oncol* 2004;22(5):777–784.

18. Herbst RS, Prager D, Hermann R, et al. TRIBUTE: a phase III trial of erlotinib hydrochloride (OSI-774) combined with carboplatin and paclitaxel chemotherapy in advanced non-small-cell lung cancer. *J Clin Oncol* 2005;23(25):5892–5899.

19. Tsao MS, Sakurada A, Cutz JC, et al. Erlotinib in lung cancer - molecular and clinical predictors of outcome. *N Engl J Med* 2005;353(2):133–144.

20. Mok TS, Wu YL, Thongprasert S, et al. Gefitinib or carboplatin-paclitaxel in pulmonary adenocarcinoma. *N Engl J Med* 2009;361(10):947–957.

21. Schaller JL, Burkland GA. Case report: rapid and complete control of idiopathic hypereosinophilia with imatinib mesylate. *MedGenMed* 2001;3(5):9.

22. Ault P, Cortes J, Koller C, et al. Response of idiopathic hypereosinophilic syndrome to treatment with imatinib mesylate. *Leuk Res* 2002;26(9):881–884.

23. Cools J, DeAngelo DJ, Gotlib J, et al. A tyrosine kinase created by fusion of the PDGFRA and FIP1L1 genes as a therapeutic target of imatinib in idiopathic hypereosinophilic syndrome. *N Engl J Med* 2003;348(13):1201–1214.

24. Golub TR, Barker GF, Lovett M, et al. Fusion of PDGF receptor beta to a novel ets-like gene, tel, in chronic myelomonocytic leukemia with t(5;12) chromosomal translocation. *Cell* 1994;77(2):307–316.

25. Apperley JF, Gardembas M, Melo JV, et al. Response to imatinib mesylate in patients with chronic myeloproliferative diseases with rearrangements of the platelet-derived growth factor receptor beta. *N Engl J Med* 2002;347(7):481–487.

26. Rutkowski P, Van Glabbeke M, Rankin CJ, et al. Imatinib mesylate in advanced dermatofibrosarcoma protuberans: pooled analysis of two phase II clinical trials. *J Clin Oncol* 2010;28(10):1772–1779.

27. Davies H, Bignell GR, Cox C, et al. Mutations of the BRAF gene in human cancer. *Nature* 2002;417(6892):949–954.

28. Baxter EJ, Scott LM, Campbell PJ, et al., Acquired mutation of the tyrosine kinase JAK2 in human myeloproliferative disorders. *Lancet* 2005;365(9464):1054–1061.

29. James C, Ugo V, Le Couédic JP, et al. A unique clonal JAK2 mutation leading to constitutive signalling causes polycythaemia vera. *Nature* 2005;434(7037):1144–1148.

30. Levine RL, Wadleigh M, Cools J, et al. Activating mutation in the tyrosine kinase JAK2 in polycythemia vera, essential thrombocythemia, and myeloid metaplasia with myelofibrosis. *Cancer Cell* 2005;7(4):387–397.

31. Samuels Y, Wang Z, Bardellli A, et al. High frequency of mutations of the PIK3CA gene in human cancers. *Science* 2004;304(5670):554.

32. International Cancer Genome Consortium, Hudson TJ, Anderson W, et al. International network of cancer genome projects. *Nature* 2010;464(7291):993–998.

33. Vogelstein B, Papadopoulos N, Velculescu VE, et al. Cancer genome landscapes. *Science* 2013;339(6127):1546–1558.

34. Lawrence MS, Stojanov P, Mermel CH, et al. Discovery and saturation analysis of cancer genes across 21 tumour types. *Nature* 2014;505(7484):495–501.

35. Eisen T, Ahmad T, Flaherty KT, et al. Sorafenib in advanced melanoma: a Phase II randomised discontinuation trial analysis. *Br J Cancer* 2006;95(5):581–586.

36. Solit DB, Garraway LA, Pratilas CA, et al. BRAF mutation predicts sensitivity to MEK inhibition. *Nature* 2006;439(7074):358–362.

37. McDermott U, Sharma SV, Dowell L, et al. Identification of genotype-correlated sensitivity to selective kinase inhibitors by using high-throughput tumor cell line profiling. *Proc Natl Acad Sci U S A* 2007;104(50):19936–19941.

38. Pratilas CA, Taylor BS, Ye Q, et al. (V600E)BRAF is associated with disabled feedback inhibition of RAF-MEK signaling and elevated transcriptional output of the pathway. *Proc Natl Acad Sci U S A* 2009;106(11):4519–4524.

39. LoRusso PM, Krishnamurthi SS, Rinehart JJ, et al. Phase I pharmacokinetic and pharmacodynamic study of the oral MAPK/ERK kinase inhibitor PD-0325901 in patients with advanced cancers. *Clin Cancer Res* 2010;16(6):1924–1937.

40. Adjei AA, Cohen RB, Franklin W, et al. Phase I pharmacokinetic and pharmacodynamic study of the oral, small-molecule mitogen-activated protein kinase kinase 1/2 inhibitor AZD6244 (ARRY-142886) in patients with advanced cancers. *J Clin Oncol* 2008;26(13):2139–2146.

41. Dummer R, Chapman PB, Sosman JA, et al. AZD6244 (ARRY-142886) vs temozolomide (TMZ) in patients (pts) with advanced melanoma: An open-label, randomized, multicenter, phase II study. *J Clin Oncol* 2008;26(May 20 suppl):9033.

42. Flaherty KT, Robert C, Hersey P, et al. Improved survival with MEK inhibition in BRAF-mutated melanoma. *N Engl J Med* 2012;367(2):107–114.

43. Joseph EW, Pratilas CA, Poulikakos PI, et al. The RAF inhibitor PLX4032 inhibits ERK signaling and tumor cell proliferation in a V600E BRAF-selective manner. *Proc Natl Acad Sci U S A* 2010;107(33):14903–14908.

44. Flaherty K, Puzanov I, Sosman J, et al. Phase I study of PLX4032: proof of concept for V600E BRAF mutation as a therapeutic target in human cancer. *J Clin Oncol* 2009;27(15s):abstract 9000.

45. Flaherty KT, Puzanov I, Kim KB, et al. Inhibition of mutated, activated BRAF in metastatic melanoma. *N Engl J Med* 2010;363(9):809–819.

46. Bollag G, Hirth P, Tsai J, et al. Clinical efficacy of a RAF inhibitor needs broad target blockade in BRAF-mutant melanoma. *Nature* 2010;467(7315):596–599.

47. Hauschild A, Grob JJ, Demidov LV, et al. Dabrafenib in BRAF-mutated metastatic melanoma: a multicentre, open-label, phase 3 randomised controlled trial. *Lancet* 2012;380(9839):358–365.

48. Kwak EL, Camidge DR, Clark J, et al. Clinical activity observed in a phase I dose escalation trial of an oral c-MET and ALK inhibitor, PF-02341066. *J Clin Oncol* 2009;27(Suppl):148s.

49. Morris SW, Kirstein MN, Valentine MB, et al. Fusion of a kinase gene, ALK, to a nucleolar protein gene, NPM, in non-Hodgkin's lymphoma. *Science* 1994;263(5151):1281–1284.

50. Soda M, Choi YL, Enomoto M, et al. Identification of the transforming EML4-ALK fusion gene in non-small-cell lung cancer. *Nature* 2007;448(7153):561–566.

51. Bang Y, Kwak EL, Shaw AT, et al. Clinical activity of the oral ALK inhibitor PF-02341066 in ALK-positive patients with non-small cell lung cancer (NSCLC). *J Clin Oncol* 2010;28:18s.

52. Shaw AT, Kim DW, Nakagawa K, et al. Crizotinib versus chemotherapy in advanced ALK-positive lung cancer. *N Engl J Med* 2013;368(25):2385–2394.

53. Chen Y, Takita J, Choi YL, et al. Oncogenic mutations of ALK kinase in neuroblastoma. *Nature* 2008;455(7215):971–974.

54. Sirvent N, Hawkins AL, Moeglin D, et al. ALK probe rearrangement in a t(2;11;2)(p23;p15;q31) translocation found in a prenatal myofibroblastic fibrous lesion: toward a molecular definition of an inflammatory myofibroblastic tumor family? *Genes Chromosomes Cancer* 2001;31(1):85–90.

55. Fagin JA, Mitsiades N. Molecular pathology of thyroid cancer: diagnostic and clinical implications. *Best Pract Res Clin Endocrinol Metab* 2008;22(6):955–969.

56. Wells SA Jr, Gosnell JE, Gagel RF, et al. Vandetanib for the treatment of patients with locally advanced or metastatic hereditary medullary thyroid cancer. *J Clin Oncol* 28(5):767–772.

57. Lam ET, Ringel MD, Kloos RT, et al. Phase II clinical trial of sorafenib in metastatic medullary thyroid cancer. *J Clin Oncol* 28(14):2323–2330.

58. Kloos RT, Ringel MD, Knopp MV, et al. Phase II trial of sorafenib in metastatic thyroid cancer. *J Clin Oncol* 2009;27(10):1675–1684.

59. Schlumberger MJ, Elisei R, Bastholt L, et al. Phase II study of safety and efficacy of motesanib in patients with progressive or symptomatic, advanced or metastatic medullary thyroid cancer. *J Clin Oncol* 2009;27(23):3794–3801.

60. Kurzrock R, Cohen EE, Sherman SI, et al. Long-term results in a cohort of medullary thyroid cancer (MTC) patients (pts) in a phase I study of XL184 (BMS 907351), an oral inhibitor of MET, VEGFR2, and RET. *J Clin Oncol* 2010;28(Suppl):15s.

61. Wells SA Jr, Robinson BG, Gagel RF, et al. Vandetanib in patients with locally advanced or metastatic medullary thyroid cancer: a randomized, double-blind phase III trial. *J Clin Oncol* 2012;30(2):134–141.

62. Elisei R, Schlumberger MJ, Müller SP, et al. Cabozantinib in progressive medullary thyroid cancer. *J Clin Oncol* 2013;31(29):3639–3646.

63. Sawyers CL. Finding the next Gleevec: FLT3 targeted kinase inhibitor therapy for acute myeloid leukemia. *Cancer Cell* 2002;1(5):413–415.

64. Kelly LM, Qing L, Jeffery L, et al. FLT3 internal tandem duplication mutations associated with human acute myeloid leukemias induce myeloproliferative disease in a murine bone marrow transplant model. *Blood* 2002;99(1):310–318.

65. Stone RM, DeAngelo DJ, Klimek V, et al. Patients with acute myeloid leukemia and an activating mutation in FLT3 respond to a small-molecule FLT3 tyrosine kinase inhibitor, PKC412. *Blood* 2005;105(1):54–60.

66. Knapper S, Burnett AK, Littlewood T, et al. A phase 2 trial of the FLT3 inhibitor lestaurtinib (CEP701) as first-line treatment for older patients with acute myeloid leukemia not considered fit for intensive chemotherapy. *Blood* 2006;108(10):3262–3270.

67. Fiedler W, Serve H, Döhner H, et al. A phase 1 study of SU11248 in the treatment of patients with refractory or resistant acute myeloid leukemia (AML) or not amenable to conventional therapy for the disease. *Blood* 2005;105(3):986–993.

68. Stone RM, Fischer T, Paquette R, et al. A Phase 1b study of midostaurin (PKC412) in combination with daunorubicin and cytarabine induction and high-dose cytarabine consolidation in patients under age 61 with newly diagnosed de novo acute myeloid leukemia: overall survival of patients whose blasts have FLT3 mutations is similar to those with wild-type FLT3. Paper presented at: 2009 American Society of Hematology Annual Meeting; 2009; New Orleans, LA.

69. Zarrinkar PP, Gunawardane RN, Cramer MD, et al. AC220 is a uniquely potent and selective inhibitor of FLT3 for the treatment of acute myeloid leukemia (AML). *Blood* 2009;114(14):2984–2992.

70. Cortes J, et al. AC220, a potent, selective, second generation FLT3 receptor tyrosine kinase (RTK) inhibitor, in a first-in-human (FIH) phase 1 AML study. Paper presented at: 2009 American Society of Hematology Annual Meeting; 2009; New Orleans, LA.

71. Smith CC, Wang Q, Chin CS, et al. Validation of ITD mutations in FLT3 as a therapeutic target in human acute myeloid leukaemia. *Nature* 2012;485(7397):260–263.

72. Kaelin WG Jr. The von Hippel-Lindau tumour suppressor protein: O2 sensing and cancer. *Nat Rev Cancer* 2008;8(11):865–873.

73. Yang JC, Haworth L, Sherry RM, et al. A randomized trial of bevacizumab, an anti-vascular endothelial growth factor antibody, for metastatic renal cancer. *N Engl J Med* 2003;349(5):427–434.

**CANCER THERAPEUTICS**

74. Escudier B, Eisen T, Stadler WM, et al. Sorafenib in advanced clear-cell renal-cell carcinoma. *N Engl J Med* 2007;356(2):125–134.

75. Motzer RJ, Hutson TE, Tomczak P, et al. Sunitinib versus interferon alfa in metastatic renal-cell carcinoma. *N Engl J Med* 2007;356(2):115–124.

76. Rini BI, Wilding G, Hudes G, et al. Phase II study of axitinib in sorafenib-refractory metastatic renal cell carcinoma. *J Clin Oncol* 2009;27(27):4462–4468.

77. Sonpavde G, Hutson TE, Sternberg CN. Pazopanib, a potent orally administered small-molecule multitargeted tyrosine kinase inhibitor for renal cell carcinoma. *Expert Opin Investig Drugs* 2008;17(2):253–261.

78. Bhargava P, Esteves B, Al-Adhami M, et al. Activity of tivozanib (AV-951) in patients with renal cell carcinoma (RCC): Subgroup analysis from a phase II randomized discontinuation trial (RDT). *J Clin Oncol* 2010;28(suppl):15s.

79. Hudes G, Carducci M, Tomczak P, et al. Temsirolimus, interferon alfa, or both for advanced renal-cell carcinoma. *N Engl J Med* 2007;356(22):2271–2281.

80. Motzer RJ, Escudier B, Oudard S, et al. Efficacy of everolimus in advanced renal cell carcinoma: a double-blind, randomised, placebo-controlled phase III trial. *Lancet* 2008;372(9637):449–456.

81. McKeage K, Murdoch D, Goa FL. The sirolimus-eluting stent: a review of its use in the treatment of coronary artery disease. *Am J Cardiovasc Drugs* 2003;3(3):211–230.

82. Atkins MB, Hidalgo M, Stadler WM, et al. Randomized phase II study of multiple dose levels of CCI-779, a novel mammalian target of rapamycin kinase inhibitor, in patients with advanced refractory renal cell carcinoma. *J Clin Oncol* 2004;22(5):909–918.

83. Guertin DA, Sabatini DM. Defining the role of mTOR in cancer. *Cancer Cell* 2007;12(1):9–22.

84. Thomas GV, Tran C, Mellinghoff IK, et al. Hypoxia-inducible factor determines sensitivity to inhibitors of mTOR in kidney cancer. *Nat Med* 2006;12(1):122–127.

85. Bachelot T, Bourgier C, Cropet C, et al. Randomized phase II trial of everolimus in combination with tamoxifen in patients with hormone receptor-positive, human epidermal growth factor receptor 2-negative metastatic breast cancer with prior exposure to aromatase inhibitors: a GINECO study. *J Clin Oncol* 2012;30(22):2718–2724.

86. Baselga J, Campone M, Piccart M, et al. Everolimus in postmenopausal hormone-receptor-positive advanced breast cancer. *N Engl J Med* 2012;366(6):520–529.

87. Carver BS, Chapinski C, Wongvipat J, et al. Reciprocal feedback regulation of PI3K and androgen receptor signaling in PTEN-deficient prostate cancer. *Cancer Cell* 2011;19(5):575–586.

88. Krueger DA, Care MM, Holland K, et al. Everolimus for subependymal giant-cell astrocytomas in tuberous sclerosis. *N Engl J Med* 2010;363(19):1801–1811.

89. Iyer G, Hanrahan AL, Milowsky MI, et al. Genome sequencing identifies a basis for everolimus sensitivity. *Science* 2012;338(6104):221.

90. O'Reilly KE, Rojo F, She QB, et al. mTOR inhibition induces upstream receptor tyrosine kinase signaling and activates Akt. *Cancer Res* 2006;66(3):1500–1508.

91. Gonzalez-Angulo AM, Juric D, Argilis G, et al. Safety, pharmacokinetics, and preliminary activity of the alpha-specific PI3K inhibitor BYL719: results from the first-in-human study. *J Clin Oncol* 2013;31(15 Suppl):2531.

92. Byrd JC, Furman RR, Coutre SE, et al. Targeting BTK with ibrutinib in relapsed chronic lymphocytic leukemia. *N Engl J Med* 2013;369(1):32–42.

93. Wang ML, Rule S, Martin P, et al. Targeting BTK with ibrutinib in relapsed or refractory mantle-cell lymphoma. *N Engl J Med* 2013;369(6):507–516.

94. She QB, Halilovic E, Ye Q, et al. 4E-BP1 is a key effector of the oncogenic activation of the AKT and ERK signaling pathways that integrates their function in tumors. *Cancer Cell* 18(1):39–51.

95. Engelman JA, Chen L, Tan X, et al. Effective use of PI3K and MEK inhibitors to treat mutant Kras G12D and PIK3CA H1047R murine lung cancers. *Nat Med* 2008;14(12):1351–1356.

96. Gorre ME, Mohammed M, Ellwood K, et al. Clinical resistance to STI-571 cancer therapy caused by BCR-ABL gene mutation or amplification. *Science* 2001;293(5531):876–880.

97. Shah NP, Nicoll JM, Nagar B, et al. Multiple BCR-ABL kinase domain mutations confer polyclonal resistance to the tyrosine kinase inhibitor imatinib (STI571) in chronic phase and blast crisis chronic myeloid leukemia. *Cancer Cell* 2002;2(2):117–125.

98. Shah NP, Tran C, Lee FY, et al. Overriding imatinib resistance with a novel ABL kinase inhibitor. *Science* 2004;305(5682):399–401.

99. Talpaz M, Shah NP, Kantarjian H, et al. Dasatinib in imatinib-resistant Philadelphia chromosome-positive leukemias. *N Engl J Med* 2006;354(24):2531–2541.

100. Kantarjian H, Shah NP, Hochhaus A, et al. Dasatinib versus imatinib in newly diagnosed chronic-phase chronic myeloid leukemia. *N Engl J Med* 2010;362(24):2260–2270.

101. Sawyers CL. Even better kinase inhibitors for chronic myeloid leukemia. *N Engl J Med* 2010;362(24):2314–2315.

102. Saglio G, Kim DW, Issaragrisil S, et al. Nilotinib versus imatinib for newly diagnosed chronic myeloid leukemia. *N Engl J Med* 362(24):2251–2259.

103. Cortes JE, Kim DW, Pinilla-Ibarz J, et al. A phase 2 trial of ponatinib in Philadelphia chromosome-positive leukemias. *N Engl J Med* 2013;369(19):1783–1796.

104. Pao W, Miller VA, Politi KA, et al. Acquired resistance of lung adenocarcinomas to gefitinib or erlotinib is associated with a second mutation in the EGFR kinase domain. *PLoS Med* 2005;2(3):e73.

105. Antonescu CR, Besmer P, Guo T, et al. Acquired resistance to imatinib in gastrointestinal stromal tumor occurs through secondary gene mutation. *Clin Cancer Res* 2005;11(11):4182–4190.

106. Shah NP, Kantarjian HM, Kim DW, et al. Intermittent target inhibition with dasatinib 100 mg once daily preserves efficacy and improves tolerability in imatinib-resistant and -intolerant chronic-phase chronic myeloid leukemia. *J Clin Oncol* 2008;26(19):3204–3212.

107. Shah NP, Kasap C, Weier C, et al. Transient potent BCR-ABL inhibition is sufficient to commit chronic myeloid leukemia cells irreversibly to apoptosis. *Cancer Cell* 2008;14(6):485–493.

108. Von Hoff DD, LoRusso PM, Rudin CM, et al. Inhibition of the hedgehog pathway in advanced basal-cell carcinoma. *N Engl J Med* 2009;361(12):1164–1172.

109. Rudin CM, Hann CL, Laterra J, et al. Treatment of medulloblastoma with hedgehog pathway inhibitor GDC-0449. *N Engl J Med* 2009;361(12):1173–1178.

110. Parsons DW, Jones S, Zhang X, et al. An integrated genomic analysis of human glioblastoma multiforme. *Science* 2008;321(5897):1807–1812.

111. Mardis ER, Ding L, Dooling DJ, et al. Recurring mutations found by sequencing an acute myeloid leukemia genome. *N Engl J Med* 2009;361(11):1058–1066.

112. Ward PS, Patel J, Wise DR, et al. The common feature of leukemia-associated IDH1 and IDH2 mutations is a neomorphic enzyme activity converting alpha-ketoglutarate to 2-hydroxyglutarate. *Cancer Cell* 2010;17(3):225–234.

113. McCabe MT, Ott HM, Ganji G, et al. EZH2 inhibition as a therapeutic strategy for lymphoma with EZH2-activating mutations. *Nature* 2012;492(7427):108–112.

114. Morin RD, Johnson NA, Severson TM, et al. Somatic mutations altering EZH2 (Tyr641) in follicular and diffuse large B-cell lymphomas of germinal-center origin. *Nat Genet* 2010;42(2):181–185.

115. Bernt KM, Zhu N, Sinha AU, et al. MLL-rearranged leukemia is dependent on aberrant H3K79 methylation by DOT1L. *Cancer Cell* 2011;20(1):66–78.

116. Daigle SR, Olhava EJ, Therkelsen CA, et al. Selective killing of mixed lineage leukemia cells by a potent small-molecule DOT1L inhibitor. *Cancer Cell* 2011;20(1):53–65.

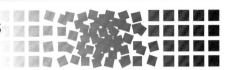

# 23 Histone Deacetylase Inhibitors and Demethylating Agents

Steven D. Gore, Stephen B. Baylin, and James G. Herman

## INTRODUCTION

The past decade has seen an explosive growth, especially at a genome-wide level, in our understanding of the role of chromatin in the normal regulation of gene expression and in the concept of the *epigenome*.[1–3] Concomitant with these advances has been the increasing appreciation of the role of epigenetic abnormalities in the progression of cancer[4–7] and the concept of the *cancer epigenome*. The translational consequences of this research include the possibilities for developing therapies in cancer that target epigenetic abnormalities. These are being explored in clinical trials and several have entered clinical practice.[4,5,7,8] Of these epigenetic abnormalities, the most thoroughly examined is the occurrence of abnormal cytosine guanine (CpG) promoter region DNA methylation and associated altered chromatin involving histone modifications, in the transcriptional silencing of genes, including a group of well-defined tumor suppressor genes.[4,5,7,8] However, targeting epigenetic processes to downregulate the action of overexpressed genes is also an emerging area of research.[9,10] This chapter describes the basis of epigenetic changes in cancer and discusses some of the latest approaches that target epigenetic abnormalities in cancer,[11] including those designed to induce the reexpression of silenced genes, for cancer therapy. The two approaches most mature in development are the inhibition of DNA methyltransferases, which mediate the abnormal promoter DNA methylation, and the inhibition of histone deacetylases, which remove histone modifications associated with active chromatin that alone, or in association with DNA methylation, are associated with transcriptional repression.[4,5,7,8] However, several exciting newer approaches are now in clinical trials and these will be mentioned.

Aberrant gene function and altered patterns of gene expression are key features of cancer.[4] Although genetic alterations remain the best characterized in the development and progression of cancer, increasingly it is appreciated that epigenetic abnormalities cooperate with genetic alterations in multiple ways to cause dysfunction of key regulatory pathways. Through genomic approaches to mutation discovery, there is growing recognition of the frequency of mutations in genes encoding for proteins that regulate the epigenome.[12] This chapter will outline the understanding of how each of these epigenetic alterations contribute to cancer and how derivation of therapeutic approaches may depend on understanding the biology of these changes.

## EPIGENETIC ABNORMALITIES AND GENE EXPRESSION CHANGES IN CANCER

Epigenetic changes are defined as heritable alterations of gene expression patterns and cell phenotypes, which are not accompanied by changes in DNA sequence.[13] This definition clearly delineates the two key features of epigenetic regulation important for an understanding of therapies described in this chapter. Specifically, in contrast to genetic alterations (point mutations, deletions,

or translocations), epigenetic changes do not alter the coding sequence of targeted genes. Thus, reversal of epigenetic changes can potentially restore the normal function of affected genes and their encoded proteins. Second, the heritable nature of epigenetic changes—that is, the ability of a cell to pass on regulation of gene expression through DNA replication—suggests that such changes, while relatively stable, can be reversed. Thus, therapeutic reprogramming of patterns of gene expression could theoretically result in a long-term change in the cancer cell phenotype, even after the inducing drugs are removed, although to date, this has not been accomplished.

The fundamental unit that determines epigenetic states is the nucleosome that contains an octamer of histone proteins around which approximately 160 base pairs of DNA are wrapped.[13] It is the positioning of these structures, and the three-dimensional aspects of their spacing, and the regulation of this process by posttranslational modifications of the constituent histones that underpins the functions of the epigenome.[13,14]

## Abnormal Gene Silencing

One key alteration in cancer, which can be associated with altered epigenetic control, is abnormal gene silencing. Normally, such silencing is fundamental and required at the level of chromatin and DNA methylation regulation for the life of multicellular eukaryotic organisms. The silencing is critical for regulating important biologic processes, including all aspects of development, differentiation, imprinting, and silencing of large chromosomal domains, including the X chromosome of female mammals.[13] For example, the diversity of structure and function of cells derived from epithelial or mesenchymal origin, ultimately differentiating into cells lining the intestine or lung or forming mature granulocytes and myocytes, result from heritable changes in gene expression that are not the result of a change in DNA sequence. Although in many species, silencing can be initiated and maintained solely by processes involving the covalent modifications of histones and other chromatin components, vertebrates utilize an additional layer of gene regulation. This process involves the only natural covalent modification of DNA in humans and is characterized by DNA cytosine methylation that occurs nearly exclusively at the fifth position of the cytosine ring in cytosines preceding guanine, the so-called CpG dinucleotide (Fig. 23.1).[13,15]

Like most biologic processes, the normal patterns of silencing can be altered, resulting in the development of disease states. Thus, activation of genes normally not expressed, or silencing of a gene that should be expressed, can contribute to the dysregulation of gene function that characterizes cancer and, when stably present, represent epigenetic alterations.[4–7] Most studies have focused on the silencing of normally expressed genes. For the purposes of understanding the rationale behind epigenetic therapy, it is important to understand the mechanisms through which such silencing occurs. Alterations in gene expression associated with epigenetic changes that give rise to a growth advantage would be expected to be selected for in the host tissue, leading to progressive dysregulated

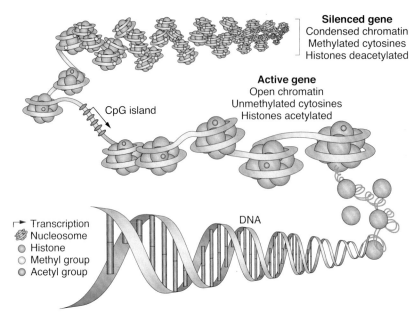

**Figure 23.1** Epigenetic regulation of gene expression. In the promoter region, gene expression is controlled by a combination of DNA methylation and chromatin configuration. In normal cells, gene expression is silenced by condensing chromatin, methylating DNA, and deacetylating histones. By contrast, active genes are those with open nucleosome spacing around the transcription start site, are unmethylated, and are associated with acetylated histones. In cancer cells, CpG islands that are rich in cytosine and guanine—and are typically unmethylated to promote gene expression—can be epigenetically silenced by hypermethylation. (Redrawn with permission from Azad N, Zahnow CA, Rudin CM, et al. The future of epigenetic therapy in solid tumours—lessons from the past. *Nat Rev Clin Oncol* 2013;10:256–266.)

growth of the tumor. Such dysregulation is commonly associated with increases in promoter region DNA methylation and is associated with repressive chromatin changes.

## Changes in DNA Methylation

The importance of abnormal cytosine methylation and gene silencing has been clearly established in the past 2 decades and been shown convincingly to be involved in cancer development.[4–7] The CpG dinucleotide, usually underrepresented in the genome, is clustered in the promoter regions of approximately 50% of human genes in regions termed *CpG islands*. These regions are largely protected from DNA methylation in normal cells, with the exception of genes on the inactive X chromosome and imprinted genes.[16] This protection is critical, because the methylation of promoter region CpG islands is associated with a loss of gene expression.[4–7] Abnormal de novo DNA methylation of gene promoter CpG islands is a very frequent abnormality in virtually all cancer types and is associated with a process that can serve as an alternative mechanism for loss of tumor suppressor gene function.[4–7] Although a limited number of classic tumor suppressor genes can be affected by this process, a patient's individual cancer may harbor hundreds of such genes.[4–7] Which of these latter genes are drivers of cancer, individually or in groups, versus those which are passengers reflecting only the widespread effects of a global epigenetic abnormality is a leading question in the field and the target of much research.[5,6] A clue to the importance of at least groups of the previous DNA hypermethylated genes may come from the fact that an inordinate number of them are involved in holding normal embryonic and adult stem cells in the self-renewal state and/or rendering such cells refractory to differentiation cues.[17,18] Normally, these genes are then in a poised expression state and can be induced to be activated or repressed as needed for changes in

cell state.[18] Abnormal promoter DNA methylation of such genes renders them more repressed and could be a factor in the fact that cancers inevitably exhibit cell populations with enhanced self-renewal or refractoriness to full differentiation.[18]

Recent studies have also suggested that DNA regions other than promoter CpG islands may undergo changes of DNA methylation in cancer. For example, non–CpG-rich sequences surrounding promoter CpG islands, termed CpG island shores, are abnormally methylated in cancers[19] and may be altered in stem cell populations.[20] Thus, the relative cancer specificity of changes of DNA methylation in multiple CpG regions makes reversal of these changes by targeting DNA methyltransferases, the enzymes that catalyze DNA methylation, logical for cancer therapeutics.

As a key example of the previous points, perhaps the most studied tumor suppressor gene for promoter hypermethylation is the *p16* gene, currently designated *CDKN2A*, a cyclin-dependent kinase inhibitor that functions in the regulation of the phosphorylation of the Rb protein. Hypermethylation associated with loss of expression of the *CDKN2A* gene has been found to be one of the most frequent alterations in neoplasia being common in the lung, head and neck, gliomas, colorectal, and breast carcinomas[21,22] and other cancer types. A member of the same gene family, *p15* or *CDKN2B*, also regulates Rb and is silenced in association with promoter methylation in many forms of leukemia and in the chronic myeloid neoplasm myelodysplastic syndrome (MDS).[23] These two previous changes are of much relevance for the clinical uses of epigenetic therapies discussed later.

As mentioned, many hundreds of genes may be inactivated in a single cancer by promoter methylation,[5,6,18,24] providing potential targets for gene reactivation using epigenetic therapies.[25–27] The latter represents one of the potential ways in which epigenetic therapy may be effective: Multiple genes and gene pathways, all

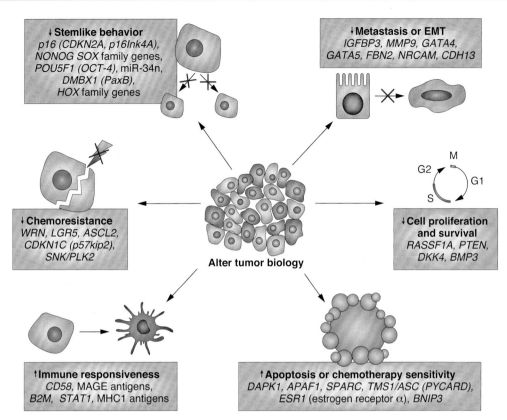

**Figure 23.2** Concurrent widespread changes in gene expression with epigenetic therapy. Anticancer efficacy of treatment with epigenetic-modulating agents is associated with extensive changes in gene expression that influence several biologic processes. Gene expression is increased through the direct reversal of epigenetic modifications of genomic DNA, whereas for cancer-promoting genes, gene expression is reduced by the regression of their regulatory genes. EMT, epithelial-membrane transition. (Redrawn with permission from Azad N, Zahnow CA, Rudin CM, et al. The future of epigenetic therapy in solid tumours—lessons from the past. *Nat Rev Clin Oncol* 2013;10:256–266.)

repressed by changes in DNA methylation and chromatin modification, can be reactivated by DNA methyltransferase inhibitors and histone deacetylase (HDAC) inhibitors (HDACi), thereby restoring normal cell cycle control, differentiation, and apoptotic signaling (Fig. 23.2).[8,26,28] In general, methylated CpG islands are not capable of the initiation of transcription unless the methylation signal can be overridden by alterations in factors that modulate chromatin, such as the removal of methylated cytosine-binding proteins. However, reversal of DNA methylation with secondary changes in histone modification or directed reversal of repressive histone modifications represent a target for epigenetic therapies.[8,26,28]

Most studies of DNA methylation, particularly in the study of cancer, have focused on CpG island promoter methylation. However, about 40% of human genes do not contain bona fide CpG islands in their promoters.[29] The primary focus on CpG islands has resulted from the clear demonstration that CpG-island promoter methylation permanently silences genes both physiologically and pathologically in mammalian cells. However, recent work has shown correlations between tissue-specific expression and methylation of non-CpG islands, including, for example, the maspin gene,[30] and as mentioned previously, regions near CpG islands,[19,20] suggesting that many additional genes could be regulated, either normally or abnormally, by changes in DNA methylation.

An exciting new area of DNA methylation research involves the role of this change in regulating gene enhancers: small DNA regions that regulate the expression of multiple target genes.[31-33] The presence of DNA methylation in these areas, which can reside considerable distances from the genes that are being regulated,

generally works together with histone modifications to mediate a repressive state for that enhancer.[31-33] The status of enhancers is also emerging as important for cancer risk states.[34]

## Chromatin in Gene Regulation

Heritable gene silencing involves the interplay between DNA methylation and histone covalent modifications. Complexes of proteins that can regulate how nucleosomes are positioned perform nucleosomal remodeling.[35-37] What was initially termed the *histone code*, with reference to how histones are modified, has emerged to be much more complex than originally envisioned. An explosion of research findings during the last several years now allows for an appreciation of how the epigenome is controlled by a complex interplay between a myriad of posttranslational histone modifications that occur on key amino acid residues of these proteins.[37] Acetylation, deacetylation, methylation, phosphorylation, and other modifications all modify chromatin structure and thereby alter gene expression.[38] Some of the enzymes that catalyze these modifications include HDACs, histone methyltransferases (HMT), and most recently, histone demethylases.[13,14,39,40] These modifications help establish heritable states at the start site of genes, but also at enhancers and other transcribed DNA regions not encoding for canonical genes. The latter areas contain noncoding RNAs (ncRNAs) and micro-RNAs (miRNAs), which play key modulatory roles for overall gene expression and protein patterns that can be altered in cancer.[41-43] Again, much research is being focused on epigenetic changes in these DNA regions, which may be important to cancer development and, potentially, to cancer management.

A link between covalent histone modifications and DNA methylation has been clearly established.[44–46] In this interaction, cytosine methylation attracts methylated DNA-binding proteins and HDACs to methylated CpG sites during chromatin compaction and gene silencing.[46,47] In addition, the DNA methylation binding protein (MBD2) interacts with the nucleosomal remodeling complex (NuRD) and directs the complex to methylated DNA.[48] This complex also binds HDACs and has recently been identified as a central player for the abnormal silencing of genes associated with promoter DNA hypermethylation in cancer.[47] Thus, the three processes of DNA cytosine methylation, histone modification, and nucleosomal remodeling are intimately linked, and alterations in these processes can result in abnormalities of gene expression in cancer-relevant genes.

## Enzymes Regulating DNA Methylation and Histone Acetylation

DNA methylation involves the covalent addition of a methyl group to the 5′ position of cytosine. In mammals, three enzymes have been shown to catalyze this transfer of a methyl group from the methyl donor S-adenosylmethionine. Most of the methyltransferase activity present in differentiated cells is derived from the expression of DNMT1.[49] This enzyme is thought to be most important in maintaining DNA methylation patterns following DNA replication and thus is referred to as a maintenance methyltransferase. However, the enzyme does possess the ability to methylate previously unmethylated DNA sequences (de novo activity).[50] In contrast, the other enzymes, DNMT3a and DNMT3b, are efficient at methylating previously unmethylated DNA and thus are considered de novo methyltransferases. Each of these enzymes possesses a similar catalytic site,[51] a fact important for the inhibition of DNMT enzymes by nucleoside analogs, discussed later in this chapter.

DNA methylation is closely associated with changes in the histone modifications. As previously discussed, histone proteins are the central components of the nucleosome, and modifications of the histone tails of core histones are associated with active or repressed chromatin.[52] Although it is beyond the scope of this chapter to fully discuss the complex series of modifications to the histone tails of histone H3 and H4, a few well-characterized modifications should be mentioned that are relevant to therapies designed to target epigenetic abnormalities in cancer. In reference to currently investigated epigenetic therapies, changes in histone acetylation are of importance. Acetylation of histones H3 and H4 at key amino acids is associated with the active chromatin present at the promoters of transcribed genes, whereas the absence of histone acetylation is associated with repressed, silenced genes.[13,14,53] Histone acetyltransferases (HAT) HDACs have opposing functions to maintain the proper level of histone acetylation for gene expression.[13,14,53] HDACs specifically deacetylate the lysine residues of the histone tails, and this deacetylation is associated with condensation of nucleosome positions in what is termed a closed chromatin formation. This scenario is key to transcriptional repression. There are four classes of HDACs.[53] Class I HDACs are characterized by their similarity to the yeast Rpd3 HDAC. In humans, this class of enzymes includes HDAC1, -2, -3, and -8. These HDACs are thought to be ubiquitously expressed in tissue throughout the body. In contrast, class II HDACs are similar to yeast Hda1 and include HDAC4, -5, -6, -7, -9, and -10, and they have a greater degree of tissue specificity. Class III HDACs are similar to yeast Sir2 and are set apart from the other classes by their dependence on nicotinamide adenine dinucleotide (NAD+) as a cofactor. Finally, class IV includes HDAC11.[53]

Of the previously listed HDACs, class I and 2 HDACs have been most closely tied to gene silencing associated with abnormal promoter DNA hypermethylation.[48] These are bound to the nucleosome remodeling complex, NuRD.[48,49] Experimental decreases in NURD, after use of a DNA demethylating agent, can augment reactivation of many abnormally silenced and DNA hypermethylated genes in colon cancer cells.[48] Manipulation of these HDACs is under study in clinical trials, with and without the use of DNA methyltransferase inhibitors, and is discussed later. Another HDAC, SIRT1 in the class III of these proteins, is also involved with gene silencing.[54,55] This deacetylase has been linked to silencing of DNA hypermethylated genes, and blocking its activity can be associated with reactivation of such genes.[55]

## Reversal of Layers of Gene Silencing

The interaction between DNA methylation and HDAC activity and repressive chromatin marks in maintaining aberrant silencing of hypermethylated genes in cancer has therapeutic implications for epigenetic therapies. Experimental evidence suggests that DNA methylation functions as a dominant event that stably establishes transcriptional repression. Inhibition of HDAC activity alone, by potent and specific HDACis, does not generally result in the reactivation of aberrantly silenced and densely hypermethylated genes in tumor cells.[56] In contrast, treatment with HDACis can reactivate densely silenced genes if the cells are first treated with demethylating drugs, such as 5-azacitidine.[56] The clinical implications of this observation are discussed in more detail in the following section (Table 23.1).

## DNA Methyltransferase Inhibitors

Originally synthesized as cytotoxic antimetabolite drugs in the 1960s,[57] azacytosine nucleosides were recognized as inhibitors of DNA methylation in the early 1980s. The inhibitors 5-azacitidine (5AC) and 2′-deoxy-5-azacytidine induced muscle, fat, and chondrocyte differentiation in mouse embryo cells, in association with a reversal of DNA methylation.[58,59] The incorporation of azacytosine nucleosides into DNA in lieu of cytosine residues was shown to be associated with inhibition of DNMT activity.[59,60] DNMT inhibition requires the incorporation of decitabine triphosphate into DNA. The incorporated azacytosine nucleoside forms an irreversible inactive adduct with DNMT. The sequential reversal of DNA methylation then results when DNA replication proceeds in the absence of active DNMT.[61] The inhibitor 5AC must be phosphorylated and converted to decitabine diphosphate by ribonucleotide reductase before it can be activated through triphosphorylation, whereas decitabine does not require ribonucleotide reductase. The inhibitor 5AC can also be incorporated into RNA. DNMT2, a misnamed protein that is actually an RNA-specific methyltransferase,[62] becomes inhibited, leading to the depletion of methylated tRNA.[60] This may contribute to the inhibition of protein synthesis and is a potential difference between azacitidine and decitabine.[63] The previous DNA methyltransferase inhibitors not only block the catalytic activities of DNMTs, but also trigger degradation of these proteins, especially DNMTs 1 and 3B.[64–68] This latter activity is potentially important for their activities for gene reexpression because each of these two proteins, experimentally, possess transcriptional repression properties independent of their DNA methylation catalytic sites.[69,70]

The azacytosine nucleosides exhibit complex dose–response characteristics. At low concentrations (0.2 to 1 μM), the *epigenetic* activities of these drugs predominate, with dose-dependent reversal of DNA methylation[71,72] and induction of terminal differentiation in some systems.[28,71] As concentrations are increased, DNA damage and apoptosis become more prominent.[28,72] Cell lines with 30-fold resistance to the cytotoxic effects of doxifluridine,

**TABLE 23.1**

**Small Molecules Targeting Epigenetic Abnormalities in Clinical Development**

| Drug | Class | Target | Dose Range | Schedule | Route of Administration |
|------|-------|--------|-----------|----------|-------------------------|
| 5-Azacitidine | Nucleoside | DNA methyl-transferase | 30–75 mg/m²/d | Daily × 7–14 d/28 d | Subcutaneous or intravenous |
| 2′-Deoxy-5-azacytidine | Nucleoside | DNA methyl-transferase | 10–45 mg/m²/d | Daily × 3–5 d/4–6 wk | Intravenous |
| SG110 | Nucleoside | DNA methyl-transferase | Being determined | Being determined | Subcutaneous |
| Valproic acid | Small chain fatty acid | Histone deacetylase (class I and II) | 25–50 mg/kg/d | Daily | Oral or intravenous |
| Vorinostat | Hydroxamic acid | Histone deacetylase (class I and II) | 400–600 mg/d | Divided doses | Oral |
| Entinostat | Benzamide | Histone deacetylase (class I) | 2–8 mg/m² | Weekly | Oral |
| Belinostat | Hydroxamic acid | Histone deacetylase (class I and II) | 600–1,000 mg/m² | Daily × 5/28 d | Intravenous |
| Romidepsin | Cyclic tetrapeptide | Histone deacetylase (class I and II) | 13–18 mg/m² | Weekly | Intravenous |
| LBH-589 | Hydroxamic acid | Histone deacetylase (class I and II) | 5–11 mg/m² | Daily × 3 | Intravenous |
| MGCD-0103 | Benzamide | Histone deacetylase (class I) | 40–125 mg/m² | Twice weekly | Oral |
| CI-994 | Benzamide | Histone deacetylase (class I) | 5–8 mg/m² | Daily | Oral |

adriamycin, cyclophosphamide (DAC) continue to reverse methylation in response to this nucleoside, suggesting that the methylation reversing and cytotoxic activities of this compound can be separated.[73] The ability of these drugs to inhibit the cell cycle, at least in part through induction of p21[WAF1/CIP1] expression, complicates the goal of reversing DNA methylation, because the latter requires DNA replication with the azacytosine nucleoside incorporated into the DNA.

The importance of low doses of the two azacytosine nucleosides to achieve a targeted therapeutic effect has been recently explored in a series of laboratory observations. Transient exposure of both leukemia and solid tumor cells to submicromolar doses induce such cells to undergo cellular reprogramming, accompanied by decreases in ability to clone in long-term self-renewal assays and to grow as explants in immune-incompetent mice.[28] These effects occur with partial genome-wide DNA demethylation and changes in gene expression in multiple pathways potentially key for driving tumorigenesis.

The pharmacokinetic properties of the two azacytosine nucleosides are also very important to consider for their clinical use. In this regard, a major potential challenge for their usage is the fact that these drugs are highly unstable in an aqueous solution, resulting in their rapid hydrolysis and resultant inactivation.[74] In clinical practice, the drugs must be administered shortly after reconstitution. The drugs are also metabolized by cytidine deaminase,[74] leading to a short half-life in plasma. When injected subcutaneously, 5AC reaches a maximal plasma concentration at 30 minutes, with a terminal half-life of 1.5 to 2.3 hours.[75,76] At the U.S. Food and Drug Administration (FDA) approved dose of 5AC (75 mg/m² administered subcutaneously daily for 7 days), peak plasma concentrations were 3 to 5 μM, which is well within the range of DNMT inhibitory concentrations.[75,76] Intravenous (IV) administration of the same dose has led to higher peak plasma concentrations (11 μM) with a shorter half-life

(approximately 22 minutes).[75] DAC given over 1 hour IV at 15 to 20 mg/m² produced plasma concentrations of 1.1 to 1.6 μM during the infusion,[77] whereas in a phase 1 study in patients with thoracic malignancies, patients were treated with escalating doses of decitabine for 72-hour IV infusions for two 35-day cycles. The maximum tolerated total dose was 60 to 75 mg/m² with neutropenia as the dose-limiting toxicity. Steady-state plasma concentrations ranged from 25 to 40 nM, which is less than those usually used to induce expression of methylated genes in tissue culture models.[78] An oral formulation of 5AC has also been studied. The oral bioavailability of oral azacitidine ranged from 6% to 20%. Nonetheless, MDS and acute myelogenous leukemia (AML) patients receiving oral azacitidine developed clinical responses similar to patients receiving parenteral azacitidine. Oral azacitidine has also been safely administered on 14-daily and 21-daily schedules repeated monthly. The extended administration of lower daily doses may provide favorable pharmacodynamics of DNA methylation reversal given the need for ongoing cell cycling to effect methylation reversal.[79]

SGI-110 is a dinucleoside that acts as a prodrug for decitabine. This drug is being studied in myelodysplasia and AML.[80]

## HISTONE DEACETYLASE INHIBITORS

The increasing recognition of the critical importance of histone modifications in regulating the transcriptional permissively of chromatin has led to intense interest in compounds that can inhibit the activity of HDAC proteins, facilitating the acetylation of lysines associated with transcriptional activation of genes. As with the DNMT inhibitors discussed previously, there are multiple, sometimes dose-dependent, effects of HDACis in preclinical studies. Some of these may truly be epigenetic, others strictly cytotoxic, and others a combination of both.[9,81–84] Some actions of HDACis may relate to altering how chromatin is central to the repair of DNA. Thus, at especially high doses, these compounds can blunt efficient repair and even induce DNA breaks.[84,85] These effects may underlie cell cycle arrest and induction of cell death as is often observed in preclinical studies of HDACis.[81–84]

Perhaps novel uses of these drugs may be inferred by results from recent studies suggesting they could be extremely powerful epigenetic therapy agents when used in proper doses, for targeted purposes, and at key time intervals. Recent studies by Settleman and colleagues[86] suggest that histone acetylation changes, and thus epigenetic mechanisms, could be a key factor for cancer therapy resistance to both targeted therapy agents and conventional chemotherapy. The mechanisms involved may involve the emergence of drug-tolerant stem-like cells.[86] In such cells, gene expression studies suggest that a protein upregulated in resistance is a histone demethylase, which diminishes a key histone modification for active transcription, H3K4methyl.[86] A very similar enzyme has been shown in other studies to be central to self-renewal of stem-like melanoma cells.[87] Key to the therapies under discussion is that, in the previous drug-resistance studies, low doses of HDACis, could reversibly reduce drug-resistant cells induced by the various anticancer drugs.[86] It is essential going forward to sort out which of these effects are dose-related off-target effects and which are desired on-target effects that can be optimized for efficacious therapy strategies.

## Types of Histone Deacetylase Inhibitors

### Small Chain Fatty Acids

The earliest report of the use of an HDACi to treat leukemia described the treatment of a child with refractory AML with intravenous sodium butyrate, with a concomitant clearance of peripheral blood blast cells and a decrement in bone marrow blasts.[88] No responses developed in a subsequent study of nine AML patients who were treated with intravenous butyrate.[89] Phase 1 studies of sodium phenylbutyrate (NaPB) in MDS and AML explored 7-day continuous infusions administered monthly or biweekly, and 21-day continuous infusions administered monthly.[90,91] At the maximum tolerated dose (375 mg per kilogram per day), the mean steady-state plasma concentration was 0.3 mM, within the range of HDAC inhibition.[90–92] Isolated patients developed hematologic improvement in response to NaPB.

Similar to NaPB, valproic acid (VPA) requires near millimolar concentrations to effectively inhibit HDACs. Of 18 patients with MDS or AML with trilineage dysplasia treated with VPA to target plasma concentrations of 0.3 to 0.7 mM, 6 patients developed hematologic improvement.[93] Of 20 elderly patients with AML treated with VPA, only 11 could remain in control long enough to be considered evaluable for response. Five had improvement in platelet counts.[94] VPA induced hematologic improvement in combination with all-transretinoic acid in two of eight patients treated with AML; a fluorescence in situ hybridization analysis showed definitive evidence of terminal differentiation of the malignant cells.[95] A larger study of this combination induced hematologic response in only 2 of 26 elderly patients with AML.[96] It appears unlikely that the small chain fatty acids will develop an important role in the treatment of malignancy given the availability of HDACis with vastly greater potency.

### Hydroxamic Acids

The FDA approved vorinostat as the first commercially available HDACi. The approval was based on activity of this agent in cutaneous T-cell lymphoma (CTCL). Thirty-three patients with a median number of five prior systemic therapy regimens received one of three dose schedules of vorinostat in a single institution study.[97] Eight patients achieved a partial response, with a median time to response of 12 weeks and a median duration of response of 15 weeks. Overall, 45% of patients had relief of pruritus. Fatigue, diarrhea, nausea, and thrombocytopenia were common toxicities. In a multicenter phase 2 trial, 74 patients with relapsed or refractory CTCL were treated with 400 mg daily.[98] Similar to the prior study, 29% of patients responded, consisting almost entirely of partial responses. Median time to response was 56 days, and median duration of response was greater than 6 months. In phase 1 trials, responses to vorinostat have developed in other non-Hodgkin's and Hodgkin's lymphoma cases.[99] More recently, in a trial combining vorinostat with carboplatin and paclitaxel in patients with untreated, advanced, non–small-cell lung cancer (NSCLC), response rates increased significantly from 12.5% to 34%, and a trend to improved progression-free survival and overall survival was observed.[100]

Panobinostat (LBH589), a cinnamic hydroxamic acid HDACi, reduced peripheral blood blast percentage but did not induce remissions in a phase 1 trial of daily times 7 oral dosing in patients with a variety of relapsed hematologic malignancies.[101] Asymptomatic changes in electrocardiographic T waves developed in 80% of treated patients. Gastrointestinal symptoms and thrombocytopenia were common. Panobinostat has recently been approved by the FDA for the treatment of multiple myeloma.[102]

## Cyclic Tetrapeptides

Romidepsin is FDA approved for the treatment of CTCL[103] and peripheral T-cell lymphoma.[104,105] Antitumor activity, including tumor lysis syndrome, was demonstrated in a phase 1 study that enrolled patients with chronic lymphocytic leukemia and AML, but no complete or partial remissions were seen.[75] The administration of romidepsin induces electrocardiographic changes, including T-wave flattening and ST-T wave depression in greater than half of the posttreatment tracings; however, no changes in serum cardiac troponin levels or left ventricular ejection fraction have been reported.[106]

## Benzamides

Entinostat, formerly known as MS-275, was administered weekly times four to patients with relapsed and refractory AML in a phase 1 study. Infections, unsteady gate, and somnolence were dose-limiting toxicities. No clinical responses developed, although improvements in neutrophil counts were observed.[107] Entinostat did not increase the response rate in patients with higher risk MDS and AML with MDS-related changes when combined with azacitidine compared to azacitidine alone.[108] Most recently, however, studies NSCLC suggest that entinostat could be a valuable therapeutic agent in solid tumors when used with established therapies. When combined with the epidermal growth factor inhibitor erlotinib, in a randomized phase 2 trial for patients with recurrent advanced NSCLC, entinostat was not efficacious alone but appeared to combine with erlotinib to benefit a group of patients whose tumors contained baseline high E-cadherin levels. Overall survival in these latter patients yielded an increased survival benefit of 9.4 versus 5.4 months.[109] Finally, entinostat significantly increased survival when combined with an aromatase inhibitor in a phase 2 trial for patients with breast cancer.[110]

## Pharmacodynamic Properties

The administration of oral vorinostat was associated with a transient increase in acetylation of histone H3 in peripheral blood lymphocytes, which peaked at 2 hours post dosing and reverted to baseline by 8 hours; similar changes were observed in the lymph node of a treated patient with lymphoma.[99] Treatment with vorinostat was associated with translocation of phosphorylated signal transducer and activator of transcription 3 (STAT-3) from nucleus to cytoplasm in responding patients and with reduced microvessel density.[97]

Similar changes in the acetylation of histones 2B and 3 were observed in peripheral blood cells from patients treated with LBH589.[101] Romidepsin induced acetylation of H3 and H4 in peripheral blood tumor cells within 4 hours of dosing[111]; of interest, p21[WAF1/CIP1] protein levels also increased, associated with an increase in acetylation of H4 at the p21 promoter (using chromatin immunoprecipitation). Treatment with entinostat led to increased acetylation of H3 and H4 in both peripheral blood and bone marrow. This increase was detectable within 8 hours and remained above baseline throughout the treatment cycle. Thus, this compound may provide the most prolonged inhibition of protein deacetylation of HDACis and is under current investigation.[107] Increases in p21[WAF1/CIP1] and activation of caspase 3 were also demonstrated in these samples.

# EPIGENETIC THERAPY FOR HEMATOLOGIC MALIGNANCIES

## DNA Methyltransferase Inhibitors

Epigenetic therapy has seen the most widespread use to date and achieved the greatest efficacy in hematologic malignancies. The therapeutic efficacy of 5AC and DAC for patients with the chronic myeloid neoplasm myelodysplasia (MDS) and AML has been well reviewed.[26,27] Their FDA approval for MDS/AML emerged only after doses were reduced, with resultant diminishing toxicities for patients. The successful development of 5AC for the treatment of MDS can be credited largely to Silverman et al.[25,112,114] in the Cancer and Leukemia Group B (CALGB). The inhibitor 5AC had successfully induced the expression of hemoglobin F in patients with sickle cell anemia.[25,112] Viewing this compound as a potential inducer of terminal differentiation, Silverman et al. conducted a series of phase 2 trials of 5AC administered as a continuous intravenous infusion or as subcutaneous injections for the treatment of MDS.[113,114] Based on significant hematologic responses, the group performed a phase 2 trial (CALGB 9221) in which patients with low- and high-risk MDS with significant hematopoietic compromise were randomly assigned to receive subcutaneous 5AC (75 mg/m² per day daily for 7 days, repeated on a 28-day cycle) or observation. Patients on the observation arm with progressive disease could cross over to receive 5AC. This study firmly established the ability of 5AC to induce hematologic improvement, and, less frequently, complete and partial responses.[113,115] The median time to development of AML (defined by 30% bone marrow blast cells) or death was greater in the 5AC arm by 9 months (21 versus 12 months); of note, the observation arm included patients who subsequently crossed over to 5AC treatment.

In a subsequent phase 3 trial (AZA001),[116] patients with higher risk myelodysplastic syndromes were randomly assigned one-to-one to receive 5AC (75 mg/m² per day for 7 days every 28 days) or conventional care (best supportive care, low-dose cytarabine, or intensive chemotherapy as selected by investigators before randomization). Three hundred fifty-eight patients were randomly assigned to receive 5AC (n = 179) or conventional care regimens (n = 179). After a median follow-up of 21.1 months (interquartile range [IQR] 15.1 to 26.9), median overall survival was 24.5 months (9.9 not reached) for the azacitidine group versus 15.0 months (5.6 to 24.1) for the conventional care group (hazard ratio [HR] 0.58; 95% confidence interval [CI], 0.43 to 0.77; p = 0.0001). At 2 years, on the basis of Kaplan-Meier estimates, 50.8% (95% CI, 42.1 to 58.8) of patients in the 5AC group were

alive compared with 26.2% (95% CI, 18.7 to 34.3) in the conventional care group (p < 0.0001). Median time to AML transformation was 17.8 months (IQR 8.6 to 36.8; 95% CI, 13.6 to 23.6) in the 5AC group compared with 11.5 months (4.9 not reached; 8.3 to 14.5) in the conventional care group (HR 0.50; 95% CI, 0.35 to 0.70; p < 0.0001). Subsequent unplanned analyses of AZA001 included an examination of elderly patients with what would now be classified as AML (blast count 20% to 30%). In these 113 patients, there remains a statistically significant improvement in survival of 24.5 months versus 16.0 months (HR 0.47; 95% CI; p = 0.0001).[117]

The early development of decitabine in MDS took place primarily in Europe under the leadership of Wijermans et al.[118,119] These investigators pursued intravenous scheduling of decitabine administered three times daily for 3 days (45 mg/m² per day total dose). This cycle was repeated every 6 weeks. Phase 2 studies suggested a response rate of approximately 50% in MDS patients. In a randomized trial of DAC versus observation, patients with International Prognostic Score risk categories intermediate 1 to high received the previously listed schedule of decitabine or observation. No crossover was allowed in this trial. Response rates reported were: complete response: 9%, partial response: 8%, and hematologic improvement: 13%.[120] A 10% induction death rate occurred, suggesting that this schedule of DAC may be more toxic than the CALGB schedule of 5AC (1% induction mortality). DAC has also been investigated in low-dose daily intravenous dosing[121] and in daily-times-five schedules. The latter appears convenient and well tolerated. A daily-times-five schedule (20 mg/m² per day) has been FDA approved[121]; 99 patients with MDS (de novo or secondary) of any French-American-British (FAB) subtype and an International Prognostic Scoring System (IPSS) score equal to or greater than 0.5 were treated, with an overall response rate of 32% (17 complete responses [CR] plus 15 marrow CRs [mCR]).[122] Among patients who improved, 82% demonstrated responses by the end of cycle two. This well-tolerated regimen allows outpatient administration and, as noted previously, provides plasma levels of decitabine that inhibit DNMTs.

The 3-day intravenous schedule of DAC has been studied in two randomized trials compared to supportive care in patients with higher risk MDS. The first trial confirmed the hematologic activity of decitabine in this patient population but failed to show an improvement in survival in the DAC-treated patients.[123] Survival was also not increased in the subsequent trial, performed by the European Organization for Research and Treatment of Cancer (EORTC).[124] The failure of the randomized decitabine trials to show a survival benefit may be partially due to study design. Both randomized trials of 5AC continued treatment until disease progression for patients who did not achieve complete remission; in fact, this meant that most patients received maintenance therapy. In contrast, both randomized trials of decitabine allowed a maximum of eight cycles of treatment. The need for maintenance therapy in patients treated with DNMT inhibitors has not been tested in prospective randomized trials. An additional difference in the conduct of the two sets of DNMT inhibitor trials involves the duration of therapy administered. The median number of cycles of treatment administered in the two randomized trials of decitabine was three, compared to nine in the azacytidine trials. This may reflect greater toxicity of the originally 3-day schedule of decitabine compared to that of the approved schedule of 5AC. Although the differences in survival may reflect differences in trial design and trial conduct, emerging data suggests that despite similarities in methylation reversal, the two drugs differ in other potentially important biologic parameters, which may contribute to clinical outcomes.[62,63,125]

Two randomized phase 3 trials have been published treating elderly AML patients (greater than 20% blasts) with decitabine, both demonstrating improvement in survival that was not statistically significant. In the European study, 233 patients received either

DAC at 15 mg/m$^2$ × 9 doses over 3 days on 42-day cycles or best supportive care. The patients received a median of 4 cycles (0 to 9), and the overall survival was improved in the decitabine-treated patients, but did not reach statistical significance (median overall survival [OS], 10.1 versus 8.5 months, respectively; HR, 0.88; 95% CI, 0.66 to 1.17; two-sided, log-rank $p$ = 0.38).[126] In the M.D. Anderson Cancer Center–led multicenter trial,[127] 485 patients 65 years or older were randomly assigned to receive decitabine 20 mg/m$^2$ per day as a 1-hour intravenous infusion for 5 consecutive days every 4 weeks or best supportive care or low-dose cytarabine (20 mg/m$^2$ per day for 10 days every 4 weeks). There was a similar improvement in OS with decitabine (7.7 months; 95% CI, 6.2 to 9.2) versus the control group (5.0 months; 95% CI, 4.3 to 6.3; $p$ = 0.108; HR, 0.85; 95% CI, 0.69 to 1.04).[127]

The azacytosine nucleosides require prolonged administration to demonstrate hematologic improvement in MDS. Median time to development of first clinical response in the CALGB studies of 5AC was three cycles; 90% of responses developed by cycle six.[114] In the phase 3 trial of decitabine, the median time to response was two cycles,[123] as also seen in the alternative regimen of decitabine.[122] It is, therefore, extremely important when treating patients with azacytosine nucleosides to commit to administering between four and six cycles of therapy before determining whether a patient is responding to treatment. Furthermore, survival benefit is seen even in patients not showing bone marrow improvement for 5AC, perhaps related to decreased transfusion requirements or delayed progression to AML.[116]

Because AML in the context of MDS is arbitrarily defined based on marrow blast count, activity of the azanucleoside analogs in AML should not be surprising. In CALGB 9221, 20 patients were reclassified upon central pathology review as meeting criteria for AML (greater than 30% blasts). Their outcomes were comparable to the overall population in the study.[115] In all three CALGB studies among patients meeting current World Health Organization (WHO) criteria for AML (greater than 20% blasts), a complete response was achieved in 9% and hematologic improvement in 26%.[114] A retrospective review of 20 patients with AML, including 8 patients with bone marrow blasts greater than 29% treated with 5AC, reported a complete remission in 4 patients, a partial response in 5, and a hematologic improvement in 3. The median duration of response was 8 months (range: 3 to 33 months).[128] DAC induced a complete hematologic response in 2 of 20 patients treated who had the blastic phase of chronic myeloid leukemia.[129] These studies suggest activity of the azacytosine nucleosides in the treatment of a subset of AML patients. Current studies do not allow for the determination of whether this subset is limited to MDS-associated AML (AML with MDS-related changes), which tends to have low white blood cell counts and have a low proliferative rate, or whether these compounds are also active for those with AML without a history of antecedent hematologic disorder. Several reports describe the sensitivity MDS and AML, characterized by abnormalities of chromosome 7 and associated with poor outcomes in response to cytarabine-based therapy to azanucleosides. In one nonrandomized retrospective study, survival of such patients following the administration of DNMT inhibitors surpassed survival in response to conventional cytotoxic chemotherapy, similar to the outcomes of AZA001.[130–132]

Although the mechanisms underlying the clinical activity of azacytosine analogs may involve reversal of gene methylation, other actions need to be considered. The administration of DAC has been shown to induce transient decrements of methylation in noncoding regions, including long interspersed nuclear element (LINE) and ALU elements.[133] Early studies that examined methylation reversal of the target gene p15$^{INK4B}$ in response to DAC showed no correlation between methylation reversal and clinical response.[134,135] Clinical responders to DAC developed significantly higher expression of this gene following treatment, and certainly key biologic roles for this gene and its low basal expression are probable. Moreover, in one study, the clinical response was closely associated with the reversal of methylation of p15 or CDH-1 during the first cycle of treatment with 5AC followed by the HDACi NaPB.[25] In that study, it was noteworthy that the administration of 5AC prior to the addition of an HDACi was associated with the induction of histone acetylation. Although the mechanism underlying this activity is unknown, histone acetylation has been observed following DNA damage due to gamma irradiation.[136] Subsequent studies have found demethylation following treatment with either DAC or 5AC[137–140] but not consistently associated with response.[137,138,140] More work will be required to answer the important mechanistic question underpinning the clinical activity of azacytosine analogs.

## Combining Inhibitors in the Treatment of Hematologic Malignancies

It is almost certain that the biggest promise of epigenetic therapy lies in strategies to combine existing and newer drugs with each other and with current chemotherapies and targeted therapies. To date, the example for existing agents is the combination of DNMT inhibitors and HDAC inhibitors based on the hypothesis from the laboratory that this paradigm leads to optimal reexpression of transcriptionally silenced genes with promoter methylation.[56,141] This in vitro treatment paradigm has led to a variety of clinical studies that have attempted to apply this concept to the treatment of hematologic malignances. Much remains to be determined with regard to its efficacy and precisely what determines this. The first study of sequential DNMT/HDAC inhibitors administered a variety of doses of 5AC for 5 to 14 days followed by 7 days of NaPB by continuous infusion at its maximum tolerated dose to patients with MDS and AML.[25] The combination was well tolerated, and clinical responses were frequent in patients receiving 5AC at 50 mg/m$^2$ per day daily for 10 days and 25 mg/m$^2$ per day daily for 14 days, with 5 of 14 patients at those dose schedules achieving complete or partial response.

In a pilot study, 10 patients with MDS or AML were treated with 5AC at 75 mg/m$^2$ per day daily times seven followed by 5 days of NaPB given at 200 mg per kilogram per day as a 1- to 2-hour infusion. Three patients developed a partial response.[142]

In a similar study, investigators at the M.D. Anderson Cancer Center treated leukemic patients with decitabine (15 mg/m$^2$ per day IV daily times 10) and concomitant VPA at a variety of doses. Of 54 patients, 12 achieved complete remission or complete remission with incomplete platelet recovery.[143] The inhibitors 5AC, VPA, and all-transretinoic acid have been administered to patients with AML and MDS. Of 33 previously untreated patients, 14 over the age of 60 years developed a complete remission or a complete remission with inadequate platelet recovery.[144] A subsequent study of 5AC and VPA suggests increased efficacy of this combination in high-risk MDS.[145]

Entinostat has been successfully combined with azacytidine in patients with myeloid malignancies.[140] The US Leukemia Intergroup recently completed a randomized phase 2 trial of this combination compared with 5AC alone. In this study, of 149 patients, the primary endpoint of hematologic normalization was statistically similar, with 32% (95% CI, 22% to 44%) of the 5AC group reaching hematologic normalization (HN) versus 27% (95% CI, 17% to 39%) in the AZA + entinostat group. Median overall survivals were 18 months for the AZA group and 13 months for the AZA + entinostat group, but were also not statistically significant.[108] In the latter study, the administration of the combination was associated with less DNA methylation reversal compared to azacitidine monotherapy, likely due to cell cycle inhibitory effects of the HDACi. This highlights the complexity of effectively targeting epigenetic gene regulation.

It remains to be established whether combination therapies are more effective than single-agent demethylating therapies.

## Epigenetically Targeted Therapy in Nonhematologic Malignancies

The efficacies that have emerged in the application of epigenetically targeted drugs to hematologic malignancies has spurred interest in using epigenetic therapy for other types of cancer. As outlined as follows, laboratory studies and clinical trials support this approach. Studies in the lab have been directed by lessons learned from therapy in hematologic malignancies, suggesting that low doses of drugs like DAC and 5AC, in the nanomolar range, may avoid excess toxicities due to off-target effects of the drugs and may maximize epigenetic effects of the agents.[28] The desired effects may require minimizing initial cellular cytotoxicity, giving tumor cells time to accrue maximal cellular reprogramming responses to the inhibition of DNMTs.[28] DAC and 5AC are effective only when they have been incorporated into DNA, after which they irreversibly inhibit DNMT catalytic activity and target these proteins for degradation.[64-68] In cell culture and mouse explants, low nanomolar doses appear to induce both human leukemic and solid tumor cells to exhibit blunting of self-renewal and tumorigenic activity of tumor stem-like cells.[28] These preclinical results suggest a key possibility that use of epigenetic therapies might inhibit these latter cell populations, which often are difficult to eradicate and are a factor in resistance to many standard cancer therapies.[146] Exhaustion of such cells over time during therapy with DAC or 5AC might explain the observation that most patients with MDS/AML take several months to reach best response.[147] Leukemic stem cells were not eliminated in one study in MDS and AML patients treated with 5AC in combination with VPA, although their frequency decreased in clinical responders.[148]

Clinical trials for common solid tumors, informed through the previous laboratory studies, have been initiated including phase 2 designs using low-dose strategies with 5AC often combined with use of histone deacetylase inhibitors. Sixty-five patients with advanced, multiply treated NSCLCs were treated with 5AC plus entinostat.[149] Only 3% of patients developed Response Evaluation Criteria (RECIST)-measureable responses; however, these two patients had durable responses, with survival of 3 to 4 years.[149] Upregulation of immunogenic pathways in NSCLC and other solid tumor cells, observed in laboratory studies, suggest a potential for sequencing DNMT inhibitors with immune checkpoint inhibitors.[150] This drug is also reported to induce antitumor responses and immune recognition in a model of pancreatic cancer.[151] Other laboratory results and emerging clinical trials also suggest the promise of combining epigenetic therapy approaches to sensitize cancers other than NSCLC to subsequent therapies. Low-dose DAC appears able to upregulate a key mediator of 5-fluorouracil (5FU) action,

uridine monophosphate (UMP) kinase, in colorectal cancer cell lines.[152] These increases correlated with a reversal of 5FU resistance. Similar to studies discussed previously, DAC plus the HDACi, trichostatin A, decreased marker identified self-renewal populations in ovarian cancer while simultaneously inducing increased sensitivity to cisplatin.[153] In advanced ovarian cancer, 5AC or DAC plus carboplatin have yielded durable responses and induced stable disease in ovarian cancer patients.[154,155] These early results are being extrapolated for verification in larger, ongoing clinical trials.

## NEW APROACHES TO EPIGENETIC THERAPY

As we have outlined previously, the emerging promise for epigenetic therapy and the future of the approaches may lie in combinatorial drug strategies. Although this is already being explored with older agents, new drugs for new targets are now entering the picture.[9,11,156-158] In these efforts, several themes we have introduced in this chapter will likely dominate.

Most epigenetic therapies will not induce, when used at truly targeting doses, immediate cytotoxic effects. Therapeutic efficacy based on cellular reprogramming may require significant time to manifest. Clinical trial designs may need adaptation so that effective therapies are not discarded due to premature response evaluations. Finally, the ultimate promise for epigenetic therapy may lie with newer drugs now entering clinical trials. Outcomes with DNMT inhibitors may be improved with alternative scheduling of oral azacitidine or through prolonged pharmacokinetics of the decitabine prodrug SGI110.[79] Also, drugs targeting other proteins including BET family bromodomain proteins are generating much excitement.[9,82,156-159] BET inhibitors may interfere with localization of the oncogene *C-MYC* to acetylated lysines in regulatory regions of target genes.[9,82,156-159] These inhibitors are now entering clinical trials. Other promising approaches include the use of inhibitors of EZH2, the enzyme in the PcG system, which catalyzes the repressive histone mark H3K27me3.[9,82,156-159] Another clinical trial underway employs targeting of the translocation in which the protein mixed lineage leukemia (MLL) is fused with several targets, such as in infant leukemias. These translocations result in abnormal recruitment of the histone methyltransferase, DOT1L, to target genes like *HOXA9*.[158] This fusion induces hypermethylation of H3K79 and abnormal activation of MLL target genes.[158,160] Very selective inhibitors of DOT1L are now in clinical trials.

Epigenetically targeted therapies continue to hold great promise that reprogramming of malignant cells could alter approaches to cancer management. Strategies to merge older drugs, which we have focused on in this chapter, with the newer agents briefly discussed in this section, will underpin future trials to test this approach.

## REFERENCES

1. Bernstein BE, Meissner A, Lander ES. The mammalian epigenome. *Cell* 2007;128:669–681.
2. Young RA. Control of the embryonic stem cell state. *Cell* 2011;144:940–954.
3. Suva ML, Riggi N, Bernstein BE. Epigenetic reprogramming in cancer. *Science* 2013;339:1567–1570.
4. Herman JG, Baylin SB. Gene silencing in cancer in association with promoter hypermethylation. *N Engl J Med* 2003;349:2042–2054.
5. Jones PA, Baylin SB. The epigenomics of cancer. *Cell* 2007;128:683–692.
6. Baylin SB, Jones PA. A decade of exploring the cancer epigenome — biological and translational implications. *Nat Rev Cancer* 2011;11:726–734.
7. Esteller M. Cancer epigenomics: DNA methylomes and histone-modification maps. *Nat Rev Genet* 2007;8:286–298.
8. Yoo CB, Jones PA. Epigenetic therapy of cancer: past, present and future. *Nat Rev Drug Discov* 2006;5:37–50.
9. Dawson MA, Kouzarides T. Cancer epigenetics: from mechanism to therapy. *Cell* 2012;150:12–27.
10. Dawson MA, Kouzarides T, Huntly BJ. Targeting epigenetic readers in cancer. *N Engl J Med* 2012;367:647–657.
11. Bradner J. New targets for hematologic malignancies. *Clin Adv Hematol Oncol* 2013;11:375–376.
12. You JS, Jones PA. Cancer genetics and epigenetics: two sides of the same coin? *Cancer Cell* 2012;22:9–20.
13. Allis C, Jenuwein T, Reinberg D. *Epigenetics*, Vol. 1. Cold Spring Harbor, NY: Cold Spring Harbor Laboratory Press; 2007.

14. Kouzarides T. Chromatin modifications and their function. *Cell* 2007;128: 693–705.

15. Baylin SB, Jones PA. Epigenetic determinants of cancer. In: Allis CD, Jenuwein T, Reinberg D, eds. *Epigenetics*. Cold Spring Harbor, NY: Cold Spring Harbor Laboratory Press; 2006: 457–476.

16. Bird AP. CpG-rich islands and the function of DNA methylation. *Nature* 1986;321:209–213.

17. Morey L, Pascual G, Cozzuto L, et al. Nonoverlapping functions of the Polycomb group Cbx family of proteins in embryonic stem cells. *Cell Stem Cell* 2012;10:47–62.

18. Easwaran H, Johnstone SE, Van Neste L, et al. A DNA hypermethylation module for the stem/progenitor cell signature of cancer. *Genome Res* 2012;22: 837–849.

19. Irizarry RA, Ladd-Acosta C, Wen B, et al. The human colon cancer methylome shows similar hypo- and hypermethylation at conserved tissue-specific CpG island shores. *Nat Genet* 2009;41:178–186.

20. Doi A, Park IH, Wen B, et al. Differential methylation of tissue- and cancer-specific CpG island shores distinguishes human induced pluripotent stem cells, embryonic stem cells and fibroblasts. *Nat Genet* 2009;41:1350–1353.

21. Herman JG, Merlo A, Mao L, et al. Inactivation of the CDKN2/p16/MTS1 gene is frequently associated with aberrant DNA methylation in all common human cancers. *Cancer Res* 1995;55:4525–4530.

22. Merlo A, Herman JG, Mao L, et al. 5′ CpG island methylation is associated with transcriptional silencing of the tumour suppressor p16/CDKN2/MTS1 in human cancers. *Nat Med* 1995;1:686–692.

23. Herman JG, Civin CI, Issa JP, et al. Distinct patterns of inactivation of p15INK4B and p16INK4A characterize the major types of hematological malignancies. *Cancer Res* 1997;57:837–841.

24. Costello JF, Fruhwald MC, Smiraglia DJ, et al. Aberrant CpG-island methylation has non-random and tumour-type-specific patterns. *Nat Genet* 2000;24:132–138.

25. Gore SD, Baylin S, Sugar E, et al. Combined DNA methyltransferase and histone deacetylase inhibition in the treatment of myeloid neoplasms. *Cancer Res* 2006;66:6361–6369.

26. Azad N, Zahnow CA, Rudin CM, et al. The future of epigenetic therapy in solid tumours—lessons from the past. *Nat Rev Clin Oncol* 2013;10:256–266.

27. Issa JP, Kantarjian HM. Targeting DNA methylation. *Clin Cancer Res* 2009;15:3938–3946.

28. Tsai HC, Li H, Van Neste L, et al. Transient low doses of DNA-demethylating agents exert durable antitumor effects on hematological and epithelial tumor cells. *Cancer Cell* 2012;21:430–446.

29. Takai D, Jones PA. Comprehensive analysis of CpG islands in human chromosomes 21 and 22. *Proc Natl Acad Sci U S A* 2002;99:3740–3745.

30. Futscher BW, Oshiro MM, Wozniak RJ, et al. Role for DNA methylation in the control of cell type specific maspin expression. *Nat Genet* 2002;31:175–179.

31. Feldmann A, Ivanek R, Murr R, et al. Transcription factor occupancy can mediate active turnover of DNA methylation at regulatory regions. *PLoS Genet* 2013;9:e1003994.

32. Aran D, Hellman A. Unmasking risk loci: DNA methylation illuminates the biology of cancer predisposition: analyzing DNA methylation of transcriptional enhancers reveals missed regulatory links between cancer risk loci and genes. *Bioessays* 2014;36:184–190.

33. Ziller MJ, Gu H, Muller F, et al. Charting a dynamic DNA methylation landscape of the human genome. *Nature* 2013;500:477–481.

34. Akhtar-Zaidi B, Cowper-Sal-lari R, Corradin O, et al. Epigenomic enhancer profiling defines a signature of colon cancer. *Science* 2012;336:736–739.

35. Kingston R, Tamkun JW. Transcriptional regulation by trithorax group. In: Allis CD, Jenuwein T, Reinberd D, eds. *Epigenetics*. Cold Spring Harbor, NY: Cold Spring Harbor Laboratory Press; 2006: 231–248.

36. Becker PB, Workman JL. Nucleosome remodeling and epigenetics. *Cold Spring Harb Perspect Biol* 2013;5.

37. Petty E, Pillus L. Balancing chromatin remodeling and histone modifications in transcription. *Trends Genet* 2013;29:621–629.

38. Jones PA. Functions of DNA methylation: islands, start sites, gene bodies and beyond. *Nat Rev Genet* 2012;13:484–492.

39. Bannister AJ, Kouzarides T. Reversing histone methylation. *Nature* 2005; 436:1103–1106.

40. Bannister AJ, Kouzarides T. Regulation of chromatin by histone modifications. *Cell Res* 2011;21:381–395.

41. Di Leva G, Garofalo M, Croce CM. MicroRNAs in cancer. *Annu Rev Pathol* 2014;9:287–314.

42. Han BW, Chen YQ. Potential pathological and functional links between long noncoding RNAs and hematopoiesis. *Sci Signal* 2013;6:re5.

43. Xi JJ. MicroRNAs in Cancer. *Cancer Treat Res* 2013;158:119–137.

44. Nan X, Ng HH, Johnson CA, et al. Transcriptional repression by the methyl-CpG-binding protein MeCP2 involves a histone deacetylase complex. *Nature* 1998;393:386–389.

45. Jones PL, Veenstra GJ, Wade PA, et al. Methylated DNA and MeCP2 recruit histone deacetylase to repress transcription. *Nat Genet* 1998;19:187–191.

46. Parry L, Clarke AR. The Roles of the Methyl-CpG Binding Proteins in Cancer. *Genes Cancer* 2011;2:618–630.

47. Lopez-Serra L, Esteller M. Proteins that bind methylated DNA and human cancer: reading the wrong words. *Br J Cancer* 2008;98:1881–1885.

48. Cai Y, Geutjes EJ, de Lint K, et al. The NuRD complex cooperates with DNMTs to maintain silencing of key colorectal tumor suppressor genes. *Oncogene* 2014;33:2157–2168.

49. Bestor TH. Cloning of a mammalian DNA methyltransferase. *Gene* 1998; 74:9–12.

50. Jair KW, Bachman KE, Suzuki H, et al. De novo CpG island methylation in human cancer cells. *Cancer Res* 2006;66:682–692.

51. Rius M, Lyko F. Epigenetic cancer therapy: rationales, targets and drugs. *Oncogene* 2012;31:4257–4265.

52. Jenuwein T, Allis CD. Translating the histone code. *Science* 2001;293: 1074–1080.

53. Bolden JE, Peart MJ, Johnstone RW. Anticancer activities of histone deacetylase inhibitors. *Nat Rev Drug Discov* 2006;5:769–784.

54. Vaquero A, Scher M, Erdjument-Bromage H, et al. SIRT1 regulates the histone methyl-transferase SUV39H1 during heterochromatin formation. *Nature* 2007;450:440–444.

55. Pruitt K, Zinn RL, Ohm JE, et al. Inhibition of SIRT1 reactivates silenced cancer genes without loss of promoter DNA hypermethylation. *PLoS Genet* 2006;2:344–352.

56. Cameron EE, Bachman KE, Myohanen S, et al. Synergy of demethylation and histone deacetylase inhibition in the re-expression of genes silenced in cancer. *Nat Genet* 1999;21:103–107.

57. Sorm F, Piskala A, Cihak A, et al. 5-Azacytidine, a new, highly effective cancerostatic. *Experientia* 1964;20:202–203.

58. Taylor SM, Jones PA. Multiple new phenotypes induced in 10T1/2 and 3T3 cells treated with 5-azacytidine. *Cell* 1979;17:771–779.

59. Jones PA, Taylor SM. Hemimethylated duplex DNAs prepared from 5-azacytidine-treated cells. *Nucleic Acids Res* 1981;9:2933–2947.

60. Lu SH, Ohshima H, Bartsch H. Recent studies on N-nitroso compounds as possible etiological factors in oesophageal cancer. *IARC Sci Publ* 1984;947–953.

61. Taylor SM, Jones PA. Mechanism of action of eukaryotic DNA methyltransferase. Use of 5-azacytosine-containing DNA. *J Mol Biol* 1982;162:679–692.

62. Schaefer M, Hagemann S, Hanna K, et al. Azacytidine inhibits RNA methylation at DNMT2 target sites in human cancer cell lines. *Cancer Res* 2009; 69:8127–8132.

63. Hollenbach PW, Nguyen AN, Brady H, et al. A comparison of azacitidine and decitabine activities in acute myeloid leukemia cell lines. *PLoS One* 2010; 5:e9001.

64. Kelly TK, De Carvalho DD, Jones PA. Epigenetic modifications as therapeutic targets. *Nat Biotechnol* 2010;28:1069–1078.

65. Ferguson AT, Vertino PM, Spitzner JR, et al. Role of estrogen receptor gene demethylation and DNA methyltransferase. DNA adduct formation in 5-aza-2′deoxycytidine-induced cytotoxicity in human breast cancer cells. *J Biol Chem* 1997;272:32260–32266.

66. Gabbara S, Bhagwat AS. The mechanism of inhibition of DNA (cytosine-5-)-methyltransferases by 5-azacytosine is likely to involve methyl transfer to the inhibitor. *Biochem J* 1995;307:87–92.

67. Santi DV, Norment A, Garrett CE. Covalent bond formation between a DNA-cytosine methyltransferase and DNA containing 5-azacytosine. *Proc Natl Acad Sci U S A* 1984;81:6993–6997.

68. Ghoshal K, Datta J, Majumder S, et al. 5-Aza-deoxycytidine induces selective degradation of DNA methyltransferase 1 by a proteasomal pathway that requires the KEN box, bromo-adjacent homology domain, and nuclear localization signal. *Mol Cell Biol* 2005;25:4727–4741.

69. Rountree MR, Bachman KE, Baylin SB. DNMT1 binds HDAC2 and a new co-repressor, DMAP1, to form a complex at replication foci. *Nat Genet* 2000;25:269–277.

70. Bachman KE, Rountree MR, Baylin SB. Dnmt3a and Dnmt3b are transcriptional repressors that exhibit unique localization properties to heterochromatin. *J Biol Chem* 2001;276:32282–32287.

71. Jones PA, Taylor SM. Cellular differentiation, cytidine analogs and DNA methylation. *Cell* 1980;20:85–93.

72. Berg T, Guo Y, Abdelkarim M, et al. Reversal of p15/INK4b hypermethylation in AML1/ETO-positive and -negative myeloid leukemia cell lines. *Leuk Res* 2007;31:497–506.

73. Flatau E, Gonzales FA, Michalowsky LA, et al. DNA methylation in 5-aza-2′-deoxycytidine-resistant variants of C3H 10T1/2 C18 cells. *Mol Cell Biol* 1984;4:2098–2102.

74. Chan KK, Giannini DD, Staroscik JA, et al. 5-Azacytidine hydrolysis kinetics measured by high-pressure liquid chromatography and 13C-NMR spectroscopy. *J Pharm Sci* 1979;68:807–812.

75. Gore SD, Weng LJ, Figg WD, et al. Impact of prolonged infusions of the putative differentiating agent sodium phenylbutyrate on myelodysplastic syndromes and acute myeloid leukemia. *Clin Cancer Res* 2002;8:963–970.

76. Yu L, Liu C, Vandeusen J, et al. Global assessment of promoter methylation in a mouse model of cancer identifies ID4 as a putative tumor-suppressor gene in human leukemia. *Nat Genet* 2005;37:265–274.

77. Blum W, Klisovic RB, Hackanson B, et al. Phase I study of decitabine alone or in combination with valproic acid in acute myeloid leukemia. *J Clin Oncol* 2007;25:3884–3891.

78. Schrump DS, Fischette MR, Nguyen DM, et al. Phase I study of decitabine-mediated gene expression in patients with cancers involving the lungs, esophagus, or pleura. *Clin Cancer Res* 2006;12:5777–5785.

79. Garcia-Manero G, Gore SD, Cogle C, et al. Phase I study of oral azacitidine in myelodysplastic syndromes, chronic myelomonocytic leukemia, and acute myeloid leukemia. *J Clin Oncol* 2011;29:2521–2527.

80. Issa JP, Roboz G, Rizzieri D, et al. Abstract LB-214: Interim results from a randomized Phase 1-2 first-in-human (FIH) study of PK/PD guided escalating doses of SGI-110, a novel subcutaneous (SQ) second generation hypomethylating

agent (HMA) in relapsed/refractory MDS and AML. *Cancer Res* 2012;72: LB–214.

81. Mund C, Lyko F. Epigenetic cancer therapy: Proof of concept and remaining challenges. *Bioessays* 2010;32:949–957.

82. Popovic R, Licht JD. Emerging epigenetic targets and therapies in cancer medicine. *Cancer Discov* 2012;2:405–413.

83. Verbrugge I, Johnstone RW, Bots M. Promises and challenges of anticancer drugs that target the epigenome. *Epigenomics* 2011;3:547–565.

84. Robert C, Rassool FV. HDAC inhibitors: roles of DNA damage and repair. *Adv Cancer Res* 2012;116:87–129.

85. Kachhap SK, Rosmus N, Collis SJ, et al. Downregulation of homologous recombination DNA repair genes by HDAC inhibition in prostate cancer is mediated through the E2F1 transcription factor. *PLoS One* 2010;5:e11208.

86. Sharma SV, Lee DY, Li B, et al. A chromatin-mediated reversible drug-tolerant state in cancer cell subpopulations. *Cell* 2010;141:69–80.

87. Villanueva J, Vultur A, Lee JT, et al. Acquired resistance to BRAF inhibitors mediated by a RAF kinase switch in melanoma can be overcome by cotargeting MEK and IGF-1R/PI3K. *Cancer Cell* 2010;18:683–695.

88. Novogrodsky A, Dvir A, Ravid A, et al. Effect of polar organic compounds on leukemic cells. Butyrate-induced partial remission of acute myelogenous leukemia in a child. *Cancer* 1983;51:9–14.

89. Miller AA, Kurschel E, Osieka R, et al. Clinical pharmacology of sodium butyrate in patients with acute leukemia. *Eur J Cancer Clin Oncol* 1987; 23:1283–1287.

90. Gore SD, Weng LJ, Zhai S, et al. Impact of the putative differentiating agent sodium phenylbutyrate on myelodysplastic syndromes and acute myeloid leukemia. *Clin Cancer Res* 2001;7:2330–2339.

91. Gore SD, Weng LJ, Figg WD, et al. Impact of prolonged infusions of the putative differentiating agent sodium phenylbutyrate on myelodysplastic syndromes and acute myeloid leukemia. *Clin Cancer Res* 2002;8:963–970.

92. DiGiuseppe JA, Weng LJ, Yu KH, et al. Phenylbutyrate-induced G1 arrest and apoptosis in myeloid leukemia cells: structure-function analysis. *Leukemia* 1999;13:1243–1253.

93. Kuendgen A, Strupp C, Aivado M, et al. Treatment of myelodysplastic syndromes with valproic acid alone or in combination with all-trans retinoic acid. *Blood* 2004;104:1266–1269.

94. Pilatrino C, Cilloni D, Messa E, et al. Increase in platelet count in older, poor-risk patients with acute myeloid leukemia or myelodysplastic syndrome treated with valproic acid and all-trans retinoic acid. *Cancer* 2005;104:101–109.

95. Fizzotti M, Cimino G, Pisegna S, et al. Detection of homozygous deletions of the cyclin-dependent kinase 4 inhibitor (p16) gene in acute lymphoblastic leukemia and association with adverse prognostic features. *Blood* 1995; 85:2685–2690.

96. Xu GL, Bestor TH, Bourc'his D, et al. Chromosome instability and immunodeficiency syndrome caused by mutations in a DNA methyltransferase gene. *Nature* 1999;402:187–191.

97. Duvic M, Talpur R, Ni X, et al. Phase 2 trial of oral vorinostat (suberoylanilide hydroxamic acid, SAHA) for refractory cutaneous T-cell lymphoma (CTCL). *Blood* 2007;109:31–39.

98. Olsen EA, Kim YH, Kuzel TM, et al. Phase IIb multicenter trial of vorinostat in patients with persistent, progressive, or treatment refractory cutaneous T-cell lymphoma. *J Clin Oncol* 2007;25:3109–3115.

99. O'Connor OA, Heaney ML, Schwartz L, et al. Clinical experience with intravenous and oral formulations of the novel histone deacetylase inhibitor suberoylanilide hydroxamic acid in patients with advanced hematologic malignancies. *J Clin Oncol* 2006;24:166–173.

100. Ramalingam SS, Maitland ML, Frankel P, et al. Carboplatin and Paclitaxel in combination with either vorinostat or placebo for first-line therapy of advanced non-small-cell lung cancer. *J Clin Oncol* 2010;28:56–62.

101. Giles F, Fischer T, Cortes J, et al. A phase I study of intravenous LBH589, a novel cinnamic hydroxamic acid analogue histone deacetylase inhibitor, in patients with refractory hematologic malignancies. *Clin Cancer Res* 2006; 12:4628–4635.

102. Richardson PG, Hungria VTM, Yoon S-S, et al. Panorama 1: A randomized, double-blind, phase 3 study of panobinostat or placebo plus bortezomib and dexamethasone in relapsed or relapsed and refractory multiple myeloma. *ASCO Meeting Abstracts* 2014;32:8510.

103. Piekarz RL, Robey R, Sandor V, et al. Inhibitor of histone deacetylation, depsipeptide (FR901228), in the treatment of peripheral and cutaneous T-cell lymphoma: a case report. *Blood* 2001;98:2865–2868.

104. Coiffier B, Pro B, Prince HM, et al. Romidepsin for the treatment of relapsed/refractory peripheral T-cell lymphoma: pivotal study update demonstrates durable responses. *J Hematol Oncol* 2014;7:11.

105. Coiffier B, Pro B, Prince HM, et al. Results from a pivotal, open-label, phase II study of romidepsin in relapsed or refractory peripheral T-cell lymphoma after prior systemic therapy. *J Clin Oncol* 2012;30:631–636.

106. Piekarz RL, Frye AR, Wright JJ, et al. Cardiac studies in patients treated with depsipeptide, FK228, in a phase II trial for T-cell lymphoma. *Clin Cancer Res* 2006;12:3762–3773.

107. Gojo I, Jiemjit A, Trepel JB, et al. Phase 1 and pharmacologic study of MS-275, a histone deacetylase inhibitor, in adults with refractory and relapsed acute leukemias. *Blood* 2007;109:2781–2790.

108. Prebet T, Sun Z, Figueroa ME, et al. Prolonged administration of azacitidine with or without entinostat for myelodysplastic syndrome and acute myeloid leukemia with myelodysplasia-related changes: results of the US Leukemia Intergroup Trial E1905. *J Clin Oncol* 2014;32:1242–1248.

109. Witta SE, Jotte RM, Konduri K, et al. Randomized phase II trial of erlotinib with and without entinostat in patients with advanced non-small-cell lung cancer who progressed on prior chemotherapy. *J Clin Oncol* 2012;30:2248–2255.

110. Yardley DA, Ismail-Khan RR, Melichar B, et al. Randomized phase II, double-blind, placebo-controlled study of exemestane with or without entinostat in postmenopausal women with locally recurrent or metastatic estrogen receptor-positive breast cancer progressing on treatment with a nonsteroidal aromatase inhibitor. *J Clin Oncol* 2013;31:2128–2135.

111. Byrd JC, Marcucci G, Parthun MR, et al. A phase 1 and pharmacodynamic study of depsipeptide (FK228) in chronic lymphocytic leukemia and acute myeloid leukemia. *Blood* 2005;105:959–967.

112. Charache S, Dover G, Smith K, et al. Treatment of sickle cell anemia with 5-azacytidine results in increased fetal hemoglobin production and is associated with nonrandom hypomethylation of DNA around the gamma-delta-beta-globin gene complex. *Proc Natl Acad Sci U S A* 1983;80:4842–4846.

113. Silverman LR, Holland JF, Weinberg RS, et al. Effects of treatment with 5-azacytidine on the in vivo and in vitro hematopoiesis in patients with myelodysplastic syndromes. *Leukemia* 1993;7:21–29.

114. Silverman LR, McKenzie DR, Peterson BL, et al. Further analysis of trials with azacitidine in patients with myelodysplastic syndrome: studies 8421, 8921, and 9221 by the Cancer and Leukemia Group B. *J Clin Oncol* 2006;24:3895–3903.

115. Silverman LR, Demakos EP, Peterson BL, et al. Randomized controlled trial of azacitidine in patients with the myelodysplastic syndrome: a study of the Cancer and Leukemia Group B. *J Clin Oncol* 2002;20:2429–2440.

116. Fenaux P, Mufti GJ, Hellstrom-Lindberg E, et al. Efficacy of azacitidine compared with that of conventional care regimens in the treatment of higher-risk myelodysplastic syndromes: a randomised, open-label, phase III study. *Lancet Oncol* 2009;10:223–232.

117. Fenaux P, Mufti GJ, Hellstrom-Lindberg E, et al. Azacitidine prolongs overall survival compared with conventional care regimens in elderly patients with low bone marrow blast count acute myeloid leukemia. *J Clin Oncol* 2010;28: 562–569.

118. Wijermans P, Lubbert M, Verhoef G, et al. Low-dose 5-aza-2'-deoxycytidine, a DNA hypomethylating agent, for the treatment of high-risk myelodysplastic syndrome: a multicenter phase II study in elderly patients. *J Clin Oncol* 2000;18:956–962.

119. Wijermans PW, Krulder JW, Huijgens PC, et al. Continuous infusion of low-dose 5-Aza-2'-deoxycytidine in elderly patients with high-risk myelodysplastic syndrome. *Leukemia* 1997;11:1–5.

120. Kantarjian HM, O'Brien S, Cortes J, et al. Results of decitabine (5-aza-2'deoxycytidine) therapy in 130 patients with chronic myelogenous leukemia. *Cancer* 2003;98:522–528.

121. Kantarjian H, Oki Y, Garcia-Manero G, et al. Results of a randomized study of 3 schedules of low-dose decitabine in higher-risk myelodysplastic syndrome and chronic myelomonocytic leukemia. *Blood* 2007;109:52–57.

122. Steensma DP, Baer MR, Slack JL, et al. Multicenter study of decitabine administered daily for 5 days every 4 weeks to adults with myelodysplastic syndromes: the alternative dosing for outpatient treatment (ADOPT) trial. *J Clin Oncol* 2009;27:3842–3848.

123. Kantarjian H, Issa JP, Rosenfeld CS, et al. Decitabine improves patient outcomes in myelodysplastic syndromes: results of a phase III randomized study. *Cancer* 2006;106:1794–1803.

124. WijerMans P, Suciu S, Baila L, et al. Low-dose decitabine versus best supportive care in elderly patients with intermediate or high risk MDS not eligible for intensive chemotherapy: final results of the randomized phase III study (06011) of the EORTC Leukemia and German MDS Study Groups. *ASH Annual Meeting Abstracts* 2008;112:226.

125. Flotho C, Claus R, Batz C, et al. The DNA methyltransferase inhibitors azacitidine, decitabine and zebularine exert differential effects on cancer gene expression in acute myeloid leukemia cells. *Leukemia* 2009;23:1019–1028.

126. Lübbert M, Suciu S, Baila L, et al. Low-dose decitabine versus best supportive care in elderly patients with intermediate- or high-risk myelodysplastic syndrome (MDS) ineligible for intensive chemotherapy: final results of the randomized phase III study (06011) of the European Organisation for Research and Treatment of Cancer Leukemia Group and the German MDS Study Group. *J Clin Oncol* 2011;29:1987–1996.

127. Kantarjian HM, Thomas XG, Dmoszynska A, et al. Multicenter, randomized, open-label, phase III trial of decitabine versus patient choice, with physician advice, of either supportive care or low-dose cytarabine for the treatment of older patients with newly diagnosed acute myeloid leukemia. *J Clin Oncol* 2012;30:2670–2677.

128. Sudan N, Rossetti JM, Shadduck RK, et al. Treatment of acute myelogenous leukemia with outpatient azacitidine. *Cancer* 2006;107:1839–1843.

129. Kantarjian HM, O'Brien SM, Keating M, et al. Results of decitabine therapy in the accelerated and blastic phases of chronic myelogenous leukemia. *Leukemia* 1997;11:1617–1620.

130. Ruter B, Wijermans P, Claus R, et al. Preferential cytogenetic response to continuous intravenous low-dose decitabine (DAC) administration in myelodysplastic syndrome with monosomy 7. *Blood* 2007;110:1080–1082.

131. Raj K, John A, Ho A, et al. CDKN2B methylation status and isolated chromosome 7 abnormalities predict responses to treatment with 5-azacytidine. *Leukemia* 2007;21:1937–1944.

132. Ravandi F, Issa JP, Garcia-Manero G, et al. Superior outcome with hypomethylating therapy in patients with acute myeloid leukemia and high-risk myelodysplastic syndrome and chromosome 5 and 7 abnormalities. *Cancer* 2009;115:5746–5751.

CANCER THERAPEUTICS

133. Yang AS, Doshi KD, Choi SW, et al. DNA methylation changes after 5-aza-2'-deoxycytidine therapy in patients with leukemia. *Cancer Res* 2006;66:5495–5503.

134. Yang AS, Estecio MR, Doshi K, et al. A simple method for estimating global DNA methylation using bisulfite PCR of repetitive DNA elements. *Nucleic Acids Res* 2004;32:e38.

135. Daskalakis M, Nguyen TT, Nguyen C, et al. Demethylation of a hypermethylated P15/INK4B gene in patients with myelodysplastic syndrome by 5-Aza-2'-deoxycytidine (decitabine) treatment. *Blood* 2002;100:2957–2964.

136. Bakkenist CJ, Kastan MB. DNA damage activates ATM through intermolecular autophosphorylation and dimer dissociation. *Nature* 2003;421:499–506.

137. Borthakur G, Ahdab SE, Ravandi F, et al. Activity of decitabine in patients with myelodysplastic syndrome previously treated with azacitidine. *Leuk Lymphoma* 2008;49:690–695.

138. Shen L, Kantarjian H, Guo Y, et al. DNA methylation predicts survival and response to therapy in patients with myelodysplastic syndromes. *J Clin Oncol* 2010;28:605–613.

139. Figueroa ME, Skrabanek L, Li Y, et al. MDS and secondary AML display unique patterns and abundance of aberrant DNA methylation. *Blood* 2009;114:3448–3458.

140. Fandy TE, Herman JG, Kerns P, et al. Early epigenetic changes and DNA damage do not predict clinical response in an overlapping schedule of 5-azacytidine and entinostat in patients with myeloid malignancies. *Blood* 2009;114:2764–2773.

141. Schuebel KE, Chen W, Cope L, et al. Comparing the DNA hypermethylome with gene mutations in human colorectal cancer. *PLoS Genet* 2007;3:1709–1723.

142. Maslak P, Chanel S, Camacho LH, et al. Pilot study of combination transcriptional modulation therapy with sodium phenylbutyrate and 5-azacytidine in patients with acute myeloid leukemia or myelodysplastic syndrome. *Leukemia* 2006;20:212–217.

143. Garcia-Manero G, Kantarjian HM, Sanchez-Gonzalez B, et al. Phase I/II study of the combination of 5-aza-2'-deoxycytidine with valproic acid in patients with leukemia. *Blood* 2006;108:3271–3279.

144. Soriano AO, Yang H, Faderl S, et al. Safety and clinical activity of the combination of 5-azacytidine, valproic acid, and all-trans retinoic acid in acute myeloid leukemia and myelodysplastic syndrome. *Blood* 2007;110:2302–2308.

145. Voso MT, Santini V, Finelli C, et al. Valproic acid at therapeutic plasma levels may increase 5-azacytidine efficacy in higher risk myelodysplastic syndromes. *Clin Cancer Res* 2009;15:5002–5007.

146. Sharma S, Kelly TK, Jones PA. Epigenetics in cancer. *Carcinogenesis* 2010;31:27–36.

147. Silverman LR, Fenaux P, Mufti GJ, et al. Continued azacitidine therapy beyond time of first response improves quality of response in patients with higher-risk myelodysplastic syndromes. *Cancer* 2011;117:2697–2702.

148. Craddock C, Quek L, Goardon N, et al. Azacitidine fails to eradicate leukemic stem/progenitor cell populations in patients with acute myeloid leukemia and myelodysplasia. *Leukemia* 2013;27:1028–1036.

149. Juergens RA, Wrangle J, Vendetti FP, et al. Combination epigenetic therapy has efficacy in patients with refractory advanced non-small cell lung cancer. *Cancer Discov* 2011;1: 598–607.

150. Wrangle J, Wang W, Koch A, et al. Alterations of immune response of Non-Small Cell Lung Cancer with Azacytidine. *Oncotarget* 2013;4:2067–2079.

151. Shakya R, Gonda TA, Quante M, et al. Hypomethylating therapy in an aggressive stroma-rich model of pancreatic carcinoma. *Cancer Res* 2013;73: 885–896.

152. Humeniuk R, Menon LG, Mishra PJ, et al. Decreased levels of UMP kinase as a mechanism of fluoropyrimidine resistance. *Mol Cancer Ther* 2009;8: 1037–1044.

153. Meng F, Sun G, Zhong M, et al. Anticancer efficacy of the combination of low-dose cisplatin and trichostatin A or 5-aza-2'-deoxycytidine in ovarian cancer cells. Paper presented at: 2012 ASCO Annual Meeting; 2012; Chicago, IL.

154. Matei D, Fang F, Shen C, et al. Epigenetic resensitization to platinum in ovarian cancer. *Cancer Res* 2012;72:2197–2205.

155. Fu S, Hu W, Iyer R, et al. Phase 1b-2a study to reverse platinum resistance through use of a hypomethylating agent, azacitidine, in patients with platinum-resistant or platinum-refractory epithelial ovarian cancer. *Cancer* 2011;117:1661–1669.

156. Chung CW, Coste H, White JH, et al. Discovery and characterization of small molecule inhibitors of the BET family bromodomains. *J Med Chem* 2011;54:3827–3838.

157. Bernt KM, Zhu N, Sinha AU, et al. MLL-rearranged leukemia is dependent on aberrant H3K79 methylation by DOT1L. *Cancer Cell* 2011;20:66–78.

158. Daigle SR, Olhava EJ, Therkelsen CA, et al. Selective killing of mixed lineage leukemia cells by a potent small-molecule DOT1L inhibitor. *Cancer Cell* 2011;20:53–65.

159. Spannhoff A, Hauser AT, Heinke R, et al. The emerging therapeutic potential of histone methyltransferase and demethylase inhibitors. *ChemMedChem* 2009;4:1568–1582.

160. Okada Y, Feng Q, Lin Y, et al. hDOT1L links histone methylation to leukemogenesis. *Cell* 2005;121:167–178.

# 24 Proteasome Inhibitors

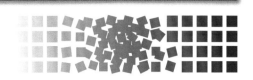

Christopher J. Kirk, Brian B. Tuch, Shirin Arastu-Kapur, and Lawrence H. Boise

## BIOCHEMISTRY OF THE UBIQUITIN-PROTEASOME PATHWAY

The ubiquitin proteasome system is involved in the degradation of more than 80% of cellular proteins, including those that control cell-cycle progression, apoptosis, DNA repair, and the stress response.[1] A key step in this process is the *tagging* of proteins targeted for degradation with multiple copies of ubiquitin, a 76–amino acid protein whose primary sequence and structure is highly conserved in organisms ranging from yeasts to mammals.[2,3] Once polyubiquitinated, proteins targeted for degradation bind to the 26S proteasome, a holoenzyme composed of two 19S regulatory complexes capping a central 20S proteolytic core. The 20S core is a hollow "barrel" consisting of four stacked heptameric rings. The subunits of the rings are classified as either β subunits (outer two rings) or β subunits (inner two rings). The 19S regulatory complex consists of a lid that recognizes ubiquitinated protein substrates with high fidelity, and a base that contains six adenosine triphosphatases, unfolds protein substrates, removes the polyubiquitin tag, and threads them into the catalytic chamber of the 20S particle in an adenosine triphosphate–dependent manner.[4,5] Unlike typical proteases, the 20S proteasome in eukaryotic cells contains multiple proteolytic activities resulting in the cleavage of protein targets after many different amino acids. In most cells, the 20S core particle contains the catalytic subunits β5 (PSMB5), β1 (PSMB1), and β2 (PSMB2), accounting for chymotrypsinlike (CT-L), caspaselike (C-L), and trypsinlike (T-L) activities, respectively, each differing in their substrate preference.[6] However, in cells of hematopoietic origin, such as lymphocytes and monocytes, the proteasome catalytic subunits are encoded by homologous gene products: LMP7 (PSMB8), LMP2 (PSMB9), and MECL-1 (PSMB10).[7] These immunoproteasome subunits are also induced in nonhematopoietic cells following exposure to inflammatory cytokines such as interferon-γ (IFN-γ) and tumor necrosis factor alpha (TNF-α).[8] In the immunoproteasome, the 19S regulatory complex can be replaced with proteasome activators such as PA28, whose expression is also induced in cells following exposure to IFN-γ. Hybrid proteasomes, both for the catalytic subunits and regulatory particles, have been described.[9]

Given its key role in maintaining cellular homeostasis, the ubiquitin proteasome system appeared to be an unlikely target for pharmaceutical intervention. However, a variety of groundbreaking studies in the 1990s suggested that inhibitors of proteasome function might prove to be viable therapeutic agents.[10] Initial studies used substrate-related peptide aldehydes to investigate the proteolytic functions and specificity of the proteasome.[11] In vitro and in vivo studies with these inhibitors demonstrated their ability to induce apoptosis as well as inhibit tumor growth.[12–15] It was subsequently discovered that several natural products with antitumor activity exert their action via proteasome inhibition, providing additional rationale for the development of selective proteasome inhibitors (PIs).[16,17]

## PROTEASOME INHIBITORS

### Chemical Classes of Proteasome Inhibitors in Clinical Development

As of the writing of this overview, six different proteasome inhibitors comprising three distinct chemical classes have been tested in clinical trials (Table 24.1) and include: (1) dipeptide boronic acids, (2) peptide epoxy ketones, and (3) β-lactones.[18,19] Bortezomib (PS-341, Velcade), a dipeptide boronic acid, was developed by Millennium Pharmaceuticals (Cambridge, MA) and was the first PI approved for clinical use.[20] Two additional dipeptide boronic acids have entered clinical development, ixazomib/MLN 9708 (Millennium), currently in phase III studies, and delanzomib/CEP-18770 (Teva Pharmaceuticals; Frazer, PA), the clinical development of which has been halted. Carfilzomib (Onyx Pharmaceuticals; San Francisco, CA), a tetrapeptide epoxy ketone, received U.S. Food and Drug Administration (FDA) approval in 2012.[21] A second peptide epoxy ketone proteasome inhibitor, oprozomib (Onyx), entered clinical study in 2010. The third class of proteasome inhibitors, β-lactones, is represented by NPI-0052 (salinosporamide A [Marizomib]) and is currently being developed by Nereus Pharmaceuticals, Inc. (San Diego, CA). The initial approvals for both bortezomib and carfilzomib were in multiple myeloma (MM), a plasma cell neoplasm and the second most common hematologic cancer. However, the activity of PIs in other B-cell neoplasms has resulted in an expansion of the clinical utilization of this drug class.

### Preclinical Activity of Proteasome Inhibitors

Each of the three classes of inhibitors has a distinct chemical mechanism of proteasome inhibition.[22] Peptide boronates form stable but reversible tetrahedral intermediates with the γ-hydroxyl (γ-OH) group of the catalytic N-terminal threonine of the proteasome active sites.[23,24] β-lactones also interact with this γ-OH, but form a completely irreversible interaction.[25] Similarly, peptide epoxy ketones form irreversible covalent adducts with the active site threonine but do so via a dual covalent adduction of γ-OH group and the free amine.[26] This interaction is highly specific for N-terminal threonine-containing hydrolases and renders peptide epoxy ketones the most selective proteasome inhibitors yet described.[27,28]

The primary targets of these PIs within the constitutive and immunoproteasomes are the CT-L subunits, β5 and LMP7, respectively. Despite accounting for less than 50% of total protein turnover by the proteasome, these subunits are essential for cell survival.[29] In MM cell lines, inhibiting both subunits (β5 and LMP7) is necessary and sufficient for tumor cell death.[30] Cytotoxicity of other tumor cell types requires the inhibition of multiple active sites beyond the CT-L activity. The combination of inhibitors specific for either the T-L or C-L activities, which have no cytotoxic activity on their own, augments the cytotoxic potential of the CT-L–specific inhibitors.[31,32]

## TABLE 24.1

**Proteasome Inhibitors in Clinical Development**

| Agent | Other Names | Drug Class | Stage of Development | Tumor Types | Route of Administration | Dose Levels | Schedule of Administration |
|---|---|---|---|---|---|---|---|
| Bortezomib | Velcade PS-341 | Peptide boronate | FDA/EMEA approved | Multiple myeloma, mantle cell lymphoma | Intravenous, subcutaneous | 1.3 mg/m$^2$ | Days 1, 4, 8, & 11 (21-day cycle) |
| Ixazomib | MLN 9708 MLN 2238 | Peptide boronate | Phase III | Multiple myeloma, AL, amyloidosis | Oral | 4 mg | Once weekly (21-day cycle) |
| Delanzomib | CEP-18770 | Peptide boronate | Phase I (discontinued) | Multiple myeloma | Intravenous | 0.1–1.8 mg/m$^2$ | Days 1, 4, 8, & 11 (21-day cycle) |
| Carfilzomib | Kyprolis PR-171 | Peptide epoxy ketone | FDA approved, phase III | Multiple myeloma | Intravenous | 20/27 mg/m$^2$ | Days 1, 2, 8, 9, 15, & 16 (28-day cycle) |
| Oprozomib | ONX 0912 PR-047 | Peptide epoxy ketone | Phase I/II | Multiple myeloma | Oral | 150–240 mg (dose escalation ongoing) | Days 1, 2, 8, & 9 (14-day cycle) Days 1–5 (14-day cycle) |
| Marizomib | NPI-0052 Salinosporamide A | β-lactone | Phase II | Multiple myeloma | Intravenous | 0.075–0.6 mg/m$^2$ | Days 1, 4, 8, & 11 (21-day cycle) |

EMEA, European Medicines Agency; AL, amyloid light chain.

Given its status as the first proteasome inhibitor approved for marketed use, the antitumor potential and preclinical activity of other proteasome inhibitors have generally been compared to bortezomib.[19] Carfilzomib showed equivalent antitumor activity to bortezomib in vitro against a panel of tumor cell lines under standard culture conditions but was >10-fold more potent at inducing tumor cell death when cells were exposed to drug for a 1-hour pulse, which mimics the pharmacokinetics of both compounds.[33] MLN2238 (the active agent of ixazomib) was active in the same mouse models of human tumors as bortezomib, but demonstrated greater levels of proteasome inhibition in the tumors.[34] In biochemical assays of proteasome activity, delanzomib had an identical potency and subunit activity profile to bortezomib, but in tumor cytotoxicity assays, potency relative to bortezomib was 2- to 10-fold less.[35] In addition, delanzomib appeared to be less cytotoxic than bortezomib to normal cells and had a differential effect on cytokine release in bone marrow stromal cells, suggesting a different pharmacologic activity. Oprozomib is 10-fold less potent than carfilzomib in proteasome activity assays, but showed similar antitumor activity in mouse tumor models.[36,37] Marizomib displayed greater potency against the non–CT-L active sites of the proteasome than bortezomib.[38] Interestingly, this agent synergized with bortezomib in killing tumor cells in vitro.[39] All of the second-generation inhibitors have shown activity in tumor cells made resistant to bortezomib and/or MM cells isolated from patients relapsed from bortezomib-based therapies[35,36,40–42]

The inhibition of tumor cells with proteasome inhibitors induces cell death via the induction of apoptosis through death effector caspase activation.[10] Although the mechanism underlying the induction of cell death remains to be fully elucidated, extensive research suggests a complex interplay of multiple pathways. PIs have been shown to affect the half-life of the *BH3-only* members of the Bcl-2 family, specifically BH3–interacting-domain death agonist (Bid) and Bcl-2 interacting killer (Bik).[43] Moreover the BH3-only protein NOXA is upregulated at the transcription level by PIs.[44–48] Proteasome inhibition also upregulates the expression of several key cell-cycle checkpoint proteins that include p53 (an inducer of G0/G1 cell-cycle arrest through accumulation of the cyclin-dependent kinase [CDK] inhibitor p27); the CDK inhibitor p21;

mammalian cyclins A, B, D, and E; and transcription factors E2F and Rb.[49,50] The transcription factor nuclear factor kappa B (NF-κB), an important regulator of cell survival and cytokine/growth factor production,[51] is also affected by proteasome inhibition in multiple ways. The net effect on NF-κB signaling is not consistent across various assays and cell lines, and its relative importance in the antitumor effects of PIs remains unclear. Although it is interesting to note that patients whose myeloma harbor NF-κB–activating mutations (~20%) respond better to bortezomib than those without NF-κB–activating mutations.[52–54] In MM cell lines, there is growing evidence that the major determinant of sensitivity to proteasome inhibition is the relative load of protein flux to the proteasome.[55–57] These data suggest that induction of the terminal unfolded protein response may drive cell death. Whether proteotoxic stress induced cell death reflects sensitivity to proteasome inhibitors in other tumor types remains to be determined.

## Pharmacokinetics and Pharmacodynamics of Proteasome Inhibitors in Animals

Following intravenous (IV) administration to animals and humans, proteasome activity is inhibited in a dose-dependent fashion within minutes; however, PIs such as bortezomib and carfilzomib are also rapidly cleared from circulation.[55,56,58–61] Recovery of proteasome activity in animals occurs in tissues with a half-life of approximately 24 hours, mirroring the recovery time of cells exposed to sublethal concentrations of PIs in vitro and likely reflecting new protein synthesis.[33,62]

## PROTEASOME INHIBITORS IN CANCER

### Clinical Activity of Bortezomib

Bortezomib is typically administered on days 1, 4, 8, and 11 of a 3-week cycle either as an IV bolus or subcutaneous administration. Increasing doses of bortezomib inhibit proteasome activity in blood in a dose-dependent fashion, reaching a maximum of 74% inhibition at a dose of 1.38 mg/m$^2$. Daily dosing schedules in animal studies have been associated with severe toxicity and have not been attempted in humans. In clinical trials, thrombocytopenia and peripheral neuropathy (PN) were common adverse events.[20,63,64] Bortezomib has shown remarkable single-agent antitumor activity in a wide range of B-cell neoplasms, including MM, non Hodgkin lymphoma (NHL), and Waldenström macroglobulinemia (WM). In 2003, bortezomib was approved by the FDA for use as a single agent for the treatment of patients with MM following two prior therapies and who demonstrated disease progression with their most recent therapy. The primary efficacy data for this approval was derived from the SUMMIT trial in which 202 patients with heavily pretreated disease were treated with bortezomib at 1.3 mg/m$^2$.[65] In this trial, the overall response rate (ORR), defined as patients achieving at least a 50% reduction in serum or urine levels of the myeloma M protein, was 35%. This clinical trial was supported by the CREST trial, in which the activity of 1.3 mg/m$^2$ dose was determined to be superior to a dose of 1.0 mg/m$^2$.[66] Bortezomib is also active as a single agent in earlier stage MM patient populations. A single-agent ORR of 38%, with a 6% complete response (CR) rate, was seen in the phase III APEX study in early relapsed MM, with a time to progression (TTP) of 6.2 months and a median duration of response of 8 months.[67] In this study, the major grade 3 and 4 toxicities were PN, 12%; dysesthesia and related symptoms, 8% to 10%; anemia, 8%; diarrhea, 8%; neutropenia, 14%; and fatigue, 12%. In the frontline setting, bortezomib demonstrated a single-agent response rate of 41% (5% CR rate).[68]

Bortezomib is also approved for newly diagnosed MM in combination with velcade, melphalan and prednisone (VMP). The phase III VISTA trial evaluated VMP in patients with untreated MM who were ineligible for high-dose therapy.[69] The addition of bortezomib to the melphalan prednisone (MP) backbone significantly improved response rates in this setting with an ORR of 71% for VMP (including 30% CR) versus 35% (with only 4% CR) for MP.[52] VMP was associated with a TTP of ~24 months, compared with ~16.6 months with MP. After a 5-year follow-up, there was a 31% reduced risk of death for the VMP group versus MP-treated patients.[70]

Bortezomib has also shown promise when combined with other agents in relapsed and refractory MM patients. The combination of bortezomib with pegylated doxorubicin (Doxil, Centocor Ortho Biotech Products, L.P.; Horsham, PA) resulted in an ORR of 79% in relapsed patients, and toxicities were similar to those observed with each agent administered separately.[71] A phase III study in 646 patients with relapsed and refractory MM compared this treatment with bortezomib alone; the combination produced a 44% ORR and extended the TTP from 6 to 9.3 months.[72,73] The combination of bortezomib with revlimid, lenalidomide and dexamethasone (Rd), a standard of care in the treatment of MM, resulted in an ORR of 64% and a median duration of response of 8.7 months.[74] This activity is striking given that 53% of patients had received prior bortezomib and 75% of patients had received prior thalidomide, a closely related analog of lenalidomide. Other agents tested in combination with bortezomib include vorinostat, the anti-CS1 mAb, elotuzumab, the Hsp90 inhibitor tanespimycin, and the Akt inhibitor perifosine.[75]

Frontline combinations with bortezomib in MM patients have shown high ORRs with a notable improvement in CR rates. In longer term studies, CR rates with bortezomib-based combinations have been shown to be associated with improved clinical outcomes.[63,64] A community-based phase IIIb study evaluating bortezomib + dexamethasone (VD) versus bortezomib + thalidomide + dexamethasone (VTD) versus VMP found similar ORR (60%, 70%, and 52%, respectively) and CR rates (13%, 18%, and 15%, respectively).[63] Bortezomib + melphalan + prednisone + thalidomide (VMPT) followed by bortezomib + thalidomide (VT) maintenance resulted in a superior CR rate compared with VMP with no maintenance (34% versus 21%) and improved 2-year progression-free survival (70% versus 58.2%).[64] A protocol modification in this trial involved changing from twice weekly

to weekly bortezomib administration, which yielded similar TTP but reduced the incidence (21% versus 43%) and severity of PN (2% grade 3/4 versus 14%).[64] The bortezomib, lenalidomide, and dexamethasone combination in newly diagnosed MM resulted in a ORR of 100% in 66 patients, 29% of whom achieved a CR.[76]

Bortezomib has also shown activity in other hematologic cancers, most notably mantle cell lymphoma (MCL).[77,78] As a single agent in 155 relapsed and refractory MCL patients, bortezomib yielded an ORR of 33% (8% CR), a median duration of response of 9.2 months, and a TTP of 6.2 months.[78] Toxicities observed were similar to those seen in patients with MM and included thrombocytopenia, PN, and fatigue. When bortezomib was used to treat both newly diagnosed and refractory MCL, a response rate of 46% was observed in both populations,[77] leading to FDA approval late in 2006.

Bortezomib has been tested in a variety of solid tumors in phase I and II studies.[79] Partial responses (PR) were reported in 8% of patients with refractory non–small-cell lung cancer (NSCLC), although the TTP was 1.5 months.[80] Exacerbation of PN was common. Bortezomib was subsequently tested in combination with paclitaxel, irinotecan, and gemcitabine/carboplatin; however, results have not been encouraging. Bortezomib continues to be tested in combination with other agents in a variety of tumor types.[81,82]

Recent clinical activity and preclinical data suggest that proteasome inhibition may extend to nononcology applications. Single-agent bortezomib therapy in kidney transplant patients undergoing antibody-mediated rejection resulted in a reduction of donor-specific antibodies and improved renal function.[83] In mouse models of lupus nephritis, bortezomib resulted in a reduction of pathogenic plasma cells and the prevention of disease progression.[84] These data suggest that PIs may be useful in a wide range of B-cell–mediated diseases. However, toxicities with bortezomib, particularly PN, may prevent wider application of this particular agent.

## Carfilzomib

Parallel phase I studies of carfilzomib have been conducted in patients with multiple tumor types, and two phase I dose-finding studies targeting B-cell malignancies have been completed. The first study used daily IV bolus dosing with doses up to 20 mg/m$^2$ for 5 consecutive days followed by 9 days of rest and resulted in substantial inhibition of proteasome activity.[85] In the second study, carfilzomib was administered daily for 2 days for 3 consecutive weeks (days 1, 2, 8, 9, 15, and 16), followed by 12 days of recovery.[86] Hematologic toxicities were the most frequent adverse events, observed along with transient, noncumulative elevations in serum creatinine, usually with increases in serum urea nitrogen and consistent with a *prerenal* etiology. New onset PN was infrequent. Among 20 evaluable patients (including bortezomib-refractory patients), 4 PRs and 1 minor response were seen. Responses were also durable, lasting more than 1 year in some cases. Although the maximum tolerated dose of carfilzomib was not established in this study, a dose of 20 mg/m$^2$ was initially selected for the phase II studies.

Based on the phase I studies, an open-label, single-arm, phase II study of single-agent carfilzomib in relapsed and refractory MM was initiated in 2007.[87,88] Carfilzomib was administered as an IV bolus on the twice-weekly dose schedule. Patients enrolled in the initial phase of the study (003-A0) had received a median of five prior therapies, and 78% of patients had grade 1/2 PN at entry.[87] Among 39 evaluable patients in 003-A0, 10 (26%) achieved a minor response or better, including 5 PRs, and 16 additional patients with stable disease. Based on new safety information from phase I studies, the protocol was amended and the carfilzomib dose was escalated to 27 mg/m$^2$ after the first cycle (003-A1).[89] In this trial, 266 patients were enrolled and all patients had previously been treated with an immunomodulatory agent (IMiD) and bortezomib and were refractory to their last therapy. An ORR of 24% with a median duration of response of 8 months was reported. Adverse events were predominantly hematopoietic (thrombocytopenia, lymphopenia, and anemia) and there was a <1% rate of grade 3 PN, despite 77% having a history of PN. Based on these findings, carfilzomib was granted conditional approval by the FDA in 2012 for the treatment of patients with relapsed and refractory myeloma who had received prior bortezomib and IMiD therapy.

The parallel PX-171-004 trial enrolled patients with relapsed MM following one to three prior treatments and who may have been refractory to one or more of these therapies.[90,91] Of the 155 patients enrolled in this trial, 120 had not received prior bortezomib-based therapy. In patients with relapsed disease, non-hematologic and hematologic toxicity profiles were similar. Despite high rates of baseline PN, reports of worsening neuropathic symptoms were infrequent (2% incidence of grade 3 and no grade 4 events). Carfilzomib demonstrated considerable activity in bortezomib-naïve patients, inducing PR or better in 46% of 54 evaluable patients at 20 mg/m$^2$ and 53% of patients at 27 mg/m$^2$.[91] The response rate in patients previously exposed to bortezomib was lower (18%).[90] Responses across groups are durable, typically 8 to 9 months.[90,91]

Based on findings in animal studies in which a 30-minute infusion of carfilzomib resulted in reduced toxicities,[61] the effect of infusional administration was tested in patients with relapsed and refractory myeloma. In a dose escalation study, PX-171-007, the MTD dose of carfilzomib was determined to be 56 mg/m$^2$, more than twice the dose used in the studies described previously. In a cohort of 24 patients receiving this dose and who had received a median of five prior lines of therapy (including two prior bortezomib-containing regimens), the ORR was 60%.[92] This enhanced efficacy also correlated with a greater level of inhibition of all three subunits of the immunoproteasome measured in isolated peripheral blood mononuclear cells (Lee S, et al., unpublished).[93] This same dose and infusion time is currently being explored in a phase III trial of nearly 900 patients comparing carfilzomib plus low-dose dexamethasone (Cd) to bortezomib plus low-dose dexamethasone (Vd) in MM patients with relapsed disease.

Trials of carfilzomib in combination with other agents in MM have been initiated, including a phase Ib/II safety and efficacy study of carfilzomib in combination with lenalidomide and low-dose dexamethasone (CRd) in relapsed and/or refractory MM. At the maximum planned dose, the ORR was 77% with a median duration of response of 22 months.[94] The CRd combination is now being tested in an international, multicenter, randomized, open-label phase III study in comparison with lenalidomide and low-dose dexamethasone (Rd) in approximately 780 patients with relapsed MM following one to three prior therapies. The CRd regimen has also been explored in newly diagnosed MM patients.[95] When carfilzomib is combined with Rd at a dose of 36 mg/m$^2$, 62% of the 53 patients treated achieved a CR. In addition, 20 of 21 patients analyzed for signs of minimal residual disease (MRD), utilizing multiparameter flow cytometry were determined to be free of MRD.

## Ixazomib

Initial clinical studies of ixazomib involved dose escalation studies in patients with hematologic malignancies and explored both weekly and twice weekly dosing schedules.[96,97] Oral administration resulted in potent proteasome inhibition of ~65%. Clinical activity in patients with relapsed MM was 16%.[98] In patients with newly diagnosed MM, ixazomib plus lenalidomide and low-dose dexamethasone resulted in an ORR of 93% with 24% achieving a CR.[99] This combination is also being investigated in a phase III trial comparing this to Rd in patients with relapsed MM.

## Oprozomib

Initial clinical testing of oprozomib in patients with solid tumors investigated a dosing schedule consisting of a 14-day cycle with once daily administration for 5 consecutive days.[100] In patients with relapsed and/or refractory B-cell neoplasms, two dosing schedules are being utilized: the schedule described previously and one involving 2 consecutive days of dosing repeated weekly.[101] Proteasome inhibition following the administration of oprozomib reached >80% and clinical activity was noted in patients with MM and WM. In patients receiving the 5 consecutive day schedule, 5 of 19 MM patients (26%) and 8 of 10 WM patients (80%) achieved a partial response or better. Exploration of the dose and schedule continues as a single agent and in combination with other anti-MM therapies.

## Biomarkers for Proteasome Inhibitors

As described previously, PI-based therapies have proven highly effective in the treatment of MM and other B-cell neoplasms. Given that response rates in single-agent trials are generally <50%, there would be a distinct clinical benefit to identify those patients most likely to respond to proteasome inhibition prior to treatment initiation. Gene expression analysis from bone marrow–derived MM tumor cells from 169 bortezomib-treated patients and 70 dexamethasone-treated patients revealed a 100-gene signature that provided a stratification for patients likely to respond that performed better than standard staging systems.[102] However, this signature provided only a modest increase in predictive power for treatment with bortezomib versus dexamethasone. More recently, Keats et al.[54] reanalyzed this dataset based on a pathway analysis of NF-κB and the realization that TRAF3, a key regulatory of the noncanonical NF-κB pathway, is a tumor suppressor in MM cell lines. They found a dramatic enrichment for response to bortezomib in patients with low levels of TRAF3 expression. However, these data remain to be validated in a separate sample set. A transcriptomic analysis of samples derived from single-agent carfilzomib trials suggest that patients with the highest level of immunoglobulin heavy chain expression were the most sensitive to carfilzomib therapy.[103] Similar findings were noted in the expression data from bortezomib-treated patients described previously.[103] These data are supported by phenotypic data from patients progressing on bortezomib-based therapy, in which resistance to bortezomib was associated with a dedifferentiated (and lower immunoglobulin expressing) B-cell phenotype.[104] Taken together, these findings suggest that biomarkers, potentially those involving an analysis of protein load of immunoglobulin expression, may be developed to predict those patients most likely to respond to PIs.

**REFERENCES**

1. Ciechanover A. Intracellular protein degradation: from a vague idea thru the lysosome and the ubiquitin-proteasome system and onto human diseases and drug targeting. *Biochim Biophys Acta* 2012;1824:3–13.
2. Kopp F, Hendil KB, Dahlmann B, et al. Subunit arrangement in the human 20S proteasome. *Proc Natl Acad Sci U S A* 1997;94:2939–2944.
3. Wilkinson KD. Ubiquitination and deubiquitination: targeting of proteins for degradation by the proteasome. *Semin Cell Dev Biol* 2000;11:141–148.
4. Braun BC, Glickman M, Kraft R, et al. The base of the proteasome regulatory particle exhibits chaperone-like activity. *Nat Cell Biol* 1999;1:221–226.
5. Groll M, Ditzel L, Lowe J, et al. Structure of 20S proteasome from yeast at 2.4 A resolution. *Nature* 1997;386:463–471.
6. Borissenko L, Groll M. 20S proteasome and its inhibitors: crystallographic knowledge for drug development. *Chem Rev* 2007;107:687–717.
7. Kloetzel PM, Ossendorp F. Proteasome and peptidase function in MHC-class-I-mediated antigen presentation. *Curr Opin Immunol* 2004;16:76–81.
8. Griffin TA, Nandi D, Cruz M, et al. Immunoproteasome assembly: cooperative incorporation of interferon gamma (IFN-gamma)-inducible subunits. *J Exp Med* 1998;187:97–104.

9. Tanahashi N, Murakami Y, Minami Y, et al. Hybrid proteasomes. Induction by interferon-gamma and contribution to ATP-dependent proteolysis. *J Biol Chem* 2000;275:14336–14345.

10. Adams J. The proteasome: a suitable antineoplastic target. *Nat Rev Cancer* 2004;4:349–360.

11. Vinitsky A, Michaud C, Powers JC, et al. Inhibition of the chymotrypsin-like activity of the pituitary multicatalytic proteinase complex. *Biochemistry* 1992;31:9421–9428.

12. Orlowski RZ, Eswara JR, Lafond-Walker A, et al. Tumor growth inhibition induced in a murine model of human Burkitt's lymphoma by a proteasome inhibitor. *Cancer Res* 1998;58:4342–4348.

13. Imajoh-Ohmi S, Kawaguchi T, Sugiyama S, et al. Lactacystin, a specific inhibitor of the proteasome, induces apoptosis in human monoblast U937 cells. *Biochem Biophys Res Commun* 1995;217:1070–1077.

14. Shinohara K, Tomioka M, Nakano H, et al. Apoptosis induction resulting from proteasome inhibition. *Biochem J* 1996;317:385–388.

15. Delic J, Masdehors P, Omura S, et al. The proteasome inhibitor lactacystin induces apoptosis and sensitizes chemo- and radioresistant human chronic lymphocytic leukaemia lymphocytes to TNF-alpha-initiated apoptosis. *Br J Cancer* 1998;77:1103–1107.

16. Meng L, Mohan R, Kwok BH, et al. Epoxomicin, a potent and selective proteasome inhibitor, exhibits in vivo antiinflammatory activity. *Proc Natl Acad Sci U S A* 1999;96:10403–10408.

17. Meng L, Kwok BH, Sin N, et al. Eponemycin exerts its antitumor effect through the inhibition of proteasome function. *Cancer Res* 1999;59:2798–2801.

18. Dick LR, Fleming PE. Building on bortezomib: second-generation proteasome inhibitors as anti-cancer therapy. *Drug Discov Today* 2010;15:243–249.

19. Kirk CJ. Discovery and development of second-generation proteasome inhibitors. *Semin Hematol* 2012;49:207–214.

20. Bross PF, Kane R, Farrell AT, et al. Approval summary for bortezomib for injection in the treatment of multiple myeloma. *Clin Cancer Res* 2004;10:3954–3964.

21. Herndon TM, Deisseroth A, Kaminskas E, et al. U.S. Food and Drug Administration approval: carfilzomib for the treatment of multiple myeloma. *Clin Cancer Res* 2013;19:4559–4563.

22. Bennett MK, Kirk CJ. Development of proteasome inhibitors in oncology and autoimmune diseases. *Curr Opin Drug Discov Devel* 2008;11:616–625.

23. Adams J, Behnke M, Chen S, et al. Potent and selective inhibitors of the proteasome: dipeptidyl boronic acids. *Bioorg Med Chem Lett* 1998;8:333–338.

24. Groll M, Berkers CR, Ploegh HL, et al. Crystal structure of the boronic acid-based proteasome inhibitor bortezomib in complex with the yeast 20S proteasome. *Structure* 2006;14:451–456.

25. Groll M, Huber R, Potts BC. Crystal structures of Salinosporamide A (NPI-0052) and B (NPI-0047) in complex with the 20S proteasome reveal important consequences of beta-lactone ring opening and a mechanism for irreversible binding. *J Am Chem Soc* 2006;19:5136–5141.

26. Groll M, Kim KB, Kairies N, et al. Crystal structure of epoxomicin: 20S proteasome reveals a molecular basis for selectivity of a' b'-epoxyketone proteasome inhibitors. *J Am Chem Soc* 2000;122:1237–1238.

27. Kisselev AF, van der Linden WA, Overkleeft HS. Proteasome inhibitors: an expanding army attacking a unique target. *Chem Biol* 2012;19:99–115.

28. Arastu-Kapur S, Anderl JL, Kraus M, et al. Nonproteasomal targets of the proteasome inhibitors bortezomib and carfilzomib: a link to clinical adverse events. *Clin Cancer Res* 2011;17:2734–2743.

29. Kisselev AF, Callard A, Goldberg AL. Importance of the different proteolytic sites of the proteasome and the efficacy of inhibitors varies with the protein substrate. *J Biol Chem* 2006;281:8582–8590.

30. Parlati F, Lee SJ, Aujay M, et al. Carfilzomib can induce tumor cell death through selective inhibition of the chymotrypsin-like activity of the proteasome. *Blood* 2009;114:3439–3447.

31. Britton M, Lucas MM, Downey SL, et al. Selective inhibitor of proteasome's caspase-like sites sensitizes cells to specific inhibition of chymotrypsin-like sites. *Chem Biol* 2009;16:1278–1289.

32. Mirabella AC, Pletnev AA, Downey SL, et al. Specific cell-permeable inhibitor of proteasome trypsin-like sites selectively sensitizes myeloma cells to bortezomib and carfilzomib. *Chem Biol* 2011;18:608–618.

33. Demo SD, Kirk CJ, Aujay MA, et al. Antitumor activity of PR-171, a novel irreversible inhibitor of the proteasome. *Cancer Res* 2007;67:6383–6391.

34. Kupperman E, Lee EC, Cao Y, et al. Evaluation of the proteasome inhibitor MLN9708 in preclinical models of human cancer. *Cancer Res* 2010;70:1970–1980.

35. Piva R, Ruggeri B, Williams M, et al. CEP-18770: A novel, orally active proteasome inhibitor with a tumor-selective pharmacologic profile competitive with bortezomib. *Blood* 2008;111:2765–2775.

36. Chauhan D, Singh AV, Aujay M, et al. A novel orally active proteasome inhibitor ONX 0912 triggers in vitro and in vivo cytotoxicity in multiple myeloma. *Blood* 2010;116:4906–4915.

37. Zhou HJ, Aujay MA, Bennett MK, et al. Design and synthesis of an orally bioavailable and selective peptide epoxyketone proteasome inhibitor (PR-047). *J Med Chem* 2009;52:3028–3038.

38. Chauhan D, Catley L, Li G, et al. A novel orally active proteasome inhibitor induces apoptosis in multiple myeloma cells with mechanisms distinct from Bortezomib. *Cancer Cell* 2005;8:407–419.

39. Chauhan D, Singh A, Brahmandam M, et al. Combination of proteasome inhibitors bortezomib and NPI-0052 trigger in vivo synergistic cytotoxicity in multiple myeloma. *Blood* 2008;111:1654–1664.

40. Chauhan D, Tian Z, Zhou B, et al. In vitro and in vivo selective antitumor activity of a novel orally bioavailable proteasome inhibitor MLN9708 against multiple myeloma cells. *Clin Cancer Res* 2011;17:5311–5321.

41. Kuhn DJ, Chen Q, Voorhees PM, et al. Potent activity of carfilzomib, a novel, irreversible inhibitor of the ubiquitin-proteasome pathway, against preclinical models of multiple myeloma. *Blood* 2007;110:3281–3290.

42. Suzuki E, Demo S, Deu E, et al. Molecular mechanisms of bortezomib resistant adenocarcinoma cells. *PLoS One* 2011;6:e27996.

43. Zhang HG, Wang J, Yang X, et al. Regulation of apoptosis proteins in cancer cells by ubiquitin. *Oncogene* 2004;23:2009–2015.

44. Fernandez Y, Verhaegen M, Miller TP, et al. Differential regulation of noxa in normal melanocytes and melanoma cells by proteasome inhibition: therapeutic implications. *Cancer Res* 2005;65:6294–6304.

45. Nikiforov MA, Riblett M, Tang WH, et al. Tumor cell-selective regulation of NOXA by c-MYC in response to proteasome inhibition. *Proc Natl Acad Sci U S A* 2007;104:19488–19493.

46. Qin JZ, Ziffra J, Stennett L, et al. Proteasome inhibitors trigger NOXA-mediated apoptosis in melanoma and myeloma cells. *Cancer Res* 2005;65:6282–6293.

47. Wang Q, Mora-Jensen H, Weniger MA, et al. ERAD inhibitors integrate ER stress with an epigenetic mechanism to activate BH3-only protein NOXA in cancer cells. *Proc Natl Acad Sci U S A* 2009;106:2200–2205.

48. Mannava S, Zhuang D, Nair JR, et al. KLF9 is a novel transcriptional regulator of bortezomib- and LBH589-induced apoptosis in multiple myeloma cells. *Blood* 2012;119:1450–1458.

49. Koepp DM, Harper JW, Elledge SJ. How the cyclin became a cyclin: regulated proteolysis in the cell cycle. *Cell* 1999;97:431–434.

50. Pagano M, Tam SW, Theodoras AM, et al. Role of the ubiquitin-proteasome pathway in regulating abundance of the cyclin-dependent kinase inhibitor p27. *Science* 1995;269:682–685.

51. Wan F, Lenardo MJ. The nuclear signaling of NF-kappaB: current knowledge, new insights, and future perspectives. *Cell Res* 2010;20:24–33.

52. Annunziata CM, Davis RE, Demchenko Y, et al. Frequent engagement of the classical and alternative NF-kappaB pathways by diverse genetic abnormalities in multiple myeloma. *Cancer Cell* 2007;12:115–130.

53. Chapman MA, Lawrence MS, Keats JJ, et al. Initial genome sequencing and analysis of multiple myeloma. *Nature* 2011;471:467–472.

54. Keats JJ, Fonseca R, Chesi M, et al. Promiscuous mutations activate the noncanonical NF-kappaB pathway in multiple myeloma. *Cancer Cell* 2007;12:131–144.

55. Meister S, Schubert U, Neubert K, et al. Extensive immunoglobulin production sensitizes myeloma cells for proteasome inhibition. *Cancer Res* 2007;67:1783–1792.

56. Obeng EA, Carlson LM, Gutman DM, et al. Proteasome inhibitors induce a terminal unfolded protein response in multiple myeloma cells. *Blood* 2006;107:4907–4916.

57. Shabaneh TB, Downey SL, Goddard AL, et al. Molecular basis of differential sensitivity of myeloma cells to clinically relevant bolus treatment with bortezomib. *PLoS One* 2013;8:e56132.

58. Papadopoulos KP, Burris HA III, Gordon M, et al. A phase I/II study of carfilzomib 2-10-min infusion in patients with advanced solid tumors. *Cancer Chemother Pharmacol* 2013;72:861–868.

59. Papandreou CN, Daliani DD, Nix D, et al. Phase I trial of the proteasome inhibitor bortezomib in patients with advanced solid tumors with observations in androgen-independent prostate cancer. *J Clin Oncol* 2004;22:2108–2121.

60. Wang Z, Yang J, Kirk C, et al. Clinical pharmacokinetics, metabolism, and drug-drug interaction of carfilzomib. *Drug Metab Dispos* 2013;41:230–237.

61. Yang J, Wang Z, Fang Y, et al. Pharmacokinetics, pharmacodynamics, metabolism, distribution, and excretion of carfilzomib in rats. *Drug Metab Dispos* 2011;39:1873–1882.

62. Meiners S, Heyken D, Weller A, et al. Inhibition of proteasome activity induces concerted expression of proteasome genes and de novo formation of mammalian proteasomes. *J Biol Chem* 2003;278:21517–21525.

63. Lonial S, Waller EK, Richardson PG, et al. Risk factors and kinetics of thrombocytopenia associated with bortezomib for relapsed, refractory multiple myeloma. *Blood* 2005;106:3777–3784.

64. Richardson PG, Briemberg H, Jagannath S, et al. Frequency, characteristics, and reversibility of peripheral neuropathy during treatment of advanced multiple myeloma with bortezomib. *J Clin Oncol* 2006;24:3113–3120.

65. Richardson PG, Barlogie B, Berenson J, et al. A phase 2 study of bortezomib in relapsed, refractory myeloma. *N Engl J Med* 2003;348:2609–2617.

66. Jagannath S, Barlogie B, Berenson J, et al. A phase 2 study of two doses of bortezomib in relapsed or refractory myeloma. *Br J Haematol* 2004;127:165–172.

67. Richardson PG, Sonneveld P, Schuster MW, et al. Bortezomib or high-dose dexamethasone for relapsed multiple myeloma. *N Engl J Med* 2005;352:2487–2498.

68. Jagannath S, Brian D, Wolf JL, et al. A phase 2 study of bortezomib as first-line therapy in patients with multiple myeloma. *Blood* 2004;104:333.

69. San Miguel JF, Schlag R, Khuageva NK, et al. Bortezomib plus melphalan and prednisone for initial treatment of multiple myeloma. *N Engl J Med* 2008;359:906–917.

70. San Miguel JF, Schlag R, Khuageva NK, et al. Persistent overall survival benefit and no increased risk of second malignancies with bortezomib-melphalan-prednisone versus melphalan-prednisone in patients with previously untreated multiple myeloma. *J Clin Oncol* 2013;31:448–455.

71. Orlowski RZ, Voorhees PM, Garcia RA, et al. Phase 1 trial of the proteasome inhibitor bortezomib and pegylated liposomal doxorubicin in patients with advanced hematologic malignancies. *Blood* 2005;105:3058–3065.

72. Orlowski RZ, Nagler A, Sonneveld P, et al. Randomized phase III study of pegylated liposomal doxorubicin plus bortezomib compared with bortezomib alone in relapsed or refractory multiple myeloma: combination therapy improves time to progression. *J Clin Oncol* 2007;25:3892–3901.

73. Sonneveld P, Hajek R, Nagler A, et al. Combined pegylated liposomal doxorubicin and bortezomib is highly effective in patients with recurrent or refractory multiple myeloma who received prior thalidomide/lenalidomide therapy. *Cancer* 2008;112:1529–1537.

74. Richardson PG, Xie W, Jagannath S, et al. A phase II trial of lenalidomide, bortezomib and dexamethasone in patients with relapsed and relapsed/refractory myeloma. *Blood* 2014;123:1461–1469.

75. Kapoor P, Ramakrishnan V, Rajkumar SV. Bortezomib combination therapy in multiple myeloma. *Semin Hematol* 2012;49:228–242.

76. Richardson PG, Weller E, Lonial S, et al. Lenalidomide, bortezomib, and dexamethasone combination therapy in patients with newly diagnosed multiple myeloma. *Blood* 2010;116:679–686.

77. Belch A, Kouroukis CT, Crump M, et al. A phase II study of bortezomib in mantle cell lymphoma: the National Cancer Institute of Canada Clinical Trials Group trial IND.150. *Ann Oncol* 2007;18:116–121.

78. Fisher RI, Bernstein SH, Kahl BS, et al. Multicenter phase II study of bortezomib in patients with relapsed or refractory mantle cell lymphoma. *J Clin Oncol* 2006;24:4867–4874.

79. Milano A, Iaffaioli RV, Caponigro F. The proteasome: a worthwhile target for the treatment of solid tumours? *Eur J Cancer* 2007;43:1125–1133.

80. Fanucchi MP, Fossella FV, Belt R, et al. Randomized phase II study of bortezomib alone and bortezomib in combination with docetaxel in previously treated advanced non-small-cell lung cancer. *J Clin Oncol* 2006;24:5025–5033.

81. Ramaswamy B, Phelps MA, Baiocchi R, et al. A dose-finding, pharmacokinetic and pharmacodynamic study of a novel schedule of flavopiridol in patients with advanced solid tumors. *Invest New Drugs* 2012;30:629–638.

82. Luu T, Chow W, Lim D, et al. Phase I trial of fixed-dose rate gemcitabine in combination with bortezomib in advanced solid tumors. *Anticancer Res* 2010;30:167–174.

83. Everly MJ, Everly JJ, Susskind B, et al. Bortezomib provides effective therapy for antibody- and cell-mediated acute rejection. *Transplantation* 2008; 86:1754–1761.

84. Neubert K, Meister S, Moser K, et al. The proteasome inhibitor bortezomib depletes plasma cells and protects mice with lupus-like disease from nephritis. *Nat Med* 2008;14:748–755.

85. O'Connor OA, Stewart AK, Vallone M, et al. A phase 1 dose escalation study of the safety and pharmacokinetics of the novel proteasome inhibitor carfilzomib (PR-171) in patients with hematologic malignancies. *Clin Cancer Res* 2009;15: 7085–7091.

86. Alsina M, Trudel S, Furman RR, et al. A phase I single-agent study of twice-weekly consecutive-day dosing of the proteasome inhibitor carfilzomib in patients with relapsed or refractory multiple myeloma or lymphoma. *Clin Cancer Res* 2012;18:4830–4840.

87. Jagannath S, Vij R, Stewart AK, et al. An open-label single-arm pilot phase II study (PX-171-003-A0) of low-dose, single-agent carfilzomib in patients with relapsed and refractory multiple myeloma. *Clin Lymphoma Myeloma Leuk* 2012;12:310–318.

88. Siegel DS, Martin T, Wang M, et al. A phase 2 study of single-agent carfilzomib (PX-171-003-A1) in patients with relapsed and refractory multiple myeloma. *Blood* 2012;120:2817–2825.

89. Siegel DS, Martin T, Wang M, et al. Results of PX-171-003-A1, an open-label, single-arm, phase 2 (Ph 2) study of carfilzomib (CFZ) in patients (pts) with relapsed and refractory multiple myeloma (MM). *Blood* 2012;120:2817–2825.

90. Vij R, Siegel DS, Jagannath S, et al. An open-label, single-arm, phase 2 study of single-agent carfilzomib in patients with relapsed and/or refractory multiple myeloma who have been previously treated with bortezomib. *Br J Haematol* 2012;158:739–748.

91. Vij R, Wang M, Kaufman JL, et al. An open-label, single-arm, phase 2 (PX-171-004) study of single-agent carfilzomib in bortezomib-naive patients with relapsed and/or refractory multiple myeloma. *Blood* 2012;119:5661–5670.

92. Papadopoulos K, Capua Siegel DS, Singhal SB, et al. Phase 1b evaluation of the safety and efficacy of a 30-minute IV infusion of carfilzomib in patients with relapsed and/or refractory multiple myeloma. *Blood* 2010;116:3024.

93. Lee SJ, Levitsky K, Parlati F, et al. Clinical activity of carfilzomib correlates with inhibition of multiple proteasome subunits: application of a novel pharmacodynamics assay. (In press).

94. Wang M, Martin T, Bensinger W, et al. Phase 2 dose-expansion study (PX-171-006) of carfilzomib, lenalidomide, and low-dose dexamethasone in relapsed or progressive multiple myeloma. *Blood* 2013;122:3122–3128.

95. Jakubowiak AJ, Dytfeld D, Griffith KA, et al. A phase 1/2 study of carfilzomib in combination with lenalidomide and low-dose dexamethasone as a frontline treatment for multiple myeloma. *Blood* 2012;120:1801–1809.

96. Richardson PG, Baz R, Wang L, et al. Investigational agent MLN9708, an oral proteasome inhibitor, in patients (Pts) with relapsed and/or refractory multiple myeloma (MM): results from the expansion cohorts of a phase 1 dose-escalation study. *Blood* 2011;118:301.

97. Richardson PG, Spencer A, Cannell P, et al. Phase 1 clinical evaluation of twice-weekly marizomib (NPI-0052), a novel proteasome inhibitor, in patients with relapsed/refractory multiple myeloma (MM). *Blood* 2011;118:302.

98. Roy V, Reeder C, LaPlant BR, et al. Phase 2 trial Of single agent MLN9708 in patients with relapsed multiple myeloma not refractory to bortezomib. *Blood* 2013;122:1944.

99. Hofmeister CC, Rosenbaum CA, Htut M, et al. Twice-weekly oral MLN9708 (ixazomib citrate), an investigational proteasome inhibitor, in combination with lenalidomide (len) and dexamethasone (dex) in patients (pts) with newly diagnosed multiple myeloma (MM): final phase 1 results and phase 2 data. *Blood* 2013;122:535.

100. Papadopoulos KP, Mendelson DS, Tolcher AW, et al. A phase I, open-label, dose-escalation study of the novel oral proteasome inhibitor (PI) ONX 0912 in patients with advanced refractory or recurrent solid tumors. *Blood* 2011;29:3075.

101. Kaufman JL, Siegel DS, Vij R, et al. Clinical profile of single-agent modified-release oprozomib tablets in patients (pts) with hematologic malignancies: updated results from a multicenter, open-label, dose escalation phase 1b/2 study. *Blood* 2013;122:3184.

102. Mulligan G, Mitsiades C, Bryant B, et al. Gene expression profiling and correlation with outcome in clinical trials of the proteasome inhibitor bortezomib. *Blood* 2007;109:3177–3188.

103. Loehr A, Degenhardt JD, Kwei KA, et al. Immunoglobulin expression is a major determinant of patient sensitivity to proteasome inhibitors. *Blood* 2013;122:1903.

104. Leung-Hagesteijn C, Erdmann N, Cheung G, et al. Xbp1s-negative tumor B cells and pre-plasmablasts mediate therapeutic proteasome inhibitor resistance in multiple myeloma. *Cancer Cell* 2013;24:289–304.

# 25 Poly (ADP-ribose) Polymerase Inhibitors

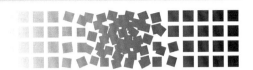

Alan Ashworth

## INTRODUCTION

Cancer cells may harbor defects in DNA repair pathways leading to genomic instability. This can foster tumorigenesis but also provides a weakness that can be exploited therapeutically. Tumors with compromised ability to repair double-strand DNA breaks by homologous recombination, including those with defects in the *BRCA1* and *BRCA2* genes, are highly sensitive to blockade of the repair of DNA single-strand breaks, via the inhibition of the enzyme poly(ADP-ribose) (PARP). This provides the basis for a *synthetic lethal* approach to cancer therapy, which is showing considerable promise in the clinic.

## CELLULAR DNA REPAIR PATHWAYS

DNA is continually damaged by environmental exposures and endogenous activities, such as DNA replication and cellular free-radical generation, which cause diverse lesions including base modifications, double-strand breaks (DSB), single-strand breaks (SSB), and intrastrand and interstrand cross-links.[1] These aberrations are repaired by distinct repair pathways, which are coordinated to maintain the stability and integrity of the genome. This faithful repair of DNA damage is an essential prerequisite for the maintenance of genomic integrity and cellular and organismal viability. Where one DNA strand is affected and the intact complementary strand is available as a template, the base-excision repair (BER), nucleotide-excision repair, or mismatch repair pathways are used and these pathways are highly efficient at repairing damage. DSBs, more problematic than SSBs because the complementary strand is not available as a template, are repaired by the homologous recombination (HR) or nonhomologous end-joining (NHEJ) pathways.[1]

Endogenous base damage, including SSBs, is the most common DNA aberration and it has been estimated that the average cell may repair 10,000 such lesions every day. BER is an important pathway for the repair of SSBs and involves the sensing of the lesion followed by the recruitment of a number of other proteins. PARP-1 (poly[ADP]ribose polymerase) is a critical component of the major "short-patch" BER pathway. PARP is an enzyme, discovered over 40 years ago,[2] that produces large branched chains of poly(ADP) ribose (PAR) from $NAD^+$. In humans, there are 17 members of the PARP gene family but most of these are poorly characterized.[3,4] The abundant nuclear protein PARP-1 senses and binds to DNA nicks and breaks, resulting in activation of catalytic activity causing poly(ADP)ribosylation of PARP-1 itself as well as other acceptor proteins including histones. This modification may signal the recruitment of other components of DNA repair pathways as well as modify their activity. The highly negatively charged PAR that is produced around the site of damage may also serve as an antirecombinogenic factor. In addition to the BER pathway PARP enzymes have been implicated in numerous cellular pathways.[3,4]

Two main DSB repair pathways are available within eukaryotic cells: NHEJ and HR.[5,6] HR can be further subdivided into the gene conversion (GC) and single-strand annealing (SSA) subpathways.[1]

Both GC and SSA rely on sequence homology for repair whereas NHEJ uses no, or little, homology.[2,3] NHEJ is the most important pathway for the repair of DSBs during $G_0$, $G_1$, and early S phases of the cell cycle, although it is likely active throughout the cell cycle.[7,8] This form of DSB repair usually results in changes in DNA sequence at the break site and, occasionally, in the joining of previously unlinked DNA molecules, potentially resulting in gross chromosomal rearrangements such as translocations.[9] GC uses a homologous sequence, preferably the sister chromatid, as a template to resynthesize the DNA surrounding the DSB, and therefore generally results in accurate repair of the break. Repair by GC is critically dependent on the recombinase function of RAD51 and is facilitated by a number of other proteins. SSA also involves the use of homologous sequences for the repair of DSBs, but unlike GC, SSA is RAD51-independent and involves the annealing of DNA strands formed after resection at the DSB. The detailed mechanism of SSA is still obscure but it frequently results in the loss of one of the homologous sequences and deletion of the intervening sequence.[9] SSA is a potentially important pathway of mutagenesis because a significant fraction of mammalian genomes consist of repetitive elements. GC and SSA are cell-cycle regulated and are most active in S-$G_2$ phases of the cell cycle.[10]

## THE DEVELOPMENT OF PARP INHIBITORS

PARP inhibitors were originally developed as chemopotentiators, which are agents that enhance the effects of DNA damage—a common mechanism of action of drugs used to treat cancer. The rationale was that inhibition of the repair of chemotherapy-induced DNA damage might give greater efficacy. Early studies using relatively nonspecific PARP inhibitors such as 3-aminobenzamide, demonstrated potential synergy with alkylating agents.[11] Subsequent studies with more potent PARP inhibitors demonstrated synergy with temozolomide, an observation that was taken into a clinical trial with AG014699,[12] a PARP inhibitor developed by Pfizer. This agent is now being developed by Clovis. Although the major focus of this chapter is the use of PARP inhibitors in synthetic lethal therapeutic strategies, their use in chemopotentiation in combination with chemotherapy remains under active investigation, as described later.

## *BRCA1* AND *BRCA2* MUTATIONS AND DNA REPAIR

Heterozygous germline mutations in the *BRCA1* and *BRCA2* genes confer a high risk of breast (up to 85% lifetime risk) and ovarian (10% to 40%) cancer in addition to a significantly increased risk of pancreatic, prostate, and male breast cancer.[13] The genes have been classified as tumor suppressors, because the wild-type *BRCA* allele is frequently lost in tumors, a phenomenon that occurs by a variety of mechanisms. The *BRCA1* and *BRCA2* genes encode large proteins that likely function in multiple cellular pathways, including transcription, cell-cycle regulation, and the maintenance of genome integrity. However, the roles of BRCA1 and BRCA2 in DNA repair have been best documented.[14]

BRCA1- and BRCA2-deficient cells are highly sensitive to ionizing radiation and display chromosomal instability, which is likely to be a direct consequence of unrepaired DNA damage.[14] The similar genomic instability in BRCA1- and BRCA2-deficient cells and the interaction of both BRCA1 and BRCA2 with RAD51 suggested a functional link between the three proteins in the RAD51-mediated DNA damage repair process. However, although BRCA2 is directly involved in RAD51-mediated repair, affecting the choice between GC and SSA, BRCA1 acts upstream of these pathways[15]; both GC and SSA are reduced in BRCA1-deficient cells, placing BRCA1 before the branch point of GC and SSA.[15]

BRCA1 has a role in signaling DNA damage and cell-cycle checkpoint regulation,[14,15] whereas BRCA2 has a more direct role in DNA repair itself. BRCA2 is thought to promote genomic stability through a role in the error-free repair of DSBs by GC via association with RAD51. Aberrations in BRCA2-deficient cells arise at least in part by the use of the SSA pathway. NHEJ, however, is apparently unaffected in BRCA2-deficient cells.[14,15] Loss of BRCA2, therefore, results in the repair of DSBs by preferential utilization of an error-prone mechanism, which potentially explains the apparent chromosome instability associated with BRCA2 deficiency.[15]

The physical interaction between BRCA2 and RAD51 is essential for error-free DSB repair. BRCA2 is required for the localization of RAD51 to sites of DNA damage, where RAD51 forms the nucleoprotein filament required for recombination. The foci of the RAD51 protein are apparent in the nucleus after certain forms of DNA damage and these likely represent sites of repair by HR; BRCA2-deficient cells do not form RAD51 foci in response to DNA damage.[15] Two different domains within BRCA2 interact with RAD51, the eight BRC repeats in the central part of the protein and a distinct domain, TR2, at the C-terminus.[16]

## PARP-1 INHIBITION AS A SYNTHETIC LETHAL THERAPEUTIC STRATEGY FOR THE TREATMENT OF BRCA-DEFICIENT CANCERS

Synthetic lethality is defined as the situation when a mutation in either of two genes individually has no effect, but combining the mutations leads to death.[17] This effect was first described and studied in genetically tractable organisms such as *Drosophila* and yeast.[17,18] This effect can arise because of a number of different gene–gene interactions. Examples include two genes in separate semiredundant or cooperating pathways, and two genes acting in the same pathway where loss of both critically affects flux through the pathway. The implication is that targeting one of these genes in a cancer where the other is defective should be selectively lethal to the tumor cells but not toxic to the normal cells. In principle, this should lead to a large therapeutic window.[19] The original suggestion that the concept of synthetic lethality could be used in the selection or development of cancer therapeutics came from Hartwell et al.,[18] and from experiments performed in yeast. Synthetic lethal screens have now been performed in a number of model organisms[20] and in human cells,[21] and these have revealed multiple potential gene–gene interactions, some of which could be exploited clinically. However, synthetic lethal therapies have not been clinically used until recently, when evidence has been provided for PARP-1 inhibition as a potential synthetic lethal approach for the treatment of BRCA-mutation–associated cancers.

PARP-1 inhibition causes failure of the repair of SSB lesions but does not affect DSB repair.[22] However, a persistent DNA SSB encountered by a DNA replication fork will cause stalling of the fork and may result in either fork collapse or the formation of a DSB.[23] Therefore, the loss of PARP-1 increases the formation of

DNA lesions that might be repaired by GC. As a loss of function of either BRCA1 or BRCA2 impairs GC,[14,15] a loss of PARP-1 function in a BRCA1- or BRCA2-defective background could result in the generation of replication-associated DNA lesions normally repaired by sister chromatid exchange. If so, this might lead to cell-cycle arrest and/or cell death. Therefore, PARP inhibitors could be selectively lethal to cells lacking functional BRCA1 or BRCA2 but might be minimally toxic to normal cells. This would indicate a synthetic lethal interaction between PARP and BRCA1 or BRCA2. Exemplifying this principle, potent inhibitors of PARP were applied to cells deficient in either BRCA1 or BRCA2. Cell survival assays showed that cell lines lacking wild-type BRCA1 or BRCA2 were extremely sensitive to these agents compared with heterozygous mutant or wild-type cells.[24,25]

To explain these observations, a model was proposed whereby persistent single-strand gaps in DNA caused by PARP inhibition when encountered by a replication fork might trigger fork arrest, collapse, and/or a DSB.[26] Alternatively, PARP-1 trapped on DNA by the inhibition of enzyme activity might also cause a fork collapse. Normally, these DSBs would be repaired by RAD51-dependent GC.[14,15] However, in the absence of BRCA1 or BRCA2, the replication fork cannot be restarted and collapses, causing persistent chromatid breaks. When repaired by the alternative error-prone DSB repair mechanisms of SSA or NHEJ, large numbers of chromatid aberrations would be induced, leading to cell lethality.[26] The idea that the defect in GC is being targeted in BRCA-deficient cells is supported by the demonstration that deficiency in other genes implicated in HR also confers sensitivity to PARP inhibitors.[27] This further suggests that this approach may be more widely applicable in the treatment of sporadic cancers with impairments of the HR pathway or BRCAness[28] (see the following).

## INITIAL CLINICAL RESULTS TESTING SYNTHETIC LETHALITY OF PARP INHIBITORS AND BRCA MUTATION

Phase I studies[29] established that olaparib (AstraZeneca, London, UK; formerly KU-0059436, KuDOS Pharmaceuticals, Cambridge, UK) could be administered safely as a single agent at a dose of 400 mg twice per day. Side effects were classified as mild and were unlike those typically experienced with cytotoxic chemotherapy. Significant and durable responses were observed in patients with germ-line BRCA1 or BRCA2 mutations and breast ovary or prostate cancer. Of the 19 mutation carriers enrolled, 9 had an objective response defined by Response Evaluation Criteria in Sold Tumors (RECIST) criteria and 12 had stable disease for more than 4 months in duration. A similar magnitude of clinical responses was observed in an expanded cohort.[30] These observations are impressive because the cohort had been heavily pretreated and most were resistant to a wide range of chemotherapies.[29,30]

Phase II studies were subsequently performed in advanced breast and ovarian cancers arising in BRCA1 and BRCA2 mutation carriers.[31,32] The reported response rate was 41% in the breast study and 52% in the ovarian group; both groups had been heavily pretreated. Again, the drug was well tolerated. Another study of BRCA1/2 carriers with ovarian cancer compared olaparib with pegylated liposomal doxorubicin (PLD).[33] There was no significant difference in the response rates, but there were some differences in the patient characteristics and an unexpectedly high rate of response to PLD.

There are also reports of responses to PARP inhibitors in BRCA2 mutation carriers with prostate[34] and pancreatic[35] cancer. A number of other PARP inhibitors are in clinical development (Table 25.1), and some of these have shown efficacy in the treatment of cancers arising in BRCA1 or BRCA2 mutation carriers.[36,37]

**CANCER THERAPEUTICS**

## TABLE 25.1

**PARP Inhibitors in Late Stage Clinical Development**

| Agent | Company | Phase III Trials |
|---|---|---|
| Olaparib | AstraZeneca (formerly KuDOS) | BRCA-mutant ovarian cancer |
| Niraparib | Tesaro (formerly Merck) | Platinum sensitive ovarian cancer BRCA-mutant breast cancer |
| Rucaparib | Clovis (formerly Pfizer) | Platinum sensitive ovarian cancer |
| Veliparib | AbbVie (formerly Abbot) | Undisclosed |
| BMN673 | BioMarin (formerly Lead) | BRCA-mutant breast cancer |

Adapted from Garber, K. PARP inhibitors bounce back. *Nat Rev Drug Discov* 2013;12:725–727.

## THE USE OF PARP INHIBITORS IN SPORADIC CANCERS

Germline mutations in BRCA1 or BRCA2 are relatively common in hereditary breast and ovarian cancer. However, inactivation of BRCA genes by mutation in sporadic cancers is rare, at least in breast cancer, which may seem to limit the application of PARP inhibitors to a wider range of patients. However, many tumors display features in common with BRCA-deficient tumors, including similar defects in DNA repair due to either epigenetic mutation of BRCA1, such as promoter methylation, or mutation of other components of BRCA-associated pathways.[28] This BRCAness may make these tumors also susceptible to PARP inhibition.[28] For example, phosphatase and tensin homolog (PTEN) mutations, which occur with a frequency estimated at 50% to 80% in sporadic tumors,[38] may cause PARP inhibitor sensitivity in preclinical models, possibly because PTEN-null cells display BRCAness phenotypes, such as the inability to efficiently repair certain forms of DNA damage.[39]

Traditional histopathologic methods and, more recently, gene expression profiling approaches have shown the phenotypic overlap between triple-negative breast cancers, basal-like breast cancers, and BRCA1 familial breast cancers.[40,41] In gene expression profiling studies, it has been observed that BRCA1 familial cancers strongly segregate with basal-like tumors and share features such as high-grade and pushing margins.[28,40,41] Although the overlap is not absolute, it leads to the hypothesis that there may be a subset of sporadic breast cancers that exhibits features of BRCAness, including deficiencies in HR and that may be susceptible to treatment with drugs such as PARP inhibitors.[26]

There have been several studies of PARP inhibitors in sporadic ovarian cancer. A study by Lederman[42] showed in a maintenance study following the response to platinum therapy a significant benefit in terms of progression-free survival (PFS) of olaparib compared to placebo. This was even more pronounced when the subgroup of BRCA mutation carriers were examined.[43] In both cases, the overall survival (OS) advantage was less than the PFS, but in the case of the BRCA mutation group, this reached statistical significance. Gelmon[44] also showed activity in sporadic ovarian cancer. In contrast, a study in sporadic triple-negative breast cancer failed to observe any benefit, although the study was small and the patients were heavily pretreated.[44]

Iniparib (initially reported as a PARP inhibitor) showed an overall survival benefit in a Phase II trial of triple-negative breast cancer in combination with gemcitabine and carboplatin compared with chemotherapy alone.[45] However, a subsequent Phase III study showed no improvement in PFS.[45] The reasons for this are uncertain, but significant questions have been raised about whether iniparib is indeed a bona fide PARP inhibitor. Therefore, it is now generally conceded that studies of iniparib have no implications for PARP inhibitors as a drug class.[46]

Which population of patients lacking a BRCA1 or BRCA2 mutation might benefit from PARP inhibitors remains unclear. This is likely to require the development of a clinical test to identify prospectively tumors with intrinsic sensitivity. Presently, most efforts are directed at developing assays of DNA repair deficiency.[47]

## MECHANISMS OF RESISTANCE TO PARP INHIBITORS

Resistance to targeted therapy frequently occurs, but it was unclear how resistance might arise to a synthetic lethal therapy.[48] Potential mechanisms of resistance to PARP inhibitors have, however, been elucidated both directly in vitro, in mouse models, and in the clinic.[48] An in vitro model for resistance was developed by producing cells from the highly PARP inhibitor–sensitive BRCA2-deficient cell line CAPAN1, which carries a c.6174delT BRCA2 frameshift mutation. CAPAN1 cells cannot form damage-induced RAD51 foci, are defective for HR, and are extremely sensitive to treatment with PARP inhibitors.[49] PARP inhibitor–resistant clones were highly resistant (over 1,000-fold) to the drug and were also cross-resistant to the DNA cross-linking agent cisplatin, but not to the microtubule-stabilizing drug docetaxel. PARP inhibitors and cisplatin both exert their effects on BRCA-deficient cells by increasing the frequency of misrepaired DSBs in the absence of effective HR. Therefore, this observation indicates that the resistance of PARP inhibitor–resistant clones to PARP inhibitors might be because of restored HR. This contention was supported by the acquisition in PARP inhibitor–resistant clone cells of the ability to form RAD51 foci after PARP inhibitor treatment or exposure to irradiation.

DNA sequencing of PARP inhibitor–resistant clones revealed the unexpected presence of novel BRCA2 alleles that resulted in the elimination of the c.6174delT mutation and restoration of an open reading frame.[49] Therefore, in this case, resistance arises because of gain of function mutations in the synthetic lethal partner (BRCA2) rather than the direct drug target (PARP). Alternative mechanisms of PARP inhibitor resistance have also been described.[48] A mouse model of BRCA1-associated mammary gland cancer demonstrated the efficacy of olaparib in vivo and was used to study mechanisms of resistance.[50] Resistance seemed to be caused by the upregulation of ABCB1a/b, which encode P-glycoprotein pumps; this effect could be reversed with the P-glycoprotein inhibitor tariquidar. In addition, other alterations in DNA repair pathways have been proposed to compensate for BRCA1 deficiency resulting in PARP inhibitor deficiency.[48]

Studies of the mechanisms of resistance to PARP inhibitors in patient material are still at an early stage. Initial studies addressed the mechanism of resistance to platinum salts in BRCA mutation carriers. Cisplatin and carboplatin are part of the standard of care for the treatment of ovarian cancer, including individuals with BRCA1 or BRCA2 mutations. Platinum salts are thought to exert their BRCA-selective effects by a similar mechanism to PARP inhibitors.[15] Clinical observations suggest that BRCA mutation carriers with ovarian cancer usually respond better to these agents than patients without BRCA mutations[51,52]; however, resistance does eventually occur. To investigate this effect, BRCA1 and BRCA2 have been sequenced in tumor material from mutation carriers.[49,53] These studies revealed mutations in BRCA1 or BRCA2 that restored the open reading frame and likely contributed to platinum resistance. These observations suggest that specific mutations in BRCA1 or BRCA2 and sensitivity to therapeutics in cell lines and patients can be suppressed by intragenic deletion. Presumably, these mutations occur randomly and are then selected for by differential drug sensitivity. Therefore, the best use of these agents is likely to be earlier in the disease process when the disease burden is smaller, which will reduce the probability of resistance based on stochastic genetic reversion. Recently, similar observations of revertant *BRCA* alleles were made in two patients who became resistant after an initial response to olaparib.[54] Although preliminary, these results suggest that this mechanism is responsible for at least some of the clinical resistance observed. Doubtless, as with other targeted therapies, multiple resistance mechanisms will be implicated as further patients are studied.[48]

## PROSPECTS

Currently, the treatments for cancers arising in carriers of *BRCA1* or *BRCA2* mutations are the same as those that occur sporadically matched for tumor pathology and age of onset. However, tumors in *BRCA1* or *BRCA2* mutation carriers lack wild-type *BRCA1* or *BRCA2*, but normal tissues retain a single wild-type copy of the relevant gene. This is a potentially targetable alteration that provides the basis for new mechanism-based approaches to the treatment of cancer. The biochemical difference in capacity to carry out HR between the tumor and normal tissues, in a *BRCA1* or

*BRCA2* carrier, provides the rationale for this approach. Inhibiting the DNA repair protein PARP results in the generation of specific DNA lesions that require BRCA1 and BRCA2 specialized repair function(s) for their removal. Preclinical data indicate that tumors defective in wild-type BRCA1 or BRCA2 could be much more sensitive to PARP inhibition than unaffected heterozygous tissues, providing a potentially large therapeutic window. The safety and efficacy of this approach is currently being tested in clinical trials, which, if successful, may lead to registration for routine clinical use of one or more PARP inhibitors.[37]

Synthetic lethality by combinatorial targeting of DNA repair pathways may have usefulness as a therapeutic approach beyond familial cancers. The majority of solid tumors also exhibit genomic instability and aneuploidy. This suggests that pathways involved in the maintenance of genomic stability are dysfunctional in a significant proportion of neoplastic disorders.[47] Understanding which specialized DNA damage response and repair pathways are abrogated in sporadic tumor subtypes may allow for the development of therapies that target the residual repair pathways on which the cancer, but not normal tissue, is now completely dependent. These potential therapies may significantly improve response rates while causing fewer treatment-related toxicities. However, these approaches may be associated with mechanism-associated resistance, and careful consideration of their optimal use will be required.

## REFERENCES

1. Hoeijmakers JH. Genome maintenance mechanisms for preventing cancer. *Nature* 2001;411:366–374.
2. Chambon P, Weill JD, Mandel P. Nicotinamide mononucleotide activation of new DNA-dependent polyadenylic acid synthesizing nuclear enzyme. *Biochem Biophys Res Commun* 1963;11:39–43.
3. Amé JC, Spenlehauer C, de Murcia G. The PARP superfamily. *Bioessays* 2004;26:882–893.
4. Otto H, Reche PA, Bazan F, et al. In silico characterization of the family of PARP-like poly(ADP-ribosyl)transferases (pARTs). *BMC Genomics* 2005;6:139.
5. van Gent DC, Hoeijmakers JH, Kanaar R. Chromosomal stability and the DNA double-stranded break connection. *Nat Rev Genet* 2001;2:196–206.
6. Shin DS, Chahwan C, Huffman JL, et al. Structure and function of the double-strand break repair machinery. *DNA Repair (Amst)* 2004;3: 863–873.
7. Takata M, Sasaki MS, Sonoda E, et al. Homologous recombination and non-homologous end-joining pathways of DNA double-strand break repair have overlapping roles in the maintenance of chromosomal integrity in vertebrate cells. *EMBO J* 1998;17:5497–5508.
8. Rothkamm K, Krüger I, Thompson LH, et al. Pathways of DNA double-strand break repair during the mammalian cell cycle. *Mol Cell Biol* 2003;23: 5706–5715.
9. Stark JM, Pierce AJ, Oh J, et al. Genetic steps of mammalian homologous repair with distinct mutagenic consequences. *Mol Cell Biol* 2004;24: 9305–9316.
10. Elliott B, Richardson C, Jasin M. Chromosomal translocation mechanisms at intronic alu elements in mammalian cells. *Mol Cell* 2005;17:885–894.
11. Durkacz BW, Omidiji O, Gray DA, et al. (ADP-ribose)n participates in DNA excision repair. *Nature* 1980;283(5747):593–596.
12. Tertoli L, Graziani G. Chemosensitisation by PARP inhibitors in cancer therapy. *Pharmacol Res* 2005;52:25–33.
13. Wooster R, Weber BL. Breast and ovarian cancer. *N Engl J Med* 2003;348: 2339–2347.
14. Gudmundsdottir K, Ashworth A. The roles of BRCA1 and BRCA2 and associated proteins in the maintenance of genomic stability. *Oncogene* 2006;25: 5864–5874.
15. Tutt AN, Lord CJ, McCabe N, et al. Exploiting the DNA repair defect in BRCA mutant cells in the design of new therapeutic strategies for cancer. *Cold Spring Harb Symp Quant Biol* 2005;70:139–148.
16. Lord CJ, Ashworth A. RAD51, BRCA2 and DNA repair: a partial resolution. *Nat Struct Mol Biol* 2007;14:461–462.
17. Dobzhansky T. Genetics of natural populations: Xiii. Recombination and variability in populations of *Drosophila pseudoobscura*. *Genetics* 1946;31:269–290.
18. Hartwell LH, Szankasi P, Roberts CJ, et al. Integrating genetic approaches into the discovery of anticancer drugs. *Science* 1997;278:1064–1068.
19. Kaelin WG Jr. The concept of synthetic lethality in the context of anticancer therapy. *Nat Rev Cancer* 2005;5:689–698.
20. Ooi SL, Pan X, Peyser BD, et al. Global synthetic-lethality analysis and yeast functional profiling. *Trends Genet* 2006;22:56–63.
21. Iorns E, Lord CJ, Turner N, et al. Utilizing RNA interference to enhance cancer drug discovery. *Nat Rev Drug Discov* 2007;6:556–568.

22. Noël G, Giocanti N, Fernet M, et al. Poly(ADP-ribose) polymerase (PARP-1) is not involved in DNA double-strand break recovery. *BMC Cell Biol* 2003;4:7.
23. Haber JE. DNA recombination: the replication connection. *Trends Biochem Sci* 1999;24:271–275.
24. Farmer H, McCabe N, Lord CJ, et al. Targeting the DNA repair defect in BRCA mutant cells as a therapeutic strategy. *Nature* 2005;434:917–921.
25. Bryant HE, Schultz N, Thomas HD, et al. Specific killing of BRCA2-deficient tumours with inhibitors of poly(ADP-ribose) polymerase. *Nature* 2005;434: 913–917.
26. Ashworth A. A synthetic lethal therapeutic approach: PARP inhibitors for the treatment of cancers deficient in double-strand break repair. *J Clin Oncol* 2008;26:3785–3790.
27. McCabe N, Turner NC, Lord CJ, et al. Deficiency in the repair of DNA damage by homologous recombination and sensitivity to poly(ADP-ribose) polymerase inhibition. *Cancer Res* 2006;66:8109–8115.
28. Turner N, Tutt A, Ashworth A. Hallmarks of 'BRCAness' in sporadic cancers. *Nat Rev Cancer* 2004;4:814–819.
29. Fong PC, Boss DS, Yap TA, et al. Inhibition of poly(ADP-ribose) polymerase in tumors from BRCA mutation carriers. *N Engl J Med* 2009;361:123–134.
30. Fong PC, Yap TA, Boss DS, et al. Poly(ADP)-ribose polymerase (PARP) inhibition: frequent durable responses in BRCA carrier ovarian cancer correlating with platinum-free interval. *J Clin Oncol* 2010;28:2512–2519.
31. Audeh MW, Carmichael J, Penson RT, et al. Oral poly(ADP-ribose) polymerase inhibitor olaparib in patients with *BRCA1* or *BRCA2* mutations and recurrent ovarian cancer: a proof-of-concept trial. *Lancet* 2010;376:245–251.
32. Tutt A, Robson M, Garber JE, et al. Oral poly(ADP-ribose) polymerase inhibitor olaparib in patients with *BRCA1* or *BRCA2* mutations and advanced breast cancer: a proof-of-concept trial. *Lancet* 2010;376:235–244.
33. Kaye SB, Lubinski J, Matulonis U, et al. Phase II, open-label, randomized, multicenter study comparing the efficacy and safety of olaparib, a poly (ADP-ribose) polymerase inhibitor, and pegylated liposomal doxorubicin in patients with BRCA1 or BRCA2 mutations and recurrent ovarian cancer. *J Clin Oncol* 2012;30:372–379.
34. Sandhu SK, Omlin A, Hylands L et al. Poly (ADP-ribose) polymerase (PARP) inhibitors for the treatment of advanced germline BRCA2 mutant prostate cancer. *Ann Oncol* 2013;24:1416–1418.
35. Fogelman DR, Wolff RA, Kopetz S, et al. Evidence for the efficacy of Iniparib, a PARP–1 inhibitor, in BRCA2-associated pancreatic cancer. *Anticancer Res* 2011;31:1417–1420.
36. Maxwell KN, Domchek SM. Cancer treatment according to BRCA1 and BRCA2 mutations *Nat Rev Clin Oncol* 2012;9:520–528.
37. Garber K. PARP inhibitors bounce back. *Nat Rev Drug Discov* 2013;12: 725–727.
38. Salmena L, Carracedo A, Pandolfi PP. Tenets of PTEN tumor suppression. *Cell* 2008;133:403–414.
39. Mendes-Pereira AM, Martin SA, Brough R, et al. Synthetic lethal targeting of PTEN mutant cells with PARP inhibitors. *EMBO Mol Med* 2009;1:315–322.
40. Foulkes WD, Stefansson IM, Chappuis PO, et al. Germline BRCA1 mutations and a basal epithelial phenotype in breast cancer. *J Natl Cancer Inst* 2003;95:1482–1485.

41. Turner NC, Reis-Filho JS. Basal-like breast cancer and the BRCA1 phenotype. *Oncogene* 2006;25:5846–5853.

42. Ledermann J, Harter P, Gourley C, et al. Olaparib maintenance therapy in platinum-sensitive relapsed ovarian cancer. *N Engl J Med* 2012;366:1382–1392.

43. Ledermann JA, Harter P, Gourley C. Olaparib maintenance therapy in patients with platinum-sensitive relapsed serous ovarian cancer (SOC) and a BRCA mutation (BRCAm). *J Clin Oncol* 2013;31 (suppl; abstr 5505).

44. Gelmon KA, Tischkowitz M, Mackay H, et al. Olaparib in patients with recurrent high-grade serous or poorly differentiated ovarian carcinoma or triple-negative breast cancer: a phase 2, multicentre, open-label, non-randomised study. *Lancet Oncol* 2011;12:852–861.

45. O'Shaughnessy J, Osborne C, Pippen J, et al. Iniparib plus chemotherapy in metastatic triple-negative breast cancer. *N Engl J Med* 2011;3:205–214.

46. Mateo J, Ong M, Tan DS, et al. Appraising iniparib, the PARP inhibitor that never was—what must we learn? *Nat Rev Clin Oncol* 2013;10:688–696.

47. Lord CJ, Ashworth A. The DNA damage response and cancer therapy. *Nature* 2012;481:287–294.

48. Lord CJ, Ashworth A. Mechanisms of resistance to therapies targeting BRCA-mutant cancers. *Nat Med* 2013;19:1381–1388.

49. Edwards S, Brough R, Lord CJ, et al. Resistance to therapy caused by intragenic deletion in BRCA2. *Nature* 2008;451(7182):1111–1115.

50. Rottenberg S, Jaspers JE, Kersbergen A, et al. High sensitivity of BRCA1-deficient mammary tumors to the PARP inhibitor AZD2281 alone and in combination with platinum drugs. *Proc Natl Acad Sci U S A* 2008;105:17079–17084.

51. Cass I, Baldwin RL, Varkey T, et al. Improved survival in women with BRCA-associated ovarian carcinoma. *Cancer* 2003;97:2187–2195.

52. Pal T, Permuth-Wey J, Kapoor R, et al. Improved survival in BRCA2 carriers with ovarian cancer. *Fam Cancer* 2007;6:113–119.

53. Sakai W, Swisher EM, Karlan BY, et al. Secondary mutations as a mechanism of cisplatin resistance in BRCA2-mutated cancers. *Nature* 2008;451:1116–1120.

54. Barber LJ, Sandhu S, Chen L, et al. Secondary mutations in BRCA2 associated with clinical resistance to a PARP inhibitor. *J Pathol* 2013;229:422–429.

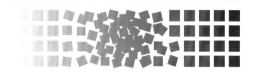

# 26 Miscellaneous Chemotherapeutic Agents

M. Sitki Copur, Scott Nicholas Gettinger, Sarah B. Goldberg, and
Hari A. Deshpande

## HOMOHARRINGTONINE AND OMACETAXINE

Homoharringtonine and its congener, harringtonine, are cephalotaxine esters isolated from the evergreen tree *Cephalotaxus hainanensis*, which are distributed throughout southern and northeastern China. The two differ only by a single methylene group, but both have a similar activity against murine leukemia.[1] The primary action of homoharringtonine appears to be the inhibition of protein synthesis and chain elongation through binding to 80S ribosome in eukaryotic cells.[2] DNA effects may also be important, involving a block in progression of cells from G1 phase into S phase and from G2 phase into M phase.[3] Homoharringtonine exhibits a triphasic plasma decay with a terminal half-life of 65.3 hours and apparent volume of distribution of 2.4 L/kg.[4] In early phase I studies, homoharringtonine was administered as a 10 to 360 minute infusion daily for 10 days.[5] Dose-limiting cardiovascular toxicity with hypotension began 4 or more hours after drug administration, which was alleviated by interrupting the infusion or by fluid administration and prolonging the duration of administration. Initial clinical studies with homoharringtonine in China showed activity against acute myeloid leukemia (AML) and chronic phase chronic myeloid leukemia (CML).[6] Variable activity was observed in the initial series of phase II trials in pediatric and adult patients with acute leukemia. In early studies of homoharringtonine, a continuous intravenous (IV) infusion at 2.5 mg/m$^2$ per day for 10 to 14 days per month induced complete hematologic and cytogenetic responses in 72% and 31% of patients, respectively, with chronic phase CML.[7]

The greater availability of homoharringtonine led to its further testing and the development of a semisynthetic cephalotaxine ester, omacetaxine mepesuccinate.[2] The mechanism of action of omacetaxine includes inhibition of protein synthesis and is independent of direct Bcr-Abl binding. In vitro, it reduces protein levels of the Bcr-Abl oncoprotein and Mcl-1, an antiapoptotic B-cell lymphoma 2 (Bcl-2) family member. The antileukemic effect of omacetaxine is not affected by the presence of mutations in Bcr-Abl.[8] Omacetaxine is absorbed following subcutaneous administration of 1.25 mg/m$^2$ twice daily for 11 days with a mean half-life of 6 hours, and a volume of distribution of 141 +/−93.4 L. A phase 2 trial assessed the efficacy of omacetaxine in CML patients with T315I and tyrosine–kinase inhibitor failure. Patients received subcutaneous omacetaxine 1.25 mg/m$^2$ twice daily on days 1 through 14, every 28 days until hematologic response or a maximum of 6 cycles, and then days 1 through 7 every 28 days as maintenance. Complete hematologic response was achieved in 77%, with a median response duration of 9.1 months. Of patients, 23% achieved a major cytogenetic response, including a complete cytogenetic response in 16%. Hematologic toxicity included thrombocytopenia (76%), neutropenia (44%), and anemia (39%) and was typically manageable by dose reduction. Nonhematologic adverse events were mostly grade 1/2 and included infection, diarrhea, and nausea.[9]

## L-ASPARAGINASE

L-Asparaginase (L-asparagine aminohydrolase, EC 3.5.1.1), which catalyzes the hydrolysis of the essential amino acid L-asparagine to L-aspartic acid and ammonia, is a naturally occurring enzyme in some microorganisms.[10,11] Although cancer cells depend on an exogenous source of L-asparagine for survival, normal cells can synthesize asparagine. In addition to the depletion of L-asparagine, it may exert its antitumor activity through a glutaminase effect, depleting essential glutamine stores and leading to the inhibition of DNA biosynthesis. It comes in three preparations, two of which are native forms purified from bacterial sources, *Escherichia coli* and *Erwinia carotovora*. A third preparation, pegylated (PEG)-L-asparaginase, is a chemically modified form of the enzyme in which native *E. coli* L-asparaginase has been covalently conjugated to polyethylene glycol.[12]

After an intramuscular (IM) injection, peak plasma levels, approximately one-half of those achieved with IV administration, are reached within 14 to 24 hours. Plasma protein binding is 30%. The pharmacokinetics vary depending on the source of the enzyme.[13] Pharmacokinetic studies in newly diagnosed children with acute lymphocytic leukemia (ALL) have shown peak serum concentrations in the range of 1 to 10 IU/mL in 24 to 48 hours of a single dose of 2,500 to 25,000 IU/m$^2$ of the enzyme derived from *E. coli*. After a single dose of 25,000 IU/m$^2$, peak serum levels are reached within 24 hours. PEG-L-asparaginase, when administered at a dose of 2,500 IU/m$^2$, achieves peak drug levels at 72 to 96 hours and has a significantly longer half-life (5.7 days) than the *E. coli* L-asparaginase preparation.[13] Clinical trials have demonstrated the efficacy, safety, and tolerability of PEG-L-asparaginase administered intramuscularly, subcutaneously, or intravenously as part of multiagent chemotherapy regimens in the management of newly diagnosed and relapsed pediatric and adult ALL. L-Asparaginase can antagonize antineoplastic effects of methotrexate if given concurrently or immediately before. These two drugs should be administered sequentially at least 24 hours apart. L-Asparaginase has also been shown to inhibit the metabolic clearance of vincristine and can result in increased neurotoxicity. Toxicity is less pronounced if L-asparaginase is administered after vincristine. Hypersensitivity reactions occur in up to 25% of patients as a skin rash and urticaria or serious anaphylactic reactions. The risk increases with repeat exposure, and as a single-agent use without steroids. PEG-L-asparaginase is less immunogenic than the native nonpegylated forms of the enzyme. A number of other side effects are observed that are secondary to the inhibitory effects of L-asparaginase on cellular protein synthesis. Decreased serum levels of insulin, key lipoproteins, and albumin have been reported. L-Asparaginase can cause alterations in thyroid function tests as early as 2 days after an administered dose, possibly secondary to a reduction in the serum levels of thyroxine-binding globulin. Alterations in coagulation parameters with prolonged thrombin time, prothrombin time, and partial thromboplastin time have been observed. Patients treated with L-asparaginase are at an increased risk for bleeding or thromboembolic events.[14] L-Asparaginase is contraindicated in patients with a prior history of pancreatitis, because there is a 10% incidence of acute pancreatitis. Neurologic toxicity includes lethargy, confusion, agitation, hallucinations, and/or coma. In contrast to the other anticancer agents used to treat ALL, myelosuppression is rare.

# BLEOMYCIN

Bleomycin is a glycopeptide antibiotic produced by the bacterium *Streptomyces verticillus*. The most active chemotherapeutical forms are bleomycin $A_2$ and $B_2$.[15] The effect of bleomycin is cell cycle specific, because its main effects are mediated in the $G_2$ and M phases of the cell cycle.[16] The exact mechanism for DNA strand scission has been suggested to be due to bleomycin's chelating of metal ions (primarily iron) and producing a pseudoenzyme that reacts with oxygen to produce superoxide- and hydroxide-free radicals, thus cleaving DNA. Alternatively, bleomycin may bind at specific sites in the DNA strand and induce scission by abstracting the hydrogen atom from the base, resulting in strand cleavage as the base undergoes a Criegee-type rearrangement, or bleomycin may form an alkali-labile lesion.[17] Bleomycin is used in the treatment of Hodgkin lymphoma (as a component of the ABVD and BEACOPP regimen), squamous cell carcinomas, and testicular cancer; in the treatment of plantar warts,[18] as a means of effecting pleurodesis,[19] as well as an intralesional agent with electrochemotherapy in the management of cutaneous malignancies.[20]

The oral bioavailability is poor. It must be administered via IV or IM routes. The initial distribution half-life is 10 to 20 minutes with a terminal half-life of 3 hours. Bleomycin can be administered via the intracavitary route to control malignant pleural effusions or ascites, or both. Approximately 45% to 55% of an administered intracavitary dose of bleomycin is absorbed into the systemic circulation. Elimination is primarily via the kidneys, and approximately 60% to 70% of an administered dose is excreted unchanged in the urine. Dose reductions are required if creatinine clearance is less than 25 mL per minute.

Bleomycin-induced pneumonitis, the dose-limiting toxicity of the drug, occurs in 10% of patients, and is dependent on the cumulative dose.[21] The risk increases in patients older than 70 years and in those who receive a total cumulative dose greater than 400 U. In addition, patients with an underlying lung disease, prior irradiation to the chest or mediastinum, and exposure to high concentrations of inspired oxygen are at increased risk. Increased use of granulocyte colony-stimulating factor (G-CSF) has been paralleled by an increased incidence of bleomycin-induced pulmonary toxicity. The exacerbating effects of G-CSFs seem to be associated with a marked infiltration of activated neutrophils along with the lung injury caused by the direct effects of bleomycin.[22,23] In a retrospective review, 18% of a total of 141 patients with Hodgkin lymphoma treated with a bleomycin-containing regimen developed pulmonary toxicity. G-CSF use was one of the key factors associated with the development of this complication, and omission of bleomycin had no impact on clinical outcomes.[24] Similarly the combination of brentuximab vedotin and ABVD was associated with excessive pulmonary toxicity, indicating that brentuximab vedotin and bleomycin should not be used together.[25]

Patients with bleomycin-induced pulmonary toxicity may present with cough, dyspnea, dry inspiratory crackles, and infiltrates on chest radiograph. Pulmonary function testing is the most sensitive approach to monitor patients, and pulmonary function tests should be obtained at baseline and before each cycle of therapy, with a specific focus on the carbon monoxide diffusion capacity and vital capacity. A decrease greater than 15% in either diffusion capacity of carbon monoxide or vital capacity should mandate immediate discontinuation of bleomycin. Early clinical trials and isolated case reports suggest that bleomycin-induced acute hypersensitivity reactions occur in 1% of patients with lymphoma and less than 0.5% of those with solid tumors. The reactions are mainly characterized by high-grade fever, chills, hypotension, and, in a few cases, cardiovascular collapse, which

can lead to death. The exact mechanism of these reactions is unclear, but is thought to be related to the release of endogenous pyrogens from the host cells. Supportive care, including hydration, steroids, antipyretics, and antihistamines, may resolve the symptoms.

Clinicians should monitor their patients for any signs and symptoms of acute hyperpyrexic reactions during bleomycin administration. Because the onset of the reactions can occur with any dose of bleomycin and at any time, routine test dosing does not seem to predict when drug reactions may occur.[26] Mucocutaneous toxicity presents as mucositis, erythema, hyperpigmentation, induration, hyperkeratosis, and skin peeling, which may progress to ulceration, and usually develops in the 2nd and 3rd week of treatment and after a cumulative dose of 150 to 200 U of the drug. Levels of bleomycin hydrolase are relatively low in lung and skin tissue, perhaps offering an explanation as to why these normal tissues are more adversely affected by bleomycin. Myelosuppression and immunosuppression are relatively mild. In rare cases, vascular events, including myocardial infarction, stroke, and Raynaud phenomenon, have been reported.

# PROCARBAZINE

Originally prepared as a monoamine oxidase inhibitor, procarbazine is a prodrug, which after oxidation of the hydrazine in the liver, undergoes a complex enzymatic and chemical breakdown to its alkylating and methylating species.[27,28] The precise mechanism of action is uncertain, but may involve damaging the DNA, RNA or transfer RNA, and the inhibition of protein synthesis. Procarbazine is a cell-cycle phase-nonspecific antineoplastic agent. This agent was initially approved by the U.S. Food and Drug Administration (FDA) in 1969 as part of the MOPP (mechlorethamine, vincristine, procarbazine, and prednisone) regimen for the treatment of Hodgkin lymphoma. Since then, it has also demonstrated clinical activity in non-Hodgkin lymphoma, cutaneous T-cell lymphoma, and brain tumors.

Procarbazine is rapidly and completely absorbed from the gastrointestinal tract. Following oral administration, peak drug levels are reached within 10 to 15 minutes. Procarbazine crosses the blood–brain barrier and rapidly equilibrates between plasma and cerebrospinal fluid after oral administration. Peak cerebrospinal fluid drug concentrations are reached within 30 to 90 minutes after drug administration. The biologic half-life of procarbazine hydrochloride in both plasma and cerebrospinal fluid is approximately 1 hour. Procarbazine is metabolized to active and inactive metabolites by chemical breakdown in an aqueous solution and the liver microsomal P-450 system. Approximately 70% of procarbazine is excreted in urine within 24 hours, and less than 5% to 10% of the drug is eliminated in an unchanged form.[29,30]

A careful food and drug history is required before starting a patient on procarbazine therapy, because there are several potential drug–drug and drug–food interactions. Patients should avoid tyramine-containing foods, such as dark beer, wine, cheese, yogurt, bananas, and smoked foods. Procarbazine produces a disulfiramlike reaction with concurrent use of alcohol. Acute hypertensive reactions may occur with coadministration of tricyclic antidepressants and sympathomimetic drugs. Concurrent use of procarbazine with antihistamines and other central nervous system (CNS) depressants can result in CNS and/or respiratory depression.

Dose-limiting toxicity is myelosuppression, more commonly thrombocytopenia, and the nadir in platelet count is generally observed at 4 weeks. Patients with glucose-6-phosphate dehydrogenase deficiency can develop hemolytic anemia while receiving procarbazine therapy. Stepwise dose increments over the first few days of drug administration may minimize gastrointestinal intolerance. On rare occasions, procarbazine may induce interstitial pneumonitis, which mandates the discontinuation of therapy. Azoospermia and infertility after treatment with MOPP can be attributed, in part, to procarbazine. Procarbazine is associated with an increased risk of secondary malignancies, especially acute leukemia.

## VISMODEGIB

Vismodegib (Erivedge, GDC-0449, Genentech) is a first-in-class, small-molecule inhibitor of the Hedgehog pathway. It binds to and inhibits smoothened, a transmembrane protein that is involved in Hedgehog signaling.[31] Pharmacodynamic downmodulation in the Hedgehog pathway was shown by a 90% decrease in transcription factor Gli1 mRNA in basal-cell carcinoma biopsy specimens of patients treated for a month. One-month vismodegib treatment also significantly reduced tumor proliferation, as assessed by Ki-67 expression, but did not change apoptosis, as assessed by cleaved caspase 3. The extent of Gli1 downmodulation does not seem to correlate with pharmacokinetic levels of vismodegib in individual patients. Vismodegib is absorbed from the gastrointestinal tract, with an oral bioavailability of 32%. Food does not affect drug exposure. Elimination is mainly hepatic, with excretion in feces. The median steady-state concentration is not changed by increasing the dose from 150 mg to 270 mg, and the median time to steady state is 14 days. The half-life is estimated at 8 days after a single dose. Intermittent doses (e.g., three times per week or once per week) were associated with a decrease of 50% and 80% in effective plasma levels of unbound drug, respectively, thus reinforcing the recommended dose and schedule of 150 mg orally daily.[32] Vismodegib is approved for the treatment of adults with metastatic basal-cell carcinoma that has recurred following surgery or in those who are not candidates for surgery and who are not candidates for radiation.[33]

No dose-limiting toxic effects or grade 5 events have been observed. However, 54% of patients receiving vismodegib discontinued the medication owing to side effects, and only one out of give eligible patients was able to continue vismodegib for 18 months. Abdominal pain, fatigue, weight loss, dysgeusia, and anorexia were reasons for discontinuation of the drug. When vismodegib was withdrawn, dysgeusia and muscle cramps ceased within 1 month, and scalp and body hair started to regrow within 3 months. Other side effects reported include hyponatremia, dyspnea, muscle spasm, atrial fibrillation, aspiration, back pain, corneal abrasion, dehydration, keratitis, lymphopenia, pneumonia, urinary tract infection, and a prolonged QT interval.[34]

## ADO-TRASTUZUMAB EMTANSINE

Ado-trastuzumab emtansine (T-DM1), is a HER2-targeted antibody-drug conjugate (ADC). It is a novel compound composed of trastuzumab, a stable thioether linker, and DM1. DM1, a derivative of maytansine, is a microtubule polymerization inhibitor with activity similar to that of vinca alkaloids. T-DM1 is taken up into cells after binding to HER2, allowing for cytotoxic drug delivery specifically to cells overexpressing HER2. It has a drug-to-antibody ratio of approximately 3.5:1. T-DM1 is administered intravenously every 3 weeks and has been tested in a phase I trial at doses ranging from 0.3 to 4.8 mg/kg. The maximally tolerated dose is 3.6 mg/kg, which was the dose used in further phase II–III trials. T-DM1 is metabolized by the liver, via CYP3A4/5, and has a half-life of 3.5 days.[35]

T-DM1 is approved for use in patients with metastatic HER2-positive breast cancer who have received prior trastuzumab and a taxane. This approval was based on the results of the EMILIA trial, which randomized 991 patients with HER2-positive unresectable, locally advanced or metastatic breast cancer to T-DM1 3.6 mg/kg IV every 21 days or lapatinib 1,250 mg daily plus capecitabine 1,000 mg/m[2] on days 1 through 14 every 21 days. All patients were previously treated with trastuzumab and a taxane. T-DM1 resulted in a progression-free survival of 9.6 months compared to 6.4 months for lapatinib plus capecitabine (hazard ratio [HR] 0.65; 95% confidence interval [CI] 0.55 to 0.77; p <0.001). The response rate and overall survival was also higher with T-DM1 compared to lapatinib plus capecitabine.[36]

Although maytansine itself is associated with significant toxicity, T-DM1 is very well tolerated overall, which is likely due to the targeted nature of the compound. Side effects from T-DM1 include thrombocytopenia, hepatotoxicity, hypersensitivity/infusion

reactions, and cardiotoxicity. Nausea, fatigue, headaches, and anemia are also common. The left ventricular ejection fraction should be monitored prior to and at least every 3 months during therapy because of the potential for cardiac dysfunction.

## SIROLIMUS AND TEMSIROLIMUS

Sirolimus (rapamycin) was isolated from the soil bacteria *Streptomyces hygroscopicus*, in the mid 1970s.[37] This bacterial macrolide later became the preferred immunosuppressant for kidney transplantation, because it was mildly immunosuppressive; however, in contrast to cyclosporine A, it did not enhance tumor incidence.[38] Sirolimus is the prototypic inhibitor of the mammalian target of rapamycin (mTOR), a serine/threonine protein kinase that is a highly conserved regulatory protein involved in cell-cycle progression, proliferation, and angiogenesis.[39] Signaling pathways both upstream and downstream of mTOR have been shown to be commonly dysregulated in cancer. mTOR functions through two main mechanisms, depending on the presence and activity of the mTOR-associated protein complexes, mTORC1 and mTORC2. Sirolimus and its analog compounds, temsirolimus and everolimus, form a complex with the FK-binding protein (FKBP) and inhibit activation of a subset of mTOR proteins residing within mTORC1. In contrast, mTORC2 holds mTOR in a form that is not as readily inhibited by these rapamycin analogs, and upregulation of mTORC2 may represent a mechanism by which resistance can develop to this class of compounds.

Temsirolimus (CCI-779), a novel functional ester of sirolimus, is a water-soluble dihydroxymethyl propionic acid compound that rapidly undergoes hydrolysis to sirolimus after IV administration, reaching peak concentrations within 0.5 to 2.0 hours.[40] This drug is widely distributed in tissues, and steady-state drug levels are reached in 7 to 8 days. Temsirolimus is metabolized primarily in the liver by CYP3A4 microsomal enzymes to yield sirolimus as the main metabolite. The terminal half-life of temsirolimus is 17 hours, whereas that of sirolimus is approximately 55 hours. When bound to temsirolimus, mTOR is unable to phosphorylate the key protein translation factors, such as 4E-BP1 and S6K1, leading to translational inhibition of several critical regulatory proteins involved in cell-cycle control. Several other cellular proteins involved in the regulation of angiogenesis, such as hypoxia-inducible factor-1α (HIF-1α) and vascular endothelial growth factor (VEGF), are suppressed through mTOR inhibition by temsirolimus.

Phase I studies of temsirolimus have investigated various schedules and doses, ranging from 7.5 mg to 220 mg given as weekly 30-minute infusions.[40] A phase II study in patients with cytokine-refractory renal cell cancer (RCC) investigated the efficacy and safety of three different dose levels (25 mg, 75 mg, and 250 mg, respectively) administered on a weekly schedule. This study showed promising antitumor activity for all three dose levels with no significant difference in efficacy or toxicity.[41] As a result, the 25-mg dose was eventually selected as the monotherapy dose for further study. A phase III randomized trial compared interferon, temsirolimus, and the combination of the two agents in previously untreated patients with advanced RCC who had at least three of six poor prognostic features.[42] Once-weekly IV temsirolimus, 25 mg, prolonged the median overall survival of patients with poor prognostic features by 49% from 7.3 months (95% CI, 6.1 to 8.8 months) in the interferon arm to 10.9 months (95% CI, 8.6 to 12.7 months) in the temsirolimus arm (P = .008). The temsirolimus arm also had a prolonged median progression-free survival of 5.5 months compared to 3.1 months in the interferon arm (P <.001). Moreover, temsirolimus was effective for both clear cell and non–clear cell histologies.[43,44]

Mantle cell lymphoma was the first hematologic malignancy in which mTOR inhibition was explored as a treatment strategy. The rationale for this approach was that mantle cell lymphoma is characterized by overexpression of cyclin D1, which is a cyclin whose expression appears to be tightly regulated by mTOR signaling. The early-phase clinical trials of temsirolimus showed promising activity against non-Hodgkin lymphomas, multiple myeloma, and myeloid leukemias, with some evidence of success thus far.[45]

In terms of the safety profile, the most common adverse events associated with temsirolimus were asthenia and fatigue, dry skin with acneiform skin rash, nausea/vomiting, mucositis, and anorexia. Hyperlipidemia with increased serum triglycerides and/or cholesterol as well as hyperglycemia occur in up to 90% of patients. Allergic, hypersensitivity reactions have been observed in about 10% of patients, and pulmonary toxicity, presenting as increased cough, dyspnea, fever, and pulmonary infiltrates, is a relatively rare event, occurring in less than 1% of patients. However, the risk of pulmonary toxicity increases in patients with an underlying pulmonary disease.[46]

## EVEROLIMUS

Everolimus (RAD001) is an orally active hydroxyethyl ether analog of rapamycin that contains a 2-hydroxyethyl chain substitution. This molecule is significantly more water soluble than sirolimus. As with sirolimus and temsirolimus, everolimus targets mTOR by forming a complex with mTOR and FKBP, resulting in inhibition of mTOR activity. Few data are available regarding the actual differences in the ability of temsirolimus and everolimus to inhibit mTOR. One preclinical in vitro study showed that the binding of everolimus to FKBP was approximately threefold weaker than that of sirolimus.[47] In vivo studies, however, have documented similar efficacy of the two agents in terms of immunosuppressive activity as well as antitumor activity. In preclinical models, the administration of everolimus results in the inhibition of mTOR, similar to what has been observed with the other rapamycin analogs.[48] In terms of clinical pharmacology, peak drug levels are achieved within 1 to 2 hours after oral administration, and food with a high fat content reduces oral bioavailability by up to 20%. This compound is metabolized in the liver, mainly by the CYP3A4 system, and six main metabolites have been identified. In general, these metabolites are less active than the parent compound. Elimination is mainly hepatic with excretion in feces, and caution should be used in patients with moderate liver impairment (Child-Pugh class B).[49] In this setting, the daily dose of drug should be reduced to 5 mg. In patients with severe liver dysfunction (Child-Pugh class C), the use of this drug is contraindicated.

Encouraging clinical activity was initially observed in phase 1/2 trials in patients with non–small-cell lung, gastric, and esophageal cancers, sarcomas, pancreatic neuroendocrine tumors, as well as hematologic malignancies.[50–53] Presently, everolimus is indicated and approved for the treatment of adults with advanced RCC after failure with sunitinib or sorafenib; advanced hormone receptor-positive, HER2-negative breast cancer in combination with exemestane; and progressive unresectable, locally advanced, or metastatic neuroendocrine tumors of pancreatic origin (PNET).[54,55] The recommended dose of everolimus for these indications is 10 mg taken orally once daily.

The safety profile of everolimus is similar to what has been observed with temsirolimus. The most common adverse events include asthenia and fatigue, dry skin with acneiform skin rash, nausea/vomiting, mucositis, and anorexia. Hyperlipidemia with increased serum triglycerides and/or cholesterol as well as hyperglycemia occur in up to 90% of patients. Allergic, hypersensitivity reactions have been observed in about 10% of patients, and pulmonary toxicity, presenting as increased cough, dyspnea, fever, and pulmonary infiltrates, are a relatively rare event, occurring in less than 1% of patients. However, the risk of pulmonary toxicity increases in patients with an underlying pulmonary disease.

## THALIDOMIDE, LENALIDOMIDE, AND POMALIDOMIDE

Thalidomide and its amino-substituted analogs, lenalidomide and pomalidomide, are small-molecule glutamic acid derivatives that possess a wide range of biologic properties, including immunomodulating, antiangiogenic, and epigenetic effects. They are classified as class I (non–phosphodiesterase-4 inhibitory) immunomodulatory drugs (IMiDs). Although their primary mechanism of activity against malignancy is uncertain, it is believed that IMiDs exert their anticancer effects both directly on cancer cells and indirectly via effects on the tumor microenvironment and host antitumor immunity. Specific mechanisms include the inhibition of nuclear factor kappa B (NF-κB) transcriptional activity in malignant cells with a resultant decrease in the production of anti-apoptotic molecules; the inhibition of surface adhesion molecule expression on both multiple myeloma cells and bone marrow stromal cells; the inhibition of the production and release of various growth factors (including vascular endothelial growth factor, basic fibroblast growth factor, tumor necrosis factor alpha, and interleukin [IL] 6) that regulate angiogenesis and tumor cell proliferation; and costimulation of IL-2 and interferon gamma (IFN-γ) release with T-helper 1 subset skewing and augmentation of cytotoxic T-cell and natural killer cell effector function.[56,57] Unlike thalidomide, both lenalidomide and pomalidomide result in cell cycle arrest and apoptosis of myeloma cells in vitro, believed in part to be related to epigenetic effects.[58] They are also more potent stimulators of IL-2 and INF-γ production and T-cell proliferation than thalidomide, and appear to additionally inhibit T-regulatory cells.[57] Clinically, lenalidomide has activity in patients with thalidomide-resistant multiple myeloma, and pomalidomide has additional activity in patients with lenalidomide-resistant disease.[59,60] Recently, the protein cereblon (cerebral protein with lon protease), a highly conserved E3 ligase, was recognized as a primary target of IMiDs teratogenic effect, and appears to be an important target of IMiD anticancer activity.[61–63] Efforts are currently under way to evaluate the expression of Cereblon as a predictive biomarker of response to IMiDs.[63] Due to the potential risk of significant teratogenicity, thalidomide, lenalidomide, and pomalidomide can only be prescribed by licensed prescribers who are registered in restricted distribution programs.

### Thalidomide

Thalidomide (2-[2,6-dioxopiperidin-3-yl]-2,3-dihydro-1H-isoindole-1,3-dione; Thalomid) is a synthetic glutamic acid derivative that was initially synthesized in 1953. It was used widely in Europe between 1956 and 1962 as a sleeping aid and antiemetic for pregnant women before it was discovered to cause severe congenital malformations. Initial reports of its efficacy in multiple myeloma were published in 1999, and the 200-mg daily dose combined with pulse dexamethasone (40-mg daily dose on days 1 through 4, 9 through 12, and 17 through 20 on a 28-day schedule) was approved by the FDA in 2006 for newly diagnosed multiple myeloma. The use of thalidomide has dropped precipitously in the United States with the FDA approval of more efficacious and less toxic therapies for myeloma. Thalidomide is poorly soluble, and it is absorbed slowly from the gastrointestinal tract, reaching peak plasma concentration in 3 to 6 hours, with 55% to 66% bound to plasma proteins. The exact metabolic route and fate of thalidomide is not known. Thalidomide does not appear to be hepatically metabolized, but rather undergoes spontaneous nonenzymatic hydrolysis in plasma to multiple metabolites, with a half-life of elimination ranging from 5 to 7 hours. These metabolites are believed to be responsible for the antitumor effects of thalidomide. Less than 1% is excreted into the urine as unchanged drug.[64]

Thalidomide frequently causes drowsiness, constipation, and fatigue. Peripheral neuropathy is a common and potentially severe and irreversible side effect occurring in up to 30% of patients. Increased incidences of venous thromboembolic events, such as deep venous thrombosis and pulmonary embolus, have also been observed with thalidomide, particularly when used in combination with dexamethasone or anthracycline-based chemotherapy. Patients who are appropriate candidates may benefit from concurrent prophylactic anticoagulation or aspirin treatment.[65] Other side effects of thalidomide include rash, nausea, dizziness, orthostatic hypotension, bradycardia, and mood changes. In 2013, additional alerts were released linking thalidomide to an increased risk of developing second primary malignancies (both acute myelogenous leukemia and myelodysplastic syndrome) and arterial thromboembolic events.

## Lenalidomide

Lenalidomide (3-[4-amino-1-oxo-2,3-dihydro-1H-isoindol-2-yl]piperidine-2,6-dione; Revlimid) is a thalidomide derivative that shares the immunomodulatory and antineoplastic properties of its parent compound. However, lenalidomide appears to be more potent in vitro with less nonhematologic toxicities in clinical studies. It initially received FDA approval (10-mg daily dose) in 2005 for the treatment of patients with transfusion-dependent anemia secondary to low or intermediate risk myelodysplastic syndromes associated with a deletion 5q cytogenetic abnormality, with or without additional cytogenetic abnormalities. In 2006, lenalidomide (25-mg daily dose on days 1 through 21 of a 28-day cycle) in combination with dexamethasone (40-mg daily dose on days 1 through 4, 9 through 12, and 17 through 20 on each 28-day cycle for the first four cycles, then 40 mg daily on days 1 through 4 every 28 days) was approved by the FDA for the treatment of patients with multiple myeloma who had received at least one prior therapy for multiple myeloma. In 2013, lenalidomide 25 mg daily (days 1 through 21 on repeated 28-day cycles) was additionally approved for use in refractory mantle cell lymphoma (after relapse/ progression on two lines of therapy, one of which contained bortezomib). Lenalidomide is administered orally and is rapidly absorbed from the gastrointestinal tract. Maximum plasma concentration is reached 0.625 to 1.5 hours after dosing, with approximately 30% bound to plasma proteins. The half-life of elimination is approximately 3 hours, with little information currently available concerning metabolism. Approximately 70% of an administered dose is excreted unchanged by the kidneys.[66]

Compared with thalidomide, lenalidomide is associated with less sedation, constipation, and peripheral neuropathy. However, myelosuppression in the form of neutropenia and thrombocytopenia can be dose limiting. As with thalidomide, the incidence of thromboembolic events is significant with the combination of dexamethasone and lenalidomide. A pooled analysis of 691 patients enrolled in two randomized studies reported a 12% incidence of thrombotic or thromboembolic events with the combination, compared with 4% with dexamethasone alone.[67]

## Pomalidomide

Pomalidomide (4-amino-2-[2,6-dioxopiperidin-3-yl]-2,3-dihydro-1H-isoindole-1,3-dione; Pomalyst) is another thalidomide derivative designed to be more portent and less toxic than both thalidomide and lenalidomide. It is currently FDA approved (4-mg once daily dose orally on days 1 through 21 of a 28-day cycle, with or without dexamethasone) for use in patients with progressive multiple myeloma who have received at least two prior therapies, including lenalidomide and bortezomib. Pomalidomide is administered orally and is rapidly absorbed. Maximum plasma concentration is reached 2 to 3 hours after ingestion, with approximately 12% to 44% protein binding.[68] The half-life of elimination is between 7.5 and 9.5 hours. Pomalidomide is metabolized in the liver, via CYP1A2/CYP3A4 (major) and CYP2C19/CYP2D6 (minor), and excretion occurs primarily through the kidneys (73%; 2% as unchanged drug).

Like lenalidomide, pomalidomide is better tolerated than thalidomide at approved doses with less constipation, fatigue, and neuropathy.[69] The primary toxicity appreciated in myeloma trials has been myelosuppression, particularly neutropenia, which can be dose limiting. The risk of thromboembolic events is similar to that seen with thalidomide and lenalidomide. Unlike thalidomide or lenalidomide, dermatologic toxicity is rare with pomalidomide. A summary of the characteristics of the miscellaneous drugs mentioned in this chapter is provided in Table 26.1. A summary of all hematology oncology drug approvals since the last edition of the textbook can be viewed in Table 26.2.

| **TABLE 26.1** | | | | |
|---|---|---|---|---|
| **Miscellaneous Chemotherapeutic Agents** | | | | |
| | **Main Therapeutic Uses** | **Clinical Pharmacology** | **Major Toxicities** | **Notes** |
| **Omacetaxine** | CML | Mean half-life of 6 h after subcutaneous injection | Thrombocytopenia, anemia, nausea, diarrhea | Efficacy shown in Bcr-Abl–mutated CML |
| **L-Asparaginase** | Pediatric and adult ALL | Peak concentration 7–12 h after IV administration; 30% plasma protein binding; PEG form has longer half-life of 5.7 days; antagonize effects of methotrexate if given before or concurrently | Hypersensitivity reactions, alterations in thyroid function, prolonged PT/PTT, decreased levels of vitamin K–dependent factors, acute pancreatitis | Myelosuppression is rare; hypersensitivity reaction risk increases with repeated exposure and when used as single agent; PEG form is less immunogenic |
| **Bleomycin** | Hodgkin disease, neoplastic pleural effusion, non-Hodgkin lymphoma, squamous cell carcinoma of cervix, squamous cell carcinoma of nasopharynx, squamous cell carcinoma of penis, squamous cell carcinoma of the head and neck, squamous cell carcinoma of vulva, testicular cancer | Terminal half-life of 3h; can be given intracavitary; 45%–55% of intracavitary dose absorbed systemically; elimination via kidneys if CrCl <25–35 mL/min dose reduction required | Pulmonary toxicity dose-limiting; more if age >70 y; cumulative dose >400 U; acute hypersensitivity reactions rare (1%); mucositis, erythema, hyperpigmentation | Not myelosuppressive; immunosuppressive; metabolizing enzyme; bleomycin hydrolase enzyme low in lung and skin tissue; G-CSF use seems to exacerbate pulmonary toxicity |

*(continued)*

**TABLE 26.1**

## Miscellaneous Chemotherapeutic Agents *(continued)*

| | Main Therapeutic Uses | Clinical Pharmacology | Major Toxicities | Notes |
|---|---|---|---|---|
| **Procarbazine** | Hodgkin lymphoma | Rapid complete oral absorption; peak concentration, 10–15 min; crosses blood–brain barrier; half-life 1 h; several drug–drug and food–drug interactions; metabolized by hepatic microsomal P-450 system; 70% excreted in urine | Dose-limiting toxicity is myelosuppression, more commonly thrombocytopenia nadir at 4 wk; G-6PD–deficient patients can develop hemolytic anemia, nausea, vomiting, diarrhea, flulike symptoms, peripheral neuropathy, hypersensitivity reactions | Avoid tyramine-containing foods; disulfiramlike reaction with concurrent alcohol use; hypertensive reaction with concurrent tricyclic antidepressant use; increased risk for azoospermia/infertility and secondary malignancy |
| **Vismodegib** | Basal cell carcinoma of the skin | Oral bioavailability 32%; not affected by food | No dose limiting toxicity; abdominal pain, fatigue, weight loss, dysgeusia | Hedgehog-signaling pathway inhibitor |
| **Ado-trastuzumabemtansine** | Advanced HER2-positive breast cancer | Peak concentration near the end of infusion metabolized by CYP3A4/5; half-life, 3.5 days | Thrombocytopenia, hepatotoxicity, cardiac toxicity fatigue, nausea | Monitor cardiac function |
| **Temsirolimus** | Advanced renal cancer | Peak concentration, 0.5–2 h; widely distributed in tissues; steady-state levels reached in 7–8 d; half-life, 17 h | Asthenia, fatigue, dry skin, acneiform skin rash, mucositis, anorexia, hyperlipidemia, hyperglycemia | Efficacy shown for both clear cell and non–clear-cell histologies; efficacy in hematologic malignancies (mantle cell lymphoma, non-Hodgkin lymphoma, multiple myeloma) |
| **Everolimus** | Advanced renal cell carcinoma, breast cancer, pancreatic neuroendocrine tumor | Peak concentration, 1–2 hr; reduced bioavailability with high fat content food; metabolized by CYP3A4 system; mainly hepatic excretion | Asthenia, dry skin, nausea, vomiting, mucositis, hyperlipidemia, hyperglycemia, allergic hypersensitivity reaction, pulmonary toxicity | Contraindicated in Child-Pugh class C patients; encouraging activity in gastric, non–small-cell, lung, esophageal cancers, sarcomas; approved for organ rejection prophylaxis |
| **Thalidomide** | Multiple myeloma, erythema nodosum leprosum | Oral absorption slow; peak concentration, 3–6 h; 55%–66% bound to plasma proteins; half-life, 5–7 h; spontaneous nonenzymatic hydrolysis in plasma | Drowsiness, constipation, fatigue, skin rash, increased risk for thromboembolic complications | Pregnancy category X; may be present in semen; serious skin reactions including Stevens-Johnson syndrome |
| **Lenalidomide** | Low-to-intermediate risk myelodysplastic syndrome associated with 5q deletion, multiple myeloma | Rapid oral absorption; peak concentration, 0.6–1.5 h; half-life, 3 h; 70% excreted unchanged by kidneys | Less sedation, drowsiness, constipation than thalidomide; myelosuppression; thromboembolic events; peripheral neuropathy | Pregnancy category X; caution in patients with renal function impairment; neutropenia; thrombocytopenia may be dose limiting |
| **Pomalidomide** | Multiple myeloma who have received at least two prior therapies | Rapid oral absorption; peak concentration, 2–3 h; half-life, 7.5 h | Myelosuppression; thromboembolic events; skin toxicity rare | Better tolerated than thalidomide; effective in prior bortezomib- and lenalidomide-receiving patients |

PT, prothrombin time; PTT, partial thromboplastin time; CrCl, creatinine clearance.

CANCER THERAPEUTICS

## TABLE 26.2

### U.S. Food And Drug Administration Hematology Oncology Drug Approvals 2010–2013

| Drug/Manufacturer | Indication | Approval Date |
| --- | --- | --- |
| Sorafenib (NEXAVAR tablets, Bayer Healthcare Pharmaceuticals Inc.) | For the treatment of locally recurrent or metastatic, progressive, differentiated thyroid carcinoma (DTC) refractory to radioactive iodine treatment. | November 22, 2013 |
| Crizotinib (Xalkori, Pfizer, Inc.) capsules | For the treatment of patients with metastatic non–small-cell lung cancer (NSCLC) whose tumors are anaplastic lymphoma kinase (ALK) positive as detected by an FDA-approved test. | November 20, 2013 |
| Ibrutinib (IMBRUVICA, Pharmacyclics, Inc.) | For the treatment of patients with mantle cell lymphoma (MCL) who have received at least one prior therapy. | November 13, 2013 |
| Obinutuzumab (GAZYVA injection, for intravenous use, Genentech, Inc.; previously known as GA101) | For use in combination with chlorambucil for the treatment of patients with previously untreated chronic lymphocytic leukemia (CLL). | November 1, 2013 |
| Pertuzumab injection (PERJETA, Genentech, Inc.) | For use in combination with trastuzumab and docetaxel for the neoadjuvant treatment of patients with HER2-positive, locally advanced, inflammatory, or early stage breast cancer (either greater than 2 cm in diameter or node positive) as part of a complete treatment regimen for early breast cancer. | September 30, 2013 |
| Paclitaxel protein-bound particles (albumin-bound) (Abraxane for injectable suspension, Abraxis BioScience, LLC, a wholly owned subsidiary of Celgene Corporation) | In combination with gemcitabine for the first-line treatment of patients with metastatic adenocarcinoma of the pancreas. | September 6, 2013 |
| Afatinib (Gilotrif tablets, Boehringer Ingelheim Pharmaceuticals, Inc.) | For the first-line treatment of patients with metastatic NSCLC whose tumors have epidermal growth factor receptor (EGFR) exon 19 deletions or exon 21 (L858R) substitution mutations as detected by an FDA-approved test. The safety and efficacy of afatinib have not been established in patients whose tumors have other EGFR mutations. | July 12, 2013 |
| Denosumab (Xgeva injection, for subcutaneous use, Amgen Inc.) | For the treatment of adults and skeletally mature adolescents with a giant cell tumor of bone that is unresectable or where surgical resection is likely to result in severe morbidity. | June 13, 2013 |
| Lenalidomide capsules (REVLIMID, Celgene Corporation) | For the treatment of patients with MCL whose disease has relapsed or progressed after two prior therapies, one of which included bortezomib. | June 5, 2013 |
| Trametinib (MEKINIST tablet, GlaxoSmithKline, LLC) | For the treatment of patients with unresectable or metastatic melanoma with BRAF V600E or V600K mutation as detected by an FDA-approved test. | May 29, 2013 |
| Dabrafenib (TAFINLAR capsule, GlaxoSmithKline, LLC) | For the treatment of patients with unresectable or metastatic melanoma with BRAF V600E mutation as detected by an FDA-approved test. | May 29, 2013 |
| Radium Ra 223 dichloride (Xofigo Injection, Bayer HealthCare Pharmaceuticals Inc.) | For the treatment of patients with castration-resistant prostate cancer, symptomatic bone metastases, and no known visceral metastatic disease. | May 15, 2013 |
| Erlotinib (Tarceva, Astellas Pharma Inc.) | For the first-line treatment of metastatic NSCLC patients whose tumors have EGFR exon 19 deletions or exon 21 (L858R) substitution mutations. | May 14, 2013 |
| Ado-trastuzumab emtansine (KADCYLA for injection, Genentech, Inc.) | For use as a single agent for the treatment of patients with HER2-positive, metastatic breast cancer who previously received trastuzumab and a taxane, separately or in combination. | February 22, 2013 |
| Pomalidomide (POMALYST capsules, Celgene Corporation) | For the treatment of patients with multiple myeloma who have received at least two prior therapies, including lenalidomide and bortezomib, and have demonstrated disease progression on or within 60 days of completion of the last therapy. | February 8, 2013 |

(continued)

**TABLE 26.2**

**U.S. Food And Drug Administration Hematology Oncology Drug Approvals 2010–2013** *(continued)*

| Drug/Manufacturer | Indication | Approval Date |
|---|---|---|
| Doxorubicin hydrochloride liposome injection (Sun Pharma Global FZE), a generic version of DOXIL Injection (doxorubicin hydrochloride liposome; Janssen Products, L.P.) | For the treatment of ovarian cancer in patients whose disease has progressed or recurred after platinum-based chemotherapy and for AIDS-related Kaposi sarcoma after failure of prior systemic chemotherapy or intolerance to such therapy. | February 4, 2013 |
| Bevacizumab (Avastin, Genentech U.S., Inc.) | For use in combination with fluoropyrimidine–irinotecan- or fluoropyrimidine–oxaliplatin-based chemotherapy for the treatment of patients with metastatic colorectal cancer (mCRC) whose disease has progressed on a first-line bevacizumab-containing regimen. | January 23, 2013 |
| Ponatinib (Iclusig tablets, ARIAD Pharmaceuticals, Inc.) | For the treatment of adult patients with chronic phase, accelerated phase, or blast phase chronic myeloid leukemia (CML) that is resistant or intolerant to prior tyrosine–kinase inhibitor (TKI) therapy or Philadelphia chromosome–positive acute lymphoblastic leukemia (Ph+ ALL) that is resistant or intolerant to prior TKI therapy. | December 17, 2012 |
| Abiraterone acetate (Zytiga Tablets, Janssen Biotech, Inc.) | In combination with prednisone for the treatment of patients with metastatic castration-resistant prostate cancer. | December 10, 2012 |
| Cabozantinib (COMETRIQ capsules, Exelixis, Inc.) | For the treatment of patients with progressive metastatic medullary thyroid cancer (MTC).Cabozantinib is a small molecule that inhibits the activity of multiple tyrosine kinases, including RET, MET, and VEGF receptor 2. | November 29, 2012 |
| Omacetaxine mepesuccinate (SYNRIBO for injection, for subcutaneous use, Teva Pharmaceutical Industries Ltd.) | For the treatment of adult patients with chronic or accelerated phase CML with resistance and/or intolerance to two or more TKIs. | October 26, 2012 |
| Paclitaxel protein-bound particles for injectable suspension, albumin-bound (ABRAXANE for injectable suspension; Abraxis Bioscience a wholly owned subsidiary of Celgene Corporation) | For use in combination with carboplatin for the initial treatment of patients with locally advanced or metastatic NSCLC who are not candidates for curative surgery or radiation therapy. | October 11, 2012 |
| Regorafenib (Stivarga tablets, Bayer HealthCare Pharmaceuticals, Inc.) | For the treatment of patients with mCRC who have been previously treated with fluoropyrimidine-, oxaliplatin-, and irinotecan-based chemotherapy, an anti-VEGF therapy, and, if KRAS wild-type, an anti-EGFR therapy. | September 27, 2012 |
| Bosutinib tablets (Bosulif, Pfizer, Inc.) | for the treatment of chronic, accelerated, or blast phase Ph+ CML in adult patients with resistance or intolerance to prior therapy. | September 4, 2012 |
| Enzalutamide (XTANDI Capsules, Medivation, Inc., and Astellas Pharma US, Inc.) | For the treatment of patients with metastatic castration-resistant prostate cancer who have previously received docetaxel. | August 31, 2012 |
| Everolimus tablets for oral suspension (Afinitor Disperz, Novartis Pharmaceuticals Corp.) | For the treatment of pediatric and adult patients with tuberous sclerosis complex (TSC) who have subependymal giant cell astrocytoma (SEGA) that requires therapeutic intervention, but that cannot be curatively resected. | August 30, 2012 |
| Vincristine sulfate LIPOSOME injection (Marqibo, Talon Therapeutics, Inc.) | For the treatment of adult patients with Ph- ALL in second or greater relapse or whose disease has progressed following two or more antileukemia therapies. | August 9, 2012 |
| Ziv-aflibercept injection (ZALTRAP, Sanofi U.S., Inc.) | For use in combination with 5-fluorouracil, leucovorin, irinotecan (FOLFIRI) for the treatment of patients with mCRC that is resistant to or has progressed following an oxaliplatin-containing regimen. | August 3, 2012 |
| Everolimus tablets (Afinitor, Novartis Pharmaceuticals Corporation) | For the treatment of postmenopausal women with advanced hormone receptor–positive, HER2-negative breast cancer in combination with exemestane, after failure of treatment with letrozole or anastrozole. | July 20, 2012 |

*(continued)*

TABLE 26.2

**U.S. Food And Drug Administration Hematology Oncology Drug Approvals 2010–2013 (continued)**

| Drug/Manufacturer | Indication | Approval Date |
|---|---|---|
| Carfilzomib injection (Kyprolis, Onyx Pharmaceuticals) | For the treatment of patients with multiple myeloma who have received at least two prior therapies, including bortezomib and an immunomodulatory agent, and have demonstrated disease progression on or within 60 days of the completion of the last therapy. | July 20, 2012 |
| Cetuximab (Erbitux, ImClone LLC, a wholly owned subsidiary of Eli Lilly and Co.) | For use in combination with FOLFIRI for first-line treatment of patients with K-ras mutation-negative (wild-type), EGFR-expressing mCRC as determined by FDA-approved tests for this use. | July 9, 2012 |
| Pertuzumab injection (PERJETA, Genentech, Inc.) | For use in combination with trastuzumab and docetaxel for the treatment of patients with HER2-positive metastatic breast cancer who have not received prior anti-HER2 therapy or chemotherapy for metastatic disease. | June 8, 2012 |
| Pazopanib tablets (VOTRIENT, a registered Trademark of GlaxoSmithKline) | For the treatment of patients with advanced soft tissue sarcoma (STS) who have received prior chemotherapy. | April 26, 2012 |
| Everolimus (Afinitor tablets, Novartis) | For the treatment of adults with renal angiomyolipoma, associated with TSC who do not require immediate surgery. | April 26, 2012 |
| Imatinib mesylate tablets (Gleevec, Novartis Pharmaceuticals) | For the adjuvant treatment of adult patients following complete gross resection of Kit (CD117)-positive gastrointestinal stromal tumors (GIST). | January 31, 2012 |
| Vismodegib (ERIVEDGE Capsule, Genentech, Inc.) | For the treatment of adults with metastatic basal cell carcinoma or with locally advanced basal cell carcinoma that has recurred following surgery or who are not candidates for surgery and who are not candidates for radiation. | January 30, 2012 |
| Axitinib tablets (Inlyta, Pfizer, Inc.) | For the treatment of advanced renal cell carcinoma after failure of one prior systemic therapy. | January 27, 2012 |
| Glucarpidase injection (Voraxaze, BTG International Inc.) | For the treatment of toxic plasma methotrexate concentrations ($> 1$ $\mu$mol/L) in patients with delayed methotrexate clearance due to impaired renal function. | January 17, 2012 |
| Asparaginase *Erwinia chrysanthemi* (Erwinaze, injection, EUSA Pharma [USA], Inc.) | As a component of a multiagent chemotherapeutic regimen for the treatment of patients with ALL who have developed hypersensitivity to *E. coli*–derived asparaginase. | November 18, 2011 |
| Ruxolitinib (Jakafi oral tablets, Incyte Corporation) | For the treatment of intermediate and high risk myelofibrosis, including primary myelofibrosis, postpolycythemia vera myelofibrosis, and postessential thrombocythemia myelofibrosis. | November 16, 2011 |
| Cetuximab (Erbitux, ImClone LLC, a wholly-owned subsidiary of Eli Lilly and Company) | In combination with platinum-based therapy plus 5-fluorouracil (5-FU) for the first-line treatment of patients with recurrent locoregional disease and/or metastatic squamous cell carcinoma of the head and neck (SCCHN). | November 7, 2011 |
| Eculizumab (Soliris, Alexion, Inc.) | For the treatment of pediatric and adult patients with atypical hemolytic uremic syndrome (aHUS). | September 23, 2011 |
| Denosumab (Prolia, Amgen Inc.) | As a treatment to increase bone mass in patients at high risk for fracture receiving androgen-deprivation therapy (ADT) for nonmetastatic prostate cancer or adjuvant aromatase inhibitor (AI) therapy for breast cancer. | September 16, 2011 |
| Crizotinib (XALKORI Capsules, Pfizer Inc.) | For the treatment of patients with locally advanced or metastatic NSCLC that is ALK-positive as detected by an FDA-approved test. | August 26, 2011 |

*(continued)*

**TABLE 26.2**

**U.S. Food And Drug Administration Hematology Oncology Drug Approvals 2010–2013 (continued)**

| Drug/Manufacturer | Indication | Approval Date |
|---|---|---|
| Brentuximab vedotin (Adcetris for injection, Seattle Genetics, Inc.) | For treatment of patients with Hodgkin lymphoma after failure of autologous stem cell transplant (ASCT) or after failure of at least two prior multiagent chemotherapy regimens in patients who are not ASCT candidates and treatment of patients with systemic anaplastic large cell lymphoma (ALCL) after failure of at least one prior multiagent chemotherapy regimen. | August 19, 2011 |
| Vemurafenib tablets (ZELBORAF, Hoffmann-La Roche Inc.) | For the treatment of patients with unresectable or metastatic melanoma with the BRAFV600E mutation as detected by an FDA-approved test. | August 17, 2011 |
| Sunitinib (Sutent capsules, Pfizer, Inc.) | For the treatment of progressive, well-differentiated pancreatic neuroendocrine tumors (pNET) in patients with unresectable, locally advanced, or metastatic disease. | May 20, 2011 |
| Everolimus (Afinitor tablets, Novartis Pharmaceuticals Corporation) | For the treatment of progressive PNET in patients with unresectable, locally advanced, or metastatic disease. | May 5, 2011 |
| Abiraterone acetate (Zytiga tablets, Centocor Ortho Biotech, Inc.) | For use in combination with prednisone for the treatment of patients with metastatic castration-resistant prostate cancer (mCRPC) who have received prior chemotherapy containing docetaxel. | April 28, 2011 |
| Vandetanib tablets (Vandetanib tablets, AstraZeneca Pharmaceuticals LP) | For the treatment of symptomatic or progressive medullary thyroid cancer in patients with unresectable, locally advanced, or metastatic disease. | April 6, 2011 |
| Peginterferon alfa-2b (Sylatron, Schering Corporation, Kenilworth, NJ 07033) | For the treatment of patients with melanoma with microscopic or gross nodal involvement within 84 days of definitive surgical resection including complete lymphadenectomy. | March 29, 2011 |
| Ipilimumab injection (YERVOY, Bristol-Myers Squibb Company) | For the treatment of unresectable or metastatic melanoma. | March 25, 2011 |
| Rituximab (Rituxan, Genentech, Inc.) | For maintenance therapy in patients with previously untreated follicular, CD-20 positive, B-cell non-Hodgkin lymphoma who achieve a response to rituximab in combination with chemotherapy. | January 28, 2011 |
| Eribulin mesylate (Halaven injection, Eisai Inc.) | For the treatment of patients with metastatic breast cancer who have previously received an anthracycline and a taxane in either the adjuvant or metastatic setting, and at least two chemotherapeutic regimens for the treatment of metastatic disease. | November 15, 2010 |
| Everolimus (Afinitor, Novartis), an mTOR inhibitor | For patients with SEGA associated with tuberous sclerosis (TS) who require therapy but who are not candidates for surgical resection. | October 29, 2010 |
| Dasatinib (Sprycel, Bristol-Myers Squibb) | For the treatment of newly diagnosed adult patients with Ph+ CML in chronic phase (CP-CML). | October 28, 2010 |
| Trastuzumab (Herceptin, Genentech, Inc.) | In combination with cisplatin and a fluoropyrimidine (capecitabine or 5-FU), for the treatment of patients with HER2-overexpressing metastatic gastric or gastroesophageal (GE) junction adenocarcinoma, who have not received prior treatment for metastatic disease. | October 20, 2010 |
| Nilotinib (Tasigna capsules, Novartis Pharmaceuticals Corporation) | For the treatment of adult patients with newly diagnosed Ph+ CP-CML. | June 17, 2010 |
| Cabazitaxel (Jevtana injection, Sanofi-Aventis) | For use in combination with prednisone for treatment of patients with metastatic hormone-refractory prostate cancer (mHRPC) previously treated with a docetaxel-containing regimen. | June 17, 2010 |

**CANCER THERAPEUTICS**

# REFERENCES

1. Powell RG, Weisleder D, Smith CR, et al. Antitumor alkaloids from *Cephalotaxus harringtonia* structure and activity. *J Pharm Sci* 1972;61:1227–1230.
2. Huang MT. Harringtonine, an inhibitor of initiation of protein biosynthesis. *Mol Pharmacol* 1975;11:511–519.
3. Baaske DM, Heinstein P. Cytotoxicity and cell cycle specificity of homoharrintonine. *Antimicrob Agents Chemother* 1977;12:298–300.
4. Savaraj N, Lu K, Dimery I, et al. Clinical pharmacology of homoharringtonine. *Cancer Treat Rep* 1986;70:1403–1407.
5. Neidhart JA, Young DC, Derocher D, et al. Phase I trial of homoharringtonine. *Cancer Treat Rep* 1983;67:801–804.
6. Grem JL, Cheson BD, King SA, et al. Cephalotoxine esters: antileukemic advance of therapeutic failure. *J Natl Cancer Inst* 1988;80:1095–1103.
7. O'Brien S, Kantarjian H, Keating M, et al. Homoharringtonine therapy indices responses in patients with chronic myelogenous leukemia in late chronic phase. *Blood* 1995;86:3322–3326.
8. Legros L, Hayette S, Nicolini FE, et al. BCR-ABL(T315I) transcript disappearance in an imatinib-resistant CML patient treated with homoharringtonine: a new therapeutic challenge? *Leukemia* 2007;21(10):2204–2206.
9. Jorge Cortes J, Lipton JF, Rea D, et al. Phase 2 study of subcutaneous omacetaxine mepesuccinate after TKI failure in patients with chronic-phase CML with T315I mutation. *Blood* 2012;120:2573–2580.
10. Labrou NE, Papageorgiou AC, Avramis VI. Structure-function relationships and clinical applications of L-Asparaginases. *Curr Med Chem* 2010;17:2183–2195.
11. Verma N, Kumar K, Kaur G, et al. L-Asparaginase: a promising chemotherapeutic agent. *Crit Rev Biotechnol* 2007;27:45–62.
12. Zeidan A, Wang ES, Wetzler M. Pegasparaginase: where do we stand? *Expert Opin Biol Ther* 2009;9:111–119.
13. Avramis VI, Panosyan EH. Pharmacokinetic/pharmacodynamic relationships of asparaginase formulations: the past, the present and recommendations for the future. *Clin Pharmacokinet* 2005;44:367–393.
14. Appel IM, Hop WC, Pieters R. Changes in hypercoagulability by asparaginase: a randomized study between two asparaginases. *Blood Coagul Fibrinolysis* 2006;17:139–146.
15. Evans WE, Yee GC, Crom WR, et al. Clinical pharmacology of bleomycin and cisplatin. *Head Neck Surg* 1981;4:98–110.
16. Chen J, Stubbe J. Bleomycins: towards better therapeutics. *Nat Rev Cancer* 2005;2:102–112.
17. Hecht SM. Bleomycin: new perspectives on the mechanism of action. *J Nat Prod* 2000;63:158–168.
18. Lewis TG, Nydorf ED. Intralesional bleomycin for warts: a review. *J Drugs Dermatol* 2006;5:499–504.
19. Shaw P, Agarwal R. Pleurodesis for malignant pleural effusions. *Cochrane Database Syst Rev* 2004;(1):CD002916.
20. Good LM, Miller MD, High WA. Intralesional agents in the management of cutaneous malignancy: a review. *J Am Acad Dermatol* 2011;64:413–422
21. Kawai K, Akaza H. Bleomycin-induced pulmonary toxicity in chemotherapy for testicular cancer. *Expert Opin Drug Saf* 2003;2:587–596.
22. Azulay E, Herigault S, Levame M, et al. Effect of granulocyte colony-stimulating factor on bleomycin-induced acute lung injury and pulmonary fibrosis. *Crit Care Med* 2003;31:1442–1448.
23. Adachi K, Suzuki M, Sugimoto T, et al. Effects of granulocyte colony-stimulating factor on the kinetics of inflammatory cells in the peripheral blood and pulmonary lesions during the development of bleomycin-induced lung injury in rats. *Exp Toxicol Pathol* 2003;55:21–32.
24. Martin WG, Ristow KM, Habermann TM, et al. Bleomycin pulmonary toxicity has a negative impact on the outcome of patients with Hodgkin's lymphoma. *J Clin Oncol* 2005;23:7614–7620.
25. Younes A, Connors JM, Park SI et al. Brentuximab vedotin combined with ABVD or AVD for patients with newly diagnosed Hodgkin's lymphoma: a phase 1, open-label, dose-escalation study. *Lancet Oncol* 2013;14:1348–1356.
26. Lam MS. The need for routine bleomycin test dosing in the 21st century. *Ann Pharmacother* 2005;39:1897–1902.
27. Swaffar DS, Horstman MG, Jaw JY, et al. Methylazoxyprocarbazine, the active escoubet-lozach responsible for the anticancer activity of procarbazine against L1210 leukemia. *Cancer Res* 1989;49:2442–2447.
28. Patterson LH, Murray GI. Tumour cytochrome P450 and drug activation. *Curr Pharm Des* 2002;8:1335–1347.
29. Swaffar DS, Pomerantz SC, Harker WG, et al. Non-enzymatic activation of procarbazine to active cytotoxic species. *Oncol Res* 1992;4:49–58.
30. Preiss R, Baumann F, Regenthal R, et al. Plasma kinetics of procarbazine and azo-procarbazine in humans. *Anticancer Drugs* 2006;17:75–80.
31. Von Hoff DD, LoRusso PM, Rudin CM, et al. Inhibition of the hedgehog pathway in advanced basal-cell carcinoma. *N Engl J Med* 2009;361:1164–1172.
32. Rudin CM. Vismodegib. *Clin Cancer Res* 2012;18:1–5.
33. U.S. Food and Drug Administation. News & Events: FDA News Release: FDA approves new treatment for most common types of skin cancer. http://www.fda.gov/NewsEvents/Newsroom/PressAnnouncements/ucm289545.htm. Published January 30, 2012. Updated January 31, 2012.
34. Tang JY, Mackay-Wiggan JM, Aszterbaum M, et al. Inhibiting the Hedgehog pathway in patients with the basal-cell nevus syndrome. *N Engl J Med* 2012;366:2180–2188.
35. Krop IE, Beeram M, Modi S, et al. Phase I study of trastuzumab-DM1, an HER2 antibody-drug conjugate, given every 3 weeks to patients with HER2-positive metastatic breast cancer. *J Clin Oncol* 2010;28:2698–2704.
36. Verma S, Miles D, Gianni L, et al. Trastuzumab emtansine for HER2-positive advanced breast cancer. *N Engl J Med* 2012;367:1783–1791.
37. Sehgal SN, Baker H, Vézina C. Rapamycin (AY-22,989), a new antifungal antibiotic. II. Fermentation, isolation and characterization. *J Antibiot (Tokyo)* 1975;28:727–732.
38. Sehgal SN, Molnar-Kimber K, Ocain TD, et al. Rapamycin: a novel immunosuppressive macrolide. *Med Res Rev* 1994;14:1–22.
39. Wullschleger S, Loewith R, Hall MN. TOR signaling in growth and metabolism. *Cell* 2006;124:471–484.
40. Raymond E, Alexandre J, Faivre S, et al. Safety and pharmacokinetics of escalated doses of weekly intravenous infusion of CCI-779, a novel mTOR inhibitor in patients with cancer. *J Clin Oncol* 2004;22:2336–2347.
41. Zeng Z, Sarbassov dos D, Samudio IJ, et al. Rapamycin derivatives reduce mTORC2 signaling and inhibit AKT activation in AML. *Blood* 2007;109:3509–3512.
42. Kapoor A, Figlin RA. Targeted inhibition of mammalian target of rapamycin for the treatment of advanced renal cell carcinoma. *Cancer* 2009;115:3618–3630.
43. Atkins MB, Hidalgo M, Stadler WM, et al. Randomized phase II study of multiple dose levels of CCI-779, a novel mammalian target of rapamycin kinase inhibitor, in patients with advanced refractory renal cell carcinoma. *J Clin Oncol* 2004;22:909–918.
44. Hudes G, Carducci M, Tomczak P, et al. Temsirolimus, interferon alfa, or both for advanced renal-cell carcinoma. *N Engl J Med* 2007;356:2271–2281.
45. Smith SM, van Besien K, Karrison T, et al. Temsirolimus has activity in non-mantle cell non-Hodgkin's lymphoma subtypes: The University of Chicago phase II consortium. *J Clin Oncol* 2010;28:4740–4746.
46. Duran I, Siu LL, Oza AM, et al. Characterization of the lung toxicity of the cell cycle inhibitor temsirolimus. *Eur J Cancer* 2006;42:1875–1880.
47. Schuler W, Sedrani R, Cottens S, et al. SDZ RAD, a new rapamycine derivative: pharmacological properties in vitro and in vivo. *Transplantation* 1997;64:36–42.
48. Dudkin L, Dilling MB, Cheshire PJ, et al. Biochemical correlates of mTOR inhibition by the rapamycin ester CCI-779 and tumor growth inhibition. *Clin Cancer Res* 2001;7:1758–1764.
49. Kirchner GI, Meier-Wiedenbach I, Manns MP. Clinical pharmacokinetics of everolimus. *Clin Pharmacokinet* 2004;43:83–95.
50. Doi T, Muro K, Boku N, et al. Multicenter phase II study of everolimus in patients with previously treated metastatic gastric cancer. *J Clin Oncol* 2010;28:1904–1910.
51. Yao JC, Lombard-Bohas C, Baudin E, et al. Daily oral everolimus activity in patients with metastatic pancreatic neuroendocrine tumors after failure of cytotoxic chemotherapy: a phase II trial. *J Clin Oncol* 2010;28:69–76.
52. Yee KW, Zeng Z, Konopleva M, et al. Phase I/II study of the mammalian target of rapamycin inhibitor everolimus(RAD001) in patients with relapsed or refractory hematological malignancies. *Clin Cancer Res* 2008;12:5165–5173.
53. Okuno S. Mammalian target of rapamycin inhibitors in sarcomas. *Curr Opin Oncol* 2006;18:360–362.
54. Yao JC, Shah MH, Ito T, et al. Everolimus for advanced pancreatic neuroendocrine tumors. *N Engl J Med* 2011;364:514–523.
55. Baselga J, Campone M, Piccart M, et al. Everolimus in postmenopausal hormone-receptor-positive advanced breast cancer. *N Engl J Med* 2012;366:520–529.
56. Shortt J, Hsu AK, Johnstone RW. Thalidomide-analogue biology: immunological, molecular and epigenetic targets in cancer therapy. *Oncogene* 2013;32:4191–4202.
57. Zhu YX, Kortuem KM, Stewart AK. Molecular mechanism of action of immune-modulatory drugs thalidomide, lenalidomide and pomalidomide in multiple myeloma. *Leuk Lymphoma* 2013;54:683–687.
58. Escoubet-Lozach L, Lin IL, Jensen-Pergakes K, et al. Pomalidomide and lenalidomide induce p21 WAF-1 expression in both lymphoma and multiple myeloma through a LSD1-mediated epigenetic mechanism. *Cancer Res* 2009;69:7347–7356.
59. Madan S, Lacy MQ, Dispenzieri A, et al. Efficacy of retreatment with immunomodulatory drugs (IMiDs) in patients receiving IMiDs for initial therapy of newly diagnosed multiple myeloma. *Blood* 2011;118:1763–1765.
60. Lacy MQ, Tefferi A. Pomalidomide therapy for multiple myeloma and myelofibrosis: an update. *Leuk Lymphoma* 2011;52:560–566.
61. Ito T, Ando H, Suzuki T, et al. Identification of a primary target of thalidomide teratogenicity. *Science* 2010;327:1345–1350.
62. Zhu YX, Braggio E, Shi CX, et al. Cereblon expression is required for the antimyeloma activity of lenalidomide and pomalidomide. *Blood* 2011;118:4771–4779.
63. Lopez-Girona A, Mendy D, Ito T, et al. Cereblon is a direct protein target for immunomodulatory and antiproliferative activities of lenalidomide and pomalidomide. *Leukemia* 2012;26:2326–2335.
64. Schuster SR, Kortuem KM, Zhu YX, et al. Cereblon expression predicts response, progression free and overall survival after pomalidomide and

dexamethasone therapy in multiple myeloma. *ASH Ann Meeting Abstracts* 2012;120:194.

65. Bennett CL, Angelotta C, Yarnold PR, et al. Thalidomide- and lenalidomide-associated thromboembolism among patients with cancer. *JAMA* #2006;296:2558–2560.

66. Rao KV. Lenalidomide in the treatment of multiple myeloma. *Am J Health Syst Pharm* 2007;64:1799–1807.

67. Lenalidomide. Drugs@FDA. Food and Drug Administration Web site. http://www.accessdata.fda.gov/drugsatfda_docs/label/2009/021880s006s016s017lbl.pdf. Published December 2008.

68. Pomalidomide. Drugs@FDA. Food and Drug Administration Web site. http://www.accessdata.fda.gov/drugsatfda_docs/label/2013/204026lbl.pdf. Revised February 2013.

69. Lacy MQ, McCurdy AR. Pomalidomide. *Blood* 2013;122:2305–2309.

# 27 Hormonal Agents

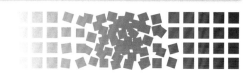

Matthew P. Goetz, Charles Erlichman, Charles L. Loprinzi, and Manish Kohli

## INTRODUCTION

Hormonal agents are commonly used as a treatment of hormonally responsive cancers, such as breast, prostate, or endometrial carcinomas. Other uses for some hormonal therapies include the treatment of paraneoplastic syndromes, such as carcinoid syndrome, and symptoms caused by cancer, including anorexia. This chapter discusses the major hormonal agents for such therapy, first with an overview of their use in practice, then with more detailed pharmacologic information regarding them (Table 27.1).

## SELECTIVE ESTROGEN RECEPTOR MODULATORS

### Tamoxifen

Tamoxifen continues to be an important hormonal therapy for the prevention and treatment of breast cancer worldwide. The continued importance of tamoxifen is reflected in the fact that it is the only hormonal agent approved by the U.S. Food and Drug Administration (FDA) for the prevention of premenopausal breast cancer,[1] the treatment of ductal carcinoma in situ (DCIS),[2] and the treatment of surgically resected premenopausal estrogen receptor (ER)–positive breast cancer.[3]

The standard daily dose of tamoxifen is 20 mg, and the optimal duration depends on the underlying clinical setting. Although the recommended duration in the prevention and DCIS settings is 5 years, recently published prospective studies have demonstrated that for the adjuvant treatment of invasive breast cancer, a duration of 10 years (compared to 5 years) further reduced the risk of breast cancer mortality and improved overall survival.[4]

The most common toxicity from tamoxifen is hot flashes, affecting approximately 50% of treated women. These hot flashes are of varying intensity and duration. Tamoxifen-induced hot flashes appear to increase over the first 3 months of therapy and then plateau. They appear to be more prominent in women with a history of hot flashes or estrogen replacement use. Tamoxifen-induced hot flashes can be ameliorated by a number of different pharmacotherapies, including low doses of megestrol[5]; antidepressants such as venlafaxine,[6] desvenlafaxine,[7] citalopram,[8] escitalopram,[9] and paroxetine[10]; and the anticonvulsant drugs gabapentin[11] and pregabalin.[12] There is evidence that drugs that inhibit CYP2D6 (e.g., paroxetine) alter the metabolic activation of tamoxifen to endoxifen, a critical metabolite associated with in vivo tamoxifen efficacy.[13]

The estrogenic properties of tamoxifen are responsible for both beneficial and deleterious side effects. Tamoxifen increases the incidence of endometrial cancer in postmenopausal (but not premenopausal) women, with the increase in the annual incidence of endometrial cancer being approximately 2.58 (ratio of incidence rates).[14] The absolute risk depends on the duration of tamoxifen administration. For women who receive 10 years of adjuvant tamoxifen, the cumulative risk is 3.1% (mortality, 0.4%) versus 1.6% (mortality, 0.2%) for 5 years of tamoxifen.[4] The incidence of a rarer form of uterine cancer, uterine sarcoma, is also increased after tamoxifen use.[15] This form of endometrial cancer comprises approximately 15% of all uterine malignancies that develop after tamoxifen use.[15] Beneficial estrogenic effects from tamoxifen include a decrease in total cholesterol[16] and the preservation of bone density in postmenopausal women.[17] In premenopausal women, however, tamoxifen has a negative effect on bone density.[18] Although most patients do not complain of vaginal symptoms, a few complain of vaginal dryness, whereas others have increased vaginal secretions and discharge, the latter of which is an indication of the estrogenic activity of tamoxifen on the vagina. In the Arimidex, Tamoxifen, Alone or in Combination (ATAC) trial, a commonly observed tamoxifen side effect was vaginal bleeding, leading to a higher hysterectomy rate for patients randomized to tamoxifen (5%) compared to anastrozole (1%).[19] An uncommon effect from tamoxifen is retinal toxicity. This drug can also increase the risk of cataracts. However, no difference in the rate of vision-threatening ocular toxicity has been seen among prospectively treated tamoxifen patients.[20] Tamoxifen predisposes patients to thromboembolic phenomena, especially if used with concomitant chemotherapy. Depression has also been described, but the association with tamoxifen is not clear. Although liver cancers have been noted in laboratory animals, there is no established association between tamoxifen and liver cancers in humans.

### Pharmacology

Tamoxifen acts by blocking estrogen stimulation of breast cancer cells, inhibiting both translocation and nuclear binding of the ER. This alters transcriptional and posttranscriptional events mediated by this receptor.[21] Tamoxifen has agonistic, partial agonistic, or antagonistic effects depending on the species, tissue, or endpoints that have been assessed. Additionally, there are marked differences between the antiproliferative properties of tamoxifen and its metabolites.[22]

Resistance to tamoxifen can be intrinsic or acquired, and the potential mechanisms for this resistance are reviewed in the following paragraphs. At each step of the signal transduction pathway with which tamoxifen or its metabolites interferes, there is the potential for an alteration in response. The most important factor appears to be the level of ER, which is highly predictive for a response to tamoxifen. Tamoxifen is ineffective in ER-negative breast cancer. Although decreased or absent expression of the progesterone receptor (PR) is associated with a worse prognosis, the relative risk reduction in tamoxifen-treated patients is the same regardless of the presence or absence of the PR.

Following binding to the ER, subsequent translocation of the tamoxifen/ER complex to the nucleus and binding to an estrogen-response element may occur. This binding prevents transcriptional activation of estrogen-responsive genes. Laboratory and clinical data have demonstrated that ER-positive breast cancers that overexpress HER2 may be less responsive to tamoxifen and

**TABLE 27.1**

**Overview of Major Hormonal Agents Used in Cancer**

| Class of Drug | Individual Drug | Dose | Route of Delivery | Frequency of Delivery |
|---|---|---|---|---|
| Selective estrogen receptor modulator | Tamoxifen | 20 mg | Oral | Once daily |
| | Toremifene | 60 mg | Oral | Once daily |
| | Raloxifene | 60 mg | Oral | Once daily |
| Aromatase inhibitor | Anastrozole | 1 mg | Oral | Once daily |
| | Letrozole | 2.5 mg | Oral | Once daily |
| | Exemestane | 25 mg | Oral | Once daily |
| Estrogen receptor downregulator | Fulvestrant | 500 mg | IM | Once monthly |
| Luteinizing hormone releasing hormone agonist | Goserelin | 7.5 | IM | Once monthly[a] |
| | Leuprolide | 3.6 | IM | Once monthly[a] |
| GnRH antagonist | Degarelix | 240 mg loading dose | SC | 80 mg SC monthly maintenance dose |
| Antiandrogen | Flutamide | 250 mg | Oral | Three times daily |
| | Bicalutamide | 50 mg | Oral | Once daily |
| | Nilutamide | 300 mg for 30 d then 150 mg | Oral | Once daily |
| Cytochrome P45017 alpha inhibitors | Abiraterone Acetate | 1,000 mg (four 250 mg capsules) | Oral | Once Daily |
| AR "super antagonists" | Enzalutamide | 160–240 mg | Oral | Daily |
| Androgen | Fluoxymesterone | 10 mg | Oral | Twice daily |
| Estrogen | Estradiol | 10 mg | Oral | Up to three times daily |
| Somatostatin analog | Octreotide | Varies | SC or IV | Up to three times daily[b] |
| Progestational agents | Megestrol | Varies | Oral | Once daily |
| | Medroxyprogesterone acetate | Varies | Oral or IM | Varies |

[a] Longer acting depot preparations (every 3 months) are available.
[b] Depot formulations are available.
IM, intramuscular; SC, subcutaneous; GnRH, gonadotropin-releasing hormone; CYP, cytochrome P-450; AR, androgen receptor.

to hormonal therapy in general.[23–26] In these tumors, ligand-independent activation of the ER by mitogen-activated protein kinase (MAPK) pathways may contribute to resistance.[27–29] In addition, the expression of AIB1, an estrogen-receptor coactivator, has been associated with tamoxifen resistance in patients whose breast cancers overexpress HER2.[30] In some cases, resistance may result from a decrease or loss of ER expression.[31,32] Although mutations in the ER ligand binding domain (LBD) are rare in newly diagnosed breast cancer, ER mutations are present in up to 20% of recurrent breast cancers.[33–36] These mutations lead to a conformational change in the LBD, which mimics the conformation of activated ligand-bound receptor and constitutive, ligand-independent transcriptional activity, resulting in resistance to hormonal therapy. Preclinical studies suggest that some of these mutations, although insensitive to aromatase inhibitors, retain sensitivity to higher dose selective estrogen-receptor modulators (SERM), such as endoxifen, as well as fulvestrant.[35]

The carcinogenic potential of tamoxifen has been recognized in rat studies[37–39] and in humans (endometrial cancer).[40] It has been proposed that the generation of reactive intermediates that bind covalently to macromolecules underlies the process. Such reactive intermediates have been demonstrated in vitro.[40–43] In addition, the induction of covalent DNA adducts in rat livers treated with tamoxifen has been reported.[44] Both constitutive and inducible cytochrome P-450 (CYP) enzymes have been implicated in the formation of metabolites with tamoxifen,[45,46] and the flavone-containing monooxygenase has been implicated in the formation of the N-oxide of tamoxifen. Reactive intermediates from

such metabolic steps are being evaluated for their carcinogenic potential in vitro and in vivo.

Multiple studies to evaluate tumor gene expression profiling have identified gene expression patterns or specific genes associated with resistance to tamoxifen therapy. A commonly utilized gene expression assay, Oncotype DX 21 gene assay (Genomic Health, Redwood City, California), measures the expression of genes known to be involved in estrogen signaling (e.g., ER, PR), HER2, proliferation (e.g., Ki-67), and others. In multiple different data sets, the recurrence score has been associated with a higher risk of breast cancer recurrence in patients treated with hormonal therapy (e.g., tamoxifen or aromatase inhibitors) without concomitant chemotherapy.[47–49]

The pharmacokinetics of tamoxifen is complex. The chemical structure and metabolic pathway of tamoxifen are shown in Figure 27.1. Metabolic activation of tamoxifen is associated with greater pharmacologic activity. The two most active tamoxifen metabolites are 4-hydroxytamoxifen (4-OH tamoxifen) and 4-OH-N-desmethyltamoxifen (endoxifen). A series of studies carried out to characterize endoxifen pharmacology have demonstrated that it has equivalent potency in vitro to 4-hydroxytamoxifen in ER-$\alpha$ and -beta (ER-$\beta$) binding,[50] for the suppression of ER-dependent human breast cancer cell line proliferation,[22,50] and in global ER-responsive gene expression.[51] A recent study suggests that endoxifen's effect on the ER may differ from 4-hydroxytamoxifen based on the observation of ER-$\alpha$ degradation.[52]

In women who receive tamoxifen at a dose of 20 mg per day, plasma endoxifen steady-state concentrations are generally 6 to

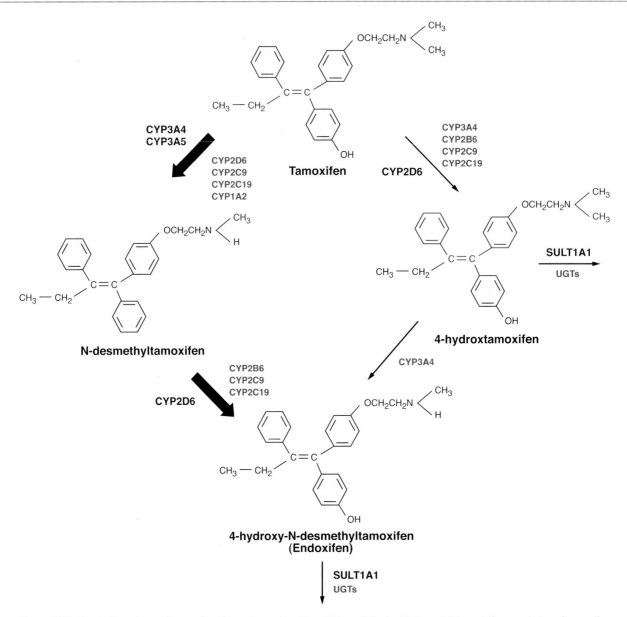

**Figure 27.1** Metabolic pathway of tamoxifen biotransformation. (From Sideras K, Ingle JN, Ames MM, et al. Coprescription of tamoxifen and medications that inhibit CYP2D6. *J Clin Oncol* 2010;28:2768–2776.)

10 times higher than 4-hydroxytamoxifen.[53] Although the metabolism of tamoxifen to 4-OH-tamoxifen is catalyzed by multiple enzymes, endoxifen is formed predominantly by the CYP2D6-mediated oxidation of N-desmethyltamoxifen, the most abundant tamoxifen metabolite (see Fig. 27.1).[54] Multiple clinical studies have demonstrated that common *CYP2D6* genetic variation (leading to low or absent CYP2D6 activity) or the drug-induced inhibition of CYP2D6 significantly lowers endoxifen concentrations.[53,55] The *CYP2D6* gene is highly polymorphic, with more than 70 major alleles with four well-defined phenotypes: poor metabolizers (PM), intermediate metabolizers (IM), extensive metabolizers (EM), and ultrarapid metabolizers (UM).

The clinical studies to evaluate the association between *CYP2D6* polymorphisms and tamoxifen outcomes have yielded conflicting results. Initial[56] and follow-up data[57,58] demonstrated that CYP2D6 PM had an approximately two- to threefold higher risk of breast cancer recurrence (compared to CYP2D6 EM) and these data led an FDA special emphasis panel to recommend a tamoxifen label change to incorporate data that the *CYP2D6* genotype was an important biomarker associated with tamoxifen

efficacy.[5] However, this label change has been delayed, in part because of conflicting data from secondary analyses of 5-year tamoxifen prospective trials (ATAC,[59] BIG 1-98,[60] and ABCSG8[61]) as well as meta-analyses,[62] which demonstrate that the *CYP2D6* genotype is associated with tamoxifen efficacy when tamoxifen is administered as monotherapy for the adjuvant treatment of postmenopausal, ER-positive breast cancer. Additional support for the importance of endoxifen concentrations came from a secondary analysis of a prospective study, which demonstrated a higher risk of recurrence for women with low endoxifen concentrations.[13]

Many drugs are known to inhibit CYP2D6 activity. In tamoxifen-treated women, the coadministration of potent CYP2D6 inhibitors, such as paroxetine, converts a patient with normal CYP2D6 metabolism to a phenotypic PM.[63] Many other clinically important drugs have been reported to inhibit the CYP2D6 enzyme system, but their effects on tamoxifen metabolism have not been prospectively studied. As with the data regarding *CYP2D6* genotype, the data regarding CYP2D6 inhibitors has additionally been controversial, including two studies that reported opposite findings with regard to CYP2D6 inhibitor use and breast cancer recurrence or death.[64,65] Although the *CYP2D6* data remain controversial, we conclude that until results from prospective adjuvant studies are available, women should be counseled regarding the potential impact of the *CYP2D6* genotype on the effectiveness of adjuvant tamoxifen, and potent CYP2D6 inhibitors should be avoided. Additional caution should be used with drugs that induce CYP3A, such as rifampicin, as a these drugs have been demonstrated to substantially reduce (up to 86%) the concentrations of tamoxifen and its metabolites.[66]

Strategies to overcome low endoxifen concentrations include dose escalation of tamoxifen to 40 mg per day, which has been demonstrated to significantly increase endoxifen concentrations,[67,68] as well as the direct administration of endoxifen itself. The latter strategy is ongoing in multiple different clinical trials, and early reports suggest clinical activity in aromatase inhibitors (AI)-resistant breast cancer.[69]

Following the metabolic activation of tamoxifen, the hydroxylated metabolites undergo both glucuronidation and sulfation. Peak plasma levels of tamoxifen (maximum concentration [Cmax]) are seen 3 to 7 hours after oral administration. Assuming an oral bioavailability of 30%, the volume of distribution has been calculated to be 20 L/kg, and plasma clearance ranges from 1.2 to 5.1 L per hour.[70] The terminal half-life of tamoxifen has been reported to range between 4 and 11 days.[71,72] The elimination half-life of tamoxifen increases with successive doses, which is consistent with saturable kinetics.[71,73] The drug's distribution in tissues is extensive. Levels of the parent drug and metabolites have been reported to be higher in tissue than in plasma in animal studies.[74,75] Reports of tamoxifen concentrations 10- to 60-fold higher than plasma concentrations in the liver, lungs, brain, pancreas, skin, and bones are reported.[76,77] Elevated levels of tamoxifen with biliary obstruction have been reported.[78]

Tamoxifen has been reported to interact with warfarin,[73,79–81] digitoxin, phenytoin,[82] and medroxyprogesterone.[73] Tamoxifen-induced activation of human transcription factor pregnane X receptor (hPXR), resulting in the induction of CYP3A4, may increase the elimination of concomitantly administered CYP3A substrates,[83] such as anastrozole.[84]

## Toremifene

Toremifene is an agent similar to tamoxifen. It is available in the United States for the treatment of patients with metastatic breast cancer, and is approved in other countries for the adjuvant treatment of ER-positive breast cancer. Clinical trials have demonstrated no difference in either disease-free or overall survival when toremifene was compared with tamoxifen for the treatment of ER-positive breast cancer,[85,86] and evidence exists for major cross-resistance between tamoxifen and toremifene.[87,88]

## Pharmacology

Toremifene is an antiestrogen with a chemical structure that differs from that of tamoxifen by the substitution of a chlorine for a hydrogen atom that is retained when toremifene undergoes metabolism.[89] Like tamoxifen, toremifene is metabolized by CYP3A,[90] with a secondary metabolism to form hydroxylated metabolites that appear to have similar binding affinities to 4-OH tamoxifen.[89,91] The importance of these metabolites or the role of metabolism to the hydroxylated metabolites is unknown, but may play a role given the structural similarity of toremifene to tamoxifen. Although the oral bioavailability has not been defined, toremifene's oral absorption appears to be good. The time to peak plasma concentrations after oral administration ranges from 1.5 to 6.0 hours,[92] with the terminal half-lives for toremifene and one metabolite, 4-hydroxytoremifene, being 5 to 6 days.[93,94] The apparent clearance is 5.1 L per hour. The terminal half-life for the major metabolite, N-desmethyltoremifene, is 21 days.[95] The time to reach plasma steady-state concentrations is 1 to 5 weeks. Plasma protein binding is more than 99%. As with tamoxifen, toremifene is present at higher concentrations in tissues compared to plasma with a high apparent volume of distribution (958 L). Seventy percent of the drug is excreted in feces as metabolites. Studies in patients with impaired liver function or those on anticonvulsants known to induce CYP3A have demonstrated that hepatic dysfunction decreases the clearance of toremifene and N-desmethyltoremifene,[95] whereas those patients on anticonvulsants had an increased clearance. Although toremifene appeared to be less carcinogenic than tamoxifen in preclinical models,[43,96,97] of the rates of endometrial cancer in the adjuvant studies have been similar to tamoxifen.[85]

## Raloxifene

Raloxifene is an estrogen agonist and antagonist originally developed to treat osteoporosis. Large placebo-controlled randomized trials demonstrated reduced rates of osteoporosis and a reduction in new breast cancers in treated women, leading to the development of a second-generation breast cancer chemoprevention trial (National Surgical Adjuvant Breast and Bowel Project, NSAPB P2) in which raloxifene was compared with tamoxifen in high-risk postmenopausal women. In this study, tamoxifen was superior to raloxifene in terms of both invasive and noninvasive cancer events, but was associated with a higher risk of thromboembolic events and endometrial cancer.[98]

## Pharmacology

Raloxifene is partially estrogenic in bone[99] and lowers cholesterol.[100] It is antiestrogenic in mammary tissue[101,102] and uterine tissue.[103]

The pharmacokinetics of raloxifene have been studied principally in postmenopausal women.[104–106] Pharmacokinetic parameters of raloxifene show considerable interindividual variation. Limited information is available on the pharmacokinetics of raloxifene in individuals with hepatic impairment, renal impairment, or both.

Raloxifene is rapidly absorbed from the gastrointestinal tract. Because raloxifene undergoes extensive first-pass glucuronidation, oral bioavailability of unchanged drug is low. Although approximately 60% of an oral dose is absorbed, the absolute bioavailability as unchanged raloxifene is only 2%. However, systemic availability of raloxifene may be greater than that indicated in bioavailability studies, because circulating glucuronide conjugates are converted back to the parent drug in various tissues.

After the oral administration of a single 120- or 150-mg dose of raloxifene hydrochloride, peak plasma concentrations of raloxifene and its glucuronide conjugates are achieved at 6 hours and 1 hour, respectively. After the oral administration of radiolabeled raloxifene, less than 1% of total circulating radiolabeled material in plasma represents the parent drug.

Results of a single-dose study in patients with liver dysfunction indicate that plasma raloxifene concentrations correlate with serum bilirubin concentrations and are 2.5 times higher than individuals with normal hepatic function. In postmenopausal women who received raloxifene in clinical trials, plasma concentrations of raloxifene and the glucuronide conjugates in those with renal impairment (i.e., estimated creatinine clearance values as low as 23 mL per minute) were similar to values in women with normal renal function.

Raloxifene and its monoglucuronide conjugates are more than 95% bound to plasma proteins. Raloxifene binds to albumin and $\alpha_1$-acid glycoprotein. Raloxifene undergoes extensive first-pass metabolism to the glucuronide conjugates raloxifene 4'-glucuronide, 6-glucuronide, and 6,4'-diglucuronide. UGT1A1 and -1A8 have been found to catalyze the formation of both the 6-β-and 4'-β-glucuronides, whereas UGT1A10 formed only the 4'-β-glucuronide.[107] The metabolism of raloxifene does not appear to be mediated by CYP enzymes (such as CYP2D6), because metabolites other than glucuronide conjugates have not been identified.

The plasma elimination half-life of raloxifene at steady state averages 32.5 hours (range, 15.8 to 86.6 hours). Raloxifene is excreted principally in feces as an unabsorbed drug and via biliary elimination as glucuronide conjugates, which, subsequently, are metabolized by bacteria in the gastrointestinal tract to the parent drug. After oral administration, less than 0.2% of a raloxifene dose is excreted as the parent compound and less than 6% as glucuronide conjugates in urine.

## Fulvestrant

Fulvestrant is an ER antagonist that has no known agonist activity and results in ER downregulation.[108–111] Like tamoxifen, fulvestrant competitively binds to the ER but with a higher affinity—approximately 100 times greater than that of tamoxifen,[108,112–114]—thus preventing endogenous estrogen from exerting its effect in target cells.

Results from two phase III clinical trials using the 250 mg per month dose demonstrated fulvestrant to be as effective as anastrozole in the treatment of postmenopausal women with advanced hormone receptor–positive breast cancer previously treated with antiestrogen therapy (mainly tamoxifen).[112–116] In the setting of first-line hormone-responsive metastatic breast cancer, a randomized phase III clinical trial to compare tamoxifen to fulvestrant (250 mg per month) demonstrated no differences in response or time to progression.[117] Because of pharmacology data (discussed in the following paragraphs), the 500 mg per day dose was developed. A randomized trial comparing the 250 mg per month with 500 mg per month dose demonstrated a 4-month improvement in median overall survival advantage for the higher dose.[118] For this reason, the higher dose is now the standard recommended dose.

Fulvestrant is well tolerated. The most common drug-related events (greater than 10% incidence) from the randomized phase III studies were injection-site reactions and hot flashes. Common events (1% to 10% incidence) included asthenia, headache, and gastrointestinal disturbances such as nausea, vomiting, and diarrhea, with minor gastrointestinal disturbances being the most commonly described adverse event.

### Pharmacology

Fulvestrant is a steroidal molecule derived from $E_2$ with an alkylsulphonyl side chain in the 7-$\alpha$ position (Fig. 27.2). Because fulvestrant is poorly soluble and has low and unpredictable oral bioavailability, a parenteral formulation of fulvestrant was developed in an attempt to maximize delivery of the drug.[111] The intramuscular formulation provides prolonged release of the drug over several weeks. The pharmacokinetics of three different single doses of fulvestrant (50, 125, and 250 mg) have been published.[111] In this phase I/II multicenter study, postmenopausal women with primary breast cancer who were awaiting curative surgery received either fulvestrant, tamoxifen, or placebo. After single intramuscular injections of fulvestrant, the time of maximal concentration ($t_{max}$) ranged from 2 to 19 days, with the median being 7 days for each dose group. At the interval of 28 days, Cmin values were two- to fivefold lower than the Cmax values. For most patients in the 125- and 250-mg dose groups, significant levels of fulvestrant were still measurable 84 days after administration. Pharmacokinetic modeling of the pooled data from the 250-mg cohort was best described by a two-compartment model in which a longer terminal phase began approximately 3 weeks after administration. Because of the long time needed to reach a steady state, the 500-mg loading dose regimen was prospectively studied and determined to be superior to the 250 mg per month dose, both in terms of steady state concentrations achieved within 1 month[119] as well as progression-free and overall survival.[118]

## AROMATASE INHIBITORS

At menopause, the synthesis of ovarian hormones ceases. However, estrogen continues to be converted from androgens (produced by the adrenal glands) by aromatase, an enzyme of the CYP superfamily. Aromatase is the enzyme complex responsible for the final step in estrogen synthesis via the conversion of androgens, androstenedione and testosterone, to estrogens, estrone ($E_1$) and $E_2$. This biologic pathway served as the basis for the development of the antiaromatase class of compounds. Alterations in aromatase expression have been implicated in the pathogenesis of estrogen-dependent disease, including breast cancer, endometrial cancer, and endometriosis. The importance of this enzyme is also highlighted by the fact that selective aromatase inhibitors are commonly used as first-line therapy for the treatment of postmenopausal women with estrogen-responsive breast cancer. Aminoglutethimide was the first clinically used aromatase inhibitor. When it became available, it was used to cause a *medical adrenalectomy*. Because of the lack of selectivity for aromatase and the resultant suppression of aldosterone and cortisol, aminoglutethimide is no longer recommended for treating metastatic breast cancer. Aminoglutethimide is also occasionally used to try to reverse excess hormone production by adrenocortical cancers.[120]

Aromatase (cytochrome P-450 19 [CYP19]) is encoded by the CYP19 gene, which is highly polymorphic. Some of these variants are functionally important[121] and may have clinical significance.[122,123]

Aromatase inhibitors have been classified in a number of different ways, including first, second, and third generation; steroidal and nonsteroidal; and reversible (ionic binding) and irreversible (suicide inhibitor, covalent binding).[124] The nonsteroidal aromatase inhibitors include aminoglutethimide (first generation), rogletimide and fadrozole (second generation), and anastrozole, letrozole, and vorozole (third generation). The steroidal aromatase inhibitors include formestane (second generation) and exemestane (third generation).

Steroidal and nonsteroidal aromatase inhibitors differ in their modes of interaction with, and their inactivation of, the aromatase enzyme. Steroidal inhibitors compete with the endogenous

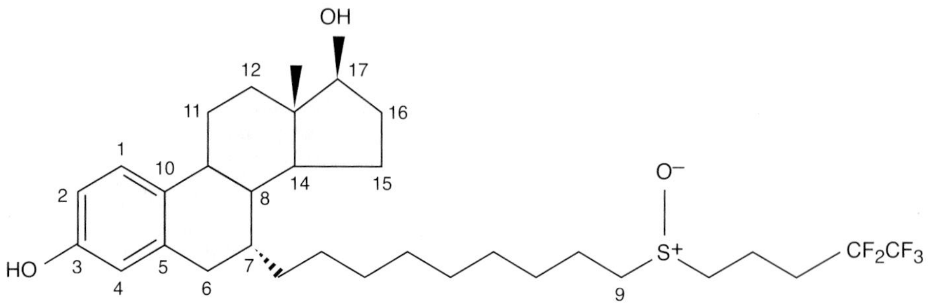

**Figure 27.2** Structure of fulvestrant.

substrates, androstenedione and testosterone, for the active site of the enzyme and are processed into intermediates that bind irreversibly to the active site, causing irreversible enzyme inhibition.[19] Nonsteroidal inhibitors also compete with the endogenous substrates for access to the active site, where they then form a reversible bond to the heme iron atom so that enzyme activity can recover if the inhibitor is removed; however, inhibition is sustained whenever the inhibitor is present.[19]

## Letrozole and Anastrozole

Both letrozole and anastrozole have been extensively studied in the metastatic and adjuvant settings. When compared to tamoxifen, both letrozole and anastrozole have demonstrated superior response rates and progression-free survival in the metastatic setting.[124,125] In the adjuvant setting, two trials have been performed and demonstrated superiority in terms of relapse-free survivals of both anastrozole (ATAC)[126] and letrozole (BIG 1-98).[127] Additionally, anastrozole has been studied in a sequential approach, and the sequence of tamoxifen followed by anastrozole is superior to 5 years of tamoxifen alone.[128] Anastrozole has recently been compared to placebo in women at an increased risk of developing breast cancer and was demonstrated to significantly reduce the incidence of invasive breast cancer.[129]

The side effects of both anastrozole and letrozole are similar and include arthralgias and myalgias in up to 50% of patients. Both letrozole and anastrozole are associated with a higher rate of bone fracture, compared with the tamoxifen.[130] At the present time, minimal long-term (longer than 5 years) clinical data regarding the effect of aromatase inhibitors on bones are available. When offering anastrozole for extended periods of time to patients with early breast cancer, attention to bone health is paramount, and bone density should be monitored in all patients. Prospective studies have demonstrated that bisphosphonates prevent aromatase-inhibitor–induced bone loss and a meta-analysis presented at the 2013 San Antonio Breast Cancer Symposium demonstrated that bisphosphonates reduce bone recurrences and prolong overall survival. Therefore, bisphosphonates should be considered in AI-treated patients, both in those with and without an increased risk of bone fractures.

A meta-analysis of toxicities comparing aromatase inhibitors with tamoxifen has demonstrated a 30% increase in grade 3 and 4 cardiac events with aromatase inhibitors.[131] However, prospective data demonstrate no differences in myocardial events comparing anastrozole with placebo, although an increase in hypertension was observed.[129]

No impact has been seen with anastrozole on adrenal steroidogenesis at up to 10 times the clinically recommended dose.[132] Although letrozole may decrease basal and adrenocorticotropic hormone–stimulated cortisol synthesis,[133,134] the clinical effect appears to be minimal. Aromatase inhibitors appear to have differential effects on lipids. In a study of over 900 patients with metastatic disease, anastrozole showed no marked effect on lipid profiles compared with baseline.[135] Conversely, the administration of letrozole in women with advanced breast cancer resulted in significant increases in total cholesterol and low-density lipoprotein, from baseline, after 8 and 16 weeks of therapy.[136] In the Breast International Group 1-98 trial, more women who received letrozole experienced grade 1 hypercholesterolemia compared to women who received tamoxifen.[127]

Letrozole is a nonsteroidal aromatase inhibitor with a high specificity for the inhibition of estrogen production (Fig. 27.3). Letrozole is 180 times more potent than aminoglutethimide as an inhibitor of aromatase in vitro. Aldosterone production in vitro is inhibited by concentrations 10,000 times higher than those required for inhibition of estrogen synthesis.[137,138] In a normal male volunteer study, letrozole was shown to decrease $E_2$ and serum $E_1$ levels to 10% of baseline with a single 3-mg dose. In phase I

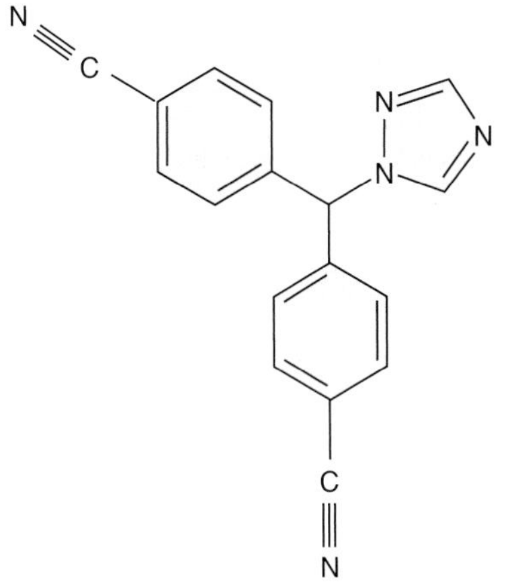

**Figure 27.3** Structure of letrozole.

studies, letrozole caused a significant decline in plasma $E_1$ and $E_2$ within 24 hours of a single oral dose of 0.1 mg.[139,140] After 2 weeks of treatment, the blood levels of $E_2$, $E_1$, and estrone sulfate were suppressed 95% or more from baseline. This continued over the 12 weeks of therapy. There was no apparent alteration in plasma levels of cortisol and aldosterone with letrozole or after corticotropin stimulation.[139] In postmenopausal women with advanced breast cancer, the drug did not have any effect on follicle-stimulating hormone (FSH), luteinizing hormone (LH), thyrotropin (previously thyroid-stimulating hormone), cortisol, 17-α-hydroxyprogesterone, androstenedione, or aldosterone blood concentrations.[141,142]

Anastrozole is a nonsteroidal aromatase inhibitor that is 200-fold more potent than aminoglutethimide.[143] No effect on the adrenal glands has been detected. In human studies, the $t_{max}$ is 2 to 3 hours after oral ingestion.[144] Elimination is primarily via hepatic metabolism, with 85% excreted by that route and only 10% excreted unchanged in urine. The main circulating metabolite is triazole after cleavage of the two rings in anastrozole by N-dealkylation. Linear pharmacokinetics have been observed in the dose range of 1 to 20 mg and do not change with repeat dosing. The terminal half-life is approximately 50 hours, and steady-state concentrations are achieved in approximately 10 days with once-a-day dosing and are three to four times higher than peak concentrations after a single dose. Plasma protein binding is approximately 40%.[145] In one study, anastrozole 1 mg and 10 mg daily, inhibited in vivo aromatization by 96.7% and 98.1%, respectively, and plasma $E_1$ and $E_2$ levels were suppressed 86.5% and 83.5%, respectively, regardless of dose.[146] Thus, 1 mg of anastrozole achieves near maximal aromatase inhibition and plasma estrogen suppression in breast cancer patients.

A recent prospective study to evaluate the pharmacokinetics of anastrozole (1 mg per day) demonstrated large interindividual variations in plasma anastrozole and anastrozole metabolite concentrations, as well as pretreatment and postdrug plasma $E_1$, $E_2$, and $E_1$ conjugate and estrogen precursor (androstenedione and testosterone) concentrations.[147] Further research is needed to determine the basis for the wide variability in the pharmacokinetics of anastrozole and whether these findings are clinically relevant.

## Exemestane

Exemestane has a steroidal structure and is classified as a type 1 aromatase inhibitor, also known as an *aromatase inactivator*, because it irreversibly binds with and permanently inactivates the enzyme.[134] Exemestane has been compared to tamoxifen in both the metastatic and adjuvant settings. In the setting of tamoxifen-refractory metastatic breast cancer, exemestane is superior to megestrol acetate, as demonstrated in a phase III trial in which improvements in both median time to tumor progression and median survival were observed.[148] In the adjuvant setting, the international exemestane study compared 2 to 3 years of tamoxifen with 2 to 3 years of exemestane in women who had previously competed 2 to 3 years of adjuvant tamoxifen. In this trial, a switch to exemestane resulted in superior disease-free and overall survival in the hormone receptor–positive subtype. Furthermore, exemestane has been compared with the nonsteroidal agent anastrozole in the adjuvant treatment of ER-positive breast cancer, and there were no differences in disease-free or overall survival.[149] Finally, exemestane has been compared to placebo in patients at increased risk of breast cancer, and a significant reduction in the risk of developing invasive breast cancer was observed.[150]

## Side Effects of Exemestane

Although preclinical studies have suggested that exemestane prevented bone loss in ovariectomized rats,[151] the Intergroup Exemestane adjuvant trial still demonstrated a higher rate of bone fracture for patients randomized to the exemestane arm and there were no differences in fracture rates comparing anastrozole with exemestane.[149] Side effects, including arthralgias and myalgias, appear to be similar to the other AIs. With regard to steroidogenesis, no impact on either cortisol or aldosterone levels was seen in a small study after the administration of exemestane for 7 days.[152] Finally, exemestane has weak androgenic properties, and its use at higher doses has been associated with steroidal-like side effects, such as weight gain and acne.[153,154] However, these side effects have not been observed with the FDA-approved dose (25 mg per day).[155]

## Pharmacology

Exemestane is administered once daily by mouth, with the recommended daily dose being 25 mg. The time needed to reach maximal $E_2$ suppression is 7 days,[156] and its half-life is 27 hours.[157] At daily doses of 10 to 25 mg, exemestane suppresses estrogen concentrations to 6% to 15% of pretreatment levels. This activity is more pronounced than that produced by formestane and comparable to that produced by the nonsteroidal AIs, anastrozole and letrozole.[158–160] Exemestane does not appear to affect cortisol or aldosterone levels when evaluated after 7 days of treatment based on dose-ranging studies, including doses from 0.5 to 800 mg.[152] Exemestane is metabolized by CYP3A4.[134] Although drug–drug interactions have not been formally reported for exemestane, there is the potential for interactions with drugs that affect CYP3A4.[134]

# GONADOTROPIN-RELEASING HORMONE ANALOGS

Gonadotropin-releasing hormone (GnRH) analogs result in a *medical orchiectomy* in men and are used as a means of providing androgen ablation for hormone-sensitive and castration refractory metastatic prostate cancer.[161] Because the initial agonist activity of GnRH analogs can cause a *tumor flare* from temporarily increased androgen levels, concomitant use of the antiandrogen flutamide or bicalutamide has been used to prevent this effect. GnRH analogs can also cause tumor regressions in hormonally responsive breast cancers[162] and have received FDA approval for the treatment of metastatic breast cancer in premenopausal women. Data suggest that these drugs may be useful as adjuvant therapy of premenopausal women with resected breast cancer.[163] The use of these drugs in combination with tamoxifen or exemestane in premenopausal women with primary breast cancer is the subject of large, ongoing, international clinical trials. The primary toxicities of GnRH analogs are secondary to the ablation of sex steroid

concentrations and include hot flashes, sweating, and nausea.[164] These symptoms can be reversed with low doses of progesterone analogs.[5] In males treated with GnRH analogs for prostate cancer, an alternate strategy of intermittent schedule of GnRH administration may result in improved tolerability and quality of life, with comparable efficacy compared with continuous GnRH analog administration in well-selected advanced prostate cancer patient cohorts.[165] However, in a recent trial comparing intermittent with continuous androgen ablation in newly diagnosed metastatic hormone sensitive prostate cancer patients, a greater risk for death from an intermittent strategy could not be conclusively ruled out although intermittent therapy resulted in small improvements in quality of life.[166]

GnRH analogs available for clinical use include goserelin[167,168] and leuprolide.[169] Both are available in depot intramuscular preparations to be given at monthly intervals. The recommended monthly dose of leuprolide is 7.5 mg and of goserelin is 3.6 mg. There are also longer acting depot preparations to be administered every 3, 4, 6, and 12 months.

## Pharmacology

Analogs of the decapeptide GnRH[167,169,170] have been synthesized by modifications of position 6 in which the l-glycine has been exchanged for a d-amino acid and the C-terminal amino acid has been either replaced by an ethylamide or substituted for a modified amino acid. These changes increase the affinity of the analog for the GnRH receptor and decrease the susceptibility to enzymatic degradation. There is an amino acid structure of GnRH with the substitutions for leuprolide and goserelin. Initial administration of these compounds results in stimulation of gonadotropin release. However, prolonged administration has led to profound inhibition of the pituitary–gonadal axis.[170] Plasma $E_2$ and progesterone are consistently suppressed to postmenopausal or castrate levels after 2 to 4 weeks of treatment with goserelin or leuprolide.[164,171] These drugs are administered intramuscularly or subcutaneously in a parenteral sustained-release microcapsule preparation, because parenteral administration of the parent drug is otherwise associated with rapid clearance. The GnRH analogs are metabolized in the liver, kidney, hypothalamus, and pituitary gland by neutral peptidase cleavage of the peptide bond between the tyrosine in the 5 position and the amino acid in position 6 and by a postproline-cleaving enzyme that cleaves the peptide bond between proline in the 9 position and the glycine-$NH_2$ in the 10 position. Substitutions at the glycine 6 position and modification of the C-terminal make these analogs more resistant to this enzymatic cleavage.

Leuprolide is approximately 80 to 100 times more potent than endogenous GnRH. It induces castrate levels of testosterone in men with prostate cancer within 3 to 4 weeks of drug administration after an initial sharp increase in LH and FSH. The mechanisms of action include pituitary desensitization after a reduction in pituitary GnRH receptor binding sites and possibly a direct antitumor effect in ER-positive human breast cancer cells.[169] The depot form results in a dose rate of 210 $\mu$g per day of leuprolide. Peak concentrations of the depot form, achieved approximately 3 hours after drug administration, have been reported to range between 13.1 and 54.5 $\mu$g/L. There appears to be a linear increase in the area under the curve (AUC) for doses of 3.75, 7.5, and 15.0 mg in the depot form. The parenteral bioavailability of subcutaneously injected leuprolide is 94%. The volume of distribution ranges from 27.4 to 37.1 L. In human studies, leuprolide urinary excretion as a metabolite was the primary route of clearance.

Goserelin is approximately 100 times more potent than the naturally occurring GnRH. Like leuprolide, it causes the stimulation of LH and FSH acutely, and with subsequent administration, GnRH receptor numbers decrease, and the pituitary becomes desensitized with decreasing LH and FSH levels. Castrate levels of testosterone are achieved within 1 month. In women, goserelin inhibits ovarian androgen production, but serum levels of dehydroepiandrosterone sulfate and, to a lesser extent, androstenedione, are preserved. In vitro, goserelin has demonstrated antitumor activity in estrogen-dependent MCF7 human breast cancer cells and LNCaP2 prostate cancer cells. The drug is released at a continuous mean rate of 120 μg per day in the depot form, with peak concentrations in the range of 2 to 3 μg/L achieved. The mean volume of distribution in six patients has been reported to be 13.7 L,[172] which is consistent with extracellular fluid volume. Goserelin is principally excreted in the urine, with a mean total body clearance of 8 L per hour in patients with normal renal function. The total body clearance is reduced by approximately 75%, with renal dysfunction and the elimination half-life increased two- or threefold. However, dose adjustment for renal insufficiency does not appear to be necessary. The 5 to 10 hexapeptide and the 4 to 10 hexapeptide were detected in urine in animal studies.[173] The terminal half-life of goserelin is approximately 5 hours after subcutaneous injection. Protein binding is low, and no known drug interactions have been documented.

# GONADOTROPIN-RELEASING HORMONE ANTAGONISTS

Modification to the structure of GnRH has resulted in the development of GnRH antagonist compounds that are currently being used in the treatment of prostate cancer. Abarelix was initially approved by the FDA in 2003 as the first depot-injectable GnRH antagonist, but was subsequently withdrawn in 2005. Degarelix is a synthetically modified compound with GnRH antagonist activity that was approved for use by the FDA in 2008 for the management of prostate cancer.[174] Its effect in prostate cancer treatment is to block the GnRH receptor, and thereby prevent the trigger for the production of LH, which mediates androgen synthesis. In contrast to GnRH analogs, degarelix does not cause *tumor flare* symptoms secondary to temporary increased androgen production. A large randomized clinical trial demonstrated that degarelix was associated with a rapid and sustained reduction in serum testosterone, prostate-specific antigen (PSA), FSH, and LH levels, with a loading dose of 240 mg subcutaneously, followed by a monthly maintenance dose of 80 mg[175] with comparable efficacy to leuprolide.[176] The most common side effects (greater than 10%) were hot flashes and pain at the injection site[176] when patients were provided degarelix for a 12-month period. It is unknown if degarelix will have a similar chronic side effect profile known to be associated with long-term GnRH analog use.

## Pharmacology

The recommended loading dose of degarelix is 240 mg, administered as two injections of 120 mg each subcutaneously. Monthly maintenance doses of 80 mg as a 20 mg/mL solution is started 28 days after the loading dose. In an analysis of pharmacokinetic/pharmacodynamic (PK/PD) properties of degarelix in 60 healthy males, after a single subcutaneous dose, a terminal half life of 47 days was observed.[177] PK properties of degarelix have been evaluated when administered as a subcutaneous depot of drug as a gel in six different doses to 48 healthy males and when administered intravenously. Using data from several clinical trials, the rate of drug diffusion from subcutaneous administration results in detectable drug up to 60 days after a single dose compared to less than 4 days when the drug is injected intravenously.

# ANTIANDROGENS

## Flutamide

The antiandrogen flutamide is used in men with metastatic prostate cancer either as initial therapy, combined with GnRH analog

administration, or when the metastatic prostate cancer is unresponsive, despite androgen ablation therapy. The recommended dose is 250 mg by mouth three times a day. In patients whose prostate cancer is growing despite flutamide use, stopping flutamide can sometimes cause a flutamide-withdrawal response.

The most common toxicity seen with flutamide is diarrhea, with or without abdominal discomfort. Gynecomastia, which can be tender, frequently occurs in men who are not receiving concomitant androgen ablation therapy.[178] Flutamide can rarely cause hepatotoxicity, a condition that is reversible if detected early, but this toxicity can also be fatal.[179] There is no accepted, clinically recommended testing schedule to screen for flutamide-induced hepatotoxicity other than being aware of this phenomenon and testing for liver function if hepatic symptoms develop.

## Pharmacology

Flutamide is a pure antiandrogen with no intrinsic steroidal activity.[180] Flutamide's mechanism of action is as an androgen-receptor antagonist. This binding prevents dihydrotestosterone binding and subsequent translocation of the androgen-receptor complex into the nuclei of cells. Because it is a pure antiandrogen, it acts only at the cellular level. The administration of flutamide alone leads to increased LH and FSH production and a concomitant increase in plasma testosterone and $E_2$ levels. Plasma protein binding ranges between 94% and 96% for flutamide and between 92% and 94% for 2-hydroxyflutamide, its major metabolite. When the drug is administered three times a day, steady state levels are achieved by day 6. The elimination half-life at steady state is 7.8 hours, and 2-hydroxyflutamide achieves concentrations 50 times higher than the parent drug at steady state and has equal or greater potency than that of flutamide.[180] The elimination half-life for the metabolite is 9.6 hours. The high plasma concentrations of 2-hydroxyflutamide, as compared with flutamide, suggest that the therapeutic benefits of flutamide are mediated primarily through its active metabolite.[181]

## Bicalutamide

Bicalutamide is another nonsteroidal antiandrogen that has been approved by the FDA for use in the United States. The recommended dose is one 50-mg tablet per day. One randomized trial reported that bicalutamide compared favorably with flutamide in patients with advanced prostate cancer.[182] Bicalutamide appears to be relatively well tolerated and is associated with a lower incidence of diarrhea than is flutamide.

## Pharmacology

Bicalutamide has a binding affinity to the androgen receptor in the rat prostate that is four times greater than that of 2-hydroxyflutamide.[183,184] In vivo, bicalutamide caused a marked inhibition of growth of accessory sex organs in rats, with a potency 5 to 10 times greater than that of flutamide. Unlike flutamide, bicalutamide did not cause a significant increase in LH or testosterone in rats. In humans, the drug has a long plasma half-life of 5 to 7 days, so it may be administered on a weekly schedule. Pharmacokinetics of the drug showed a dose-dependent increase in mean peak plasma concentrations, and the AUC increased linearly with the dose. The half-life of bicalutamide in humans was approximately 6 days, and the drug clearance was not saturable at plasma concentrations up to 1,000 ng/mL. Daily dosing of the drug led to an approximately tenfold accumulation after 12 weeks of administration. In contrast to results in rats, serum concentrations of testosterone and LH increased significantly from baseline at all dose levels tested in humans. Whereas serum FSH concentrations remained essentially unchanged, the median serum $E_2$ concentrations increased significantly.[185]

## Nilutamide

Nilutamide represents the third variation of an antiandrogen available for use in patients with prostate cancer. The observation of unique toxicities, night blindness, and pulmonary toxicity has limited its use.

# NOVEL ANTIANDROGENS

Although testosterone depletion remains an unchallenged standard for advanced stage hormone-sensitive disease, evidence has emerged that *castration-recurrent* prostate cancer remains androgen receptor (AR) dependent and is neither *hormone refractory* nor *androgen independent*, which were commonly used terms to define the progression of advanced stage disease following androgen deprivation therapy. Recognition of AR functioning despite the paucity of circulating androgens is evidenced by the elevation of AR messenger RNA in castration-recurrent tumor tissue relative to androgen-dependent tumors and reexpression of some androgen-regulated genes during clinical castration resistance. Recently, the AR axis has been the focus of therapeutic targeting.

## Abiraterone Acetate

After the failure of initial androgen manipulation with GnRH analogs and peripheral antiandrogens, prostate cancer continues to respond to a variety of second- and third-line hormonal interventions. Based on this observation, CYP17, a key enzyme in androgen and estrogen synthesis, was targeted using ketoconazole, which is a weak, reversible, and nonspecific inhibitor of CYP17 resulting in modest antitumor activity of short durability. More recently, abiraterone, a more potent (i.e., 20 times more than ketoconazole), selective, and irreversible inhibitor of CYP17, has been investigated in castration-recurrent prostate cancer, and significant objective responses have been observed.[186] Chemically, it is a 3-pyridyl steroid pregnenolone–derived compound available in an oral prodrug form of abiraterone acetate. Its main toxicity is from symptoms of mineralocorticoid excess (including hypokalemia, hypertension, and fluid overload), because continuous CYP17 blockade results in raising adrenocorticotrophic hormone (ACTH) levels that increase steroid levels upstream of CYP17, including corticosterone and deoxycorticosterone. These adverse effects are best avoided by the coadministration of steroids.

The established dose of abiraterone is 1,000 mg a day (four 250 mg tablets). Following oral administration of abiraterone acetate, the median time to maximum plasma abiraterone concentrations is 2 hours. At the dose of 1,000 mg daily, steady state values (mean ± standard deviation [SD]) of Cmax were 226 ± 178 ng/mL and of AUC were 1173 ± 690 ng.hr/mL. Abiraterone is highly bound (>99%) to the human plasma proteins, albumin and alpha-1 acid glycoprotein. The apparent steady state volume of distribution (mean ± SD) is 19,669 ± 13,358 L. No major deviation from dose proportionality was observed in the dose range of 250 mg to 1,000 mg. However, the exposure was not significantly increased when the dose was doubled from 1,000 to 2,000 mg (8% increase in mean AUC). The two main circulating metabolites of abiraterone in human plasma are abiraterone sulfate (inactive) and N-oxide abiraterone sulfate (inactive), which each account for about 43% of exposure. CYP3A4 and SULT2A1 are enzymes involved in the formation and conjugation of N-oxide abiraterone.

## Enzalutamide

Enzalutamide is a new diarylthiohydantoin compound that binds AR with an affinity that is several-fold greater than the antiandrogens bicalutamide and flutamide. This class of novel AR inhibitor also disrupts the nuclear translocation of AR and impairs DNA binding to androgen response elements and the recruitment of coactivators.[187] In early clinical trials, promising results have been observed in castrate refractory and chemotherapy-resistant settings. The major metabolite of enzalutamide is N-desmethyl enzalutamide, and CYP2C8 is responsible for the formation of the active metabolite, N-desmethyl enzalutamide. Enzalutamide pharmacokinetics, in the studied dose range between 30 mg to 480 mg, exhibited a linear, two-compartmental model with first-order kinetics. In patients with mCRPC, the mean (% coefficient of variation [CV]) predose Cmin values for enzalutamide and N-desmethyl enzalutamide were 11.4 (25.9%) µg/mL and 13.0 (29.9%) µg/mL, respectively. Enzalutamide is mainly metabolized by CYP2C8 and CYP3A4. Doses ranging from 30 to 600 mg daily have been evaluated, with dose-limiting toxicities including fatigue, seizure, asthenia, anemia, and arthralgia occurring at higher dose levels. At present, enzalutamide has been approved for treating advanced castrate-recurrent prostate cancer[188] after a failure of docetaxel chemotherapy at a dose of 160 mg (four, 40 mg oral capsules). Clinical trials are ongoing to evaluate the efficacy of enzalutamide in castrate-recurrent patients who are chemotherapy naïve.

## Galeterone and Orteronel

Novel CYP17 inhibitors that are more selective for 17,20-lyase over 17 α-hydroxylase are currently being developed. Orteronel (TAK-700) is an example of a highly selective 17,20 lyase, which is currently undergoing phase III clinical trials in a pre- and post-chemotherapy castrate-recurrent setting after the failure of androgen-deprivation therapy.[189] Other novel agents being developed include galeterone, which is an inhibitor of CYP 17 α-hydroxylase and C17,20 lyase. Survival mechanisms of prostate cancer cells targeted by galeterone include its binding to AR, competitive inhibition of testosterone binding, and a reduction in the quantity of AR protein within the prostate cancer cells. It can also enhance the degradation of constitutively active splice variants. Therefore, taken together, it diminishes the ability of the cells to respond to the low levels of androgenic growth signals. This agent is currently in early clinical safety and efficacy testing for advanced stage prostate cancer.

# OTHER SEX STEROID THERAPIES

## Fluoxymesterone

Fluoxymesterone is an androgen that has been used in women with metastatic breast cancer who have hormonally responsive cancers and who have progressed on other hormonal therapies such as tamoxifen, an aromatase inhibitor, or megestrol acetate. The usual dose is 10 mg given twice daily. Although the overall response rate is low for fluoxymesterone used in this clinical situation,[190] there are some patients who have substantial antitumor responses lasting for months or even years.

Toxicities associated with fluoxymesterone are those that would be expected with an androgen: hirsutism, male-pattern baldness, voice lowering (hoarseness), acne, enhanced libido, and erythrocytosis. Fluoxymesterone can also cause elevated liver function test results in some patients and, rarely, has been associated with hepatic neoplasms.

## Pharmacology

Fluoxymesterone is a chlorinated synthetic analog of testosterone with potent androgenic and anabolic activity in humans. Limited pharmacologic information is available on this agent. Colburn,[191] using a radioimmunoassay, studied two patients after a single oral administration of a 50-mg dose. Peak serum concentrations were achieved between 1 and 3 hours after administration, with the average peak concentrations being 335 ng/mL. By 5 hours after drug administration, serum levels had declined to approximately 50% of the peak concentration. Urinary excretion of a 10-mg dose can be detected for 24 hours, and at least 6-hydroxy, 4-ene, 3-β, and 11-hydroxy metabolites of fluoxymesterone have been detected.[192]

## Estrogens: Diethylstilbestrol and Estradiol

Diethylstilbestrol (DES) had been the primary hormonal therapy for postmenopausal metastatic breast cancer. Randomized comparative trials demonstrated it had a similar response rate to that of tamoxifen.[193,194] However, based on these trials, DES use was supplanted by tamoxifen, primarily because DES has more toxicity. DES is occasionally used in metastatic breast cancer patients who have hormonally sensitive cancers that have failed to respond to multiple other hormonal therapies. The usual dose in this situation is 15 mg per day, either as a single dose or as divided doses. DES was also used as androgen ablation therapy in men with metastatic prostate cancer.[195] Doses of approximately 3 mg per day result in testosterone levels that are seen in an anorchid state.

DES toxicities include nausea and vomiting, breast tenderness, and a darkening of the nipple–areolar complex. DES increases the risk of thromboembolic phenomenon, which may result in life-threatening complications. Although DES is not clinically available in the United States, similar antitumor effects and toxicities are seen with estradiol, with a target dose of 10 mg by mouth three times a day. The pharmacology of $E_2$ has been extensively described elsewhere.[196]

## Medroxyprogesterone and Megestrol

Medroxyprogesterone and megestrol are 17-OH-progesterone derivatives differing in a double bond between C6 and C7 positions in megestrol. Historically, megestrol was used as a hormonal agent for patients with advanced breast cancer, usually at a total daily dose of 160 mg. Additionally, it is still used for the treatment of hormonally responsive metastatic endometrial cancer, at a dose of 320 mg per day. In addition, doses of 160 mg per day are occasionally used as a hormonal therapy for prostate cancer.[197] Megestrol has also been extensively evaluated for the treatment of anorexia/cachexia related to cancer or AIDS.[198–201] Various dosages ranging from 160 to 1,600 mg per day have been used. A prospective study has demonstrated a dose–response relationship with doses up to 800 mg per day.[202] Low dosages of megestrol (20 to 40 mg per day) have been shown to be an effective means of reducing hot flashes in women with breast cancer and in men who have undergone androgen ablation therapy.[5] Although megestrol had historically been commonly administered four times per day, the long terminal half-life supports once-per-day dosing.

Megestrol is a relatively well-tolerated medication, with its most prominent side effects being appetite stimulation and resultant weight gain. Although these may be beneficial effects in patients with anorexia/cachexia, they can be important problems in patients with breast or endometrial cancers. Another side effect of megestrol acetate is the marked suppression of adrenal steroid production by suppression of the pituitary–adrenal axis.[203] Although this appears to be asymptomatic in the majority of patients, reports suggest that this adrenal suppression can cause clinical problems in some patients.[204] This drug has been abruptly stopped for decades without the recognition of untoward sequelae in patients, and it seems reasonable to continue this practice. Nonetheless, if Addisonian signs or symptoms develop after drug discontinuation, corticosteroids should be administered.

Furthermore, if patients who receive megestrol have a significant infection, experience trauma, or undergo surgery, then corticosteroid coverage should be administered. There appears to be a slightly increased incidence of thromboembolic phenomena in patients receiving megestrol alone.[202] This risk appears to be higher if megestrol is administered with concomitant cytotoxic therapy.[205] There are conflicting reports regarding megestrol-causing edema.[206] If it does, the edema is generally minimal and easily handled with a mild diuretic. Megestrol may cause impotence in some men.[207] The incidence of this is controversial, although it is generally agreed that this is a reversible situation. Megestrol can cause menstrual irregularities, the most prominent of which is withdrawal menstrual bleeding within a few weeks of drug discontinuation.[5] Although nausea and vomiting have sometimes been attributed as a toxicity of this drug, there are data to demonstrate that this drug has antiemetic properties.[200,201,205] In terms of magnitude, megestrol appears to decrease both nausea and vomiting in advanced-stage cancer patients by approximately two thirds.

Medroxyprogesterone has many of the same properties, clinical uses, and toxicities as megestrol acetate. It has never been commonly used in the United States for the treatment of breast cancer but has been used more in Europe. Medroxyprogesterone is available in 2.5- and 10-mg tablets and in injectable formulations of 100 and 400 mg/L. Dosing for the treatment of metastatic breast or prostate cancer has commonly been 400 mg per week or more and 1,000 mg per week or more for metastatic endometrial cancer. Injectable or daily oral doses have been used for controlling hot flashes.

## Pharmacology

The exact mechanism of antitumor effect of medroxyprogesterone and megestrol is unclear. These drugs have been reported to suppress adrenal steroid synthesis,[208] suppress ER levels,[209] alter tumor hormone metabolism,[210] enhance steroid metabolism,[211] and directly kill tumor cells.[212] In addition, progestins may influence some growth factors,[213] suppress plasma estrone sulfate formation, and, at high concentrations, inhibit P-glycoprotein.

The oral bioavailability of these progestational agents is unknown, although absorption appears to be poor for medroxyprogesterone relative to megestrol.

The terminal half-life for megestrol is approximately 14 hours,[214,215] with a $t_{max}$ of 2 to 5 hours after oral ingestion.[216] The AUC for a single megestrol dose of 160 mg is between 2.5- and 8-fold higher than that for single-dose medroxyprogesterone at 1,000 mg with a radioactive dose of megestrol; 50% to 78% is found in the urine after oral administration, and 8% to 30% is found in the feces.

Metabolism and excretion of medroxyprogesterone have been incompletely characterized. In humans, 20% to 50% of a [$^3$H]medroxyprogesterone dose is excreted in the urine and 5% to 10% in the stool after intravenous administration.[217–219] Metabolism of medroxyprogesterone occurs via hydroxylation, reduction, demethylation, and combinations of these reactions.[220] The major urinary metabolite is a glucuronide. Less than 3% of the dose is excreted as unconjugated medroxyprogesterone in humans. Clearance of medroxyprogesterone has been reported to range between 27 and 70 L per hour.[219] The initial volume of distribution is between 4 and 8 L in humans. The mean terminal half-life is 60 hours. The $t_{max}$ for medroxyprogesterone occurs 2 to 5 hours after oral administration. Medroxyprogesterone appears to be concentrated in the small intestine, the colon, and in adipose tissue in human autopsy studies.[221] Drug interactions of medroxyprogesterone have been reported with aminoglutethimide, which decreases plasma medroxyprogesterone levels.[222] Medroxyprogesterone may reduce the concentration of the N-desmethyltamoxifen metabolite concentration. Progestational agents also may increase plasma warfarin levels.[223] These reports are consistent with CYP3A being the site of interaction.

# OTHER HORMONAL THERAPIES

## Octreotide

Octreotide is a somatostatin analog that is administered for the treatment of carcinoid syndrome and other hormonal excess syndromes associated with some pancreatic islet cell cancers and acromegaly. Response rates (measured in terms of a reduction in diarrhea and flushing) are high and can last for several months to years. Occasionally, antitumor responses temporarily related to octreotide are seen with these tumors. Octreotide may be useful to alleviate 5-fluorouracil–associated diarrhea.[224-226]

Octreotide can be administered intravenously or subcutaneously. Initial doses of 50 µg are given two to three times on the first day. The dose is titrated upward, with a usual daily dose of 300 to 450 µg per day for most patients. A depot preparation is available, allowing doses to be administered at monthly intervals. Octreotide is generally well tolerated overall. It appears to cause more toxicity in acromegalic patients, with such problems as bradycardia, diarrhea, hypoglycemia, hyperglycemia, hypothyroidism, and cholelithiasis.

## Pharmacology

Octreotide is an 8-amino acid synthetic analog of the 14-amino acid peptide somatostatin.[227] Octreotide has a similar high affinity for somatostatin receptors, as does its parent compound, with a concentration that inhibits the receptor by 50% in the subnanomolar range. Octreotide inhibits insulin, glucagon, pancreatic polypeptide, gastric inhibitory polypeptide, and gastrin secretion. It has a much longer duration of action than the parent compound because of its greater resistance to enzymatic degradation. Its absorption after subcutaneous administration is rapid, and bioavailability is 100% after subcutaneous injection. Peak concentrations of 4 µg/L after a 100-µg dose occur within 20 to 30 minutes of subcutaneous injection and are 20% to 40% of the corresponding intravenous injection. Both peak concentration and AUC for octreotide increase linearly with dose. The total body clearance in healthy volunteers is 9.6 L per hour. Hepatic metabolism of octreotide accounts for 30% to 40% of the drug's disposition, and 11% to 20% is excreted unchanged in the urine. The volume of distribution ranges between 18 and 30 L, and the terminal half-life is reported to be between 72 and 98 minutes. Sixty-five percent of the drug is protein bound primarily to the lipoprotein fraction.[227,228] Because of the short half-life, classic octreotide is administered subcutaneously two or three times per day.[229] A slow-release form of octreotide, designed for once-per-month administration, controls the symptoms of carcinoid syndrome at least as well as three-times-per-day octreotide.[230]

# REFERENCES

1. Fisher B, Costantino JP, Wickerham DL, et al. Tamoxifen for the prevention of breast cancer: current status of the National Surgical Adjuvant Breast and Bowel Project P-1 study. J Natl Cancer Inst 2005;97:1652–1662.
2. Fisher B, Dignam J, Wolmark N, et al. Tamoxifen in treatment of intraductal breast cancer: National Surgical Adjuvant Breast and Bowel Project B-24 randomised controlled trial. Lancet 1999;353:1993–2000.
3. Colleoni M, Gelber S, Goldhirsch A, et al. Tamoxifen after adjuvant chemotherapy for premenopausal women with lymph node-positive breast cancer: International Breast Cancer Study Group Trial 13-93. J Clin Oncol 2006;24:1332–1341.
4. Davies C, Pan H, Godwin J, et al. Long-term effects of continuing adjuvant tamoxifen to 10 years versus stopping at 5 years after diagnosis of oestrogen receptor-positive breast cancer: ATLAS, a randomised trial. Lancet 2013;381:805–816.
5. Loprinzi CL, Michalak JC, Quella SK, et al. Megestrol acetate for the prevention of hot flashes. N Engl J Med 1994;331:347–352.
6. Loprinzi CL, Kugler JW, Sloan JA, et al. Venlafaxine in management of hot flashes in survivors of breast cancer: a randomised controlled trial. Lancet 2000;356:2059–2063.
7. Archer DF, Dupont CM, Constantine GD, et al. Desvenlafaxine for the treatment of vasomotor symptoms associated with menopause: a double-blind, randomized, placebo-controlled trial of efficacy and safety. Am J Obstet Gynecol 2009;200:238.e1–238e10.
8. Barton DL, LaVasseur BI, Sloan JA, et al. Phase III, placebo-controlled trial of three doses of citalopram for the treatment of hot flashes: NCCTG trial N05C9. J Clin Oncol 2010;28:3278–3283.
9. Freeman EW, Guthrie KA, Caan B, et al. Efficacy of escitalopram for hot flashes in healthy menopausal women: a randomized controlled trial. JAMA 2011;305:267–274.
10. Stearns V, Beebe KL, Iyengar M, et al. Paroxetine controlled release in the treatment of menopausal hot flashes: a randomized controlled trial. JAMA 2003;289:2827–2834.
11. Pandya KJ, Morrow GR, Roscoe JA, et al. Gabapentin for hot flashes in 420 women with breast cancer: a randomised double-blind placebo-controlled trial. Lancet 2005;366:818–824.
12. Loprinzi CL, Qin R, Balcueva EP, et al. Phase III, randomized, double-blind, placebo-controlled evaluation of pregabalin for alleviating hot flashes, N07C1. J Clin Oncol 2010;28:641–647.
13. Madlensky L, Natarajan L, Tchu S, et al. Tamoxifen metabolite concentrations, CYP2D6 genotype, and breast cancer outcomes. Clin Pharmacol Ther 2011;89:718–725.
14. Tamoxifen for early breast cancer: an overview of the randomised trials. Early Breast Cancer Trialists' Collaborative Group. Lancet 1998;351:1451–1467.
15. Wickerham DL, Fisher B, Wolmark N, et al. Association of tamoxifen and uterine sarcoma. J Clin Oncol 2002;20:2758–2760.
16. Dewar JA, Horobin JM, Preece PE, et al. Long term effects of tamoxifen on blood lipid values in breast cancer. BMJ 1992;305:225–226.
17. Love RR, Mazess RB, Barden HS, et al. Effects of tamoxifen on bone mineral density in postmenopausal women with breast cancer. N Engl J Med 1992;326:852–856.
18. Powles TJ, Hickish T, Kanis JA, et al. Effect of tamoxifen on bone mineral density measured by dual-energy x-ray absorptiometry in healthy premenopausal and postmenopausal women. J Clin Oncol 1996;14:78–84.
19. Buzdar A, Howell A, Cuzick J, et al. Comprehensive side-effect profile of anastrozole and tamoxifen as adjuvant treatment for early-stage breast cancer: long-term safety analysis of the ATAC trial. Lancet Oncol 2006;7:633–643.
20. Gorin MB, Day R, Costantino JP, et al. Long-term tamoxifen citrate use and potential ocular toxicity. Am J Ophthalmol 1998;125:493–501.
21. Tonetti DA, Jordan VC. Possible mechanisms in the emergence of tamoxifen-resistant breast cancer. Anticancer Drugs 1995;6:498–507.
22. Lim YC, Desta Z, Flockhart DA, et al. Endoxifen (4-hydroxy-N-desmethyl-tamoxifen) has anti-estrogenic effects in breast cancer cells with potency similar to 4-hydroxy-tamoxifen. Cancer Chemother Pharmacol 2005;55:471–478.
23. Benz CC, Scott GK, Sarup JC, et al. Estrogen-dependent, tamoxifen-resistant tumorigenic growth of MCF-7 cells transfected with HER2/neu. Breast Cancer Res Treat 1993;24:85–95.
24. Borg A, Baldetorp B, Ferno M, et al. ERBB2 amplification is associated with tamoxifen resistance in steroid-receptor positive breast cancer. Cancer Lett 1994;81:137–144.
25. Houston SJ, Plunkett TA, Barnes DM, et al. Overexpression of c-erbB2 is an independent marker of resistance to endocrine therapy in advanced breast cancer. Br J Cancer 1999;79:1220–1226.
26. Lipton A, Ali SM, Leitzel K, et al. Serum HER-2/neu and response to the aromatase inhibitor letrozole versus tamoxifen. J Clin Oncol 2003;21:1967–1972.
27. Bunone G, Briand PA, Miksicek RJ, et al. Activation of the unliganded estrogen receptor by EGF involves the MAP kinase pathway and direct phosphorylation. Embo J 1996;15:2174–2183.
28. Kato S, Endoh H, Masuhiro Y, et al. Activation of the estrogen receptor through phosphorylation by mitogen-activated protein kinase. Science 1995;270:1491–1494.
29. Pietras RJ, Arboleda J, Reese DM, et al. HER-2 tyrosine kinase pathway targets estrogen receptor and promotes hormone-independent growth in human breast cancer cells. Oncogene 1995;10:2435–2446.
30. Osborne CK, Bardou V, Hopp TA, et al. Role of the estrogen receptor coactivator AIB1 (SRC-3) and HER-2/neu in tamoxifen resistance in breast cancer. J Natl Cancer Inst 2003;95:353–361.
31. Encarnacion CA, Ciocca DR, McGuire WL, et al. Measurement of steroid hormone receptors in breast cancer patients on tamoxifen. Breast Cancer Res Treat 1993;26:237–246.
32. Watts CK, Handel ML, King RJ, et al. Oestrogen receptor gene structure and function in breast cancer. J Steroid Biochem Mol Biol 1992;41:529–536.
33. Zhang QX, Borg A, Wolf DM, et al. An estrogen receptor mutant with strong hormone-independent activity from a metastatic breast cancer. Cancer Res 1997;57:1244–1249.
34. Toy W, Shen Y, Won H, et al. ESR1 ligand-binding domain mutations in hormone-resistant breast cancer. Nat Genet 2013;45:1439–1445.
35. Robinson DR, Wu YM, Vats P, et al. Activating ESR1 mutations in hormone-resistant metastatic breast cancer. Nat Genet 2013;45:1446–1451.

36. Merenbakh-Lamin K, Ben-Baruch N, Yeheskel A, et al. D538G mutation in estrogen receptor-alpha: a novel mechanism for acquired endocrine resistance in breast cancer. *Cancer Res* 2013;73:6856–6864.

37. Fendl KC, Zimniski SJ. Role of tamoxifen in the induction of hormone-independent rat mammary tumors. *Cancer Res* 1992;52:235–237.

38. Williams GM. Tamoxifen experimental carcinogenicity studies: implications for human effects. *Proc Soc Exp Biol Med* 1995;208:141–143.

39. Williams GM, Iatropoulos MJ, Djordjevic MV, et al. The triphenylethylene drug tamoxifen is a strong liver carcinogen in the rat. *Carcinogenesis* 1993;14: 315–317.

40. Rutqvist LE, Johansson H, Signomklao T, et al. Adjuvant tamoxifen therapy for early stage breast cancer and second primary malignancies. Stockholm Breast Cancer Study Group. *J Natl Cancer Inst* 1995;87:645–651.

41. Mani C, Kupfer D. Cytochrome P-450-mediated activation and irreversible binding of the antiestrogen tamoxifen to proteins in rat and human liver: possible involvement of flavin-containing monooxygenases in tamoxifen activation. *Cancer Res* 1991;51:6052–6058.

42. Mani C, Pearce R, Parkinson A, et al. Involvement of cytochrome P4503A in catalysis of tamoxifen activation and covalent binding to rat and human liver microsomes. *Carcinogenesis* 1994;15:2715–2720.

43. Styles JA, Davies A, Lim CK, et al. Genotoxicity of tamoxifen, tamoxifen epoxide and toremifene in human lymphoblastoid cells containing human cytochrome P450s. *Carcinogenesis* 1994;15:5–9.

44. Han XL, Liehr JG. Induction of covalent DNA adducts in rodents by tamoxifen. *Cancer Res* 1992;52:1360–1363.

45. Mani C, Hodgson E, Kupfer D. Metabolism of the antimammary cancer antiestrogenic agent tamoxifen. II. Flavin-containing monooxygenase-mediated N-oxidation. *Drug Metab Dispos* 1993;21:657–661.

46. Mani C, Gelboin HV, Park SS, et al. Metabolism of the antimammary cancer antiestrogenic agent tamoxifen. I. Cytochrome P-450-catalyzed N-demethylation and 4-hydroxylation. *Drug Metab Dispos* 1993;21:645–656.

47. Albain KS, Barlow WE, Shak S, et al. Prognostic and predictive value of the 21-gene recurrence score assay in postmenopausal women with node-positive, oestrogen-receptor-positive breast cancer on chemotherapy: a retrospective analysis of a randomised trial. *Lancet Oncol* 2010;11:55–65.

48. Dowsett M, Cuzick J, Wale C, et al. Prediction of risk of distant recurrence using the 21-gene recurrence score in node-negative and node-positive postmenopausal patients with breast cancer treated with anastrozole or tamoxifen: a TransATAC study. *J Clin Oncol* 2010;28:1829–1834.

49. Paik S, Shak S, Tang G, et al. A multigene assay to predict recurrence of tamoxifen-treated, node-negative breast cancer. *N Engl J Med* 2004;351:2817–2826.

50. Johnson MD, Zuo H, Lee KH, et al. Pharmacological characterization of 4-hydroxy-N-desmethyl tamoxifen, a novel active metabolite of tamoxifen. *Breast Cancer Res Treat* 2004;85:151–159.

51. Lim YC, Li L, Desta Z, et al. Endoxifen, a secondary metabolite of tamoxifen, and 4-OH-tamoxifen induce similar changes in global gene expression patterns in MCF-7 breast cancer cells. *J Pharmacol Exp Ther* 2006;318:503–512.

52. Wu X, Hawse JR, Subramaniam M, et al. The tamoxifen metabolite, endoxifen, is a potent antiestrogen that targets estrogen receptor alpha for degradation in breast cancer cells. *Cancer Res* 2009;69:1722–1727.

53. Jin Y, Desta Z, Stearns V, et al. CYP2D6 genotype, antidepressant use, and tamoxifen metabolism during adjuvant breast cancer treatment. *J Natl Cancer Inst* 2005;97:30–39.

54. Desta Z, Ward BA, Soukhova NV, et al. Comprehensive evaluation of tamoxifen sequential biotransformation by the human cytochrome P450 system in vitro: prominent roles for CYP3A and CYP2D6. *J Pharmacol Exp Ther* 2004;310:1062–1075.

55. Stearns V, Johnson MD, Rae JM, et al. Active tamoxifen metabolite plasma concentrations after coadministration of tamoxifen and the selective serotonin reuptake inhibitor paroxetine. *J Natl Cancer Inst* 2003;95:1758–1764.

56. Goetz MP, Rae JM, Suman VJ, et al. Pharmacogenetics of tamoxifen biotransformation is associated with clinical outcomes of efficacy and hot flashes. *J Clin Oncol* 2005;23:9312–9318.

57. Schroth W, Antoniadou L, Fritz P, et al. Breast cancer treatment outcome with adjuvant tamoxifen relative to patient CYP2D6 and CYP2C19 genotypes. *J Clin Oncol* 2007;25:5187–5193.

58. Schroth W, Goetz MP, Hamann U, et al. Association between CYP2D6 polymorphisms and outcomes among women with early stage breast cancer treated with tamoxifen. *JAMA* 2009;302:1429–1436.

59. Rae JM, Drury S, Hayes DF, et al. CYP2D6 and UGT2B7 genotype and risk of recurrence in tamoxifen-treated breast cancer patients. *J Natl Cancer Inst* 2012;104:452–460.

60. Regan MM, Leyland-Jones B, Bouzyk M, et al. CYP2D6 genotype and tamoxifen response in postmenopausal women with endocrine-responsive breast cancer: the breast international group 1-98 trial. *J Natl Cancer Inst* 2012;104:441–451.

61. Goetz MP, Suman VJ, Hoskin TL, et al. CYP2D6 metabolism and patient outcome in the Austrian Breast and Colorectal Cancer Study Group trial (ABCSG) 8. *Clin Cancer Res* 2013;19:500–507.

62. Province MA, Goetz MP, Brauch H, et al. CYP2D6 Genotype and adjuvant tamoxifen: meta-analysis of heterogeneous study populations. *Clin Pharmacol Ther* 2014;95:216–227.

63. Borges S, Desta Z, Li L, et al. Quantitative effect of CYP2D6 genotype and inhibitors on tamoxifen metabolism: implication for optimization of breast cancer treatment. *Clin Pharmacol Ther* 2006;80:61–74.

64. Dezentje VO, van Blijderveen NJ, Gelderblom H, et al. Effect of concomitant CYP2D6 inhibitor use and tamoxifen adherence on breast cancer recurrence in early-stage breast cancer. *J Clin Oncol* 2010;28:2423–2429.

65. Kelly CM, Juurlink DN, Gomes T, et al. Selective serotonin reuptake inhibitors and breast cancer mortality in women receiving tamoxifen: a population based cohort study. *BMJ* 2010;340:c693.

66. Binkhorst L, van Gelder T, Loos WJ, et al. Effects of CYP induction by rifampicin on tamoxifen exposure. *Clin Pharmacol Ther* 2012;92:62–67.

67. Irvin WJ Jr., Walko CM, Weck KE, et al. Genotype-guided tamoxifen dosing increases active metabolite exposure in women with reduced CYP2D6 metabolism: a multicenter study. *J Clin Oncol* 2011;29:3232–3239.

68. Kiyotani K, Mushiroda T, Imamura CK, et al. Dose-adjustment study of tamoxifen based on CYP2D6 genotypes in Japanese breast cancer patients. *Breast Cancer Res Treat* 2012;131:137–145.

69. Goetz MP, Suman VA, Reid JR, et al. A first-in-human phase I study of the tamoxifen (TAM) metabolite, Z-endoxifen hydrochloride (Z-Endx) in women with aromatase inhibitor (AI) refractory metastatic breast cancer (MBC) (NCT01327781). *Cancer Res* 2013;73(24 Suppl): Abstract nr PD3-4.

70. Lien EA, Anker G, Lonning PE, et al. Decreased serum concentrations of tamoxifen and its metabolites induced by aminoglutethimide. *Cancer Res* 1990;50:5851–5857.

71. Adam HK, Patterson JS, Kemp JV. Studies on the metabolism and pharmacokinetics of tamoxifen in normal volunteers. *Cancer Treat Rep* 1980;64: 761–764.

72. Patterson JS, Settatree RS, Adam HK, et al. Serum concentrations of tamoxifen and major metabolite during long-term nolvadex therapy, correlated with clinical response. *Eur J Cancer Suppl* 1980;1:89–92.

73. Camaggi CM, Strocchi E, Canova N, et al. Medroxyprogesterone acetate (MAP) and tamoxifen (TMX) plasma levels after simultaneous treatment with 'low' TMX and 'high' MAP doses. *Cancer Chemother Pharmacol* 1985;14: 229–231.

74. Lien EA, Solheim E, Lea OA, et al. Distribution of 4-hydroxy-N-desmethyl-tamoxifen and other tamoxifen metabolites in human biological fluids during tamoxifen treatment. *Cancer Res* 1989;49:2175–2183.

75. Lien EA, Solheim E, Ueland PM. Distribution of tamoxifen and its metabolites in rat and human tissues during steady-state treatment. *Cancer Res* 1991;51:4837–4844.

76. Daniel P, Gaskell SJ, Bishop H, et al. Determination of tamoxifen and biologically active metabolites in human breast tumours and plasma. *Eur J Cancer Clin Oncol* 1981;17:1183–1189.

77. Robinson SP, Langan-Fahey SM, Johnson DA, et al. Metabolites, pharmacodynamics, and pharmacokinetics of tamoxifen in rats and mice compared to the breast cancer patient. *Drug Metab Dispos* 1991;19:36–43.

78. DeGregorio MW, Wiebe VJ, Venook AP, et al. Elevated plasma tamoxifen levels in a patient with liver obstruction. *Cancer Chemother Pharmacol* 1989;23:194–195.

79. Lodwick R, McConkey B, Brown AM. Life threatening interaction between tamoxifen and warfarin. *Br Med J (Clin Res Ed)* 1987;295:1141.

80. Ritchie LD, Grant SM. Tamoxifen-warfarin interaction: the Aberdeen hospitals drug file. *BMJ* 1989;298:1253.

81. Tenni P, Lalich DL, Byrne MJ. Life threatening interaction between tamoxifen and warfarin. *BMJ* 1989;298:93.

82. Rabinowicz AL, Hinton DR, Dyck P, et al. High-dose tamoxifen in treatment of brain tumors: interaction with antiepileptic drugs. *Epilepsia* 1995;36: 513–515.

83. Desai PB, Nallani SC, Sane RS, et al. Induction of cytochrome P450 3A4 in primary human hepatocytes and activation of the human pregnane X receptor by tamoxifen and 4-hydroxytamoxifen. *Drug Metab Dispos* 2002;30:608–612.

84. Dowsett M, Cuzick J, Howell A, et al. Pharmacokinetics of anastrozole and tamoxifen alone, and in combination, during adjuvant endocrine therapy for early breast cancer in postmenopausal women: a sub-protocol of the 'Arimidex and tamoxifen alone or in combination' (ATAC) trial. *Br J Cancer* 2001;85:317–324.

85. Pagani O, Gelber S, Price K, et al. Toremifene and tamoxifen are equally effective for early-stage breast cancer: first results of International Breast Cancer Study Group Trials 12-93 and 14-93. *Ann Oncol* 2004;15:1749–1759.

86. Hayes DF, Van Zyl JA, Hacking A, et al. Randomized comparison of tamoxifen and two separate doses of toremifene in postmenopausal women with metastatic breast cancer. *J Clin Oncol* 1995;13:2556–2566.

87. Stenbygaard LE, Herrstedt J, Thomsen JF, et al. Toremifene and tamoxifen in advanced breast cancer—a double-blind cross-over trial. *Breast Cancer Res Treat* 1993;25:57–63.

88. Vogel CL, Shemano I, Schoenfelder J, et al. Multicenter phase II efficacy trial of toremifene in tamoxifen-refractory patients with advanced breast cancer. *J Clin Oncol* 1993;11:345–350.

89. Kangas L. Review of the pharmacological properties of toremifene. *J Steroid Biochem* 1990;36:191–195.

90. Berthou F, Dreano Y, Belloc C, et al. Involvement of cytochrome P450 3A enzyme family in the major metabolic pathways of toremifene in human liver microsomes. *Biochem Pharmacol* 1994;47:1883–1895.

91. Simberg NH, Murai JT, Siiteri PK. In vitro and in vivo binding of toremifene and its metabolites in rat uterus. *J Steroid Biochem* 1990;36:197–202.

92. Kohler PC, Hamm JT, Wiebe VJ, et al. Phase I study of the tolerance and pharmacokinetics of toremifene in patients with cancer. *Breast Cancer Res Treat* 1990;16 Suppl:S19–S26.

93. Tominaga T, Abe O, Izuo M. A phase I study of toremifene. *Breast Cancer Res Treat* 1990;16 (Suppl):27.

94. Wiebe VJ, Benz CC, Shemano I, et al. Pharmacokinetics of toremifene and its metabolites in patients with advanced breast cancer. *Cancer Chemother Pharmacol* 1990;25:247–251.

**CANCER THERAPEUTICS**

95. Anttila M, Laakso S, Nylanden P, et al. Pharmacokinetics of the novel antiestrogenic agent toremifene in subjects with altered liver and kidney function. *Clin Pharmacol Ther* 1995;57:628–635.

96. Hard GC, Iatropoulos MJ, Jordan K, et al. Major difference in the hepatocarcinogenicity and DNA adduct forming ability between toremifene and tamoxifen in female Crl:CD(BR) rats. *Cancer Res* 1993;53:4534–4541.

97. Montandon F, Williams GM. Comparison of DNA reactivity of the polyphenylethylene hormonal agents diethylstilbestrol, tamoxifen and toremifene in rat and hamster liver. *Arch Toxicol* 1994;68:272–275.

98. Vogel VG, Costantino JP, Wickerham DL, et al. Update of the National Surgical Adjuvant Breast and Bowel Project Study of Tamoxifen and Raloxifene (STAR) P-2 Trial: Preventing Breast Cancer. *Cancer Prev Res (Phila)* 2010;3:696–706.

99. Delmas PD, Balena R, Confravreux E, et al. Bisphosphonate risedronate prevents bone loss in women with artificial menopause due to chemotherapy of breast cancer: a double-blind, placebo-controlled study. *J Clin Oncol* 1997;15:955–962.

100. Draper MW, Flowers DE, Huster WJ, et al. A controlled trial of raloxifene (LY139481) HCl: impact on bone turnover and serum lipid profile in healthy postmenopausal women. *J Bone Miner Res* 1996;11:835–842.

101. Anzano MA, Peer CW, Smith JM, et al. Chemoprevention of mammary carcinogenesis in the rat: combined use of raloxifene and 9-cis-retinoic acid. *J Natl Cancer Inst* 1996;88:123–125.

102. Gottardis MM, Jordan VC. Antitumor actions of keoxifene and tamoxifen in the N-nitrosomethylurea-induced rat mammary carcinoma model. *Cancer Res* 1987;47:4020–4024.

103. Black LJ, Jones CD, Falcone JF. Antagonism of estrogen action with a new benzothiophene derived antiestrogen. *Life Sci* 1983;32:1031–1036.

104. Allerheiligen S, Geiser J, Knadler M. Raloxifen (RAL) pharmacokinetics and the associated endocrine effects in premenopausal women treated during the follicular, ovulatory, and luteal phases of the menstrual cycle. *Pharmaceut Res* 1996;13:S430.

105. Forgue ST, Rudy AC, Knadler MP. Raloxifene pharmacokinetics in healthy postmenopausal women. *Pharmaceut Res* 1996;13:S430.

106. Ni L, Allerheiligen S, Basson R. Pharacokinetics of raloxifene in men and postmenopausal women volunteers. *Pharmaceut Res* 1996;13:S430.

107. Kemp DC, Fan PW, Stevens JC. Characterization of raloxifene glucuronidation in vitro: contribution of intestinal metabolism to presystemic clearance. *Drug Metab Dispos* 2002;30:694–700.

108. Coopman P, Garcia M, Brunner N, et al. Anti-proliferative and anti-estrogenic effects of ICI 164,384 and ICI 182,780 in 4-OH-tamoxifen-resistant human breast-cancer cells. *Int J Cancer* 1994;56:295–300.

109. Howell A, DeFriend DJ, Robertson JF, et al. Pharmacokinetics, pharmacological and anti-tumour effects of the specific anti-oestrogen ICI 182780 in women with advanced breast cancer. *Br J Cancer* 1996;74:300–308.

110. Howell A, Osborne CK, Morris C, et al. ICI 182,780 (Faslodex): development of a novel, "pure" antiestrogen. *Cancer* 2000;89:817–825.

111. Robertson JF, Odling-Smee W, Holcombe C, et al. Pharmacokinetics of a single dose of fulvestrant prolonged-release intramuscular injection in postmenopausal women awaiting surgery for primary breast cancer. *Clin Ther* 2003;25:1440–1452.

112. Piccart M, Parker LM, Pritchard KI. Oestrogen receptor downregulation: an opportunity for extending the window of endocrine therapy in advanced breast cancer. *Ann Oncol* 2003;14:1017–1025.

113. Wakeling AE, Bowler J. Steroidal pure antioestrogens. *J Endocrinol* 1987;112:R7–R10.

114. Wakeling AE, Dukes M, Bowler J. A potent specific pure antiestrogen with clinical potential. *Cancer Res* 1991;51:3867–3873.

115. Howell A, Robertson JF, Quaresma Albano J, et al. Fulvestrant, formerly ICI 182,780, is as effective as anastrozole in postmenopausal women with advanced breast cancer progressing after prior endocrine treatment. *J Clin Oncol* 2002;20:3396–3403.

116. Osborne CK, Pippen J, Jones SE, et al. Double-blind, randomized trial comparing the efficacy and tolerability of fulvestrant versus anastrozole in postmenopausal women with advanced breast cancer progressing on prior endocrine therapy: results of a North American trial. *J Clin Oncol* 2002;20:3386–3395.

117. Howell A, Robertson JF, Abram P, et al. Comparison of fulvestrant versus tamoxifen for the treatment of advanced breast cancer in postmenopausal women previously untreated with endocrine therapy: a multinational, double-blind, randomized trial. *J Clin Oncol* 2004;22:1605–1613.

118. Leo AD, Jerusalem G, Petruzelka L, et al. Final overall survival: fulvestrant 500 mg vs 250 mg in the randomized CONFIRM trial. *J Natl Cancer Inst* 2014;106:djt337.

119. McCormack P, Sapunar F. Pharmacokinetic profile of the fulvestrant loading dose regimen in postmenopausal women with hormone receptor-positive advanced breast cancer. *Clin Breast Cancer* 2008;8:347–351.

120. Schteingart DE, Cash R, Conn JW. Amino-glutethimide and metastatic adrenal cancer. Maintained reversal (six months) of Cushing's syndrome. *JAMA* 1996;198:1007–1010.

121. Ma CX, Adjei AA, Salavaggione OE, et al. Human aromatase: gene resequencing and functional genomics. *Cancer Res* 2005;65:11071–11082.

122. Colomer R, Monzo M, Tusquets I, et al. A single-nucleotide polymorphism in the aromatase gene is associated with the efficacy of the aromatase inhibitor letrozole in advanced breast carcinoma. *Clin Cancer Res* 2008;14:811–816.

123. Wang L, Ellsworth KA, Moon I, et al. Functional genetic polymorphisms in the aromatase gene CYP19 vary the response of breast cancer patients to neoadjuvant therapy with aromatase inhibitors. *Cancer Res* 2010;70:319–328.

124. Goss PE, Ingle JN, Martino S, et al. A randomized trial of letrozole in postmenopausal women after five years of tamoxifen therapy for early-stage breast cancer. *N Engl J Med* 2003;349:1793–1802.

125. Mouridsen H, Gershanovich M, Sun Y, et al. Phase III study of letrozole versus tamoxifen as first-line therapy of advanced breast cancer in postmenopausal women: analysis of survival and update of efficacy from the International Letrozole Breast Cancer Group. *J Clin Oncol* 2003;21:2101–2109.

126. Howell A, Cuzick J, Baum M, et al. Results of the ATAC (Arimidex, Tamoxifen, Alone or in Combination) trial after completion of 5 years' adjuvant treatment for breast cancer. *Lancet* 2005;365:60–62.

127. Thurlimann B, Keshaviah A, Coates AS, et al. A comparison of letrozole and tamoxifen in postmenopausal women with early breast cancer. *N Engl J Med* 2005;353:2747–2757.

128. Jakesz R, Jonat W, Gnant M, et al. Switching of postmenopausal women with endocrine-responsive early breast cancer to anastrozole after 2 years' adjuvant tamoxifen: combined results of ABCSG trial 8 and ARNO 95 trial. *Lancet* 2005;366:455–462.

129. Cuzick J, Sestak I, Forbes JF, et al. Anastrozole for prevention of breast cancer in high-risk postmenopausal women (IBIS-II): an international, double-blind, randomised placebo-controlled trial. *Lancet* 2014;383:1041–1048.

130. Baum M, Budzar AU, Cuzick J, et al. Anastrozole alone or in combination with tamoxifen versus tamoxifen alone for adjuvant treatment of postmenopausal women with early breast cancer: first results of the ATAC randomised trial. *Lancet* 2002;359:2131–2139.

131. Amir E, Seruga B, Nira S, et al. Toxicity of adjuvant endocrine therapy in postmenopausal breast cancer patients: a systematic review and meta-analysis. *J Natl Cancer Inst* 2011;103:1299–1309.

132. Plourde PV, Dyroff M, Dukes M. Arimidex: a potent and selective fourth-generation aromatase inhibitor. *Breast Cancer Res Treat* 1994;30:103–111.

133. Bisagni G, Cocconi G, Scaglione F, et al. Letrozole, a new oral non-steroidal aromatase inhibitor in treating postmenopausal patients with advanced breast cancer. A pilot study. *Ann Oncol* 1996;7:99–102.

134. Buzdar AU. Pharmacology and pharmacokinetics of the newer generation aromatase inhibitors. *Clin Cancer Res* 2003;9:468S–472S.

135. Dewar JA, Nabholtz JM, Bonneterre J, et al. The effect of anastrozole (Arimidex) on serum lipids: data from a randomized comparison of anastrozole (AN) versus tamoxifen (TAM) in postmenopausal (PM) women with advanced breast cancer (ABC). *Breast Cancer Res Treat* 2000;64:51.

136. Elisaf MS, Bairaktari ET, Nicolaides C, et al. Effect of letrozole on the lipid profile in postmenopausal women with breast cancer. *Eur J Cancer* 2001;37:1510–1513.

137. Bhatnagar AS, Hausler A, Schieweck K. Inhibition of aromatase in vitro and in vivo by aromatase inhibitors. *J Enzyme Inhib* 1990;4:179–186.

138. Bhatnagar AS, Hausler A, Schieweck K, et al. Highly selective inhibition of estrogen biosynthesis by CGS 20267, a new non-steroidal aromatase inhibitor. *J Steroid Biochem Mol Biol* 1990;37:1021–1027.

139. Demers LM. Effects of Fadrozole (CGS 16949A) and Letrozole (CGS 20267) on the inhibition of aromatase activity in breast cancer patients. *Breast Cancer Res Treat* 1994;30:95–102.

140. Lipton A, Demers LM, Harvey HA, et al. Letrozole (CGS 20267). A phase I study of a new potent oral aromatase inhibitor of breast cancer. *Cancer* 1995;75:2132–2138.

141. Iveson TJ, Smith IE, Ahern J, et al. Phase I study of the oral nonsteroidal aromatase inhibitor CGS 20267 in postmenopausal patients with advanced breast cancer. *Cancer Res* 1993;53:266–270.

142. Trunet PF, Muller PH, Bhatnagar A. Phase I study in healthy male volunteers with the non-steroidal aromatase inhibitor GCS 20267. *Eur J Cancer* 1990;26:173.

143. Dukes M, Edwards PN, Large M, et al. The preclinical pharmacology of "Arimidex" (anastrozole; ZD1033)—a potent, selective aromatase inhibitor. *J Steroid Biochem Mol Biol* 1996;58:439–445.

144. Yates RA, Dowsett M, Fisher GV, et al. Arimidex (ZD1033): a selective, potent inhibitor of aromatase in postmenopausal female volunteers. *Br J Cancer* 1996;73:543–548.

145. Lonning PE, Geisler J, Dowsett M. Pharmacological and clinical profile of anastrozole. *Breast Cancer Res Treat* 1998;49:S53–S57.

146. Geisler J, King N, Dowsett M, et al. Influence of anastrozole (Arimidex), a selective, non-steroidal aromatase inhibitor, on in vivo aromatisation and plasma oestrogen levels in postmenopausal women with breast cancer. *Br J Cancer* 1996;74:1286–1291.

147. Ingle JN, Buzdar AU, Schaid DJ, et al. Variation in anastrozole metabolism and pharmacodynamics in women with early breast cancer. *Cancer Res* 2010;70:3278–3286.

148. Kaufmann M, Bajetta E, Dirix LY, et al. Exemestane is superior to megestrol acetate after tamoxifen failure in postmenopausal women with advanced breast cancer: results of a phase III randomized double-blind trial. The Exemestane Study Group. *J Clin Oncol* 2000;18:1399–1411.

149. Goss PE, Ingle JN, Pritchard KI, et al. Exemestane versus anastrozole in postmenopausal women with early breast cancer: NCIC CTG MA.27—a randomized controlled phase III trial. *J Clin Oncol* 2013;31:1398–1404.

150. Goss PE, Ingle JN, Ales-Martinez JE, et al. Exemestane for breast-cancer prevention in postmenopausal women. *N Engl J Med* 2011;364:2381–2391.

151. Goss PE, Grynpas M, Qi S, et al. The effects of exemestane on bone and lipids in the ovariectomized rat. *Breast Cancer Res Treat* 2001;69:224.

152. Evans TR, Di Salle E, Ornati G, et al. Phase I and endocrine study of exemestane (FCE 24304), a new aromatase inhibitor, in postmenopausal women. *Cancer Res* 1992;52:5933–5939.

153. Bajetta E, Zilembo N, Noberasco C, et al. The minimal effective exemestane dose for endocrine activity in advanced breast cancer. *Eur J Cancer* 1997;33:587–591.

154. Michaud LB, Buzdar AU. Risks and benefits of aromatase inhibitors in postmenopausal breast cancer. *Drug Saf* 1999;21:297–309.

155. Coombes RC, Hall E, Gibson LJ, et al. A randomized trial of exemestane after two to three years of tamoxifen therapy in postmenopausal women with primary breast cancer. *N Engl J Med* 2004;350:1081–1092.

156. Demers LM, Lipton A, Harvey HA. The efficacy of CGS 20267 in suppressing estrogen biosynthesis in patients with advanced stage breast cancer. *J Steroid Biochem Mol Biol* 1993;44:687–691.

157. Spinelli R, Jannuzzo MG, Poggesi I, et al. Pharmacokinetics (PK) of Aromasin (Exemestane, EXE) after single and repeated doses in healthy postmenopausal volunteers (HPV). *Eur J Cancer* 1999;35:S295.

158. Buzdar A, Howell A. Advances in aromatase inhibition: clinical efficacy and tolerability in the treatment of breast cancer. *Clin Cancer Res* 2001;7:2620–2635.

159. Johannessen DC, Engan T, Di Salle E, et al. Endocrine and clinical effects of exemestane (PNU 155971), a novel steroidal aromatase inhibitor, in postmenopausal breast cancer patients: a phase I study. *Clin Cancer Res* 1997;3:1101–1108.

160. Jones S, Vogel C, Arkhipov A, et al. Multicenter, phase II trial of exemestane as third-line hormonal therapy of postmenopausal women with metastatic breast cancer. Aromasin Study Group. *J Clin Oncol* 1999;17:3418–3425.

161. Ahmann FR, Citrin DL, deHaan HA, et al. Zoladex: a sustained-release, monthly luteinizing hormone-releasing hormone analogue for the treatment of advanced prostate cancer. *J Clin Oncol* 1987;5:912–917.

162. Corbin A. From contraception to cancer: a review of the therapeutic applications of LHRH analogues as antitumor agents. *Yale J Biol Med* 1982;55:27–47.

163. Kaufmann M, Jonat W, Blamey R, et al. Survival analyses from the ZEBRA study. Goserelin (Zoladex) versus CMF in premenopausal women with node-positive breast cancer. *Eur J Cancer* 2003;39:1711–1717.

164. Harvey HA, Lipton A, Max DT, et al. Medical castration produced by the GnRH analogue leuprolide to treat metastatic breast cancer. *J Clin Oncol* 1985;3:1068–1072.

165. Abrahamsson PA. Potential benefits of intermittent androgen suppression therapy in the treatment of prostate cancer: a systematic review of the literature. *Eur Urol* 2010;57:49–59.

166. Hussain M, Tangen CM, Berry DL, et al. Intermittent versus continuous androgen deprivation in prostate cancer. *N Engl J Med* 2013;368:1314–1325.

167. Brogden RN, Faulds D. Goserelin. A review of its pharmacodynamic and pharmacokinetic properties and therapeutic efficacy in prostate cancer. *Drugs Aging* 1995;6:324–343.

168. Vogelzang NJ, Chodak GW, Soloway MS, et al. Goserelin versus orchiectomy in the treatment of advanced prostate cancer: final results of a randomized trial. Zoladex Prostate Study Group. *Urology* 1995;46:220–226.

169. Plosker GL, Brogden RN. Leuprorelin. A review of its pharmacology and therapeutic use in prostatic cancer, endometriosis and other sex hormone-related disorders. *Drugs* 1994;48:930–967.

170. Nillius SJ. *The Therapeutic Uses of Gonadotropin-Releasing Hormone and Its Analogues*. London: Butterworth; 1981.

171. Klijn JG, DeJong FH, Blankenstein MA. Anti-tumor and endocrine effects of chronic LHRH agonist treatment (buserelin) with or without tamoxifen in premenopausal metastatic breast cancer. *Breast Cancer Res Treat* 1984;4:209.

172. Clayton RN, Bailey LC, Cottam J, et al. A radioimmunoassay for GnRH agonist analogue in serum of patients with prostate cancer treated with D-Ser (tBu)6 AZA Gly10 GnRH. *Clin Endocrinol (Oxf)* 1985;22:453–462.

173. Chrisp P, Goa KL. Goserelin. A review of its pharmacodynamic and pharmacokinetic properties, and clinical use in sex hormone-related conditions. *Drugs* 1991;41:254–288.

174. Samant MP, Hong DJ, Croston G, et al. Novel gonadotropin-releasing hormone antagonists with substitutions at position 5. *Biopolymers* 2005;80:386–391.

175. Van Poppel H, Tombal B, de la Rosette JJ, et al. Degarelix: a novel gonadotropin-releasing hormone (GnRH) receptor blocker—results from a 1-yr, multicentre, randomised, phase 2 dosage-finding study in the treatment of prostate cancer. *Eur Urol* 2008;54:805–813.

176. Klotz L, Boccon-Gibod L, Shore ND, et al. The efficacy and safety of degarelix: a 12-month, comparative, randomized, open-label, parallel-group phase III study in patients with prostate cancer. *BJU Int* 2008;102:1531–1538.

177. Steinberg M. Degarelix: a gonadotropin-releasing hormone antagonist for the management of prostate cancer. *Clin Ther* 2009;31:2312–2331.

178. Brogden RN, Clissold SP. Flutamide. A preliminary review of its pharmacodynamic and pharmacokinetic properties, and therapeutic efficacy in advanced prostatic cancer. *Drugs* 1989;38:185–203.

179. Wysowski DK, Freiman JP, Tourtelot JB, et al. Fatal and nonfatal hepatotoxicity associated with flutamide. *Ann Intern Med* 1993;118:860–864.

180. Brogden RN, Chrisp P. Flutamide. A review of its pharmacodynamic and pharmacokinetic properties, and therapeutic use in advanced prostatic cancer. *Drugs Aging* 1991;1:104–115.

181. Radwanski E, Perentesis G, Symchowicz S, et al. Single and multiple dose pharmacokinetic evaluation of flutamide in normal geriatric volunteers. *J Clin Pharmacol* 1989;29:554–558.

182. Schellhammer PF, Sharifi R, Block NL, et al. A controlled trial of bicalutamide versus flutamide, each in combination with luteinizing hormone-releasing hormone analogue therapy, in patients with advanced prostate carcinoma. Analysis of time to progression. CASODEX Combination Study Group. *Cancer* 1996;78:2164–2169.

183. Furr BJ. Casodex (ICI 176,334)—a new, pure, peripherally-selective anti-androgen: preclinical studies. *Horm Res* 1989;32:69.

184. Furr BJ. Casodex: preclinical studies. *Eur Urol* 1990;18:2.

185. Kennealey GT, Furr BJ. Use of the nonsteroidal anti-androgen Casodex in advanced prostatic carcinoma. *Urol Clin North Am* 1991;18:99–110.

186. Attard G, Reid AH, A'Hern R, et al. Selective inhibition of CYP17 with abiraterone acetate is highly active in the treatment of castration-resistant prostate cancer. *J Clin Oncol* 2009;27:3742–3748.

187. Tran C, Ouk S, Clegg NJ, et al. Development of a second-generation antiandrogen for treatment of advanced prostate cancer. *Science* 2009;324:787–790.

188. Scher HI, Fizazi K, Saad F, et al. Increased survival with enzalutamide in prostate cancer after chemotherapy. *N Engl J Med* 2012;367:1187–1197.

189. Zhu H, Garcia JA. Targeting the adrenal gland in castration-resistant prostate cancer: a case for orteronel, a selective CYP-17 17,20-lyase inhibitor. *Curr Oncol Rep* 2013;15:105–112.

190. Kennedy BJ. Hormonal therapies in breast cancer. *Semin Oncol* 1974;1:119–130.

191. Colburn WA. Radioimmunoassay for fluoxymesterone (Halotestin). *Steroids* 1975;25:43–52.

192. Kammerer RC, Merdink JL, Jagels M, et al. Testing for fluoxymesterone (Halotestin) administration to man: identification of urinary metabolites by gas chromatography-mass spectrometry. *J Steroid Biochem* 1990;36:659–666.

193. Ingle JN, Ahmann DL, Green SJ, et al. Randomized clinical trial of diethylstilbestrol versus tamoxifen in postmenopausal women with advanced breast cancer. *N Engl J Med* 1981;304:16–21.

194. Stewart HJ, Forrest AP, Gunn JM, et al. The tamoxifen trial - a double-blind comparison with stilboestrol in postmenopausal women with advanced breast cancer. *Eur J Cancer* 1980;Suppl 1:83–88.

195. Byar DP. Proceedings: The Veterans Administration Cooperative Urological Research Group's studies of cancer of the prostate. *Cancer* 1973;32:1126–1130.

196. Loose-Mitchell DS, Stancel GM. *Estrogens and Progestins*. 10 ed. New York: McGraw-Hill; 2001.

197. Bonomi P, Pessis D, Bunting N, et al. Megestrol acetate used as primary hormonal therapy in stage D prostatic cancer. *Semin Oncol* 1985;12:36–39.

198. Bruera E, Macmillan K, Kuehn N, et al. A controlled trial of megestrol acetate on appetite, caloric intake, nutritional status, and other symptoms in patients with advanced cancer. *Cancer* 1990;66:1279–1282.

199. Feliu J, Gonzalez-Baron M, Berrocal A, et al. Usefulness of megestrol acetate in cancer cachexia and anorexia. A placebo-controlled study. *Am J Clin Oncol* 1992;15:436–440.

200. Loprinzi CL, Ellison NM, Schaid DJ, et al. Controlled trial of megestrol acetate for the treatment of cancer anorexia and cachexia. *J Natl Cancer Inst* 1990;82:1127–1132.

201. Tchekmedyian NS, Hickman M, Siau J, et al. Megestrol acetate in cancer anorexia and weight loss. *Cancer* 1992;69:1268–1274.

202. Loprinzi CL, Michalak JC, Schaid DJ, et al. Phase III evaluation of four doses of megestrol acetate as therapy for patients with cancer anorexia and/or cachexia. *J Clin Oncol* 1993;11:762–767.

203. Loprinzi CL, Jensen MD, Jiang NS, et al. Effect of megestrol acetate on the human pituitary-adrenal axis. *Mayo Clin Proc* 1992;67:1160–1162.

204. Leinung MC, Liporace R, Miller CH. Induction of adrenal suppression by megestrol acetate in patients with AIDS. *Ann Intern Med* 1995;122:843–845.

205. Rowland KM Jr., Loprinzi CL, Shaw EG, et al. Randomized double-blind placebo-controlled trial of cisplatin and etoposide plus megestrol acetate/placebo in extensive-stage small-cell lung cancer: a North Central Cancer Treatment Group study. *J Clin Oncol* 1996;14:135–141.

206. Loprinzi CL, Johnson PA, Jensen M. Megestrol acetate for anorexia and cachexia. *Oncology* 1992;49:46–49.

207. Von Roenn JH, Armstrong D, Kotler DP, et al. Megestrol acetate in patients with AIDS-related cachexia. *Ann Intern Med* 1994;121:393–399.

208. Alexieva-Figusch J, Blankenstein MA, Hop WC, et al. Treatment of metastatic breast cancer patients with different dosages of megestrol acetate; dose relations, metabolic and endocrine effects. *Eur J Cancer Clin Oncol* 1984;20:33–40.

209. Tseng L, Gurpide E. Effects of progestins on estradiol receptor levels in human endometrium. *J Clin Endocrinol Metab* 1975;41:402–404.

210. Gurpide E, Tseng L, Gusberg SB. Estrogen metabolism in normal and neoplastic endometrium. *Am J Obstet Gynecol* 1977;129:809–816.

211. Gordon GG, Altman K, Southren AL, et al. Human hepatic testosterone A-ring reductase activity: effect of medroxyprogesterone acetate. *J Clin Endocrinol Metab* 1971;32:457–461.

212. Allegra JC, Kiefer SM. Mechanisms of action of progestational agents. *Semin Oncol* 1985;12:3–5.

213. Ewing TM, Murphy LJ, Ng ML, et al. Regulation of epidermal growth factor receptor by progestins and glucocorticoids in human breast cancer cell lines. *Int J Cancer* 1989;44:744–752.

214. Adlercreutz H, Eriksen PB, Christensen MS. Plasma concentration of megestrol acetate and medroxyprogesterone acetate after single oral administration to healthy subjects. *J Pharm Biomed Anal* 1983;1:153.

215. Martin F, Adlercreutz H, eds. *Aspects of Megestrol Acetate and Medroxyprogesterone Acetate Metabolism*. New York: Raven Press; 1977.

216. Gaver RC, Pittman KA, Reilly CM, et al. Bioequivalence evaluation of new megestrol acetate formulations in humans. *Semin Oncol* 1985;12:17–19.

217. Fotherby K, Kamyab S, Littleton P. Metabolism of synthetic progestational compounds in humans. *J Reprod Fertil* 1968;5:51–61.

218. Fukushima DK, Ievin J, Liang JS, et al. Isolation and partial synthesis of a new metabolite of medroxyrogesterone acetate. *Steroids* 1979;34: 57–72.

219. Utaaker E, Lundgren S, Kvinnsland S, et al. Pharmacokinetics and metabolism of medroxyprogesterone acetate in patients with advanced breast cancer. *J Steroid Biochem* 1988;31:437–441.

220. Sturm G, Haberlein H, Bauer T, et al. Mass spectrometric and high-performance liquid chromatographic studies of medroxyprogesterone acetate metabolites in human plasma. *J Chromatogr* 1991;562:351–362.

221. Pannuti F, Camaggi CM, Strocchi E, eds. *Medroxyprogesterone Acetate Pharmacokinetics*. New York: Raven Press; 1984.

222. Lundgren S, Lonning PE, Aakvaag A, et al. Influence of aminoglutethimide on the metabolism of medroxyprogesterone acetate and megestrol acetate in postmenopausal patients with advanced breast cancer. *Cancer Chemother Pharmacol* 1990;27:101–105.

223. Lundgren S, Kvinnsland S, Utaaker E, et al. Effect of oral high-dose progestins on the disposition of antipyrine, digitoxin, and warfarin in patients with advanced breast cancer. *Cancer Chemother Pharmacol* 1986;18:270–275.

224. Cascinu S, Fedeli A, Fedeli SL, et al. Control of chemotherapy-induced diarrhoea with octreotide in patients receiving 5-fluorouracil. *Eur J Cancer* 1992;28:482–483.

225. Cascinu S, Fedeli A, Fedeli SL, et al. Octreotide versus loperamide in the treatment of fluorouracil-induced diarrhea: a randomized trial. *J Clin Oncol* 1993;11:148–151.

226. Gebbia V, Carreca I, Testa A, et al. Subcutaneous octreotide versus oral loperamide in the treatment of diarrhea following chemotherapy. *Anticancer Drugs* 1993;4:443–445.

227. Harris AG. Somatostatin and somatostatin analogues: pharmacokinetics and pharmacodynamic effects. *Gut* 1994;35:S1–S4.

228. Chanson P, Timsit J, Harris AG. Clinical pharmacokinetics of octreotide. Therapeutic applications in patients with pituitary tumours. *Clin Pharmacokinet* 1993;25:375–391.

229. Marbach P, Briner U, Lemaire M. From somatostatin to Sandostatin: pharmacodynamics and pharmacokinetics. *Digestion* 1993;54:9–13.

230. Rubin J, Ajani J, Schirmer W, et al. Octreotide acetate long-acting formulation versus open-label subcutaneous octreotide acetate in malignant carcinoid syndrome. *J Clin Oncol* 1999;17:600–606.

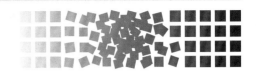

# 28  Antiangiogenesis Agents

Cindy H. Chau and William Douglas Figg, Sr.

## INTRODUCTION

Blood vessels are indispensable for tumor growth and metastasis, and the formation of a new network of blood vessels from the existing vasculature, termed *angiogenesis*, is one of the essential hallmarks of cancer development.[1] Indeed, it was over 70 years ago that the existence of tumor-derived factors responsible for promoting new vessel growth was postulated,[2] and that tumor growth is essentially dependent on vascular induction and the development of a neovascular supply.[3] By the late 1960s, Dr. Judah Folkman and colleagues[4] had begun the search for a tumor angiogenesis factor. In the 1971 landmark report, Folkman[5] proposed that inhibition of angiogenesis by means of holding tumors in a nonvascularized dormant state would be an effective strategy to treat human cancer, and hence laid the groundwork for the concept behind the development of *antiangiogenesis* agents. This fostered the search for angiogenic factors, regulators of angiogenesis, and antiangiogenic molecules over the next few decades and shed light on angiogenesis as an important therapeutic target for the treatment of cancer and other diseases.

A decade has passed since the regulatory approval of the first antiangiogenic drug bevacizumab, and while initial results were regarded as highly promising, clinical evidence indicated that antiangiogenic therapy also had limitations. Successful development and clinical translation of this novel class of agents depends on the complete understanding of the biology of angiogenesis and the regulatory proteins that govern this angiogenic process, topics that have been covered in greater detail in another section of this textbook. This chapter will briefly review the mechanisms underlying tumor angiogenesis followed by an in-depth discussion of antiangiogenic therapy, the modes of action of angiogenesis inhibitors, and the successes and challenges of this treatment modality.

## UNDERSTANDING THE ANGIOGENIC PROCESS

### Angiogenic Switch and Regulatory Proteins

Tumor development and progression depend on angiogenesis. Recruitment of new blood vessels to the tumor site is required for the delivery of nutrients and oxygen to the cancerous growths and for the removal of waste products.[6] Cancer cells promote angiogenesis at an early stage of tumorigenesis, beginning with the release of molecules that send signals to the surrounding normal host tissue and stimulate the migration of microvascular endothelial cells (EC) in the direction of the angiogenic stimulus. These angiogenic factors not only mediate EC migration, but also EC proliferation and microvessel formation in tumors undergoing the switch to the angiogenic phenotype.[7] Experimental evidence for this *angiogenic switch* was observed when hyperplastic islets in transgenic mice (RIP-Tag model) switch from small (<1 mm), white microscopic dormant tumors to red, rapidly growing tumors.[7] Dormant tumors have been discovered during autopsies of individuals who died of causes other than cancer.[8] These autopsy studies suggest that the vast majority of microscopic in situ cancers never switch to the angiogenic phenotype during a normal lifetime. Such incipient tumors are usually not neovascularized and can remain harmless to the host for long periods of time as microscopic lesions that are in a state of dormancy.[9,10] These nonangiogenic tumors cannot expand beyond the initial microscopic size and cannot become clinically detectable, lethal tumors until they have switched to the angiogenic phenotype[11-13] through neovascularization and/or blood vessel cooption.[14] Depending on the tumor type and the environment, this switch can occur at different stages of the tumor progression pathway and ultimately depends on a net balance of positive and negative regulators. Thus, the angiogenic phenotype may result from the production of growth factors by tumor cells and/or the downregulation of negative modulators.

Changes in this angiogenic balance affecting the levels of activator and inhibitor molecules dictate whether an EC will be in a quiescent or an angiogenic state. Normally, the inhibitors predominate, thereby blocking growth. Once the balance shifts in favor of the angiogenic state, proangiogenic factors prompts the activation, growth, and division of vascular ECs, resulting in the formation of new blood vessels. Activated ECs produce and release matrix metalloproteinases (MMP) into the surrounding tissue to break down the extracellular matrix to allow the ECs to migrate and organize themselves into hollow tubes that eventually evolve into a mature network of blood vessels. Proangiogenic factors or positive regulators of angiogenesis include vascular endothelial growth factor (VEGF), basic fibroblast growth factor (PlGF), platelet-derived growth factor (PDGF), placental growth factor, transforming growth factor-β, pleiotrophins, and others.[15] Activation of the hypoxia-inducible factor 1 (HIF-1) via tumor-associated hypoxic conditions is also involved in the upregulation of several angiogenic factors.[16] The angiogenic switch also involves the downregulation of angiogenesis suppressor proteins, which include endostatin, angiostatin, thrombospondin, and others.[17,18] Most notably, however, is the link between many oncogenes and angiogenesis and the significant role oncogenes play in driving the angiogenic switch.[19,20] These proangiogenic oncogenes not only induce the expression of stimulators, but may also downregulate inhibitors of angiogenesis.[21]

### Endogenous Inhibitors of Angiogenesis

The infrequency of microscopic in situ tumors that actually undergo the angiogenic switch (<1%) suggests that naturally occurring endogenous inhibitors exist in the body to defend against the angiogenic switch in pathologic conditions and to limit physiologic angiogenesis.[9] These circulating endogenous inhibitors could also prevent microscopic metastases from growing into visible tumors. Early studies by Langer et al.[22,23] demonstrated the possible existence of such inhibitors through the extraction of a functional inhibitor from cartilage, a tissue that is poorly vascularized. Since then, dozens of endogenous angiogenesis inhibitors have been identified, some of which are listed in Table 28.1.[17,18,24] Many of the endogenous inhibitors of angiogenesis that have been discovered to date are proteolytically cleaved fragments of larger proteins that are members of either the clotting/coagulation system

TABLE 28.1

**Examples of Endogenous Inhibitors of Angiogenesis**

Alphastatin

Angiostatin

Antithrombin III (cleaved)

Arrestin

Canstatin

Endostatin

Interferon alpha/beta (IFN-α/β)

2-Methoxyestradiol (2-ME)

Pigment epithelial-derived factor (PEDF)

Platelet factor 4 (PF-4)

Tetrahydrocortisol-S

Thrombospondin 1

Tissue inhibitor of metalloproteinase 2 (TIMP-2)

Tumstatin

Vasohibin

or members of the extracellular matrix family of glycoproteins. Endostatin is the most well-studied endogenous angiogenesis inhibitor.[25,26] Other potent endogenous angiogenesis inhibitors include thrombospondin-1[27] and tumstatin.[28] The discovery of vasohibin, an endogenous inhibitor that is selectively induced in ECs by proangiogenic stimulatory growth factors such as VEGF, demonstrated the existence of an intrinsic and EC-specific feedback inhibitor control mechanism,[29,30] whereas most endogenous inhibitors of angiogenesis are extrinsic to ECs. More recently, a second endothelium-produced negative regulator of angiogenesis has been discovered, the Dll4-Notch signaling system.[31,32] Both intrinsic factors have since been shown to control tumor angiogenesis by an autoregulatory or negative-feedback mechanism. The Dll4-Notch axis has emerged as a critical regulator of tumor angiogenesis, and inhibitors of this pathway (e.g., demcizumab, the anti-Dll4 monoclonal antibody) are currently being investigated in early phase trials of solid tumors.[33]

Perhaps the most compelling genetic evidence that endogenous inhibitors suppress pathologic angiogenesis was observed in studies using mice deficient in tumstatin, endostatin, or thrombospondin 1 (TSP-1).[34] These experiments demonstrate that normal physiologic levels of the inhibitors can retard the tumor growth and that their absence leads to enhanced angiogenesis and increased tumor growth by two- to threefold, strongly suggesting that endogenous inhibitors of angiogenesis can act as endothelium-specific tumor suppressors. The connection between a tumor suppressor protein and angiogenesis is best illustrated by the classic tumor suppressor p53. p53 inhibits angiogenesis by increasing the expression of TSP-1[35] by repressing VEGF[36] and basic fibroblast growth factor–binding protein,[37] and by degrading HIF-1,[38] which blocks the downstream induction of VEGF expression. New evidence suggests that p53 also indirectly downregulates VEGF expression via the retinoblastoma pathway in a p21-dependent manner during sustained hypoxia.[39] Furthermore, p53-mediated inhibition of angiogenesis may also occur in part via the antiangiogenic activity of endostatin and tumstatin.[40] This landmark finding clearly demonstrates that p53 not only controls cell proliferation, but can also repress tumor angiogenesis through enzymatic mobilization of these endogenous angiogenesis inhibitor proteins to prevent ECs from being recruited into the dormant, microscopic tumors, thereby preventing the switch to the angiogenic phenotype.[41] The discovery that these endogenous angiogenesis inhibitors can suppress the growth of primary tumors

raises the possibility that such inhibitors might also be able to slow tumor metastasis. Indeed, the inhibition of angiogenesis by angiostatin significantly reduced the rate of metastatic spread.

## DRUG DEVELOPMENT OF ANGIOGENESIS INHIBITORS

The first angiogenesis inhibitor was reported in 1980 and involved the low-dose administration of interferon α (IFN-α).[42–44] Over the next decade, several compounds were discovered to have potent antiangiogenic activity, including protamine and platelet factor 4,[45] trahydrocortisol,[46] and the fumagillin analog TNP-470.[47] The proof of concept that targeting angiogenesis is an effective strategy for treating cancer came with the approval of the first angiogenesis inhibitor, bevacizumab, by the U.S. Food and Drug Administration (FDA). Since then, several antiangiogenic agents have received FDA approval for cancer treatment (Table 28.2), and three additional agents (pegaptanib, ranibizumab, and aflibercept) are approved for the treatment of wet age-related macular degeneration.

### Rationale for Antiangiogenic Therapy

Antiangiogenic therapy stems from the fundamental concept that tumor growth, invasion, and metastasis are angiogenesis dependent; thus, blocking blood vessel recruitment to starve primary and metastatic tumors is a rational approach. The microvascular EC recruited by a tumor has become an important second target in cancer therapy. Unlike the cancer cell (the primary target of cytotoxic chemotherapy), which is genetically unstable with unpredictable mutations, the genetic stability of ECs may make them less susceptible to acquired drug resistance.[48] Moreover, ECs in the microvascular bed of a tumor may support 50 to 100 tumor cells. Coupling this amplification potential together with the lower toxicity of most angiogenesis inhibitors results in the use of antiangiogenic therapy, which should be significantly less toxic than conventional chemotherapy. However, the variable responses of antiangiogenic therapy observed in different tumor types and the fact that angiogenesis inhibitors have not delivered the benefits initially envisaged suggest that the precise mechanism of action of angiogenesis inhibitors is complex and remains incompletely understood.

### Modes of Action of Antiangiogenic Agents

Various strategies for the development of antiangiogenic drugs have been investigated over the years, with these agents being classified into several different categories depending on their modes of action. Some inhibit ECs directly, whereas others inhibit the angiogenesis signaling cascade or block the ability of ECs to break down the extracellular matrix. Inhibitors may block one main angiogenic protein, two or three angiogenic proteins, or have a broad-spectrum effect by blocking a range of angiogenic regulators that can be located in both the tumor and ECs.[49] In some cases, the antiangiogenic activity is discovered as a secondary function after the drug has received regulatory approval for a different primary function. For example, bortezomib is a proteasome inhibitor that is approved for multiple myeloma and was later found to possess antiangiogenic activity via inhibiting VEGF. Some small-molecule drugs may display their antiangiogenic activity through inducing the expression of endogenous angiogenesis inhibitors such as celecoxib, a cyclooxygenase-2 (COX-2) inhibitor, which inhibits angiogenesis by increasing levels of endostatin.[25]

Some drugs possess antiangiogenic properties but with mechanisms that are not completely understood, such as thalidomide and its analogs, lenalidomide and pomalidomide, referred to as immunomodulatory drugs. Thalidomide was originally shown to inhibit angiogenesis by D'Amato et al.[50] in 1994 and this was subsequently confirmed in several different in vitro and ex vivo

**TABLE 28.2**

**Antiangiogenic Agents that Have Received U.S. Food and Drug Administration Approval for Cancer Treatment**

| Drug | Class | Mechanism (Cellular Targets) | Year of Approval | Indications | Dosages |
|---|---|---|---|---|---|
| Bevacizumab (Avastin) | Anti-VEGF mAB | VEGF | 2004 | First- and second-line metastatic CRC | 5 mg/kg IV q2wk + bolus IFL; 10 mg/kg IV q2wk + FOLFOX4 |
| | | | 2006 | First-line NSCLC | 15 mg/kg IV q3wk + carboplatin/paclitaxel |
| | | | 2009 | Second-line GBM | 10 mg/kg IV q2wk |
| | | | 2009 | Metastatic RCC | 10 mg/kg IV q2wk + IFN |
| | | | 2013 | Second-line metastatic CRC (after prior bevacizumab-containing regimen) | 5 mg/kg IV q2wk or 7.5 mg/kg IV q3wk + fluoropyrimidine–irinotecan or fluoropyrimidine-oxaliplatin–based regimen |
| Ziv-aflibercept (Zaltrap, VEGF Trap) | Anti-VEGF mAB | VEGFA, VEGFB, PIGF1, PIGF2 | 2012 | Metastatic CRC (after prior oxaliplatin-containing regimen) | 4 mg/kg IV q2wk (1-hr infusion) |
| Sorafenib (Nexavar, BAY439006) | Small-molecule TKI | VEGFR2, VEGFR3, PDGFR, FLT3, c-Kit | 2005 / 2007 / 2013 | Advanced RCC / Unresectable HCC / RAI-refractory DTC | 400 mg PO bid (w/o food) / 400 mg PO bid (w/o food) / 400 mg PO bid (w/o food) |
| Sunitinib (Sutent, SU11248) | Small-molecule TKI | VEGFR1, VEGFR2, VEGFR3, PDGFR, FLT3, c-Kit, RET | 2006 / 2006 / 2011 | Imatinib-resistant or -intolerant GIST / Advanced RCC / Advanced pNET | 50 mg PO qd, 4 wk on/2 wk off / 50 mg PO qd, 4 wk on/2 wk off / 37.5 mg PO qd |
| Pazopanib (Votrient) | Small-molecule TKI | VEGFR1, VEGFR2, VEGFR3, PDGFR, Itk, Lck, c-Fms | 2009 / 2012 | Advanced RCC / Advanced soft tissue sarcoma | 800 mg PO qd (w/o food) / 800 mg PO qd (w/o food) |
| Vandetanib (Caprelsa) | Small molecule TKI | RET, VEGFR, EGFR, BRK, TIE2 | 2011 | Advanced MTC | 300 mg PO qd |
| Axitinib (Inlyta) | Small molecule TKI | VEGFR1, VEGFR2, VEGFR3 | 2012 | Advanced RCC (after failure of prior therapy) | 5 mg PO bid |
| Cabozantinib (XL184, Cometriq) | Small molecule TKI | MET, VEGFR2, RET, KIT, AXL, FLT3 | 2012 | Progressive, metastatic MTC | 140 mg PO qd (w/o food) |
| Regorafenib (Stivarga) | Small molecule TKI | RET, VEGFR1, VEGFR2, VEGFR3, TIE2, KIT, PDGFR | 2012 / 2013 | Previously treated metastatic CRC / GIST | 160 mg PO qd × 21days (q28-day cycle) / 160 mg PO qd × days 1–21 (q28-day cycle) |
| Temsirolimus (Torisel) | mTOR inhibitor | mTOR | 2007 | Advanced RCC | 25 mg IV qwk (infused over 30–60 min) |
| Everolimus (Afinitor, RAD-001)[a] | mTOR inhibitor | mTOR | 2009 | Second-line advanced RCC (after VEGFR TKI failure) | 10 mg PO qd |
| | | | 2010 | SEGA associated w/TSC | 4.5 mg/m$^2$ PO qd |
| | | | 2011 | pNET | 10 mg PO qd |
| | | | 2012 | Advanced HR+, HER2- breast cancer | 10 mg PO qd |
| | | | 2012 | AML associated w/TSC | 10 mg PO qd |

[a] Afinitor Disperz (everolimus tablets for oral suspension) was approved in 2012 for children aged 1 and older who have SEGA + TSC.
mAB, monoclonal antibody; CRC, colorectal cancer; IV, intravenous; IFL, irinotecan, 5-fluorouracil, and leucovorin; FOLFOX4, 5-flourouracil, leucovorin, and oxaliplatin; NSCLC, non–small-cell lung cancer; GBM, glioblastoma multiforme; RCC, renal cell carcinoma; VEGFA, vascular endothelial growth factor A; PIGF, placental growth factor; TKI, tyrosine–kinase inhibitor; VEGFR, VEGF receptor; PDGFR, platelet-derived growth factor receptor; FLT, Fms-like tyrosine kinase; c-Kit, stem cell factor receptor; HCC, hepatocellular carcinoma; RAI, radioactive iodine; DTC, differentiated thyroid carcinoma; PO, orally; RET, glial cell line-derived neurotrophic factor receptor; pNET, pancreatic neuroendocrine tumor; GIST, gastrointestinal stromal tumor; qd, every day; Itk, interleukin-2 receptor inducible T-cell kinase; Lck, leukocyte-specific protein tyrosine kinase; c-Fms, transmembrane glycoprotein receptor tyrosine kinase; bid, twice daily; EGFR, epidermal growth factor receptor; BRK, protein tyrosine kinase 6; MTC, medullary thyroid cancer; mTOR, mammalian target of rapamycin; SEGA, subependymal giant cell astrocytoma; TSC, tuberous sclerosis complex; HR, hormone receptor; HER2, human epidermal growth factor receptor 2; AML, angiomyolipoma.

assays.[51–54] Interestingly, unlike other mechanisms of action, the antiangiogenic activity of thalidomide is believed to require enzymatic activation. The extent to which the antiangiogenic properties of thalidomide and its analogs play a role in its antimyeloma activity is not clearly understood. Several mechanisms have been proposed that involve the downregulation of cytokines in EC, the inhibition of EC proliferation, the decrease in the level of circulating ECs, or the modulation of adhesion molecules between the multiple myeloma cells and the endogenous bone marrow stromal cells, thereby decreasing the production of VEGF and interleukin 6 (IL-6).[55–59] The immunomodulatory agents are discussed in greater detail in another section of this textbook. Examples of the various types of angiogenesis inhibitors are highlighted in Table 28.3.

Drugs with antiangiogenic activity may be classified as either direct or indirect angiogenesis inhibitors. A direct angiogenesis inhibitor blocks vascular ECs from proliferating, migrating, or increasing their survival in response to proangiogenic proteins. They target the activated endothelium directly and inhibit multiple angiogenic proteins. Examples of direct angiogenesis inhibitors include many of the endogenous inhibitors of angiogenesis, such as endostatin, angiostatin, and TSP-1. Indirect angiogenesis inhibitors decrease or block expression of a tumor cell product, neutralize the tumor product itself, or block its receptor on ECs. The limitation to indirect inhibitors is that, over time, tumor cells may acquire mutations that lead to increased expression of other proangiogenic proteins that are not blocked by the indirect inhibitor. This may give the appearance of drug resistance and warrants the addition of a second antiangiogenic agent, one that would target the expression of these upregulated proangiogenic proteins. Examples of drugs that interfere with the angiogenesis-signaling pathway include the anti-VEGF monoclonal antibodies and small-molecule tyrosine–kinase inhibitors. These drugs target the major signaling pathways in tumor angiogenesis: VEGF, PDGF, and their respective receptors, as well as other growth factors and/or signaling pathways.

VEGF (also known as vascular permeability factor) is a potent proangiogenic growth factor and its expression is upregulated by most cancer cell types. It stimulates EC proliferation, migration, and survival as well as induces increased vascular permeability. The different forms of VEGF bind to transmembrane receptor tyrosine kinases (RTK) on ECs: VEGFR1 (Flt-1), VEGFR2 (KDR/Flk-1 or kinase insert domain receptor/fetal liver kinase 1), or VEGFR3 (Flt-4).[60] This results in receptor dimerization, activation, and autophosphorylation of the tyrosine–kinase domain, thereby triggering downstream signaling pathways. Other signaling molecules that may represent attractive therapeutic targets include PDGF and the angiopoietins (Ang1, Ang2). PDGF-B/PDGF receptor (R)-β plays an important role in the recruitment of pericytes and maturation of the microvasculature.[61] Ang2, which binds the Tie-2 receptor, is mostly expressed in tumor-induced neovasculature, whereby its selective inhibition results in reduced EC proliferation.[62] The angiopoietins are also involved in lymphangiogenesis, the formation of new lymphatic vessels, which plays a key role in tumor metastasis. An increased Ang2/Ang1 ratio correlates with tumor angiogenesis and poor prognosis in many cancers, thus making the angiopoietins an attractive therapeutic target. Angiopoietin inhibitors are currently under investigation in the preclinical and clinical setting.

Other strategies for targeting angiogenesis involve the tumor microenvironment. Breakdown of the extracellular matrix is required to allow ECs to migrate into surrounding tissues and proliferate into new blood vessels; thus, drugs that target MMPs, enzymes that catalyze the breakdown of the matrix, can also inhibit angiogenesis. However, clinical development of MMP inhibitors (MMPI) has yielded disappointing results.[63–66]

Integrins are cell surface adhesion molecules that play an essential role in cell–cell and cell–matrix adhesion as well as in transmitting signals important for cell migration, invasion, proliferation, and survival. The involvement of integrin in tumor angiogenesis was demonstrated in studies that show the β-4 subunit of integrin promoting endothelial migration and invasion.[67] Agents that target integrins (inhibitors of $\alpha_v\beta_3$ and $\alpha_v\beta_5$) have been evaluated as potential therapeutic options and include etaracizumab, cilengitide, and intetumumab. However, all three integrin inhibitors have proven to be largely ineffective in various early and late stage cancer trials.[68–73] In summary, the downstream effects of antiangiogenic agents, in addition to blocking angiogenesis, may involve inducing vessel regression, promoting sensitization to radiotherapy and chemotherapy by depriving ECs of VEGF's prosurvival signals, and inhibiting the recruitment of proangiogenic bone marrow–derived cells as well as reducing the self-renewal capability of cancer stem cells.[74]

## CLINICAL UTILITY OF APPROVED ANTIANGIOGENIC AGENTS IN CANCER THERAPY

The following section reviews the current FDA-approved angiogenesis inhibitors (Table 28.2). These agents include: (1) the monoclonal anti-VEGF antibodies (bevacizumab and ziv-aflibercept); (2) small-molecule tyrosine–kinase inhibitors (TKI) (sorafenib, sunitinib, pazopanib, vandetanib, axitinib, cabozantinib, and regorafenib); and (3) the mammalian target of rapamycin (mTOR) inhibitors (temsirolimus and everolimus), as examples of drugs that possess antiangiogenic activity. Other approved drugs that also inhibit angiogenesis as a secondary function, such as thalidomide, are discussed in greater detail in another section of this textbook and are presented in Table 28.3.

### Anti-VEGF Therapy

#### Bevacizumab

Bevacizumab is a recombinant humanized anti–VEGF-A monoclonal antibody that received FDA approval in February 2004 for use in combination therapy with fluorouracil-based regimens for

---

### TABLE 28.3

**Examples of Drugs that Possess Antiangiogenic Activity or Inhibit Angiogenesis as a Secondary Function**

| Drug | Class |
|------|-------|
| Cetuximab<br>Panitumumab<br>Trastuzumab | EGFR/HER monoclonal antibodies |
| Gefitinib<br>Erlotinib | EGFR small-molecule tyrosine–kinase receptor inhibitors |
| Everolimus<br>Temsirolimus | mTOR inhibitors |
| Thalidomide<br>Lenalidomide<br>Pomalidomide | Immunomodulatory agents |
| Belinostat (PXD101)<br>LBH589<br>Vorinostat (SAHA) | HDAC inhibitors |
| Celecoxib | COX-2 inhibitors |
| Bortezomib | Proteasome inhibitors |
| Zoledronic acid | Bisphosphonates |
| Rosiglitazone | PPAR-γ agonists |
| Doxycycline | Antibiotic |

EGFR, epidermal growth factor receptor; mTOR, mammalian target of rapamycin HDAC, histone deacetylase; COX-2, cyclooxygenase-2; PPAR, peroxisome proliferator–activated receptor.

metastatic colorectal cancer. Bevacizumab binds VEGF and prevents the interaction of VEGF to its receptors (Flt-1 and KDR) on the surface of ECs. It is the first antiangiogenic agent clinically proven to extend survival following a large, randomized, double-blind, phase III study in which bevacizumab was administered in combination with bolus irinotecan, 5-fluorouracil, and leucovorin (IFL) as first-line therapy for metastatic colorectal cancer (CRC).[75] In 2006, its approval extended to first- or second-line treatment of patients with metastatic carcinoma of the colon or rectum. This recommendation is based on the demonstration of a statistically significant improvement in overall survival (OS) in patients receiving bevacizumab plus FOLFOX4 (5-flourouracil, leucovorin, and oxaliplatin) when compared to those receiving FOLFOX4 alone. In January 2013, it was further approved to treat mCRC for second-line treatment when used with fluoropyrimidine-based (combined with irinotecan or oxaliplatin) chemotherapy after disease progression following a first-line treatment with a bevacizumab-containing regimen based on clinical benefits observed in the randomized phase III study (ML18147).[76] Despite the benefit in the metastatic setting, the addition of bevacizumab did not improve clinical outcomes in the adjuvant setting in CRC.[77,78] In 2006, bevacizumab received an additional approval for use in combination with carboplatin and paclitaxel, and is indicated for first-line treatment of patients with unresectable, locally advanced, recurrent, or metastatic nonsquamous, non–small-cell lung cancer (NSCLC) based on the demonstration of a statistically significant improvement in OS in patients in the bevacizumab arm compared to those receiving chemotherapy alone.[79] In February 2008, the FDA granted a conditional, accelerated approval for bevacizumab to be used in combination with paclitaxel for the treatment of patients who have not received chemotherapy for metastatic human epidermal growth factor receptor 2 (*HER2*)-negative breast cancer. However, additional clinical trials were conducted and the new data showed only a small effect on progression free survival (PFS) without evidence of an improvement in OS or a clinical benefit to patients sufficient to outweigh the risks; thus, the FDA rescinded its approval and removed the breast cancer indication from the drug's label in November 2011.[80–82] This controversial decision continues to be debated with ongoing subgroup analyses to identify patients who would likely benefit from bevacizumab.

Bevacizumab received another accelerated approval as a single agent for patients with glioblastoma multiforme (GBM) with progressive disease following therapy in May 2009. The approval was based on the demonstration of durable objective response rates observed in two single-arm trials, AVF3708g and NCI 06-C-0064E.[83] Currently, no data have shown whether bevacizumab improves disease-related symptoms or survival in people previously treated for GBM. Moreover, phase III trials of bevacizumab in newly diagnosed GBM (RTOG 8025 and AVAglio) have shown a 3- to 4-month improvement of PFS, but no OS advantage over the standard of care.[84] The AVAglio trial improved patients' quality of life, whereas the RTOG 0825 did not and instead increased the burden of symptoms with a negative impact on cognition. Although these two studies showed that bevacizumab had a modest benefit as the initial therapy for GBM, it remained effective to treat recurrences where treatment options are limited. In July 2009, bevacizumab was approved for use in combination with IFN-α for the treatment of patients with metastatic renal cell carcinoma (RCC). Results from the AVOREN trial demonstrated a 5-month improvement in median PFS in patients treated with bevacizumab plus IFN-α-2a versus IFN-α-2a plus placebo.[85] Another phase III trial (CALGB 90206) of bevacizumab plus IFN-α versus IFN-α monotherapy was conducted in patients with previously untreated, metastatic clear cell RCC. Median PFS was 8.4 months versus 4.9 months in favor of the bevacizumab arm.[86] Both studies did not demonstrate a statistically significant advantage in OS.[87,88]

Clinical studies of bevacizumab in combination with oxaliplatin-containing and 5-fluorouracil–based regimens have shown that combination therapy is well tolerated with toxicity not being

substantially greater than that of the chemotherapy alone.[89] Side effects included grade 3 hypertension, grade 1 or 2 proteinuria, a slight increase (less than two percentage points) in grade 3 or 4 bleeding, and impaired surgical wound healing in patients who underwent surgery during treatment with bevacizumab. However, potentially life-threatening events (e.g., arterial and venous thromboembolic events, gastrointestinal perforation, hemoptysis, risk of ovarian failure) have occurred in some patients, thus requiring close patient monitoring in individuals who are at greater risk of adverse events.[90] In a recent meta-analysis of RCTs, bevacizumab in combination with chemotherapy or biologic therapy, compared with chemotherapy alone, was associated with increased treatment-related mortality.[91]

Although four phase III randomized studies have demonstrated improvements in PFS for ovarian cancer (OC)—two first-line trials (GOG 218 and ICON7) and two in recurrent OC [*platinum-resistant* (AURELIA Trial) or *platinum-sensitive* (OCEANS Trial)]—the role of bevacizumab in OC remains controversial. Bevacizumab is approved for use in combination with chemotherapy in the first- and second-line treatment of advanced OC in Europe, but it is not currently licensed in the United States for this indication. Mature OS data and predictive biomarkers are key to defining the subsets of patients who will most like benefit from this therapy. More recently, a randomized, phase III trial (GOG240) has demonstrated for the first time that bevacizumab can prolong OS and PFS for women with advanced, recurrent, or persistent cervical cancer that was not curable with standard chemotherapy. At the time of writing, there are currently over 400 actively recruiting, ongoing trials investigating the clinical benefits of bevacizumab in combination with chemotherapeutic regimens or as adjuvant therapy in various stages and types of cancer (http://clinicaltrial.gov).

### Ziv-aflibercept

Ziv-aflibercept (previously known as aflibercept or VEGF Trap) is a recombinant humanized fusion protein of the extracellular domains of VEGF receptor 1 (VEGFR1) and VEGFR2 with the constant region (Fc) of human immunoglobulin (Ig)G1 that binds to VEGF-A, VEGF-B, PlGF1, and PlGF2, thereby preventing these ligands from binding to and activating their cognate receptors.[92] Ziv-aflibercept has a higher VEGF-A binding affinity and more potent blockade of VEGFR1 or VEGFR2 activation than bevacizumab.[93] In tumor models, ziv-aflibercept exerts its antiangiogenic effects through regressing tumor vasculature and size, remodeling or normalizing surviving vasculature, and inhibiting ascites formation.[94] In August 2012, ziv-aflibercept received regulatory approval for use in combination with 5-fluorouracil, leucovorin, and irinotecan (FOLFIRI) for the treatment of patients with metastatic CRC that is resistant to or that has progressed following treatment with an oxaliplatin-containing regimen. Results from the pivotal phase III VELOUR trial showed that ziv-aflibercept plus FOLFIRI statistically and significantly improved PFS (median PFS, 6.90 versus 4.67 months, respectively), OS (median OS, 13.50 versus 12.06 months, respectively), and overall response rates (19% versus 11.1%, respectively) relative to placebo plus FOLFIRI.[95] Toxicities related to ziv-aflibercept were consistent with those expected from the anti-VEGF drug class. The frequency of vascular-related adverse events appeared to be higher with ziv-aflibercept than bevacizumab treatment when compared across trials. Current clinical data are insufficient to directly compare ziv-aflibercept and bevacizumab in the first- or second-line setting for metastatic CRC.

### Tyrosine–Kinase Inhibitor Therapy

#### Sorafenib

Sorafenib is a small-molecule Raf kinase and VEGF receptor kinase (VEGFR2 and VEGFR3) inhibitor. It has been shown to

CANCER THERAPEUTICS

exhibit broad-spectrum effects on multiple targets (PDGF receptor (PDGFR), stem cell factor (c-KIT) receptor, p38) that affect the maintenance of the tumor vasculature and angiogenesis.[96] In December 2005, the FDA granted approval for sorafenib, which is considered the first multikinase inhibitor, for the treatment of patients with advanced RCC. Safety and efficacy of sorafenib was proven in the largest randomized phase III study conducted in advanced RCC that showed prolong PFS in favor of sorafenib.[97,98] In November 2007, sorafenib was approved for the treatment of patients with unresectable hepatocellular carcinoma (HCC) based on the study results in patients with advanced HCC who had not received previous systemic treatment. Median survival and the time to radiologic progression were nearly 3 months longer for patients treated with sorafenib than for those given placebo.[99] In November 2013, sorafenib received a new indication under the FDA's priority review program for the treatment of locally recurrent or metastatic, progressive differentiated thyroid carcinoma (DTC) refractory to radioactive iodine (RAI) treatment based on positive results from the phase III DECISION trial. Treatment with sorafenib improved PFS (the primary endpoint of the trial) by 41% compared with placebo (10.8 versus 5.8 months, respectively; hazard ratio [HR], 0.587, 95% confidence interval [CI] [0.454 to 0.758]; p <0.0001).[100] The overall response rates were 12% for patients who received sorafenib versus 1% for the placebo arm. Although only about 5% to 15% of thyroid cancer patients become refractory to RAI, no standard treatments are available and, thus, sorafenib is the first agent specifically approved for RAI-resistant DTC. Sorafenib was generally well tolerated with a predictable safety profile. Common adverse events include diarrhea, rash/desquamation, fatigue, hand–foot skin reaction, alopecia, and nausea/vomiting. Grade 3/4 adverse events were 38% for sorafenib versus 28% for placebo. Sorafenib-induced hypertension occurred in patients with metastatic RCC. The treatment-related hypertension was noted to be a class effect observed not only with VEGFR inhibitors, but also with the VEGF monoclonal antibody as well.[90] No significant relationship between previously described mediators of blood pressure and the magnitude of increase was found in a study evaluating the mechanism of sorafenib-induced hypertension in patients.[101]

## Sunitinib

Sunitinib (SU11248) is a small-molecule, multitargeted TKI that exhibits potent antitumor and antiangiogenic activity and inhibits VEGFR-1, -2, -3, c-KIT, PDGFR; FLT-3; colony-stimulating factor receptor type 1 receptor; and the glial cell line–derived neurotrophic factor receptor. It was rationally designed and chosen for its high bioavailability and its nanomolar-range potency against the antiangiogenic RTKs. Sunitinib received its first U.S. regulatory approval in 2006 for the treatment of gastrointestinal stromal tumor (GIST) after disease progression on, or intolerance to, imatinib and accelerated approval for the treatment of advanced RCC.[102] Sunitinib demonstrated significant efficacy (prolonged median time to progression) in imatinib-resistant or -intolerant GIST in a randomized phase III trial.[103] The accelerated approval for RCC was based on durable partial responses, with a response rate of 26% to 37%, and a median duration of response of 54 weeks from two phase II, single-arm trials of patients with cytokine-refractory RCC.[104] The accelerated approval was converted to regular approval in 2007 following confirmation of an improvement in PFS and OS in a phase III trial of sunitinib for first-line treatment of patients with treatment-naïve, metastatic RCC.[105,106] In May 2011, the drug received a new indication for the treatment of progressive, well-differentiated pancreatic neuroendocrine tumors (pNET) in patients with unresectable, locally advanced, or metastatic disease. The randomized phase III trial was discontinued early after the independent data monitoring committee observed more serious adverse events and deaths in the placebo group as well as a difference in PFS favoring sunitinib. The median PFS for patients treated with sunitinib was 10.2 months,

compared with 5.4 months for patients treated with placebo (HR, 0.427, 95% CI, 0.271 to 0.673], p <0.001).[107] Common adverse effects, including diarrhea, mucositis, asthenia, skin abnormalities, and altered taste, were more common in patients receiving sunitinib. In addition, a decrease in left ventricular ejection fraction and severe hypertension were also more commonly reported in the sunitinib arm. Grade 3 or 4 treatment-emergent adverse events were reported in 56% versus 51% of patients on sunitinib versus placebo, respectively.

## Pazopanib

Pazopanib is a second-generation, multitargeted TKI that binds to VEGFR-1, -2, -3, PDGFR-α and -β, c-KIT, and several other key proteins responsible for angiogenesis, tumor growth, and cell survival. Pazopanib exhibited in vivo and in vitro activity against tumor growth, and early clinical trials demonstrated potent antitumor and antiangiogenic activity.[108] A phase III clinical trial in treatment-naïve and cytokine-pretreated patients with advanced and/or metastatic RCC showed a significant improvement in PFS and tumor response compared with placebo,[109] leading to the approval of pazopanib in the United States in October 2009. A recent, randomized phase III trial (COMPARZ) compared the efficacy and safety of pazopanib and sunitinib as first-line therapy involving patients with metastatic RCC and demonstrated that both pazopanib and sunitinib have similar efficacy, but the safety and quality-of-life profiles favor pazopanib.[110] In April 2012, pazopanib was approved for the treatment of patients with metastatic nonadipocytic soft tissue sarcoma who have received prior chemotherapy following a phase III trial that demonstrated a statistically significant improvement in PFS. The median PFS was 4.6 months for patients receiving pazopanib versus 1.6 months for the placebo arm.[111] The drug is generally well tolerated, with the most common adverse events being diarrhea, fatigue, anorexia, hypertension, and hair depigmentation, as well as laboratory abnormalities in elevated aspartate aminotransferase and alanine aminotransferase. Pazopanib has shown clinical activity in a variety of tumors, including breast cancer, thyroid cancer, HCC, and cervical cancer.[112] Ongoing phase II and III trials are further evaluating pazopanib in these malignancies.

## Vandetanib

Vandetanib is an oral, small-molecule TKI that inhibits the activity of RET kinase, VEGFR, epidermal growth factor receptor (EGFR), protein tyrosine kinase 6 (BRK), TIE2, members of the ephrin (EPH) receptors kinase family, and members of the Src family of tyrosine kinases.[113] Vandetanib reduced endothelial cell migration, proliferation, survival, and angiogenesis in vitro, and it decreased tumor vessel permeability and inhibited tumor growth and metastasis in vivo. In April 2011, vandetanib received U.S. regulatory approval for the treatment of symptomatic or progressive medullary thyroid cancer (MTC) in patients with unresectable, locally advanced, or metastatic disease. Until the approval of vandetanib, no systemic therapy was approved for the treatment of unresectable MTC, making it the first molecularly targeted agent approved for this disease. Results of a randomized phase III trial of patients with unresectable, locally advanced, or metastatic MTC demonstrated statistically significant and clinically meaningful improvements in PFS for vandetanib compared with placebo (HR, 0.46; 95% CI, 0.31 to 0.69; p <0.001).[114] Common grade 3 and 4 toxicities (>5%) were diarrhea and/or colitis, hypertension and hypertensive crisis, fatigue, hypocalcemia, rash, and corrected QT interval (QTc) prolongation. Given the toxicity profile, which includes QTc prolongation and sudden death, vandetanib is only available through a restricted distribution program. Vandetanib is also the first targeted drug to show evidence of efficacy in a randomized phase II trial in patients with locally advanced or metastatic differentiated thyroid carcinoma,[115] and a phase III trial is currently underway. Early phase studies are also being conducted in solid tumors, including GIST and kidney and pancreatic cancers.

## Axitinib

Axitinib is a potent and selective second-generation inhibitor of VEGFR-1, -2, and -3. The in vitro half-maximal inhibitory concentration (IC50) of axitinib is 10-fold lower for the VEGF family of receptors than for other TKIs such as pazopanib, sunitinib, or sorafenib.[116] In January 2012, axitinib received approval for the treatment of advanced RCC after the failure of one prior systemic therapy based on a phase III trial (AXIS) comparing the efficacy and safety of axitinib versus sorafenib as a second-line treatment for metastatic RCC.[117,118] The median PFS was 6.7 months with axitinib compared to 4.7 months with sorafenib (HR, 0.67; 95% CI, 0.54, 0.81; one-sided p <0.0001). This improvement in PFS was greater in the cytokine-pretreated subgroup in comparison with the sunitinib-pretreated subgroup. The most frequent adverse events with axitinib were diarrhea (all grade), hypertension (all grade), fatigue, decreased appetite, nausea, and dysphonia. Moreover, hypertension, nausea, dysphonia, and hypothyroidism were more common with axitinib, whereas palmar–plantar erythrodysesthesia, alopecia, and rash were more frequent with sorafenib. A phase III trial (AGILE) comparing axitinib with sorafenib as first-line therapy in patients with treatment-naïve metastatic RCC demonstrated no significant difference in median PFS between patients treated with axitinib or sorafenib.[119] Additionally, axitinib is being studied as a single agent as well as in combination with chemotherapy across several tumor types including HCC, NSCLC, and pancreatic and thyroid cancers.

## Cabozantinib

Cabozantinib (XL184) is a small-molecule TKI with potent activity toward the MET receptor and VEGFR2, as well as a number of other receptor tyrosine kinases, including RET, KIT, AXL, and FLT-3. MET is the only known receptor for hepatocyte growth factor (HGF), and its signaling activity plays a key role in tumorigenic growth, metastasis, and therapeutic resistance. The dysregulated expression and/or activation of MET and HGF have been implicated in the development of numerous human cancers including glioma; melanoma; and hepatocellular, renal, gastric, pancreatic, prostate, ovarian, breast, and lung cancers, and is often correlated with poor prognosis.[120] Recent studies have determined that the MET pathway plays an important role in the development of resistance to VEGF pathway inhibition and that the use of VEGFR inhibitors, such as sunitinib, sorafenib, or a VEGFR2-targeting antibody, can result in the development of an aggressive tumor phenotype characterized by increased invasiveness and metastasis.[121–123] Thus, there is an advantage to targeting both the MET and VEGF pathways to disrupt angiogenesis, tumorigenesis, and cancer progression. In November 2012, cabozantinib received U.S. regulatory approval for progressive metastatic MTC based on the phase III trial that demonstrated a statistically significant PFS prolongation for the cabozantinib-treatment arm.[124] The estimated median PFS was 11.2 months for cabozantinib versus 4.0 months for placebo (HR, 0.28; 95% CI, 0.19 to 0.40; p <0.001). Manageable toxicities included diarrhea, palmar–plantar erythrodysesthesia, decreased weight and appetite, nausea, and fatigue. Cabozantinib has been effective against several solid cancers, including MTC, breast, NSCLC, melanoma, and liver cancer, and is currently being studied in clinical trials in a number of tumor types, with the most significant results observed in the reduction of bone metastatic lesions in castration-resistant prostate cancer.[125]

## Regorafenib

Regorafenib is a small-molecule TKI of multiple membrane-bound and intracellular kinases including RET, VEGFR1, VEGFR2, VEGFR3, KIT, PDGFR-α, PDGFR-β, FGFR1, FGFR2, TIE2, DDR2, TrkA, Eph2A, RAF-1, BRAF, BRAFV600E, SAPK2, PTK5, and Abl pathways.[126] Regorafenib is structurally related to sorafenib and differs from the latter by the presence of a fluorine atom in the center phenyl ring, resulting in higher inhibitory potency against various proangiogenic receptors than sorafenib, including VEGFR2 and FGFR1. In September 2012, regorafenib was approved for the treatment of patients with mCRC who have been previously treated with fluoropyrimidine-, oxaliplatin-, and irinotecan-based chemotherapy, with an anti-VEGF therapy, and if KRAS wild type, with an anti-EGFR therapy. The phase III CORRECT trial that resulted in approval of the drug demonstrated a median OS of 6.4 months in the regorafenib group versus 5.0 months in the placebo group (HR, 0.77; 95% CI, 0.64 to 0.94; one-sided p = 0.0052).[127] Regorafenib is the first TKI with survival benefits in mCRC that has progressed after all standard therapies. In February 2013, it received another indication for the treatment of patients with locally advanced, unresectable, or metastatic GIST who have been previously treated with imatinib and sunitinib. This was based on positive findings of the phase III GRID trial that demonstrated a median PFS of 4.8 months for regorafenib and 0.9 months for placebo (HR, 0.27, 95% CI, 0.19 to 0.39; p <0.0001).[128] In both studies, regorafenib provided significant improvements in PFS to highly refractory patient populations who have progressed on standard treatments. The most common adverse events that were grade 3 or higher and related to regorafenib were hand–foot skin reaction, fatigue, diarrhea, hypertension, and rash or desquamation. Its clinical development as a single agent or in combination with standard chemotherapeutic agents in various malignant tumors is ongoing and includes a phase III trial in patients with HCC whose disease has progressed after treatment with sorafenib.

## mTOR Inhibitors

The mTOR pathway is a central component of the PI3K/Akt signaling pathway and a regulator of many biologic processes that are essential for angiogenesis, cell proliferation, and metabolism.[129] Inhibition of the mTOR kinase prevents downstream signaling via the Akt pathway, resulting in inhibition of protein translation and cell growth. mTOR plays a key role in angiogenesis and specifically regulates the expression of HIF-1, which is upregulated by the loss of the von Hippel–Lindau gene in RCC. In May 2007, temsirolimus was approved for the treatment of advanced RCC. Efficacy and safety were demonstrated in a phase III study in previously untreated patients (n = 626) with poor risk features of metastatic RCC assigned to one of three treatment arms: IFN-α alone, temsirolimus 25 mg alone, or the combination of temsirolimus (15 mg) and IFN-α.[130] Single-agent temsirolimus was associated with a statistically significant improvement in OS when compared with IFN; the addition of temsirolimus to IFN did not improve OS. The results of the phase III INTORSECT trial compared the efficacy of temsirolimus and sorafenib in the second-line treatment of metastatic RCC after disease progression on sunitinib demonstrated that temsirolimus did not improve survival over sorafenib in the second-line setting.[131] The significant OS difference in favor of sorafenib (stratified HR, 1.31; 95% CI, 1.05 to 1.63; two-sided p = 0.01) suggested that VEGFR inhibition may be a better option than mTOR inhibitors for patients progressing on sunitinib. The most common adverse reactions that occurred were rash, asthenia, mucositis, nausea, edema, and anorexia. Rare, but serious adverse reactions associated with temsirolimus included interstitial lung disease, bowel perforation, and acute renal failure.

Everolimus (RAD001) was approved in March 2009 for patients with advanced RCC whose disease had progressed on VEGFR-targeted therapy (sunitinib or sorafenib). Efficacy was demonstrated in a phase 3 trial that study met its primary endpoint with a median PFS of 4.9 and 1.9 months in the everolimus and placebo arms, respectively (HR, 0.33; p <0.0001).[132] Everolimus is also indicated for

CANCER THERAPEUTICS

subependymal giant cell astrocytoma (SEGA) associated with tuberous sclerosis complex (TSC), renal angiomyolipoma with TSC, progressive neuroendocrine tumors of pancreatic origin, and advanced hormone receptor-positive, HER2-negative breast cancer in combination with exemestane.[133] The most common adverse reactions were stomatitis, infections, asthenia, fatigue, cough, and diarrhea. The most common grade 3/4 adverse reactions were infections, dyspnea, fatigue, stomatitis, dehydration, pneumonitis, abdominal pain, and asthenia. Both temsirolimus and everolimus are currently being evaluated in phase I through III studies of various cancer types. By downregulating HIF-1 in the tumor cell, mTOR inhibitors may complement the effects of TKIs at the level of the EC; thus, the combination of mTOR inhibitors with other targeted agents such as bevacizumab or sorafenib/sunitinib are also being investigated.

## On the Horizon: Anti-VEGFR2 Monoclonal Antibody

Ramucirumab (IMC-1121B) is a fully human IgG1 monoclonal antibody that binds with high affinity to the extracellular VEGF-binding domain of VEGFR-2. In a phase III trial (REGARD), ramucirumab monotherapy conferred a statistically significant benefit in OS and PFS compared to placebo in patients with advanced gastric or gastroesophageal junction adenocarcinoma in the second-line setting with an acceptable safety profile.[134] The survival advantage is the first to be elicited by a single-agent biologic treatment in this setting and, based on these findings, the FDA has assigned a priority review designation for ramucirumab. An ongoing phase III trial (RAINBOW) of ramucirumab in combination with chemotherapy as second-line treatment for patients with advanced gastric cancer is currently underway, and preliminary results demonstrated the trial met both its primary (OS) and secondary (PFS) endpoints. In April 2014, the U.S. FDA approved ramucirumab for use as a single agent for the treatment of patients with advanced or metastatic, gastric or gastroesophageal junction adenocarcinoma with disease progression on or after prior treatment with fluoropyrimidine- or platinum-containing chemotherapy. The recommended ramucirumab dose and schedule is 8 mg/kg administered as a 60-minute intravenous infusion every 2 weeks. The drug also marginally improved survival in the second-line treatment of NSCLC in an ongoing phase III (REVEL) trial.

## COMBINATION THERAPIES

Tumor angiogenesis is a highly complex process involving multiple growth factors and their receptor signaling pathways. Based on current evidence, with a few exceptions, effective therapy will probably rely on a combinatorial approach that involves targeting multiple pathways simultaneously. However, a recent study has demonstrated that simultaneous inhibition of the VEGF and EGF pathways in combination with chemotherapy shortens rather than prolongs PFS as compared to inhibition of the VEGF pathway alone in combination with chemotherapy.[135] Whether other targeted agents exhibit beneficial effects when combined with VEGF inhibitors remains to be investigated. Moreover, a number of studies have shown that antiangiogenic agents in combination with chemotherapy or radiotherapy result in additive or synergistic effects. Several models have been proposed to explain the mechanism responsible for this potentiation, keying in on the chemosensitizing effects of antiangiogenic therapy.[136] One hypothesis is that antiangiogenic therapy may normalize the tumor vasculature, thus resulting in improved oxygenation, better blood perfusion, and consequently, improved delivery of chemotherapeutic drugs.[137] A second model suggests that chemotherapy delivered at low doses and at close, regular intervals with no extended drug-free break periods preferentially damages ECs in the tumor neovasculature,[138,139] and suppresses circulating endothelial progenitor cells.[140,141] This regimen, also called metronomic

chemotherapy, sustains antiangiogenic activity and reduces acute toxicity.[142] Thus, the efficacy of metronomic chemotherapy may increase when administered in combination with specific antiangiogenic drugs. Another model addresses the use of antiangiogenic drugs to slow down tumor cell repopulation between successive cycles of cytotoxic chemotherapy.[143] This model underscores the importance of timing and sequence in achieving the maximal therapeutic benefit from combination therapies. In fact, a preclinical study in murine tumor models demonstrated that the administration of sunitinib markedly reduced chemotherapy-induced bone marrow toxicity, suggesting that the sequential treatment regimen (delivery of antiangiogenics followed by chemotherapy) showed superior survival benefits compared with the simultaneous administration of two drugs.[144] Finally, other mechanisms that might also contribute to the synergism include angiogenesis inhibitor–induced tumor blood vessel regression, the prevention of tumor coopting of vessels from surrounding healthy tissues, and the formation of abnormal vessels in the tumor microenvironment.[145] Nevertheless, it remains a challenge to determine why bevacizumab has proved largely ineffective as a single agent, whereas VEGF RTK inhibitors have repeatedly failed in randomized phase III trials when used in combination with chemotherapy. Furthermore, an additional challenge is to determine the optimal dose and duration of antiangiogenic drugs as well as the impact of drug sequencing in combination regimens. Studies are warranted to delineate the discrepancy of bevacizumab's efficacy in the macrometastatic versus micrometastatic disease settings.[146,147]

## BIOMARKERS OF ANTIANGIOGENIC THERAPY

Antiangiogenic therapy has created a need to develop effective biomarkers to assess the activity of these inhibitors. Biomarkers of tumor angiogenesis activity are important to guide clinical development of these agents and to select patients most likely to benefit from this approach. Although there are currently no validated biomarkers for clinically assessing the efficacy of or selecting patients who will respond to antiangiogenic therapies, a number of candidate markers, including tissue, imaging, and circulating biomarkers, are emerging that need to be prospectively validated.[148,149] Several avenues are currently being investigated and include tumor biopsy analysis, microvessel density, noninvasive vascular imaging modalities (positron-emission tomography, dynamic contrast-enhanced magnetic resonance imaging), and measuring circulating biomarkers (levels of angiogenic factors in serum, plasma, urine, or circulating ECs and their precursors).[150–152] Recent research efforts have focused on identifying genetic and toxicity biomarkers to predict which patients will benefit from anti-VEGF/VEGFR therapy and identify patients at risk of adverse events. The existence of VEGF single-nucleotide polymorphisms (SNP) and their association with clinical outcomes may be predictive of patient response to bevacizumab. A recent study identified a locus in VEGFR1 that correlated with increased VEGFR1 expression and poor bevacizumab treatment outcomes.[153] Moreover, a breast cancer study (E2100) reported the VEGF-2578 AA and VEGF-1154 AA genotypes predicted an improved median OS, whereas the VEGF-634 CC and VEGF-1498 TT genotypes predicted protection from grade 3/4 hypertension in the combination-treatment arm.[154] The degree of hypertension can serve as a predictive biomarker of survival in patients after bevacizumab or TKI treatment. Although an association between hypertension and anti-VEGF therapy has been described, the clinical implications of this association and the predictive value of hypertension remains to be validated prospectively. A retrospective analysis of hypertension and efficacy outcomes was conducted in seven large phase III trials (n = 6,486 patients) and, in six of seven studies, early treatment-related blood pressure increase was neither predictive of clinical benefit from bevacizumab nor prognostic for the course of the disease.[155] However, one study (AVF2107g) showed early increased blood pressure was associated with longer PFS and OS. Because genetics play a significant role in modifying the risk of hypertension,[156] it remains to be determined whether polymorphisms in the VEGF/VEGFR pathway may function as potential biomarkers to predict the association between treatment-related hypertension and response to anti-VEGF therapy, as previously implicated in the E2100 trial.[154] Other biomarkers of response include elevated VEGF and placental growth factor levels,[148,152] whereas biomarkers of resistance, including circulating basic fibroblast growth factor, stromal cell-derived factor 1α, and viable circulating endothelial cells, increased when tumors escaped treatment.[157] A first prospective biomarker study (MERiDiAN) in metastatic breast cancer is currently underway to evaluate the impact of bevacizumab in patients stratified for plasma short VEGF-A isoforms. If validated, these findings could help identify which subgroup of patients should receive antiangiogenic therapy and could lead the way to possible future tailoring of individualized antiangiogenic therapy.

## RESISTANCE TO ANTIANGIOGENIC THERAPY

Despite a decade of trials with angiogenesis inhibitors, clinical experience reveals that VEGF-targeted therapy often prolongs the survival of cancer patients by only months because tumors elicit evasive resistance.[145,158] Resistance to VEGF inhibitors may be observed in late-stage tumors when tumors regrow during treatment after an initial period of growth suppression from these antiangiogenic agents. This resistance involves the reactivation of tumor angiogenesis and increased expression of other proangiogenic factors. As the disease progresses, it is possible that redundant pathways might be implicated, with VEGF being replaced by other angiogenic pathways, warranting the addition of a second angiogenesis inhibitor that would target these secondary growth factors and/or their activated receptor pathways, or the use of a multitargeted TKI antiangiogenic drug (e.g., sunitinib, sorafenib).

However, resistance to these drugs eventually occurs, implicating the existence of additional pathways mediating resistance to antiangiogenic therapies. Moreover, tumor cells bearing genetic alterations of the *p53* gene may display a lower apoptosis rate under hypoxic conditions, which might reduce their reliance on vascular supply and, therefore, their responsiveness to antiangiogenic therapy.[159] The selection and overgrowth of tumor-variant cells that are hypoxia resistant and, thus, less dependent[159] on angiogenesis and vasculature remodeling, resulting in vessel stabilization,[160] could also explain the resistance to antiangiogenic drugs. Other possible mechanisms for acquired resistance include tumor vessels becoming less sensitive to antiangiogenic agents, tumor regrowth via rebound revascularization, and vessel cooption.[161-166] Perhaps one of the most intriguing findings is that, although ECs are assumed to be genetically stable, they may under some circumstances harbor genetic abnormalities and thus acquire resistance as well.[167,168]

Recent studies report that VEGF-targeted therapies not only induce primary tumor shrinkage and inhibit tumor progression, but can also initiate mechanisms that increase malignancy to promote tumor invasiveness and metastasis.[122,123,169] These mechanisms of resistance to antiangiogenic therapy involve tumor- and host-mediated pathways and may allow for differential efficacy in different stages of disease progression.[163] Specifically, antiangiogenic drug–resistance mechanisms involve pathways mediated by the tumor, whether intrinsic or acquired in response to therapy or by the host, which is either responding directly to therapy or indirectly to tumoral cues. Taken together, antiangiogenic therapy can enhance tumor invasiveness and metastasis to facilitate and/or accelerate disease in microscopic tumors and, hence, reduce OS benefit. Understanding the mechanisms of resistance, whether intrinsic or acquired, after exposure to antiangiogenic drug treatment is essential for developing strategies that will allow for optimal exploitation of VEGF inhibitors. It is equally important to identify biomarkers of drug resistance and factors mediating this resistance because the development of reliable biomarkers can be invaluable to monitor the development of evasive resistance to angiogenesis inhibitors.

# REFERENCES

1. Hanahan D, Weinberg RA. Hallmarks of cancer: the next generation. *Cell* 2011;144:646–674.
2. Ide AG, Baker NH, Warren SL. Vascularization of the Brown Pearce rabbit epithelioma transplant as seen in the transparent ear chamger. *Am J Roentgenol* 1939;42:891–899.
3. Algire GH, Chalkley HW, Legallais FY, et al. Vascular reactions of normal and malignant tissues in vivo. I. Vascular reactions of mice to wounds and to normal and neoplastic transplants. *J Natl Cancer Inst* 1945;6:73–85.
4. Folkman J, Merler E, Abernathy C, et al. Isolation of a tumor factor responsible for angiogenesis. *J Exp Med* 1971;133:275–288.
5. Folkman J. Tumor angiogenesis: therapeutic implications. *N Engl J Med* 1971;285:1182–1186.
6. Papetti M, Herman IM. Mechanisms of normal and tumor-derived angiogenesis. *Am J Physiol Cell Physiol* 2002;282:C947–C970.
7. Hanahan D, Folkman J. Patterns and emerging mechanisms of the angiogenic switch during tumorigenesis. *Cell* 1996;86:353–364.
8. Black WC, Welch HG. Advances in diagnostic imaging and overestimations of disease prevalence and the benefits of therapy. *N Engl J Med* 1993;328:1237–1243.
9. Folkman J, Kalluri R. Cancer without disease. *Nature* 2004;427:787.
10. Weidner N, Semple JP, Welch WR, et al. Tumor angiogenesis and metastasis—correlation in invasive breast carcinoma. *N Engl J Med* 1991;324:1–8.
11. Holmgren L, O'Reilly MS, Folkman J. Dormancy of micrometastases: balanced proliferation and apoptosis in the presence of angiogenesis suppression. *Nat Med* 1995;1:149–153.
12. Naumov GN, Bender E, Zurakowski D, et al. A model of human tumor dormancy: an angiogenic switch from the nonangiogenic phenotype. *J Natl Cancer Inst* 2006;98:316–325.
13. Udagawa T, Fernandez A, Achilles EG, et al. Persistence of microscopic human cancers in mice: alterations in the angiogenic balance accompanies loss of tumor dormancy. *Faseb J* 2002;16:1361–1370.
14. Holash J, Maisonpierre PC, Compton D, et al. Vessel cooption, regression, and growth in tumors mediated by angiopoietins and VEGF. *Science* 1999;284:1994–1998.
15. Relf M, LeJeune S, Scott PA, et al. Expression of the angiogenic factors vascular endothelial cell growth factor, acidic and basic fibroblast growth factor, tumor growth factor beta-1, platelet-derived endothelial cell growth factor, placenta growth factor, and pleiotrophin in human primary breast cancer and its relation to angiogenesis. *Cancer Res* 1997;57:963–969.
16. Carmeliet P, Dor Y, Herbert JM, et al. Role of HIF-1alpha in hypoxia-mediated apoptosis, cell proliferation and tumour angiogenesis. *Nature* 1998;394:485–490.
17. Folkman J. Endogenous angiogenesis inhibitors. *Apmis* 2004;112:496–507.
18. Nyberg P, Xie L, Kalluri R. Endogenous inhibitors of angiogenesis. *Cancer Res* 2005;65:3967–3979.
19. Rak J, Yu JL. Oncogenes and tumor angiogenesis: the question of vascular "supply" and vascular "demand". *Semin Cancer Biol* 2004;14:93–104.
20. Bottos A, Bardelli A. Oncogenes and angiogenesis: a way to personalize antiangiogenic therapy? *Cell Mol Life Sci* 2013;70:4131–4140.
21. Rak J, Yu JL, Klement G, et al. Oncogenes and angiogenesis: signaling three-dimensional tumor growth. *J Investig Dermatol Symp Proc* 2000;5:24–33.
22. Langer R, Brem H, Falterman K, et al. Isolations of a cartilage factor that inhibits tumor neovascularization. *Science* 1976;193:70–72.
23. Langer R, Conn H, Vacanti J, et al. Control of tumor growth in animals by infusion of an angiogenesis inhibitor. *Proc Natl Acad Sci U S A* 1980;77:4331–4335.
24. Ribatti D. Endogenous inhibitors of angiogenesis: a historical review. *Leuk Res* 2009;33:638–644.
25. Folkman J. Antiangiogenesis in cancer therapy—endostatin and its mechanisms of action. *Exp Cell Res* 2006;312:594–607.
26. Karamouzis MV, Moschos SJ. The use of endostatin in the treatment of solid tumors. *Expert Opin Biol Ther* 2009;9:641–648.
27. Lawler J. Thrombospondin-1 as an endogenous inhibitor of angiogenesis and tumor growth. *J Cell Mol Med* 2002;6:1–12.
28. Maeshima Y, Manfredi M, Reimer C, et al. Identification of the anti-angiogenic site within vascular basement membrane-derived tumstatin. *J Biol Chem* 2001;276:15240–15248.
29. Kerbel RS. Vasohibin: the feedback on a new inhibitor of angiogenesis. *J Clin Invest* 2004;114:884–886.
30. Sato Y. The vasohibin family: a novel family for angiogenesis regulation. *J Biochem* 2013;153:5–11.

31. Noguera-Troise I, Daly C, Papadopoulos NJ, et al. Blockade of Dll4 inhibits tumour growth by promoting non-productive angiogenesis. *Nature* 2006;444:1032–1037.

32. Ridgway J, Zhang G, Wu Y, et al. Inhibition of Dll4 signalling inhibits tumour growth by deregulating angiogenesis. *Nature* 2006;444:1083–1087.

33. Kuhnert F, Kirshner JR, Thurston G. Dll4-Notch signaling as a therapeutic target in tumor angiogenesis. *Vasc Cell* 2011;3:20.

34. Sund M, Hamano Y, Sugimoto H, et al. Function of endogenous inhibitors of angiogenesis as endothelium-specific tumor suppressors. *Proc Natl Acad Sci U S A* 2005;102:2934–2939.

35. Dameron KM, Volpert OV, Tainsky MA, et al. Control of angiogenesis in fibroblasts by p53 regulation of thrombospondin-1. *Science* 1994;265:1582–1584.

36. Zhang L, Yu D, Hu M, et al. Wild-type p53 suppresses angiogenesis in human leiomyosarcoma and synovial sarcoma by transcriptional suppression of vascular endothelial growth factor expression. *Cancer Res* 2000;60:3655–3661.

37. Sherif ZA, Nakai S, Pirollo KF, et al. Downmodulation of bFGF-binding protein expression following restoration of p53 function. *Cancer Gene Ther* 2001;8:771–782.

38. Ravi R, Mookerjee B, Bhujwalla ZM, et al. Regulation of tumor angiogenesis by p53-induced degradation of hypoxia-inducible factor 1alpha. *Genes Dev* 2000;14:34–44.

39. Farhang Ghahremani M, Goossens S, Nittner D, et al. p53 promotes VEGF expression and angiogenesis in the absence of an intact p21-Rb pathway. *Cell Death Differ* 2013;20:888–897.

40. Teodoro JG, Parker AE, Zhu X, et al. p53-mediated inhibition of angiogenesis through up-regulation of a collagen prolyl hydroxylase. *Science* 2006;313:968–971.

41. Folkman J. Tumor suppression by p53 is mediated in part by the antiangiogenic activity of endostatin and tumstatin. *Sci STKE* 2006;2006:pe35.

42. Brouty-Boye D, Zetter BR. Inhibition of cell motility by interferon. *Science* 1980;208:516–518.

43. Dvorak HF, Gresser I. Microvascular injury in pathogenesis of interferon-induced necrosis of subcutaneous tumors in mice. *J Natl Cancer Inst* 1989;81:497–502.

44. Sidky YA, Borden EC. Inhibition of angiogenesis by interferons: effects on tumor- and lymphocyte-induced vascular responses. *Cancer Res* 1987;47:5155–5161.

45. Taylor S, Folkman J. Protamine is an inhibitor of angiogenesis. *Nature* 1982; 297:307–312.

46. Crum R, Szabo S, Folkman J. A new class of steroids inhibits angiogenesis in the presence of heparin or a heparin fragment. *Science* 1985;230:1375–1378.

47. Ingber D, Fujita T, Kishimoto S, et al. Synthetic analogues of fumagillin that inhibit angiogenesis and suppress tumour growth. *Nature* 1990;348:555–557.

48. Kerbel RS. Inhibition of tumor angiogenesis as a strategy to circumvent acquired resistance to anti-cancer therapeutic agents. *Bioessays* 1991;13:31–36.

49. Folkman J. Angiogenesis: an organizing principle for drug discovery? *Nat Rev Drug Discov* 2007;6:273–286.

50. D'Amato RJ, Loughnan MS, Flynn E, et al. Thalidomide is an inhibitor of angiogenesis. *Proc Natl Acad Sci U S A* 1994;91:4082–4085.

51. Bauer KS, Dixon SC, Figg WD. Inhibition of angiogenesis by thalidomide requires metabolic activation, which is species-dependent. *Biochem Pharmacol* 1998;55:1827–1834.

52. Figg WD. The 2005 Leon I. Goldberg Young Investigator Award Lecture: development of thalidomide as an angiogenesis inhibitor for the treatment of androgen-independent prostate cancer. *Clin Pharmacol Ther* 2006;79:1–8.

53. Kenyon BM, Browne F, D'Amato RJ. Effects of thalidomide and related metabolites in a mouse corneal model of neovascularization. *Exp Eye Res* 1997;64:971–978.

54. Price DK, Ando Y, Kruger EA, et al. 5'-OH-thalidomide, a metabolite of thalidomide, inhibits angiogenesis. *Ther Drug Monit* 2002;24:104–110.

55. Dredge K, Marriott JB, Macdonald CD, et al. Novel thalidomide analogues display anti-angiogenic activity independently of immunomodulatory effects. *Br J Cancer* 2002;87:1166–1172.

56. Gupta D, Treon SP, Shima Y, et al. Adherence of multiple myeloma cells to bone marrow stromal cells upregulates vascular endothelial growth factor secretion: therapeutic applications. *Leukemia* 2001;15:1950–1961.

57. Ng SS, Gutschow M, Weiss M, et al. Antiangiogenic activity of N-substituted and tetrafluorinated thalidomide analogues. *Cancer Res* 2003;63:3189–3194.

58. Zhang H, Vakil V, Braunstein M, et al. Circulating endothelial progenitor cells in multiple myeloma: implications and significance. *Blood* 2005;105: 3286–3294.

59. De Sanctis JB, Mijares M, Suarez A, et al. Pharmacological properties of thalidomide and its analogues. *Recent Pat Inflamm Allergy Drug Discov* 2010;4:144–148.

60. Ferrara N, Gerber HP, LeCouter J. The biology of VEGF and its receptors. *Nat Med* 2003;9:669–676.

61. Lindahl P, Johansson BR, Leveen P, et al. Pericyte loss and microaneurysm formation in PDGF-B-deficient mice. *Science* 1997;277:242–245.

62. Oliner J, Min H, Leal J, et al. Suppression of angiogenesis and tumor growth by selective inhibition of angiopoietin-2. *Cancer Cell* 2004;6:507–516.

63. Fingleton B. MMPs as therapeutic targets—still a viable option? *Semin Cell Dev Biol* 2008;19:61–68.

64. Roy R, Yang J, Moses MA. Matrix metalloproteinases as novel biomarkers and potential therapeutic targets in human cancer. *J Clin Oncol* 2009;27:5287–5297.

65. Shi ZG, Li JP, Shi LL, et al. An updated patent therapeutic agents targeting MMPs. *Recent Pat Anticancer Drug Discov* 2012;7:74–101.

66. Gialeli C, Theocharis AD, Karamanos NK. Roles of matrix metalloproteinases in cancer progression and their pharmacological targeting. *FEBS J* 2011;278:16–27.

67. Nikolopoulos SN, Blaikie P, Yoshioka T, et al. Integrin beta4 signaling promotes tumor angiogenesis. *Cancer Cell* 2004;6:471–483.

68. Bradley DA, Daignault S, Ryan CJ, et al. Cilengitide (EMD 121974, NSC 707544) in asymptomatic metastatic castration resistant prostate cancer patients: a randomized phase II trial by the prostate cancer clinical trials consortium. *Invest New Drugs* 2011;29:1432–1440.

69. Desgrosellier JS, Cheresh DA. Integrins in cancer: biological implications and therapeutic opportunities. *Nat Rev Cancer* 2010;10:9–22.

70. Hersey P, Sosman J, O'Day S, et al. A randomized phase 2 study of etaracizumab, a monoclonal antibody against integrin alpha(v)beta(3), + or − dacarbazine in patients with stage IV metastatic melanoma. *Cancer* 2010;116: 1526–1534.

71. Heidenreich A, Rawal SK, Szkarlat K, et al. A randomized, double-blind, multicenter, phase 2 study of a human monoclonal antibody to human alphanu integrins (intetumumab) in combination with docetaxel and prednisone for the first-line treatment of patients with metastatic castration-resistant prostate cancer. *Ann Oncol* 2013;24:329–336.

72. O'Day S, Pavlick A, Loquai C, et al. A randomised, phase II study of intetumumab, an anti-alphav-integrin mAb, alone and with dacarbazine in stage IV melanoma. *Br J Cancer* 2011;105:346–352.

73. Stupp R, Hegi M, Gorlia T, et al. Standard chemoradiotherapy ± cilengitide in newly diagnosed glioblastoma (GBM): updated results and subgroup analyses of the international randomized phase III CENTRIC trial (EORTC trial #26071-22072/Canadian Brain Tumor Consortium). Program and abstracts presented at: 2013 European Cancer Congress; 2013; Amsterdam.

74. Ellis LM, Hicklin DJ. VEGF-targeted therapy: mechanisms of anti-tumour activity. *Nat Rev Cancer* 2008;8:579–591.

75. Hurwitz H, Fehrenbacher L, Novotny W, et al. Bevacizumab plus irinotecan, fluorouracil, and leucovorin for metastatic colorectal cancer. *N Engl J Med* 2004;350:2335–2342.

76. Bennouna J, Sastre J, Arnold D, et al. Continuation of bevacizumab after first progression in metastatic colorectal cancer (ML18147): a randomised phase 3 trial. *Lancet Oncol* 2013;14:29–37.

77. Allegra CJ, Yothers G, O'Connell MJ, et al. Phase III trial assessing bevacizumab in stages II and III carcinoma of the colon: results of NSABP protocol C-08. *J Clin Oncol* 2011;29:11–16.

78. de Gramont A, Van Cutsem E, Schmoll HJ, et al. Bevacizumab plus oxaliplatin-based chemotherapy as adjuvant treatment for colon cancer (AVANT): a phase 3 randomised controlled trial. *Lancet Oncol* 2012;13:1225–1233.

79. Sandler A, Gray R, Perry MC, et al. Paclitaxel-carboplatin alone or with bevacizumab for non-small-cell lung cancer. *N Engl J Med* 2006;355:2542–2550.

80. Miles DW, Chan A, Dirix LY, et al. Phase III study of bevacizumab plus docetaxel compared with placebo plus docetaxel for the first-line treatment of human epidermal growth factor receptor 2-negative metastatic breast cancer. *J Clin Oncol* 2010;28:3239–3247.

81. Robert NJ, Dieras V, Glaspy J, et al. RIBBON-1: randomized, double-blind, placebo-controlled, phase III trial of chemotherapy with or without bevacizumab for first-line treatment of human epidermal growth factor receptor 2-negative, locally recurrent or metastatic breast cancer. *J Clin Oncol* 2011;29:1252–1260.

82. Brufsky AM, Hurvitz S, Perez E, et al. RIBBON-2: a randomized, double-blind, placebo-controlled, phase III trial evaluating the efficacy and safety of bevacizumab in combination with chemotherapy for second-line treatment of human epidermal growth factor receptor 2-negative metastatic breast cancer. *J Clin Oncol* 2011;29:4286–4293.

83. Cohen MH, Shen YL, Keegan P, et al. FDA drug approval summary: bevacizumab (Avastin) as treatment of recurrent glioblastoma multiforme. *Oncologist* 2009;14:1131–1138.

84. Soffietti R, Trevisan E, Ruda R. What have we learned from trials on antiangiogenic agents in glioblastoma? *Expert Rev Neurother* 2014;14:1–3.

85. Escudier B, Pluzanska A, Koralewski P, et al. Bevacizumab plus interferon alfa-2a for treatment of metastatic renal cell carcinoma: a randomised, double-blind phase III trial. *Lancet* 2007;370:2103–2111.

86. Rini BI, Halabi S, Rosenberg JE, et al. Bevacizumab plus interferon alfa compared with interferon alfa monotherapy in patients with metastatic renal cell carcinoma: CALGB 90206. *J Clin Oncol* 2008;26:5422–5428.

87. Escudier B, Bellmunt J, Negrier S, et al. Phase III trial of bevacizumab plus interferon alfa-2a in patients with metastatic renal cell carcinoma (AVOREN): final analysis of overall survival. *J Clin Oncol* 2010;28:2144–2150.

88. Rini BI, Halabi S, Rosenberg JE, et al. Phase III trial of bevacizumab plus interferon alfa versus interferon alfa monotherapy in patients with metastatic renal cell carcinoma: final results of CALGB 90206. *J Clin Oncol* 2010;28: 2137–2143.

89. Hurwitz H, Saini S. Bevacizumab in the treatment of metastatic colorectal cancer: safety profile and management of adverse events. *Semin Oncol* 2006;33:S26–S34.

90. Chen HX, Cleck JN. Adverse effects of anticancer agents that target the VEGF pathway. *Nat Rev Clin Oncol* 2009;6:465–477.

91. Ranpura V, Hapani S, Wu S. Treatment-related mortality with bevacizumab in cancer patients: a meta-analysis. *JAMA* 2011;305:487–494.

92. Holash J, Davis S, Papadopoulos N, et al. VEGF-Trap: a VEGF blocker with potent antitumor effects. *Proc Natl Acad Sci U S A* 2002;99:11393–11398.

93. Papadopoulos N, Martin J, Ruan Q, et al. Binding and neutralization of vascular endothelial growth factor (VEGF) and related ligands by VEGF Trap, ranibizumab and bevacizumab. *Angiogenesis* 2012;15:171–185.

94. Gaya A, Tse V. A preclinical and clinical review of aflibercept for the management of cancer. *Cancer Treat Rev* 2012;38:484–493.

95. Van Cutsem E, Tabernero J, Lakomy R, et al. Addition of aflibercept to fluorouracil, leucovorin, and irinotecan improves survival in a phase III randomized trial in patients with metastatic colorectal cancer previously treated with an oxaliplatin-based regimen. *J Clin Oncol* 2012;30:3499–3506.

96. Wilhelm SM, Carter C, Tang L, et al. BAY 43-9006 exhibits broad spectrum oral antitumor activity and targets the RAF/MEK/ERK pathway and receptor tyrosine kinases involved in tumor progression and angiogenesis. *Cancer Res* 2004;64:7099–7109.

97. Escudier B, Eisen T, Stadler WM, et al. Sorafenib in advanced clear-cell renal-cell carcinoma. *N Engl J Med* 2007;356:125–134.

98. Escudier B, Eisen T, Stadler WM, et al. Sorafenib for treatment of renal cell carcinoma: Final efficacy and safety results of the phase III treatment approaches in renal cancer global evaluation trial. *J Clin Oncol* 2009;27:3312–3318.

99. Llovet JM, Ricci S, Mazzaferro V, et al. Sorafenib in advanced hepatocellular carcinoma. *N Engl J Med* 2008;359:378–390.

100. Brose MS, Nutting C, Jarzab B, et al. Sorafenib in locally advanced or metastatic patients with radioactive iodine refractory differentiated thyroid cancer: the phase III DECISION trial. *J Clin Oncol* 2013;31.

101. Veronese ML, Mosenkis A, Flaherty KT, et al. Mechanisms of hypertension associated with BAY 43-9006. *J Clin Oncol* 2006;24:1363–1369.

102. Goodman VL, Rock EP, Dagher R, et al. Approval summary: sunitinib for the treatment of imatinib refractory or intolerant gastrointestinal stromal tumors and advanced renal cell carcinoma. *Clin Cancer Res* 2007;13:1367–1373.

103. Demetri GD, van Oosterom AT, Garrett CR, et al. Efficacy and safety of sunitinib in patients with advanced gastrointestinal stromal tumour after failure of imatinib: a randomised controlled trial. *Lancet* 2006;368:1329–1338.

104. Motzer RJ, Michaelson MD, Redman BG, et al. Activity of SU11248, a multitargeted inhibitor of vascular endothelial growth factor receptor and platelet-derived growth factor receptor, in patients with metastatic renal cell carcinoma. *J Clin Oncol* 2006;24:16–24.

105. Motzer RJ, Hutson TE, Tomczak P, et al. Sunitinib versus interferon alfa in metastatic renal-cell carcinoma. *N Engl J Med* 2007;356:115–124.

106. Motzer RJ, Hutson TE, Tomczak P, et al. Overall survival and updated results for sunitinib compared with interferon alfa in patients with metastatic renal cell carcinoma. *J Clin Oncol* 2009;27:3584–3590.

107. Raymond E, Dahan L, Raoul JL, et al. Sunitinib malate for the treatment of pancreatic neuroendocrine tumors. *N Engl J Med* 2011;364:501–513.

108. Kumar R, Knick VB, Rudolph SK, et al. Pharmacokinetic-pharmacodynamic correlation from mouse to human with pazopanib, a multikinase angiogenesis inhibitor with potent antitumor and antiangiogenic activity. *Mol Cancer Ther* 2007;6:2012–2021.

109. Sternberg CN, Davis ID, Mardiak J, et al. Pazopanib in locally advanced or metastatic renal cell carcinoma: results of a randomized phase III trial. *J Clin Oncol* 2010;28:1061–1068.

110. Motzer RJ, Hutson TE, Cella D, et al. Pazopanib versus sunitinib in metastatic renal-cell carcinoma. *N Engl J Med* 2013;369:722–731.

111. van der Graaf WT, Blay JY, Chawla SP, et al. Pazopanib for metastatic soft-tissue sarcoma (PALETTE): a randomised, double-blind, placebo-controlled phase 3 trial. *Lancet* 2012;379:1879–1886.

112. Schutz FA, Choueiri TK, Sternberg CN. Pazopanib: Clinical development of a potent anti-angiogenic drug. *Crit Rev Oncol Hematol* 2011;77:163–171.

113. Thornton K, Kim G, Maher VE, et al. Vandetanib for the treatment of symptomatic or progressive medullary thyroid cancer in patients with unresectable locally advanced or metastatic disease: U.S. Food and Drug Administration drug approval summary. *Clin Cancer Res* 2012;18:3722–3730.

114. Wells SA, Jr., Robinson BG, Gagel RF, et al. Vandetanib in patients with locally advanced or metastatic medullary thyroid cancer: a randomized, double-blind phase III trial. *J Clin Oncol* 2012;30:134–141.

115. Leboulleux S, Bastholt L, Krause T, et al. Vandetanib in locally advanced or metastatic differentiated thyroid cancer: a randomised, double-blind, phase 2 trial. *Lancet Oncol* 2012;13:897–905.

116. Gross-Goupil M, Francois L, Quivy A, et al. Axitinib: a review of its safety and efficacy in the treatment of adults with advanced renal cell carcinoma. *Clin Med Insights Oncol* 2013;7:269–277.

117. Rini BI, Escudier B, Tomczak P, et al. Comparative effectiveness of axitinib versus sorafenib in advanced renal cell carcinoma (AXIS): a randomised phase 3 trial. *Lancet* 2011;378:1931–1939.

118. Motzer RJ, Escudier B, Tomczak P, et al. Axitinib versus sorafenib as second-line treatment for advanced renal cell carcinoma: overall survival analysis and updated results from a randomised phase 3 trial. *Lancet Oncol* 2013;14:552–562.

119. Hutson TE, Lesovoy V, Al-Shukri S, et al. Axitinib versus sorafenib as first-line therapy in patients with metastatic renal-cell carcinoma: a randomised open-label phase 3 trial. *Lancet Oncol* 2013;14:1287–1294.

120. Graveel CR, Tolbert D, Vande Woude GF. MET: a critical player in tumorigenesis and therapeutic target. *Cold Spring Harb Perspect Biol* 2013;5.

121. Shojaei F, Lee JH, Simmons BH, et al. HGF/c-Met acts as an alternative angiogenic pathway in sunitinib-resistant tumors. *Cancer Res* 2010;70:10090–10100.

122. Ebos JM, Lee CR, Cruz-Munoz W, et al. Accelerated metastasis after short-term treatment with a potent inhibitor of tumor angiogenesis. *Cancer Cell* 2009;15:232–239.

123. Paez-Ribes M, Allen E, Hudock J, et al. Antiangiogenic therapy elicits malignant progression of tumors to increased local invasion and distant metastasis. *Cancer Cell* 2009;15:220–231.

124. Elisei R, Schlumberger MJ, Muller SP, et al. Cabozantinib in progressive medullary thyroid cancer. *J Clin Oncol* 2013;31:3639–3646.

125. Smith DC, Smith MR, Sweeney C, et al. Cabozantinib in patients with advanced prostate cancer: results of a phase II randomized discontinuation trial. *J Clin Oncol* 2013;31:412–429.

126. Strumberg D, Schultheis B. Regorafenib for cancer. *Expert Opin Investig Drugs* 2012;21:879–889.

127. Grothey A, Van Cutsem E, Sobrero A, et al. Regorafenib monotherapy for previously treated metastatic colorectal cancer (CORRECT): an international, multicentre, randomised, placebo-controlled, phase 3 trial. *Lancet* 2013;381:303–312.

128. Demetri GD, Reichardt P, Kang YK, et al. Efficacy and safety of regorafenib for advanced gastrointestinal stromal tumours after failure of imatinib and sunitinib (GRID): an international, multicentre, randomised, placebo-controlled, phase 3 trial. *Lancet* 2013;381:295–302.

129. Gibbons JJ, Abraham RT, Yu K. Mammalian target of rapamycin: discovery of rapamycin reveals a signaling pathway important for normal and cancer cell growth. *Semin Oncol* 2009;36 Suppl 3:S3–S17.

130. Hudes G, Carducci M, Tomczak P, et al. Temsirolimus, interferon alfa, or both for advanced renal-cell carcinoma. *N Engl J Med* 2007;356:2271–2281.

131. Hutson TE, Escudier B, Esteban E, et al. Randomized phase III trial of temsirolimus versus sorafenib as second-line therapy after sunitinib in patients with metastatic renal cell carcinoma. *J Clin Oncol* 2014;32:760–767.

132. Motzer RJ, Escudier B, Oudard S, et al. Efficacy of everolimus in advanced renal cell carcinoma: a double-blind, randomised, placebo-controlled phase III trial. *Lancet* 2008;372:449–456.

133. Lebwohl D, Anak O, Sahmoud T, et al. Development of everolimus, a novel oral mTOR inhibitor, across a spectrum of diseases. *Ann N Y Acad Sci* 2013;1291:14–32.

134. Fuchs CS, Tomasek J, Yong CJ, et al. Ramucirumab monotherapy for previously treated advanced gastric or gastro-oesophageal junction adenocarcinoma (REGARD): an international, randomised, multicentre, placebo-controlled, phase 3 trial. *Lancet* 2014;383:31–39.

135. Tol J, Koopman M, Cats A, et al. Chemotherapy, bevacizumab, and cetuximab in metastatic colorectal cancer. *N Engl J Med* 2009;360:563–572.

136. Kerbel RS. Antiangiogenic therapy: a universal chemosensitization strategy for cancer? *Science* 2006;312:1171–1175.

137. Jain RK. Normalization of tumor vasculature: an emerging concept in antiangiogenic therapy. *Science* 2005;307:58–62.

138. Browder T, Butterfield CE, Kraling BM, et al. Antiangiogenic scheduling of chemotherapy improves efficacy against experimental drug-resistant cancer. *Cancer Res* 2000;60:1878–1886.

139. Klement G, Baruchel S, Rak J, et al. Continuous low-dose therapy with vinblastine and VEGF receptor-2 antibody induces sustained tumor regression without overt toxicity. *J Clin Invest* 2000;105:R15–R24.

140. Bertolini F, Paul S, Mancuso P, et al. Maximum tolerable dose and low-dose metronomic chemotherapy have opposite effects on the mobilization and viability of circulating endothelial progenitor cells. *Cancer Res* 2003;63:4342–4346.

141. Mancuso P, Colleoni M, Calleri A, et al. Circulating endothelial-cell kinetics and viability predict survival in breast cancer patients receiving metronomic chemotherapy. *Blood* 2006;108:452–459.

142. Kerbel RS, Kamen BA. The anti-angiogenic basis of metronomic chemotherapy. *Nat Rev Cancer* 2004;4:423–436.

143. Hudis CA. Clinical implications of antiangiogenic therapies. *Oncology (Williston Park)* 2005;19:26–31.

144. Zhang D, Hedlund EM, Lim S, et al. Antiangiogenic agents significantly improve survival in tumor-bearing mice by increasing tolerance to chemotherapy-induced toxicity. *Proc Natl Acad Sci U S A* 2011;108:4117–4122.

145. Kerbel RS. Tumor angiogenesis. *N Engl J Med* 2008;358:2039–2049.

146. Mountzios G, Pentheroudakis G, Carmeliet P. Bevacizumab and micrometastases: Revisiting the preclinical and clinical rollercoaster. *Pharmacol Ther* 2014;141:117–124.

147. Ebos JM, Kerbel RS. Antiangiogenic therapy: impact on invasion, disease progression, and metastasis. *Nat Rev Clin Oncol* 2011;8:210–221.

148. Jain RK, Duda DG, Willett CG, et al. Biomarkers of response and resistance to antiangiogenic therapy. *Nat Rev Clin Oncol* 2009;6:327–338.

149. Murukesh N, Dive C, Jayson GC. Biomarkers of angiogenesis and their role in the development of VEGF inhibitors. *Br J Cancer* 2010;102:8–18.

150. Davis DW, McConkey DJ, Abbruzzese JL, et al. Surrogate markers in antiangiogenesis clinical trials. *Br J Cancer* 2003;89:8–14.

151. Wehland M, Bauer J, Magnusson NE, et al. Biomarkers for anti-angiogenic therapy in cancer. *Int J Mol Sci* 2013;14:9338–9364.

152. Lambrechts D, Lenz HJ, de Haas S, et al. Markers of response for the antiangiogenic agent bevacizumab. *J Clin Oncol* 2013;31:1219–1230.

153. Lambrechts D, Claes B, Delmar P, et al. VEGF pathway genetic variants as biomarkers of treatment outcome with bevacizumab: an analysis of data from the AViTA and AVOREN randomised trials. *Lancet Oncol* 2012;13:724–733.

154. Schneider BP, Wang M, Radovich M, et al. Association of vascular endothelial growth factor and vascular endothelial growth factor receptor-2 genetic polymorphisms with outcome in a trial of paclitaxel compared with paclitaxel plus bevacizumab in advanced breast cancer: ECOG 2100. *J Clin Oncol* 2008;26:4672–4678.

155. Hurwitz HI, Douglas PS, Middleton JP, et al. Analysis of early hypertension and clinical outcome with bevacizumab: results from seven phase III studies. *Oncologist* 2013;18:273–280.

156. Levy D, Ehret GB, Rice K, et al. Genome-wide association study of blood pressure and hypertension. *Nat Genet* 2009;41:677–687.

157. Batchelor TT, Sorensen AG, di Tomaso E, et al. AZD2171, a pan-VEGF receptor tyrosine kinase inhibitor, normalizes tumor vasculature and alleviates edema in glioblastoma patients. *Cancer Cell* 2007;11:83–95.

158. Sennino B, McDonald DM. Controlling escape from angiogenesis inhibitors. *Nat Rev Cancer* 2012;12:699–709.

159. Yu JL, Rak JW, Coomber BL, et al. Effect of p53 status on tumor response to antiangiogenic therapy. *Science* 2002;295:1526–1528.

160. Glade Bender J, Cooney EM, Kandel JJ, et al. Vascular remodeling and clinical resistance to antiangiogenic cancer therapy. *Drug Resist Updat* 2004;7:289–300.

161. Bergers G, Hanahan D. Modes of resistance to anti-angiogenic therapy. *Nat Rev Cancer* 2008;8:592–603.

162. Crawford Y, Ferrara N. Tumor and stromal pathways mediating refractoriness/resistance to anti-angiogenic therapies. *Trends Pharmacol Sci* 2009;30:624–630.

163. Ebos JM, Lee CR, Kerbel RS. Tumor and host-mediated pathways of resistance and disease progression in response to antiangiogenic therapy. *Clin Cancer Res* 2009;15:5020–5025.

164. Kerbel RS, Yu J, Tran J, et al. Possible mechanisms of acquired resistance to anti-angiogenic drugs: implications for the use of combination therapy approaches. *Cancer Metastasis Rev* 2001;20:79–86.

165. Shojaei F, Ferrara N. Role of the microenvironment in tumor growth 'and in refractoriness/resistance to anti-angiogenic therapies. *Drug Resist Updat* 2008;11:219–230.

166. Sweeney CJ, Miller KD, Sledge GW Jr. Resistance in the anti-angiogenic era: nay-saying or a word of caution? *Trends Mol Med* 2003;9:24–29.

167. Hida K, Hida Y, Amin DN, et al. Tumor-associated endothelial cells with cytogenetic abnormalities. *Cancer Res* 2004;64:8249–8255.

168. Streubel B, Chott A, Huber D, et al. Lymphoma-specific genetic aberrations in microvascular endothelial cells in B-cell lymphomas. *N Engl J Med* 2004;351:250–259.

169. Loges S, Mazzone M, Hohensinner P, et al. Silencing or fueling metastasis with VEGF inhibitors: antiangiogenesis revisited. *Cancer Cell* 2009;15:167–170.

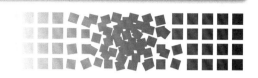

# 29 Monoclonal Antibodies

Hossein Borghaei, Matthew K. Robinson, Gregory P. Adams, and Louis M. Weiner

## INTRODUCTION

Antibody-based therapeutics are important components of the cancer therapeutic armamentarium. Early antibody therapy studies attempted to explicitly target cancers based on the structural and biologic properties that distinguish neoplastic cells from their normal counterparts. The immunogenicity and inefficient effector functions of the first-generation murine monoclonal antibodies (MAb) that were evaluated in clinical trials limited their effectiveness.[1–3] Patients developed human antimouse antibody (HAMA) responses against the therapeutic agents that rapidly cleared it from the body and limited the number of times the therapy could be administered. The development of engineered chimeric, humanized, and fully human MAbs has identified a number of important and useful applications for antibody-based cancer therapy. Currently, the U.S. Food and Drug Administration (FDA) has approved 14 MAbs and MAb-conjugates for the treatment of cancer (Table 29.1) and many more are under evaluation in late-stage clinical trials.[4] Antibodies provide an important means by which to exploit the immune system by specifically recognizing and directing antitumor responses.

Antibodies are produced by B cells and arise in response to exposures to a variety of structures, termed antigens, as a result of a series of recombinations of V, D, and J germline genes. Immunoglobulin-G (IgG) molecules are most commonly employed as the working backbones of current therapeutic monoclonal antibodies, although various other isotypes of antibodies have specialized functions (e.g., IgA molecules play important roles in mucosal immunity, IgE molecules are involved in anaphylaxis). The advent of hybridoma technology by Kohler and Milstein[5] made it possible to produce large quantities of antibodies with high purity and monospecificity for a single binding region (epitope) on an antigen.

The mechanisms that antibody-based therapeutics employ to elicit antitumor effects include focusing components of the patient's immune system to attack tumor cells[6,7] and methods to alter signal transduction pathways that drive tumor progression.[8,9] Antibody-based conjugates employ the targeting specificity of antibodies to deliver toxic compounds, such as chemotherapeutics, specifically to the tumor sites.

## IMMUNOGLOBULIN STRUCTURE

### Structural and Functional Domains

An IgG molecule is typically divided into three domains consisting of two identical antigen-binding (Fab) domains connected to an effector or Fc domain by a flexible hinge sequence. Figure 29.1 shows the structure of an IgG molecule. IgG antibodies are comprised of two identical light chains and two identical heavy chains, with the chains joined by disulfide bonds, resulting in a bilaterally symmetrical complex. The Fab domains mediate the binding of IgG molecules to their cognate antigens and are composed of an intact light chain and half of a heavy chain. Each chain in the Fab domain is further divided into variable and constant regions, with the variable region containing hypervariable, or complementarity determining regions (CDR) in which the antigen-contact residues reside. The light and heavy chain variable regions each contain three CDRs (CDR1, CDR2, and CDR3). All six CDRs form the antigen-binding pocket and are collectively defined in immunologic terms as the idiotype of the antibody. In the majority of cases, the variable heavy chain CDR3 plays a dominant role in binding.[10]

The different isotypes of immunoglobulins are defined by the structure and function of their Fc domains. The Fc domain, composed of the CH2 and CH3 regions of the antibody's heavy chains, is the critical determinant of how an antibody mediates effector functions, transports across cellular barriers, and persists in circulation.[7,11]

## MODIFIED ANTIBODY-BASED MOLECULES

Advances in antibody engineering and molecular biology have facilitated the development of many novel antibody-based structures with unique physical and pharmacokinetic properties (see Fig. 29.1). These include chimeric human-murine antibodies with human-constant regions and murine-variable regions,[12] humanized antibodies in which murine CDR sequences have been grafted into human IgG molecules, and entirely human antibodies derived from human hybridomas and, more recently, from transgenic mice expressing human immunoglobulin genes.[13] An accepted naming scheme based on "stems" was developed by the World Health Organization's International Nonproprietary Names (INN) for pharmaceuticals and is employed in the United States (Table 29.2). Engineering has also facilitated the development of antibody-based fragments. In addition to the classic, enzymatically derived Fab and F(ab′)₂ molecules, a plethora of promising IgG-derivatives have been developed that retain antigen-binding properties of intact antibodies (see Fig. 29.1; for review see Robinson et al.[14]). The basic building block for these molecules is the 25 kDa, monovalent single-chain Fv (scFv) that is comprised of the variable domains ($V_H$ and $V_L$) of an antibody fused together with a short peptide linker. Novel, bispecific antibody-based structures can facilitate binding to two tumor antigens or bridge tumor cells with immune effector cells to focus antibody-dependent cell-mediated cytotoxicity (ADCC) or killing by T cells. An example of the former is MM-111, a bispecific gene-fused molecule composed of an anti-HER2 scFv connected to an anti-HER3 scFv via a modified form of human serum albumin.[15] Examples of the latter mechanism include small scFv-based bispecific T-cell engagers (BiTE) such as the anti-CD3/anti-CD19 molecule blinatumomab[16] and larger MAb-based antibodies such as catumaxomab, a rat/mouse anti-CD3/EpCAM bispecific MAb produced via quadroma technology.[17] Both classes of bispecifics endow selectivity and targeting properties that are not obtainable with natural antibody formats.

## TABLE 29.1

### FDA Approved Antibodies for the Treatment of Cancer

| Generic Name (Trade Name) | Origin | Isotype (Conjugate) | Indication | Target | Initial Approval |
|---|---|---|---|---|---|
| **Unconjugated MAbs** | | | | | |
| Rituximab (Rituxan) | Chimeric | IgG1 | NHL | CD20 | 1997 |
| Trastuzumab (Herceptin) | Humanized | IgG1 | BrCa | HER2 | 1998 |
| Alemtuzumab (Campath-1H) | Humanized | IgG1 | CLL | CD52 | 2001 |
| Cetuximab (Erbitux) | Chimeric | IgG1 | CRC, SCCHN | EGFR | 2004 |
| Bevacizumab (Avastin) | Humanized | IgG1 | CRC, NSCLC, RCC, GBM | VEGF | 2004 |
| Panitumumab (Vectibix) | Human (XenoMouse) | IgG2 | CRC | EGFR | 2006 |
| Ofatumumab (Arzerra) | Human (XenoMouse) | IgG1 | CLL | CD20 | 2009 |
| Denosumab (Prolia/Xgeva) | Human | IgG2 | Metastasis-related SREs, ADT/AI-associated osteoporosis, GCT | RANKL | 2010 |
| Pertuzumab (Perjeta) | Humanized | IgG1 | BrCa | HER2 | 2012 |
| **Immunoconjugates** | | | | | |
| Gemtuzumab ozogamicin (Mylotarg) | Humanized | IgG4 (calicheamicin) | AML | CD33 | 2000[a] |
| Ibritumomab tiuxetan (Zevalin) | Murine | IgG1 ($^{90}$Y) | NHL | CD20 | 2002 |
| Tositumomab (Bexxar) | Murine | IgG2A ($^{131}$I) | NHL | CD20 | 2003 |
| Brentuximab vedotin (Adcetris) | Chimeric | IgG1 (MMAE) | HL, sALCL | CD30 | 2011 |
| Ado-trastuzumab emtansine (Kadcyla) | Humanized | IgG1 (DM1) | BrCa | HER2 | 2013 |

[a] Withdrawn from the US market in June 2010.
NHL, non-Hodgkin lymphoma; BrCa, breast cancer; CLL, chronic lymphocytic leukemia; CRC, colorectal cancer; SCCHN, squamous cell carcinoma of head and neck; EGFR, epidermal growth factor receptor; NSCLC, non–small-cell lung cancer; RCC, renal cell carcinoma; GBM, glioblastoma multiforme; VEGF, vascular endothelial growth factor; SREs, skeletal-related events; ADT, androgen deprivation therapy; AI, aromatase inhibitor; GCT, giant cell tumor; RANKL, RANK ligand; AML, acute myelogenous leukemia; $^{90}$Y, yttrium-90; $^{131}$I, iodine-131; MMAE, Monomethyl auristatin E; HL, Hodgkin lymphoma; sALCL, systemic anaplastic large-cell lymphoma.

## IgG

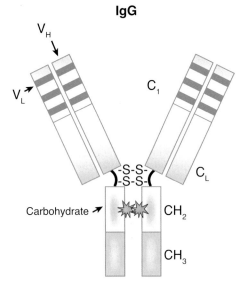

**Figure 29.1** Structure of an IgG. C, constant; V, variable; H, heavy chain; L, light chain.

## TABLE 29.2

### Rules for Naming MAb for the Treatment of Cancer

The International Nonproprietary Names (INN) for monoclonal antibodies (MAbs) are composed of "stems" that indicate their origin, specificity, and modifications. The names include a random prefix to provide distinction from other names, a substem indicating the target specificity (-t[u]- for tumor), a substem indicating the species of origin (see the following) and a suffix (-*mab*), which indicates the presence of an immunoglobulin variable domain.

| Substem Indication of the Species on Which the Immunoglobulin Sequence Is Based | |
|---|---|
| -o- | mouse |
| -xi- | chimeric |
| -zu- | humanized |
| -xizu- | chimeric/humanized |
| -u- | human |

# FACTORS REGULATING ANTIBODY-BASED TUMOR TARGETING

## Antibody Size

Nonuniform distribution of systemically administered antibody is generally observed in biopsied specimens of solid tumors. Heterogeneous tumor blood supply limits uniform antibody delivery to tumors, and elevated interstitial pressures in the center of tumors oppose inward diffusion.[18] This high interstitial pressure slows the diffusion of molecules from their vascular extravasation site in a size-dependent manner.[19,20] The relatively large transport distances in the tumor interstitium also substantially increase the time required for large IgG macromolecules to reach target cells.[21]

## Tumor Antigens

Access to the target antigen is undoubtedly a critical determinant of therapeutic effect of antibody-based applications. Such access is regulated by the heterogeneity of antigen expression by tumor cells. Shed antigen in the serum, tumor microenvironment, or both may saturate the antibody's binding sites and prevent binding to the cell surface. Alternatively, a rapid internalization of an antibody/antigen complex, although critical for antibody–drug conjugates (ADC), may deplete the quantity of cell surface MAb capable of initiating ADCC or cytotoxic signal transduction events. Finally, target antigens are normally *tumor associated* rather than *tumor specific*. Tumor-specific antigens are both highly desirable and rare. Typically, such antigens arise as a result of unique tumor-based genetic recombinations, such as clonal immunoglobulin idiotypes expressed on the surface of B-cell lymphomas.[22]

Antibody affinity for its target antigen has complex effects on tumor targeting. The *binding-site barrier* hypothesis postulates that antibodies with extremely high affinity for target antigen would bind irreversibly to the first antigen encountered upon entering the tumor, which would limit the diffusion of the antibody into the tumor and accumulate instead in regions surrounding the tumor vasculature.[23,24] Similarly, in tumor spheroids, the in vitro penetration of engineered antibodies is primarily limited by internalization and degradation.[25] The valence of an antibody molecule can increase the functional affinity of the antibody through an avidity effect.[26–28]

## Half-Life/Clearance Rate

The concentration of intact IgG in mammalian serum is maintained at constant levels with half-lives of IgGs measured in days. This homeostasis is regulated in part by the major histocompatibility complex (MHC)-class I–related Fc receptor, FcRn (n = neonatal), a saturable, pH-dependent salvage mechanism that regulates quality and quantity of IgG in serum. This mechanism can be exploited via mutations in the Fc portion of an IgG to modulate IgGs pharmacokinetics.[29,30] Indeed, multiple strategies have been developed to increase the serum persistence of antibody-based fragments and other classes of protein therapeutics.[14,31]

## Glycosylation

IgGs undergo N-linked glycosylation at the conserved Asn residue at position 297 within the $C_H2$ domain of the constant region. Glycosylation status of the residue has long been known to impact the ability of IgGs to bind effector ligands such as FcγR and C1q, which, in turn, affects their ability to participate in Fc-mediated functions such as ADCC and complement-dependent cytotoxicity (CDC).[32–34] The glycosylation of MAbs can be altered to increase ADCC by producing them in a cell line engineered to express β(1,4)-N-acetylglucosaminyltransferase III (GnTIII), the enzyme

required to add the bisecting GlcNAc residues.[33] Defucosylation of antibody Fc domains is also associated with enhanced ADCC, and in a recently completed multicenter phase II trial of a defucosylated anti-CC chemokine receptor 4 (CCR4), MAb was associated with meaningful antitumor activity, including complete responses and enhanced progression-free survival (PFS).[35]

# UNCONJUGATED ANTIBODIES

The majority of monoclonal antibodies approved for clinical use display intrinsic antitumor effects that are mediated by one or more of the following mechanisms.

## Cell-Mediated Cytotoxicity

As components of the immune system, effector cells such as natural killer (NK) cells and monocytes/macrophages represent natural lines of defense against oncologically transformed cells. These effector cells express Fcγ receptors (FcγR) on their cell surfaces, which interact with the Fc domain of IgG molecules. This family is comprised of three classes (type I, II, and III) that are further divided into subclasses (IIa/IIb and IIIa/IIIb).[36] Recognition of transformed cells by immune effector cells leads to cell-mediated killing through processes such as ADCC and phagocytosis, as shown in Figure 29.2, and can be mediated by FcγRI (CD64), a high affinity receptor capable of binding to monomeric IgG, or FcγRII (CD32) and FcγRIII (CD16), which are low affinity receptors that preferentially bind multimeric complexes of IgG. Signaling through type I, IIa, and IIIa receptors results in the activation of effector cells due to associated immunoreceptor tyrosine-based activation motifs (ITAM), whereas the engagement of type IIb receptors inhibits cell activation through associated immunoreceptor tyrosine-based inhibitory motifs (ITIM).[36] Clinical results support the idea that ADCC can play a role in the efficacy of antibody-based therapies. Naturally occurring polymorphisms in FcγRs alter their affinity for human IgG1 and have been linked to clinical response.[37,38] A polymorphism in the FCGR3A gene results in either a valine or phenylalanine at position 158 of FcγRIIIa. Human IgG1 binds more strongly to FcγRIIIa-158V than FcγRIIIa-158F, and likewise to NK cells from individuals that are either homozygous for 158F or heterozygous for this polymorphism.[39] The FcγRIIIa-158v was a predictor of early response and was associated with improved PFS.

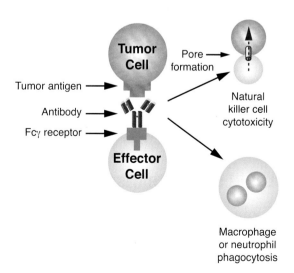

**Figure 29.2** Antibody-dependent cellular cytotoxicity. The antibody engages the tumor antigen and the Fc domain binds to cellular Fc receptors to bridge effector and target cells. This bridging induces effector cell activation, resulting in natural killer cell cytotoxicity or phagocytosis by neutrophils, monocytes, or macrophages.

A second polymorphism, FcγRIIa-131H/R, did not predict early response but was an independent predictor of time to progression (TTP).[38] Taken together, these data suggest that modulating the affinity of MAbs for FcγRIIIa, FcγRIIa, or both may increase the efficacy of therapeutic MAbs.

Each class of FcγR exhibits a characteristic specificity for IgG subclasses.[40] Many groups have focused on modifying the Fc domain of IgGs to optimize the engagement of subclasses of FcγR and the induction of ADCC, based on the findings of Shields et al.,[29] who performed a series of mutagenesis experiments to map the residues required for IgG1-FcγR interaction. Antibodies such as ocrelizumab, a humanized version of rituximab, have increased binding to low affinity FcγRIIIa variants and are now in clinical trials.

An alternative to modifying the Fc region of MAbs is to create bispecific antibodies (bsAbs) that recognize both a tumor-associated antigen and a *trigger antigen* present on the surface of an immune effector cell.[43] Simultaneous engagement of both antigens can redirect the cytotoxic potential of the effector cell against the tumor.[41–43] Such antibodies are capable of eliciting effector function against tumor cell lines in vitro and in animal models. Two HER-2 directed bispecific antibodies, 2B1 and MDX-H210, have been tested in phase I clinical trials.[44,45]

Bispecific antibodies have a number of distinctive properties, including flexible choices of cytotoxic trigger molecules,[46] recruitment of effector function in the presence of excess IgG,[42] and custom tailoring of the affinity of the bsAb to match effector cell characteristics. These advantages have been facilitated by improved methods of bsAb production.[47] BiTE antibodies represent a novel class of bispecific, single-chain Fv antibodies.[48] Promising results have been seen in early phase clinical trials with at least two BiTE antibodies, one of which, blinatumomab, targets CD19/CD3.[49] Promising phase I results have also been reported in an interim analysis of an anti-EpCAM/anti-CD3 MT110 BiTE in the setting of advanced lung and gastrointestinal tumors.[50]

### Complement-Dependent Cytotoxicity

In addition to cell-mediated killing (see previous), MAbs can recruit the complement cascade to kill cells via CDC. Although IgM is the most effective isotype for complement activation, it is not widely used in clinical oncology. Similar to ADCC, the human IgG subclass used to construct a therapeutic MAb dictates its ability to elicit CDC; IgG1 is extremely efficient at fixing complement, in contrast to IgG2 and IgG4.[51] Antibodies activate complement through the classical pathway, by engaging multiple C1q to trigger activation of a cascade of serum proteases, which kill the antibody-bound cells.[52,53] The anti-CD20 MAb rituximab has been found to depend in part on CDC for its *in vivo* efficacy.[54] Antibody engineering approaches have identified residues in the $C_H2$ domain of the Fc region that either suppress or enhance the ability of rituximab to bind C1q and activate CDC.[55] The ability to manipulate complement fixation through engineering approaches warrants *in vivo* testing to determine the impact of these changes on the efficacy and toxicity of MAbs.

### ALTERING SIGNAL TRANSDUCTION

Growth factor receptors represent a well-established class of targets for therapeutic intervention. Normal signaling through these receptors often leads to mitogenic and prosurvival responses. Unregulated signaling, as seen in a number of common cancers due to receptor overexpression, promotes tumor cell growth and insensitivity to chemotherapeutic agents. Clinically relevant MAbs can modulate signaling through their target receptors to normalize cell growth rates and sensitize tumor cells to cytotoxic agents. The binding of cetuximab or panitumumab to the epidermal growth factor receptor (EGFR) physically blocks ligand binding[56] and

prevents the receptor from assuming the extended conformation required for dimerization.[57] Pertuzumab binds to the dimerization domain of HER-2, thereby sterically inhibiting subsequent receptor heterodimerization with other ligand-bound family members.[58] Alternatively, signaling through growth factor receptors can be indirectly modified by MAbs that bind to activating ligands, as is seen with the anti–vascular endothelial growth factor (VEGF) MAb, bevacizumab.[59]

## IMMUNOCONJUGATES

MAbs that are not capable of directly eliciting antitumor effects, either by altering signal transduction or directing immune system cells, can still be effective against tumors by delivering cytotoxic payloads. MAbs have been employed to deliver a wide variety of agents, including chemotherapy, toxins, radioisotopes, and cytokines (for review see Adams and Weiner[60]). In theory, the appropriate combination of toxic agents and MAbs could lead to a synergistic effect. For example, delivery of a therapeutic radioisotope by a MAb would be significantly enhanced if, by binding to its target antigen, the MAb also activated a signaling event that increased the target cell's sensitivity to ionizing radiation.

Catalytic toxins derived from plants catalytic toxins derived from plants (e.g., ricin) and microorganisms (e.g., Pseudomonas) represent two classes of cytotoxic agent that have been investigated for their utility in immunoconjugate strategies.[61] Although there are promising preclinical studies,[62] few successful clinical trials have been reported using this approach. In a phase I clinical trial in hairy cell leukemia patients who were resistant to cladribine, 11 of 16 patients exhibited complete remissions with minimal side effects with an anti-CD22 immunotoxin with a truncated form of *Pseudomonas exotoxin*.[63] Clinical trials with other immunotoxins have been associated with unacceptable neurotoxicity[64] and life-threatening vascular leak syndrome.[65]

Immunocytokine fusions have also been investigated as an approach to direct the patient's immune response to his or her own tumor.[66] A number of cytokines have been incorporated into antibody-based constructs, including interleukin-2 (IL-2),[67,68] interferon γ (IFN-γ),[69] tumor necrosis factor α (TFN-α),[69] VEGF,[70] and IL-12.[71]

### Antibody–Drug Conjugates

The first ADC, gemtuzumab ozogamicin (Mylotarg), was approved by the FDA in 2000 for the treatment of patients with relapsed CD33-positive acute myeloid leukemia, but was voluntarily withdrawn from the US market by its manufacturer in 2010 after a confirmatory phase III trial (SWOG S0106) recommended, based on results of a planned interim analysis, that Mylotarg randomizations be terminated due to a lack of efficacy in the presence of enhanced toxicity.[72] Although two additional randomized trials[73,74] suggested that some patient populations may benefit from Mylotarg therapy, the drug remains off the market in the United States.

The majority of ADCs under development employ potent cytotoxic agents that block the polymerization of tubulin (e.g., auristatins or maytansines) or damage DNA (e.g., calicheamicins or pyrrolobenzodiazepines) by employing a variety of linkers and conjugation strategies.[75]

A variety of ADCs specific for a wide range of oncology targets are currently in clinical evaluation, with the majority of the more advanced agents being tested in the setting of diffuse malignancies.[76] The majority of these employ auristatins or maytansines as their payloads. Early observations suggest that cumulative, dose-related peripheral sensory neuropathy can result when auristatins are conjugated to an antibody via a cleavable linker, and dose-limiting thrombocytopenia can result when auristatins and maytansinoids are conjugated to the antibody via an uncleavable linker.[76,77]

Two ADCs are now approved for use in clinical practice. Ado-trastuzumab emtansine (T-DM1, Kadcyla), an ADC composed of the anti-HER2 MAb trastuzumab linked to DM1,[78] is now approved for the treatment of patients with refractory HER2/neu expressing breast cancers. The other, brentuximab vedotin (SGN-35, Adcetris), is an ADC consisting of the anti-CD30 chimeric MAb cAC10 that is linked to three to five molecules of the microtubule-disrupting agent Monomethyl auristatin E. At this point, this drug is approved for use in patients with recurrent systemic anaplastic large cell lymphoma. The clinical data associated with both of these ADCs will be discussed in subsequent sections of this chapter.

Antibodies also can be used to target liposome-encapsulated drugs[79] and other cytotoxic agents, such as antisense RNA[80] or radionuclides to tumors.

## Radioimmunoconjugates

Two anti-CD20 radioimmunoconjugates have been FDA approved for radioimmunotherapy (RIT) of non-Hodgkin lymphoma (NHL). Ibritumomab (Zevalin) and tositumomab (Bexxar) are murine MAbs labeled with yttrium-90 ($^{90}$Y) and iodine-131 ($^{131}$I), respectively. Both are associated with impressive clinical efficacy.[81,82] Although these radioimmunoconjugates are effective therapeutics, cumbersome logistics surrounding their administration have significantly limited their use. Despite significant preclinical evidence supporting the use of RIT for solid malignancies, clinical results have not demonstrated consistent antitumor activity.[60]

## ANTIBODIES APPROVED FOR USE IN SOLID TUMORS

### Trastuzumab

Trastuzumab (Herceptin) is a humanized IgG1[83] that targets domain IV of the HER2/ErbB2 member of the EGFR/ErbB family of receptor tyrosine kinases. Gene amplification as judged by fluorescence in situ hybridization (FISH) with concomitant overexpression of HER2 protein measured by immunohistochemistry (IHC) is seen in approximately 25% of breast cancers.[84,85] HER2 amplification and overexpression is now recognized to also be a critical driver in a subset (7% to 34%) of gastric cancers.[86] Trastuzumab inhibits tumor cell growth by binding to HER2 and blocking the unregulated HER2 signaling that is associated with its high level overexpression.

Trastuzumab became the first FDA-approved monoclonal antibody for the treatment of solid tumors based on a series of studies carried out in the setting of HER2-positive metastatic breast cancer.[87,88] A subsequent phase III trial investigating trastuzumab in combination with cytotoxic chemotherapy demonstrated an improved response rate compared to chemotherapy alone, from 25.0% to 57.3% with a taxane regimen.[89]

Trastuzumab is also approved for use in the adjuvant setting based on an approximately 50% reduction in recurrence after 1 year in multiple phase III trials.[90–92] Myocardial dysfunction, seen with anthracycline therapy, was observed with increased frequency in patients receiving antibody alone[93] or with doxorubicin or epirubicin.

Recognition of HER2 as a driver in a subset of gastric cancers led to an open-label, randomized, phase III trial (ToGA) that investigated the addition of trastuzumab to standard of care chemotherapy[94] and showed increased median overall survival with higher levels of HER2 expression. A study by Gomez-Martin et al.[95] in 99 patients with metastatic gastric cancer being treated with first-line trastuzumab plus chemotherapy identified a mean HER2/CEP17 ratio of 4.7 to be an optimal cut-off to discriminate between trastuzumab-sensitive and refractory patients.

### Pertuzumab

Pertuzumab (Perjeta) is a humanized IgG1 MAb that binds to domain II of HER2 and blocks ligand-dependent dimerization of HER2 with other members of the EGFR family.[96] Pertuzumab, in combination with trastuzumab and docetaxel, is approved for use as first-line therapy in HER2-positive metastatic breast cancer patients. Use of the combination is also approved for the treatment of HER2-positive, locally advanced, inflammatory, or high-risk early breast cancer (>2 cm node negative or node positive) in the neoadjuvant setting.

FDA-approval of pertuzumab was based on results of a phase III trial (CLEOPATRA) of 808 patients with locally recurrent, unresectable, or metastatic breast cancer randomized to receive trastuzumab plus docetaxel with or without the addition of pertuzumab. Inclusion of pertuzumab increased the independently assessed PFS by 6.1 months from 12.4 to 18.5 (hazard ratio [HR], 0.62 (95% confidence interval [CI], 0.51, 0.75], p <0.0001], with a trend toward improved overall survival[97] that reached statistical significance (p = 0.0008) after an additional year of follow-up.[98] The addition of pertuzumab did increase rates of grade 3 adverse events (AE), but it did not adversely affect cardiac function. Accelerated approval was granted for use of pertuzumab in combination with trastuzumab and docetaxel for the neoadjuvant treatment of high-risk early-stage breast cancer. This approval was based on results from a four-arm, open-label phase II study of 417 patients randomized to receive trastuzumab plus docetaxel, pertuzumab plus docetaxel, pertuzumab plus trastuzumab, or the triple combination. The triple combination improved the pathologic complete response (pCR) rate by 17.8% over the trastuzumab plus docetaxel arm (39.3% versus 21.5%) in the pertuzumab arm.[99] Follow-up studies to confirm a correlation between pCR and long-term clinical benefit are ongoing.

### Cetuximab

Cetuximab (Erbitux) targets the EGFR. This chimeric IgG1 binds to domain III of the EGFR, with roughly a tenfold higher affinity than either EGF or transforming growth factor α (TGF-α) ligands and thereby inhibits ligand-induced activation of this tyrosine kinase receptor. Cetuximab may also function to downregulate EGFR-dependent signaling by stimulating EGFR internalization.[100] Cetuximab is approved for the treatment of colorectal cancer (CRC) and, more recently, for the treatment of squamous cell cancer of the head and neck (SCCHN).

The efficacy and safety of cetuximab against CRC was demonstrated alone and in combination with irinotecan in a phase II, multicenter, randomized, and controlled trial of 329 patients.[101] The combination of irinotecan plus cetuximab increased both the overall response and the median duration of response as compared to cetuximab alone. Additionally, patients with irinotecan refractory disease responded to treatment with the combination regimen. Recent studies in patients with colorectal cancers have indicated that patients with KRAS mutations in codon 12 or 13 should not receive anti-EGFR therapy.[101,102]

An international, multicenter, phase III trial comparing definitive radiotherapy to radiotherapy plus cetuximab in SCCHN demonstrated that EGFR blockade with radiotherapy significantly reduced the risk of locoregional failure by 32% and the risk of death by 26%. In advanced stage non–small-cell lung cancer (NSCLC) expressing EGFR, the combination of cetuximab and standard doublet chemotherapy (cisplatin plus vinorelbine) was studied in a prospective randomized phase III trial.[103] The addition of cetuximab was associated with a slight, but statistically significant, benefit in overall survival over chemotherapy alone (median overall survival 10.1 versus 11.3 months). A similar study using the carboplatin plus paclitaxel backbone in combination with cetuximab did not meet its primary endpoint of improved PFS, although cetuximab-treated patients exhibited higher objective response rates.[104] Therefore, the benefit of adding cetuximab to standard chemotherapy for patients with advanced NSCLC is unclear.

## Panitumumab

Panitumumab (Vectibix) is a fully human IgG2 monoclonal antibody that binds to EGFR. Similar to cetuximab, panitumumab inhibits EGFR activation by blocking the binding of EGF and TGF-α. However, it does so by binding to EGFR with a higher affinity than cetuximab ($5 \times 10^{-11}$ M versus $1 \times 10^{-10}$ M). As previously mentioned, the IgG2 class of antibodies does not induce activation of the immune system cell via the Fc-receptor mechanism, so panitumumab's primary action appears to be interference with EGFR–ligand interactions.

A phase III trial of 463 patients with metastatic colorectal cancer compared panitumumab plus best supportive care (BSC) to BSC alone.[105] A partial-response rate of 8% and a stable-disease rate of 28% were reported for the panitumumab arm compared with a 10% stable-disease rate in the best supportive care arm of the study. As with cetuximab, patients with metastatic colorectal cancers who have KRAS mutations in codons 12 or 13 are not routinely offered therapy with panitumumab.[106]

## Bevacizumab

Bevacizumab (Avastin or rhuMAb VEGF) is a humanized monoclonal antibody targeting VEGF. VEGF is a critical determinant of tumor angiogenesis, a process that is a necessary component of tumor invasion, growth, and metastasis. VEGF expression by invasive tumors has been shown to correlate with vascularity and cellular proliferation and is prognostic for several human cancers.[107–109] Interestingly, the inhibition of VEGF signaling via bevacizumab treatment may normalize tumor vasculature, promoting a more effective delivery of chemotherapy agents.[110] Bevacizumab is approved for use as a first-line therapy for metastatic colorectal cancer and NSCLC when given in combination with appropriate cytotoxic chemotherapy regimens. Phase III clinical trials leading to the approval of bevacizumab for the treatment of colorectal cancer demonstrated improved response rates from 35% to 45% compared to fluorouracil (5-FU)–based chemotherapy alone. Enhanced response durations and improved patient survival were seen in patients treated with chemotherapy plus bevacizumab as compared to patients receiving chemotherapy alone.[111] A survival benefit was also seen in the setting of NSCLC. A randomized phase III trial (ECOG 4599) of paclitaxel and carboplatin with or without bevacizumab in patients with advanced nonsquamous NSCLC led to a significant improvement in median survival (12.5 months versus 10.2 months; p = 0.0075) for patients in the bevacizumab arm,[112] with significantly higher response rates. A higher incidence of bleeding was associated with bevacizumab (4.5% versus 0.7%). Five of 10 treatment-related deaths occurred as a result of hemoptysis, all in the bevacizumab arm.

A phase III trial randomized 722 patients with metastatic breast cancer with no prior chemotherapy for advanced disease to either paclitaxel or paclitaxel and bevacizumab.[113] PFS was significantly better in the paclitaxel plus bevacizumab arm (median, 11.8 versus 5.9 months; HR for progression, 0.60; p <0.001) with an increased response rate (36.9% versus 21.2%, p <0.001). Overall survival, however, was similar.

In contrast,[114] in a randomized phase III trial, capecitabine/bevacizumab increased response rates compared with capecitabine alone in 462 anthracycline and taxane pretreated metastatic breast cancer patients but did not meet its primary endpoint of improved PFS. Overall survival and time to deterioration in quality of life were comparable in both treatment groups.

Bevacizumab has not demonstrated activity in the adjuvant colorectal and breast cancer settings.[115,116] There was no improvement in overall survival between the two groups and the rate of invasive disease-free survival was also not significantly different between the treatment groups.

Bevacizumab is also approved for the management of recurrent glioblastomas based on results of phase II studies.[117]

## Ado-Trastuzumab Emtansine

Ado-trastuzumab emtansine (T-DM1, Kadcyla) is an ADC composed of the anti-HER2 MAb trastuzumab linked to DM1, a highly potent derivative of maytansine, through a stable thioether linker.[78]

Based on two single-agent phase II trials of T-DM1[118,119] that demonstrated single-agent activity in the setting of metastatic breast cancer, two separate phase III studies were conducted. The 991 patient EMILIA trial demonstrated that T-DM1 significantly prolongs both PFS and overall survival as compared to a regimen of lapatinib plus capecitabine when used in the setting of metastatic breast cancer that had progressed after treatment with trastuzumab plus a taxane.[120] Grade 3 and worse AEs were lower in the T-DM1 arm (200, 40.8%) as compared to the lapatinib plus capecitabine arm (278, 57%). Results are still awaited from the ongoing MARIANNE trial that is assessing first-line efficacy and safety of T-DM1 alone and T-DM1 plus pertuzumab versus trastuzumab plus taxane (NCT01120184).

## Denosumab

Denosumab (Xgeva) is a fully human IgG2 RANK ligand (RANKL) neutralizing antibody. Denosumab is FDA-approved for use in adults and skeletally mature adolescents who have either surgically unsalvageable giant cell tumors of the bone (GCTB) or where resection is anticipated to result in severe morbidity. Approval was based in part on two open-label, phase II trials examining subcutaneous administration of 120 mg q4 week with additional loading doses on days 8 and 15 of the first cycle.[121,122] Serious adverse events were seen in 9% of patients (n = 25). Of 187 patients, 47 (25%) exhibited partial objective responses based on modified Response Evaluation Criteria in Solid Tumors (RECIST) criteria.

Denosumab is also approved in for use in two supportive care settings based on three randomized, double-blind, placebo-controlled phase III trials evaluating its efficacy versus zoledronic acid[123–125] to reduce bone metastasis-related skeletal-related events (SRE). Based on data from two phase III trials, a second formulation and dosing schedule of denosumab is approved to increase bone mass in prostate cancer[126] and breast cancer[127] patients at high risk for bone fracture due to hormone-ablation therapies.

# ANTIBODIES USED IN HEMATOLOGIC MALIGNANCIES

## Rituximab

Rituximab (Rituxan) is a chimeric anti-CD20 monoclonal antibody that was the first MAb to be approved by the FDA for use in human malignancy.[128,129] Studies have shown that multiple doses can be safely administered, and in vitro studies have demonstrated multiple mechanisms by which anti-CD20 antibodies can lead to cell death.[130] Efficacy of rituximab monotherapy is well established.[131]

Rituximab has been tested in conjunction with chemotherapy based on supportive preclinical data.[132,133] The combination of rituximab with cyclophosphamide, doxorubicin, vincristine, and prednisolone (CHOP) resulted in a 95% overall response rate (55% complete response, 40% partial response) among 40 patients with low-grade or follicular B-cell non–Hodgkin lymphoma, with molecular complete remissions observed.[134] A long-term study of elderly patients with previously untreated diffuse large-cell lymphoma randomized to either CHOP chemotherapy plus rituximab (R-CHOP) or CHOP alone demonstrated a significant improvement in event-free survival, PFS, disease-free survival, and overall survival for the combination arm.[135] No significant differences in long-term toxicity were noted.

Low-grade B-cell lymphoma patients possessing the 158V/V polymorphism in FcγRIII experience superior response rates and outcomes when treated with rituximab.[37,38] These findings signify that antibody Fc domain::Fc receptor interactions underlie at least some of the clinical benefit of rituximab, and indicate a possible role for ADCC that depends on such interactions.

A combination of active agents (such as lenalidomide and thalidomide) that are also immune modulating may be additive with rituximab,[136] and perhaps synergize by increasing ADCC.[137] Cytokines such as interleukin-2 (IL-2), IL-12, or IL-15 and myeloid growth factors may also enhance therapeutic antibody activity as suggested by preclinical data demonstrating that IL-2 can promote NK cell proliferation and activation and can enhance rituximab activity[138] and clinical efficacy.[139,140] Myeloid growth factors, in combination with rituximab, may also activate ADCC.[141] Alternative approaches to induce effector cell activity by combining Toll-like receptors (TLR) agonists, such as CpG oligonucleotides, have been investigated.[142] Altering the balance of proapoptotic and antiapoptotic signals could generate more rituximab-induced cytotoxicity. BCL-2 downregulation by antisense oligonucleotides was found to enhance rituximab efficacy in preclinical testing.[143,144] However, small molecules that bind to the BH-3 domain common to many members of the BCL-2 family of proteins may be better therapeutic agents.[145–147]

## Ofatumumab

The anti-CD20 ofatumumab[148] is a fully human antibody that binds an epitope on CD20 distinct from that bound by rituximab and is engineered for better complement activation, although it induces less ADCC. Ofatumumab has received regulatory approval for the treatment of patients with fludarabine-refractory chronic lymphocytic leukemia (CLL). In a recently reported, planned interim analysis that included 138 CLL patients with treatment-refractory disease or bulky (>5 cm) lymphadenopathy, treatment with ofatumumab led to an overall response rate (primary endpoint) of 47% in patients with bulky disease and 5% in patients refractory to both alemtuzumab and fludarabine.[149]

Additional humanized anti-CD20 antibodies (veltuzumab[150] and ocrelizumab) are under development.

## Alemtuzumab

Alemtuzumab (Campath-1H) targets the CD52 glycopeptide, which is highly expressed on T and B lymphocytes. It has been tested as a therapeutic agent for CLL and promyelocytic leukemias, as well as other non–Hodgkin lymphomas.

## Brentuximab Vedotin

Brentuximab vedotin (SGN-35, Adcetris) is an ADC consisting of the anti-CD30 chimeric MAb cAC10 that is linked to three to five molecules of the microtubule-disrupting agent Monomethyl auristatin E (MMAE). MMAE is a highly potent derivative of dolastatin. Linkage of MMAE to cAC10 occurs through a protease-cleavable linter.[151] Brentuximab vedotin is approved for treating systemic, chemotherapy-refractory anaplastic large-cell lymphomas (sALCL). It is also approved to treat patients with Hodgkin lymphoma who have progressed after an autologous stem cell transplant (ASCT). Patients ineligible for ASCT must have failed two prior multidrug chemotherapy regimens.

Brentuximab vedotin received accelerated approval in 2011 based in part on the results of two phase II trials. In a multicenter trial conducted by Pro et al.,[152] 58 patients with relapsed or refractory sALCL received brentuximab vedotin (1.8 mg per kilogram per week), and 86% of patients achieved objective response. Complete responses occurred in 57% of patients, with a median duration of 13.2 months. An additional 17 patients (29%) had partial responses. Median overall response was 12.6 months. Most common grade 3 and 4 adverse events (AE) were neutropenia (21%), thrombocytopenia (14%), and peripheral sensory neuropathy (12%). A similar trial, in Hodgkin lymphoma, was reported by Younes et al.[153] Patients (n = 102) that had failed ASCT received brentuximab vedotin on the same schedule as listed previously and were assessed for the objective response rate. In this setting, 75% of patients had objective responses, with 34% being complete remissions. The median duration of complete responses was 20.5 months, and 31 patients were progression free after a median follow-up of 1.5 years. Phase III trials to assess the known risk of neuropathy (AETHERA) and to confirm overall clinical benefit seen in the phase II trials (ECHELON-2, or ClinicalTrials.gov Identifier NCT01712490) are ongoing.

## CONCLUSION

In the 35 years since Kohler and Milstein first developed the hybridoma technology that enabled antibody-based therapeutics, the field has made remarkable progress. Numerous antibody-based molecules are currently in clinical trials and many more are in development. Multiple therapeutic antibodies have a proven clinical benefit and have been licensed by the FDA. The thoughtful application of advances in cancer biology and antibody engineering suggest that this progress will continue.

**CANCER THERAPEUTICS**

## REFERENCES

1. Badger CC, Anasetti C, Davis J, et al. Treatment of malignancy with unmodified antibody. *Pathol Immunopathol Res* 1987;6:419–434.
2. Khazaeli MB, Conry RM, Lobuglio AF. Human immune-response to monoclonal-antibodies. *J Immunother Emphasis Tumor Immunol* 1994;15:42–52.
3. Lee J, Fenton BM, Koch CJ, et al. Interleukin 2 expression by tumor cells alters both the immune response and the tumor microenvironment. *Cancer Res* 1998;58:1478–1485.
4. Reichert JM, Dhimolea E. The future of antibodies as cancer drugs. *Drug Discov Today* 2012;17:954–963.
5. Kohler G, Milstein C. Continuous cultures of fused cells secreting antibody of predefined specificity. *Nature* 1975;256:495–497.
6. Houghton AN, Mintzer D, Cordon-Cardo C, et al. Mouse monoclonal IgG3 antibody detecting GD3 ganglioside: a phase I trial in patients with malignant melanoma. *Proc Natl Acad Sci U S A* 1985;82:1242–1246.
7. Steplewski Z, Lubeck MD, Koprowski H. Human macrophages armed with murine immunoglobulin G2a antibodies to tumors destroy human cancer cells. *Science* 1983;221:865–867.
8. Trauth BC, Klas C, Peters AM, et al. Monoclonal antibody-mediated tumor regression by induction of apoptosis. *Science* 1989;245:301–305.
9. Yang XD, Jia XC, Corvalan JR, et al. Eradication of established tumors by a fully human monoclonal antibody to the epidermal growth factor receptor without concomitant chemotherapy. *Cancer Res* 1999;59:1236–1243.

10. Komissarov AA, Calcutt MJ, Marchbank MT, et al. Equilibrium binding studies of recombinant anti-single-stranded DNA Fab. Role of heavy chain complementarity-determining regions. *J Biol Chem* 1996;271:12241–12246.
11. Ghetie V, Popov S, Borvak J, et al. Increasing the serum persistence of an IgG fragment by random mutagenesis. *Nat Biotechnol* 1997;15:637–640.
12. LoBuglio AF, Wheeler RH, Trang J, et al. Mouse/human chimeric monoclonal antibody in man: kinetics and immune response. *Proc Natl Acad Sci U S A* 1989;86:4220–4224.
13. Kudo T, Saeki H, Tachibana T. A simple and improved method to generate human hybridomas. *J Immunol Methods* 1991;145:119–125.
14. Robinson MK, Weiner LM, Adams GP. Improving monoclonal antibodies for cancer therapy. *Drug Dev Res* 2004;61:172–187.
15. Denlinger CS, Beeram M, Tolcher AW, et al. A phase I/II and pharmacologic study of MM-111 in patients with advanced, refractory HER2-positive (HER2+) cancers. *J Clin Oncol* 2010;28:15s.
16. Nagorsen D, Bargou R, Ruttinger D, et al. Immunotherapy of lymphoma and leukemia with T-cell engaging BiTE antibody blinatumomab. *Leuk Lymphoma* 2009;50:886–891.
17. Goere D, Flament C, Rusakiewicz S, et al. Potent immunomodulatory effects of the trifunctional antibody catumaxomab. *Cancer Res* 2013;73:4663–4673.
18. Jain RK. Transport of molecules in the tumor interstitium: a review. *Cancer Res* 1987;47:3039–3051.

19. Jain RK. Physiological barriers to delivery of monoclonal antibodies and other macromolecules in tumors. *Cancer Res* 1990;50:814s–819s.

20. Jain RK, Baxter LT. Mechanisms of heterogeneous distribution of monoclonal antibodies and other macromolecules in tumors: significance of elevated interstitial pressure. *Cancer Res* 1988;48:7022–7032.

21. Jain RK. Transport of molecules across tumor vasculature. *Cancer Metastasis Rev* 1987;6:559–593.

22. Miller RA, Maloney DG, Warnke R, et al. Treatment of B-cell lymphoma with monoclonal anti-idiotype antibody. *N Engl J Med* 1982;306:517–522.

23. Fujimori K, Covell DG, Fletcher JE, et al. A modeling analysis of monoclonal antibody percolation through tumors: a binding site barrier. *J Nucl Med* 1990;31:1191–1198.

24. Rudnick SI, Lou J, Shaller CC, et al. Influence of affinity and antigen internalization on the uptake and penetration of Anti-HER2 antibodies in solid tumors. *Cancer Res* 2011;71:2250–2259.

25. Thurber GM, Wittrup KD. Quantitative spatiotemporal analysis of antibody fragment diffusion and endocytic consumption in tumor spheroids. *Cancer Res* 2008;68:3334–3341.

26. Adams GP, Tai MS, McCartney JE, et al. Avidity-mediated enhancement of in vivo tumor targeting by single-chain Fv dimers. *Clin Cancer Res* 2006;12:1599–1605.

27. Wolff EA, Schreiber GJ, Cosand WL, et al. Monoclonal antibody homodimers: enhanced antitumor activity in nude mice. *Cancer Res* 1993;53:2560–2565.

28. Werlen RC, Lankinen M, Offord RE, et al. Preparation of a trivalent antigen-binding construct using polyoxime chemistry: improved biodistribution and potential for therapeutic application. *Cancer Res* 1996;56:809–815.

29. Shields RL, Namenuk AK, Hong K, et al. High resolution mapping of the binding site on human IgG1 for Fc gamma RI, Fc gamma RII, Fc gamma RIII, and FcRn and design of IgG1 variants with improved binding to the Fc gamma R. *J Biol Chem* 2001;276:6591–6604.

30. Kenanova V, Olafsen T, Crow DM, et al. Tailoring the pharmacokinetics and positron emission tomography imaging properties of anti-carcinoembryonic antigen single-chain Fv-Fc antibody fragments. *Cancer Res* 2005;65:622–631.

31. McDonagh CF, Huhalov A, Harms BD, et al. Antitumor activity of a novel bispecific antibody that targets the ErbB2/ErbB3 oncogenic unit and inhibits heregulin-induced activation of ErbB3. *Mol Cancer Ther* 2012;11:582–593.

32. Lund J, Takahashi N, Pound JD, et al. Multiple interactions of IgG with its core oligosaccharide can modulate recognition by complement and human Fc gamma receptor I and influence the synthesis of its oligosaccharide chains. *J Immunol* 1996;157:4963–4969.

33. Umana P, Jean-Mairet J, Moudry R, et al. Engineered glycoforms of an antineuroblastoma IgG1 with optimized antibody-dependent cellular cytotoxic activity. *Nat Biotechnol* 1999;17:176–180.

34. Wright A, Morrison SL. Effect of glycosylation on antibody function: implications for genetic engineering. *Trends Biotechnol* 1997;15:26–32.

35. Ishida T, Joh T, Uike N, et al. Defucosylated anti-CCR4 monoclonal antibody (KW-0761) for relapsed adult T-cell leukemia-lymphoma: a multicenter phase II study. *J Clin Oncol* 2012;30:837–842.

36. Raghavan M, Bjorkman PJ. Fc receptors and their interactions with immunoglobulins. *Annu Rev Cell Dev Biol* 1996;12:181–220.

37. Cartron G, Dacheux L, Salles G, et al. Therapeutic activity of humanized anti-CD20 monoclonal antibody and polymorphism in IgG Fc receptor FcgammaRIIIa gene. *Blood* 2002;99:754–758.

38. Weng WK, Levy R. Two immunoglobulin G fragment C receptor polymorphisms independently predict response to rituximab in patients with follicular lymphoma. *J Clin Oncol* 2003;21:3940–3947.

39. Koene HR, Kleijer M, Algra J, et al. Fc gammaRIIIa-158V/F polymorphism influences the binding of IgG by natural killer cell Fc gammaRIIIa, independently of the Fc gammaRIIIa-48L/R/H phenotype. *Blood* 1997;90:1109–1114.

40. Gessner JE, Heiken H, Tamm A, et al. The IgG Fc receptor family. *Ann Hematol* 1998;76:231–248.

41. Keler T, Graziano RF, Mandal A, et al. Bispecific antibody-dependent cellular cytotoxicity of HER2/neu-overexpressing tumor cells by Fcgamma receptor type I-expressing effector cells. *Cancer Res* 1997;57:4008–4014.

42. Weiner LM, Holmes M, Richeson A, et al. Binding and cytotoxicity characteristics of the bispecific murine monoclonal antibody 2B1. *J Immunol* 1993;151:2877–2886.

43. Shalaby MR, Shepard HM, Presta L, et al. Development of humanized bispecific antibodies reactive with cytotoxic lymphocytes and tumor cells overexpressing the HER2 protooncogene. *J Exp Med* 1992;175:217–225.

44. Valone FH, Kaufman PA, Guyre PM, et al. Phase Ia/Ib trial of bispecific antibody MDX-210 in patients with advanced breast or ovarian cancer that overexpresses the proto-oncogene HER-2/neu. *J Clin Oncol* 1995;13:2281–2292.

45. Weiner LM, Clark JI, Davey M, et al. Phase I trial of 2B1, a bispecific monoclonal antibody targeting c-erbB-2 and FcgammaRIII. *Cancer Res* 1995;55:4586–4593.

46. Liu MA, Kranz DM, Kurnick JT, et al. Heteroantibody duplexes target cells for lysis by cytotoxic T lymphocytes. *Proc Natl Acad Sci U S A* 1985;82:8648–8652.

47. Carter P. Bispecific human IgG by design. *J Immunol Methods* 2001;248:7–15.

48. Mack M, Riethmuller G, Kufer P. A small bispecific antibody construct expressed as a functional single-chain molecule with high tumor cell cytotoxicity. *Proc Natl Acad Sci U S A* 1995;92:7021–7025.

49. Bargou R, Leo E, Zugmaier G, et al. Tumor regression in cancer patients by very low doses of a T cell-engaging antibody. *Science* 2008;321:974–977.

50. Fiedler W, Hönemann D, Ritter B, et al. Safety and pharmacology of the EpCAM/CD3-bispecific BiTE antibody MT110 in patients with metastatic colorectal, gastric, and lung cancer. *Eur J Cancer* 2009;7:136–137.

51. Presta LG. Engineering antibodies for therapy. *Curr Pharm Biotechnol* 2002;3:237–256.

52. Makrides SC. Therapeutic inhibition of the complement system. *Pharmacol Rev* 1998;50:59–87.

53. Walport MJ. Complement, First of two parts. *N Engl J Med* 2001;344:1058–1066.

54. Di Gaetano N, Cittera E, Nota R, et al. Complement activation determines the therapeutic activity of rituximab in vivo. *J Immunol* 2003;171:1581–1587.

55. Idusogie EE, Presta LG, Gazzano-Santoro H, et al. Mapping of the C1q binding site on Rituxan, a chimeric antibody with a human IgG1 Fc. *J Immunol* 2000;164:4178–4184.

56. Sunada H, Magun BE, Mendelsohn J, et al. Monoclonal antibody against epidermal growth factor receptor is internalized without stimulating receptor phosphorylation. *Proc Natl Acad Sci U S A* 1986;83:3825–3829.

57. Li S, Schmitz KR, Jeffrey PD, et al. Structural basis for inhibition of the epidermal growth factor receptor by cetuximab. *Cancer Cell* 2005;7:301–311.

58. Franklin MC, Carey KD, Vajdos FF, et al. Insights into ErbB signaling from the structure of the ErbB2-pertuzumab complex. *Cancer Cell* 2004;5:317–328.

59. Presta LG, Chen H, O'Connor SJ, et al. Humanization of an anti-vascular endothelial growth factor monoclonal antibody for the therapy of solid tumors and other disorders. *Cancer Res* 1997;57:4593–4599.

60. Adams GP, Weiner LM. Monoclonal antibody therapy of cancer. *Nat Biotechnol* 2005;23:1147–1157.

61. Reiter Y, Pastan I. Recombinant Fv immunotoxins and Fv fragments as novel agents for cancer therapy and diagnosis. *Trends Biotechnol* 1998;16:513–520.

62. Kreitman RJ, Wang QC, FitzGerald DJ, et al. Complete regression of human B-cell lymphoma xenografts in mice treated with recombinant anti-CD22 immunotoxin RFB4(dsFv)-PE38 at doses tolerated by cynomolgus monkeys. *Int J Cancer* 1999;81:148–155.

63. Kreitman RJ, Wilson WH, Bergeron K, et al. Efficacy of the anti-CD22 recombinant immunotoxin BL22 in chemotherapy-resistant hairy-cell leukemia. *N Engl J Med* 2001;345:241–247.

64. Pai LH, Bookman MA, Ozols RF, et al. Clinical evaluation of intraperitoneal Pseudomonas exotoxin immunoconjugate OVB3-PE in patients with ovarian cancer. *J Clin Oncol* 1991;9:2095–2103.

65. Baluna R, Vitetta ES. Vascular leak syndrome: a side effect of immunotherapy. *Immunopharmacology* 1997;37:117–132.

66. Lode HN, Xiang R, Becker JC, et al. Immunocytokines: a promising approach to cancer immunotherapy. *Pharmacol Ther* 1998;80:277–292.

67. Hornick JL, Khawli LA, Hu P, et al. Pretreatment with a monoclonal antibody/interleukin-2 fusion protein directed against DNA enhances the delivery of therapeutic molecules to solid tumors. *Clin Cancer Res* 1999;5:51–60.

68. Lode HN, Xiang R, Duncan SR, et al. Tumor-targeted IL-2 amplifies T cell-mediated immune response induced by gene therapy with single-chain IL-12. *Proc Natl Acad Sci U S A* 1999;96:8591–8596.

69. Sharifi J, Khawli LA, Hu P, et al. Generation of human interferon gamma and tumor necrosis factor alpha chimeric TNT-3 fusion proteins. *Hybrid Hybridomics* 2002;21:421–432.

70. Halin C, Niesner U, Villani ME, et al. Tumor-targeting properties of antibody-vascular endothelial growth factor fusion proteins. *Int J Cancer* 2002;102:109–116.

71. Halin C, Rondini S, Nilsson F, et al. Enhancement of the antitumor activity of interleukin-12 by targeted delivery to neovasculature. *Nature Biotechnol* 2002;20:264–269.

72. Petersdorf SH, Kopecky KJ, Slovak M, et al. A phase 3 study of gemtuzumab ozogamicin during induction and postconsolidation therapy in younger patients with acute myeloid leukemia. *Blood* 2013;121:4854–4860.

73. Burnett AK, Hills RK, Milligan D, et al. Identification of patients with acute myeloblastic leukemia who benefit from the addition of gemtuzumab ozogamicin: results of the MRC AML15 trial. *J Clin Oncol* 2011;29:369–377.

74. Castaigne S, Pautas C, Terre C, et al. Effect of gemtuzumab ozogamicin on survival of adult patients with de-novo acute myeloid leukaemia (ALFA-0701): a randomised, open-label, phase 3 study. *Lancet* 2012;379:1508–1516.

75. Ducry L, Stump B. Antibody-drug conjugates: linking cytotoxic payloads to monoclonal antibodies. *Bioconjug Chem* 2010;21:5–13.

76. Lambert JM. Drug-conjugated antibodies for the treatment of cancer. *Br J Clin Pharmacol* 2013;76:248–262.

77. van de Donk NW, Dhimolea E. Brentuximab vedotin. *MAbs* 2012;4:458–465.

78. LoRusso PM, Weiss D, Guardino E, et al. Trastuzumab emtansine: a unique antibody-drug conjugate in development for human epidermal growth factor receptor 2-positive cancer. *Clin Cancer Res* 2011;17:6437–6447.

79. Park JW, Hong K, Kirpotin DB, et al. Anti-HER2 immunoliposomes: enhanced efficacy attributable to targeted delivery. *Clin Cancer Res* 2002;8:1172–1181.

80. Rodriguez M, Coma S, Noe V, et al. Development and effects of immunoliposomes carrying an antisense oligonucleotide against DHFR RNA and directed toward human breast cancer cells overexpressing HER2. *Antisense Nucleic Acid Drug Dev* 2002;12:311–325.

81. Juweid ME. Radioimmunotherapy of B-cell non-Hodgkin's lymphoma: from clinical trials to clinical practice. *J Nucl Med* 2002;43:1507–1529.

82. Witzig TE, White CA, Wiseman GA, et al. Phase I/II trial of IDEC-Y2B8 radioimmunotherapy for treatment of relapsed or refractory CD20(+) B-cell non-Hodgkin's lymphoma. *J Clin Oncol* 1999;17:3793–3803.

83. Carter P, Presta L, Gorman CM, et al. Humanization of an anti-p185HER2 antibody for human cancer therapy. *Proc Natl Acad Sci U S A* 1992;89: 4285–4289.

84. Slamon DJ, Clark GM, Wong SG, et al. Human breast cancer: correlation of relapse and survival with amplification of the HER-2/neu oncogene. *Science* 1987;235:177–182.

85. Dawood S, Broglio K, Buzdar AU, et al. Prognosis of women with metastatic breast cancer by HER2 status and trastuzumab treatment: an institutional-based review. *J Clin Oncol* 2010;28:92–98.

86. Tanner M, Hollmen M, Junttila TT, et al. Amplification of HER-2 in gastric carcinoma: association with Topoisomerase IIalpha gene amplification, intestinal type, poor prognosis and sensitivity to trastuzumab. *Ann Oncol* 2005;16:273–278.

87. Baselga J, Tripathy D, Mendelsohn J, et al. Phase II study of weekly intravenous recombinant humanized anti-p185HER2 monoclonal antibody in patients with HER2/neu-overexpressing metastatic breast cancer. *J Clin Oncol* 1996;14:737–744.

88. Cobleigh MA, Vogel CL, Tripathy D, et al. Multinational study of the efficacy and safety of humanized anti-HER2 monoclonal antibody in women who have HER2-overexpressing metastatic breast cancer that has progressed after chemotherapy for metastatic disease. *J Clin Oncol* 1999;17:2639–2648.

89. Slamon D, Leyland-Jones B, Shak S, et al. Addition of Herceptin™ (humanized anti-HER2 antibody) to first line chemotherapy for HER2 overexpressing metastatic breast cancer (HER21/MBC) markedly increases anticancer activity: a randomized multinational controlled phase III trial. *Proc Am Soc Clin Oncol* 1998;17:A377.

90. Piccart-Gebhart MJ, Procter M, Leyland-Jones B, et al. Trastuzumab after adjuvant chemotherapy in HER2-positive breast cancer. *N Engl J Med* 2005;353:1659–1672.

91. Romond EH, Perez EA, Bryant J, et al. Trastuzumab plus adjuvant chemotherapy for operable HER2-positive breast cancer. *N Engl J Med* 2005;353:1673–1684.

92. Smith I, Procter M, Gelber RD, et al. 2-year follow-up of trastuzumab after adjuvant chemotherapy in HER2-positive breast cancer: a randomised controlled trial. *Lancet* 2007;369:29–36.

93. Ewer MS, Gibbs HR, Swafford J, et al. Cardiotoxicity in patients receiving transtuzumab (Herceptin): primary toxicity, synergistic or sequential stress, or surveillance artifact? *Semin Oncol* 1999;26:96–101.

94. Bang YJ, Van Cutsem E, Feyereislova A, et al. Trastuzumab in combination with chemotherapy versus chemotherapy alone for treatment of HER2-positive advanced gastric or gastro-oesophageal junction cancer (ToGA): a phase 3, open-label, randomised controlled trial. *Lancet* 2010;376:687–697.

95. Gomez-Martin C, Plaza JC, Pazo-Cid R, et al. Level of HER2 gene amplification predicts response and overall survival in HER2-positive advanced gastric cancer treated with trastuzumab. *J Clin Oncol* 2013;10:4445–4452.

96. Agus DB, Akita RW, Fox WD, et al. Targeting ligand-activated ErbB2 signaling inhibits breast and prostate tumor growth. *Cancer Cell* 2002;2:127–137.

97. Baselga J, Cortes J, Kim SB, et al. Pertuzumab plus trastuzumab plus docetaxel for metastatic breast cancer. *N Engl J Med* 2012;366:109–119.

98. Swain SM, Kim SB, Cortes J, et al. Pertuzumab, trastuzumab, and docetaxel for HER2-positive metastatic breast cancer (CLEOPATRA study): overall survival results from a randomised, double-blind, placebo-controlled, phase 3 study. *Lancet Oncol* 2013;14:461–471.

99. Gianni L, Pienkowski T, Im YH, et al. Efficacy and safety of neoadjuvant pertuzumab and trastuzumab in women with locally advanced, inflammatory, or early HER2-positive breast cancer (NeoSphere): a randomised multicentre, open-label, phase 2 trial. *Lancet Oncol* 2012;13:25–32.

100. Waksal HW. Role of an anti-epidermal growth factor receptor in treating cancer. *Cancer Metastasis Rev* 1999;18:427–436.

101. Van Cutsem ELI, D'haens G. KRAS status and efficacy in the first-line treatment of patients with metastatic colorectal cancer (metastatic CRC) treated with FOLFIRI with or without cetuximab: The CRYSTAL experience. Abstract 2. *J Clin Oncol* 2008;26:5s.

102. Bokemeyer CBI, Hartmann JT. KRAS status and efficacy of first-line treatment of patients with metastatic colorectal (metastatic CRC) with FOLFOX with or without cetuximab: The OPUS experience. Abstract 4000. *J Clin Oncol* 2008;26:178s.

103. Pirker R, Pereira JR, Szczesna A, et al. Cetuximab plus chemotherapy in patients with advanced non-small-cell lung cancer (FLEX): an open-label randomised phase III trial. *Lancet* 2009;373:1525–1531.

104. Lynch TJ, Patel T, Dreisbach L, et al. Cetuximab and first-line taxane/carboplatin chemotherapy in advanced non-small-cell lung cancer: results of the randomized multicenter phase III trial BMS099. *J Clin Oncol* 2010;28: 911–917.

105. Gibson TB, Ranganathan A, Grothey A. Randomized phase III trial of panitumumab, a fully human anti-epidermal growth factor receptor monoclonal antibody, in metastatic colorectal cancer. *Clin Colorectal Cancer* 2006;6: 29–31.

106. Amado RG, Wolf M, Peeters M, et al. Wild-type KRAS is required for panitumumab efficacy in patients with metastatic colorectal cancer. *J Clin Oncol* 2008;26:1626–1634.

107. Brown LF, Berse B, Jackman RW, et al. Expression of vascular permeability factor (vascular endothelial growth factor) and its receptors in breast cancer. *Hum Pathol* 1995;26:86–91.

108. Obermair A, Kohlberger P, Bancher-Todesca D, et al. Influence of microvessel density and vascular permeability factor/vascular endothelial growth factor expression on prognosis in vulvar cancer. *Gynecol Oncol* 1996;63:204–209.

109. Takahashi Y, Tucker SL, Kitadai Y, et al. Vessel counts and expression of vascular endothelial growth factor as prognostic factors in node-negative colon cancer. *Arch Surg* 1997;132:541–546.

110. Jain RK. Normalization of tumor vasculature: an emerging concept in antiangiogenic therapy. *Science* 2005;307:58–62.

111. Hurwitz H, Fehrenbacher L, Novotny W, et al. Bevacizumab plus irinotecan, fluorouracil, and leucovorin for metastatic colorectal cancer. *N Engl J Med* 2004;350:2335–2342.

112. Sandler A, Gray R, Perry MC, et al. Paclitaxel-carboplatin alone or with bevacizumab for non-small-cell lung cancer. *N Engl J Med* 2006;355:2542–2550.

113. Miller K, Wang M, Gralow J, et al. Paclitaxel plus bevacizumab versus paclitaxel alone for metastatic breast cancer. *N Engl J Med* 2007;357:2666.

114. Miller KD, Chap LI, Holmes FA, et al. Randomized phase III trial of capecitabine compared with bevacizumab plus capecitabine in patients with previously treated metastatic breast cancer. *J Clin Oncol* 2005;23: 792–799.

115. Allegra CJ, Yothers G, O'Connell MJ, et al. Initial safety report of NSABP C-08: A randomized phase III study of modified FOLFOX6 with or without bevacizumab for the adjuvant treatment of patients with stage II or III colon cancer. *J Clin Oncol* 2009;27:3385–3390.

116. Cameron D, Brown J, Dent R, et al. Adjuvant bevacizumab-containing therapy in triple-negative breast cancer (BEATRICE): primary results of a randomised, phase 3 trial. *Lancet Oncol* 2013;14:933–942.

117. Kreisl TN, Kim L, Moore K, et al. Phase II trial of single-agent bevacizumab followed by bevacizumab plus irinotecan at tumor progression in recurrent glioblastoma. *J Clin Oncol* 2009;27:740–745.

118. Burris HA 3rd, Rugo HS, Vukelja SJ, et al. Phase II study of the antibody drug conjugate trastuzumab-DM1 for the treatment of human epidermal growth factor receptor 2 (HER2)-positive breast cancer after prior HER2-directed therapy. *J Clin Oncol* 2011;29:398–405.

119. Krop IE, LoRusso P, Miller KD, et al. A phase II study of trastuzumab emtansine in patients with human epidermal growth factor receptor 2-positive metastatic breast cancer who were previously treated with trastuzumab, lapatinib, an anthracycline, a taxane, and capecitabine. *J Clin Oncol* 2012;30: 3234–3241.

120. Verma S, Miles D, Gianni L, et al. Trastuzumab emtansine for HER2-positive advanced breast cancer. *N Engl J Med* 2012;367:1783–1791.

121. Thomas D, Carriere P, Jacobs I. Safety of denosumab in giant-cell tumour of bone. *Lancet Oncol* 2012;11:815.

122. Chawla S, Henshaw R, Seeger L, et al. Safety and efficacy of denosumab for adults and skeletally mature adolescents with giant cell tumour of bone: interim analysis of an open-label, parallel-group, phase 2 study. *Lancet Oncol* 2013;14:901–908.

123. Fizazi K, Carducci M, Smith M, et al. Denosumab versus zoledronic acid for treatment of bone metastases in men with castration-resistant prostate cancer: a randomised, double-blind study. *Lancet* 2011;377:813–822.

124. Henry DH, Costa L, Goldwasser F, et al. Randomized, double-blind study of denosumab versus zoledronic acid in the treatment of bone metastases in patients with advanced cancer (excluding breast and prostate cancer) or multiple myeloma. *J Clin Oncol* 2011;29:1125–1132.

125. Stopeck AT, Lipton A, Body JJ, et al. Denosumab compared with zoledronic acid for the treatment of bone metastases in patients with advanced breast cancer: a randomized, double-blind study. *J Clin Oncol* 2010;28:5132–5139.

126. Smith MR, Egerdie B, Hernandez Toriz N, et al. Denosumab in men receiving androgen-deprivation therapy for prostate cancer. *N Engl J Med* 2009;361: 745–755.

127. Ellis GK, Bone HG, Chlebowski R, et al. Randomized trial of denosumab in patients receiving adjuvant aromatase inhibitors for nonmetastatic breast cancer. *J Clin Oncol* 2008;26:4875–4882.

128. Maloney D, Grillo-López A, Bodkin D, et al. IDEC-C2B8: results of a phase I multiple-dose trial in patients with relapsed non-Hodgkin's lymphoma. *J Clin Oncol* 1997;15:3266–3274.

129. Maloney D, Grillo-López A, White C, et al. IDEC-C2B8 (Rituximab) anti-CD20 monoclonal antibody therapy in patients with relapsed low-grade non-Hodgkin's lymphoma. *Blood* 1997;90:2188–2195.

130. Shan D, Ledbetter J, Press O. Signaling events involved in anti-CD20-induced apoptosis of malignant human B cells. *Cancer Immunol Immunother* 2000;48:673–683.

131. Coiffier B, Haioun C, Ketterer N, et al. Rituximab (anti-CD20 monoclonal antibody) for the treatment of patients with relapsing or refractory aggressive lymphoma: a multicenter phase II study. *Blood* 1998;92:1927–1932.

132. Czuczman MS, Grillo-López AJ, White CA, et al. Treatment of patients with low-grade B-cell lymphoma with the combination of chimeric anti-CD20 monoclonal antibody and CHOP chemotherapy. *J Clin Oncol* 1999;17: 268–276.

133. Demidem A, Lam T, Alas S, et al. Chimeric anti-CD20 (IDEC-C2B8) monoclonal antibody sensitizes a B cell lymphoma cell line to cell killing by cytotoxic drugs. *Cancer Biother Radiopharm* 1997;12:177–186.

134. Gribben JG, Freedman A, Woo SD, et al. All advanced stage non-Hodgkin's lymphomas with a polymerase chain reaction amplifiable breakpoint of bcl-2 have residual cells containing the rearrangement at evaluation and after treatment. *Blood* 1991;78:3275–3280.

135. Feugier P, Van Hoof A, Sebban C, et al. Long-term results of the R-CHOP study in the treatment of elderly patients with diffuse large B-cell lymphoma: a study by the Groupe d'Etude des Lymphomes de l'Adulte. *J Clin Oncol* 2005;23:4117–4126.

CANCER THERAPEUTICS

136. Kaufmann H, Raderer M, Wohrer S, et al. Antitumor activity of rituximab plus thalidomide in patients with relapsed/refractory mantle cell lymphoma. *Blood* 2004;104:2269–2271.

137. Reddy N, Hernandez-Ilizaliturri FJ, Deeb G, et al. Immunomodulatory drugs stimulate natural killer-cell function, alter cytokine production by dendritic cells, and inhibit angiogenesis enhancing the anti-tumour activity of rituximab in vivo. *Br J Haematol* 2008;140:36–45.

138. Hooijberg E, Sein JJ, van den Berk PC, et al. Eradication of large human B cell tumors in nude mice with unconjugated CD20 monoclonal antibodies and interleukin 2. *Cancer Res* 1995;55:2627–2634.

139. Friedberg JW, Neuberg D, Gribben JG, et al. Combination immunotherapy with rituximab and interleukin 2 in patients with relapsed or refractory follicular non-Hodgkin's lymphoma. *Br J Haematol* 2002;117:828–834.

140. Khan KD, Emmanouilides C, Benson DM Jr., et al. A phase 2 study of rituximab in combination with recombinant interleukin-2 for rituximab-refractory indolent non-Hodgkin's lymphoma. *Clin Cancer Res* 2006;12:7046–7053.

141. van der Kolk LE, Grillo-López AJ, Baars JW, et al. Treatment of relapsed B-cell non-Hodgkin's lymphoma with a combination of chimeric anti-CD20 monoclonal antibodies (rituximab) and G-CSF: final report on safety and efficacy. *Leukemia* 2003;17:1658–1664.

142. Warren TL, Dahle CE, Weiner GJ. CpG oligodeoxynucleotides enhance monoclonal antibody therapy of a murine lymphoma. *Clin Lymphoma* 2000;1:57–61.

143. Smith MR, Jin F, Joshi I. Enhanced efficacy of therapy with antisense BCL-2 oligonucleotides plus anti-CD20 monoclonal antibody in scid mouse/human lymphoma xenografts. *Mol Cancer Ther* 2004;3:1693–1699.

144. Ramanarayanan J, Hernandez-Ilizaliturri FJ, Chanan-Khan A, et al. Pro-apoptotic therapy with the oligonucleotide Genasense (oblimersen sodium) targeting Bcl-2 protein expression enhances the biological anti-tumour activity of rituximab. *Br J Haematol* 2004;127:519–530.

145. van Delft MF, Wei AH, Mason KD, et al. The BH3 mimetic ABT-737 targets selective Bcl-2 proteins and efficiently induces apoptosis via Bak/Bax if Mcl-1 is neutralized. *Cancer Cell* 2006;10:389–399.

146. Paoluzzi L, Gonen M, Gardner JR, et al. Targeting Bcl-2 family members with the BH3 mimetic AT-101 markedly enhances the therapeutic effects of chemotherapeutic agents in in vitro and in vivo models of B-cell lymphoma. *Blood* 2008;111:5350–5358.

147. Nguyen M, Marcellus RC, Roulston A, et al. Small molecule obatoclax (GX15-070) antagonizes MCL-1 and overcomes MCL-1-mediated resistance to apoptosis. *Proc Natl Acad Sci U S A* 2007;104:19512–19517.

148. Coiffier B, Lepretre S, Pedersen LM, et al. Safety and efficacy of ofatumumab, a fully human monoclonal anti-CD20 antibody, in patients with relapsed or refractory B-cell chronic lymphocytic leukemia: a phase 1-2 study. *Blood* 2008;111:1094–1100.

149. Wierda WG, Kipps TJ, Mayer J, et al. Ofatumumab as single-agent CD20 immunotherapy in fludarabine-refractory chronic lymphocytic leukemia. *J Clin Oncol* 2010;28:1749–1755.

150. Stein R, Qu Z, Chen S, et al. Characterization of a new humanized anti-CD20 monoclonal antibody, IMMU-106, and its use in combination with the humanized anti-CD22 antibody, epratuzumab, for the therapy of non-Hodgkin's lymphoma. *Clin Cancer Res* 2004;10:2868–2878.

151. Senter PD, Sievers EL. The discovery and development of brentuximab vedotin for use in relapsed Hodgkin lymphoma and systemic anaplastic large cell lymphoma. *Nat Biotechnol* 2012;30:631–637.

152. Pro B, Advani R, Brice P, et al. Brentuximab vedotin (SGN-35) in patients with relapsed or refractory systemic anaplastic large-cell lymphoma: results of a phase II study. *J Clin Oncol* 2012;30:2190–2196.

153. Younes A, Gopal AK, Smith SE, et al. Results of a pivotal phase II study of brentuximab vedotin for patients with relapsed or refractory Hodgkin's lymphoma. *J Clin Oncol* 2012;30:2183–2189.

# 30 Assessment of Clinical Response

Antonio Tito Fojo and Susan E. Bates

## INTRODUCTION

Approaches to response assessments have become increasingly important over the past decade as the drug development pipeline has steadily increased in volume. In 2012, an estimated 981 medicines were in development for cancer, and the number is certainly higher today.[1] The challenge is, first, how to measure the activity of an agent in the research setting, and, second, how to measure activity in the standard of care setting.

The "modern era" of drug development began in 1976 when 16 experienced oncologists treating lymphoma gathered to decide what would be considered a reliable measure of response to a therapy.[2] Each oncologist measured 12 *simulated tumor masses* employing *usual clinical methods* (i.e., calipers or rulers). A principal goal was to identify the amount of shrinkage that *could not* be ascribed to operator error and that *would not* be found if a *placebo* was administered. Moertel and Hanley recommended that *to avoid error, a 50% reduction in the product of perpendicular diameters be employed as the criterion for efficacy.*[2] It was from this beginning that our current methodologies of response assessment evolved. The important point to note is that the decision to use a 50% reduction in the product of perpendicular diameters as a measure of efficacy was made so as to reduce error and *not because it represented a value that conferred clinical benefit.*

### From Calipers and Rulers in Lymphoma to the Bidimensional World Health Organization Criteria

In 1981, five years after the Moertel and Hanley report,[2] a World Health Organization (WHO) initiative developed standardized approaches for the "reporting of response, recurrence and disease-free interval."[3] The WHO criteria, like Moertel and Hanley, recommended that malignant disease be measured in two dimensions. Complete response (CR) was defined as the disappearance of all known disease, and a partial response (PR) was scored if there occurred a "50% decrease in the sum of the products of the perpendicular diameters of the multiple lesions." Thus, the 50% reduction initially chosen as an operationally optimal value became institutionalized as the threshold for declaring efficacy in the majority of cancers. This measure of efficacy was perpetuated in 2000 with the now widely used Response Evaluation Criteria in Solid Tumors (RECIST), but shifting to one dimension.[4] The authors noted "the definition of a partial response, in particular, is an arbitrary convention—there is no inherent meaning for an individual patient of a 50% decrease in overall tumor load." Nevertheless, the threshold chosen—a 30% reduction in one dimension—was comparable in volume to the 50% decrease in the sum of the products of the perpendicular diameters and thus perpetuated the 1976 standard. In spite of its arbitrary origins, the 50% reduction has held up over time. But the major impact of the WHO criteria was that it marked the beginning of a common language of response. These criteria have been revisited and refined over time, as technology

and medicine advanced. Table 30.1 compares the WHO criteria with those of RECIST 1.0 and RECIST 1.1 and three modifications of RECIST, whereas Figure 30.1 provides a visual presentation of the RECIST threshold required to qualify as response or progression.[3–9]

## ASSESSING RESPONSE

### RECIST 1.1

The RECIST 1.0 guidelines were updated as RECIST 1.1 in 2009, with a number of differences between the two response criteria highlighted. RECIST 1.1 preserves the same categories of response found in RECIST 1.0:

- Complete response: Complete disappearance of all disease
- Partial response: ≥30% reduction in the sum of the longest diameter of target lesions
- Stable disease: Change not meeting criteria for response or progression
- Progression: ≥20% increase in the sum of the longest diameter of target lesions

However, a decade of experience with RECIST identified several problems with the criteria, some of which could be corrected. In RECIST 1.0, minimum size varied between 1 and 2 cm depending on technique; in RECIST 1.1, a 1-cm lesion is the minimum measurable. In RECIST 1.0, 10 lesions were to be measured, 5 per organ; RECIST 1.1 reduced that to 5 lesions, 2 per organ. Response criteria in RECIST 1.0 did not address lymph nodes; in RECIST 1.1, lymph nodes decreasing to <1 cm in their short axis could constitute a complete response. Disease progression in nontarget disease was further defined to indicate that in addition to a 20% increase in target lesions over the smallest sum on study, there must be an absolute increase of 5 mm, and that an increase of a single nontarget lesion should not trump an overall disease status assessment based on target lesions.

### Variations of the RECIST Criteria

The RECIST criteria have been widely used for standardizing the reporting of clinical trial results and have improved reproducibility. However, the increasing precision and codification of RECIST has led to recognition of its limitations. For example, there are unique challenges in central nervous system (CNS) disease, relating response to tumor size measurements based on contrast enhancement. Pseudoprogression refers to an increase in contrast enhancement due to a transient increase in vascular permeability after irradiation, whereas pseudoresponse is a decrease in contrast enhancement that may occur due to a reduction in vascular permeability following corticosteroids or an antiangiogenic agent such as bevacizumab.[10–12] The McDonald criteria, traditionally used in determining glioma response based

**TABLE 30.1**

**Key Features of Response Criteria**

| | WHO[3] | RECIST 1.0[4] | RECIST 1.1[5] | CNS RANO Criteria[7] | RECIST Mesothelioma[8] | RECIST Immunotherapy[9] |
|---|---|---|---|---|---|---|
| **Dimension** | Uni- and bidimensional | Unidimensional | Unidimensional | Bidimensional | Unidimensional | Bidimensional |
| **Measurable Lesion** | Not defined | Longest diameter, ≥20 mm with most modalities; ≥10 mm with spiral CT | Longest diameter ≥10 mm on CT or on skin if using calipers; ≥20 mm if using CXR | Two perpendicular diameters of contrast enhancing lesions ≥10 mm | Tumor thickness perpendicular to chest wall or mediastinum, measured in two positions at three levels on transverse cuts of CT scan | Longest perpendicular diameters |
| **Measurable Lymph Nodes** | Not defined | Not defined | ≥15 mm short axis | — | — | — |
| **Disease Burden to be Assessed at Baseline** | All (not specified) | Measurable target lesions up to 10 total (5 per organ); other lesions nontarget | Measurable target lesions up to 5 total (2 per organ); other lesions nontarget | Two to five lesions in patients with several lesions | Pleural disease in perpendicular diameter; nodal, subcutaneous, and other bidimensional lesions measured unidimensionally as per the RECIST criteria | 5 lesions per organ, up to 10 visceral lesions and five cutaneous lesions |
| **Sum** | *Sum of the products* of bidimensional diameters or sum of linear unidimensional diameters | Sum of longest diameters of all measurable lesions | Sum of the longest diameters of target lesions with only exception use of short axis for lymph nodes | Sum of the products of perpendicular diameters of all measurable enhancing target lesions | Sum of the six measurements defines a pleural unidimensional measure | SPD with new lesions incorporated into baseline; tumor burden = $SPD_{index\ lesions} + SPD_{new\ lesions}$ |
| **Complete Response** | Disappearance all known disease | Disappearance all known disease | Disappearance all known disease; lymph nodes <10 mm | — | Disappearance all target lesions with no evidence of tumor elsewhere | Disappearance all lesions in two consecutive observations |
| **Partial Response** | ≥50% decrease | ≥30% decrease; all other no evidence of progression | ≥30% decrease; all other disease, no evidence of progression | ≥50% reduction; stable or decreased steroid use compared to baseline | ≥30% reduction in total tumor measurement | ≥50% decrease compared with baseline in two observations |
| **Response Confirmation?** | ≥4 weeks apart | ≥4 weeks apart | ≥4 weeks apart (if response primary end point); no, if secondary endpoint | ≥4 weeks apart | Repeat on two occasions ≥4 weeks apart | ≥4 weeks apart |

*(continued)*

**TABLE 30.1**

**Key Features of Response Criteria** *(continued)*

| | WHO[3] | RECIST 1.0[4] | RECIST 1.1[5] | CNS RANO Criteria[7] | RECIST Mesothelioma[8] | RECIST Immunotherapy[9] |
|---|---|---|---|---|---|---|
| **Progressive Disease** | ≥25% increase in size of one or more measurable lesions or appearance of new lesions | ≥20% increase, taking as reference smallest sum in study; or appearance of new lesions | ≥20% increase, with absolute increase ≥5 mm, taking as reference smallest sum in study; or appearance of new lesions | ≥25%, or any new lesions | ≥20% increase in the total tumor measurement over the nadir measurement, or the appearance of one or more new lesions | ≥25% increase compared with nadir confirmed ≥4 weeks apart; up to five new lesions (≥5 × 5 mm) per organ incorporated into tumor burden |
| | Nonmeasurable disease: Estimated increase of ≥25% | Nonmeasurable disease: unequivocal progression | Nonmeasurable disease: unequivocal progression | Nonmeasurable disease: >5 mm increase in maximal diameter; ≥25% increase in SPD; or significant increase in nonenhancing lesions on same or lower dose of corticosteroids | — | New, nonmeasurable lesions (i.e., <5 × 5 mm) do not define progression |
| **Stable Disease** | Stable disease or non-PR and non-PD ≥4 weeks | Non-PR, non-PD; minimum time defined by protocol | Non-PR, non-PD; minimum time defined by protocol | — | Non-PR, non-PD | Non-irPR, non-irPD |

CXR, Chest X-ray; SPD, sum of products of two largest perpendicular diameters; PD, progressive disease; irPR, immune-related partial response; irPD, immune-related progressive disease.

on two-dimensional measurements, have been recently updated as part of the Response Assessment in Neuro-Oncology (RANO) response criteria and extended to include a response assessment for metastatic CNS disease.[7,13]

Other examples where RECIST is limited include mesothelioma, gastrointestinal stromal tumors (GIST), hepatocellular cancers, among others. The pleural disease of mesothelioma increases in depth while following the pleural surface. GIST tumors may remain unchanged in size after treatment, whereas the center of the tumor mass undergoes necrosis, and progression may occur in the remaining rim.[14] Hepatocellular cancers are often treated with local–regional therapy in which the goal is tumor necrosis and treatment failure occurs in surviving viable tumor.[15] Different

strategies have emerged to quantify these diseases, including modifications of RECIST, quantifying positron-emission tomography (PET) imaging, and biomarker criteria, as will be discussed. The RECIST adaptation for mesothelioma, growing along the pleural surface, is to measure the diameter perpendicular to the chest wall or mediastinum, and to measure at three levels.[8] The adaptation for hepatocellular cancer following local therapy is measurement of the longest diameter of the tumor that shows enhancement on the arterial phase of the scan, bypassing the dense, homogeneous Lipiodol-containing necrotic area.[15]

Investigators have also observed that following immunotherapy, tumor lesions may increase in size due to the increased infiltration of T cells, even meeting criteria for RECIST-defined progressive

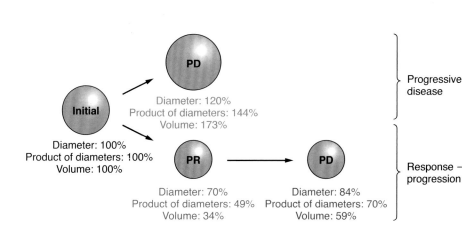

**Figure 30.1** RECIST thresholds in three parameters: diameter, product of diameters, and volume. In the figure, spheres meeting RECIST criteria for progressive disease (PD) and for PR are shown with the percentage relative to the baseline calculated for each parameter. To meet the threshold for PD, the longest diameter must increase to 120%, which is equivalent to a 144% increase in the product of the perpendicular diameters and a 173% increase in the volume of a sphere. Although PR definitions are almost identical to those employed with WHO, RECIST has a higher threshold to meet PD.[6]

disease (PD). Previously radiographically undetectable lesions may appear. Departing from conventional RECIST, which defines any new lesion as PD, the immune response criteria allow the appearance of new lesions, adding them to the total tumor burden.[9] An increase in total tumor burden of >25% relative to baseline or nadir is required to define PD.

## International Working Group Criteria for Lymphoma

Revised guidelines for lymphoma assessment were promulgated by the International Working Group (IWG) in 2007.[16] These guidelines incorporated 18F-fluorodeoxyglucose (FDG)-PET assessments in metabolically active lymphomas.[16] Although a CR requires the complete disappearance of detectable disease, a post-treatment residual mass is permitted if it is negative on FDG-PET and was positive at baseline. For lymphomas that are not consistently FDG avid, or if FDG avidity is unknown, a CR requires that nodes >1.5 cm before therapy regress to <1.5 cm, and nodes that were 1.1 to 1.5 cm in long axis and >1.0 cm in the short axis shrink to ≤1.0 cm in short axis. The definition of PR resembles the WHO criteria, in that a ≥50% decrease in the sum of the product of the diameters in up to six nodal masses or in hepatic or splenic nodules must be documented. Although RECIST 1.1 now includes lymph node assessment, the IWG criteria remain the assessment method typically used in lymphoma clinical trials.

# ALTERNATE RESPONSE CRITERIA

The previous examples represent attempts to more accurately measure tumor burden. Evolving imaging technology enabling volumetric measurements of tumor masses may eventually resolve some of these problems, but effective therapeutic agents are required to enable validation and utilization of response assessment tools. The lack of an agent that can mediate substantial tumor shrinkage underlies the concept of *clinical benefit response* (CBR) as an endpoint in pancreatic cancer. Clinical benefit was defined as a combination of improvement in pain, performance status, and weight; the assessment of CBR supported the U.S. Food and Drug Administration (FDA) approval of gemcitabine in pancreatic cancer.[17,18] Better therapies for pancreatic cancer that result in tumor shrinkage or eradication should include and then eclipse clinical benefit.

Response criteria may be specific to a particular disease or clinical setting. Some diseases by their nature require specific strategies for response assessment.

## Severity-Weighted Assessment Tool Score in Cutaneous T-Cell Lymphoma

Cutaneous T-cell lymphoma (CTCL) is a disease that can involve the entire epidermis, or comprise individual skin lesions varying widely in severity rather than size. The severity-weighted assessment tool (SWAT) assigns a factor for skin lesion severity—patch, plaque, or tumor—multiplies this factor by the percent of skin involved with each lesion type and then adds these together. This complex system formed the basis of the FDA approval of vorinostat for CTCL.[19]

## Pathologic Complete Response in Breast Cancer

One unique response endpoint is the assessment of breast cancer treated in the neoadjuvant setting. The purpose of neoadjuvant therapy is to improve survival, render locally advanced cancer amenable to surgery, or to aid in breast conservation. In that setting, the absence of cancer cells in resected breast tissue has been used to define a pathologic complete response (pCR). The rate of pCR has been proposed as a surrogate endpoint for event-free survival (EFS) or overall survival (OS) to support approval of new agents or combinations of agents tested in clinical trials.[20] In a pooled analysis of 11,955 patients enrolled on 12 neoadjuvant trials, individual patients with pCR had improved EFS and OS.[21] However, at the trial level, pCR rates did not correlate with EFS or OS, a problem likely due to heterogeneity of breast cancer subtypes among the trials. Despite this, pCR rates were recently used to support the approval of pertuzumab and trastuzumab in the neoadjuvant setting.[21,22]

## Computed Tomography-Based Tumor Density

One approach, often called the Choi criteria, advocates assessing tumor response in GIST, renal cell cancer, or hepatocellular cancer based on density on computed tomography (CT) scans (Table 30.2). This variation was prompted by the evident response to treatment with imatinib but with minimal tumor shrinkage.[23] The Choi criteria are still considered exploratory in GIST,[24,25] and it is too soon to know of benefits in other histologies.[26,27] Further study should determine its utility, although it will likely be confined to specific tumor types with specific drugs.

## FDG-PET

Although widely used in clinical practice, FDG-PET has become part of standardized response criteria for clinical trials only in lymphoma (see Table 30.2). In solid tumors, FDG-PET can aid in the detection of new or recurrent sites of disease, and can be used as an adjunct during assessments for disease progression when using RECIST criteria.[5] Although FDG uptake is a powerful diagnostic tool and its uptake reflects a tumor's metabolic activity, it has some limitations: Some tumors have variable FDG avidity; differences can occur due to variations in patient activity, carbohydrate intake, blood glucose, and timing; and there are several benign sources of uptake, including inflammatory and postsurgical sites. Multiple methods of quantitating FDG-PET and assessing response have been proposed, but to date there is no consensus, particularly regarding the definition of a metabolic response.[28–33]

The two most widely used response criteria—the European Organisation for the Research and Treatment of Cancer (EORTC) criteria and PET Response Criteria in Solid Tumors (PERCIST) (see Table 30.2)—have been evaluated in specific disease types, but unifying FDG-PET response criteria remains a challenge in anticancer drug development.[28,30] We would note that, as shown in Figure 30.1, a 30% reduction in the diameter of a sphere—the magnitude of change required to score a response according to RECIST—represents a 65% decrease in volume. If an standardized uptake value (SUV) decrease is directly equated to a volume decrease, a reduction of 25% translates to a 10% reduction in diameter, a value that likely constitutes an insufficient response.

## Serum Biomarkers of Response

The ideal response assessment method is an assay that could measure tumor quantity by a simple blood test (see Table 30.2). Circulating protein biomarkers have been identified and studied for several decades for screening, early detection of recurrent disease, determining prognosis, selecting therapy, and monitoring response to therapy. These serum tumor markers are to be distinguished from the assays determining the presence of an overexpressed or mutated molecular target. With the successful launch of therapies against such molecular targets, there has been increased interest in the assays needed to select therapy for individual patients (predictive biomarkers). The analytical and clinical validation of such assays, along with determination of their clinical utility, has created a new regulatory paradigm known as *companion diagnostics*.[34,35] This investment in the development of predictive markers for companion diagnostics has reduced the focus on protein biomarkers of treatment response relative to older literature.

As a result, there are few clinically validated biomarkers of response.[36] In addition to issues regarding sensitivity and specificity, their use and development has also been hindered by the often

## TABLE 30.2

### Alternate Response Criteria: Biomarkers

| Criterion | Baseline | Response | Progression |
|---|---|---|---|
| CA-125 in ovarian cancer (GCIG criteria)[43] | CA 125 >2× ULN | CA 125 decline ≥50% confirmed at 28 days | 2× nadir OR 2× ULN if normalized on therapy on two occasions 1 wk apart |
| PSA in prostate cancer (PSA WG1)[45,a] | PSA ≥5 ng/mL and documentation of two consecutive increases in PSA 1 wk apart | PSA decline of 50% from baseline (measured twice 3–4 wks apart) | After decrease from baseline, a 50% increase AND an increase ≥5 ng/mL, or back to baseline, whichever is lower |
| PSA in prostate cancer (PCWG2)[46,a] | PSA ≥2.0 ng/mL; estimate pretreatment PSA-DT: Need ≥3 values ≥4 wks apart | Report percent change from baseline (rise or fall) at 12 weeks, and separately, the maximal change (rise or fall) at any time using a waterfall plot | PSA increase ≥25% and absolute increase by ≥2 ng/mL above the nadir, confirmed by a second value ≥3 wks later (i.e., confirmed rising trend) OR PSA increase ≥25% and ≥2 ng/mL above baseline >12 wks |
| hCG and AFP in testicular cancer[50–51] | | Decrease consistent with marker half-life: 2–3 d for hCG, 5–7 d for AFP | Rising levels usually indicate need to change therapy |
| **Choi Criteria for CT Imaging** | | | |
| Choi criteria[24–27] | | ≥10% decrease in tumor size OR ≥15% reduction in tumor density | An increase in tumor size ≥10% and does not meet criteria of PR by tumor attenuation on CT |
| **FDG-PET Criteria** | | | |
| EORTC criteria[29–31] | ROI should be drawn, SUV calculated | **CMR:** Complete resolution of uptake **PMR:** SUV reduction ≥25% **SMD:** SUV increase <25% and decrease <15% | **PMD:** SUV increase >25% in regions defined on baseline, or appearance of new FDG-avid lesions |
| PERCIST criteria[29] | SUL peak >1.5× normal liver | **CMR:** Complete resolution of uptake **PMR:** SUL reduction ≥30% | **PMD:** SUL increase >30% in regions defined on baseline, or appearance of new FDG avid lesions |

[a] Guidelines for PSA assessment have evolved from those of the PSAWG1, where responses were dichotomized based on the percent decline, to those in the PCWG2 where PSA response is considered a continuous variable. Recently, emphasis has shifted to assessing PSA doubling time.
CA-125, cancer antigen 125; GCIG, Gynecologic Cancer InterGroup; ULN, upper limit of normal; PSA, prostate-specific antigen; PSAWG1, PSA Working Group 1; PCWG2, Prostate Cancer Working Group 2; PSA-DT, PSA-doubling time; hCG, human chorionic gonatropin; AFP, alpha-fetoprotein; EORTC, European Organisation for the Research and Treatment of Cancer; ROI, regions of interest; SUV, standardized uptake value; CMR, complete metabolic response; PMR, partial metabolic response; SMD, stable metabolic disease; PMD, progressive metabolic disease; PERCIST, PET response criteria in solid tumors; SUL, SUV normalized to lean body mass.

limited efficacy of therapies; response biomarkers are of little value without highly effective primary and salvage therapies. For example, a recent clinical trial indicates that in *asymptomatic patients* with ovarian cancer whose only evidence of disease progression is an isolated rising CA-125, nothing is gained by instituting treatment before there is other evidence of progression.[37,38]

- **Cancer Antigen 125 (CA-125):** Despite recognized limitations, CA-125 is widely used. For example, the Gynecologic Cancer InterGroup (GCIG) criteria have evolved to help determine whether a patient's tumor has responded to therapy.[39–41] Response is defined as a 50% decline from an elevated baseline value, whereas progression is defined as a doubling over the nadir or the upper limit of normal.[42] In clinical practice, CA-125 levels are followed as part of standard management, but making clinical decisions on marker changes alone is not recommended.[43]
- **Prostate-Specific Antigen (PSA):** Similar issues have confronted investigators caring for patients with prostate cancer. The PSA Working Group 1 (PCWG1) guidelines, first published in

1999, established PSA criteria, particularly for use in patients with disease that was difficult to quantify.[44] There followed a second working group (PCWG2) that recommended plotting the percent PSA change for each patient in a waterfall plot so as to avoid creating a dichotomous variable from the changes in PSA.[45] PCWG2 also recommended keeping patients on trial until evidence of a change in clinical status—either symptomatic or radiographic progression. The latter addressed concerns with patients in whom PSA changes did not reflect clinical status, particularly those with transient increases in the first 12 weeks of a new therapy.

- **Human Chorionic Gonadotropin (hCG) and alpha fetoprotein (AFP):** Because testicular cancer is a highly curable disease with validated biomarkers, outcome assessment has focused on the rapid detection of patients whose tumors have a poor response to therapy. Because both markers have relatively short half-lives—2 to 3 days for hCG and 5 to 7 days for serum AFP—the rate of decline can be determined. Various methods have demonstrated that a rapid decline or early normalization of marker levels is indicative of a good outcome, without any one method achieving widespread acceptance.[46–48] Nonetheless, the 2010 American Society of Clinical Oncology (ASCO) guidelines on serum tumor markers concluded there was still insufficient evidence to recommend changing therapy solely on the basis of a slow marker decline.[49] Rising levels after two cycles of therapy (outside the first week of treatment when rises can be due to tumor lysis) can be considered an indication to change the treatment plan.[49,50]

## Circulating Tumor Cells and Circulating Tumor DNA

Two response endpoints under recent investigation show a potential to detect the impact of therapy. One is the measurement of circulating tumor cells (CTC) in the bloodstream, enriched by one or more capture strategies, including one that has received FDA approval.[51] The number of CTCs in the blood has been shown to be prognostic, with higher levels conferring a poor prognosis, and to correlate with a response to therapy. A second approach is the determination of levels of circulating tumor DNA (ctDNA) in the blood. This is detected by quantitating the number of DNA molecules carrying a given mutation or gene rearrangement in the blood, typically detected through targeted sequencing of common mutations, or of a previously identified *mutation signature* or gene rearrangement. The amount of ctDNA appears to correlate with tumor burden, increases with stage, and in one study, was deemed more sensitive than CTC detection.[52–54] Whether these tests will ultimately prove to be more sensitive and accurate than the serum biomarkers discussed previously remains to be determined. Because targeted sequencing can be very sensitive, one concern is that false-positive ctDNA detection may occur after treatment, or intermittently in the setting of enlarging tumor masses. At the least, detection of CTCs and ctDNA is advancing our understanding of cancer biology, as studies reveal evidence of metastatic heterogeneity, clonal heterogeneity, and emergence of resistance mutations in clinical samples.

## DETERMINING OUTCOME

The response measures described previously represent different approaches to quantitate tumor burden. What happens after those data are obtained varies depending on the clinical setting. In the community, less emphasis is placed on strict criteria. In the setting of a clinical trial, tumor size is measured and the response categorized. For FDA submission, these are but factors in the risk-benefit equation needed for drug approvals. The FDA conveys full approval to new agents based on true *clinical benefit* (i.e., an improvement in a *survival* endpoint or symptom relief).[55] Surrogates for clinical benefit, such as response rate, may support either regular approval or accelerated approval, depending on the setting.

## Overall Response Rate, Duration of Response, and Stable Disease

Overall response rate (ORR) is the proportion of patients with a tumor size reduction of a predefined amount for a minimum time period. The FDA has generally defined ORR as the sum of PRs and CRs. Although OS remains the gold standard, ORR is often used both in drug development and in clinical practice to indicate antitumor efficacy of a given therapy. Table 30.3 summarizes the attributes and drawbacks of using ORR as a method of assessment. Using standardized definitions of response, it has been shown that ORR often correlates with OS, although ORR usually explains only a fraction of the variability of the survival

benefits.[56–58] Equally important, however, is the duration of response, a value that is measured from the time of initial response until documented tumor progression, and which assumes added importance when ORR is the endpoint for regulatory approval.

Unlike PR and CR, the FDA has generally not been willing to include *stable disease (SD)*, defined as shrinkage that qualifies as neither response nor progression, as part of the ORR, feeling it is often indicative of the underlying disease biology rather than a drug's therapeutic effect.[55,59] Nevertheless, in reporting data, investigators are increasingly using the term *CBR*, which includes CR + PR + SD and which is a misuse of the term *clinical benefit* because neither CR, PR, or SD are *objective tumor findings* that address the true *clinical benefit* of a therapy.[58,60] In the absence of standardized definitions for SD that are shown to effect meaningful changes in a clinical outcome, SD should not be used as a response endpoint. A better approach is to use nondichotomized response assessments, such as the waterfall plot or one of the kinetic analyses, discussed later.

## Progression-Free Survival, Time to Progression, and Time to Treatment Failure

In cancer drug development, one usually finds ORR assessed as an indicator of activity in phase II trials, whereas randomized phase III trials rely on other endpoints such as progression-free survival (PFS) and time to progression (TTP) (see Table 30.3). Although PFS and TTP attempt to assess efficacy in close proximity to a therapy, they score outcomes differently and are not interchangeable. TTP is defined as the time from randomization to *the time of disease progression*.[55] *In TTP analyses, deaths are censored either at the time of death or at an earlier visit.* In contrast, PFS is defined from the time of randomization to the time of *disease progression or death*. Although patients who discontinue trial participation for adverse events might be censored in both analyses, patients who die while on study are censored only in the TTP analysis. Those who favor TTP argue that if a patient dies without their tumor meeting criteria for progression, one cannot accurately estimate when progression might have occurred, so the data should be censored. However, those who favor PFS argue that, in some cases, death might be an adverse effect of the therapy. High-dose therapies represent an example of why PFS might be a preferable (regulatory) endpoint. If in a given tumor there is evidence of a dose-response relationship for an active drug, then high doses may have a greater response. However, such high doses may also be responsible for a greater number of deaths. Assessing only those who survive the high dose therapy and ignoring those who die (i.e., TTP) may lead to the conclusion that the high-dose therapy is more effective. The balance sheet that includes death (i.e., PFS) would clearly demonstrate this efficacy came at too great a price.

Although many have argued that PFS and TTP should be acceptable endpoints for cancer clinical trials, in the majority of tumors there is no convincing evidence PFS is a surrogate for OS, and in those where there is some evidence, its value is arguable.[61] Table 30.3 presents the attributes and drawbacks of PFS and TTP. Note that the definition of progression is often difficult, particularly in some tumor types, and that investigator bias can influence PFS and TTP. Problems with ascertainment bias and censoring, depicted in Figure 30.2, can also impact outcomes.

Alternate endpoints include time to treatment failure (TTF), defined as a composite endpoint measuring time from randomization to discontinuation of treatment for any reason, including disease progression, treatment toxicity, and death. The FDA has not recommended TTF as a regulatory endpoint for drug approval. However, the high rates of censoring due to toxicity seen in phase III clinical trails may lead to a reassessment of this position given that most can agree that not only is efficacy important, but so too is tolerability, and TTF can capture both of these attributes.

**TABLE 30.3**

**A Comparison of Important Cancer Approval Endpoints**

| Regulatory Evidence | Endpoints | Advantages | Disadvantages |
|---|---|---|---|
| **Clinical benefit** used for regular approvals | Overall survival (OS) | ■ Universally accepted direct measure of clinical benefit<br>■ Easily measured<br>■ Includes treatment-related mortality that can obscure benefit in a subset<br>■ Precisely measured; unambiguous<br>■ Not dependent on assessment intervals | ■ May involve larger studies<br>■ May require long follow-up<br>■ May be affected by crossover and/or sequential therapies<br>■ Includes noncancer deaths |
| | Symptom endpoints (patient-reported outcomes) | ■ Patient perspective of direct clinical benefit | ■ Blinding is often difficult<br>■ Data are frequently missing or incomplete<br>■ Clinical significance of small changes is unknown<br>■ Multiple analyses<br>■ Lack of validated instruments |
| **Surrogates** used for accelerated approvals or regular approvals | Disease-free survival (DFS) | ■ Smaller sample size and shorter follow-up necessary compared with survival studies | ■ Not statistically validated as surrogate for survival in all settings<br>■ Not precisely measured; subject to assessment bias, particularly in open-label studies<br>■ Definitions vary among studies |
| | Objective response rate (ORR) | ■ Can be assessed in single-arm studies<br>■ Assessed earlier and in smaller studies compared with survival studies<br>■ Effect attributable to drug, not natural history | ■ Not a direct measure of benefit<br>■ Not a comprehensive measure of drug activity<br>■ Only a subset of patients who benefit |
| | Complete response (CR) | ■ Can be assessed in single-arm studies<br>■ Durable complete responses can represent clinical benefit<br>■ Assessed earlier and in smaller studies compared with survival studies<br>■ Definition of progressive disease (PD) identifies uniform time to end treatment and data capture | ■ Not a direct measure of benefit in all cases<br>■ Not a comprehensive measure of drug activity<br>■ Small subset of patients with benefit<br>■ Requires prospective, consistent definition. Meaningful response durations not standardized<br>■ Definition of PD is arbitrary without evidence it actually represents end of benefit period |
| | Progression-free survival (PFS) or time to progression (TTP)[a] | ■ Smaller sample size and shorter follow-up necessary compared with survival studies<br>■ Measurement of stable disease included<br>■ Not confounded by crossover or subsequent therapies<br>■ Generally based on objective and quantitative assessment | ■ Statistically validated as surrogate for survival only in some settings<br>■ Not precisely measured; subject to assessment bias particularly in open-label studies<br>■ Definitions vary among studies; little agreement on magnitude of difference that constitutes clinical benefit<br>■ Requires frequent and consistent radiological or other assessments<br>■ Involves balanced timing of assessments among treatment arms |

[a] Progression-free survival includes all deaths; time to progression censors deaths that occur before progression.
Adapted from U.S. Department of Health and Human Services, Food and Drug Administration, Center for Drug Evaluation and Research (CDER), Center for Biologics Evaluation and Research (CBER). *Guidance from Industry. Clinical Trial Endpoints for the Approval of Cancer Drugs and Biologics.* 2007. http://www.fda.gov/downloads/Drugs/.../Guidances/ucm071590.pdf.

**CANCER THERAPEUTICS**

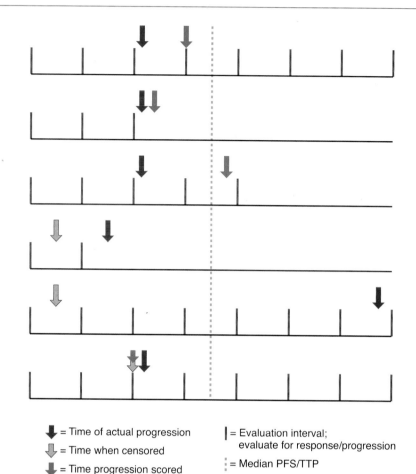

**Prespecified evaluation interval**
*Ideally, disease progression is reported at a prespecified evaluation interval*

**Ascertainment (evaluation) bias**
*An earlier evaluation leads to earlier scoring of progression (e.g., concern for symptoms prompt earlier evaluation)*

**Ascertainment (evaluation) bias**
*A later evaluation leads to delay in scoring progression (e.g., evaluation delayed by toxicity or treatment delays)*

**Censoring bias**
*Patient whose disease would have progressed quickly is censored early. Here censoring is "beneficial."*

**Censoring bias**
*Patient whose disease would have progressed late is censored early. Here censoring is "detrimental."*

**Informative censoring**
*Central review cannot score progression with available data. Although progression had been scored, the data is instead censored centrally. This is usually "beneficial."*

↓ = Time of actual progression
↓ = Time when censored
↓ = Time progression scored

| = Evaluation interval; evaluate for response/progression
⋮ = Median PFS/TTP

**Figure 30.2** The potential problems encountered when PFS is used as an endpoint. Ideally, as depicted at the *top*, response assessment will be conducted at a prespecified time. However, the date at which progression is scored may suffer from either ascertainment or censoring bias. Ascertainment bias can occur if either an evaluation occurs before the prespecified date or if it is delayed. For example, a clinician concerned about a patient who is not experiencing side effects and has likely been randomized to placebo may be more inclined to investigate symptoms early and document progression before the prespecified time, while delaying the evaluation of a patient randomized to the experimental arm who experiences some toxicity. Similarly, censoring—an increasing problem in randomized trials—may impact the outcome of a given study arm by either censoring patients who would experience early progression (beneficial impact) or censoring those who would have remained progression free for a long time (detrimental impact). Finally, informative censoring can occur when independent radiologic review cannot concur with an investigator's assessment of progression and censors the patient. This outcome is usually beneficial, because a patient who is very close to experiencing progression is censored. (Adapted from Villaruz LC, Socinski MA. The clinical viewpoint: definitions, limitations of RECIST, practical considerations of measurement. *Clin Cancer Res* 2013;19:2629–2636.)

## Overall Survival

Defined as the time from randomization to death, OS has been considered the gold standard of clinical trial endpoints (see Table 30.3). In part, this is so because it is unambiguous and does not suffer from interpretation bias. An additional advantage of the survival endpoint is that it can balance the effect of therapies with high treatment-related mortality even if tumor control is substantially better with the new treatment. However, some worry that because patients may receive multiple lines of therapy following the clinical trial, the results may be confounded by those subsequent therapies. The latter concern is often cited as the reason why an advantage in PFS/TTP *disappears* when one looks to OS. But as a review of clinical trials confirms,[62] the magnitude of the difference does not disappear, only the statistical validity (Fig. 30.3).[63,64]

When evaluating a randomized controlled trial, it is important that the OS as well as the PFS analyses are always by intention to treat (ITT). In an ITT analysis, often described as *once randomized, always analyzed*, all patients assigned to a group at the time of randomization are analyzed regardless of what occurred

subsequently.[65] An ITT analysis avoids the bias introduced by omitting dropouts and noncompliant patients that can negate randomization and overestimate clinical effectiveness.

## Kaplan–Meier Plots

In a typical clinical trial, data are often presented as a Kaplan–Meier plots. In discrete time intervals, the number of patients in each group who are progression free and alive (PFS analysis) or alive (OS analysis) at the end of the interval are counted and divided by the total number of patients in that group at the beginning of the time interval. One excludes from this calculation patients censored for a reason other than progressive disease or death during the same interval. This has the advantage that it allows one to include censored patients in estimates of the probability of PFS or OS up to the point when they were censored (i.e., they are excluded only beyond the point of censoring). In most clinical trials, a fraction of patients are typically censored.

In constructing the Kaplan–Meier plot, probabilities are calculated for each interval of time. The probability of surviving

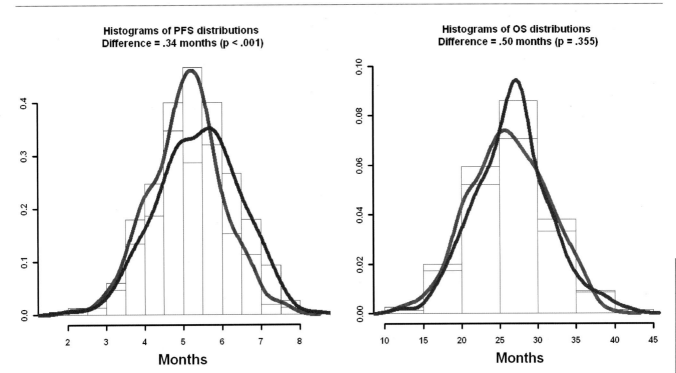

**Figure 30.3** Hypothetical distribution of PFS and OS data demonstrating the *disappearance of PFS benefit*. Because chemotherapy does not exert a lasting effect on the underlying tumor biology and because PFS is a shorter interval (measured in increments, not daily as is OS) PFS differences often disappear. The *hypothetical example* shown illustrates this phenomenon. The *left panel* shows a histogram of PFS distributions with a difference of 0.34 months that nevertheless achieves statistical significance over the short interval when PFS is measured. The *right panel* depicts similar histograms for OS captured over a longer time period. Despite a larger absolute difference of 0.5 months, the OS difference does not reach statistical significance. For these hypothetical curves, random number generated data sets (with normal distribution), histograms, and density plots were generated using R version 2.11.1 (2010-05-31).[75] The differences were deliberately chosen to be small, but a similar disappearance can also occur with larger differences. As can be seen, what disappears is not the absolute benefit, but the statistical validity.

progression free or being counted as a survivor to the end of any interval of assessment is the product of the probabilities of surviving in all the preceding assessment intervals multiplied by the probability for the interval of interest. One might ask to what extent the two curves in each study differ. One measure that is of value is the median PFS or OS—a value calculated in most studies from a Kaplan–Meier plot.

## Hazard Ratios

Increasingly, however, hazard ratios are cited in preference to the more traditional measures of efficacy such as the median PFS and median OS. *However, because a hazard ratio is a value that has no dimensions, it has very limited value, informing the reader only with regard to the reliability and uniformity of the data.* It does not quantify the magnitude of the benefit. A physician and, especially, a patient want to know the magnitude of the benefit (i.e., the extent to which a life will be prolonged), not what a dimensionless hazard ratio is. By definition, the *hazard ratio* is a ratio of the *hazard rates*. The hazard rate quantifies the likelihood that a patient will experience a *hazardous event* or a hazard during a defined interval of observation, and this is expressed as a rate or percent. For example, if during a given period of observation 20 of 100 patients receiving a reference or control therapy experience progression or death, their hazard rate during this interval is 0.2 (20/100). If during this same interval, only 10 of the 100 patients receiving the experimental therapy experience progression or death, their hazard rate is 0.1 (10/100). In this simple example, the hazard ratio for the interval, calculated as *the ratio of the hazard rates* is 0.5 (0.1/0.2) and indicates the likelihood of experiencing a hazardous event is reduced by 50% in the experimental arm. As commonly presented, and as this simple example illustrates, the lower the

hazard ratio, the better the experimental therapy. To determine whether the hazard ratio has statistical significance, one can (1) use a log-rank test to show that the null hypothesis that the two treatments lead to the same survival probabilities is wrong, or (2) use a parametric approach writing a regression model and fitting the data to the model so that one can establish the hazard ratio for the whole trial and its statistical significance. In many cases, the Cox proportional hazard model is used. Although the ideal hazard ratio would capture the differential benefit throughout the period of study, in practice, the extremes depicted in a Kaplan–Meier plot may not be analyzed.

## Forest Plots

Interest in determining whether there is heterogeneity in a treatment effect, such that better outcomes occur in some subgroups, has led to the use of Forest plots to display treatment effects across subgroups. Although simple in concept, these plots are subject to error because subgroups are composed of smaller numbers and the confidence intervals are therefore wider than those for the entire group. The most common presentation includes a vertical line at the *no effect point* (e.g., a hazard ratio of 1.0), with symbols of varying size representing the subgroups, each with its confidence interval depicted by a line that stretches from the symbol to both sides (the symbol size is usually proportional to the size of the subgroup). If the confidence interval for a subgroup crosses the no effect point, this is commonly interpreted (not necessarily correctly) as a lack of effect in the subgroup. *The information one seeks from a Forest plot is whether the effect size for different subgroups varies significantly from the main effect, which is determined by a test for heterogeneity.*[66]

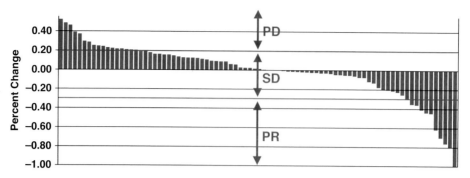

**Figure 30.4** Example of a waterfall plot demonstrating for each patient the maximum benefit obtained with the study therapy. Those to the *left* represent patients whose tumors increased, and those on the *right* represent patients whose tumors regressed. The *vertical red lines* at +20% and -30% define the boundaries of stable disease according to RECIST. Ideally, all responses should be confirmed after a period of at least 4 weeks. The example shown is of patients with renal cell carcinoma treated with the microtubule targeting agent ixabepilone. (From Huang H, Menefee M, Edgerly M, et al. A phase II clinical trial of ixabepilone [Ixempra; BMS-247550; NSC 710428], an epothilone B analog, in patients with metastatic renal cell carcinoma. *Clin Cancer Res* 2010;16:1634–1641.)

## Beyond Dichotomized Data

### Quality of Life

The assessment of cancer patients enrolled on a clinical trial can be said to consist of two sets of endpoints: cancer outcomes and patient outcomes. Cancer outcomes measure the response of the tumor to treatment, the duration of the response, the symptom-free period, and the early recognition of relapse. In contrast, patient outcomes assess the benefit achieved with a given therapy by measuring the increase in survival and the quality of life (QOL) before and after therapy. Unfortunately, physicians tend to concentrate on cancer-related outcomes, often neglecting assessments of QOL. Although a QOL assessment in clinical settings is possible with currently available instruments, there must be continued development and refinement of these instruments. Such development must focus not only on extracting valuable information in an unbiased manner, but also and equally important, developing an instrument that is user friendly and will be completed in a high percentage of encounters.

### Waterfall Plots

The arbitrary nature of the 50% cutoff set by Moertel and Hanley and its evolution to the current RECIST threshold of 30%

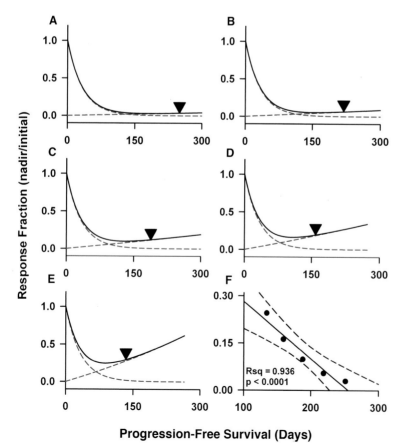

**Progression-Free Survival (Days)**

**Figure 30.5** The effect of the growth rate constant, *g*, on two commonly reported clinical values: maximum tumor shrinkage and PFS. Tumor measurements obtained in patients can be analyzed mathematically. **(A–E)** The *black line* depicts idealized clinical data using tumor quantities measured as patients received chemotherapy. Actually, clinical measurements comprise concurrent tumor regression *(dashed red line)* and growth *(dashed blue line)* that can be described by a rate constant and a first order kinetic equation, $f(t) = \exp^{(-d \cdot t)} + \exp^{(g \cdot t)} - 1$, where *exp* is the base of the natural logarithm, $e = 2.7182\ldots$, and *f* is the percent change in tumor measurement at time *t*, normalized to the value when treatment began. The rate constant *d* accounts for exponential decrease, whereas the rate constant *g* accounts for exponential growth occurring during treatment.[68,69] To demonstrate the correlation between the growth rate, tumor shrinkage and PFS, the *same* regression rate (*d*) has been modeled in panels *A* through *E*, whereas the growth rate constant, *g*, *increases* in each successive panel. The *black triangles* depict the point at which tumor size is 20% above the nadir (RECIST definition of PD). As the growth rate increases (i.e., faster tumor growth) from **A** to **E**, the nadir is reached sooner, and the depth of the nadir is less. **(F)** The correlation between PFS and maximum tumor shrinkage (nadir) is shown, plotting the correlation between PFS and response fraction, which is defined as the ratio of nadir to initial value.[68,69] Although idealized plots are given, the curves are based firmly on data obtained from patients enrolled on clinical trials.

reduction in the size of the maximum diameter raises valid queries as to why 30% is valuable and not 29% or 25%. On this background, waterfall plots such as the one shown in Figure 30.4 have become increasingly popular because they depict the benefit or lack thereof in all patients as a continuum of response, rather than a dichotomized response rate.[67] Waterfall plots can be generated from any quantitative assessment. If ctDNA or tumor cells prove to be as quantitative as hoped, the maximum decline could be plotted as a waterfall plot.

## Growth Kinetics

Efforts to quantify tumor kinetic parameters from clinical data have been investigated in recent years. Different equations have been applied to describe the two-phase curve based on tumor size as observed in most solid tumor trials, where there is first shrinkage followed by regrowth (Fig. 30.5). These models show exponential tumor shrinkage after treatment, followed by tumor regrowth that is either exponential or linear and have been shown to correlate with OS and to discriminate effective therapies as well as individual patients within trials.[68–73] A major advantage is that more of the data are used, relative to dichotomized response assessment, and regression or growth rates can be determined even in patients who are censored in a Kaplan–Meier analysis. Equations that model both regression and growth rates confirm the clinical intuition that resistant disease is emerging even as overall tumor volume is reduced. Further, "the strategy of studying tumor growth kinetics circumvents one weakness of 'progression criteria,' which is that they inherently dichotomize a complex biological process that may be better characterized using a continuous function."[74] As shown in Figure 30.5, the response of a tumor to a therapy is exemplified by the nadir, the time to the nadir, and the time to progression or PFS, and these are all are all dependent on the growth rate.

## REFERENCES

1. America's Biopharmaceutical Research Companies. *Medicines in Development for Cancer*. PhRMA Web site. http://www.phrma.org/sites/default/files/pdf/phrmamedicinesindevelopmentcancer2012.pdf.
2. Moertel CG, Hanley JA. The effect of measuring error on the results of therapeutic trials in advanced cancer. *Cancer* 1976;38:388–394.
3. Miller AB, Hoogstraten B, Staquet M, et al. Reporting results of cancer treatment. *Cancer* 1981;47:207–214.
4. Therasse P, Arbuck SG, Eisenhauer EA, et al. New guidelines to evaluate the response to treatment in solid tumors. European Organization for Research and Treatment of Cancer, National Cancer Institute of the United States, National Cancer Institute of Canada. *J Natl Cancer Inst* 2000;92:205–216.
5. Eisenhauer EA, Therasse P, Bogaerts J, et al. New response evaluation criteria in solid tumours: revised RECIST guideline (version 1.1). *Eur J Cancer* 2009;45:228–247.
6. Mazumdar M, Smith A, Schwartz LH. A statistical simulation study finds discordance between WHO criteria and RECIST guideline. *J Clin Epidemiol* 2004;57:358–365.
7. Wen PY, Macdonald DR, Reardon DA, et al. Updated response assessment criteria for high-grade gliomas: response assessment in neuro-oncology working group. *J Clin Oncol* 2010;28:1963–1972.
8. Byrne MJ, Nowak AK. Modified RECIST criteria for assessment of response in malignant pleural mesothelioma. *Ann Oncol* 2004;15:257–260.
9. Wolchok JD, Hoos A, O'Day S, et al. Guidelines for the evaluation of immune therapy activity in solid tumors: immune-related response criteria. *Clin Cancer Res* 2009;15:7412–7420.
10. Quant EC, Wen PY. Response assessment in neuro-oncology. *Curr Oncol Rep* 2011;13:50–56.
11. Hawkins-Daarud A, Rockne RC, Anderson AR, et al. Modeling tumor-associated edema in gliomas during anti-angiogenic therapy and its impact on imageable tumor. *Front Oncol* 2013;3:66.
12. Fink J, Born D, Chamberlain MC. Pseudoprogression: relevance with respect to treatment of high-grade gliomas. *Curr Treat Options Oncol* 2011;12:240–252.
13. Lin NU, Lee EQ, Aoyama H, et al. Challenges relating to solid tumour brain metastases in clinical trials, part 1: patient population, response, and progression. A report from the RANO group. *Lancet Oncol* 2013;14:e396–e406.
14. Mabille M, Vanel D, Albiter M, et al. Follow-up of hepatic and peritoneal metastases of gastrointestinal tumors (GIST) under Imatinib therapy requires different criteria of radiological evaluation (size is not everything!!!). *Eur J Radiol* 2009;69:204–208.
15. Liu L, Wang W, Chen H, et al. EASL- and mRECIST-evaluated responses to combination therapy of sorafenib with transarterial chemoembolization predict survival in patients with hepatocellular carcinoma. *Clin Cancer Res* 2014;20:1623–1631.
16. Cheson BD, Pfistner B, Juweid ME, et al. Revised response criteria for malignant lymphoma. *J Clin Oncol* 2007;25:579–586.
17. Bernhard J, Dietrich D, Scheithauer W, et al. Clinical benefit and quality of life in patients with advanced pancreatic cancer receiving gemcitabine plus capecitabine versus gemcitabine alone: a randomized multicenter phase III clinical trial—SAKK 44/00-CECOG/PAN.1.3.001. *J Clin Oncol* 2008;26:3695–3701.
18. Burris HA, Moore MJ, Andersen J, et al. Improvements in survival and clinical benefit with gemcitabine as first-line therapy for patients with advanced pancreas cancer: a randomized trial. *J Clin Oncol* 1997;15:2403–2413.
19. Mann BS, Johnson JR, He K, et al. Vorinostat for treatment of cutaneous manifestations of advanced primary cutaneous T-cell lymphoma. *Clin Cancer Res* 2007;13:2318–2322.
20. von Minckwitz G, Untch M, Blohmer JU, et al. Definition and impact of pathologic complete response on prognosis after neoadjuvant chemotherapy in various intrinsic breast cancer subtypes. *J Clin Oncol* 2012;30:1796–1804.
21. Cortazar P, Zhang L, Untch M, et al. Pathological complete response and long-term clinical benefit in breast cancer: the CTNeoBC pooled analysis. *Lancet* 2014 [Epub ahead of print].
22. Bardia A, Baselga J. Neoadjuvant therapy as a platform for drug development and approval in breast cancer. *Clin Cancer Res* 2013;19:6360–6370.
23. Choi H, Charnsangavej C, Faria SC, et al. Correlation of computed tomography and positron emission tomography in patients with metastatic gastrointestinal stromal tumor treated at a single institution with imatinib mesylate: proposal of new computed tomography response criteria. *J Clin Oncol* 2007;25:1753–1759.
24. Schramm N, Englhart E, Schlemmer M, et al. Tumor response and clinical outcome in metastatic gastrointestinal stromal tumors under sunitinib therapy: comparison of RECIST, Choi and volumetric criteria. *Eur J Radiol* 2013;82:951–958.
25. Dudeck O, Zeile M, Reichardt P, et al. Comparison of RECIST and Choi criteria for computed tomographic response evaluation in patients with advanced gastrointestinal stromal tumor treated with sunitinib. *Ann Oncol* 2011;22:1828–1833.
26. Ronot M, Bouattour M, Wassermann J, et al. Alternative response criteria (Choi, European Association for the Study of the Liver, and Modified Response Evaluation Criteria in Solid Tumors [RECIST]) versus RECIST 1.1 in patients with advanced hepatocellular carcinoma treated with sorafenib. *Oncologist* 2014. http://prostatecancer.theoncologist.com/article/alternative-response-criteria-choi-european-association-study-liver-and-modified-response.
27. van der Veldt AA, Meijerink MR, van den Eertwegh AJ, et al. Choi response criteria for early prediction of clinical outcome in patients with metastatic renal cell cancer treated with sunitinib. *Br J Cancer* 2010;102:803–809.
28. Wahl RL, Jacene H, Kasamon Y, et al. From RECIST to PERCIST: evolving considerations for PET response criteria in solid tumors. *J Nucl Med* 2009;50:122S–150S.
29. Shankar LK, Hoffman JM, Bacharach S, et al. Consensus recommendations for the use of 18F-FDG PET as an indicator of therapeutic response in patients in National Cancer Institute Trials. *J Nucl Med* 2006;47:1059–1066.
30. Young H, Baum R, Cremerius U, et al. Measurement of clinical and subclinical tumour response using [18F]-fluorodeoxyglucose and positron emission tomography: review and 1999 EORTC recommendations. European Organization for Research and Treatment of Cancer (EORTC) PET Study Group. *Eur J Cancer* 1999;35:1773–1782.
31. Kramer-Marek G, Capala J. Can PET imaging facilitate optimization of cancer therapies? *Curr Pharm Des* 2012;18:2657–2669.
32. Niederkohr RD, Greenspan BS, Prior JO, et al. Reporting guidance for oncologic 18F-FDG PET/CT imaging. *J Nucl Med* 2013;54:756–761.
33. Liu Y, Litière S, de Vries EG, et al. The role of response evaluation criteria in solid tumour in anticancer treatment evaluation: results of a survey in the oncology community. *Eur J Cancer* 2014;50:260–266.
34. Rubin EH, Allen JD, Nowak JA, et al. Developing precision medicine in a global world. *Clin Cancer Res* 2014;20:1419–1427.
35. Parkinson DR, McCormack RT, Keating SM. Evidence of clinical utility: an unmet need in molecular diagnostics for cancer patients. *Clin Cancer Res* 2014;20:1428–1444.
36. Buyse M, Sargent DJ, Grothey A, et al. Biomarkers and surrogate end points—the challenge of statistical validation. *Nat Rev Clin Oncol* 2010;7:309–317.
37. Karam AK, Karlan BY. Ovarian cancer: the duplicity of CA125 measurement. *Nat Rev Clin Oncol* 2010;7:335–339.

38. Rustin GJ, van der Burg ME, Griffin CL, et al. Early versus delayed treatment of relapsed ovarian cancer (MRC OV05/EORTC 55955): a randomised trial. *Lancet* 2010;376:1155–1163.

39. Vergote I, Rustin GJ, Eisenhauer EA, et al. Re: new guidelines to evaluate the response to treatment in solid tumors [ovarian cancer]. Gynecologic Cancer Intergroup. *J Natl Cancer Inst* 2000;92:1534–1535.

40. Guppy AE, Rustin GJ. CA125 response: can it replace the traditional response criteria in ovarian cancer? *Oncologist* 2002;7:437–443.

41. Rustin GJ, Quinn M, Thigpen T, et al. Re: New guidelines to evaluate the response to treatment in solid tumors (ovarian cancer). *J Natl Cancer Inst* 2004; 96:487–488.

42. Rustin GJ, Vergote I, Eisenhauer E, et al. Definitions for response and progression in ovarian cancer clinical trials incorporating RECIST 1.1 and CA 125 agreed by the Gynecological Cancer Intergroup (GCIG). *Int J Gynecol Cancer* 2011;21:419–423.

43. Eisenhauer EA. Optimal assessment of response in ovarian cancer. *Ann Oncol* 2011;22:viii49–viii51.

44. Bubley GJ, Carducci M, Dahut W, et al. Eligibility and response guidelines for phase II clinical trials in androgen-independent prostate cancer: recommendations from the Prostate-Specific Antigen Working Group. *J Clin Oncol* 1999;17:3461–3467.

45. Scher HI, Halabi S, Tannock I, et al. Design and end points of clinical trials for patients with progressive prostate cancer and castrate levels of testosterone: recommendations of the Prostate Cancer Clinical Trials Working Group. *J Clin Oncol* 2008;26:1148–1159.

46. Mazumdar M, Bajorin DF, Bacik J, et al. Predicting outcome to chemotherapy in patients with germ cell tumors: the value of the rate of decline of human chorionic gonadotrophin and alpha-fetoprotein during therapy. *J Clin Oncol* 2001;19:2534–2541.

47. Fizazi K, Culine S, Kramar A, et al. Early predicted time to normalization of tumor markers predicts outcome in poor-prognosis nonseminomatous germ cell tumors. *J Clin Oncol* 2004;22:3868–3876.

48. Toner GC. Early identification of therapeutic failure in nonseminomatous germ cell tumors by assessing serum tumor marker decline during chemotherapy: still not ready for routine clinical use. *J Clin Oncol* 2004;22:3842–3845.

49. Gilligan TD, Seidenfeld J, Basch EM, et al. American Society of Clinical Oncology Clinical Practice Guideline on uses of serum tumor markers in adult males with germ cell tumors. *J Clin Oncol* 2010;28:3388–3404.

50. Albers P, Albrecht W, Algaba F, et al. EAU guidelines on testicular cancer: 2011 update. *Eur Urol* 2011;60:304–319.

51. Yap T, Lorente D, Omlin A, et al. Circulating tumor cells: a multifunctional biomarker. *Clin Cancer Res* 2014;20:2553–2568.

52. Dawson SJ, Tsui DW, Murtaza M, et al. Analysis of circulating tumor DNA to monitor metastatic breast cancer. *N Engl J Med* 2013;368:1199–1209.

53. Punnoose EA, Atwal S, Liu W, et al. Evaluation of circulating tumor cells and circulating tumor DNA in non-small cell lung cancer: association with clinical endpoints in a phase II clinical trial of pertuzumab and erlotinib. *Clin Cancer Res* 2012; 18:2391–2401.

54. Bettegowda C, Sausen M, Leary RJ, et al. Detection of circulating tumor DNA in early- and late-stage human malignancies. *Sci Transl Med* 2014;6:224ra24.

55. Pazdur R. Endpoints for assessing drug activity in clinical trials. *Oncologist* 2008;13:19–21.

56. Buyse M, Thirion P, Carlson RW, et al. Relation between tumour response to first-line chemotherapy and survival in advanced colorectal cancer: a meta-analysis. Meta-Analysis Group in Cancer. *Lancet* 2000;356:373–378.

57. Bruzzi P, Del Mastro L, Sormani MP, et al. Objective response to chemotherapy as a potential surrogate end point of survival in metastatic breast cancer patients. *J Clin Oncol* 2005;23:5117–5125.

58. Vidaurre T, Wilkerson J, Simon R, et al. Stable disease is not preferentially observed with targeted therapies and as currently defined has limited value in drug development. *Cancer J* 2009;15:366–373.

59. McKee AE, Farrell AT, Pazdur R, et al. The role of the U.S. Food and Drug Administration review process: clinical trial endpoints in oncology. *Oncologist* 2010;15:13–18.

60. Ohorodnyk P, Eisenhauer EA, Booth CM. Clinical benefit in oncology trials: is this a patient-centred or tumour-centred end-point? *Eur J Cancer* 2009; 45:2249–2252.

61. Buyse M. Use of meta-analysis for the validation of surrogate endpoints and biomarkers in cancer trials. *Cancer J* 2009;15:421–425.

62. Wilkerson J, Fojo T. Progression-free survival is simply a measure of a drug's effect while administered and is not a surrogate for overall survival. *Cancer J* 2009;15:379–385.

63. Reck M, von Pawel J, Zatloukal P, et al. Overall survival with cisplatin-gemcitabine and bevacizumab or placebo as first-line therapy for nonsquamous non-small-cell lung cancer: results from a randomised phase III trial (AVAiL). *Ann Oncol* 2010;21:1804–1809.

64. Hortobagyi GN, Gomez HL, Li RK, et al. Analysis of overall survival from a phase III study of ixabepilone plus capecitabine versus capecitabine in patients with MBC resistant to anthracyclines and taxanes. *Breast Cancer Res Treat* 2010; 122:409–418.

65. Hennekens C, Buring J. *Epidemiology in Medicine.* 1st ed. Boston: Little, Brown and Co.; 1987.

66. Cuzick J. Forest plots and the interpretation of subgroups. *Lancet* 2005;365:1308.

67. Huang H, Menefee M, Edgerly M, et al. A phase II clinical trial of ixabepilone (Ixempra; BMS-247550; NSC 710428), an epothilone B analog, in patients with metastatic renal cell carcinoma. *Clin Cancer Res* 2010;16:1634–1641.

68. Stein WD, Gulley JL, Schlom J, et al. Tumor regression and growth rates determined in five intramural NCI prostate cancer trials: the growth rate constant as an indicator of therapeutic efficacy. *Clin Cancer Res* 2011;17:907–917.

69. Stein WD, Wilkerson J, Kim ST, et al. Analyzing the pivotal trial that compared sunitinib and IFN-α in renal cell carcinoma, using a method that assesses tumor regression and growth. *Clin Cancer Res* 2012;18:2374–2381.

70. Maitland ML, Wu K, Sharma MR, et al. Estimation of renal cell carcinoma treatment effects from disease progression modeling. *Clin Pharmacol Ther* 2013;93:345–351.

71. Claret L, Girard P, Hoff PM, et al. Model-based prediction of phase III overall survival in colorectal cancer on the basis of phase II tumor dynamics. *J Clin Oncol* 2009;27:4103–4108.

72. Claret L, Gupta M, Han K, et al. Evaluation of tumor-size response metrics to predict overall survival in Western and Chinese patients with first-line metastatic colorectal cancer. *J Clin Oncol* 2013;31:2110–2114.

73. Wang Y, Sung C, Dartois C, et al. Elucidation of relationship between tumor size and survival in non-small-cell lung cancer patients can aid early decision making in clinical drug development. *Clin Pharmacol Ther* 2009;86:167–174.

74. Oxnard GR, Morris MJ, Hodi FS, et al. When progressive disease does not mean treatment failure: reconsidering the criteria for progression. *J Natl Cancer Inst* 2012;104:1534–1541.

75. Team RDC. R: A language and environment for statistical computing. R Foundation for Statistical Computing. Vienna, Austria: R Foundation for Statistical Computing, 2010. http://www.r-project.org.

## PART IV

# Cancer Prevention and Screening

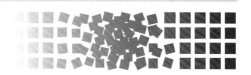

# 31 Tobacco Use and the Cancer Patient

Graham W. Warren, Benjamin A. Toll, Irene M. Tamí-Maury, and Ellen R. Gritz

## INTRODUCTION

Tobacco is commonly described as the largest preventable cause of cancer. Over 50 years ago, tobacco was increasingly recognized as the primary cause of lung cancer, with definitive recognition for tobacco use as a causative factor in the seminal 1964 U.S. Surgeon General's Report (SGR) on Smoking and Health.[1] Recent editions of the SGR have described the widespread adverse health effects of tobacco on a spectrum of diseases, including as a causative agent for a spectrum of cancers.[2,3] Tobacco use is an addiction usually initiated in youth prior to the age of 18 and is driven by the highly addictive drug, nicotine.[4] As related to the cancer patient, considerable work has been conducted to associate tobacco use with the risk of developing cancer and how tobacco cessation can substantially reduce cancer risks. However, there is a relative paucity of effort that has been put forth to identify the effects of smoking on outcomes for cancer patients or to establish methods to help cancer patients quit smoking. Fortunately, in recent years, the importance of tobacco use by the cancer patient has been increasingly recognized as an important health behavior, including a National Cancer Institute (NCI)–sponsored conference on tobacco use in 2010, a joint sponsored NCI–American Association of Cancer Research (AACR)–sponsored workshop at the Institute of Medicine in 2012, and recent recommendations by the AACR and the American Society of Clinical Oncology (ASCO) to address tobacco use in cancer patients.[5,6] The recently released 2014 SGR now provides substantial evidence behind the effects of smoking by cancer patients with the following conclusions[7]:

1. In cancer patients and survivors, the evidence is sufficient to infer a causal relationship between cigarette smoking and adverse health outcomes. Quitting smoking improves the prognosis of cancer patients.
2. In cancer patients and survivors, the evidence is sufficient to infer a causal relationship between cigarette smoking and increased all-cause mortality and cancer-specific mortality.
3. In cancer patients and survivors, the evidence is sufficient to infer a causal relationship between cigarette smoking and increased risk for second primary cancers known to be caused by cigarette smoking, such as lung cancer.
4. In cancer patients and survivors, the evidence is suggestive but not sufficient to infer a causal relationship between cigarette smoking and the risk of recurrence, poorer response to treatment, and increased treatment-related toxicity.

The overall objective of this chapter is to discuss tobacco use by cancer patients, the clinical effects of smoking in cancer patients, methods to address tobacco use by cancer patients, and areas of needed research.

## NEUROBIOLOGY OF TOBACCO DEPENDENCE

Nicotine is the primary addictive component of tobacco that increases extracellular concentrations of dopamine in the nucleus accumbens and stimulates the mesolimbic dopaminergic system,[8,9] resulting in nicotine's rewarding effect experienced by tobacco users.[10–12] Dopaminergic neurotransmission may also be involved in the assignment of incentive salience, or stimulus for a pleasure based reward, to tobacco use–related environmental cues[13,14] that may become conditioned reinforcers of tobacco use behaviors. For example, an individual who smokes while drinking their morning coffee may associate coffee, or even holding a coffee cup in their hand, with the reward from smoking. Thus, cigarette smoking is directly linked to external nontobacco-based behavioral stimuli. Activation of the nucleus accumbens has further been implicated in drug reinstatement or relapse.[15,16] Individuals who have quit tobacco use for years have restarted a tobacco habit simply by sitting next to a smoker and being exposed to secondhand smoke. Substantial work has been conducted on the addictive nature of tobacco and nicotine, and readers are referred to several comprehensive reviews on this topic.[9,12,17]

## TOBACCO USE PREVALENCE AND THE EVOLUTION OF TOBACCO PRODUCTS

Much of the discussion on tobacco use epidemiology and carcinogenesis is presented in Chapter 4. In brief, the prevalence of cigarette smoking among adults in the United States decreased to 19.0% as compared with 22.8% in 2001, but it did not meet the *Healthy People 2010* objective to reduce smoking prevalence to 12%.[18,19] There have been substantial changes in the landscape of tobacco use over time as a direct consequence of cigarette-centered policies and regulations aiming to reduce the harmful effects and number of deaths caused by smoking.[20–22] Under this new landscape, novel and reemergent noncigarette tobacco products such as cigars, cigarillos, snuff, chewing tobacco, water pipes (hookahs), and other forms of tobacco consumption have been growing in demand as a consequence of aggressive and sophisticated marketing by the tobacco industry.[23] Consumption patterns have also changed due to efforts by the tobacco industry to make cigarettes appear safer, such as low tar or filtered cigarettes, and the inclusion of flavoring (menthol, vanilla, fruits, etc.).[24] Although these efforts may have changed consumption patterns, they have not reduced cancer risk. Large patient cohorts demonstrate that the introduction of low tar and filtered cigarettes actually increased risk by promoting deeper inhalation and higher rates of addiction with no reductions in cancer risk,[24,25] resulting in subsequent changes in lung cancer from centrally located squamous cell cancers to peripherally located nonsquamous cell cancers.

The relatively recent introduction of electronic cigarettes (i.e., e-cigarettes, e-cigs, nicotine vaporizers, or electronic nicotine delivery systems [ENDS]) is noteworthy. These electronic or battery-powered devices activate a heating element that vaporizes a liquid solution contained in a cartridge, and then the user inhales this vapor. Levels of nicotine as well as other chemical additives and flavors in the cartridge are uncertain and vary according to the brand.[26] Although there are no research studies that have evaluated the potential harmful effects of the use of e-cigarettes for cancer patients,[27] organizations such as the World Health Organization have already expressed concerns about the safety of these increasingly popular products.[28,29] To date, e-cigarettes have not been approved by the U.S. Food and Drug Administration (FDA) as therapeutic devices to aid in quitting smoking.[26] Readers are referred to a recent editorial on the use of e-cigarettes by cancer patients[27]; however, it will likely be several years before evidence-based health information is available.

## TOBACCO USE BY THE CANCER PATIENT

The prevalence of current smoking among long-term adult cancer survivors appears to have declined in the past decade,[30] but data suggest higher rates of smoking among cancer survivors than in the general population.[30–32] These data are often biased by the fact that assessments in cancer patients may not include cancer patients who were current smokers at the time of death. As a result, estimates of smoking rates in cancer survivors may be misleading and may underestimate true tobacco use patterns for cancer patients. Furthermore, alternative tobacco products are often not assessed in cancer patients. Data from the Childhood Cancer Survivor Study and the 2009 Behavioral Risk Factor Surveillance System indicate that approximately 3% to 8% of cancer survivors use smokeless tobacco products.[33,34] Patients may be attracted to these alternative products due to less social stigma and the nonevidence-based perception that these products are healthier alternatives compared to cigarette smoking.

Continued tobacco use by cancer patients often represents a combined failure by the patient to recognize the need to stop smoking even after a cancer diagnosis and the effort by health-care providers to address tobacco use with evidence-based assessments and tobacco cessation support. Approximately 30% of all cancer patients use tobacco at the time of cancer diagnosis with higher rates in traditionally tobacco-related disease sites, such as head and neck or lung cancers, and lower rates in traditionally nontobacco-related disease sites, such as breast or prostate cancers.[35–44] However, findings from several studies indicate that cancer patients are receptive to smoking cessation interventions even as they continue to smoke.[35,38,45–50]

A cancer diagnosis can be used as a window of opportunity, or *teachable moment*, to intervene and provide assistance in the quitting process.[51] A recent study in 12,000 cancer patients, including 2,700 patients who smoked, capitalized on the teachable moment and demonstrated that less than 3% of patients who were contacted by the cessation program rejected tobacco cessation assistance.[45] However, only 1.2% of patients who received a mailed invitation participated in the program. This highlights the idea that patients may be interested in quitting, but methods such as mailed tobacco cessation information may not yield effective participation by cancer patients. Once enrolled, patients and clinicians must realize that although relapses in the general population usually occur within 1 week of cessation, relapses in cancer patients may be delayed due to cancer treatment–related variables such as surgical or other posttreatment healing.[52] Consequently, it is important to continue offering tobacco assessments and cessation support for cancer survivorship efforts.

### Defining Tobacco Use by the Cancer Patient

In dealing with tobacco use by cancer patients, it is important to note that virtually all of the evidence associating tobacco with cancer treatment outcomes deals with smoking. Few studies report associations between other forms of tobacco use (e.g., smokeless, cigars, cigarillos) and outcomes in cancer patients. Furthermore, the definition of smoking across published studies varies substantially.[53] In studies of cancer patients, smoking has been defined as current (e.g., smoking after diagnosis, at diagnosis, in the weeks

before diagnosis, within the 12 months prior to diagnosis, after diagnosis, within the past 10 years), former (e.g., recent, intermediate-, or long-term quit for 1 month, 3 month, 6 month, 12 month, 2 years, 5 years, 10 years), never, quitting after diagnosis, and according to exposure (e.g., multiple pack year cutoffs, Brinkman index, years of smoking, years of smoking within a predefined period of time such as 5 years prior to diagnosis). Though the nonstandard method of addressing tobacco use in cancer patients has been observed in several reports,[54–57] there are no current standard recommendations for the definition of tobacco use by any national organization. There are four primary categories for smoking status:

1. **Never smoking** is typically defined as having smoked less than 100 cigarettes in a person's lifetime and no current cigarette use. These patients are generally considered as a reference group in many studies. Categories 2 through 4 require that a person has smoked at least 100 cigarettes in their lifetime.
2. **Former smoking** is typically defined as no current cigarette use, usually within the past year.
3. **Recent smoking** (or recent quit) is generally defined as having stopped smoking within the recent past, typically for a period of 1 week to 1 year.
4. **Current smoking** is typically defined as smoking one or more cigarettes per day every day or some days.

*Ever* smoking is a combination of categories 2 through 4 (i.e., former, recent, and current smokers) that has been used to report negative associations between smoking and cancer outcomes in a number of studies.[58–70] Defining smoking according to *ever* smoking status limits the ability to interpret the effects of current smoking on a clinical outcome, and nothing can be done to address a prior tobacco use history. However, defining exposure according to *current* smoking status allows for the analysis of potentially reversible effects as well as for the potential implementation of smoking cessation to prevent the adverse outcomes of smoking on cancer patients. The primary focus for the remainder of this chapter will be on *current* smoking and will include a discussion of methods to address tobacco use with the cancer patient through accurate assessments and structured tobacco cessation support.

## THE CLINICAL EFFECTS OF SMOKING ON THE CANCER PATIENT

Cancer treatment is generally defined according to disease site, stage, treatment type (e.g., surgery, chemotherapy [CT], radiotherapy [RT], or biologic therapy), and primary treatment objective, such as cure or palliation. A comprehensive discussion of the effects of smoking on cancer patients is beyond the scope of a single chapter, but the 2014 SGR provides an excellent evidence base, concluding that "the evidence is sufficient to infer a causal relationship between cigarette smoking and adverse health outcomes."[7] Overall, approximately 75% to 80% of studies in the SGR demonstrated a negative association between smoking and outcome, with approximately 65% to 70% of studies demonstrating statistically significant negative associations. This chapter will provide an illustrative review of studies that demonstrate the adverse effects of tobacco across disease sites and treatment modalities (e.g., surgery, CT, RT), and effects will be discussed across the categories of *mortality*, *recurrence and cancer-related mortality*, *toxicity*, and *risk of a second primary cancer*. Evidence for the benefits of smoking cessation will also be presented within each section.

### The Effect of Smoking on Overall Mortality

Substantial evidence demonstrates that current smoking by cancer patients increases the risk of overall mortality across virtually all cancer disease sites and for all treatment modalities. Currently smoking significantly increased the risk of overall mortality by between 17% to 38% as compared with never, former, and recent quit smokers in a large cohort of patients across 13 disease sites.[71] Similar but larger observations were noted in elderly current smokers from a separate cohort (hazard ratio [HR], 1.72, 95% confidence interval [CI], 1.23 to 2.42).[72] A large analysis of over 20,000 patients treated with surgery demonstrated that current smoking increased mortality by 62% in gastrointestinal cancer patients and by 50% in thoracic cancer patients with a nonsignificant trend in urologic cancer patients.[73] Several larger studies with at least 500 patients demonstrated that current smoking increases mortality in head and neck cancer,[74–77] breast cancer,[78–81] gastrointestinal cancers,[82,83] prostate cancer,[84–87] renal cancer,[88] gynecologic cancers,[89,90] and lung cancer.[91–102] Smaller studies demonstrate similar effects for hematolymphoid cancers such as leukemia and lymphoma.[103,104] Studies suggest that the effects of current smoking on mortality may be dose and time dependent, with higher risks in heavier smokers[105,106] and lesser risks in patients whose time since quitting was longer.[105]

Whereas many reports rely on retrospective chart reviews, several prospective studies demonstrate that current smoking increases mortality.[71] Browman et al.[107] was one of the first prospective studies to demonstrate that current smoking increased mortality by 2.3-fold in patients who continued to smoke during RT as compared with nonsmokers. Results from Radiation Therapy Oncology Group (RTOG) 9003 and 0129 cooperative group trials demonstrated that current smoking increased mortality in advanced head and neck cancer patients treated with RT or concurrent chemoradiotherapy (CRT),[108] with a similar effect noted in 165 cervical cancer patients treated with CRT.[109] In the randomized retinoid chemoprevention trial of 1,190 early stage head and neck cancer patients, current smoking increased mortality by 2.5-fold.[110]

Numerous studies have demonstrated that current smoking increases overall mortality as compared with former and never smokers combined.[72,75,76,101,102,107,108] The adverse effects of smoking compared with former and never smokers not only reflect the negative effects of smoking on mortality as a whole, but also demonstrate that the effects of smoking are reversible. Current smoking increased mortality risk as compared with patients who quit within the year[71] or 1 to 3 months prior to diagnosis.[111,112] Furthermore, in 284 limited-stage small-cell lung cancer patients, patients who quit smoking at or following a cancer diagnosis had a 45% reduction in mortality as compared with current smokers.[113] These studies suggest that the effects of smoking on mortality are reversible.

Collectively, these studies provide significant data associating current smoking with increased overall mortality across most disease sites, tumor stages, treatment modalities, and in both traditionally tobacco-related as well as nontobacco-related cancers. The potential significance of smoking is perhaps best exemplified by Bittner et al.,[114] who analyzed causes of death in prostate cancer patients and demonstrated that more than 90% died of causes other than prostate cancer, but that current smoking increased the risks of non–prostate cancer deaths between 3- and 5.5-fold. As a result, tobacco use and cessation may be of paramount importance to cancers with high cure rates, such as prostate cancer or breast cancer, simply because patients may be at the most risk of death from noncancer-related causes such as heart disease, pulmonary disease, or other diseases related to smoking and tobacco use.

## The Effect of Smoking on Cancer Recurrence and Cancer-Related Mortality

The primary objective of cancer therapy is to cure cancer and prevent recurrence. However, smoking has been shown to increase cancer recurrence and cancer-related mortality. Across a broad spectrum of cancer patients, current smoking increased cancer mortality as compared with former and never smokers.[71] Current smoking has been shown to increase cancer mortality in patients with head and neck cancer,[108,115–118] breast cancer,[78,119]

gastrointestinal cancers,[82,120,121] prostate cancer,[41,84,122] gynecologic cancers,[89,90,106,123–125] and lung cancer.[126] Cancer recurrence, whether local or metastatic, is a key driver behind cancer-related mortality. Several studies demonstrate that current smoking increases the risk of recurrence and decreases response across multiple disease sites.[76,84,107,127,128] The effects of smoking on increasing recurrence or cancer-related mortality have also been reported in several relatively rare cancers.[120,129] In a remarkable report of patients with recurrent head and neck cancers treated with salvage surgery, continued smoking after salvage treatment continued to increase the risk of yet another recurrence by 42%.[130] The striking nature of this last study highlights the continued risks even in recurrent cancer patients and the resilience with which some cancer patients will continue to smoke.

The effects of smoking are also noted in premalignant lesions. In patients with high-grade vulvar intraepithelial neoplasia, current smoking increased the risk of persistent disease after therapy by 30-fold.[131] In a prospective trial of progesterone to treat cervical intraepithelial neoplasia (CIN), current smoking increased the risk of progression as compared with former and never smokers combined.[132] A prospective trial of 516 low-grade cervical intraepithelial neoplasia patients demonstrated that current smoking decreased response by 36%, although a similar effect was also noted in former smokers.[133]

As noted with overall mortality, several studies demonstrated that the effects of current smoking are worse than the effects of former smoking[76,86,89,109,127,134–136,137] and that the effects of smoking may be acutely reversible. Several studies also demonstrate that current smoking increases recurrence or cancer mortality, whereas former smoking has no significant effect.[41,78,82,84,85,119,122–124,138] The acutely reversible effects of smoking were shown by Browman et al.[139] who demonstrated that continued smoking increased the risk of cancer-related mortality by 23% as compared with patients who quit within 12 weeks of starting RT. In 284 colorectal cancer patients, smoking at the first postoperative visit increased the risk of cancer mortality by 2.5-fold as compared with all other patients suggesting that smoking after treatment significantly predict for adverse outcome.[121] In a notable study of over 1,400 prostate cancer patients treated with surgery, continued smoking 1 year after treatment increased the risk of recurrence 2.3-fold, but quitting smoking 1 year after treatment did not confer an increased risk of recurrence.[128] Chen et al.[138] demonstrate that patients who continue to smoke before and following a bladder cancer diagnosis have an increased risk of recurrence as compared with patients who quit in the year prior to diagnosis or within the first 3 months after diagnosis. The reversible effects of smoking on recurrence and mortality are consistent with observations on overall mortality and continue to emphasize the benefit of tobacco cessation for cancer patients who smoke at diagnosis.

## The Effect of Smoking on Cancer Treatment Toxicity

Discussion of the effects of smoking on cancer treatment toxicity is highly dependent upon disease site, treatment modality (e.g., surgery, CT, RT), and timing of toxicity. Across disease sites and treatments, current smoking has been shown to increase complications from surgery,[140–149] pulmonary complications,[150,151] toxicity from RT,[117,152–156] mucositis,[157] hospitalization,[158] and vasomotor symptoms.[159] One of the largest recent studies in over 20,000 gastrointestinal, pulmonary, and urologic patients demonstrates that former or current smoking increased the risk of surgical site infection, pulmonary complications, or 30-day mortality in a site-specific manner.[73] The effects of current smoking were most significant for pulmonary complications where former smoking had a lesser or nonsignificant effect. In 13,469 lung cancer patients treated with surgery, current smoking increased the risk of postoperative death with no increased risk in former smokers.[160] Current smoking increased the risk of complications, morbidity, or reoperation following esophagectomy, pancreatectomy, or colorectal surgery.[161–163] A study of 836 prostate cancer patients treated with RT demonstrated that current smoking increased abdominal cramps, rectal urgency, diarrhea, incomplete emptying, and sudden emptying between two- and nine-fold,[164] with similar effects noted in 3,489 cervical cancer patients who smoked more than 1 pack per day (PPD).[156]

Several studies have demonstrated that the effects of smoking on cancer treatment toxicity are reversible. Stopping smoking within 3 weeks of surgery reduced wound healing complications in esophageal cancer patients treated with surgery and reconstruction.[165] In 393 T1 laryngeal cancer patients treated with RT, quitting smoking after diagnosis reduced laryngeal complications as compared with continued smoking.[152] In a large study of 7,990 lung cancer patients from the Society of Thoracic Surgeons Database, current smoking increased the risk of pulmonary complications by 80% and hospital mortality 3.5-fold.[151] However, smoking cessation for 2 weeks eliminated the risks for pulmonary complications, and cessation for 1 month eliminated risks for hospital mortality. Vaporciyan et al.[166] also showed that current smoking increased the risk of pulmonary complications 2.7-fold as compared with smoking cessation for at least 1 month prior to surgery. In a striking example of the potentially reversible effects of smoking in 205 head and neck cancer patients treated with RT,[167] 43% of smoking patients treated in the morning experienced Grade 3+ mucositis compared with 72% of smokers treated in the afternoon (p = 0.04). These data suggest that reducing smoking overnight may yield a clinical benefit in reduced toxicity. Whereas all toxicity may not be acutely reversed, these encouraging data show that patients can make clinically meaningful improvements in their health and or cancer treatment within a short time frame by quitting smoking.

## The Effect of Smoking on Risk of Second Primary Cancer

Several studies have reported the effects of smoking on the risk of developing a second primary cancer. Park et al.[168] reported on over 14,000 male cancer patients and demonstrated that current smoking increased the risk of developing a second tobacco-related primary cancer twofold, with no increased risk in former smokers. A higher risk was observed in in head and neck cancer patients who smoked more than 10 cigarettes per day, with no increased risk in lighter smokers.[169] Kinoshita et al.[170] showed an 82% increased risk of developing a second primary in gastric cancer patients who are current smokers with no increased risk in former smokers. In the phase III randomized trial of isotretinoin for the prevention of a second primary tumor in 1,190 head and neck cancer patients, current smoking increased the risk of a second primary by 2.2-fold with a nonsignificant trend of 1.6-fold in former smokers.[110] Notably, 39% of patients who reported quitting within the previous year were biochemically confirmed smokers.[171] As a result, these data collectively suggest that some of the increased risk may be biased by continued smoking in patients who deny smoking by self-report.

The effects of smoking on the risk of a second primary cancer are also noted in nontobacco-related cancers and in long-term survivors. In 835 breast cancer patients, smoking increased the risk for the development of lung metastases after breast cancer by more than threefold.[172] Ford et al.[173] demonstrated that breast cancer patients who were former smokers had a threefold increased risk of developing lung cancer, but that current smokers had a 13-fold increased risk. In nearly 1,100 estrogen receptor (ER)-positive breast cancer patients, current smokers had a 1.8-fold increased risk of developing a second contralateral breast cancer, and current smokers at most recent follow-up had a 2.2-fold increased risk, but former smoking at the diagnosis or most recent follow-up had no increased risk.[174] In 2,700 5-year survivors of testicular cancer,

current smokers had a 1.8-fold increased risk of developing a second primary as compared with all other survivors.[175]

There are some studies suggesting that smoking, combined with cytotoxic therapy, may have an additive or synergistic effect on the risk of developing a second primary cancer. In 9,780 prostate cancer patients from the Cancer of the Prostate Strategic Urologic Research Endeavor (CaPSURE) study, RT increased the risk of bladder cancer by 1.6-fold, smoking increased the risk by 2.1-fold, and smoking combined with RT increased risk by 3.7-fold.[176] In ER-positive breast cancer patients, treatment with RT had no significant effect on the risk of developing a contralateral breast cancer, but RT combined with current smoking increased the risk of contralateral cancer by ninefold.[173] In a detailed analysis of Hodgkin lymphoma patients, nonheavy smokers (defined as never, former, and less than one PPD) had a second primary relative risk of between fourfold and sevenfold when treated with CT or RT as compared with patients who received no RT or CT.[177] However, heavy smokers had a sixfold increased risk in the absence of RT and CT and a 17- to 49-fold increased risk when combined with RT and/or CT. These observations suggest that smoking combined with cytotoxic cancer therapy may complement the risk of developing a second primary cancer perhaps through the promotion of mutations induced by CT and/or RT in the presence of tobacco smoke. The potential mechanisms of this effect have not been tested or defined at this time, but the mechanism of tobacco-induced carcinogenesis in prior reports[3] supports these observations.

## Human Papilloma Virus, Epidermal Growth Factor Receptor, Anaplastic Lymphoma Kinase, Programmed Cell Death Protein 1, and Smoking

Data over the past decade has shown that head and neck cancers that are human papilloma virus (HPV) positive are known to have an improved prognosis as compared with HPV-negative tumors.[178] Patients who have HPV-positive tumors typically have increased p16 expression and often respond better to conventional cancer therapy, including RT and CT. Many HPV-positive patients are never smokers or have a lighter smoking history. However, smoking was an independent adverse risk factor for both overall and cancer-related mortality with a 1% increase in risk per pack-year smoked.[178] Current smoking increased cancer mortality approximately fivefold even in p16-positive patients treated with surgery.[115] Smoking also increased the risk of developing second primary cancer in both HPV-positive and HPV-negative patients.[179] As a consequence, the presence of HPV does not appear to negate the adverse effects of smoking.

A similar effect is noted in lung cancer patients with epidermal growth factor receptor (EGFR)-mutated or anaplastic lymphoma kinase (ALK)-mutated tumors. As with HPV-positive head and neck cancer patients, lung cancer patients who are light or never smokers have a higher rate of EGFR-positive tumors that may respond to biologic therapy using EGFR tyrosine–kinase inhibitors. At this time, most information regarding EGFR-based therapy for lung cancer reports on the effects of ever smoking demonstrating that ever smokers have a decreased response to EGFR therapy. Early, large, randomized trials demonstrate that Tarceva (erlotinib) and Iressa (gefitinib) provide survival and tumor control benefits specifically in never smokers.[180,181] A very similar pattern is noted for ALK-positive patients with a much higher incidence in never smokers and high response rate to the ALK kinase inhibitor crizotinib.[182] Paik et al.[183] have described the importance of driver mutations in EGFR, ALK, and KRAS demonstrating that smokers have a higher preponderance for K-ras drivers, whereas nonsmokers tend to have EGFR or ALK driver mutations. In general, patients who are smokers may be best served with conventional cancer treatments rather than these biologic therapies, but randomized controlled trials confirming this suggestion are lacking at this time.

Although there are essentially no biologic therapies that have shown to have a better response in smokers, there are exciting data presented at the 2013 European CanCer Organization (ECCO) annual conference, suggesting that anti–programmed cell death protein 1 (PD-1)–based therapies may have a better response rate in smokers.[184] These very preliminary data have yet to be replicated or expanded into randomized trials, but if expanded trials prove effective, they may represent one of the only cancer treatments that may specifically benefit smokers.

### Summarizing the Clinical Effects of Smoking on the Cancer Patient

Smoking by cancer patients increases mortality, toxicity, recurrence, and the risk of a second primary cancer. There are four important conclusions, and a fifth implied conclusion, to the evidence previously presented:

1. One or more adverse effects of smoking affect all cancer disease sites.
2. One or more adverse effects of smoking affect all treatment modalities.
3. The effects of current smoking are distinct from an ever or former smoking history.
4. Several lines of evidence demonstrate that many of the effects of smoking are reversible.

Although substantial data demonstrate that smoking by cancer patients increases the risk for one or more outcomes, the largest limitations are the lack of standard tobacco use definitions, the lack of assessing tobacco use in cancer patients at follow-up, and the lack of structured tobacco cessation for cancer patients. Importantly, patients may further misrepresent tobacco use. Several studies suggest that approximately 30% of cancer patients who smoke deny tobacco use.[171,185,186] Marin et al.[187] exemplify the importance of an accurate assessment, demonstrating that patients who self-reported smoking had no significant risk associated with surgical complications; however, biochemical confirmation of smoking significantly increased the risk of surgical wound complications. This highlights the potential discrepancy between the effects of smoking based on subjective versus biochemically confirmed assessments. Due to this discrepancy, the *fifth implied conclusion* is that the adverse effects of smoking and the benefits of cessation may be more pronounced than currently reported in the literature.

## ADDRESSING TOBACCO USE BY THE CANCER PATIENT

### National Oncology Association Statements and Clinical Practice Guidelines

Professional societies are taking leadership roles in recognizing the need to assess patients' tobacco use and to examine the effects of tobacco use in medical treatment, including the important role of tobacco cessation. The American Medical Association (AMA) passed a resolution supporting documentation of smoking behavior in clinical trials, from trial registration through treatment, follow-up, and to end of the study or death.[188] The Oncology Nursing Society (ONS) has also advocated for assessment and cessation.[189,190] Both the AACR[5,191] and ASCO[6,192] have issued policy statements specifically addressing tobacco use in cancer patients, detailing that clinicians have a responsibility to address tobacco use, that all patients should be screened, that all patients who use tobacco should receive evidence-based tobacco cessation support, and that tobacco use should be included in clinical practice and research. These provide strong counsel to address tobacco use in the general population as well as in cancer patients.

### Smoking Cessation Guidelines

Overall, the approach to tobacco cessation for the cancer patient is very similar to the approach for the general population. However, there are a few specific details that are important to consider when approaching the cancer patient who smokes. It is important to recognize that virtually all newly diagnosed cancer patients are faced with a life-changing diagnosis that will require intensive treatment approaches. Treatments, toxicity, and outcomes differ according to disease site and treatment modality. Whereas some cancer patients may have a curable cancer, others may have incurable cancer. Smoking in cancer patients is also often associated with comorbid psychiatric diseases, such as depression, that may affect dependence.[193] The urgency of cessation is also important to consider. If smoking decreases the efficacy of cancer treatment, then every effort should be made to stop tobacco use as soon as possible rather than choosing a quit date several weeks or months after a cancer diagnosis. Patients may also be burdened with a "stigma" associated with certain tobacco-related cancers,[193–197] where they may be viewed by others, or themselves, as causing their cancer due to tobacco use. As a result, the rationale and motivation for quitting tobacco use likely differs among cancer patients, but there is a consistent theme that exists. (1) All patients should be asked about tobacco use with structured assessments; (2) all patients who use tobacco or are at risk for relapse should be offered evidence-based cessation support; and 3) tobacco assessment and cessation support should occur at the time of diagnosis, during treatment, and during follow-up for all cancer patients.

Empiric treatment of tobacco use by cancer patients is fundamentally supported by Public Health Service (PHS) Guidelines that are based on evidence from tobacco cessation efforts in noncancer patients. Originally issued in 1996 and renewed in 2008, *The Clinical Practice Guideline: Treating Tobacco Use and Dependence* is a PHS-sponsored, evidence-based guideline designed to assist health-care providers in delivering and supporting effective smoking cessation treatment.[198,199] The basic recommendation states that clinicians should consistently identify, document, and treat every tobacco user seen in a health-care setting. Details of cessation support range from brief to intensive intervention, but emphasize that consistent repeated cessation support and even brief counseling are effective methods to assist patients with stopping tobacco use. It is important to note that physician-delivered interventions significantly increase long-term abstinence rates.[199] Included are newer effective medication options and strong support for counseling and the use of quit lines as effective intervention strategies. As described in the PHS Guidelines, the principal steps in conducting effective smoking cessation interventions are referred to as The 5 A's:

1. *Ask* about tobacco use for every patient.
2. *Advise* every tobacco user to quit.
3. *Assess* the willingness of patients to quit.
4. *Assist* patients with quitting through counseling and pharmacotherapy.
5. *Arrange* follow-up cessation support, preferably within the first week after the quit date.

There is a strong evidence base for these interventions as documented in the clinical practice guideline.[199]

### Implementing Smoking Cessation Into Clinical Practice

An algorithm is provided to guide clinicians in implementing the five A's into clinical cancer care (Fig. 31.1).[5,45,194,199] Included in the algorithm are suggested questions that are useful to accurately assess tobacco use by cancer patients where patients can generally be divided into *current*, *former*, or *never* smokers. The first step (ASK) is to inquire about and document tobacco use behaviors for every

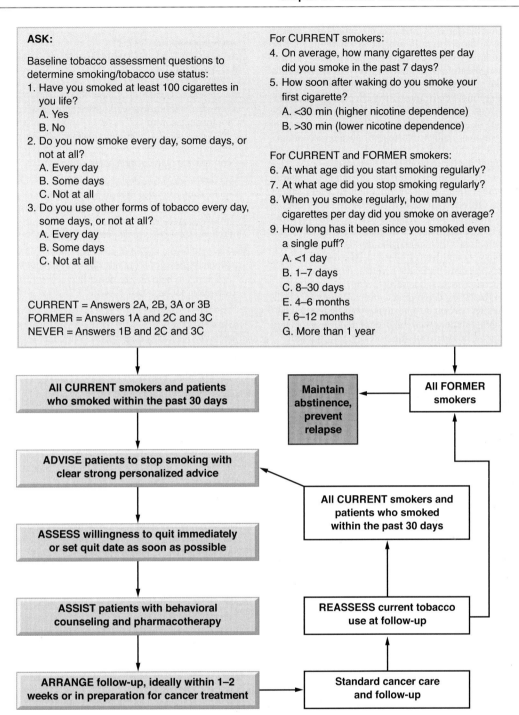

**ASK:**

Baseline tobacco assessment questions to determine smoking/tobacco use status:

1. Have you smoked at least 100 cigarettes in you life?
   A. Yes
   B. No
2. Do you now smoke every day, some days, or not at all?
   A. Every day
   B. Some days
   C. Not at all
3. Do you use other forms of tobacco every day, some days, or not at all?
   A. Every day
   B. Some days
   C. Not at all

CURRENT = Answers 2A, 2B, 3A or 3B
FORMER = Answers 1A and 2C and 3C
NEVER = Answers 1B and 2C and 3C

For CURRENT smokers:
4. On average, how many cigarettes per day did you smoke in the past 7 days?
5. How soon after waking do you smoke your first cigarette?
   A. <30 min (higher nicotine dependence)
   B. >30 min (lower nicotine dependence)

For CURRENT and FORMER smokers:
6. At what age did you start smoking regularly?
7. At what age did you stop smoking regularly?
8. When you smoke regularly, how many cigarettes per day did you smoke on average?
9. How long has it been since you smoked even a single puff?
   A. <1 day
   B. 1–7 days
   C. 8–30 days
   E. 4–6 months
   F. 6–12 months
   G. More than 1 year

**All CURRENT smokers and patients who smoked within the past 30 days**

**ADVISE patients to stop smoking with clear strong personalized advice**

**ASSESS willingness to quit immediately or set quit date as soon as possible**

**ASSIST patients with behavioral counseling and pharmacotherapy**

**ARRANGE follow-up, ideally within 1–2 weeks or in preparation for cancer treatment**

**Maintain abstinence, prevent relapse**

**All FORMER smokers**

**All CURRENT smokers and patients who smoked within the past 30 days**

**REASSESS current tobacco use at follow-up**

**Standard cancer care and follow-up**

**Figure 31.1** This 5 A's screening and smoking cessation treatment schema for cancer patients may be integrated into clinical oncology practice.

patient at every visit including follow-up visits. Whereas a more comprehensive evaluation is necessary at the first consult, only updates to current tobacco use are needed at follow-up. Including smoking status assessments as a "vital sign" for all patients significantly increases the identification and treatment for patients.[200] Tobacco-use status stickers on paper charts or an automated reminder system for electronic records can increase compliance with tobacco assessments.[45] With the recent Meaningful Use standards that were implemented in 2011, hospitals using an electronic medical record (EMR) are essentially required to document tobacco use.[201] A recent report utilized the EMR to implement mandatory tobacco assessments in cancer patients demonstrating that just a few questions at the initial evaluation and at follow-up could yield high referral.

Less than 1% of referrals were delayed when assessments were repeated on a monthly basis rather than at every clinic visit.[45] These findings reduce the clinical burden and patient fatigue associated with repeated assessments as frequently as every day such as in patients who are treated with daily RT or CT.

At the time of this chapter release, there were no national guidelines for implementation of specific questions to assess tobacco use in cancer patients. However, Figure 31.1 provides effective questions for assessing tobacco use in cancer patients based on advice from published reports.[5,45,194,199] Current, former, and never smokers are identified in a structured manner. Patients who use tobacco within the past 30 days should have structured support to quit tobacco use, maintain abstinence, and prevent relapse.

Although not explicitly stated by any specific guidelines, asking about tobacco use in family members of cancer patients may be important because family members often support cancer patients during and following treatment, but continued smoking by family members can make quitting much more difficult.[202–204]

*Advising* is the second step in promoting effective tobacco cessation that involves giving clear, strong, and personalized advice to stop tobacco use. This advice should include the importance of quitting smoking, such as explicit information on the risks of continued smoking and the benefits of cessation for cancer treatment outcomes and overall health regardless of cancer diagnosis. This includes a discussion of how it is not "too late" to quit and that quitting will in fact benefit their cancer treatment efficacy and cancer outcome.[5] Patients can also consider the cost savings of stopping a smoking habit. Clinicians must be particularly sensitive to avoid contributing to any perceived blame for the patient's illness.[195–197,205] Clinicians must remember that most patients started smoking in adolescence and did not completely understand the risks associated with tobacco use. At the same time, the severe addiction associated with chronic tobacco use makes it difficult to stop.

The next step is *assessing* dependence and willingness to quit. Asking "How soon after waking do you smoke your first cigarette?" assesses nicotine dependence, with high dependence associated with a shorter interval between waking and the first cigarette.[206] Nicotine dependence is predictive of smoking cessation outcomes and can be used as a good indicator of the intensity of cessation treatment needed, such as the need for pharmacotherapy.[207,208] Determining the patient's motivation and interest in quitting are critical parameters that influence the types of intervention strategies to be employed. Different strategies for quitting are based on the transtheoretical model of change and motivational interviewing stance, which recognizes that unique intervention messages and strategies are needed to optimally promote smoking cessation based on a patient's readiness to quit smoking.[209,210] In the general population, recommendations encourage that clinicians set a target quit date within 30 days. However, for cancer patients, the reader is encouraged to consider an urgent need to stop smoking immediately. If patients are unable to quit immediately, then patients should be encouraged to immediately reduce tobacco use and to set a quit date as soon as possible based on the typical need to start cancer treatment in the immediate future.

*Assisting* patients with smoking cessation involves clinicians helping the patient design and implement a specific quit plan or broadly enhancing the motivation to quit tobacco. Promoting an effective quit strategy for cancer patients should consist of (1) setting a quit date (immediately or as soon as possible), (2) removing all tobacco-related products from the environment (e.g., cigarettes, ashtrays, lighters), (3) requesting support from family and friends, (4) discussing challenges to quitting, and (5) discussing or prescribing pharmacotherapy where appropriate. Patients should also be provided information on cessation support services (Table 31.1). In the cancer setting, patients can also be informed that smoking cessation is a critical component of cancer care over which they have complete control, thereby conferring some personal control over their cancer care.

Patients who are unwilling to quit should continue to receive repeated assessments and counseling to help motivate patients to quit smoking. These patients should be encouraged to make immediate reductions in tobacco use and work toward abstinence as soon as possible. Clinician education, reassurance, and gentle encouragement can help them to consider changing their smoking behaviors. Specific strategies include discussing the personal relevance of smoking and benefits to cessation, providing support and acknowledging the difficulty of quitting, educating patients about the positive consequences of quitting smoking, and discussing available pharmacologic methods to assist with quitting.[211] The emphasis should be placed on patient autonomy to quit. Motivational strategies for patients unwilling to quit can be employed (e.g., asking open-ended questions, providing affirmations,

## TABLE 31.1

### Additional Tobacco Cessation Resources for Patients and Clinicians[a]

American Association for Cancer Research
Information about the adverse effects of tobacco and advocacy for tobacco control
(http://www.aacr.org/home/public–media/science-policy–government-affairs/science-policy–government-affairs-committee/tobacco-and-cancer.aspx)

American Cancer Society
A national cancer organization providing brochures and fact sheets on the health effects of tobacco and resources for smoking cessation
(http://www.cancer.org/cancer/cancercauses/tobaccocancer/)

American Legacy Foundation
A national independent public health foundation offering programs to help people quit and resources about the health effects of tobacco use
(http://www.legacyforhealth.org/)

American Society of Clinical Oncology
Resources for tobacco cessation with an emphasis on cancer patients
(http://www.asco.org/practice-research/tobacco-cessation-and-control-resources)

Centers for Disease Control and Prevention
A collection of online resources, information, and materials about quitting tobacco use
(http://www.cdc.gov/TOBACCO/)

North American Quitline Consortium
Information on local and national cessation quitlines, 1-800-QUIT-NOW
(http://www.naquitline.org/)

Smoking Cessation Leadership Center
A collaborative dedicated to disseminating knowledge about the health effects of tobacco and assistance in cessation
(http://smokingcessationleadership.ucsf.edu/)

Smokefree.gov
Tips and resources for people trying to stop smoking
(http://smokefree.gov/)

Tobacco Free Nurses
An organization aimed at engaging nurses in tobacco cessation efforts
(http://www.tobaccofreenurses.org/)

U.S. Department of Health & Human Services, Surgeon General.gov
Tobacco use and cessation information from the Surgeon General
(http://www.surgeongeneral.gov/initiatives/tobacco/index.html)

World Health Organization
An international organization tasked with implementing and monitoring public health with a focus on tobacco control
(http://www.who.int/topics/tobacco/en/)

[a] Current as of December 2013.

reflective listening, summarizing).[198,210,212,213] Table 31.2 provides suggested methods to help clinicians promote tobacco cessation.

The final step in a clinician-delivered smoking cessation intervention involves *arranging* a follow-up contact with the patient. Ideally, cancer patients will follow an immediate quit strategy and follow-up should occur preferably within 1 to 2 weeks. However, a short-term follow-up may also benefit patients who are reluctant to quit smoking. The clinician must remember that a new cancer diagnosis is stressful and patients may rely on continued smoking to

## TABLE 31.2

**Select Treatment Strategies Used for Tobacco Cessation Treatments**

Provide and monitor the use of nicotine replacement or other pharmacotherapy.

Provide education regarding the health effects of tobacco use and its addictive and relapsing nature.

Identify and change environmental and psychological cues for tobacco use.

Generate alternative behaviors for tobacco use.

Assist in optimization of social support for cessation efforts and address tobacco use in family members.

Prevent relapse including the identification of future high-risk situations and plans for specific behaviors in those situations.

Provide motivational interventions as needed throughout treatment.

Identify relaxation techniques such as guided imagery and progressive muscle relaxation.

Provide behavioral strategies to address depressed mood (e.g., increasing pleasurable activities).

Provide crisis intervention including appropriate referrals and emergency intervention if indicated.

Recognize and congratulate patients on success with reducing and/or quitting smoking.

relieve stress, but after absorbing the psychological effects of a new cancer diagnosis, patients may be more receptive to smoking cessation. During follow-up, clinicians should congratulate patients on successful cessation efforts, discuss accomplishments and setbacks, and assess pharmacotherapy use and problems. Patients should not be criticized for returning to smoking; rather, it is critical to create a supportive environment for patients to communicate progress, failure, and personal needs. Framing relapses as a learning experience can be helpful, and patients should be encouraged to set another quit date. Referrals to a psychologist or professionally trained smoking cessation counselor should be considered for patients with numerous unsuccessful quit attempts, comorbid depression, anxiety, additional substance abuse disorders, or inadequate social support.

Clinicians who are not well versed in tobacco cessation should realize that smoking is an extremely difficult addiction to overcome and should recognize the clinical pattern associated with cessation. As patients stop smoking, many will experience symptoms of withdrawal, including dry or sore throat, constipation, cravings to smoke, irritability, anxiety, trouble concentrating, restlessness, increased appetite, depression, and insomnia. In the first few weeks, patients may also report an increase in mucous secretions from the airways, a cough, and other upper respiratory tract symptoms. Patients and clinicians should realize that tobacco cessation requires a concerted effort, may require repeated attempts, and symptoms will not resolve immediately. Clinicians should counsel patients on a repeated basis, recognize success, and provide repeated assistance if patients relapse.

## Pharmacologic Treatment for Smoking Cessation

The principles of pharmacotherapy to help patients quit smoking are fundamentally based on reducing the craving associated with nicotine withdrawal. Nicotine replacement therapy (NRT), in the form of patches, lozenges, inhalers, sprays, and gum, varenicline (Chantix), and bupropion (Zyban) are the three principal first-line pharmacotherapies recommended for use either alone or in combination according to PHS Guidelines.[199] Table 31.3 presents information on these first-line agents. Nicotine is the primary addictive substance in tobacco and NRT facilitates smoking cessation by reducing craving and withdrawal that smokers experience during abstinence. NRT also weans smokers off nicotine by providing a lower level and, in some cases, slower infusion of nicotine than smoking.[214] Strong evidence from over 100 randomized clinical trials support the use of NRT to increase the odds of quitting approximately twofold as compared with placebo.[215] Pooled analyses demonstrate that 17% of smokers receiving NRT were able to quit versus 10% with placebo after at least 6 months. Recent evidence further shows that combination therapy, or dual NRT (such as a nicotine patch and lozenge), is a very effective smoking cessation therapy that produces high quit rates.[216,217] Data suggest that activation of the nicotinic acetylcholine receptor (nAChR) may promote tumor development,[218] but evidence suggests that the negative aspects of smoking outweigh these concerns.[219,220] Furthermore, there are no clinical trials reporting negative outcomes for NRT in cancer patients as related to mortality or recurrence. Studies also demonstrate that NRT is not associated with an increased risk of carcinogenesis in the general population.[221,222] As a result, NRT should be used as a clinically proven method to help cancer patients stop smoking.

Antidepressants have been studied as non-nicotine–based pharmacotherapy in part due to depression and psychiatric disease being comorbid conditions in smokers.[223] Bupropion (Zyban) is currently the only FDA-approved antidepressant for the treatment of tobacco dependence.[199] Bupropion inhibits the reuptake of both dopamine and norepinephrine, thereby increasing dopamine and norepinephrine concentrations in the mesolimbic systems.[12,224] Bupropion also antagonizes the nAChR, thereby lowering the rewarding effects of nicotine.[225] Should an abstinent smoker relapse, bupropion may function to reduce the pleasure of cigarette smoking experienced by the smoker[226] and help to prevent further relapse. A meta-analysis found that smokers who received bupropion were twice as likely as those who received placebo to have achieved long-term abstinence at either a 6- or 12-month follow-up.[227]

Varenicline (Chantix) is a α4β2 nAChR partial agonist that produces sustained dopamine release in the mesolimbic system that received FDA approval for treating tobacco dependence in 2006. Sustained dopamine release maintains a normal systemic level of the neurotransmitter, which helps to reduce craving and withdrawal during abstinence.[228] Varenicline also antagonizes the rewarding effects of nicotine. Because varenicline attenuates the pleasure smokers experience from smoking, it may decrease motivation to smoke and protect them from relapse. One of the initially reported randomized clinical trials that compared varenicline (2 mg), bupropion (300 mg), and placebo showed that varenicline was superior to bupropion and placebo, with overall continuous abstinence rates between 10% to 23%.[229] A meta-analysis demonstrated that the 1-mg daily dose approximately doubled, whereas the 2-mg daily dose approximately tripled the likelihood of long-term abstinence at 6 months as compared to placebo.[199] As a result, the 1-mg daily dose can be considered as an alternative should the patient experience significant dose-related side effects. Several meta-analyses have shown that varenicline is superior to bupropion and placebo in the general population.[230–233]

In July 2009, the FDA issued a warning after reports that some patients attempting to quit smoking while using varenicline or bupropion experienced unusual changes in behavior, depressed mood, worsening of depression, or had thoughts of suicide. This has prompted recommendations that health-care providers elicit information about a patient's psychiatric history prior to prescribing varenicline or bupropion to closely monitor changes in mood and behavior during the course of treatment. However,

TABLE 31.3

**First-Line Pharmacotherapy Agents for the Treatment of Nicotine Depedence**

| Agent | Dose | Mechanism | Use |
|---|---|---|---|
| **Nicotine Replacement** | | | |
| Transdermal (patches) | 16 h or 24 h<br>7, 14, or 21 mg<br>1 patch/d | Steady state NRT to reduce craving and withdrawal | 6–10 CPD: 14 mg daily × 8 wks then 7 mg daily × 2 wks<br>>10 CPD: 21 mg daily × 6 wks, then 14 mg × 2 wks, then 7 mg × 2 wks |
| Gum | 2 or 4 mg<br>Max: 24 pieces/d | Short-term NRT to reduce craving and withdrawal | First cigarette >30 min after waking: 2 mg PO q1–2 hr<br>First cigarette <30 min after waking: 4 mg PO q1–2 hr |
| Lozenge | 2 or 4 mg<br>Max: 20 lozenges/d | Short-term NRT to reduce craving and withdrawal | 1st cigarette >30 min after waking: 2 mg PO q1–2 hr<br>1st cigarette <30 min after waking: 4 mg PO q1–2 hr |
| Nasal spray | 0.5 mg/spray<br>Max: 10 sprays/hr or 80 sprays/d | Short-term NRT to reduce craving and withdrawal | 1 spray/nostril q1–5 hr |
| Inhaler | 4 mg/cartridge<br>Max: 16 cartridges/d | Short-term NRT to reduce craving and withdrawal | 1 cartridge inhaled over 20 min q1.5–6 hr |
| Bupropion (Zyban) | 150 mg | Block nicotinic receptors and reduces reward | 1 tablet daily × 3 d, then 1 tablet twice daily for 7–12 wks |
| Varenicline (Chantix) | 0.5 or 1 mg | Dopaminergic reward and partial nicotinic receptor antagonist | 0.5 mg daily × 3 d, then 0.5 mg twice daily × 3 d, then 1 mg twice daily |

CPD, cigarettes per day; PO, by mouth; NRT, nicotine replacement therapy.

updated recent safety studies examining very large databases (one database of N = 119,546, one database of N = 35,800) regarding safety have shown no difference in neuropsychiatric side effects between varenicline or bupropion as compared to NRT and no increased risk of depression.[234,235] Another prospective study showed no adverse events when treating participants with current or past major depression and also showed higher abstinence rates for the varenicline group as compared to placebo at weeks 9 to 52 (20.3% versus 10.4%, p <0.001).[236] Varenicline should be considered a viable cessation pharmacotherapy for cancer patients.

The clinical practice guideline also identifies two non-nicotine–based medications—clonidine and nortriptyline—as second-line pharmacotherapies for tobacco dependence. A second-line agent is used when a smoker cannot use first-line medications due to either contraindications or lack of effectiveness. Both clonidine, an antihypertensive, and nortriptyline, a tricyclic antidepressant, have been shown to effectively assist smokers achieve abstinence.[227,237] Unfortunately, many patients who quit will eventually relapse, and rates of long-term abstinence remain low. Because smoking poses enormous health risks to individuals and their families, even a modest reduction in smoking may translate into a significant impact on public health. Clinicians should continue to encourage recalcitrant smokers to stop tobacco use and use pharmacotherapy where appropriate with repeated quit attempts.

## Empirically Tested Cessation Interventions with Cancer Patients

The overwhelming majority of cessation research has been performed in the general population, but there are several studies that have been performed in cancer patients. Gritz et al.[238] conducted the first physician- or dentist-delivered randomized cessation

intervention comparison in 186 newly diagnosed head and neck cancer patients. Patients were treated with either minimal advice or an enhanced intervention with trained clinicians consisting of strong personalized advice to stop smoking, a contracted quit date, tailored written materials, and booster advice sessions. No significant differences were found between treatments, but a 70.2% continuous abstinence rate was found at 12-month follow-up regardless of treatment condition, suggesting that many cancer patients can benefit from brief physician-delivered advice. A later study by Schnoll et al.,[239] comparing cognitive behavioral treatment with standardized health education advice, also failed to find significant differences in quit rates. All patients received NRT, and quit rates in both groups approached 50% at 1-month follow-up and 40% at 3-month follow-up.

Additional studies, ranging from 15 to 80 patients, examined nurse-delivered cessation interventions for a variety of cancer patients. The lowest cessation rates were found with a single session intervention: a 21% cessation rate in the intervention group versus 14% in the usual care group 6 weeks' postintervention.[240] Higher cessation rates were associated with a more intensive intervention consisting of three inpatient visits, supplementary materials, and five postdischarge follow-up contacts. Additional studies demonstrate higher cessation rates with more intensive intervention (40% to 75%) as compared with usual care (43% to 50%), suggesting more intensive interventions may yield higher cessation rates.[241–243] In general, more intense interventions appear to be more efficacious, but even brief advice is important to achieve tobacco cessation.

In a randomized trial of 432 cancer patients coordinated by the Eastern Cooperative Oncology Group (ECOG) with a physician-delivered intervention (comprised of cessation advice, optional NRT, and written materials) or usual care (unstructured advice from physicians), there were no significant intervention effects and generally low abstinence rates (12% to 15%

at 6 to 12 months).[244] However, patients with head and neck or lung cancer were significantly more likely to have quit smoking compared to patients with tumors that were not smoking related. Analyses of outcomes from the Mayo Clinic Nicotine Dependence Center found that although lung cancer patients were more likely to achieve 6-month tobacco abstinence than controls (22% versus 14%), no significant differences were observed after adjusting for covariates.[245] Garces et al.[246] also found no significant differences in abstinence rates between head and neck cancer patients and controls (33% versus 26%). However, higher abstinence rates were found for both head and neck and lung cancer patients treated within 3 months of diagnosis compared to those treated for more than 3 months after the diagnosis, emphasizing the potential importance of the *teachable moment* at the time of the cancer diagnosis.

The potential importance of addressing smoking combined with considering comorbid disease has been noted in a few studies. In a randomized head and neck cancer patients of usual care versus 9 to 11 sessions of a nurse-administered intervention consisting of cognitive-behavioral therapy and medications, targeting comorbid smoking, drinking, and depression significantly increased quit rates at 6-month follow-up for the intervention group compared to the usual control group (47% versus 31%, p <0.05).[247] In a randomized trial of 246 cancer patients treated with 9 weeks of NRT with or without bupropion, there was no significant difference with the addition of bupropion to NRT, but in patients with depressive symptoms, bupropion increased abstinence rates, lowered withdrawal, and improved quality of life.[248] Patients without depression symptoms did equally well when treated with bupropion versus transdermal nicotine and counseling alone.

Patient recruitment has been a problem noted by some studies, including 5.5 years to accrue 246 patients with telephone screening of over 7,500 potential patients.[249] A pilot trial of varenicline in thoracic oncology patients required screening 1,130 patients to accrue 49 participants randomized to a 12-week course of either varenicline or placebo paired with a behavioral counseling platform of seven sessions.[250] A randomized trial of 185 smoking cancer patients comparing the efficacy of a hospital-based standard care smoking cessation model versus standard care augmented by a behavioral tapering regimen via a handheld device before inpatient hospitalization for cancer surgery demonstrated no difference in quit rates (both 32%,).[251] However, over 29,000 patients were screened to conduct a randomized clinical trial with a smoking cancer patient population. These studies highlight the potential difficulty recruiting participants who smoke, including considerations for the importance of medical comorbidity in guiding smoking cessation treatment, patient mix (multiple tumor sites), treatment status (awaiting treatment to completed treatment), variation in stage of disease, and considering how psychiatric conditions such as depression reflect the difficulty of conducting research in the oncology setting and the importance of these variables in future studies.

Although accruing patients to intervention trials may seem discouraging, several studies demonstrate the benefit of counseling over self-help. Emmons et al.[252] conducted a randomized controlled trial in 796 young adult survivors of pediatric cancer that included six calls, tailored and targeted written materials, and optional NRT as compared with self-help. Significantly higher quit rates were found in the counseling group compared to the self-help group at all reported follow-up time points, including 12 months (15% versus 9%; p <0.01). A randomized trial of a motivational interviewing-based smoking cessation intervention in a south Australian hospital was delivered over a 3-month period, consisted of multiple contacts with a trained counselor, and provided supplementary material tailored to cancer patients with NRT.[253] The control group received brief advice to quit and generic supplementary material. Quit rates did not differ by treatment group (5% to 6% at 3-month follow-up), but the intervention group was significantly more likely to report attempts to quit smoking.

## Current Tobacco Assessment and Cessation Support by Oncologists

Access to cessation support is critical to address tobacco use by cancer patients. A recent survey of 58 NCI-designated cancer centers indicated that about 80% reported a tobacco use program available to their patients and about 60% routinely offered educational materials, but less than 50% had a designated individual who provided services.[254] A recent survey of over 1,500 members of the International Association for the Study of Lung Cancer (IASLC)[255] and a parallel study of 1,197 ASCO members[256] observed that approximately 90% of physicians believe that tobacco affects outcomes, tobacco cessation should be a standard part of cancer care, and approximately 80% regularly advise patients to stop using tobacco, but only approximately 40% discuss medications or assist with quitting. Dominant perceived barriers to cessation support were patient resistance to treatment, an inability to get patients to quit, a lack of cessation resources, and a lack of clinician education. These data showed that even motivated clinicians are not regularly providing tobacco cessation support. A recent survey of 155 actively accruing cooperative group clinical trials further demonstrated that only 29% of active trials collected any tobacco use information, 4.5% collected any tobacco use information at follow-up, and none addressed tobacco cessation.[55] Few oncology meetings offer educational workshops or talks, and they are often poorly attended when they are offered.[257] Collectively, these data demonstrate that oncologists are not regularly providing cessation support and that we are not capturing tobacco use information that may be critical to understanding the effects of tobacco on cancer treatment outcomes.

More in-person talks as well as written and Web-based training should be made available, as well as new approaches that move from the traditional 5 A's model delivered by a single professional to referral systems that efficiently connect tobacco users to multiple resources for tobacco cessation.[258-260] The ASCO *Prevention Curriculum* has a chapter devoted to educating oncology healthcare professionals on the evaluation and treatment of tobacco use.[215] Innovative curricula, such as the Texas Tobacco Outreach Education Program (TOEP), are available and can facilitate program development in other states.[261] However, specialty programs in tobacco cessation treatment that are based in cancer centers and other medical centers are valuable resources that need to be further developed.

Addressing tobacco use in cancer patients may be approached in a systematic and efficient manner. A recent report highlighted the potential utility of automated tobacco assessment and smoking cessation using structured assessments in the EMR where all patients were automatically referred to a dedicated cessation program consisting of phone-based cessation support.[45] In 2,700 patients referred for cessation support, half received only a mailing and only 1% contacted the cessation program. However, in the arm with at least five phone call attempts made by the cessation service, 81% of patients were successfully contacted and only 3% refused cessation support. Furthermore, assessments implemented every 4 weeks, rather than more frequent assessments every 2 weeks, resulted in delayed cessation referrals in less than 1% of smokers. This is the first report to try and identify clinically efficient mechanisms of addressing tobacco use that may be useful in clinical practice or research that may be an effective method of increasing patient participation in cessation support, but substantial work is needed to assess who may benefit from low versus high intensity support in such a program.

## Examples of Model Tobacco Treatment Programs

Several dedicated tobacco treatment programs at cancer centers have been developed. Table 31.4 contrasts the core elements of

**TABLE 31.4**

**Attributes of Prototypical Tobacco Treatment Programs**

| Attribute | MDACC | RPCI | Yale | MSKCC |
|---|---|---|---|---|
| Tobacco assessment of all patients (EMR) | Yes | Yes | Yes | Yes |
| Automatic referral of all patients | Yes | Yes | No | Yes |
| In-person counseling | Yes | No | Yes | Yes |
| Telephone counseling | Yes | Yes | No | Yes |
| Medications prescribed | Yes | No | Yes | Yes |
| Biochemical confirmation (CO) testing | Yes | No | Yes | No |
| Free to patient | Yes | Yes | No | Yes |
| Third-party payment | No | No | Yes | Yes |
| Research studies of new treatments | Yes | Yes | Yes | Yes |

MDACC, M.D. Anderson Cancer Center, Houston, TX; RPCI, Roswell Park Cancer Institute, Buffalo, NY; Yale, Yale University Hospital, Smilow Cancer Center, New Haven, CT; MSKCC, Memorial Sloan Kettering Cancer Center, New York, NY.

four active model programs at the end of 2013 (University of Texas M.D. Anderson Cancer Center, Roswell Park Cancer Institute, Yale Cancer Center, and Memorial Sloan Kettering Cancer Center), each of which employ different methods to help cancer patients quit smoking. All programs follow the evidence-based 5 A's model described previously from PHS Guidelines.[199] All programs were made available to patients at their respective medical centers and are now designed to evaluate and treat all patients who self-report current tobacco use. Importantly, not all cancer centers can treat smoking cessation in the same manner. Financing of a cessation program is critical and may include institutional funds, state funds, research funds, and third-party billing. Notably, given the broad spectrum of adverse health effects associated with smoking, cancer centers should carefully consider the potential health benefits and cost savings associated with tobacco cessation due to reductions in treatment complications and recurrence associated with smoking by cancer patients. There is no one "correct" way to create and sustain a tobacco treatment program at a cancer center, but at the very least and consistent with evidence, rigorous behavioral counseling should be provided and, if possible, medication management as well.

## FUTURE CONSIDERATIONS

### Research Considerations

The past several years have shown a surge in activities identifying the effects of tobacco in cancer patients and increasing awareness is being developed for cessation support at cancer centers as well as through several national organizations. There are three fundamental areas of research that need to be expanded:

1. *Evaluating the effects of tobacco use and cessation on clinical cancer outcomes.* The 2014 SGR concluded that smoking caused adverse outcomes in cancer patients,[7] but several limitations remain. Tobacco-use definitions should be standardized and implemented at diagnosis, during treatment, and follow-up. Biochemical confirmation with cotinine or exhaled carbon monoxide may improve the accuracy of tobacco assessment in at-risk groups such as current smokers who are trying to quit or patients who reported quitting in the past year.[171,185,186,262] Although smoking is the predominant form of tobacco consumption, all tobacco products should be considered. A further understanding of the effects of tobacco on the efficacy and toxicity of cancer treatment, tumor response, quality of life, survival, recurrence,

compliance, second primary, and noncancer-related comorbidity is needed. All cancer disease sites and stages are important to consider.

2. *Understanding the effects of tobacco and cessation on cancer biology.* Although not a primary focus of this chapter, tobacco and tobacco-related products increase tumor growth, angiogenesis, migration, invasion and metastasis and decrease response to conventional cancer treatments such as CT and RT. These and other areas are important to consider, including the potential effects on immune-related therapy and vaccine development. *In vivo* models of exposure and cancer response are not well developed, yet are critical to this research area. Work is also needed to assess the effect of emerging tobacco-related products such as e-cigarettes.

3. *Advance understanding of models to increase access to cessation support and increase efficacy of tobacco cessation methods for cancer patients.* This diverse area includes assessing the timing of intervention, intensity, duration, follow-up, and the potential effects of harm-reduction strategies. Cessation pharmacology requires additional consideration in combination with unique approaches to motivational and behavioral counseling in cancer patients. Significant work is needed to disseminate evidence-based cessation support and to assess the cost-effectiveness of different cessation strategies, particularly with regard to improving the cost of cancer care as a whole. Preventing relapse and evaluating the safety of transition to alternative products such as e-cigarettes is equally important and increasingly complex with the addition of new tobacco-related products. Identifying and addressing barriers to effective cessation support is also needed. As related to the cancer patient, clinicians and cessation specialists should consider how their research relates to cancer care. Taking advantage of new integrated medical management systems presents a significant opportunity to improve cessation support access as well as to develop a more effective tracking of patient outcomes.

### Policy Implications and Systematic Issues

Several national and international organizations have emphasized the importance of tobacco assessments and cessation for the general population and for cancer patients that include tools to evaluate tobacco use at diagnosis, during treatment, and follow-up appointments, as well as routine support for smoking cessation.[5,6,188–191] In 2012, ASCO, with the contribution of the American Legacy Foundation, published a Tobacco Cessation Toolkit for the oncology setting.[263] This evidence-based guideline intends to help oncology providers integrate tobacco cessation strategies into their patient care. Utilization of the EMR and standardized, automated systems for more efficacious and efficient access to tobacco cessation support has also been suggested,[45] but requires participation by clinicians, institutions, insurers, and health departments. Not only should providers be aware of the need for tobacco cessation and available interventions, but health-care institutions must also build such treatment into their overall system of care. Thus, the identification of patients who smoke or use any alternative tobacco product, referral or direct treatment by providers, billing and reimbursement for treatment provided, and consistent efforts from professional oncology organizations are critically important.[257] The

tremendous public health burden from tobacco-related disability and death has not been countered by a proportional level of funding in tobacco control, cancer treatment research, or public advocacy. Researchers, clinicians, and advocates must come together to persuade policy makers to increase funding in tobacco-related research, treatment, and policy initiatives on behalf of healthy individuals and patients. A united front is critically needed in support of a common agenda that includes both increased tobacco-control efforts and additional funding for disease-related research and treatment. With clinical rationale, guidelines, and advocacy in place, the final steps in effective tobacco control and improving health outcomes are to implement these recommendations into practice.

## REFERENCES

1. U.S. Department of Health, Education, and Welfare. *Smoking and Health: Report of the Advisory Committee to the Surgeon General of the Public Health Service.* PHS Publication No. 1103. Washington, D.C.: U.S. Department of Health, Education, and Welfare, Public Health Service, Center for Disease Control; 1964.
2. Office of the Surgeon General, Office on Smoking and Health. *The Health Consequences of Smoking. A Report of the Surgeon General.* Atlanta: Centers for Disease Control and Prevention; 2004.
3. Centers for Disease Control and Prevention, National Center for Chronic Disease Prevention and Health Promotion, Office on Smoking and Health. *How Tobacco Smoke Causes Disease: The Biology and Behavioral Basis for Smoking-Attributable Disease: A Report of the Surgeon General.* Atlanta: Centers for Disease Control and Prevention; 2010.
4. U.S. Department of Health and Human Services. *The Health Consequences of Smoking: Nicotine Addiction. A Report of the Surgeon General.* DHHS Publication No. (CDC) 88-8406. Atlanta: U.S. Department of Health and Human Services, Public Health Service, Centers for Disease Control, National Center for Chronic Disease Prevention and Health Promotion, Office on Smoking and Health; 1988.
5. Toll BA, Brandon TH, Gritz ER, et al. Assessing tobacco use by cancer patients and facilitating cessation: an American Association for Cancer Research policy statement. *Clin Cancer Res* 2013;19:1941–1948.
6. Hanna N, Mulshine J, Wollins DS, et al. Tobacco cessation and control a decade later: American society of clinical oncology policy statement update. *J Clin Oncol* 2013;31:3147–3157.
7. U.S. Department of Health and Human Services. *The Health Consequences of Smoking—50 Years of Progress: A Report of the Surgeon General.* Atlanta: U.S. Department of Health and Human Services, Centers for Disease Control and Prevention, National Center for Chronic Disease Prevention and Health Promotion, Office on Smoking and Health; 2014.
8. Brunzell DH. Preclinical evidence that activation of mesolimbic alpha 6 subunit containing nicotinic acetylcholine receptors supports nicotine addiction phenotype. *Nicotine Tob Res* 2012;14:1258–1269.
9. Benowitz NL. Nicotine addiction. *N Engl J Med.* 2010;362:2295–2303.
10. Nestler EJ. Is there a common molecular pathway for addiction? *Nat Neurosci* 2005;8:1445–1449.
11. Dani JA, De Biasi M. Cellular mechanisms of nicotine addiction. *Pharmacol Biochem Behav* 2001;70:439–446.
12. Balfour DJ. The neurobiology of tobacco dependence: a preclinical perspective on the role of the dopamine projections to the nucleus accumbens. *Nicotine Tob Res* 2004;6:899–912.
13. Berridge KC, Robinson TE. What is the role of dopamine in reward: hedonic impact, reward learning, or incentive salience? *Brain Res Brain Res Rev* 1998;28:309–369.
14. Schultz W. Multiple dopamine functions at different time courses. *Annu Rev Neurosci* 2007;30:259–288.
15. Kalivas PW, McFarland K. Brain circuitry and the reinstatement of cocaine-seeking behavior. *Psychopharmacology* 2003;168:44–56.
16. Dani JA, Balfour DJK. Historical and current perspective on tobacco use and nicotine addiction. *Trends Neurosci* 2011;34:383–439.
17. Di Chiara G. Role of dopamine in the behavioural actions of nicotine related to addiction. *Eur J Pharmacol* 2000;393:295–314.
18. Centers for Disease Control and Prevention. Current cigarette smoking among adults—United States, 2011. *MMWR Morb Mortal Wkly Rep* 2012;61:889–894.
19. Centers for Disease Control and Prevention. Cigarette smoking among adults—United States, 2001. *MMWR Morb Mortal Wkly Rep* 2003;52:953–956.
20. Smokefree Laws and Policies. American Lung Association Web site. http://www.lungusa2.org/slati/smokefree_laws.php. Accessed November 25, 2013.
21. Tobacco Policy Project/State Legislated Actions on Tobacco Issues (SLATI). American Lung Association Web site. http://www.lungusa2.org/slati. Accessed November 25, 2013.
22. Tobacco Taxes. American Lung Association Web site. http://www.lungusa2.org/slati/tobacco_taxes.php. Accessed November 25, 2013.
23. Tobacco Situation and Outlook Report, U.S. Department of Agriculture, U.S. Census 1880-2005.

24. Warren GW, Cummings KM. Tobacco and lung cancer: risks, trends, and outcomes in patients with cancer. In: *American Society of Clinical Oncology 2013 Educational Book.* 201; 359–364. ASCO University Web site. http://meetinglibrary.asco.org//content/200-132. Accessed November 25, 2013.
25. Thun MJ, Carter BD, Feskanich D, et al. 50-year trends in smoking-related mortality in the United States. *N Engl J Med.* 2013;368:351–364.
26. U.S. Food and Drug Administration. Summary of Results: Laboratory Analysis of Electronic Cigarettes Conducted by FDA. U.S. Food and Drug Administration Web site. http://www.fda.gov/NewsEvents/PublicHealthFocus/ucm173146.htm. Accessed November 25, 2013.
27. Cummings KM, Dresler CM, Field JK, et al. E-cigarettes and cancer patients. *J Thorac Oncol* 2014;9:438–441.
28. Kuschner WG, Reddy S, Mehrotra N, et al. Electronic cigarettes and thirdhand tobacco smoke: two emerging health care challenges for the primary care provider. *Int J Gen Med* 2011;4:115–120.
29. WHO Study Group on Tobacco Product Regulation. WHO Study Group on Tobacco Product Regulation. Report on the scientific basis of tobacco product regulation: third report of a WHO study group. *World Health Organ Tech Rep Ser* 2009;(955):1–41.
30. National Cancer Institute. Cancer Trends Progress Report – 2011/2012 Update. Nation Cancer Institute Web site. http://progressreport.cancer.gov. Published August 2012. Accessed November 25, 2013.
31. Bellizzi KM, Rowland JH, Jeffery DD, et al. Health behaviors of cancer survivors: examining opportunities for cancer control intervention. *J Clin Oncol* 2005;23:8884–8893.
32. Coups EJ, Ostroff JS. A population-based estimate of the prevalence of behavioral risk factors among adult cancer survivors and noncancer controls. *Prev Med* 2005;40:702–711.
33. Klosky JL, Hum AM, Zhang N, et al. Smokeless and dual tobacco use among males surviving childhood cancer: a report from the Childhood Cancer Survivor Study. *Cancer Epidemiol Biomarkers Prev* 2013;22:1025–1029.
34. Underwood JM, Townsend JS, Tai E, et al. Persistent cigarette smoking and other tobacco use after a tobacco-related cancer diagnosis. *J Cancer Surviv* 2012;6:333–344.
35. Walker MS, Vidrine DJ, Gritz ER, et al. Smoking relapse during the first year after treatment for early-stage non-small-cell lung cancer. *Cancer Epidemiol Biomarkers Prev* 2006;15:2370–2377.
36. Gritz ER. Smoking and smoking cessation in cancer patients. *Br J Addict* 1991;86:549–554.
37. Lippman SM, Lee JJ, Karp DD, et al. Randomized phase III intergroup trial of isotretinoin to prevent second primary tumors in stage I non-small-cell lung cancer. *J Natl Cancer Inst* 2001;93:605–618.
38. Ostroff JS, Jacobsen PB, Moadel AB, et al. Prevalence and predictors of continued tobacco use after treatment of patients with head and neck cancer. *Cancer* 1995;75:569–576.
39. Hickey K, Do KA, Green A. Smoking and prostate cancer. *Epidemiol Rev* 2001;23:115–125.
40. Plaskon LA, Penson DF, Vaughan TL, et al. Cigarette smoking and risk of prostate cancer in middle-aged men. *Cancer Epidemiol Biomarkers Prev* 2003;12:604–609.
41. Watters JL, Park Y, Hollenbeck A, et al. Cigarette smoking and prostate cancer in a prospective US cohort study. *Cancer Epidemiol Biomarkers Prev* 2009;18:2427–2435.
42. Alberg AJ, Singh S, May JW, et al. Epidemiology, prevention, and early detection of breast cancer. *Curr Opin Oncol* 2000;12:515–520.
43. Johnson KC, Miller AB, Collishaw NE, et al. Active smoking and secondhand smoke increase breast cancer risk: the report of the Canadian Expert Panel on Tobacco Smoke and Breast Cancer Risk (2009). *Tob Control* 2011;20:e2.
44. Breast Cancer Family Registry; Kathleen Cuningham Consortium for Research into Familial Breast Cancer (Australasia); Ontario Cancer Genetics Network (Canada). Smoking and risk of breast cancer in carriers of mutations in BRCA1 or BRCA2 aged less than 50 years. *Breast Cancer Res Treat* 2008;109:67–75.
45. Warren GW, Marshall JR, Cummings KM, et al. Automated tobacco assessment and cessation support for cancer patients. *Cancer* 2014;120:562–569.
46. Centers for Disease Control and Prevention. Cigarette smoking among adults—United States, 2004. *MMWR Morb Mortal Wkly Rep* 2005;54:1121–1124.

47. Centers for Disease Control and Prevention. Tobacco use among adults—United States, 2005. *MMWR Morb Mortal Wkly Rep* 2006;55:1145–1148.

48. Gritz ER, Nisenbaum R, Elashoff RE, et al. Smoking behavior following diagnosis in patients with stage I non-small cell lung cancer. *Cancer Causes Control* 1991;2:105–112.

49. Chen AM, Vazquez E, Courquin J, et al. Tobacco use among long-term survivors of head and neck cancer treated with radiation therapy. *Psychooncology* 2014;23:190–194.

50. Ostroff J, Garland J, Moadel A, et al. Cigarette smoking patterns in patients after treatment of bladder cancer. *J Cancer Educ* 2000;15:86–90.

51. McBride CM, Emmons KM, Lipkus IM. Understanding the potential of teachable moments: the case of smoking cessation. *Health Educ Res* 2003;18:156–170.

52. Gritz ER, Schacherer C, Koehly L, et al. Smoking withdrawal and relapse in head and neck cancer patients. *Head Neck* 1999;21:420–427.

53. Warren GW, Marshall JR, Cummings KM. Smoking, cancer treatment, and design of clinical trials. *Proc AACR* 2013;54:594.

54. Parsons A, Daley A, Begh R, et al. Influence of smoking cessation after diagnosis of early stage cancer on prognosis: systematic review of observational studies with meta-analysis. *BMJ* 2010;340:b5569.

55. Peters EN, Torres E, Toll BA, et al. Tobacco assessment in actively accruing National Cancer Institute Cooperative Group Program Clinical Trials. *J Clin Oncol* 2012;30:2869–2875.

56. Land SR. Methodologic barriers to addressing critical questions about tobacco and cancer prognosis. *J Clin Oncol* 2012;30:2030–2032.

57. Gritz ER, Dresler C, Sarna L. Smoking, the missing drug interaction in clinical trials: ignoring the obvious. *Cancer Epidemiol Biomarkers Prev* 2005;14:2287–2293.

58. Yu GP, Ostroff JS, Zhang ZF, et al. Smoking history and cancer patient survival: a hospital cancer registry study. *Cancer Detect Prev* 1997;21:497–509.

59. Dahlstrom KR, Calzada G, Hanby JD, et al. An evolution in demographics, treatment, and outcomes of oropharyngeal cancer at a major cancer center: a staging system in need of repair. *Cancer* 2012;119:81–89.

60. Molina MA, Cheung MC, Perez EA, et al. African American and poor patients have a dramatically worse prognosis for head and neck cancer: an examination of 20,915 patients. *Cancer* 2008;113:2797–2806.

61. Dragun AE, Huang B, Tucker TC, et al. Disparities in the application of adjuvant radiotherapy after breast-conserving surgery for early stage breast cancer: impact on overall survival. *Cancer* 2011;117:2590–2598.

62. Bostrom PJ, Alkhateeb S, Trottier G, et al. Sex differences in bladder cancer outcomes among smokers with advanced bladder cancer. *BJU Int* 2011;109:70–76.

63. Kroeger N, Klatte T, Birkhäuser FD, et al. Smoking negatively impacts renal cell carcinoma overall and cancer-specific survival. *Cancer* 2011;118:1795–1802.

64. Marks DI, Ballen K, Logan BR, et al. The effect of smoking on allogeneic transplant outcomes. *Biol Blood Marrow Transplant* 2009;15:1277–1287.

65. Gridelli C, Ciardiello F, Gallo C, et al. First-line erlotinib followed by second-line cisplatin-gemcitabine chemotherapy in advanced non-small-cell lung cancer: the TORCH randomized trial. *J Clin Oncol* 2012;30:3002–3011.

66. Maeda R, Yoshida J, Ishii G, et al. Influence of cigarette smoking on survival and tumor invasiveness in clinical stage IA lung adenocarcinoma. *Ann Thorac Surg* 2012;93:1626–1632.

67. Maeda R, Yoshida J, Ishii G, et al. The prognostic impact of cigarette smoking on patients with non-small cell lung cancer. *J Thorac Oncol* 2011;6:735–742.

68. Janjigian YY, McDonnell K, Kris MG, et al. Pack-years of cigarette smoking as a prognostic factor in patients with stage IIIB/IV nonsmall cell lung cancer. *Cancer* 2010;116:670–675.

69. Toyooka S, Takano T, Kosaka T, et al. Epidermal growth factor receptor mutation, but not sex and smoking, is independently associated with favorable prognosis of gefitinib-treated patients with lung adenocarcinoma. *Cancer Sci* 2008;99:303–308.

70. Kawai H, Tada A, Kawahara M, et al. Smoking history before surgery and prognosis in patients with stage IA non-small-cell lung cancer—a multicenter study. *Lung Cancer* 2005;49:63–70.

71. Warren GW, Kasza K, Reid M, et al. Smoking at diagnosis and survival in cancer patients. *Int J Cancer* 2013;132:401–410.

72. Kvale E, Ekundayo OJ, Zhang Y, et al. History of cancer and mortality in community-dwelling older adults. *Cancer Epidemiol* 2011;35:30–36.

73. Gajdos C, Hawn MT, Campagna EJ, et al. Adverse effects of smoking on postoperative outcomes in cancer patients. *Ann Surg Oncol* 2012;19:1430–1438.

74. Duffy SA, Ronis DL, McLean S, et al. Pretreatment health behaviors predict survival among patients with head and neck squamous cell carcinoma. *J Clin Oncol* 2009;27:1969–1975.

75. Farshadpour F, Kranenborg H, Calkoen EV, et al. Survival analysis of head and neck squamous cell carcinoma: influence of smoking and drinking. *Head Neck* 2011;33:817–823.

76. Meyer F, Bairati I, Fortin A, et al. Interaction between antioxidant vitamin supplementation and cigarette smoking during radiation therapy in relation to long-term effects on recurrence and mortality: a randomized trial among head and neck cancer patients. *Int J Cancer* 2008;122:1679–1683.

77. Shen GP, Xu FH, He F, et al. Pretreatment lifestyle behaviors as survival predictors for patients with nasopharyngeal carcinoma. *PLoS One* 2012;7:e36515.

78. Dal Maso L, Zucchetto A, Talamini R, et al. Effect of obesity and other lifestyle factors on mortality in women with breast cancer. *Int J Cancer* 2008;123:2188–2194.

79. Hellmann SS, Thygesen LC, Tolstrup JS, et al. Modifiable risk factors and survival in women diagnosed with primary breast cancer: results from a prospective cohort study. *Eur J Cancer Prev* 2010;19:366–673.

80. Holmes MD, Murin S, Chen WY, et al. Smoking and survival after breast cancer diagnosis. *Int J Cancer* 2007;120:2672–2677.

81. Sagiv SK, Gaudet MM, Eng SM, et al. Active and passive cigarette smoke and breast cancer survival. *Ann Epidemiol* 2007;17:385–393.

82. Phipps AI, Baron J, Newcomb PA. Prediagnostic smoking history, alcohol consumption, and colorectal cancer survival: the Seattle Colon Cancer Family Registry. *Cancer* 2011;117:4948–4957.

83. Huang XE, Tajima K, Hamajima N, et al. Effects of dietary, drinking, and smoking habits on the prognosis of gastric cancer. *Nutr Cancer* 2000;38:30–36.

84. Kenfield SA, Stampfer MJ, Chan JM, et al. Smoking and prostate cancer survival and recurrence. *JAMA* 2011;305:2548–2555.

85. Merrick GS, Butler WM, Wallner KE, et al. Androgen-deprivation therapy does not impact cause-specific or overall survival after permanent prostate brachytherapy. *Int J Radiat Oncol Biol Phys* 2006;65:669–677.

86. Pickles T, Liu M, Berthelet E, et al. The effect of smoking on outcome following external radiation for localized prostate cancer. *J Urol* 2004;171:1543–1546.

87. Taira AV, Merrick GS, Butler WM, et al. Long-term outcome for clinically localized prostate cancer treated with permanent interstitial brachytherapy. *Int J Radiat Oncol Biol Phys* 2011;79:1336–1342.

88. Sweeney C, Farrow DC. Differential survival related to smoking among patients with renal cell carcinoma. *Epidemiology* 2000;11:344–346.

89. Coker AL, DeSimone CP, Eggleston KS, et al. Smoking and survival among Kentucky women diagnosed with invasive cervical cancer: 1995–2005. *Gynecol Oncol* 2009;112:365–369.

90. Modesitt SC, Huang B, Shelton BJ, et al. Endometrial cancer in Kentucky: the impact of age, smoking status, and rural residence. *Gynecol Oncol* 2006;103:300–306.

91. Poullis M, McShane J, Shaw M, et al. Smoking status at diagnosis and histology type as determinants of long-term outcomes of lung cancer patients. *Eur J Cardiothorac Surg* 2012;43:919–924.

92. Kawaguchi T, Tamiya A, Tamura A, et al. Chemotherapy is beneficial for elderly patients with advanced non-small-cell lung cancer: analysis of patients aged 70–74, 75–79, and 80 or older in Japan. *Clin Lung Cancer* 2012;13:442–447.

93. Pirker R, Pereira JR, Szczesna A, et al. Prognostic factors in patients with advanced non-small cell lung cancer: data from the phase III FLEX study. *Lung Cancer* 2012;77:376–382.

94. Ferketich AK, Niland JC, Mamet R, et al. Smoking status and survival in the national comprehensive cancer network non-small cell lung cancer cohort. *Cancer* 2013;119:847–853.

95. Chansky K, Sculier JP, Crowley JJ, et al. The International Association for the Study of Lung Cancer Staging Project: prognostic factors and pathologic TNM stage in surgically managed non-small cell lung cancer. *J Thorac Oncol* 2009;4:792–801.

96. Myrdal G, Lamberg K, Lambe M, et al. Regional differences in treatment and outcome in non-small cell lung cancer: a population-based study (Sweden). *Lung Cancer* 2009;63:16–22.

97. Saito-Nakaya K, Nakaya N, Akechi T, et al. Marital status and non-small cell lung cancer survival: the Lung Cancer Database Project in Japan. *Psychooncology*. 2008;17:869–876.

98. Zhou W, Heist RS, Liu G, et al. Smoking cessation before diagnosis and survival in early stage non-small cell lung cancer patients. *Lung Cancer* 2006;53:375–380.

99. Tsao AS, Liu D, Lee JJ, et al. Smoking affects treatment outcome in patients with advanced nonsmall cell lung cancer. *Cancer* 2006;106:2428–2436.

100. Ebbert JO, Williams BA, Sun Z, et al. Duration of smoking abstinence as a predictor for non-small-cell lung cancer survival in women. *Lung Cancer* 2005;47:165-172.

101. Tammemagi CM, Neslund-Dudas C, Simoff M, et al. Smoking and lung cancer survival: the role of comorbidity and treatment. *Chest* 2004;125:27–37.

102. Nordquist LT, Simon GR, Cantor A, et al. Improved survival in never-smokers vs current smokers with primary adenocarcinoma of the lung. *Chest* 2004;126:347–351.

103. Ehlers SL, Gastineau DA, Patten CA, et al. The impact of smoking on outcomes among patients undergoing hematopoietic SCT for the treatment of acute leukemia. *Bone Marrow Transplant* 2011;46:285–290.

104. Geyer SM, Morton LM, Habermann TM, et al. Smoking, alcohol use, obesity, and overall survival from non-Hodgkin lymphoma: a population-based study. *Cancer* 2010;116:2993–3000.

105. Deleyiannis FW, Thomas DB, Vaughan TL, et al. Alcoholism: independent predictor of survival in patients with head and neck cancer. *J Natl Cancer Inst* 1996;88:542–549.

106. Ngô C, Alran S, Plancher C, et al. Outcome in early cervical cancer following pre-operative low dose rate brachytherapy: a ten-year follow up of 257 patients treated at a single institution. *Gynecol Oncol* 2011;123:248–252.

107. Browman GP, Wong G, Hodson I, et al. Influence of cigarette smoking on the efficacy of radiation therapy in head and neck cancer. *N Engl J Med* 1993;328:159–163.

108. Gillison ML, Zhang Q, Jordan R, et al. Tobacco smoking and increased risk of death and progression for patients with p16-positive and p16-negative oropharyngeal cancer. *J Clin Oncol* 2012;30:2102–2111.

109. Waggoner SE, Darcy KM, Fuhrman B, et al. Association between cigarette smoking and prognosis in locally advanced cervical carcinoma treated with chemoradiation: a Gynecologic Oncology Group study. *Gynecol Oncol* 2006;103:853–858.

110. Khuri FR, Lee JJ, Lippman SM, et al. Randomized phase III trial of low-dose isotretinoin for prevention of second primary tumors in stage I and II head and neck cancer patients. *J Natl Cancer Inst* 2006;98:441–450.

111. Karvonen-Gutierrez CA, Ronis DL, Fowler KE, et al. Quality of life scores predict survival among patients with head and neck cancer. *J Clin Oncol* 2008;26:2754–2760.

112. Sardari Nia P, Weyler J, Colpaert C, et al. Prognostic value of smoking status in operated non-small cell lung cancer. *Lung Cancer* 2005;47:351–359.

113. Chen J, Jiang R, Garces YI, et al. Prognostic factors for limited-stage small cell lung cancer: a study of 284 patients. *Lung Cancer* 2010;67:221–226.

114. Bittner N, Merrick GS, Galbreath RW, et al. Primary causes of death after permanent prostate brachytherapy. *Int J Radiat Oncol Biol Phys* 2008;72:433–440.

115. Haughey BH, Sinha P. Prognostic factors and survival unique to surgically treated p16+ oropharyngeal cancer. *Laryngoscope* 2012;122:S13– S33.

116. Kawakita D, Hosono S, Ito H, et al. Impact of smoking status on clinical outcome in oral cavity cancer patients. *Oral Oncol* 2012;48:186–191.

117. Chen AM, Chen LM, Vaughan A, et al. Tobacco smoking during radiation therapy for head-and-neck cancer is associated with unfavorable outcome. *Int J Radiat Oncol Biol Phys* 2011;79:414–419.

118. Junor E, Kerr G, Oniscu A, et al. Benefit of chemotherapy as part of treatment for HPV DNA-positive but p16-negative squamous cell carcinoma of the oropharynx. *Br J Cancer* 2012;106:358–365.

119. Manjer J, Andersson I, Berglund G, et al. Survival of women with breast cancer in relation to smoking. *Eur J Surg* 2000;166:852–858.

120. Kountourakis P, Correa AM, Hofstetter WL, et al. Combined modality therapy of cT2N0M0 esophageal cancer: the University of Texas M. D. Anderson Cancer Center experience. *Cancer* 2011;117:925–930.

121. Munro AJ, Bentley AH, Ackland C, et al. Smoking compromises cause-specific survival in patients with operable colorectal cancer. *Clin Oncol (R Coll Radiol)* 2006;18:436–440.

122. Gong Z, Agalliu I, Lin DW, et al. Cigarette smoking and prostate cancer-specific mortality following diagnosis in middle-aged men. *Cancer Causes Control* 2008;19:25–31.

123. Kjaerbye-Thygesen A, Frederiksen K, Hogdall EV, et al. Smoking and overweight: negative prognostic factors in stage III epithelial ovarian cancer. *Cancer Epidemiol Biomarkers Prev* 2006;15:798–803.

124. Nagle CM, Bain CJ, Webb PM. Cigarette smoking and survival after ovarian cancer diagnosis. *Cancer Epidemiol Biomarkers Prev* 2006;15:2557–2560.

125. Wright JD, Li J, Gerhard DS, et al. Human papillomavirus type and tobacco use as predictors of survival in early stage cervical carcinoma. *Gynecol Oncol* 2005;98:84–91.

126. Sardari Nia P, Van Marck E, Weyler J, et al. Prognostic value of a biologic classification of non-small-cell lung cancer into the growth patterns along with other clinical, pathological and immunohistochemical factors. *Eur J Cardiothorac Surg* 2010;38:628–636.

127. Hoff CM, Grau C, Overgaard J. Effect of smoking on oxygen delivery and outcome in patients treated with radiotherapy for head and neck squamous cell carcinoma—a prospective study. *Radiother Oncol* 2012;103:38–44.

128. Joshu CE, Mondul AM, Meinhold CL, et al. Cigarette smoking and prostate cancer recurrence after prostatectomy. *J Natl Cancer Inst* 2011;103:835–838.

129. Mai SK, Welzel G, Haegele V, et al. The influence of smoking and other risk factors on the outcome after radiochemotherapy for anal cancer. *Radiat Oncol* 2007;2:30.

130. Kim AJ, Suh JD, Sercarz JA, et al. Salvage surgery with free flap reconstruction: factors affecting outcome after treatment of recurrent head and neck squamous carcinoma. *Laryngoscope* 2007;117:1019–1023.

131. Khan AM, Freeman-Wang T, Pisal N, et al. Smoking and multicentric vulval intraepithelial neoplasia. *J Obstet Gynaecol* 2009;29:123–125.

132. Hefler L, Grimm C, Tempfer C, et al. Treatment with vaginal progesterone in women with low-grade cervical dysplasia: a phase II trial. *Anticancer Res* 2010;30:1257–1261.

133. Matsumoto K, Oki A, Furuta R, et al. Tobacco smoking and regression of low-grade cervical abnormalities. *Cancer Sci* 2010;101:2065–2073.

134. Fleshner N, Garland J, Moadel A, et al. Influence of smoking status on the disease-related outcomes of patients with tobacco-associated superficial transitional cell carcinoma of the bladder. *Cancer* 1999;86:2337–2345.

135. Ioffe YJ, Elmore RG, Karlan BY, et al. Effect of cigarette smoking on epithelial ovarian cancer survival. *J Reprod Med* 2010;55:346–350.

136. Schlumbrecht MP, Sun CC, Wong KN, et al. Clinicodemographic factors influencing outcomes in patients with low-grade serous ovarian carcinoma. *Cancer* 2011;117:3741–3749.

137. Fortin A, Wang CS, Vigneault E. Influence of smoking and alcohol drinking behaviors on treatment outcomes of patients with squamous cell carcinomas of the head and neck. *Int J Radiat Oncol Biol Phys* 2009;74:1062–1069.

138. Chen CH, Shun CT, Huang KH, et al. Stopping smoking might reduce tumour recurrence in nonmuscle-invasive bladder cancer. *BJU Int* 2007;100:281–286.

139. Browman GP, Mohide EA, Willan A, et al. Association between smoking during radiotherapy and prognosis in head and neck cancer: a follow-up study. *Head Neck* 2002;24:1031–1037.

140. Clark JR, McCluskey SA, Hall F, et al. Predictors of morbidity following free flap reconstruction for cancer of the head and neck. *Head Neck* 2007;29:1090–1101.

141. Little SC, Hughley BB, Park SS. Complications with forehead flaps in nasal reconstruction. *Laryngoscope.* 2009;119:1093–1099.

142. Patel RS, McCluskey SA, Goldstein DP, et al. Clinicopathologic and therapeutic risk factors for perioperative complications and prolonged hospital stay in free flap reconstruction of the head and neck. *Head Neck* 2010;32:1345–1353.

143. Baumann DP, Lin HY, Chevray PM. Perforator number predicts fat necrosis in a prospective analysis of breast reconstruction with free TRAM, DIEP, and SIEA flaps. *Plast Reconstr Surg* 2010;125:1335–1341.

144. Goodwin SJ, McCarthy CM, Pusic AL, et al. Complications in smokers after postmastectomy tissue expander/implant breast reconstruction. *Ann Plast Surg* 2005;55:16–19.

145. Bertelsen CA, Andreasen AH, Jorgensen T, et al. Anastomotic leakage after anterior resection for rectal cancer: risk factors. *Colorectal Dis* 2010;12:37–43.

146. Cooke DT, Lin GC, Lau CL, et al. Analysis of cervical esophagogastric anastomotic leaks after transhiatal esophagectomy: risk factors, presentation, and detection. *Ann Thorac Surg* 2009;88:177–184.

147. Richards CH, Platt JJ, Anderson JH, et al. The impact of perioperative risk, tumor pathology and surgical complications on disease recurrence following potentially curative resection of colorectal cancer. *Ann Surg* 2011;254:83–89.

148. Nickelsen TN, Jorgensen T, Kronborg O. Lifestyle and 30-day complications to surgery for colorectal cancer. *Acta Oncol* 2005;44:218–223.

149. Begum FD, Hogdall E, Christensen IJ, et al. Serum tetranectin as a preoperative indicator for postoperative complications in Danish ovarian cancer patients. *Gynecol Oncol* 2010;117:446–450.

150. Joo YH, Sun DI, Cho JH, et al. Factors that predict postoperative pulmonary complications after supracricoid partial laryngectomy. *Arch Otolaryngol Head Neck Surg* 2009;135:1154–1157.

151. Mason DP, Subramanian S, Nowicki ER, et al. Impact of smoking cessation before resection of lung cancer: a Society of Thoracic Surgeons General Thoracic Surgery Database study. *Ann Thorac Surg* 2009;88:362–370.

152. van der Voet JC, Keus RB, Hart AA, et al. The impact of treatment time and smoking on local control and complications in T1 glottic cancer. *Int J Radiat Oncol Biol Phys* 1998;42:247–255.

153. Wedlake LJ, Thomas K, Lalji A, et al. Predicting late effects of pelvic radiotherapy: is there a better approach? *Int J Radiat Oncol Biol Phys* 2010;78:1163–1170.

154. Hocevar-Boltezar I, Zargi M, Strojan P. Risk factors for voice quality after radiotherapy for early glottic cancer. *Radiother Oncol* 2009;93:524–529.

155. Lilla C, Ambrosone CB, Kropp S, et al. Predictive factors for late normal tissue complications following radiotherapy for breast cancer. *Breast Cancer Res Treat* 2007;106:143–150.

156. Eifel PJ, Jhingran A, Bodurka DC, et al. Correlation of smoking history and other patient characteristics with major complications of pelvic radiation therapy for cervical cancer. *J Clin Oncol* 2002;20:3651–3657.

157. Wuketich S, Hienz SA, Marosi C. Prevalence of clinically relevant oral mucositis in outpatients receiving myelosuppressive chemotherapy for solid tumors. *Support Care Cancer* 2012;20:175–183.

158. Zevallos JP, Mallen MJ, Lam CY, et al. Complications of radiotherapy in laryngopharyngeal cancer: effects of a prospective smoking cessation program. *Cancer* 2009;115:4636–4644.

159. Gold EB, Flatt SW, Pierce JP, et al. Dietary factors and vasomotor symptoms in breast cancer survivors: the WHEL Study. *Menopause* 2006;13:423–433.

160. Cheung MC, Hamilton K, Sherman R, et al. Impact of teaching facility status and high-volume centers on outcomes for lung cancer resection: an examination of 13,469 surgical patients. *Ann Surg Oncol* 2009;16:3–13.

161. Zingg U, Smithers BM, Gotley DC, et al. Factors associated with postoperative pulmonary morbidity after esophagectomy for cancer. *Ann Surg Oncol* 2011;18:1460–1468.

162. Kelly KJ, Greenblatt DY, Wan Y, et al. Risk stratification for distal pancreatectomy utilizing ACS-NSQIP: preoperative factors predict morbidity and mortality. *J Gastrointest Surg* 2011;15:250–259.

163. Merkow RP, Bilimoria KY, Cohen ME, et al. Variability in reoperation rates at 182 hospitals: a potential target for quality improvement. *J Am Coll Surg.* 2009;209:557–564.

164. Alsadius D, Hedelin M, Johansson KA, et al. Tobacco smoking and long-lasting symptoms from the bowel and the anal-sphincter region after radiotherapy for prostate cancer. *Radiother Oncol* 2011;101:495–501.

165. Kuri M, Nakagawa M, Tanaka H, et al. Determination of the duration of preoperative smoking cessation to improve wound healing after head and neck surgery. *Anesthesiology* 2005;102:892–896.

166. Vaporciyan AA, Merriman KW, Ece F, et al. Incidence of major pulmonary morbidity after pneumonectomy: association with timing of smoking cessation. *Ann Thorac Surg* 2002;73:420–425.

167. Bjarnason GA, Mackenzie RG, Nabid A, et al. Comparison of toxicity associated with early morning versus late afternoon radiotherapy in patients with head-and-neck cancer: a prospective randomized trial of the National Cancer Institute of Canada Clinical Trials Group (HN3). *Int J Radiat Oncol Biol Phys* 2009;73:166–172.

168. Park SM, Lim MK, Jung KW, et al. Prediagnosis smoking, obesity, insulin resistance, and second primary cancer risk in male cancer survivors: National Health Insurance Corporation Study. *J Clin Oncol* 2007;25:4835–4843.

169. Leon X, del Prado Venegas M, Orus C, et al. Influence of the persistence of tobacco and alcohol use in the appearance of second neoplasm in patients with a head and neck cancer. A case-control study. *Cancer Causes Control* 2009;20:645–652.

170. Kinoshita Y, Tsukuma H, Ajiki W, et al. The risk for second primaries in gastric cancer patients: adjuvant therapy and habitual smoking and drinking. *J Epidemiol* 2000;10:300–304.

171. Khuri FR, Kim ES, Lee JJ, et al. The impact of smoking status, disease stage, and index tumor site on second primary tumor incidence and tumor recurrence in the head and neck retinoid chemoprevention trial. *Cancer Epidemiol Biomarkers Prev* 2001;10:823–829.

CANCER PREVENTION AND SCREENING

172. Scanlon EF, Suh O, Murthy SM, et al. Influence of smoking on the development of lung metastases from breast cancer. *Cancer* 1995;75:2693–2699.

173. Ford MB, Sigurdson AJ, Petrulis ES, et al. Effects of smoking and radiotherapy on lung carcinoma in breast carcinoma survivors. *Cancer* 2003;98:1457–1464.

174. Li CI, Daling JR, Porter PL, et al. Relationship between potentially modifiable lifestyle factors and risk of second primary contralateral breast cancer among women diagnosed with estrogen receptor-positive invasive breast cancer. *J Clin Oncol* 2009;27:5312–5318.

175. van den Belt-Dusebout AW, de Wit R, Gietema JA, et al. Treatment-specific risks of second malignancies and cardiovascular disease in 5-year survivors of testicular cancer. *J Clin Oncol* 2007;25:4370–4378.

176. Boorjian S, Cowan JE, Konety BR, et al. Cancer of the Prostate Strategic Urologic Research Endeavor Investigators. Bladder cancer incidence and risk factors in men with prostate cancer: results from Cancer of the Prostate Strategic Urologic Research Endeavor. *J Urol* 2007;177:883–887.

177. Travis LB, Gospodarowicz M, Curtis RE, et al. Lung cancer following chemotherapy and radiotherapy for Hodgkin's disease. *J Natl Cancer Inst* 2002;94:182–192.

178. Ang KK, Harris J, Wheeler R, et al. Human papillomavirus and survival of patients with oropharyngeal cancer. *N Engl J Med* 2010;363:24–35.

179. Peck BW, Dahlstrom KR, Gan SJ, et al. Low risk of second primary malignancies among never smokers with human papillomavirus-associated index oropharyngeal cancers. *Head Neck* 2012;35:794–799.

180. Herbst RS, Prager D, Hermann R, et al. TRIBUTE: a phase III trial of erlotinib hydrochloride (OSI-774) combined with carboplatin and paclitaxel chemotherapy in advanced non-small-cell lung cancer. *J Clin Oncol* 2005;23:5892–5899.

181. Thatcher N, Chang A, Parikh P, et al. Gefitinib plus best supportive care in previously treated patients with refractory advanced non-small-cell lung cancer: results from a randomised, placebo-controlled, multicentre study (Iressa Survival Evaluation in Lung Cancer). *Lancet* 2005;366:1527–1537.

182. Kwak EL, Bang YJ, Camidge DR, et al. Anaplastic lymphoma kinase inhibition in non-small-cell lung cancer. *N Engl J Med* 2010;363:1693–1703.

183. Paik PK, Johnson ML, D'Angelo SP, et al. Driver mutations determine survival in smokers and never-smokers with stage IIIB/IV lung adenocarcinomas. *Cancer* 2012;118:5840–5847.

184. Soria JC, Cruz C, Bahleda R, et al. Clinical activity, safety and biomarkers of PD-L1 blockade in non-small cell lung cancer (NSCLC): additional analyses from a clinical study of the engineered antibody MPDL3280A (anti-PDL1). Presented at: 2013 European Cancer Congress 2013; 2013; Amsterdam.

185. Morales N, Romano M, Cummings KM, et al. Accuracy of self-reported tobacco use in newly diagnosed cancer patients. *Cancer Causes Control* 2013;24:1223–1230.

186. Warren GW, Arnold SM, Valentino JP, et al. Accuracy of self-reported tobacco assessments in a head and neck cancer treatment population. *Radiother Oncol* 2012;103:45–48.

187. Marin VP, Pytynia KB, Langstein HN, et al. Serum cotinine concentration and wound complications in head and neck reconstruction. *Plast Reconstr Surg* 2008;121:451–457.

188. American Medical Association. Tobacco use or exposure as a variable in clinical research (Resolution 424, A-06).www.ama-assn.org.ama1/pub/upload/nm/475/bot479i406.pdf.

189. Sarna L, Bialous SA. Nursing and tobacco cessation: setting a research agenda. Reports from a national conference. In: *Nursing Research*. Philadelphia: Lippincott Williams & Wilkins; 2006: 4S.

190. Sarna L, Bialous SA, Chan S, et al. International symposia: global perspectives on nursing involvement in tobacco control. Presented in: Oncology Nursing Society, 28th Annual Congress Syllabus, May 1–4, 2003, Denver, Colorado. Denver: Oncology Nursing Society; 2003: 112.

191. Viswanath K, Herbst RS, Land SR, et al. Tobacco and cancer: an American Association for Cancer research policy statement. *Cancer Res* 2010;70(17):3419–3430.

192. American Society of Clinical Oncology. American Society of Clinical Oncology policy statement update: tobacco control—Reducing cancer incidence and saving lives. 2003. *J Clin Oncol* 2003;21:2777–2786.

193. Gritz ER, Fingeret MC, Vidrine DJ, et al. Successes and failures of the teachable moment: smoking cessation in cancer patients. *Cancer* 2006;106:17–27.

194. Gritz ER, Dresler C, Sarna L. Smoking, the missing drug interaction in clinical trials: ignoring the obvious. *Cancer Epidemiol Biomarkers Prev* 2005;14:2287–2293.

195. Chappel A, Ziebland S, McPherson A. Stigma, shame, and blame experienced by patients with lung cancer: qualitative study. *BMJ* 2004;328:1470.

196. LoConte NK, Else-Quest NM, Eickhoff J, et al. Assessment of guilt and shame in patients with non-small-cell lung cancer compared with patients with breast and prostate cancer. *Clin Lung Cancer* 2008;9:171–178.

197. Wassenaar TR, Eickhoff JC, Jarzemsky DR, et al. Differences in primary care clinicians' approach to non-small cell lung cancer patients compared with breast cancer. *J Thorac Oncol* 2007;2:722–728.

198. Fiore MC, Bailey WC, Cohen SJ, et al. *Quick Reference Guide for Clinicians. Treating Tobacco Use and Dependence.* Rockville, MD: U.S. Department of Health and Human Services, Public Health Services; 2000. http://health.state.tn.us/Downloads/TQL_Quick%20Reference.pdf. Accessed November 25, 2013.

199. Fiore MC, Jaén CR, Baker TB, et al. *Treating Tobacco Use and Dependence: 2008 Update.* Rockville, MD: U.S. Department of Health and Human Services; 2008. http://www.ncbi.nlm.nih.gov/books/NBK63952/. Accessed November 25, 2013.

200. Fiore MC, Jorenby DE, Schensky AE, et al. Smoking status as the new vital sign: effect on assessment and intervention in patients who smoke. *Mayo Clin Proc* 1995;70:209–213.

201. Blumenthal D, Tavenner M. The "meaningful use" regulation for electronic health records. *N Engl J Med* 2010;363:501–504.

202. Couple approaches to smoking cessation. In: Schmaling KB, Sher TG, eds. *The Psychology of Couples and Illness: Theory, Research, & Practice.* Washington, D.C.: American Psychological Association; 2000: 311–336.

203. Homish GG, Leonard KE. Spousal influence on smoking behaviors in a US community sample of newly married couples. *Soc Sci Med* 2005;61:2557–2567.

204. Hemsing N, Greaves L, O'Leary R, et al. Partner support for smoking cessation during pregnancy: a systematic review. *Nicotine Tob Res* 2012;14:767–776.

205. Tod AM, Joanne R. Overcoming delay in the diagnosis of lung cancer: a qualitative study. *Nurs Stan* 2010;24:35–43.

206. Fagerstrom KO, Schneider NG. Measuring nicotine dependence: a review of the Fagerstrom Tolerance Questionnaire. *J Behav Med* 1989;12:159–182.

207. Baker TB, Piper ME, Bolt DM, et al. Time to first cigarette in the morning smoking as an index of ability to quit smoking: implications for nicotine dependence. *Nicotine Tob Res* 2007;9:S555–S570.

208. Ferguson JA, Patten CA, Schroeder DR, et al. Predictors of 6-month tobacco abstinence among 1224 cigarette smokers treated for nicotine dependence. *Addict Behav* 2003;28:1203–1218.

209. Prochaska JO, DiClemente CC. Stages and processes of self-change of smoking: toward an integrative model of change. *J Consult Clin Psychol* 1983;51:390–395.

210. Prokhorov AV, Hudmon KS, Gritz ER. Promoting smoking cessation among cancer patients: a behavioral model. *Oncology (Williston Park)* 1997;11:1807–1813.

211. Toll BA, Rojewski AM, Duncan L, et al. "Quitting smoking will benefit your health": the evolution of clinician messaging to encourage tobacco cessation. *Clin Cancer Res* 2014;20:301–309.

212. Miller WR, Rose GS. Toward a theory of motivational interviewing. *Am Psychol* 2009;64:527–537.

213. Gritz ER, Fingeret MC, Vidrine DJ. Tobacco control in the oncology setting. In: Brawley OW, Khuri FR, Rock CL, eds. *ASCO Cancer Prevention Curriculum.* Alexandria, VA: American Society of Clinical Oncology; 2007.

214. Henningfield JE, Keenan RM. Nicotine delivery kinetics and abuse liability. *J Consult Clin Psychol* 1993;61:743–750.

215. Silagy C, Lancaster T, Stead L, et al. Nicotine replacement therapy for smoking cessation. *Cochrane Database Syst Rev* 2004;(3):CD000146.

216. Piper M, Smith S, Schlam T, et al. A randomized placebo-controlled clinical trial of 5 smoking cessation pharmacotherapies. *Arch Gen Psychiatry* 2009;66:1253–1262.

217. Smith S, McCarthy D, Japuntich S, et al. Comparative effectiveness of 5 smoking cessation pharmacotherapies in primary care clinics. *Arch Intern Med* 2009;169:2148–2155.

218. Warren GW, Singh AK. Nicotine and lung cancer. *J Carcinog* 2013;12:1–8.

219. Myles PS, Iacono GA, Hunt JO, et al. Risk of respiratory complications and wound infection in patients undergoing ambulatory surgery: smokers versus nonsmokers. *Anesthesiology* 2002;97:842–847.

220. Sørensen L, Hørby J, Friis E, et al. Smoking as a risk factor for wound healing and infection in breast cancer surgery. *Eur J Surg Oncol* 2002;28:815–820.

221. Jorgensen ED, Zhao H, Traganos F, et al. DNA damage response induced by exposure of human lung adenocarcinoma cells to smoke from tobacco- and nicotine-free cigarettes. *Cell Cycle* 2010;9:2170–2176.

222. Murray RP, Connett JE, Zapawa LM. Does nicotine replacement therapy cause cancer? Evidence from the Lung Health Study. *Nicotine Tob Res* 2009;11:1076–1082.

223. Hughes JR, Stead LF, Lancaster T. Nortriptyline for smoking cessation: a review. *Nicotine Tob Res* 2005;7:491–499.

224. Ascher JA, Cole JO, Colin JN, et al. Bupropion: a review of its mechanism of antidepressant activity. *J Clin Psychiatry* 1995;56:395–401.

225. Fryer JD, Lukas RJ. Noncompetitive functional inhibition at diverse, human nicotinic acetylcholine receptor subtypes by bupropion, phencyclidine, and ibogaine. *J Pharmacol Exp Ther* 1999;288:88–92.

226. Cryan JF, Bruijnzeel AW, Skjei KL, et al. Bupropion enhances brain reward function and reverses the affective and somatic aspects of nicotine withdrawal in the rat. *Psychopharmacology* 2003;168:347–358.

227. Hughes JR, Stead LF, Lancaster T. Antidepressants for smoking cessation. *Cochrane Database Syst Rev* 2003;(2):CD000031.

228. Coe JW, Brooks PR, Vetelino MG, et al. Varenicline: an alpha4beta2 nicotinic receptor partial agonist for smoking cessation. *J Med Chem* 2005;48:3474–3477.

229. Jorenby DE, Hays JT, Rigotti NA, et al. Efficacy of varenicline, an alpha4beta2 nicotinic acetylcholine receptor partial agonist, vs placebo or sustained-release bupropion for smoking cessation: a randomized controlled trial. *JAMA* 2006;296:56–63.

230. Cahill K, Stead LF, Lancaster T. Nicotine receptor partial agonists for smoking cessation. *Cochrane Database Syst Rev* 2012;4:CD006103.

231. Hoogendoorn M, Welsing P, Rutten-van Mölken MP. Cost-effectiveness of varenicline compared with bupropion, NRT, and nortriptyline for smoking cessation in the Netherlands. *Curr Med Res Opin* 2008;24:51–61.

232. Linden K, Jormanainen V, Linna M, et al. Cost effectiveness of varenicline versus bupropion and unaided cessation for smoking cessation in a cohort of Finnish adult smokers. *Curr Med Res Opin* 2010;26:549–560.

233. Zimovetz EA, Wilson K, Samuel M, et al. A review of cost-effectiveness of varenicline and comparison of cost-effectiveness of treatments for major smoking-related morbidities. *J Eval Clin Pract* 2011;17:288–297.

234. Gibbons RD, Mann JJ. Varenicline, smoking cessation, and neuropsychiatric adverse events. *Am J of Psychiatry* 2013;170:1460–1467.

235. Thomas KH, Martin RM, Davies NM, et al. Smoking cessation treatment and risk of depression, suicide, and self harm in the Clinical Practice Research Datalink: prospective cohort study. *BMJ* 2013;347:f5704.

236. Anthenelli RM, Morris C, Ramey TS, et al. Effects of varenicline on smoking cessation in adults with stably treated current or past major depression: a randomized trial. *Ann Intern Med* 2013;159:390–400.

237. Gourlay SG, Stead LF, Benowitz NL. Clonidine for smoking cessation. *Cochrane Database Syst Rev* 2004;(3):CD000058.

238. Gritz ER, Carr CR, Rapkin D, et al. Predictors of long-term smoking cessation in head and neck cancer patients. *Cancer Epidemiol Biomarkers Prev* 1993;2:261–270.

239. Schnoll RA, Rothman RL, Wielt DB, et al. A randomized pilot study of cognitive-behavioral therapy versus basic health education for smoking cessation among cancer patients. *Ann Behav Med* 2005;30:1–11.

240. Griebel B, Wewers ME, Baker CA. The effectiveness of a nurse-managed minimal smoking-cessation intervention among hospitalized patients with cancer. *Oncol Nurs Forum* 1998;25:897–902.

241. Wewers ME, Bowen JM, Stanislaw AE, et al. A nurse-delivered smoking cessation intervention among hospitalized postoperative patients—influence of a smoking-related diagnosis: a pilot study. *Heart Lung* 1994;23:151–156.

242. Wewers ME, Jenkins L, Mignery T. A nurse-managed smoking cessation intervention during diagnostic testing for lung cancer. *Oncol Nurs Forum* 1997;24:1419–1422.

243. Stanislaw AE, Wewers ME. A smoking cessation intervention with hospitalized surgical cancer patients: a pilot study. *Cancer Nurs* 1994;17:81–86.

244. Schnoll RA, Zhang B, Rue M, et al. Brief physician-initiated quit-smoking strategies for clinical oncology settings: a trial coordinated by the Eastern Cooperative Oncology Group. *J Clin Oncol* 2003;21:355–365.

245. Sanderson Cox L, Patten CA, Ebbert JO, et al. Tobacco use outcomes among patients with lung cancer treated for nicotine dependence. *J Clin Oncol* 2002;20:3461–3469.

246. Garces YI, Schroeder DR, Nirelli LM, et al. Tobacco use outcomes among patients with head and neck carcinoma treated for nicotine dependence: a matched-pair analysis. *Cancer* 2004;101:116–124.

247. Duffy SA, Ronis DL, Valenstein M, et al. A tailored smoking, alcohol, and depression intervention for head and neck cancer patients. *Cancer Epidemiol Biomarkers Prev* 2006;15:2203–2208.

248. Schnoll RA, Martinez E, Tatum KL, et al. A bupropion smoking cessation clinical trial for cancer patients. *Cancer Causes Control* 2010;21:811–820.

249. Martinez E, Tatum KL, Weber DM, et al. Issues related to implementing a smoking cessation clinical trial for cancer patients. *Cancer Causes Control* 2009;20:97–104.

250. Park ER, Japuntich S, Temel J, et al. A smoking cessation intervention for thoracic surgery and oncology clinics: a pilot trial. *J Thorac Oncol* 2011;6:1059–1065.

251. Ostroff JS, Burkhalter JE, Cinciripini PM, et al. Randomized trial of a presurgical scheduled reduced smoking intervention for patients newly diagnosed with cancer. *Health Psychol* 2013 [Epub ahead of print].

252. Emmons KM, Puleo E, Park E, et al. Peer-delivered smoking counseling for childhood cancer survivors increases rate of cessation: the partnership for health study. *J Clin Oncol* 2005;23:6516–6523.

253. Wakefield M, Olver I, Whitford H, et al. Motivational interviewing as a smoking cessation intervention for patients with cancer: randomized controlled trial. *Nurs Res* 2004;53:396–406.

254. Goldstein AO, Ripley-Moffitt CE, Pathman DE, et al. Tobacco use treatment at the U.S. National Cancer Institute's designated Cancer Centers. *Nicotine Tob Res* 2013;15:52–58.

255. Warren GW, Marshall JR, Cummings KM, et al. Practice patterns and perceptions of thoracic oncology providers on tobacco use and cessation in cancer patients. *J Thorac Oncol* 2013;8:543–548.

256. Warren GW, Marshall JR, Cummings KM, et al. Addressing tobacco use in cancer patients: a survey of American Society of Clinical Oncology (ASCO) members. *J Oncol Pract* 2013;9:258–262.

257. Gritz ER, Sarna L, Dresler C, et al. Building a united front: aligning the agendas for tobacco control, lung cancer research, and policy. *Cancer Epidemiol Biomarkers Prev* 2007;16:859–863.

258. Vidrine JI, Shete S, Cao Y, et al. Ask-Advise-Connect: a new approach to smoking treatment delivery in health care settings. *JAMA Intern Med* 2013;173:458–464.

259. Bernstein SL, Jearld S, Prasad D, et al. Rapid implementation of a smokers' quitline fax referral service in an urban area. *J Health Care Poor Underserved* 2009;20:55–63.

260. Sarna L, Bialous SA, Ong MK, et al. Increasing nursing referral to telephone quitlines for smoking cessation using a web-based program. *Nurs Res* 2012;61:433–440.

261. Stancic N, Mullen PD, Prokhorov AV, et al. Continuing medical education: what delivery format do physicians prefer? *J Contin Educ Health Prof* 2003;23:162–167.

262. Society for Research on Nicotine and Tobacco Committee on Biochemical Verification. Biochemical verification of tobacco use and cessation. *Nicotine Tob Res* 2002;4:149–159.

263. American Society of Clinical Oncology. Tobacco Cessation Guide: for Oncology Providers. ASCO Web site. http://www.asco.org/sites/default/files/tobacco_cessation_guide.pdf. Accessed November 25, 2013.

**CANCER PREVENTION AND SCREENING**

# 32 Role of Surgery in Cancer Prevention

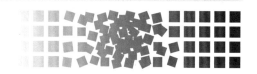

José G. Guillem, Andrew Berchuck, Jeffrey F. Moley, Jeffrey A. Norton, Sheryl G. A. Gabram-Mendola, and Vanessa W. Hui

## INTRODUCTION

Since the heritable component of some cancer predispositions has been linked to mutations in specific genes, clinical interventions have been formulated for mutation carriers within affected families. The primary interventions for mutation carriers for highly penetrant syndromes, such as multiple endocrine neoplasia (MEN), familial adenomatous polyposis (FAP), hereditary nonpolyposis colorectal cancer (CRC), and hereditary breast and ovarian cancer syndromes, are primarily surgical. This chapter is divided into five sections addressing breast (S.G.A.G.), gastric (J.N.), ovarian and endometrial (A.B.), and MENs (J.F.M.) and colorectal (J.G.G., V.W.H.). For each, the clinical and genetic indications and timing of prophylactic surgery and its efficacy, when known, are provided.

Prophylactic surgery in hereditary cancer is a complex process, requiring a clear understanding of the natural history of the disease and variance of penetrance, a realistic appreciation of the potential benefit and consequence of a risk-reducing procedure in an otherwise potentially healthy individual, and the long-term sequelae of such surgical intervention, as well as the individual patient's and family's perception of surgical risk and anticipated benefit.

## PATIENTS AT HIGH RISK FOR BREAST CANCER

### Identification of Patients at Risk

A detailed family history is the most important tool for identifying individuals at increased risk for hereditary cancers. The US Preventive Services Task Force updated their recommendation for risk assessment, genetic counseling, and genetic testing for asymptomatic women who have not been diagnosed with a *BRCA*-related cancer. In this update, the use of a risk screening tool is highly recommended to identify appropriate patients for referral for genetic counseling.[1] The American Society of Clinical Oncology has also updated the policy on genetic and genomic testing for cancer susceptibility, and this update includes information on genetic tests of uncertain clinical utility and direct-to-consumer marketing, both of which impact the practice of oncology and preventive medicine.[2] Historically, genetic counseling and testing were offered by health-care providers. However, with the advent of direct-to-consumer marketing, individuals may obtain tests and receive results directly from a company. The American Society of Clinical Oncology still endorses pre- and posttest counseling for thorough disclosure of the impact of testing. Before any woman considers risk-reduction surgery such as bilateral mastectomy or salpingo-oophorectomy, referral to a high-risk or genetic screening program is desirable, as women often overestimate their actual breast cancer risk.[3]

The most common cancer syndromes that place women at risk for breast cancer are *BRCA1*[4] and *BRCA2*[5] gene mutations. Other less common syndromes are listed in Table 32.1.[6,7]

Following referral for genetic assessment, three groups of patients emerge.[8] The first consists of those women who have undergone genetic testing and have been found to harbor a mutated gene associated with high penetrance for breast cancer. Given that the possibility of developing breast cancer in this group may be as high as 90%, there is a role for enhanced surveillance or risk-reduction surgery. The American Cancer Society has published guidelines for magnetic resonance imaging (MRI) screening as a method for enhanced surveillance.[9] Women in this first group qualify for such screening, which can be offered annually but scheduled at 6-month intervals with screening mammography to increase the rate of identifying interval cancers. Alternatively, simultaneous screening with MRI and mammography to compare one modality with the other on an annual basis may also be offered. Another choice for this group of women is to pursue bilateral risk-reduction mastectomy with an option for immediate reconstruction. Bilateral salpingo-oophorectomy for *BRCA1* and *BRCA2* mutation carriers may also be considered, as this procedure has been shown to reduce breast cancer risk by almost 50%.[8,10] This is especially true for *BRCA2* mutation carriers, who tend to develop hormone receptor–positive breast cancers.

The second group consists of women with strong family histories suggestive of hereditary breast cancer who test negative for both the *BRCA1* and *BRCA2* mutations as well as the other described syndromes. In this group, there may not have been a family member with cancer who was tested for the mutation. Therefore, a negative test does not necessarily indicate that a woman's risk is equivalent to that of the general population.[7] There may also be an undetected mutation in such a family, indicating the possibility of higher-than-average risk for that particular woman. These women may or may not qualify for enhanced surveillance with MRI screening,[9] and accurate assessment of their risk may require the use of other risk prediction tools,[3] in addition to evaluating for the presence of lobular carcinoma in situ, atypical lobular hyperplasia, or atypical ductal hyperplasia, and determining if a more intensive surveillance regimen is necessary based on heterogeneously or extremely dense breast tissue on mammography.

The third group consists of women with a strong family history of breast cancer, who for various reasons, have chosen not to pursue genetic testing. These individuals may have other health-related problems, psychological concerns, cost issues, or they may fear perceived medical insurance discrimination. Women in all groups can be educated that with passage of the Genetic Information Nondiscrimination Act in 2008, significant advances have occurred that protect patients from discrimination by employers and health insurers.[11]

Women in the second and third groups may still qualify for bilateral risk-reduction mastectomy and immediate reconstruction. Often, women who elect this path are influenced by their family history or by witnessing breast and/or ovarian cancer deaths in close family members, giving them a significant fear of a breast or ovarian cancer diagnosis. For women in all three groups, the decision of whether to pursue risk-reducing surgery is difficult. Often, the expertise of a cancer clinical psychologist or psychiatrist

**TABLE 32.1**

**Hereditary Carcinoma Syndromes Including Breast Cancer**

| Syndrome | Chromosome/Gene | Primary Carcinoma | Secondary Carcinoma | Breast Cancer Penetrance |
|---|---|---|---|---|
| Familial breast cancer/ovarian cancer syndrome | 17g21; *BRCA1* Autosomal dominant | Breast cancer, ovarian cancer | Colon, prostate | 60%–80% |
| Familial breast cancer/ovarian cancer syndrome | 13q12; *BRCA2* Autosomal dominant | Breast cancer, ovarian cancer | Male breast cancer, endometrial, prostate, oropharyngeal, pancreatic | 60%–80% |
| Li-Fraumeni syndrome | 17p13.1 and 22q12.1; *TP53* and *CHEK2* Autosomal dominant | Soft tissue cancers (including breast) | Soft tissue sarcoma, leukemia, osteosarcoma, melanoma, colon, pancreas, adrenal syndrome, cortex, and brain tumors | 50%–85% (for all types of cancers in this syndrome) |
| PTEN hamartoma syndrome (Cowden's) | 10q23.31; *PTEN* mutation Autosomal dominant | Breast cancer | Thyroid (follicular) and endometrial carcinoma | 25%–50% |
| Peutz-Jeghers syndrome | 19p13.3; *STK11* Autosomal dominant | Gastrointestinal cancers | Esophagus, stomach, small intestine, large bowel, pancreas, lung, ovary, endometrial | 29% |
| Diffuse gastric cancer | 16q22.1; *CDH1* Autosomal dominant | Diffuse gastric cancer | Colorectal, lobular breast cancer | 39% (lobular breast cancer) |
| Louis-Bar syndrome | 11q22.3; *ATM* Autosomal recessive | Leukemia and lymphoma | Ovarian, breast, gastric, melanoma, leiomyomas, sarcomas | 38% (for all types of cancers in the syndrome) |

PTEN, phosphatase and tensin homolog.
Data from Lux MP, Fasching PA, Beckmann MW. Hereditary breast and ovarian cancer: review and future perspectives. *J Mol Med* 2006;84:16–28; and Shannon KM, Chittenden A. Genetic testing by cancer site: breast. *Cancer J* 2012;18:310–319.

is enlisted, as risk-reduction mastectomy involves an irreversible procedure with body image and sexual implications.[8]

Updated in 2007, the Society of Surgical Oncology published a position statement on the role of prophylactic mastectomy for patients at high risk for breast cancer, as well as those patients recently diagnosed with breast cancer who are considering contralateral prophylactic breast surgery.[12] For women at high risk, indications fall into three broad categories: presence of a mutation in *BRCA* or other susceptible genes, strong family history with no demonstrable mutation, and histologic risk factors (biopsy-proven atypical ductal hyperplasia, atypical lobular hyperplasia, or lobular carcinoma in situ especially in patients with a strong family history of breast cancer). Recommendations for patients with recently diagnosed breast cancer are similar in that they include the indications for high-risk individuals previously noted, as well as future surveillance challenges for the opposite breast (clinically and mammographically dense breast tissue or diffuse, indeterminate microcalcifications in the contralateral breast). Another important consideration is the need for symmetry in patients with large, ptotic, or disproportionately sized contralateral breasts.

## Surgical Issues and Technique

In a single institution's 33-year experience,[13] the risk for breast cancer in both moderate- and high-risk groups of women based on family history was reduced by at least 89% for women who underwent bilateral prophylactic mastectomy. From a technical perspective, in this study, women either had a subcutaneous mastectomy (removal of the majority of breast tissue with sparing of the nipple–areola complex) or total mastectomy (removal of the entire breast through the nipple–areola complex). Most of the recurrences occurred in women undergoing a subcutaneous mastectomy. However, this was the most frequent procedure performed at that time and thus may have contributed to the number of increased recurrences.

Another surgical option for high-risk women is bilateral salpingo-oophorectomy. Among a cohort of women with *BRCA1* and *BRCA2* mutations, this procedure has been associated with a lower risk of mortality from both breast and ovarian cancer.[10] As an additional benefit, this procedure also decreases the risk of breast cancer in this patient population, likely through the mechanism of decreasing hormonal exposure at a younger age.

Contemporary surgical procedures for risk-reducing bilateral mastectomy include total mastectomy, skin-sparing mastectomy (preservation of the skin envelope by removal of the entire breast through a circumareolar incision around the nipple–areola complex), subcutaneous mastectomy, areola-sparing mastectomy (removal of the nipple while sparing the areola), and nipple-sparing mastectomy (removal of entire breast and nipple core tissue but preservation of nipple–areolar skin).[14] Given advances in reconstructive nipple–areolar techniques, it appears that total mastectomy with or without skin-sparing methods reduces the risk of breast cancer to the greatest extent with reasonable cosmesis. More limited and long-term follow-up data are available on areola- and nipple-sparing techniques. The potential limitations of these procedures are distortion of the nipple–areola complex and lack of sensitivity after breast tissue has been completely removed.[8]

Immediate reconstruction is offered to patients and performed in the vast majority undergoing bilateral risk-reduction mastectomy. Choices of reconstruction include a bilateral pedicled or free tissue transverse rectus abdominis muscle flap, a free bilateral deep inferior epigastric perforator flap or superficial inferior epigastric artery flap, bilateral latissimus flaps with or without implant or expanders, or bilateral implant or expander placement alone.[14] Although tissue flap transfer gives a more natural appearance and texture to the reconstructed site, individual body contour drives the ultimate plan for reconstruction. The decision about the type of reconstruction should be made by the plastic surgeon with input from the surgical oncologist, especially for the group of women with breast cancer desiring bilateral mastectomies who may require adjuvant radiation for treatment.

Although the risk reduction is dramatic for bilateral mastectomy, residual breast tissue may be left behind, especially with skin-sparing procedures. Patients should be educated that careful chest wall surveillance is recommended after such a procedure. Local recurrences after bilateral implant reconstruction are reliably detected by clinical examination. Recurrences after reconstruction with autologous tissue present most commonly on the skin 50% to 72% of the time and are detectable by physician examination.[15] Nonpalpable deeper recurrences in this setting are less common, and use of mammography image surveillance may be indicated, especially if significant breast tissue was left behind unintentionally during the bilateral mastectomy procedure. At times, an initial "screening" mammogram may be performed, if significant residual breast tissue is suspected; this should occur well after all healing has taken place to delineate the amount of visible breast tissue on imaging. This drives future decisions of whether to follow a patient with imaging. Finally, all patients should be instructed to return for clinical breast examination with the health provider if any change is noted on the reconstructed breasts, regardless of imaging plan.

Although risk-reduction bilateral mastectomy may be exceedingly beneficial for high-risk women, especially for those testing positive for *BRCA1*, *BRCA2*, or other deleterious mutations, or belonging to a family afflicted with a cancer syndrome, they are never emergent procedures. Along with risk-reduction bilateral salpingo-oophorectomy, risk-reduction bilateral mastectomy resides at the far end of the spectrum of an individual's choices.[16] These procedures should be offered only after appropriate genetic counseling and accurate assessment of a woman's actual risk for breast and ovarian cancer. An in-depth consultation with the patient and her family members is necessary prior to proceeding with an operative plan.

## HEREDITARY DIFFUSE GASTRIC CANCER

Gastric cancer is the fourth most common cause of cancer worldwide and is the second leading cause of cancer mortality.[17] Although environmental agents, including *Helicobacter pylori* and diet, are the primary risk factors for this disease, approximately 10% of gastric cancers are a result of familial clustering.[18,19] Histologically, gastric cancers may be classified as either intestinal or diffuse types. The intestinal type histopathology is linked to environmental factors and advanced age. The diffuse type occurs in younger patients and is associated with a familial predisposition. Because of

a decrease in intestinal-type gastric cancers, the overall incidence of gastric cancer has declined significantly in the past 50 years. However, the incidence of diffuse gastric cancer (DGC), which is also called signet ring cell or linitis plastica, has remained stable and, by some reports, may be increasing.

Hereditary DGC (HDGC) is a genetic cancer susceptibility syndrome defined by one of the following: (1) two or more documented cases of DGC in first- or second-degree relatives, with at least one diagnosed before the age of 50; or (2) three or more cases of documented DGC in first- or second-degree relatives, independent of age of onset. The average age of onset of HDGC is 38, and the pattern of inheritance is autosomal dominant.[20] Figure 32.1 shows a pedigree with HDGC.

In 1998, inactivating germline mutations in the E-cadherin gene *CDH1* were identified in three Maori families, each with multiple cases of poorly differentiated DGC.[21] The *CDH1* mutations in these families were inherited in an autosomal dominant pattern, with incomplete but high penetrance. Onset of clinically apparent cancer was early, with the youngest affected individual dying of DGC at the age of 14.[21] Since then, germline mutations of *CDH1* have been identified in 30% to 50% of all patients with HDGC.[19,22] More than 50 mutations have been recognized across diverse ethnic backgrounds, including European, African American, Pakistani, Japanese, Korean, and others.[19] In addition to gastric cancers, germline *CDH1* mutations are associated with increased risk of lobular carcinoma of the breast, and this was the first manifestation of a *CDH1* mutation in one series.[23] *CDH1* is, to date, the only gene implicated in HDGC. Penetrance of DGC in patients carrying a *CDH1* mutation is estimated at 70% to 80%, but may be higher. The need for a systematic study of specimens is supported by recent work by Gaya et al.[24] in which initial total gastrectomy specimens were reported as negative, but detailed sectioning and analysis showed invasive carcinoma.

*CDH1* is localized on chromosome 16q22.1 and encodes the calcium-dependent cell adhesion glycoprotein E-cadherin. Functionally, E-cadherin impacts maintenance of normal tissue morphology and cellular differentiation. It is hypothesized that *CDH1* acts as a tumor suppressor gene in HDGC, with loss of function leading to loss of cell adhesion and subsequently to proliferation, invasion, and metastases. Figure 32.2 shows the *CDH1* mutation for the pedigree depicted in Figure 32.1.

The germline *CDH1* mutation is most frequently a truncating mutation. Germline missense mutations are causative in a few HDGC kindreds, but are more often clinically insignificant. In vitro assays for cellular invasion and aggregation may predict the functional impact of missense mutations to aid in this distinction.[22] Within the gastric mucosa, the "second hit" leading to complete loss of E-cadherin function results from *CDH1* promoter methylation, as has been described in sporadic gastric cancer.[25]

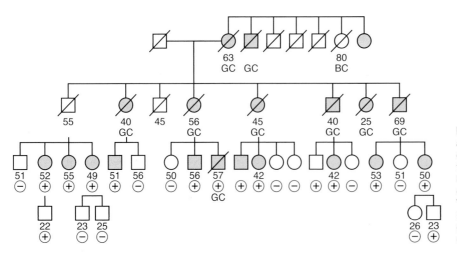

**Figure 32.1** A family pedigree showing autosomal dominant inheritance of gastric cancer. Individual mutation testing results for the codon 1003 CDH1 mutation are indicated by + or −. Individuals affected with gastric cancer are *shaded*. (From Norton JA, Ham CM, Van Dam J, et al. CDH1 truncating mutations in the E-cadherin gene: an indication for total gastrectomy to treat hereditary diffuse gastric cancer. *Ann Surg* 2007;245:873.)

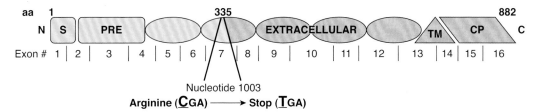

**Figure 32.2** The mutation in this kindred is located in the central region of the E-cadherin gene that codes for the extracellular cadherin domains of the protein containing calcium-binding motifs important in the adhesion process. The C → T transition in exon 7 of nucleotide 1003 results in a premature stop codon (R335X), producing truncated peptides that lack the transmembrane and cytoplasmic β-catenin–binding domains essential for tight cell-cell adhesion. *Black* area indicates truncated portion of peptide. N, N-terminus; C, C-terminus; S, signal peptide; PRE, precursor sequence; TM, transmembrane domain; CP, cytoplasmic domain. (From Norton JA, Ham CM, Van Dam J, et al. CDH1 truncating mutations in the E-cadherin gene: an indication for total gastrectomy to treat hereditary diffuse gastric cancer. *Ann Surg* 2007;245:873.)

It remains unclear whether specific *CDH1* mutations are associated with distinctive phenotypic characteristics or rates of penetrance, although this may become apparent as more recurrent mutations are recognized. To date, most mutations identified have been novel and distributed throughout *CDH1*. Recognition of recurrent mutations has usually resulted from independent events; however, there is evidence for the role of founder effects in certain kindreds.[22] At present, it is also unclear whether patients with HDGC without detectable *CDH1* mutations have mutation of a different gene or merely a *CDH1* mutation that has gone unrecognized.

New recommended screening criteria for *CDH1* mutations are as follows:

1. Families with one or more cases of DGC
2. Individuals with DGC before the age of 40 years without a family history
3. Families or individuals with cases of DGC (one case below the age of 50 years) and lobular breast cancer
4. Cases where pathologists detect in situ signet ring cells or pagetoid spread of signet ring cells adjacent to diffuse type gastric cancer[18,26]

As in other familial cancer syndromes, genetic counseling should take place prior to genetic testing so that the family understands the potential impact of the results. After obtaining informed consent, a team comprising a geneticist, gastroenterologist, surgeon, and oncologist should discuss the possible outcomes of testing and the management options associated with each. Genetic testing should first be performed on a family member with HDGC or on a tissue sample if no affected relative is living. In addition to direct sequencing, multiplex ligation-dependent probe amplification is recommended to test for large genomic rearrangements. If a *CDH1* mutation is identified, asymptomatic family members may proceed with genetic testing, preferably by the age of 20.[19] If no mutation is identified in the family member with DGC, the value of testing asymptomatic relatives is low.

Among individuals found to carry a germline *CDH1* mutation, clinical screening is problematic. Histologically, DGC is characterized by multiple infiltrates of malignant signet ring cells, which may underlie normal mucosa.[27] Because these malignant foci are small in size and widely distributed, they are difficult to identify via random endoscopic biopsy. Chromoendoscopy and positron emission tomography have reportedly been used, but the clinical utility of these tools in early detection remains unproven. Lack of a sensitive screening test for HDGC makes early diagnosis extremely challenging. By the time patients are symptomatic and present for treatment, many have diffuse involvement of the stomach or linitis plastica, and rates of mortality are high. Published case reports describe patients who have presented with extensive DGC despite recent normal endoscopy and negative biopsies.[28] The 5-year survival rate for individuals who develop clinically apparent DGC is only 10%, with the majority dying before age 40.

Because of high cancer penetrance, poor outcome, and inadequacy of clinical screening tools for HDGC, prophylactic total gastrectomy is recommended as a management option for asymptomatic carriers of *CDH1* mutations.[18] Although total gastrectomy is performed with prophylactic intent in these cases, most specimens have been found to contain foci of diffuse signet ring cell cancer.[19,28,29] Foci of DGC have been identified even in patients who have undergone extensive negative screening, including high-resolution computed tomography, positron emission tomography scan, chromoendoscopy-guided biopsies, and endoscopic ultrasonography.[19] However, HGDC in asymptomatic *CDH1* carriers is usually completely resected by prophylactic gastrectomy, as pathologic analyses of resected specimens have shown only T1N0 disease.

Because these signet ring cell cancers are multifocal and distributed throughout the entire stomach, especially in the cardia,[30] prophylactic gastrectomy should include the entire stomach, and the surgeon must transect the esophagus and not the proximal stomach. Furthermore, it should be performed by a surgeon experienced in the technical aspects of the procedure and familiar with HDGC. In asymptomatic patients, lymph node metastases have not been observed; therefore, D2 lymph node resection is not necessary. The optimal timing of prophylactic gastrectomy in individuals with *CDH1* mutations is unknown, but recent consensus recommendations indicate that age 20 is reasonable.[18]

Although it is a potentially lifesaving procedure, prophylactic gastrectomy for *CDH1* mutation carries significant risks that must be considered. Overall mortality for total gastrectomy is estimated to be as high as 2% to 4%, although it is estimated to be 1% when performed prophylactically. Patients must also be aware that there is a nearly 100% risk of long-term morbidity associated with this procedure, including diarrhea, dumping, weight loss, and difficulty eating.[19] A recent study of the effects of prophylactic gastrectomy for *CDH1* mutation demonstrated that physical and mental function were normal at 12 months, but specific digestive issues were recognized. Overall, 70% had diarrhea, 63% fatigue, 81% eating discomfort, 63% reflux, 45% eating restrictions, and 44% had altered body image, suggesting that this operation impacted negatively on quality of life.[31] Because of these complications and the fact that lymph node spread has not been observed, some recommend vagus-preserving gastrectomy done either open or laparoscopically. In addition, because the penetrance of *CDH1* mutations is incomplete, some patients who undergo prophylactic gastrectomy would never have gone on to develop clinically significant gastric cancer. Prophylactic gastrectomy has, in fact, been performed on several patients reported to show no evidence of gastric cancer on pathology.[29]

Some individuals with *CDH1* mutations choose not to pursue prophylactic gastrectomy. These individuals should undergo careful surveillance, including biannual chromoendoscopy with biopsies, beginning when they are at least 10 years younger than the youngest family member with DGC was at time of diagnosis. It is recommended that any endoscopically visible lesion is targeted and that six random biopsies are taken from the following regions: antrum, transitional zone, body, fundus, and cardia. Careful white-light examination with targeted and random biopsies combined with detailed histopathology can identify early lesions and help to inform decision making with regard to gastrectomy.[32] Additionally, because women with *CDH1* mutations have a nearly 40% lifetime risk of developing lobular breast carcinoma, they should be carefully screened with annual mammography and breast MRI starting at age 35.[23] They should also do monthly self-examinations and have a breast examination by a physician every 6 months. The same surveillance recommendations are probably appropriate for HDGC families without identifiable *CDH1* mutations, although no current guidelines for this exist.

The emergence of gene-directed gastrectomy as a treatment strategy for patients with HDGC represents the culmination of a successful collaboration between molecular biologists, geneticists, oncologists, gastroenterologists, and surgeons. It is anticipated that the recognition of similar molecular markers in other familial cancer syndromes will transform the approach to the early diagnosis and treatment of a variety of tumors.

## SURGICAL PROPHYLAXIS OF HEREDITARY OVARIAN AND ENDOMETRIAL CANCER

### Hereditary Ovarian Cancer (*BRCA1, BRCA2*)

Inherited mutations in *BRCA1* and *BRCA2* strongly predispose women to breast cancer and to high-grade serous cancers of the ovary, fallopian tube, and peritoneum.[33,34] About two-thirds are due to *BRCA1* mutations and one-third *BRCA2* mutations, and these account for about 15% to 20% of high-grade serous cases. The lifetime risk of these gynecologic cancers increases from a baseline of 1.5% to about 15% to 25% in *BRCA2* carriers and 30% to 60% in *BRCA1* carriers.[33,34] *BRCA1/2* mutations are rare in most populations (<1 in 500 individuals); one notable exception is the Ashkenazi Jewish population, in which the carrier frequency is 1 in 40.[35] *BRCA1*-associated cases peak in the 50s and *BRCA2*-associated cancers in the 60s.[36] In addition to *BRCA1/2* mutations, germline mutations in a number of other genes in the homologous recombination DNA repair pathway confer high penetrance susceptibility to ovarian cancer (e.g., *RAD51C, RAD51D, BRIP1, PALB2*).[37] This has led to the development of more comprehensive cancer genetic testing panels that are increasingly being used to identify women who are candidates for risk-reducing salpingo-oophorectomy (RRSO).

Genetic testing for inherited high-penetrance mutations in *BRCA1/2* and other genes should be discussed with women who have a significant family history of early onset breast cancer and/or cancers of the ovary, fallopian tube, or peritoneum. Involvement of a genetic counselor prior to testing is helpful, as they have expertise in managing the inherent clinical and social issues. Most *BRCA1/2* mutations involve base deletions or insertions in the coding sequence or splice sites that encode truncated protein products that are clearly dysfunctional. Less frequently, disease-causing mutations may occur that alter a single amino acid, though most of these missense variants represent innocent polymorphisms. The clinical significance of missense mutations can sometimes be elucidated by determining whether they segregate with cancer in other family members. In addition, genomic rearrangements may occur that inactivate *BRCA1* or *BRCA2*, and identification of such alterations requires molecular testing beyond sequencing.

Penetrance of ovarian cancer is not 100% in those with clearly deleterious *BRCA1/2* mutations, but presently it is not possible to provide more precise personalized risk estimates to guide the use of RRSO. However, common variants have been discovered in other genes that appear to affect the risk of ovarian cancer in *BRCA1/2* carriers.[38] Based on the known ovarian cancer risk–modifying loci, it has been reported that the 5% of *BRCA1* carriers at lowest risk have a lifetime risk of ≤28% of developing ovarian cancer, whereas the 5% at highest risk have a ≥63% lifetime risk. In the future, when modifier loci are more completely catalogued, more precise estimates of cancer risk may be provided to individual patients who are considering RRSO.

As about 20% of women with high-grade serous ovarian cancers have *BRCA1/2* mutations, it has been suggested that all of these women undergo genetic testing regardless of family history.[39] Mutational analysis in women with these cancers may increasingly become standard practice as the cost of genetic testing declines. Testing may also be driven by the availability of poly(ADP-ribose) polymerase inhibitor therapy for women whose cancers have germline or sporadic mutations in genes such as *BRCA1/2* and others that are involved in homologous recombination DNA repair.

RRSO is strongly recommended in women who carry *BRCA1/2* mutations because of the high mortality rate of ovarian cancer and the lack of effective screening and prevention approaches. Although screening with pelvic ultrasound and serum CA125 is generally recommended for *BRCA1/2* carriers during their 20s and 30s, it is not proven to reduce ovarian cancer mortality because even early stage high-grade cancers have a very high mortality. Oral contraceptives reduce the risk of ovarian cancer in the general population and appear to have a similar effect in *BRCA1/2* carriers, but this must be balanced against concerns regarding increased breast cancer risks.

The past practice of performing RRSO based solely on family history has been replaced by reliance on genetic testing. Clinical management of women with a strong family history in whom a deleterious germline mutation is not found, or those with variants of uncertain significance, should be resolved on a case-by-case basis. RRSO may be deemed appropriate in some cases, despite the absence of a clearly deleterious mutation. Fortunately, the risk of hereditary ovarian cancer does not rise dramatically until the mid-30s in women with *BRCA1* mutations and the 40s for women with *BRCA2* mutations.[36] As a result, most women are able to complete childbearing prior to undergoing RRSO. It is advisable for *BRCA1* carriers to undergo RRSO around age 35, as there is a 4% risk of ovarian cancer being discovered clinically or at the time of RRSO by age 40.[10] *BRCA2* carriers may choose to delay surgery into their 40s due to their lower risk of ovarian cancer, but this could diminish the protection against breast cancer that is afforded by RRSO. If a mutation carrier, particularly a *BRCA1* carrier, chooses to pursue fertility into her 40s, then she should be counseled that she is at considerable risk of developing a life-threatening cancer that is largely preventable.

Several studies have provided evidence of the efficacy of RRSO. In one early study of *BRCA1/2* carriers, RRSO reduced the rate of breast and ovarian cancer by 75% over several years of follow-up.[40] A separate study in 2002 examined outcome in 551 *BRCA1/2* carriers from various registries.[41] Among 259 women who had undergone RRSO, 6 (2.3%) were found to have stage I ovarian cancer at the time of the procedure and 2 (0.8%) subsequently developed serous peritoneal carcinoma. Among the controls, 58 (20%) women developed ovarian cancer after a mean follow-up of 8.8 years. With the exclusion of the six women whose cancers were diagnosed at surgery, RRSO reduced ovarian cancer risk by 96%. More recently, in 2014, an international registry study of over 5,783 subjects with median follow-up of 5.6 years found that RRSO reduced ovarian, tubal, and peritoneal cancer risk by 80%.[36] There was an estimated lifetime risk of primary peritoneal cancer after RRSO of about 4% for *BRCA1* carriers and 2% for *BRCA2* carriers.[36] The risk of death from all causes was reduced by 77%. A prospective cohort study noted that RRSO was associated with reduction in breast cancer–specific (hazard ratio [HR] = 0.44; 95% confidence interval [CI] = 0.26 to 0.76), ovarian cancer–specific (HR = 0.21; 95% CI = 0.06 to 0.80), and all-cause mortality (HR = 0.40; 95% CI = 0.26 to 0.61).[10]

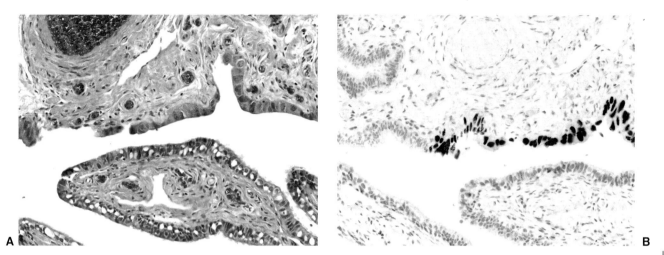

**Figure 32.3** Hematoxylin and eosin **(A)** and immunohistochemical staining **(B)** demonstrating overexpression of mutant *TP53* in serous carcinoma in situ of the fallopian tube from a *BRCA1* mutation carrier who underwent risk-reducing bilateral salpingo-oophorectomy.

Removal of the ovaries, as internal organs, usually has little effect on body image and self-esteem, and most *BRCA1/2* mutation carriers elect to undergo RRSO. Insurance payers will almost always pay for RRSO in proven mutation carriers.

RRSO can be performed laparoscopically in most women, with discharge to home the same day. If a laparoscopic approach is problematic due to obesity or adhesions, the surgery can be performed through a small lower abdominal incision. Morbidity including bleeding, infection, and damage to the urinary or gastrointestinal tracts can occur, but the incidence of serious complications is very low. As the fallopian tubes and ovaries are small discrete organs, they are relatively easy to remove completely. Attention should be paid to transecting the ovarian artery and vein proximal to the ovary and tube so that remnants are not left behind. This involves opening the pelvic sidewall peritoneum, visualizing the ureter, and then isolating the ovarian blood supply. If there are adhesions between the adnexa and adjacent structures, careful dissection should be performed to ensure complete removal of the ovaries and fallopian tubes. If the uterus is not removed, care should be taken to remove the entire fallopian tube. A small portion of the tube inevitably will be left in the cornu of the uterus, but the risk of fallopian tube cancer developing in such remnants appears to be negligible.

Though there is not strong evidence that *BRCA1/2* mutations increase uterine cancer risk, many women elect to have the uterus removed as part of the surgical procedure because they have completed their family or have other gynecologic indications. Although the addition of a hysterectomy may increase operative time, blood loss, surgical complications, and hospital stay, it usually can be performed laparoscopically and serious adverse outcomes are infrequent. Furthermore, the likelihood of future exposure to tamoxifen in the context of breast cancer prevention or treatment, which increases endometrial cancer risk two- to three-fold, also argues for concomitant hysterectomy. Women who receive hormone replacement therapy after surgery will require a progestin along with estrogen to protect against the development of endometrial cancer if the uterus is not removed.

In younger women, surgical menopause after RRSO is associated with vasomotor symptoms, vaginal atrophy, decreased libido, and an accelerated onset and incidence of osteoporosis and cardiovascular disease. In premenopausal women who do not have a personal history of breast cancer, estrogen replacement can be administered to ameliorate many of the deleterious effects of premature menopause. Systemic estrogen levels are lower in oophorectomized premenopausal women taking hormone replacement than if the ovaries had been left in place. The therapeutic benefit of oophorectomy in women with breast cancer has long been

appreciated, and more recent studies support the contention that RRSO reduces the risk of breast cancer by about half in *BRCA1/2* carriers.[42] However, a meta-analysis showed that while RRSO was strongly protective against estrogen receptor–positive breast cancer (HR = 0.22), there was no protection against estrogen receptor–negative breast cancer.[42] Many carriers are identified after developing early onset breast cancer, and this group represents the most difficult in which to balance the potential risks and benefits of estrogen replacement therapy.

Early stage high-grade serous cancers and in situ lesions with *TP53* mutations have been identified in the fallopian tubes of some RRSO specimens (Fig. 32.3). This has led to a paradigm shift in which it is now thought that most high-grade serous cancers found in the ovary, fallopian tube, and peritoneum are derived from cells that originate in the tubal fimbria.[43] The frequency of occult malignancies has varied between reports, but appears to be about 3%.[43] In view of this, the pelvis and peritoneal cavity should be examined carefully. Malignant cells also have been found in peritoneal cytologic specimens, and washings of the pelvis should be obtained when performing RRSO. The pathologist should be informed of the indication for surgery and serial sections of the fallopian tubes should be performed to look for the presence of early lesions. Patients found to have occult invasive high-grade serous cancers should be treated with chemotherapy after surgery. Those with in situ lesions appear to have a good outcome without chemotherapy.[44]

Cases of peritoneal serous carcinoma indistinguishable from ovarian cancer have been observed years after RRSO, but the origin of these cancers is unclear. Some may represent recurrences of occult ovarian or tubal cancers. In this regard, retrospective examination of the ovaries and fallopian tubes sometimes has revealed primary cancers that were not originally recognized. In contrast, some of these cancers likely arise directly from fallopian tube cells that have implanted in the peritoneum and subsequently become malignant. Patients who undergo RRSO should be made aware of their residual risk of peritoneal cancer, but there is no evidence that continued surveillance using CA125 and/or ultrasound is beneficial.

## HEREDITARY ENDOMETRIAL CANCER (LYNCH SYNDROME)

Although Lynch syndrome (LS, also known as hereditary nonpolyposis CRC syndrome) typically manifests as familial clustering of early onset CRC, there is also an increased incidence of several other types of cancers—most notably endometrial cancer in women.[45] About 3% of endometrial cancers are attributable to inherited mutations in the DNA mismatch repair (MMR) genes that cause LS. Most often, *MSH2* and *MLH1* are implicated, but mutations in *MSH6* and *PMS2* also occur.[45] The risk of ovarian cancer is also significantly increased in LS, but to a lesser degree than in *BRCA1/2* mutation carriers, and accounts for only about 1% of all ovarian cancers.

Cells in which one of the LS genes have been inactivated exhibit a phenomenon called microsatellite instability (MSI).[46] This occurs as DNA mismatches cause shortening or lengthening of repetitive DNA sequences and these mismatches go unrepaired. This results in generation of alleles in the cancer that contain a greater or lesser number of repeats than are present in normal cells from that individual. MSI occurs in most LS-associated colorectal and endometrial cancers.[46] However, MSI is found in about 20% of sporadic cancers that arise in these organs, and in most cases is caused by silencing of the *MLH1* gene due to promoter hypermethylation. Screening strategies for identification of MMR gene alterations in families with LS-associated cancers include analysis of tumor tissue for MSI and/or loss of DNA MMR gene expression using immunohistochemistry (IHC).[46] In cancers with MSI or loss of expression of one of the MMR genes, or in families with pedigrees suggestive of LS, these genes can be sequenced to identify disease-causing mutations, most of which cause truncated protein products.[47] Although it has been suggested that it may be cost-effective to do these tests on all endometrial cancers, this approach has not been widely adopted.[47]

The risk of a woman who carries a LS mutation developing endometrial cancer ranges from 20% to 60% in various reports.[45,48] The risk of ovarian cancer is increased to about 5% to 12%. Whereas the mean age of women with sporadic endometrial cancers is in the early 60s, cancers that arise in association with LS are often diagnosed before menopause, with the average age in the 40s. The clinical features of these endometrial cancers are similar to those of most sporadic cases (well-differentiated, endometrioid histology, early stage), and survival is about 90%. The mean age of onset of ovarian cancer in LS is in the early 40s, and the clinical features of these cancers are generally more favorable than in sporadic cases. They usually are identified at an early stage, are well- or moderately differentiated, have favorable survival, and some occur in the setting of a synchronous endometrial cancer.

Recommendations for screening and risk-reducing surgery in LS are better established for CRC than for extracolonic malignancies.[49] Transvaginal ultrasound has been proposed as a screening test for endometrial cancer (and ovarian cancer), but its efficacy is unproven.[50] Endometrial biopsy is the most sensitive means of diagnosing endometrial cancer, and it has been suggested that this should be employed periodically beginning around age 30 to 35. However, there are no published studies demonstrating that this approach prevents endometrial cancer deaths compared to simply performing a biopsy if abnormal uterine bleeding occurs.

Most experts believe that risk-reducing hysterectomy has a role in the management of some women with LS because of the high incidence of endometrial cancer. The risk of endometrial cancer is low during the prime reproductive years, and the uterus does not serve a vital function once childbearing has been completed. In view of the increased risk of ovarian cancer in LS, concomitant bilateral salpingo-oophorectomy should also be considered. One study demonstrated that there were no cases of endometrial or ovarian cancer in 61 LS carriers who underwent risk-reducing hysterectomy and bilateral salpingo-oophorectomy, while endometrial cancer occurred in 33% and ovarian cancer in 5% who retained their uterus and ovaries.[51] Despite the low risk of death from gynecologic cancers in LS, cost-effectiveness analyses of various approaches suggest that risk-reducing hysterectomy and salpingo-oophorectomy leads to both the lowest cost and the greatest increase in quality-adjusted life-years.[52] Estrogen replacement after removal of the ovaries in premenopausal women with LS is not contraindicated, as there is no evidence that this adversely affects the incidence of other cancers.

Many women with LS elect to undergo risk-reducing colectomy, which provides an opportunity to perform concomitant hysterectomy. Hysterectomy in concert with colectomy, either via laparoscopy or laparotomy, does not greatly increase operative time or surgical complications. If an endometrial biopsy has not been performed preoperatively, an intraoperative inspection of the uterine cavity and possibly frozen section should be performed to exclude the presence of cancer. If cancer is found in the uterus, surgical staging—including sampling of the regional lymph nodes—should be considered in addition to hysterectomy.[53] It is also appropriate to discuss risk-reducing hysterectomy with LS carriers who do not elect to undergo prophylactic colectomy. The operative approach (vaginal versus laparotomy versus laparoscopy) can be determined based on the presence or absence of uterine pathology (e.g., myomas), whether the patient has had prior abdominal surgery, and whether the ovaries are also to be removed.

## GYNECOLOGIC CANCER RISK IN VERY RARE HEREDITARY CANCER SYNDROMES

Several very rare hereditary cancer syndromes also increase the risk of gynecologic cancers, and some of these women could potentially benefit from risk-reducing surgery to remove the ovaries and/or uterus. Peutz-Jeghers syndrome is characterized by intestinal polyps and an increased risk of colorectal and breast cancers. This rare syndrome is due to inherited mutations in the *STK11* gene. Affected women also have an increased risk of ovarian sex cord–stromal tumors with annular tubules and adenoma malignum of the cervix. Li-Fraumeni syndrome is caused by inherited mutations in the *TP53* gene, and carriers are predisposed to a number of types of cancers including sarcomas and breast cancer. The risk of ovarian cancer is increased as well, but is not a major cause of cancer in these families. Cowden syndrome is due to germline *PTEN* mutations and increases the risk of several malignancies including breast, thyroid, mucocutaneous, and endometrial cancers. Finally, small cell carcinoma of the ovary, hypercalcemic type, is due to mutations in the *SMARCA4* gene. These highly lethal ovarian cancers occur at a very young age (median 24 years) and present difficult challenges related to timing of RRSO. There are no well-accepted evidence-based guidelines for early detection and prevention of gynecologic cancers in these very rare hereditary cancer syndromes. An awareness of the risk and natural history of gynecologic cancers in these families provides a basis for counseling individual patients.

## MULTIPLE ENDOCRINE NEOPLASIA TYPE 2

### Gene Carriers

The MEN type 2 syndromes include MEN 2A, MEN 2B, and familial (non-MEN) medullary thyroid carcinoma (FMTC).[54-56] These are autosomal dominant inherited syndromes caused by germline mutations in the *RET* proto-oncogene. Their hallmark is the development of multifocal bilateral medullary thyroid carcinoma (MTC) associated with C-cell hyperplasia. MTCs arise from the thyroid C-cells, also called parafollicular cells. C-cells secrete the hormone calcitonin, a specific tumor marker for MTC. A slow-growing tumor in most cases, MTC causes significant morbidity and death in patients with uncontrolled local or metastatic spread. Large tumor burden is associated with diarrhea and flushing. In the MEN 2 syndromes, there is almost complete penetrance of MTC. Other features are variably expressed, with incomplete penetrance (summarized in Table 32.2).

In MEN 2A, all patients develop MTC. Approximately 42% of affected patients also develop pheochromocytomas, associated with adrenal medullary hyperplasia. Hyperparathyroidism develops in

**TABLE 32.2**

**Clinical Features of Sporadic Medullay Thyroid Carcinoma, Multiple Endocrine Neoplasia 2A, Multiple Endocrine Neoplasia 2B, and Familial Medullary Thyroid Carcinoma**

| Clinical Setting | Features of MTC | Inheritance Pattern | Associated Abnormalities | Genetic Defect |
|---|---|---|---|---|
| Sporadic MTC | Unifocal | None | None | Somatic *RET* mutations in >20% of tumors |
| MEN 2A | Multifocal, bilateral | Autosomal dominant | Pheochromocytomas, hyperparathyroidism, cutaneous lichen amyloidosis, Hirshprung's disease | Germline missense mutations in extracellular cysteine codons of *RET* |
| MEN 2B | Multifocal, bilateral | Autosomal dominant | Pheochromocytomas, mucosal neuromas, megacolon, skeletal abnormalities | Germline missense mutation in tyrosine kinase domain of *RET* |
| FMTC | Multifocal, bilateral | Autosomal dominant | None | Germline missense mutations in extracellular or intracellular cysteine codons of *RET* |

MTC, medullary thyroid carcinoma; MEN, multiple endocrine neoplasia; FMTC, familial medullary thyroid carcinoma.

10% to 35%. Cutaneous lichen amyloidosis and Hirschsprung's disease are infrequently associated with MEN 2A.[57-60]

MEN 2B appears to be the most aggressive form of hereditary MTC. In MEN 2B, MTC develops in all patients at a very young age (infancy). All affected individuals develop neural gangliomas, particularly in the mucosa of the digestive tract, conjunctiva, lips, and tongue; 40% to 50% develop pheochromocytomas. Patients with MEN 2B may also have megacolon, skeletal abnormalities, and markedly enlarged peripheral nerves. They do not develop hyperparathyroidism.

FMTC is characterized by development of MTC in the absence of any other endocrinopathies. MTC in these patients has a more indolent clinical course. Some individuals with FMTC may never manifest clinical evidence (i.e., symptoms or a lump in the neck), although biochemical testing and histologic evaluation of the thyroid demonstrates MTC.[55,56]

## *RET* Genotype-Phenotype Correlations

Mutations in the *RET* proto-oncogene are responsible for MEN 2A, MEN 2B, and FMTC.[61-64] This gene encodes a transmembrane tyrosine kinase protein.[57,65] The mutations that cause the MEN 2 syndromes are activating gain-of-function mutations affecting constitutive activation of the protein. This is unusual among hereditary cancer syndromes, which are usually caused by loss-of-function mutations in the predisposition gene (e.g., familial polyposis, *BRCA1* and 2, von Hippel-Lindau, and MEN 1). More than 30 missense mutations have been described in patients affected by the MEN 2 syndromes (Fig. 32.4).

There is a relationship between the type of inherited *RET* mutation and presentation of MTC. The most virulent form is seen in patients with MEN 2B. These patients most commonly have a germline mutation in codon 918 of *RET* (ATG->ACG), although other mutations have been described (codon 883 and 922). As noted previously, MTC in MEN 2B has an extremely early age of onset (infancy). Despite its distinctive clinical appearance and associated gastrointestinal difficulties, the disease is often not detected until the patient develops a neck mass. Metastatic spread is usually present at the time of initial treatment, and calcitonin levels often remain elevated postoperatively.

MTC has a variable course in patients with MEN 2A, similar to that of sporadic MTC. Codon 634 and 618 mutations are the most common *RET* mutations associated with MEN 2A, although

mutations at other codons are also observed (see Fig. 32.4). Some patients do extremely well for many years, even with distant metastases, while others develop inanition, symptomatic liver, lung or skeletal metastases, as well as disabling diarrhea. Recurrence in the central neck, with invasion of the airway or great vessels, may cause death.

In patients with FMTC, MTC is usually indolent. These individuals most commonly have mutations of codons 609, 611, 618, 620, 768, 804, or 891, although mutations of other codons have been identified (see Fig. 32.4). Many patients with FMTC are cured by thyroidectomy alone, and even those with persistent elevation of calcitonin levels do well for many years. Occasionally, patients with FMTC survive into the seventh or eighth decade without clinical signs of disease, although pathologic examination of the thyroid will reveal MTC or C-cell hyperplasia.[66]

## Risk-Reducing Thyroidectomy in *RET* Mutation Carriers

Genetic counseling and informed consent should be obtained prior to genetic testing. Specific issues that should be covered in genetic counseling sessions include explaining the patterns of heritability, likelihood of expression of different tumors, their prevention and treatment, insurability, nonpaternity, survivor guilt, and others.

It has been shown that *RET* mutation carriers may harbor foci of MTC in the thyroid gland, even when calcitonin levels are normal.[67] While the age of onset and rate of disease progression may differ, the lifetime penetrance of MTC is near 100% in carriers of *RET* mutations associated with MEN 2 syndromes. At-risk individuals who are found to have inherited a *RET* gene mutation are therefore candidates for thyroidectomy, regardless of their plasma calcitonin levels.

The best option for prevention of MTC in *RET* mutation carriers is complete surgical resection prior to malignant transformation. Prophylactic thyroidectomy prior to the development of MTC is the goal in these patients. A number of studies have demonstrated improved biochemical cure rates and/or decreased recurrence rates from early thyroidectomy, performed after positive screening by calcitonin testing or *RET* mutation testing.[68-70]

MEN 2B mutations are the highest risk level, designated level III (see Fig. 32.4).[55,71] Patients with MEN 2B have the most aggressive form of MTC, with invasive disease reported in patients <1 year of age. These patients should have preventative surgery

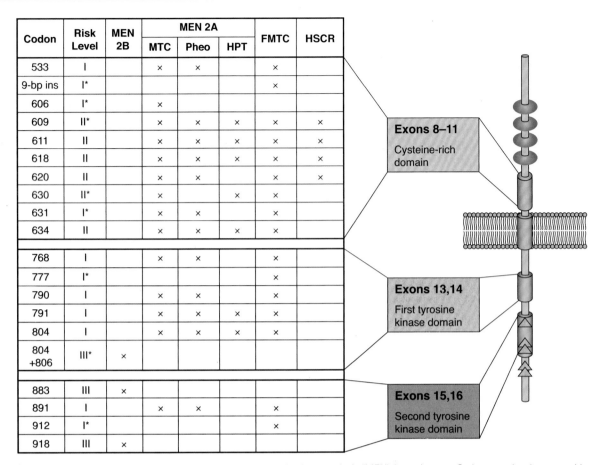

| Codon | Risk Level | MEN 2B | MEN 2A | | | FMTC | HSCR |
|---|---|---|---|---|---|---|---|
| | | | MTC | Pheo | HPT | | |
| 533 | I | | × | × | | × | |
| 9-bp ins | I* | | | | | × | |
| 606 | I* | | × | | | | |
| 609 | II* | | × | × | × | × | × |
| 611 | II | | × | × | × | × | × |
| 618 | II | | × | × | × | × | × |
| 620 | II | | × | × | | × | × |
| 630 | II* | | × | | × | × | |
| 631 | I* | | × | × | | × | |
| 634 | II | | × | × | × | × | |
| 768 | I | | × | × | | × | |
| 777 | I* | | | | | × | |
| 790 | I | | × | × | | × | |
| 791 | I | | × | × | × | × | |
| 804 | I | | × | × | × | × | |
| 804 +806 | III* | × | | | | | |
| 883 | III | × | | | | | |
| 891 | I | | × | × | | × | |
| 912 | I* | | | | | × | |
| 918 | III | × | | | | | |

**Figure 32.4** *RET* mutation sites associated with multiple endocrine neoplasia (MEN) 2 syndromes. Codons previously reported in association with MEN-2 syndromes are listed by structural domain within the RET protein. Risk level is based on consensus guidelines or more recent clinical reports. Previously reported phenotypes for each codon are shown. MTC, medullary thyroid carcinoma; Pheo, pheochromocytoma; HPT, hyperparathyroidism; FMTC, familial medullary thyroid carcinoma; HSCR, Hirschsprung's disease. *Asterisk* indicates risk level based on recent clinical reports not available at publication of the consensus guidelines. (From Traugott AL, Moley JF. The RET protooncogene. *Cancer Treat Res* 2010;153:303–319.)

early in the first year of life, if possible. Identification and preservation of parathyroid glands can be extremely difficult in these infants, due to their small size, translucent appearance, and the presence of exuberant thymic and perithyroidal nodal tissue. These procedures should be performed by surgeons experienced in parathyroid and/or pediatric thyroid operations.

Patients with MEN 2A with mutations in codons 634, 620, 618, and 611 are also considered high risk (level II).[55,71] Patients with level II mutations should undergo a total thyroidectomy at 5 to 6 years of age. There is evidence that the risk of lymph node metastasis is very low in patients with MEN 2A under the age of 8, with normal calcitonin levels. Central lymph node dissection is associated with higher risk of hypoparathyroidism, and recurrent laryngeal nerve injury and should be reserved for patients with elevated calcitonin levels.

A larger subset of *RET* mutations, associated with MEN 2A and/or FMTC, is considered the lowest risk (level I).[55,71] These include mutations at codons 768, 790, 791, 804, and 891. For patients with low-risk level I mutations, total thyroidectomy is recommended before age 5 to 10 years. This decision, however, regarding ideal age at preventative thyroidectomy in low-risk mutation carriers, is currently being reviewed, and may be driven by additional clinical data such as the basal or stimulated serum calcitonin level.[72,73] There are no guidelines at present that address the issue of timing of surgery based on calcitonin level, and at present, pentagastrin (the primary calcitonin secretagogue used in testing) is not available in the United States. It is anticipated that within a decade, there will

be enough published data to direct timing of interventions based upon this information. As with the level II mutations, the need for central lymph node dissection should be guided by calcitonin levels and clinical features of the patient and kindred.

Until recently, some groups recommended total thyroidectomy with central neck lymph node dissection and total parathyroidectomy with autotransplantation for all *RET* mutation carriers. Recent studies and personal experience, however, have demonstrated an extremely low likelihood of nodal metastases in patients with MEN 2A or FMTC younger than 8 years of age, and in patients with a normal calcitonin level.[70] Our current strategy is to leave the parathyroid in situ in these patients, if possible.[74] Often, however, the desired complete removal of thyroid tissue results in compromise of parathyroid blood supply. In these situations, autotransplantation of devascularized parathyroid is required. We routinely remove and autotransplant the parathyroid if a central node dissection is done. In parathyroid autotransplantation, parathyroid glands are sliced into 1 mm × 3 mm fragments and autotransplanted into individual muscle pockets in the muscle of the nondominant forearm in patients with MEN 2A, or in the sternocleidomastoid muscle in patients with FMTC or MEN 2B. Patients are maintained on calcium and vitamin D supplementation for 4 to 8 weeks postoperatively.

In a recent series of thyroidectomies performed in 50 individuals with MEN 2A (identified by genetic screening), total thyroidectomy and central node dissection with parathyroidectomy and parathyroid autografting were performed in all patients (Fig. 32.5).[70]

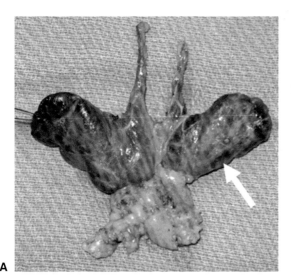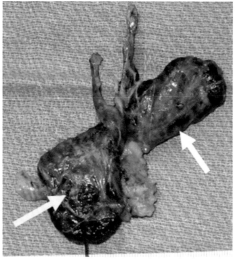

**Figure 32.5** Total thyroidectomy specimen with attached central nodes from a patient with germline *RET* mutation and elevated calcitonin levels. Note small visible foci of medullary thyroid carcinoma (*arrows*).

All autografts functioned, but three patients required supplemental calcium. The percentage of individuals requiring calcium supplementation following parathyroidectomy with parathyroid autografting reportedly ranges from 0% to 18%. Parathyroidectomy should be performed in all patients showing gross parathyroid enlargement or biochemical evidence of parathyroid disease at time of surgery. The operating surgeon should have expertise in preservation of parathyroid function. It is important that the surgeon performing an operative procedure for MTC be familiar with the techniques described here. If not, the patient should be referred to a center where these procedures are routinely performed.

Some patients with MEN 2 will be found to have elevated calcitonin levels prior to thyroidectomy. This is usually associated with medullary thyroid carcinoma or C-cell hyperplasia in the gland, and may be associated with lymph node metastases. Much has been written about the correlation between preoperative calcitonin levels and extent of nodal involvement. It has been suggested that preoperative calcitonin level may guide the extent of node dissection. In a study of 300 European patients with MTC, node metastases were not identified when the preoperative basal calcitonin level was <20 pg/ml.[75] Involvement of nodal groups was correlated with basal calcitonin level as follows: ipsilateral central and lateral neck nodes (basal calcitonin >20 pg/ml), contralateral central nodes (basal calcitonin >50 pg/ml), contralateral lateral neck nodes (basal calcitonin >200 pg/ml), and mediastinal nodes (basal calcitonin >500 pg/ml). Based upon these findings, this group (who also wrote the European guidelines) recommends thyroidectomy only if basal calcitonin is <20 pg/ml, ipsilateral central and lateral neck dissection if the calcitonin is 20 to 50 pg/ml, and contralateral central neck dissection if the basal calcitonin is 50 to 200 pg/ml, with the addition of contralateral lateral neck dissection if the calcitonin is 200 to 500 pg/ml. Most experts agree that sternotomy with mediastinal neck dissection should be reserved for patients with image evidence of mediastinal disease. In contrast, most North American surgeons rely heavily upon preoperative ultrasound imaging to map the extent of nodal involvement and determine extent of surgery based upon calcitonin and imaging results.[55,74,76]

### Follow-up

Following thyroidectomy, thyroid hormone replacement is required for life. Patients may need several weeks of oral calcium and vitamin D until parathyroid function recovers. Intermittent calcitonin testing may be done to monitor for persistent or recurrent

MTC. The importance of regular monitoring of patients' compliance with thyroid medication following thyroidectomy should not be underestimated. Children and teenagers are frequently noncompliant, and this can be determined by routine measurement of thyroid-stimulating hormone levels. Continued noncompliance can result in growth problems. Occasionally, local human services agencies may need to be involved in particularly difficult cases.

The term "biochemical cure" is used to refer to patients with normal calcitonin levels after surgery for MTC. Complete postoperative normalization of calcitonin has been associated with decreased long-term risk of MTC recurrence, though the evidence is less clear for a survival benefit. A persistent or recurrent elevation in calcitonin indicates residual or recurrent MTC and warrants additional investigation by imaging. However, as most MTC has a fairly indolent course, patients with biochemical evidence of recurrent disease may not have corollary imaging findings for some time.

### Conclusions

Identification of *RET* gene mutations in individuals at risk for developing hereditary forms of MTC has simplified management, expanding the scope of indications for surgical intervention. Patients who carry this mutation can be offered operative treatment at a very young age, hopefully before the cancer has developed or spread, and those identified as not having the mutation are spared further genetic and biochemical screening. This achievement marks a new paradigm in surgery: the indication that an operation be performed based on the results of a genetic test. As in the decision to perform any surgical procedure, meticulous preparation and detailed discussion with patient and family must precede the final recommendation. It is also important that the patient and family be involved in preoperative discussions with genetic counselors. Postoperative follow-up for compliance with thyroid medication is important, especially in children and teenagers who are still growing and developing into adults.

## FAMILIAL ADENOMATOUS POLYPOSIS, *MYH*-ASSOCIATED POLUPOSIS, AND LYNCH SYNDROME

Inherited CRC syndromes with multiple adenomatous polyps include FAP, *MYH*-associated polyposis (MAP), and LS. In some cases, the diagnosis is suspected because of a striking family history

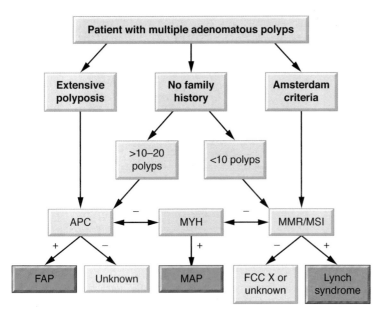

**Figure 32.6** Schematic demonstrating the potential genetic workup for a patient with multiple adenomatous colorectal polyps and suspected of having an inherited colorectal cancer syndrome. APC, adenomatous polyposis coli; MMR, mismatch repair; MSI, microsatellite instability; FAP, familial adenomatous polyposis; MAP, *MYH*-associated polyposis; FCC X, familial colorectal cancer syndrome X.

of CRC, while in others, suspicion arises from a very young onset of CRC or florid polyposis.

Although adenomatous polyp burden and family history may suggest one syndrome over another, an initial negative genetic test result should be followed by further evaluation for other syndromes. For example, in clinical practice, a negative adenomatous polyposis coli (APC) gene test in a patient with a suspected CRC syndrome is followed by reflex testing for MAP and LS, as shown in Figure 32.6.

FAP is an autosomal dominant syndrome that accounts for <1% of the annual CRC burden, is caused by mutations in the tumor-suppressor *APC* gene. It is characterized by the presence of ≥100 adenomatous polyps in the colorectum, nearly 100% penetrance, and an inevitable risk of CRC if prophylactic colectomy is not performed.[8,77] Patients with a less severe form known as attenuated FAP (AFAP) usually present with <100 colorectal adenomas that tend to be proximally located. MAP is an autosomal recessive syndrome that often presents phenotypically as attenuated polyposis. While an estimated 2% of the general population are mono-allelic carriers of a mutated base-excision-repair *MUTYH* (*MYH*) gene, biallelic germline mutations may account for 9% to 18% of patients with FAP or AFAP phenotypes who have no demonstrable *APC* mutation.[78–80]

LS accounts for 1% to 4% of all newly diagnosed CRC and is attributable to a germline mutation in one of the DNA MMR genes (*MLH1*, *MSH2*, *MSH6*, and *PMS2*).[81–83] Epigenetic silencing of the *MSH2* gene via a 3′-end deletion in *EPCAM* (*TACSTD1*), a neighbor of *MSH2* that plays a role in cell adhesion, also accounts for 20% to 25% of all suspected *MSH2* cases and 1% to 6% of LS cases overall.[84–86] LS is characterized by early age-of-onset CRC, predominance of lesions proximal to the splenic flexure, an increased rate of metachronous CRC, and a unique spectrum of benign and malignant extracolonic tumors. Lifetime risk of CRC in patients with LS may be as high as 80%.[83,87] MSI reflects a deficiency in DNA repair secondary to MMR gene mutation and is a hallmark feature of LS-associated tumors.

Variability in penetrance, phenotypic expression, and certainty of disease development mandate distinctly different surgical approaches in these three syndromes, including the type and timing of risk-reducing colon and rectal surgery.[88]

## Familial Adenomatous Polyposis

Surveillance of at-risk family members should begin around age 10 to 15 years with an annual colonoscopy or flexible sigmoidoscopy.[89]

At-risk individuals who belong to families with an AFAP phenotype should undergo colonoscopic screening every 2 to 3 years starting in their late teens. Informative genetic testing is possible in families with a demonstrated *APC* mutation, and mutations are detected in most pedigrees. However, approximately 25% of patients with FAP will have a de novo *APC* mutation.[87] Severity of polyposis should be established during colonoscopy, as the timing of surgery and the risk of developing colorectal is dependent on the extent of polyp burden. Patients with mild polyposis and a correspondingly lower CRC risk can undergo surgery in their late teens. Patients with severe polyposis, a high degree of dysplasia, multiple adenomas >5 mm in size, and symptoms (bleeding, persistent diarrhea, anemia, failure to thrive, psychosocial stress, etc.) should undergo risk-reducing colorectal surgery as soon as is practical after diagnosis.[90,91] However, in carefully selected, fully asymptomatic patients who have small adenomas but a strong family history of aggressive abdominal desmoid disease, consideration can be given to delaying prophylactic colectomy, as the risk of desmoid-related complication may be greater than the risk of CRC development.

The three current surgical options for patients with FAP are total proctocolectomy (TPC) with permanent ileostomy, total colectomy with ileorectal anastomosis (IRA), and proctocolectomy with ileal pouch-anal anastomosis (IPAA). IPAA can be a double-stapled, end-of-pouch-to-anus anastomosis, which may leave behind approximately 1 cm of anal transition zone. An alternative approach, which is preferred when there is carpeting of the anal transition zone with adenomas, is to perform a mucosal stripping of the anal transition zone down to the dentate line followed by a hand-sewn per anal anastomosis of pouch to the dentate line. Selection of the optimal procedure for an individual patient is based on several factors, including characteristics of the FAP syndrome within the patient and family, differences in likely postoperative functional outcome, preoperative anal sphincter status, and patient preference.[8]

TPC with permanent ileostomy, although rarely chosen as a primary procedure, is used in patients with invasive cancer involving the sphincters or levator complex, or patients for whom an IPAA is not technically feasible (secondary to desmoid disease and foreshortening of the small bowel mesentery, making it surgically impossible to bring the ileal pouch to the anus) nor likely to lead to good function such as massive obesity or weak anal sphincters. However, TPC is occasionally chosen as a primary procedure by patients who perceive that their lifestyle would be compromised by the frequent bowel movements (five to six per day) sometimes associated with the IPAA procedure.

In addition to these issues, the key in deciding between an IPAA and an IRA is based primarily on the risk of rectal cancer development if the rectum is left in situ. The risk of rectal cancer following IRA may range from 3% to 10% at 10 years, while the risk for a secondary proctectomy for uncontrolled rectal polyposis ranges from 10% to 61% at 20 years following initial colectomy with IRA.[92–94] The magnitude of risk in an individual patient is, however, related to the overall extent of colorectal polyposis. IRA may be considered for patients with <1,000 colorectal polyps (including those with attenuated FAP) and <20 rectal adenomas, as these individuals have a relatively low risk of developing rectal cancer.[88,93] Patients with severe rectal (>20 adenomas) or colonic (>1,000 adenomas) polyposis, an adenoma >3 cm, or an adenoma with severe dysplasia should ideally undergo a risk-reducing procedure that will include a proctectomy.[90,91,93]

The risk of secondary rectal excision, due to uncontrollable rectal polyposis or rectal cancer, may be estimated by identifying the specific location of the causative APC mutation. Patients with mutations located between codons 1250 and 1464 have been shown to have a six-fold increased risk of developing rectal cancer, compared to those with mutations prior to codon 1250 or after codon 1464 (mean number of rectal polyps 42 versus 22, respectively).[8,92] Although the use of the genotype-phenotype relationship to guide patient management may be appealing,[92] it is important to recognize the variability of phenotypic expression that exists even among members of the same family. This suggests that at the current time, the choice between an IRA and an IPAA should be based primarily on clinical (rather than genetic) grounds.[90]

The risk of polyp and cancer development following primary surgery is not limited to patients undergoing IRA. In patients undergoing IPAA, neoplasia may occur at the site of ileal pouch anastomosis; the frequency appears to be greater after stapled anastomosis (28% to 31%) than after mucosectomy and hand-sewn anastomosis (10% to 14%).[95] In the case of neoplasia developing at the anal transition zone after a stapled anastomosis, transanal mucosectomy may be performed, followed by advancement of the pouch to the dentate line. Of additional concern is the development of adenomatous polyps in the ileal pouch, which occurs in approximately 45% of patients by 10-year follow-up.[96] Consequently, depending on polyp burden, lifetime endoscopic surveillance of the rectal remnant (after IRA) every 6 to 12 months or the ileal pouch (after IPAA) every 1 to 3 years is required following either procedure.[89]

Another important consideration in choosing between IPAA and IRA is postoperative bowel function and quality of life. Some studies have associated IPAA with higher frequency of both daytime and nocturnal bowel movements, higher incidence of passive incontinence and incidental soiling, and greater postoperative morbidity.[97] However, long-term follow-up demonstrates a comparable quality of life following IPAA for FAP relative to the patient's preoperative baseline.[98] Therefore, although the choice of procedure must be carefully individualized, because of the risk of rectal cancer associated with IRA, the authors favor IPAA for most patients with FAP whenever feasible. However, an IRA should be considered in specific circumstances, such as when there is mild rectal polyposis (as in AFAP), or a young patient with rectal sparing who is not interested in undergoing the multiple procedures that accompany an IPAA and diverting loop ileostomy, or a young woman interested in having children and trying to avoid the decreased fecundity associated with an IPAA procedure.[99] The use of minimally invasive techniques such as laparoscopy may reduce the risk of infertility associated with IPAA.[100,101] Though a diverting loop ileostomy should be performed in all IPAA procedures, it is not always feasible due to a number of anatomic factors such as body habitus.

Endoscopic surveillance of the rectal segment at 6- to 12-month intervals after the index surgery is recommended, with subsequent surveillance frequencies dependent on the number and size of adenomas observed.[89] Although small (<5 mm) scattered adenomas can be safely observed or removed with biopsy forceps, polyps >5 mm should be removed by snare. However, repeated fulguration and polypectomy over many years can lead to difficulty with subsequent polypectomy, reduced rectal compliance, and difficulty identifying flat cancers in the background of scar tissue. The development of severe dysplasia and/or villous adenomas not amenable to endoscopic removal is indication for proctectomy.

### Long-Term Considerations from Extracolonic Manifestations

Despite the reduced risk of CRC-related death following prophylactic colectomy, patients with FAP are still at increased risk of mortality from both rectal cancer and other causes relative to the general population. The three main causes of death following IRA are progression of desmoid disease, stomach and duodenal cancer, and perioperative mortality. Additional FAP-related extraintestinal manifestations include epidermoid cysts, supernumerary teeth, osteomas of the jaw and/or skull, congenital hypertrophy of the retinal pigment epithelium, cancers of the hepatopancreatobiliary tract and genitourinary tract, and thyroid cancer.[102–104]

### Desmoids

Desmoids may occur in 10% to 25% of patients with FAP.[105,106] Unlike those found in the general population, FAP-associated desmoids tend to be intra-abdominal and arise following abdominal surgery.[106,107] Although conflicting reports exist, it appears that female patients, those with extracolonic manifestations of FAP, a positive family history of desmoids, and APC mutations located at 3′ of codon 1440 are at increased risk of developing desmoids.[106,108,109] These tumors often involve the small bowel mesentery as well as the retroperitoneum and are often life-threatening due to invasion or compression of adjacent viscera. Further, recurrence and morbidity rates are high following attempted resection, with recurrent disease often more aggressive than the initial desmoid. Estimated 5-year overall survival for patients with intra-abdominal desmoids causing severe symptoms such as significant pain and septic fistula/abscess, diameter >20 cm or rapidly growing, and/or need for parenteral nutrition is only 53%.[107] Therefore, desmoid resection is evaluated on an individualized case-by-case basis with surgery reserved for highly select cases.

Desmoids that involve the small bowel mesentery may preclude the formation of an IPAA secondary to foreshortening of the small bowel mesentery, especially in patients undergoing proctectomy after an initial IRA.[110] Surgery for intra-abdominal and abdominal wall desmoids should be reserved for limited disease where the likelihood of clear margins is high.

In symptomatic cases where resection of an intra-abdominal desmoid may not be feasible, intestinal bypass or ureteral stenting may be necessary to alleviate bowel or urinary obstruction secondary to mass effect. In addition to surgical intervention, several medical options with variable efficacy are available for the management of desmoid disease and include nonsteroidal anti-inflammatory drugs (e.g., sulindac), selective estrogen receptor modulators (e.g., tamoxifen), immunomodulators (e.g., imatinib, sorafenib, interferon), doxorubin-based cytotoxic chemotherapy, and radiation.

### *MYH*-Associated Polyposis

MAP should be suspected in patients with >10 colorectal adenomas, a weak history of CRC, and no family history of FAP. The diagnosis is confirmed by *MUTYH* (*MYH*) gene testing.[80,88]

Depending on the polyp burden, the management of the colon and rectum of a patient with a biallelic *MYH* mutation can be endoscopic or surgical. If the polyp burden is limited and an endoscopic approach is pursued, colonoscopy should be performed every 1 to 3 years.[87,89] If the polyp burden is not amenable to an endoscopic approach at the time of diagnosis, then a resection is indicated. In most cases in which surgery is deemed necessary, an IRA is sufficient. However, if rectal polyposis is severe, an IPAA may be indicated. Indications for surgery following an endoscopic surveillance program include increasing polyp size or number, or worsening histology.

Extracolonic manifestations of MAP are similar to FAP and include osteomas, desmoids, congenital hypertrophy of the retinal pigment epithelium, as well as cancers of the thyroid, ovary, bladder, sebaceous gland, and breast. In addition, patients with MAP are also at a 4% lifetime risk of developing duodenal cancer and require upper endoscopies every 1 to 3 years beginning as early as ages 18 to 20 years and starting no later than ages 30 to 35 years.[87,89,111]

## Lynch Syndrome

Due to the discordance associated with the term hereditary nonpolyposis colorectal cancer, the use of this term has largely been abandoned with reversion back to the eponym LS, which refers to individuals with a predisposition to CRC and other malignancies as a result of a germline MMR mutation.[112] Overall, CRC occurs in up to 80% of patients with LS by their mid-40s.[8,82] Endometrial cancer occurs in 40% to 60%, gastric cancer in 11% to 19%, urinary tract cancer in 5% to 18%, and ovarian cancer in 9% to 15% of affected individuals.[8,82,87]

The Amsterdam criteria and revised Bethesda guidelines[113] (Table 32.3) are used in clinical practice to identify patients at risk for LS who require further genetic evaluation. The Amsterdam criteria, which led to the identification of the LS-causing MMR gene mutations require that there be:

- Three relatives (one a first-degree relative of the other two) with colorectal, endometrial, stomach, ovary, small bowel, ureteral/renal pelvis, brain, hepatobiliary, and/or sebaceous cancer;
- In two or more successive generations;
- With at least one case of cancer diagnosed before the age of 50;
- And that FAP as a diagnosis is excluded.[114]

Though the Amsterdam criteria can be used clinically to identify potential patients with LS, using it alone will result in identification of only 42% of LS mutation carriers.[115] Families meeting Amsterdam criteria but lacking an MMR mutation are referred to as having "familial colorectal cancer type X" and appear to have a lower incidence of colorectal and extracolonic cancers than those with a LS germline MMR mutation (see Fig. 32.6). Of note, they have an increased incidence of left-sided and nonmucinous microsatellite stable tumors.[77,88]

Patients with CRC who belong to pedigrees suspicious for LS should be offered screening by IHC for loss of MMR protein expression or by MSI analysis. As the sensitivity of IHC testing for loss of MMR protein expression is comparable to MSI testing, either approach can be pursued.[112] However, IHC testing is less expensive and can also identify a specific MMR protein loss, which can help target subsequent germline testing. Routine IHC testing for loss of MMR protein in individuals younger than 50 years at the time of CRC diagnosis is feasible and has led to the identification of patients with LS who might otherwise have been missed.[116,117] Patients with MSI-high tumors should undergo testing for germline MMR mutations in *MSH2*, *MLH1*, *MSH6*, and *PMS2*. Reflex IHC and/or MSI testing on all newly diagnosed CRC has been advocated by some expert groups and has been successfully implemented at some institutions.[83,112,118] However, a majority of cancer programs nationwide currently do not have a protocol for reflex testing for LS, citing lack of institutional protocols as well as fear of nonreimbursement.[119] As such, a unified move toward universal testing remains some time away. In families for which tumor tissue is not available, initial germline testing may be considered though the financial burden is not insignificant, with the cost of finding a single LS carrier measuring approximately $58,000 (compared to the $5,000 spent in finding a single LS carrier using IHC screening).[120] As in FAP, a mutation in an affected individual must be established for testing in at-risk individuals to be conclusive.

In lieu of universal testing, several predictive models such as the MMRpredict, MMRpro, and PREMM$_{1,2,6}$ have been devised in order to assess an individual's likelihood of harboring LS.[115,121,122] These models quantify an individual's risk for carrying an *MLH1*, *MSH2, or MSH6* germline mutation by using clinical characteristics such as age at onset of CRC and/or other LS-associated cancers, location of CRC, family history, history of synchronous or metachronous CRC, among others. A study of these predictive models demonstrated that they all performed better than the revised Bethesda guidelines in terms of identifying patients with germline mutations for LS.[123] The MMRpredict model appeared to have to be the best predictor, with a sensitivity and specificity for LS of 94% and 91%, respectively. Other validation studies, however, have not demonstrated the superiority of MMRpredict compared to the other aforementioned models.[124,125] It appears that the use of clinical characteristics in combination with MSI or MMR protein expression status in predictive models may potentially improve our ability to establish LS diagnoses in patients with CRC. However, the practicality and applicability of these tools in a clinical setting requires further assessment.

Although development of CRC in LS is not a certainty, the 80% lifetime risk, the 16% to 30% risk of metachronous CRC, and the possibly accelerated adenoma-to-carcinoma sequence mandate consideration of prophylactic surgical options.[82,87,126–129] Patients with LS who have a CRC or more than one advanced adenoma should be offered the options of prophylactic total colectomy with IRA or segmental colectomy with annual postoperative surveillance colonoscopy. Careful surveillance is also necessary after total colectomy and IRA, as the risk of high-risk adenomas and cancer in the retained rectum at a median of 104 months are 11% and 8%, respectively.[126] Although there has been no study demonstrating an improved survival for patients with LS undergoing total colectomy and IRA versus segmental colectomy, mathematical models suggest a slight survival benefit for total colectomy and IRA, especially for individuals under the age of 30.[130,131] In addition, because of increased rates of metachronous CRC development and the risk of multiple abdominal surgeries

---

## TABLE 32.3

### The Revised Bethesda Guidelines for Testing Colorectal Tumors for Microsatellite Instability

Tumors from individuals should be tested for MSI in the following situations:

1. Colorectal cancer diagnosed in a patient who is <50 y of age.
2. Presence of synchronous, metachronous colorectal, or other HNPCC-associated tumors,[a] regardless of age.
3. Colorectal cancer with the MSI-H[b] histology[c] diagnosed in a patient who is <60 y of age.[d]
4. Colorectal cancer diagnosed in one or more first-degree relatives with an HNPCC-related tumor, with one of the cancers being diagnosed under age 50 years.
5. Colorectal cancer diagnosed in two or more first- or second-degree relatives with HNPCC-related tumors, regardless of age.

MSI, microsatellite instability; HNPCC, hereditary nonpolyposis colorectal cancer; MSI-H, microsatellite instability–high.
[a] HNPCC-related tumors include colorectal, endometrial, stomach, ovarian, pancreas, ureter and renal pelvis, biliary tract, and brain (usually glioblastoma as seen in Turcot syndrome) tumors, sebaceous gland adenomas and keratoacanthomas in Muir-Torre syndrome, and carcinoma of the small bowel.
[b] MSI-H in tumors refers to changes in two or more of the five National Cancer Institute–recommended panels of microsatellite markers.
[c] Presence of tumor-infiltrating lymphocytes, Crohn's-like lymphocytic reaction, mucinous/signet ring differentiation, or medullary growth pattern.
[d] There was no consensus among the workshop participants on whether to include the age criteria in guideline 3; participants voted to keep <60 years of age in the guidelines.
From Umar A, Boland CR, Terdiman JP, et al. Revised Bethesda Guidelines for hereditary nonpolyposis colorectal cancer (Lynch syndrome) and microsatellite instability. *J Natl Cancer Inst* 2004;96:261–268.

in those undergoing a segmental resection, a total colectomy and IRA has emerged as the procedure of choice for the index cancer, with consideration for TPC in cases where a high risk of metachronous rectal cancer can be predicted.[126–128] Targeted genetic testing approaches—such as the single amplicon MSH2 A636P mutation test in Ashkenazi Jewish patients with CRC—have demonstrated how a rapid and inexpensive preoperative genetic test can help direct the extent of colon resection.[132]

LS mutation carriers with a normal colon and without a history of CRC may also be offered prophylactic colectomy in highly select situations. One rationale for this approach is the similarity of lifetime cancer risk between patients with APC and MMR gene mutations, and the fact that total abdominal colectomy with IRA produces less functional disturbance than the prophylactic procedure recommended for FAP (TPC with IPAA). However, an alternate strategy for these individuals is surveillance by colonoscopy, which is cost-effective and greatly reduces the rate of CRC development and overall mortality.[133] There is a risk of CRC development in the interval between colonoscopies, though most interval cancers tend to be early stage.[134,135] As such, given that metachronous CRC may develop in as short a duration as a median of 11.3 months,[136] the recommended interval for surveillance colonoscopies is now every 1 to 2 years.[89] While prophylactic colectomy is not routinely recommended, it may be indicated in highly select patients for whom colonoscopic surveillance is not technically possible or in those who refuse to undergo regular surveillance. A decision analysis model suggests that prophylactic subtotal colectomy at age 25 may offer a survival benefit of 1.8 years, compared with surveillance colonoscopy. The benefit of prophylactic colectomy decreases when surgery is delayed until later in life and is negligible when performed at the time of cancer development.[137] Thus, the decision between prophylactic surgery and surveillance for a gene-positive unaffected individual is based on many factors including penetrance of disease in the

family, early age-of-onset in affected family members, functional and quality-of-life considerations, and likelihood of compliance with surveillance. Table 32.4 lists some of the pros and cons of a prophylactic colectomy for germline mutation carriers for LS without a history of CRC. Patients with LS and an index rectal cancer should be offered the options of TPC with IPAA or anterior proctosigmoidectomy with primary reconstruction.[128,138] The rationale for TPC is the 10% to 15% associated risk of metachronous colon cancer in the remaining colon following the index rectal cancer. Choosing between the two procedures depends, in part, on the patient's willingness to undergo intensive surveillance of the retained proximal colon, as well as issues regarding quality of life and bowel function.

---

**TABLE 32.4**

**Prophylactic Total Abdominal Colectomy and Ileorectal Anastomosis for Lynch Syndrome Patients without Cancer**

**Pros**

- Elimination of colon cancer risk
- Elimination of need for surveillance colonoscopy
- Alleviating patient anxiety over the prospect of colon cancer development

**Cons**

- Persistence of risk of rectal cancer development
- Rectum still requires flexible endoscopic surveillance
- Patient anxiety of prospect of rectal cancer persists
- Possible altered bowel function
- Risk of surgery and possible associated complications

---

CANCER PREVENTION AND SCREENING

## REFERENCES

1. Moyer VA, US Preventive Services Task Force. Risk Assessment, Genetic Counseling, and Genetic Testing for BRCA-Related Cancer in Women: U.S. Preventive Services Task Force Recommendation Statement. *Ann Intern Med* 2014;160.
2. Robson ME, Storm CD, Weitzel J, et al. American Society of Clinical Oncology policy statement update: genetic and genomic testing for cancer susceptibility. *J Clin Oncol* 2010;28:893–901.
3. Amir E, Freedman OC, Seruga B, et al. Assessing women at high risk of breast cancer: a review of risk assessment models. *J Natl Cancer Inst* 2010;102:680–691.
4. Miki Y, Swensen J, Shattuck-Eidens D, et al. A strong candidate for the breast and ovarian cancer susceptibility gene BRCA1. *Science* 1994;266:66–71.
5. Wooster R, Neuhausen SL, Mangion J, et al. Localization of a breast cancer susceptibility gene, BRCA2, to chromosome 13q12-13. *Science* 1994;265:2088–2090.
6. Lux MP, Fasching PA, Beckmann MW. Hereditary breast and ovarian cancer: review and future perspectives. *J Mol Med* 2006;84:16–28.
7. Shannon KM, Chittenden A. Genetic testing by cancer site: breast. *Cancer J* 2012;18:310–319.
8. Guillem JG, Wood WC, Moley JF, et al. ASCO/SSO review of current role of risk-reducing surgery in common hereditary cancer syndromes. *J Clin Oncol* 2006; 24:4642–4660.
9. Saslow D, Boetes C, Burke W, et al. American Cancer Society guidelines for breast screening with MRI as an adjunct to mammography. *CA Cancer J Clin* 2007;57:75–89.
10. Domchek SM, Friebel TM, Singer CF, et al. Association of risk-reducing surgery in BRCA1 or BRCA2 mutation carriers with cancer risk and mortality. *JAMA* 2010;304:967–975.
11. US Equal Employment Opportunity Commission. Genetic information discrimination. http://www.eeoc.gov/laws/types/genetic.cfm. Accessed January 2, 2014.
12. Society of Surgical Oncology. Position statement on prophylactic mastectomy. http://www.surgonc.org/practice-policy/practice-management/consensus-statements/position-statement-on-prophylactic-mastectomy. Accessed February 1, 2014.
13. Hartmann LC, Schaid DJ, Woods JE, et al. Efficacy of bilateral prophylactic mastectomy in women with a family history of breast cancer. *N Engl J Med* 1999;340:77–84.
14. Eldor L, Spiegel A. Breast reconstruction after bilateral prophylactic mastectomy in women at high risk for breast cancer. *Breast J* 2009;15:S81–S89.
15. Zakhireh J, Fowble B, Esserman LJ. Application of screening principles to the reconstructed breast. *J Clin Oncol* 2010;28:173–180.
16. Gabram SG, Dougherty T, Albain KS, et al. Assessing breast cancer risk and providing treatment recommendations: immediate impact of an educational session. *Breast J* 2009;15:S39–S45.
17. Nadauld LD, Ford JM. Molecular profiling of gastric cancer: toward personalized cancer medicine. *J Clin Oncol* 2013;31:838–839.
18. Bardram L, Hansen TV, Gerdes AM, et al. Prophylactic total gastrectomy in hereditary diffuse gastric cancer: identification of two novel CDH1 gene mutations-a clinical observational study. *Fam Cancer* 2014;13:231–242.
19. Norton JA, Ham CM, Van Dam J, et al. CDH1 truncating mutations in the E-cadherin gene: an indication for total gastrectomy to treat hereditary diffuse gastric cancer. *Ann Surg* 2007;245:873–879.
20. Lynch HT, Grady W, Suriano G, et al. Gastric cancer: new genetic developments. *J Surg Oncol* 2005;90:114–133, discussion 133.
21. Guilford P, Hopkins J, Harraway J, et al. E-cadherin germline mutations in familial gastric cancer. *Nature* 1998;392:402–405.
22. Kaurah P, MacMillan A, Boyd N, et al. Founder and recurrent CDH1 mutations in families with hereditary diffuse gastric cancer. *JAMA* 2007;297:2360–2372.
23. Benusiglio PR, Malka D, Rouleau E, et al. CDH1 germline mutations and the hereditary diffuse gastric and lobular breast cancer syndrome: a multicentre study. *J Med Genet* 2013;50:486–489.
24. Gaya DR, Stuart RC, Going JJ, et al. Hereditary diffuse gastric cancer associated with E-cadherin mutation: penetrance after all. *Eur J Gastroenterol Hepatol* 2008;20:1249–1251.
25. Lee KH, Hwang D, Kang KY, et al. Frequent promoter methylation of CDH1 in non-neoplastic mucosa of sporadic diffuse gastric cancer. *Anticancer Res* 2013;33:3765–3774.
26. Oliveira C, Sousa S, Pinheiro H, et al. Quantification of epigenetic and genetic 2nd hits in CDH1 during hereditary diffuse gastric cancer syndrome progression. *Gastroenterology* 2009;136:2137–2148.
27. Carneiro F, Huntsman DG, Smyrk TC, et al. Model of the early development of diffuse gastric cancer in E-cadherin mutation carriers and its implications for patient screening. *J Pathol* 2004;203:681–687.
28. Huntsman DG, Carneiro F, Lewis FR, et al. Early gastric cancer in young, asymptomatic carriers of germ-line E-cadherin mutations. *N Engl J Med* 2001; 344:1904–1909.
29. Suriano G, Yew S, Ferreira P, et al. Characterization of a recurrent germ line mutation of the E-cadherin gene: implications for genetic testing and clinical management. *Clin Cancer Res* 2005;11:5401–5409.

30. Rogers WM, Dobo E, Norton JA, et al. Risk-reducing total gastrectomy for germline mutations in E-cadherin (CDH1): pathologic findings with clinical implications. *Am J Surg Pathol* 2008;32:799–809.

31. Worster E, Liu X, Richardson S, et al. The impact of prophylactic total gastrectomy on health-related quality of life: a prospective cohort study. *Ann Surg* 2014;260:87–93.

32. Lim YC, di Pietro M, O'Donovan M, et al. Prospective cohort study assessing outcomes of patients from families fulfilling criteria for hereditary diffuse gastric cancer undergoing endoscopic surveillance. *Gastrointest Endosc* 2014;80:78–87.

33. Mavaddat N, Peock S, Frost D, et al. Cancer risks for BRCA1 and BRCA2 mutation carriers: results from prospective analysis of EMBRACE. *J Natl Cancer Inst* 2013;105:812–822.

34. Risch HA, McLaughlin JR, Cole DE, et al. Prevalence and penetrance of germline BRCA1 and BRCA2 mutations in a population series of 649 women with ovarian cancer. *Am J Hum Genet* 2001;68:700–710.

35. Struewing JP, Hartge P, Wacholder S, et al. The risk of cancer associated with specific mutations of BRCA1 and BRCA2 among Ashkenazi Jews. *N Engl J Med* 1997;336:1401–1408.

36. Finch AP, Lubinski J, Moller P, et al. Impact of oophorectomy on cancer incidence and mortality in women with a BRCA1 or BRCA2 mutation. *J Clin Oncol* 2014;32:1547–1553.

37. Walsh T, Casadei S, Lee MK, et al. Mutations in 12 genes for inherited ovarian, fallopian tube, and peritoneal carcinoma identified by massively parallel sequencing. *Proc Natl Acad Sci U S A* 2011;108:18032–18037.

38. Couch FJ, Wang X, McGuffog L, et al. Genome-wide association study in BRCA1 mutation carriers identifies novel loci associated with breast and ovarian cancer risk. *PLoS Genet* 2013;9:e1003212.

39. Schrader KA, Hurlburt J, Kalloger SE, et al. Germline BRCA1 and BRCA2 mutations in ovarian cancer: utility of a histology-based referral strategy. *Obstet Gynecol* 2012;120:235–240.

40. Kauff ND, Satagopan JM, Robson ME, et al. Risk-reducing salpingo-oophorectomy in women with a BRCA1 or BRCA2 mutation. *N Engl J Med* 2002;346:1609–1615.

41. Rebbeck TR, Lynch HT, Neuhausen SL, et al. Prophylactic oophorectomy in carriers of BRCA1 or BRCA2 mutations. *N Engl J Med* 2002;346:1616–1622.

42. Kauff ND, Domchek SM, Friebel TM, et al. Risk-reducing salpingo-oophorectomy for the prevention of BRCA1- and BRCA2-associated breast and gynecologic cancer: a multicenter, prospective study. *J Clin Oncol* 2008; 26:1331–1337.

43. Folkins AK, Jarboe EA, Roh MH, et al. Precursors to pelvic serous carcinoma and their clinical implications. *Gynecol Oncol* 2009;113:391–396.

44. Wethington SL, Park KJ, Soslow RA, et al. Clinical outcome of isolated serous tubal intraepithelial carcinomas (STIC). *Int J Gynecol Cancer* 2013; 23:1603–1611.

45. Bonadona V, Bonaiti B, Olschwang S, et al. Cancer risks associated with germline mutations in MLH1, MSH2, and MSH6 genes in Lynch syndrome. *JAMA* 2011;305:2304–2310.

46. Leenen CH, van Lier MG, van Doorn HC, et al. Prospective evaluation of molecular screening for Lynch syndrome in patients with endometrial cancer ≤70 years. *Gynecol Oncol* 2012;125:414–420.

47. Resnick K, Straughn JM Jr, Backes F, et al. Lynch syndrome screening strategies among newly diagnosed endometrial cancer patients. *Obstet Gynecol* 2009;114:530–536.

48. Watson P, Vasen HF, Mecklin JP, et al. The risk of endometrial cancer in hereditary nonpolyposis colorectal cancer. *Am J Med* 1994;96:516–520.

49. Koornstra JJ, Mourits MJ, Sijmons RH, et al. Management of extracolonic tumours in patients with Lynch syndrome. *Lancet Oncol* 2009;10:400–408.

50. Dove-Edwin I, Boks D, Goff S, et al. The outcome of endometrial carcinoma surveillance by ultrasound scan in women at risk of hereditary nonpolyposis colorectal carcinoma and familial colorectal carcinoma. *Cancer* 2002;94:1708–1712.

51. Schmeler KM, Lynch HT, Chen LM, et al. Prophylactic surgery to reduce the risk of gynecologic cancers in the Lynch syndrome. *N Engl J Med* 2006;354: 261–269.

52. Yang KY, Caughey AB, Little SE, et al. A cost-effectiveness analysis of prophylactic surgery versus gynecologic surveillance for women from hereditary nonpolyposis colorectal cancer (HNPCC) Families. *Fam Cancer* 2011;10:535–543.

53. Pistorius S, Kruger S, Hohl R, et al. Occult endometrial cancer and decision making for prophylactic hysterectomy in hereditary nonpolyposis colorectal cancer patients. *Gynecol Oncol* 2006;102:189–194.

54. Traugott AL, Moley JF. Multiple endocrine neoplasia type 2: clinical manifestations and management. *Cancer Treat Res* 2009;153:321–337.

55. American Thyroid Association Guidelines Task Force, Kloos RT, Eng C, et al. Medullary thyroid cancer: management guidelines of the American Thyroid Association. *Thyroid* 2009;19:565–612.

56. Wells SA Jr, Pacini F, Robinson BG, et al. Multiple endocrine neoplasia type 2 and familial medullary thyroid carcinoma: an update. *J Clin Endocrinol Metab* 2013;98:3149–3164.

57. Eng C, Clayton D, Schuffenecker I, et al. The relationship between specific RET proto-oncogene mutations and disease phenotype in multiple endocrine neoplasia type 2. International RET mutation consortium analysis. *JAMA* 1996;276:1575–1579.

58. Howe JR, Norton JA, Wells SA Jr. Prevalence of pheochromocytoma and hyperparathyroidism in multiple endocrine neoplasia type 2A: results of long-term follow-up. *Surgery* 1993;114:1070–1077.

59. Machens A, Niccoli-Sire P, Hoegel J, et al. Early malignant progression of hereditary medullary thyroid cancer. *N Engl J Med* 2003;349:1517–1525.

60. Gagel RF, Levy ML, Donovan DT, et al. Multiple endocrine neoplasia type 2A associated with cutaneous lichen amyloidosis. *Ann Intern Med* 1989; 111:802–806.

61. Santoro M, Carlomagno F, Romano A, et al. Activation of RET as a dominant transforming gene by germline mutations of MEN2A and MEN2B. *Science* 1995;267:381–383.

62. Mulligan LM, Ponder BA. Genetic basis of endocrine disease: multiple endocrine neoplasia type 2. *J Clin Endocrinol Metab* 1995;80:1989–1995.

63. Mulligan L, Kwok J, Healy C. Germ-line mutations of the RET protooncogene in multiple endocrine neoplasia type 2A (MEN 2A). *Nature* 1993; 363:458–460.

64. Donis-Keller H, Dou S, Chi D, et al. Mutations in the RET proto-oncogene are associated with MEN 2A and FMTC. *Hum Mol Genet* 1993;2:851–856.

65. Traugott AL, Moley JF. The RET Protooncogene. *Cancer Treat Res* 2010; 153:303–319.

66. Quayle FJ, Benveniste R, DeBenedetti MK, et al. Hereditary medullary thyroid carcinoma in patients greater than 50 years old. *Surgery* 2004;136:1116–1121.

67. Lips CJ, Landsvater RM, Hoppener JW, et al. Clinical screening as compared with DNA analysis in families with multiple endocrine neoplasia type 2A. *N Engl J Med* 1994;331:828–835.

68. Niccoli-Sire P, Murat A, Baudin E, et al. Early or prophylactic thyroidectomy in MEN 2/FMTC gene carriers: results in 71 thyroidectomized patients. The French Calcitonin Tumours Study Group (GETC). *Eur J Endocrinol* 1999;141:468–474.

69. Rodriguez GJ, Balsalobre MD, Pomares F, et al. Prophylactic thyroidectomy in MEN 2A syndrome: experience in a single center. *J Am Coll Surg* 2002;195: 159–166.

70. Skinner MA, Moley JA, Dilley WG, et al. Prophylactic thyroidectomy in multiple endocrine neoplasia type 2A. *N Engl J Med* 2005;353:1105–1113.

71. Brandi ML, Gagel RF, Angeli A, et al. Guidelines for diagnosis and therapy of MEN type 1 and type 2. *J Clin Endocrinol Metab* 2001;86:5658–5671.

72. Elisei R, Romei C, Renzini G, et al. The timing of total thyroidectomy in RET gene mutation carriers could be personalized and safely planned on the basis of serum calcitonin: 18 years experience at one single center. *J Clin Endocrinol Metab* 2012;97:426–435.

73. Waguespack SG, Rich TA, Perrier ND, et al. Management of medullary thyroid carcinoma and MEN2 syndromes in childhood. *Nat Rev Endocrinol* 2011;7:596–607.

74. Moley JF. Medullary thyroid carcinoma: management of lymph node metastases. *J Natl Compr Canc Netw* 2010;8:549–556.

75. Machens A, Dralle H. Biomarker-based risk stratification for previously untreated medullary thyroid cancer. *J Clin Endocrinol Metab* 2010;95:2655–2663.

76. Solorzano CC, Evans DB. Same-day ultrasound guidance in reoperations for locally recurrent papillary thyroid cancer. *Surgery* 2007;142:973–975.

77. Patel SG, Ahnen DJ. Familial colon cancer syndromes: an update of a rapidly evolving field. *Curr Gastroenterol Rep* 2012;14:428–438.

78. Aretz S, Uhlhaas S, Goergens H, et al. MUTYH-associated polyposis: 70 of 71 patients with biallelic mutations present with an attenuated or atypical phenotype. *Int J Cancer* 2006;119:807–814.

79. Russell AM, Zhang J, Luz J, et al. Prevalence of MYH germline mutations in Swiss APC mutation-negative polyposis patients. *Int J Cancer* 2006; 118:1937–1940.

80. Jasperson KW. Genetic testing by cancer site: colon (polyposis syndromes). *Cancer J* 2012;18:328–333.

81. Hampel H, Frankel WL, Martin E, et al. Screening for the Lynch syndrome (hereditary nonpolyposis colorectal cancer). *N Engl J Med* 2005;352: 1851–1860.

82. Lynch HT, Lynch PM, Lanspa SJ, et al. Review of the Lynch syndrome: history, molecular genetics, screening, differential diagnosis, and medicolegal ramifications. *Clin Genet* 2009;76:1–18.

83. Vasen HF, Blanco I, Aktan-Collan K, et al. Revised guidelines for the clinical management of Lynch syndrome (HNPCC): recommendations by a group of European experts. *Gut* 2013;62:812–823.

84. Niessen RC, Hofstra RM, Westers H, et al. Germline hypermethylation of MLH1 and EPCAM deletions are a frequent cause of Lynch syndrome. *Genes Chromosomes Cancer* 2009;48:737–744.

85. Kuiper RP, Vissers LE, Venkatachalam R, et al. Recurrence and variability of germline EPCAM deletions in Lynch syndrome. *Hum Mutat* 2011;32: 407–414.

86. Rumilla K, Schowalter KV, Lindor NM, et al. Frequency of deletions of EPCAM (TACSTD1) in MSH2-associated Lynch syndrome cases. *J Mol Diagn* 2011;13:93–99.

87. Jasperson KW, Tuohy TM, Neklason DW, et al. Hereditary and familial colon cancer. *Gastroenterology* 2010;138:2044–2058.

88. Steinhagen E, Markowitz AJ, Guillem JG. How to manage a patient with multiple adenomatous polyps. *Surg Oncol Clin N Am* 2010;19:711–723.

89. National Comprehensive Cancer Network. NCCN *Clinical Practice Guidelines in Oncology: Colorectal Cancer Screening.* http://www.nccn.org/professionals/physician_gls/pdf/colorectal_screening.pdf. Accessed February 19, 2014.

90. Vasen HF, Moslein G, Alonso A, et al. Guidelines for the clinical management of familial adenomatous polyposis (FAP). *Gut* 2008;57:704–713.

91. Church J. Familial adenomatous polyposis. *Surg Oncol Clin N Am* 2009; 18:585–598.

92. Nieuwenhuis MH, Bulow S, Bjork J, et al. Genotype predicting phenotype in familial adenomatous polyposis: a practical application to the choice of surgery. *Dis Colon Rectum* 2009;52:1259–1263.

93. Sinha A, Tekkis PP, Rashid S, et al. Risk factors for secondary proctectomy in patients with familial adenomatous polyposis. *Br J Surg* 2010;97:1710–1715.

94. Koskenvuo L, Renkonen-Sinisalo L, Jarvinen HJ, et al. Risk of cancer and secondary proctectomy after colectomy and ileorectal anastomosis in familial adenomatous polyposis. *Int J Colorectal Dis* 2014;29:225–230.

95. Remzi FH, Church JM, Bast J, et al. Mucosectomy vs. stapled ileal pouch-anal anastomosis in patients with familial adenomatous polyposis: functional outcome and neoplasia control. *Dis Colon Rectum* 2001;44:1590–1596.

96. Friederich P, de Jong AE, Mathus-Vliegen LM, et al. Risk of developing adenomas and carcinomas in the ileal pouch in patients with familial adenomatous polyposis. *Clin Gastroenterol Hepatol* 2008;6:1237–1242.

97. Aziz O, Athanasiou T, Fazio VW, et al. Meta-analysis of observational studies of ileorectal versus ileal pouch-anal anastomosis for familial adenomatous polyposis. *Br J Surg* 2006;93:407–417.

98. Fazio VW, Kiran RP, Remzi FH, et al. Ileal pouch anal anastomosis: analysis of outcome and quality of life in 3707 patients. *Ann Surg* 2013;257:679–685.

99. Rajaratnam SG, Eglinton TW, Hider P, et al. Impact of ileal pouch-anal anastomosis on female fertility: meta-analysis and systematic review. *Int J Colorectal Dis* 2011;26:1365–1374.

100. Bartels SA, D'Hoore A, Cuesta MA, et al. Significantly increased pregnancy rates after laparoscopic restorative proctocolectomy: a cross-sectional study. *Ann Surg* 2012;256:1045–1048.

101. Beyer-Berjot L, Maggiori L, Birnbaum D, et al. A total laparoscopic approach reduces the infertility rate after ileal pouch-anal anastomosis: a 2-center study. *Ann Surg* 2013;258:275–282.

102. Steinhagen E, Guillem JG, Chang G, et al. The prevalence of thyroid cancer and benign thyroid disease in patients with familial adenomatous polyposis may be higher than previously recognized. *Clin Colorectal Cancer* 2012;11:304–308.

103. Steinhagen E, Hui VW, Levy RA, et al. Results of a prospective thyroid ultrasound screening program in adenomatous polyposis patients. *Am J Surg* [ePub ahead of print].

104. Jarrar AM, Milas M, Mitchell J, et al. Screening for thyroid cancer in patients with familial adenomatous polyposis. *Ann Surg* 2011;253:515–521.

105. Giardiello FM, Burt RW, Jarvinen H, et al. Familial adenomatous polyposis. In: Bosman FT, Carneiro F, Hruban RH, et al, eds. *Classification of Tumours of the Digestive System*. Lyon: IARC Press; 2010:147–151.

106. Nieuwenhuis MH, Lefevre JH, Bulow S, et al. Family history, surgery, and APC mutation are risk factors for desmoid tumors in familial adenomatous polyposis: an international cohort study. *Dis Colon Rectum* 2011;54:1229–1234.

107. Quintini C, Ward G, Shatnawei A, et al. Mortality of intra-abdominal desmoid tumors in patients with familial adenomatous polyposis: a single center review of 154 patients. *Ann Surg* 2012;255:511–516.

108. Sinha A, Gibbons DC, Phillips RK, et al. Surgical prophylaxis in familial adenomatous polyposis: do pre-existing desmoids outside the abdominal cavity matter? *Fam Cancer* 2010;9:407–411.

109. Schiessling S, Kihm M, Ganschow P, et al. Desmoid tumour biology in patients with familial adenomatous polyposis coli. *Br J Surg* 2013;100:694–703.

110. von Roon AC, Tekkis PP, Lovegrove RE, et al. Comparison of outcomes of ileal pouch-anal anastomosis for familial adenomatous polyposis with and without previous ileorectal anastomosis. *Br J Surg* 2008;95:494–498.

111. Nieuwenhuis MH, Vogt S, Jones N, et al. Evidence for accelerated colorectal adenoma—carcinoma progression in MUTYH-associated polyposis? *Gut* 2012;61:734–738.

112. Palomaki GE, McClain MR, Melillo S, et al. EGAPP supplementary evidence review: DNA testing strategies aimed at reducing morbidity and mortality from Lynch syndrome. *Genet Med* 2009;11:42–65.

113. Umar A, Boland CR, Terdiman JP, et al. Revised Bethesda Guidelines for hereditary nonpolyposis colorectal cancer (Lynch syndrome) and microsatellite instability. *J Natl Cancer Inst* 2004;96:261–268.

114. Vasen HF, Watson P, Mecklin JP, et al. New clinical criteria for hereditary nonpolyposis colorectal cancer (HNPCC, Lynch syndrome) proposed by the International Collaborative group on HNPCC. *Gastroenterology* 1999;116:1453–1456.

115. Barnetson RA, Tenesa A, Farrington SM, et al. Identification and survival of carriers of mutations in DNA mismatch-repair genes in colon cancer. *N Engl J Med* 2006;354:2751–2763.

116. Lee-Kong SA, Markowitz AJ, Glogowski E, et al. Prospective immunohistochemical analysis of primary colorectal cancers for loss of mismatch repair protein expression. *Clin Colorectal Cancer* 2010;9:255–259.

117. Steinhagen E, Shia J, Markowitz AJ, et al. Systematic immunohistochemistry screening for Lynch syndrome in early age-of-onset colorectal cancer patients undergoing surgical resection. *J Am Coll Surg* 2012;214:61–67.

118. Heald B, Plesec T, Liu X, et al. Implementation of universal microsatellite instability and immunohistochemistry screening for diagnosing lynch syndrome in a large academic medical center. *J Clin Oncol* 2013;31:1336–1340.

119. Beamer LC, Grant ML, Espenschied CR, et al. Reflex immunohistochemistry and microsatellite instability testing of colorectal tumors for Lynch syndrome among US cancer programs and follow-up of abnormal results. *J Clin Oncol* 2012;30:1058–1063.

120. Mvundura M, Grosse SD, Hampel H, et al. The cost-effectiveness of genetic testing strategies for Lynch syndrome among newly diagnosed patients with colorectal cancer. *Genet Med* 2010;12:93–104.

121. Chen S, Wang W, Lee S, et al. Prediction of germline mutations and cancer risk in the Lynch syndrome. *JAMA* 2006;296:1479–1487.

122. Kastrinos F, Steyerberg EW, Mercado R, et al. The PREMM(1,2,6) model predicts risk of MLH1, MSH2, and MSH6 germline mutations based on cancer history. *Gastroenterology* 2011;140:73–81.

123. Green RC, Parfrey PS, Woods MO, et al. Prediction of Lynch syndrome in consecutive patients with colorectal cancer. *J Natl Cancer Inst* 2009;101:331–340.

124. Khan O, Blanco A, Conrad P, et al. Performance of Lynch syndrome predictive models in a multi-center US referral population. *Am J Gastroenterol* 2011;106:1822–1827, quiz 1828.

125. Tresallet C, Brouquet A, Julie C, et al. Evaluation of predictive models in daily practice for the identification of patients with Lynch syndrome. *Int J Cancer* 2012;130:1367–1377.

126. Kalady MF, McGannon E, Vogel JD, et al. Risk of colorectal adenoma and carcinoma after colectomy for colorectal cancer in patients meeting Amsterdam criteria. *Ann Surg* 2010;252:507–511, discussion 511–513.

127. Parry S, Win AK, Parry B, et al. Metachronous colorectal cancer risk for mismatch repair gene mutation carriers: the advantage of more extensive colon surgery. *Gut* 2011;60:950–957.

128. Kalady MF, Lipman J, McGannon E, et al. Risk of colonic neoplasia after proctectomy for rectal cancer in hereditary nonpolyposis colorectal cancer. *Ann Surg* 2012;255:1121–1125.

129. Cirillo L, Urso ED, Parrinello G, et al. High risk of rectal cancer and of metachronous colorectal cancer in probands of families fulfilling the Amsterdam criteria. *Ann Surg* 2013;257:900–904.

130. Stupart DA, Goldberg PA, Baigrie RJ, et al. Surgery for colonic cancer in HNPCC: total vs segmental colectomy. *Colorectal Dis* 2011;13:1395–1399.

131. Maeda T, Cannom RR, Beart RW Jr, et al. Decision model of segmental compared with total abdominal colectomy for colon cancer in hereditary nonpolyposis colorectal cancer. *J Clin Oncol* 2010;28:1175–1180.

132. Guillem JG, Glogowski E, Moore HG, et al. Single-amplicon MSH2 A636P mutation testing in Ashkenazi Jewish patients with colorectal cancer: role in presurgical management. *Ann Surg* 2007;245:560–565.

133. Barrow P, Hawkin M, Lalloo F, et al. Systematic review of the impact of registration and screening on colorectal cancer incidence and mortality in familial adenomatous polyposis and Lynch syndrome. *Br J Surg* 2013;100:1719–1731.

134. Vasen HF, Abdirahman M, Brohet R, et al. One to 2-year surveillance intervals reduce risk of colorectal cancer in families with Lynch syndrome. *Gastroenterology* 2010;138:2300–2306.

135. Stuckless S, Green JS, Morgenstern M, et al. Impact of colonoscopic screening in male and female Lynch syndrome carriers with an MSH2 mutation. *Clin Genet* 2012;82:439–445.

136. Engel C, Rahner N, Schulmann K, et al. Efficacy of annual colonoscopic surveillance in individuals with hereditary nonpolyposis colorectal cancer. *Clin Gastroenterol Hepatol* 2010;8:174–182.

137. Syngal S, Weeks JC, Schrag D, et al. Benefits of colonoscopic surveillance and prophylactic colectomy in patients with hereditary nonpolyposis colorectal cancer mutations. *Ann Intern Med* 1998;129:787–796.

138. Giardiello FM, Allen JI, Axilbund JE, et al. Guidelines on genetic evaluation and management of Lynch syndrome: a consensus statement by the US Multi-Society Task Force on Colorectal Cancer. *Dis Colon Rectum* 2014;57(8):1025–1048.

**CANCER PREVENTION AND SCREENING**

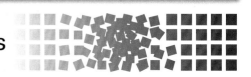

# 33 Cancer Risk–Reducing Agents

Dean E. Brenner, Scott M. Lippman, and Susan T. Mayne

## WHY CANCER PREVENTION AS A CLINICAL ONCOLOGY DISCIPLINE

Until recently, clinical oncology has been defined as a medical specialty that attempts to intervene in order to slow or reverse the final stage of the cancer process—the clonally derived, genomically damaged, invasive cell mass. Cancer is a long process, a stepwise carcinogenic progression that encompasses critical molecular events that culminate in the loss of key cellular control homeostatic functions (e.g., control of proliferation, apoptosis, invasion, angiogenesis).[1] These events occur prior to and during the morphologic changes that have historically defined neoplasia. Morphologic changes, such as subtle increases in cellular proliferation that progress to early and late precancerous lesions containing dysplastic cells, characterize the carcinogenesis process (Fig. 33.1).[1–3] Opportunities for intervention in this process can include diverse, nonpharmacologic approaches (e.g., obesity management via diet/lifestyle interventions) or pharmacologic interventions (e.g., drugs or nutrients/nonnutrient substances used as drugs) aimed at delaying or reversing the carcinogenesis process prior to or following the appearance of early morphologic changes. Cancer screening and early detection strategies (e.g., surveillance endoscopy, fecal occult blood testing, mammography) identify not only those individuals with early stage, curable malignant transformations, but also those individuals with noninvasive neoplasias who are at risk for progression to transformed invasive malignancies.

Recognizing that cancer is a continuum, oncologists are increasingly expected to be knowledgeable about a diverse array of cancer-related topics including lifestyle behaviors such as diet and exercise, risk assessment, screening, other preventive interventions, in addition to current treatments for advanced malignancy. The understanding, use, and management of interventions designed to delay or reverse the carcinogenesis process have become integral components of the this role.[4]

## DEFINING CANCER RISK–REDUCING AGENTS (CHEMOPREVENTION)

Cancer risk reduction, commonly referred to as chemoprevention, is the use of a range of interventions from drugs to isolated dietary components to whole-diet modulation to block, reverse, or prevent the development of invasive cancer.[5,6] Human cancer risk reduction asserts that one can intervene at many steps in the carcinogenic process, which occurs over many years. This prolonged latency provides opportunities to intervene at many time points and at multiple events in the carcinogenic process. Successful deployment of cancer risk–reducing agent interventions requires evidence of reduced cancer-associated incidence and/or mortality.

The concept of field carcinogenesis was first described in the early 1950s as *field cancerization* in squamous cell carcinomas of the head and neck, and subsequently ascribed to many epithelial sites. The field carcinogenesis concept is that patients have a wide surface area of precancerous or cancerous tissue change that can be detected at the gross (oral premalignant lesions, polyps), microscopic (metaplasia, dysplasia), and/or molecular (gene loss or amplification) levels. Recent molecular studies detecting profound genetic alterations in histologically normal tissue from high-risk individuals have provided strong support for the field carcinogenesis concept. The implication of the field effect is that multifocal, genetically distinct, and clonally related premalignant lesions can progress over a broad tissue region.[1] The essence of cancer risk reduction, then, is intervention within the multistep carcinogenic process and throughout a wide field.

## IDENTIFYING POTENTIAL CANCER RISK–REDUCING AGENTS

Cancer risk–reducing agent identification results from the synthesis of data from population, basic, translational, and clinical sciences. Findings from all of these disciplines are combined to contribute to the identification of agents with the potential to delay or reverse the carcinogenesis process (see Fig. 33.1).

The Hanahan and Weinberg hallmarks of malignant transformation—self-sufficiency in growth signals, insensitivity to growth-inhibitory signals, evasion of apoptosis, limitless replication potential, sustained angiogenesis, and tissue invasion and metastasis[7]—reflect the loss of cellular signaling control. The molecular damage that results in transformation is triggered by a large array of genetic and environmental stressors such as chronic inflammation, oxidation, inherited genetic mutations, and exogenous environmental exposures. Many such signaling intermediates have common functions in multiple organ sites (see Fig. 33.1). The complexity and overlap of signal transduction pathways suggests that single molecular therapeutic/preventive targets may have limited effectiveness. Interventions aimed at preventing the occurrence of or overcoming the effects of molecular defects in multiple pathways or targets may be required to arrest or reverse carcinogenesis. Using the Hanahan and Weinberg hallmarks, examples of possible targets are shown in Table 33.1.

## PRECLINICAL DEVELOPMENT OF CANCER RISK–REDUCING AGENTS

Similar to the development of therapeutic interventions, the assessment of efficacy and toxicity of single chemically synthesized entities, agents designed *in silico*, botanicals, nutrients/nonnutrient substances used as drugs for cancer risk–reducing agent efficacy proceeds through a translational paradigm that identifies efficacy in cell culture models, in live animal models, and in humans. Preclinical models that simulate the carcinogenesis process in target epithelia identify molecular biomarkers for modulation by interventions. These models can be used to identify potential toxicity of interventions and to assess the effect of interventions on the development and progression of preneoplasia/neoplasia.[8]

The U.S. National Cancer Institute's (NCI) PREVENT Cancer Preclinical Drug Development Program is a prime example of a

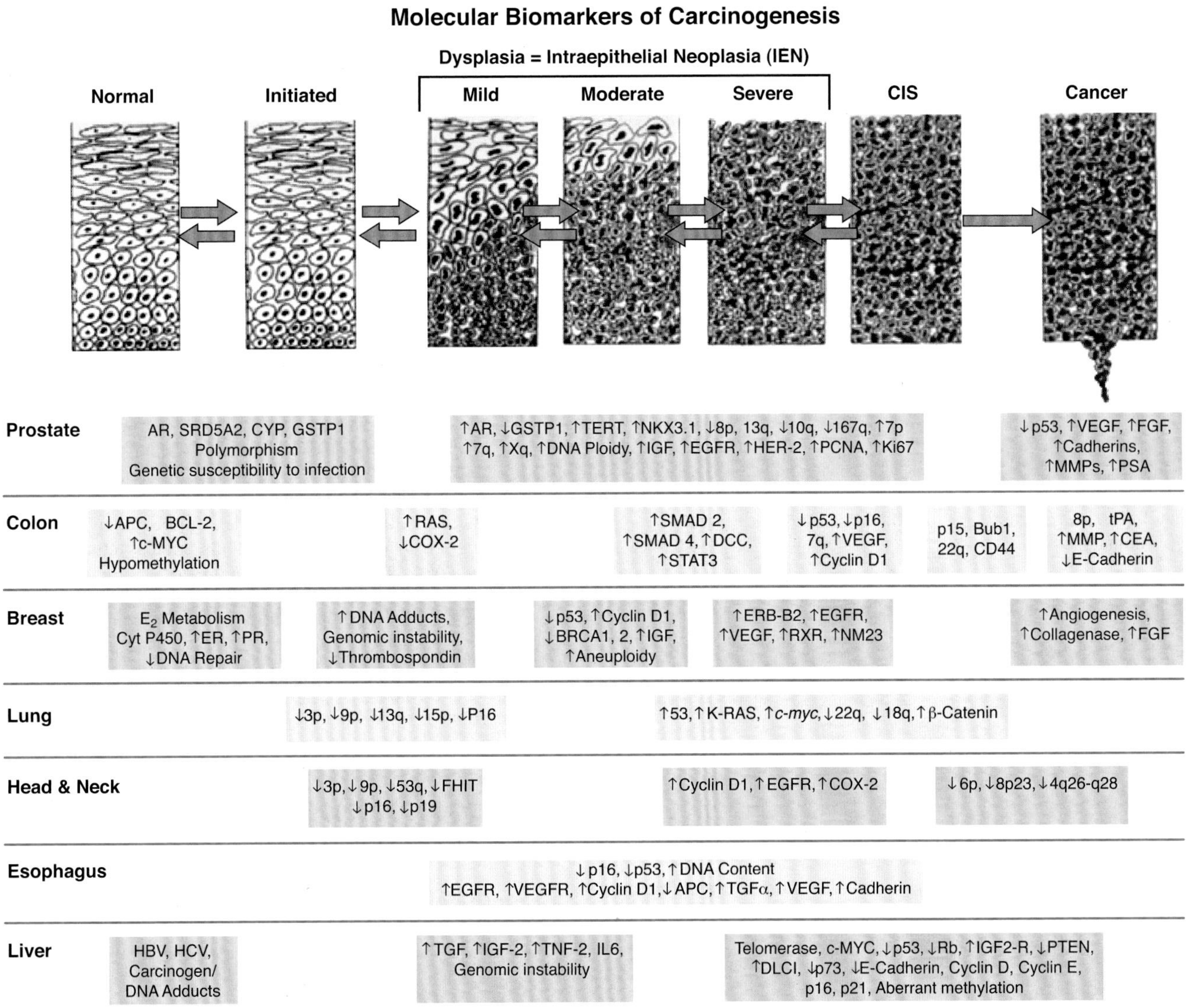

## Molecular Biomarkers of Carcinogenesis

### Dysplasia = Intraepithelial Neoplasia (IEN)

| | Normal | Initiated | Mild | Moderate | Severe | CIS | Cancer |
|---|---|---|---|---|---|---|---|
| **Prostate** | AR, SRD5A2, CYP, GSTP1 Polymorphism Genetic susceptibility to infection | | ↑AR, ↓GSTP1, ↑TERT, ↑NKX3.1, ↓8p, 13q, ↓10q, ↓167q, ↑7p ↑7q, ↑Xq, ↑DNA Ploidy, ↑IGF, ↑EGFR, ↑HER-2, ↑PCNA, ↑Ki67 | | | | ↓p53, ↑VEGF, ↑FGF, ↑Cadherins, ↑MMPs, ↑PSA |
| **Colon** | ↓APC, BCL-2, ↑c-MYC Hypomethylation | ↑RAS, ↓COX-2 | | ↑SMAD 2, ↑SMAD 4, ↑DCC, ↑STAT3 | ↓p53, ↓p16, 7q, ↑VEGF, ↑Cyclin D1 | p15, Bub1, 22q, CD44 | 8p, tPA, ↑MMP, ↑CEA, ↓E-Cadherin |
| **Breast** | E₂ Metabolism Cyt P450, ↑ER, ↑PR, ↓DNA Repair | ↑DNA Adducts, Genomic instability, ↓Thrombospondin | ↓p53, ↑Cyclin D1, ↓BRCA1, 2, ↑IGF, ↑Aneuploidy | ↑ERB-B2, ↑EGFR, ↑VEGF, ↑RXR, ↑NM23 | | | ↑Angiogenesis, ↑Collagenase, ↑FGF |
| **Lung** | | ↓3p, ↓9p, ↓13q, ↓15p, ↓P16 | | ↑53, ↑K-RAS, ↑c-myc, ↓22q, ↓18q, ↑β-Catenin | | | |
| **Head & Neck** | | ↓3p, ↓9p, ↓53q, ↓FHIT ↓p16, ↓p19 | | ↑Cyclin D1, ↑EGFR, ↑COX-2 | | ↓6p, ↓8p23, ↓4q26-q28 | |
| **Esophagus** | | | ↓p16, ↓p53, ↑DNA Content ↑EGFR, ↑VEGFR, ↑Cyclin D1, ↓APC, ↑TGFα, ↑VEGF, ↑Cadherin | | | | |
| **Liver** | HBV, HCV, Carcinogen/ DNA Adducts | | ↑TGF, ↑IGF-2, ↑TNF-2, IL6, Genomic instability | Telomerase, c-MYC, ↓p53, ↓Rb, ↑IGF2-R, ↓PTEN, ↑DLCI, ↓p73, ↓E-Cadherin, Cyclin D, Cyclin E, p16, p21, Aberrant methylation | | | |

**Figure 33.1** Genetic progression in major cancers. Carcinogenesis is driven by genetic progression. This progression is marked by the appearance of molecular biomarkers in distinctive patterns representing accumulating changes in gene expression and correlating with changes in histologic phenotype as cells move from normal through the early stages of clonal expansion to dysplasia and finally to early invasive, locally advanced, and metastatic cancer. The figure[257] shows candidate molecular biomarkers of genetic progression in seven target organs: the prostate,[300–302] the colon,[2] the breast,[303,304] the lung,[305–307] the head and neck,[308–311] the esophagus,[312,313] and the liver.[314] CIS, carcinoma in situ; AR, androgen receptor; CYP, cytochrome P-450; GSTP1, glutathione S transferase P1; TERT, telomerase reverse transcriptase; NKX3.1, NK 3 transcription factor related, locus 1 (prostate specific, androgen regulated); IGF, insulin-like growth factor; EGFR, epidermal growth factor receptor; HER-2, human epidermal growth factor receptor-2; PCNA, proliferating cell nuclear antigen; VEGF, vascular endothelial growth factor; FGF, fibroblast growth factor; MMP, matrix metalloproteinase; PSA, prostate-specific antigen; APC, adenomatous polyposis coli; BCL-2, B-cell lymphoma 2 gene, apoptosis control; c-MYC, v-myc avian myelocytomatosis viral oncogene homolog; COX-2, cyclooxygenase-2; SMAD, homolog of mothers against decapentaplegic + *C. Elegans* SMA protein; DCC, deleted in colon cancer gene; CEA, carcinoembryonic antigen; ER, estrogen receptor; PR, progesterone receptor; ERB-B2, Receptor tyrosine-protein kinase erbB-2, same as HER-2; RXR, retinoid X receptor; NM23, Nucleoside disphophate kinase A; K-RAS, Kirsten rat sarcoma viral oncogene homolog; FHIT, fragile histidine triad protein; TGFα, tumor growth factor alpha; HBV, hepatitis B virus; HCV, hepatitis C virus; TNF-2, tumor necrosis factor 2; IL6, interleukin 6; PTEN, phosphatase and tensin homolog. (Figure and revised caption from Kelloff GJ, Lippman SM, Dannenberg AJ, et al. Progress in chemoprevention drug development: the promise of molecular biomarkers for prevention of intraepithelial neoplasia and cancer—a plan to move forward. *Clin Cancer Res* 2006;12:3661–3697, published with permission from the American Association for Cancer Research.)

rational strategy to select promising agents for clinical trials through a stepwise approach of preclinical in vitro testing followed by *in vivo* screening.[8–10] This system involves several phases: biochemical prescreening assays, in vitro efficacy models, in vivo short-term screening, animal efficacy testing, and preclinical toxicology testing.

## Biochemical Prescreening Assays

Prescreening assays are a series of short-term, mechanistic assays developed to evaluate the ability of a test compound to modulate biochemical events presumed to be mechanistically linked to carcinogenesis.[8]

These in vitro assays are rapidly completed for potential cancer risk–reducing agents. Examples of such assays include carcinogen-DNA binding, prostaglandin synthesis inhibition, glutathione–S-transferase inhibition, and ornithine decarboxylase inhibition.

## In Vitro Efficacy Models

In vitro assays test the cancer risk–reducing activity of a screened compound in four epithelial cell systems (primary rat tracheal epithelial cells, human lung tumor [A427] cells, mouse mammary organ cultures [MMOC], and human foreskin epithelial cells).

**Molecular Mechanisms Common to Transforming Cells and Potential Preventive Interventions**

| Characteristics of Neoplasia | Possible Molecular Targets |
|---|---|
| ▪ Self-sufficiency in cell growth | EGFR, platelet-derived growth factor, MAPK, PI3K |
| ▪ Insensitivity to antigrowth signals | SMADs, pRb, cyclin-dependent kinases, MYC |
| ▪ Limitless replicative potential | hTERT, pRb, p53 |
| ▪ Evading apoptosis | Bcl-2, BAX, caspases, Fas, tumor necrosis factor receptor, insulin growth factor/PI3K/Akt, mTOR, p53, NF-κB, PTEN, RAS |
| ▪ Sustained angiogenesis | VEGF, basic fibroblast growth factor, integrins ($\alpha_v\beta_3$), thrombospondin-1, HIF-1α |
| ▪ Tissue invasion and metastases | MMPs, MAPK, E-cadherin |

EGFR, epidermal growth factor receptor; MAPK, mitogen-activated protein kinase; PI3K, phosphoinositide 3-kinase; SMAD, drosophila protein, mothers against decapentaplegic gene and the *Elegans* protein SMA; pRb, phosphorylated Rb protein; hTERT, human telomerase reverse transcriptase; mTOR, mammalian target of rapamycin; NF-κB, nuclear factor kappa B; PTEN, phosphatase and tensin homolog; VEGF, vascular endothelial growth factor; HIF-1α, hypoxia-inducible factor-1α; MMP, Matrix metalloproteinases. Adapted from Kelloff GJ, Lippman SM, Dannenberg AJ, et al. Progress in chemoprevention drug development: the promise of molecular biomarkers for prevention of intraepithelial neoplasia and cancer—a plan to move forward. *Clin Cancer Res* 2006;12:3661–3697 and derived from Hanahan D, Weinberg RA. The hallmarks of cancer. *Cell* 2000;100:57–70.

The assays measure the ability of potential cancer risk–reducing agents to reverse transformation in normal epithelial cells exposed to carcinogens. For example, after treatment with a carcinogen such as 7,12-demethylbenz(a)anthracene, MMOCs develop lesions similar to alveolar nodules that are considered precancerous in mouse mammary glands in vivo.[11] Pretreatment of organ cultures before carcinogen exposure measures the effect of cancer risk–reducing agents in the initiation stage of carcinogenesis, whereas treatment

after carcinogen exposure measures activity during tumor promotion. Three of these assays (using rat tracheal epithelial, A427, and MMOC cells) have shown predictive values of 76% to 83% for cancer risk–reducing agent efficacy in in vivo models.[8]

## Preclinical In Vivo Models for Cancer Risk–Reducing Agent Efficacy Testing

Animal models remain a crucial link in the efficacy assessment of cancer risk–reducing agents for epithelial cancer. Chemical carcinogenesis models provide the reproducible development of tumors in animals following the administration of a known chemical initiator or combination initiator/promoter and have been the primary in vivo screening tool for cancer risk–reducing agents (Table 33.2A).[12,13] Carcinogenesis models employing genetically engineered mice permit the interrogation of targeted pathways and the corresponding efficacy of cancer risk–reducing agents. Although useful for mechanistic studies, knockout or genetic mutational models create accelerated neoplastic progression that does not accurately recapitulate the more complex, stepwise, human carcinogenesis process. Recombinant alleles can be driven by the addition of drug-sensitive regulatory elements, such as tetracycline or tamoxifen analogs. The drug-sensitive regulatory elements achieve temporal control over a gene promoter through the administration of the drug that binds to the regulatory element. Such a system permits the inhibition or overexpression of the organ-specific gene using Cre recombinase, a site-specific DNA recombinase that targets DNA regions flanked by loxP sequences. Tables 33.2A and 2B list representative organ-specific chemical and transgenic mouse models that may be used for cancer risk–reducing agent testing.

## CLINICAL DEVELOPMENT OF CANCER RISK–REDUCING AGENTS

### Special Features of Cancer Risk–Reducing Agent Development

The clinical efficacy assessment of cancer risk–reducing agents employs phased testing (phase I to III) models used for development of drugs[14] but with crucial differences in study design and end points. Special features for the clinical development of

**Chemical Carcinogenesis Models Used for Screening of Cancer Risk–Reducing Agents for Common Epithelial Neoplasms in Animals**

| Organ Site | Species | Carcinogen | End Point |
|---|---|---|---|
| Colon | Rat, mouse | Azoxymethane (AOM) | Aberrant crypts, adenomas, adenocarcinomas |
| Lung | Mouse | N—butyl-N-(4-hydroxylbutyl)nitrosamine (NNK); benzo[a]pyrene; cigarette smoke | Adenomas, adenocarcinomas |
| | Hamster | Methylnitrosourea (MNU) | Squamous cell carcinomas |
| | Mouse | N-nitroso-tris-chloroethylurea | Squamous cell carcinomas |
| Breast | Rat | Dimethylbenz[a]anthracene (DMBA); MNU | Adenocarcinomas, adenomas |
| Prostate | Rat | MNU + testosterone | Adenocarcinomas |
| Bladder | Rat, mouse | N-butyl-N-(4-hydroxybutyl)nitrosamine (OH-BBN) | Transitional cell carcinoma |
| Pancreas | Hamster | N-nitrobis-(2-oxopropyl)amine (BOP) | Ductal carcinomas |
| Head and neck | Rat | 4-nitroquinoline-1-oxide (4-NQO) | Tongue squamous cell carcinomas |
| | Mouse | DMBA | Squamous cell carcinomas |
| Esophagus | Rat | Dimethylbenz[a]anthracene | Squamous cell carcinomas |
| | Rat | Esophagogastroduodenal anastomosis + iron | Adenocarcinomas |

Adapted from Steele VE, Lubet RA. The use of animal models for cancer chemoprevention drug development. *Semin Oncol* 2010;37:327–338.

## TABLE 33.2B

**Selected Transgenic Animal Models for Carcinogenesis Evaluation**

| Organ Site | Genes Targeted | End Point | References |
|---|---|---|---|
| Colon | *Apc, Lrig1, gp130, Stat3, Smad3, Wnt-β-catenin, villin, TGFBR2, Kras, Ink4a* | Adenomas and adenocarcinomas | (258, 259) |
| Lung | *KrasG12D, KrasG12Vgeo, PTEN, Braf*V600E, *cRaf, Egfr* L858R±T790M, *PIK3CA*, EMLA4-ALK fusion *Rb. P53* | Adenomas and adenocarcinomas  <br><br>Small cell | (260) |
| Breast | Mouse mammary tumor virus long terminal repeat promoter (MMTV) driven *BRCA1, p53, ERα*, aromatase, *TGFα, Her2/neu, wnt*, PELP-1, AIB-1 | DCIS, adenocarcinomas | (261) |
| Prostate | Probasin promotor driving SV40 large T antigen (*TRAMP/LADY*), *c-Myc, TMPRSS-ERG, Akt, Wnt-β-catenin*, androgen receptor  <br><br>*Nkx3.1, FGFR1, TGF, PTEN* | Prostate intraepithelial neoplasia, neuroendocrine tumors (TRAMP); adenocarcinomas (*c-Myc, TMPRESS-ERG, Akt, Wnt*, androgen receptor)  <br>Adenocarcinomas | (262) |
| Pancreas | *KrasG12D* alone, *LSL-Kras, PDX-1, R26Notch, Tif1γ* Combined *PDX-1, LSL-Kras, LSL-Trp53*; combined *PDX-1, Brca2, LSL-Kras Trp53; KrasG12D* on *Mist1* locus; *PDX-1, KrasG12D+ Ink4a/Arf* or *Smad4; Ptf1a, KrasG12D, TGFBR2* | Pancreatic intraepithelial neoplasia Pancreatic adenocarcinoma | (263) |

*Note:* Most models are mouse models. Such models will permit efficacy testing of specific pathway targets using single agent interventions, combinations, or multimechanism-based natural products.

cancer risk–reducing agents create the following challenges to be overcome: (1) the need for large therapeutic index (doses associated with potential toxicity of an intervention need to substantially exceed doses aimed at delaying or reversing transformation) for use in individuals who are asymptomatic yet may benefit from an extended (years) treatment course; (2) the long latency to malignant transformation (an assessment of effectiveness based on the reduction in cancer incidence requires studies lasting for years and involving thousands of participants); (3) adherence (once-daily dosing regimens using interventions that have sufficiently long half-lives may minimize the impact of a missed dose yet maintain the biologic impact on the physiologic target; minimal toxicity and strong psychological commitment to preventive goals also enhance adherence[15]); and (4) complex risk assessment for cancer (individuals with highly penetrant but infrequent, germ-line genetic susceptibility to breast and colon cancers[16,17] are excellent candidates for cancer risk–reducing agents and are likely to accept some toxicity for reduced cancer risk). For individuals at more modestly increased risk (e.g., long-term, current smokers; persons with a family history of cancer; women with mammographically dense breasts), quantitative risk assessment algorithms may be useful in the future to identify optimal cancer risk–reducing agents. The refinement of cancer risk calculators for breast,[18] colon,[19] and prostate cancer[20] promises to appropriately select high-risk individuals for cancer risk–reducing agents such that anticipated benefits exceed potential risks.

## Biomarkers as Cancer Risk–Reducing Agent Targets and Efficacy End Points

A biomarker is a characteristic that is measured and evaluated as an indicator of normal biologic processes, pathogenic processes, or pharmacologic responses to therapeutic interventions.[21] A surrogate end point for cancer prevention assumes that a measured biologic feature will predict the presence or future development of a cancer outcome.[22] Biomarkers enable a reduction in the size and duration of an intervention trial by replacing a rare or distal end point with a more frequent, proximate end point.[23] Intraepithelial

neoplasia has served and continues to serve as a biomarker for invasive malignancy (Table 33.3). Although many advocate the use of intraepithelial neoplasia-based biomarkers as regulatory surrogate end points, others caution that intraepithelial neoplasias may not serve as sufficiently robust surrogate biomarkers for cancer incidence or mortality.[24]

In order to be useful as end points for cancer risk–reducing agent efficacy testing as regulatory end points, any biomarker must have statistical accuracy, precision, and effectiveness of results[24] that demonstrate prediction of a *hard* disease end point—cancer incidence or mortality. An independent validation data set must address defined standards of validation that minimize bias in the study design and the populations studied.[25] The biomarker must be generalizable to the specific clinical or screening population (Table 33.4).

## Phases of Cancer Risk–Reducing Agent Development

*Phase I cancer risk–reducing agent trials* define an optimal cancer risk–reducing agent dose. An optimal cancer risk–reducing agent dose is one that is usually nontoxic, scheduled once daily, and modulates a tissue, cellular, or serum biomarker of drug activity (e.g., the dose of aspirin that inhibits prostaglandin production in a target tissue site). The definition of a maximum tolerated dose is not an essential end point of a phase I cancer risk–reducing agent trial. Higher, yet nontoxic doses may lower cancer risk–reducing agent efficacy. For example, β-carotene at high doses has pro-oxidant activity and may enhance the carcinogenesis process, whereas at low doses, it is a potent antioxidant and differentiating agent.[26]

*Phase II cancer risk–reducing agent trials* begin to define cancer risk–reduction efficacy. These short-term (6 months to 1 year) treatment periods gather evidence of risk reduction by assessing drug effects on tissue, cellular, or blood surrogate markers of carcinogenesis. Phase IIa trials are nonrandomized, biomarker modulation trials. Phase IIb trials are randomized, placebo-controlled trials of several hundred subjects testing, for example, whether a risk-reducing agent reduces recurrence of a previously resected intraepithelial neoplastic lesion as the primary end point. Cellular dynamic

## TABLE 33.3

**Common Intraepithelial Neoplasias**

| Epithelium | Intraepithelial Neoplasia | References |
|---|---|---|
| Colon and rectum | Adenoma | (264) |
| Lower esophagus | Barrett esophagus | (265) |
| Upper esophagus | Squamous dysplasia | (266, 267) |
| Skin: Squamous/basal cell | Actinic keratosis | (268) |
| Skin: Pigmented | Dysplastic nevus | (269) |
| Cervix | Cervical intraepithelial neoplasia | (270) |
| Head and neck | Leukoplakia/oral epithelial dysplasia | (271) |
| Prostate | Prostate intraepithelial neoplasia (PIN), intraductal carcinoma of the prostate | (272) |
| Lung | Bronchial dysplasia | (273) |
| Pancreas | Pancreatic intraepithelial neoplasia | (274) |

(e.g., proliferation, apoptotic index), biochemical, or molecular (e.g., p53, cyclin D) end points may be used as secondary end points. Preoperative or *window of opportunity trials* enroll subjects for brief study periods prior to obtaining tissue by a planned resection of an invasive neoplasm. Such designs permit the exploration of biomarker modulation in the invasive neoplasm and in contiguous epithelial fields proximal and distal to the invasive neoplasm.[27]

*Phase III cancer risk–reducing agent trials* define reduction in a hard cancer end point such as cancer incidence or mortality. Such trials, using large, higher risk populations in a randomized, double-blinded intervention, are designed to identify a standard of preventive care for a given risk population. For example, trials of tamoxifen for the reduction of breast cancer incidence,[28,29] finasteride for the reduction of prostate cancer incidence,[30] and β-carotene for the reduction of lung cancer incidence[31] serve as examples of well-conducted, definitive phase III cancer risk–reducing agent clinical trials.

Some investigators consider randomized, controlled clinical trials with an end point sufficient for regulatory review as phase III.

## TABLE 33.4

**Characteristics of Biomarkers for Use as End Points in Cancer Risk–Reducing Agent Efficacy Assessment**

- Variability of expression between phases of the carcinogenesis process
- Detected early in the carcinogenesis process
- Genetic progression or protein pathway based
- Target of modulation by preventive interventions
- Changes in biomarker linked to reduction in incident cancer of epithelial target
- Changes in biomarker linked to clinical benefit
- Can be quantified directly or via closely related activity such as a downstream target or upstream kinase
- Measurable in an accessible biosample (preferably urine, serum, saliva, stool, or breath)
- High throughput, technically feasible, analytical procedure with strong quality assurance/quality control procedures
- Cost-effective

Using such a definition, a clinical trial with an end point of reduction in adenoma recurrence is considered a phase III trial. Other investigators define phase III cancer risk–reducing agent trials as randomized, controlled clinical trials with a cancer incidence or mortality end point. This controversy causes confusion in the literature. For the purpose of clarity in this textbook, the latter definition of phase III trial is used—a prospective, randomized, controlled clinical trial with a cancer incidence or mortality end point. Randomized, controlled clinical trials with a surrogate biomarker end point such as an intraepithelial neoplasia (e.g., adenoma) are defined as phase IIb cancer risk–reducing agent trials.

# MICRONUTRIENTS

## Definition

Micronutrients comprise a large, diverse group of molecules typically ingested as part of the diet that play roles in normal human biology. This group of compounds has been investigated extensively as cancer risk–reducing agents in purified forms (i.e., supplements), as components of multiagent cocktails, and occasionally, as components of food extracts/other mixtures. Although retinoids are not micronutrients per se, they are related to retinol (vitamin A) and share certain properties with carotenoids, which are diet derived and, therefore, included along with micronutrients.

## Retinoids, Carotenoids, and Antioxidant Nutrients

### Overview and Mechanisms

Retinoids are the natural derivatives and synthetic analogs of vitamin A.[32] Cancer risk–reduction intervention studies have evaluated the parent compound (retinol, typically given as retinyl acetate or palmitate), naturally occurring retinoids such as all-trans–retinoic acid (ATRA) and 13-cis-retinoic acid (13cRA), and also synthetic retinoids such as etretinate and fenretinide (4-hydroxy[phenyl]retinamide [4HPR]). These agents have been of interest for cancer risk reduction for decades. Mechanistically, retinoids have been shown to modulate cellular growth and differentiation, as well as apoptosis.[32] A large body of research indicates that retinoids have activity in the promotion and progression phases of carcinogenesis, including extensive evidence of efficacy in the setting of premalignant lesions, leading to their evaluation in human Phase III trials. Nuclear retinoic acid receptors mediate many of the retinoid-signaling effects; however, retinoids interact with other signaling pathways, such as estrogen signaling in breast cancer.[33]

Carotenoids are a group of naturally occurring plant pigments, only some of which are found in appreciable levels in the human diet and human tissues, including beta-carotene, alpha-carotene, lycopene, lutein, and β-cryptoxanthin.[34] Of these, the most widely studied carotenoids for cancer risk reduction are beta-carotene and lycopene. Beta-carotene has the highest pro–vitamin A activity of the carotenoids, but alpha-carotene and β-cryptoxanthin also possess pro–vitamin A activity. Other carotenoids, such as lycopene, do not possess vitamin A activity but are known to have potent antioxidant activity, particularly with regard to singlet oxygen quenching.[35] Furthermore, eccentric cleavage products of beta-carotene,[36] as well as other non-pro–vitamin A carotenoids such as lycopene (e.g., apocarotenals, apocarotenoic acids) appear to be biologically active and may also act via retinoid-signaling pathways.[37]

Because of the known antioxidant function of carotenoids, they are often studied for risk-reducing efficacy in combination with other antioxidant nutrients, especially vitamins E and C and selenium (sometimes as a cocktail, versus placebo). Thus, we will consider this group of nutrients first, followed by other micronutrients that are thought to act via different mechanisms and/or pathways.

## Epidemiology

A large body of literature indicates that people who consume greater amounts of carotenoids from foods (primarily fruits and vegetables) and people with higher serum or plasma levels of various carotenoids have a lower risk for various cancers.[38] In particular, according to the systematic review of the literature conducted by the World Cancer Research Fund/American Institute for Cancer Research,[38] foods containing carotenoids are "probably" associated with lower risks of cancers of the mouth/pharynx/larynx and lung; foods containing beta-carotene are "probably" associated with lower risks of cancers of the esophagus; and foods containing lycopene are "probably" associated with lower risks of prostate cancer. Preformed retinol intake is inconsistently associated with risks of various cancers but that, in part, likely reflects confounding, because dietary sources of preformed retinol primarily include foods of animal origin (e.g., liver, eggs, milk). Vitamin C in the diet comes primarily from the consumption of fruits and vegetables; therefore, vitamin C and carotenoids often trend together in epidemiologic findings. Vitamin E, in contrast, is found in different foods, especially nuts, seeds, and vegetable oils; intake and blood concentrations are somewhat inconsistently associated with cancer risk.[39] Selenium, being a trace mineral, is difficult to measure in the diet, but higher selenium status has been associated with a lower risk of certain cancers, although the results are not entirely consistent.[39]

## Preclinical In Vivo Models

In preclinical models, retinoids induce differentiation as well as arrest proliferation[33] of various cancers, making them attractive agents for cancer risk reduction.[40] The International Agency for Research on Cancer reviewed the preclinical research involving beta-carotene, concluding that there was "sufficient" evidence of cancer preventive activity, particularly involving mouse skin tumor models and the hamster buccal pouch model.[41] Notably, there was inconsistent evidence of efficacy in respiratory tract models. Lycopene has been evaluated in numerous cell culture systems and in a variety of models of prostate carcinogenesis, including chemically induced, orthotopic implantation, transgenic, and xenotransplantation, with mixed evidence of efficacy.[42] Evidence, primarily from cell culture studies, suggests that lycopene metabolites may be at least partially responsible for anticarcinogenic activity.[37]

## Clinical Trials: Retinoids, Carotenoids, and Antioxidant Nutrients

Retinoids, carotenoids, and antioxidant nutrients have been evaluated in the setting of preneoplasia/neoplasia in many different organ sites, as will be discussed. Of the many clinical trials of retinoids and carotenoids/other antioxidant nutrients, key trials with cancer incidence/recurrence as primary outcomes are tabulated (see Tables 33.5 and 33.6) and reviewed.

### Clinical Efficacy in the Upper Airway

Many trials of cancer risk–reducing agents have been done in the setting of squamous cell carcinomas of the head and neck, in large part because of the substantial clinical problem of relatively high rates of recurrences and second primary tumors in curatively treated cancer patients. Early work demonstrated that high-dose 13cRA (50 to 100 mg/m² per day) produced no significant differences in disease recurrence (local, regional, or distant) but significantly lowered the rate of second primary invasive neoplasms,[43] with the benefits persisting for at least 5 years.[44] Substantial retinoid toxicity, however, including skin dryness and peeling, cheilitis, conjunctivitis, and hypertriglyceridemia, was evident in a large proportion of patients. Subsequent trials thus used lower doses of retinoids (13cRA or a synthetic retinoid, etretinate), but failed to show efficacy in reducing second primary tumor formation (Table 33.5).[45,46]

Supplemental beta-carotene has also been studied as a single agent and in combination with other agents for the prevention of second primary cancers of the mouth and throat (Table 33.6). One trial of beta-carotene alone observed no harm or benefit[47]; another observed nonsignificantly fewer second head and neck cancers but more lung cancers[48]; and a third gave beta-carotene with α-tocopherol (400 IU per day).[49] In the third trial, beta-carotene was discontinued early due to adverse findings from lung cancer prevention trials (see the following); however, after a median follow-up of 6.5 years, all-cause mortality was increased, which the authors attributed to the supplemental α-tocopherol. As will be discussed later, adverse effects of antioxidant nutrients are not limited to head and neck cancer patients; potential mechanisms for adverse effects are discussed further.

### Clinical Efficacy in the Lung (Lower Airway)

**Reversal of Metaplasia or Dysplasia.** Active smokers and recent quitters have multiple preinvasive metaplastic and dysplastic lesions in the pulmonary tree. Most of these lesions resolve upon smoking cessation, but some remain and progress to invasive neoplasms. Unfortunately, micronutrient or retinoid interventions have not demonstrated preventive efficacy in most rigorous trials in patients with early lesions. For example, a US trial randomized 755 asbestos workers to receive beta-carotene (50 mg per day) and retinol (25,000 IU every other day) versus placebo; sputum atypia was not reduced after 5 years.[50] As another example, eligible smokers with lung metaplasia or dysplasia were randomized to 6 months of 13cRA or placebo. The extent of metaplasia decreased similarly (in approximately 50% of subjects) in both study arms.[51] Only smoking cessation was associated with a significant reduction in the metaplasia index during the 6-month intervention.

**Prevention of Invasive Neoplasms.** Large, phase III efficacy trials of beta-carotene plus other micronutrients for primary prevention of lung cancer have been completed, as summarized in Table 33.6. The Alpha-Tocopherol, Beta-carotene (ATBC) Trial involved 29,133 men from Finland who were heavy cigarette smokers at entry.[52] In a two-by-two factorial design, participants were randomized to receive either supplemental α-tocopherol, beta-carotene, the combination, or placebo. Unexpectedly, participants receiving beta-carotene (alone or in combination with α-tocopherol) had a statistically significant 18% increase in lung cancer incidence and an 8% increase in total mortality relative to participants receiving placebo. α-Tocopherol had no effect.

The finding of an increased incidence of lung cancer in the beta-carotene–supplemented smokers was replicated in the Carotene and Retinol Efficacy Trial (CARET), a large randomized trial of supplemental beta-carotene plus retinol versus placebo in asbestos workers and smokers.[53] This trial was terminated early, but, at the time of termination, overall lung cancer incidence was increased by 28% in the supplemented subjects and total mortality was also increased by 17%. In contrast, the Physicians' Health Study (PHS) of supplemental beta-carotene versus placebo in 22,071 male US physicians reported no significant effect—positive or negative—of 12 years of supplementation of beta-carotene on total cancer, lung cancer, or cardiovascular disease (see Table 33.6).[54] Two other trials involving supplemental beta-carotene alone (the Women's Health Study[55]) or with other antioxidant nutrients (the Medical Research Council/British Heart Foundation Heart Protection Study[56]) on overall cancer incidence also failed to observe efficacy.

**Prevention of Second Primary Invasive Neoplasms.** EUROSCAN was a multicenter trial employing a two-by-two factorial design to test retinyl palmitate and N-acetylcysteine (also a compound with known antioxidant activity) in preventing second primary invasive neoplasms in patients with early stage cancers

**Larger, Randomized Trials of Retinoids in Human Cancer Risk Reduction with Cancer Outcomes[a,b]**

| Population | Drug (Dose) | End Point | Outcomes | References |
|---|---|---|---|---|
| United States, prior HNSCC | 13cRA (50–100 mg/m²/d) | Second primary tumor | Significant reduction in second primary tumors at 32 and 55 mos; however, substantial toxicity | (43, 44) |
| France, prior HNSCC | Etretinate (50/25 mg/d) | Second primary tumor | No difference | (46) |
| United States, prior HNSCC | 13cRA (30 mg/d) | Second primary tumor | No difference | (45) |
| Europe, prior HNSCC, NSCLC | Vitamin A (300,000/150,000 IU/d) +/− N-acetylcysteine | Second primary tumor | No difference | (57) |
| United States, Prior NSCLC | 13cRA (30 mg/d) | Second primary tumor | No difference, but second primary tumors were lower in nonsmokers on drug but higher in smokers on drug | (58) |
| Italy, prior breast cancer | 4HPR (200 mg/d) No treatment | Contralateral breast cancer | Nonsignificant reduction; premenopausal women did better but opposite in postmenopausal women | (60) |
| United States, prior BCC | 13cRA (10 mg/d) | Second basal cell carcinoma | No difference | (65) |
| United States, prior actinic keratosis | Retinol (25,000 IU/d) | Skin cancer incidence | Reduction in squamous cell carcinomas but not basal cell carcinomas | (67) |
| United States, prior BCC/SCC of the skin | 13cRA (5–10 mg/d) Retinol (25,000 IU/d) | Second skin cancer | No significant difference for either agent | (66) |
| Netherlands, renal transplant patients | Acitretin (30 mg/d) | Skin cancer | Significant reduction | (64) |
| United States, aggressive SCC of the skin | 13cRA (1 mg/kg/d) + interferon alpha | Second primary tumors and tumor recurrences | No effect | (275) |
| United States, prior bladder TCC | Megadose vitamins (40,000 IU retinol/d) versus RDA vitamins | Recurrence | Significant reduction in recurrence | (73) |
| United States, prior bladder TCC | 4HPR (200 mg/d) | Recurrence | No difference | (72) |

[a] Trials of retinoids that also included beta-carotene are listed under Table 33.2 only.
[b] Versus placebo unless otherwise indicated.
HNSCC, head and neck squamous cell carcinoma; NSLC, non–small-cell lung cancer; BCC, basal cell carcinoma; TCC, transitional cell carcinoma; RDA, recommended dietary allowance.

of the head and neck or lung. None of the interventions reduced second airway primary invasive neoplasms.[57] The Lung Intergroup Trial randomized patients with surgically resected lung cancer to 13cRA versus placebo and found no significant differences between the two arms in second primary tumors.[58] Notably, smoking status modified the effect of the 13cRA intervention, which was harmful in current smokers yet beneficial in former smokers.

Thus, phase III trials of both carotenoids/antioxidants and retinoids indicate that these agents overall do not reduce the risk of developing invasive lung cancers, nor do they prevent the development of second primary invasive neoplasms. However, the finding that former smokers seemed to benefit from both 13cRA[58] and beta-carotene[53] is intriguing. Mechanistic work suggests this interaction is real rather than chance (see the following), suggesting that (1) risk-reduction in smokers is especially challenging,[59] and (2) trials in former smokers may merit consideration.

### Clinical Efficacy in the Breast

Moon et al.[40] first showed that fenretinide was a promising cancer risk–reducing agent for the breast, having a high therapeutic index and synergistic interaction with tamoxifen in mammary carcinogenesis model studies. This laboratory work led to a large-scale randomized trial of fenretinide (versus no treatment) for 5 years to prevent contralateral breast cancer in women aged 30 to 70 years with a history of resected early breast cancer and no prior adjuvant therapy.[60] The intervention produced no significant overall effect, although fenretinide reduced contralateral and ipsilateral breast cancer rates in premenopausal women, with an opposite (adverse) trend observed in postmenopausal women. The reduced incidence of second breast cancer in premenopausal patients persisted with longer follow-up.[61]

Retinoid X receptor (RXR)–selective retinoids are also being evaluated in preclinical and clinical studies. Ongoing work suggests that combination treatment may represent a promising new strategy to suppress both estrogen receptor–negative and estrogen receptor–positive breast tumors, and the combination of retinoids with antiestrogens may be particularly effective.[62]

### Clinical Efficacy in the Skin

Retinoids have been widely studied for cancer risk–reducing efficacy in skin. Early work was done in patients who have substantial skin cancer risk either due to xeroderma pigmentosum or medication-induced immunosuppression for transplants. For example, 13cRA reduced skin cancer by 63% in patients with

**TABLE 33.6**

## Randomized Trials of Antioxidant Nutrients in Human Cancer Risk Reduction with Cancer Outcomes[a]

| Population | Drug (Dose) | End Point | Outcomes | References |
|---|---|---|---|---|
| United States, prior head/neck cancer | Beta-carotene (50 mg/d) | Second primary head and neck cancers | Nonsignificant reduction in second head and neck cancer, increase in lung cancer | (48) |
| Italy, prior head/neck cancer | Beta-carotene (75 mg/d) for 3 mos with 1 mo off | Second primary head and neck cancers | No effect on second primary tumors, nonsignificant decrease in death | (47) |
| Canada, prior head/neck cancer | 30 mg beta-carotene/d + 400 IU vitamin E/d | Deaths | Beta-carotene discontinued, mortality increased at end of trial | (49) |
| Finland, male smokers | 20 mg beta-carotene/d +/− 50 mg vitamin E/d | Lung cancer | Lung cancer increased with beta-carotene, no effect vitamin E | (52) |
| United States, smokers and asbestos workers | Beta-carotene (30 mg/d) + retinol (25,000 IU/d) | Lung cancer | Lung cancer increased with beta-carotene + vitamin A | (53) |
| United States, resected stage I non–small-cell lung cancer | Selenized yeast, 200 μg/d versus placebo | Second primary cancer | No effect | (276) |
| United States, male physicians | Beta-carotene (50 mg every other day) | Total cancer | No effect | (54) |
| United States, female health professionals | Beta-carotene (50 mg/every other day) | All cancers | No effect | (55) |
| United Kingdom, adults at risk for coronary heart disease | 20 mg beta-carotene/d + 600 mg vitamin E/d + 250 mg vitamin C/d | Total cancers | No effect | (56) |
| United States, prior skin cancer | 50 mg beta-carotene/d | Second skin cancer | No effect | (68) |
| Australia | Beta-carotene (30 mg/d) | Incident squamous cell skin cancer incident basal cell skin cancer | No effect | (69) |
| United States, prior skin cancer | 200 μg selenium/d | Second skin cancer | No effect, with longer follow-up became adverse | (70) |
| Linxian County, China, general population | 15 mg beta-carotene/d + 30 mg vitamin E/d + 50 μg selenium/d | Stomach cancer death Esophageal cancer death | Significant decrease in stomach cancer death; no effect on esophageal cancer death | (75) |
| Linxian County, China, esophageal dysplasia | Multivitamin/multimineral + 15 mg beta-carotene/d | Stomach cancer death Esophageal cancer death | No effect | (78) |
| United States, males | 200 μg selenium/d +/− 400 IU vitamin E/d | Prostate cancer incidence | No effect; with longer follow-up vitamin E became adverse | (84) |
| United States, male physicians II | 500 mg vitamin C/d + 400 IU vitamin E every other day | Prostate cancer incidence, total cancer incidence | No effect | (86) |

[a] All versus placebo.

xeroderma pigmentosum; however, severe, acute mucocutaneous toxicity with the 13cRA occurred.[63] Also, the preventive effect of the retinoid was lost after stopping retinoid therapy. In renal transplant patients, acitretin (30 mg per day) reduced the numbers of premalignant lesions, the number of patients with skin cancer, and the cumulative number of skin cancers.[64]

In lower risk populations, low-dose 13cRA (10 mg per day)[65] and retinol or 13cRA alone did not reduce the recurrence of basal or squamous cell skin cancers,[66] although retinol alone reduced squamous but not basal cell carcinomas in patients with prior actinic keratoses.[67]

Beta-carotene (50 mg per day), in a randomized trial did not reduce the recurrence of nonmelanoma skin cancers.[68] Consistent with findings in the lung, the risk was increased by 44% in current smokers randomized to beta-carotene but not in never smokers randomized to beta-carotene as compared with placebo.

Supplemental beta-carotene (30 mg per day) also did not prevent basal cell carcinoma or squamous cell carcinoma of the skin in an Australian trial.[69]

Clark et al.[70] randomized patients with a history of nonmelanoma skin cancer to 200 μg per day selenium or placebo.[70] Selenium did not reduce the incidence of second skin cancers; a further report of this trial with longer follow-up[71] indicated that there was instead a significant increase in total nonmelanoma skin cancer (hazard ratio [HR] = 1.17; 95% confidence interval [CI], 1.02 to 1.34) and squamous cell skin cancer (HR = 1.25; 95% CI, 1.03 to 1.51).

### Clinical Efficacy in the Bladder

A trial of fenretinide (200 mg per day orally for 12 months) versus placebo was conducted for preventing tumor recurrence in patients with nonmuscle-invasive bladder transitional cell carcinoma after transurethral resection with or without adjuvant intravesical bacillus Calmette-Guérin; recurrence rates were similar in both groups.[72] Another trial randomized 65 patients with biopsy-confirmed transitional cell carcinoma of the bladder to a multivitamin (recommended dietary allowance [RDA] levels) alone or supplemented with 40,000 IU retinol, 100 mg pyridoxine, 2,000 mg ascorbic acid, 400 U of α-tocopherol, and 90 mg zinc.[73] The 5-year estimate of tumor recurrence was 91% in the RDA arm versus 41% in the higher-dose nutrient arm ($p = 0.0014$).

### Clinical Efficacy in the Cervix

Randomized trials include four with beta-carotene (alone or with other antioxidant nutrients), and five with retinoids. Only one of these trials, involving ATRA,[74] found a significant treatment effect. This trial administered a 0.372% ATRA solution by collagen sponge in a cervical cap delivery system. There was a higher complete response rate in the ATRA group (43%) than the placebo group (27%; $p = 0.041$) among the 141 patients with moderate dysplasia; no significant differences in dysplasia regression rates between the two study arms were detected in patients with severe dysplasia. The investigators experienced substantial losses to follow-up in this patient population.

### Clinical Efficacy in the Esophagus and Stomach

Certain regions of China (Huixian and Linxian) have strikingly high incidence rates of esophageal and gastric cancers. Two trials were done in Linxian County; one was a general population trial that tested the efficacy of four different nutrient combinations at inhibiting the development of esophageal and gastric cancers.[75] Those who were given the combination of beta-carotene, vitamin E, and selenium had a 13% reduction in total cancer deaths, a 4% reduction in esophageal cancer deaths, and a 21% reduction in gastric cancer deaths (see Table 33.6). None of the other nutrient combinations reduced gastric or esophageal cancer deaths significantly in this trial. The treatment benefit has been shown to persist for 10 years postintervention, with greater efficacy seen in participants under age 55 years.[76] This finding stands in contrast to most other antioxidant nutrient supplement intervention trials, suggesting that the applicability of these results for populations with adequate nutritional status and for other tumor sites may be limited.[77]

The other Linxian trial evaluated a multivitamin/multimineral preparation plus beta-carotene (15 mg per day) in residents with esophageal dysplasia.[78] There was no clear evidence of efficacy, although confidence intervals were wide.

### Clinical Efficacy in the Colon/Rectum

Of the randomized trials aimed at the prevention of recurrent colorectal adenomas with micronutrients that have been completed, some used beta-carotene alone[79] or with other nonmicronutrient interventions.[80] Others evaluated beta-carotene with and without supplemental vitamins C and E.[81] None of the trials observed benefit with supplementation. A subsequent report from one trial noted that alcohol intake and cigarette smoking modified the efficacy of beta-carotene.[82] Among nonsmokers and nondrinkers, beta-carotene was associated with a significant decrease in the risk of one or more recurrent adenomas (relative risk [RR] = 0.56). Among persons who smoked and also drank more than one alcoholic drink per day, beta-carotene significantly increased the risk of recurrent adenoma (RR = 2.07).

### Clinical Efficacy in the Prostate

Because oxidative stress may play a role in the etiology of prostate cancer, several antioxidant nutrients, including vitamin E, selenium, and lycopene, have been of interest for preventing prostate cancer. The largest trial to date of these nutrients is the Selenium and Vitamin E Cancer Prevention Trial (SELECT), which tested selenium and vitamin E in a two-by-two factorial design for the primary prevention of prostate cancer. Despite preliminary indications of prostate cancer risk–reducing efficacy for selenium (from a trial of selenium for skin cancer[70]) and vitamin E (from a trial of vitamin E to prevent lung cancer[83]), there was no evidence of efficacy.[84] With extended follow-up, the nonsignificant adverse effect of vitamin E became significantly adverse.[85] Negative/neutral findings also were reported for vitamins E and C and prostate and total cancer in the PHS II randomized controlled trial.[86]

The carotenoid lycopene has generated much interest with regard to prostate cancer risk, and several intervention trials have been conducted based on lycopene supplements. These studies have been small, short term, based on intermediate end points, and often lack adequate control groups. The use of a tomato sauce–based intervention is arguably a better approach to evaluate, based on animal data indicating that tomato powder (which includes lycopene along with other phytochemicals), but not lycopene alone, was effective at inhibiting prostate carcinogenesis.[87]

### Mechanisms for Ineffective Retinoid and Carotenoid Cancer Risk–Reducing Activity

There are now a number of trials demonstrating that supplemental beta-carotene/retinoids given to current smokers can produce increases rather than reductions in cancer incidence. In tobacco users, beta-carotene and other carotenoids may produce oxidative carotenoid breakdown products that alter retinoid metabolism and signaling pathways, along with pro-oxidation.[88] For retinoids such as 13cRA, smoking may induce genetic and epigenetic changes in the lung that affect retinoid activity; for example, tobacco smoking can affect RAR-β expression.[58] The adverse effects of supplemental nutrients are not limited to smokers; α-tocopherol increased rather than reduced prostate cancer in SELECT (which had relatively few smokers) and selenium increased prostate cancer among men without a baseline selenium deficiency.[89] This may be a consequence of the relatively high doses used in SELECT,[77] but certainly calls into question the notion that reducing oxidative stress is a pivotal cancer risk–reduction strategy, even in nonsmokers.

It has become clear that reactive oxygen species (ROS), such as hydrogen peroxide, can act as important physiologic regulators of intracellular signaling pathways.[90,91] Data in mouse models have shown that vitamin E accelerates lung tumor growth by disrupting the ROS–p53 axis, potentially by removing oxidative damage to DNA, which can serve as a potent stimulus for p53 activation.[92] Although some of the large cancer risk–reducing trials may have failed in their primary objective, they may indirectly contribute to a clearer understanding of cancer biology, leading to the recognition that the role of oxidative stress and ROS in human disease is much more nuanced than originally hypothesized.[93]

As for the retinoids, these agents are generally too toxic to be used as single agents for risk-reducing efficacy; however, a major area of ongoing research is examining retinoids (low doses) given in combination with other agents, especially those that regulate the epigenome, such histone deacetylase (HDAC) inhibitors.[33]

### Folic Acid and Other B Vitamins

**Overview and Mechanisms.** Folate is a water-soluble B vitamin found in foods, whereas folic acid is the synthetic form found in supplements and fortified foods. Adequate folate is critical for DNA methylation, repair, and synthesis.[94,95] The methylation status of genes can play a key role in gene silencing and gene expression, lending plausibility to the idea that folate could be a key nutrient in regulating cell growth and proliferation.

**Epidemiology.** Epidemiologic studies have linked low folate intake with higher risk of several cancers, most notably colorectal cancer.[96] Long-term use of multivitamin supplements, which are a major source of folate and other B vitamins, has been associated with a reduction in the risk of colon cancer in some studies, including recent (postfortification) findings.[97–99] Supporting an anticancer role of folate is that genotypes for methylene tetrahydrofolate reductase, an enzyme known to be involved in folate metabolism, predict the risk of colon cancer dependent on folate intake or status.[100] Vitamin B$_6$ has been less studied in relation to cancer than folate, but some epidemiologic studies suggest that vitamin B$_6$ may be important for colorectal cancer.[101,102] A higher risk of cancer related to deficiencies of these vitamins has been suggested for alcohol drinkers.[103]

**Clinical Trials: Folic Acid and B Vitamins.** Risk-reducing efficacy for supplemental folic acid has been primarily evaluated in the setting of prevention of recurrent colorectal adenomas (i.e., in patients with prior adenomas). Of six randomized trials of folic acid, two small trials reported suggestions of benefit of folic acid supplementation.[104,105] However, benefits were not observed in two much larger trials, the Aspirin/Folate Polyp Prevention Study (AFPPS) (dose: 1 mg of folic acid daily)[106] and the United Kingdom Colorectal Adenoma Prevention (ukCAP) trial (dose: 500 µg of folic acid daily).[107] AFPPS found indications of an increased risk for advanced lesions and multiple adenomas with prolonged treatment and follow-up. A third large trial, the Nurses Health Study/Health Professionals Follow-up Study (NHS/HPFS) folic acid polyp prevention trial, showed no overall risk reduction.[108] The most recent trial, done in a Chinese population >50 years of age,[109] reported that 1 mg folic acid per day reduced sporadic colorectal adenomas when compared with no intervention (not a placebo-controlled study). One possible explanation for the discrepancy of the Chinese trial versus North American and European trials is the baseline plasma folate status. In the Chinese trial, the mean baseline folate concentration of 5 ng/mL[109] was half of the reported 10 ng/mL in a United States trial,[106] where folate fortification of the food supply occurs.

## Calcium and Vitamin D

**Overview and Mechanisms.** There are two major forms of vitamin D: ergocalciferol (D$_2$) and cholecalciferol (D$_3$). Vitamin D$_2$ is absorbed through dietary sources such as fortified milk products, and D$_3$ is synthesized via ultraviolet (UV) B light isomerization of 7-dehydrocholestrol in the epidermis.[110] Vitamin D$_3$ is converted to calcitriol (1, 25-[OH]$_2$ D$_3$) in a two-step process requiring both hepatic and renal hydroxylation. Calcitriol binds to the vitamin D receptor, which translocates to the nucleus and binds to multiple gene promoter sites. Through this mechanism, vitamin D regulates cytoplasmic signaling pathways that impact cellular differentiation and growth through proteins such as Ras and mitogen-activated protein kinase (MAPK), protein lipase A, prostaglandins, cyclic adenosine monophosphate (AMP), protein kinase A, and phosphatidyl inositol 3 kinase.[110] 1,25(OH)$_2$D$_3$ regulates cellular proliferation and apoptosis. For example, 1,25(OH)$_2$D$_3$ can induce cleavage of caspase 3, poly (ADP-ribose) polymerase (PARP), and MAPK, leading to apoptosis. 1,25(OH)$_2$D$_3$ inhibits the expression and phosphorylation of Akt, a key regulator of cellular proliferation. The differentiation properties of 1,25(OH)$_2$D$_3$ are mediated through transcriptional activation of the CDK inhibitor p21. The effects of vitamin D on multiple signal transduction pathways operational in cancer cells are reviewed by Deeb et al.[111]

**Epidemiology.** Observational epidemiologic studies have shown a relatively consistent inverse association between low calcium intake, including that from supplements, and increased colorectal and colon cancer risk.[112,113] Vitamin D exposure is typically assessed by measuring 25(OH)vitamin D in plasma because exposure is derived not only from diet and supplements, but also from cutaneous synthesis following dermal exposure to UV radiation. A large number of observational studies have evaluated the association between vitamin D status and cancer risk, as systematically reviewed by the Agency for Healthcare Research and Quality (AHRQ).[114] The evidence is inconsistent for most cancer sites, with the exception of studies showing that individuals with lower blood vitamin D levels have a higher risk of colorectal cancer or adenoma. Although some observational studies have reported that higher serum vitamin D is associated with lower breast cancer risk, the association is inconsistent.[114,115] Also, there are some studies suggesting high serum vitamin D is associated with increases in certain cancers, particularly pancreatic cancer.[116]

### Clinical Trials: Calcium and Vitamin D

*Clinical Efficacy in the Colon.* Baron et al.[117] randomized subjects with a recent history of colorectal adenomas to either calcium carbonate (1,200 mg per day of elemental calcium) or placebo. Results showed significant benefit for the calcium arm (adjusted RR = 0.81; 95% CI, 0.67 to 0.99; $p$ = 0.04). In a smaller, similar study of calcium gluconolactate and carbonate (2 g elemental calcium daily), the adjusted odds ratio (OR) for adenoma recurrence was 0.66 (95% CI, 0.38 to 1.17; $p$ = 0.16) for calcium treatment,[118] and while not statistically significant, it was similar to the data of Baron et al.[117]

In the largest trial of calcium and vitamin D with primary cancer end points (e.g., colon, breast), the US Women's Health Initiative (WHI) evaluated the combination of 400 IU of vitamin D per day plus 1,000 mg of calcium per day in 36,282 postmenopausal women. For colon cancer, there was no benefit observed,[119] although the mean baseline intake of calcium was already very high (more than 1,151 mg per day). With regard to vitamin D as a single agent, there was also no suggestion of benefit for colon cancer incidence in a 5-year British trial of vitamin D (100,000 IU every 4 months) that reported colon cancer incidence,[120] although this was not a primary end point.

*Clinical Efficacy in the Breast.* Vitamin D has received considerable attention for a possible role in the prevention of breast cancer,[121] although no trials have yet investigated vitamin D as a single agent for breast cancer risk reduction. The large WHI trial gave a combination of calcium and vitamin D, as noted previously, and there was no significant effect of this combination on breast cancer risk (HR, 0.96; 95% CI, 0.85 to 1.09).[122] Lappe et al.[123] conducted a trial that examined the relation between calcium plus vitamin D (1,100 IU per day) supplementation (versus calcium alone or placebo) in 1,179 healthy postmenopausal women in Nebraska.[123] Although fracture was the primary outcome of the trial, total cancer incidence was reportedly lower in the calcium plus vitamin D group, although the number of end points was very small (n = 50 total cancers observed during the follow-up). An ongoing randomized trial of vitamin D and omega-3 fatty acids (the VITamin D and OmegA-3 TriaL [VITAL]) among 20,000 participants is expected to provide more definitive data on a possible role of vitamin D in the prevention of breast and other cancers.[124]

## Summary and Conclusion: Micronutrients

Certain agents, including the retinoids, beta-carotene, folic acid, calcium plus vitamin D, vitamin E, and selenium, have received substantial attention for a possible role in reducing the risk of cancer in humans. As reviewed herein, some of the trials have observed statistically significant reductions in the risk of the primary end point (e.g., retinoids in skin carcinogenesis models, calcium in colorectal adenomas, antioxidant nutrients in Linxian, China, for gastric cancer prevention), whereas others have observed statistically significant increases in the risk of the primary end points (beta-carotene and retinoid lung cancer prevention trials in smokers, vitamin E and prostate cancer, selenium and nonmelanoma skin cancer). Considering the completed trials, there is clear evidence against the general use of nutrient *supplements* for cancer prevention, which is the conclusion also reached by the World Cancer Research Fund/American Institute for Cancer Research.[38] Note that there is no evidence that food sources of these nutrients increase risk.

Having noted that, there are other key themes emerging from this growing body of research. One such theme is that nutrient supplementation may be of benefit to some but not all. One such population that may benefit includes persons who are low in the nutrient of interest at baseline.[77] This was initially suggested in the Linxian Country trial (done in a micronutrient-deficient population), with growing support from subgroup analyses of several completed trials.[77] However, the hypothesis that nutrient supplementation can reduce cancer risk in subgroups selected based on inadequate nutritional status has, to date, not been formally evaluated in intervention trials.

Another consistent theme is that lifestyle factors (e.g., smoking) and genetics (polymorphisms) may determine who is most likely to benefit from supplementation. Trial data will likely be increasingly mined to identify genetic profiles associated with both better outcomes (risk prediction) and response to intervention.[125,126] Ultimately, a more personalized approach to cancer risk reduction may emerge, consistent with the movement toward a more personalized approach for cancer treatment.

Finally, nearly all of these trials initiate intervention with older adults (who are more likely to develop cancer end points during the follow-up); but, animal models suggest that the timing of exposure may likely be quite relevant. For example, folic acid may protect against initiation, but may also promote the proliferation of existing neoplasms.[127] Thus, the dose, form (food versus supplement), timing, and nutritional and lifestyle characteristics may all be relevant in affecting the efficacy of risk-reducing interventions involving nutrients and related substances. Further research, drawing upon newer tools now available through the field of nutritional genomics, will be needed to gain greater clarity on the heterogeneous biologic effects observed in nutrient-based risk reduction.

# ANTI-INFLAMMATORY DRUGS

## Mechanism

Nonsteroidal anti-inflammatory drugs (NSAIDs) represent a class of drugs that reduce cellular inflammation through multiple mechanisms, the most prominent of them being the modulation of eicosanoid metabolism.[128] Eicosanoids are metabolites of dietary fatty acids, primarily linoleic acid. Linoleic acid is metabolized to arachidonic acid, which is stored in the lipid membrane and, once mobilized from the membrane, further metabolized by prostaglandin-H synthases (PGHS) 1 and 2 to $PGD_2$, $PGE_2$, $PGF_{2\alpha}$, $PGI_2$, or thromboxane $A_2$ ($TxA_2$) by specific synthases. Leukotriene pathways involve the conversion of arachidonic acid to leukotriene $A_4$ by 5-lipoxygenase and subsequent hydrolysis of leukotriene $A_4$ to other downstream leukotrienes. Newly formed prostaglandins function primarily through binding to prostaglandin receptors (EP receptors), releasing coupled G-proteins to elicit responses in the same or neighboring cells.[129]

Prostaglandins (PG) play crucial roles in controlling cellular proliferation, apoptosis, cellular invasiveness, and angiogenesis and in modulating immunosuppression.[129] Because $PGE_2$ is the most abundant PG in tumors, reducing local concentrations of $PGE_2$ may be a pivotal cancer preventive strategy.[129]

PGHS-independent mechanisms of NSAID action may, at least in part, explain NSAID preventive efficacy.[130] A diverse group of NSAIDs inhibit apoptosis via multiple mechanisms. Among the more prominent of these mechanisms is the inhibition of cyclic guanosine monophosphate (cGMP) phosphodiesterase activity, attenuation of beta-catenin mRNA through suppressing transcription of the *CTNNB1* gene, and activation of c-Jun N-terminal kinase 1.[130] NSAIDs activate peroxisome proliferator–activated receptor (PPAR)γ, leading to increased E-cadherin

expression and reduced colony formation in vitro, while reducing PPARδ, leading to reduced resistance to apoptosis.[130] Selective cyclooxygenase 2 (COX-2) inhibitors inhibit Akt signaling and induce apoptosis of human colorectal and prostate cancer cells in vitro in a COX-2–independent manner via the inhibition of phosphoinositide-dependent kinase-1 (PDK-1). NSAIDs inhibit nuclear factor kappa B (NF-κB) at pharmacologic concentrations and key cellular proliferation signaling intermediates such as activator protein 1 (AP-1) and other intermediates of the MAPK pathway.[130] The impact of NSAIDs on carcinogenic events driven by these upstream pathways in humans as opposed to preliminary in vitro or in vivo models remains unclear.

## Epidemiology

Pooled analyses of 34 controlled trials of aspirin 75 mg to 100 mg daily (69,224 participants), conducted primarily for cardiovascular disease reduction, observed reduced cancer deaths (OR, 0.63; 95% CI, 0.49 to 0.82). Most of the benefit occurred after 5 years follow-up.[131] In a pooled analysis of 150 case control and 45 cohort studies, in addition to a reduced risk of death from colorectal cancer (OR, 0.58; 95% CI, 0.44 to 0.78), chronic and frequent (once daily or more) use of aspirin also reduced the risk of death from esophageal (OR, 0.58; 95% CI, 0.44 to 0.76), gastric (OR, 0.61; 95% CI, 0.40 to 0.93), and breast (OR, 0.81; 95% CI, 0.72 to 0.93) cancers.[132] An analysis of 662,624 men and women enrolled in the American Cancer Society's Cancer Prevention Study II found that aspirin taken at least 16 times per month over a 6-year period conferred a 40% reduced risk of colorectal cancer mortality.[133] Both the 46,363 male patients of the Health Professional Study[134] and the 82,911 patients of the Nurse's Health Study[135] suggest that prolonged use (>10 years) of 325 mg of aspirin twice weekly or more reduces colorectal cancer risk (RR, 0.77; 95% CI, 0.67 to 0.88, from the Nurse's Health Study). Daily NSAID intake is associated with a 40% reduction (OR, 0.56; 95% CI, 0.43 to 0.73) in the risk of esophageal adenocarcinoma.[136]

## Evidence in Preclinical In Vivo Carcinogenesis Models

NSAIDs, including aspirin, indomethacin, piroxicam, sulindac, ibuprofen, and ketoprofen, suppress colonic tumorigenesis induced chemically (1,2-dimethylhydrazine or its metabolites) or transgenically ($Min^+$).[137,138] The selective COX-2 inhibitors were the most efficacious colon tumorigenesis inhibitors in both chemical and transgenic rodent models.[139,140] In preclinical models, NSAIDs affect the onset and progression of cancers in the stomach, skin, breast, lung, prostate, and urinary bladder, although the evidence is more limited than for colon cancers.[141]

## Clinical Trials

Key clinical trials of NSAIDs for the prevention of colorectal cancer are summarized in Table 33.7. Sulindac reduced the size and number of preexisting adenomas in patients with familial adenomatous polyposis but did not suppress the development of new adenomas,[142] whereas the selective COX-2 inhibitor, celecoxib, suppressed the development of new adenomatous polyps in patients with familial adenomatous polyposis.[143] Although these results are promising, reports of invasive neoplasms developing in familial adenomatous polyposis patients being treated with sulindac[144] raise the question of whether NSAIDs preferentially alter the formation or regression of those adenomas less likely to progress to invasive adenocarcinomas, as compared to those more likely to progress.

Randomized, double-blinded placebo controlled trials of NSAIDs as cancer risk–reducing agents for colorectal adenocarcinoma (see Table 33.7) have confirmed that aspirin suppresses

**TABLE 33.7**

### Summary of Clinical Trials of Nonsteroidal Anti-Inflammatory Drugs as Colorectal Cancer Risk–Reducing Agents

| Population | Drug (Dose), Duration | Phase | Endpoint | Outcome | References |
|---|---|---|---|---|---|
| *Gene Associated* | | | | | |
| Familial adenomatous polyposis (FAP) | Sulindac (300–400 mg/d, divided doses) | IIb | Polyp regression | Colorectal and duodenal polyps regressed in ~50% | (277, 278) (279) |
| Hereditary nonpolyposis colon cancer (Lynch syndrome) | Aspirin 600 mg/d, resistant starch | III | Cancer | ≥2 yr, hazard ratio (HR) colon cancer 0.41; 95% CI, 0.19–0.86; all cancers Incidence rate ratio 0.37; 95% CI, 0.18–0.78; no effect of starch | (280, 281) |
| *Sporadic Risk* | | | | | |
| Previous adenomatous polyps, healthy subjects | Aspirin (40, 81, 325, 650 mg once per day) | I, IIa | Dose-biomarker | Aspirin dose of 81 mg daily sufficient to suppress colorectal mucosal prostaglandin $E_2$ | (282–284) |
| Previous adenomatous polyps | Sulindac (300 mg), 4 mos | IIb | Polyp regression | Sulindac did not significantly decrease the number or size of polyps | (146) |
| Previous adenomatous polyps | Piroxicam (7.5 mg), 2 yr | IIb | Polyp recurrence | Colorectal mucosal $PGE_2$ reduced in piroxicam treated arm, unacceptable toxicity | (145) |
| Prior colorectal cancer | Aspirin (325 mg once per day), 3 yr | IIb | Polyp recurrence | Aspirin use associated with delayed development of adenomatous polyps | (285) |
| Previous adenomatous polyps | Aspirin (81 mg once per day or 325 mg once per day) and/or folate, 3 yr | IIb | Polyp recurrence | Low-dose aspirin reduced the recurrence of adenomatous polyps | (286) |
| Previous adenomatous polyps | Celecoxib and rofecoxib | IIb | Polyp recurrence | Celecoxib and rofecoxib reduced the recurrence of adenomatous polyps, unacceptable toxicity | (148–150) |

adenoma recurrence in patients previously treated for adenomas or for cancer. Neither sulindac nor piroxicam alone suppressed adenoma formation in high-risk, sporadic populations at tolerable doses.[145,146] Sulindac, in combination with difluoromethylornithine, has potent colorectal anticarcinogenesis effects.[147] Selective COX-2 inhibitors (celecoxib, rofecoxib) reduce the recurrence of adenomas by one-third in all patients previously treated for adenomas and by one-half in patients with previously resected large (≥1 cm) adenomas,[148–150] but they are too toxic as cancer risk–reducing agents due to their cardiovascular toxicity.[151,152] Although most NSAIDs (piroxicam, indomethacin) have sufficient gastrointestinal (GI) toxicity to reduce their acceptability as cancer risk–reducing agents,[153,154] the long-term administration of low-dose aspirin in vascular prevention trials demonstrates acceptable GI toxicity.[155]

Up to 40% of individuals screened for colorectal neoplasms will have an adenomatous polyp detected and removed, yet only 10% of these lesions will progress to invasive neoplasms. To date, prospective NSAID trials of only 2 to 3 years cannot substitute for cancer incidence or mortality end points. Given the 10-year latency between adenoma formation and a cancer event, prospective trials sufficiently powered to detect colorectal cancer incidence end points are unlikely in the future.[156] Alternatively, a follow-up of patients randomized on trials of aspirin in the prevention of vascular events in the 1980s and 1990s offers secondary analysis opportunities. In a pooled analysis of three prospective vascular end point cohort studies, 20-year low-dose aspirin treatments reduced cancer deaths from all solid tumors (OR, 0.69; CI, 0.54 to 0.88) and from lung and esophageal adenocarcinomas (OR, 0.66; CI, 0.56 to 0.77).[155] Despite this, the U.S. Preventive Services Task Force (USPSTF) does not recommend the use of aspirin or NSAIDs as cancer risk–reducing agents for normal risk populations, preferring adherence to colorectal cancer screening recommendations (fecal occult blood testing and endoscopy).[153,154,157]

Minimal prospective cancer risk reduction data are available at other epithelial organ sites. Ketorolac, given as a 1% rinse solution, did not reduce the size or histology of leukoplakia lesions.[158] Celecoxib reduces the Ki67 labeling index and increases the expression of nuclear survivin without significantly changing the cytoplasmic survivin in bronchial biopsies of smokers.[159] Cancer prevention trials of aspirin as interventions for delaying progression from intraepithelial neoplasias in other epithelial sites remain ongoing for the lower esophagus.[136] No prospective, randomized trials or data are available for breast, prostate, or gynecologic cancer prevention.

## EPIGENETIC TARGETING AGENTS (SELECTIVE ESTROGEN RECEPTOR MODULATORS, 5α-STEROID REDUCTASE INHIBITORS, POLYAMINE INHIBITORS)

Posttranslational pathway targets remain a fertile source of chemopreventive strategies. Phase III data support cancer risk–reduction agent efficacy of selective estrogen receptor modulators (SERM) and 5α-steroid reductase inhibitors for breast and prostate cancer prevention, respectively. Inhibitors of the polyamine pathway may be useful preventives for colorectal cancer.

### Selective Estrogen Receptor Modulators

#### Mechanism

SERMs function as estrogen receptor (ER) agonists and antagonists depending on the SERM structure and target tissue. Predominant ERα receptors occur in the human uterus, cortical bone, and the liver; whereas predominant ERβ receptors occur in blood vessels, cancellous bone, the whole brain, and immune cells.[160,161] During carcinogenesis, the amount of ERα increases while the amount of ERβ decreases in breast tissues.[162] Ideally, a desirable SERM for cancer prevention will function as an antiestrogen in the breast and uterus, but a partial estrogen agonist in skeletal, cardiovascular, central nervous system (CNS), GI tract, and vaginal tissues. In addition, an ideal SERM will not have procoagulant effects and will not cause perimenopausal symptoms such as hot flashes.[162]

Tamoxifen. Tamoxifen is a triphenylethylene compound developed for the treatment of ER-positive breast cancer in the 1960s and 1970s.[163,164] Tamoxifen inhibits the initiation and promotion phases of breast carcinogenesis in the dimethylbenzanthracene chemical carcinogenesis model.[164,165] When tamoxifen binds to ERβ, which then binds to an AP-1 type gene promoter, it functions as an estrogen agonist. When bound to ERα, which binds to an estrogen response element (ERE) target gene promoter, tamoxifen functions as an estrogen antagonist.[162,166] Tamoxifen has estrogen antagonist effects in the human breast; partial estrogen agonist effects in bone, the cardiovascular system, and CNS; and predominant estrogen agonist effects in the uterus, liver, and vagina. The estrogen agonist effects in the liver and uterus result in tamoxifen's toxicities of thromboembolism and endometrial cancer, respectively. The clinical finding that tamoxifen reduces the incidence of contralateral second primary breast cancers during adjuvant treatment regimens catalyzed the push for its development as a cancer risk–reduction agent.[167,168]

Raloxifene. The benzothiophene structure of raloxifene confers a different tissue-specific ER-binding profile than the triphenylethylene tamoxifen. Raloxifene has greater estrogen agonist activity in bone but reduced estrogen agonist activity in the uterus. Raloxifene was studied for the treatment and prevention of osteoporosis in a large, pivotal trial (the Multiple Outcomes of Raloxifene Evaluation [MORE]) and was found to reduce the rate of vertebral fracture as compared to placebo in postmenopausal women.[169]

Lasofoxifene and Arzoxifene. Lasofoxifene and arzoxifene are third-generation SERMs developed as more potent blockers of bone resorption with the goal of reducing the risk of fractures, breast cancer, and heart disease while minimizing the SERM-induced risk of endometrial hyperplasia in postmenopausal women. Both agents proved potent in vitro and in preliminary clinical trials for bone fracture prevention.[170–173]

## Selective Estrogen Receptor Modulators as Risk-Reducing Agents for Breast Cancer Prevention

Efficacy. Table 33.8 summarizes the phase III data for SERM-based breast cancer–risk reduction. In a systematic review of MEDLINE and Cochrane databases through December, 2012, the USPSTF identified seven trials of tamoxifen or raloxifene that showed a reduced incidence of invasive breast cancer by 7 to 9 cases in 1,000 women over 5 years compared to placebo.[174] Tamoxifen is more effective than raloxifene; it reduces breast cancer incidence more than raloxifene by 5 cases in 1,000 women. Both drugs reduce the incidence of ER-positive breast cancer, but neither reduces the risk of ER-negative breast cancer. Neither drug reduced breast cancer–specific or all cause mortality rates. Based on benefit–risk models, women with estimated 5-year risks of breast cancer of 3% or greater are likely to benefit from treatment.[175] Using similar

---

### TABLE 33.8

**Phase III, Randomized, Controlled Clinical Trials of SERMs for the Prevention of Breast Cancer**

| Study | Drug and Daily Dose | N = | Treatment Duration (Years) | Entry Criteria | Overall Outcome HR (95% CI) | References |
|---|---|---|---|---|---|---|
| NSABP P-1 | Tamoxifen 20 mg Placebo | 13,388 | 5 | Gail model: 5 yr predicted risk of ≥1.66% | 0.52 (0.42–0.64) | (28,287) |
| IBIS-I | Tamoxifen 20 mg Placebo | 7,139 | 5 | >Twofold relative risk | 0.72 (0.58–0.90) | (288) |
| Marsden | Tamoxifen 20 mg Placebo | 2,471 | 8 | Family history | 0.87 (0.63–1.21) | (289) |
| Italian | Tamoxifen 20 mg Placebo | 5,408 | 5 | Normal risk, hysterectomy | 0.67 (0.59–0.76) | (290) |
| NSABP P-2 (STAR) | Raloxifene 60 mg Tamoxifen 20 mg | 19,747 | 5 | Gail model: 5 yr predicted risk of ≥1.66% | RR Raloxifene versus tamoxifen 1.02 (0.81–1.28) | (29) |
| MORE/CORE | Raloxifene 60 mg Placebo Raloxifene 120 mg Placebo | 7,705 6,511 | 5 | Normal risk, postmenopausal with osteoporosis | 0.42 (0.29–0.60) | (291,292) |
| RUTH | Raloxifene 60 mg Placebo | 10,101 | 5 | Normal risk, postmenopausal with risk of coronary heart disease | 0.67(0.47–0.96) | (179) |
| PEARL | Lasofoxifene 0.5 mg Lasofoxifene 0.25 mg Placebo | 8,856 | 5 | Normal risk, postmenopausal, with osteoporosis | 0.25 mg: 0.82 (0.45–1.49) 0.5 mg: 0.21 (0.05–0.55) | (170) |
| GENERATIONS | Arzoxifene 20 mg Placebo | 9,354 | 4 | Normal risk, postmenopausal, with osteoporosis | 0.42 (0.25–0.68) | (172) |

Table and data adapted from Cuzick J, Sestak I, Bonanni B, et al. Selective oestrogen-receptor modulators in prevention of breast cancer: an updated meta-analysis of individual participant data. *Lancet* 2013;381:1827–1834.

analysis methods as the USPSTF, the American Society of Clinical Oncology recommends the use of tamoxifen (20 mg per day orally for 5 years) or raloxifene (60 mg per day orally for 5 years) "in premenopausal women who are age ≥35 years with a 5-year projected absolute breast cancer risk ≥1.66% according to the NCI Breast Cancer Risk Assessment Tool (or equivalent measures), or with lobular carcinoma in situ."[176] Tamoxifen reduces the risk of in situ (preinvasive) breast neoplasms (lobular carcinoma in situ, ductal carcinoma in situ) by 50%.[177,178] The reduction during treatment persists for at least 5 years after treatment.[177,178] Raloxifene does not reduce the risk of in situ breast neoplasms.

Data from two trials designed to evaluate the safety and efficacy of lasofoxifene (PEARL)[170,171] and arzoxifene (GENERATIONS)[172,173] as bone fracture preventives have been analyzed for breast cancer–risk reduction. Their effect at reducing breast cancer incidence was captured in secondary analyses (see Table 33.8). Neither lasofoxifene nor arzoxifene have been evaluated in phase III randomized controlled breast cancer prevention trials. Arzoxifene development has been discontinued in the United States.

Toxicity Profiles. Tamoxifen causes a twofold increase in the risk of endometrial adenocarcinoma (RR, 2.13; 95% CI, 1.36 to 3.32) and is related to more benign gynecologic conditions, uterine bleeding, and surgical procedures than the placebo controls, whereas raloxifene did not increase the risk for endometrial cancer or uterine bleeding.[174] Tamoxifen causes a twofold increase in thromboembolic events (RR, 1.93; 95% CI, 1.41 to 2.64), whereas raloxifene causes a 60% increase in risk of venous thromboembolism (RR, 1.60; 95% CI, 1.15 to 2.23).[174] Raloxifene does not differ from tamoxifen in risk of fractures, other cancers, or cardiovascular events.[177] Raloxifene's lower risk of endometrial adenocarcinomas compared to tamoxifen needs to be weighed against the increased risk of stroke seen in in the MORE/CORE trials (see Table 33.8).[179] Raloxifene's effectiveness in the community may also be compromised by its poor bioavailability (2%) due to rapid phase II enzyme metabolism in the gut and liver,[180] whereas tamoxifen is more bioavailable and has active metabolites that permit a prolonged drug effect. Missed raloxifene doses may potentially compromise efficacy and prevention outcomes in widespread, community use.

Aromatase Inhibitors. In adjuvant clinical trials for breast cancer, aromatase inhibitors (anastrozole, exemestane, letrozole) given after 5 years of tamoxifen enhance the reduction of breast cancer recurrence in the contralateral breast compared to tamoxifen alone.[181] In a phase I cancer risk–reducing agent trial, letrozole reduced the Ki-67 proliferation index of breast epithelial cells aspirated from high-risk women.[182] Exemestane reduced the overall risk of ER-positive invasive breast cancer (Table 33.9). It did not reduce the risk of noninvasive breast neoplasms or ER-negative breast cancer.[183] Exemestane has no increased risk of venous thromboembolism, endometrial cancer, fracture, or cataract,[183] but losses in bone mineral density and cortical thickness of the distal tibia and radius occurred after 2 years of treatment despite calcium and vitamin D supplementation.[184] The results of the

International Breast Cancer Intervention Study II (IBIS-II), comparing anastrozole with placebo, are similar to those reported for exemestane.[185] Compared to exemestane, anastrozole decreases the incidence of ductal carcinoma in situ (DCIS), whereas exemestane does not. Neither aromatase inhibitor increased survival compared to placebo controls. The American Society of Clinical Oncology recommends exemestane for breast cancer prevention in addition to tamoxifen and raloxifene.

Use Counseling. Despite the widespread evidence of breast cancer preventive efficacy for tamoxifen and raloxifene, only 3% to 20% of eligible high-risk women agree to take tamoxifen for primary prevention.[186] The low willingness of eligible women to take tamoxifen for 5 years demonstrates the issue of risk benefit for cancer risk–reducing agents. Women with high short-term risk (5 year Gail risk of >3%)—for example, those with ER-positive atypical hyperplasia, lobular carcinoma in situ, and the majority of non–high-grade ductal carcinoma in situ lesions—have an acceptable risk to benefit ratio and are the most likely to benefit from a 5-year cancer risk–reducing agent intervention with a SERM.[175,176] The toxicity profile of aromatase inhibitors differs from SERMs. Although aromatase inhibitors may have a more favorable risk to benefit profile than SERMs, long-term outcomes and toxicity experience for aromatase inhibitor risk-reducing agent intervention are not available to date. In the National Surgical Adjuvant Breast and Bowel Project, tamoxifen-treated women with a *BRCA2* mutation but not a *BRCA1* mutation had reduced cancer incidence,[187] but subsequent data from another group have found reduced cancer risk in women with both BRCA mutations.[188] Data remain insufficient to recommend the use of SERMs for risk reduction in women with BRCA mutations.

## 5α-Steroid Reductase Inhibitors

### Mechanism

Prostate cancers require androgens to proliferate and evade apoptosis. The primary nuclear androgen responsible for the maintenance of epithelial function is dihydrotestosterone. The testes and adrenal gland synthesize dihydrotestosterone by the conversion of testosterone by 5α-steroid reductase types 1 and 2 isozymes. Dihydrotestosterone binds to intracellular androgen receptors to form a complex that binds to DNA hormone response elements controlling cellular proliferation and apoptosis. Finasteride, a selective, competitive inhibitor of type 2 5α-steroid reductase,[189] inhibits proliferation in the transformed prostate cell. In the 3,2'-dimethyl-4-aminobiphenyl (DMAB), methylnitrosourea (MNU), and testosterone chemical carcinogenesis models in rats, finasteride reduces prostate tumor incidence by close to six-fold. Finasteride appears to be more effective in the promotion phase of prostate carcinogenesis.[190] Dutasteride inhibits both 5α-steroid reductase inhibitor[190] types 1 and 2 isoforms and has similar anticarcinogenesis activity in preclinical models to finasteride.

## TABLE 33.9

**Phase III, Randomized, Controlled Clinical Trials of Aromatase Inhibitors for the Prevention of Breast Cancer**

| Study | Drug and Daily Dose | N = | Treatment Duration (Years) | Entry Criteria | Overall Outcome HR (95% CI) | References |
|---|---|---|---|---|---|---|
| MAP.3 | Exemestane 25 mg Placebo | 4,560 | 5 | Gail model 5 yr predicted risk of ≥2.3% | 0.35 (0.18–0.70) | (183) |
| IBIS-II | Anastrozole 1 mg Placebo | 3,851 | 5 | RR twofold higher than general population or Tyrer-Cuzick 10-yr risk >5% | 0.47 (0.32–0.68) | (185) |

TABLE 33.10

**Phase III, Randomized, Controlled Clinical Trials of 5α-Steroid Reductase Inhibitors for the Prevention of Prostate Cancer**

| Study | Drug and Daily Dose | N = | Treatment Duration (Years) | Entry Criteria | Overall Outcome HR (95% CI) | References |
|---|---|---|---|---|---|---|
| PCPT | Finasteride 5 mg Placebo | 18,880 | 7 | Age ≥55 y, PSA ≤3 ng/mL | 0.70 (0.65–0.76) | (30, 193) |
| REDUCE | Dutaseride 0.5 mg Placebo | 6,729 | 4 | Age 50–75 y, PSA 2.5–10.0 ng/mL, core biopsies within 6 mos | RR = 0.77 (0.70–0.85) | (192) |

PSA, prostate specific antigen.

## Cancer Risk–Reducing Agent Activity

Randomized, placebo-controlled cancer incidence end point risk-reducing agent clinical trials demonstrated that finasteride and dutasteride reduced the incidence of prostate cancer by approximately 22% (Table 33.10).[30,191,192] Patients who are treated with either drug yet progress to transformed neoplasms develop more tumors of a high Gleason grade (7 to 10) compared to the placebo arm (22%). After 18 years of follow-up, no significant differences in overall survival or survival after prostate cancer diagnosis were found in the finasteride-treated group compared to the placebo-treated group.[193] Sexual function side effects (e.g., erectile dysfunction, loss of libido, gynecomastia) were more common in the finasteride- or dutasteride-treated groups.[30,192]

The 5α-steroid reductase inhibitors, finasteride and dutasteride, prevent or delay carcinogenesis progression in the prostate, yet progression of high-grade lesions is unaffected. Use of finasteride for a period of 7 years reduced the incidence of prostate cancer but did not significantly affect mortality.[193] Increasing the diagnosis of low-grade prostate cancer through prostate-specific antigen (PSA) testing or intervention with a drug with a minimal toxicity profile without reducing mortality is of no benefit and "all forms of therapy cause considerable burden to the patient and to society."[193]

# SIGNAL TRANSDUCTION MODIFIERS

Both cancer therapy and cancer prevention have investigated drugs that modify specific targets in signal transduction pathways. Although the emphasis in drug development has focused on cancer treatment, interventions aimed at modulating signal transduction pathways promise new approaches to interventions in the carcinogenic process. Because of the complexity of signaling systems, the inhibition of single targets may not be effective or may cause unacceptable toxicity.

## Difluoromethylornithine

### Mechanism

Polyamines (spermidine, spermine, and the diamine, putrescine) are required to maintain cellular growth and function.[194] In mammalian cells, polyamine inhibition by genetic mutation or pharmaceutical agents is associated with virtual cessation in cellular growth. Difluoromethylornithine (DFMO) is an enzyme-activated irreversible inhibitor of ornithine decarboxylase (which is trans-activated by the c-MYC oncogene and cooperates with the RAS oncogene in malignant transformation).[195]

### Evidence in Preclinical In Vivo Carcinogenesis Models

Extensive preclinical data has found that DFMO prevents tumor promotion in a variety of systems, including skin, mammary, colon, cervical, and bladder carcinogenesis models.[194] Synergistic

or additive activity with retinoids, butylated hydroxyanisole, tamoxifen, piroxicam, and fish oil has been demonstrated with low concentrations of DFMO.[194]

### Clinical Trials

In phase I prevention trials, DFMO at a dose of 0.5 mg/m$^2$ per day reduced tissue polyamines in the colon and skin[196,197] and causes regression of cervical intraepithelial neoplasia when used topically,[198] but does not reduce tissue polyamines or other biomarkers of cellular proliferation in the human breast.[199] As a single agent, DFMO has anticarcinogenic activity for nonmelanoma skin cancers, primarily basal cell carcinoma. In combination with an NSAID (sulindac), DFMO reduced adenoma recurrences, suggesting a synergistic reduction of colorectal cancer risk (Table 33.11). Preliminary data suggest some cancer risk–reducing agent activity for the lower esophagus and the prostate (see Table 33.11).[200]

## Statins

### Mechanism

Statins are hydroxyl-3-methylglutaryl coenzyme A (HMG-CoA) reductase inhibitors that inhibit the conversion of HMG-CoA to mevalonate, a cholesterol precursor. The statins are a class of medications with similar structures but with variable moieties that can result in hydrophilic forms (e.g., pravastatin, rosuvastatin) and lipophilic forms (e.g., lovastatin, simvastatin, fluvastatin, atorvastatin).[201] Statins decrease the risk of cancer in preclinical studies by inhibiting RAS- and RHO-mediated cell proliferation, upregulating cell cycle inhibitors (e.g., p21 and p27), and inducing apoptosis of transformed cells and the inhibition of angiogenesis.[202]

### Evidence in Preclinical In Vivo Carcinogenesis Models

Lipophilic statins delay progression of pancreatic intraepithelial neoplasias and the growth of pancreatic carcinoma xenografts. Atorvastatin alone and in combination with NSAIDs reduced colonic adenoma and adenocarcinoma incidence and multiplicity by half in rodent transgenic and chemical carcinogenesis models. Lovastatin reduced lung adenoma multiplicity but not incidence.[201]

### Clinical Trials

Although several large trials of pravastatin or simvastatin on cardiovascular disease risk with cancer as secondary end points have shown no benefit for reducing cancer risk with follow-ups between 18 months to 4 years, these trials were not adequately powered to examine cancer end points.[201] Several case control studies evaluating statin effects have shown a significant association with lower risk of colorectal adenocarcinoma with odds ratios ranging from 0.53 to 0.91 for arzoxifene. A secondary analysis of a celecoxib prevention trial demonstrated no statin protection against colorectal

**TABLE 33.11**

### Summary of Clinical Trials of Difluoromethylornithine as a Cancer Risk–Reducing Agent

| Population | Dose per Day, Duration | Phase | Endpoint | Outcome | References |
|---|---|---|---|---|---|
| Low risk bladder cancer (Ta. T1. Grades 1 or 2) | 1 gm versus placebo × 1 year | III | Bladder cancer recurrence | Did not prevent or delay recurrence | (293) |
| Prostate risk: men with family history prostate cancer, age 35–70 yr | 500 mg versus placebo × 1 yr | IIb | Prostate volume, polyamines, PSA | 10-fold reduction of prostate size increase over 1 yr compared to placebo, PSA reduction not significant | (294) |
| Nonmelanoma skin cancer | 500 mg/m² versus placebo × 4–5 y | III | New nonmelanoma skin cancers | Lower rate of basal cell carcinomas per year (0.28 versus 0.40); persistent reduction in nonmelanoma skin cancers, not statistically significant | (295, 296) |
| Colon adenomas | DFMO: 500 mg Sulindac: 150 mg versus placebo × 3 y | IIb | Adenoma recurrence | RR for adenoma recurrence for DFMO/sulindac treatment 5 0.30 (0.18–0.49) | (147) |

PSA, prostate specific antigen.

neoplasms.[203] The Women's Health Initiative (prospective longitudinal cohort of 159,319 women) found that lovastatin was associated with a lower risk of developing colorectal cancer (HR = 0.62; 95% CI, 0.39 to 0.99).[204] Prospective longitudinal studies have shown mixed results. The PHS reported statin use was inversely associated with prostate cancer (adjusted RR, 0.51),[205] whereas the Nurse's Health Study showed no association with risk of breast cancer.[206] Interventional trials to determine statin preventive efficacy for colon and breast cancer are ongoing.[201] Statins may be effective risk-reducing agents in individuals with the A/A variant of the predominant T/T genotype of rs12654264 of the HMG-CoA reductase gene.[207]

## Bisphosphonates

### Mechanism

Bisphosphonates are pyrophosphate analogs with a central phosphorus-carbon-phosphorus bond that resists bone degradation preventing bone loss and fractures. Second- and third-generation amino bisphosphonates (pamidronic, alendronic, risedronic, ibandronic, and zoledronic acids) inhibit farnesyl diphosphate synthase downstream of HMG-CoA reductase, leading to decreased posttranslational prenylation of GTP-binding proteins such as RAS and Rho. Amino bisphosphonates inhibit cell proliferation, angiogenesis, and cell cycle arrest while inducing apoptosis.[201]

### Evidence in In Vivo Preclinical and Clinical Models

HER2-transgenic mice treated with zoledronic acid had increased tumor-free survival and overall survival. Zoledronic acid suppressed bone, lung, and liver metastases when treated prior to an injection of breast cancer cells.[201] The short-term use of bisphosphonates is associated with reduced breast cancer incidence in case control studies[208,209] and prospective cohort studies (HR = 0.68; 95% CI, 0.52 to 0.88 in a prospective cohort study).[210] Randomized trials of amino-bisphosphonates in postmenopausal women with breast cancer treated for 1 year have found a reduction of breast cancer risk in the contralateral breast (HR = 0.39; 95% CI, 0.18 to 0.88).[211] Case control data suggesting a bisphosphonate-associated reduction in colorectal cancer risk have not been confirmed by prospective cohort studies (i.e., Women's Health Initiative, Nurse's Health Study).[201]

## Metformin

### Mechanism

Metformin, an oral antidiabetic drug in the biguanide class, is the first-line drug of choice for the treatment of type 2 diabetes.[212] Cancers are more common in diabetics and obese individuals than their normal weight and normoglycemic counterparts, leading to the hypothesis that elevated serum insulin concentrations promote cancer risk.[213,214] Insulin and insulin-like growth factors (IGF1 and 2) stimulate cellular DNA synthesis, proliferation, and tumor growth through phosphoinositide-3 kinase (PI3K), mammalian target of rapamycin (mTOR), and the RAS-MAPK signaling pathways.[213] Metformin activates the adenosine monophosphate-activated protein kinase (AMPK) via LKB1, a protein-threonine kinase that has tumor-suppressor activity.[201] Metformin anticarcinogenesis activity appears to be broad and includes downregulation of erbB-2 and epidermal growth factor receptor (EGFR) expression, inhibiting the phosphorylation of erbB family members, IGF1R, Akt, mTOR, and STAT3 in vivo. Low doses of metformin inhibit the self-renewal/proliferation of cancer stem cells in breast, colon, and pancreatic models.[215,216]

### Evidence in Preclinical In Vivo Carcinogenesis Models

Metformin reduces tobacco carcinogen–induced tumors in mice, and pancreatic premalignant and malignant tumors in hamsters.[201] However, metformin's anticarcinogenic activity appears dependent on the dose and the induced carcinogenesis process. Metformin promoted carcinogenesis in MNU-induced rat breast cancers, MMTV-Neu ER-negative breast cancers, OH-BBN induced bladder cancer, and Min⁺ mouse intestinal tumors using nonobese rodents.[217] Metformin cancer risk–reducing agent effects may be limited to obesity- and diabetes-associated carcinogenesis mechanisms.

### Clinical Trials

Two large retrospective cohort studies have shown that metformin therapy is associated with a reduced risk of solid tumors by 25% to 30%.[201] The Women's Health Imitative observed a lower incidence of invasive breast cancer in metformin-treated women with type 2 diabetes mellitus.[218] Phase II window of opportunity randomized trials have shown reduced proliferation and increased apoptosis in resected tissue of breast cancer patients.[201]

### Diet-Derived Natural Products

#### Mechanism

Polyphenolic phytochemicals, such as curcumin, resveratrol, epigallocatechin gallate (EGCG), genistein, and ginger, are attractive as cancer risk–reducing agents for their low toxicity and multimechanism anticarcinogenic properties. They have anti-inflammatory activity, in part through scavenging of ROS, modulation of protein kinase signal transduction pathways (e.g., STAT-3, HER2/neu, MAPK, and Akt), and downstream inhibition of eicosanoid synthesis potentially due to upstream inhibition of NF-κB and PPAR or direct blockade or inhibition of eicosanoid-metabolizing enzymes.[219–221] Curcumin, and presumably other polyphenolics, downregulate stem cell driver signaling systems Wnt, Hedgehog, and Notch with subsequent reductions of breast, pancreatic, and colonic stem cell self-renewal.[222,223]

Omega-3 fatty acids (derived from marine products) compete with omega-6 fatty acid substrates for eicosanoid-metabolizing enzymes with subsequent tissue reduction of these inflammatory mediators.[224,225] These fatty acids have other diverse anticarcinogenic mechanisms (e.g., G-protein inhibition, changes in membrane physical characteristics that alter transmembrane signaling protein dynamics) that make them attractive as cancer risk–reducing agents.[226,227]

Whole berries, black raspberries, and strawberries contain mixtures of multiple anticarcinogenic compounds such as ellagic acid, anthocyanins, and tocopherols.[228] Research-grade berries are grown in a standardized cultivation environment and assayed for key components to ensure year-to-year reproducibility despite yearly climatologic variation. Berries have potent stabilization of methylation properties in addition to the expected anti-inflammatory and antioxidative properties associated with the prominent components.[229,230]

**Preclinical and Clinical Anticarcinogenesis Efficacy.** Diverse diet-derived natural products have moderate-to-strong anticarcinogenic effects in both chemical and transgenic rodent carcinogenesis models (Table 33.12). Phase I clinical trials of curcumin detected little parent compound in plasma or tissues, raising the possibility of biologically active conjugates or deconjugation at the target site.[231–233] Resveratrol's plasma bioavailability exceeds that of curcumin and ginger, and partitions into human colon tissue at 10-fold concentrations compared to plasma.[219,234,235] No natural products have been studied in large prospective, cancer incidence risk–reduction trials. Using intraepithelial biomarker end points in human phase II trials, berry formulations reduce esophageal dysplasia and oral leukoplakia.[236,237] Curcumin reduces the number of colon aberrant crypt foci in human smokers.[238]

### ANTI-INFECTIVES

Many infectious agents are known causes of human cancers, including the human hepatitis viruses, hepatitis B virus (HBV) and hepatitis C virus (HCV) for hepatocellular carcinoma[239]; *Helicobacter pylori* for gastric adenocarcinoma[240]; human papilloma viruses (HPV) for cervical, anal, vulva, penis, and oral cavity and pharynx carcinomas[241]; herpes virus-8 for Kaposi sarcoma[242]; Epstein-Barr virus for Burkitt and other lymphomas[243]; liver flukes for cholangiocarcinoma[244]; and schistosomes for bladder carcinoma.[245] The success of the HPV vaccine at reducing the incidence of intraepithelial neoplasia of the cervix is one example that demonstrates the potential of immunochemoprevention for epithelial targets for which an etiologic agent can be identified.

### *Helicobacter pylori*

Intestinal-type gastric adenocarcinoma arises through a multistep process that begins with chronic gastritis initiated by *H. pylori*, progressing through gastric mucosal atrophy, intestinal metaplasia to dysplasia, and ultimately, to adenocarcinoma.[246] *H. pylori* infects 50% of the world's population.[240] Infection occurs early in life, remains quiescent, and may be associated with chronic gastritis of variable intensity but with minimal symptoms. Although the majority of *H. pylori* organisms remain in the gastric mucous layer, 10% adhere to the gastric mucosa through adhesion *BabA*, an outer membrane protein that binds to the Lewis-B histo-blood group antigen.[240] Progression to atrophic gastritis and peptic ulcer disease (occurs in 10% to 15% of infected individuals) requires other bacterial and host cofactors.[245,246] Infection with *H. pylori* is associated with an OR of 2.7 to 6.0 for gastric cancer; *CagA* increases this risk by 20- to 40-fold. The risk of developing gastric adenocarcinoma with an *H. pylori* infection is estimated to be 1% to 3%.[245,246]

The eradication of *H. pylori* with antibiotics and anti-inflammatory agents—for example, amoxicillin, metronidazole, and bismuth subsalicylate—increases the rate of regression of nonmetaplastic gastric atrophy and intestinal metaplasia in geographically diverse regions.[247,248] A combination of a 2-week course of a proton pump inhibitor (omeprazole) and an antibiotic (amoxicillin) reduced the risk of gastric cancer in a high-risk population in China (OR = 0.61; (95% CI, 0.36 to 0.96) for 14.7 years after the treatment.[249] The sequence of giving proton pump inhibitors and antibiotic therapy does not alter the treatment outcome. In addition to contributing to gastric cancer risk, *H. pylori* infections may also contribute to pancreatic cancer risk.[250] Because *H. pylori* infections are so widespread, mass eradication campaigns in high-risk regions are being considered.[251] However, complicating this is that *H. pylori* infections have also been associated with a reduced risk of both esophageal adenocarcinoma and gastric cardia carcinoma.[252]

## MULTIAGENT APPROACHES TO CANCER RISK REDUCTION

In the transition to molecularly targeted interventions, combinations of targets that logically address critical carcinogenic pathways may have greater efficacy than single agents. For example, previously demonstrated interactive signaling of EGFRs and COX-2 experiments in Min+ mice[253] demonstrates cancer preventive synergism. Combining atorvastatin with selective or nonselective COX inhibitors enhanced the inhibition of azoxymethane-induced colon carcinogenesis in F344 rats and reduced the dose of the combined drugs required to achieve a reduction of colon carcinogenesis.[254]

DFMO plus sulindac inhibited adenoma formation in a phase IIb trial of 375 patients with a prior history of adenomas followed for 36 months (see Table 33.11).[147] Cardiovascular-adverse outcomes were higher in DFMO/sulindac-treated patients who had preexisting high baseline cardiovascular risk; however, the cardiovascular-adverse events were similar to placebo in moderate or low cardiovascular risk patients.[255] Using IGF-1 as a biomarker, Guerrieri-Gonzaga et al.[256] showed that the combination of low-dose tamoxifen with low-dose fenretinide is safe but not synergistic. As more data accumulate from in vivo models, combined drugs aimed at specific targets in coordinated signaling pathways will enter clinical biomarker-based trials. Optimal doses, toxicity, and biomarker modulation data will select those combinations useful for risk reduction trials and, ultimately, generalized use in at-risk populations.

**TABLE 33.12**

**Selected Diet-Derived Natural Products with Cancer Risk–Reducing Activity**

| Nutritional Extract | Source | Mechanisms | In Vivo Anticarcinogenesis Efficacy | Human Trials | References |
|---|---|---|---|---|---|
| Curcumin ([1E,6E]-1,7-bis-[4-hydroxy-3-methoxyphenyl]-1,6-heptadiene-3,5-dione/ diferuloylmethane) | Turmeric, rhizome of *Curcuma longa* | Inhibits: $PGE_2$ synthesis via direct binding to COX-2 and through inhibition of NF-κB; angiogenesis. ErbB2 transduction; PI3K-Akt transduction; Inhibits stem cell self renewal Agonist: vitamin D receptor | Colon, breast, skin | Phase I: Poor bioavailability due to biotransformation in gut, enterohepatic cycling of metabolites; Phase IIa: reduced aberrant crypt foci | (219, 238) |
| Resveratrol (3,5,4′-trihydroxy-trans-stilbene) | Grapes, mulberries, peanuts, and *Cassia quinquangulata* plants | Inhibits: Carcinogen activation via inhibition of phase I isozyme, eicosanoids via direct binding; NF-κB; Nrf2. Acts as a caloric restriction mimetic, activates the histone deacetylase SIRT1 and AMPK | Colorectal, breast, pancreas, skin, and prostate | Phase I: 1 g dose generated peak concentration ~2 μM, conjugates 10-fold higher; resveratrol tissue concentrations 10-fold higher than plasma; Phase IIa: Small reduction in IGF-1 and IGFBP-1 | (220, 234) |
| Ginger (gingerols, paradols, shagaols) | Rhizome of *Zingiber officinale* | Induces apoptosis via caspase-3 mechanisms; Inhibits NF-κB activation and downstream COX-2 expression; reduces iNOS expression and ornithine decarboxylase activity | Colon, breast, skin, oral cavity, liver | Phase I: 2 g dose nontoxic; Phase IIa: Small reductions in $PGE_2$, increased Bax in upper colon crypt | (235, 297, 298) |
| Green tea (epigallocatechin gallate, other catechins) | Green tea extract | Inhibits: PI3K-Akt transduction, IGF-1, IGFBP-3; NK-κB; catenin reduces methylation via inhibition of DNA methyltransferase 1 | Lung, prostate, skin, colorectal | Phase IIa: 500–1,000 mg/m$^2$ × 12 wk reduced oral premalignant lesions in 50%; Phase IIb: 2.5 g × 1 yr reduced colorectal adenoma recurrence by 50% | (221) |
| Omega-3 fatty acids (eicosapentaenoic acid; docosahexaenoic acid) | Fish oil | Reduction of inflammation via eicosanoid reduction; direct binding to G receptor proteins; PPAR activation; induction of anti-inflammatory lipid mediators (resolvins, protectins, maresins) | Colon, breast, prostate | Phase II: 4–7 mg/d reduced colon adenomas in familial adenomatous polyposis; ongoing trials for sporadic; extensive case control studies | (226, 299) |
| Berries | Black raspberries, strawberries | Reduction of methylation via inhibition of methyltransferases, re-regulated Wnt; inhibits NF-κB; inhibits cyclooxygenases; inhibits proliferation | Esophageal squamous cell, colon, skin | Phase IIb: Freeze dried strawberries reduced esophageal dysplasia; Phase IIa: Blackberry gel reduced leukoplakia | (228, 229, 236, 237) |

IGFBP-1, insulin growth factor binding protein-1; iNOS, inducible isoform of nitric oxide synthase.

# REFERENCES

1. Vogelstein B, Papadopoulos N, Velculescu VE, et al. Cancer genome landscapes. *Science* 2013;339:1546–1558.
2. Fearon ER, Vogelstein B. A genetic model for colorectal tumorigenesis. *Cell* 1990;61:759–767.
3. Sidransky D. Emerging molecular markers of cancer. *Nat Rev Cancer* 2002;2:210–219.
4. Lippman SM, Levin B, Brenner DE, et al. Cancer prevention and the American Society of Clinical Oncology. *J Clin Oncol* 2004;22:3848–3851.
5. Wattenberg L. Chemoprevention of cancer. *Cancer Res* 1985;45:1–8.
6. Greenwald P, Kelloff G. The role of chemoprevention in cancer control. *IARC Scientific Publications (Lyon)* 1996;139:13–22.
7. Hanahan D, Weinberg RA. The hallmarks of cancer. *Cell* 2000;100:57–70.
8. Steele VE, Boone CW, Lubet RA, et al. Preclinical drug development paradigms for chemopreventives. *Hematol Oncol Clin North Am* 1998;12:943–961.
9. Perloff M, Steele VE. Early-phase development of cancer prevention agents: challenges and opportunities. *Cancer Prev Res (Phila)* 2013;6:379–383.
10. National Cancer Institute. PREVENT Cancer Preclinical Drug Development Program. National Cancer Institute Web site. http://prevention.cancer.gov/programs-resources/programs/prevent. Accessed December 7, 2013.
11. Mehta RG, Naithani R, Huma L, et al. Efficacy of chemopreventive agents in mouse mammary gland organ culture (MMOC) model: a comprehensive review. *Curr Med Chem.* 2008;15:2785–2825.
12. Hoenerhoff MJ, Hong HH, Ton TV, et al. A review of the molecular mechanisms of chemically induced neoplasia in rat and mouse models in National Toxicology Program bioassays and their relevance to human cancer. *Toxicol Pathol* 2009;37:835–848.
13. Steele VE, Lubet RA. The use of animal models for cancer chemoprevention drug development. *Semin Oncol* 2010;37:327–338.
14. Shureiqi I, Reddy P, Brenner DE. Chemoprevention: general perspective. *Crit Rev Oncol Hematol* 2000;33:157–167.
15. Becker M. Adherence to prescribed therapies. *Med Care* 1985;23:539–554.
16. Miki Y, Swensen J, Shattuck-Eidens D, et al. A strong candidate for the breast and ovarian cancer susceptibility gene BRCA1. *Science* 1994;266:66–71.
17. Powell SM, Petersen GM, Krush AJ, et al. Molecular diagnosis of familial adenomatous polyposis. *N Engl J Med* 1993;329:1982–1987.
18. Meads C, Ahmed I, Riley RD. A systematic review of breast cancer incidence risk prediction models with meta-analysis of their performance. *Breast Cancer Res Treat* 2012;132:365–377.
19. Kastrinos F, Steyerberg EW, Balmana J, et al. Comparison of the clinical prediction model PREMM(1,2,6) and molecular testing for the systematic identification of Lynch syndrome in colorectal cancer. *Gut* 2013;62:272–279.
20. Ankerst DP, Boeck A, Freedland SJ, et al. Evaluating the PCPT risk calculator in ten international biopsy cohorts: results from the Prostate Biopsy Collaborative Group. *World J Urol* 2012;30:181–187.
21. National Institutes of Health, U.S. Food and Drug Administration. *Biomarkers and Surrogate Endpoints: Advancing Clinical Research and Applications.* Bethesda, MD: National Insitutes of Health; 1999.
22. Schatzkin A, Freedman LS, Schiffman MH, et al. Validation of intermediate end points in cancer research. *J Natl Cancer Inst* 1990;82:1746–1752.
23. Prentice R. Surrogate endpoints in clinical trials: definition and operational criteria. *Statistics Med* 1989;8:431–440.
24. Ransohoff DF. Rules of evidence for cancer molecular-marker discovery and validation. *Nat Rev Cancer* 2004;4:309–314.
25. Pepe MS, Feng Z, Janes H, et al. Pivotal evaluation of the accuracy of a biomarker used for classification or prediction: standards for study design. *J Natl Cancer Inst* 2008;100:1432–1438.
26. Pryor WA, Stahl W, Rock CL. Beta carotene: from biochemistry to clinical trials. *Nutr Rev* 2000;58:39–53.
27. Brenner DE, Hawk E. Trials and tribulations of interrogating biomarkers to define efficacy of cancer risk reductive interventions. *Cancer Prev Res (Phila)* 2013;6:71–73.
28. Fisher B, Costantino J, Wickerham D, et al. Tamoxifen for prevention of breast cancer: report of the National Surgical Adjuvant Breast and Bowel Project P-1 study. *J Natl Cancer Inst* 1998;90:1371–1388.
29. Vogel VG, Costantino JP, Wickerham DL, et al. Update of the National Surgical Adjuvant Breast and Bowel Project Study of Tamoxifen and Raloxifene (STAR) P-2 Trial: Preventing breast cancer. *Cancer Prev Res (Phila)* 2010;3:696–706.
30. Thompson IM, Goodman PJ, Tangen CM, et al. The influence of finasteride on the development of prostate cancer. *N Engl J Med* 2003;349:215–224.
31. Omenn G, Goodman G, Thornquist M, et al. Effects of a combination of beta carotene and vitamin A on lung cancer and cardiovascular disease. *N Engl J Med* 1996;334:1150–1155.
32. Lotan R. Retinoids in cancer chemoprevention. *Faseb J* 1996;10:1031–1039.
33. Tang X-H, Gudas LJ. Retinoids, retinoic acid receptors, and cancer. *Annu Rev Pathol* 2011;6:345–364.
34. Khachik F, Beecher, G, Smith JC Jr. Lutein, lycopene, and their oxidative metabolites in chemoprevention of cancer. *J Cell Biochem* 1995;22:236–246.
35. Di Mascio P, Kaiser S, Sies H. Lycopene as the most efficient biological carotenoid singlet oxygen quencher. *Arch Biochem Biophys* 1989;274:532–538.
36. Eroglu A, Hruszkewycz DP, dela Sena C, et al. Naturally occurring eccentric cleavage products of provitamin A beta-carotene function as antagonists of retinoic acid receptors. *J Biol Chem* 2012;287:15886–15895.
37. Ford NA, Erdman JW Jr. Are lycopene metabolites metabolically active? *Acta Biochim Pol* 2012;59:1–4.
38. World Cancer Research Fund, American Institute for Cancer Research. *Food, Nutrition, Physical Activity, and the Prevention of Cancer: A Global Perspective.* Washington, DC: AICR; 2007.
39. Panel on Dietary Antioxidants and Related Compounds, Subcommittees on Upper Reference Levels of Nutrients and Interpretation and Uses of DRIs, Standing Committee on the Scientific Evaluation of Dietary Reference Intakes, Food and Nutrition Board, Institute of Medicine. *Dietary Reference Intakes for Vitamin C, Vitamin E, Selenium, and Carotenoids.* Washington, DC: National Academy Press; 2000.
40. Moon RC, Mehta RG, Rao KVN. Retinoids and cancer in experimental animals. In: Sporn MB, Roberts AB, Goodman DS, eds., *The Retinoids.* 2nd ed. New York: Raven Press; 1994: 573–595.
41. International Agency for Research on Cancer World Health Organization. *Carotenoids.* Lyon: International Agency for Research on Cancer; 1998.
42. Holzapfel NP, Holzapfel BM, Champ S, et al. The potential role of lycopene for the prevention and therapy of prostate cancer: from molecular mechanisms to clinical evidence. *Int J Mol Sci* 2013;14:14620–14646.
43. Hong WK, Lippman SM, Itri LM, et al. Prevention of second primary tumors with 13cRA in squamous-cell carcinoma of the head and neck. *N Engl J Med* 1990;323:795–801.
44. Benner SE, Pajak TF, Lippman SM, et al. Prevention of second primary tumors with isotretinoin in patients with squamous cell carcinoma of the head and neck: long term follow-up. *J Natl Cancer Inst* 1994;86:140–141.
45. Khuri FR, Lee JJ, Lippman SM, et al. Randomized phase III trial of low-dose isotretinoin for prevention of second primary tumors in stage I and II head and neck cancer patients. *J Natl Cancer Inst* 2006;98:441–450.
46. Bolla M, Lefur R, Ton Van J, et al. Prevention of second primary tumours with etretinate in squamous cell carcinoma of the oral cavity and oropharynx. Results of a multicentric double-blind randomised study. *Eur J Cancer* 1994;30A:767–772.
47. Toma S, Bonelli L, Sartoris A, et al. beta-carotene supplementation in patients radically treated for stage I-II head and neck cancer: results of a randomized trial. *Oncol Rep* 2003;10:1895–1901.
48. Mayne ST, Cartmel B, Baum M, et al. Randomized trial of supplemental beta-carotene to prevent second head and neck cancer. *Cancer Res* 2001;61:1457–1463.
49. Bairati I, Meyer F, Jobin E, et al. Antioxidant vitamins supplementation and mortality: a randomized trial in head and neck cancer patients. *Int J Cancer* 2006;119:2221–2224.
50. McLarty JW, Holiday DB, Girard WM, et al. Beta-carotene, vitamin A and lung cancer chemoprevention: results of an intermediate endpoint study. *Am J Clin Nutr* 1995;62:1431S–1438S.
51. Lee JS, Lippman SM, Benner SE, et al. Randomized placebo-controlled trial of isotretinoin in chemoprevention of bronchial squamous metaplasia. *J Clin Oncol* 1994;12:937–945.
52. The Alpha-Tocopherol Beta Carotene Cancer Prevention Study Group. The effect of vitamin E and beta carotene on the incidence of lung cancer and other cancers in male smokers. *N Engl J Med* 1994;330:1029–1035.
53. Omenn GS, Goodman G, Thornquist M, et al. Chemoprevention of lung cancer: the beta-Carotene and Retinol Efficacy Trial (CARET) in high-risk smokers and asbestos-exposed workers. *IARC Sci Publ* 1996;67–85.
54. Hennekens CH, Buring JE, Manson JE, et al. Lack of effect of long-term supplementation with beta carotene on the incidence of malignant neoplasms and cardiovascular disease. *N Engl J Med* 1996;334:1145–1149.
55. Lee IM, Cook NR, Manson JE, et al. Beta-carotene supplementation and incidence of cancer and cardiovascular disease: the Women's Health Study. *J Natl Cancer Inst* 1999;91:2102–2106.
56. Heart Protection Study Collaborative Group. MRC/BHF Heart Protection Study of antioxidant vitamin supplementation in 20,536 high-risk individuals: a randomised placebo-controlled trial. *Lancet* 2002;360:23–33.
57. van Zandwijk N, Dalesio O, Pastorino U, et al. EUROSCAN, a randomized trial of vitamin A and N-acetylcysteine in patients with head and neck cancer or lung cancer. For the European Organization for Research and Treatment of Cancer Head and Neck and Lung Cancer Cooperative Groups. *J Natl Cancer Inst* 2000;92:977–986.
58. Lippman SM, Lee JJ, Karp DD, et al. Randomized phase III intergroup trial of isotretinoin to prevent second primary tumors in stage I non-small-cell lung cancer. *J Natl Cancer Inst* 2001;93:605–618.
59. Mayne ST, Lippman SM. Cigarettes: a smoking gun in cancer chemoprevention. *J Natl Cancer Inst* 2005;97:1319–1321.
60. Veronesi U, De Palo G, Marubini E, et al. Randomized trial of fenretinide to prevent second breast malignancy in women with early breast cancer. *J Natl Cancer Inst* 1999;91:1847–1856.
61. De Palo G, Mariani L, Camerini T, et al. Effect of fenretinide on ovarian carcinoma occurrence. *Gynecol Oncol* 2002;86:24–27.
62. Uray IP, Brown PH. Chemoprevention of hormone receptor-negative breast cancer: new approaches needed. *Recent Results Cancer Res* 2011;188:147–162.
63. Kraemer KH, DiGiovanna JJ, Moshell AN, et al. Prevention of skin cancer in xeroderma pigmentosum with the use of oral isotretinoin. *N Engl J Med* 1988;318:1633–1637.
64. Bouwes Bavinck JN, Tieben LM, Van Der Woude FJ, et al. Prevention of skin cancer and reduction of keratotic skin lesions during acitretin therapy in renal

transplant recipients: a double-blind, placebo-controlled study. *J Clin Oncol* 1995;13:1933–1938.

65. Tangrea JA, Edwards BK, Taylor PR, et al. Long-term therapy with low-dose isotretinoin for prevention of basal cell carcinoma: a multicenter clinical trial Isotretinoin-Basal Cell Carcinoma Study Group. *J Natl Cancer Inst* 1992;84:328–332.

66. Levine N, Moon TE, Cartmel B, et al. Trial of retinol and isotretinoin in skin cancer prevention: a randomized, double-blind, controlled trial. Southwest Skin Cancer Prevention Study Group. *Cancer Epidemiol Biomarkers Prev* 1997;6:957–961.

67. Moon TE, Levine N, Cartmel B, et al. Effect of retinol in preventing squamous cell skin cancer in moderate-risk subjects: a randomized, double-blind, controlled trial. Southwest Skin Cancer Prevention Study Group. *Cancer Epidemiol Biomarkers Prev* 1997;6:949–956.

68. Greenberg ER, Baron JA, Stukel TA, et al. A clinical trial of beta carotene to prevent basal-cell and squamous-cell cancers of the skin. The Skin Cancer Prevention Study Group. *N Engl J Med* 1990;323:789–895.

69. Green A, Williams G, Neale R, et al. Daily sunscreen application and beta-carotene supplementation in prevention of basal-cell and squamous-cell carcinomas of the skin: a randomised controlled trial. *Lancet* 1999;354:723–729.

70. Clark LC, Combs GF Jr, Turnbull BW, et al. Effects of selenium supplementation for cancer prevention in patients with carcinoma of the skin. A randomized controlled trial. Nutritional Prevention of Cancer Study Group. *JAMA* 1996;276:1957–1963.

71. Duffield-Lillico AJ, Slate EH, Reid ME, et al. Nutritional Prevention of Cancer Study Group. Selenium supplementation and secondary prevention of nonmelanoma skin cancer in a randomized trial. *J Natl Cancer Inst* 2003;95:1477–1481.

72. Sabichi AL, Lerner SP, Atkinson EN, et al. Phase III prevention trial of fenretinide in patients with resected non-muscle-invasive bladder cancer. *Clin Cancer Res* 2008;14:224–229.

73. Lamm DL, Riggs DR, Shriver JS, et al. Megadose vitamins in bladder cancer: a double-blind clinical trial. *J Urol* 1994;151:21–26.

74. Meyskens FL Jr, Surwit E, Moon TE, et al. Enhancement of regression of cervical intraepithelial neoplasia II (moderate dysplasia) with topically applied all-trans-retinoic acid: a randomized trial. *J Natl Cancer Inst* 1994; 86:539–543.

75. Blot WJ, Li JY, Taylor PR, et al. Nutrition intervention trials in Linxian, China: supplementation with specific vitamin/mineral combinations, cancer incidence, and disease-specific mortality in the general population. *J Natl Cancer Inst* 1993;85:1483–1492.

76. Qiao YL, Dawsey SM, Kamangar F, et al. Total and cancer mortality after supplementation with vitamins and minerals: follow-up of the Linxian General Population Nutrition Intervention Trial. *J Natl Cancer Inst* 2009;101:507–518.

77. Mayne ST, Ferrucci LM, Cartmel B. Lessons learned from randomized clinical trials of micronutrient supplementation for cancer prevention. *Annu Rev Nutr* 2012;32:369–390.

78. Li JY, Taylor PR, Li B, et al. Nutrition intervention trials in Linxian, China: multiple vitamin/mineral supplementation, cancer incidence, and disease-specific mortality among adults with esophageal dysplasia. *J Natl Cancer Inst* 1993;85:1492–1498.

79. Kikendall JW, Mobarhan S, Nelson R, et al. Oral beta carotene does not reduce the recurrence of colorectal adenomas [Abstract]. *Am J Gastroenterol* 1991;36:1356.

80. MacLennan R, Macrae F, Bain C, et al. Randomized trial of intake of fat, fiber, and beta carotene to prevent colorectal adenomas. *J Natl Cancer Inst* 1995;87:1760–1766.

81. Greenberg ER, Baron JA, Tosteson TD, et al. A clinical trial of antioxidant vitamins to prevent colorectal adenoma. Polyp Prevention Study Group. *N Engl J Med* 1994;331:141–147.

82. Baron JA, Cole BF, Mott L, et al. Neoplastic and antineoplastic effects of beta-carotene on colorectal adenoma recurrence: results of a randomized trial. *J Natl Cancer Inst* 2003;95:717–722.

83. Heinonen OP, Albanes D, Virtamo J, et al. Prostate cancer and supplementation with alpha-tocopherol and beta-carotene: incidence and mortality in a controlled trial. *J Natl Cancer Inst* 1998;90:440–446.

84. Lippman SM, Klein EA, Goodman PJ, et al. Effect of selenium and vitamin E on risk of prostate cancer and other cancers: the Selenium and Vitamin E Cancer Prevention Trial (SELECT). *JAMA* 2009;301:39–51.

85. Klein EA, Thompson IM Jr, Tangen CM, et al. Vitamin E and the risk of prostate cancer: the Selenium and Vitamin E Cancer Prevention Trial (SELECT). *JAMA* 2011;306:1549–1556.

86. Gaziano JM, Glynn RJ, Christen WG, et al. Vitamins E and C in the prevention of prostate and total cancer in men: the Physicians' Health Study II randomized controlled trial. *JAMA* 2009;301:52–62.

87. Boileau TW, Liao Z, Kim S, et al. Prostate carcinogenesis in N-methyl-N-nitrosourea (NMU)-testosterone-treated rats fed tomato powder, lycopene, or energy-restricted diets. *J Natl Cancer Inst* 2003;95:1578–1586.

88. Goralczyk R. Beta-carotene and lung cancer in smokers: review of hypotheses and status of research. *Nutr Cancer* 2009;61:767–774.

89. Kristal AR, Darke AK, Morris JS, et al. Baseline Selenium Status and Effects of Selenium and Vitamin E Supplementation on Prostate Cancer Risk. *J Natl Cancer Inst* 2014:106:djt456.

90. Stone JR, Yang S. Hydrogen peroxide: a signaling messenger. *Antioxid Redox Signal* 2006;8:243–270.

91. Finkel T. Signal transduction by reactive oxygen species. *J Cell Biol* 2011; 194:7–15.

92. Sayin V, Ibrahim M, Larsson E, et al. Antioxidants accelerate lung cancer progression in mice. *Sci Transl Med* 2014;6:ra15.

93. Mayne ST. Oxidative stress, dietary antioxidant supplements, and health: is the glass half full or half empty? *Cancer Epidemiol Biomarkers Prev* 2013; 22:2145–2147.

94. Duthie SJ, Narayanan S, Blum S, et al. Folate deficiency in vitro induces uracil misincorporation and DNA hypomethylation and inhibits DNA excision repair in immortalized normal human colon epithelial cells. *Nutr Cancer* 2000;37:245–251.

95. Blount BC, Mack MM, Wehr CM, et al. Folate deficiency causes uracil misincorporation into human DNA and chromosome breakage: implications for cancer and neuronal damage. *Proc Natl Acad Sci U S A* 1997;94:3290–3295.

96. Giovannucci E. Epidemiologic studies of folate and colorectal neoplasia: a review. *J Nutr* 2002;132:2350S–2355S.

97. White E, Shannon JS, Patterson RE. Relationship between vitamin and calcium supplement use and colon cancer. *Cancer Epidemiol Biomarkers Prev* 1997;6:769–774.

98. Jacobs EJ, Connell CJ, Patel AV, et al. Multivitamin use and colon cancer mortality in the Cancer Prevention Study II cohort (United States). *Cancer Causes Control* 2001;12:927–934.

99. Gibson TM, Weinstein SJ, Pfeiffer RM, et al. Pre- and postfortification intake of folate and risk of colorectal cancer in a large prospective cohort study in the United States. *Am J Clin Nutr* 2011;94:1053–1062.

100. Chen J, Giovannucci E, Kelsey, K, et al. A methylenetetrahydrofolate reductase polymorphism and the risk of colorectal cancer. *Cancer Res* 1996;56:4862–4864.

101. Larsson S, Giovannucci, E, Wolk A. Vitamin A intake, alcohol consumption, and colorectal cancer: a longitudinal population-based cohort of women. *Gastroenterology* 2005;128:1830–1837.

102. Wei E, Giovannucci E, Selhub J, et al. Plasma vitamin B6 and the risk of colorectal cancer and adenoma in women. *J Natl Cancer Inst* 2005;97:684–692.

103. Giovannucci E, Rimm EB, Ascherio A, et al. Alcohol, low-methionine-low-folate diets, and risk of colon cancer in men. *J Natl Cancer Inst* 1995;87:265–273.

104. Jaszewski R, Misra S, Tobi M, et al. Folic acid supplementation inhibits recurrence of colorectal adenomas: a randomized chemoprevention trial. *World J Gastroenterol* 2008;14:4492–4498.

105. Paspatis GA, Karamanolis DG. Folate supplementation and adenomatous colonic polyps. *Dis Colon Rectum* 1994;37:1340–1341.

106. Cole BF, Baron JA, Sandler RS, et al. Folic acid for the prevention of colorectal adenomas: a randomized clinical trial. *JAMA* 2007;297:2351–2359.

107. Logan RF, Grainge MJ, Shepherd VC, et al. Aspirin and folic acid for the prevention of recurrent colorectal adenomas. *Gastroenterology* 2008;134:29–38.

108. Wu K, Platz EA, Willett WC, et al. A randomized trial on folic acid supplementation and risk of recurrent colorectal adenoma. *Am J Clin Nutr* 2009;90: 1623–1631.

109. Gao Q-Y, Chen H-M, Chen Y-X, et al. Folic acid prevents the initial occurrence of sporadic colorectal adenoma in Chinese older than 50 years of age: a randomized clinical trial. *Cancer prevention research (Phila)* 2013;6:744–752.

110. Ramnath N, Kim S, Christensen PJ. Vitamin D and lung cancer. *Expert Rev Respir Med* 2011;5:305–309.

111. Deeb KK, Trump DL, Johnson CS. Vitamin D signalling pathways in cancer: potential for anticancer therapeutics. *Nat Rev Cancer* 2007;7:684–700.

112. McCullough M, Robertson AS, Rodriguez C, et al. Calcium, vitamin D, dairy products, and risk of colorectal cancer in the cancer prevention study II nutrition cohort (United States). *Cancer Causes Control* 2003;14:1–12.

113. Wu K, Willett WC, Fuchs CS, et al. Calcium intake and risk of colon cancer in women and men. *J Natl Cancer Inst* 2002;94:437–446.

114. Chung M, Balk EM, Brendel M, et al. *Vitamin D and Calcium: A Systematic Review of Health Outcomes.* Evidence Report No. 183 (Prepared by the Tufts Evidence-based Practice Center). Rockville, MD: Agency for Healthcare Research and Quality; 2009.

115. World Health Organization, International Agency for Research on Cancer. Vitamin D and Cancer. Working Group Reports, Volume 5. Lyon, France: IARC; 2008.

116. Stolzenberg-Solomon RZ, Jacobs EJ, Arslan AA, et al. Circulating 25-hydroxyvitamin D and risk of pancreatic cancer: Cohort Consortium Vitamin D Pooling Project of Rarer Cancers. *Am J Epidemiol* 2010;172:81–93.

117. Baron J, Beach M, Mandel JS, et al. Calcium supplements for the prevention of colorectal adenomas. The Calcium Polyp Prevention Study Group. *N Engl J Med* 1999;340:101–107.

118. Bonithon-Kopp C, Kronborg O, Giacosa A, et al. Calcium and fibre supplementation in prevention of colorectal adenoma recurrence: a randomized intervention trial. *Lancet* 2000;356:1300–1306.

119. Wactawski-Wende J, Kotchen JM, Anderson GL, et al. Calcium plus vitamin D supplementation and the risk of colorectal cancer. *N Engl J Med* 2006; 354:684–696.

120. Trivedi DP, Doll R, Khaw KT. Effect of four monthly oral vitamin D3 (cholecalciferol) supplementation on fractures and mortality in men and women living in the community: randomised double blind controlled trial. *BMJ* 2003; 326:469.

121. Cui Y, Rohan TE. Vitamin D, calcium, and breast cancer risk: a review. *Cancer Epidemiol Biomarkers Prev* 2006;15:1427–1437.

122. Chlebowski RT, Johnson KC, Kooperberg C, et al. Calcium plus vitamin D supplementation and the risk of breast cancer. *J Natl Cancer Inst* 2008;100: 1581–1591.

123. Lappe JM, Travers-Gustafson D, Davies KM, et al. Vitamin D and calcium supplementation reduces cancer risk: results of a randomized trial. *Am J Clin Nutr* 2007;85:1586–1591.

124. Manson JE, Bassuk SS, Lee IM, et al. The VITamin D and OmegA-3 TriaL (VITAL): rationale and design of a large randomized controlled trial of vitamin D and marine omega-3 fatty acid supplements for the primary prevention of cancer and cardiovascular disease. *Contemp Clin Trials* 2012;33: 159–171.

125. Wu X, Spitz MR, Lee JJ, et al. Novel susceptibility loci for second primary tumors/recurrence in head and neck cancer patients: large-scale evaluation of genetic variants. *Cancer Prev Res (Phila)* 2009;2:617–624.

126. Platz EA. Is prostate cancer prevention with selenium all in the genes? *Cancer Prev Res (Phila)* 2010;3:576–578.

127. Miller JW, Ulrich CM. Folic acid and cancer—where are we today? *Lancet* 2013;381:974–976.

128. Thun MJ, Henley SJ, Patrono C. Nonsteroidal anti-inflammatory drugs as anticancer agents: mechanistic, pharmacologic, and clinical issues. *J Natl Cancer Inst* 2002;94:252–266.

129. Wang D, Mann JR, DuBois RN. The role of prostaglandins and other eicosanoids in the gastrointestinal tract. *Gastroenterology* 2005;128:1445–1461.

130. Gurpinar E, Grizzle WE, Piazza GA. COX-Independent Mechanisms of Cancer Chemoprevention by Anti-Inflammatory Drugs. *Front Oncol* 2013;3:181.

131. Rothwell PM, Wilson M, Price JF, et al. Effect of daily aspirin on risk of cancer metastasis: a study of incident cancers during randomised controlled trials. *Lancet* 2012;379:1591–1601.

132. Rothwell PM, Price JF, Fowkes FG, et al. Short-term effects of daily aspirin on cancer incidence, mortality, and non-vascular death: analysis of the time course of risks and benefits in 51 randomised controlled trials. *Lancet* 2012;379:1602–1612.

133. Thun MJ, Namboodiri MM, Heath C Jr. Aspirin use and reduced risk of fatal colon cancer. *N Engl J Med* 1991;325:1593–1596.

134. Chan AT, Giovannucci EL, Meyerhardt JA, et al. Aspirin dose and duration of use and risk of colorectal cancer in men. *Gastroenterology* 2008;134:21–28.

135. Chan AT, Giovannucci EL, Meyerhardt JA, et al. Long-term use of aspirin and nonsteroidal anti-inflammatory drugs and risk of colorectal cancer. *JAMA* 2005;294:914–923.

136. Liao LM, Vaughan TL, Corley DA, et al. Nonsteroidal anti-inflammatory drug use reduces risk of adenocarcinomas of the esophagus and esophagogastric junction in a pooled analysis. *Gastroenterology* 2012;142:442–452.

137. Pollard M, Luckert PH. Effect of indomethacin on intestinal tumor induced in rats by the acetate derivative of dimethylnitrosamine. *Science* 1981;214:558–559.

138. Jacoby RF, Marshall DJ, Newton MA, et al. Chemoprevention of spontaneous intestinal adenomas in the Apc Min mouse model by the nonsteroidal anti-inflammatory drug piroxicam. *Cancer Res* 1996;56:710–714.

139. Kawamori T, Rao C, Seibert K, et al. Chemopreventive effect of celecoxib, a specific cyclooxygenase-2 inhibitor on colon carcinogenesis. *Cancer Res* 1998;58:409–412.

140. Oshima M, Dinchuk JE, Kargman SL. Suppression of intestinal polyposis in Apc delta 716 knockout ice by inhibition of cyclooxygenase 2 (COX-2). *Cell* 1996;87:803–809.

141. Anderson WF, Umar A, Viner JL, et al. The role of cyclooxygenase inhibitors in cancer prevention. *Curr Pharm Des* 2002;8:1035–1062.

142. Giardiello FM, Yang VW, Hylind LM, et al. Primary chemoprevention of familial adenomatous polyposis with sulindac. *N Engl J Med* 2002;346:1054–1059.

143. Steinbach G, Lynch PM, Phillips RK. The effect of celecoxib, a cyclooxygenase-2 inhibitor, in familial adenomatous polyposis. *N Engl J Med* 2000;342:1946–1952.

144. Thorson AG, Lynch HT, Smyrk TC. Rectal cancer in FAP patient after sulindac. *Lancet* 1994;343:180.

145. Calaluce R, Earnest DL, Heddens D, et al. Effects of piroxicam on prostaglandin E2 levels in rectal mucosa of adenomatous polyp patients: a randomized phase IIb trial. *Cancer Epidemiol Biomarkers Prev* 2000;9:1287–1292.

146. Ladenheim J, Garcia G, Titzer D, et al. Effects of sulindac on sporadic colonic polyps. *Gastroenterology* 1995;108:1083–1087.

147. Meyskens FL Jr, McLaren CE, Pelot D, et al. Difluoromethylornithine plus sulindac for the prevention of sporadic colorectal adenomas: a randomized placebo-controlled, double-blind trial. *Cancer Prev Res (Phila)* 2008;1:32–38.

148. Arber N, Eagle CJ, Spicak J, et al. Celecoxib for the prevention of colorectal adenomatous polyps. *N Engl J Med* 2006;355:885–895.

149. Bertagnolli MM, Eagle CJ, Zauber AG, et al. Celecoxib for the prevention of sporadic colorectal adenomas. *N Engl J Med* 2006;355:873–884.

150. Baron JA, Sandler RS, Bresalier RS, et al. A randomized trial of rofecoxib for the chemoprevention of colorectal adenomas. *Gastroenterology* 2006;131: 1674–1682.

151. Bresalier RS, Sandler RS, Quan H, et al. Cardiovascular events associated with rofecoxib in a colorectal adenoma chemoprevention trial. *N Engl J Med* 2005; 352:1092–1102.

152. Solomon SD, McMurray JJ, Pfeffer MA, et al. Cardiovascular risk associated with celecoxib in a clinical trial for colorectal adenoma prevention. *N Engl J Med* 2005;352:1071–1080.

153. Rostom A, Dube C, Lewin G, et al. Nonsteroidal anti-inflammatory drugs and cyclooxygenase-2 inhibitors for primary prevention of colorectal cancer: a systematic review prepared for the U.S. Preventive Services Task Force. *Ann Intern Med* 2007;146:376–389.

154. Dube C, Rostom A, Lewin G, et al. The use of aspirin for primary prevention of colorectal cancer: a systematic review prepared for the U.S. Preventive Services Task Force. *Ann Intern Med* 2007;146:365–375.

155. Rothwell PM, Fowkes FG, Belch JF, et al. Effect of daily aspirin on long-term risk of death due to cancer: analysis of individual patient data from randomised trials. *Lancet* 2011;377:31–41.

156. Rothwell PM. Aspirin in prevention of sporadic colorectal cancer: current clinical evidence and overall balance of risks and benefits. *Recent Results Cancer Res* 2013;191:121–142.

157. U.S. Preventive Services Task Force. Routine aspirin or nonsteroidal anti-inflammatory drugs for the primary prevention of colorectal cancer: U.S. Preventive Services Task Force recommendation statement. *Ann Intern Med* 2007; 146:361–364.

158. Mulshine JL, Atkinson JC, Greer RO, et al. Randomized, double-blind, placebo-controlled phase IIb trial of the cyclooxygenase inhibitor ketorolac as an oral rinse in oropharyngeal leukoplakia. *Clin Cancer Res* 2004;10:1565–1573.

159. Mao JT, Fishbein MC, Adams B, et al. Celecoxib decreases Ki-67 proliferative index in active smokers. *Clin Cancer Res* 2006;12:314–320.

160. Bord S, Horner A, Beavan S, et al. Estrogen receptors alpha and beta are differentially expressed in developing human bone. *J Clin Endocrinol Metab* 2001;86:2309–2314.

161. Kuiper GG, Carlsson B, Grandien K, et al. Comparison of the ligand binding specificity and transcript tissue distribution of estrogen receptors alpha and beta. *Endocrinology* 1997;138:863–870.

162. Fabian CJ, Kimler BF. Selective estrogen-receptor modulators for primary prevention of breast cancer. *J Clin Oncol* 2005;23:1644–1655.

163. Jordan VC. SERMs: meeting the promise of multifunctional medicines. *J Natl Cancer Inst* 2007;99:350–356.

164. Jordan VC. Tamoxifen (ICI46,474) as a targeted therapy to treat and prevent breast cancer. *Br J Pharmacol* 2006;147:S269–S276.

165. Jordan VC. Effect of tamoxifen (ICI 46,474) on initiation and growth of DMBA-induced rat mammary carcinomata. *Eur J Cancer* 1976;12:419–424.

166. Jordan VC. Chemoprevention of breast cancer with selective oestrogen-receptor modulators. *Nat Rev Cancer* 2007;7:46–53.

167. Cuzick J, Baum M. Tamoxifen and contralateral breast cancer. *Lancet* 1985;2:282.

168. Fisher B, Redmond C. New perspective on cancer of the contralateral breast: a marker for assessing tamoxifen as a preventive agent. *J Natl Cancer Inst* 1991;83:1278–1280.

169. Ettinger B, Black DM, Mitlak BH, et al. Reduction of vertebral fracture risk in postmenopausal women with osteoporosis treated with raloxifene: results from a 3-year randomized clinical trial. Multiple Outcomes of Raloxifene Evaluation (MORE) Investigators. *JAMA* 1999;282:637–645.

170. LaCroix AZ, Powles T, Osborne CK, et al. Breast cancer incidence in the randomized PEARL trial of lasofoxifene in postmenopausal osteoporotic women. *J Natl Cancer Inst* 2010;102:1706–1715.

171. Cummings SR, Ensrud K, Delmas PD, et al. Lasofoxifene in postmenopausal women with osteoporosis. *N Engl J Med* 2010;362:686–696.

172. Cummings SR, McClung M, Reginster JY, et al. Arzoxifene for prevention of fractures and invasive breast cancer in postmenopausal women. *J Bone Miner Res* 2011;26:397–404.

173. Powles TJ, Diem SJ, Fabian CJ, et al. Breast cancer incidence in postmenopausal women with osteoporosis or low bone mass using arzoxifene. *Breast Cancer Res Treat* 2012;134:299–306.

174. Nelson HD, Smith ME, Griffin JC, et al. Use of medications to reduce risk for primary breast cancer: a systematic review for the U.S. Preventive Services Task Force. *Ann Intern Med* 2013;158:604–614.

175. Moyer VA. Medications for risk reduction of primary breast cancer in women: U.S. Preventive Services Task Force recommendation statement. *Ann Intern Med* 2013;159:698-708.

176. Visvanathan K, Hurley P, Bantug E, et al. Use of pharmacologic interventions for breast cancer risk reduction: American Society of Clinical Oncology clinical practice guideline. *J Clin Oncol* 2013;31:2942–2962.

177. Vogel VG, Costantino JP, Wickerham DL, et al. Carcinoma in situ outcomes in National Surgical Adjuvant Breast and Bowel Project Breast Cancer Chemoprevention Trials. *J Natl Cancer Inst Monogr* 2010;2010:181–186.

178. Cuzick J, Sestak I, Bonanni B, et al. Selective oestrogen receptor modulators in prevention of breast cancer: an updated meta-analysis of individual participant data. *Lancet* 2013;381:1827–1834.

179. Barrett-Connor E, Mosca L, Collins P, et al. Effects of raloxifene on cardiovascular events and breast cancer in postmenopausal women. *N Engl J Med* 2006;355:125–137.

180. Snyder KR, Sparano N, Malinowski JM. Raloxifene hydrochloride. *Am J Health Syst Pharm* 2000;57:1669–1675.

181. Goss PE, Ingle JN, Martino S, et al. A randomized trial of letrozole in postmenopausal women after five years of tamoxifen therapy for early-stage breast cancer. *N Engl J Med* 2003;349:1793–1802.

182. Fabian CJ, Kimler BF, Zalles CM, et al. Reduction in proliferation with six months of letrozole in women on hormone replacement therapy. *Breast Cancer Res Treat* 2007;106:75–84.

183. Goss PE, Ingle JN, Ales-Martinez JE, et al. Exemestane for breast-cancer prevention in postmenopausal women. *N Engl J Med* 2011;364:2381–2391.

184. Cheung AM, Tile L, Cardew S, et al. Bone density and structure in healthy postmenopausal women treated with exemestane for the primary prevention of breast cancer: a nested substudy of the MAP.3 randomised controlled trial. *Lancet Oncol* 2012;13:275–284.

185. Cuzick J, Sestak I, Forbes JF, et al. Anastrozole for prevention of breast cancer in high-risk postmenopausal women (IBIS-II): an international, double-blind, randomised placebo-controlled trial. *Lancet* 2014;383:1041–1048.

186. Waters EA, McNeel TS, Stevens WM, et al. Use of tamoxifen and raloxifene for breast cancer chemoprevention in 2010. *Breast Cancer Res Treat* 2012;134:875–880.

187. King MC, Wieand S, Hale K, et al. Tamoxifen and breast cancer incidence among women with inherited mutations in BRCA1 and BRCA2: National Surgical Adjuvant Breast and Bowel Project (NSABP-P1) Breast Cancer Prevention Trial. *JAMA* 2001;286:2251–2256.

188. Gronwald J, Tung N, Foulkes WD, et al. Tamoxifen and contralateral breast cancer in BRCA1 and BRCA2 carriers: an update. *Int J Cancer* 2006; 118:2281–2284.

189. Hess-Wilson JK, Knudsen KE. Endocrine disrupting compounds and prostate cancer. *Cancer Lett* 2006;241:1–12.

190. Andriole G, Bostwick D, Civantos F, et al. The effects of 5alpha-reductase inhibitors on the natural history, detection and grading of prostate cancer: current state of knowledge. *J Urol* 2005;174:2098–2104.

191. Thompson IM, Tangen CM, Goodman PJ, et al. Chemoprevention of prostate cancer. *J Urol* 2009;182:499–507.

192. Andriole GL, Bostwick DG, Brawley OW, et al. Effect of dutasteride on the risk of prostate cancer. *N Engl J Med* 2010;362:1192–1202.

193. Thompson IM Jr, Goodman PJ, Tangen CM, et al. Long-term survival of participants in the prostate cancer prevention trial. *N Engl J Med* 2013;369: 603–610.

194. Gerner EW, Meyskens FL Jr. Polyamines and cancer: old molecules, new understanding. *Nat Rev Cancer* 2004;4:781–792.

195. Meyskens FL Jr, Gerner EW. Development of difluoromethylornithine (DFMO) as a chemoprevention agent. *Clin Cancer Res* 1999;5:945–951.

196. Love R, Carbone P, Verma A, et al. Randomized phase I chemoprevention dose seeking study of alpha-difluoromethylornithine. *J Natl Cancer Inst* 1993;85: 732–737.

197. Alberts DS, Dorr RT, Einspahr JG, et al. Chemoprevention of human actinic keratoses by topical 2-(difluoromethyl)-dl-ornithine. *Cancer Epidemiol Biomarkers Prev* 2000;9:1281–1286.

198. Meyskens FL Jr, Surwit E, Moon TE, et al. Enhancement of regression of cervical intraepithelial neoplasia II (moderate dysplasia) with topically applied all-trans-retinoic acid: randomized trial. *J Natl Cancer Inst* 1994;86: 539–543.

199. Fabian CJ, Kimler BF, Brady DA, et al. A phase II breast cancer chemoprevention trial of oral alpha-difluoromethylornithine: breast tissue, imaging, and serum and urine biomarkers. *Clin Cancer Res* 2002;8:3105–3117.

200. Jeter JM, Alberts DS. Difluoromethylornithine: the proof is in the polyamines. *Cancer Prev Res (Phila)* 2012;5:1341–1344.

201. Gronich N, Rennert G. Beyond aspirin-cancer prevention with statins, metformin and bisphosphonates. *Nat Rev Clin Oncol* 2013;10:625–642.

202. Moyad MA. Why a statin and/or another proven heart healthy agent should be utilized in the next major cancer chemoprevention trial: part II. *Urologic Oncol* 2004;22:472–477.

203. Bertagnolli MM, Hsu M, Hawk ET, et al. Statin use and colorectal adenoma risk: results from the adenoma prevention with celecoxib trial. *Cancer Prev Res (Phila)* 2010;3:588–596.

204. Simon MS, Rosenberg CA, Rodabough RJ, et al. Prospective analysis of association between use of statins or other lipid-lowering agents and colorectal cancer risk. *Ann Epidemiol* 2012;22:17–27.

205. Platz EA, Leitzmann MF, Visvanathan K, et al. Statin drugs and risk of advanced prostate cancer. *J Natl Cancer Inst* 2006;98:1819–1825.

206. Eliassen AH, Colditz GA, Rosner B, et al. Serum lipids, lipid-lowering drugs, and the risk of breast cancer. *Arch Intern Med* 2005;165:2264–2271.

207. Lipkin SM, Chao EC, Moreno V, et al. Genetic variation in 3-hydroxy-3-methylglutaryl CoA reductase modifies the chemopreventive activity of statins for colorectal cancer. *Cancer Prev Res (Phila)* 2010;3:597–603.

208. Rennert G. Bisphosphonates: beyond prevention of bone metastases. *J Natl Cancer Inst* 2011;103:1728–1729.

209. Rennert G, Pinchev M, Rennert HS. Use of bisphosphonates and risk of postmenopausal breast cancer. *J Clin Oncol* 2010;28:3577–3581.

210. Chlebowski RT, Chen Z, Cauley JA, et al. Oral bisphosphonate use and breast cancer incidence in postmenopausal women. *J Clin Oncol* 2010;28: 3582–3590.

211. Monsees GM, Malone KE, Tang MT, et al. Bisphosphonate use after estrogen receptor-positive breast cancer and risk of contralateral breast cancer. *J Natl Cancer Inst* 2011;103:1752–1760.

212. Kirpichnikov D, McFarlane SI, Sowers JR. Metformin: an update. *Ann Intern Med* 2002;137:25–33.

213. Pollack MN. Insulin, insulin-like growth factors, insulin resistance, and neoplasia. *Am J Clin Nutr* 2007;86:s820–s822.

214. Evans JM, Donnelly LA, Emslie-Smith AM, et al. Metformin and reduced risk of cancer in diabetic patients. *BMJ* 2005;330:1304–1305.

215. Zhu P, Davis M, Blackwelder A, et al. Metformin selectively targets tumor initiating cells in erbB-2 overexpressing breast cancer models. *Cancer Prev Res (Phila)* 2014;7:199–210.

216. Lonardo E, Cioffi M, Sancho P, et al. Metformin targets the metabolic achilles heel of human pancreatic cancer stem cells. *PLoS One* 2013;8:e76518.

217. Grubbs C, Clapper M, Reid J, et al. *Metformin Promotes Tumorigenesis in Animal Models of Cancer Prevention.* Washington, DC: American Association for Cancer Research; 2013.

218. Chlebowski RT, McTiernan A, Wactawski-Wende J, et al. Diabetes, metformin, and breast cancer in postmenopausal women. *J Clin Oncol* 2012;30: 2844–2852.

219. Heger M, van Golen RF, Broekgaarden M, et al. The molecular basis for the pharmacokinetics and pharmacodynamics of curcumin and its metabolites in relation to cancer. *Pharmacol Rev* 2014;66:222–307.

220. Whitlock NC, Baek SJ. The anticancer effects of resveratrol: modulation of transcription factors. *Nutr Cancer* 2012;64:493–502.

221. Lambert JD. Does tea prevent cancer? Evidence from laboratory and human intervention studies. *Am J Clin Nutr* 2013;98:1667S–1675S.

222. Kakarala M, Brenner DE, Korkaya H, et al. Targeting breast stem cells with the cancer preventive compounds curcumin and piperine. *Breast Cancer Res Treat* 2010;122:777–785.

223. Norris L, Karmokar A, Howells L, et al. The role of cancer stem cells in the anti-carcinogenicity of curcumin. *Mol Nutr Food Res* 2013;57:1630–1637.

224. Zou H, Yuan C, Dong L, et al. Human cyclooxygenase-1 activity and its responses to COX inhibitors are allosterically regulated by nonsubstrate fatty acids. *J Lipid Res* 2012;53:1336–1347.

225. Wada M, Delong CJ, Hong YH, et al. Enzymes and receptors of prostaglandin pathways with arachidonic acid- vs. eicosapentaenoic acid-derived substrates and products. *J Biol Chem* 2007;282:22254–22266.

226. Laviano A, Rianda S, Molfino A, et al. Omega-3 fatty acids in cancer. *Curr Opin Clin Nutr Metab Care* 2013;16:156–161.

227. Cockbain AJ, Toogood GJ, Hull MA. Omega-3 polyunsaturated fatty acids for the treatment and prevention of colorectal cancer. *Gut* 2012;61:135–149.

228. Stoner GD, Wang LS, Casto BC. Laboratory and clinical studies of cancer chemoprevention by antioxidants in berries. *Carcinogenesis* 2008;29:1665–1674.

229. Wang LS, Dombkowski AA, Seguin C, et al. Mechanistic basis for the chemopreventive effects of black raspberries at a late stage of rat esophageal carcinogenesis. *Mol Carcinog* 2011;50:291–300.

230. Wang LS, Kuo CT, Stoner K, et al. Dietary black raspberries modulate DNA methylation in dextran sodium sulfate (DSS)-induced ulcerative colitis. *Carcinogenesis* 2013;34:2842–2850.

231. Ireson C, Orr S, Jones DJ, et al. Characterization of metabolites of the chemopreventive agent curcumin in human and rat hepatocytes and in the rat in vivo, and evaluation of their ability to inhibit phorbol ester-induced prostaglandin E2 production. *Cancer Res* 2001;61:1058–1064.

232. Ireson CR, Jones DJ, Orr S, et al. Metabolism of the cancer chemopreventive agent curcumin in human and rat intestine. *Cancer Epidemiol Biomarkers Prev* 2002;11:105–111.

233. Vareed SK, Kakarala M, Ruffin MT, et al. Pharmacokinetics of curcumin conjugate metabolites in healthy human subjects. *Cancer Epidemiol Biomarkers Prev* 2008;17:1411–1417.

234. Gescher A, Steward WP, Brown K. Resveratrol in the management of human cancer: how strong is the clinical evidence? *Ann N Y Acad Sci* 2013;1290:12–20.

235. Stoner GD. Ginger: is it ready for prime time? *Cancer Prev Res (Phila)* 2013;6:257–262.

236. Stoner GD, Wang LS. Chemoprevention of esophageal squamous cell carcinoma with berries. *Top Curr Chem* 2013;329:1–20.

237. Mallery SR, Zwick JC, Pei P, et al. Topical application of a bioadhesive black raspberry gel modulates gene expression and reduces cyclooxygenase 2 protein in human premalignant oral lesions. *Cancer Res* 2008;68:4945–4957.

238. Carroll RE, Benya RV, Turgeon DK, et al. Phase IIa clinical trial of curcumin for the prevention of colorectal neoplasia. *Cancer Prev Res (Phila)* 2011;4: 354–364.

239. Seeff LB, Hoofnagle JH. Epidemiology of hepatocellular carcinoma in areas of low hepatitis B and hepatitis C endemicity. *Oncogene* 2006;25:3771–3777.

240. Fox JG, Wang TC. Inflammation, atrophy, and gastric cancer. *J Clin Invest* 2007;117:60–69.

241. Saslow D, Castle PE, Cox JT, et al. American Cancer Society Guideline for human papillomavirus (HPV) vaccine use to prevent cervical cancer and its precursors. *CA Cancer J Clin* 2007;57:7–28.

242. Mohanna S, Maco V, Bravo F, et al. Epidemiology and clinical characteristics of classic Kaposi's sarcoma, seroprevalence, and variants of human herpesvirus 8 in South America: a critical review of an old disease. *Int J Infect Dis* 2005;9:239–250.

243. Castillo JJ, Reagan JL, Bishop KD, et al. Viral lymphomagenesis: from pathophysiology to the rationale for novel therapies. *Br J Haematol* 2014;165: 300–315.

244. Al-Bahrani R, Abuetabh Y, Zeitouni N, et al. Cholangiocarcinoma: risk factors, environmental influences and oncogenesis. *Ann Clin Lab Sci* 2013;43: 195–210.

245. Mostafa MH, Sheweita SA, O'Connor PJ. Relationship between schistosomiasis and bladder cancer. *Clin Microbiol Rev* 1999;12:97–111.

246. Zivny J, Wang TC, Yantiss R, et al. Role of therapy or monitoring in preventing progression to gastric cancer. *J Clin Gastroenterol* 2003;36:S50–S60.

247. Correa P, Fontham ET, Bravo JC, et al. Chemoprevention of gastric dysplasia: randomized trial of antioxidant supplements and anti-helicobacter pylori therapy. *J Natl Cancer Inst* 2000;92:1881–1888.

248. Wong BC, Zhang L, Ma JL, et al. Effects of selective COX-2 inhibitor and Helicobacter pylori eradication on precancerous gastric lesions. *Gut* 2012;61:812–818.

249. Ma JL, Zhang L, Brown LM, et al. Fifteen-year effects of Helicobacter pylori, garlic, and vitamin treatments on gastric cancer incidence and mortality. *J Natl Cancer Inst* 2012;104:488–492.

250. Risch HA, Lu L, Kidd MS, et al. Helicobacter pylori seropositivities and risk of pancreatic carcinoma. *Cancer Epidemiol Biomarkers Prev* 2014;23: 172–178.

251. Mazzoleni LE, Francesconi CF, Sander GB. Mass eradication of *Helicobacter pylori*: feasible and advisable? *Lancet* 2011;378:462–464.

252. Whiteman DC, Parmar P, Fahey P, et al. Association of Helicobacter pylori infection with reduced risk for esophageal cancer is independent of environmental and genetic modifiers. *Gastroenterology* 2010;139:73–83.

**CANCER PREVENTION AND SCREENING**

253. Torrance CJ, Jackson PE, Montgomery E, et al. Combinatorial chemoprevention of intestinal neoplasia. *Nat Med* 2000;6:1024–1028.

254. Reddy BS, Wang CX, Kong AN, et al. Prevention of azoxymethane-induced colon cancer by combination of low doses of atorvastatin, aspirin, and celecoxib in F 344 rats. *Cancer Res* 2006;66:4542–4546.

255. Zell JA, Pelot D, Chen WP, et al. Risk of cardiovascular events in a randomized placebo-controlled, double-blind trial of difluoromethylornithine plus sulindac for the prevention of sporadic colorectal adenomas. *Cancer Prev Res (Phila)* 2009;2:209–212.

256. Guerrieri-Gonzaga A, Robertson C, Bonanni B, et al. Preliminary results on safety and activity of a randomized, double-blind, 2 x 2 trial of low-dose tamoxifen and fenretinide for breast cancer prevention in premenopausal women. *J Clin Oncol* 2006;24:129–135.

257. Kelloff GJ, Lippman SM, Dannenberg AJ, et al. Progress in chemoprevention drug development: the promise of molecular biomarkers for prevention of intraepithelial neoplasia and cancer—a plan to move forward. *Clin Cancer Res* 2006;12:3661–3697.

258. Washington MK, Powell AE, Sullivan R, et al. Pathology of rodent models of intestinal cancer: progress report and recommendations. *Gastroenterology* 2013;144:705–717.

259. Nandan MO, Yang VW. Genetic and chemical models of colorectal cancer in mice. *Curr Colorectal Cancer Rep* 2010;6:51–59.

260. Kwon MC, Berns A. Mouse models for lung cancer. *Mol Oncol* 2013;7:165–177.

261. Kirma NB, Tekmal RR. Transgenic mouse models of hormonal mammary carcinogenesis: advantages and limitations. *J Steroid Biochem Mol Biol* 2012;131:76–82.

262. Irshad S, Abate-Shen C. Modeling prostate cancer in mice: something old, something new, something premalignant, something metastatic. *Cancer Metastasis Rev* 2013;32:109–122.

263. Herreros-Villanueva M, Hijona E, Cosme A, et al. Mouse models of pancreatic cancer. *World J Gastroenterol* 2012;18:1286–1294.

264. Winawer SJ, Zauber AG, Ho MN, et al. Prevention of colorectal cancer by colonoscopic polypectomy. The National Polyp Study Workgroup. *N Engl J Med* 1993;329:1977–1981.

265. Spechler S. Barrett's esophagus. *Semin Oncol* 1994;21:431–437.

266. Shen O, Liu S, Dawsey S, et al. Cytologic screening for esophageal cancer: results from 12,877 subjects from a high risk population in China. *Int J Cancer* 1993;54:185–188.

267. Taylor P, Li B, Dawsey S, et al. Prevention of esophageal cancer: the nutrition intervention trials in Linxian, China. Linxian Nutrition Intervention Trials Study Group. *Cancer Res* 1994;54:2029s–2031s.

268. Sober A, Burstein J. Precursors to skin cancer. *Cancer* 1995;75:645–650.

269. Tucker M, Halpern A, Holly E, et al. Clinically recognized dysplastic nevi. A central risk factor for cutaneous melanoma. *JAMA* 1997;277:1439–1444.

270. Gustafsson L, Adami H-O. Natural history of cervical neoplasia:consistent results obtained by an identification technique. *Br J Cancer* 1989;60:132–137.

271. Cawson R. Premalignant lesions in the mouth. *Br Med Bull* 1975;31:164–180.

272. Zhou M. Intraductal carcinoma of the prostate: the whole story. *Pathology* 2013; 45:533–539.

273. Saccomanno G, Archer VE, Auerbach O, et al. Development of carcinoma of the lung as reflected in exfoliated cells. *Cancer* 1974;33:256–270.

274. Cooper CL, O'Toole SA, Kench JG. Classification, morphology and molecular pathology of premalignant lesions of the pancreas. *Pathology* 2013;45:286–304.

275. Brewster AM, Lee JJ, Clayman GL, et al. Randomized trial of adjuvant 13-cis-retinoic acid and interferon alfa for patients with aggressive skin squamous cell carcinoma. *J Clin Oncol* 2007;25:1974–1978.

276. Karp DD, Lee SJ, Keller SM, et al. Randomized, double-blind, placebo-controlled, phase III chemoprevention trial of selenium supplementation in patients with resected stage I non-small-cell lung cancer: ECOG 5597. *J Clin Oncol* 2013;31:4179–4187.

277. Labayle D, Fischer D, Vielh P. Sulindac causes regression of rectal polyps in familial adenomatous polyposis. *Gastroenterology* 1991;101:635–639.

278. Giardiello FM, Hamilton SR, Krush AJ, et al. Treatment of colonic and rectal adenomas with sulindac in familial adenomatous polyposis. *N Engl J Med* 1993;328:1313–1316.

279. Nugent KP, Farmer KC, Sipgelman AD, et al. Randomized controlled trial of the effect of sulindac on duodenal and rectal polyposis and cell proliferation in patients with familial adenomatous polyposis. *Br J Surg* 1993;80: 1618–1619.

280. Mathers JC, Movahedi M, Macrae F, et al. Long-term effect of resistant starch on cancer risk in carriers of hereditary colorectal cancer: an analysis from the CAPP2 randomised controlled trial. *Lancet Oncol* 2012;13:1242–1249.

281. Burn J, Gerdes AM, Macrae F, et al. Long-term effect of aspirin on cancer risk in carriers of hereditary colorectal cancer: an analysis from the CAPP2 randomised controlled trial. *Lancet* 2011;378:2081–2087.

282. Ruffin MT, Krishnan K, Rock CL, et al. Suppression of human colorectal mucosal prostaglandins: determining the lowest effective aspirin dose. *J Natl Cancer Inst* 1997;89:1152–1160.

283. Krishnan K, Ruffin MT, Normolle D, et al. Colonic mucosal prostaglandin E2 and cyclooxygenase expression before and after low aspirin doses in subjects at high risk or at normal risk for colorectal cancer. *Cancer Epidemiol Biomarkers Prev* 2001;10:447–453.

284. Sample D, Wargovich M, Fischer SM, et al. A dose-finding study of aspirin for chemoprevention utilizing rectal mucosal prostaglandin E(2) levels as a biomarker. *Cancer Epidemiol Biomarkers Prev* 2002;11:275–279.

285. Sandler RS, Halabi S, Baron JA, et al. A randomized trial of aspirin to prevent colorectal adenomas in patients with previous colorectal cancer. *N Engl J Med* 2003;348:883–890.

286. Baron JA, Cole BF, Sandler RS, et al. A randomized trial of aspirin to prevent colorectal adenomas. *N Engl J Med* 2003;348:891–899.

287. Fisher B, Costantino JP, Wickerham DL, et al. Tamoxifen for the prevention of breast cancer: current status of the National Surgical Adjuvant Breast and Bowel Project P-1 study. *J Natl Cancer Inst* 2005;97:1652–1662.

288. Cuzick J, Forbes JF, Sestak I, et al. Long-term results of tamoxifen prophylaxis for breast cancer—96-month follow-up of the randomized IBIS-I trial. *J Natl Cancer Inst* 2007;99:272–282.

289. Powles TJ, Ashley S, Tidy A, et al. Twenty-year follow-up of the Royal Marsden randomized, double-blinded tamoxifen breast cancer prevention trial. *J Natl Cancer Inst* 2007;99:283–290.

290. Veronesi U, Maisonneuve P, Rotmensz N, et al. Tamoxifen for the prevention of breast cancer: Late results of the Italian randomzied tamoxifen prevention trial among women with hysterectomy. *J Natl Cancer Inst* 2007;99:727–737.

291. Cauley JA, Norton L, Lippman ME, et al. Continued breast cancer risk reduction in postmenopausal women treated with raloxifene: 4-year results from the MORE trial. Multiple outcomes of raloxifene evaluation. *Breast Cancer Res Treat* 2001;65:125–134.

292. Martino S, Cauley JA, Barrett-Connor E, et al. Continuing outcomes relevant to Evista: breast cancer incidence in postmenopausal osteoporotic women in a randomized trial of raloxifene. *J Natl Cancer Inst* 2004;96: 1751–1761.

293. Messing E, Kim KM, Sharkey F, et al. Randomized prospective phase III trial of difluoromethylornithine vs placebo in preventing recurrence of completely resected low risk superficial bladder cancer. *J Urol* 2006;176:500–504.

294. Simoneau AR, Gerner EW, Nagle R, et al. The effect of difluoromethylornithine on decreasing prostate size and polyamines in men: results of a year-long phase IIb randomized placebo-controlled chemoprevention trial. *Cancer Epidemiol Biomarkers Prev* 2008;17:292–299.

295. Bailey HH, Kim K, Verma AK, et al. A randomized, double-blind, placebo-controlled phase 3 skin cancer prevention study of (alpha)-difluoromethylornithine in subjects with previous history of skin cancer. *Cancer Prev Res (Phila)* 2010;3:35–47.

296. Kreul SM, Havighurst T, Kim K, et al. A phase III skin cancer chemoprevention study of DFMO: long-term follow-up of skin cancer events and toxicity. *Cancer Prev Res (Phila)* 2012;5:1368–1374.

297. Zick SM, Ruffin MT, Djuric Z, et al. Quantitation of 6-, 8- and 10-gingerols and 6-shogaol in human plasma by high-performance liquid chromatography with electrochemical detection. *Int J Biomed Sci* 2010;6:233–240.

298. Zick SM, Turgeon DK, Vareed SK, et al. Phase II study of the effects of ginger root extract on eicosanoids in colon mucosa in people at normal risk for colorectal cancer. *Cancer Prev Res (Phila)* 2011;4:1929–1937.

299. Hull MA. Nutritional agents with anti-inflammatory properties in chemoprevention of colorectal neoplasia. *Recent Results Cancer Res* 2013;191:143–156.

300. Nelson WG, De Marzo AM, Isaacs WB. Prostate cancer. *N Engl J Med* 2003;349:366–381.

301. von Knobloch R, Konrad L, Barth PJ, et al. Genetic pathways and new progression markers for prostate cancer suggested by microsatellite allelotyping. *Clin Cancer Res* 2004;10:1064–1073.

302. Palapattu GS, Sutcliffe S, Bastian PJ, et al. Prostate carcinogenesis and inflammation: emerging insights. *Carcinogenesis* 2005;26:1170–1181.

303. Dontu G, Liu S, Wicha MS. Stem cells in mammary development and carcinogenesis: implications for prevention and treatment. *Stem Cell Rev* 2005;1: 207–213.

304. Liu S, Dontu G, Mantle ID, et al. Hedgehog signaling and Bmi-1 regulate self-renewal of normal and malignant human mammary stem cells. *Cancer Res* 2006;66:6063–6071.

305. Wistuba II, Lam S, Behrens C, et al. Molecular damage in the bronchial epithelium of current and former smokers. *J Natl Cancer Inst* 1997;89: 1366–1373.

306. Massion PP, Carbone DP. The molecular basis of lung cancer: molecular abnormalities and therapeutic implications. *Respir Res* 2003;4:12.

307. Mao C, Koutsky LA, Ault KA, et al. Efficacy of human papillomavirus-16 vaccine to prevent cervical intraepithelial neoplasia: a randomized controlled trial. *Obstet Gynecol* 2006;107:18–27.

308. Califano J, van der Riet P, Westra W, et al. Genetic progression model for head and neck cancer: implications for field cancerization. *Cancer Res* 1996;56: 2488–2492.

309. Califano J, Westra WH, Meininger G, et al. Genetic progression and clonal relationship of recurrent premalignant head and neck lesions. *Clin Cancer Res* 2000;6:347–352.

310. Braakhuis BJ, Tabor MP, Kummer JA, et al. A genetic explanation of Slaughter's concept of field cancerization: evidence and clinical implications. *Cancer Res* 2003;63:1727–1730.

311. Ha PK, Benoit NE, Yochem R, et al. A transcriptional progression model for head and neck cancer. *Clin Cancer Res* 2003;9:3058–3064.

312. Barrett MT, Sanchez CA, Prevo LJ, et al. Evolution of neoplastic cell lineages in Barrett oesophagus. *Nat Genet* 1999;22:106–109.

313. Reid BJ, Levine DS, Longton G, et al. Predictors of progression to cancer in Barrett's esophagus: baseline histology and flow cytometry identify low- and high-risk patient subsets. *Am J Gastroenterol* 2000;95:1669–1676.

314. Thorgeirsson SS, Grisham JW. Molecular pathogenesis of human hepatocellular carcinoma. *Nat Genet* 2002;31:339–346.

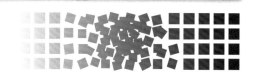

# 34 Cancer Screening

Otis W. Brawley and Howard L. Parnes

## INTRODUCTION

Cancer screening refers to a test or examination performed on an asymptomatic individual. The goal is not simply to find cancer at an early stage, nor is it to diagnose as many patients with cancer as possible. The goal of cancer screening is to prevent death and suffering from the disease in question through early therapeutic intervention.

The assumption that early detection improves outcomes can be traced back to the concept that cancer inexorably progresses from a small, localized, primary tumor to local–regional spread, to distant metastases and death. This linear model of disease progression predicts that early intervention would reduce cancer mortality.

Cancer screening was an element of the "periodic physical examination," as espoused by the American Medical Association in the 1920s.[1] It consisted of palpation to find a mass or enlarged lymph nodes and auscultation to find a rub or abnormal sound. Today, screening has grown to include radiologic testing, the measurement of serum markers of disease, and even molecular testing. A positive screening test leads to further diagnostic testing, which might lead to a cancer diagnosis.

The intuitive appeal of early detection accounts for the emphasis that has long been placed on screening. However, it is not widely understood that screening tests are always associated with some harm (e.g., anxiety, financial costs) and may actually cause substantial harm (e.g., invasive follow-up diagnostic or therapeutic procedures). Because screening is, by definition, done in healthy people, all early detection tests should be carefully studied and their risk–benefit ratio determined before they are adopted for widespread usage.

Screening is a public health intervention. However, some draw a distinction between screening an individual within the doctor–patient relationship and mass screening, a program aimed at screening a large population. The latter may involve advertising campaigns to encourage people to be screened for a particular cancer at a shopping mall or at a community event, such as state fair.

Screening may be either *opportunistic* (i.e., a patient sees a health-care provider who chooses to screen or not to screen) or *programmatic*. Programmatic refers to a standardized approach with algorithms for screening and follow-up as well as recall of patients for regular routine screening with quality control measures. Programmatic screening is usually more effective.

## PERFORMANCE CHARACTERISTICS

The degree to which a screening test can discriminate between individuals with and without a particular disease is described by its performance characteristics. These include the a test's sensitivity, specificity, positive predictive value (PPV), and negative predictive value (NPV) (Table 34.1). It should be noted that these measures relate to the accuracy of a screening test;

they do not provide any information regarding a test's efficacy or effectiveness.

- Sensitivity is the proportion of persons designated positive by the screening test among all individuals who have the disease: true positive (TP)/(TP + false negative [FN]).
- Specificity is the proportion of persons designated negative by the screening test among all individuals who do not have the disease: true negative TN/(TN + false positive [FP]).
- Positive predictive value is the proportion of individuals with a positive screening test who have the disease: (TP)/(TP + FP).
- Negative predictive value is the proportion of individuals with a negative screening test who do not have the disease: (TN)/(TN + false negative [FN]).[2]

For a given screening test, sensitivity and specificity are inversely related. For example, as one lowers the threshold for considering a serum prostate-specific antigen (PSA) level to represent a *positive* screen, the sensitivity of the test increases and more cancers will be detected. This increased sensitivity comes at the cost of decreased specificity (i.e., more men without cancer will have *positive* screenings tests and, therefore, will be subjected to unnecessary diagnostic procedures).

Some screening tests, such as mammograms, are more subjective and operator dependent than others. For this reason, the sensitivity and specificity of screening mammography varies among radiologists. For a given radiologist, the lower his or her threshold for considering a mammogram to be suspicious, the higher the sensitivity and lower the specificity will be for them. However, mammography can have both a higher sensitivity and higher specificity in the hands of a more experienced versus a less experienced radiologist.

As opposed to sensitivity and specificity, the PPV and NPV of a screening test are dependent on disease prevalence. PPV is also highly responsive to small increases in specificity. As shown in Table 34.2, given a disease prevalence of 5 cases per 1,000 (0.005), the PPV of a hypothetical screening test increases dramatically as specificity goes from 95% to 99.9%, but only marginally as sensitivity goes from 80% to 95%. Given a disease prevalence of only 1 per 10,000 (0.0001), the PPV of the same test is poor even at high sensitivity and specificity. The positive association between breast cancer prevalence and age is the major reason why screening mammography is a better test (higher PPV) for women aged 50 to 59 than for women 40 to 49 years of age.

## ASSESSING SCREENING TESTS AND OUTCOMES

### Screening Test Results

*Lead time bias* occurs whenever screening results in an earlier diagnosis than would have occurred in the absence of screening.

## Performance Characteristics of a Screening Test

Sensitivity is the proportion designated positive by the screening test among all individuals who have the disease.

$$\frac{TP}{TP + FN}$$

Specificity is the proportion designated negative by the screening test among all those who do not have the disease.

$$\frac{TN}{TN + FP}$$

Positive predictive value is the proportion of individuals with a positive test who have the disease.

$$\frac{TP}{TP + FP}$$

Negative predictive value is the proportion of individuals with a negative test negative who do not have the disease.

$$\frac{TN}{TN + FN}$$

TP, true positive, the condition present and the test is positive; FN, false negative, the condition is present and the test is negative; FP, false positive, the condition is absent and the test is positive; TN, true negative, the condition is absent and test is negative.

Because survival is measured *from the time of diagnosis*, an earlier diagnosis, by definition, increases survival. Unless an effective intervention is available, lead time bias has no impact on the natural history of a disease and death will occur at the same time it would have in the absence of early detection (Fig. 34.1).

*Length bias* is a function of the biologic behavior of a cancer. Slower growing, less aggressive cancers are more likely to be detected by a screening test than faster growing cancers, which are more likely to be diagnosed due to the onset of symptoms between scheduled screenings (interval cancers). Length bias has an even greater effect on survival statistics than lead time bias (Fig. 34.2).

*Overdiagnosis* is an extreme form of length bias and represents pure harm. It refers to the detection of tumors, often through highly sensitive modern imaging modalities and other diagnostic tests, that fulfill the histologic criteria for malignancy

## Positive Predictive Value Given Varying Sensitivity and Specificity and Prevalence

| Prevalence 0.005 | | Sensitivity % | | |
|---|---|---|---|---|
| | | 80 | 90 | 95 |
| Specificity % | 95 | 7 | 8 | 9 |
| | 99 | 29 | 31 | 32 |
| | 99.9 | 80 | 82 | 83 |
| Prevalence 0.0001 | | Sensitivity % | | |
| | | 80 | 90 | 95 |
| Specificity % | 95 | 0.2 | 0.2 | 2.0 |
| | 99 | 0.8 | 0.9 | 0.9 |
| | 99.9 | 0.7 | 8.0 | 9.0 |

PPV improves dramatically in response to small changes in specificity. Changes in specificity influence PPV much more than changes in sensitivity. Note the influence of prevalence on PPV. Screening tests do not perform as well in populations with a low prevalence of disease.

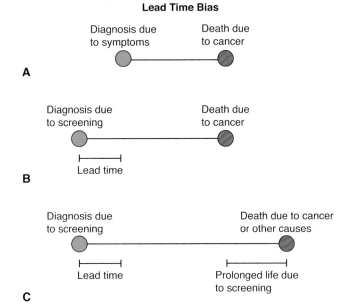

**Lead Time Bias**

**Figure 34.1** Survival is the time from cancer diagnosis to death. **(A)** Lead time bias occurs when screening results in an earlier diagnosis. Without screening, a patient is diagnosed with cancer due to symptoms. **(B)** With screening, the patient is often diagnosed earlier. When screening and treatment do not prolong life, the screened patient can have a longer survival solely due to the earlier diagnosis. The survival increase is pure lead time bias. **(C)** When screening and treatment are beneficial, the patient is diagnosed before the onset of symptoms and the patient lives beyond the point in which death would have occurred without screening.

but are not biologically destined to harm the patient (see Fig. 34.2).

There are two categories of overdiagnosis: the detection of histologically defined *cancers* not destined to metastasize or harm the patient, and the detection of cancers not destined to metastasize or cause harm *in the life span of the specific patient*. The importance of this second category is illustrated by the widespread practice in the United States of screening elderly patients with limited life expectancies, who are thus unlikely to benefit from early cancer diagnosis.

Overdiagnosis occurs with many malignancies, including lung, breast, prostate, renal cell, melanoma, and thyroid cancers.[3] Neuroblastoma provides one of the most striking examples of overdiagnosis.[4] Urine vanillylmandelic acid (VMA) testing is a highly sensitive screening test for the detection of this pediatric disease. After screening programs in Germany, Japan, and Canada showed marked increases in the incidence of this disease without a concomitant decline in mortality, it was noticed that nearby areas that did not screen had similar death rates with lower incidence.[4,5] It is now appreciated that screen-detected neuroblastomas have a very good prognosis with minimal or no treatment. Many actually regress spontaneously.

*Stage shift*—i.e., a cancer diagnosis at an earlier stage than would have occurred in the absence of screening—is necessary, but not sufficient, for a screening test to be effective in terms of reducing mortality. Both lead time bias and length bias contribute to this phenomenon. Although it is tempting to speculate that diagnosis at an earlier stage must confer benefit, this is not necessarily the case. For example, a substantial proportion of men treated with radical prostatectomy for what appears to be a localized prostate cancer relapse after undergoing surgery. Conversely, some men who are treated with definitive therapy would never have gone on to develop metastatic disease in the absence of treatment.

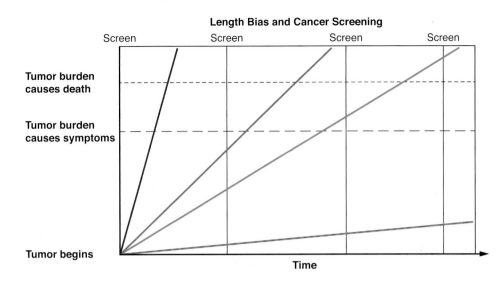

**Figure 34.2** Length bias and cancer screening. The *red line* is indicative of a fast-growing tumor that is not amenable to regular screening. The *blue line* is indicative of a fast-growing tumor that can be diagnosed by screening or later by symptoms; death may possibly be prevented by treatment. The *green line* is a slower growing but potentially deadly cancer that can be detected by symptoms or several screenings and treated, possibly preventing death. The *orange line* is indicative of a very slow growing tumor that would never cause death and would never need treatment despite being screen detected. This is classic overdiagnosis.

*Selection bias* occurs when enrollees in a clinical study differ from the general population. In fact, people who voluntarily participate in clinical trials tend to be healthier than the general population, perhaps due to a greater interest in health and healthcare research. Screening studies tend to enroll individuals healthier than the general population. This so-called *healthy volunteer effect*[6,7] can introduce a powerful bias if not adequately controlled for by randomization procedures.

## Assessing Screening Outcomes

The usual primary goal of cancer screening is to reduce mortality from the disease in question (a reduction in disease-specific mortality). Screening studies generally do not have sufficient statistical power to assess the impact of screening for a specific malignancy on overall mortality. (Lung cancer screening provides an exception to this rule; see the following.) As discussed previously, the fact that a screening test increases the percentage of people diagnosed with early stage cancer and decreases that of late stage cancer (stage shift) is not equivalent to proof of mortality reduction. Further, due to the healthy volunteer effect, case control and cohort studies cannot provide definitive evidence of mortality benefit. Prospective, randomized clinical trials are required to address this issue. In such trials, volunteers are randomized to be screened or not and are then followed longitudinally to determine if there is a difference in disease-specific or overall mortality.

A reduction in mortality rates or in the risk of death is often stated in terms of relative risk. However, this method of reporting may be misleading. It is preferable to report both the relative and absolute reduction in mortality. For example, the European Randomized Study of Screening for Prostate Cancer (ERSPC) showed that screening reduced the risk of prostate cancer death by 20%. However, this translates into only 1 prostate cancer death averted per 1,000 men screened (5 prostate cancer deaths per 1,000 men not screened versus 4 prostate cancer deaths per 1,000 men screened) and a relatively modest lifetime reduction in the absolute risk of prostate cancer death of only 0.6%, from 3.0% to 2.4%.[8]

# PROBLEMS WITH RANDOMIZED TRIALS

It is important to acknowledge that even prospective, randomized trials can have serious methodologic shortcomings. For example, imbalances caused by flaws in the randomization scheme can prejudice the outcome of a trial. Other flaws include so-called *drop-in* or *contamination*, in which some participants on the control arm get the intervention. Patients on the intervention arm may also

drop out of the study. Both drop-ins and drop-outs reduce the statistical power of a clinical trial.

In the United States, it is now considered standard to obtain informed consent before randomization takes place. However, there have been several published studies that randomized participants from rosters of eligible subjects such as census lists. In these trials, informed consent was obtained after randomization and only among those randomized to the screening arm of the study. Those randomized to the control arm were not contacted, and indeed, did not know they were in a clinical trial. They were followed through national death registries. Although the study was analyzed on an intent-to-screen basis, this method can still introduce biases. For example, only patients on the intervention arm had access to the screening facility and staff for counseling and treatment if diagnosed; those in the control group were more likely to be treated in the community as opposed to high-volume centers of excellence and were less likely to be treated with surgery and more likely to be treated with hormones alone than those on the screened arm. The study arms would also tend to differ in their knowledge of the disease, which may contribute to an overestimate of the benefits of a screening test.[9]

Virtually every screening test is a balance between known harms and potential benefits. The most important risk of screening is the detection and subsequent treatment of a cancer that would never have come to clinical detection or harmed the patient in the absence of screening (i.e., overdiagnosis and overtreatment). Treatment can cause emotional and physical morbidity and even death.[10] Even when screening has a net mortality benefit, there can be considerable harm. For example, in the recent randomized trial of spiral lung computed tomography (CT) scan, approximately 27,000 current smokers and former smokers were given three annual low-dose CT scans. More than 20% had a *positive* screening CT scan, necessitating further testing. About 1,000 subsequently underwent invasive diagnostic procedures and 16 deaths were reported within 60 days of the procedure.[11] It is not known how many of these deaths were directly related to the screening.

It can be dangerous to extrapolate estimates of benefit from one population to another. In particular, studies showing that a radiographic test is beneficial to average risk individuals may not mean that it is beneficial to a population at high risk, and vice versa. For example, women at high risk for breast cancer due to an inherited mutation of a DNA repair gene may be at higher risk for radiation-induced cancer from mammographies compared to the general population; a screening test (e.g., spiral lung CT scan), shown to be efficacious in a high-risk population of heavy smokers may result in net harm if applied to a low or average risk population.

# SCREENING GUIDELINES AND RECOMMENDATIONS

A number of organizations develop cancer screening recommendations or guidelines. These organizations use varying methods. The Institute of Medicine (IOM) has released two reports to establish standards for developing trustworthy clinical practice guidelines and conducting systematic evidence reviews that serve as their basis.[12,13] The U.S. Preventive Services Task Force (USPSTF) and the American Cancer Society (ACS) are two organizations that issue respected and widely used cancer guidelines (Table 34.3). Both have changed their methods to comply with the IOM standards.

The USPSTF is a panel of experts in prevention and evidence-based medicine.[14] They are primary care providers specializing in internal medicine, pediatrics, family practice, gynecology and obstetrics, nursing, and health behavior. The task force process begins by conducting an extensive structured scientific evidence review. The task force then develops recommendations for primary care clinicians and health-care systems. They adhere to some of the highest standards for recommending a screening test. They are very much concerned with the question, "Does the evidence supporting a screening test demonstrate that the benefits outweigh its harms?"

The ACS guidelines date back to the 1970s. The current process for making guidelines involves commissioning academics to do an independent systematic evidence review. A single generalist group digests the evidence review, listens to public input, and writes the guidelines. The ACS panel tries to clearly articulate the benefits, limitations, and harms associated with a screening test.[15]

# BREAST CANCER

Mammographies, clinical breast examinations (CBE) by a health-care provider, and breast self-examinations (BSE) have long been advocated[16] for the early detection of breast cancer. In recent years, ultrasound, magnetic resonance imaging (MRI), and other technologies have been added to the list of proposed screening modalities.

Mammographic screening was first advocated in the 1950s. The Health Insurance Plan (HIP) Study was the first prospective, randomized clinical trial to formally assess its value in reducing death from breast cancer. In this study, started in 1963, about 61,000 women were randomized to three annual mammograms with clinical breast examination versus no screening, which was the standard practice at that time. HIP first reported that mammography reduced breast cancer mortality by 30% at about 10 years after study entry. With 18 years of follow-up, those in the screening arm had a 25% lower breast cancer mortality rate.[16]

Nine additional prospective randomized studies have been published. These studies provide the basis for the current consensus that screening women 40 to 75 years of age does reduce the relative risk of breast cancer death by 10% to 25%. The 10 studies demonstrate that the risk–benefit ratio is more favorable for women over 50 years of age. Mammography has also been shown to be operator dependent, with better performance characteristics (higher sensitivity and specificity and lower FP rates) reported by high-volume centers (Table 34.4).

It is important to note that every one of these studies has some flaws and limitations. They vary in the questions asked and their findings. The Canadian screening trial suggests mammographies and clinical breast examinations do not decrease risk of death for woman aged 40 to 49 and that mammographies add nothing to CBEs for women age 50 to 59 years.[17] On the other extreme, the Kopparberg Sweden study suggests that mammographies are associated with a 32% reduction in the risk of death for women aged 40 to 74 years.[18]

To date, no study has shown that BSEs decrease mortality. BSEs have been studied in two large randomized trials. In one, approximately 266,000 Chinese women were randomized to receive intensive BSE instruction with reinforcements and reminders compared to a control group receiving no instruction on BSE. At 10 years of follow-up, there was no difference in mortality, but the intervention arm had a significantly higher incidence of benign breast lesions diagnosed and breast biopsies preformed. In the second study, 124,000 Russian women were randomized to monthly BSEs versus no BSEs. There was no difference in mortality rates, despite the BSE group having a higher proportion of early stage tumors and a significant increase in the proportion of cancer patients surviving 15 years after diagnosis.

Ultrasonography is primarily used in the diagnostic evaluation of a breast mass identified by palpation or mammography. There is little evidence to support the use of ultrasound as an initial screening test. This modality is highly operator dependent and time consuming, with a high rate of FP findings.[19] An MRI is used for screening women at elevated breast cancer risk due to BRCA1 and BRCA2 mutations, Li-Fraumeni syndrome, Cowden disease, or a very strong family history. MRI is more sensitive but less specific than mammography, leading to a high FP rate and more unnecessary biopsies, especially among young women.[20] The impact of MRI breast screening on breast cancer mortality has not yet been determined.

Thermography, an infrared imaging technology, has some advocates as a breast cancer screening modality despite a lack of evidence from several small cohort studies.[21] Nipple aspirate cytology and ductal lavage have also been suggested as possible screening methods. Both should be considered experimental at this time.[22]

## Effectiveness of Breast Cancer Screening

Breast cancer screening has been associated with a dramatic rise in breast cancer incidence. At the same time, there has been a dramatic decrease in breast cancer mortality rates. However, in the United States and Europe, incidence-by-stage data show a dramatic increase in the proportion of early stage cancers without a concomitant decrease in the incidence of regional and metastatic cancers.[23] These findings are at odds with the clinical trials data and raise questions regarding the extent to which early diagnosis is responsible for declining breast cancer mortality rates.

From 1976 to 2008, the incidence of early-stage breast cancer for American women aged 40 and older increased from 112 to 234 per 100,000. This is a rise of 122 cases per 100,000, whereas the absolute decrease in late-stage cancers was only 8 cases per 100,000 (from 102 to 94 cases per 100,000). These data raise questions regarding the magnitude of benefit, as well as the potential risks, of breast cancer screening. The discrepancy between the magnitude of the increase of early disease and the decrease of late-stage cancer and cancer mortality suggests that a proportion of invasive breast cancers diagnosed by screening represents overdiagnosis. These data suggest that overdiagnosis accounts for up to 31% of all breast cancers diagnosed by screening.[24] Others have estimated that up to 50% of breast cancers detected by screening mammography are overdiagnosed cancers. In an exhaustive review of the screening literature, a panel of experts concluded that overdiagnosis does exist and estimated it to be 11% to 19% of breast cancers diagnosed by screening.[25]

A confounding factor with regard to the mortality benefits of breast cancer screening is the improvement that has occurred in breast cancer treatment over this period of time. The effects of the advances in therapy are supported by cancer modeling studies. Indeed, the Cancer Intervention and Surveillance Modeling Network (CISNET), supported by the U.S. National Cancer Institute (NCI), has estimated that two-thirds of the observed breast cancer mortality reduction is attributable to modern therapy, rather than to screening.[26]

TABLE 34.3

**Screening Recommendations for Normal-Risk Asymptomatic Subjects**

| Cancer Type | Test or Procedure | American Cancer Society | U.S. Preventive Services Task Force |
|---|---|---|---|
| Breast | Self-examination | Women ≥20 years: Breast self-exam is an option | "D" |
| | Clinical examination | Women 20–39 years: Perform every 3 years<br>Women ≥40 years: Perform annually | Women ≥40 years: "I" (as a stand alone without mammography) |
| | Mammography | Women ≥40 years: Screen annually for as long as the woman is in good health | Women 40–49 years: The decision should be an individual one, and take patient context/values into account ("C")<br>Women 50–74 years: Every 2 years ("B")<br>Women ≥75 years: "I" |
| | MRI | Women >20% lifetime risk of breast cancer: Screen with MRI plus mammography annually<br>Women 15%–20% lifetime risk of breast cancer: Discuss option of MRI plus mammography annually<br>Women <15% lifetime risk of breast cancer: Do not screen annually with MRI | "I" |
| Cervical | Pap test (cytology) | Women ages 21–29 years: Screen every 3 years<br><br>Women 30–65 years: Acceptable approach to screen with cytology every 3 years (see HPV test)<br><br>Women <21 years: No screening<br>Women >65 years: No screening following adequate negative prior screening<br>Women after total hysterectomy for noncancerous causes: Do not screen | Women ages 21–65 years: Screen every 3 years ("A")<br><br>Women <21 years: "D"<br>Women >65 years, with adequate, normal prior Pap screenings: "D"<br><br><br><br>Women after total hysterectomy for noncancerous causes: "D" |
| | HPV test | Women <30 years: Do not use HPV testing<br>Women ages 30–65 years: Preferred approach to screen with HPV and cytology cotesting every 5 years (see Pap test)<br>Women >65 years: No screening following adequate negative prior screening<br>Women after total hysterectomy for noncancerous causes: Do not screen | Women ages 30–65 years: Screen in combination with cytology every 5 years if woman desires to lengthen the screening interval (see Pap test) ("A")<br>Women <30 years: "D"<br>Women >65 years, with adequate, normal prior Pap screenings: "D"<br>Women after total hysterectomy for noncancerous causes: "D" |
| Colorectal | Sigmoidoscopy | Adults ≥50 years: Screen every 5 years<br>Note: For all CRC screening tests, stop screening when benefits are unlikely due to life-limiting comorbidity. | Adults 50–75 years: Every 5 years in combination with high-sensitivity fecal occult blood testing (FOBT) every 3 years ("A")[a]<br>Adults 76–85 years: "C"<br>Adults ≥85 years: "D" |
| | Fecal occult blood testing (FOBT) | Adults ≥50 years: Screen every year with high sensitivity guaiac based FOBT or fecal immunochemical test (FIT) only | Adults 50–75 years: Annually, for high-sensitivity FOBT ("A")<br>Adults 76–85 years: "C"<br>Adults ≥85 years: "D" |
| | Colonoscopy | Adults ≥50 years: Screen every 10 years | Adults 50–75 years: every 10 years ("A")<br>Adults 76–85 years: "C"<br>Adults ≥85 years: "D" |
| | Fecal DNA testing | Adults ≥50 years: Screen, but interval uncertain | "I" |
| | Fecal immunochemical testing (FIT) | Adults ≥50 years: Screen every year | "I" |
| | CT colonography | Adults ≥50 years: Screen every 5 years | "I" |
| Lung | Complete skin examination by clinician or patient | Men and women, 55–74 years, with ≥30 pack-year smoking history, still smoking or have quit within past 15 years: Discuss benefits, limitations, and potential harms of screening. Only perform screening in facilities with the right type of CT scanner and with high expertise/specialists. | "I" ("B" draft recommendation issued for public comment in July 2013) |

*(continued)*

**TABLE 34.3**

**Screening Recommendations for Normal-Risk Asymptomatic Subjects** *(continued)*

| Cancer Type | Test or Procedure | American Cancer Society | U.S. Preventive Services Task Force |
|---|---|---|---|
| Ovary | CA-125<br>Transvaginal ultrasound | There is no sufficiently accurate test proven effective in the early detection of ovarian cancer. For women at high risk of ovarian cancer and/or who have unexplained, persistent symptoms, the combination of CA-125 and transvaginal ultrasound with pelvic exam may be offered. | "D"<br>"D" |
| Prostate | Prostate-specific antigen (PSA) | Starting at age 50, men should talk to a doctor about the pros and cons of testing so they can decide if testing is the right choice for them. If African American or have a father or brother who had prostate cancer before age 65, men should have this talk starting at age 45. How often they are tested will depend on their PSA level. | Men, all ages: "D" |
|  | Digital rectal examination (DRE) | As for PSA; if men decide to be tested, they should have the PSA blood test with or without a rectal exam. | No individual recommendation |
| Skin | Complete skin examination by clinician or patient | Self-examination monthly; clinical exam as part of routine cancer-related checkup | "I" |

*Note:* Summary of the screening procedures recommended for the general population by the American Cancer Society and the U.S. Preventive Services Task Force. These recommendations refer to asymptomatic persons who have no risk factors for the cancer, other than age or gender.
[a] USPSTF lettered recommendations are defined as follows:
"A": The USPSTF recommends the service, because there is high certainty that the net benefit is substantial.
"B": The USPSTF recommends the service, because there is high certainty that the net benefit is moderate or moderate certainty that the net benefit is moderate to substantial.
"C": The USPSTF recommends selectively offering or providing this service to individual patients based on professional judgment and patient preferences. There is at least moderate certainty that the net benefit is small.
"D": The USPSTF recommends against the service, because there is moderate or high certainty that the service has no net benefit or that the harms outweigh the benefits.
"I": The USPSTF concludes that the current evidence is insufficient to assess the balance of benefits and harms of the service.

Questions have also been raised regarding the quality of the randomized screening trials that demonstrated the mortality benefits of mammography and clinical breast examination because these trials suffered from a variety of design flaws. In some, randomization methods were suboptimal, others reported varying numbers of participants over the years, and still others had substantial contamination (drop-ins). Perhaps more importantly, most trials were started and concluded before the widespread use of more advanced mammographic technology, before the modern era of adjuvant therapy, and before the advent of targeted therapy.

Although randomized control trials (RCT) remain the gold standard for assessing the benefits of a clinical intervention, they cannot take into account improvements in both treatment and patient awareness that occurred over time. For this reason, observational and modeling studies can provide important, complementary information.

One systematic review of 17 published population-based and cohort studies compared breast cancer mortality in groups of women aged 50 to 69 years who started breast cancer screening at different times. Although these studies are subject to methodologic limitations, only four suggested that breast cancer screening reduced the relative risk of breast cancer mortality by 33% or more and five suggested no benefit from screening. The review concluded that breast cancer screening likely reduces the risk of breast cancer death by no more than 10%.[27]

Even with these limitations, a systematic review of the data sponsored by the USPSTF concluded that regular mammography reduces breast cancer mortality in women aged 40 to 74 years.[28] The task force also concluded that the benefits of mammography are most significant in women aged 50 to 74 years.

## Screening Women Age 40 to 49

Experts disagree about the utility of screening women in their forties. In the HIP Randomized Control Trial, women who entered at age 40 to 49 years had a mortality benefit at 18 years of follow-up. However, to a large extent, the mortality benefit among those aged 45 to 49 years at entry was driven by breast cancers diagnosed after they reached age 50 years.[16]

Mammography, like all screening tests, is more efficient (higher PPV) for the detection of disease in populations with higher disease prevalence (see Table 34.2). Mammography is, therefore, a better test in women age 50 to 59 years than it is among women age 40 to 49 years because the risk of breast cancer increases with age. Mammography is also less optimal in women age 40 to 49 years compared to women 50 to 59 years of age for the following reasons:

- A larger proportion have increased breast density, which can obscure lesions (lower sensitivity).
- Younger women are more likely to develop aggressive, fast-growing breast cancers that are diagnosed between regular screening visits. By definition, these *interval cancers* are not screen detected.[29]

The USPSTF meta-analysis of eight large randomized trials suggested a 15% relative reduction in mortality (relative risk [RR], 0.85; 95% confidence interval [CI], 0.75 to 0.96) from mammography screening for women aged 40 to 49 years after 11 to 20 years of follow-up. This is equivalent to a needing to invite 1,904 women to screenings over 10 years to prevent one breast cancer death. Studies, however, show that more than half of women aged 40 to 49 years screened annually over a 10-year period will have an FP mammogram necessitating further evaluation, often including biopsy. In addition, estimates of overdiagnosis in this group range from 10% to 40% of diagnosed invasive cancers.[30]

In an effort to decrease FP rates, some have suggested screening every 2 years rather than yearly. Comparing biennial with annual screening, the CISNET Model consistently shows that biennial screening of women ages 40 to 70 only marginally decreases the number of lives saved while halving the false positive rate.[29] Notably, the Swedish two-county trial, which had a planned 24-month screening interval (the actual interval was 33 months) reported one

**TABLE 34.4**

**Randomized Controlled Trials**

| Study | Randomization | Sample Size | Intervention and Age at Entry | Follow-up | Finding |
|---|---|---|---|---|---|
| Health Insurance Plan, United States 1963[a,b] | Individual | 60,565–60,857 | MMG and CBE for 3 years Age 40–64 years | 18 years | RR 0.77 (95% CI: 0.61–0.97) |
| Malmo, Sweden 1976[c,d] | Individual | 42,283 | Two-view MMG every 18–24 months × 5 Age 45–69 years | 12 years | RR 0.81 (95% CI: 0.62–1.07) |
| Ostergotland (County E of Two-County Trial) Sweden 1977[e–g] | Geographic cluster | 38,405–39,034 study 37,145–37,936 control | Three single-view MMG every 2 years women, Age 40–50 years Every 33 months women, Age 50–74 | 12 years | RR 0.82 (95% CI: 0.64–1.05) |
| Kopparberg (County W of Two-County Trial) Sweden 1977[e–g] | Geographic cluster | 38,562–39,051 intervention 18,478–18,846 control | Three single-view MMG every 2 years women, Age 40–50 years Every 33 months women, Age 50–74 years | 12 years | RR 0.68 (95% CI: 0.52–0.89) |
| Edinburgh, United Kingdom[h] | Cluster by physician practice | 23,266 study 21,904 control | Initially, two-view MMG and CBE Then annual CBE with single-view MMG years 3, 5, and 7, Age 45–64 years | 10 years | RR 0.84 (95% CI: 0.63–1.12) |
| NBSS-1, Canada 1980[i,j] | Individual | 25,214 study (100% screened after entry CBE) 25,216 control | Annual two-view MMG and CBE for 4–5 years, Age 40–49 years | 13 years | RR 0.97 (95% CI: 0.74–1.27) |
| NBSS-2, Canada 1980[i,j] | Individual | 19,711 study (100% screened after entry CBE) 19,694 control | Annual two-view MMG and CBE versus CBE, Age 50–59 years | 11–16 years (mean 13 years) | RR 1.02 (95% CI: 0.78–1.33) |
| Stockholm, Sweden 1981[k] | Cluster by birth date | 40,318–38,525 intervention group 19,943–20,978 control group | Single view MMG every 28 months × 2 Age 40–64 years | 8 years | RR 0.80 (95%) CI: 0.53–1.22) |
| Gothenberg, Sweden 1982[d] | Complex | 21,650 invited 29,961 control | Initial two-view MMG, then single-view MMG every 18 months × 4 Single read first three rounds, then double-read, Age 39–59 years | 12–14 years | RR 0.79 (95% CI 0.58–1.08) In the evaluation phase RR 0.77 (95% CI 0.60–1.00) In follow-up phase |
| Age Trial[l] | Individual | 160,921 (53,884 invited; 106,956 not invited) | Invited group aged 48 and younger offered annual screening by MMG (double-view first screen, then single mediolateral oblique view thereafter); 68% accepted screening on the first screen an 69% and 70% were reinvited (81% attended at least one screen) Age 39–41 years | 10.7 years | RR 0.83 (95% CI: 0.66–1.04) |

[a] Shapiro S, Venet W, Strax P, et al. Ten- to fourteen-year effect of screening on breast cancer mortality. *J Natl Cancer Inst* 1982;69:349–355.
[b] Shapiro S. Periodic screening for breast cancer: the HIP Randomized Controlled Trial. Health Insurance Plan. *J Natl Cancer Inst Monogr* 1997:27–30.
[c] Andersson I, Aspegren K, Janzon L, et al. Mammographic screening and mortality from breast cancer: the Malmo mammographic screening trial. *BMJ* 1988;297:943–948.
[d] Nystrom L, Rutqvist LE, Wall S, et al. Breast cancer screening with mammography: overview of Swedish randomised trials. *Lancet* 1993;341:973–978.
[e] Tabar L, Fagerberg CJ, Gad A, et al. Reduction in mortality from breast cancer after mass screening with mammography. Randomised trial from the Breast Cancer Screening Working Group of the Swedish National Board of Health and Welfare. *Lancet* 1985;1:829–832.
[f] Tabar L, Fagerberg G, Duffy SW, Day NE. The Swedish two county trial of mammographic screening for breast cancer: recent results and calculation of benefit. *J Epidemiol Community Health* 1989;43:107–114.
[g] Tabar L, Fagerberg G, Duffy SW, et al. Update of the Swedish two-county program of mammographic screening for breast cancer. *Radiol Clin North Am* 1992;30:187–210.
[h] Roberts MM, Alexander FE, Anderson TJ, et al. Edinburgh trial of screening for breast cancer: mortality at seven years. *Lancet* 1990;335:241–246.
[i] Miller AB, To T, Baines CJ, Wall C. The Canadian National Breast Screening Study-1: breast cancer mortality after 11 to 16 years of follow-up. A randomized screening trial of mammography in women age 40 to 49 years. *Ann Intern Med* 2002;137:305–312.
[j] Miller AB, Wall C, Baines CJ, et al. Twenty five year follow-up for breast cancer incidence and mortality of the Canadian National Breast Screening Study: randomised screening trial. *BMJ* 2014;348–366.
[k] Frisell J, Eklund G, Hellstrom L, et al. Randomized study of mammography screening—preliminary report on mortality in the Stockholm trial. *Breast Cancer Res Treat* 1991;18:49–56.
[l] Moss SM, Cuckle H, Evans A, et al. Effect of mammographic screening from age 40 years on breast cancer mortality at 10 years' follow-up: a randomised controlled trial. *Lancet* 2006;368:2053–2060.

of the greatest reductions in breast cancer mortality among the RCTs conducted to date.

## Screening Women at High Risk

There is interest in creating risk profiles as a way of reducing the inconveniences and harms of screening. It might be possible to identify women who are at greater risk of breast cancer and refocus screening efforts on those most likely to benefit.

Risk factors for breast cancer include the following:

- Extremely dense breasts on mammography or a first-degree relative with breast cancer are each associated with at least a twofold increase in breast cancer risk
- Prior benign breast biopsy, second-degree relatives with breast cancer, or heterogeneously dense breasts each increase risk 1.5- to twofold
- Current oral contraceptive use, nulliparity, and age at first birth 30 years and older increase risk 1- to 1.5-fold.[31]

Importantly, these are risk factors for breast cancer diagnosis, not breast cancer mortality. Few studies have assessed the association between these factors and death from breast cancer; however, reproductive factors and breast density have been shown to have limited influence on breast cancer mortality.[32,33]

Genetic testing for *BRCA1* and *BRCA2* mutations and other markers of breast cancer risk has identified a group of women at high risk for breast cancer. Unfortunately, when to begin and the optimal frequency of screening have not been defined. Mammography is less sensitive at detecting breast cancers in women carrying *BRCA1* and *BRCA2* mutations, possibly because such cancers occur in younger women in whom mammography is known to be less sensitive.

MRI screening may be more sensitive than mammography in women at high risk, but specificity is lower. MRIs are associated with both an increase in FP and an increase in the detection of smaller cancers, which are more likely to be biologically indolent. The impact of MRIs on breast cancer mortality with or without concomitant use of mammographies has not been evaluated in a randomized controlled trial.

## Breast Density

It is well established that mammogram sensitivity is lower in women with heterogeneously dense or very dense breasts.[29,32] However, at this time, there are no clear guidelines regarding whether or how screening algorithms should take breast density into account.

In the American College of Radiology's Imaging Network (ACRIN)/NCI 666 Trial, breast ultrasound was offered to women with increased mammographic breast density and, if either test was positive, they were referred for a breast biopsy.[34] The radiologists performing the ultrasounds were not aware of the mammographic findings. Mammography detected 7.6 cancers per 1,000 women screened; ultrasound increased the cancer detection rate to 11.8 per 1,000. However, the PPV for mammography alone was 22.6%, whereas the PPV for mammography with ultrasound was only 11.2%.

It has yet to be determined whether supplemental imaging reduces breast cancer mortality in women with increased breast density. Although it continues to be strongly advocated by some, systematic reviews have concluded that the evidence is currently insufficient to recommend for or against this approach.[35] There are also a number of barriers to supplemental imaging, including inconsistent insurance coverage, lack of availability in many communities, concerns about cost-effectiveness (particularly with regard to MRI), and the increased FP rate associated with supplemental imaging leading to unnecessary biopsies.[36]

Newer technologies may improve screening accuracy for women with dense breasts. Compared to conventional mammography, full field digital mammography (FFDM) appears to have less FPs. This could reduce the number of women needing supplemental imaging and biopsies.[37] Digital breast tomosynthesis (DBT) uses x-rays and a digital detector to generate cross-sectional images of the breasts. Data are limited, but compared to mammograms, DBT appears to offer increased sensitivity and a reduction in the recall rates.[38] Another potential supplementary imaging modality currently under investigation is three-dimensional (3-D) automated breast ultrasound, and having screening ultrasounds performed by technologists rather than radiologists.

## Ductal Carcinoma In Situ

The incidence of noninvasive ductal carcinoma in situ (DCIS) has increased more than fivefold since 1970 as a direct consequence of widespread screening mammographies.[39] DCIS is a heterogeneous condition with low- and intermediate-grade lesions taking a decade or more to progress. Nevertheless, women with this diagnosis are uniformly subjected to treatment. A better understanding of this entity and an increased ability to predict its biologic behavior may enable more judicious, personalized treatment of DCIS.

There is little evidence that the early detection and aggressive treatment of low- and intermediate-grade DCIS reduces breast cancer mortality. The standard of care for all grades of DCIS is lumpectomy with radiation or mastectomy, followed by tamoxifen for 5 years. Interestingly, patterns of care studies indicate that mastectomy rates are increasing,[40] and that women are more often choosing double mastectomies for the treatment of DCIS.[41] Genomic characterization will hopefully lead to the identification of a subset of noninvasive cancers that can be treated less aggressively or even observed.

## Harms

The harms and disadvantages of mammography screening include overdiagnosis, FP tests, FN tests, and the possibility of radiation-induced breast cancer.

The fact that mammography screening has increased the incidence of localized disease without a significant change in metastatic disease at the time of diagnosis suggests that there is some degree of overdiagnosis. The risk of overdiagnosis is greatest at the first screening[3] and varies with patient age, tumor type, and grade of disease.

FP screening tests lead to substantial inconvenience and anxiety in addition to unnecessary invasive biopsies with their attendant complications. In the United States, about 10% of all women screened for breast cancer are called back for additional testing, and less than half of them will be diagnosed with breast cancer.[39] The risk of a FP mammogram is greater for women under the age of 50.[37]

FN tests delay diagnosis and provide false reassurance. They are more common in younger women and in women with dense breasts.[42,43] Certain histologic subtypes are also more difficult to see on mammogram. Mucinous and lobular tumors and rapidly growing tumors tend to blend in with normal breast architecture.[44]

A typical screening mammogram provides approximately 4 mSv of radiation. It has been estimated that annual mammographies will cause up to 1 case of breast cancer per 1,000 women screened from age 40 to age 80 years. Radiation exposure at younger ages causes a greater risk of breast cancer.[45] There is also concern that ionizing radiation from mammographies might disproportionately increase the breast cancer risk for women with certain *BRCA1* or *BRCA2* mutations, because these genes are related to DNA repair.[46]

## Recommendations

### Women at Average Risk

The ACS and most other medical groups recommend that average risk women undergo a CBE every 3 years starting at age 20 and that women 40 years of age and over should undergo CBEs and screening mammograms annually. Women should be informed of the benefits, limitations, and harms associated with breast cancer screening. A mammography will not detect all breast cancers, and some breast cancers detected with mammographies may still have a poor prognosis. The harms associated with breast cancer screening also include the potential for FP results, causing substantial anxiety. When abnormal findings cannot be resolved with additional imaging, a biopsy is required to rule out the possibility of breast cancer. A majority of biopsies are benign. Finally, some breast cancers detected by a mammography may be biologically indolent, meaning they would not have caused a problem or have been detected in a woman's lifetime had she not undergone a mammography.

The USPSTF, the American College of Physicians, and the Canadian Task Force on the Periodic Health Examination recommend routine screening beginning at age 50 years.[30,47,48] For women aged 40 to 49 years of age, these groups advise physicians to enter into a discussion with the patient. The physician and patient should take into account individual risks and concerns before deciding to screen.[47]

An Advisory Committee on Cancer Prevention in the European Union recommends that women between the ages of 50 and 69 years be offered mammogram screening in an organized screening program with quality assurance.[49] This committee says women aged 40 to 49 years should be advised of the potential harms of screening and, if mammographic screening is offered, it should be performed with strict quality standards and double reading.

### Women at High Risk

The ACS has issued guidelines for women who were known or likely carriers of a *BRCA* mutation and other rarer high-risk genetic syndromes, or at high risk for other reasons.[50] Annual screening mammographies and MRIs starting at age 30 is recommended for women:

- With a known *BRCA* mutation
- Who are untested but have a first-degree relative with a *BRCA* mutation
- Who had been treated with radiation to the chest for Hodgkin disease
- Who have an approximately 20% to 25% or greater lifetime risk of breast cancer based on specialized breast cancer risk estimation models.

## COLON CANCER SCREENING

Colorectal cancer screening with the rigid sigmoidoscope dates back to the late 1960s. The desire to examine the entire colon led to the use of a barium enema and the development of fecal occult blood tests. With the development of fiber optics, flexible sigmoidoscopies and, later, colonoscopies were employed. Today, fecal occult blood testing (FOBT), stool DNA testing, flexible sigmoidoscopies, colonoscopies, and CT colonographies and, occasionally, barium enemas are all used in colorectal cancer screening. MRI colonoscopy is in development.

Screening examinations of the colon and rectum can find cancer early, but also find precancerous polyps. Randomized trials have demonstrated that endoscopic polypectomies reduce the incidence of colorectal cancer by about 20%.[51–53]

*FOBT* was the first colorectal screening test studied in a prospective randomized clinical trial. The Minnesota Colon Cancer Control Study randomized 46,551 adults to one of three arms: annual FOBTs, biennial screening, or usual care. A rehydrated guaiac test was used. With 13 years of follow-up, the annual screened arm had a 33% relative reduction in colorectal cancer mortality compared to the usual care group.[54] At 18 years of follow-up, the biennially screened group had a 21% reduction in colorectal cancer

mortality.[55] This study would subsequently show that stool blood testing was associated with a 20% reduction in colon cancer incidence.[51] These results were confirmed by two other randomized trials.[56,57] A reduction in colon cancer–specific mortality persisted in the Minnesota trial through 30 years of follow-up. Overall mortality was not affected.

Rehydration increases the sensitivity of FOBT at the expense of lowering specificity.[58] Indeed, rehydrated specimens have a very high FP rate. Overall, 1% to 5% of FOBTs are positive, but only 2% to 10% of those with a positive FOBT have cancer.

*Fecal immunochemical tests* (FIT) are stool tests that do not react to hemoglobin in dietary products. They appear to have higher sensitivity and specificity for colorectal cancer when compared to nonrehydrated FOBT tests.[59]

*Fecal DNA* testing is an emerging modality. These tests look for DNA sequences specific to colorectal polyps and colorectal cancer. They may have increased sensitivity and specificity compared to FOBT. Although fecal DNA tests appear to find cancer, the body of evidence on their ability to reduce colorectal cancer mortality is limited due to a lack of study. This test has been intermittently available.

*Flexible sigmoidoscopies* are, of course, limited to an examination of the rectum and sigmoid colon. A prospective randomized trial of once-only flexible sigmoidoscopies demonstrated a 23% reduction in colorectal cancer incidence and a 31% reduction in colorectal cancer mortality after a median 11.2 years of follow-up.[60] In the NCI's Prostate, Lung, Colorectal, and Ovarian Cancer Screening Trial (PLCO), there was a 21% reduction in colorectal cancer incidence and a 26% reduction in colorectal cancer mortality with two sigmoidoscopies done 3 to 5 years apart compared with the usual care group after a median follow-up of 11.9 years.[53] In both studies, there was no effect on proximal lesions (i.e., right and transverse colon) due to the limited reach of the scope. It is estimated that flexible sigmoidoscopies can find 60% to 80% of cancers and polyps found by colonoscopies.[61]

In two meta-analyses of five randomized controlled trials of sigmoidoscopies, there was an 18% relative reduction in colorectal cancer incidence and a 28% relative reduction in colorectal cancer mortality.[62,63] Participants ranged in age from 50 to 74 years. Follow-up ranged from 6 to 13 years.

The *colonoscopy* has become the preferred screening method of many, although there have been no prospective, randomized trials of colonoscopy screening. A positive FOBT, FIT, fecal DNA test, or sigmoidoscopy warrants a follow-up diagnostic colonoscopy. Perhaps the best support for colonoscopy screening is indirect evidence from the Minnesota Colon Cancer Control Study, which required that all participants with a positive stool blood test have diagnostic imaging of the entire colon. In the Minnesota study, more than 40% of those screened annually eventually received a colonoscopy. One can also make the argument that the sigmoidoscopy studies indirectly support the efficacy of colonoscopy screening, although it can be argued that embryologic and epidemiologic evidence indicate that the right and left colon are biologically distinct and, therefore, the mortality benefits from sigmoidoscopies do not constitute proof that a colonoscopy would similarly reduce mortality from proximal colon lesions.

In studies involving repeat colonoscopies by a second physician, 21% of all adenomas were missed, including 26% of 1 to 5 mm adenomas and 2% of adenomas 10 mm or more in length.[64] Other limitations of colonoscopies include the inconvenience of the bowel preparation and the risk of bowel perforation (about 3 out of 1,000 procedures, overall, with nearly all of the risk among patients who undergo colonoscopic polypectomies). The cost of the procedure and the limited number of physicians who can do the procedure are also of concern.

A *CT colonography* or *virtual* colonoscopy allows a physician to visually reproduce the endoscopic examination on a computer screen. A CT colonography involves the same prep as a colonoscopy, but is less invasive. It might have a higher compliance rate.

In experienced hands, the sensitivity of a CT colonography for the detection of polyps ≥6 mm appears to be comparable to that of a colonoscopy. In a meta-analysis of 30 studies, 2-D and 3-D CT colonographies performed equally well.[65]

The disadvantages of a CT colonography include the fact that it requires a colonic prep and a finding on CT requires a follow-up diagnostic colonoscopy. The rate of extracolonic findings of uncertain significance is high (~15% to 30%), and each one must be evaluated, thereby contributing to additional expense and potential morbidity. The long-term, cumulative radiation risk of repeated colonography screenings is also a concern.

## Current Recommendations

The ACS, the American College of Gastroenterology, the American Gastroenterological Association, the American Society for Gastrointestinal Endoscopy, and the American College of Radiology have issued joint colorectal cancer guidelines. These groups consider FOBT, FIT, rigid and flexible sigmoidoscopies, colonoscopies, and CT colonographies to all be reasonable screening methodologies.

They recommend the following: (1) Screening modalities be chosen based on personal preference and access, and (2) average risk adults should begin colorectal cancer screening at age 50 years with *one* of the following options:

1. Annual high sensitivity FOBT or FIT
2. A flexible sigmoidoscopy every 5 years
3. A colonoscopy every 10 years
4. A double contrast barium enema every 5 years
5. A CT colonography every 5 years

No test is of unequivocal superiority. Patient preferences should be incorporated into screening in order to increase compliance. The guidelines also stress that a single screening examination is far from optimal and that patients should be in a program of regular screening.

Although some colorectal cancers are diagnosed in persons under the age of 50 years, screening persons age 40 to 49 years has low yield.[66] The guidelines also state that patients with less than a 10-year life expectancy should not be screened.

The USPSTF issued colorectal cancer screening guidelines in 2008.[67] The guidelines were based on a systematic literature review and decision models. The task force concluded that three screening strategies appear to be equivalent for adults age 50 to 75 years:

1. An annual FOBT with a sensitive test
2. A flexible sigmoidoscopy every 5 years, with a sensitive FOBT every 3 years
3. A colonoscopy every 10 years

The task force recommends that patients age 76 to 85 years be evaluated individually for screening. They found "insufficient evidence" to recommend CT colonographies or fecal DNA testing.

### Patients at Increased Risk of Colorectal Cancer

Patients can have higher than average risk of colorectal cancer due to familial or hereditary factors and clinical conditions such as inflammatory bowel disease. These patients technically undergo surveillance and not screening. Nevertheless, there are few clinical studies to guide recommendations. Guidelines have been created based on professional opinion and an understanding of the biology of colorectal cancer (Table 34.5).[68]

## OTHER CANCERS OF THE GASTROINTESTINAL TRACT

There are no widely accepted screening guidelines for cancers of the esophagus, stomach, pancreas, and liver. However, surveillance is advocated for some patients at high risk.

### Esophageal Cancer Screening

Esophageal cancer screening has centered on endoscopic examinations for those at high risk due to chronic, severe gastroesophageal reflux disease.[69] Some physicians advocate routine endoscopic surveillance of patients with Barrett esophagus. At this time, there is no evidence that such surveillance is effective at reducing cancer mortality.

---

**TABLE 34.5**

**Colon Cancer Screening Recommendations for People with Familial or Inherited Risk**

| Familial Risk Category | Screening Recommendation |
| --- | --- |
| First-degree relative[a] affected with *colorectal cancer* or an *adenomatous polyp* at age ≥60 years, or two second-degree relatives[b] affected with colorectal *cancer* | Same as average risk but starting at age 40 years |
| Two or more first-degree relatives with *colon cancer*, or a single first-degree relative with *colon cancer* or *adenomatous polyps* diagnosed at an age <60 years | Colonoscopy every 5 years, beginning at age 40 years or 10 years younger than the earliest diagnosis in the family, whichever comes first |
| One second-degree or any third-degree relative[b,c] with *colorectal cancer* | Same as average risk |
| Gene *carrier* or *at risk* for familial adenomatous polyposis[d] | Sigmoidoscopy annually, beginning at age 10–12 years[e] |
| Gene carrier or at risk for HNPCC | Colonoscopy, every 1–2 years, beginning at age 20–25 years or 10 years younger than the earliest case in the family, whichever comes first |

[a] First-degree relatives include patients, siblings, and children.
[b] Second-degree relatives include grandparents, aunts, and uncles.
[c] Third-degree relatives include great-grandparents and cousins.
[d] Includes the subcategories of familial adenomatous polyposis, Gardner syndrome, some Turcot syndrome families, and attenuated adenomatous polyposis coli (AAPC).
[e] In AAPC, colonoscopy should be used instead of sigmoidoscopy because of the preponderance of proximal colonic adenomas. Colonoscopy screening in AAPC should probably begin in the late teens or early 20s.
HNPCC, hereditary nonpolyposis colon cancer.
From Winawer S, Fletcher R, Rex D, et al. Colorectal cancer screening and surveillance: clinical guidelines and rationale: update based on new evidence. *Gastroenterology* 2003;124:544–560, with permission.

## Gastric Cancer Screening

Barium-meal photofluorography, serum pepsinogen, and gastric endoscopy have been proposed as screening methods for the early detection of gastric cancer. There are no randomized trials evaluating the impact of these modalities on gastric cancer mortality. Indeed, screening with barium-meal photofluorography has been studied in high-risk populations for more than 40 years without clear evidence of benefit.

Time-trend analysis and case control studies of gastric endoscopy have suggested a decrease in gastric cancer mortality among those at high risk in screened versus unscreened individuals; however, a large observational study in a high-risk population failed to demonstrate a benefit.[70,71]

Although widespread gastric screenings cannot be advocated, there may be justification for endoscopic screenings of high-risk populations. Candidates for screening might include elderly individuals with atrophic gastritis or pernicious anemia, patients who have had partial gastrectomy,[72] those with a history of sporadic adenomas, and patients with familial adenomatous polyposis or hereditary nonpolyposis colon cancer.

## Pancreatic Cancer Screening

At this time, there are no data from prospective clinical trials to support a role for pancreatic cancer screening. Some patients with an extensive family history have undergone periodic CT scanning of the abdomen, but this approach has not been shown to reduce pancreatic cancer mortality. There is an ongoing search for screening biomarkers. There is a need to follow large cohorts prospectively after collecting and storing biologic samples to identify biomarkers of risk.[73]

## Liver Cancer Screening

Screening for liver cancer or hepatocellular carcinoma (HCC) has focused on very high-risk individuals, such as those with cirrhosis.[54] To date, trial results are unreliable due to small study sizes and a lack of randomization.

Serum alpha-fetoprotein (AFP), a fetal-specific glycoprotein antigen, is an HCC tumor marker used in screening. It is not specific to HCC because it may be elevated in hepatitis, pregnancy, and some germ cell tumors. AFP has variable sensitivity and has not been tested in any randomized clinical trial with a mortality end point.

In one prospective, 16-year, population-based observational study, screening was done on 1,487 Alaska natives with chronic hepatis B virus (HBV) infection. The survival of those with screen-detected HCC was compared with a historical group of clinically diagnosed HCC patients.[74] With a target of AFP determination every 6 months, there was a 97% sensitivity and 95% specificity for HCC. Such high sensitivity and specificity have not been found in other studies. It is not known if AFP screening decreases HCC mortality.[75]

Hepatic ultrasound has been used as an additional method for detection of HCC. This procedure is operator dependent with variable sensitivity and specificity. Ultrasound screening is commonly used in patients with hepatitis and cirrhosis.[76,77]

Interest in CT scanning has grown due to the limitations of AFP and ultrasound. CT scans may be a more sensitive test for HCC than ultrasound or AFP.[75]

# GYNECOLOGIC CANCER

## Cervical Cancer Screening

Dr. George Papanicolaou first introduced the Pap smear or Pap test in the early 1940s. The test was widely adopted based on its ability to identify squamous premalignancies and malignancies (from the ectodermal cervix) and glandular dysplasia and adenocarcinomas (from the endocervix). It is, however, more sensitive at detecting squamous lesions.

The Pap test was introduced before the advent of the prospective, randomized clinical trial and, therefore, has never been so tested. However, a number of observational studies over the past 60 years support the effectiveness of this screening test.[78,79] Multiple ecologic studies have shown an inverse correlation between the introduction of Pap testing in a given country and reductions in both cervical cancer incidence and mortality.[80] Importantly, mortality reductions in these studies have been proportional to the intensity of screening. In one series, more than half of women diagnosed with cervical cancer either had never had a Pap test or had not been screened within 5 years of diagnosis.[80]

Cervical cytology has evolved over the years. The original Pap smear used an ectocervical spatula to apply a specimen ("smear") to glass slides. It later included an endocervical brush. The smear was fixed, stained, and manually examined under a microscope. That method is still used today, but a liquid-based/thin-layer system capable of being analyzed by computer is gaining in popularity.[81]

Human papillomavirus (HPV) 16 and 18 are the cause of more than 70% of cervical cancers. Thirteen other HPV subtypes are known to be associated with cervical cancer. With increasing understanding of the role of HPV in cervical disease, interest in developing tests to determine the presence of HPV DNA and RNA has grown. HPV screening can be used along with cytology (*cotesting*), in response to an abnormal cytologic test (*reflexive testing*), or as a stand-alone test. One advantage of the liquid-based/thin-layer tests over the older smears is that it makes reflexive testing easier to perform. An abnormal cytology screen can be objectively verified by testing for the presence of the HPV virus without calling the patient back.

HPV testing is especially useful because of its negative predictive value. Although a positive test for HPV infection is not diagnostic of cervical disease, a negative HPV test strongly suggests that the abnormal Pap does not represent a premalignant condition.

The utility of the HPV test is limited in younger women because one-third or more of women in their 20s have active cervical infections at any given time. The overwhelming majority of these infections and resultant dysplasia will regress and resolve within 8 to 24 months. For women over the age of 30, screening for the presence of HPV DNA or RNA appears to be superior to cytology in identifying women at risk for cervical dysplasia and cancer.[82] An HPV infection in women over the age of 30 is more likely to be persistent and clinically significant.[83] The risk of cervical cancer also increases with age, and most cervical cancer deaths occur in women over 50 years of age.

### Cytologic Terminology

The terminology of the Pap smear has changed over time. The traditional cytologic categories were mild, moderate, and severe dysplasia and carcinoma in situ. *Mild* correlated with cervical intraepithelial neoplasia (CIN)1 histology on biopsy; *moderate* usually indicated CIN2; and *severe* dysplasia indicated CIN3 or carcinoma in situ.

There was some subjectivity and some overlap, especially in the area of mild and moderate dysplasia. The NCI sponsored the development of the Bethesda system in 1988. This system provides an assessment of the adequacy of the cervical specimen and a way of categorizing and describing the Pap smear findings. It more effectively and uniformly communicates cytology results from the laboratory to the patient caregiver. The Bethesda system was modified in 1991 and again in 2001.[84] Today, more than 40 international professional societies have endorsed the Bethesda system.

The Bethesda system recognizes both squamous and glandular cytologic abnormalities.

Squamous cell abnormalities include:

- Atypical squamous cells (ASC), which are categorized as either:
  - Of undetermined significance (ASC-US)
  - Cannot exclude high-grade squamous intraepithelial lesions (ASC-H)
- Low-grade squamous intraepithelial lesion (LSIL), which correlates with histologic CIN1
- High-grade squamous intraepithelial lesion (HSIL), which correlates with histologic CIN2, CIN3, and carcinoma in situ

Glandular cell abnormalities (features suggestive of adenocarcinoma) include:

- Atypical glandular cells (AGC): endocervical, endometrial, or not otherwise specified
- AGCs, favor neoplastic
- Endocervical or not otherwise specified
- Endocervical adenocarcinoma in situ (AIS)
- Adenocarcinoma

ASCs differ from normal cells but do not meet criteria for LSIL or HSIL. A small proportion of ASC-US smears are from CIN1 lesions; a smaller proportion are from CIN2 or 3. LSILs are usually due to a transient HPV infection. HSILs are more likely to be due to a persistent HPV infection and are more likely to progress to cervical cancer than LSILs.

The Lower Anogenital Squamous Terminology (LAST) project of the College of American Pathology and the American Society for Colposcopy and Cervical Pathology has proposed that histologic cervical findings be described using the same terminology as cytologic findings.[85]

Women under the age of 30 who have not received the HPV vaccine have a high incidence of HPV infection[86] and the highest prevalence of CIN. However, the overwhelming majority of these HPV infections and associated CIN will spontaneously regress.[87,88] Due to the high regression rates, cervical screening and treatment in women aged 20 to 24 years appear to have little or no impact on the incidence of invasive cervical cancer. It is estimated that about 6% of CIN1 lesions progress to CIN3, and 10% to 20% of CIN3 lesions progress to invasive cancer.[89]

The Atypical Squamous Cells of Undetermined Significance (ASCUS)-LSIL Triage Study (ALTS) evaluated women with abnormal Pap smears.[90] The investigators concluded that women with ASC-US should be tested for HPV. Those who are HPV positive should receive a colposcopy. In addition, because most women with LSIL or HSIL had an HPV infection, an immediate colposcopy and a biopsy of lesions was recommended.[91] HPV DNA testing is very sensitive for identifying CIN2 or worse pathology. Among women 30 to 69 years of age, the sensitivity of the Pap test with HPV testing was 95% compared with 55% for the Pap test alone.[92]

## Performance Characteristics of Cervical Cytology

The sensitivity of cytology varies and is a function of the adequacy of the cervical specimen. It is also affected by the age of the woman and the experience of the cytologist. The addition of HPV testing increases the number of women referred for a colposcopy. Not surprisingly, sensitivity is improved by serial examinations over time versus a single screen.

## Screening Recommendations

Cervical screening, like other screening tests, is associated with some degree of overdiagnosis as evidenced by the phenomenon of spontaneous regression (see previous) and, therefore, potential harm from overtreatment, such as cervical incompetence, which may reduce fertility and the ability to carry a pregnancy to term. Because dysplasia takes years to progress to cervical cancer,

increasing the screening interval can reduce overdiagnosis and excessive treatment without decreasing screening efficacy.

In 2012, the ACS, the American Society for Colposcopy and Cervical Pathology (ASCCP), and the American Society for Clinical Pathology (ASCP) issued joint screening guidelines.[93] These guidelines recommend different surveillance strategies and options based on a woman's age, screening history, risk factors, and choice of screening tests. The following are the recommendations for a woman at average risk.

- Screening for cervical cancer should begin at 21 years of age. Women aged 21 to 29 years should receive cytology screening (with either conventional cervical cytology smears or liquid-based cytology) every 3 years. HPV testing should not be performed in this age group (although it can be used to follow-up a diagnosis of ASC-US). Women under 21 years of age should not be screened regardless of their age of sexual initiation.
- For women aged 30 to 65 years, the preferred approach is to be screened every 5 years with both HPV testing and cytology (*cotesting*). It is also acceptable to continue screening every 3 years with cytology alone.
- Women should discontinue screening after age 65 years if they have had three consecutive negative cytology tests or two consecutive negative HPV test results within the 10-year period before ceasing screening, with the most recent test occurring within the last 5 years.
- Women who have undergone a hysterectomy for noncancerous conditions do not need to undergo cervical cancer screening.
- Women, regardless of age, should NOT be screened annually by any screening method.
- Women who have received HPV vaccinations should still be screened according to the previously listed schedule.

## Screening in Low Resource Countries

Cytology and HPV testing is not widely available in much of the world. Cervical cancer remains a leading cause of death in many of these areas. Visual inspection of the cervix is a low-tech method of screening that is now recognized as having the potential to save thousands of lives per year. A clustered, randomized trial in India compared one-time cervical visual inspection and immediate colposcopy, biopsy, and/or cryotherapy (where indicated) versus counseling on cervical cancer deaths in women aged 30 to 59 years. After 7 years of follow-up, the age-standardized rate of death due to cervical cancer was 39.6 per 100,000 person-years in the intervention group versus 56.7 per 100,000 person-years in unscreened controls.[94,95] This was the first prospective randomized clinical trial to evaluate cervical cancer screening.

## Ovarian Cancer Screening

Modalities proposed for ovarian cancer screening include the bimanual pelvic examination, serum CA-125 antigen measurement, and transvaginal ultrasound (TVU). The bimanual pelvic examination is subjective and not very reproducible, but serum CA-125 can be objectively measured. Unfortunately, CA-125 is neither sensitive nor specific. It is elevated in only about half of women with ovarian cancer and may be elevated in a number of nonmalignant diseases (e.g., diverticulosis, endometriosis, cirrhosis, normal menstruation, pregnancy, uterine fibroids).[96–98] TVU has shown poor performance in the detection of ovarian cancer in average and high-risk women.[99] There is interest in the analysis of serum proteomic patterns, but this should be considered experimental.[100,101]

The combination of CA-125 and TVU has been assessed in two large, prospective randomized trials. The U.S. trial, the Prostate Lung Colorectal and Ovarian trial (PLCO), enrolled

78,216 women of average risk age 55 to 74 years.[102,103] Participants were randomized to receive annual examinations with CA-125 (at entry and then annually for 5 years) and TVU (at entry and then annually for 3 years) (n = 39,105), or usual care (n = 39,111). Participants were followed for a maximum of 13 years, with mortality from ovarian cancer as the main study outcome. At the conclusion of the study, the number of deaths from ovarian cancer was similar in each group. There were 3.1 ovarian cancer deaths per 10,000 women years in the screened group versus 2.6 deaths per 10,000 women years in the control group (RR = 1.18; 95% CI, 0.82 to 1.71).[103]

The U.K. Collaborative Trial of Ovarian Cancer Screening (UKCTOCS) is a randomized trial assessing the efficacy of CA-125 and TVU in more than 200,000 postmenopausal women. In this trial, CA-125 is being used as a first-line test and TVU as a follow-up test using a risk of ovarian cancer algorithm (ROCA).[104] The ROCA measures changes in CA-125 over time rather than using a predefined cut point.[105] ROCA is believed to improve sensitivity for smaller tumors without measurably increasing the FP rate. A mortality assessment is expected in 2015.[106]

No organization currently recommends screening average risk women for ovarian cancer. In 2012, the USPSTF recommended against screening for ovarian cancer, concluding that there was "adequate evidence" that (1) annual screening with TVU and CA-125 does not reduce ovarian cancer mortality and (2) screening for ovarian cancer can lead to important harms, mainly surgical interventions in women without ovarian cancer.[107]

### Women at High Risk for Ovarian Cancer

Although no study has shown a mortality benefit for ovarian cancer screening of high-risk individuals, a National Institutes of Health (NIH) consensus panel concluded that it was prudent for women with a known hereditary ovarian cancer syndrome, such as *BRCA1/2* mutations or HNPCC, to have annual rectovaginal pelvic examinations, CA-125 determinations, and TVU until childbearing is completed or at least until age 35 years, at which time a prophylactic bilateral oophorectomy is recommended.[108]

### Endometrial Cancer Screening

There is insufficient evidence to recommend endometrial cancer screening either for women at average risk or for those at increased risk due to a history of unopposed estrogen therapy, tamoxifen therapy, late menopause, nulliparity, infertility or failure to ovulate, obesity, diabetes, or hypertension.[109] The ACS recommends that women be informed about the symptoms of endometrial cancer—in particular, vaginal bleeding and spotting—after the onset of menopause. Women should be encouraged to immediately report these symptoms to their physician.

### Women at High Risk for Endometrial Cancer

Women with a suspected autosomal-dominant predisposition to colon cancer (e.g. Lynch syndrome), should consider undergoing an annual endometrial biopsy to evaluate endometrial histology, beginning at age 35 years.[110,111] This is based only on *expert opinion*, given the paucity of clinical trial data. Women should be informed about the potential benefits, harms, and limitations of testing for early endometrial cancer.

## LUNG CANCER SCREENING

Lung cancer screening programs using chest radiographs (CXR) and sputum cytology began in the late 1940s.[112] An evaluation of these programs showed that screening led to the diagnosis of an increased number of cancers, an increased proportion of early stage cancers, and a larger proportion of screen-diagnosed patients surviving more than 5 years.

These findings led many to advocate for mass lung cancer screening, whereas others called for a prospective, randomized trial with a lung cancer mortality endpoint.[113] The Mayo Lung Project (MLP), which began in 1971, was such a trial. More than 9,200 male smokers were enrolled and randomized to either have sputum cytology collected and CXRs done every 4 months for 6 years or to have these same tests performed annually.

At 13 years of follow-up, there were more early stage cancers in the intensively screened arm (n = 99) than in the control arm (n = 51), but the number of advanced tumors was nearly identical (107 versus 109, respectively).[114] Despite an increase in 5-year survival (35% versus 15%) intensive screening was not associated with a reduction in lung cancer mortality (3.2 versus 3.0 deaths per 1,000 person-years, respectively).[115]

The impact of screening on cancer incidence persisted through nearly 20 years of follow-up. There were 585 lung cancers diagnosed on the intensive screening arm versus 500 on the control arm (p = 0.009) and intensive screening continued to be associated with a significant increase in disease-specific survival. However, a concomitant decrease in lung-cancer mortality did not emerge with long-term follow-up (4.4 lung cancer deaths per 1,000 person-years in the intensively screened arm versus 3.9 per 1,000 person-years in the control arm).[116] This suggests that some lung cancers diagnosed by screening would not have resulted in death had they not been detected (i.e., overdiagnosis).[116]

Two other large, randomized studies of CXR and sputum cytology were conducted in the United States during the same time period. All three studies evaluated different screening schedules rather than screening versus no screening. Paradoxically, a meta-analysis of the three studies found that more frequent screening was associated with an increase (albeit not statistically significant), rather than a decrease, in lung cancer mortality when compared with less frequent screening.[117] A study conducted in Czechoslovakia in the 1980s also failed to show a reduction in lung cancer mortality with CXR screening.[118]

More recently, the NCI conducted the PLCO trial at 10 sites across the United States. This was a prospective, randomized trial of nearly 155,000 men and women, aged 55 to 74 years. Participants were randomized to receive annual, single-view, posteroanterior CXRs for 4 years versus routine care. With 13 years of follow-up, no significant difference in lung cancer mortality was observed. A total of 1,213 lung cancer deaths occurred on the intervention arm versus 1,230 in the control group (RR, 0.99; 95% CI, 0.87 to 1.22).[119]

*Low-dose computerized tomography (LDCT)* is an appealing technology for lung cancer screening. It uses an average of 1.5 mSv of radiation to perform a lung scan in 15 seconds. A conventional CT scan uses 8 mSv of radiation and takes several minutes. The LDCT image is not as sharp as the conventional image, but sensitivity and specificity for the detection of lung lesions are similar.

As in the early chest radiograph trials, a number of single-arm LDCT studies reported a substantial increase in the number of early stage lung cancers diagnosed. These studies also demonstrated that 5-year survival rates were increased in screened compared to unscreened populations.

These findings led to the conduct of several randomized trials of LDCT for the early detection of lung cancer. The largest, longest, and first to report a mortality end point is the National Lung Screening Trial (NLST). In this trial, approximately 53,000 persons were randomized to receive three annual LDCT scans or single-view posteroanterior CXRs. Eligible participants were current and former smokers between 55 and 74 years of age at the time of randomization with at least a 30 pack-year smoking history; former smokers were eligible if they had quit smoking within the previous 15 years.

With a median follow-up of 6.5 years, 13% more lung cancers were diagnosed and a 20% (95% CI, 6.8 to 26.7; p = 0.004) relative reduction in lung cancer mortality was observed in the LDCT arm compared to the CXR arm.[11] This corresponds to rates of death from lung cancer of 247 and 309 per 100,000 person-years, respectively.[11] Another important finding from the NLST was a 6.7% (95% CI, 1.2 to 13.6; p = 0.02) decrease in death from any cause in the LDCT group.

NLST participants were at high risk for developing lung cancer based on their smoking history. Indeed, 25% of all participant deaths were due to lung cancer. A further analysis of the NLST shows that screening prevented the greatest number of lung cancer deaths among participants who were at the highest risk but prevented very few deaths among those at the lowest risk. These findings provide empirical support for risk-based screening.[120]

LDCT screening is clearly promising, but there are some notable caveats. The risk of a FP finding in the first screen was 21%. Overall, after three CT scans, 39.1% of participants had at least one positive screening result. Of those who screened positive, the FP rate was 96.4% in the LDCT group.[11] Positive results require additional workup, which can include conventional CT scans, a needle biopsy, bronchoscopy, mediastinoscopy, or thoracotomy. These diagnostic procedures are associated with anxiety, expense, and complications (e.g., pneumo- or hemothorax after a lung biopsy). In the LDCT study arm, there were 16 deaths within 60 days of an invasive diagnostic procedure. Of the 16 deaths, 6 ultimately did not have cancer. Although it is not known whether these deaths were directly caused by the invasive procedure, such findings do give pause. Although the radiation dose from LDCT is low, the possibility that this screening test could cause radiation-induced cancers is at least a theoretical concern. The possibility of this long-term phenomenon will have to be assessed in future analyses.

The CXR lung screening studies suggested that there is a reservoir of biologically indolent lung cancer and that a percentage of screen-detected lung cancers represent overdiagnosis. The estimated rate of overdiagnosis in the long-term follow-up of the Mayo Lung Study and the other CXR studies was 17 to 18.5%.[121] Similarly, it is estimated that 18.5% of the cancers diagnosed on the LDCT arm of the NLST represented overdiagnosis.[122]

There are estimates that widespread, high-quality screening has the potential to prevent 12,000 lung cancer deaths per year in the United States.[123] However, the NLST was performed at 33 centers specifically chosen for their expertise in the screening, diagnosis, and treatment of lung cancer. It is not known whether the widespread adoption of LDCT lung cancer screening will result in higher complication rates and a less favorable risk–benefit ratio.

Although LDCT lung cancer screening should clearly be considered for those at high risk of the disease, those at lower risk are equally likely to suffer the harms associated with screening but less likely to reap the benefits.

Following the announcement of the NLST results, the ACS, the American College of Chest Physicians (AACP), the American Society of Clinical Oncology (ASCO), and the National Comprehensive Cancer Network (NCCN) recommended that clinicians should initiate a discussion about lung cancer screening with patients who would have qualified for the trial. That is:

- Age 55 to 74 years
- At least a 30 pack-year smoking history
- Currently smoke or have quit within the past 15 years
- Relatively good health

Core elements of this discussion should include the benefits, uncertainties, and harms associated with screening for lung cancer with LDCT. Adults who choose to be screened should enter an organized screening program at an institution with expertise in LDCT screening, with access to a multidisciplinary team skilled in the evaluation, diagnosis, and treatment of abnormal lung lesions. If such a program is not available, the risks of harm due to screening may be greater than the benefits.[124,125] The guidelines recommend an annual LDCT screening with the caveat that participants in NLST had only three annual screens.

The USPSTF guidelines give LDCT a grade B recommendation, concluding that there is moderate certainty that annual screening for lung cancer with LDCT is of moderate net benefit in asymptomatic persons at high risk for lung cancer based on age, total cumulative exposure to tobacco smoke, and years since quitting.

## PROSTATE CANCER SCREENING

Hugh Hampton Young first advocated the early detection of prostate cancer with a careful digital rectal examination (DRE) in 1903. Screening for prostate cancer with the DRE and serum PSA was first advocated in the mid 1980s and became commonplace by 1992. PSA screening is directly responsible for prostate cancer becoming the most common nonskin cancer in American men.

PSA is a glycoprotein produced almost exclusively by the epithelial component of the prostate gland. This protein was discovered in the late 1970s, and a serum test to measure circulating levels was developed in the early 1980s. Although PSA is prostate specific, it is not prostate cancer specific and may be elevated in a variety of conditions (e.g., benign prostatic hyperplasia, inflammation and following trauma to the gland, the presence of prostate cancer).

The PSA test has been widely advocated for prostate cancer screening because it is objective, easily measured, reproducible, noninvasive, and inexpensive. Although PSA screening increases the detection of potentially curable disease, there is substantial debate about the overall utility of the test. This is because PSA screening introduces substantial lead time and length bias as well as being associated with a high FN and FP rates and having a low positive predictive value. The prostate cancer conundrum was best summarized by the distinguished urologist, Willet Whitmore when he said, "Is cure necessary for those in whom it is possible? Is cure possible for those in whom it is necessary?"[126]

Observational studies suggest that the problem of prostate cancer overdiagnosis precedes the PSA era. In a landmark analysis with 20-year follow-up, only a small proportion of 767 men, diagnosed with localized prostate cancer in the 1970s and early 1980s and followed expectantly, died from prostate cancer: 4% to 7% of those with Gleason 2 to 4 tumors, 6% to 11% of those with Gleason 5 disease, and 18% to 30% of men with Gleason 6 cancer.[127]

Although obviously present in the pre-PSA era, overdiagnosis increased substantially after the introduction of PSA screening. This is illustrated by an examination of the prostate cancer incidence and mortality rates in Washington state and Connecticut. Due to the earlier uptake of PSA screening, the incidence of prostate cancer in Washington increased to twice that of Connecticut during the 1990s. However, mortality rates remained similar throughout the decade and, in fact, have remained similar to this day. The Surveillance, Epidemiology, and End Results (SEER) cancer registries show that, over the last 2 decades, a larger proportion of men living in western Washington have been diagnosed with prostate cancer and definitively treated, without a concomitant reduction in prostate cancer mortality compared to that of men living in Connecticut.[128]

Additional evidence of the potential for overdiagnosis comes from the unexpectedly large number of men diagnosed with prostate cancer in the Prostate Cancer Prevention Trial (PCPT). The PCPT was a prospective, randomized, placebo-controlled trial of finasteride for prostate cancer prevention. Men were screened annually during this trial, and those who had not been diagnosed with prostate cancer after 7 years on-study were asked to undergo an end-of-study prostate biopsy. Of 4,692 men on the placebo arm whose prostate cancer status had been determined by biopsy or transurethral resection (TURP), 24.4% were diagnosed with prostate cancer. Given that the lifetime risk of prostate cancer mortality in the United States is less than 3%, it is clear that many men harbor indolent prostate cancer and, therefore, are at risk of being overdiagnosed.

The unexpectedly high rate of positive end-of-study biopsies in men with PSA levels less than or equal to 4.0 ng/mL provided a more accurate assessment of disease prevalence and thus a more accurate assessment of PSA sensitivity than was previously possible. Of the 2,950 men on the placebo arm of the PCPT with PSA levels consistently less than or equal to 4 ng/mL who underwent end-of-study biopsies, 449 (15.2%) were diagnosed with prostate cancer. Accordingly, a PSA level <4.0 ng/mL is more likely to be a *false* negative. Because Sensitivity = True Positives / (True Positives + False Negatives), a higher FN rate means a lower sensitivity at any given PSA threshold. This has prompted some to advocate using a lower PSA threshold for recommending biopsies. However, although lowering the PSA threshold from 4.0 to 2.5 ng/mL increases the sensitivity from 24% to 42.8%, it reduces specificity from 92.7% to an unacceptably low 80%.[129]

In the PCPT, cancer was found on end-of-study biopsies at all PSA levels (e.g., including 10% of biopsies in men with PSA levels between 0.6 and 1.0 ng/mL and 6% of biopsies in men with PSA levels between 0 and 0.6 were positive), suggesting a continuum of prostate cancer risk and no cut point with simultaneously high sensitivity and high specificity. High-grade disease was also documented at all PSA levels, albeit at an overall frequency of only 2.3% of men with PSAs <4 ng/mL.[130,131]

## Does Prostate Cancer Treatment Prevent Deaths?

In order for screening to work, treatment has to work. The first prospective, randomized studies showing that any prostate cancer treatment saves lives were published in the late 1990s. These studies demonstrated an overall survival benefit for the addition of long-term androgen deprivation to radiation therapy in men with locally advanced, high-risk prostate cancer.[132]

The value of surgery for localized disease was assessed by the Scandinavian Prostate Cancer Group 4 study (SPCG-4). In this trial, 695 men with clinically localized prostate cancer were prospectively randomized to receive radical prostatectomy (RP) or watchful waiting (WW). In the expectant management group, hormonal therapy was given at the time of symptomatic metastases. About 60% of those enrolled had low-grade, 23% had moderate-grade, 5% had high-grade tumors, and 12% had tumors of unknown grade. At a median follow-up of 12.8 years, the RP group had significantly lower overall (RR 0.75; p = 0.007) and prostate cancer–specific mortality (RR 0.62; p = 0.01), with 14.6% of the PR group and 20.7% of the WW group having died of prostate cancer. The number needed to treat or prevent one prostate cancer death was 15. The survival benefit associated with RP was similar before and after 9 years of follow-up and for men with low and high-risk disease. However, a subset analysis suggested that the mortality benefit of surgery was limited to men less than 65 years of age. An important limitation of this trial is that 75% of the study participants had palpable disease, only 12% had nonpalpable disease, and only 5% of the cancers had been screen detected. It is, therefore, difficult to apply these data to the US prostate cancer population, which is dominated by nonpalpable, screen-detected disease.[133]

In contrast to the SPCG-4, the Prostate Intervention versus Observation Trial (PIVOT) was conducted in the United States during the early PSA era. In this study, 731 men with screen-detected prostate cancer were randomized to receive RP or WW. Of the participants, 50% had nonpalpable disease and, using established criteria for PSA levels, grade, and tumor stage, 43% of men had low-risk, 36% had intermediate-risk, and 21% had high-risk prostate cancer. With a median follow-up of 12 years, during which time 48.4% (354 of 731) of the study participants had died, RP was associated with statistically insignificant 2.9% and 2.6% absolute reductions in overall and prostate cancer–specific mortality,

respectively. Subgroup analyses suggested mortality benefits for men with PSA values greater than 10 ng/mL and for those with intermediate- and high-risk disease.[134]

## The Prospective Randomized Screening Trials

The PLCO Cancer Screening Trial was a multicenter, phase III trial conducted in the United States by the NCI. In this trial, nearly 77,000 men age 55 to 74 years were randomized to receive annual PSA testing for 6 years or usual care. At 13 years of follow-up, a nonsignificant increase in cumulative prostate cancer mortality was observed among men randomized to annual screening (RR, 1.09; 95% CI, 0.87 to 1.36).[135] The most important limitation of this trial was the high rate of PSA testing among men randomized to the control arm. This *drop-in* or *contamination* served to reduce the statistical power of the study to detect differences in outcome between the two arms. It has also been argued that, due to the high rate of PSA screening on the control arm, PLCO effectively compared regular prostate cancer screening to opportunistic screening rather than comparing screening to no screening.

The ERSPC is a multicenter trial initiated in 1991 in the Netherlands and Belgium; five additional European countries joined between 1994 and 1998.[136,137] The frequency of PSA testing was every 4 years in all countries except Sweden, in which it was every 2 years. The study results were initially reported in 2009 and updated in 2012.[136,137] Although the overall analysis of 182,160 men, aged 50 to 74, did not show a reduction in prostate cancer–specific mortality, screening was associated with a significant decrease in prostate cancer mortality in the prespecified core age group, 55 to 69 years, which included 162,243 men. After a median follow-up of 11 years, a 21% relative reduction of prostate cancer death (RR, 0.79; 95% CI, 0.68 to 0.91) was observed in this group. In absolute terms, prostate cancer mortality was reduced from 5 to 4 men per 1,000 screened and 37 men had to be diagnosed to avert one prostate cancer death. It remains to be seen whether the benefits of screening will increase with continued follow-up.

The recruitment and randomization procedures of the ERSPC differed among countries. Notably, potential participants in Finland, Sweden, and Italy were identified from population registries and underwent randomization *before* written informed consent was obtained. In some trials, men on the control arm were not aware they were in the study. Therefore, men on the intervention arm in these countries were more likely to be cared for at high-volume referral centers. This may have contributed to the higher proportion of men on the screening arm, with clinically localized cancer being treated with RPs.[138]

In a separate report on 20,000 men randomized to screening or a control group in Göteborg, Sweden, there was a 40% (95% CI, 1.50 to 1.80) risk reduction at 14 years of follow-up.[139] They reported 293 (95% CI, 177 to 799) needed to be screened and 12 needed to be diagnosed in order to prevent one prostate cancer death. Three-fourths of the men in this report and 89% of the prostate cancer deaths were included in the published ERSPC analysis. Given this, these data do not constitute independent evidence of the efficacy of prostate cancer screening.

The other site to report separately was in Finland. A total of 80,144 men were randomized to a screening or usual care arm. At 12 years after randomization, there was no statistical difference in risk of prostate cancer death (hazard ratio [HR] = 0.85; 95% CI, 0.69 to 1.04).[140] Possible explanations as to why Sweden and Finland would have such different outcomes include differences in the frequency of screening (every 2 years versus every 4 years, respectively) and the higher background rate of death from prostate cancer in the control group in the Goteborg cohort. Given that the mortality data from these two cohorts have been largely included in the ERSPC analyses, they do not provide independent evidence of the efficacy of prostate cancer screening.

**CANCER PREVENTION AND SCREENING**

The decline in prostate cancer mortality in the United States since the introduction of PSA screening 2 decades ago is often offered as evidence supporting a mortality benefit for prostate cancer screening. However, prostate cancer mortality rates have also declined in many countries that have not widely adopted screening.[141] Thus, it is likely that improvements in treatment have contributed, at least in part, to the observed decline in prostate cancer mortality. Another possible contributing factor may be the World Health Organization (WHO) algorithm for adjudicating cause of death. A change occurred just as mortality rates began to go up in the late 1970s, and WHO changed back to the older algorithm in 1991 when prostate cancer mortality began declining in many countries.[142] All of these factors, including a beneficial effect from screening, may be contributing to the declining prostate cancer mortality rates in the United States.

### Screening Recommendations

The topic of prostate cancer screening tends to evoke strong emotional reactions. Although the intuitive appeal of early detection is undeniable and screening may save some lives, the magnitude of the mortality reduction is relatively small, whereas the harms associated with screening can be substantial. Whether the potential benefits outweigh the known harms is a question that each man must answer for himself based on his individual preferences.

Several professional organizations in the United States, Europe, and Canada have recently reviewed the screening data and issued screening guidelines. All acknowledge that legitimate concerns remain regarding the risk–benefit ratio of prostate cancer screening. There is also general agreement that prostate cancer screening should only be done in the context of fully informed consent and that men should know that experts do not agree as to whether the benefits of screening for this disease outweigh the harms. Most recommend against mass screening in public meeting places, malls, churches, etc.

In 2009, the American Urological Association (AUA) PSA Best Practice Statement was published, which stated, "Given the uncertainty that PSA testing results in more benefit than harm, a thoughtful and broad approach to PSA is critical. Patients need to be informed of the risks and the benefits of testing before it is undertaken. The risks of over-detection and over-treatment should be included in this discussion."[143]

In 2010, the ACS updated their guidelines, stating that the balance of benefits and harms related to prostate cancer early detection are uncertain and the existing evidence is insufficient to support a recommendation for or against the routine use of PSA screening.[144] The ACS called for discussion and shared decision making within the physician–patient relationship.

The most recent 2012 USPSTF guidelines recommend against the use of PSA screening on the basis that there is moderate certainty that the harms of PSA testing outweigh the benefits and, on that basis, recommended against PSA-based screening for all men.[14] The task force did acknowledge that some men will continue to request screening and some physicians will continue to offer it. Like the ACS and AUA, they state that screening under such circumstances should respect patient preferences.

In 2013, the AUA conducted a systematic review of over 300 studies. They recommended against screening men younger than 40 years of age, and against screening average-risk men age 40 to 54 years, most men over 70 years of age, and men with a life expectancy of less than 10 to 15 years. They recommend that screening decisions be individualized for higher risk men ages 40 to 54 years and men over 70 years of age who are in excellent health. They placed primacy on shared decision making versus physician judgments about the balance of benefits and harms at the population level.[145] Even for men aged 55 to 69 years, the AUA concluded that the quality of evidence for benefits associated with screening was moderate, whereas the quality of the evidence for harm was high. They recommended shared decision making for this group, in whom they have concluded the benefits may outweigh the harm.

## SKIN CANCER SCREENING

Assessments of skin cancer screening have focused on melanoma end points with very little attention to screening for nonmelanoma skin cancer. A systematic review of skin cancer screening studies examining the available evidence through mid 2005 concluded that direct evidence of improved health outcomes associated with skin cancer screening is lacking.[146]

No randomized, clinical trial of skin cancer screening has been attempted. However, several observational studies have suggested that melanoma screening might reduce mortality. For example, a decrease in melanoma mortality did occur after a Scottish campaign to promote awareness of the signs of suspicious skin lesions and encourage early self-referral. However, uncontrolled, ecologic studies such as this provide a relatively low level of evidence, because it is not possible to determine whether the observed mortality reduction was due to screening or other factors.

More recently, the Skin Cancer Research to Provide Evidence for Effectiveness of Screening project, or SCREEN project, compared a region of Germany in which intensive skin cancer screening was performed to areas of Germany without intensive screening. Approximately 360,000 residents of the Schleswig-Holstein region aged 20 years and older participated. They chose either to be screened by a nondermatologist physician trained in skin examinations or by a dermatologist. Almost 16,000 biopsies were performed and 585 melanomas were diagnosed. Overall, 1 in 23 participants had an excisional skin biopsy and 620 persons needed to be screened to detect one melanoma. This screening effort led to a 16% and 38% increase in melanoma incidence among men and women, respectively, compared to 2 years earlier. The melanoma incidence rate returned to preprogram levels after the program ended. Of the screen-detected melanomas, 90% were less than 1 mm thick. Screening was performed in 2003 to 2004, and melanoma mortality in this region subsequently declined. In 2008, it was nearly 50% lower in both men and women compared to the rest of Germany.[147,148]

### Recommendations of Experts

Skin cancer screening recommendations are based on *expert opinion*, given the absence of a randomized clinical trial data and limited observational studies. The ACS recommends monthly skin self-examinations and a yearly clinical skin examination as part of a routine cancer-related checkup.[149] The USPSTF finds insufficient evidence to recommend for or against either routine skin cancer screening of the general population by primary care providers or counseling patients to perform periodic skin self-examinations. The task force does recommend that clinicians "remain alert" for skin lesions with malignant features when performing a physical examination for other purposes, particularly in high-risk individuals. The American Academy of Dermatology recommends that persons at highest risk (i.e., those with a strong family history of melanoma and multiple atypical nevi), perform frequent self-examination and seek a professional evaluation of the skin at least once per year.[150]

High-risk individuals are persons with multiple nevi or atypical moles. There is consensus they should be educated about the need for frequent surveillance by a trained health-care provider beginning at an early age. In the United States, Australia, and Western Europe, Caucasian men age 50 years and over account for nearly half of all melanoma cases. There is some discussion that melanoma early detection efforts should be focused on this population.

# REFERENCES

1. Collen MF, Dales LG, Friedman GD, et al. Multiphasic checkup evaluation study. 4. Preliminary cost benefit analysis for middle-aged men. *Prev Med* 1973; 2:236–246.
2. Prorok PC, Kramer BS, Gohagan JK. Screening theory and study design: the basics. In: Kramer B, Prorok P, eds. *Cancer Screening*. New York: Marcel Dekker; 1999: 29–53.
3. Welch HG, Black WC. Overdiagnosis in cancer. *J Natl Cancer Inst* 2010; 102:605–613.
4. Yamamoto K, Hayashi Y, Hanada R, et al. Mass screening and age-specific incidence of neuroblastoma in Saitama Prefecture, Japan. *J Clin Oncol* 1995;13:2033–2038.
5. Woods WG, Gao RN, Shuster JJ, et al. Screening of infants and mortality due to neuroblastoma. *N Engl J Med* 2002;346:1041–1046.
6. Friedman GD, Collen MF, Fireman BH. Multiphasic Health Checkup Evaluation: a 16-year follow-up. *J Chronic Dis* 1986;39:453–463.
7. Pinsky PF, Miller A, Kramer BS, et al. Evidence of a healthy volunteer effect in the prostate, lung, colorectal, and ovarian cancer screening trial. *Am J Epidemiol* 2007;165:874–881.
8. Boyle P, Brawley OW. Prostate cancer: current evidence weighs against population screening. *CA Cancer J Clin* 2009;59:220–224.
9. Autier P, Boyle P, Buyse M, et al. Is FOB screening really the answer for lowering mortality in colorectal cancer? *Recent Results Cancer Res* 2003;163: 254–263.
10. de Boer AG, Taskila T, Ojajarvi A, et al. Cancer survivors and unemployment: a meta-analysis and meta-regression. *JAMA* 2009;301:753–762.
11. Aberle DR, Adams AM, Berg CD, et al. Reduced lung-cancer mortality with low-dose computed tomographic screening. *N Engl J Med* 2011;365: 395–409.
12. Eden J, Levit L, Berg A, et al., eds. *Finding What Works in Health Care: Standards for Systematic Reviews*. Washington DC: The National Academies Press; 2011.
13. Graham R, Mancher M, Wolman DM, et al. Medicine CoSfDTCPGIo. Washington, DC: The National Academies; 2011.
14. Moyer VA. Screening for prostate cancer: U.S. Preventive Services Task Force recommendation statement. *Ann Intern Med* 2012;157:120–134.
15. Brawley O, Byers T, Chen A, et al. New American Cancer Society process for creating trustworthy cancer screening guidelines. *JAMA* 2011;306:2495–2499.
16. Shapiro S. Periodic screening for breast cancer: the HIP Randomized Controlled Trial. Health Insurance Plan. *J Natl Cancer Inst Monogr* 1997;27–30.
17. Miller AB, Wall C, Baines CJ, et al. Twenty five year follow-up for breast cancer incidence and mortality of the Canadian National Breast Screening Study: randomised screening trial. *BMJ* 2014;348:g366.
18. Tabar L, Fagerberg G, Duffy SW, et al. Update of the Swedish two-county program of mammographic screening for breast cancer. *Radiol Clin North Am* 1992;30: 187–210.
19. Moy L, Slanetz PJ, Moore R, et al. Specificity of mammography and US in the evaluation of a palpable abnormality: retrospective review. *Radiology* 2002;225:176–181.
20. Lord SJ, Lei W, Craft P, et al. A systematic review of the effectiveness of magnetic resonance imaging (MRI) as an addition to mammography and ultrasound in screening young women at high risk of breast cancer. *Eur J Cancer* 2007;43:1905–1917.
21. Wishart GC, Campisi M, Boswell M, et al. The accuracy of digital infrared imaging for breast cancer detection in women undergoing breast biopsy. *Eur J Surg Oncol* 2010;36:535–540.
22. Dooley WC, Ljung BM, Veronesi U, et al. Ductal lavage for detection of cellular atypia in women at high risk for breast cancer. *J Natl Cancer Inst* 2001;93:1624–1632.
23. Autier P, Boniol M, Middleton R, et al. Advanced breast cancer incidence following population-based mammographic screening. *Ann Oncol* 2011;22:1726–1735.
24. Bleyer A, Welch HG. Effect of three decades of screening mammography on breast-cancer incidence. *N Engl J Med* 2012;367:1998–2005.
25. Marmot MG, Altman DG, Cameron DA, et al. The benefits and harms of breast cancer screening: an independent review. *Br J Cancer* 2013;108:2205–2240.
26. Berry DA, Cronin KA, Plevritis SK, et al. Effect of screening and adjuvant therapy on mortality from breast cancer. *N Engl J Med* 2005;353:1784–1792.
27. Harris R, Yeatts J, Kinsinger L. Breast cancer screening for women ages 50 to 69 years a systematic review of observational evidence. *Prev Med* 2011;53: 108–114.
28. Nelson HD, Tyne K, Naik A, et al. Screening for breast cancer: an update for the U.S. Preventive Services Task Force. *Ann Intern Med* 2009;151:727–737.
29. Mandelblatt JS, Cronin KA, Bailey S, et al. Effects of mammography screening under different screening schedules: model estimates of potential benefits and harms. *Ann Intern Med* 2009;151:738–747.
30. U.S. Preventive Services Task Force. Screening for breast cancer: U.S. Preventive Services Task Force recommendation statement. *Ann Intern Med* 2009;151:716–726.
31. Nelson HD, Zakher B, Cantor A, et al. Risk factors for breast cancer for women aged 40 to 49 years: a systematic review and meta-analysis. *Ann Intern Med* 2012;156:635–648.
32. Barnett GC, Shah M, Redman K, et al. Risk factors for the incidence of breast cancer: do they affect survival from the disease? *J Clin Oncol* 2008;26: 3310–3316.
33. Gierach GL, Ichikawa L, Kerlikowske K, et al. Relationship between mammographic density and breast cancer death in the Breast Cancer Surveillance Consortium. *J Natl Cancer Inst* 2012;104:1218–1227.
34. Berg WA, Blume JD, Cormack JB, et al. Combined screening with ultrasound and mammography vs mammography alone in women at elevated risk of breast cancer. *JAMA* 2008;299:2151–2163.
35. Gartlehner G, Thaler K, Chapman A, et al. Mammography in combination with breast ultrasonography versus mammography for breast cancer screening in women at average risk. *Cochrane Database Syst Rev* 2013;4:CD009632.
36. Tice JA, O'Meara ES, Weaver DL, et al. Benign breast disease, mammographic breast density, and the risk of breast cancer. *J Natl Cancer Inst* 2013;105: 1043–1049.
37. Kerlikowske K, Hubbard RA, Miglioretti DL, et al. Comparative effectiveness of digital versus film-screen mammography in community practice in the United States: a cohort study. *Ann Intern Med* 2011;155:493–502.
38. Haas BM, Kalra V, Geisel J, et al. Comparison of tomosynthesis plus digital mammography and digital mammography alone for breast cancer screening. *Radiology* 2013;269:694–700.
39. Rosenberg RD, Yankaskas BC, Abraham LA, et al. Performance benchmarks for screening mammography. *Radiology* 2006;241:55–66.
40. Gomez SL, Lichtensztajn D, Kurian AW, et al. Increasing mastectomy rates for early-stage breast cancer? Population-based trends from California. *J Clin Oncol* 2010;28:e155–e157.
41. Tuttle TM, Jarosek S, Habermann EB, et al. Increasing rates of contralateral prophylactic mastectomy among patients with ductal carcinoma in situ. *J Clin Oncol* 2009;27:1362–1367.
42. Rosenberg RD, Hunt WC, Williamson MR, et al. Effects of age, breast density, ethnicity, and estrogen replacement therapy on screening mammographic sensitivity and cancer stage at diagnosis: review of 183,134 screening mammograms in Albuquerque, New Mexico. *Radiology* 1998;209:511–518.
43. Kerlikowske K, Grady D, Barclay J, et al. Effect of age, breast density, and family history on the sensitivity of first screening mammography. *JAMA* 1996;276: 33–38.
44. Porter PL, El-Bastawissi AY, Mandelson MT, et al. Breast tumor characteristics as predictors of mammographic detection: comparison of interval- and screen-detected cancers. *J Natl Cancer Inst* 1999;91:2020–2028.
45. Ronckers CM, Erdmann CA, Land CE. Radiation and breast cancer: a review of current evidence. *Breast Cancer Res* 2005;7:21–32.
46. Pijpe A, Andrieu N, Easton DF, et al. Exposure to diagnostic radiation and risk of breast cancer among carriers of BRCA1/2 mutations: retrospective cohort study (GENE-RAD-RISK). *BMJ* 2012;345:e5660.
47. Qaseem A, Snow V, Sherif K, et al. Screening mammography for women 40 to 49 years of age: a clinical practice guideline from the American College of Physicians. *Ann Intern Med* 2007;146:511–515.
48. Tonelli M, Connor Gorber S, Joffres M, et al. Recommendations on screening for breast cancer in average-risk women aged 40-74 years. *CMAJ* 2011;183: 1991–2001.
49. Recommendations on cancer screening in the European Union. Advisory Committee on Cancer Prevention. *Eur J Cancer* 2000;36:1473–1478.
50. Saslow D, Boetes C, Burke W, et al. American Cancer Society guidelines for breast screening with MRI as an adjunct to mammography. *CA Cancer J Clin* 2007;57:75–89.
51. Mandel JS, Church TR, Bond JH, et al. The effect of fecal occult-blood screening on the incidence of colorectal cancer. *N Engl J Med* 2000;343: 1603–1607.
52. Nishihara R, Wu K, Lochhead P, et al. Long-term colorectal-cancer incidence and mortality after lower endoscopy. *N Engl J Med* 2013;369: 1095–1105.
53. Schoen RE, Pinsky PF, Weissfeld JL, et al. Colorectal-cancer incidence and mortality with screening flexible sigmoidoscopy. *N Engl J Med* 2012;366: 2345–2357.
54. Mandel JS, Bond JH, Church TR, et al. Reducing mortality from colorectal cancer by screening for fecal occult blood. Minnesota Colon Cancer Control Study. *N Engl J Med* 1993;328:1365–1371.
55. Mandel JS, Church TR, Ederer F, et al. Colorectal cancer mortality: effectiveness of biennial screening for fecal occult blood. *J Natl Cancer Inst* 1999;91:434–437.
56. Hardcastle JD, Chamberlain JO, Robinson MH, et al. Randomised controlled trial of faecal-occult-blood screening for colorectal cancer. *Lancet* 1996;348: 1472–1477.
57. Kronborg O, Fenger C, Olsen J, et al. Randomised study of screening for colorectal cancer with faecal-occult-blood test. *Lancet* 1996;348:1467–1471.
58. Ahlquist DA, Wieand HS, Moertel CG, et al. Accuracy of fecal occult blood screening for colorectal neoplasia. A prospective study using Hemoccult and HemoQuant tests. *JAMA* 1993;269:1262–1267.
59. Levin B, Brooks D, Smith RA, et al. Emerging technologies in screening for colorectal cancer: CT colonography, immunochemical fecal occult blood tests, and stool screening using molecular markers. *CA Cancer J Clin* 2003;53:44–55.
60. Atkin WS, Edwards R, Kralj-Hans I, et al. Once-only flexible sigmoidoscopy screening in prevention of colorectal cancer: a multicentre randomised controlled trial. *Lancet* 2010;375:1624–1633.
61. Levin TR. Flexible sigmoidoscopy for colorectal cancer screening: valid approach or short-sighted? *Gastroenterol Clin North Am* 2002;31:1015–1029.

**CANCER PREVENTION AND SCREENING**

62. Littlejohn C, Hilton S, Macfarlane GJ, et al. Systematic review and meta-analysis of the evidence for flexible sigmoidoscopy as a screening method for the prevention of colorectal cancer. *Br J Surg* 2012;99:1488–1500.

63. Elmunzer BJ, Hayward RA, Schoenfeld PS, et al. Effect of flexible sigmoidoscopy-based screening on incidence and mortality of colorectal cancer: a systematic review and meta-analysis of randomized controlled trials. *PLoS Med* 2012;9:e1001352.

64. van Rijn JC, Reitsma JB, Stoker J, et al. Polyp miss rate determined by tandem colonoscopy: a systematic review. *Am J Gastroenterol* 2006;101:343–350.

65. Rosman AS, Korsten MA. Meta-analysis comparing CT colonography, air contrast barium enema, and colonoscopy. *Am J Med* 2007;120:203–210.

66. Imperiale TF, Wagner DR, Lin CY, et al. Using risk for advanced proximal colonic neoplasia to tailor endoscopic screening for colorectal cancer. *Ann Intern Med* 2003;139:959–965.

67. U.S. Preventive Services Task Force. Screening for colorectal cancer: U.S. Preventive Services Task Force recommendation statement. *Ann Intern Med* 2008;149:627–637.

68. Winawer S, Fletcher R, Rex D, et al. Colorectal cancer screening and surveillance: clinical guidelines and rationale-Update based on new evidence. *Gastroenterology* 2003;124:544–560.

69. Quintero E, Castells A, Bujanda L, et al. Colonoscopy versus fecal immunochemical testing in colorectal-cancer screening. *N Engl J Med* 2012;366:697–706.

70. Murakami R, Tsukuma H, Ubukata T, et al. Estimation of validity of mass screening program for gastric cancer in Osaka, Japan. *Cancer* 1990;65:1255–1260.

71. Kampschoer GH, Fujii A, Masuda Y. Gastric cancer detected by mass survey. Comparison between mass survey and outpatient detection. *Scand J Gastroenterol* 1989;24:813–817.

72. Stael von Holstein C, Eriksson S, Huldt B, et al. Endoscopic screening during 17 years for gastric stump carcinoma. A prospective clinical trial. *Scand J Gastroenterol* 1991;26:1020–1026.

73. Shaukat A, Mongin SJ, Geisser MS, et al. Long-term mortality after screening for colorectal cancer. *N Engl J Med* 2013;369:1106–1114.

74. McMahon BJ, Bulkow L, Harpster A, et al. Screening for hepatocellular carcinoma in Alaska natives infected with chronic hepatitis B: a 16-year population-based study. *Hepatology* 2000;32:842–846.

75. Chalasani N, Horlander JC Sr, Said A, et al. Screening for hepatocellular carcinoma in patients with advanced cirrhosis. *Am J Gastroenterol* 1999;94:2988–2993.

76. Sherman M, Peltekian KM, Lee C. Screening for hepatocellular carcinoma in chronic carriers of hepatitis B virus: incidence and prevalence of hepatocellular carcinoma in a North American urban population. *Hepatology* 1995;22:432–438.

77. Dodd GD 3rd, Miller WJ, Baron RL, et al. Detection of malignant tumors in end-stage cirrhotic livers: efficacy of sonography as a screening technique. *AJR Am J Roentgenol* 1992;159:727–733.

78. Laara E, Day NE, Hakama M. Trends in mortality from cervical cancer in the Nordic countries: association with organised screening programmes. *Lancet* 1987;1:1247–1249.

79. Christopherson WM, Lundin FE Jr, Mendez WM, et al. Cervical cancer control: a study of morbidity and mortality trends over a twenty-one-year period. *Cancer* 1976;38:1357–1366.

80. Janerich DT, Hadjimichael O, Schwartz PE, et al. The screening histories of women with invasive cervical cancer, Connecticut. *Am J Public Health* 1995;85:791–794.

81. Sawaya GF, McConnell KJ, Kulasingam SL, et al. Risk of cervical cancer associated with extending the interval between cervical-cancer screenings. *N Engl J Med* 2003;349:1501–1509.

82. Sankaranarayanan R, Nene BM, Shastri SS, et al. HPV screening for cervical cancer in rural India. *N Engl J Med* 2009;360:1385–1394.

83. Vesco KK, Whitlock EP, Eder M, et al. In: *Screening for Cervical Cancer: A Systematic Evidence Review for the US Preventive Services Task Force*. Rockville, MD: Agency for Healthcare Research and Quality; 2011.

84. Solomon D, Davey D, Kurman R, et al. The 2001 Bethesda System: terminology for reporting results of cervical cytology. *JAMA* 2002;287:2114–2119.

85. Darragh TM, Colgan TJ, Thomas Cox J, et al. The Lower Anogenital Squamous Terminology Standardization project for HPV-associated lesions: background and consensus recommendations from the College of American Pathologists and the American Society for Colposcopy and Cervical Pathology. *Int J Gynecol Pathol* 2013;32:76–115.

86. Ho GY, Bierman R, Beardsley L, et al. Natural history of cervicovaginal papillomavirus infection in young women. *N Engl J Med* 1998;338:423–428.

87. Holowaty P, Miller AB, Rohan T, et al. Natural history of dysplasia of the uterine cervix. *J Natl Cancer Inst* 1999;91:252–258.

88. Richardson H, Kelsall G, Tellier P, et al. The natural history of type-specific human papillomavirus infections in female university students. *Cancer Epidemiol Biomarkers Prev* 2003;12:485–490.

89. Melnikow J, Nuovo J, Willan AR, et al. Natural history of cervical squamous intraepithelial lesions: a meta-analysis. *Obstet Gynecol* 1998;92:727–735.

90. Cox JT, Schiffman M, Solomon D. Prospective follow-up suggests similar risk of subsequent cervical intraepithelial neoplasia grade 2 or 3 among women with cervical intraepithelial neoplasia grade 1 or negative colposcopy and directed biopsy. *Am J Obstet Gynecol* 2003;188:1406–1412.

91. Guido R, Schiffman M, Solomon D, et al. Postcolposcopy management strategies for women referred with low-grade squamous intraepithelial lesions or human papillomavirus DNA-positive atypical squamous cells of undetermined significance: a two-year prospective study. *Am J Obstet Gynecol* 2003;188:1401–1405.

92. Mayrand MH, Duarte-Franco E, Rodrigues I, et al. Human papillomavirus DNA versus Papanicolaou screening tests for cervical cancer. *N Engl J Med* 2007;357:1579–1588.

93. Saslow D, Solomon D, Lawson HW, et al. American Cancer Society, American Society for Colposcopy and Cervical Pathology, and American Society for Clinical Pathology screening guidelines for the prevention and early detection of cervical cancer. *CA Cancer J Clin* 2012;62:147–172.

94. Sankaranarayanan R, Esmy PO, Rajkumar R, et al. Effect of visual screening on cervical cancer incidence and mortality in Tamil Nadu, India: a cluster-randomised trial. *Lancet* 2007;370:398–406.

95. Szarewski A. Cervical screening by visual inspection with acetic acid. *Lancet* 2007;370:365–366.

96. Johnson CC, Kessel B, Riley TL, et al. The epidemiology of CA-125 in women without evidence of ovarian cancer in the Prostate, Lung, Colorectal and Ovarian (PLCO) Screening Trial. *Gynecol Oncol* 2008;110:383–389.

97. Duffy MJ, Bonfrer JM, Kulpa J, et al. CA125 in ovarian cancer: European Group on Tumor Markers guidelines for clinical use. *Int J Gynecol Cancer* 2005;15:679–691.

98. Moss EL, Hollingworth J, Reynolds TM. The role of CA125 in clinical practice. *J Clin Pathol* 2005;58:308–312.

99. Fishman DA, Cohen L, Blank SV, et al. The role of ultrasound evaluation in the detection of early-stage epithelial ovarian cancer. *Am J Obstet Gynecol* 2005;192:1214–1221.

100. Kobayashi E, Ueda Y, Matsuzaki S, et al. Biomarkers for screening, diagnosis, and monitoring of ovarian cancer. *Cancer Epidemiol Biomarkers Prev* 2012;21:1902–1912.

101. Ren J, Cai H, Li Y, et al. Tumor markers for early detection of ovarian cancer. *Expert Rev Mol Diagn* 2010;10:787–798.

102. Prorok PC, Andriole GL, Bresalier RS, et al. Design of the Prostate, Lung, Colorectal and Ovarian (PLCO) Cancer Screening Trial. *Control Clin Trials* 2000;21:273S–309S.

103. Buys SS, Partridge E, Black A, et al. Effect of screening on ovarian cancer mortality: the Prostate, Lung, Colorectal and Ovarian (PLCO) Cancer Screening Randomized Controlled Trial. *JAMA* 2011;305:2295–2303.

104. Menon U, Gentry-Maharaj A, Hallett R, et al. Sensitivity and specificity of multimodal and ultrasound screening for ovarian cancer, and stage distribution of detected cancers: results of the prevalence screen of the UK Collaborative Trial of Ovarian Cancer Screening (UKCTOCS). *Lancet Oncol* 2009;10:327–340.

105. Drescher CW, Shah C, Thorpe J, et al. Longitudinal screening algorithm that incorporates change over time in CA125 levels identifies ovarian cancer earlier than a single-threshold rule. *J Clin Oncol* 2013;31:387–392.

106. Sharma A, Apostolidou S, Burnell M, et al. Risk of epithelial ovarian cancer in asymptomatic women with ultrasound-detected ovarian masses: a prospective cohort study within the UK collaborative trial of ovarian cancer screening (UKCTOCS). *Ultrasound Obstet Gynecol* 2012;40:338–344.

107. Moyer VA. Screening for ovarian cancer: U.S. Preventive Services Task Force reaffirmation recommendation statement. *Ann Intern Med* 2012;157:900–904.

108. NIH consensus conference. Ovarian cancer. Screening, treatment, and follow-up. NIH Consensus Development Panel on Ovarian Cancer. *JAMA* 1995;273:491–497.

109. Smith RA, von Eschenbach AC, Wender R, et al. American Cancer Society guidelines for the early detection of cancer: update of early detection guidelines for prostate, colorectal, and endometrial cancers. Also: update 2001—testing for early lung cancer detection. *CA Cancer J Clin* 2001;51:38–75.

110. Burke W, Petersen G, Lynch P, et al. Recommendations for follow-up care of individuals with an inherited predisposition to cancer. I. Hereditary nonpolyposis colon cancer. Cancer Genetics Studies Consortium. *JAMA* 1997;277:915–919.

111. Gull B, Karlsson B, Milsom I, et al. Can ultrasound replace dilation and curettage? A longitudinal evaluation of postmenopausal bleeding and transvaginal sonographic measurement of the endometrium as predictors of endometrial cancer. *Am J Obstet Gynecol* 2003;188:401–408.

112. Scanman CL. Follow-up study of lung cancer suspects in a mass chest X-ray survey. *N Engl J Med* 1951;244:541–544.

113. Croswell JM, Ransohoff DF, Kramer BS. Principles of cancer screening: lessons from history and study design issues. *Semin Oncol* 2010;37:202–215.

114. Fontana RS, Sanderson DR, Taylor WF, et al. Early lung cancer detection: results of the initial (prevalence) radiologic and cytologic screening in the Mayo Clinic study. *Am Rev Respir Dis* 1984;130:561–565.

115. Fontana RS, Sanderson DR, Woolner LB, et al. Screening for lung cancer. A critique of the Mayo Lung Project. *Cancer* 1991;67:1155–1164.

116. Marcus PM, Bergstralh EJ, Zweig MH, et al. Extended lung cancer incidence follow-up in the Mayo Lung Project and overdiagnosis. *J Natl Cancer Inst* 2006;98:748–756.

117. Manser R, Wright G, Hart D, et al. Surgery for early stage non-small cell lung cancer. *Cochrane Database Syst Rev* 2005:CD004699.

118. Kubik A, Parkin DM, Khlat M, et al. Lack of benefit from semi-annual screening for cancer of the lung: follow-up report of a randomized controlled trial on a population of high-risk males in Czechoslovakia. *Int J Cancer* 1990;45:26–33.

119. Oken MM, Hocking WG, Kvale PA, et al. Screening by chest radiograph and lung cancer mortality: the Prostate, Lung, Colorectal, and Ovarian (PLCO) randomized trial. *JAMA* 2011;306:1865–1873.

120. Kovalchik SA, Tammemagi M, Berg CD, et al. Targeting of low-dose CT screening according to the risk of lung-cancer death. *N Engl J Med* 2013;369:245–254.

121. Kubik AK, Parkin DM, Zatloukal P. Czech Study on Lung Cancer Screening: post-trial follow-up of lung cancer deaths up to year 15 since enrollment. *Cancer* 2000;89:2363–2368.

122. Patz EF Jr, Pinsky P, Gatsonis C, et al. Overdiagnosis in low-dose computed tomography screening for lung cancer. *JAMA Intern Med* 2014;174:269–274.

123. Ma J, Ward EM, Smith R, et al. Annual number of lung cancer deaths potentially avertable by screening in the United States. *Cancer* 2013;119: 1381–1385.

124. Wender R, Fontham ET, Barrera E Jr, et al. American Cancer Society lung cancer screening guidelines. *CA Cancer J Clin* 2013;63:107–117.

125. Bach PB, Mirkin JN, Oliver TK, et al. Benefits and harms of CT screening for lung cancer: a systematic review. *JAMA* 2012;307:2418–2429.

126. Montie JE, Smith JA. Whitmoreisms: memorable quotes from Willet F. Whitmore, Jr, M.D. *Urology* 2004;63:207–209.

127. Albertsen PC, Hanley JA, Fine J. 20-year outcomes following conservative management of clinically localized prostate cancer. *JAMA* 2005;293:2095–2101.

128. Lu-Yao G, Albertsen PC, Stanford JL, et al. Screening, treatment, and prostate cancer mortality in the Seattle area and Connecticut: fifteen-year follow-up. *J Gen Intern Med* 2008;23:1809–1814.

129. Thompson IM, Chi C, Ankerst DP, et al. Effect of finasteride on the sensitivity of PSA for detecting prostate cancer. *J Natl Cancer Inst* 2006;98:1128–1133.

130. Thompson IM, Pauler DK, Goodman PJ, et al. Prevalence of prostate cancer among men with a prostate-specific antigen level < or =4.0 ng per milliliter. N *Engl J Med* 2004;350:2239–2246.

131. Thompson IM, Ankerst DP, Chi C, et al. Operating characteristics of prostate-specific antigen in men with an initial PSA level of 3.0 ng/ml or lower. *JAMA* 2005;294:66–70.

132. Widmark A, Klepp O, Solberg A, et al. Endocrine treatment, with or without radiotherapy, in locally advanced prostate cancer (SPCG-7/SFUO-3): an open randomised phase III trial. *Lancet* 2009;373:301–308.

133. Bill-Axelson A, Holmberg L, Ruutu M, et al. Radical prostatectomy versus watchful waiting in early prostate cancer. *N Engl J Med* 2011;364: 1708–1717.

134. Wilt TJ, Brawer MK, Jones KM, et al. Radical prostatectomy versus observation for localized prostate cancer. *N Engl J Med* 2012;367:203–213.

135. Andriole GL, Crawford ED, Grubb RL 3rd, et al. Prostate cancer screening in the randomized Prostate, Lung, Colorectal, and Ovarian Cancer Screening Trial: mortality results after 13 years of follow-up. *J Natl Cancer Inst* 2012;104:125–132.

136. Schroder FH, Hugosson J, Roobol MJ, et al. Screening and prostate-cancer mortality in a randomized European study. *N Engl J Med* 2009;360:1320–1328.

137. Schroder FH, Hugosson J, Roobol MJ, et al. Prostate-cancer mortality at 11 years of follow-up. *N Engl J Med* 2012;366:981–990.

138. Wolters T, Roobol MJ, Steyerberg EW, et al. The effect of study arm on prostate cancer treatment in the large screening trial ERSPC. *Int J Cancer* 2010;126:2387–2393.

139. Hugosson J, Carlsson S, Aus G, et al. Mortality results from the Goteborg randomised population-based prostate-cancer screening trial. *Lancet Oncol* 2010;11: 725–732.

140. Kilpelainen TP, Tammela TL, Malila N, et al. Prostate cancer mortality in the Finnish randomized screening trial. *J Natl Cancer Inst* 2013;105: 719–725.

141. Center MM, Jemal A, Lortet-Tieulent J, et al. International variation in prostate cancer incidence and mortality rates. *Eur Urol* 2012;61:1079–1092.

142. Boyle P. Screening for prostate cancer: have you had your cholesterol measured? *BJU Int* 2003;92:191–199.

143. Greene KL, Albertsen PC, Babaian RJ, et al. Prostate specific antigen best practice statement: 2009 update. *J Urol* 2009;182:2232–2241.

144. Wolf AM, Wender RC, Etzioni RB, et al. American Cancer Society guideline for the early detection of prostate cancer: update 2010. *CA Cancer J Clin* 2010;60:70–98.

145. Carter HB. American Urological Association (AUA) guideline on prostate cancer detection: process and rationale. *BJU Int* 2013;112:543–547.

146. Wolff T, Tai E, Miller T. Screening for skin cancer: an update of the evidence for the U.S. Preventive Services Task Force. *Ann Intern Med* 2009;150: 194–198.

147. Katalinic A, Waldmann A, Weinstock MA, et al. Does skin cancer screening save lives?: an observational study comparing trends in melanoma mortality in regions with and without screening. *Cancer* 2012;118:5395–5402.

148. Breitbart EW, Waldmann A, Nolte S, et al. Systematic skin cancer screening in Northern Germany. *J Am Acad Dermatol* 2012;66:201–211.

149. Smith RA, Brooks D, Cokkinides V, et al. Cancer screening in the United States, 2013: a review of current American Cancer Society guidelines, current issues in cancer screening, and new guidance on cervical cancer screening and lung cancer screening. *CA Cancer J Clin* 2013;63:88–105.

150. U.S. Preventive Services Task Force. Screening for skin cancer: U.S. Preventive Services Task Force recommendation statement. *Ann Intern Med* 2009;150: 188–193.

# 35 Genetic Counseling

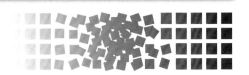

Ellen T. Matloff and Danielle C. Bonadies

## INTRODUCTION

Clinically based genetic testing has evolved from an uncommon analysis ordered for the rare hereditary cancer family to a widely available tool ordered on a routine basis to assist in surgical and radiation decision making, chemoprevention, and surveillance of the patient with cancer, as well as management of the entire family. The evolution of this field has created a need for accurate cancer genetic counseling and risk assessment. Extensive coverage of this topic by the media, including Angelina Jolie's public disclosure of her BRCA1+ status in May 2013, and widespread advertising by commercial testing laboratories have further fueled the demand for counseling and testing.

Cancer genetic counseling is a communication process between a health-care professional and an individual concerning cancer occurrence and risk in his or her family.[1] The process, which may include the entire family through a blend of genetic, medical, and psychosocial assessments and interventions, has been described as a bridge between the fields of traditional oncology and genetic counseling.[1]

The goals of this process include providing the client with an assessment of individual cancer risk, while offering the emotional support needed to understand and cope with this information. It also involves deciphering whether the cancers in a family are likely to be caused by a mutation in a cancer gene and, if so, *which one*. There are >30 hereditary cancer syndromes, many of which can be caused by mutations in different genes. Therefore, testing for these syndromes can be complicated. Advertisements by genetic testing companies bill genetic testing as a simple process that can be carried out by health-care professionals with no training in this area; however, there are many genes involved in cancer, the interpretation of the test results is often complicated, the risk of result misinterpretation is great and associated with potential liability, and the emotional and psychological ramifications for the patient and family can be powerful.[2,3] A few hours of training by a company generating a profit from the sale of these tests does not adequately prepare providers to offer their own genetic counseling and testing services.[4] Furthermore, the delegation of genetic testing responsibilities to office staff and, recently, mammography technicians, is alarming and likely presents a huge liability for these ordering physicians, their practices, and their institutions.[5,6] *Providers should proceed with caution before taking on the role of primary genetic counselor for their patients.*

Counseling about hereditary cancers differs from *traditional* genetic counseling in several ways. Clients seeking cancer genetic counseling are rarely concerned with reproductive decisions, which are often the primary focus in traditional genetic counseling, but are instead seeking information about their own and other relatives' chances of developing cancer.[1] Additionally, the risks given are not absolute but change over time as the family and personal history changes and the patient ages. The risk reduction options available are often radical (e.g., chemoprevention or prophylactic surgery), and are not appropriate for every patient at every age. The surveillance and management plan must be tailored to the

patient's age, childbearing status, menopausal status, risk category, ease of screening, and personal preferences and will likely change over time with the patient. The ultimate goal of cancer genetic counseling is to help the patient reach the decision best suited to her personal situation, needs, and circumstances.

There are now a significant number of referral centers across the country specializing in cancer genetic counseling, and the numbers are growing. However, some experts insist that the only way to keep up with the overwhelming demand for counseling will be to educate more physicians and nurses in cancer genetics. The feasibility of adding another specialized and time-consuming task to the clinical burden of these professionals is questionable, particularly with average patient encounters of 19.5 and 21.6 minutes for general practitioners and gynecologists, respectively.[7,8] A more practical goal is to better educate clinicians in the area of risk assessment so that they can screen their patient populations for individuals at high risk for hereditary cancer and refer them on to comprehensive counseling and testing programs. Access to genetic counseling is no longer an issue because there are now internet, phone, and satellite-based telemedicine services available (Table 35.1), with most major health insurance companies now covering these services[9–11] and several requiring them.[12]

## WHO IS A CANDIDATE FOR CANCER GENETIC COUNSELING?

Only 5% to 10% of most cancer is thought to be caused by single mutations within autosomal-dominant inherited cancer susceptibility genes.[13] The key for clinicians is to determine which patients are at greatest risk to carry a hereditary mutation. There are seven critical risk factors in hereditary cancer (Table 35.2). The first is early age of cancer onset. This risk factor, *even in the absence of a family history,* has been shown to be associated with an increased frequency of germline mutations in many types of cancers.[14] The second risk factor is the presence of the same cancer in multiple affected relatives on the same side of the pedigree. These cancers do not need to be of similar histologic type in order to be caused by a single mutation. The third risk factor is the clustering of cancers known to be caused by a single gene mutation in one family (e.g., breast/ovarian/pancreatic cancer or colon/uterine/ovarian cancers). The fourth risk factor is the occurrence of multiple primary cancers in one individual. This includes multiple primary breast or colon cancers as well as a single individual with separate cancers known to be caused by a single gene mutation (e.g., breast and ovarian cancer in a single individual). Ethnicity also plays a role in determining who is at greatest risk to carry a hereditary cancer mutation. Individuals of Jewish ancestry are at increased risk to carry three specific BRCA1/2 mutations.[15] The presence of a cancer that presents unusually—in this case, breast cancer in a male—represents a sixth risk factor and is important even when it is the only risk factor present. Finally, the last risk factor is pathology. Certain types of cancer are overrepresented in hereditary cancer families. For example, medullary and triple negative breast

## TABLE 35.1

**How to Find a Genetic Counselor for Your Patient**

**American Board of Genetic Counselors**

https://abgcmember.goamp.com/Net/ABGCWcm/Find_
Counselor/ABGCWcm/PublicDir.aspx?hkey=0ad511c0-
d9e9-4714-bd4b-0d73a59ee175

http://bit.ly/1kzTbk9

*Directory of board-certified genetic counselors*

**InformedDNA**

www.informeddna.com

(800) 975-4819

*A nationwide network of independent genetic counselors
that use telephone and internet technology to bring genetic
counseling to patients and providers. Covered by many
insurance companies.*

**National Society of Genetic Counselors**

www.nsgc.org (click "Find a Counselor" button)

(312) 321-6834

*For a listing of genetic counselors in your area who specialize
in cancer.*

**National Cancer Institute Cancer Genetics Services Directory**

www.cancer.gov/cancertopics/genetics/directory

(800) 4-CANCER

*A free service designed to locate providers of cancer risk
counseling and testing services.*

cancers (where the estrogen, progesterone and Her2 receptors are all negative, often abbreviated ER-/PR-/Her2) are overrepresented in *BRCA1* families,[16,17] and the National Comprehensive Cancer Network (NCCN) BRCA testing guidelines now include individuals diagnosed with a triple negative breast cancer <age 60 years.[18] However, breast cancer patients without these pathologic findings are *not* necessarily at lower risk to carry a mutation. In contrast, patients with a borderline or mucinous ovarian carcinoma are at lower risk to carry a *BRCA1* or *BRCA2* mutation[19] and may instead

## TABLE 35.2

**Risk Factors that Warrant Genetic Counseling for
Hereditary Cancer Syndromes**

1. Early age of onset (e.g., <50 years for breast, colon, and
   uterine cancer)

2. Multiple family members on the same side of the pedigree
   with the same cancer

3. Clustering of cancers in the family known to be caused
   by a single gene mutation (e.g., breast/ovarian/pancreatic;
   colon/uterine/ovarian; colon cancer/polyps/desmoid tumors/
   osteomas)

4. Multiple primary cancers in one individual (e.g., breast/ovarian
   cancer; colon/uterine; synchronous/metachronous colon
   cancers; <15 gastrointestinal polyps; <5 hamartomatous or
   juvenile polyps)

5. Ethnicity (e.g., Jewish ancestry for breast/ovarian cancer
   syndrome)

6. Unusual presentation of cancer/tumor (e.g., breast cancer in
   a male; medullary thyroid cancer; retinoblastoma; even one
   sebaceous carcinoma or adenoma)

7. Pathology (e.g., triple negative [ER/PR/Her-2] breast cancer
   <60; medullary breast cancers are overrepresented in
   women with hereditary breast and ovarian cancer; a colon
   tumor with an abnormal microsatellite instability (MSI) or
   immunohistochemistry (IHC) result increases the risk for a
   hereditary colon cancer syndrome)

carry a mutation in a different gene. It is already well-established that medullary thyroid carcinoma, sebaceous adenoma or carcinoma, adrenocortical carcinoma before the age of 25 years, and multiple adenomatous, hamartomatous, or juvenile colon polyps are indicative of other rare hereditary cancer syndromes.[11,20] These risk factors should be viewed in the context of the entire family history, and must be weighed in proportion to the number of individuals who have not developed cancer. The risk assessment is often limited in families that are small or have few female relatives; in such families, a single risk factor may carry more weight.

A less common, but extremely important, finding is the presence of unusual physical findings or birth defects that are known to be associated with rare hereditary cancer syndromes. Examples include benign skin findings, autism, large head circumference[20,21] and thyroid disorders in Cowden syndrome, odontogenic keratocysts in Gorlin syndrome,[22] and desmoid tumors or dental abnormalities in familial adenomatous polyposis (FAP).[23] These and other findings should prompt further investigation of the patient's family history and consideration of a referral to genetic counseling.

In this chapter, the breast/ovarian cancer counseling session with a female patient will serve as a paradigm by which all other sessions may follow broadly.

## COMPONENTS OF THE CANCER GENETIC COUNSELING SESSION

### Precounseling Information

Before coming in for genetic counseling, the counselee should be informed about what to expect at each visit, and what information he/she should collect ahead of time. The counselee can then begin to collect medical and family history information and pathology reports that will be essential for the genetic counseling session.

### Family History

An accurate family history is undoubtedly one of the most essential components of the cancer genetic counseling session. Optimally, a family history should include at least three generations; however, patients do not always have this information. For each individual affected with cancer, it is important to document the exact diagnosis, age at diagnosis, treatment strategies, and environmental exposures (i.e., occupational exposures, cigarettes, other agents).[24] The current age of the individual, laterality, and occurrence of any other cancers must also be documented. Cancer diagnoses should be confirmed with pathology reports whenever possible. A study by Love et al.[25] revealed that individuals accurately reported the primary site of cancer only 83% of the time in their first degree relatives with cancer, and 67% and 60% of the time in second and third degree relatives, respectively. It is common for patients to report a uterine cancer as an ovarian cancer, or a colon polyp as an invasive colorectal cancer. These differences, although seemingly subtle to the patient, can make a tremendous difference in risk assessment. Individuals should be asked if there are any consanguineous (inbred) relationships in the family, if any relatives were born with birth defects or mental retardation, and whether other genetic diseases run in the family (e.g., Fanconi anemia, Cowden syndrome), because these pieces of information could prove to be important in reaching a diagnosis.

The most common misconception in family history taking is that somehow a maternal family history of breast, ovarian, or uterine cancer is more significant than a paternal history. Conversely, many still believe that a paternal history of prostate cancer is more significant than a maternal history. Few cancer genes discovered thus far are located on the sex chromosomes and, therefore, both maternal and paternal history are significant and must be explored thoroughly. It has also become necessary to elicit the spouse's personal and family history of cancer. This has bearing on the cancer status of common children, but may also determine if children are at increased risk for a serious recessive genetic disease such as Fanconi anemia.[26] Children who inherit two copies of a BRCA2 mutation (one from each parent) are now known to have this serious disorder characterized by defective DNA repair and high rates of birth defects, aplastic anemia, leukemia, and solid tumors.[26] Patients should be encouraged to report changes in their family history over time (e.g., new cancer diagnoses, genetic testing results in relatives), because this may change their risk assessment and counseling.

A detailed family history should also include genetic diseases, birth defects, mental retardation, multiple miscarriages, and infant deaths. A history of certain recessive genetic diseases (e.g., ataxia telangiectasia, Fanconi anemia) can indicate that healthy family members who carry just one copy of the genetic mutation may be at increased risk to develop cancer.[26,27] Other genetic disorders, such as hereditary hemorrhagic telangiectasia, can be associated with a hereditary cancer syndrome caused by a mutation in the same gene—in this case, juvenile polyposis.[28]

### Dysmorphology Screening

Congenital anomalies, benign tumors, and unusual dermatologic features occur in a large number of hereditary cancer predisposition syndromes. Examples include osteomas of the jaw in FAP, palmar pits in Gorlin syndrome, and papillomas of the lips and mucous membranes in Cowden syndrome. Obtaining an accurate past medical history of benign lesions and birth defects, and screening for such dysmorphology can greatly impact diagnosis, counseling, and testing. For example, BRCA1/2 testing is inappropriate in a patient with breast cancer who has a family history of thyroid cancer and the orocutaneous manifestations of Cowden syndrome.

### Risk Assessment

Risk assessment is one of the most complicated components of the genetic counseling session. It is crucial to remember that risk assessment changes over time as the person ages and as the health statuses of their family members change. Risk assessment can be broken down into three separate components.

- What is the chance that the counselee will develop the cancer observed in his/her family (or a genetically related cancer such as ovarian cancer due to a family history of breast cancer)?
- What is the chance that the cancers in this family are caused by a single gene mutation?
- What is the chance that we can identify the gene mutation in this family with our current knowledge and laboratory techniques?

Cancer clustering in a family may be due to genetic and/or environmental factors, or may be coincidental because some cancers are very common in the general population.[29] Although inherited factors may be the primary cause of cancers in some families, in others, cancer may develop because an inherited factor increases the individual's susceptibility to environmental carcinogens. It is also possible that members of the same family may be exposed to similar environmental exposures due to shared geography or patterns in behavior and diet that may increase the risk of cancer.[30] Therefore, it is important to distinguish the difference between a familial pattern of cancer (due to environmental factors or chance) and a hereditary pattern of cancer (due to a shared genetic mutation). Emerging research is also evaluating the role and clinical utility of more common low-penetrance susceptibility genes and single nucleotide polymorphisms (SNP) that may account for a proportion of familial cancers.[31]

Several models are available to calculate the chance that a woman will develop breast cancer, including the Gail and Claus models.[32,33] Computer-based models are also available to help determine the chance that a BRCA mutation will be found in a family.[34] At first glance, many of these models appear simple and easy to use, and it may be tempting to exclusively rely on these models to assess cancer risk. However, each model has its strengths and weaknesses, and the counselor needs to understand the limitations well and know which are validated, which are considered problematic, when a model will not work on a particular patient, or when another genetic syndrome should be considered. For example, none of the existing models are able to factor in other risks that may be essential in hereditary risk calculation (e.g., a sister who was diagnosed with breast cancer after radiation treatment for Hodgkin disease).

The risk of a detectable mutation will also vary based on cancer history and the degree of relationship to an affected family member. For example, family members with early-onset breast cancer have a higher likelihood of testing positive than unaffected family members. Therefore, the risk assessment process should include a discussion of which family member is the best candidate for testing.

### DNA Testing

DNA testing is now available for a variety of hereditary cancer syndromes. However, despite misrepresentation by the media, testing is feasible for only a small percentage of individuals with cancer. DNA testing offers the important advantage of presenting clients with *actual risks* instead of the empiric risks derived from risk calculation models. DNA testing can be very expensive; full sequencing and rearrangement testing of the BRCA1/2 genes currently averages $2,500, and full panel testing costs up to $7,000 per patient. Importantly, testing should begin in an affected family member whenever possible to maximize scientific accuracy. Most insurance companies now cover cancer genetic testing in families where the test is medically indicated.

One of the most crucial aspects of DNA testing is accurate result ordering and interpretation. Unfortunately, errors in ordering and interpretation are the greatest risk of genetic testing and are very common.[35] Emerging data reveal that between 30% to 50% of genetic tests are ordered inappropriately, which is problematic for patients, clinicians, and insurers.[36–38] Recent data demonstrate that many medical providers have difficulty interpreting even basic pedigrees and genetic test results.[33–35] Additional studies have demonstrated that an inaccurate interpretation of genetic testing has been shown to result in inappropriate medical management recommendations, unnecessary prophylactic surgeries, a massive waste of health-care dollars, psychosocial distress, and false reassurance for patients.[2,3]

Interpretations are becoming increasingly complicated as more tests and gene panels become available. For example, one study demonstrated that approximately 25% of high-risk families that were BRCA1 and BRCA2 negative by commercially available sequencing were found to carry a deletion or duplication in one of these genes, or a mutation in another gene.[39]

This is particularly concerning in an era in which testing companies are canvassing physicians, and now mammography technicians, and encouraging them to perform their own counseling and testing. The potential impact of test results on the patient and his/her family is great and, therefore, accurate interpretation of the results is paramount. Professional groups have recognized this and have adopted standards encouraging clinicians to refer patients to genetics experts to ensure proper ordering and interpretation of genetic tests. The U.S. Preventive Services Task Force recommends that women whose family history is suggestive of a BRCA mutation be referred for genetic counseling before being offered genetic testing.[40] The American College of Surgeons' Commission on Cancer standards include "cancer risk assessment, genetic counseling and testing services provided to patients either on site or by referral, by a qualified genetics professional."[4] In an effort to reduce errors, some insurance companies are requiring genetic counseling by a certified genetic counselor before testing for hereditary breast or colon cancer syndromes.[12]

Results can fall into a few broad categories. It is important to note that a negative test result can actually be interpreted in three different ways, detailed in #2, #3, and #4, which follows.

1. Deleterious mutation "positive." When a deleterious mutation in a well-known cancer gene is discovered, the cancer risks for the patient and her family are relatively straightforward. However, with the development of multigene panels and the inclusion of many lesser known genes, the risks of detecting a mutation within a gene whose cancer risks are ill defined and medical management options unknown is much greater. Even for well-known genes, the risks are not precise and should be presented to patients as a risk range.[41,42] When a true mutation is found, it is critical to test both parents (whenever possible) to determine from which side of the family the mutation is originating, even when the answer appears obvious.
2. True negative. An individual does not carry the deleterious mutation found in her family, which ideally, has been proven to segregate with the cancer family history. In this case, the patient's cancer risks are usually reduced to the population risks.
3. Negative. A mutation was not detected, and the cancers in the family are not likely to be hereditary based on the personal and family history assessment. For example, a patient is diagnosed with breast cancer at age 38 years and comes from a large family with no other cancer diagnoses and relatives who died at old ages of other causes.
4. Uninformative. A mutation cannot be found in affected family members of a family in which the cancer pattern appears to be hereditary; there is likely an undetectable mutation within the gene, or the family carries a mutation in a different gene. If, for example, the patient developed breast cancer at age 38 years, has a father with breast cancer, and has a paternal aunt who developed breast and ovarian cancers before age 50 years, a negative test result would be almost meaningless. It would simply mean that the family has a mutation that could not be identified with our current testing methods or a mutation in another cancer gene. The entire family would be followed as high risk.
5. Variant of uncertain significance. A genetic change is identified, the significance of which is unknown. It is possible that this change is deleterious or completely benign. It may be helpful to test other *affected* family members to see if the mutation segregates with disease in the family. If it does not segregate, the variant is less likely to be significant. If it does, the variant is more likely to be significant. Other tools, including a splice site predictor, in conjunction with data on species conservation and amino acid difference scores, can also be helpful in determining the likelihood that a variant is significant. It is rarely helpful (and can be detrimental) to test *unaffected* family members for such variants. The rates of variants of uncertain significance vary greatly depending on the reporting protocols of the lab and the genes analyzed. Creation of open databases through a nationwide movement called Free the Data will likely improve variant reporting for all laboratories.

In order to pinpoint the mutation in a family, an affected individual most likely to carry the mutation should be tested first whenever possible. This is most often a person affected with the cancer in question at the earliest age. Test subjects should be selected with care, because it is possible for a person to develop sporadic cancer in a hereditary cancer family. For example, in an early-onset breast cancer family, it would not be ideal to first test a woman diagnosed with breast cancer at age 65 years because she may represent a sporadic case.

If a mutation is detected in an affected relative, other family members can be tested for the same mutation with a great degree of accuracy. Family members who do not carry the mutation found in their family are deemed true negative. Those who are found to carry the mutation in their family will have more definitive information about their risks to develop cancer. This information can be crucial in assisting patients in decision making regarding surveillance and risk reduction.

If a mutation is not identified in the affected relative, it usually means that either the cancers in the family are (1) not hereditary, or (2) caused by an undetectable mutation or a mutation in a different gene. A careful review of the family history and the risk factors will help to decipher whether interpretation 1 or 2 is more likely. Additional genetic testing may need to be ordered at this point. In cases in which the cancers appear hereditary and no mutation is found, DNA banking should be offered to the proband for a time in the future when improved testing may become available. A letter indicating exactly who in the family has access to the DNA should accompany the banked sample.

The genetic counseling result disclosure session should also include a detailed discussion of which other family members would benefit from genetic counseling and testing and referral information. This can apply not only to families who have been found to carry a deleterious mutation, but may also prove useful in other families (e.g., test a higher risk relative or determine segregation of a variant within a family).

The penetrance of mutations in cancer susceptibility genes is also difficult to interpret. Initial estimates derived from high-risk families provided very high cancer risks for *BRCA1* and *BRCA2* mutation carriers.[43] More recent studies done on populations that were not selected for family history have revealed lower penetrances.[44] Because exact penetrance rates cannot be determined for individual families at this time, and because precise genotype/phenotype correlations remain unclear, it is prudent to provide patients with a range of cancer risk and to explain that their risk probably falls somewhere within this spectrum. This can prove challenging for genes that lack published long-term data on cancer associations and risks.

Female carriers of *BRCA1* and *BRCA2* mutations have a 50% to 85% lifetime risk to develop breast cancer and between a 15% to 60% lifetime risk to develop ovarian cancer.[15,42,43] It is important to note that the classification "ovarian cancer" also includes cancer of the fallopian tubes and primary peritoneal carcinoma.[44,45] *BRCA2* carriers also have an increased lifetime risk of male breast cancer, pancreatic cancer, and possibly, melanoma.[46,47]

## Options for Surveillance, Risk Reduction, and Tailored Treatment

The cancer risk counseling session is a forum to provide counselees with information, support, options, and hope. Mutation carriers can be offered: earlier and more aggressive surveillance, chemoprevention, and/or prophylactic surgery. Detailed management options for *BRCA* carriers are discussed in this chapter.

Surveillance recommendations are evolving with newer techniques and additional data. At this time, it is recommended that individuals at increased risk for breast cancer, particularly those who carry a *BRCA* mutation, have annual mammograms beginning at age 25 years, with a clinical breast exam by a breast specialist, a yearly breast magnetic resonance imaging (MRI) with a clinical breast exam by a breast specialist, and a yearly clinical breast exam by a gynecologist.[48,49] It is suggested that the mammogram and MRI be spaced out around the calendar year so that some intervention is planned every 6 months. Recent data suggest that MRI may be safer and more effective in *BRCA* carriers <40 years of age and may someday replace mammograms in this population.[50]

*BRCA* carriers may take a selective estrogen-receptor modulator (SERM) or aromatase inhibitor in hopes of reducing their risks of developing breast cancer. These medications have been proven effective in women at increased risk due to a positive family history of breast cancer.[51–53] There are limited data on the effectiveness of such medications in unaffected *BRCA* carriers[54–56]; however, there are some data to suggest that *BRCA* carriers taking tamoxifen as treatment for a breast cancer reduce their risk of a contralateral breast cancer.[57] Additionally, the majority of *BRCA2* carriers who develop breast cancer develop an estrogen-positive form of the disease,[58] and it is hoped that this population will respond especially well to chemoprevention. Further studies in this area are necessary before drawing conclusions about the efficacy of chemoprevention in this population. Prophylactic bilateral mastectomy reduces the risk of breast cancer by >90% in women at high-risk for the disease.[59] Before genetic testing was available, it was not uncommon for entire generations of cancer families to have at-risk tissues removed without knowing if they were *personally* at increased risk for their familial cancer. Fifty percent of unaffected individuals in hereditary cancer families will *not* carry the inherited predisposition gene and can be spared prophylactic surgery or invasive high-risk surveillance regimens. Therefore, it is clearly not appropriate to offer prophylactic surgery until a patient is referred for genetic counseling and, if possible, testing.[60]

Women who carry *BRCA1* mutations are also at increased risk to develop second contralateral and ipsilateral primaries of the breast.[61] These data bring into question the option of breast conserving surgery in women at high risk to develop a second primary within the same breast. For this reason, the *BRCA1/2* carrier status can have a profound impact on surgical decision making,[62] and many patients have genetic counseling and testing immediately after diagnosis and before surgery or radiation therapy. Those patients who test positive and opt for prophylactic mastectomy can often be spared radiation and the resulting side effects that can complicate reconstruction. Approximately 30% to 60% of previously irradiated patients who later opt for mastectomy with reconstruction report significant complications or unfavorable cosmetic results.[62,63]

Women who carry *BRCA1/2* mutations are also at increased risk to develop ovarian, fallopian tube, and primary peritoneal cancer, even if no one in their family has developed these cancers. Surveillance for ovarian cancer includes transvaginal ultrasounds and CA-125 testing; however, the effectiveness of such surveillance in detecting ovarian cancers at early, more treatable stages has not been proven in any population. Oral contraceptives reduce the risk of ovarian cancer in all women, including *BRCA* carriers.[64] Recent data indicate that the impact of this intervention on increasing breast cancer risk, if any, is low.[56,65] Given the difficulties in screening and in the treatment of ovarian cancer, the risk/benefit analysis likely favors the use of oral contraceptives in young carriers of *BRCA1/2* mutations[30] who are not yet ready to have their ovaries removed. Prophylactic bilateral salpingo-oophorectomy (BSO) is currently the most effective means to reduce the risk of ovarian cancer and is recommended to *BRCA1/2* carriers by the age of 35 to 40 or when childbearing is complete.[66] Specific operative and pathologic protocols have been developed for this prophylactic surgery.[67] In *BRCA1/2* carriers whose pathologies come back normal, this surgery is highly effective at reducing the subsequent risk of ovarian cancer.[68] A decision analysis, comparing various surveillance and risk-reducing options available to *BRCA* carriers, has shown an increase in life expectancy if BSO is pursued by age 40.[69] Emerging data indicate that most ovarian cancers begin in the fallopian tube, and that salpingectomy may someday be sufficient in reducing ovarian cancer risk in young women; however, more data are needed before this option is offered to patients outside of clinical trials.[70] A relatively small percentage of women who pursue BSO may develop primary peritoneal carcinoma.[44,71] There has been some debate about whether *BRCA1/2* carriers should also opt for total abdominal hysterectomy (TAH) due to the fact that small stumps of the fallopian tubes remain after BSO alone. The question of whether *BRCA* carriers are at increased risk for uterine serous papillary carcinoma (USPC) has also been raised.[72–74] If a relationship does exist between *BRCA* mutations and uterine

cancer, the risk appears to be low and not elevated over that of the general population.[75] Removing the uterus may make it possible for a *BRCA* carrier to take unopposed estrogen or tamoxifen in the future without the risk of uterine cancer, but this surgery is associated with a longer recovery time and has more side effects than does BSO alone. Each patient should be counseled about the pros and cons of each procedure and the risks associated with premature menopause before having surgery.[76]

A secondary, but important, reason for female *BRCA* carriers to consider prophylactic oophorectomy is that it also significantly reduces the risk of a subsequent breast cancer, particularly if they have this surgery before menopause.[77,78] The reduction in breast cancer risk remains even if a healthy premenopausal carrier elects to take low-dose hormone-replacement therapy (HRT) after this surgery.[79] Early data suggest that tamoxifen, in addition to premenopausal oophorectomy, in *BRCA* carriers may have little additional benefit in terms of breast cancer risk reduction.[80] Research is needed in balancing quality of life issues secondary to estrogen deprivation with cancer risk reduction in these young female *BRCA1/2* carriers.

New developments are also emerging in the treatment and, possibly, the prevention of *BRCA*-related cancers. Early data revealed that breast and ovarian cancers in *BRCA* carriers were particularly sensitive to treatment with poly adenosine diphosphate (ADP)-ribose polymerases (PARP) inhibitors in combination with chemotherapy.[81,82] New trials are focusing on which chemotherapeutic regimens are most effective in mutation carriers. More data are needed on larger cohorts of patients and are currently being studies in multiple clinical trials.

Genetic counseling and testing is also available for dozens of cancer syndromes, including Lynch syndrome, von Hippel-Lindau syndrome, multiple endocrine neoplasias, and familial adenomatous polyposis. Surveillance and risk reduction for patients who are known mutation carriers for such conditions may decrease the associated morbidity and mortality of these syndromes.

## Follow-up

A follow-up letter to the patient is a concrete means of documenting the information conveyed in the sessions so that the patient and his/her family members can review it over time. This letter should be sent to the patient and health-care professionals to whom the patient has granted access to this information. A follow-up phone call and/or counseling session may also be helpful, particularly in the case of a positive test result. Some programs provide patients with an annual or biannual newsletter updating them on new information in the field of cancer genetics or patient support groups. It is now recommended that patients return for follow-up counseling sessions months, or even years, after their initial consult to discuss advances in genetic testing and changes in surveillance and risk reduction options. This can be beneficial for individuals who have been found to carry a hereditary predisposition, for those in whom a syndrome/mutation is suspected but yet unidentified, and for those who are ready to move forward with genetic testing. Follow-up counseling is also recommended for patients whose life circumstances have changed (e.g., preconception, after childbearing is complete), who are preparing for prophylactic surgery, or who are ready to discuss the family genetics with their children.

## ISSUES IN CANCER GENETIC COUNSELING

### Psychosocial Issues

The psychosocial impact of cancer genetic counseling cannot be underestimated. Just the process of scheduling a cancer risk counseling session may be quite difficult for some individuals with a family history who are not only frightened about their own cancer risk, but also are reliving painful experiences associated with the cancer of their loved ones.[13] Counselees may be faced with an onslaught of emotions, including anger, fear of developing cancer, fear of disfigurement and dying, grief, lack of control, negative body image, and a sense of isolation.[24] Some counselees wrestle with the fear that insurance companies, employers, family members, and even future partners will react negatively to their cancer risks. For many, it is a double-edged sword as they balance their fears and apprehensions about dredging up these issues with the possibility of obtaining reassuring news and much needed information.

A person's perceived cancer risk is often dependent on many "nonmedical" variables. They may estimate that their risk is higher if they look like an affected individual, or share some of their personality traits.[24] Their perceived risks will vary depending on if their relatives were cancer survivors or died painful deaths from the disease. Many people wonder not *if* they are going to get cancer, but *when*.

The counseling session is an opportunity for individuals to express why they believe they have developed cancer, or why their family members have cancer. Some explanations may revolve around family folklore, and it is important to listen to and address these explanations rather than dismiss them.[24] In doing this, the counselor will allow the clients to alleviate their greatest fears and to give more credibility to the medical theory. Understanding a patient's perceived cancer risk is important, because that fear may *decrease* surveillance and preventive health-care behaviors.[83] For patients and families who are moving forward with DNA testing, a referral to a mental health-care professional is often very helpful. Genetic testing has an impact not only on the patient, but also on his/her children, siblings, parents, and extended relatives. This can be overwhelming for an individual and the family, and should be discussed in detail prior to testing.

To date, studies conducted in the setting of pre- and post-genetic counseling have revealed that, at least in the short term, most patients do not experience adverse psychological outcomes after receiving their test results.[84,85] In fact, preliminary data have revealed that individuals in families with known mutations who seek testing seem to fare better psychologically at 6 months than those who avoid testing.[84] Among individuals who learn they are *BRCA* mutation carriers, anxiety and distress levels appear to increase slightly after receiving their test results but returned to pre-test levels in several weeks.[86] Although these data are reassuring, it is important to recognize that genetic testing is an individual decision and will not be right for every patient or every family.

## Presymptomatic Testing in Children

Presymptomatic testing in children has been widely discussed, and most concur that it is appropriate only when the onset of the condition regularly occurs in childhood or if there are useful interventions that can be applied.[87] For example, genetic testing for mutations in the *BRCA* genes and other adult-onset diseases is generally limited to individuals who are >18 years of age. The American College of Medical Genetics states that if the "medical or psychosocial benefits of a genetic test will not accrue until adulthood . . . genetic testing generally should be deferred."[88] In contrast, the DNA-based diagnosis of children and young adults at risk for hereditary medullary thyroid carcinoma (MTC) is appropriate and has improved the management of these patients.[89] DNA-based testing for MTC is virtually 100% accurate and allows at-risk family members to make informed decisions about prophylactic thyroidectomy. FAP is a disorder that occurs in childhood and in which mortality can be reduced if detection is presymptomatic.[90] Testing is clearly indicated in these instances.

Questions have been raised about the parents' right to demand testing for adult-onset diseases, and this is now happening regularly

with direct-to-consumer tests and whole exome testing of children.[91] The risks of such testing to the child, and the child's right *not* to be tested must be considered. Whenever childhood testing is not medically indicated, it is preferable that testing decisions are postponed until the children are adults and can decide for themselves whether to be tested.

## Confidentiality

The level of confidentiality surrounding cancer genetic testing is paramount due to concerns of genetic discrimination. Careful consideration should be given to the confidentially of family history information, pedigrees, genetic test results, pathology reports, and the carrier status of other family members as most hospitals and clinicians transition to electronic medical records systems. The goal of electronic records is to share information about the patient with his/her entire health-care team. However, genetics is a unique specialty that involves the whole family. Patient's charts often contain Health Insurance Portability and Accountability Act (HIPAA)–protected health information and genetic test results for many other family members. This information may not be appropriate to enter into an electronic record. The unique issues of genetics services need to be considered when designing electronic medical record standards.

Confidentiality of test results *within* a family can also be of issue, because genetic counseling and testing often reveals the risk statuses of family members other than the patient. Under confidentiality codes, the patient needs to grant permission before at-risk family members can be contacted. For this reason, many programs have built in a "share information with family members" clause to their informed consent documents. It has been questioned whether or not a family member could sue a health-care professional for negligence if they were identified at high risk yet not informed.[92] Most recommendations have stated that the burden of confidentiality lies between the provider and the patient. However, more recent recommendations state that confidentiality *should* be violated if the potential harm of not notifying other family members outweighs the harm of breaking a confidence to the patient.[93] There is no patent solution for this difficult dilemma, and situations must be considered on a case-by-case basis with the assistance of the in-house legal department and ethics committee.

## Insurance and Discrimination Issues

When genetic testing for cancer predisposition first became widely available, the fear of health insurance discrimination by both patients and providers was one of the most common concerns.[94,95] It appears that the risks of health insurance discrimination were overstated and that almost no discrimination by health insurers has been reported.[96] HIPAA banned the use of genetic information as a preexisting condition.[97,98] In May of 2008, Congress passed the Genetic Information Nondiscrimination Act (GINA, HR 493), which provides broad protection of an individual's genetic information against health insurance and employment discrimination.[99] In addition, the Heath Care and Education Reconciliation Act of 2010 (HR 4872) prohibits group health plans from denying insurance based on preexisting conditions and from increasing premiums based on health status.[100] Health-care providers can now more confidently reassure their patients that genetic counseling and testing will not put them at risk of losing group or individual health insurance.

More and more patients are choosing to submit their genetic counseling and/or testing charges to their health insurance companies. In the past few years, more insurance companies have agreed to pay for counseling and/or testing,[101] perhaps in light of data that show these services reduce errors related to ordering and interpreting genetic testing and that decision analyses have revealed subsequent prophylactic surgeries to be cost effective.[102] The risk of life or disability insurance discrimination, however, is more realistic. Patients should be counseled about such risks before they pursue genetic testing.

## Reproductive Issues

Reproductive technology in the form of preimplantation genetic diagnosis, prenatal testing, or sperm sorting are options[103] for men and women with a hereditary cancer syndrome, but are requested by few patients for adult-onset conditions in which there are viable options for surveillance and risk reduction. Importantly, if a BRCA2 carrier is considering having a child, it is important to assess the spouse's risk of also carrying a BRCA2 mutation. If the spouse is of Jewish ancestry or has a personal or family history of breast, ovarian, or pancreatic cancer, BRCA testing should be considered and a discussion of the risk of Fanconi anemia in a child with two BRCA2 mutations should take place.[104]

## RECENT ADVANCES AND FUTURE DIRECTIONS

Cancer genetic counseling and testing were thrust into the national spotlight in the spring of 2013 when Hollywood icon Angelina Jolie publically disclosed that she was a BRCA1 carrier. One month later the Supreme Court unanimously ruled against gene patents. Referrals for genetic testing spiked across the country and have not returned to baseline levels at most centers. Within hours of the ruling, other labs began offering less expensive and more comprehensive BRCA testing, dramatically changing the marketplace of genetic testing for hereditary breast cancer.

All laboratories that have entered the BRCA marketplace have done so by including BRCA1 and BRCA2 in gene panels. These panels simultaneously analyze groups of genes that contribute to increased risk for breast, colon, ovarian, uterine, and other cancers. The cost of this technology continues to decrease with some multigene panels costing just a few hundred dollars *less* than traditional BRCA testing (~$4,000). Some panels include only well-known genes (e.g., p53, APC, MLH1), although many include lesser known genes (e.g., BRIP1, NBN, MRE11A) for which cancer risks are ill defined and medical management options are unknown. Because testing for these genes is new to the clinical setting, it is expected to take several years to compile accurate cancer risk estimates and appropriate recommendations for surveillance and risk reduction. Furthermore, the rate of *variants of uncertain significance* will likely be more common in the lesser known genes. These changes have increased the complexity of genetic testing exponentially. In response, several state and one national insurance company have mandated genetic counseling by certified providers before they will cover cancer genetic testing. In a surprising response, the American Society of Clinical Oncology (ASCO) opposed this insurer's decision, despite more than a decade's worth of data demonstrating that the majority of physicians do not have the time or expertise to offer genetic counseling and testing[38,105-108]. The AMA will decide whether to back the ASCO resolution in June 2014.

Some companies are now offering direct-to-consumer (DTC) genetic testing via websites. The accuracy of some of these DTC genetic tests are in question, and the leading company, 23andMe, has recently come under fire by the U.S. Food and Drug Administration.[105]

Maintaining high standards for thorough genetic counseling, informed consent, and accurate result interpretation will be paramount in reducing potential risks and maximizing the benefits of genetic technology in the next century.

## REFERENCES

1. Peters J. Breast cancer genetics: relevance to oncology practice. *Cancer Control* 1995;2:195–208.
2. Brierley KL, Campfield D, Ducaine W, et al. Errors in delivery of cancer genetics services: implications for practice. *Conn Med* 2010;74:413–423.
3. Brierley KL, Blouch E, Cogswell W, et al. Adverse events in cancer genetic testing: medical, ethical, legal, and financial implications. *Cancer J* 2012;18: 303–309.
4. American College of Surgeons, Commission on Cancer: Cancer Program Standards 2012: Ensuring Patient-Centered Care. http://www.facs.org/cancer/coc/programstandards2012.html Accessed on December 3, 2012.
5. Yale Cancer Genetic Counseling Program. Mammography techs ordering their own genetic testing? It appears our suspicion was correct. yalecancergeneticcounseling.blogspot.com October 2, 2013. http://yalecancergenetic counseling.blogspot.com/2013/10/mammography-techs-ordering-their-own.html
6. Lubin IM, Caggana M, Constantin C, et al. Ordering molecular genetic tests and reporting results: practices in laboratory and clinical settings. *J Mol Diagn* 2008;10:459–468.
7. Weeks WB, Wallace AE. Time and money: a retrospective evaluation of the inputs, outputs, efficiency, and incomes of physicians. *Arch Intern Med* 2003;163(8):944–948.
8. Doksum T, Bernhardt BA, Holtzman NA. Does knowledge about the genetics of breast cancer differ between nongeneticist physicians who do or do not discuss or order BRCA testing? *Genet Med* 2003;5:99–105.
9. Rosenthal ET. Shortage of genetics counselors may be anecdotal, but need is real. *Oncology Times* 2007;29:34–36.
10. Informed Medical Decisions. Adult Genetics: Genetic counseling for your health concerns. Available at: http://www.informeddna.com/index.php/patients/adult-genetics.html. Accessed August 24, 2009.
11. Informed Medical Decisions. News: Aetna Press Release: Aetna to offer access to confidential telephonic cancer genetic counseling to health plan members. Available at: http://www.informeddna.com/images/stories/news_articles/aetna%20press%20release%20bw.pdf. Accessed August 24, 2009.
12. Schneider, ME. Cigna to require counseling for some genetic tests. Internal Medicine News Digital Network. July 26, 2013. http://www.internalmedicine news.com/single-view/cigna-to-require-counseling-for-some-genetic-tests/efd4f421df8b46ba2208da423adf198d.html
13. Claus E, Schildkraut J, Thompson W, et al. The genetic attributable risks of breast and ovarian cancer. *Cancer* 1996;77:2318–2324.

14. Loman N, Johannsson O, Kristoffersson U. Family history of breast and ovarian cancers and BRCA1 and BRCA2 mutations in a population-based series of early-onset breast cancer. *J Natl Cancer Inst* 2001;93:1215.
15. Struewing J, Hartge P, Wacholder S. The risk of cancer associated with specific mutations of BRCA1 and BRCA2 among Ashkenazi Jews. *N Engl J Med* 1997;336:1401–1408.
16. Eisinger F, Jacquemier J, Charpin C, et al. Mutations at BRCA1: the medullary breast carcinoma revisited. *Cancer Res* 1998;58:1588–1592.
17. Kandel M, Stadler Z, Masciari S, et al. Prevalence of BRCA1 mutations in triple negative breast cancer. Paper presented at: 2006 42nd Annual ASCO Meeting; 2006; Atlanta, GA.
18. National Comprehensive Cancer Network Clinical Guidelines in Oncology: Genetics/Familial High-Risk Assessment - Breast and Ovarian Cancer. http://www.nccn.org/professionals/physician_gls/f_guidelines.asp#detection Accessed November 2, 2012.
19. Risch H, McLaughlin J, Cole D, et al. Population BRCA1 and BRCA2 mutation frequencies and cancer penetrances: a kin-cohort study in Ontario, Canada. *JNCI* 2006;98:1694–706.
20. Matloff E, Brierley K, Chimera C. A clinician's guide to hereditary colon cancer. *Cancer J* 2004;10(5):280–287.
21. Pilarski R. Cowden syndrome: a critical review of the clinical literature. *J Genet Couns* 2009 Feb;18:13–27.
22. Varga EA, Pastore M, Prior T, et al. The prevalence of PTEN mutations in a clinical pediatric cohort with autism spectrum disorders, developmental delay, and macrocephaly. *Genet Med* 2009;11:111–117.
23. Gorlin R. Nevoid basal-cell carcinoma syndrome. *Medicine* 1987;66(2): 98–113.
24. Schneider K. *Counseling About Cancer: Strategies for Genetic Counseling*. 2nd ed. Wiley-Liss; 2001.
25. Love R, Evan A, Josten D. The accuracy of patient reports of a family history. *J Chronic Dis* 1985;38(4):289–293.
26. Alter B, Rosenberg P, Brody L. Clinical and molecular features associated with biallelic mutations in FANCD1/BRCA2. *J Med Genet* 2007;44:1–9.
27. Thompson D, Duedal S, Kirner J, et al. Cancer risks and mortality in heterozygous ATM mutation carriers. *J Natl Cancer Inst* 2005;97:813–822.
28. Korzenik J, Chung D, Digumarthy S, at al. Case 33-2005: a 43 year-old man with lower gastrointestinal bleeding. *N Engl J Med* 2005;353:1836–1844.
29. American Cancer Society. *Cancer Facts and Figures 2009*. Atlanta, GA: American Cancer Society; 2009.

30. Olopade O, Weber B. Breast cancer genetics: toward molecular characterization of individuals at increased risk for breast cancer. Part II. PPO Updates 1998;12:1–8.

31. Stratton MR, Rahman N. The emerging landscape of breast cancer susceptibility. *Nat Genet* 2008;40:17–22.

32. Gail M, Brinton L, Byar D. Projecting individualized probabilities of developing breast cancer for white females who are being examined annually. *J Natl Cancer Inst* 1989;81:1879–1886.

33. Claus E, Risch N, Thompson W. Autosomal dominant inheritance of early-onset breast cancer. *Cancer* 1994;73:643.

34. Parmigiani G, Berry D, Aguilar O. Determining carrier probabilities for breast cancer susceptibility genes BRCA1 and BRCA2. *Am J Hum Genet* 1998;62:145–158.

35. Friedman S. *Thoughts from FORCE: Comments Submitted to the Secretary's Advisory Committee on Genetics Health and Society.* http://facingourrisk.wordpress.com/2008/12/03/comments-submitted-to-the-secretarys-advisory-committee-on-genetics-health-and-society/. Accessed April 6, 2010.

36. UnitedHealth. *Personalized Medicine: Trends and Prospects for the New Science of Genetic Testing and Molecular Diagnostics.* Working Paper 7. Minnetonka, MN: UnitedHealth Center for Health Reform & Modernization; March 2012.

37. ARUP Laboratories. *Value of Genetic Counselors in the Laboratory.* Salt Lake City: ARUP Laboratories; March 2011.

38. Plon SE, Cooper HP, Parks B, et al. Genetic testing and cancer risk management recommendations by physicians for at-risk relatives. *Genet Med* 2011;13:148–154.

39. Walsh T. *More Than 25% of Breast Cancer Families with Wild-Type Results from Commercial Genetic Testing of BRCA1 and BRCA2 Are Resolved by BROCA Sequencing of All Known Breast Cancer Genes.* Paper presented at: 2013 American Society of Human Genetics Meeting Session #19; 2013; Boston, MA.

40. U.S. Preventive Services Task Force. *Genetic Risk Assessment and BRCA Mutation Testing for Breast and Ovarian Cancer Susceptibility.* Rockville, MD: Agency for Healthcare Research and Quality; 2013. http://www.uspreventiveservicestaskforce.org/uspstf12/brcatest/brcatestfinalrs.htm. Accessed June 2, 2014.

41. King MC, Marks JH, Mandell JB, et al. Breast and ovarian cancer risks due to inherited mutations in BRCA1 and BRCA2. *Science* 2003;302:643–646.

42. Antoniou A, Pharoah PD, Narod S, et al. Average risks of breast and ovarian cancer associated with BRCA1 or BRCA2 mutations detected in case Series unselected for family history: a combined analysis of 22 studies. *Am J Hum Genet* 2003;72:1117–1130.

43. Ford D, Easton D, Bishop D, et al. Risks of cancer in BRCA1 mutation carriers. *Lancet* 1994;343:692–695.

44. Piver M, Jishi M, Tsukada Y. Primary peritoneal carcinoma after prophylactic oophorectomy in women with a family history of ovarian cancer. *Cancer* 1993;71:2751–2755.

45. Aziz S, Kuperstein G, Rosen B. A genetic epidemiological study of carcinoma of the fallopian tube. *Gynecol Oncol* 2001;80:341–345.

46. van Asperen C, Brohet R, Meijers-Heijboer, et al. Cancer risks in BRCA2 families: estimates for sites other than breast and ovary. *J Med Genet* 2005;42:711–719.

47. Breast Cancer Linkage Consortium. Cancer risks in BRCA2 mutation carriers. *J Natl Cancer Inst* 1999;91:1310–1316.

48. Warner E, Plewes D, Hill K, et al. Surveillance of BRCA1 and BRCA2 mutation carriers with magnetic resonance imaging, ultrasound, mammography, and clinical breast examination. *JAMA* 2004;202:1317–1325.

49. Kriege M, Brekelmans CT, Boetes C, et al. Efficacy of MRI and mammography for breast-cancer screening in women with a familial or genetic predisposition. *N Engl J Med* 2004;29:351:427–437.

50. Kuhl C, Weigel S, Schrading S, et al. Prospective multicenter cohort study to refine management recommendations for women at elevated familial risk of breast cancer: the EVA Trial. *J Clin Oncol* 2010:1450–1457.

51. Powles T, Ashley S, Tidy A, et al. Twenty-year follow-up of the Royal Marsden randomized, double-blinded tamoxifen breast cancer prevention trial. *J Natl Cancer Inst* 2007;99:283–290.

52. Cuzick J, Forbes J, Sestak I, et al. Long-term results of tamoxifen prophylaxis for breast cancer: 96 month follow-up of the randomized IBIS-I trial. *J Natl Cancer Inst* 2007;99:272–282.

53. Goss PE, Ingle JN, Alés-Martínez JE, et al. Exemestane for breast-cancer prevention in postmenopausal women. *N Engl J Med* 2011;364:2381.

54. Fisher B, Constantino J, Wickerman D. Tamoxifen for the prevention of breast cancer: report of the National Surgical Adjuvant Breast and Bowel Project P-1 Study. *J Natl Cancer Inst* 1998;90:1371–1388.

55. King M, Wieand S, Hale K. Tamoxifen and breast cancer incidence among women with inherited mutations in BRCA1 and BRCA2. *JAMA* 2001;286:2251–2256.

56. Narod S, Brunet J, Ghadirian P. Tamoxifen and risk of contralateral breast cancer in BRCA1 and BRCA2 mutation carriers: a case-control study. *Lancet* 2000;356:1876–1881.

57. Phillips KA, Milne RL, Rookus MA, et al. Tamoxifen and risk of contralateral breast cancer for BRCA1 and BRCA2 mutation carriers. *J Clin Oncol* 2013;31:3091–3099.

58. Lakhani S, van de Vijver M, Jacquemier J, et al. The pathology of familial breast cancer: predictive value of immunohistochemical markers estrogen receptor, progesterone receptor, HER-2, and p53 in patients with mutations in BRCA1 and BRCA2. *J Clin Oncol* 2002;20:2310–2318.

59. Hartmann L, Schaid D, Woods J. Efficacy of bilateral prophylactic mastectomy in women with a family history of breast cancer. *N Engl J Med* 1999;340:77–84.

60. Matloff E. The breast surgeon's role in BRCA1 and BRCA2 testing. *Am J Surg* 2000;180:294–298.

61. Turner B, Harold E, Matloff E, et al. BRCA1/BRCA2 germline mutations in locally recurrent breast cancer patients after lumpectomy and radiation therapy: Implications for breast-conserving management in patients with BRCA1/BRCA2 mutations. *J Clin Oncol* 1999;17:3017–3024.

62. Contant CM, et al. Clinical experience of prophylactic mastectomy followed by immediate breast reconstruction in women at hereditary risk of breast cancer (HBOC) or a proven BRCA1 or BRCA2 germ-line mutation. *Eur J Surg Oncol* 2002;28:627–632.

63. Forman DL, Chiu J, Restifo RJ, et al. Breast reconstruction in previously irradiated patients using tissue expanders and implants: a potentially unfavorable result. *Ann Plast Surg* 1998;40:360–363.

64. McLaughlin J, Risch H, Lubinski J, et al. Reproductive risk factors for ovarian cancer in carriers of BRCA1 or BRCA2 mutations: a case-control study. *Lancet* 2007;8:26–34.

65. Milne R, Knight J, John E, et al. Oral contraceptive use and risk of early-onset breast cancer in carriers and noncarriers of BRCA1 and BRCA2 mutations. *Cancer Epidemiol Biomarkers Prev* 2005;14:350–356.

66. Domchek S, Friebel T, Neuhausen S, et al. Mortality reduction after risk-reducing bilateral salpingo-oophorectomy in a prospective cohort of BRCA1 and BRCA2 mutation carriers. *Lancet Oncol* 2006;7:223–229.

67. Powel CB, Kenley E, Chen LM, et al. Risk-reducing salpingo-oophorectomy in BRCA mutation carriers: role of serial sectioning in the detection of occult malignancy. *J Clin Oncol* 2005;23:127–132.

68. Finch A, Beiner M, Lubinski J, et al. Salpingo-oophorectomy and the risk of ovarian, fallopian tube, and peritoneal cancers in women with a BRCA1 or BRCA2 mutation. *JAMA* 2006;296:185–192.

69. Kurian AW, Sigal BM, Plevritis SK. Survival analysis of cancer risk reduction strategies for BRCA1/2 mutation carriers. *J Clin Oncol* 2010;10;28:222–231.

70. Kwon JS, Tinker A, Pansegrau G, et al. Prophylactic salpingectomy and delayed oophorectomy as an alternative for BRCA mutation carriers. *Obstet Gynecol* 2013;121:14–24.

71. American College of Obstetricians and Gynecologists. ACOG committee opinion. Breast–ovarian cancer screening. Number 176, October 1996. Committee on Genetics. The American College of Obstetricians and Gynecologists. *Int J Gynaecol Obstet* 1997;56:82–83.

72. Hornreich G, Beller U, Lavie O. Is uterine serous papillary carcinoma a BRCA1 related disease? Case report and review of the literature. *Gynecol Oncol* 1999;75(2):300–304.

73. Levine D, Lin P, Barakat R. Risk of endometrial carcinoma associated with BRCA mutation. *Gynecol Oncol* 2001;80(3):395–398.

74. Goshen R, Chu W, Elit L. Is uterine papillary serous adenocarcinoma a manifestation of the hereditary breast-ovarian cancer syndrome? *Gynecol Oncol* 2000;79(3):477–481.

75. Boyd J. The breast, ovarian, and other cancer genes. *Gynecol Oncol* 2001; 80(3):337–340.

76. Campfield Bonadies D, Moyer A, Matloff ET. What I wish I'd known before surgery: BRCA carriers' perspectives after bilateral salipingo-oophorectomy. *Fam Cancer* 2011;10:79–85.

77. Rebbeck T, Lynch H, Neuhausen S, et al. Prophylactic oophorectomy in carriers of BRCA1 or BRCA2 mutations. *N Engl J Med* 2002;346:1616–1622.

78. Kauff N, Satagopan J, Robson M, et al. Risk-reducing salpingo-oophorectomy in women with a BRCA1 or BRCA2 mutation. *N Engl J Med* 2002;346:1609–1615.

79. Rebbeck T, Friebel T, Wagner T, et al. Effect of short-term hormone replacement therapy on breast cancer risk reduction after bilateral prophylactic oophorectomy in BRCA1 and BRCA2 mutation carriers: the PROSE study group. *J Clin Oncol* 2005;23:7804–7810.

80. Gronwald J, Tung N, Foulkes W, et al. Tamoxifen and contralateral breast cancer in BRCA1 and BRCA2 carriers: an update. *Int J Cancer* 2006;118:2281–2284.

81. Fong PC, Boss DS, Yap TA, et al. Inhibition of Poly (ADPRibose) Polymerase in Tumors from BRCA Mutation Carriers. *N Engl J Med* 2009;361:1–12.

82. Inglhart JD, Silver DP. Synthetic lethality – a new direction in cancer-drug development. *N Engl J Med* 2009;361:1–3.

83. Kash K, Holland J, Halper M, et al. Psychological distress and surveillance behaviors of women with a family history of breast cancer. *J Natl Cancer Inst* 1992;84:24–30.

84. Lerman C, Hughes C, Lemon S. What you don't know can hurt you: adverse psychologic effects in members of BRCA1-linked and BRCA2-linked families who decline genetic testing. *J Clin Oncol* 1998;16:1650–1654.

85. Croyle R, Smith K, Botkin J. Psychological responses to BRCA1 mutation testing: preliminary findings. *Health Psychol* 1997;16:63–72.

86. Hamilton JG, Lobel M, Moyer A. Emotional distress following genetic testing for hereditary breast and ovarian cancer: a meta-analytic review. *Health Psychol* 2009;28:510–518.

87. Clayton E. Removing the shadow of the law from the debate about genetic testing of children. *Am J Med Genet* 1995;57:630–634.

88. ASHG/ACMG. Points to consider: ethical, legal, and psychosocial implications of genetic testing in children and adolescents. American Society of Human Genetics Board of Directors, American College of Medical Genetics Board of Directors. *Am J Hum Genet* 1995;57:1233–1241.

89. Ledger G, Khosia S, Lindor N, et al. Genetic testing in the diagnosis and management of multiple endocrine neoplasia type II. *Ann Intern Med* 1995; 122:118–124.

CANCER PREVENTION AND SCREENING

90. Rhodes M, Bradburn D. Overview of screening and management of familial adenomatous polyposis. *Br J Surg* 1992;33:125–123.

91. Howard HC, Avard D, Borry P. Are the kids really all right? Direct-to-consumer genetic testing in children: are company policies clashing with professional norms? *Eur J Hum Genet* 2011;19:1122–1126.

92. Tsoucalas C. Legal aspects of cancer genetics - screening, counseling, and registers. In: Lynch H, Kullander S, eds. *Cancer Genetics in Women*. Vol I. Boca Raton, FL: CRC Press, Inc.; 1987:9.

93. American Society of Human Genetics. ASHG Statement: professional disclosure of familial genetic information. *Am J Hum Genet* 1998;62:474–483.

94. Bluman L, Rimer B, Berry D. Attitudes, knowledge, and risk perceptions of women with breast and/or ovarian cancer considering testing for BRCA1 and BRCA2. *J Clin Oncol* 1999; 17:1040–1046.

95. Matloff E, Shappell H, Brierley K, et al. What would you do? Specialists' perspectives on cancer genetic testing, prophylactic surgery and insurance discrimination. *J Clin Oncol* 2000;18:2484–2492.

96. Hall MA, Rich SS. Patients' fear of genetic discrimination by health insurers: the impact of legal protections *Genet Med* 2000:2:214–221.

97. Leib JR, Hoodfar E, Larsen Haidle J, Nagy R. The new genetic privacy law. *Community Oncol* 2008;5:351–354.

98. Hudson KL, Holohan JD, Collins FS. Keeping pace with the times — the Genetic Information Nondiscrimination Act of 2008. *N Engl J Med* 2008;358:2661–2663.

99. The Genetic Information Nondiscrimination Act of 2008 (H.R. 493). Library of Congress Web site. http://beta.congress.gov/bill/110th-congress/house-bill/493. Accessed June 2, 2014.

100. The Health Care and Education Affordability Reconciliation Act of 2010 (H.R. 4872). Library of Congress Web site. http://beta.congress.gov/bill/111th-congress/house-bill/4872: Accessed June 2, 2014.

101. Manley S, Pennell R, Frank T. Insurance coverage of BRCA1 and BRCA2 sequence analysis. *J Genet Couns* 1998;7:A462.

102. Grann V, Whang W, Jabcobson J, et al. Benefits and costs of screening Ashkenazi Jewish women for BRCA1 and BRCA2. *J Clin Oncol* 1999;17: 494–500.

103. Offit K, Kohut K, Clagett B, et al. Cancer genetic testing and assisted reproduction. *J Clin Oncol* 2006;24:4775–4782.

104. Offit K, Levran O, Mullaney B, et al. Shared genetic susceptibility to breast cancer, brain tumors, and Fanconi anemia. *J Natl Cancer Inst* 2003;95(20): 1548–1551.

105. Greendale K, Pyeritz RE. Empowering primary care health professionals in medical genetics: How soon? How fast? How far? *Am J Med Genet* 2001;106:223–232.

106. Wilkins-Haug L, Hill LD, Power ML, et al. Gynecologists' training, knowledge, and experiences in genetics: a survey. *Obstet Gynecol* 2000;95:421–424.

107. Wood ME, Stockdale A, Flynn BS. Interviews with primary care physicians regarding taking and interpreting the cancer family history. *Fam Pract* 2008; 25:334–340.

108. Bellcross CA, Kolor K, Goddard K, et al. Awareness and utilization of BRCA1/2 testing among U.S. primary care physicians. *Am J Prev Med* 2011;40:61–66.

109. Pollack A. F.D.A. Orders genetic testing firm to stop selling DNA analysis service. *New York Times*. November 25, 2013. http://www.nytimes.com/2013/11/26/business/fda-demands-a-halt-to-a-dna-test-kits-marketing.html?_r=0

## PART V

# Cancers of the Genitourinary System

# Molecular Biology
# of Kidney Cancer

W. Marston Linehan and Laura S. Schmidt

## INTRODUCTION

Kidney cancer or renal cell carcinoma (RCC) affects more than 271,000 people annually worldwide, resulting in 116,000 deaths each year.[1] A variety of risk factors, including obesity, hypertension, tobacco smoking, and certain occupational exposures, have been shown to increase one's risk for developing RCC. Our current understanding of the molecular genetics of kidney cancer has come from studies of families with an inherited predisposition to develop renal tumors. Individuals with a family history of RCC have a 2.5-fold greater chance for developing renal cancer during their lifetimes[2] and comprise about 4% of all RCCs.

Kidney cancer is not a single disease, but rather is classified into tumor subtypes based on histology.[3] Over the past 2 decades, studies of families with inherited renal carcinoma enabled the identification of five inherited renal cancer syndromes and their predisposing genes (Table 36.1), which implicate diverse biologic pathways in renal cancer tumorigenesis.[4] The von Hippel-Lindau (VHL) tumor suppressor gene was discovered in 1993.[5] Subsequently, activating mutations were identified in the MET protooncogene in patients with hereditary papillary renal carcinoma (HPRC).[6] More recently, germ-line mutations in the gene for Krebs cycle enzyme fumarate hydratase (FH), responsible for hereditary leiomyomatosis and renal cell carcinoma (HLRCC),[7] and in FLCN, the gene for Birt–Hogg–Dubé (BHD) syndrome, were identified.[8] Germ-line mutations in the genes encoding subunits B, C, and D of another Krebs cycle enzyme, succinate dehydrogenase (SDHB/SDHC/SDHD), have been found in patients with familial renal cancer.[9–11] Discovery of the genes for the inherited forms of renal cancer has enabled the development of diagnostic genetic tests for presymptomatic diagnosis and improved prognosis for at-risk individuals.

## VON HIPPEL-LINDAU DISEASE

Von Hippel-Lindau (VHL) disease is an autosomal-dominant inherited multisystem neoplastic disorder that is characterized by clear cell renal tumors, retinal angiomas, central nervous system hemangioblastomas, tumors of the adrenal gland (pheochromocytoma), endolymphatic sac and pancreatic islet cell, and cysts in the pancreas and kidney. VHL occurs in about 1 in 36,000 and develops during the 2nd to 4th decades of life with nearly 70% penetrance by age 60. Bilateral, multifocal renal tumors with clear cell histology develop in 25% to 45% of VHL patients[12] that can have metastatic potential when they reach 3 cm.

### Genetics of VHL

Loss of heterozygosity (LOH) on chromosome 3p in clear cell renal tumors suggested the location of a predisposing gene for RCC.[13] Positional cloning in VHL kindreds defined the disease locus to chromosome 3p25-26, leading to the cloning of the VHL gene in 1993.[5] VHL is a tumor suppressor gene in which both copies of VHL must be inactivated for tumor initiation. Germ-line VHL mutations that predispose individuals to VHL encompass the entire mutation spectrum, including large deletions, protein-truncating mutations, and missense mutations that exchange the amino acid in the VHL protein. Over 700 different VHL mutations have been identified in more than 945 VHL families worldwide. Mutations are located throughout the entire gene with the exception of the first 35 residues in the acidic domain.[12] With the development of new methods for detection of deletions, VHL mutation detection rates are approaching 100%.[14,15] VHL subclasses based on the predisposition to develop pheochromocytomas and a high or low risk of RCC have been established with clear genotype–phenotype associations emerging.[16]

## Gene Mutated in Renal Cancer Families with Chromosome 3p Translocations

In 1979, Cohen et al.[17] described a family with a constitutional t(3;8)(p14;q24) balanced translocation that cosegregated with bilateral multifocal clear cell renal tumors. Loss of the derivative chromosome carrying the 3p segment and different somatic mutations in the remaining copy of VHL were identified in the tumors from this translocation family. Based on these data, Schmidt et al.[18] proposed a three-step tumorigenesis model in 3p translocation families: (1) inheritance of the constitutional translocation, (2) loss of the derivative chromosome bearing 3p25, and (3) mutation of the remaining copy of VHL, resulting in inactivation of both copies of VHL and predisposing individuals to clear cell RCC. A number of chromosome 3 translocation families have been described.[19,20] Loss of the derivative chromosome concomitant with the somatic mutation of the remaining copy of VHL in these families provides strong evidence for the three-step tumorigenesis model and implicates VHL loss in clear cell RCC that develops in chromosome 3 translocation kindreds.

## Gene for Sporadic Clear Cell Kidney Cancer

Somatic mutation of the VHL gene with associated loss of the wild-type allele is found in a high percentage of tumors from patients with clear cell kidney cancer.[21] Nickerson et al.[22] recently identified mutation or methylation of the VHL gene in 92% of clear cell kidney cancers. The VHL gene mutation is not found in papillary, chromophobe, collecting duct, medullary, or other types of kidney cancer.

## Function of the VHL Protein

The most well-understood function of the VHL protein pVHL is the substrate recognition site for the hypoxia-inducible factor

## TABLE 36.1

### Hereditary Renal Cancer Syndromes

| Syndrome | Chromosome Location | Predisposing Gene | Histology | Frequency of Gene Mutations | |
|---|---|---|---|---|---|
| | | | | Germ Line | Sporadic RCC |
| Von Hippel-Lindau (VHL) disease | 3p25 | VHL | Clear cell | 100%[14] | 92%[22] |
| Hereditary papillary renal carcinoma type 1 (HPRC) | 7q31 | MET | Type 1 papillary | 100%[6,41,42] | 13%[45] |
| Birt-Hogg-Dubé syndrome (BHD) | 17p11.2 | FLCN | Chromophobe, hybrid | 90%[65] | 11%[76] |
| Hereditary leiomyomatosis and renal cell carcinoma (HLRCC) | 1q42–43 | FH | Type 2 papillary | 93%[105] | TBD |
| Succinate dehydrogenase (SDH)–associated familial renal cancer | 1p35–36 1q23.3 11q23 | SDHB SDHC SDHD | Clear cell, chromophobe, oncocytic neoplasm | TBD | TBD |
| Tuberous sclerosis complex (TSC) | 9q34 16p13.3 | TSC1 TSC2 | Angiomyolipoma, all histologies | 80%–90% | TBD |

TBD, to be determined.

(HIF)-α family of transcription factors targeting them for ubiquitin-mediated proteasomal degradation (Fig. 36.1).[16] pVHL binds through its α domain to elongin C and forms an E3 ubiquitin ligase complex with elongin B, cullin-2, and Rbx-1. Under normal oxygen conditions, HIF-α becomes hydroxylated on critical prolines by a family of HIF prolyl hydroxylases (PHD) that require α-ketoglutarate, molecular oxygen, ascorbic acid, and iron as cofactors. pVHL then binds to hydroxylated HIF-α through its β domain, targeting HIF-α for ubiquitylation by the E3 ligase complex. Under hypoxic conditions when PHDs are unable to function or when pVHL is mutated—thereby altering its binding to HIF-α or elongin C—HIF-α cannot be recognized by pVHL. HIF-α accumulates and transcriptionally upregulates a number of genes important in blood vessel development (EPO, VEGF), cell proliferation (PDGFβ, TGFα), and glucose metabolism

(GLUT-1).[16] HIF-α–dependent upregulation of target genes involved in neovascularization provides an explanation for the increased vascularity of central nervous system (CNS) hemangioblastomas and clear cell renal tumors in VHL. Germ-line VHL mutations frequently occur in the pVHL binding domains for HIF-α and elongin C.[23] HIF-2α (rather than HIF-1α) stabilization appears to be critical for renal tumor development.[24,25] Additional HIF-independent functions for pVHL have been reported,[12,16,26] including an increase of p53 activity through the suppression of MDM2-mediated ubiquitination and nuclear export,[27] modulation of nuclear factor κ B (NF-κB) through casein kinase 2 binding and inhibitory phosphorylation of NF-κB agonist CARD9,[28] microtubule stabilization,[29] maintenance of primary cilium,[30] and extracellular matrix formation affecting cell–cell adhesion.[31,32]

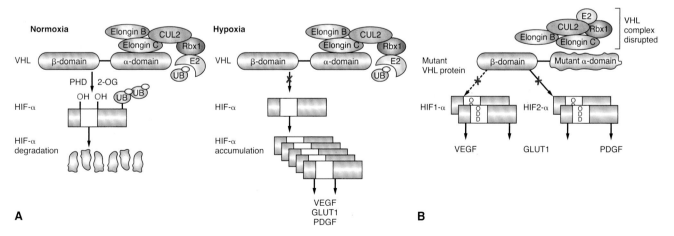

**Figure 36.1** The von Hippel-Lindau (VHL) E3 ubiquitin ligase complex targets hypoxia-inducible factor (HIF)-α for ubiquitin-mediated degradation. **(A)** Under normal oxygen conditions, HIF-α is hydroxylated on critical prolines by HIF prolyl hydroxylase (PHD), requiring molecular oxygen, α-ketoglutarate (2-OG), and iron as cosubstrates. The VHL protein (pVHL) can then recognize and bind hydroxylated HIF-α, enabling ubiquitylation by the VHL E3 ligase complex and degradation by the proteasome. Under hypoxic conditions, PHD is unable to function properly, pVHL cannot recognize HIF-α, and HIF-α accumulates, leading to the upregulation of HIF-target genes (VEGF, GLUT1, PDGF) that support tumor growth and neovascularization. **(B)** When VHL is mutated and pVHL is unable to bind HIF-α, HIF-α stabilization leads to transcriptional upregulation of HIF target genes. (From Linehan WM, Srinivasan R, Schmidt LS. The genetic basis of kidney cancer: a metabolic disease. Nat Rev Urol 2010;7:277–285.)

## Additional Genes for Clear Cell Kidney Cancer

Studies using next-generation sequencing approaches to identify the genetic basis of clear cell kidney cancer have revealed a considerable number of genetic alterations in chromatin remodeling genes important for the maintenance of chromatin states. Significantly mutated genes identified in sporadic clear cell kidney cancer in addition to *VHL* include *PBRM1*, a subunit of the PBAF SWI/SNF chromatin remodeling complex (41%),[33] histone methyl transferase *SETD2* (4%)[34] histone demethylases *JARID1C* (*KDM5C*; 3%)[35] and *UTX* (*KMD6A*; 3%),[35] and the novel tumor suppressor gene, BAP1 (15%),[36] a histone deubiquitinase. *BAP1* is also mutated, albeit rarely, in the germ line of inherited clear cell kidney cancer families[37,38] and is associated with poor survival outcome.[39]

## HEREDITARY PAPILLARY RENAL CARCINOMA TYPE 1

HPRC is an autosomal-dominant hereditary cancer syndrome in which affected individuals are at risk for the development of multifocal, bilateral papillary type 1 kidney cancer.[40] HPRC develops in the 5th and 6th decades, with age-dependent penetrance estimated at 67% by 60 years of age[41]; however, early-onset HPRC has been described.[42] This rare disorder has been reported in less than 40 kindreds worldwide.[40]

### Genetics of Hereditary Papillary Renal Carcinoma: *MET* Proto-oncogene

In 1995, Zbar et al.[43] described 10 families in which multifocal, bilateral papillary renal tumors were inherited in an autosomal-dominant fashion and suggested that these families might represent a hereditary counterpart to sporadic papillary tumors. Schmidt et al.[6] localized the HPRC disease locus to chromosome 7q31.1-34 by genetic linkage analysis. Because the trisomy of chromosome 7 was described as a hallmark feature of papillary renal tumors,[44] a gain-of-function oncogene seemed a likely candidate disease gene; in fact, germ-line missense mutations were identified in the tyrosine-kinase domain of the *MET* protooncogene located at 7q31 in affected HPRC family members.[6] Mutations of the *MET* gene have been detected in 13% of sporadic papillary renal tumors.[6,45] Further studies to determine the role of *MET* and related genes in papillary type 1 kidney cancer are currently under way.

### Hereditary Papillary Renal Carcinoma: Functional Consequences of *MET* Mutations

The *MET* protooncogene encodes the hepatocyte growth factor/scatter factor (HGF/SF) receptor tyrosine kinase. Binding of ligand HGF to MET triggers autophosphorylation of critical tyrosines in the intracellular tyrosine kinase domain, subsequent phosphorylation of tyrosines in the multifunctional docking site, and recruitment of a variety of transducers of downstream signaling cascades that regulate cellular programs leading to cell growth, branching morphogenesis, differentiation, and "invasive growth."[46] Although MET overexpression has been demonstrated in a number of epithelial cancers,[47] HPRC was the first cancer syndrome for which germ-line *MET* mutations were identified. The missense *MET* mutations in HPRC are constitutively activating without ligand stimulation, display oncogenic potential in vitro,[48,49] and are predicted by molecular modeling to stabilize active MET kinase.[50] Nonrandom duplication of the chromosome 7 bearing the mutant *MET* allele was demonstrated in papillary renal tumors from HPRC patients[51] and may represent the second step in HPRC tumor pathogenesis. The presence of two copies of mutant *MET* may give kidney cells a proliferative growth advantage and lead to tumor progression.

## XP11.2 TRANSLOCATION RENAL CELL CANCER

Xp11.2 translocation renal cell carcinomas, typically presenting with papillary architecture and clear or eosinophilic cytoplasm, are rare tumors in adults (1.6%), but are the cause of 20% to 45% of renal cancers in children and young adults. Translocations involving Xp11.2 and 1q21.2 associated with sporadic papillary renal carcinoma, and first described in a 2-year-old child,[52] generate a fusion between a novel gene, *PRCC*, and the basic helix-loop-helix-leucine zipper transcription factor gene, *TFE3*, a member of the microphthalmia (MiT) family of transcription factors.[53] The encoded fusion protein, PRCC-TFE3, acts as a stronger transcriptional activator than native TFE3, and a loss of the majority of native TFE3 transcripts is observed in these tumors. This deregulation of normal TFE3 transcriptional control caused by the chromosomal translocation may be important to the development of sporadic papillary renal cell carcinoma.[54,55] Xp11.2 translocation renal cell carcinomas involving at least five different TFE3 gene fusions and resulting in deregulation of TFE3 transcription activity have been described, including *NonO-TFE3*, *PSF-TFE3*, *CLTC-TFE3*, and *ASPL-TFE3*.[56] Tsuda et al.[57] have shown that these TFE3 fusion proteins are strong transcriptional activators of the *MET* gene, resulting in inappropriate MET-directed cell proliferation and invasive growth. Given the physiologic consequences of TFE3 fusion protein expression, therapeutic targeting of MET may be an effective treatment for Xp11.2 translocation renal tumors.

The fusion of another member of the MiT family, *TFEB*, with the *Alpha* gene has been described in renal tumors harboring t(6;11)(p21;q13) chromosomal translocation.[58] The first case of renal cancer involving a third MiT family member, *MITF*, was recently reported, in which an activating *MITF* mutation was identified in the germ-line of family members affected with renal tumors.[59]

## BIRT-HOGG-DUBÉ SYNDROME

BHD syndrome is a rare autosomal-dominant inherited cancer syndrome characterized by benign tumors of the hair follicle (fibrofolliculoma), pulmonary cysts and spontaneous pneumothorax, and a sevenfold increased risk for renal cancers.[60–63] Fibrofolliculomas and lung cysts are the most common manifestations (>85%) of BHD patients.[64–66] Renal tumors with variable histologies develop in about 30% of BHD-affected individuals (median age, 48 to 50 years), most frequently chromophobe renal carcinoma and hybrid oncocytic tumors.[64,67] Metastases may develop from BHD renal tumors, but they are uncommon.

### Genetics of Birt-Hogg-Dubé Syndrome: Folliculin Gene

A genetic linkage analysis performed in BHD kindreds led to the localization of the disease locus on the short arm of chromosome 17[68,69] and the identification of the BHD gene, *FLCN*.[8] Almost all BHD-associated *FLCN* mutations are predicted to truncate the BHD protein, folliculin, including insertion or deletion, nonsense, and splice-site mutations,[8,64,65,70] but recently, several missense mutations located in conserved amino acid residues and partial gene deletions have been described.[65,71–73] The mutation detection rate in several large BHD cohorts approached 90%, and germ-line mutations were distributed throughout the entire length of the *FLCN* gene with no clear genotype–phenotype correlations.[64,65,74] Vocke et al.[75] identified second "hit" somatic mutations or LOH in 70% of renal tumors from BHD patients, supporting a role for *FLCN* as a tumor suppressor gene that predisposes individuals to renal tumors when both copies are inactivated. *FLCN* mutations have

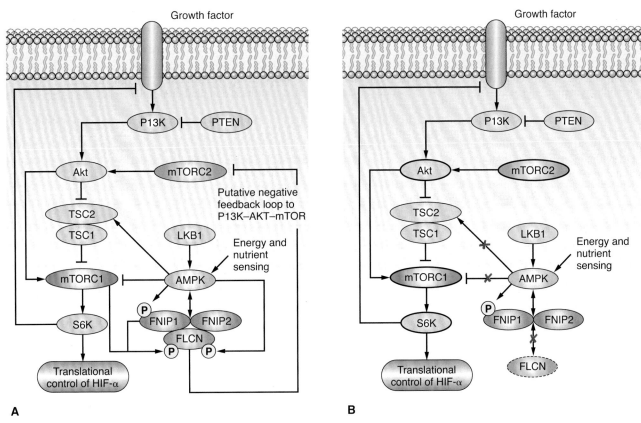

**Figure 36.2** The putative Birt-Hogg-Dubé gene (*FLCN*) pathway. **(A)** *FLCN* binds through FNIP1/2 to AMP–activated protein kinase (AMPK) and may become phosphorylated by AMPK or by a rapamycin-sensitive kinase (i.e., mTOR). **(B)** When *FLCN* is inactivated and, presumably, FLCN protein is absent, mTOR is dysregulated, potentially driving kidney tumor formation in BHD patients. (From Linehan WM, Srinivasan R, Schmidt LS. The genetic basis of kidney cancer: a metabolic disease. *Nat Rev Urol* 2010;7:277–285.)

been found infrequently in chromophobe renal cell carcinomas (11%),[76] and only rarely in other histologic variants of RCC.[77–79]

## Function of the Birt-Hogg-Dubé Protein: Folliculin

The *FLCN* gene encodes a novel protein, folliculin (FLCN), with no characteristic functional domains. Baba et al.[80] identified a novel FLCN-interacting protein, FNIP1, and showed that FNIP1 interacts with the γ subunit of 5′ adenosine monophosphate (AMP)–activated protein kinase (AMPK), an energy sensor in cells that negatively regulates mammalian target of rapamycin (mTOR), the master switch for protein translation and cell proliferation, through TSC1/2.[81,82] A second folliculin interacting protein, FNIP2, was subsequently identified that displayed similar biochemical properties to FNIP1.[83,84] FLCN, through FNIP1/2, may play a role in the regulation of the AMPK-TSC1/2–mTOR signaling pathway (Fig. 36.2). Published data from in vivo models and BHD renal tumors, supporting mTOR activation[85,86] as well as mTOR inhibition[87–89] as a consequence of *FLCN* inactivation, has led to the hypothesis that the mechanism by which FLCN interacts with and modulates mTOR is context dependent.[89]

Additional functional roles for FLCN in transforming growth factor β (TGF-β) signaling,[90,91] modulation of HIF-α and its target genes,[92] ciliogenesis,[93] peroxisome proliferator-activated receptor γ coactivator 1α (PGC-1α) regulation and mitochondrial biogenesis,[94,95] cell–cell adhesion,[96,97] exit from embryonic stem cell pluripotency,[98] and regulation of lysosome function through cytoplasmic sequestration of the transcription factors TFE3[99] and TFEB[100] have been reported. The resolution of C-terminal FLCN crystal structure has demonstrated structural homology to the

DENN domain, which has guanine exchange factor (GEF) activity toward RabGTPases.[101] Two recent reports have shown FLCN/FNIP1/FNIP2 interaction with RagGTPases and proposed a role of this complex in amino acid sensing for mTOR activation.[100,102] In addition to a role for FNIP1 in facilitating FLCN interaction with AMPK, *Fnip1* knockout mice displayed a defect in pro- to preB cell differentiation demonstrating a unique requirement for the FLCN-FNIP1 complex in B-cell development.[103]

## HEREDITARY LEIOMYOMATOSIS AND RENAL CELL CARCINOMA

HLRCC is an autosomal-dominant inherited disorder that predisposes individuals to the development of skin and uterine leiomyomas and an aggressive form of type 2 papillary renal carcinoma. Fewer than 150 HLRCC families have been reported worldwide.[104,105] Renal tumors, which are often unilateral and solitary,[104,106] may develop with early age of onset in 15% to 25% of affected individuals[104,105] and can be aggressive, metastasize, and cause death within 5 years of diagnosis.

### Genetics of Hereditary Leiomyomatosis and Renal Cell Carcinoma: Fumarate Hydratase Gene

A genetic linkage analysis localized the HLRCC disease locus to chromosome 1q42-43,[107] but an association with renal cancer was not appreciated until Launonen et al.[108] demonstrated a linkage to chromosome 1q in two Finnish multiple cutaneous and uterine leiomyomata (MCUL) kindreds with solitary, highly aggressive papillary type 2 renal tumors. The disorder was renamed *hereditary leiomyomatosis and renal cell carcinoma* and the locus was subsequently mapped to a 1.6-Mb region of 1q42. Germ-line mutations were identified in the fumarate hydratase (*FH*) gene, a Krebs cycle enzyme that converts fumarate to malate in HLRCC-affected family members.[7] *FH* mutations in HLRCC include missense, frameshift, nonsense, and splice-site mutations, as well as partial and complete gene deletions.[104,106,109,110] Missense mutations are the most common (57%) and occur mainly at evolutionarily conserved residues.[106,109,110] Mutations are found throughout the entire length of the *FH* gene excluding exon 1, which encodes a mitochondrial signal peptide, and no clear genotype–phenotype associations have been reported.[104] *FH* acts as a classic tumor suppressor gene with a loss or somatic mutation of the wild-type *FH* allele at high frequency in renal tumors and skin and uterine leiomyomata.[7] *FH* mutations are rarely detected in sporadic uterine and skin leiomyomata or sporadic RCCs.[111]

## Functional Consequences of Fumarate Hydratase Mutations

*FH* mutations reduce FH activity by 20% to 80%[7,109,112] in lymphoblastoid cell lines from HLRCC patients. HLRCC-associated missense mutations significantly lowered FH activity compared to truncating mutations,[109] suggesting that mutant FH monomers might act in a dominant negative manner to alter proper conformation of FH tetramers. Loss of FH activity in HLRCC leads to accumulation of fumarate and, to a lesser extent, succinate, due to a block in the Krebs cycle.[113,114] Pollard et al.[113] have confirmed that the accumulation of fumarate and succinate resulted in the elevation of HIF-1α and HIF-target genes (*VEGF*, *BNIP*), and increased microvessel density[115] in HLRCC-associated uterine fibroids. Isaacs et al.[114] showed that stabilization of HIF-1α resulted from the competitive inhibition of the HIF PHD co-substrate, α-ketoglutarate, by fumarate accumulation, leading to the abrogation of PHD function and release of HIF-1α from proteasomal degradation. This pseudohypoxic drive, resulting from loss of FH activity, HIF-1α stabilization, and upregulation of HIF-inducible genes, contributes to the aggressive nature of HLRCC-associated renal tumors (Fig. 36.3). Xiao et al.[116] have demonstrated that accumulated fumarate and succinate can act as competitive inhibitors of multiple α-ketoglutarate–dependent dioxygenases, including histone demethylases and the ten-eleven translocation (TET) family of 5-methylcytosine hydroxylases leading to more global alterations in histone and DNA methylation. Additionally, Sudarshan et al.[117] showed that *FH* mutations in an HLRCC-derived cell line led to glucose-mediated generation of

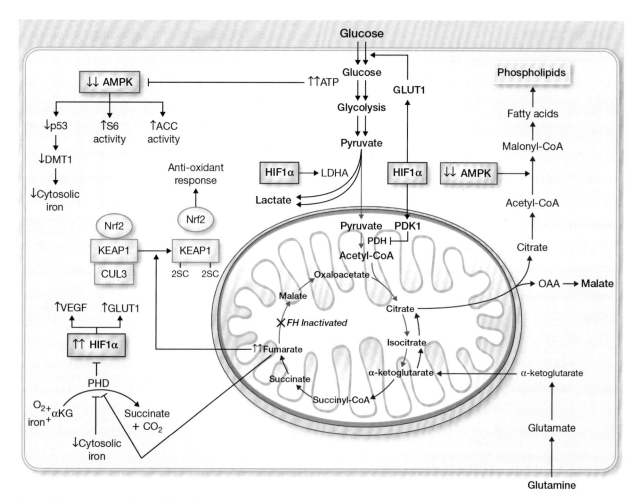

**Figure 36.3** Fumarate hydratase (FH)–deficient kidney cancer, an aggressive form of type 2 papillary kidney cancer, is found in patients affected with the hereditary cancer syndrome, HLRCC. FH-deficient kidney cancer is characterized by a metabolic shift to aerobic glycolysis. Mitochondrial function is impaired by a decrease in FH function, and the cell depends on aerobic glycolysis for adenosine triphosphate (ATP) production needed for rapid growth. The increased ATP leads to decreased activation of AMPK, which results in increased mTOR/phosphoS6 activity and increased Acetyl CoA carboxylase (ACC)/fatty acid production. Increased fumarate, a result of decreased fumarate hydratase activity, inhibits HIF PHD, resulting in increased HIF1α levels. The increased fumarate also inhibits KEAP1 activity, resulting in increased Nrf2 transcriptional activity that is critical for the survival of these cells, which are characterized by high oxidative stress. (From Linehan WM, Rouault TA. Molecular pathways: fumarate hydratase-deficient kidney cancer: targeting the Warburg effect in cancer. *Clin Cancer Res* 2013;19:3345–3352.)

reactive oxygen species (ROS) and ROS-dependent HIF-1α stabilization, supporting an alternate mechanism by which pseudohypoxic drive could support renal tumorigenesis in HLRCC. Further, Sullivan et al.[118] determined that the increase in ROS was due to the succination of antioxidant glutathione by accumulated fumarate (see the following) to produce the oncometabolite succinated glutathione, an alternate substrate to glutathione reductase, resulting in a decrease in NADPH levels, enhanced ROS and HIF1-α activation.

Recent in vivo and in vitro evidence supports a role for fumarate accumulation in activation of the nuclear factor (erythroid-derived 2)–like 2 (Nrf2)-mediated antioxidant signaling pathway.[119] Kelch-like erythroid-derived Cap-n-Collar homology (ECH)–associated protein 1 (KEAP1), an electrophile sensor and substrate recognition site for cullin-3 (CUL3)–based E3 ubiquitin ligase, binds to Nrf transcription factors under low electrophile conditions facilitating interactions with CUL3 for ubiquitin-mediated degradation. However, intracellular accumulated fumarate in FH-deficient kidney cancer (HLRCC) reacts with exposed cysteines on the KEAP1 protein (*succination*), resulting in a conformational change that inhibits KEAP1–Nrf2 binding (see Fig. 36.3). Consequently Nrf2 becomes available for transcriptional activation of its target genes that are regulated through antioxidant response elements (ARE) in their promoters.[120,121] In support of this model, somatic inactivating mutations in *KEAP1* and *CUL3*, and activating mutations in *NRF2*, have been identified in sporadic papillary RCC type 2.[122] Inhibiting upregulated Nrf2-target genes (i.e., heme oxygenase1 [HMOX1], which is important for heme oxygenation)[123] that promote cancer cell survival may provide a novel therapeutic approach to HLRCC and sporadic PRCC2 treatment.

Finally, cells normally generate energy through the Krebs cycle coupled to oxidative phosphorylation, but FH-deficient kidney cancer cells lack the enzyme to convert fumarate to malate, resulting in a block in the Krebs cycle. Mullen et al.[124] showed that FH-deficient kidney cancer cells that lack a fully functional electron transport chain use glutamine-dependent reductive carboxylation via isocitrate dehydrogenases 1 and 2 to produce acetyl coenzyme A (CoA) for lipid synthesis and Krebs cycle intermediates. Metabolic reprogramming of FH-deficient kidney cancer cells enables the elevated production of ribose from glucose via increased flux through the pentose phosphate pathway to meet the high demand for nucleotides.[125]

## FAMILIAL RENAL CANCER: SUCCINATE DEHYDROGENASE GENE

Bilateral multifocal renal tumors with early onset (<40 years of age) have been reported in the setting of hereditary head and neck paragangliomas (HPGL) and adrenal or extra-adrenal pheochromocytomas.[9] Most frequently, a unique form of oncocytic RCC develops; however, clear cell RCC, chromophobe RCC, papillary type 2 RCC, and renal oncocytoma have been described.[126–128]

### Genetics of Familial Renal Cancer: Succinate Dehydrogenase Subunit B and D Mutations

Germ-line mutations in the gene encoding succinate dehydrogenase subunit D (SDHD) were initially associated with HPGL

and later with familial and sporadic pheochromocytomas.[129,130] Subsequently, inactivating mutations in *SDHB* were found in kindreds with familial pheochromocytoma only and with HPGL, and in one case of sporadic pheochromocytoma.[131] Later, early onset clear cell RCC was diagnosed in two individuals with HPGL and germ-line *SDHB* mutations.[9] Renal carcinomas with various histologies have been reported in patients with germ-line missense, frameshift, and nonsense mutations in *SDHB, C,* and *D*.[10,11,126–128,132]

### Functional Consequences of Succinate Dehydrogenase Subunit B and D Mutations

Mutational inactivation of the *SDH* gene results in reduced SDH enzyme activity and the accumulation of succinate in renal tumors. In a mechanism similar to *FH* mutations in HLRCC (see Fig. 36.3), the accumulation of succinate serves to competitively inhibit α-ketoglutarate and block PHD activity.[113,114] In the absence of PHD, HIF-α accumulates and drives transcriptional activation of HIF-α target genes that support tumor neovascularization, growth, and invasion.

## TUBEROUS SCLEROSIS COMPLEX

The tuberous sclerosis complex (TSC) is a multisystem, autosomal-dominant disorder affecting both children and adults and is characterized by facial angiofibromas, renal angiomyolipomas, lymphangiomyomatosis of the lung, and disabling neurologic manifestations. The disease is phenotypically heterogeneous, and many patients have only minimal symptoms of disease.[133]

The predominant renal manifestations in TSC are bilateral multifocal angiomyolipomas (AML), benign tumors composed of abnormal vessels, immature smooth muscle cells, and fat cells. The lifetime risk of renal cancer in TSC patients is 2% to 3%, which is similar to the general population.[133] The most common histologic type of renal tumor is clear cell; however, there are rare reports of papillary RCCs, chromophobe RCCs, and oncocytoma in TSC patients.[133] TSC is caused by mutations in one of two genes—*TSC1* that encodes hamartin[134] or *TSC2* that encodes tuberin[135]—leading to a loss of TSC1/2-negative regulation of mTOR signaling.[81,82,136] Drug therapy targeting the mTOR pathway may be most effective for treating TSC-associated AMLs and renal tumors.[137]

## CONCLUSION

Twelve renal cancer predisposing genes—*VHL, MET, FLCN, TFE3, TFEB, MITF, TSC1, TSC2, PTEN, FH, SDHB,* and *SDHD*—have been identified mainly through studies of inherited renal cancer syndromes, including VHL, HPRC, BHD, HLRCC, SDH-related familial renal cancer, and TSC (Fig. 36.4). These studies have provided valuable insight into the genetic events that lead to the development of renal tumors and the biochemical mechanisms that contribute to their progression and, ultimately, in some cases, to metastasis. These findings have enabled the development of diagnostic genetic testing and provided the foundation for the development of targeted therapeutic agents for patients with the common form of sporadic kidney cancer.

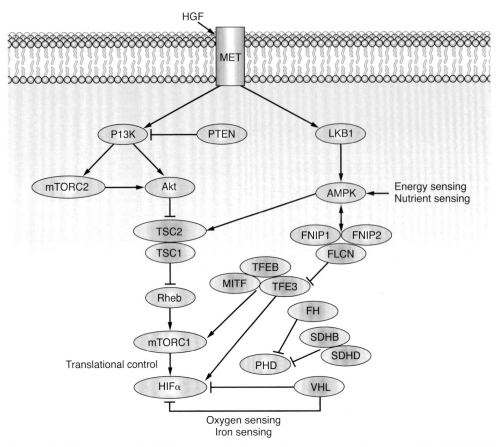

**Figure 36.4** The genetic basis of kidney cancer. Twelve renal cancer predisposing genes—*VHL, MET, FLCN, TFE3, TFEB, MITF, TSC1, TSC2, PTEN, FH, SDHB,* and *SDHD*— have been identified mainly through studies of inherited kidney cancer syndromes. These genes interact through common oxygen, iron, nutrient, and energy sensing pathways and demonstrate that kidney cancer is fundamentally a metabolic disease. Our understanding of the molecular mechanisms by which these genes interact in these pathways has enabled the development of targeted therapeutic agents to benefit kidney cancer patients. (From Linehan WM, Ricketts CJ. The metabolic basis of kidney cancer. *Semin Cancer Biol* 2013;23:46–55.)

# REFERENCES

1. Ferlay J, Shin HR, Bray F, et al. Estimates of worldwide burden of cancer in 2008: GLOBOCAN 2008. *Int J Cancer* 2010;127:2893–2917.
2. Heck JE, Charbotel B, Moore LE, et al. Occupation and renal cell cancer in Central and Eastern Europe. *Occup Environ Med* 2010;67:47–53.
3. Kovacs G, Akhtar M, Beckwith BJ, et al. The Heidelberg classification of renal cell tumours. *J Pathol* 1997;183:131–133.
4. Linehan WM, Srinivasan R, Schmidt LS. The genetic basis of kidney cancer: a metabolic disease. *Nat Rev Urol* 2010;7:277–285.
5. Latif F, Tory K, Gnarra JR, et al. Identification of the von Hippel-Lindau disease tumor suppressor gene. *Science* 1993;260:1317–1320.
6. Schmidt LS, Duh FM, Chen F, et al. Germline and somatic mutations in the tyrosine kinase domain of the MET proto-oncogene in papillary renal carcinomas. *Nat Genet* 1997;16:68–73.
7. Tomlinson IP, Alam NA, Rowan AJ, et al. Germline mutations in FH predispose to dominantly inherited uterine fibroids, skin leiomyomata and papillary renal cell cancer. *Nat Genet* 2002;30:406–410.
8. Nickerson ML, Warren MB, Toro JR, et al. Mutations in a novel gene lead to kidney tumors, lung wall defects, and benign tumors of the hair follicle in patients with the Birt-Hogg-Dubé syndrome. *Cancer Cell* 2002;2:157–164.
9. Vanharanta S, Buchta M, McWhinney SR, et al. Early-onset renal cell carcinoma as a novel extraparaganglial component of SDHB-associated heritable paraganglioma. *Am J Hum Genet* 2004;74:153–159.
10. Ricketts CJ, Shuch B, Vocke CD, et al. Succinate dehydrogenase kidney cancer: an aggressive example of the Warburg effect in cancer. *J Urol* 2012; 188:2063–2071.
11. Malinoc A, Sullivan M, Wiech T, et al. Biallelic inactivation of the SDHC gene in renal carcinoma associated with paraganglioma syndrome type 3. *Endocr Relat Cancer* 2012;19:283–290.
12. Nordstrom-O'Brien M, van der Luijt RB, van Rooijen E, et al. Genetic analysis of von Hippel-Lindau disease. *Hum Mutat* 2010;31:521–537.
13. Zbar B, Brauch H, Talmadge C, et al. Loss of alleles of loci on the short arm of chromosome 3 in renal cell carcinoma. *Nature* 1987;327:721–724.
14. Stolle C, Glenn GM, Zbar B, et al. Improved detection of germline mutations in the von Hippel-Lindau disease tumor suppressor gene. *Hum Mutat* 1998;12:417–423.
15. Cho HJ, Ki CS, Kim JW. Improved detection of germline mutations in Korean VHL patients by multiple ligation-dependent probe amplification analysis. *J Korean Med Sci* 2009;24:77–83.
16. Kaelin WG Jr. The von Hippel-Lindau tumour suppressor protein: O2 sensing and cancer. *Nat Rev Cancer* 2008;8:865–873.
17. Cohen AJ, Li FP, Berg S, et al. Hereditary renal-cell carcinoma associated with a chromosomal translocation. *N Engl J Med* 1979;301:592–595.
18. Schmidt LS, Li F, Brown RS, et al. Mechanism of tumorigenesis of renal carcinomas associated with the constitutional chromosome 3;8 translocation. *Cancer J Sci Am* 1995;1:191–195.
19. Melendez B, Rodriguez-Perales S, Martinez-Delgado B, et al. Molecular study of a new family with hereditary renal cell carcinoma and a translocation t(3;8)(p13;q24.1). *Hum Genet* 2003;112:178–185.
20. Bodmer D, van den Hurk W, van Groningen JJ, et al. Understanding familial and non-familial renal cell cancer. *Hum Mol Genet* 2002;11:2489–2498.
21. Gnarra JR, Tory K, Weng Y, et al. Mutations of the VHL tumour suppressor gene in renal carcinoma. *Nat Genet* 1994;7:85–90.
22. Nickerson ML, Jaeger E, Shi Y, et al. Improved identification of von Hippel-Lindau gene alterations in clear cell renal tumors. *Clin Cancer Res* 2008;14:4726–4734.
23. Stebbins CE, Kaelin WG, Pavletich NP. Structure of the VHL-ElonginC-ElonginB complex: implications for VHL tumor suppressor function. *Science* 1999;284:455–461.
24. Kondo K, Klco J, Nakamura E, et al. Inhibition of HIF is necessary for tumor suppression by the von Hippel-Lindau protein. *Cancer Cell* 2002;1:237–246.

25. Maranchie JK, Vasselli JR, Riss J, et al. The contribution of VHL substrate binding and HIF1-alpha to the phenotype of VHL loss in renal cell carcinoma. *Cancer Cell* 2002;1:247–255.
26. Li M, Kim WY. Two sides to every story: the HIF-dependent and HIF-independent functions of pVHL. *J Cell Mol Med* 2011;15:187–195.
27. Roe JS, Kim H, Lee SM, et al. p53 stabilization and transactivation by a von Hippel-Lindau protein. *Mol Cell* 2006;22:395–405.
28. Yang H, Minamishima YA, Yan Q, et al. pVHL acts as an adaptor to promote the inhibitory phosphorylation of the NF-kappaB agonist Card9 by CK2. *Mol Cell* 2007;28:15–27.
29. Hergovich A, Lisztwan J, Barry R, et al. Regulation of microtubule stability by the von Hippel-Lindau tumour suppressor protein pVHL. *Nat Cell Biol* 2003;5:64–70.
30. Lutz MS, Burk RD. Primary cilium formation requires von Hippel-Lindau gene function in renal-derived cells. *Cancer Res* 2006;66:6903–6907.
31. Kurban G, Duplan E, Ramlal N, et al. Collagen matrix assembly is driven by the interaction of von Hippel-Lindau tumor suppressor protein with hydroxy-lated collagen IV alpha 2. *Oncogene* 2008;27:1004–1012.
32. Tang N, Mack F, Haase VH, et al. pVHL function is essential for endothelial extracellular matrix deposition. *Mol Cell Biol* 2006;26:2519–2530.
33. Varela I, Tarpey P, Raine K, et al. Exome sequencing identifies frequent mutation of the SWI/SNF complex gene PBRM1 in renal carcinoma. *Nature* 2011;469:539–542.
34. Guo G, Gui Y, Gao S, et al. Frequent mutations of genes encoding ubiquitin-mediated proteolysis pathway components in clear cell renal cell carcinoma. *Nat Genet* 2011;12:1–3.
35. Dalgliesh GL, Furge K, Greenman C, et al. Systematic sequencing of renal carcinoma reveals inactivation of histone modifying genes. *Nature* 2010;463:360–363.
36. Pena-Llopis S, Vega-Rubin-de-Celis S, Liao A, et al. BAP1 loss defines a new class of renal cell carcinoma. *Nat Genet* 2012;44:751–759.
37. Farley MN, Schmidt LS, Mester JL, et al. A novel germline mutation in BAP1 predisposes to familial clear-cell renal cell carcinoma. *Mol Cancer Res* 2013;11:1061–1071.
38. Popova T, Hebert L, Jacquemin V, et al. Germline BAP1 mutations predispose to renal cell carcinomas. *Am J Hum Genet* 2013;92:974–980.
39. The Cancer Genome Atlas Research Network. Comprehensive molecular characterization of clear cell renal cell carcinoma. *Nature* 2013;499:43–49.
40. Dharmawardana PG, Giubellino A, Bottaro DP. Hereditary papillary renal carcinoma type I. *Curr Mol Med* 2004;4:855–868.
41. Schmidt LS, Junker K, Weirich G, et al. Two North American families with hereditary papillary renal carcinoma and identical novel mutations in the MET proto-oncogene. *Cancer Res* 1998;58:1719–1722.
42. Schmidt LS, Nickerson ML, Angeloni D, et al. Early onset hereditary papillary renal carcinoma: germline missense mutations in the tyrosine kinase domain of the Met proto-oncogene. *J Urol* 2004;172:1256–1261.
43. Zbar B, Glenn GM, Lubensky IA, et al. Hereditary papillary renal cell carcinoma: clinical studies in 10 families. *J Urol* 1995;153:907–912.
44. Kovacs G, Fuzesi L, Emanual A, et al. Cytogenetics of papillary renal cell tumors. *Genes Chromosomes Cancer* 1991;3:249–255.
45. Schmidt LS, Junker K, Nakaigawa N, et al. Novel mutations of the MET proto-oncogene in papillary renal cell carcinomas. *Oncogene* 1999;18:2343–2350.
46. Gentile A, Trusolino L, Comoglio PM. The Met tyrosine kinase receptor in development and cancer. *Cancer Metastasis Rev* 2008;27:85–94.
47. Birchmeier C, Birchmeier W, Gherardi E, et al. Met, metastasis, motility and more. *Nat Rev Mol Cell Biol* 2003;4:915–925.
48. Jeffers M, Schmidt LS, Nakaigawa N, et al. Activating mutations for the met tyrosine kinase receptor in human cancer. *Proc Natl Acad Sci U S A* 1997;94:11445–11450.
49. Jeffers M, Fiscella M, Webb CP, et al. The mutationally activated Met receptor mediates motility and metastasis. *Proc Natl Acad Sci U S A* 1998;95:14417–14422.
50. Miller M, Ginalski K, Lesyng B, et al. Structural basis of oncogenic activation caused by point mutations in the kinase domain of the MET proto-oncogene: modeling studies. *Proteins* 2001;44:32–43.
51. Zhuang Z, Park WS, Pack S, et al. Trisomy 7 - harboring non-random duplication of the mutant MET allele in hereditary papillary renal carcinomas. *Nat Genet* 1998;20:66–69.
52. de Jong B, Molenaar IM, Leeuw JA, et al. Cytogenetics of a renal adenocarcinoma in a 2-year-old child. *Cancer Genet Cytogenet* 1986;21:165–169.
53. Sidhar SK, Clark J, Gill S, et al. The t(X;1)(p11.2;q21.2) translocation in papillary renal carcinoma fuses a novel gene PRCC to the TFE3 transcription factor gene. *Hum Mol Genet* 1996;5:1333–1338.
54. Weterman MJ, van Groningen JJ, Jansen A, et al. Nuclear localization and transactivating capacities of the papillary renal cell carcinoma-associated TFE3 and PRCC (fusion) proteins. *Oncogene* 2000;19:69–74.
55. Weterman MA, van Groningen JJ, den HA, et al. Transformation capacities of the papillary renal cell carcinoma-associated PRCCTFE3 and TFE3PRCC fusion genes. *Oncogene* 2001;20:1414–1424.
56. Armah HB, Parwani AV. Xp11.2 translocation renal cell carcinoma. *Arch Pathol Lab Med* 2010;134:124–129.
57. Tsuda M, Davis IJ, Argani P, et al. TFE3 fusions activate MET signaling by transcriptional up-regulation, defining another class of tumors as candidates for therapeutic MET inhibition. *Cancer Res* 2007;67:919–929.
58. Davis IJ, Hsi BL, Arroyo JD, et al. Cloning of an Alpha-TFEB fusion in renal tumors harboring the t(6;11)(p21;q13) chromosome translocation. *Proc Natl Acad Sci U S A* 2003;100:6051–6056.
59. Bertolotto C, Lesueur F, Giuliano S, et al. A SUMOylation-defective MITF germline mutation predisposes to melanoma and renal carcinoma. *Nature* 2011;480:94–98.
60. Birt AR, Hogg GR, Dubé WJ. Hereditary multiple fibrofolliculomas with trichodiscomas and acrochordons. *Arch Dermatol* 1977;113:1674–1677.
61. Toro JR, Glenn G, Duray P, et al. Birt-Hogg-Dubé syndrome: a novel marker of kidney neoplasia. *Arch Dermatol* 1999;135:1195–1202.
62. Zbar B, Alvord WG, Glenn GM, et al. Risk of renal and colonic neoplasms and spontaneous pneumothorax in the Birt-Hogg-Dubé syndrome. *Cancer Epidemiol Biomarkers Prev* 2002;11:393–400.
63. Menko FH, van Steensel MA, Giraud S, et al. Birt-Hogg-Dubé syndrome: diagnosis and management. *Lancet Oncol* 2009;10:1199–1206.
64. Schmidt LS, Nickerson ML, Warren MB, et al. Germline BHD-mutation spectrum and phenotype analysis of a large cohort of families with Birt-Hogg-Dubé syndrome. *Am J Hum Genet* 2005;76:1023–1033.
65. Toro JR, Wei MH, Glenn GM, et al. BHD mutations, clinical and molecular genetic investigations of Birt-Hogg-Dubé syndrome: a new series of 50 families and a review of published reports. *J Med Genet* 2008;45:321–331.
66. Toro JR, Pautler SE, Stewart L, et al. Lung cysts, spontaneous pneumothorax and genetic associations in 89 families with Birt-Hogg-Dubé syndrome. *Am J Respir Crit Care Med* 2007;175:1044–1053.
67. Pavlovich CP, Walther MM, Eyler RA, et al. Renal tumors in the Birt-Hogg-Dubé syndrome. *Am J Surg Pathol* 2002;26:1542–1552.
68. Schmidt LS, Warren MB, Nickerson ML, et al. Birt-Hogg-Dubé syndrome, a genodermatosis associated with spontaneous pneumothorax and kidney neoplasia, maps to chromosome 17p11.2. *Am J Hum Genet* 2001;69:876–882.
69. Khoo SK, Bradley M, Wong FK, et al. Birt-Hogg-Dubé syndrome: mapping of a novel hereditary neoplasia gene to chromosome 17p12-q11.2. *Oncogene* 2001;20:5239–5242.
70. Leter EM, Koopmans AK, Gille JJ, et al. Birt-Hogg-Dubé syndrome: clinical and genetic studies of 20 families. *J Invest Dermatol* 2008;128:45–49.
71. Benhammou JN, Vocke CD, Santani A, et al. Identification of intragenic deletions and duplication in the FLCN gene in Birt-Hogg-Dubé syndrome. *Genes Chromosomes Cancer* 2011;50:466–477.
72. Kluger N, Giraud S, Coupier I, et al. Birt-Hogg-Dubé syndrome: clinical and genetic studies of 10 French families. *Br J Dermatol* 2010;162:527–537.
73. Kunogi M, Kurihara M, Ikegami TS, et al. Clinical and genetic spectrum of Birt-Hogg-Dubé syndrome patients in whom pneumothorax and/or multiple lung cysts are the presenting feature. *J Med Genet* 2010;47:281–287.
74. Lim DH, Rehal PK, Nahorski MS, et al. A new locus-specific database (LSDB) for mutations in the folliculin (FLCN) gene. *Hum Mutat* 2010;31:E1043–E1051.
75. Vocke CD, Yang Y, Pavlovich CP, et al. High frequency of somatic frameshift BHD gene mutations in Birt-Hogg-Dubé-associated renal tumors. *J Natl Cancer Inst* 2005;97:931–935.
76. Gad S, Lefevre SH, Khoo SK, et al. Mutations in BHD and TP53 genes, but not in HNF1beta gene, in a large series of sporadic chromophobe renal cell carcinoma. *Br J Cancer* 2007;96:336–340.
77. da Silva NF, Gentle D, Hesson LB, et al. Analysis of the Birt-Hogg-Dubé (BHD) tumour suppressor gene in sporadic renal cell carcinoma and colorectal cancer. *J Med Genet* 2003;40:820–824.
78. Khoo SK, Kahnoski K, Sugimura J, et al. Inactivation of BHD in sporadic renal tumors. *Cancer Res* 2003;63:4583–4587.
79. Nagy A, Zoubakov D, Stupar Z, et al. Lack of mutation of the folliculin gene in sporadic chromophobe renal cell carcinoma and renal oncocytoma. *Int J Cancer* 2004;109:472–475.
80. Baba M, Hong SB, Sharma N, et al. Folliculin encoded by the BHD gene interacts with a binding protein, FNIP1, and AMPK, and is involved in AMPK and mTOR signaling. *Proc Natl Acad Sci U S A* 2006;103:15552–15557.
81. Inoki K, Corradetti MN, Guan KL. Dysregulation of the TSC-mTOR pathway in human disease. *Nat Genet* 2005;37:19–24.
82. Inoki K, Li Y, Xu T, et al. Rheb GTPase is a direct target of TSC2 GAP activity and regulates mTOR signaling. *Genes Dev* 2003;17:1829–1834.
83. Hasumi H, Baba M, Hong SB, et al. Identification and characterization of a novel folliculin-interacting protein FNIP2. *Gene* 2008;415:60–67.
84. Takagi Y, Kobayashi T, Shiono M, et al. Interaction of folliculin (Birt-Hogg-Dubé gene product) with a novel Fnip1-like (FnipL/Fnip2) protein. *Oncogene* 2008;27:5339–5347.
85. Baba M, Furihata M, Hong SB, et al. Kidney-targeted Birt-Hogg-Dubé gene inactivation in a mouse model: Erk1/2 and Akt-mTOR activation, cell hyperproliferation, and polycystic kidneys. *J Natl Cancer Inst* 2008;100:140–154.
86. Hasumi Y, Baba M, Ajima R, et al. Homozygous loss of BHD causes early embryonic lethality and kidney tumor development with activation of mTORC1 and mTORC2. *Proc Natl Acad Sci U S A* 2009;106:18722–18727.
87. van Slegtenhorst M, Khabibullin D, Hartman TR, et al. The Birt-Hogg-Dubé and tuberous sclerosis complex homologs have opposing roles in amino acid homeostasis in Schizosaccharomyces pombe. *J Biol Chem* 2007;282:24583–24590.
88. Hudon V, Sabourin S, Dydensborg AB, et al. Renal tumour suppressor function of the Birt-Hogg-Dubé syndrome gene product folliculin. *J Med Genet* 2010;47:182–189.
89. Hartman TR, Nicolas E, Klein-Szanto A, et al. The role of the Birt-Hogg-Dubé protein in mTOR activation and renal tumorigenesis. *Oncogene* 2009;28:1594–1604.

CANCERS OF THE GENITOURINARY SYSTEM

90. Cash TP, Gruber JJ, Hartman TR, et al. Loss of the Birt-Hogg-Dubé tumor suppressor results in apoptotic resistance due to aberrant TGFbeta-mediated transcription. *Oncogene* 2011;30:2534–2546.

91. Hong SB, Oh H, Valera VA, et al. Tumor suppressor FLCN inhibits tumorigenesis of a FLCN-null renal cancer cell line and regulates expression of key molecules in TGF-beta signaling. *Molecular Cancer* 2010;9:160.

92. Preston RS, Philp A, Claessens T, et al. Absence of the Birt-Hogg-Dubé gene product is associated with increased hypoxia-inducible factor transcriptional activity and a loss of metabolic flexibility. *Oncogene* 2011;30:1159–1173.

93. Luijten MN, Basten SG, Claessens T, et al. Birt-Hogg-Dubé syndrome is a novel ciliopathy. *Hum Mol Genet* 2013;22:4383–4397.

94. Klomp JA, Petillo D, Niemi NM, et al. Birt-Hogg-Dubé renal tumors are genetically distinct from other renal neoplasias and are associated with up-regulation of mitochondrial gene expression. *BMC Med Genomics* 2010;3:59.

95. Hasumi H, Baba M, Hasumi Y, et al. Regulation of mitochondrial oxidative metabolism by tumor suppressor FLCN. *J Natl Cancer Inst* 2012;104:1750–1764.

96. Nahorski MS, Seabra L, Straatman-Iwanowska A, et al. Folliculin interacts with p0071 (plakophilin-4) and deficiency is associated with disordered RhoA signalling, epithelial polarization and cytokinesis. *Hum Mol Genet* 2012;21:5268–5279.

97. Medvetz DA, Khabibullin D, Hariharan V, et al. Folliculin, the product of the Birt-Hogg-Dubé tumor suppressor gene, interacts with the adherens junction protein p0071 to regulate cell-cell adhesion. *PLoS One* 2012;7:e47842.

98. Betschinger J, Nichols J, Dietmann S, et al. Exit from pluripotency is gated by intracellular redistribution of the bHLH transcription factor Tfe3. *Cell* 2013;153:335–347.

99. Hong SB, Oh H, Valera VA, et al. Inactivation of the FLCN tumor suppressor gene induces TFE3 transcriptional activity by increasing its nuclear localization. *PLoS ONE* 2010;5:e15793.

100. Petit CS, Roczniak-Ferguson A, Ferguson SM. Recruitment of folliculin to lysosomes supports the amino acid-dependent activation of Rag GTPases. *J Cell Biol* 2013;202:1107–1122.

101. Nookala RK, Langemeyer L, Pacitto A, et al. Crystal structure of folliculin reveals a hidDENN function in genetically inherited renal cancer. *Open Biol* 2012;2:120071.

102. Tsun ZY, Bar-Peled L, Chantranupong L, et al. The folliculin tumor suppressor is a GAP for the RagC/D GTPases that signal amino acid levels to mTORC1. *Mol Cell* 2013;52:495–505.

103. Baba M, Keller JR, Sun HW, et al. The folliculin-FNIP1 pathway deleted in human Birt-Hogg-Dubé syndrome is required for murine B-cell development. *Blood* 2012;120:1254–1261.

104. Kiuru M, Launonen V. Hereditary leiomyomatosis and renal cell cancer (HLRCC). *Curr Mol Med* 2004;4:869–875.

105. Wei MH, Toure O, Glenn GM, et al. Novel mutations in FH and expansion of the spectrum of phenotypes expressed in families with hereditary leiomyomatosis and renal cell cancer. *J Med Genet* 2006;43:18–27.

106. Toro JR, Nickerson ML, Wei MH, et al. Mutations in the fumarate hydratase gene cause hereditary leiomyomatosis and renal cell cancer in families in North America. *Am J Hum Genet* 2003;73:95–106.

107. Alam NA, Bevan S, Churchman M, et al. Localization of a gene (MCUL1) for multiple cutaneous leiomyomata and uterine fibroids to chromosome 1q42.3-q43. *Am J Hum Genet* 2001;68:1264–1269.

108. Launonen V, Vierimaa O, Kiuru M, et al. Inherited susceptibility to uterine leiomyomas and renal cell cancer. *Proc Natl Acad Sci U S A* 2001;98:3387–3392.

109. Alam NA, Rowan AJ, Wortham NC, et al. Genetic and functional analyses of FH mutations in multiple cutaneous and uterine leiomyomatosis, hereditary leiomyomatosis and renal cancer, and fumarate hydratase deficiency. *Hum Mol Genet* 2003;12:1241–1252.

110. Bayley JP, Launonen V, Tomlinson IP. The FH mutation database: an online database of fumarate hydratase mutations involved in the MCUL (HLRCC) tumor syndrome and congenital fumarase deficiency. *BMC Med Genet* 2008;9:20.

111. Kiuru M, Lehtonen R, Arola J, et al. Few FH mutations in sporadic counterparts of tumor types observed in hereditary leiomyomatosis and renal cell cancer families. *Cancer Res* 2002;62:4554–4557.

112. Pithukpakorn M, Wei MH, Toure O, et al. Fumarate hydratase enzyme activity in lymphoblastoid cells and fibroblasts of individuals in families with hereditary leiomyomatosis and renal cell cancer. *J Med Genet* 2006;43:755–762.

113. Pollard PJ, Briere JJ, Alam NA, et al. Accumulation of Krebs cycle intermediates and over-expression of HIF1alpha in tumours which result from germline FH and SDH mutations. *Hum Mol Genet* 2005;14:2231–2239.

114. Isaacs JS, Jung YJ, Mole DR, et al. HIF overexpression correlates with biallelic loss of fumarate hydratase in renal cancer: novel role of fumarate in regulation of HIF stability. *Cancer Cell* 2005;8:143–153.

115. Pollard P, Wortham N, Barclay E, et al. Evidence of increased microvessel density and activation of the hypoxia pathway in tumours from the hereditary leiomyomatosis and renal cell cancer syndrome. *J Pathol* 2005;205:41–49.

116. Xiao M, Yang H, Xu W, et al. Inhibition of alpha-KG-dependent histone and DNA demethylases by fumarate and succinate that are accumulated in mutations of FH and SDH tumor suppressors. *Genes Dev* 2012;26:1326–1338.

117. Sudarshan S, Sourbier C, Kong HS, et al. Fumarate hydratase deficiency in renal cancer induces glycolytic addiction and HIF-1 alpha stabilization by glucose-dependent generation of reactive oxygen species. *Mol Cell Biol* 2009;15:4080–4090.

118. Sullivan LB, Garcia-Martinez E, Nguyen H, et al. The proto-oncometabolite fumarate binds glutathione to amplify ROS-dependent signaling. *Mol Cell* 2013;51:236–248.

119. Kansanen E, Kuosmanen SM, Leinonen H, et al. The Keap1-Nrf2 pathway: Mechanisms of activation and dysregulation in cancer. *Redox Biol* 2013;1:45–49.

120. Ooi A, Wong JC, Petillo D, et al. An antioxidant response phenotype shared between hereditary and sporadic type 2 papillary renal cell carcinoma. *Cancer Cell* 2011;20:511–523.

121. Adam J, Hatipoglu E, O'Flaherty L, et al. Renal cyst formation in Fh1-deficient mice is independent of the Hif/Phd pathway: roles for fumarate in KEAP1 succination and Nrf2 signaling. *Cancer Cell* 2011;20:524–537.

122. Ooi A, Dykema K, Ansari A, et al. CUL3 and NRF2 mutations confer an NRF2 activation phenotype in a sporadic form of papillary renal cell carcinoma. *Cancer Res* 2013;73:2044–2051.

123. Frezza C, Zheng L, Folger O, et al. Haem oxygenase is synthetically lethal with the tumour suppressor fumarate hydratase. *Nature* 2011;477:225–228.

124. Mullen AR, Wheaton WW, Jin ES, et al. Reductive carboxylation supports growth in tumour cells with defective mitochondria. *Nature* 2011;481:385–388.

125. Yang Y, Lane AN, Fan TW, et al. Metabolic reprogramming for producing energy and reducing power in Fumarate Hydratase null cells from hereditary leiomyomatosis renal cell carcinoma. *PLoS One* 2013;8:e72179.

126. Srirangalingam U, Walker L, Khoo B, et al. Clinical manifestations of familial paraganglioma and phaeochromocytomas in succinate dehydrogenase B (SDH-B) gene mutation carriers. *Clin Endocrinol (Oxf)* 2008;69:587–596.

127. Henderson A, Douglas F, Perros P, et al. SDHB-associated renal oncocytoma suggests a broadening of the renal phenotype in hereditary paragangliomatosis. *Fam Cancer* 2009;8:257–260.

128. Ricketts C, Woodward ER, Killick P, et al. Germline SDHB mutations and familial renal cell carcinoma. *J Natl Cancer Inst* 2008;100:1260–1262.

129. Astuti D, Douglas F, Lennard TW, et al. Germline SDHD mutation in familial phaeochromocytoma. *Lancet* 2001;357:1181–1182.

130. Pawlu C, Bausch B, Neumann HP. Mutations of the SDHB and SDHD genes. *Fam Cancer* 2005;4:49–54.

131. Astuti D, Latif F, Dallol A, et al. Gene mutations in the succinate dehydrogenase subunit SDHB cause susceptibility to familial pheochromocytoma and to familial paraganglioma. *Am J Hum Genet* 2001;69:49–54.

132. Ricketts CJ, Forman JR, Rattenberry E, et al. Tumor risks and genotype-phenotype-proteotype analysis in 358 patients with germline mutations in SDHB and SDHD. *Hum Mutat* 2010;31:41–51.

133. Crino PB, Nathanson KL, Henske EP. The tuberous sclerosis complex. *N Engl J Med* 2006;355:1345–1356.

134. van Slegtenhorst M, de Hoogt R, Hermans C, et al. Identification of the tuberous sclerosis gene TSC1 on chromosome 9q34. *Science* 1997;277:805–808.

135. The European Chromosome 16 Tuberous Sclerosis Consortium. Identification and characterization of the tuberous sclerosis gene on chromosome 16. *Cell* 1993;75:1305–1315.

136. Shaw RJ, Bardeesy N, Manning BD, et al. The LKB1 tumor suppressor negatively regulates mTOR signaling. *Cancer Cell* 2004;6:91–99.

137. Bissler JJ, McCormack FX, Young LR, et al. Sirolimus for angiomyolipoma in tuberous sclerosis complex or lymphangioleiomyomatosis. *N Engl J Med* 2008;358:140–151.

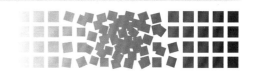

# 37 Cancer of the Kidney

Brian R. Lane, Daniel J. Canter, Brian I. Rini, and Robert G. Uzzo

## INTRODUCTION

Cancer of the kidney is neither common enough to cause a large percentage of cancer-related deaths nor uncommon enough to be considered an "orphan" malignancy. In that context, the progress made in uncovering the genetic basis of renal cell carcinoma (RCC), its molecular pathways, and the approval of novel therapies to perturb those pathways over the last decade is indeed remarkable. Over a relatively short time, the management options for localized kidney cancer have evolved from near universal acceptance of open radical nephrectomy (RN) to the routine use of minimally invasive partial nephrectomy (PN), thermal ablation (TA), and active surveillance (AS). Concurrently, metastatic RCC has progressed from marginally treatable, with a low incidence of spontaneous and/or immune-induced durable regression, to overall response rates (complete response + partial response + stable disease) of >50% and a near doubling of cancer-specific survival. Looking forward, it is anticipated that kidney cancer will soon become a chronic disorder as we better understand the biologic heterogeneity and systemic therapies for RCC. Herein, we review the current and rapid evolution in our understanding and management of cancer of the kidney.

## EPIDEMIOLOGY, DEMOGRAPHICS, AND RISK FACTORS

Kidney cancer accounts for approximately 2% of malignancies worldwide with about 300,000 cases diagnosed per year and 100,000 deaths.[1] Data suggest the incidence of RCC is more common in industrialized countries, which may be related to increased incidental detection. In the United States, tumors of the kidney account for 3% to 4% of all cancer diagnoses with an estimated 65,000 cases and 14,000 deaths.[2] There is a male-to-female predominance with the lifetime risk of a RCC diagnosis of 1:69 in men and 1:116 in women.[3] While kidney cancer remains predominantly a tumor of the elderly (median age at diagnosis of 65 years), the number of new kidney cancer cases appears to be rising in younger individuals.[2] This may be explained by either the increasing use of noninvasive imaging in younger patients[4–6] or perhaps true biologic differences in the disease.[7] Similarly, racial differences have also been described with increased rates and decreased survival noted in African Americans and improved survival in Asian populations.[8] Whether this represents differences in health-care access or disease biology is unclear.

The most commonly cited risk factors for the development of RCC include smoking, obesity, and hypertension.[9] The data regarding smoking as a risk factor for RCC appear strong. In a meta-analysis evaluating 19 case control studies and 5 cohort studies, Hunt et al.[10] found a 38% increased risk in current and former smokers, noting not only a dose-risk relationship, but also an abatement of risk with smoking cessation >10 years. The relationship between obesity and RCC is less well studied, although the epidemiology seems to point to a causal association. In a quantitative review of the literature between 1966 and 1998, Renehan et al.[11]

calculated a relative risk of 1.07 per increase in unit body mass index and concluded that nearly a third of RCC cases may be attributable to obesity. Data suggesting a stronger association of obesity and RCC in women lead to hypotheses that the relationship may be due to dysregulation of sex hormones, insulin metabolism, or the immune system.[3] The relationship between hypertension and RCC is based largely upon retrospective and/or population-based epidemiologic data. In an analysis of 13 case controlled studies, Grossman et al.[12] noted hypertensive patients exhibited a pooled odds ratio of 1.75 of having RCC. While there may be a relationship between severity and duration of hypertension, given the limits of the data, if such an association exists it is difficult to ascertain.[3] Finally, exposure to chronic diuretics,[13] nonsteroidal analgesics,[14] and tricholorethylene, a cleaning agent, have all been associated with an increased risk of RCC.[3]

While screening for kidney and other potentially lethal diseases is enticing, a risk benefit analysis argues against it given the low overall prevalence of RCC in the general population. One large study, in which over 200,000 adults were screened for abdominal malignancy with ultrasound, found only 192 cases of RCC (0.09%).[15] Screening has, therefore, been proposed in target populations, including individuals with familial RCC syndromes such as von Hippel-Lindau disease (VHL) and those on hemodialysis, who are known to be more likely to be diagnosed with RCC. In patients on dialysis, while there appears to be an increased incidence of RCC in the native kidneys or even in a transplanted allograft, this may be due to their medical follow-up. Indeed, most patients with end-stage renal disease will have been "screened" during the evaluation and management of their renal failure/allograph, making the reasons for this association difficult to dissect. This is distinctively different than an emerging population of patients with increased genetic risk for cancer, but whose kidneys have not yet been imaged. In families who carry known mutations in the genes responsible for VHL, hereditary papillary RCC, hereditary leiomyoma RCC, Birt-Hogg-Dubé syndrome (BHD), potentially tuberous sclerosis, and/or autosomal dominant polycystic kidney disease, a renal ultrasound may be an inexpensive, low-risk, and judicious means of targeted screening. The initial timing, frequency, and effectiveness of screening in these at-risk populations are not yet established.

## PATHOLOGY OF RENAL CELL CARCINOMA

Pathologic classifications assist in diagnosis and prognosis, and inform therapy. Most pathologic classifications emphasize a tumor's morphology and histology—although, increasingly they are incorporating genetic characteristics.[16] There are 10 tumor subtypes in the current World Health Organization classification system for RCC (Table 37.1). The major histologic variants include clear cell, papillary, chromophobe, and collecting duct tumors, which account for 90% to 95% of renal carcinomas,[17] although less common subtypes and an "unclassified" category also exist. Uncommon subtypes of RCC, not included in the World Health Organization classification, include tubulocystic carcinoma, clear

**TABLE 37.1**

**2004 World Health Organization Classification of Sporadic Renal Cell Carcinoma with Genetic and Clinical Correlates**

| Type | Genetics | Clinical |
|---|---|---|
| ccRCC (70% to 80%) | Deletion, mutation or methylation of 3p25-26 (VHL) | Most common variant<br>Prognosis predicted by stage and grade |
| Multilocular cystic ccRCC (uncommon) | Deletion, mutation, or methylation of 3p25-26 (VHL) | Variant of ccRCC<br>Distant metastases uncommon |
| Papillary RCC (10% to 15%) | Gain of 7 or 17 (trisomy or tetrasomy), loss of Y, deletion of 9p. Mutations of 7q31 when associated with hereditary papillary RCC | 10% to 15% of RCC<br>95% + 5-year cancer-specific survival in type I papillary RCC<br>Response to tyrosine-kinase inhibitors less robust |
| Chromophobe RCC (3% to 5%) | Extensive chromosomal loss of Y, 1, 2, 6, 10, 13, 17, 21 Mutations of 17p11.2 when associated with BHD | 5% of RCC<br>Affects men and women equally with overall excellent prognosis |
| Collecting duct carcinoma (Bellini tumor) (<1%) | Highly variable<br>Losses of 1q, 6p, 8p, 9p, 13q, 19q, 21q | Male preponderance (2:1)<br>Mean age 55<br>Microscopically high grade, may resemble urothelial spectrum of cancers,<br>Overall poor prognosis |
| Renal medullary carcinoma (rare) | Not defined | Associated with sickle cell trait<br>Aggressive and lethal within 12 mo<br>Mean age 19 y<br>Male>female |
| Xp11 translocation carcinoma (rare) | Translocation of TFE3 gene on XP11.2 | Children and young adults<br>May present at advanced state and act more aggressively in adults |
| Renal carcinoma associated with neuroblastoma (rare) | Not defined | Morphologically and microscopically similar to ccRCC |
| Mucinous tubular and spindle cell carcinoma (rare) | Not defined | Female preponderance (4:1)<br>Rarely metastasize |
| Unclassified RCC (1% to 3%) | Varied | Generally poor prognosis |

ccRCC, clear cell renal cell carcinoma; RCC, renal cell carcinoma.
Adapted from Deng FM, Melamed J, Zhou M. Pathology of renal cell carcinoma. In: Libertino JA, ed. In *Renal Cancer: Contemporary Management*. New York: Springer; 2013:51–69.

cell tubulopapillary RCC, thyroid-like follicular carcinoma, and acquired cystic disease–associated RCC. The relatively rapid movement in RCC toward molecular classification follows advances in our molecular understanding of these variants and may soon supplant simple morphologic classification.

Other pathologically relevant variables in RCC include nuclear grade, sarcomatoid and rhabdoid differentiation, tumor necrosis, and vascular invasion. Nuclear grade usually follows the Fuhrman grading system[18] and is most often and best used for clear cell RCC (ccRCC) as the prognostic value in non-ccRCC remains largely unproven. Sarcomatoid differentiation exists in 5% of RCC and can be seen in any subtype. As such it is not considered a distinct entity, but rather a high-grade or poorly differentiated component. The presence and extent of micro- or macronecrosis has been correlated with prognosis in ccRCC.[19] Micro- or macrovascular invasion is thought to be a requisite step toward systemic disease; however, correlation between the extent of invasion and prognosis remains imprecise.

## DIFFERENTIAL DIAGNOSIS AND STAGING

Most patients with RCC present with an incidental, radiographically detected renal mass (Fig. 37.1). While symptoms including microscopic or gross hematuria, flank pain, gastrointestinal disturbances and/or pain, bleeding or systemic disturbances related to metastases may lead to the diagnosis, the use of routine cross-sectional imaging has led to the more common scenario of

an incidentally detected renal mass. While the suspicion for RCC may be high in cases such as these, RCC is a pathologic/tissue diagnosis, not a clinical one (Fig. 37.2). Proper radiographic evaluation of a renal mass requires a pre- and postcontrast computed tomography or magnetic resonance imaging (MRI) to assess enhancement.[20] Duplex ultrasound, renal mass biopsy, and noncontrast diffusion-weighted MRI with antibody drug conjugates mapping may be useful adjunctive tests in various clinical settings. deoxy-2[18F]fluoro-d-glucose positron emission tomography exhibits a low sensitivity for the diagnosis of RCC and is therefore not recommended for the evaluation of RCC. ImmunoPET with G-250 using an iodine-labeled antibody against carbonic anhydrase IX (CA-IX), which is known to be overexpressed in ccRCC, exhibits near 90% sensitivity and specificity for this RCC subtype.[21]

The differential diagnosis of the renal mass is broad and includes a long list of benign, malignant, and inflammatory conditions. Clinical and radiographic features can assist the astute clinician in narrowing down the diagnosis of the renal mass, particularly for benign and inflammatory lesions. Cystic lesions, for example, are frequently benign,[22] and fat-containing solid lesions are most commonly found to be angiomyolipomas (also benign). About 20% of enhancing renal masses and 15% of surgically removed masses are nonmalignant, with the most common diagnoses being oncocytoma and fat-poor angiomyolipoma.[23–25] Young to middle-aged women, in particular, are more likely to have benign pathology, as high as 40% in some series, while the likelihood of malignancy gradually decreases with age in men.[24,26] Tumor size is the most

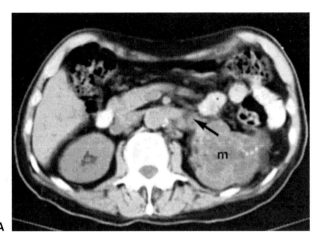 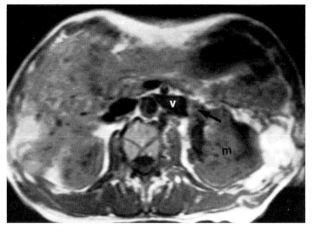

**Figure 37.1** Cross-sectional imaging of kidney cancer using computed tomography and magnetic resonance imaging. **(A)** Contrast-enhanced computed tomography imaging (parenchymal phase) reveals a left renal mass with tumor thrombus within the left renal vein. **(B)** Magnetic resonance imaging in the same patient shows that the renal vein thrombus extends within the renal vein, but not to the confluence with the inferior vena cava (level 0 thrombus). m, mass; v, vein.

important determinant of pathology and biologic aggressiveness with larger tumors more likely to be high grade, locally invasive, and/or of adverse histologic subtype.[23,24,27] Incorporation of readily available features can allow the physician to provide an individualized risk of cancer (ranging between ~50% and ~99%), but a certain diagnosis requires pathologic confirmation.[24,28] The most accurate nomogram currently available gives estimates of preoperative prediction of tumor histology with an area under the curve of 0.76 and high-grade malignancy with an area under the curve of 0.73.[28]

Percutaneous renal mass sampling is now being performed with increased regularity at many centers.[29] There is a strong rationale for biopsy when the findings will change management, such as when there is reason to suspect lymphoma/leukemia or abscess or to guide systemic therapy for metastatic disease. Even for clinically localized renal tumors, conventional renal mass biopsy can provide a definitive diagnosis in 80% to 90% of cases, and the ability to subtype and grade RCC can increase with the use of immunohistochemical and other molecular analyses.[30,31] Therefore, renal mass sampling should be considered in patients with enhancing renal masses who are candidates for a wide range of management strategies.[30–34] However, younger, healthier patients who are unwilling to accept the uncertainty associated with renal mass biopsy as well as elderly, frail patients who will be managed conservatively (independent of biopsy results) should still be managed without a biopsy.

Clinical and pathologic staging systems provide a basis of standardized communication, comparison, and prognostication. They are used to communicate risk for treatment decision making and clinical trials planning. There have been several staging systems for RCC proposed. The most widely used is version 7 of the TNM (tumor, node, metastasis) staging system of the American Joint Committee on Cancer and the Union for International Cancer Control, updated in 2010 (Table 37.2). It distinguishes T1a from T1b and T2a from T2b based on tumor size.[35] Additionally, adrenal involvement was changed from pathologic stage T3a to T4 and venous invasion was separated into renal vein/segmental branches (T3a) and inferior vena cava (IVC) below (T3b) or above the diaphragm (T3c). Nodal and metastatic disease are only classified as negative (N0/M0) or positive (N1/M1). Other potential prognostic features of the primary tumor not included in the TNM classification include necrosis, urothelial involvement, microvascular invasion and molecular features. Review of these and other prognostic features of RCC are available.[36]

## HEREDITARY KIDNEY CANCER SYNDROMES, GENETICS, AND MOLECULAR BIOLOGY

While most renal cancers are believed to occur sporadically, familial clusters have led to the discovery of at least seven RCC susceptible syndromes (Table 37.3). It is estimated that approximately 4% of RCC have a hereditary basis.[37] In these cases, in addition to a provocative family history, tumors tend to be bilateral,

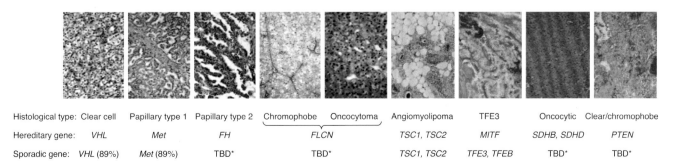

| Histological type: | Clear cell | Papillary type 1 | Papillary type 2 | Chromophobe | Oncocytoma | Angiomyolipoma | TFE3 | Oncocytic | Clear/chromophobe |
|---|---|---|---|---|---|---|---|---|---|
| Hereditary gene: | VHL | Met | FH | FLCN | | TSC1, TSC2 | MITF | SDHB, SDHD | PTEN |
| Sporadic gene: | VHL (89%) | Met (89%) | TBD* | TBD* | | TSC1, TSC2 | TFE3, TFEB | TBD* | TBD* |

**Figure 37.2** Human renal epithelial neoplasms. Renal cortical tumors do not conform to a single pathology. There are a number of different tumor subtypes that display the full range of oncologic activity, ranging from benign to indolent to aggressive. Each histologic type is characterized by distinct gross and microscopic appearance, gene associated with their familial forms, and genetic changes commonly detected in sporadic cases. (Used with permission from Linehan WM, Ricketts CJ. The metabolic basis of kidney cancer. *Semin Cancer Biol* 2013;23:46–55.)

**TABLE 37.2**

**International Tumor, Node, Metastasis Staging System for Renal Cell Carcinoma and Survival Rates**

| *T: Primary Tumor* | | Five-Year Survival (%) |
|---|---|---|
| TX | Primary tumor cannot be assessed | |
| T0 | No evidence of primary tumor | |
| T1a | Tumor ≤4 cm and confined to the kidney | 90–100 |
| T1b | Tumor >4 cm and ≤7 cm and confined to the kidney | 80–90 |
| T2a | Tumor >7 cm and ≤10 cm and confined to the kidney | 65–80 |
| T2b | Tumor >10 cm and confined to the kidney | 50–70 |
| T3a | Tumor grossly extends into the renal vein or its segmental (muscle containing) branches, or tumor invades perirenal and/or renal sinus fat but not beyond Gerota fascia | 40–65 |
| T3b | Tumor grossly extends into the vena cava below the diaphragm | 30–50 |
| T3c | Tumor grossly extends into the vena cava above the diaphragm or invades the wall of the vena cava | 20–40 |
| T4 | Tumor invades beyond Gerota fascia (including contiguous extension into the ipsilateral adrenal gland) | 0–20 |

| *N: Regional Lymph Nodes* | | |
|---|---|---|
| NX | Regional lymph nodes cannot be assessed | |
| N0 | No regional lymph nodes metastasis | |
| N1 | Metastasis in regional lymph node(s) | 0–20 |

| *M: Distant Metastases* | | |
|---|---|---|
| MX | Distant metastasis cannot be assessed | |
| M0 | No distant metastasis | |
| M1 | Distant metastasis present | 0–10 |

| *Stage Grouping* | | | |
|---|---|---|---|
| Stage I | T1 | N0 | M0 |
| Stage II | T2 | N0 | M0 |
| Stage III | T3 | Any N | M0 |
| | T1 or T2 | N1 | M0 |
| Stage IV | T4 | Any N | M0 |
| | Any T | Any N | M1 |

Modified from American Joint Committee on Cancer. Edge S, Byrd DR, Compton CC, et al, eds. *AJCC Cancer Staging Manual.* 7th ed. New York: Springer-Verlag; 2010. Data from Hafez KS, Fergany AF, Novick AC. Nephron sparing surgery for localized renal cell carcinoma: impact of tumor size on patient survival, tumor recurrence, and TNM staging. *J Urol* 1999;162(6): 1930-1933; Leibovich BC, Cheville JC, Lohse CM, et al. Cancer specific survival for patients with pT3 renal cell carcinoma—can the 2002 primary tumor classification be improved? *J Urol* 2005;173(3):716–719; Thompson RH, Cheville JC, Lohse CM, et al. Reclassification of patients with pT3 and pT4 renal cell carcinoma improves prognostic accuracy. *Cancer* 2005;104:53–60; Lane BR, Kattan MW. Prognostic models and algorithms in renal cell carcinoma. *Urol Clin North Am* 2008;35:613–625; Campbell L, Nuttall R, Griffiths D, et al. Activated extracellular signal-regulated kinase is an independent prognostic factor in clinically confined renal cell carcinoma. *Cancer* 2009; 115:3457–3467; Martinez-Salamanca JI, Huang WC, Millán I, et al; International Renal Cell Carcinoma-Venous Thrombus Consortium. Prognostic impact of the 2009 UICC/AJCC TNM staging system for renal cell carcinoma with venous extension. *Eur Urol* 2011;59:120–127; Haddad H, Rini BL. Current treatment considerations in metastatic renal cell carcinoma. *Curr Treat Options Oncol* 2012;13:212–229.

multifocal, and arise at an early age of onset. Importantly, the study of hereditary kidney cancer has dramatically changed our understanding of the genetic and molecular basis of RCC and has led to the development of effective, approved therapeutic agents as similar cytogenetic and molecular alterations appear to be shared between sporadic and hereditary RCC (see Fig. 37.2).[38]

The molecular alterations in RCC appear to converge on similar pathways involved in dysregulated oxygen sensing/angiogenesis, iron metabolism, and energy/nutrient sensing.[39,40] The predominant genetic and molecular defects in RCC known to date include VHL loss of function (ccRCC), neurofibromatosis type 2 loss of function (ccRCC), MET gain of function (papillary type I RCC), NRF2 gain of function and alterations in fumarate hydratase (papillary type II RCC), CCND1 gain of function and folliculin loss of function (oncocytoma/chromophobe RCC), and MiTF-TFE3 gain of function (translocation RCC). Additionally, inactivation of chromatin modifying proteins including *PBRM1*, *BAP1*, and histone methylases/demethylases, as well as inactivation of electron transporters, may represent early or common events in multiple subtypes.[41] While important, the associations of these aberrant pathways with various subtypes of RCC likely represent an overly simplified model of renal tumor development.[42] A variety of small nucleotide mutations, structural mutations, and large chromosomal abnormalities characterizes RCC, with as many as 5 to 70 small somatic mutations found in individual renal tumor cells.[42] Moreover, variable gene expressions may reflect differences in cell types from which RCC originates, suggesting that genetic aberrations require a specific cellular context for dysregulated growth. The development of rapid sequencers continues to redefine the molecular characterization of RCC from which a genetic profile/classification is emerging with important implications for the development of the next generation of targeted therapeutic molecules.[43,44]

## Von Hippel-Lindau Disease

VHL is a syndrome characterized by the development of highly vascular tumors of the retina, central nervous system, pancreas, adrenal, and kidney (ccRCC). It is inherited in an autosomal dominant fashion with an incidence of 1:35,000.[39] Loss of VHL function (3p25.1) by genetic or epigenetic means in a classic tumor suppressor fashion is the known cause. In an established genotype-phenotype relationship, type 1 VHL (absence of pheochromocytoma) is due to germline deletions, insertions, and nonsense mutations, whereas type II VHL (with pheochromocytoma) is associated with missense mutations.[45] Between 25% to 60% of patients with VHL develop bilateral multifocal cystic and solid RCC, which represents a common cause of death (Fig. 37.3). Management of renal tumors in patients with VHL now includes surveillance of smaller tumors (<3 cm) and resection of larger ones (>3 cm) by PN with the goal of preventing metastases and optimizing renal function by "resetting the biologic clock" through appropriately timed surgeries.[46] The goal of complete tumor removal with wide negative surgical margins is less appropriate for these patients where management of localized lesions supplants cure.[39,46] Patients should be evaluated and followed by a team of clinicians familiar with the complexities of multisystem genetic disorders.

## Hereditary Papillary Renal Cell Carcinoma

Hereditary papillary RCC is perhaps the least common familial RCC syndrome, with manifestations that appear to only affect the kidney. Affected individuals develop bilateral multifocal type I papillary RCC due to mutations in the *MET* gene located at 7q31. MET is a tyrosine kinase receptor with hepatocyte growth factor as its ligand.[47] The syndrome is transmitted in an autosomal dominant fashion and tumors usually appear after the age of 30.[39] As with VHL, management of renal tumors recognizes the need to remove larger lesions and observe smaller ones. While no size cutoff for intervention has been established, the biology of type I papillary RCC appears to be more indolent that ccRCC,

| TABLE 37.3 | | |
|---|---|---|
| **Familial Renal Cell Carcinoma Syndromes** | | |
| **Syndrome** | **Gene (Chromosome)** | **Major Clinical Manifestations** |
| von Hippel-Lindau | *VHL* gene (3p25-26) | Clear cell RCC<br>Retinal angiomas<br>Central nervous system hemangioblastomas<br>Pheochromocytoma<br>Other tumors |
| Hereditary papillary RCC | *c-met* proto-oncogene (7q31) | Multiple, bilateral type 1 papillary RCCs |
| Familial leiomyomatosis and RCC | *Fumarate hydratase* (1q42-43) | Type 2 papillary RCC<br>Collecting duct RCC<br>Leiomyomas of skin or uterus<br>Uterine leiomyosarcomas |
| Birt-Hogg-Dubé | *Folliculin* (17p11) | Multiple chromophobe RCC, hybrid oncocytic tumor, oncocytomas<br>Occasional clear cell (occasionally)<br>Papillary RCC (occasionally)<br>Facial fibrofolliculomas<br>Lung cysts<br>Spontaneous pneumothorax |
| Succinate dehydrogenase RCC | Succinate dehydrogenase complex subunits: *SDHB* (1p36.1-35) or *SDHD* (11q23) | Chromophobe, clear cell, type 2 papillary RCC, oncocytoma<br>Paragangliomas (benign and malignant)<br>Papillary thyroid carcinoma |
| Tuberous sclerosis | *TSC1* (9q34) or *TSC2* (16p13) | Multiple renal angiomyolipomas<br>Clear cell RCC (occasionally)<br>Renal cysts/polycystic kidney disease<br>Cutaneous angiofibromas<br>Pulmonary lymphangiomyomatosis |
| PTEN hamartoma tumor syndrome (Cowden syndrome) | *PTEN* (10q23) | Breast tumors (malignant and benign)<br>Epithelial thyroid carcinoma<br>Papillary RCC or other histology |

PTEN, phosphatase and tensin homolog; RCC, renal cell carcinoma.
Adapted from Linehan WM, Walther MM, Zbar B. The genetic basis of cancer of the kidney. *J Urol* 2003; 170(6 Pt 1):2163-2172. and Linehan WM, Ricketts CJ. The metabolic basis of kidney cancer. *Semin Cancer Biol* 2013;23:46–55.

suggesting the risk of death from kidney cancer in these patients is low. Again, PN with renal preservation is emphasized despite the diffuse micro- and macromultifocality of these lesions.

## Birt-Hogg-Dubé Syndrome

BHD is characterized by cutaneous fibrofolliculomas, a 50-fold increased risk of pneumothorax, and bilateral multifocal solid renal tumors. It is an autosomal dominant disorder with an incidence of around 1:200,000. Linkage analysis has mapped the gene for BHD (*folliculin*), a tumor suppressor, to 17p11.2. Folliculin is thought to be a downstream effector of activated protein kinase and mammalian target of rapamycin (mTOR).[39] Renal tumors associated with BHD are more indolent in nature, occurring in approximately 20% of individuals, with <5% developing metastases. While the histology of renal tumors associated with BHD is most often chromophobe RCC, oncocytoma, or hybrids of both, clear cell or papillary tumors may rarely occur as well.

## Hereditary Leiomyomatosis Renal Cell Carcinoma

Hereditary leiomyomatosis RCC is also characterized by dermatologic manifestations. Patients with HLRCC exhibit cutaneous leiomyomas, early onset of uterine fibroids, macronodular adrenal hyperplasia, and kidney cancer. Linkage analysis has localized the HLRCC gene (*fumarate hydratase*), a key Kreb cycle enzyme, to 1p42.3 (FN).[48]

Renal tumors in HLRCC tend to be aggressive and lethal. The most common histology observed is type II (eosinophilic) papillary RCC.[39] Unlike other hereditary forms of RCC, given the aggressive nature of these tumors, AS with delayed intervention is not recommended.

## TREATMENT OF LOCALIZED RENAL CELL CARCINOMA

Greater use of cross-sectional imaging has contributed to earlier detection of RCC in many cases.[2,49,50] Between 50% to 70% of RCC are detected incidentally,[51] and the majority are "small renal masses (SRM)," or clinically localized renal cortical tumors up to 4 cm in size. Our perspectives about treatment of clinical T1 renal masses have changed substantially in the past 20 years. While all had been presumed to be malignant and managed aggressively, we now recognize the tremendous biologic heterogeneity of these lesions, and multiple management strategies are now available, including RN, PN, TA, and AS.[52–57] Once controversial, elective PN is now accepted as a standard of care, based in part on the appreciation of the deleterious renal functional consequences of RN (Fig. 37.4).[53,55,58] Ongoing analysis of the relative merits of PN, RN, and other management strategies has produced vibrant literature over the past few years.[46,59–62] Both the American Urologic Association (AUA) and the European Association of Urology have released guidelines for the management of localized renal masses in recent years providing a robust analysis of the available studies.[9,63–67] Each approach has associated risks and benefits, and no one approach is best in all circumstances

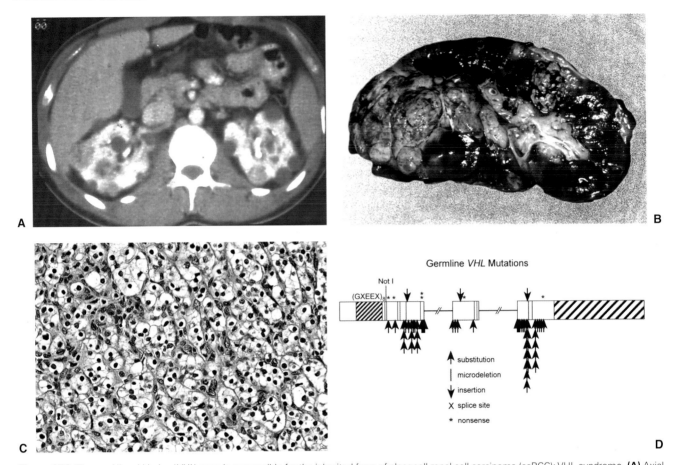

**Figure 37.3** The von Hippel-Lindau (*VHL*) gene is responsible for the inherited form of clear cell renal cell carcinoma (ccRCC): VHL syndrome. **(A)** Axial computed tomography image showing multifocal and bilateral renal tumors and cysts. **(B)** Gross image of nephrectomy specimen showing typical yellow-gold appearance of ccRCC present in multiple portions of this kidney from a patient with VHL. **(C)** Histologic appearance of ccRCC, showing the clearing of the cytoplasm around the darker nuclei typical of these "clear cells." **(D)** Structure of the VHL gene with sites of point mutations and truncations indicated. (Used with permission from Linehan and colleagues' prior work. DeVita VT, Lawrence TS, Rosenberg SA, et al, eds. *DeVita, Hellman, and Rosenberg's Cancer: Principles and Practice of Oncology.* 9th ed. Philadelphia, PA: Lippincott Williams & Wilkins; 2011.)

(Table 37.4). The involvement of an urologist with expertise in the management of RCC is essential for selection of the optimal strategy based on the individual features of each patient and tumor.

## Radical Nephrectomy for Renal Cell Carcinoma

The objective of surgical therapy for RCC is to excise all of the cancer with an adequate surgical margin. Simple nephrectomy was practiced for many decades, but was replaced by RN when Robson and colleagues (1969) established this procedure as the "gold standard" approach for localized RCC.[68] "RN" as currently practiced may be better termed "total nephrectomy," as it often omits several of the components of the original, "radical" nephrectomy, which always included extrafascial nephrectomy, adrenalectomy, and extended lymphadenectomy from the crus of the diaphragm to the aortic bifurcation. Perifascial dissection is still routinely practiced for larger tumors, as ≥25% of these tumors extend into the perinephric fat.[69,70] Removal of the ipsilateral adrenal gland is no longer recommended, unless there is suspicion of direct invasion of the gland by tumor or a radiographically or clinically suspicious adrenal tumor, because of the similar propensity of RCC to metastasize to the ipsilateral or contralateral adrenal gland.[71–73] Finally, extended lymphadenectomy has been shown to be of no benefit for patients with clinically localized RCC and remains controversial for those with higher-risk disease.[74–77]

RN is still a preferred option for many patients with localized RCC, such as those with very large tumors (most clinical T2 tumors) or the relatively limited subgroup of patients with clinical T1 tumors that are not amenable to nephron-sparing approaches.[78] The surgical approach for RN depends on the size and location of the tumor, as well as the patient's habitus and medical/surgical history. For locally advanced disease and/or bulky lymphadenopathy, an open surgical approach using either an extended subcostal, midline, or thoracoabdominal incision is generally used.[79]

Current minimally invasive approaches allow all of the essential steps of RN to be performed, with the associated benefits of shorter convalescence and reduced morbidity.[80–83] Laparoscopic RN is now established as a preferred approach for moderate to large volume tumors (≤10 cm to 12 cm), without invasion of adjacent organs, with limited (or no) venous involvement, and having manageable (or no) lymphadenopathy. Therefore, a minimally invasive approach is suitable for most patients with renal tumors, even including some patients with features previously thought to mandate open RN.

On the other hand, RN has fallen out of favor for smaller renal tumors due to concerns about chronic kidney disease (CKD), and it should only be performed when necessary in this population.[53,58,78,84] Several studies have shown an increased risk of CKD on longitudinal follow-up after RN.[58,85,86] Huang et al. first reported that 26% of patient populations with a small renal mass, normal opposite kidney, and "normal" serum creatinine had preexisting grade 3 CKD (estimated glomerular filtration rate [eGFR] <60 ml/min per 1.73 m²). After surgery, stage 3b or higher CKD (eGFR <45 ml/min per 1.73 m²) was more common after RN than PN (36% versus 5%, $p$ <0.001). CKD has been proven to lead to increased rates of cardiovascular events and death, with

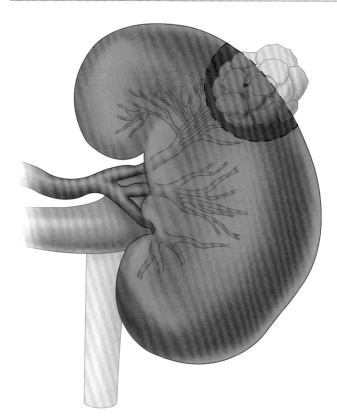

**Figure 37.4** Partial nephrectomy. The intention of kidney-sparing surgery, or "nephron-sparing surgery," is to achieve complete local resection of the tumor while leaving as much functioning parenchyma in the involved kidney as possible. An assessment of volume preservation can be made by accounting for both the amount of parenchyma replaced by tumor and the adjacent uninvolved parenchyma removed or devascularized during the procedure.[61] The amount of volume preservation and the quality of the functioning renal remnant are the most important determinants of renal function after renal surgery. Partial nephrectomy and other kidney-sparing alternatives provide definite renal functional benefits that must be weighed against the potential for increased risk of cancer recurrence, when compared with radical nephrectomy.[287] (Artwork courtesy of Kristen Tobert.)

proportionally greater impact with higher CKD stage (and lower GFR). For example, in a population-based study of >1 million subjects, the relative death rates were 1.2, 1.8, 3.2, and 5.9 for eGFR (ml/min per 1.73 m$^2$) of 45 to 60, 30 to 45, 15 to 30, and <15, respectively, even after controlling for hypertension, diabetes, and other potential confounding factors.[87] Coupled with the biologic heterogeneity of small renal masses, many of which will never lead to compromised survival, the potential negative consequences of RN on renal function have highlighted the importance of nephron-sparing approaches.[53,58,72,88–90]

## Partial Nephrectomy for Renal Cell Carcinoma

Kidney-sparing surgery for renal tumors was first described by Czerny in 1890; however, significant morbidity limited its use for the next half century.[91] Vermooten (1950) revisited the concept of local excision with a margin of normal parenchyma for encapsulated and peripherally located renal tumors.[92] The use of PN for RCC has subsequently been stimulated by experience with renal vascular surgery for other conditions, advances in renal imaging, growing numbers of incidentally discovered small renal masses, greater appreciation of the deleterious effects of CKD, introduction of minimally invasive techniques, and encouraging long-term survival in patients undergoing this form of treatment during the

last 50 years.[93–95] Kidney-sparing surgery entails complete local resection of the tumor while leaving the largest possible amount of normal functioning parenchyma in the involved kidney (see Fig. 37.4).

Initially described for patients with an "absolute" indication for kidney-sparing surgery or for the "elective" indication of a small renal tumor in the setting of a normal contralateral kidney, PN is now strongly considered whenever preservation of renal function is potentially important. Common indications include conditions that pose a threat to future renal function, such as hypertension, diabetes mellitus, peripheral or coronary artery disease, or nephrolithiasis, and patients with baseline CKD, an abnormal contralateral kidney, or those with multifocal or familial RCC.[96,97] PN is generally considered feasible for the vast majority of localized renal masses <5 cm in size and often for tumors ≥7 cm by those with expertise with kidney-sparing surgery.[98–101] Particularly for those with a strong rationale for nephron-sparing surgery, PN can even be performed for tumors that deeply invest the renal vascular structures or with limited venous thrombus, but such procedures clearly carry higher perioperative morbidity.[95,102] Local recurrence rates after PN for imperative indications have averaged 3% to 5% or higher in historical series.[103] The decision to perform a PN in such circumstances should be individualized, weighing the potential increased technical and oncologic risks of such an operation with the renal functional consequences of RN (see Fig. 37.4).

PN clearly leads to improved functional outcomes, when compared with RN, even for complicated situations.[104,105] Temporary or permanent renal replacement therapy has been reported to be necessary in <5% of patients undergoing PN in a solitary kidney and is rarely needed for patients with a functioning contralateral kidney.[106,107] In fact, the vast majority of patients will avoid permanent dialysis, even following multiple surgeries for multiple tumors in both kidneys, so long as at least 30% of a well-functioning remnant kidney is preserved.[95] For situations in which PN is deemed impossible, RN with ensuing hemodialysis is sometimes necessary, but presurgical therapy with a tyrosine-kinase inhibitor is an alternative approach that has proven successful in some patients.[108–111]

For patients with clinical T1 renal masses, local recurrence rates are 1% to 2% after PN and most commonly located distant from the initial resection. Cancer-free survival is achieved in well above 90% of patients.[104] The contralateral kidney is also at risk for metachronous disease, which also occurs in 1% to 2% of patients, even with contemporary imaging modalities. This provides further rationale to avoid unnecessary RN for tumors amenable to nephron-sparing surgery. The goal of PN is resection of all grossly appreciated tumor with negative microscopic surgical margins; this is generally performed with a thin rim of normal parenchyma based on prior literature indicating that margin width is immaterial.[67,112–117] Some centers now routinely perform enucleation of renal tumors with excellent oncologic outcomes, although enthusiasm for more widespread use of this approach has been tempered by the somewhat higher recurrence rate among patients with RCC with positive margins and the propensity of some RCC subtypes to invade the pseudocapsule that is generally present.

Within the last decade, substantial progress has been made with minimally invasive PN, which is now the most commonly performed procedure for small renal masses. Laparoscopic PN, with or without robotic assistance, is performed according to the same principles as open PN. Margin status and oncologic outcomes with laparoscopic and open PN appear equivalent in series of patients in which patients were selected appropriately for each of these approaches.[101,118] Although early to intermediate experience with laparoscopic PN suggested increased urologic complications compared with open RN,[119] subsequent experience with pure laparoscopic PN and more prevalent use of robotic PN have substantially reduced perioperative morbidity.[104,120–125] Tumor complexity remains a major predictor for intraoperative and postoperative complications, regardless of surgical approach, and open PN should be considered for particularly challenging situations.[126]

**TABLE 37.4**

## Treatments for Localized Renal Cell Carcinoma

| | Advantages | Disadvantages | Main Indications |
|---|---|---|---|
| **ORN** | Traditional surgical approach for renal cancer, effective in removing tumor with surrounding structures and lymph nodes when indicated | Morbidity of surgical incision (flank, subcostal, midline, thoracoabdominal) <br> Renal functional implications of removing entire kidney (average 35% decrease in GFR) | Large tumor (>12 cm) <br> Locally advanced tumor <br> Bulky adenopathy |
| **MIRN** | Reproducible and effective surgery for most localized renal tumors <br> Minimally invasive surgery, with decreased pain, morbidity and convalescence compared to ORN | Many tumors up to 7 cm can be treated with PN <br> Renal functional implications of removing entire kidney (average 35% decrease in GFR) | Medium to large tumor (up to 10 to 12 cm) <br> High tumor complexity |
| **OPN** | Oncologic outcomes appear similar to RN, although selection biases limit this conclusion <br> Maximizes renal functional preservation when performed with precise tumor excision and judicious use of regional hypothermia | Morbidity of flank incision (bulge, longer recovery) <br> Potential for local recurrence due to incomplete excision or de novo tumors in the renal remnant | Small to medium tumors (up to 7 cm and occasionally larger) <br> Moderate to high-complexity tumors |
| **MIPN** | Kidney-sparing surgery, with preservation of renal function when warm ischemia kept to limited duration (<20 to 25 min) <br> Minimally invasive surgery, with decreased pain, morbidity, and convalescence compared to OPN | Higher complication rate for high complexity tumors and in less-experienced hands <br> Positive surgical margins and local recurrence rates may be higher in such situations | Small renal masses (up to 5 cm and occasionally larger) <br> Low to moderate (and selected high) complexity tumors |
| **TA** | Kidney-sparing approach, with renal functional benefits versus RN <br> Can be performed outside of OR (percutaneous) or with minimally invasive approach (laparoscopic) <br> For small (<3 cm) tumors, provides comparable control of metastasis to PN and RN | Relatively high rate of local failure <br> Imprecision of histopathologic diagnosis <br> Increased and challenging radiographic follow-up | Prior ipsilateral surgery for renal tumor <br> Poorer surgical candidates unwilling to undergo surveillance |
| **AS** | Least invasive and kidney-sparing of all strategies <br> Most SRMs have limited oncologic potential and can be safely managed with initial short interval follow-up imaging <br> Intensity of surveillance can be tailored to patient and tumor characteristics | Tumor remains in place and untreated <br> Oncologic nature of tumor unknown (without biopsy) | Poor surgical candidates <br> Limited life expectancy |

ORN, open radical nephrectomy; GFR; glomerular filtration rate; MIRN, minimally invasive radical nephrectomy; OPN, open partial nephrectomy; RN, radical nephrectomy; MIPN, minimally invasive partial nephrectomy; TA, thermal ablation; OR, operating room; PN, partial nephrectomy; AS, active surveillance; SRM, small renal mass.

## Thermal Ablation of Renal Cell Carcinoma

TA, including renal cryosurgery and radiofrequency ablation (RFA) have emerged as alternative kidney-sparing treatments for patients with small (<3 cm) renal tumors.[127,128] Both can be administered percutaneously or with laparoscopic exposure and thus offer the potential for reduced morbidity and more rapid recovery compared with extirpative approaches.[128,129] In general, the long-term efficacy of TA has not been well established when compared to surgical excision, and current data suggest that the local recurrence rates are somewhat higher than that reported with extirpative approaches.[55,63] Another concern has been the lack of accurate histologic and pathologic information obtained with these modalities because the treated lesion is left in situ.

The ideal candidates for TA are patients with advanced age and/or significant comorbidities who prefer a proactive approach (over surveillance), but are not optimal candidates for conventional surgery, patients with local recurrence after previous kidney-sparing surgery, and patients with hereditary renal cancer who present with multifocal lesions for which multiple PNs might be cumbersome.[55] Patient preference must also be considered as some patients not fitting these criteria may select TA after balanced counseling about the current status of these modalities.[130,131] Tumor size is an important factor in patient selection because the current technology does not allow for reliable treatment of lesions >4 cm and success rates appear to be highest for tumors <2.5 cm to 3 cm.[132–135]

Clinical experience and follow-up of patients after renal cryosurgery suggests successful local control in about 90% of patients, although many studies provide limited and often incomplete, follow-up.[136–140] Diagnosis of local recurrence after TA can be challenging because evolving fibrosis within the tumor bed can be difficult to differentiate from residual cancer. In general, central or nodular enhancement within the tumor bed on extended follow-up has been considered diagnostic of local recurrence and the clinical experience with cryoablation has thus far supported this.[141,142] Other findings that suggest local recurrence include failure of the treated lesion to regress over time, a progressive increase in size of an ablated neoplasm, new nodularity in or around the treated zone, or satellite or port site lesions.[143] If these features are found, biopsy and possible retreatment should be considered. The AUA guidelines for surveillance after TA include cross-sectional scanning (computed tomography or MRI) with and without intravenous contrast at 3 and 6 months following ablative therapy and annually with chest X-ray for 5 years thereafter.[143]

More mature data from a limited number of studies now provide encouraging outcomes for smaller tumors, particularly those <3 cm, yet the cumulative experience continues to suggest that local control after cryoablative therapy remains suboptimal when compared to surgical excision.[55,138] The 5-year local recurrence rates in two series were 8% to 9%,[52,144] which is significantly higher than the 1% to 2% consistently reported with surgical excision of analogous small renal masses.[53] Other concerns with TA relate to surgical salvage and potential morbidity. Most local recurrences can be salvaged with repeat ablation, but some patients with progressive disease eventually require surgical extirpation. Nguyen and colleagues (2008b) have shown that PN and minimally invasive approaches are occasionally precluded in this setting due to the extensive fibrotic reaction induced by TA.[78] As expected, the incidence of treatment failure or complications after TA correlates with tumor size and complexity.[145]

The experience with RFA has been even more variable, likely related to surgeon experience, the availability of different platforms for the procedure, and inability to monitor treatment progress.[128] Local control after RFA is estimated to be 80% to 90%, although the definitions of local recurrence within the literature have been inconsistent.[53,55] Although loss of enhancement on cross-sectional imaging within the lesion has generally been accepted as an indicator of success, viable cancer cells have been detected at biopsy of the tumor bed even in the absence of enhancement on the MRI 6 months after treatment.[142] The issue of potential false-negative and false-positive imaging findings after TA remains a concern, and more strict definitions of local control after TA were recently advocated by an AUA guidelines panel.[143,146] The technology for RFA continues to improve with most contemporary series reporting relatively low rates of local recurrence. Some patients require repeat treatments to achieve local control, which is an infrequent event with cryoablation and rarely required with conventional surgical treatments for localized RCC.[128] One recent series documented local control in 91% of 179 patients with biopsy proven RCC at median follow-up of 27 months.[135] Some RFA series report even more encouraging results, particularly for tumors <3 cm diameter,[132] but others have reported 5-year local recurrence rates as high as 39%.[147]

Complications from ablation are uncommon, but have included acute renal failure, stricture of the ureteropelvic junction, necrotizing pancreatitis, and lumbar radiculopathy; therefore, careful and judicious selection of patients is essential.[128] Direct comparisons between cryoablation and RFA are inevitable, but perhaps unfair because RFA is earlier in its development and recent reports suggest great promise.[128,132] Other new technologies, such as high-intensity focused ultrasound and frameless, image-guided radiosurgical treatments (CyberKnife), are also under development and may allow extracorporeal treatment of small renal tumors in the future.[148–150] However, at present cell kill with these modalities is not sufficiently reliable and they should still be considered developmental.[151]

## Active Surveillance of Clinically Localized Renal Cell Carcinoma

The concept of overdiagnosis and overtreatment of kidney cancers is a relatively new concept. The risks and consequences associated with unnecessary treatment of low-risk RCC are an unintentional, yet underappreciated harm associated with incidental detection of these tumors. While early detection leads to "cure," lead time biases in reported surgical series and the growing recognition that some localized renal tumors exhibit an indolent natural history have challenged the "find it, excise it" practice pattern. As the data emerge, AS remains a rational therapeutic option, particularly in the elderly or infirm where competing health, surgical, or renal functional risks may exceed that of the tumor's biology.[152,153]

Objectifying and comparing the risks of treatment (excision/ablation) versus AS remains difficult as the data upon which competing risks models are based remain largely retrospective and incomplete.[28] Nonetheless, data have emerged to suggest

that radiographically localized small renal masses, most of which are RCC,[154,152] exhibit slow linear/volumetric growth (0.3 cm/year on average) with a low metastatic potential (1.1% to 1.4%) over the first 24 to 36 months following diagnosis.[154,152] Moreover, in patients with localized small renal tumors at diagnosis, the risk of metastases appears to be related to both the size of the primary tumor and perhaps more importantly the growth kinetics of the lesion.[155] Interestingly, as many as 20% to 30% of small renal tumors exhibit zero radiographic growth over the initial 24 months following diagnosis.[55] Given these data, the practice of AS with delayed intervention informed by an objective assessment of risk in the elderly, infirm, and/or well-informed is emerging.[156] This practice is a calculated risk accepted by the patient and managed by the physician. Percutaneous biopsy and emerging biologic and genetic markers will continue to improve the decision-making process. In the meantime, AS remains a viable option for highly motivated patients and highly engaged physicians.

### Follow-Up for Localized Renal Cell Carcinoma

Follow-up for cancer survivors focuses broadly on early detection of cancer recurrence. With earlier diagnosis of many cancers and a longer length of life after diagnosis and treatment, an increasing number of survivors remain under the care of cancer specialists and primary care physicians. Wide variations in recommended practice have led to the development of guidelines by various organizations. The AUA released guidelines for follow-up of clinically localized RCC in 2013 that reflect a consistent approach that also takes into account the heterogeneity of the population of cancer survivors (Table 37.5).[143] Clinicians should be aware that in managing adult cancer survivors they are not only looking for RCC recurrence, but also monitoring for secondary malignancy and the effects of cancer treatment, implementing therapies to prevent recurrences or new tumors, understanding the consequences of cancer and its treatment effects, and coordinating the overall care between cancer specialists and the primary care physician to meet each individual's needs.

## TREATMENT OF LOCALLY ADVANCED RENAL CELL CARCINOMA

### Surgery for Tumor Thrombus in the Inferior Vena Cava

Renal tumors are unique in their ability to form tumor thrombi that can propagate from the ipsilateral renal vein into the IVC and extend as far as the patient's right atrium. Approximately 4% to 10% of patients who present with renal masses will have a concomitant tumor thrombus. The level of tumor thrombus is classified as level 0 (thrombus limited to the renal vein), level I (thrombus extending into the inferior vena cava ≤2 cm above the renal vein), level II (thrombus extending into the inferior vena cava >2 cm above the renal vein, but below the hepatic veins), level III (thrombus extending into the inferior vena cava to or above the level of the hepatic veins, but still remaining below the diaphragm), and level IV (thrombus extending into the inferior vena cava and above the level of the diaphragm) (Fig. 37.5). A tumor thrombus should be suspected in patients with a renal tumor who also have new onset lower extremity edema, an isolated right-sided varicocele or one that does not collapse with recumbency, dilated superficial abdominal veins, proteinuria, pulmonary embolism, right atrial mass, or nonfunction of the involved kidney.

Five-year cancer-specific survival for patients with RCC and venous extension ranges from 45% to 70%, and surgical therapy in the form of RN and IVC thrombectomy can be curative. Interestingly, many patients with vena cava extension will present

**Guidelines for Follow-Up of Clinically Localized Renal Cell Carcinoma**

| Follow-up Measure | Recommendation |
|---|---|
| Physical exam and history | History and physical examination directed at detecting signs and symptoms of metastatic spread or local progression |
| Laboratory testing | Basic laboratory testing including blood urea nitrogen/creatinine, urinalysis and estimated glomerular filtration rate for all patients<br>Progressive renal insufficiency should prompt nephrology referral<br>Complete blood count, lactate dehydrogenase, liver function tests, alkaline phosphatase, and serum calcium per discretion of the physician |
| Abdominal imaging | Obtain a baseline abdominal scan (CT or magnetic resonance imaging) within 3 to 6 mo following surgery, and periodically thereafter based on individual risk factors (e.g., every 6 mo for 3 y for moderate to high-risk RCC)<br>Perform site-specific imaging as symptoms warrant<br>Imaging beyond 5 y may be performed at the discretion of the clinician |
| Chest imaging | Low-risk RCC: Chest X-ray annually for 3 y and only as clinically indicated beyond that time period<br>Moderate to high-risk RCC: baseline chest CT 3 to 6 mo after surgery with continued imaging (chest X-ray or CT) every 6 mo for at least 3 y<br>Imaging beyond 5 y is optional and should be based on individual patient characteristic and tumor risk factors |
| Bone scan | Elevated alkaline phosphatase, clinical symptoms such as bone pain, and/or radiographic findings suggestive of a bony neoplasm should prompt a bone scan<br>Bone scan should not be performed in the absence of these signs and symptoms |
| Central nervous system imaging | Acute neurologic signs should lead to prompt neurologic cross-sectional imaging of the head or spine based on localized symptoms |

CT, computed tomography; RCC, renal cell carcinoma.
Adapted from Donat SM, Diaz M, Bishoff JT, et al. Follow-up for clinically localized renal neoplasms: AUA guideline. *J Urol* 2013;190:407–416.

without metastatic disease.[157,158] The prognostic significance of IVC thrombus level has been controversial. Most studies suggest that the incidence of locoregional or systemic progression is higher in patients with level III-IV IVC thrombus, which may account for the reduced survival reported in this subgroup in some series.[159–162] Other series have shown that any IVC involvement is worse than renal vein involvement without distinction with regard to IVC level; in these series, other factors, such as nodal or metastatic involvement and tumor grade, have more impact on overall survival (OS).[163,164] Despite this debate, patients with any tumor thrombus

level can be cured with surgical resection, even level IV, in the absence of metastases and other adverse features.[165–168]

More recent series have re-evaluated the clinical variables predictive of survival after surgery for patients with tumor thrombi. In a single institutional series of 99 patients, median survival for patients with level I/II tumor thrombus was 6.6 years compared to 1.4 years for patients with level III/IV tumor thrombi. Higher level of tumor thrombus ([III/IV versus I/II], hazard ratio [HR] = 1.84 95% confidence interval [CI] = 1.03 to 3.30, $p = 0.041$) and the presence of metastatic disease at the time of surgery (HR = 2.97, 95% CI = 1.65 to 5.36, $p <0.001$) both portended a worse OS on multivariate analysis.[169] Other investigators have examined the impact of tumor histology on clinical and pathologic outcomes in patients with venous tumor extension. Authors at the Mayo Clinic found that patients with non–clear cell histology presented with a significantly larger tumor size, greater rate of lymph node disease, higher nuclear grade, and more frequent sarcomatoid differentiation.[170] As a result of these clinical and pathologic variables, these patients had a considerably worse 5-year cancer-specific survival as compared with patients with clear cell histology ($p = 0.03$).[170] Similarly, a recent international multi-institutional retrospective study analyzed the role of tumor histology on survival in patients undergoing RN and caval thrombectomy. In this series of 1,774 patients, the overall 5-year cancer-specific survival was 53.4%.[171] In this series' multivariable analysis, papillary histology (HR = 1.62, 95% CI = 1.01 to 2.61, $p <0.05$), fat invasion (HR = 1.49, 95% CI = 1.10 to 2.03, $p <0.01$), and thrombus level ($p <0.01$) were all independent predictors of a poor cancer-specific survival.[171] In contrast to the Mayo series, when the authors restricted their analysis to only N0M0 patients, thrombus level and papillary histology were still significantly associated with a decreased cancer-specific survival.[170,171]

Surgery remains an integral part in the treatment paradigm for patients with tumor venous extension because of the sequelae of such vascular involvement. The surgical approach and technique to treat these challenging tumors are tailored to the level of IVC thrombus, but uniformly begin with careful mobilization of the kidney and early ligation of the arterial blood supply.[164,172,173] With an increasing tumor thrombus level, more advanced surgical techniques are required for vasculature control and complete tumor extirpation, including veno-venous bypass and cardiopulmonary bypass potentially with hypothermic circulatory arrest for some cases. Specifically for level III and level IV thrombi, a multidisciplinary surgical team is often required for advanced surgical maneuvers, including a liver surgeon to aid in mobilization of the liver and exposure of the intrahepatic IVC and a vascular and/or cardiac surgeon if bypass is required.

Despite the surgical ability to resect these tumor thrombi, perioperative mortality rates associated with RN and IVC thrombectomy have been reported to be as high as 5% to 10% in some series, depending on patient comorbidities and tumor characteristics.[164,166] Although there may be a palliative role for surgery in some patients with metastasis who experience severe disability from intractable edema, ascites, cardiac dysfunction, or associated local symptoms such as abdominal pain and hematuria, most such patients will not benefit due to risk of perioperative morbidity and limited life expectancy.[174,175]

## Lymphadenectomy

The need for extensive lymphadenectomy in patients undergoing RN remains a subject of debate. Despite the fact that multiple prior studies have shown a survival benefit with a lymph node dissection performed at the time of nephrectomy,[75,176,177] a recent randomized trial failed to show a distinct advantage.[74] Although this trial represents level I evidence, its generalizability is limited since the trial included many patients at low risk for nodal metastasis (81% of patients had grade 1 or 2 tumors and 72% had organ-confined

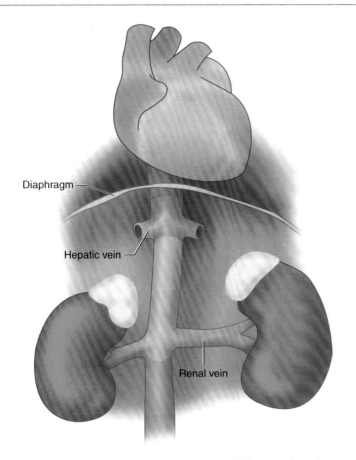

Diaphragm

Hepatic vein

Renal vein

**Prognostic and surgical staging systems of IVC tumor thrombus**

| Anatomic landmark | Staging systems | | | | |
|---|---|---|---|---|---|
| | TNM | Neves | Novick | Hinman | Robson |
| RV | T3b | 0 | I | I | IIIa |
| IVC <2 cm above RV | | I | II | | |
| IVC >2 cm above RV and below hepatic veins | | II | | | |
| IVC above hepatic veins and below diaphragm | | III | III | II | |
| IVC above diaphragm | T3c | IV | IV | III | |

**Figure 37.5** Classification of renal cell carcinoma venous tumor thrombi. Level 0 (*green*): Thrombus within main renal vein (RV) or its branches and not reaching into the inferior vena cava (IVC). Level I (*yellow*): IVC thrombus is present within the IVC, <2 cm above renal vein. Level II (*orange*): IVC thrombus extends along the IVC, but not to the level of the main hepatic veins. Level III (*purple*): IVC thrombus extends within the IVC above the level of the main hepatic veins, but below the diaphragm. Level IV (*red*): IVC thrombus extends above the diaphragm, near to or into the right atrium and occasionally beyond. TNM, tumor, node, metastasis. (Reproduced with permission from Pouliot F, Shuch B, Larochelle JC, et al. Contemporary management of renal tumors with venous tumor thrombus. *J Urol* 2010;184:833–841.)

disease).[74] Furthermore, in the entire cohort, lymph node metastases were present in only 4% of patients undergoing complete lymph node dissection.[74] Based on this trial, a compelling argument for lymph node dissection in patients with clinically localized RCC cannot be supported.

Of greater impact is the study from Blute and colleagues[164] who elucidated pathologic features associated with increased risk for nodal metastases: tumor grade (grade 3 or 4), presence of a sarcomatoid component, tumor size ≥10 cm, tumor stage pT3 or pT4, and histologic tumor necrosis. Based on this study and a subsequent prospective evaluation of this approach, patients with two or more of these risk factors should be considered for extensive lymph node dissection incorporating the ipsilateral renal hilar

region, the ipsilateral great vessel, and the interaortocaval region. This dissection should extend from the crus of the diaphragm to the common iliac artery. In a retrospective study, 45% of patients had positive lymph nodes outside of the renal hilar region, mandating a broader template.[177] Finally, a recently published retrospective study of 1,983 patients treated for RCC assessed the factors predictive of lymph node invasion and/or progression. In this study, the overall prevalence of lymph node invasion was 6.1% and the clinical factors that were independently predictive of lymph node involvement were tumor stage (T3-T4), clinical nodal status, the presence of metastatic disease, and tumor size as a continuous variable.[178] Using these variables, the authors created a nomogram that calculates a patient's probability of having lymph node disease at the time of nephrectomy or in disease follow-up.[178] It appears fair to conclude that a lymph node dissection is not routinely needed for organ-confined disease; however, the presence of multiple adverse pathologic features (e.g., large tumor size, locally advanced disease, etc.) seems to favor performing a lymph node dissection that is more extensive than simply the hilar region.

## ADJUVANT THERAPY FOR RENAL CELL CARCINOMA

Although a significant proportion of patients can be considered to be cured or in remission after surgical treatment for nonmetastatic RCC, distant metastases are detected in 20% to 35% and local recurrence in 2% to 5% of patients.[54,94] Patients with locally advanced RCC and other high-risk features are at greater risk of recurrence and various predictive tools can be used to provide an individualized estimate.[54] Despite the significant likelihood of recurrence in patients with poor-risk features, no therapy has ever been shown to be of benefit in the adjuvant setting. Prior trials have evaluated hormone therapy, radiotherapy, immunotherapy, and tumor vaccines, all with essentially negative results. Based on the significant antitumor activity of targeted molecular therapies in advanced RCC, a number of randomized trials evaluating the ability of these agents to prevent metastasis have completed enrollment and results of these trials can be expected as early as 2015 (Table 37.6).

## SURGICAL MANAGEMENT OF ADVANCED RENAL CELL CARCINOMA

### Cytoreductive Nephrectomy

Approximately 30% to 40% of patients will present with metastatic or advanced RCC.[179] For these patients, multimodal therapy, which includes surgery, has produced improved progression-free survival (PFS) and OS. The National Comprehensive Cancer Network Guidelines for kidney cancer list cytoreductive nephrectomy (CN) with or without metastasectomy prior to systemic treatment as the primary treatment option for patients with stage IV RCC.[180] The data supporting this recommendation come from three randomized trials demonstrating a survival benefit for patients who received systemic immunotherapy with interferon (IFN)-alfa after surgical removal of the primary tumor.[181–183] Flanigan et al.[181] found the median survival of 120 patients assigned to surgery followed by IFN-alfa to be 11.1 months compared to 8.1 months in 121 patients assigned to IFN-alfa alone ($p = 0.05$). Similarly, Mickisch et al.[183] found time to progression (5 months versus 3 months) and median duration of survival to be better in patients randomized to surgery plus IFN-alfa compared to those randomized to IFN-alfa alone. Combining the survival data from all these trials resulted in a median survival of 13.6 months versus 7.8 months for patients undergoing surgery in addition to IFN-alfa as compared to IFN-alfa alone.[181,183–185]

More recent data accounting for the current use of targeted therapies as first-line systemic therapy for patients with metastatic RCC have confirmed the survival advantage associated with CN. In one retrospective study, patients ($n = 201$) who underwent CN had an independent statistically significant survival advantage as compared to patients ($n = 113$) who did not (HR = 0.68; 95% CI = 0.46 to 0.99, $p = 0.04$).[186] This survival advantage was present even when adjusting for contemporary adverse prognostic risk factors (e.g., performance status, time from diagnosis to therapy initiation, anemia, hypercalcemia, neutrophilia, and thrombocytosis).[187] Despite these promising results, other studies have shown that CN may not confer a survival advantage in patients with non–clear cell histology, especially those with sarcomatoid features.[172,188,189] Fortunately, a prospective study evaluating the benefit of surgery in combination with sunitinib versus sunitinib alone is currently ongoing in patients with metastatic RCC.

Although the use of laparoscopic/minimally invasive techniques in patients with advanced disease can potentially provide a less invasive and less morbid method for cytoreduction as preparation for administration of systemic therapies, CN is still not without risk, and surgical risk assessment needs to be considered preoperatively. According to prior reports, patients that are most

## TABLE 37.6

**Clinical Trials of Adjuvant Treatment for Nonmetastatic Renal Call Carcinoma**

| Trial | Study Groups | Treatment Duration | Inclusion Criteria |
|---|---|---|---|
| ASSURE: Adjuvant Sorafenib or Sunitinib for Unfavorable Renal Cell Carcinoma | Sunitinib vs. sorafenib vs. placebo | 1 y | Clear cell and non–clear cell RCC eligible pT1b and G3-4; pT2/pT3/pT4; N1 if complete dissection performed |
| SORCE: Sorafenib for Patients with Resected Primary Renal Cell Carcinoma | Sorafenib (for 1 or 3 y) vs. placebo | 3 y | Clear cell and non–clear cell RCC eligible Mayo Clinic progression score 3–11 |
| S-TRAC: Sunitinib vs. Placebo for the Treatment of Patients at high risk for Recurrent Renal Cell Cancer | Sunitinib vs. placebo | 1 y | Clear cell predominant histology eligible High-risk RCC according to UISS |
| EVEREST: Everolimus for Renal Cancer Ensuing Surgical Therapy | Everolimus vs. placebo | 1 y | Clear cell and non–clear cell RCC eligible pT1b and G3-4; pT2/pT3/pT4; N1 if complete dissection performed |
| ATLAS: Adjuvant Axitinib Treatment of Renal Cancer | Axitinib vs. placebo | 3 y | Clear cell predominant (>50%) eligible pT2 and G3-4; pT3a and >4 cm; pT3b/pT3c/pT4; N1 |
| PROTECT: Pazopanib as an Adjuvant Treatment for Locally Advanced Renal Cell Carcinoma | Pazopanib vs. placebo | 1 y | Clear cell predominant (>50%) eligible pT2 and G3-4; pT3/pT4; N1 |

RCC, renal cell carcinoma; pT: pathologic T stage; G: Fuhrman nuclear grade; . UISS: University of California, Los Angeles, integrated staging system.
Source: Zisman A, Pantuck AJ, Chao DH, et al. Renal cell carcinoma with tumor thrombus: is cytoreductive nephrectomy for advanced disease associated with an increased complication rate? *J Urol* 2002;168:962–967.

likely to benefit from CN are those patients with lung-only metastatic disease, good prognostic features as defined by Motzer (or other) criteria, and a good performance status.[175,190] Conversely, predictors of short survival for patients with advanced RCC include an elevated serum lactate dehydrogenase (LDH; >1.5 times upper limit of normal), a hemoglobin level <lower limit of normal, a corrected serum calcium level >10 mg/dl, an interval of <1 year from original diagnosis to the start of systemic therapy, a Karnofsky performance score ≤70, and two or more sites of organ metastasis.[191] However, the challenge associated with these risk criteria is that they mostly account for the risk associated with the disease and do not consider the perioperative risk to the patient, which is not insignificant.

For example, Abdollah et al.[192] identified 17,688 patients within the Florida Inpatient Database that underwent nephrectomy between the years 1999 to 2008. They identified 1,063 (6%) patients who underwent a CN and found that these patients were more likely to have a longer length of stay (8.4 versus 5.7 days, $p$ <0.001), a secondary surgical procedure (28.3% versus 10%, $p$ <0.001), an in-hospital mortality (2.4% versus 0.9%, $p$ <0.001), and a postoperative complication (26.5% versus 18.9%, $p$ <0.001). In this report, increasing age was predictive of increasing in-hospital mortality and complications for patients undergoing CN. A similar analysis was conducted by Trinh et al[193] using the Nationwide Inpatient Sample registry. Thirty one percent of the study population ($n$ = 16,285) experienced a perioperative complication, and patients ≥75 years old who had a comorbidity score ≥3 were more likely to experience a complication after CN (both $p$ <0.001).[193] Of the patients ($n$ = 4,974) that experienced an adverse event, 5% ($n$ = 245 patients) died during their hospitalization.[193] Finally, it is worth noting that despite the survival advantage garnered from a CN followed by targeted therapy, it is not universally received. In a single institutional study from the Fox Chase Cancer Center, only 69.5% of patients actually received systemic therapy after surgery.[194] The most common reason in this study for patients not to receive systemic therapy was rapid disease progression, which occurred in 30% of patients. Also, there were eight perioperative deaths, accounting for 19% of patients who did not receive systemic treatment.[194]

In summary, CN offers patients with metastatic RCC a survival advantage and the National Comprehensive Cancer Network Guidelines recommend a CN for patients with an Eastern Cooperative Oncology Group performance status <2 who have no evidence of brain metastasis.[180] Despite these recommendations, recent data has shown that surgical risk associated with CN is not insignificant, especially in the elderly and comorbid, and should be weighed against the patient's disease biology (presence of poor-risk disease) before reflexively proceeding with surgery.

## Surgical Management of Recurrent and Metastatic Disease

Approximately one-third of patients initially diagnosed with RCC will present with metastatic disease.[179] An additional 40% of patients that present with localized disease will ultimately develop metastatic disease.[179,195] As these statistics illustrate, the biology of RCC is unique and variable and as such the treatment of patients with metastatic RCC is as well. In patients with diffuse metastatic disease, metastatectomy is not routinely used for therapeutic purposes. However, for the subset of patients who either present with or develop low-volume, radiographically solitary, or limited metastases, whether it be synchronous or metachronous, resection is often an integral part of the treatment paradigm and can confer a survival advantage.[180,196,197] Complete metastasectomy has been associated with a two-fold reduction in the risk of death from RCC.[162]

Of the approximately 30% of patients with RCC who present with metastases, only 1.5% to 3.5% have a solitary metastasis.[198]

Patients with a solitary synchronous metastatic lesion have decreased survival when compared with patients who develop metastasis after the primary tumor is removed.[199] Nevertheless, surgical resection of metastatic disease either alone or in combination with immunotherapy/targeted therapy has been shown to be curative or to confer a survival advantage compared to patients who did not undergo consolidative metastasectomy. However, these data must be interpreted in the context that only a small subset of patients will be optimal candidates for surgical extirpation of metastatic lesions. In a large series from the Mayo Clinic, 887 patients were identified with multiple metastatic sites of disease from RCC who underwent surgical resection. Of this large cohort, only 125 (14%) patients underwent a complete resection of their metastatic disease, whereas 698 (78.7%) patients had died of RCC at a median of 1.2 years after the first occurrence of their metastatic disease.[200] In this analysis, the authors demonstrated that complete surgical resection of metastatic disease, across all subgroups, was predictive of improved survival. For example, the median RCC specific and OS for patients who underwent complete metastatectomy were 4.8 and 4.0 years, respectively.[200] Comparative RCC-specific and OS rates for patients where complete surgical resection was not achieved were 1.3 and 1.3 years, respectively. Also, patients experienced an improved survival if they underwent complete surgical resection regardless of metastatic sites (lung versus nonlung, $p$ <0.001), number of metastatic sites ($p$ <0.001), and timing of metastatic disease—synchronous ($p$ <0.001) and asynchronous ($p$ = 0.002).[200] Finally, on multivariate analysis, patients in whom surgery did not achieve a complete metastasectomy were almost three times more likely to die of RCC (HR = 2.91; 95% CI = 2.17 to 3.90, $p$ <0.001).[200] In this series, approximately half of the patients (45.6%) received some form of systemic therapy during their treatment course and the receipt of systemic therapy was associated with a significant improvement in survival only in patients who did not undergo complete metastasectomy, highlighting the importance of surgery in the treatment of metastatic/recurrent RCC.[200]

In patients treated with immunotherapy, there are multiple retrospective series demonstrating that patients who underwent metastasectomy had better outcomes than those who did not undergo resection of metastatic sites. In these series, 24% to 100% of patients were disease free 1 to 4 years postsurgery.[201–206] More recent data in patients who have received targeted therapies has shown similar results, albeit in small patient cohorts. In a retrospective, multi-institutional study, only 22 patients with metastatic RCC who underwent metastasectomy after targeted therapy were identified. At a median follow-up of 42 weeks after surgery, 50% of patients had experienced a tumor recurrence; however, only one patient died of RCC 105 weeks after surgery.[207]

Surgical management of recurrent and metastatic RCC plays an important role in the treatment paradigm of this group of patients and appears to confer a survival advantage in retrospective series. However, not all patients will ultimately be optimal surgical candidates and the ability to achieve a complete surgical resection is paramount in helping to guide preoperative surgical decision making.

## SYSTEMIC THERAPY FOR ADVANCED RENAL CELL CARCINOMA

### Prognostic Factors

Clinical characteristics have been extensively studied as potential prognostic factors in metastatic RCC. Performance status is a measure of overall well-being and is the most consistently reported factor associated with survival in advanced RCC, while other demographic features, such as age, gender, and race, are of limited value.[208–211] Some studies have found the presence of visceral (i.e., lung, liver, and adrenal), bone, and brain metastases to be associated with poor survival,[208,211,212] whereas others have found no relationship between these sites and prognosis.[210,213] A more reliable finding is the number of metastatic sites present, which provides a rough estimate of tumor burden. Most studies have found that patients with higher number of metastatic sites (more than two) are independently associated with at least two-fold greater probability of death. Similarly, patients with a short interval from initial RCC diagnosis to metastases have been found to have a worse outcome, likely as a reflection of faster-growing disease.[209,211,214,215] Those with synchronous metastases have outcomes intermediate between those with metastases developing within 1 year of diagnosis and those with asynchronous metastases that develop later.[216] Investigators have evaluated the effects of several laboratory parameters in patients with advanced RCC. Erythrocyte sedimentation rate, C-reactive protein, hemoglobin, white blood cell, and platelet parameters have been evaluated. Elevated erythrocyte sedimentation rate and C-reactive protein were consistently found to be independent poor prognostic factors.[64,214,217,218] Patients with thrombocytosis (defined as platelet counts >400,000/µL), another potential marker of inflammation, have been reported to have a negative impact on survival mostly in patients with localized RCC. Studies overall have been inconsistent in the metastatic setting, especially when other markers of inflammation were considered. Anemia has also consistently been found to be an independent prognostic factor for an adverse outcome. Patients with pretreatment hemoglobin below the lower limit of laboratory normal values were found to have twice the risk of death compared with patients with normal hemoglobin in several large studies.[210,211] The mechanism of effect of such blood parameters is unknown—whether these markers reflect an underlying inflammatory disease and/or somehow contribute to the disease process itself is unclear. Other biochemical factors that have been implicated in RCC prognosis include pretreatment serum LDH and calcium (corrected for albumin), while serum alkaline phosphatase, creatinine, gamma glutamyltransefrease, and triglycerides have not been found to have prognostic value. Corrected serum calcium >10 mg/dL and LDH >1.5 times the upper limit of normal have been associated with a two- to three-fold higher risk of death, respectively.[210,211,214]

## Prognostic Schema

Using the previously identified variables, investigators have combined these variables to stratify patients into "risk groups" to predict outcome. Such schema serve to aid in individual patient counseling, stratify patients for randomized clinical trial entry, and aid in interpretation of nonrandomized clinical trials (Table 37.7). The most commonly employed schema from Memorial Sloan-Kettering Cancer Center was developed from patients treated with IFN-based regimens.[219] This schema uses Eastern Cooperative Oncology Group performance status, anemia, LDH, corrected serum calcium, and time from diagnosis to metastatic disease to segregate patients into three risk groups. This schema is still widely used today despite the limited IFN use currently and has been shown to also segregate patients treated with newer agents. More recent efforts have developed prognostic variables and risk groups based on patients treated with targeted agents. This schema uses hemoglobin, corrected calcium, performance status, and time from diagnosis to treatment, but additionally neutrophil and platelet count.[187] Both Memorial Sloan-Kettering Cancer Center and Heng criteria are used to describe patient populations treated in the targeted therapy era.

## Predictive Markers

With the shift in systemic therapy for RCC to molecularly targeted agents, looking at the molecular characteristics of tumors

| TABLE 37.7 | | |
|---|---|---|
| **Prognostic System in Metastatic Renal Cell Carcinoma** | | |
| **Schema** | **Factors** | **Comments** |
| MSKCC[215] | ▪ Low Karnofsky performance status<br>▪ High lactate dehydrogenase<br>▪ Low serum hemoglobin<br>▪ High corrected serum calcium<br>▪ Time from initial RCC diagnosis to start of therapy <1 y | Developed from patients with metastatic RCC patients treated with IFN-based therapy on clinical trials at MSKCC |
| Heng et al.[187] | ▪ Low Karnofsky performance status<br>▪ Low serum hemoglobin<br>▪ High corrected serum calcium<br>▪ Time from initial RCC diagnosis to start of therapy <1 y<br>▪ Elevated neutrophils<br>▪ Elevated platelets | Developed from retrospective data for a global multicenter consortium of patients receiving targeted therapy for metastatic RCC |

MSKCC, Memorial Sloan-Kettering Cancer Center; RCC, renal cell carcinoma; IFN, interferon.

has occurred to identify additional prognostic factors. VHL gene status has been investigated for an association with clinical outcome. Over multiple retrospective series and prospective trials, VHL status (and other VHL pathway elements, such as hypoxia-inducible factor expression) has not been consistently associated with response to vascular endothelial growth factor (VEGF)-targeted agents.[220–222] CA-IX, a member of the carbonic anhydrase family, regulates pH during hypoxia and is a product of the hypoxia inducible transcription factor (HIF) complex overexpression. The vast majority of ccRCC tumor samples stain positive for CA-IX and high CA-IX staining (>85% staining by immunohistochemical analysis) was found to be an independent favorable prognostic indicator of survival in patients with metastatic ccRCC.[223] Retrospective data initially suggested CA-IX to be potentially associated with response to high-dose interleukin (IL)-2.[224] However, the prospective SELECT trial failed to confirm this finding and thus there remain no predictive biomarkers to identify the small percentage of patients who will have a complete response to high-dose IL-2.[225] Single nucleotide polymorphisms, which are natural variations in tumor and/or germline DNA sequences, have also been investigated in relation to targeted therapy efficacy and toxicity in RCC.[226–228] While several retrospective series have found associations between single nucleotide polymorphisms associated with the VEGF pathway and/or drug metabolism with outcome, none have been consistent or robust enough to currently affect clinical practice. Finally, clinical markers, such as treatment-induced hypertension, have been explored. Several retrospective data sets have identified a strong association of treatment-induced hypertension and clinical outcome in response to VEGF-targeting agents.[229,230] This has been identified across mechanism of agent and including non-RCC diseases.[231] The precise biologic mechanism underlying this observation remains to be elucidated. In addition, this observation requires treatment of all patients initially and as a result does not spare ineffective therapy for patients who will not benefit.

## Systemic Therapy

Although several active agents now exist for metastatic RCC (as discussed subsequently), they are considered noncurative for the majority of patients and thus require chronic therapy. Thus, benefits must be weighed against the toxicity, time commitment, and cost. There exists a subset of patients with metastatic RCC with low-volume slow-growing disease in which withholding systemic therapy until radiographic progression has occurred may be a reasonable approach. Further investigation into this strategy is ongoing.

Historically, progestational agents such as medroxyprogesterone acetate were investigated in metastatic RCC.[232,233] These reports documented some tumor regression and symptom reduction, largely applied to a very advanced, symptomatic population of RCC patients. Multicenter randomized trials demonstrate uniformly low response rates.[234] In the current era, progestational agents may be useful for symptom palliation, but do not appear to have any significant antitumor effects.

Due to success in other solid tumors, chemotherapy for advanced RCC has been extensively studied during the last four decades. A summary of clinical trials from 1983 to 1993 noted a 6% overall response rate in 4,093 patients with advanced RCC.[235] Another report of 51 published phase 2 clinical trials ($n = 1,347$) involving 33 chemotherapeutic agents noted an overall response rate of 5.5%.[236] Combinations of 5-fluorouracil and analogues with gemcitabine have produced modestly higher response rates, on the order of 10% to 15%.[237,238] Similarly, the addition of chemotherapy to cytokine regimens has not resulted in significant benefit over cytokines alone when investigated in phase 3 trials.[239,240] A report of 18 metastatic RCC patients with sarcomatoid histologic features and/or rapidly progressing disease treated with doxorubicin and gemcitabine noted a 28% objective response rate (ORR), potentially identifying a subset of patients with RCC where chemotherapy may have some utility.[241] Overall, chemotherapy currently has little to no role in the treatment of metastatic RCC pending further study of novel chemotherapeutic agents or combinations, or perhaps through additional patient selection efforts.

## Immunotherapy

IL-2 and IFN had been the standard of care for patients with metastatic RCC until the development of targeted therapy. These agents are nonspecific cytokines that presumably have an antitumor effect through stimulation of an antitumor immune response that is not adequate in the patient prior to therapy. Specific insights into mechanism(s) of action are still lacking after decades of use and further clinical and/or molecular markers to predict benefit are lacking.

Bolus high-dose intravenous IL-2 treatment, as initially described many years ago, leads to sustained responses in a small subset of patients.[242] However, later randomized trials failed to demonstrate a benefit over lower-dose cytokine regimens for the entire cohort, likely reflecting the small number of patients benefitting.[243,244] The durable complete remissions that occur in 5% to 7% of patients, however, served as the basis for US Food and Drug Administration (FDA) approval of high-dose IL-2 in the United States in 1992.[245–247] Thus, given the noncurative nature of targeted therapy and considering only a small fraction of patients are eligible for this toxic treatment, IL-2 remains a viable treatment option for patients with ccRCC and a good performance status.

IFN (given only in low doses in RCC) has also been employed. While never approved by the FDA specifically for this indication, two large randomized trials demonstrated that IFN improved OS compared with medroxyprogesterone[234] or vinblastine.[248] IFN thus was a community standard for metastatic RCC prior to targeted therapy and served as the comparator arm in many trials. Single-agent IFN is generally no longer used. As noted in the following, IFN combined with bevacizumab is a currently approved regimen for metastatic RCC, although in practice many oncologists use bevacizumab monotherapy as the IFN likely adds some benefit, but significantly more toxicity. Multiple attempts over many decades to improve on the modest effects of IL-2 and IFN, including combinations of cytokines, combinations with chemotherapy, and cytokine sequencing, have failed.[249–252]

## Investigational Immunotherapy

RCC has long been considered responsive to immune manipulation due to the modest response to cytokines noted previously. Additional efforts are ongoing to expand the application of immunotherapy. Specifically, IMA901, a vaccine composed of multiple tumor-associated peptides, has been found to be safe and to induce antitumor immunity in patients with metastatic RCC.[253] Based in part on data that sunitinib may favorably modulate the immune repertoire,[254] a phase 3 trial that randomized patients with metastatic RCC to sunitinib alone or sunitinib in combination with IMA901 has completed accrual. In addition, an autologous dendritic cell vaccine derived from primary patient tumor-specific antigens demonstrated favorable results in phase 2 studies and is currently in phase 3 testing.[255]

In addition, checkpoint inhibitors, agents that stimulate antitumor immunity by releasing the natural "brake" of the immune system, have entered clinical testing in metastatic RCC with promising initial results.[256,257] Nivolumab, which binds to programmed death receptor 1 is one such checkpoint inhibitor. A phase I expansion RCC cohort reported a 30% ORR associated with durable responses even after therapy was stopped. Additional phase II trials and a phase III registration trial are ongoing. In addition, several anti–programmed death receptor 1 agents and antibodies against its ligand, PD-L1, are being investigated in metastatic RCC.

### Vascular Endothelial Growth Factor–Targeted Therapy

RCC presents a unique clinical setting for the application of antiangiogenic approaches. Through mutations in the *VHL* gene and/or other genetic events that result in the deregulated expression of the hypoxia inducible transcription factors, HIF-1α and/or HIF-2α, a large cohort of hypoxia-responsive genes is induced, including VEGF as one of the classic transcriptional targets.[258] There is a direct link between *VHL* mutation and upregulation of angiogenesis-promoting proteins, including VEGF and platelet-derived growth factor (PDGF). Thus, increased expression of these proteins and the consequences of that increased expression are central events in the development of most RCC tumors. VEGF is the major factor responsible for tumor angiogenesis. Several treatment strategies have thus been investigated in metastatic RCC to block components of the angiogenic signaling pathway components, such as VEGF.

### Sunitinib

Sunitinib (Sutent, Pfizer Inc., New York, NY) is an oral drug with in vitro and cellular inhibitory activity against several related protein tyrosine kinase receptors, including PDGF-receptor-beta, stem cell factor receptor (KIT), and Fms-like tyrosine kinase-3 (FLT-3), as well as VEGF receptors 1, 2, and 3.[259,260] Sunitinib was initially studied in metastatic RCC in two sequential phase 2 trials in cytokine-refractory patients that demonstrated an ORR of approximately 40% with a combined median PFS of 8.2 months (Table 37.8).[261,262] The most common adverse events with sunitinib are fatigue, diarrhea, mucositis, hand-foot syndrome, and hypertension. A phase 3 randomized trial of first-line sunitinib versus IFN-alfa in 750 patients with metastatic ccRCC showed statistically significant improvements in ORR and PFS with sunitinib compared with IFN. Median PFS as assessed by an

## Summary of Target Agents in Metastatic Renal Cell Carcinoma

| Treatment | Response Rate | Progression-Free Survival | Overall Survival |
|---|---|---|---|
| *VEGF Receptor Inhibitors* | | | |
| Sunitinib | 30% to 47% | 9.5 to 11 mo in treatment-naïve patients<br>8.4 mo in cytokine refractory patients | 29.3 mo in untreated patients |
| Pazopanib | 30% | 8.4 to 9.2 mo<br>(11.1 mo in treatment-naïve patients) | 28.4 mo in untreated patients |
| Sorafenib | 2% to 10% | 5.7 to 9 mo in treatment-naïve patients<br>5.5 mo in treatment-refractory patients | 17.8 to 19.2 mo in treatment-refractory patients |
| Axitinib | 19% | 6.7 mo (second-line) | 20.1 mo in treatment-refractory patients |
| *VEGF Ligand-Binding Agents* | | | |
| Bevacizumab | 10% to 13% as monotherapy<br>26% to 31% in combination<br>with IFNA | 8.5 mo in treatment-naïve patients as monotherapy<br>8.5 to 10.2 mo in treatment-naïve patients in combination with IFNA<br>4.8 mo in cytokine-refractory patients | 18.3 to 23.3 mo |
| *mTOR-Inhibiting Agents* | | | |
| Temsirolimus | 7% to 9% | 3.7 mo (vs. 1.9 mo for IFNA monotherapy; $p = 0.0001$) in treatment-naïve patients<br>5.8 mo in treatment-refractory patients | 10.9 mo (vs. 7.3 mo for IFNA; $p = 0.008$) |
| Everolimus | 1% | 4.9 mo (vs. 1.9 mo for placebo-treated patients) in refractory patients | 14.8 mo (vs. 14.4 mo for placebo-treated patients; $p = 0.177$) |

VEGF, vascular endothelial growth factor; IFNA, interferon-alfa; mTOR, mammalian target of rapamycin.

independent review was 11 months in the sunitinib arm versus 5 months in the IFN arm, and ORR was 31% versus 6%, respectively ($p < 0.000001$; see Table 37.8).[263] Median OS was 26.4 months for sunitinib versus 21.8 months for IFN ($p = 0.051$).[264] The OS data are a reflection of not only sunitinib activity, but several other active drugs that patients received upon progression, resulting in notably prolonged median survival times compared to historical controls. Sunitinib was approved by the FDA as monotherapy for advanced RCC in January 2006 and remains an initial standard of care in metastatic RCC.

### Pazopanib

Pazopanib is an oral multitargeted tyrosine kinase inhibitor that targets VEGF receptors 1 to 3, PDGF receptor, and c-kit. A phase 2 study initially designed as a randomized discontinuation study was revised to an open-label study based on the response rate of a planned interim analysis. This study evaluated 255 patients with metastatic RCC who received pazopanib 800 mg once daily; 69% had no prior treatment and 31% had received one prior treatment. The overall response rate was 35%, the median PFS was 52 weeks, and the median duration of response was 68 weeks. The main adverse effects were diarrhea and fatigue, and the most common grade 3-4 side effect was hypertension. Alanine transaminase and aspartate transaminase elevation occurred in 54% of patients. In October 2009, the FDA approved pazopanib for the treatment of metastatic RCC, based on the results of a phase 3 trial. This study evaluated 435 patients with advanced ccRCC with either no previous treatment or with one prior cytokine treatment. Patients were randomized (2:1) to receive pazopanib 800 mg daily or placebo. The response rate for patients treated with pazopanib was 30% and the median duration of response was 58.7 weeks. Median PFS was 9.2 months in the pazopanib group and 4.2 months in the placebo group (HR = 0.46; $p < 0.0001$; see Table 37.8). PFS was prolonged in both treatment naïve patients (11.1 months versus 2.8 months;

$p < 0.0001$) and in cytokine-pretreated patients (7.4 months versus 4.2 months; $p < 0.001$).

Pazopanib has been further studied in a noninferiority study compared to sunitinib in the front-line treatment of metastatic RCC (COMPARZ study).[265] Over 1,100 patients with previously untreated ccRCC were randomized to either pazopanib or sunitinib (1:1) in a noninferiority design. Median PFS was 9.5 months with sunitinib and 8.4 months with pazopanib, with a hazard ratio of 1.047 (95% CI = 0.898 to 1.220). The upper bound of the confidence interval was $<1.25$, satisfying the predefined boundary for noninferiority. OS was approximately 29 months in both arms. Certain toxicities were more common with sunitinib including fatigue and hand-foot syndrome, while pazopanib produced greater hepatic abnormalities. This trial demonstrated that both sunitinib and pazopanib are appropriate front-line treatment options in metastatic RCC and that a differing toxicity profile may allow the physician to tailor therapy to each individual patient.

### Sorafenib

Sorafenib (Nexavar, Bayer Pharmaceuticals and Onyx, Leverkusen, Germany) is an oral multikinase inhibitor that inhibits VEGF receptors 1 to 3, PDGF-receptor-beta, and the serine threonine kinase Raf-1, which acts through the RAF/MEK/ERK signaling pathway and plays a role in cellular proliferation and tumorigenesis.[266,267] In an initial sorafenib trial, metastatic RCC patients ($n = 202$) were treated with 12 weeks of continuous oral sorafenib 400 mg bid and patients with tumor burden increase or decrease within 25% of baseline were randomized to placebo or to continuation of sorafenib. A PFS advantage of 24 versus 6 weeks ($p = 0.0087$) was demonstrated in the randomized cohort of 65 patients at 12 weeks postrandomization.[268] A subsequent 905 patient, placebo-controlled, randomized trial of sorafenib 400 mg bid in treatment-refractory, metastatic RCC reported a PFS advantage in the sorafenib arm of 5.5 months versus 2.8 months for placebo ($p < 0.000001$; see Table 37.8). A 2% RECIST-defined ORR was seen in the sorafenib arm, but 74% of patients overall had some degree of tumor burden shrinkage thus accounting for the PFS benefit. The median OS was 19.3 months for patients in the sorafenib group and 15.9 months for patients in the placebo group (HR = 0.77; 95% CI = 0.63 to 0.95; $p = 0.02$), which did not reach prespecified statistical boundaries for significance.[269] Common toxicity in the sorafenib trials has included dermatologic (hand-foot syndrome), fatigue, diarrhea, and hypertension. Sorafenib was approved by the FDA as monotherapy for advanced RCC in December 2005. A randomized phase 2 trial of sorafenib versus IFN in untreated metastatic RCC failed to demonstrate a difference in median PFS between the two treatment arms.[270] Sorafenib has thus assumed a small, salvage role in the treatment of metastatic RCC.

### Bevacizumab

Bevacizumab (Avastin, Genentech, South San Francisco, CA) is a monoclonal antibody that binds and neutralizes circulating VEGF protein.[271] The activity of this agent in RCC was initially identified by small randomized trials.[272,273] Two phase 3 trials were subsequently reported and led to FDA approval of bevacizumab plus IFN for advanced RCC. One phase 3 trial randomized 649 untreated patients with metastatic RCC to treatment with IFN (Roferon, Roche, Basel, Switzerland) plus placebo infusion or to IFN plus bevacizumab infusion 10 mg/kg every 2 weeks.[274] A significant advantage for bevacizumab plus IFN was observed for ORR (31% versus 13%, $p < 0.0001$) and PFS (10.2 months versus 5.4 months, $p < 0.0001$; see Table 37.8). A second multicenter phase 3 trial, conducted in the United States and Canada through the Cancer and Leukemia Group B, was nearly identical in design with the exception of lacking a placebo infusion and not requiring prior nephrectomy.[275] In this trial, the median PFS was 8.5 months in patients receiving bevacizumab plus IFN (95% CI = 7.5 to 9.7) versus 5.2 months (95% CI = 3.1 to 5.6) for IFN monotherapy ($p < 0.0001$; see Table 37.8). Also, among patients with measurable disease, the ORR was higher in patients treated with bevacizumab plus IFN (25.5%) than for IFN monotherapy (13.1%; $p < 0.0001$). OS data are similar to the other agents with a numerical advantage in median survival not meeting statistical significance, reflecting the large proportion of patents who receive subsequent active therapy. The contribution of IFN to the antitumor effect of this regimen is unclear at present, although preliminary results indicate a longer PFS and higher response rate than expected with bevacizumab monotherapy.[272] Combination IFN and bevacizumab therapy is more toxic than either as monotherapy, notable for fatigue, anorexia, hypertension, and proteinuria. Thus, the use of IFN with bevacizumab requires evaluation of the risk/benefit ratio for each patient.

### Axitinib

Axitinib is a potent VEGF receptor family inhibitor studied in several setting in metastatic RCC. Initial studies in cytokine- and sorafenib-refractory patients demonstrated objective responses and disease control, which prompted further development.[276,277] The phase 3 AXIS trial randomized 723 patients with metastatic RCC (refractory to either sunitinib, cytokines, bevacizumab, or temsirolimus) to axitinib or sorafenib.[278] The median PFS was 6.7 months for axitinib versus 4.7 months for sorafenib (HR for disease progression or death of 0.665 [95% CI = 0.544 to 0.812]; $p < 0.0001$). ORR was 19.4% versus 9.4% with axitinib and sorafenib, respectively. This trial resulted in FDA approval of axitinib for previously treated metastatic RCC. A separate trial examined axitinib versus sorafenib in the front-line setting.[279] Despite a numerical advantage for PFS for axitinib, this trial did not meet its stringent predefined efficacy endpoint, and thus axitinib is largely used in the second-line setting in RCC.

## Mammalian Target of Rapamycin–Targeted Therapy

### Temsirolimus

Temsirolimus is an inhibitor of mTOR, a molecule implicated in multiple tumor-promoting intracellular signaling pathways, including regulation of transcription factors involved in VEGF expression, such as HIF.[280] A phase 2 trial in patients with treatment-refractory, metastatic RCC randomized 111 patients to temsirolimus at one of multiple dose levels (25 mg, 75 mg, or 250 mg intravenously weekly).[281] The ORR was 7% with additional patients demonstrating minor responses (see Table 37.8). Retrospective assignment of risk criteria to patients in this study identified a poor-prognosis group with a median OS of 8.2 months compared to 4.9 months for historical IFN-treated patients.[215] Loss of phosphatase and tensin homolog and/or activation of Akt (upstream regulators of the mTOR expression) may be more common in poor-risk patients and thereby potentially increase the relevance of mTOR-targeted therapy in this subgroup.

A subsequent randomized phase 3 trial was conducted in patients with metastatic RCC ($n = 626$) and three or more adverse risk features as defined by existing prognostic schema (see Table 37.7).[211,215] Patients were randomized equally to receive IFN (18 million units subcutaneously) three times a week, temsirolimus 25 mg intravenously weekly, or temsirolimus 15 mg intravenously weekly and IFN (6 million units subcutaneously) three times a week. The primary study endpoint was OS and the study was powered to compare each of the temsirolimus arms to the IFN arm. Both temsirolimus-containing arms demonstrated a PFS advantage versus IFN (3.7 months for each arm versus 1.9 months; $p = 0.0001$ for temsirolimus monotherapy and $p = 0.0019$ for temsirolimus plus IFN). Patients treated with temsirolimus monotherapy had a statistically longer survival than those treated with IFN alone (10.9 months versus 7.3 months, $p = 0.0069$). OS of patients treated with IFN and temsirolimus + IFN were not statistically different (7.3 months versus 8.4 months, $p = 0.6912$). Even though temsirolimus has demonstrated activity in poor-risk RCC, it is not clear that this agent has more activity than the VEGF-targeted agents in this subset, as VEGF-targeted agents have shown activity, albeit in limited subsets, in poor-risk patients.

### Everolimus

Everolimus is an oral rapamycin analogue that inhibits mTOR. A phase 3 study evaluated 410 patients previously treated with sorafenib, sunitinib, or both who were randomized (2:1) to receive everolimus 10 mg once daily or placebo.[282] PFS was significantly longer in the everolimus group (HR = 0.30, 95% CI = 0.22 to 0.40; $p < 0.0001$). Median PFS in the everolimus group was 4.9 months versus 1.9 months in the placebo group. Partial response in the everolimus group occurred in 1% of the patients, and 63% (versus 32% in the placebo group) had disease stabilization for at least 56 days. Most common adverse effects of everolimus were stomatitis, rash, fatigue, asthenia, and diarrhea. Stomatitis, fatigue, infection, and pneumonitis were the most common grade 3/4 toxicities. On the basis of these results, everolimus was approved for the treatment of metastatic RCC refractory to sunitinib and/or sorafenib.

A recent trial (RECORD-3) randomized 471 patients with previously untreated metastatic RCC to either sunitinib or everolimus, with crossover at progression.[283] This trial, reported to date only in abstract form, demonstrated an advantage to sunitinib in response rate (27% versus 8%), PFS (10.7 months versus 7.9 months), and OS (32 months versus 22 months). In addition, all subsets examined (non–clear cell, clear cell, and prognostic groups) favored sunitinib. These data support the use of everolimus only in a refractory setting and confirm a hypothesis that VEGF targeting is a superior initial strategy for RCC therapy.

## Second-Line Therapy

As noted previously, axitinib has been studied and FDA-approved as second-line therapy in metastatic RCC with a PFS advantage over sorafenib. Still debated is the role of everolimus versus a VEGF agent in this setting. The INTORSECT trial randomized patients with metastatic RCC refractory to prior sunitinib to receive either temsirolimus or sorafenib.[284] Although there was no significant difference in PFS (approximately 4 months in both arms), an OS advantage to sorafenib was observed. These data lend support to the hypothesis that continued VEGF targeting is of benefit in metastatic RCC, although no PFS advantage was demonstrated and the mTOR inhibitor used in this trial had not been specifically shown to have benefits in this setting.

## Current Status of Systemic Therapy in Metastatic Renal Cell Carcinoma

Of note, several trials have been conducted attempting to combine the targeted therapies discussed previously. None have demonstrated an advantage over monotherapy, in large part due to excessive toxicity in the combination arms.[285,286] Sunitinib and pazopanib are the most commonly used front-line agents based in large part on the COMPARZ efficacy data as well as their tolerability and oral formulation. There is no proven sequence of agents or ability to predict response to any given agent, and thus the current

standard of care is an empiric sequence of targeted therapy monotherapy, notwithstanding the select patient who initially receives high-dose IL-2.

## CONCLUSION AND FUTURE DIRECTIONS

The last 20 years have seen a tremendous increase in our understanding of the tumor biology of the heterogeneous tumors within the family of renal cancers. Insights beginning with the clinical observation of the hypervascularity of these tumors, continuing with rigorous scientific investigation of familial cases of RCC, and culminating in the development of treatments based on the VEGF pathway, have made the last decade a rich period of expansion in treatment options for RCC. With increasing availability of next generation sequencing, the potential for subsequent discoveries to advance our understanding of and therapies for this often lethal malignancy remains considerable. Through multidisciplinary explorations of these fascinating neoplasms, renal cancer can continue to pace oncologic discoveries for the next 20 years as well.

## ACKNOWLEDGMENTS

The authors would like to thank Sabrina Noyes for administrative support and technical editing.

# REFERENCES

1. Ferlay J, Shin HR, Bray F, et al. Estimates of worldwide burden of cancer in 2008: GLOBOCAN 2008. *Int J Cancer* 2010;127:2893–2917.
2. Siegel R, Naishadham D, Jemal A. Cancer statistics, 2013. *CA Cancer J Clin* 2013;63:11–30.
3. Lipsky MJ, Deibert CM, McKiernan JM. Epidemiology, screening, and clinical staging. In: Libertino JA, ed. *Renal Cancer: Contemporary Management.* New York: Springer Science + Business Media; 2013:1–18.
4. Luciani LG, Cestari R, Tallarigo C. Incidental renal cell carcinoma-age and stage characterization and clinical implications: study of 1092 patients (1982–1997). *Urology* 2000;56:58–62.
5. Decastro GJ, McKiernan JM. Epidemiology, clinical staging, and presentation of renal cancer. *Urol Clin North Am* 2008;35:581–592; vi.
6. Kummerlin IP, ten Kate FJ, Wijkstra H, et al. Changes in the stage and surgical management of renal tumours during 1995-2005: an analysis of the Dutch national histopathology registry. *BJU Int* 2008;102:946–951.
7. Verhoest G, Veillard D, Guille F, et al. Relationship between age at diagnosis and clinicopathologic features of renal cell carcinoma. *Eur Urol* 2007;51:1298–1304; discussion 1304–1305.
8. Stafford HS, Saltzstein SL, Shimasaki S, et al. Racial/ethnic and gender disparities in renal cell carcinoma incidence and survival. *J Urol* 2008;179:1704–1708.
9. Ljungberg B, Campbell SC, Choo HY, et al. The epidemiology of renal cell carcinoma. *Eur Urol* 2011;60:615–621.
10. Hunt JD, van der Hel OL, McMillan GP, et al. Renal cell carcinoma in relation to cigarette smoking: meta-analysis of 24 studies. *Int J Cancer* 2005;114:101–108.
11. Renehan AG, Tyson M, Egger M, et al. Body-mass index and incidence of cancer: a systematic review and meta-analysis of prospective observational studies. *Lancet* 2008;371:569–578.
12. Grossman E, Messerli FH, Boyko V, et al. Is there an association between hypertension and cancer mortality? *Am J Med* 2002;112:479–486.
13. Grossman E, Messerli FH, Goldbourt U. Antihypertensive therapy and the risk of malignancies. *Eur Heart J* 2001;22:1343–1352.
14. Cho E, Curhan G, Hankinson SE, et al. Prospective evaluation of analgesic use and risk of renal cell cancer. *Arch Intern Med* 2011;171:1487–1493.
15. Mihara S, Kuroda K, Yoshioka R, et al. Early detection of renal cell carcinoma by ultrasonographic screening—based on the results of 13 years screening in Japan. *Ultrasound Med Biol* 1999;25:1033–1039.
16. Algaba F, Akaza H, Lopez-Beltran A, et al. Current pathology keys of renal cell carcinoma. *Eur Urol* 2011;60:634–643.
17. Deng F-M, Melamed J, Zhou M. Pathology of renal cell carcinoma. In: Libertino JA, ed. *Renal Cancer: Contemporary Management.* New York: Springer Science + Business Media; 2013:51–69.
18. Fuhrman SA, Lasky LC, Limas C. Prognostic significance of morphologic parameters in renal cell carcinoma. *Am J Surg Pathol* 1982;6:655–663.
19. Cheville JC, Lohse CM, Zincke H, et al. Comparisons of outcome and prognostic features among histologic subtypes of renal cell carcinoma. *Am J Surg Pathol* 2003;27:612–624.
20. Kang SK, Chandarana H. Contemporary imaging of the renal mass. *Urol Clin North Am* 2012;39:161–170.
21. Divgi CR, Uzzo RG, Gatsonis C, et al. Positron emission tomography/computed tomography identification of clear cell renal cell carcinoma: results from the REDECT trial. *J Clin Oncol* 2013;31:187–194.
22. Bosniak MA. The Bosniak renal cyst classification: 25 years later. *Radiology* 2012;262:781–785.
23. Corcoran AT, Russo P, Lowrance WT, et al. A review of contemporary data on surgically resected renal masses—benign or malignant? *Urology* 2013;81:707–713.
24. Lane BR, Babineau D, Kattan MW, et al. A preoperative prognostic nomogram for solid enhancing renal tumors 7 cm or less amenable to partial nephrectomy. *J Urol* 2007;178:429–434.
25. Lane BR, Aydin H, Danforth TL, et al. Clinical correlates of renal angiomyolipoma subtypes in 209 patients: classic, fat poor, tuberous sclerosis associated and epithelioid. *J Urol* 2008;180:836–843.
26. Eggener SE, Rubenstein JN, Smith ND, et al. Renal tumors in young adults. *J Urol* 2004;171:106–110.
27. Frank I, Blute ML, Cheville JC, et al. Solid renal tumors: an analysis of pathological features related to tumor size. *J Urol* 2003;170:2217–2220.
28. Kutikov A, Smaldone MC, Egleston BL, et al. Anatomic features of enhancing renal masses predict malignant and high-grade pathology: a preoperative nomogram using the RENAL Nephrometry score. *Eur Urol* 2011;60:241–248.
29. Halverson SJ, Kunju LP, Bhalla R, et al. Accuracy of determining small renal mass management with risk stratified biopsies: confirmation by final pathology. *J Urol* 2013;189:441–446.
30. Lane BR, Samplaski MK, Herts BR, et al. Renal mass biopsy—a renaissance? *J Urol* 2008;179:20–27.
31. Samplaski MK, Zhou M, Lane BR, et al. Renal mass sampling: an enlightened perspective. *Int J Urol* 2011;18:5–19.
32. Leveridge M, Musquera M, Evans A, et al. Renal cell carcinoma in the native and allograft kidneys of renal transplant recipients. *J Urol* 2011;186:219–223.
33. Schmidbauer J, Remzi M, Memarsadeghi M, et al. Diagnostic accuracy of computed tomography-guided percutaneous biopsy of renal masses. *Eur Urol* 2008;53:1003–1011.
34. Volpe A, Finelli A, Gill IS, et al. Rationale for percutaneous biopsy and histologic characterisation of renal tumours. *Eur Urol* 2012;62:491–504.
35. Edge SB, Byrd DR, Compton CC. *AJCC Cancer Staging Manual.* Vol 7. New York, NY: Springer; 2010.
36. Meskawi M, Sun M, Trinh QD, et al. A review of integrated staging systems for renal cell carcinoma. *Eur Urol* 2012;62:303–314.
37. Linehan WM, Pinto PA, Bratslavsky G, et al. Hereditary kidney cancer: unique opportunity for disease-based therapy. *Cancer* 2009;115:2252–2261.
38. Linehan WM, Ricketts CJ. The metabolic basis of kidney cancer. *Semin Cancer Biol* 2013;23:46–55.

39. Shuch B, Pinto P. Familial and hereditary syndromes. In: Libertino JA, ed. *Renal Cancer: Contemporary Management.* New York: Springer Science + Business Media; 2013:39–50.
40. Keefe SM, Nathanson KL, Rathmell WK. The molecular biology of renal cell carcinoma. *Semin Oncol* 2013;40:421–428.
41. Jonasch E, Futreal PA, Davis IJ, et al. State of the science: an update on renal cell carcinoma. *Mol Cancer Res* 2012;10:859–880.
42. Klomp J, Dykema K, Teh BT, et al. Molecular biology and genetics. In: Libertino JA, ed. *Renal Cancer: Contemporary Management.* New York: Springer Science + Business Media; 2013:19–37.
43. Zhao Q, Caballero OL, Davis ID, et al. Tumor-specific isoform switch of the fibroblast growth factor receptor 2 underlies the mesenchymal and malignant phenotypes of clear cell renal cell carcinomas. *Clin Cancer Res* 2013;19:2460–2472.
44. Cancer Genome Atlas Research Network. Comprehensive molecular characterization of clear cell renal cell carcinoma. *Nature* 2013;499:43–49.
45. Chen F, Kishida T, Yao M, et al. Germline mutations in the von Hippel-Lindau disease tumor suppressor gene: correlations with phenotype. *Hum Mutat* 1995;5:66–75.
46. Shuch B, Singer EA, Bratslavsky G. The surgical approach to multifocal renal cancers: hereditary syndromes, ipsilateral multifocality, and bilateral tumors. *Urol Clin North Am* 2012;39:133–148, v.
47. Bottaro DP, Rubin JS, Faletto DL, et al. Identification of the hepatocyte growth factor receptor as the c-met proto-oncogene product. *Science* 1991;251:802–804.
48. Ooi A, Wong JC, Petillo D, et al. An antioxidant response phenotype shared between hereditary and sporadic type 2 papillary renal cell carcinoma. *Cancer Cell* 2011;20:511–523.
49. Lipworth L, Tarone RE, McLaughlin JK. The epidemiology of renal cell carcinoma. *J Urol* 2006;176:2353–2358.
50. Miller DC, Ruterbusch J, Colt JS, et al. Contemporary clinical epidemiology of renal cell carcinoma: insight from a population based case-control study. *J Urol* 2010;184:2254–2258.
51. Silverman SG, Israel GM, Herts BR, et al. Management of the incidental renal mass. *Radiology* 2008;249:16–31.
52. Aron M, Gill IS, Boorjian SA, et al. Treatment of the 2 to 3 cm renal mass. *J Urol* 2010;184:419–422.
53. Campbell SC, Thomas AA, Rini BI, et al. Response of the primary tumor to neoadjuvant sunitinib in patients with advanced renal cell carcinoma. *J Urol* 2009;181:518–523.
54. Kim SP, Thompson RH. Approach to the small renal mass: to treat or not to treat. *Urol Clin North Am* 2012;39(2):171–179.
55. Kunkle DA, Chen DYT, Greenberg RE, et al. Metastatic progression of enhancing renal masses under active surveillance is associated with rapid interval growth of the primary tumor. *J Urol* 2008;179(4 Suppl):375.
56. Van Poppel H, Becker F, Cadeddu JA, et al. Treatment of localised renal cell carcinoma. *Eur Urol* 2011;60:662–672.
57. Volpe A, Cadeddu JA, Cestari A, et al. Contemporary management of small renal masses. *Eur Urol* 2011;60:501–515.
58. Russo P, Huang W. The medical and oncological rationale for partial nephrectomy for the treatment of T1 renal cortical tumors. *Urol Clin North Am* 2008;35:635–643; vii.
59. Van Poppel H, Da Pozzo L, Albrecht W, et al. A prospective, randomised EORTC intergroup phase 3 study comparing the oncologic outcome of elective nephron-sparing surgery and radical nephrectomy for low-stage renal cell carcinoma. *Eur Urol* 2011;59:543–552.
60. Tan HJ, Norton EC, Ye Z, et al. Long-term survival following partial vs radical nephrectomy among older patients with early-stage kidney cancer. *JAMA* 2012;307:1629–1635.
61. Tobert CM, Riedinger CB, Lane BR. Do we know (or just believe) that partial nephrectomy leads to better survival than radical nephrectomy for renal cancer? *World J Urol* 2014 (Epub ahead of print).
62. Kim SP, Thompson RH, Boorjian SA, et al. Comparative effectiveness for survival and renal function of partial and radical nephrectomy for localized renal tumors: a systematic review and meta-analysis. *J Urol* 2012;188:51–57.
63. Campbell DE, Tustin NB, Riedel E, et al. Cryopreservation decreases receptor PD-1 and ligand PD-L1 coinhibitory expression on peripheral blood mononuclear cell-derived T cells and monocytes. *Clin Vaccine Immunol* 2009;16:1648–1653.
64. Ljungberg B, Grankvist K, Rasmuson T. Serum acute phase reactants and prognosis in renal cell carcinoma. *Cancer* 1995;76:1435–1439.
65. Ljungberg B, Cowan NC, Hanbury DC, et al. EAU guidelines on renal cell carcinoma: the 2010 update. *Eur Urol* 2010;58:398–406.
66. Ljungberg B, Hanbury DC, Kuczyk MA, et al. Renal cell carcinoma guideline. *Eur Urol* 2007;51:1502–1510.
67. Campbell SC, Novick AC, Belldegrun A, et al. Guideline for management of the clinical T1 renal mass. *J Urol* 2009;182:1271–1279.
68. Robson CJ, Churchill BM, Anderson W. The results of radical nephrectomy for renal cell carcinoma. *J Urol* 1969;101:297–301.
69. Lam JS, Klatte T, Patard JJ, et al. Prognostic relevance of tumour size in T3a renal cell carcinoma: a multicentre experience. *Eur Urol* 2007;52:155–162.
70. Thompson RH, Blute ML, Krambeck AE, et al. Patients with pT1 renal cell carcinoma who die from disease after nephrectomy may have unrecognized renal sinus fat invasion. *Am J Surg Pathol* 2007;31:1089–1093.
71. Bratslavsky G, Linehan WM. Surgery: Routine adrenalectomy in renal cancer—an antiquated practice. *Nat Rev Urol* 2011;8:534–536.
72. Lane BR, Tiong HY, Campbell SC, et al. Management of the adrenal gland during partial nephrectomy. *J Urol* 2009;181:2430–2437.
73. Weight CJ, Kim SP, Lohse CM, et al. Routine adrenalectomy in patients with locally advanced renal cell cancer does not offer oncologic benefit and places a significant portion of patients at risk for an asynchronous metastasis in a solitary adrenal gland. *Eur Urol* 2011;60:458–464.
74. Blom JH, van Poppel H, Marechal JM, et al. Radical nephrectomy with and without lymph-node dissection: final results of European Organization for Research and Treatment of Cancer (EORTC) randomized phase 3 trial 30881. *Eur Urol* 2009;55:28–34.
75. Leibovich BC, Blute ML. Lymph node dissection in the management of renal cell carcinoma. *Urol Clin North Am* 2008;35:673–678; viii.
76. Patard JJ, Leray E, Rioux-Leclercq N, et al. Prognostic value of histologic subtypes in renal cell carcinoma: a multicenter experience. *J Clin Oncol* 2005;23:2763–2771.
77. Phillips CK, Taneja SS. The role of lymphadenectomy in the surgical management of renal cell carcinoma. *Urol Oncol* 2004;22:214–224.
78. Nguyen CT, Campbell SC. Salvage of local recurrence after primary thermal ablation for small renal masses. *Expert Rev Anticancer Ther* 2008;8:1899–1905.
79. Diblasio CJ, Snyder ME, Russo P. Mini-flank supra-11th rib incision for open partial or radical nephrectomy. *BJU Int* 2006;97:149–156.
80. Chung SD, Chueh SC, Lai MK, et al. Long-term outcome of hand-assisted laparoscopic radical nephroureterectomy for upper-tract urothelial carcinoma: comparison with open surgery. *J Endourol* 2007;21:595–599.
81. Kawauchi A, Yoneda K, Fujito A, et al. Oncologic outcome of hand-assisted laparoscopic radical nephrectomy. *Urology* 2007;69:53–56.
82. Miyake H, Hara I, Nakano Y, et al. Hand-assisted laparoscopic radical nephrectomy: comparison with conventional open radical nephrectomy. *J Endourol* 2007;21:429–432.
83. Nadler RB, Loeb S, Clemens JQ, et al. A prospective study of laparoscopic radical nephrectomy for T1 tumors—is transperitoneal, retroperitoneal or hand assisted the best approach? *J Urol* 2006;175:1230–1234.
84. Nakada SY. Surgical removal of small renal tumors—going, going, gone? *J Urol* 2005;174:9.
85. Huang WC, Levey AS, Serio AM, et al. Chronic kidney disease after nephrectomy in patients with renal cortical tumours: a retrospective cohort study. *Lancet Oncol* 2006;7:735–740.
86. Lane BR, Russo P, Uzzo RG, et al. Comparison of cold and warm ischemia during partial nephrectomy in 660 solitary kidneys reveals predominant role of nonmodifiable factors in determining ultimate renal function. *J Urol* 2011;185:421–427.
87. Go AS, Chertow GM, Fan D, et al. Chronic kidney disease and the risks of death, cardiovascular events, and hospitalization. *N Engl J Med* 2004;351:1296–1305.
88. Huang WC, Elkin EB, Levey AS, et al. Partial nephrectomy versus radical nephrectomy in patients with small renal tumors—is there a difference in mortality and cardiovascular outcomes? *J Urol* 2009;181:55–62.
89. Miller DC, Schonlau M, Litwin MS, et al. Renal and cardiovascular morbidity after partial or radical nephrectomy. *Cancer* 2008;112:511–520.
90. Thompson RH, Boorjian SA, Lohse CM, et al. Radical nephrectomy for pT1a renal masses may be associated with decreased overall survival compared with partial nephrectomy. *J Urol* 2008;179:468–471; discussion 472–473.
91. Herr HW. A history of partial nephrectomy for renal tumors. *J Urol* 2005;173:705–708.
92. Vermooten V. Indications for conservative surgery in certain renal tumors: a study based on the growth pattern of the cell carcinoma. *J Urol* 1950;64:200–208.
93. Chow WH, Shuch B, Linehan WM, et al. Racial disparity in renal cell carcinoma patient survival according to demographic and clinical characteristics. *Cancer* 2013;119:388–394.
94. Lane BR, Kattan MW. Prognostic models and algorithms in renal cell carcinoma. *Urol Clin North Am* 2008;35:613–625.
95. Uzzo RG, Novick AC. Nephron sparing surgery for renal tumors: indications, techniques and outcomes. *J Urol* 2001;166:6–18.
96. Campbell SC, Novick AC, Streem SB, et al. Management of renal cell carcinoma with coexistent renal artery disease. *J Urol* 1993;150:808–813.
97. Hafez KS, Krishnamurthi V, Campbell SC, et al. Contemporary management of renal cell carcinoma with coexistent renal artery disease: update of the Cleveland Clinic experience. *Urology* 2000;56:382–386.
98. Breau RH, Crispen PL, Jimenez RE, et al. Outcome of stage T2 or greater renal cell cancer treated with partial nephrectomy. *J Urol* 2010;183:903–908.
99. Long CJ, Canter DJ, Kutikov A, et al. Partial nephrectomy for renal masses >/= 7 cm: technical, oncological and functional outcomes. *BJU Int* 2012;109:1450–1456.
100. Kopp RP, Mehrazin R, Palazzi KL, et al. Survival outcomes after radical and partial nephrectomy for clinical T2 renal tumors categorized by RENAL nephrometry score. *BJU Int* 2013 (Epub ahead of print).
101. Lane BR, Golan S, Eggener S, et al. Differential use of partial nephrectomy for intermediate and high complexity tumors may explain variability in reported utilization rates. *J Urol* 2013;189:2047–2053.
102. Lane BR, Fergany AF, Linehan WM, et al. Should preservable parenchyma, and not tumor size, be the main determinant of the feasibility of partial nephrectomy? *Urology* 2010;76:608–609.
103. Fergany AF, Hafez KS, Novick AC. Long-term results of nephron sparing surgery for localized renal cell carcinoma: 10-year followup. *J Urol* 2000;163:442.

CANCERS OF THE GENITOURINARY SYSTEM

104. Lane BR, Campbell SC, Gill IS. Ten-year oncologic outcomes after laparoscopic and open partial nephrectomy. *J Urol* 2013;190:44–49.

105. Lane BR, Fergany AF, Weight CJ, et al. Renal functional outcomes after partial nephrectomy with extended ischemic intervals are better than after radical nephrectomy. *J Urol* 2010;184:1286–1290.

106. Fergany AF, Saad IR, Woo L, et al. Open partial nephrectomy for tumor in a solitary kidney: experience with 400 cases. *J Urol* 2006;175:1630–1633.

107. Ghavamian R, Cheville JC, Lohse CM, et al. Renal cell carcinoma in the solitary kidney: an analysis of complications and outcome after nephron sparing surgery. *J Urol* 2002;168:454–459.

108. Gorin MA, Ekwenna O, Soloway MS, et al. Dramatic reduction in tumor burden with neoadjuvant sunitinib prior to bilateral nephron-sparing surgery. *Urology* 2012;79:e11.

109. Kroon BK, de Bruijn R, Prevoo W, et al. Probability of downsizing primary tumors of renal cell carcinoma by targeted therapies is related to size at presentation. *Urology* 2013;81:111–115.

110. Thomas AA, Rini BI, Campbell SC. Integration of surgery and systemic therapy in the management of metastatic renal cancer. *Curr Urol Rep* 2009;10:35–41.

111. Lane BR, Derweesh IH, Kim HL, et al. Presurgical sunitinib reduces tumor size and may facilitate partial nephrectomy in patients with renal cell carcinoma. *Urology* (In press).

112. Bensalah K, Pantuck AJ, Rioux-Leclercq N, et al. Positive surgical margin appears to have negligible impact on survival of renal cell carcinomas treated by nephron-sparing surgery. *Eur Urol* 2010;57:466–471.

113. Bernhard JC, Pantuck AJ, Wallerand H, et al. Predictive factors for ipsilateral recurrence after nephron-sparing surgery in renal cell carcinoma. *Eur Urol* 2010;57:1080–1086.

114. Li QL, Cheng L, Guan HW, et al. Safety and efficacy of mini-margin nephron-sparing surgery for renal cell carcinoma 4-cm or less. *Urology* 2008;71:924–927.

115. Marszalek M, Carini M, Chlosta P, et al. Positive surgical margins after nephron-sparing surgery. *Eur Urol* 2012;61:757–763.

116. Sundaram V, Figenshau RS, Roytman TM, et al. Positive margin during partial nephrectomy: does cancer remain in the renal remnant? *Urology* 2011;77:1400–1403.

117. Yossepowitch O, Thompson RH, Leibovich BC, et al. Positive surgical margins at partial nephrectomy: predictors and oncological outcomes. *J Urol* 2008;179:2158–2163.

118. Lane BR, Gill IS. Five year outcomes of laparoscopic partial nephrectomy. *J Urol* 2007;177:70–74.

119. Gill IS, Kavoussi LR, Lane BR, et al. Comparison of 1,800 laparoscopic and open partial nephrectomies for single renal tumors. *J Urol* 2007;178:41–46.

120. Dulabon LM, Kaouk JH, Haber GP, et al. Multi-institutional analysis of robotic partial nephrectomy for hilar versus nonhilar lesions in 446 consecutive cases. *Eur Urol* 2011;59:325–330.

121. Gill IS, Kamoi K, Aron M, et al. 800 Laparoscopic partial nephrectomies: a single surgeon series. *J Urol* 2010;183:34–41.

122. Kaouk JH, Hillyer SP, Autorino R, et al. 252 robotic partial nephrectomies: Evolving renorrhaphy technique and surgical outcomes at a single institution. *Urology* 2011;78:1338–1344.

123. Kaouk JH, Khalifeh A, Hillyer S, et al. Robot-assisted laparoscopic partial nephrectomy: step-by-step contemporary technique and surgical outcomes at a single high-volume institution. *Eur Urol* 2012;62:553–561.

124. Mullins JK, Feng T, Pierorazio PM, et al. Comparative analysis of minimally invasive partial nephrectomy techniques in the treatment of localized renal tumors. *Urology* 2012;80:316–321.

125. Turna B, Kaouk JH, Frota R, et al. Minimally invasive nephron sparing management for renal tumors in solitary kidneys. *J Urol* 2009;182:2150–2157.

126. Simhan J, Smaldone MC, Tsai KJ, et al. Perioperative outcomes of robotic and open partial nephrectomy for moderately and highly complex renal lesions. *J Urol* 2012;187:2000–2004.

127. Murphy DP, Gill IS. Energy-based renal tumor ablation: a review. *Semin Urol Oncol* 2001;19:133–140.

128. Sterrett SP, Nakada SY, Wingo MS, et al. Renal thermal ablative therapy. *Urol Clin North Am* 2008;35:397–414, viii.

129. Johnson DB, Solomon SB, Su LM, et al. Defining the complications of cryoablation and radio frequency ablation of small renal tumors: a multi-institutional review. *J Urol* 2004;172:874–877.

130. Faddegon S, Cadeddu JA. Does renal mass ablation provide adequate long-term oncologic control? *Urol Clin North Am* 2012;39:181–190.

131. Matin SF, Ahrar K. Management of small renal masses: energy-ablative therapy for small renal masses. In: Campbell SC, Rini BI, eds. *Renal Cell Carcinoma.* Vol 1. Shelton, CT: People's Medical Publishing House; 2009:81–94.

132. Atwell TD, Schmit GD, Boorjian SA, et al. Percutaneous ablation of renal masses measuring 3.0 cm and smaller: comparative local control and complications after radiofrequency ablation and cryoablation. *AJR Am J Roentgenol* 2013;200:461–466.

133. del Cura JL, Zabala R, Iriarte JI, et al. Treatment of renal tumors by percutaneous ultrasound-guided radiofrequency ablation using a multitined electrode: effectiveness and complications. *Eur Urol* 2010;57:459–465.

134. Tanagho YS, Roytman TM, Bhayani SB, et al. Laparoscopic cryoablation of renal masses: single-center long-term experience. *Urology* 2012;80:307–314.

135. Tracy CR, Raman JD, Donnally C, et al. Durable oncologic outcomes after radiofrequency ablation: experience from treating 243 small renal masses over 7.5 years. *Cancer* 2010;116:3135–3142.

136. Campbell SC, Palese MA. Laparoscopic cryoablation for a 3 cm nonhilar renal tumor. *J Urol* 2011;185:14–16.

137. Gill IS, Remer EM, Hasan WA, et al. Renal cryoablation: outcome at 3 years. *J Urol* 2005;173:1903–1907.

138. Guillotreau J, Haber GP, Autorino R, et al. Robotic partial nephrectomy versus laparoscopic cryoablation for the small renal mass. *Eur Urol* 2012;61:899–904.

139. Klatte T, Grubmuller B, Waldert M, et al. Laparoscopic cryoablation versus partial nephrectomy for the treatment of small renal masses: systematic review and cumulative analysis of observational studies. *Eur Urol* 2011;60:435–443.

140. Stein RJ, Kaouk JH. Renal cryotherapy: a detailed review including a 5-year follow-up. *BJU Int* 2007;99:1265–1270.

141. Bolte SL, Ankem MK, Moon TD, et al. Magnetic resonance imaging findings after laparoscopic renal cryoablation. *Urology* 2006;67:485–489.

142. Weight CJ, Kaouk JH, Hegarty NJ, et al. Correlation of radiographic imaging and histopathology following cryoablation and radio frequency ablation for renal tumors. *J Urol* 2008;179:1277–1281.

143. Donat SM, Diaz M, Bishoff JT, et al. Follow-up for clinically localized renal neoplasms: AUA guideline. *J Urol* 2013;190:407–416.

144. Lusch A, Graversen JA, Liss MA, et al. Ablative techniques: Radiofrequency and cryotherapy, which is the best? *Archivos Espanoles de Urologia* 2013;66:71–78.

145. Schmit GD, Thompson RH, Kurup AN, et al. Usefulness of R.E.N.A.L. nephrometry scoring system for predicting outcomes and complications of percutaneous ablation of 751 renal tumors. *J Urol* 2013;189:30–35.

146. Matin SF. Determining failure after renal ablative therapy for renal cell carcinoma: false-negative and false-positive imaging findings. *Urology* 2010;75:1254–1257.

147. Samarasekera D, Khalifeh A, Autorino R, et al. Percutaneous radiofrequency ablation versus percutaneous cryoablation: Long-term outcomes following ablation for renal cell carcinoma. *J Urol* 2013:Abstract 1795.

148. Haber GP, Crouzet S, Remer EM, et al. Stereotactic percutaneous cryoablation for renal tumors: initial clinical experience. *J Urol* 2010;183:884–888.

149. Kroeze SG, Grimbergen MC, Rehmann H, et al. Photodynamic therapy as novel nephron sparing treatment option for small renal masses. *J Urol* 2012;187:289–295.

150. Ponsky LE, Mahadevan A, Gill IS, et al. Renal radiosurgery: initial clinical experience with histological evaluation. *Surg Innov* 2007;14:265–269.

151. Castle SM, Salas N, Leveillee RJ. Initial experience using microwave ablation therapy for renal tumor treatment: 18-month follow-up. *Urology* 2011;77:792–797.

152. Lane BR, Tobert CM, Riedinger CB. Growth kinetics and active surveillance for small renal masses. *Curr Opin Urol* 2012;22:353–359.

153. Lane BR, Abouassaly R, Gao T, et al. Active treatment of localized renal tumors may not impact overall survival in patients aged 75 years or older. *Cancer* 2010;116:3119–3126.

154. Corcoran AT, Russo P, Lowrance WT, et al. A review of contemporary data on surgically resected renal masses—benign or malignant? *Urology* 2013;81:707–713.

155. Smaldone MC, Kutikov A, Egleston BL, et al. Small renal masses progressing to metastases under active surveillance: a systematic review and pooled analysis. *Cancer* 2012;118:997–1006.

156. Crispen PL, Soljic A, Stewart G, et al. Enhancing renal tumors in patients with prior normal abdominal imaging: further insight into the natural history of renal cell carcinoma. *J Urol* 2012;188:1089–1094.

157. Wotkowicz C, Wszolek MF, Libertino JA. Resection of renal tumors invading the vena cava. *Urol Clin North Am* 2008;35:657–671; viii.

158. Gettman MT, Blute ML. Update on pathologic staging of renal cell carcinoma. *Urology* 2002;60:209–217.

159. Sosa RE, Muecke EC, Vaughan ED Jr, et al. Renal cell carcinoma extending into the inferior vena cava: the prognostic significance of the level of vena caval involvement. *J Urol* 1984;132:1097–1100.

160. Quek ML, Stein JP, Skinner DG. Surgical approaches to venous tumor thrombus. *Semin Urol Oncol* 2001;19:88–97.

161. Zisman A, Wieder JA, Pantuck AJ, et al. Renal cell carcinoma with tumor thrombus extension: biology, role of nephrectomy and response to immunotherapy. *J Urol* 2003;169:909–916.

162. Leibovich BC, Cheville JC, Lohse CM, et al. Cancer specific survival for patients with pT3 renal cell carcinoma-can the 2002 primary tumor classification be improved? *J Urol* 2005;173:716–719.

163. Terakawa T, Miyake H, Takenaka A, et al. Clinical outcome of surgical management for patients with renal cell carcinoma involving the inferior vena cava. *Int J Urol* 2007;14:781–784.

164. Blute ML, Leibovich BC, Cheville JC, et al. A protocol for performing extended lymph node dissection using primary tumor pathological features for patients treated with radical nephrectomy for clear cell renal cell carcinoma. *J Urol* 2004;172:465–469.

165. Libertino JA, Zinman L, Watkins E Jr. Long-term results of resection of renal cell cancer with extension into inferior vena cava. *J Urol* 1987;137:21–24.

166. Ciancio G, Livingstone AS, Soloway M. Surgical management of renal cell carcinoma with tumor thrombus in the renal and inferior vena cava: the University of Miami experience in using liver transplantation techniques. *Eur Urol* 2007;51:988–994; discussion 994–995.

167. Glazer AA, Novick AC. Long-term followup after surgical treatment for renal cell carcinoma extending into the right atrium. *J Urol* 1996;155:448–450.

168. Granberg CF, Boorjian SA, Schaff HV, et al. Surgical management, complications, and outcome of radical nephrectomy with inferior vena cava tumor thrombectomy facilitated by vascular bypass. *Urology* 2008;72:148–152.

169. Spiess PE, Kurian T, Lin HY, et al. Preoperative metastatic status, level of thrombus and body mass index predict overall survival in patients undergoing nephrectomy and inferior vena cava thrombectomy. *BJU Int* 2012;110:E470–E474.

170. Kutikov A, Uzzo RG. The R.E.N.A.L. nephrometry score: a comprehensive standardized system for quantitating renal tumor size, location and depth. *J Urol* 2009;182:844–853.

171. Tilki D, Nguyen HG, Dall'era MA, et al. Impact of histologic subtype on cancer-specific survival in patients with renal cell carcinoma and tumor thrombus. *Eur Urol* (Epub ahead of print).

172. Shuch B, Said J, La Rochelle JC, et al. Cytoreductive nephrectomy for kidney cancer with sarcomatoid histology—is up-front resection indicated and, if not, is it avoidable? *J Urol* 2009;182:2164–2171.

173. Ciancio G, Gonzalez J, Shirodkar SP, et al. Liver transplantation techniques for the surgical management of renal cell carcinoma with tumor thrombus in the inferior vena cava: step-by-step description. *Eur Urol* 2011;59:401–406.

174. Slaton JW, Balbay MD, Levy DA, et al. Nephrectomy and vena caval thrombectomy in patients with metastatic renal cell carcinoma. *Urology* 1997;50:673–677.

175. Culp SH, Tannir NM, Abel EJ, et al. Can we better select patients with metastatic renal cell carcinoma for cytoreductive nephrectomy? *Cancer* 2010;116:3378–3388.

176. Margulis V, Master VA, Cost NG, et al. International consultation on urologic diseases and the European Association of Urology international consultation on locally advanced renal cell carcinoma. *Eur Urol* 2011;60:673–683.

177. Crispen PL, Breau RH, Allmer C, et al. Lymph node dissection at the time of radical nephrectomy for high-risk clear cell renal cell carcinoma: indications and recommendations for surgical templates. *Eur Urol* 2011;59:18–23.

178. Capitanio U, Abdollah F, Matloob R, et al. When to perform lymph node dissection in patients with renal cell carcinoma: a novel approach to the preoperative assessment of risk of lymph node invasion at surgery and of lymph node progression during follow-up. *BJU Int* 2013;112:E59–E66.

179. Smaldone MC, Fung C, Uzzo RG, et al. Adjuvant and neoadjuvant therapies in high-risk renal cell carcinoma. *Hematol Oncol Clin North Am* 2011;25:765–791.

180. Motzer RJ, Agarwal N, Beard C, et al. Kidney cancer. *J Natl Compr Canc Netw* 2011;9:960–977.

181. Flanigan RC, Salmon SE, Blumenstein BA, et al. Nephrectomy followed by interferon alfa-2b compared with interferon alfa-2b alone for metastatic renal-cell cancer. *N Engl J Med* 2001;345:1655–1659.

182. Flanigan RC, Mickisch G, Sylvester R, et al. Cytoreductive nephrectomy in patients with metastatic renal cancer: a combined analysis. *J Urol* 2004;171:1071–1076.

183. Mickisch GH, Garin A, van Poppel H, et al. Radical nephrectomy plus interferon-alfa-based immunotherapy compared with interferon alfa alone in metastatic renal-cell carcinoma: a randomised trial. *Lancet* 2001;358:966–970.

184. Polcari AJ, Gorbonos A, Milner JE, et al. The role of cytoreductive nephrectomy in the era of molecular targeted therapy. *Int J Urol* 2009;16:227–233.

185. Flanigan RC, Mickisch G, Sylvester R, et al. Cytoreductive nephrectomy in patients with metastatic renal cancer: a combined analysis. *J Urol* 2004;171:1071–1076.

186. Choueiri TK, Xie W, Kollmannsberger C, et al. The impact of cytoreductive nephrectomy on survival of patients with metastatic renal cell carcinoma receiving vascular endothelial growth factor targeted therapy. *J Urol* 2011;185:60–66.

187. Heng DY, Xie W, Regan MM, et al. Prognostic factors for overall survival in patients with metastatic renal cell carcinoma treated with vascular endothelial growth factor-targeted agents: Results From a large, multicenter study. *J Clin Oncol* 2009;27:5794–5799.

188. Kassouf W, Sanchez-Ortiz R, Tamboli P, et al. Cytoreductive nephrectomy for T4NxM1 renal cell carcinoma: the M.D. Anderson Cancer Center experience. *Urology* 2007;69:835–838.

189. Kaushik D, Linder BJ, Thompson RH, et al. The impact of histology on clinicopathologic outcomes for patients with renal cell carcinoma and venous tumor thrombus: a matched cohort analysis. *Urology* 2013;82:136–141.

190. Choueiri TK. Clinical treatment decisions for advanced renal cell cancer. *J Natl Compr Canc Netw* 2013;11:694–697.

191. Hudes G, Carducci M, Tomczak P, et al. Temsirolimus, interferon alfa, or both for advanced renal-cell carcinoma. *N Engl J Med* 2007;356:2271–2281.

192. Abdollah F, Sun M, Thuret R, et al. Mortality and morbidity after cytoreductive nephrectomy for metastatic renal cell carcinoma: a population-based study. *Ann Surg Oncol* 2011;18:2988–2996.

193. Trinh QD, Bianchi M, Hansen J, et al. In-hospital mortality and failure to rescue after cytoreductive nephrectomy. *Eur Urol* 2013;63:1107–1114.

194. Kutikov A, Uzzo RG, Caraway A, et al. Use of systemic therapy and factors affecting survival for patients undergoing cytoreductive nephrectomy. *BJU Int* 2010;106:218–223.

195. Pantuck AJ, Zisman A, Belldegrun AS. The changing natural history of renal cell carcinoma. *J Urol* 2001;166:1611–1623.

196. Eggener SE, Yossepowitch O, Kundu S, et al. Risk score and metastasectomy independently impact prognosis of patients with recurrent renal cell carcinoma. *J Urol* 2008;180:873–878; discussion 878.

197. Daliani DD, Tannir NM, Papandreou CN, et al. Prospective assessment of systemic therapy followed by surgical removal of metastases in selected patients with renal cell carcinoma. *BJU Int* 2009;104:456–460.

198. Middleton RG. Surgery for metastatic renal cell carcinoma. *J Urol* 1967;97:973–977.

199. van der Poel HG, Roukema JA, Horenblas S, et al. Metastasectomy in renal cell carcinoma: A multicenter retrospective analysis. *Eur Urol* 1999;35:197–203.

200. Alt AL, Boorjian SA, Lohse CM, et al. Survival after complete surgical resection of multiple metastases from renal cell carcinoma. *Cancer* 2011;117:2873–2882.

201. Pogrebniak HW, Haas G, Linehan WM, et al. Renal cell carcinoma: resection of solitary and multiple metastases. *Ann Thorac Surg* 1992;54:33–38.

202. Tanguay S, Swanson DA, Putnam JB Jr. Renal cell carcinoma metastatic to the lung: potential benefit in the combination of biological therapy and surgery. *J Urol* 1996;156:1586–1589.

203. Kim B, Louie AC. Surgical resection following interleukin 2 therapy for metastatic renal cell carcinoma prolongs remission. *Arch Surg* 1992;127:1343–1349.

204. Krishnamurthi V, Novick AC, Bukowski RM. Efficacy of multimodality therapy in advanced renal cell carcinoma. *Urology* 1998;51:933–937.

205. Sella A, Swanson DA, Ro JY, et al. Surgery following response to interferon-alpha-based therapy for residual renal cell carcinoma. *J Urol* 1993;149:19–21; discussion 21–22.

206. Sherry RM, Pass HI, Rosenberg SA, et al. Surgical resection of metastatic renal cell carcinoma and melanoma after response to interleukin-2-based immunotherapy. *Cancer* 1992;69:1850–1855.

207. Karam JA, Rini BI, Varella L, et al. Metastasectomy after targeted therapy in patients with advanced renal cell carcinoma. *J Urol* 2011;185:439–444.

208. Elson PJ, Witte RS, Trump DL. Prognostic factors for survival in patients with recurrent or metastatic renal cell carcinoma. *Cancer Res* 1988;48:7310–7313.

209. Palmer PA, Vinke J, Philip T, et al. Prognostic factors for survival in patients with advanced renal cell carcinoma treated with recombinant interleukin-2. *Ann Oncol* 1992;3:475–480.

210. Motzer RJ, Mazumdar M, Bacik J, et al. Survival and prognostic stratification of 670 patients with advanced renal cell carcinoma. *J Clin Oncol* 1999;17:2530–2540.

211. Mekhail TM, Abou-Jawde RM, Boumerhi G, et al. Validation and extension of the Memorial Sloan-Kettering prognostic factors model for survival in patients with previously untreated metastatic renal cell carcinoma. *J Clin Oncol* 2005;23:832–841.

212. de Forges A, Rey A, Klink M, et al. Prognostic factors of adult metastatic renal carcinoma: a multivariate analysis. *Semin Surg Oncol* 1988;4:149–154.

213. Neves RJ, Zincke H, Taylor WF. Metastatic renal cell cancer and radical nephrectomy: identification of prognostic factors and patient survival. *J Urol* 1988;139:1173–1176.

214. Atzpodien J, Royston P, Wandert T, et al. Metastatic renal carcinoma comprehensive prognostic system. *Br J Cancer* 2003;88:348–353.

215. Motzer RJ, Bacik J, Mariani T, et al. Treatment outcome and survival associated with metastatic renal cell carcinoma of non-clear-cell histology. *J Clin Oncol* 2002;20:2376–2381.

216. Leibovich BC, Blute ML, Cheville JC, et al. Prediction of progression after radical nephrectomy for patients with clear cell renal cell carcinoma: a stratification tool for prospective clinical trials. *Cancer* 2003;97:1663–1671.

217. Lopez Hänninen E, Kirchner H, Atzpodien J. Interleukin-2 based home therapy of metastatic renal cell carcinoma: risks and benefits in 215 consecutive single institution patients. *J Urol* 1996;155:19–25.

218. Fossa SD, Kramar A, Droz JP. Prognostic factors and survival in patients with metastatic renal cell carcinoma treated with chemotherapy or interferon-alpha. *Eur J Cancer* 1994;30A:1310–1314.

219. Motzer RJ, Bacik J, Murphy BA, et al. Interferon-alfa as a comparative treatment for clinical trials of new therapies against advanced renal cell carcinoma. *J Clin Oncol* 2002;20:289–296.

220. Rini BI. VEGF-targeted therapy in renal cell carcinoma: active drugs and active choices. *Curr Oncol Rep* 2006;8:85–89.

221. Choueiri TK, Vaziri SA, Jaeger E, et al. von Hippel-Lindau gene status and response to vascular endothelial growth factor targeted therapy for metastatic clear cell renal cell carcinoma. *J Urol* 2008;180:860–865.

222. Choueiri TK, Fay AP, Gagnon R, et al. The role of aberrant VHL/HIF pathway elements in predicting clinical outcome to pazopanib therapy in patients with metastatic clear-cell renal cell carcinoma. *Clin Cancer Res* 2013;19:5218–5226.

223. Bui MH, Seligson D, Han KR, et al. Carbonic anhydrase IX is an independent predictor of survival in advanced renal clear cell carcinoma: implications for prognosis and therapy. *Clin Cancer Res* 2003;9:802–811.

224. Atkins M, Regan M, McDermott D, et al. Carbonic anhydrase IX expression predicts outcome of interleukin 2 therapy for renal cancer. *Clin Cancer Res* 2005;11:3714–3721.

225. Clement JM, McDermott DF. The high-dose aldesleukin (IL-2) "select" trial: a trial designed to prospectively validate predictive models of response to high-dose IL-2 treatment in patients with metastatic renal cell carcinoma. *Clin Genitourin Cancer* 2009;7:E7–E9.

226. Xu CF, Bing NX, Ball HA, et al. Pazopanib efficacy in renal cell carcinoma: evidence for predictive genetic markers in angiogenesis-related and exposure-related genes. *J Clin Oncol* 2011;29:2557–2564.

227. Garcia-Donas J, Esteban E, Leandro-Garcia LJ, et al. Single nucleotide polymorphism associations with response and toxic effects in patients with advanced renal-cell carcinoma treated with first-line sunitinib: a multicentre, observational, prospective study. *Lancet Oncol* 2011;12:1143–1150.

228. van Erp NP, Eechoute K, van der Veldt AA, et al. Pharmacogenetic pathway analysis for determination of sunitinib-induced toxicity. *J Clin Oncol* 2009;27:4406–4412.

229. Rini BI, Basappa NS, Elson P, et al. The impact of tumor burden characteristics in patients with metastatic renal cell carcinoma treated with sunitinib. *Cancer* 2011;117:1183–1189.

230. Rini BI, Cohen DP, Lu DR, et al. Hypertension as a biomarker of efficacy in patients with metastatic renal cell carcinoma treated with sunitinib. *J Natl Cancer Inst* 2011;103:763–773.

231. Dahlberg SE, Sandler AB, Brahmer JR, et al. Clinical course of advanced non-small-cell lung cancer patients experiencing hypertension during treatment with bevacizumab in combination with carboplatin and paclitaxel on ECOG 4599. *J Clin Oncol* 2010;28:949–954.

232. Papac RJ, Ross SA, Levy A. Renal cell carcinoma: analysis of 31 cases with assessment of endocrine therapy. *Am J Med Sci* 1977;274:281–290.

233. Pizzocaro G, Di Fronzo G, Cappelletti V, et al. Hormone treatment and sex steroid receptors in metastatic renal cell carcinoma: report of a multicentric prospective study. *Tumori* 1983;69:215–220.

234. Interferon-alpha and survival in metastatic renal carcinoma: early results of a randomised controlled trial. Medical Research Council Renal Cancer Collaborators. *Lancet* 1999;353:14–17.

235. Yagoda A, Abi-Rached B, Petrylak D. Chemotherapy for advanced renal-cell carcinoma: 1983-1993. *Semin Oncol* 1995;22:42–60.

236. Buti S, Bersanelli M, Sikokis A, et al. Chemotherapy in metastatic renal cell carcinoma today? A systematic review. *Anticancer Drugs* 2013;24:535–554.

237. Rini BI, Weinberg V, Small EJ. A phase I trial of fixed dose rate gemcitabine and capecitabine in metastatic renal cell carcinoma. *Cancer* 2005;103: 553–558.

238. Stadler WM, Halabi S, Rini B, et al. A phase II study of gemcitabine and capecitabine in metastatic renal cancer: a report of Cancer and Leukemia Group B protocol 90008. *Cancer* 2006;107:1273–1279.

239. Fossa SD, Droz JP, Pavone-Macaluso MM, et al. Vinblastine in metastatic renal cell carcinoma: EORTC phase II trial 30882. The EORTC Genitourinary Group. *Eur J Cancer* 1992;28A:878–880.

240. Neidhart JA, Anderson SA, Harris JE, et al. Vinblastine fails to improve response of renal cancer to interferon alfa-n1: high response rate in patients with pulmonary metastases. *J Clin Oncol* 1991;9:832–836.

241. Nanus DM, Garino A, Milowsky MI, et al. Active chemotherapy for sarcomatoid and rapidly progressing renal cell carcinoma. *Cancer* 2004;101:1545–1551.

242. Rosenberg SA, Lotze MT, Muul LM, et al. Observations on the systemic administration of autologous lymphokine-activated killer cells and recombinant interleukin-2 to patients with metastatic cancer. *N Engl J Med* 1985;313:1485–1492.

243. McDermott DF, Regan MM, Clark JI, et al. Randomized phase III trial of high-dose interleukin-2 versus subcutaneous interleukin-2 and interferon in patients with metastatic renal cell carcinoma. *J Clin Oncol* 2005;23:133–141.

244. Yang JC, Sherry RM, Steinberg SM, et al. Randomized study of high-dose and low-dose interleukin-2 in patients with metastatic renal cancer. *J Clin Oncol* 2003;21:3127–3132.

245. Fyfe G, Fisher RI, Rosenberg SA, et al. Results of treatment of 255 patients with metastatic renal cell carcinoma who received high-dose recombinant interleukin-2 therapy. *J Clin Oncol* 1995;13:688–696.

246. Fyfe GA, Fisher RI, Rosenberg SA, et al. Long-term response data for 255 patients with metastatic renal cell carcinoma treated with high-dose recombinant interleukin-2 therapy. *J Clin Oncol* 1996;14:2410–2411.

247. Fisher RI, Rosenberg SA, Fyfe G. Long-term survival update for high-dose recombinant interleukin-2 in patients with renal cell cancer. *Cancer J Sci Am* 2000;6:S55–S57.

248. Pyrhonen S, Salminen E, Ruutu M, et al. Prospective randomized trial of interferon alfa-2a plus vinblastine versus vinblastine alone in patients with advanced renal cell cancer. *J Clin Oncol* 1999;17:2859–2867.

249. Negrier S, Escudier B, Lasset C, et al. Recombinant human interleukin-2, recombinant human interferon alfa-2a, or both in metastatic renal-cell carcinoma. Groupe Francais d'Immunotherapie. *N Engl J Med* 1998;338:1272–1278.

250. Escudier B, Chevreau C, Lasset C, et al. Cytokines in metastatic renal cell carcinoma: is it useful to switch to interleukin-2 or interferon after failure of a first treatment? Groupe Francais d'Immunotherape. *J Clin Oncol* 1999;17:2039–2043.

251. Atzpodien J, Kirchner H, Illiger HJ, et al. IL-2 in combination with IFN- alpha and 5-FU versus tamoxifen in metastatic renal cell carcinoma: long-term results of a controlled randomized clinical trial. *Br J Cancer* 2001;85:1130–1136.

252. Atzpodien J, Kirchner H, Jonas U, et al. Interleukin-2- and interferon alfa-2a-based immunochemotherapy in advanced renal cell carcinoma: a prospectively randomized trial of the German Cooperative Renal Carcinoma Chemoimmunotherapy Group (DGCIN). *J Clin Oncol* 2004;22:1188–1194.

253. Walter S, Weinschenk T, Stenzl A, et al. Multipeptide immune response to cancer vaccine IMA901 after single-dose cyclophosphamide associates with longer patient survival. *Nat Med* 2012;18:1254–1261.

254. Finke JH, Rini B, Ireland J, et al. Sunitinib reverses type-1 immune suppression and decreases T-regulatory cells in renal cell carcinoma patients. *Clin Cancer Res* 2008;14:6674–6682.

255. Pal SK, Hu A, Figlin RA. A new age for vaccine therapy in renal cell carcinoma. *Cancer J* 2013;19:365–370.

256. McDermott DF, Drake CG, Sznol M, et al. Clinical activity and safety of anti-PD-1 (BMS-936558, MDX-1106) in patients with previously treated metastatic renal cell carcinoma (mRCC). *J Clin Oncol* 2012;30(15 Suppl):4505.

257. Topalian SL, Brahmer JR, Hodi FS, et al. Anti-PD-1 (BMS-936558, MDX-1106) in patients with advanced solid tumors: Clinical activity, safety, and a potential biomarker for response. *J Clin Oncol* 2012;30(15 Suppl):CRA2509.

258. Shweiki D, Itin A, Soffer D, et al. Vascular endothelial growth factor induced by hypoxia may mediate hypoxia-initiated angiogenesis. *Nature* 1992;359:843–845.

259. Abrams TJ, Lee LB, Murray LJ, et al. SU11248 inhibits KIT and platelet-derived growth factor receptor beta in preclinical models of human small cell lung cancer. *Mol Cancer Ther* 2003;2:471–478.

260. Mendel DB, Laird AD, Xin X, et al. In vivo antitumor activity of SU11248, a novel tyrosine kinase inhibitor targeting vascular endothelial growth factor and platelet-derived growth factor receptors: determination of a pharmacokinetic/pharmacodynamic relationship. *Clin Cancer Res* 2003;9:327–337.

261. Motzer RJ, Dror Michaelson M, Redman BG, et al. Activity of SU11248, a multitargeted inhibitor of vascular endothelial growth factor receptor and platelet-derived growth factor receptor, in patients with metastatic renal cell carcinoma. *J Clin Oncol* 2006;24:16–24.

262. Motzer RJ, Rini BI, Bukowski RM, et al. Sunitinib in patients with metastatic renal cell carcinoma. *JAMA* 2006;295:2516–2524.

263. Motzer RJ, Hutson TE, Tomczak P, et al. Sunitinib versus interferon alfa in metastatic renal-cell carcinoma. *N Engl J Med* 2007;356:115–124.

264. Motzer RJ, Hudes G, Wilding G, et al. Phase I trial of sunitinib malate plus interferon-alpha for patients with metastatic renal cell carcinoma. *Clin Genitourin Cancer* 2009;7:28–33.

265. Motzer RJ, Hutson TE, Cella D, et al. Pazopanib versus sunitinib in metastatic renal-cell carcinoma. *N Engl J Med* 2013;369:722–731.

266. Lyons JF, Wilhelm S, Hibner B, et al. Discovery of a novel Raf kinase inhibitor. *Endocr Relat Cancer* 2001;8:219–225.

267. Wilhelm SM, Carter C, Tang L, et al. BAY 43-9006 exhibits broad spectrum oral antitumor activity and targets the RAF/MEK/ERK pathway and receptor tyrosine kinases involved in tumor progression and angiogenesis. *Cancer Res* 2004;64:7099–7109.

268. Ratain MJ, Eisen T, Stadler WM, et al. Phase II placebo-controlled randomized discontinuation trial of sorafenib in patients with metastatic renal cell carcinoma. *J Clin Oncol* 2006;24:2505–2512.

269. Bukowski R, Cella D, Gondek K, et al. Effects of sorafenib on symptoms and quality of life: results from a large randomized placebo-controlled study in renal cancer. *Am J Clin Oncol* 2007;30:220–227.

270. Escudier B, Eisen T, Stadler WM, et al. Sorafenib in advanced clear-cell renal-cell carcinoma. *N Engl J Med* 2007;356:125–134.

271. Presta LG, Chen H, O'Connor SJ, et al. Humanization of an anti-vascular endothelial growth factor monoclonal antibody for the therapy of solid tumors and other disorders. *Cancer Res* 1997;57:4593–4599.

272. Bukowski RM, Kabbinavar FF, Figlin RA, et al. Randomized phase II study of erlotinib combined with bevacizumab compared with bevacizumab alone in metastatic renal cell cancer. *J Clin Oncol* 2007;25:4536–4541.

273. Yang JC, Haworth L, Sherry RM, et al. A randomized trial of bevacizumab, an anti-vascular endothelial growth factor antibody, for metastatic renal cancer. *N Engl J Med* 2003;349:427–434.

274. Escudier B, Pluzanska A, Koralewski P, et al. Bevacizumab plus interferon alfa-2a for treatment of metastatic renal cell carcinoma: a randomised, double-blind phase III trial. *Lancet* 2007;370:2103–2111.

275. Rini BI, Halabi S, Rosenberg JE, et al. Bevacizumab plus interferon alfa compared with interferon alfa monotherapy in patients with metastatic renal cell carcinoma: CALGB 90206. *J Clin Oncol* 2008;26:5422–5428.

276. Rini BI, Wilding G, Hudes G, et al. Phase II study of axitinib in sorafenib-refractory metastatic renal cell carcinoma. *J Clin Oncol* 2009;27:4462–4468.

277. Rixe O, Bukowski RM, Michaelson MD, et al. Axitinib treatment in patients with cytokine-refractory metastatic renal-cell cancer: a phase II study. *Lancet Oncol* 2007;8:975–984.

278. Rini BI, Escudier B, Tomczak P, et al. Comparative effectiveness of axitinib versus sorafenib in advanced renal cell carcinoma (AXIS): a randomised phase 3 trial. *Lancet* 2011;378:1931–1939.

279. Hutson TE, Lesovoy V, Al-Shukri S, et al. Axitinib versus sorafenib as first-line therapy in patients with metastatic renal-cell carcinoma: a randomised open-label phase 3 trial. *Lancet Oncol* 2013;14:1287–1294.

280. Barthelemy P, Hoch B, Chevreau C, et al. mTOR inhibitors in advanced renal cell carcinomas: From biology to clinical practice. *Crit Rev Oncol Hematol* 2013;88:42–56.

281. Atkins MB, Hidalgo M, Stadler WM, et al. Randomized phase II study of multiple dose levels of CCI-779, a novel mammalian target of rapamycin kinase inhibitor, in patients with advanced refractory renal cell carcinoma. *J Clin Oncol* 2004;22:909–918.

282. Motzer RJ, Bukowski RM, Figlin RA, et al. Prognostic nomogram for sunitinib in patients with metastatic renal cell carcinoma. *Cancer* 2008;113:1552–1558.

283. Motzer RJ, Barrios CH, Kim TM, et al. Record-3: Phase II randomized trial comparing sequential first-line everolimus (EVE) and second-line sunitinib (SUN) versus first-line SUN and second-line EVE in patients with metastatic renal cell carcinoma (mRCC). *J Clin Oncol* 2013;31:abstr 4504.

284. Hutson TE, Escudier B, Esteban E, et al. Randomized phase III trial of temsirolimus versus sorafenib as second-line therapy after sunitinib in patients with metastatic renal cell carcinoma. *J Clin Oncol* 2014;32:760–767.

285. Rini BI, Bellmunt J, Clancy J, et al. Randomized phase IIIB trial of temsirolimus and bevacizumab versus interferon and bevacizumab in metastatic renal cell carcinoma: results from INTORACT (LBA21). *Ann Oncol* 2012;23(suppl 9):ixe1–ixe30.

286. Ravaud A, Barrios CH, Anak Ö, et al. Randomized phase II study of first-line everolimus (EVE) + bevacizumab (BEV) versus interferon alfa-2A (IFN) + BEV in patients (PTS) with metastatic renal cell carcinoma (MRCC): record-2. Abstract #7830. *Ann Oncol* 2012;23:ixe1–ixe30.

287. Weight CJ, Miller DC, Campbell SC, et al. The management of a clinical T1b renal tumor in the presence of a normal contralateral kidney: the case for nephron sparing surgery. *J Urol* 2013;189:1198–1202.

# 38 Molecular Biology of Bladder Cancer

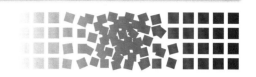

Margaret A. Knowles and Carolyn D. Hurst

## INTRODUCTION

There has been rapid progress in elucidating the molecular changes that underlie bladder cancer development. A wealth of data is now available that identifies several critical drivers of the malignant urothelial phenotype, some of which have clear potential for therapeutic targeting. Most studies have focused on urothelial carcinomas (UC), which comprise the majority (>90%) of tumors diagnosed in the Western world. This chapter will provide an overview of somatic molecular features of UC identified by genomic, epigenomic, and expression profiling. There is also much information about germline variants that confer increased risk of UC development and the reader is referred to recent reviews on this topic.[1,2]

At diagnosis, approximately 60% of UCs are noninvasive (stage Ta) papillary lesions. These commonly recur, but progression to muscle invasion is infrequent (10% to 15%) and prognosis is good. In contrast, tumors that are muscle invasive at diagnosis (≥T2) have poor prognosis (<50% survival at 5 years). Stage T1 tumors, which have penetrated the epithelial basement membrane but not invaded muscle, represent a clinically challenging and molecularly heterogeneous group with features related to each of the two major groups. The distinction of the two major groups is supported by a wealth of molecular information, and a "two-pathway" model for UC pathogenesis has long dominated thinking about this cancer type and its clinical management. Many genomic alterations and expression of specific genes relate directly to these groups and will be discussed in this context here. Global expression and epigenetic alterations show less direct relationships and will be discussed together. Importantly, recent molecular information provides strong evidence for multiple molecular subgroups that are independent of tumor grade and stage. This new molecular classification, which shows great promise of clinical relevance, is described in a separate section.

## KEY MOLECULAR ALTERATIONS IN STAGE Ta UROTHELIAL CARCINOMA

Low-grade stage Ta papillary UC ("superficial" UC) are genomically stable, often with near-diploid karyotype. Common features are activation of *FGFR1*, *FGFR3*, *PIK3CA*, and *CCND1* genes by mutation or upregulated expression and mutational inactivation of *CDKN2A*, *STAG2*, and *TSC1*. The most common event recorded to date is mutation of the promoter region of telomerase reverse transcriptase (*TERT*).

### FGF Receptors

Activating point mutations in FGF receptor 3 (*FGFR3*) are present in ≥ 70% of cases.[3] These are in hot-spot codons in exons 7, 10, and 15 (Fig. 38.1A) and are all predicted to constitutively activate the receptor.[4] Mutations are also found in urothelial papilloma, a likely precursor of superficial UC.[5] Increased expression of mutant FGFR3 is common in these tumors.[6] MicroRNAs (miRNAs) miR-99a/100, which are commonly downregulated in non–muscle-invasive (NMI)

tumors, are negative regulators of FGFR3 expression.[7] Transcriptional regulation by the p53 family member p63 has also been demonstrated.[8] In cultured normal human urothelial cells (NHUC), expression of mutant FGFR3 leads to activation of the RAS-MAPK pathway and PLCγ, leading to overgrowth of cells at confluence,[9] and suggesting a possible contribution of FGFR3 activation to urothelial hyperplasia in vivo. An alternative mechanism of FGFR3 activation in a subset of cases (2% to 5%) is chromosomal translocation to generate a fusion protein. All FGFR3 fusions identified to date show loss of the final exon of FGFR3 and fusion in-frame to *TACC3* (transforming acid coiled-coil containing protein 3), or in one case to *BAIAP2L1* (BAI1-associated protein 2-like 1) also known as IRTKS (insulin receptor tyrosine-kinase substrate).[10] It is not yet clear whether this activation mechanism is related to tumor grade or stage. These fusion proteins are highly activated and transforming oncogenes. FGF1 and FGF2 are expressed in UC tissues and cell lines,[11,12] FGF2 is detected in the urine of patients with bladder cancer,[13] and expression has been detected in the urothelial stroma.[14] Thus, it is also likely that both autocrine and paracrine FGF production contributes to FGFR3 activation in UC, particularly in those tumors with expression of wild-type protein (Fig. 38.1B).

Activation of the RAS-MAPK pathway in Ta tumors may also be achieved by mutation of one of the RAS genes (most commonly *HRAS* or *KRAS2*), and this is mutually exclusive with *FGFR3* mutation.[15] More than 80% of noninvasive bladder tumors are predicted to have RAS-MAPK pathway activation via these mechanisms (Fig. 38.2A). Compatible with this, urothelial expression of an activated Ras transgene in mice leads to hyperplasia and papillary tumors,[16] suggesting an important role for activation of the RAS-MAPK pathway in the generation of urothelial hyperplasia.

In NMI UC, *FGFR3* mutation is associated with favorable outcome.[17–19] High FGFR3 expression, normal staining pattern for CK20, and low proliferative index in papillary urothelial neoplasms of low malignant potential[20] is reported to identify tumors that do not recur.[21]

FGFR3 is considered a good therapeutic target in superficial UC, though early clinical application is most likely in muscle invasive rather than superficial UC (see the following). Several studies indicate that inhibition of mutant *FGFR3* by knockdown or inhibition using small molecules or antibodies has a profound effect on UC cell phenotype, including inhibition of xenograft growth in vivo.[22]

Upregulated expression of the related receptor FGFR1 is also found in Ta tumors.[23] No mutations have been detected, and there is infrequent gene amplification.[24] Ectopic expression of FGFR1 in NHUC in the presence of FGF2 ligand, activates the RAS-MAPK pathway and PLCγ, and promotes cell survival.[23] Currently, there is no information on the prognostic significance of these alterations.

## PIK3CA

The phosphatidylinositol-3 kinase (PI3K) pathway plays a pivotal role in signaling from receptor tyrosine kinases (Fig. 38.2A). Activating mutations of the p110α catalytic subunit (*PIK3CA*) are found in UC, most commonly in low-grade, stage Ta tumors (~25%).[25–28]

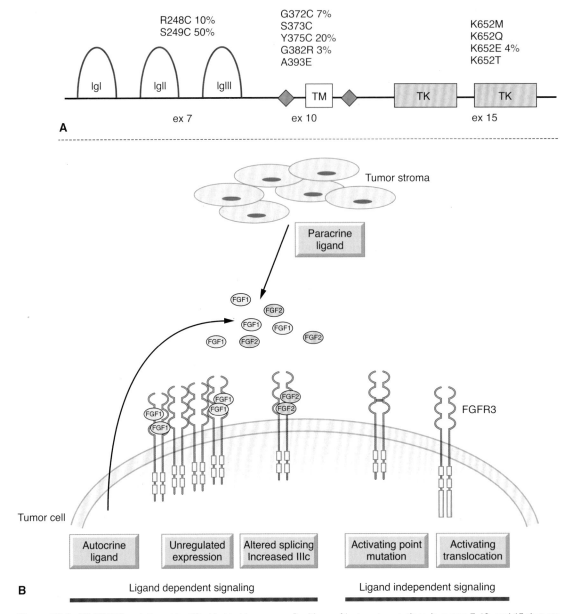

**Figure 38.1 (A)** *FGFR3* mutations identified in bladder cancer. Positions of hot-spot mutations in exons 7, 10, and 15 that are found in bladder cancer are shown in relation to protein structure. The relative frequency of the more common mutations is given as a percentage. IgI, IgII, IgIII, immunoglobulinlike domains; TM, transmembrane domain; TK, tyrosine-kinase domain. **(B)** Mechanisms of FGFR3 activation in bladder cancer. FGFR3 can be activated by ligand-dependent and -independent mechanisms. Ligand-dependent activation may be via increased expression of wild-type FGFR3, increased production of FGFs by tumor or stromal cells, with or without upregulated FGFR3 expression, or through expression of splice variants with the ability to bind a wider range of FGF ligands. Ligand independent activation can be achieved by point mutation that facilitates receptor dimerization or by the generation of fusion proteins that constitutively dimerise.

The mutation spectrum (Fig. 38.2B) differs significantly from that found in other cancers. Mutations E542K and E545K in the helical domain are most common (22% and 60%, respectively) and the kinase domain mutation H1047R, which is the most common mutation in other cancers, is less frequent. The selective pressure for helical domain mutation in UC is not fully understood. E542K and E545K forms require interaction with RAS-GTP but not binding to p85, the regulatory subunit of PI3K, whereas H1047R depends on p85 binding and is active in the absence of RAS binding.[29] This suggests potential cooperation between helical domain PIK3CA mutant proteins and events in UC that activate RAS. Compatible with this, *PIK3CA* and *FGFR3* mutations are commonly found together.[25–28] Mutant PIK3CA confers a proliferative advantage at confluence and stimulates intraepithelial movement in NHUC,

with higher activity of helical domain than kinase domain mutants in this cell context.[30] Several other mechanisms of PI3K pathway activation have been identified in UC, though none of these are common in noninvasive tumors (Table 38.1).

## STAG2

Inactivating mutations in the cohesin complex component *STAG2* (Xq25) have been identified in UC.[31–34] Mutations are most common in stage Ta tumors (20% to 36%) and are predominantly inactivating, suggesting a tumor suppressor function. The cohesin complex, which in human cells contains SMC1A, SMC3, RAD21, and either STAG2 or STAG1, mediates

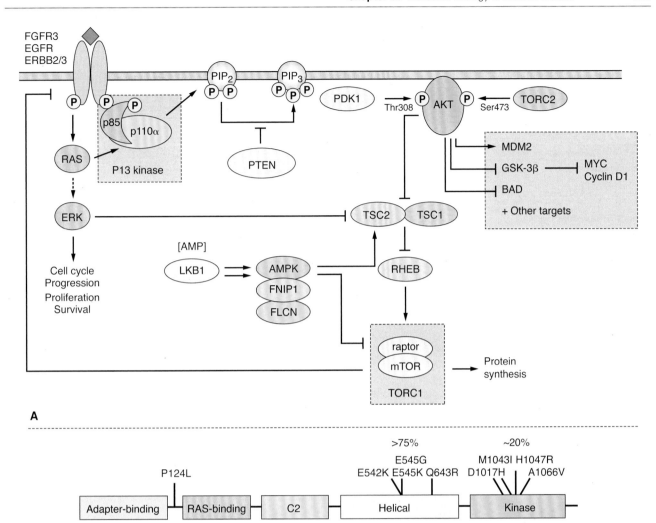

A

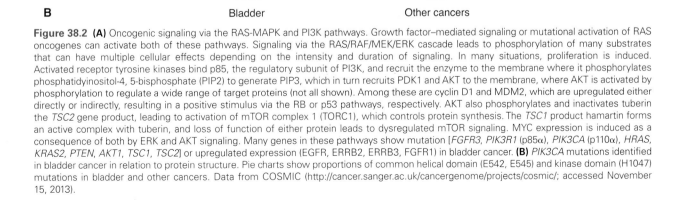

B                Bladder                Other cancers

**Figure 38.2 (A)** Oncogenic signaling via the RAS-MAPK and PI3K pathways. Growth factor–mediated signaling or mutational activation of RAS oncogenes can activate both of these pathways. Signaling via the RAS/RAF/MEK/ERK cascade leads to phosphorylation of many substrates that can have multiple cellular effects depending on the intensity and duration of signaling. In many situations, proliferation is induced. Activated receptor tyrosine kinases bind p85, the regulatory subunit of PI3K, and recruit the enzyme to the membrane where it phosphorylates phosphatidyinositol-4, 5-bisphosphate (PIP2) to generate PIP3, which in turn recruits PDK1 and AKT to the membrane, where AKT is activated by phosphorylation to regulate a wide range of target proteins (not all shown). Among these are cyclin D1 and MDM2, which are upregulated either directly or indirectly, resulting in a positive stimulus via the RB or p53 pathways, respectively. AKT also phosphorylates and inactivates tuberin the *TSC2* gene product, leading to activation of mTOR complex 1 (TORC1), which controls protein synthesis. The *TSC1* product hamartin forms an active complex with tuberin, and loss of function of either protein leads to dysregulated mTOR signaling. MYC expression is induced as a consequence of both by ERK and AKT signaling. Many genes in these pathways show mutation [*FGFR3*, *PIK3R1* (p85α), *PIK3CA* (p110α), *HRAS*, *KRAS2*, *PTEN*, *AKT1*, *TSC1*, *TSC2*] or upregulated expression (EGFR, ERRB2, ERRB3, FGFR1) in bladder cancer. **(B)** *PIK3CA* mutations identified in bladder cancer in relation to protein structure. Pie charts show proportions of common helical domain (E542, E545) and kinase domain (H1047) mutations in bladder and other cancers. Data from COSMIC (http://cancer.sanger.ac.uk/cancergenome/projects/cosmic/; accessed November 15, 2013).

TABLE 38.1

**Genetic Changes Identified in Stage Ta Bladder Tumors**

| Gene (Cytogenetic Location) | Alteration | Frequency (%) |
|---|---|---|
| **Oncogenes** | | |
| HRAS (11p15)/NRAS (1p13)/KRAS2 (12p12) | Activating mutations | 15[15,27,28,221] |
| FGFR3 (4p16) | Activating mutations | 60–80[3,222] |
| CCND1 (11q13) | Amplification/overexpression | 10–20[58,223–225] |
| PIK3CA (3q26) | Activating mutations | 27 PUNLMP; 16–30 Ta[25,26] |
| MDM2 (12q13) | Overexpression/amplification | ~30 overexpression; amplification infrequent[58,85,226] |
| **Tumor Suppressor Genes** | | |
| CDKN2A (9p21) | Homozygous deletion/mutation/methylation | HD 20–30[40,41,227,228] LOH ~60[229] |
| PTCH (9q22) | Deletion/mutation | LOH ~ 60; mutation frequency low[43,44] |
| TSC1 (9q34) | Deletion/mutation | LOH ~ 60; mutation ~12[26,27,48,230] |
| STAG2 (Xq25) | Deletion/mutation | 34–36[33,34] |
| KDM6A (Xp11) | Mutation | 10–30[31,32,140] |
| ARID1A | Mutation | 10[31,32] |
| **DNA Copy Number Changes[a]** | | |
| 8p, 10q, 11p, 11q, 13q, 17p, 18q | Deletion | >15[57,135,231,232] |
| 9p, 9q | Deletion | 46–53[57,135,231,232] |
| 1q, 20q | Gain | >15[57,135,231,232] |
| 1q13, 1q21-q24, 3p25 (including RAF1, PPARG), 3q25, 3q26, 4p16 (including FGFR3), 4q21, 5p13.3-p12, 6p22 (including E2F3, SOX4), 8p12, 8q24 (including MYC), 10q26 (including FGFR2), 11q13 (including CCND1), 11q24, 12q15 (including MDM2), 17q12-q21 (including ERBB2), 20q11-q13 (including YWHAB, MYBL2) | Amplification | Occasional[57,58,232] |

[a]Array-based comparative genomic hybridization analyses.
PUNLMP, papillary urothelial neoplasms of low malignant potential; HD, homozygous deletion; LOH, loss of heterozygosity.

cohesion between sister chromatids following DNA replication to ensure correct chromosomal segregation. Mutations in STAG2 in glioblastoma have been reported to cause aneuploidy[35] but this relationship is not apparent in UC, where most mutations have been found in low grade/stage, genomically stable tumors, and there is no association of mutation with chromosomal copy number changes.[31,34]

In addition to its well-documented functions during cell division, cohesin regulates gene expression through mechanisms involving DNA looping and interactions with transcriptional regulators such as CTCF, though evidence to date suggests that these roles are mainly related to STAG1-cohesin.[36] Functional studies are now required to elucidate the consequences of STAG2 loss of function in UC.

## Telomerase Reverse Transcriptase Gene Promoter

The most common genomic alterations identified in UC of all grades and stages are mutations in the promoter of the telomerase reverse transcriptase gene (TERT) in more than 80% of cases.[37,38] Mutations are predominantly in two hotspot positions [-124 bp (G>A) and -146 bp (G>A) relative to the ATG translational start site], and this has facilitated the design of robust methods of

detection. Examination of TERT expression in UC tissues has not revealed an effect of mutation on expression,[37] so that the functional significance of these mutations remains to be determined. Nevertheless, the ease with which these mutations can be detected in urine sediments[37,38] is likely to make a major contribution to the development of urine-based assays for detection of bladder tumors of all grades and stages.

## Other Genomic Alterations in Noninvasive Urothelial Carcinoma

These tumors are often near diploid. The most common genomic alteration is loss of heterozygosity (LOH) or copy number loss of chromosome 9, often an entire homolog. More than 50% of UC of all of grades and stages show chromosome 9 LOH. A critical region on 9p21 and at least three regions on 9q (9q22, 9q32–q33, and 9q34) have been identified. Candidate genes within these regions are CDKN2A (p16/p14ARF) and CDKN2B (p15) at 9p21,[39–42] PTCH (Gorlin syndrome gene) at 9q22,[43,44] DBC1 at 9q32–q33,[45–47] and TSC1 (tuberous sclerosis syndrome gene 1) at 9q34[26,48,49] (Table 38.1).

CDKN2A (9p21) encodes the two cell-cycle regulators, p16 and p14ARF. p16 is a negative regulator of the RB pathway and p14ARF, a negative regulator of the p53 pathway (Fig. 38.3).

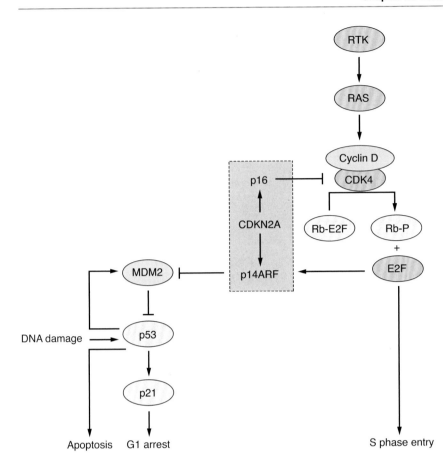

**Figure 38.3** Key interactions in the RB and p53 pathways. The *CDKN2A* locus encodes p16 and p14ARF that act as negative regulators of the RB and p53 pathways, respectively. This interrelated signaling network is central to tumor suppression via the mechanisms of cell-cycle arrest and apoptosis. Stimulation by mitogens induces cyclin D1 expression. Phosphorylation of RB1 by CDK4-cyclin D1 complexes releases E2F family members to induce expression of genes required for progression into S phase. The cyclin D-CDK4 complexes also sequester p27 and p21 (not shown). This allows formation of cyclin E-CDK2, which reinforces the inactivation of RB1. p16 negatively regulates this process by interacting with CDK4. The p53 pathway responds to stress signals (e.g., DNA damage). p21 expression is induced and this leads to cell-cycle arrest. MDM2 is a ubiquitin ligase responsible for inactivation of p53. In turn, p53 regulates MDM2 expression providing a negative feedback loop. The p53 and RB pathways are connected by p14ARF, which sequesters (inactivates) MDM2 in the nucleus and is upregulated by E2Fs and in response to mitogenic signaling. Overexpression of E2Fs and oncogenes such as *MYC* can both result in p53-triggered cell-cycle arrest via p14ARF. RTK; receptor tyrosine kinase.

Inactivation of this locus in UC is commonly by homozygous deletion (HD). LOH of 9p, HD of *CDKN2A*, and loss of expression of p16 in NMI UC is predictive of reduced recurrence-free interval.[50–52] Mouse knockout and in vitro experiments indicate that p16 and/or p14ARF may be haploinsufficient.[53,54] In human UC, this may affect the biology of approximately 45% of cases that have LOH or reduced copy number of 9p21.

On 9q, three genes are implicated. *PTCH*, the Gorlin syndrome gene (9q22), shows infrequent mutation,[44] but many tumors have reduced mRNA expression.[43] *DBC1* (9q33) shows HD in a few tumors[55] and no mutations, but is commonly silenced by hypermethylation.[45,56] *TSC1* is the best-validated 9q tumor suppressor gene. TSC1 in complex with TSC2 negatively regulates the mTOR branch of the PI3K pathway (Fig. 38.2A).

Biallelic inactivation of *TSC1* is found in 12% to 16% of UC with no relationship to grade or stage.[26,27]

## Cyclin D1

*CCND1* (11q13) is amplified in some superficial and invasive UC,[57,58] and the protein is overexpressed in an even larger number.[59,60] Overexpression in many cases may be the consequence of other alterations, such as activation of the MAPK or PI3K pathways (Fig. 38.2A). In Ta tumors, upregulated expression is associated with higher risk of progression to muscle invasion.[60]

## KEY MOLECULAR ALTERATIONS IN INVASIVE UROTHELIAL CARCINOMA

Many genomic alterations are found in muscle-invasive (MI) UC, including alterations to known genes and genomic alterations for which the target genes are currently unknown (Table 38.2).

## Oncogenes

Overexpression of EGFR, ERBB2, and/or ERBB3 is associated with higher tumor grade and stage and with clinical outcome.[61–63] *ERBB2* (17q23) is amplified in 10% to 20% and overexpressed in 10% to 50% of MI UC.[64–66] Amplification is more common in metastatic lesions than in the related primary tumor.[67] As this receptor cannot bind ligand and relies on heterodimerization with ERBB3, it is likely that ERBB3 status and/or ligand expression may have significant influence.[65,68,69] Up to 70% of MI tumors overexpress EGFR, and this is associated with poor prognosis.[61,70,71] Both ERBB2 and EGFR represent potential therapeutic targets in advanced UC.[72] These changes may activate the RAS-MAPK and/or PI3K pathways (Fig. 38.2A).

RAS gene mutation is not associated with either invasive or noninvasive disease (mutations in ~13% overall).[15] Although mice expressing mutant H-ras in the urothelium develop superficial papillary tumors rather than MI tumors,[73] in vitro experiments in human tumor cells indicate that HRAS can induce an invasive phenotype.[74] Thus, RAS mutation may contribute to development of both major forms of UC.

*PIK3CA* and *FGFR3* are mutated less frequently than in NMI UC. Approximately 15% of T2 tumors show *FGFR3* mutation.[3,6,75] However, protein expression is upregulated in 40% to 50% of nonmutant MI UC.[6] Thus FGFR3 is considered a good therapeutic target in invasive and metastatic disease and preclinical studies have shown that gene knockdown[76] or treatment with FGFR-selective small molecules and antibodies inhibits cell proliferation and tumorigenicity of UC cell lines with mutant or upregulated FGFR3.[77–79] Potential predictive biomarkers include mutation, overexpression, or detection of an FGFR3 fusion protein. The presence of FGFR3 fusion proteins in UC cell lines[10] is associated with good response to FGFR inhibitors.[77] Epithelial phenotype may provide an additional biomarker as in vitro assays indicate that

## TABLE 38.2

### Genetic Changes Identified in Invasive (Stage ≥T2) Bladder Tumors

| Gene (Cytogenetic Location) | Alteration | Frequency (%) |
|---|---|---|
| **Oncogenes** | | |
| *HRAS* (11p15)/*NRAS* (1p13)/*KRAS2* (12p12) | Activating mutations | 4–15[15,27,28,32,221] |
| *FGFR3* (4p16) | Activating mutations | 0–20[3,6,28,222,233] |
| *ERBB2* (17q) | Amplification/overexpression | 10–14 amplification 10–50 overexpression[64–66] |
| *CCND1* (11q13) | Amplification/overexpression | 10–20 amplification[223,224,234] |
| *MDM2* (12q13) | Amplification/overexpression | 4–11 amplification[85,235,236] |
| *E2F3* (6p22) | Amplification/overexpression | 9–11 amplification in ≥T1[89,91] |
| **Tumor Suppressor Genes** | | |
| *CDKN2A* (9p21) | Homozygous deletion/mutation/methylation | HD 20–30[40–42,228] LOH ~60[229] |
| *PTCH* (9q22) | Deletion/mutation | LOH ~60; mutation frequency low[43,44] |
| *TSC1* (9q34) | Deletion/mutation | LOH ~60; mutation ~12[26,27,48,230] |
| *STAG2* (Xq25) | Deletion/mutation/methylation | 9–13[31–34] |
| *TP53* (17p13) | Deletion/mutation | Mutation 50–70[237–239] |
| *RB1* (13q14) | Deletion/mutation | LOH or loss of expression 37[96,99] |
| *PTEN* (10q23) | Deletion/mutation | LOH 30–35[106–109]; mutation 17[111] |
| *ARID1A* | Mutation | ~10[32,240] |
| *KDM6A* | Mutation | 11–15[31,32] |
| *CREBBP* | Mutation | 10–15[31,32] |
| *EP300* | Mutation | 6–8[31,32] |
| **DNA Copy Number Changes[a]** | | |
| 2q, 3p, 3q, 4p, 4q, 5q, 6p, 6q, 8p, 9p, 9q, 10p, 10q, 11p, 11q, 12q, 13q, 14q, 15q, 16p, 16q, 17p, 18q, 19p, 19q, 22q | Deletion | >15[57,135,231,232] |
| 1p, 1q, 2p, 2q, 3p, 3q, 4p, 4q, 5p, 5q, 6p, 7p, 7q, 8p, 8q, 9p, 10p, 10q, 11q, 12p, 12q, 13q, 14q, 15q, 16p, 16q, 17p, 17q, 18p, 19p, 19q, 20p, 20q, 21q, 22q | Gain | >15[57,135,231,232] |
| 1q23, 3p25 (including *RAF1*, *PPARG*), 6p22 (including *E2F3*, *SOX4*), 8p12-p11.2 (including *FGFR1*, *TACC1*, *POLB*), 8q24 (including *MYC*), 8q22 (including *YWHAZ*), 11q13 (including *CCND1*), 12q15 (including *MDM2*), 17q12-q21 (including *ERBB2*), 20q12-q13.2 (including *YWHAB*, *MYBL2*), 20q13.32-q13.33 | Amplification | 3–12 [57,232] |

[a] Array-based comparative genomic hybridization analyses.
HD, homozygous deletion; LOH, loss of heterozygosity.

UC cells with epithelial phenotype have enhanced sensitivity to FGFR inhibition compared to those with mesenchymal phenotype.[80] A recent RNAi screen in UC cell lines indicated that up-regulated EGFR signaling provides a mechanism of escape from FGFR inhibition and can mediate de novo resistance. A reciprocal relationship was found when EGFR was inhibited and both in vitro and in a preclinical in vivo model, combined inhibition showed improved anti-tumor activity.[81] Thus, assessment of both FGFR3 and EGFR status may be required to predict response and combined EGFR and FGFR3 inhibition may be essential. Several clinical trials of FGFR inhibitors are now planned or in progress in advanced UC.

FGFR1 is also overexpressed in many of these cancers.[23] An increased ratio of the FGFR1-β:FGFR1-α splice variants is found in MI tumors. The β isoform, lacking the first immunoglobulin-like domain, has increased sensitivity to FGF1.[82] FGF2 stimulation of ectopically expressed FGFR1-β in some UC-derived cell lines induces an epithelial-mesenchymal transition (EMT), a major feature of which is PLCγ-mediated upregulation of COX-2.[83] This is in contrast to the effect of FGFR1 signaling in NHUC, where increased proliferation and reduced apoptosis but no EMT is induced,[23] suggesting that FGFR1 plays different roles in NMI and MI UC. Compatible with this, UC cell lines with highest FGFR1 expression show a mesenchymal (EMT) phenotype (low E-cadherin expression) and upregulated FGF2 expression, and those with epithelial phenotype show higher FGFR3 and E-cadherin and lower FGFR1.[84] In an animal model of UC metastasis using an FGFR1-dependent cell line, an FGFR inhibitor reduced the development of circulating tumor cells and metastasis but not primary tumor growth.[84] Currently, there is no information on the prognostic significance of FGFR1 upregulation, and FGFR1 has not yet been examined independently of FGFR3 as a potential therapeutic target.

Several other oncogenes are implicated in MI UC. Four to six percent have amplification of *MDM2* (12q14).[57,85,86] MDM2 regulates p53 levels, and overexpression provides an alternative mechanism to inactivate p53 function (Fig. 38.3). There is no consensus on the relationship of upregulated MDM2 to tumor grade, stage, or prognosis. MYC is upregulated in many bladder tumors, although the mechanism for this is unclear.[87] Although amplifications of 8q are found in invasive UC, MYC is not the major target. However, additional copies of the whole of 8q are common and may lead to overexpression.[24,57] MYC is also upregulated in response to other molecular events (e.g., MAPK pathway stimulation). An amplicon on 6p in 14% of MI UC and cell lines contains *E2F3*, and functional studies indicate that *E2F3* can drive urothelial cell proliferation.[88–92] E2F transcription factors interact with and are regulated by RB1 (Fig. 38.3) and in accord with this, tumors with *E2F3* amplification have RB1 or p16 inactivated.[89]

## Tumor Suppressor Genes

As in other aggressive cancers, the tumor suppressor genes *TP53*, *RB1*, *CDKN2A*, and *PTEN* are implicated in MI UC. The pathways controlled by TP53 and RB1 regulate cell-cycle progression and responses to stress (Fig. 38.3). *TP53* mutation is common in invasive UC and detection of mutation or TP53 protein accumulation is associated with poor prognosis. Although immunohistochemical detection of TP53 protein with increased half-life identifies many mutant TP53 proteins and is commonly used as a surrogate marker for mutation, some *TP53* mutations (~20%) yield unstable or truncated proteins that cannot be detected in this way. Thus, TP53 protein accumulation is not a useful prognostic marker. Two meta-analyses indicate only a small association between TP53 positivity and poor prognosis.[93,94] However, examination of both protein expression and mutation of *TP53* provides useful prognostic information.[95]

The RB pathway regulates cell-cycle progression from G1 to S phase (Fig. 38.3). HD, LOH of 13q14, and loss of RB1 protein expression are common in MI UC.[96–99] Loss of p16 expression is inversely related to positive RB1 expression,[100] and high-level p16 expression results from negative feedback in tumors with loss of RB1.[101] Thus, both loss of expression and high-level expression of p16 are associated with RB pathway deregulation, and these are adverse prognostic biomarkers found in >50% of MI tumors.[102] Interestingly, in MI UC with *FGFR3* mutation, a high frequency of *CDKN2A* HD has been reported, which may identify a progression pathway for NMI *FGFR3*-mutant tumors to muscle invasion via loss of *CDKN2A*.[103] As indicated previously, amplification and overexpression of E2F3, which is normally repressed by RB1, is associated with RB1 or p16 loss in MI tumors.[89] p16 and p14[ARF] proteins link the RB and p53 pathways (Fig. 38.3), and due to multiple regulatory feedback mechanisms, inactivation of both pathways together is predicted to have greater impact than inactivation of either pathway alone. This is borne out by the achievement of greater predictive power in studies using concurrent analyses of multiple changes that deregulate the G1 checkpoint.[102,104,105]

Altered PTEN expression is the most frequent mechanism for deregulation of the PI3K pathway in MI UC. PTEN (phosphatase and tensin homolog deleted on chromosome 10) (10q23) is a lipid and protein phosphatase whose major lipid substrate is phosphatidylinositol (3,4,5)-triphosphate (PIP3) generated by PI3K (Fig. 38.2A). *PTEN* LOH is found in 24% to 58% of invasive UC,[106–108] and copy number analysis has identified a relationship of PTEN loss to metastatic disease.[57] Mutation of the retained copy is infrequent but HD has been detected in tumor cell lines.[26,109–111] Overall, 46% of UC lines (largely derived from MI tumors) had PTEN alterations.[26] Reduced expression is common

in tumors[26,112] and is associated with TP53 alteration. Many tumors (41%) with altered TP53 show downregulation of *PTEN*, and this combined alteration is associated with poor outcome.[113] As *PTEN* is haploinsufficient in mouse models,[114] loss of one allele in UC may lead to altered phenotype. In mice, conditional deletion of *Pten* in the urothelium led to early urothelial hyperplasia[112,115] and late development of tumors resembling human papillary superficial tumors. A study that induced stochastic deletion of *p53* and/or *Pten* showed that deletion of either gene alone did not lead to tumor formation, but dual deletion led to early development of aggressive UC, with frequent metastases.[113] PTEN loss may affect proliferation, apoptosis, and migration. Reexpression in PTEN-null UC cells has revealed effects on cell chemotaxis, anchorage-independent growth, and tumor growth in vivo.[116–118] UC cell invasion can be inhibited by the protein phosphatase activity of PTEN alone.[116] Thus, loss of lipid and protein phosphatase activities of PTEN may contribute in different ways to urothelial tumorigenesis.

The *TSC1* product hamartin acts in the PI3K pathway downstream of PTEN (Fig. 38.2A), providing an alternative mechanism of pathway activation in 13% of invasive UCs that have mutational inactivation.[26,27] Whereas good response to mTOR inhibitors has been reported in some patients and UC cell lines with mutant *TSC1*, mutation alone is not a sufficient predictive biomarker.[119,120]

The Rho GDP dissociation inhibitor RhoGDI2 has been implicated as a tumor suppressor in UC. Expression is reduced in an isogenic cell line model of metastasis and low expression is associated with reduced survival in patients with UC.[121] Potential downstream effectors of RhoGDI2 are endothelin and versican, which are upregulated upon loss of RhoGDI2 expression. In an experimental model of metastasis, endothelin 1 was required for lung colonization by UC cells and pharmacologic inhibition of the endothelin axis reduced colonization.[122] RhoGDI2-regulated versican levels are implicated in enhancing macrophage recruitment and chemokine CCL1 levels.[123] As both of these proteins enhance the inflammatory response, the major role of RhoGDI2 may be to inhibit this. RhoGDI2 is phosphorylated by SRC, and this enhances its membrane localization and metastasis-suppression activity.[124] Compatible with this, and unlike the situation in many tumors, SRC levels in UC are highest in NMI tumors where RhoGDI2 function is intact.[125,126] SRC contributes to suppression of metastasis via regulation of p190Rho GAP, which in turn downregulates the activity of RHOA, RHOC, and ROCK.[127]

The WNT signaling pathway is also implicated in UC. Mutations in *APC* have been reported,[27,128] mainly in MI tumors. The frequency of mutations in *CTNNB1* is low, but altered beta-catenin expression (reduced expression or increased nuclear localization) is frequent in MI UC,[128–131] though this is not associated with *APC* mutation.[128] Other alterations in the WNT pathway include epigenetic silencing of the antagonists of WNT signaling, secreted frizzled receptor proteins,[132] and the Wnt inhibitory factor 1 (WIF1).[133]

## Other Genomic Alterations in Invasive Urothelial Carcinoma

Invasive UC is often genomically unstable, with significant genetic divergence of related tumors in the same patient over time. Array-based comparative genomic hybridization and single nucleotide polymorphism array analyses have identified many copy number alterations[57,134–137] (Table 38.2). These include numerous losses and gains in DNA copy number and many regions of high-level amplification that may contain novel oncogenes. To date, the target genes within many of these regions have not been identified. Many regions of copy number alteration show significant association with high tumor grade, stage, and/or outcome. These include amplicons at 1q21–24, 3p25, 6p22, 8p11, 8q22, 11q12, 12q15, and 17q12. Plausible candidate oncogenes within these are *PPARG* (3p25), *E2F3* and *SOX4* (6p22), *FGFR1*, *TACC1* and *POLB* (8p11), *YWHAZ* (8q22),

*CCND1* (11q12), *MDM2* (12q15), and *ERBB2* (17q12).[57,135,138,139] On 1q21–24, at least three regions have been defined, two of which contain plausible candidates (*BCL9* and *CHD1L* in one, and *MCL1*, *SETDB1*, and *HIF1B* in a second).[139] Regions of HD include 1p34, 2q36, 9p21, 11p11, 18p11, and 19q13.[57] On 9p22, *CDKN2A* is one target and two further regions of HD have been identified.[57] Candidates within the other regions are less obvious.

It is notable that some stage T1 tumors show similar profiles to MI tumors (T2 or greater), suggesting that these tumors with the ability to break through the basement membrane may be aggressive lesions. However, other T1 tumors show remarkable similarity in their copy number profiles to Ta tumors, suggesting that distinct biologic subgroups exist.[57]

## INFORMATION FROM EXOME SEQUENCING

At the time of writing, three studies have reported sequencing of whole UC exomes.[31,32,140] In total, these have sequenced 12 Ta, 41 T1, and 72 T2 tumors. In two studies, selected genes were assessed in larger sample sets to examine prevalence.[31,140] Whereas the overall numbers of tumors studied remains relatively small, several important conclusions can be drawn. The first is that UC contains a relatively high frequency of somatic single nucleotide mutations, with estimates ranging from 50 to 170 per sample on average but with wide variability between samples. Many of the mutations ($\geq$ 30%) were nonsynonymous, a large proportion of which are predicted to be damaging (~60% estimated in one study[31]). To date, significant differences in mutation rates between non-aggressive and aggressive tumors are not apparent, though it is notable that very few stage Ta tumors have been studied so far. The most common base change reported is C:G>T:A transition followed by C:G>G:A transversion.

The most significant finding is that in addition to genes already implicated in UC (*TP53*, *FGFR3*, *HRAS*, *KRAS*, *PIK3CA*, *RB1*, *TSC1*), a large number of genes involved in chromatin modification show mutation. In the largest study, 58% of tumors had mutation in chromatin remodeling genes,[32] indicating that altered regulation of chromatin is a major oncogenic driver in UC. Mutated genes include histone demethylases (*KDM6A*, *KDM5A*, *KDM5B*, *UTY*), chromatin remodeling genes (*ARID1A*, *ARID4A*), histone lysine methyltransferases (*MLL*, *MLL2*, *MLL3*, *MLL5*), histone acetyltransferases (*CREBBP*, *EP300*, *EP400*), and SWI/SNF complex-related genes (*SMARCA4*, *SMARCA1*). Many of the mutations are predicted to impair function, suggesting tumor suppressor roles. Mutations were also found in DNA repair genes including *ATM*, *FANCA*, and *ERCC2*. Overall, in MI tumors the most frequently mutated genes were *KDM6A* (30%), *TP53* (24%), *ARID1A* (15%), *CREBBP* (15%), *EP300* (13%), *HRAS* (13%), *RB1* (13%), *PIK3CA* (12%), *STAG2* (11%), and *FGFR3* (11%).[32] In all three studies, relatively large numbers of genes were mutated at low frequency, suggesting that there is considerable biologic heterogeneity.

## EPIGENETIC ALTERATIONS

Epigenetic alterations, mainly those involving DNA methylation, have been widely reported. Most studies have analyzed single genes or small series of genes.[141–144] Genome-wide analyses have identified novel candidates, some with clinicopathologic associations.[145–149] In general, hypermethylation in CpG islands is more common in MI tumors and hypomethylation in regions distinct from CpG islands in NMI tumors.[147,148] Integrated analysis of methylation and gene expression indicates that CpG island hypermethylation is associated with loss of expression and CpG methylation within genes or at transcription factor binding sites with increased expression.[149] Hypermethylation-associated disease progression biomarkers in NMI tumors include *TBX2*, *TBX3*, *TBX4*, *GATA2*, and *ZIC2*.[145,147] These genes, which encode transcription factors

involved in lineage decisions during development, are implicated in EMT, stem cell phenotype, and differentiation. In the high-risk group of T1 grade 3 tumors treated with BCG, combined methylation of *MSH6* and *THBS1* is associated with disease progression.[150] Hypermethylation of several miRNAs is associated with tumor grade and stage. Some of these have prognostic value (e.g., the miR-200 family and miR-205) and are frequently silenced in MI tumors, and this is correlated with disease progression in T1 tumors.[151]

There are many reports of improved detection of UC by analysis of methylation biomarkers in urine. Examples include a panel of five biomarkers (*MYO3A*, *CA10*, *NKX6-2*, *DBC1*, and *SOX11* or *PENK*),[152] two panels each of four biomarkers (*ZNF154*, *POU4F2*, *HOXA9*, and *EOMES*),[147] (*APC*, 2 *TERT* CpGs, and *EDNRB*),[153] one of two markers (*TWIST1* and *NID2*),[154] and one of three markers (*OTX1*, *ONECUT*, and *OSR1*), used in combination with *FGFR3* mutation.[155]

To date, chromatin modification has not been extensively studied. In UC cell lines, the active histone mark H3K9Ac and the repressive mark H3K27me3 are associated with miR-200/miR-205 expression or methylation, respectively.[151] Genomewide analysis has identified UC-specific differences in the distribution of histone marks and indicated the importance of both DNA and H3K27 methylation in gene silencing in cell lines.[156] In tumor tissues, seven genomic regions where transcriptional deregulation is independent of DNA copy number[157] were shown to be silenced by a mechanism associated with histone H3K9 and H3K27 trimethylation and histone H3K9 hypoacetylation, a pattern of silencing also found in a subgroup of UC with a carcinoma in situ (CIS)–associated expression signature.[158] With the recent identification of many mutations in chromatin remodeling genes in UC,[31,32,140] more extensive analysis of chromatin modifications and assessment of potential therapeutic opportunities are now needed.

## INFORMATION FROM EXPRESSION PROFILING

mRNA expression signatures associated with UC grade, stage, progression, nodal involvement, response to chemotherapy, and survival have been derived,[134,159–171] and some signatures have performed well in independent validation studies.[172,173] Overlap between signatures from different studies is generally low, but there is significant overlap in the cellular processes implicated.[174] Clinical application of these signatures requires the development of robust polymerase chain reaction–based assays or identification of antibodies suitable for immunohistochemistry. Already polymerase chain reaction–based gene signatures have been derived to predict progression in NMI tumors.[169,175] Recently, a novel system of classification for UC based on global analysis of expression data has been developed, and this is discussed in detail in a following section.

There are several reports of altered miRNA expression in UC.[176,177] Changes in apparently "normal" urothelium from patients with UC indicate that such alterations may occur early in disease development.[7] Global analyses using array-based methods or deep sequencing have revealed common upregulation of miRNAs in MI tumors and downregulation in NMI tumors.[7,178] Clustering analysis of miRNA data generated three clusters containing mainly Ta, T1, and T2-T4 tumors.[179] miRNAs downregulated in Ta tumors include miRs 7, 99a/100, 125b, 143, 146, 188, and 29c.[176,179,180] Many miRNA alterations are found in MI UC.[151,176,178–183] Examples include upregulation of miR-21,[7,182] which negatively regulates *TP53*,[7] and the miR-200 family, which are implicated in regulation of EMT.[184] Several miRNAs that are downregulated in MI UC (e.g., miR-145, miR-143, miR-203, miR-1, miR-133a, miR-195, and miR-125b) can induce apoptosis, reduce cell proliferation or migration in cultured UC cells, and show reciprocal expression with their targets in tumor tissues.[185–191] Upregulated miRNAs include miR-222 and miR-452, which are associated with adverse outcome.[192] Downregulation of miR-138 was shown to increase cisplatin sensitivity in UC cell lines.[193] Together, these data indicate that miRNA expression profiles may be valuable prognostic biomarkers.

## UROTHELIAL TUMOR–INITIATING CELLS

There is evidence for the existence of highly tumorigenic subpopulations of cells with stem cell–like characteristics within UC populations. As cancer stem cells in other tumor types show resistance to chemotherapy agents and are predicted to be the cause of posttreatment disease relapse, there is great interest in characterizing these cells and identifying markers that may allow specific targeting. Isolation of bladder cancer "stem" or "tumor-initiating" cells has been attempted from fresh tumor tissues and UC cell lines, using a range of assays. The putative stem cells express a range of markers including 67kD laminin receptor (67LR), CD44, CD90, ALDH1A1, and keratins 5, 14, and 17.[194,195] The majority of these are markers expressed by normal urothelial basal cells and in low-grade tumors, cells expressing these markers reside at the tumor-stromal interface.[196] Cell surface markers have been used to great effect to sort putative stem cells from mass cell populations. Cells from tumor samples that expressed CD44+, CK5+, CK20– had enhanced tumor-initiating ability compared to CD44–, CK5–, CK20+ cells and could generate tumors that contained both CD44+ and CD44– cells.[197] In UC cell lines, a subpopulation of CD44+, ALDH1A1+ cells is reported to have higher tumorigenicity than CD44–, ALDH1A1– cells, and in UC tissues higher ALDH1A1 expression was an independent prognostic factor for overall survival.[198] However, the finding that 58% of UC do not express CD44[197] has suggested that not all UC stem cells are derived from the basal compartment. Combinations of markers related to different urothelial differentiation states were found to stratify UC into clinically relevant subgroups; in each group, it was found that the least differentiated cell type showed stem cell–like characteristics.[199] This implies that UC stem cells can be derived from urothelial cells of different differentiation states. This diversity in stem cell phenotype may influence subsequent disease development and may have prognostic value.

## MOLECULAR PATHOGENESIS AND TUMOR CLONALITY

Multifocality and/or development of multiple recurrent tumors in the same patient is a common feature of UC. Although some patients develop more than one molecularly distinct tumor (oligoclonal disease),[200] most commonly tumors from the same patient are molecularly related,[201–203] with evidence for subclonal genomic evolution in different lesions.[204] Chromosome 9 LOH has been proposed as an early event in UC development as it is found in "normal" urothelium and hyperplasia in tumor-bearing patients.[205,206] Compatible with this, loss of the same allele is commonly shared by all related tumors.[207] Construction of phylogenetic trees from multiple related NMI tumors confirms the early loss of chromosome 9 with later events including 11p–, 20q+, 17p–, and 11q–.[203] Interestingly, tumors with highest genomic complexity are not necessarily the last to appear in the patient.[208,209]

Urothelial dysplasia and CIS, predicted precursors of MI UC, show frequent chromosome 9 LOH and *TP53* mutation,[210–212] and multiple other chromosomal alterations.[213] Detailed genomic mapping of cystectomy specimens has indicated that prior to detectable morphologic abnormality, large areas of urothelium show LOH of specific chromosomal regions. Areas of dysplasia showed more complex patterns of LOH, suggesting sequential evolutionary changes associated with acquisition of growth advantage. Thus, it is suggested that development of MI UC involves displacement of the normal urothelium by a molecularly altered clone, within which subclones with additional alterations arise. Six critical regions of LOH (3q22, 5q22–23, 9q21, 10q26, and 17p13) were identified.[214,215] Biallelic inactivation of *ITM2B* and *P2RY5*, genes close to *RB1*, implicate these in driving early clonal expansion.[214]

Polyclonal hypermethylation detected throughout the "normal" urothelium in tumor-bearing bladders also suggests widespread pre-malignant epigenetic "field change."[148] The genes affected, which may represent early "drivers" of UC, include ZO2, MYOD1, CDH13, and many polycomb repressive complex 2 (PRC2) targets, all of which have plausible functional significance and showed hypermethylation in the related invasive tumors.

## MULTIPLE TUMOR SUBGROUPS DEFINED BY MOLECULAR PROFILING

Bladder tumors of similar grade and stage commonly show divergent clinical behavior. In particular, stage T1 tumors show considerable molecular and clinical diversity. Until recently, molecular features have failed to explain or predict this heterogeneity. The two tumor groupings that have for so long dominated the bladder cancer literature are insufficient for this. Recent studies have begun to unravel this complexity, revealing multiple subgroups that are independent of conventional grade and stage groupings (Fig. 38.4).

Initial assessment of mRNA expression profiles of UC of all grades and stages identified the two major molecular subtypes, separated mainly though not entirely, according to grade and stage with stage T1 tumors distributed relatively equally between the two.[134,135] More recent analysis has defined additional subtypes. Five major subtypes were termed urobasal A (UroA), UroB, GU, squamous cell carcinoma–like (SCCL), and "infiltrated"[216] (Fig. 38.4A). Tumors in the latter group are highly infiltrated with nontumor cells, whereas the definition of the other groups reflects tumor cell–specific criteria. Clear differences in expression of cell cycle regulators, keratins, receptor tyrosine kinases, and cell adhesion molecules are evident. UroA and UroB subtypes express high levels of FGFR3, CCND1, and TP63; GU tumors show low levels of these proteins but high levels of ERBB2 and E-cadherin; and SCCL tumors express P-cadherin and high levels of KRT5, KRT14, and proteins involved in keratinization. These subtypes showed distinct clinical outcome. UroA had good prognosis, GU had intermediate prognosis, and SCCL and UroB, the worst prognosis. UroB tumors share epithelial characteristics with UroA tumors including *FGFR3* mutation, but they also show *TP53* mutation and are often invasive. T1 tumors appear evenly distributed between molecular subtypes.[216]

Robust assays, ideally based on immunohistochemical detection of proteins in formalin-fixed, paraffin-embedded tissues are required to apply these findings in the clinic. Immunohistochemistry of a panel of markers selected from the defined mRNA subgroup signatures has recently been assessed in combination with morphologic criteria.[217] Histopathologic and immunohistochemical profiles were examined in all subtypes except "infiltrated," with excellent correlation between mRNA and protein expression for the majority of markers. Importantly, the distribution of protein expression within the tissues also provided valuable information. For example, UroA tumors show restriction of KRT5, P-cadherin, EGFR, and CCNB1 expression to the basal cell layer, reminiscent of normal urothelium, implying retention of dependence on stromal interactions, whereas many UroB tumor show expression of these proteins in suprabasal layers. The keratin expression profile (KRT14+, KRT5+, KRT20–) of SCCL tumors is characteristic of the least differentiated class of tumor initiating cells described by Chan et al.[197] and termed "basal" in the study of Volkmer et al.[199] Their phenotype is also similar to basal-like breast carcinoma,[218] and it has been suggested that these UC could in future be defined as "basal-like."[217]

A simple classifier based on grade and urothelial differentiation pattern and expression of KRT5 and CCNB1 was able to reproduce the original genomewide expression classification with an accuracy of 0.88.[217] The three major subgroups, urobasal (UroA + UroB), GU, and SCCL, showed highly significant association with disease-specific survival. However, a simple method to distinguish UroA from the small, related UroB subset, many of which are MI, proved difficult.[217] The common features of UroA and UroB may indicate that MI UroB tumors have their origins as non-invasive

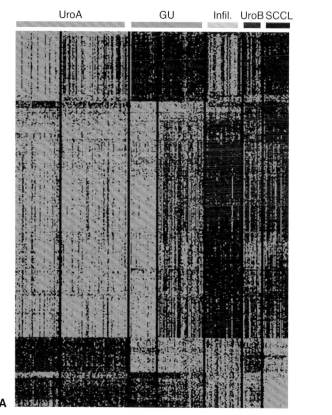
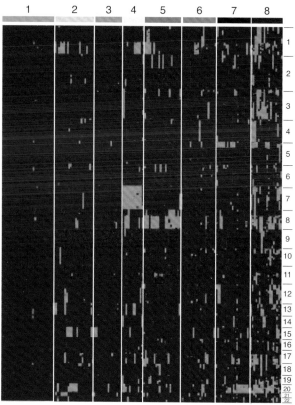

**Figure 38.4** Tumor subgroups defined by molecular profiling. **(A)** Major bladder cancer subtypes identified by mRNA expression profiling (adapted with permission from Sjodahl et al.[216]). Hierarchical cluster analysis of 308 samples generated five major tumor clusters. Each column of the heatmap represents one sample, and each row represents one gene. *Green* represents low gene expression, and *red* represents high gene expression. The five major subtypes are indicated by the *color bars* at the top of figure. GU, genomically unstable; SCCL, squamous cell carcinoma–like; UroA, urobasal A; UroB, urobasal B; Infil, "Infiltrated". **(B)** Major bladder cancer subtypes identified by array-based comparative genomic hybridization.[57] Hierarchical cluster analysis was performed using copy number data from 160 tumors. *Red* represents copy number loss, and *green* represents copy number gain. Chromosome number is shown down the right-hand side of the figure. Eight main clusters of tumors were identified, and these are indicated by the *color bars* at the top of the figure.

UroA tumors. Interestingly, UroB showed common loss of p16 expression, which as discussed previously, may represent a means by which NMI *FGFR3*-mutant tumors can progress.[103] In common with NMI tumors, UroB retains TP63 expression and may represent the aggressive subset of TP63-expressing advanced UC reported by Choi et al.[219] Further studies of this subtype are essential to allow development of a clinically applicable classification assay.

Similarly, DNA copy number and mutation status has identified multiple subgroups of tumors within the conventional grade and stage groupings[57] (Fig 38.4B), though these have not been as extensively studied as expression-based subtypes and classification signatures are not yet defined. DNA methylation profiles also identify several subtypes.[148,149,220] Four "epitypes" showed broad alignment with expression subtypes.[149] One epitype showed methylation pattern similar to immune cells and represented the heavily infiltrated group of tumors. Two others corresponded to the two major expression subtypes,[134,135] one of which contained many aggressive

tumors with upregulation of EZH2 and corresponding DNA methylation of polycomb target genes and several HOX genes, whose hypermethylation is implicated in aggressive growth of other cancer types. As for expression subtypes, these epitypes do not align absolutely with tumor grade and stage. Integration of information from all genome-wide platforms, including miRNA expression data, is now needed to provide optimum prognostic and predictive biomarkers. As DNA and miRNA are more robust molecules than RNA in formalin-fixed, paraffin-embedded specimens, a combination of these and protein biomarkers may ultimately be most useful.

## ACKNOWLEDGEMENTS

We acknowledge the valuable advice of Professor M Höglund and Dr KS Chan on the sections on tumor subgroups and urothelial tumor-initiating cells.

## REFERENCES

1. Dudek AM, Grotenhuis AJ, Vermeulen SH, et al. Urinary bladder cancer susceptibility markers. What do we know about functional mechanisms? *Int J Mol Sci* 2013;14:12346–12366.
2. Chang DW, Gu J, Wu X. Germline prognostic markers for urinary bladder cancer: obstacles and opportunities. *Urol Oncol* 2012;30:524–532.
3. Billerey C, Chopin D, Aubriot-Lorton MH, et al. Frequent FGFR3 mutations in papillary non-invasive bladder (pTa) tumors. *Am J Pathol* 2001;158: 1955–1959.
4. Ornitz DM, Itoh N. Fibroblast growth factors. *Genome Biol* 2001;2.
5. van Rhijn BWG, Montironi R, Zwarthoff EC, et al. Frequent FGFR3 mutations in urothelial papilloma. *J Pathol* 2002;198:245–251.

6. Tomlinson DC, Baldo O, Harnden P, et al. FGFR3 protein expression and its relationship to mutation status and prognostic variables in bladder cancer. *J Pathol* 2007;213:91–98.
7. Catto JW, Miah S, Owen HC, et al. Distinct microRNA alterations characterize high- and low-grade bladder cancer. *Cancer Res* 2009;69:8472–8481.
8. Sayan AE, D'Angelo B, Sayan BS, et al. p73 and p63 regulate the expression of fibroblast growth factor receptor 3. *Biochem Biophys Res Commun* 2010;394:824–828.
9. di Martino E, L'Hôte CG, Kennedy W, et al. Mutant fibroblast growth factor receptor 3 induces intracellular signaling and cellular transformation in a cell type- and mutation-specific manner. *Oncogene* 2009;28:4306–4316.

10. Williams SV, Hurst CD, Knowles MA. Oncogenic FGFR3 gene fusions in bladder cancer. *Hum Mol Genet* 2012.

11. Gan Y, Wientjes MG, Au JL. Expression of basic fibroblast growth factor correlates with resistance to paclitaxel in human patient tumors. *Pharm Res* 2006;23:1324–1331.

12. Yoshimura K, Eto H, Miyake H, et al. Messenger ribonucleic acids for fibroblast growth factors and their receptor in bladder and renal cell carcinoma cell lines. *Cancer Lett* 1996;103:91–97.

13. O'Brien TS, Smith K, Cranston D, et al. Urinary basic fibroblast growth factor in patients with bladder cancer and benign prostatic hypertrophy. *Br J Urol* 1995;76:311–314.

14. O'Brien T, Cranston D, Fuggle S, et al. Two mechanisms of basic fibroblast growth factor-induced angiogenesis in bladder cancer. *Cancer Res* 1997;57:136–140.

15. Jebar AH, Hurst CD, Tomlinson DC, et al. FGFR3 and Ras gene mutations are mutually exclusive genetic events in urothelial cell carcinoma. *Oncogene* 2005;24:5218–5225.

16. Mo L, Zheng X, Huang H-Y, et al. Hyperactivation of Ha-ras oncogene, but not Ink4a/Arf deficiency, triggers bladder tumorigenesis. *J Clin Invest* 2007;117:314–325.

17. Zieger K, Dyrskjot L, Wiuf C, et al. Role of activating fibroblast growth factor receptor 3 mutations in the development of bladder tumors. *Clin Cancer Res* 2005;11:7709–7719.

18. Hernandez S, Lopez-Knowles E, Lloreta J, et al. Prospective study of FGFR3 mutations as a prognostic factor in nonmuscle invasive urothelial bladder carcinomas. *J Clin Oncol* 2006;24:3664–3671.

19. Kompier LC, van der Aa MNM, Lurkin I, et al. The development of multiple bladder tumour recurrences in relation to the FGFR3 mutation status of the primary tumour. *J Pathol* 2009;218:104–112.

20. Eble JN, Sauter G, Epstein JI, et al. *World Health Organization Classification of Tumours. Pathology and Genetics of Tumours of the Urinary System and Male Genital Organs.* Lyon, France: IARC Press; 2004.

21. Barbisan F, Santinelli A, Mazzucchelli R, et al. Strong immunohistochemical expression of fibroblast growth factor receptor 3, superficial staining pattern of cytokeratin 20, and low proliferative activity define those papillary urothelial neoplasms of low malignant potential that do not recur. *Cancer* 2008;112:636–644.

22. di Martino E, Tomlinson DC, Knowles MA. A decade of FGF receptor research in bladder cancer: Past, present, and future challenges. *Adv Urol* 2012; 2012:429213.

23. Tomlinson DC, Lamont FR, Shnyder SD, et al. Fibroblast growth factor receptor 1 promotes proliferation and survival via activation of the mitogen-activated protein kinase pathway in bladder cancer. *Cancer Res* 2009;69:4613–4620.

24. Williams SV, Platt FM, Hurst CD, et al. High-resolution analysis of genomic alteration on chromosome arm 8p in urothelial carcinoma. *Genes Chromosomes Cancer* 2010;49:642–659.

25. López-Knowles E, Hernández S, Malats N, et al. PIK3CA mutations are an early genetic alteration associated with FGFR3 mutations in superficial papillary bladder tumors. *Cancer Res* 2006;66:7401–7404.

26. Platt FM, Hurst CD, Taylor CF, et al. Spectrum of phosphatidylinositol 3-kinase pathway gene alterations in bladder cancer. *Clin Cancer Res* 2009;15:6008–6017.

27. Sjodahl G, Lauss M, Gudjonsson S, et al. A systematic study of gene mutations in urothelial carcinoma; inactivating mutations in TSC2 and PIK3R1. *PloS One* 2011;6:e18583.

28. Kompier LC, Lurkin I, van der Aa MNM, et al. FGFR3, HRAS, KRAS, NRAS and PIK3CA mutations in bladder cancer and their potential as biomarkers for surveillance and therapy. *PloS One* 2010;5:e13821.

29. Zhao L, Vogt PK. Helical domain and kinase domain mutations in p110(alpha) of phosphatidylinositol 3-kinase induce gain of function by different mechanisms. *Proc Natl Acad Sci* 2008;105:2652–2657.

30. Ross RL, Askham JM, Knowles MA. PIK3CA mutation spectrum in urothelial carcinoma reflects cell context-dependent signaling and phenotypic outputs. *Oncogene* 2012;32:768–776.

31. Balbas-Martinez C, Sagrera A, Carrillo-de-Santa-Pau E, et al. Recurrent inactivation of STAG2 in bladder cancer is not associated with aneuploidy. *Nat Genet* 2013;45:1464–1469.

32. Guo G, Sun X, Chen C, et al. Whole-genome and whole-exome sequencing of bladder cancer identifies frequent alterations in genes involved in sister chromatid cohesion and segregation. *Nat Genet* 2013;45:1459–1463.

33. Solomon DA, Kim JS, Bondaruk J, et al. Frequent truncating mutations of STAG2 in bladder cancer. *Nat Genet* 2013;45:1428–1430.

34. Taylor C, Platt F, Hurst C, et al. Frequent inactivating mutations of STAG2 in bladder cancer are associated with low tumor grade and stage and inversely related to chromosomal copy number changes. *Hum Mol Genet* 2014;23: 1964–1974.

35. Solomon DA, Kim T, Diaz-Martinez LA, et al. Mutational inactivation of STAG2 causes aneuploidy in human cancer. *Science* 2011;333:1039–1043.

36. Cuadrado A, Remeseiro S, Gomez-Lopez G, et al. The specific contributions of cohesin-SA1 to cohesion and gene expression: implications for cancer and development. *Cell Cycle* 2012;11:2233–2238.

37. Allory Y, Beukers W, Sagrera A, et al. Telomerase reverse transcriptase promoter mutations in bladder cancer: High frequency across stages, detection in urine, and lack of association with outcome. *Eur Urol* 2014;65:360–366.

38. Hurst CD, Platt FM, Knowles MA. Comprehensive mutation analysis of the TERT promoter in bladder cancer and detection of mutations in voided urine. *Eur Urol* 2014;65:367–369.

39. Berggren P, Kumar R, Sakano S, et al. Detecting homozygous deletions in the CDKN2A(p16(INK4a))/ARF(p14(ARF)) gene in urinary bladder cancer using real-time quantitative PCR. *Clin Cancer Res* 2003;9:235–242.

40. Cairns P, Tokino K, Eby Y, et al. Homozygous deletions of 9p21 in primary human bladder tumors detected by comparative multiplex polymerase chain reaction. *Cancer Res* 1994;54:1422–1424.

41. Williamson MP, Elder PA, Shaw ME, et al. p16 (CDKN2) is a major deletion target at 9p21 in bladder cancer. *Hum Mol Genet* 1995;4:1569–1577.

42. Orlow I, Lacombe L, Hannon GJ, et al. Deletion of the p16 and p15 genes in human bladder tumors. *J Natl Cancer Inst* 1995;87:1524–1529.

43. Aboulkassim TO, LaRue H, Lemieux P, et al. Alteration of the PATCHED locus in superficial bladder cancer. *Oncogene* 2003;22:2967–2971.

44. McGarvey TW, Maruta Y, Tomaszewski JE, et al. PTCH gene mutations in invasive transitional cell carcinoma of the bladder. *Oncogene* 1998;17:1167–1172.

45. Habuchi T, Luscombe M, Elder PA, et al. Structure and methylation-based silencing of a gene (DBCCR1) within a candidate bladder cancer tumor suppressor region at 9q32-q33. *Genomics* 1998;48:277–288.

46. Nishiyama H, Hornigold N, Davies A, et al. A sequence-ready 840-kb PAC contig spanning the candidate tumor suppressor locus DBC1 on human chromosome 9q32-q33. *Genomics* 1999;59:335–338.

47. Stadler WM, Steinberg G, Yang X, et al. Alterations of the 9p21 and 9q33 chromosomal bands in clinical bladder cancer specimens by fluorescence in situ hybridization. *Clin Cancer Res* 2001;7:1676–1682.

48. Knowles MA, Habuchi T, Kennedy W, et al. Mutation Spectrum of the 9q34 Tuberous Sclerosis Gene TSC1 in Transitional Cell Carcinoma of the Bladder. *Cancer Res* 2003;63:7652–7656.

49. Pymar LS, Platt FM, Askham JM, et al. Bladder tumour-derived somatic TSC1 missense mutations cause loss of function via distinct mechanisms. *Hum Mol Genet* 2008;17:2006–2017.

50. Ploussard G, Dubosq F, Soliman H, et al. Prognostic value of loss of heterozygosity at chromosome 9p in non-muscle-invasive bladder cancer. *Urology* 2010;76:513–518.

51. Kruger S, Mahnken A, Kausch I, et al. P16 immunoreactivity is an independent predictor of tumor progression in minimally invasive urothelial bladder carcinoma. *Eur Urol* 2005;47:463–467.

52. Bartoletti R, Cai T, Nesi G, et al. Loss of P16 expression and chromosome 9p21 LOH in predicting outcome of patients affected by superficial bladder cancer. *J Surg Res* 2007;143:422–427.

53. Carnero A, Hudson JD, Price CM, et al. p16INK4A and p19ARF act in overlapping pathways in cellular immortalization. *Nat Cell Biol* 2000;2:148–155.

54. Serrano M. The INK4a/ARF locus in murine tumorigenesis. *Carcinogenesis* 2000;21:865–869.

55. Nishiyama H, Takahashi T, Kakehi Y, et al. Homozygous deletion at the 9q32–33 candidate tumor suppressor locus in primary human bladder cancer. *Genes Chromosomes Cancer* 1999;26:171–175.

56. Habuchi T, Takahashi T, Kakinuma H, et al. Hypermethylation at 9q32–33 tumour suppressor region is age-related in normal urothelium and an early and frequent alteration in bladder cancer. *Oncogene* 2001;20:531–537.

57. Hurst CD, Platt FM, Taylor CF, et al. Novel tumor subgroups of urothelial carcinoma of the bladder defined by integrated genomic analysis. *Clin Cancer Res* 2012;18:5865–5877.

58. Nord H, Segersten U, Sandgren J, et al. Focal amplifications are associated with high grade and recurrences in stage Ta bladder carcinoma. *Int J Cancer* 2010;126:1390–1402.

59. Shariat SF, Ashfaq R, Sagalowsky AI, et al. Correlation of cyclin D1 and E1 expression with bladder cancer presence, invasion, progression, and metastasis. *Hum Pathol* 2006;37:1568–1576.

60. Fristrup N, Birkenkamp-Demtroder K, Reinert T, et al. Multicenter validation of cyclin D1, MCM7, TRIM29, and UBE2C as prognostic protein markers in non-muscle-invasive bladder cancer. *Am J Pathol* 2013;182:339–349.

61. Kassouf W, Black PC, Tuziak T, et al. Distinctive expression pattern of ErbB family receptors signifies an aggressive variant of bladder cancer. *J Urol* 2008; 179:353–358.

62. Jimenez RE, Hussain M, Bianco FJ Jr, et al. Her-2/neu overexpression in muscle-invasive urothelial carcinoma of the bladder: prognostic significance and comparative analysis in primary and metastatic tumors. *Clin Cancer Res* 2001;7:2440–2447.

63. Kruger S, Weitsch G, Buttner H, et al. HER2 overexpression in muscle-invasive urothelial carcinoma of the bladder: prognostic implications. *Int J Cancer* 2002; 102:514–518.

64. Chow NH, Chan SH, Tzai TS, et al. Expression profiles of ErbB family receptors and prognosis in primary transitional cell carcinoma of the urinary bladder. *Clin Cancer Res* 2001;7:1957–1962.

65. Forster JA, Paul AB, Harnden P, et al. Expression of NRG1 and its receptors in human bladder cancer. *Br J Cancer* 2011;104:1135–1143.

66. Sauter G, Moch H, Moore D, et al. Heterogeneity of erbB-2 gene amplification in bladder cancer. *Cancer Res* 1993;53:2199–2203.

67. Fleischmann A, Rotzer D, Seiler R, et al. Her2 amplification is significantly more frequent in lymph node metastases from urothelial bladder cancer than in the primary tumours. *Eur Urol* 2011;60:350–357.

68. Memon AA, Sorensen BS, Meldgaard P, et al. The relation between survival and expression of HER1 and HER2 depends on the expression of HER3 and HER4: a study in bladder cancer patients. *Br J Cancer* 2006;94:1703–1709.

69. Amsellem-Ouazana D, Bieche I, Tozlu S, et al. Gene expression profiling of ERBB receptors and ligands in human transitional cell carcinoma of the bladder. *J Urol* 2006;175:1127–1132.

70. Mellon K, Wright C, Kelly P, et al. Long-term outcome related to epidermal growth factor receptor status in bladder cancer. *J Urol* 1995;153:919–925.

71. Neal DE, Marsh C, Bennett MK, et al. Epidermal-growth-factor receptors in human bladder cancer: comparison of invasive and superficial tumours. *Lancet* 1985;1:366–368.

72. Verdoom B, Kessler E, Flaig T. Targeted therapy in advanced urothelial carcinoma. *Oncology* 2013;27:219–226.

73. Zhang ZT, Pak J, Huang HY, et al. Role of Ha-ras activation in superficial papillary pathway of urothelial tumor formation. *Oncogene* 2001;20:1973–1980.

74. Theodorescu D, Cornil I, Sheehan C, et al. Ha-*ras* induction of the invasive phenotype results in up-regulation of epidermal growth factor receptors and altered responsiveness to epidermal growth factor in human papillary transitional cell carcinoma cells. *Cancer Res* 1991;51:4486–4491.

75. van Rhijn BWG, van der Kwast TH, Vis AN, et al. FGFR3 and P53 characterize alternative genetic pathways in the pathogenesis of urothelial cell carcinoma. *Cancer Res* 2004;64:1911–1914.

76. Tomlinson DC, Hurst CD, Knowles MA. Knockdown by shRNA identifies S249C mutant FGFR3 as a potential therapeutic target in bladder cancer. *Oncogene* 2007;26:5889–5899.

77. Lamont FR, Tomlinson DC, Cooper PA, et al. Small molecule FGF receptor inhibitors block FGFR-dependent urothelial carcinoma growth in vitro and in vivo. *Br J Cancer* 2011;104:75–82.

78. Qing J, Du X, Chen Y, et al. Antibody-based targeting of FGFR3 in bladder carcinoma and t(4;14)-positive multiple myeloma in mice. *J Clin Invest* 2009;119:1216–1229.

79. Miyake M, Ishii M, Koyama N, et al. PD173074, a selective tyrosine kinase inhibitor of FGFR3, inhibits cell proliferation of bladder cancer carrying the FGFR3 gene mutation along with up-regulation of p27/Kip1 and G1/G0 arrest. *J Pharmacol Exp Ther* 2010;332:795–802.

80. Gust KM, McConkey DJ, Awrey S, et al. Fibroblast growth factor receptor 3 is a rational therapeutic target in bladder cancer. *Mol Cancer Ther* 2013;12:1245–1254.

81. Herrera-Abreu MT, Pearson A, Campbell J, et al. Parallel RNA interference screens identify EGFR activation as an escape mechanism in FGFR3 mutant cancer. *Cancer Discovery* 2013;3:1058–1071.

82. Tomlinson DC, Knowles MA. Altered splicing of FGFR1 is associated with high tumor grade and stage and leads to increased sensitivity to FGF1 in bladder cancer. *Am J Pathol* 2010;177:2379–2386.

83. Tomlinson DC, Baxter EW, Loadman PM, et al. FGFR1-induced epithelial to mesenchymal transition through MAPK/PLCgamma/COX-2-mediated mechanisms. *PloS One* 2012;7:e38972.

84. Cheng T, Roth B, Choi W, et al. Fibroblast growth factor receptors-1 and -3 play distinct roles in the regulation of bladder cancer growth and metastasis: implications for therapeutic targeting. *PloS One* 2013;8:e57284.

85. Habuchi T, Kinoshita H, Yamada H, et al. Oncogene amplification in urothelial cancers with p53 gene mutation or MDM2 amplification. *J Natl Cancer Inst* 1994;86:1331–1335.

86. Simon R, Struckmann K, Schraml P, et al. Amplification pattern of 12q13-q15 genes (MDM2, CDK4, GLI) in urinary bladder cancer. *Oncogene* 2002;21:2476–2483.

87. Schmitz-Drager BJ, Schulz WA, Jurgens B, et al. c-myc in bladder cancer. Clinical findings and analysis of mechanism. *Urol Res* 1997;25:S45–S49.

88. Feber A, Clark J, Goodwin G, et al. Amplification and overexpression of E2F3 in human bladder cancer. *Oncogene* 2004;23:1627–1630.

89. Hurst CD, Tomlinson DC, Williams SV, et al. Inactivation of the Rb pathway and overexpression of both isoforms of E2F3 are obligate events in bladder tumours with 6p22 amplification. *Oncogene* 2008;27:2716–2727.

90. Oeggerli M, Schraml P, Ruiz C, et al. E2F3 is the main target gene of the 6p22 amplicon with high specificity for human bladder cancer. *Oncogene* 2006;25:6538–6543.

91. Oeggerli M, Tomovska S, Schraml P, et al. E2F3 amplification and overexpression is associated with invasive tumor growth and rapid tumor cell proliferation in urinary bladder cancer. *Oncogene* 2004;23:5616–5623.

92. Olsson AY, Feber A, Edwards S, et al. Role of E2F3 expression in modulating cellular proliferation rate in human bladder and prostate cancer cells. *Oncogene* 2007;26:1028–1037.

93. Malats N, Bustos A, Nascimento CM, et al. P53 as a prognostic marker for bladder cancer: A meta-analysis and review. *Lancet Oncol* 2005;6:678–686.

94. Schmitz-Drager BJ, Goebell PJ, Ebert T, et al. p53 immunohistochemistry as a prognostic marker in bladder cancer. Playground for urology scientists? *Eur Urol* 2000;38:691–699;discussion 700.

95. George B, Datar RH, Wu L, et al. p53 gene and protein status: the role of p53 alterations in predicting outcome in patients with bladder cancer. *J Clin Oncol* 2007;25:5352–5358.

96. Cairns P, Proctor AJ, Knowles MA. Loss of heterozygosity at the *RB* locus is frequent and correlates with muscle invasion in bladder carcinoma. *Oncogene* 1991;6:2305–2309.

97. Cordon-Cardo C, Wartinger D, Petrylak D, et al. Altered expression of the retinoblastoma gene product: Prognostic indicator in bladder cancer. *J Natl Cancer Inst* 1992;84:1251–1256.

98. Logothetis CJ, Xu H-J, Ro JY, et al. Altered expression of retinoblastoma protein and known prognostic variables in locally advanced bladder cancer. *J Natl Cancer Inst* 1992;84:1256–1261.

99. Xu H, Cairns P, Hu S, et al. Loss of RB protein expression in primary bladder cancer correlates with loss of heterozygosity at the RB locus and tumor progression. *Int J Cancer* 1993;53:781–784.

100. Le Frere-Belda MA, Gil Diez de Medina S, Daher A, et al. Profiles of the 2 INK4a gene products, p16 and p14ARF, in human reference urothelium and bladder carcinomas, according to pRb and p53 protein status. *Hum Pathol* 2004;35:817–824.

101. Benedict WF, Lerner SP, Zhou J, et al. Level of retinoblastoma protein expression correlates with p16 (MTS-1/INK4A/CDKN2) status in bladder cancer. *Oncogene* 1999;18:1197–1203.

102. Shariat SF, Tokunaga H, Zhou J, et al. p53, p21, pRB, and p16 expression predict clinical outcome in cystectomy with bladder cancer. *J Clin Oncol* 2004;22:1014–1024.

103. Rebouissou S, Herault A, Letouze E, et al. CDKN2A homozygous deletion is associated with muscle invasion in FGFR3-mutated urothelial bladder carcinoma. *J Pathol* 2012;227:315–324.

104. Shariat SF, Ashfaq R, Sagalowsky AI, et al. Predictive value of cell cycle biomarkers in nonmuscle invasive bladder transitional cell carcinoma. *J Urol* 2007;177:481–487.

105. Chatterjee SJ, Datar R, Youssefzadeh D, et al. Combined effects of p53, p21, and pRb expression in the progression of bladder transitional cell carcinoma. *J Clin Oncol* 2004;22:1007–1013.

106. Aveyard JS, Skilleter A, Habuchi T, et al. Somatic mutation of PTEN in bladder carcinoma. *Br J Cancer* 1999;80:904–908.

107. Cappellen D, Gil Diez de Medina S, Chopin D, et al. Frequent loss of heterozygosity on chromosome 10q in muscle-invasive transitional cell carcinomas of the bladder. *Oncogene* 1997;14:3059–3066.

108. Kagan J, Liu J, Stein JD, et al. Cluster of allele losses within a 2.5 cM region of chromosome 10 in high-grade invasive bladder cancer. *Oncogene* 1998;16:909–913.

109. Cairns P, Evron E, Okami K, et al. Point mutation and homozygous deletion of PTEN/MMAC1 in primary bladder cancers. *Oncogene* 1998;16:3215–3218.

110. Liu J, Babaian DC, Liebert M, et al. Inactivation of MMAC1 in bladder transitional-cell carcinoma cell lines and specimens. *Mol Carcinog* 2000;29:143–150.

111. Wang DS, Rieger-Christ K, Latini JM, et al. Molecular analysis of PTEN and MXI1 in primary bladder carcinoma. *Int J Cancer* 2000;88:620–625.

112. Tsuruta H, Kishimoto H, Sasaki T, et al. Hyperplasia and carcinomas in Pten-deficient mice and reduced PTEN protein in human bladder cancer patients. *Cancer Res* 2006;66:8389–8396.

113. Puzio-Kuter AM, Castillo-Martin M, Kinkade CW, et al. Inactivation of p53 and Pten promotes invasive bladder cancer. *Genes Dev* 2009;23:675–680.

114. Di Cristofano A, Pesce B, Cordon-Cardo C, et al. Pten is essential for embryonic development and tumour suppression. *Nat Genet* 1998;19:348–355.

115. Yoo LI, Liu DW, Le Vu S, et al. Pten deficiency activates distinct downstream signaling pathways in a tissue-specific manner. *Cancer Res* 2006;66:1929–1939.

116. Gildea JJ, Herlevsen M, Harding MA, et al. PTEN can inhibit in vitro organotypic and in vivo orthotopic invasion of human bladder cancer cells even in the absence of its lipid phosphatase activity. *Oncogene* 2004;23:6788–6797.

117. Tanaka M, Grossman HB. In vivo gene therapy of human bladder cancer with PTEN suppresses tumor growth, downregulates phosphorylated Akt, and increases sensitivity to doxorubicin. *Gene Ther* 2003;10:1636–1642.

118. Tanaka M, Koul D, Davies MA, et al. MMAC1/PTEN inhibits cell growth and induces chemosensitivity to doxorubicin in human bladder cancer cells. *Oncogene* 2000;19:5406–5412.

119. Iyer G, Hanrahan AJ, Milowsky MI, et al. Genome sequencing identifies a basis for everolimus sensitivity. *Science* 2012;338:221.

120. Guo Y, Chekaluk Y, Zhang J, et al. TSC1 involvement in bladder cancer: diverse effects and therapeutic implications. *J Pathol* 2013;230:17–27.

121. Griner EM, Theodorescu D. The faces and friends of RhoGDI2. *Cancer Metastasis Rev* 2012;31:519–528.

122. Said N, Smith S, Sanchez-Carbayo M, et al. Tumor endothelin-1 enhances metastatic colonization of the lung in mouse xenograft models of bladder cancer. *J Clin Invest* 2011;121:132–147.

123. Said N, Sanchez-Carbayo M, Smith SC, et al. RhoGDI2 suppresses lung metastasis in mice by reducing tumor versican expression and macrophage infiltration. *J Clin Invest* 2012;122:1503–1518.

124. Wu Y, Moissoglu K, Wang H, et al. Src phosphorylation of RhoGDI2 regulates its metastasis suppressor function. *Proc Natl Acad Sci* 2009;106:5807–5812.

125. Fanning P, Bulovas K, Saini KS, et al. Elevated expression of pp60c-src in low grade human bladder carcinoma. *Cancer Res* 1992;52:1457–1462.

126. Qayyum T, Fyffe G, Duncan M, et al. The interrelationships between Src, Cav-1 and RhoGDI2 in transitional cell carcinoma of the bladder. *Br J Cancer* 2012;106:1187–1195.

127. Thomas S, Overdevest JB, Nitz MD, et al. Src and caveolin-1 reciprocally regulate metastasis via a common downstream signaling pathway in bladder cancer. *Cancer Res* 2011;71:832–841.

128. Kastritis E, Murray S, Kyriakou F, et al. Somatic mutations of adenomatous polyposis coli gene and nuclear β-catenin accumulation have prognostic significance in invasive urothelial carcinomas: evidence for Wnt pathway implication. *Int J Cancer* 2009;124:103–108.

129. Zhu X, Kanai Y, Saito A, et al. Aberrant expression of beta-catenin and mutation of exon 3 of the beta-catenin gene in renal and urothelial carcinomas. *Pathol Int* 2000;50:945–952.

130. Kashibuchi K, Tomita K, Schalken JA, et al. The prognostic value of E-cadherin, alpha-, beta- and gamma-catenin in bladder cancer patients who underwent radical cystectomy. *Int J Urol* 2007;14:789–794.

131. Baumgart E, Cohen MS, Silva Neto B, et al. Identification and prognostic significance of an epithelial-mesenchymal transition expression profile in human bladder tumors. *Clin Cancer Res* 2007;13:1685–1694.

132. Marsit CJ, Karagas MR, Andrew A, et al. Epigenetic inactivation of SFRP genes and TP53 alteration act jointly as markers of invasive bladder cancer. *Cancer Res* 2005;65:7081–7085.

133. Urakami S, Shiina H, Enokida H, et al. Epigenetic inactivation of Wnt inhibitory factor-1 plays an important role in bladder cancer through aberrant canonical Wnt/beta-catenin signaling pathway. *Clin Cancer Res* 2006;12:383–391.

134. Lindgren D, Frigyesi A, Gudjonsson S, et al. Combined gene expression and genomic profiling define two intrinsic molecular subtypes of urothelial carcinoma and gene signatures for molecular grading and outcome. *Cancer Res* 2010;70:3463–3472.

135. Lindgren D, Sjodahl G, Lauss M, et al. Integrated genomic and gene expression profiling identifies two major genomic circuits in urothelial carcinoma. *PloS One* 2012;7:e38863.

136. Zieger K, Wiuf C, Jensen KM, et al. Chromosomal imbalance in the progression of high-risk non-muscle invasive bladder cancer. *BMC Cancer* 2009;9:149.

137. Iyer G, Al-Ahmadie H, Schultz N, et al. Prevalence and co-occurrence of actionable genomic alterations in high-grade bladder cancer. *J Clin Oncol* 2013;31:3133–3140.

138. Chekaluk Y, Wu CL, Rosenberg J, et al. Identification of nine genomic regions of amplification in urothelial carcinoma, correlation with stage, and potential prognostic and therapeutic value. *PloS One* 2013;8:e60927.

139. Eriksson P, Aine M, Sjodahl G, et al. Detailed analysis of focal chromosome arm 1q and 6p amplifications in urothelial carcinoma reveals complex genomic events on 1q, and as a possible auxiliary target on 6p. *PloS One* 2013; 8:e67222.

140. Gui Y, Guo G, Huang Y, et al. Frequent mutations of chromatin remodeling genes in transitional cell carcinoma of the bladder. *Nat Genet* 2011;43:875–878.

141. Kim WJ, Kim YJ. Epigenetic biomarkers in urothelial bladder cancer. *Expert Rev Mol Diagn* 2009;9:259–269.

142. Dudziec E, Goepel JR, Catto JW. Global epigenetic profiling in bladder cancer. *Epigenomics* 2011;3:35–45.

143. Sanchez-Carbayo M. Hypermethylation in bladder cancer: Biological pathways and translational applications. *Tumour Biol* 2012;33:347–361.

144. Hoffman AM, Cairns P. Epigenetics of kidney cancer and bladder cancer. *Epigenomics* 2011;3:19–34.

145. Kandimalla R, van Tilborg AA, Kompier LC, et al. Genome-wide analysis of CpG island methylation in bladder cancer identified TBX2, TBX3, GATA2, and ZIC4 as pTa-specific prognostic markers. *Eur Urol* 2012;61:1245–1256.

146. Marsit CJ, Houseman EA, Christensen BC, et al. Identification of methylated genes associated with aggressive bladder cancer. *PloS One* 2010;5:e12334.

147. Reinert T, Modin C, Castano FM, et al. Comprehensive genome methylation analysis in bladder cancer: Identification and validation of novel methylated genes and application of these as urinary tumor markers. *Clin Cancer Res* 2011;17:5582–5592.

148. Wolff EM, Chihara Y, Pan F, et al. Unique DNA methylation patterns distinguish noninvasive and invasive urothelial cancers and establish an epigenetic field defect in premalignant tissue. *Cancer Res* 2010;70:8169–8178.

149. Lauss M, Aine M, Sjodahl G, et al. DNA methylation analyses of urothelial carcinoma reveal distinct epigenetic subtypes and an association between gene copy number and methylation status. *Epigenetics* 2012;7:858–867.

150. Agundez M, Grau L, Palou J, et al. Evaluation of the methylation status of tumour suppressor genes for predicting bacillus Calmette-Guerin response in patients with T1G3 high-risk bladder tumours. *Eur Urol* 2011;60:131–140.

151. Wiklund ED, Bramsen JB, Hulf T, et al. Coordinated epigenetic repression of the miR-200 family and miR-205 in invasive bladder cancer. *Int J Cancer* 2011;128:1327–1334.

152. Chung W, Bondaruk J, Jelinek J, et al. Detection of bladder cancer using novel DNA methylation biomarkers in urine sediments. *Cancer Epidemiol Biomarkers Prev* 2011;20:1483–1491.

153. Zuiverloon TC, Beukers W, van der Keur KA, et al. A methylation assay for the detection of non-muscle-invasive bladder cancer (NMIBC) recurrences in voided urine. *BJU Int* 2012;109:941–948.

154. Renard I, Joniau S, van Cleynenbreugel B, et al. Identification and validation of the methylated TWIST1 and NID2 genes through real-time methylation-specific polymerase chain reaction assays for the noninvasive detection of primary bladder cancer in urine samples. *Eur Urol* 2010;58:96–104.

155. Kandimalla R, Masius R, Beukers W, et al. A 3-Plex methylation assay combined with the FGFR3 mutation assay sensitively detects recurrent bladder cancer in voided urine. *Clin Cancer Res* 2013;19:4760–4769.

156. Dudziec E, Gogol-Doring A, Cookson V, et al. Integrated epigenome profiling of repressive histone modifications, DNA methylation and gene expression in normal and malignant urothelial cells. *PloS One* 2012;7:e32750.

157. Stransky N, Vallot C, Reyal F, et al. Regional copy number-independent deregulation of transcription in cancer. *Nat Genet* 2006;38:1386–1396.

158. Vallot C, Stransky N, Bernard-Pierrot I, et al. A novel epigenetic phenotype associated with the most aggressive pathway of bladder tumor progression. *J Natl Cancer Inst* 2011;103:47–60.

159. Blaveri E, Simko JP, Korkola JE, et al. Bladder cancer outcome and subtype classification by gene expression. *Clin Cancer Res* 2005;11:4044–4055.

160. Wild PJ, Herr A, Wissmann C, et al. Gene expression profiling of progressive papillary noninvasive carcinomas of the urinary bladder. *Clin Cancer Res* 2005;11:4415–4429.

161. Dyrskjot L, Kruhoffer M, Thykjaer T, et al. Gene expression in the urinary bladder: A common carcinoma in situ gene expression signature exists disregarding histopathological classification. *Cancer Res* 2004;64:4040–4048.

162. Dyrskjot L, Thykjaer T, Kruhoffer M, et al. Identifying distinct classes of bladder carcinoma using microarrays. *Nat Genet* 2003;33:90–96.

163. Dyrskjot L, Zieger K, Kruhoffer M, et al. A molecular signature in superficial bladder carcinoma predicts clinical outcome. *Clin Cancer Res* 2005; 11:4029–4036.

164. Sanchez-Carbayo M, Socci ND, Lozano J, et al. Defining molecular profiles of poor outcome in patients with invasive bladder cancer using oligonucleotide microarrays. *J Clin Oncol* 2006;24:778–789.

165. Kim W-J, Kim E-J, Kim S-K, et al. Predictive value of progression-related gene classifier in primary non-muscle invasive bladder cancer. *Mol Cancer* 2010;9:3.

166. Lindgren D, Liedberg F, Andersson A, et al. Molecular characterization of early-stage bladder carcinomas by expression profiles, FGFR3 mutation status, and loss of 9q. *Oncogene* 2006;25:2685–2696.

167. Takata R, Katagiri T, Kanehira M, et al. Predicting response to methotrexate, vinblastine, doxorubicin, and cisplatin neoadjuvant chemotherapy for bladder cancers through genome-wide gene expression profiling. *Clin Cancer Res* 2005;11:2625–2636.

168. Als AB, Dyrskjot L, von der Maase H, et al. Emmprin and survivin predict response and survival following cisplatin-containing chemotherapy in patients with advanced bladder cancer. *Clin Cancer Res* 2007;13:4407–4414.

169. Wang R, Morris DS, Tomlins SA, et al. Development of a multiplex quantitative PCR signature to predict progression in non-muscle-invasive bladder cancer. *Cancer Res* 2009;69:3810–3818.

170. Dancik G, Aisner D, Theodorescu D. A 20 gene model for predicting nodal involvement in bladder cancer patients with muscle invasive tumors. *PLoS Currents* 2011;3:RRN1248.

171. Riester M, Taylor JM, Feifer A, et al. Combination of a novel gene expression signature with a clinical nomogram improves the prediction of survival in high-risk bladder cancer. *Clin Cancer Res* 2012;18:1323–1333.

172. Dyrskjot L, Zieger K, Real FX, et al. Gene expression signatures predict outcome in non-muscle-invasive bladder carcinoma: a multicenter validation study. *Clin Cancer Res* 2007;13:3545–3551.

173. Takata R, Katagiri T, Kanehira M, et al. Validation study of the prediction system for clinical response of M-VAC neoadjuvant chemotherapy. *Cancer Science* 2007;98:113–117.

174. Lauss M, Ringner M, Hoglund M. Prediction of stage, grade, and survival in bladder cancer using genome-wide expression data: a validation study. *Clin Cancer Res* 2010;16:4421–4433.

175. Dyrskjot L, Reinert T, Novoradovsky A, et al. Analysis of molecular intra-patient variation and delineation of a prognostic 12-gene signature in non-muscle invasive bladder cancer; technology transfer from microarrays to PCR. *Br J Cancer* 2012;107:1392–1398.

176. Catto JW, Alcaraz A, Bjartell AS, et al. MicroRNA in prostate, bladder, and kidney cancer: A systematic review. *Eur Urol* 2011;59:671–681.

177. Guancial EA, Bellmunt J, Yeh S, et al. The evolving understanding of microRNA in bladder cancer. *Urol Oncol* 2014;32:41.e31–e40.

178. Han Y, Chen J, Zhao X, et al. MicroRNA expression signatures of bladder cancer revealed by deep sequencing. *PloS One* 2011;6:e18286.

179. Veerla S, Lindgren D, Kvist A, et al. MiRNA expression in urothelial carcinomas: important roles of miR-10a, miR-222, miR-125b, miR-7 and miR-452 for tumor stage and metastasis, and frequent homozygous losses of miR-31. *Int J Cancer* 2009;124:2236–2242.

180. Dyrskjot L, Ostenfeld MS, Bramsen JB, et al. Genomic profiling of microRNAs in bladder cancer: miR-129 is associated with poor outcome and promotes cell death in vitro. *Cancer Res* 2009;69:4851–4860.

181. Gottardo F, Liu CG, Ferracin M, et al. Micro-RNA profiling in kidney and bladder cancers. *Urol Oncol* 2007;25:387–392.

182. Wszolek MF, Rieger-Christ KM, Kenney PA, et al. A MicroRNA expression profile defining the invasive bladder tumor phenotype. *Urologic Oncol* 2011;29:794–801, e791.

183. Zhu J, Jiang Z, Gao F, et al. A systematic analysis on DNA methylation and the expression of both mRNA and microRNA in bladder cancer. *PloS One* 2011;6:e28223.

184. Lamouille S, Subramanyam D, Blelloch R, et al. Regulation of epithelial-mesenchymal and mesenchymal-epithelial transitions by microRNAs. *Curr Opin Cell Biol* 2013;25:200–207.

185. Chiyomaru T, Enokida H, Tatarano S, et al. miR-145 and miR-133a function as tumour suppressors and directly regulate FSCN1 expression in bladder cancer. *Br J Cancer* 2010;102:883–891.

186. Ostenfeld MS, Bramsen JB, Lamy P, et al. miR-145 induces caspase-dependent and -independent cell death in urothelial cancer cell lines with targeting of an expression signature present in Ta bladder tumors. *Oncogene* 2010;29:1073–1084.

187. Villadsen SB, Bramsen JB, Ostenfeld MS, et al. The miR-143/-145 cluster regulates plasminogen activator inhibitor-1 in bladder cancer. *Br J Cancer* 2012;106:366–374.

188. Bo J, Yang G, Huo K, et al. microRNA-203 suppresses bladder cancer development by repressing bcl-w expression. *FEBS J* 2011;278:786–792.

189. Yoshino H, Chiyomaru T, Enokida H, et al. The tumour-suppressive function of miR-1 and miR-133a targeting TAGLN2 in bladder cancer. *Br J Cancer* 2011;104:808–818.

190. Huang L, Luo J, Cai Q, et al. MicroRNA-125b suppresses the development of bladder cancer by targeting E2F3. *Int J Cancer* 2011;128:1758–1769.

191. Lin Y, Wu J, Chen H, et al. Cyclin-dependent kinase 4 is a novel target in micoRNA-195-mediated cell cycle arrest in bladder cancer cells. *FEBS Lett* 2012;586:442–447.

192. Puerta-Gil P, Garcia-Baquero R, Jia AY, et al. miR-143, miR-222, and miR-452 are useful as tumor stratification and noninvasive diagnostic biomarkers for bladder cancer. *Am J Pathol* 2012;180:1808–1815.

193. Nordentoft I, Birkenkamp-Demtroder K, Agerbaek M, et al. miRNAs associated with chemo-sensitivity in cell lines and in advanced bladder cancer. *BMC Med Genomics* 2012;5:40.

194. Ho PL, Kurtova A, Chan KS. Normal and neoplastic urothelial stem cells: getting to the root of the problem. *Nat Rev Urol* 2012;9:583–594.

195. van der Horst G, Bos L, van der Pluijm G. Epithelial plasticity, cancer stem cells, and the tumor-supportive stroma in bladder carcinoma. *Mol Cancer Res* 2012;10:995–1009.

196. He X, Marchionni L, Hansel DE, et al. Differentiation of a highly tumorigenic basal cell compartment in urothelial carcinoma. *Stem Cells* 2009;27:1487–1495.

197. Chan KS, Espinosa I, Chao M, et al. Identification, molecular characterization, clinical prognosis, and therapeutic targeting of human bladder tumor-initiating cells. *Proc Natl Acad Sci* 2009;106:14016–14021.

198. Su Y, Qiu Q, Zhang X, et al. Aldehyde dehydrogenase 1 A1-positive cell population is enriched in tumor-initiating cells and associated with progression of bladder cancer. *Cancer Epidemiol Biomarkers Prev* 2010;19:327–337.

199. Volkmer JP, Sahoo D, Chin RK, et al. Three differentiation states risk-stratify bladder cancer into distinct subtypes. *Proc Natl Acad Sci* 2012;109:2078–2083.

200. Hafner C, Knuechel R, Zanardo L, et al. Evidence for oligoclonality and tumor spread by intraluminal seeding in multifocal urothelial carcinomas of the upper and lower urinary tract. *Oncogene* 2001;20:4910–4915.

201. Cheng L, Gu J, Ulbright TM, et al. Precise microdissection of human bladder carcinomas reveals divergent tumor subclones in the same tumor. *Cancer* 2002;94:104–110.

202. Kawanishi H, Takahashi T, Ito M, et al. High throughput comparative genomic hybridization array analysis of multifocal urothelial cancers. *Cancer Sci* 2006;97:746–752.

203. Kawanishi H, Takahashi T, Ito M, et al. Genetic analysis of multifocal superficial urothelial cancers by array-based comparative genomic hybridisation. *Br J Cancer* 2007;97:260–266.

204. Habuchi T. Origin of multifocal carcinomas of the bladder and upper urinary tract: Molecular analysis and clinical implications. *Int J Urol* 2005;12:709–716.

205. Hartmann A, Moser K, Kriegmair M, et al. Frequent genetic alterations in simple urothelial hyperplasias of the bladder in patients with papillary urothelial carcinoma. *Am J Pathol* 1999;154:721–727.

206. Obermann EC, Meyer S, Hellge D, et al. Fluorescence in situ hybridization detects frequent chromosome 9 deletions and aneuploidy in histologically normal urothelium of bladder cancer patients. *Oncol Rep* 2004;11:745–751.

207. Takahashi T, Habuchi T, Kakehi Y, et al. Clonal and chronological genetic analysis of multifocal cancers of the bladder and upper urinary tract. *Cancer Res* 1998;58:5835–5841.

208. van Tilborg AA, de Vries A, de Bont M, et al. Molecular evolution of multiple recurrent cancers of the bladder. *Hum Mol Genet* 2000;9:2973–2980.

209. Letouzé E, Allory Y, Bollet MA, et al. Analysis of the copy number profiles of several tumor samples from the same patient reveals the successive steps in tumorigenesis. *Genome Biology* 2010;11:R76.

210. Hartmann A, Schlake G, Zaak D, et al. Occurrence of chromosome 9 and p53 alterations in multifocal dysplasia and carcinoma in situ of human urinary bladder. *Cancer Res* 2002;62:809–818.

211. Spruck CH 3rd, Ohneseit PF, Gonzalez-Zulueta M, et al. Two molecular pathways to transitional cell carcinoma of the bladder. *Cancer Res* 1994;54:784–788.

212. Hopman AH, Kamps MA, Speel EJ, et al. Identification of chromosome 9 alterations and p53 accumulation in isolated carcinoma in situ of the urinary bladder versus carcinoma in situ associated with carcinoma. *Am J Pathol* 2002;161:1119–1125.

213. Rosin MP, Cairns P, Epstein JI, et al. Partial allelotype of carcinoma in situ of the human bladder. *Cancer Res* 1995;55:5213–5216.

214. Lee S, Jeong J, Majewski T, et al. Forerunner genes contiguous to RB1 contribute to the development of in situ neoplasia. *Proc Natl Acad Sci* 2007;104:13732–13737.

215. Majewski T, Lee S, Jeong J, et al. Understanding the development of human bladder cancer by using a whole-organ genomic mapping strategy. *Lab Invest* 2008;88:694–721.

216. Sjodahl G, Lauss M, Lovgren K, et al. A molecular taxonomy for urothelial carcinoma. *Clin Cancer Res* 2012;18:3377–3386.

217. Sjodahl G, Lovgren K, Lauss M, et al. Toward a molecular pathologic classification of urothelial carcinoma. *Am J Pathol* 2013;183:681–691.

218. Perou CM, Sorlie T, Eisen MB, et al. Molecular portraits of human breast tumours. *Nature* 2000;406:747–752.

219. Choi W, Shah JB, Tran M, et al. p63 expression defines a lethal subset of muscle-invasive bladder cancers. *PloS One* 2012;7:e30206.

220. Wilhelm-Benartzi CS, Koestler DC, Houseman EA, et al. DNA methylation profiles delineate etiologic heterogeneity and clinically important subgroups of bladder cancer. *Carcinogenesis* 2010;31:1972–1976.

221. Juanpere N, Agell L, Lorenzo M, et al. Mutations in FGFR3 and PIK3CA, singly or combined with RAS and AKT1, are associated with AKT but not with MAPK pathway activation in urothelial bladder cancer. *Hum Pathol* 2012;43:1573–1582.

222. Cappellen D, De Oliveira C, Ricol D, et al. Frequent activating mutations of FGFR3 in human bladder and cervix carcinomas. *Nat Genet* 1999;23:18–20.

223. Bringuier PP, Tamimi J, Schuuring E. Amplification of the chromosome 11q13 region in bladder tumours. *Urol Res* 1994;21:451.

224. Proctor A, Coombs L, Cairns J, et al. Amplification at chromosome 11q13 in transitional cell tumours of the bladder. *Oncogene* 1991;6:789–795.

225. Sgambato A, Migaldi M, Faraglia B, et al. Cyclin D1 expression in papillary superficial bladder cancer: its association with other cell cycle-associated proteins, cell proliferation and clinical outcome. *Int J Cancer* 2002;97:671–678.

226. Lianes P, Orlow I, Zhang ZF, et al. Altered patterns of MDM2 and TP53 expression in human bladder cancer. *J Natl Cancer Inst* 1994;86:1325–1330.

227. Devlin J, Keen AJ, Knowles MA. Homozygous deletion mapping at 9p21 in bladder carcinoma defines a critical region within 2cM of IFNA. *Oncogene* 1994;9:2757–2760.

228. Chapman EJ, Harnden P, Chambers P, et al. Comprehensive analysis of CDKN2A status in microdissected urothelial cell carcinoma reveals potential haploinsufficiency, a high frequency of homozygous co-deletion and associations with clinical phenotype. *Clin Cancer Res* 2005;11:5740–5747.

229. Cairns P, Shaw ME, Knowles MA. Initiation of bladder cancer may involve deletion of a tumour-suppressor gene on chromosome 9. *Oncogene* 1993;8:1083–1085.

230. Adachi H, Igawa M, Shiina H, et al. Human bladder tumors with 2-hit mutations of tumor suppressor gene TSC1 and decreased expression of p27. *J Urol* 2003;170:601–604.

231. Blaveri E, Brewer JL, Roydasgupta R, et al. Bladder cancer stage and outcome by array-based comparative genomic hybridization. *Clin Cancer Res* 2005;11:7012.

232. Heidenblad M, Lindgren D, Jonson T, et al. Tiling resolution array CGH and high density expression profiling of urothelial carcinomas delineate genomic amplicons and candidate target genes specific for advanced tumors. *BMC Med Genomics* 2008;1:3.

233. van Rhijn BW, Lurkin I, Radvanyi F, et al. The fibroblast growth factor receptor 3 (FGFR3) mutation is a strong indicator of superficial bladder cancer with low recurrence rate. *Cancer Res* 2001;61:1265–1268.

234. Zaharieva BM, Simon R, Diener PA, et al. High-throughput tissue microarray analysis of 11q13 gene amplification (CCND1, FGF3, FGF4, EMS1) in urinary bladder cancer. *J Pathol* 2003;201:603–608.

235. Lianes P, Orlow I, Zhang ZF, et al. Altered patterns of MDM2 and TP53 expression in human bladder cancer [see comments]. *J Natl Cancer Inst* 1994;86:1325–1330.

236. Ross JS, Wang K, Al-Rohil RN, et al. Advanced urothelial carcinoma: next-generation sequencing reveals diverse genomic alterations and targets of therapy. *Mod Pathol* 2014;27:271–280.

237. Habuchi T, Takahashi R, Yamada H, et al. Influence of cigarette smoking and schistosomiasis on p53 gene mutation in urothelial cancer. *Cancer Res* 1993;53:3795–3799.

238. Sidransky D, Von Eschenbach A, Tsai YC, et al. Identification of p53 gene mutations in bladder cancers and urine samples. *Science* 1991;252:706–709.

239. Fujimoto K, Yamada Y, Okajima E, et al. Frequent association of p53 gene mutation in invasive bladder cancer. *Cancer Res* 1992;52:1393–1398.

240. Balbas-Martinez C, Rodriguez-Pinilla M, Casanova A, et al. ARID1A alterations are associated with FGFR3-wild type, poor-prognosis, urothelial bladder tumors. *PloS One* 2013;8:e62483.

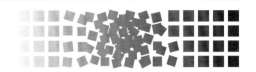

# 39 Cancer of the Bladder, Ureter, and Renal Pelvis

Adam S. Feldman, Jason A. Efstathiou, Richard J. Lee, Douglas M. Dahl,
M. Dror Michaelson, and Anthony L. Zietman

## INTRODUCTION

This chapter details the incidence, epidemiology, pathology, and treatment of cancers of the bladder, ureter, and renal pelvis. Transitional cell carcinomas (TCC) constitute 90% to 95% of all the urothelial tumors diagnosed in North America and Europe. TCCs occur throughout the lining of the urinary tract from the renal calyceal system to the proximal two-thirds of the urethra, at which point squamous epithelium predominates. In this 10th edition, cancers of the renal pelvis and ureter are grouped with bladder cancer rather than with cancers of the kidney. This is a natural fit, because approximately 90% of the urothelial cancers of the renal pelvis, ureter, and bladder are transitional cell cancers, all of which share similarities in epidemiology, pathology, biology, patterns of spread, molecular tumor markers, and treatment. The chapter presents the common characteristics of urothelial cancers in an initial section and then deals in subsequent sections with the separate characteristics of these organs. The multidisciplinary treatment of this chapter reflects the current approach to patients with these diseases.

## UROTHELIAL CANCERS

### Epidemiology

Bladder cancer is almost three times more common in males than in females and more common in whites than in blacks. In 2013, there were approximately 72,570 new cases in the United States, over a 20% increase from 20 years ago. The incidence increases with age and peaks in the 6th, 7th, and 8th decades of life.[1]

Simultaneous or subsequent development of TCC of the urethra in patients with TCC of the bladder occurs with an incidence of 6% to 16% more commonly in women than men and in those with recurrent multifocal bladder cancers, and bladder neck or trigonal involvement with either invasive cancer or carcinoma in situ (CIS).[2,3]

The incidence of ureteral TCC is 0.7 per 100,000, whereas renal pelvic TCCs have an incidence of 1 per 100,000.[4] Renal pelvic tumors constitute 5% of all renal tumors, and 90% of them are TCCs. Squamous cell carcinoma and adenocarcinoma constitute the majority of the remainder. Renal pelvic transitional cell cancers constitute 5% of all TCCs of the urinary tract. Patients who have primary TCCs of the renal pelvis or ureter have a 20% to 40% incidence of either synchronous or metachronous bladder cancer. Conversely, patients with bladder cancer have a 1% to 4% incidence of synchronous or metachronous upper tract urothelial tumors.[5,6] However, if the bladder cancer is grade 3, there is associated CIS, or the patient has failed intravesical chemotherapy, some reports suggest a doubling of the incidence of upper tract tumors.[7] Patients with Balkan nephropathy have an increased incidence of upper tract tumors; these tumors are usually low grade and multiple.[8]

Recently, aristolochic acid, a component of all *Aristolochia* plants, was identified as the etiologic agent causing Balkan nephropathy and the associated urothelial carcinoma.[9–11] In the Balkan region, the exposure seems to occur via consumption of bread made from flour contaminated with *Aristolochia clematitis* seeds.[12] There are also specific areas of Taiwan where TCC of the renal pelvis accounts for 40% of all renal tumors, whereas in other nonendemic areas, the upper tract tumors account for only 1% or 2% of renal tumors.[13] Aristolochic acid has also recently been identified as the etiology in this population due to widespread use of *Aristolochia* herbal remedies.[14,15]

Risk factors for urothelial cancer may be classified into one of three categories: (1) gene abnormalities that result in perturbations in cell cycle regulatory processes, (2) chemical exposure, or (3) chronic irritation. Those risk factors that involve genetic abnormalities include chromosome deletions or duplications, proto-oncogene expression, tumor suppressor gene mutation, and abnormalities of specific cell cycle regulatory proteins. In non–muscularis propria–invasive transitional cell cancers, deletions of part or all of chromosome 9 and alterations in the gene encoding for fibroblast growth factor receptor 3 (FGFR3) are often encountered. Inactivation of the cohesion subunit stromal antigen 2 (Stage 2), which regulates sister chromatid cohesion and segregation, is frequently found in low-grade and low-stage bladder cancer.[16–18] Other proto-oncogenes that have been implicated in bladder cancer include the RAS and p21 proteins.[19] Genetic abnormalities associated with CIS include alterations in the retinoblastoma gene (Rb), p53, and phosphatase and tensin homolog (PTEN). In muscularis propria–invasive disease, the tumor suppressor genes that have been associated with an altered biology and more aggressive behavior include the *p53* and the *Rb* gene.[20] Abnormalities in specific cell-cycle regulatory proteins such as epidermal growth factor (EGF), Ki-67, cyclin D1, metalloproteinase (MMP), and tissue inhibition of metalloproteinase (TIMP) have also been implicated.[20–25] At this time, there is no single molecular marker that is capable of predicting the tumor with a high degree of accuracy, which may result in muscularis propria invasion or distant metastases.

Chemical exposure has perhaps the most epidemiologic evidence to support it as an inciting agent. Aromatic amines, aniline dyes, and nitrites and nitrates have all been implicated. There are genetic polymorphisms that appear to increase the susceptibility of affected patients exposed to carcinogens. N-acetyltransferase, which detoxifies nitrosamines and glutathione-S transferase, which conjugates reactive chemicals, have been implicated in increasing the risk for the development of bladder cancer in patients so afflicted. Tobacco use carries with it, for those who continue to smoke, a threefold increased risk of developing bladder cancer, and even ex-smokers have a twofold increased risk.[26] Numerous reports have shown strong associations between the development of both bladder and upper tract TCCs with industrial contact to chemicals, plastics, coal, tar, and asphalt, and aristolochic acid, as discussed previously. Cyclophosphamide administration over the long term, particularly in patients who have upper tract or bladder outlet obstructions, results in an increased risk of bladder cancer. These cancers, when discovered, tend to be particularly aggressive. Coffee, tea, analgesics, alcohol, and artificial sweeteners have not been shown to act as independent risk factors.

Chronic irritants include catheters, recurrent urinary track infections, *Schistosoma haematobium*, and irradiation. Chronic irritation due to indwelling catheters associated with chronic infection increases the risk for the development of squamous cell carcinoma; a *S. haematobium* infestation results in an increased risk of squamous cell and TCCs; pelvic irradiation also carries with it an increased risk of developing a urothelial cancer.

There are many studies that suggest high water consumption, vitamin intake, and various diets as beneficial in preventing bladder cancer. However, none of these have shown any clear benefit with respect to prevention.

## Screening and Early Detection

Screening has not been particularly useful in the detection of bladder cancer and the most recent statement from the U.S. Preventive Services Task Force concludes that the current data are insufficient to make a definitive recommendation on screening for bladder cancer in asymptomatic adults.[27] The only test of proven usefulness is a urinalysis to detect microhematuria. If significant microhematuria is detected, then specific diagnostic studies are performed. When individuals are screened, 4% to 20% are found to have microhematuria. Of those with microhematuria, 0.5% to 8.1% have bladder tumors.[28–30] In these particular studies, high-grade disease was identified in 2.4% to 3.5% of those presenting with dipstick microhematuria, and invasive disease was identified in 0.4% to 1%. Although one of these studies suggests that routine screening results in a reduced mortality from bladder cancer, the data are unconvincing due to a lack of randomization and likely significant selection bias.[30] Others have suggested that screening in high-risk populations increases the early detection rate of high-grade cancers. Early treatment of these would be expected to be associated with an increased survival, although this hypothesis in this group of patients has not been substantiated. Screening does not generally improve the detection rate of low-grade tumors because the methods used for screening have a large number of false-negative findings for low-grade tumors. When urothelial cancer is suspected, noninvasive screening may be performed using cytology, nuclear matrix protein, telomerase, or fluorescence in situ hybridization analysis, but the definitive diagnosis is made only by cystoscopy and biopsy.

Cytology has been regarded as the gold standard for noninvasive screening of urine for bladder cancer. It has a sensitivity of 40% to 60% and specificity in excess of 90%. Nuclear matrix protein[31] fibrin or fibrinogen degradation products,[32] urinary bladder cancer antigen,[33] and basic fetoprotein[34] have all been compared with cytology in bladder cancer screening studies. Other methods used include fluorescence in situ hybridization,[35] microsatellite analysis of free DNA,[36] and telomerase reverse transcriptase determination.[37] Unfortunately, all of these tests have a sensitivity that ranges from only 40% to 75% with a specificity of 50% to 90%, thus making it impossible to eliminate the need for cystoscopy by the use of these tests.[38] These urinary biomarkers have not been studied yet for sensitivity and specificity in detecting upper tract TCCs.

Cytology remains the preferred bladder tumor marker for specificity[39]; however, many of the other bladder tumor markers have a better sensitivity.[40]

## Pathology

More than 90% of the TCCs throughout the lining of the urinary tract occur in the urinary bladder and of the remaining 10%, most are in the renal pelvis and fewer than 2% are in the ureter and urethra. Squamous cell carcinomas, defined by the presence of keratinization, account for 5% of bladder tumors. Other, even less common bladder tumor types include adenocarcinoma and undifferentiated carcinoma variants such as small-cell carcinoma, giant-cell carcinoma, and lymphoepitheliomas.[41–43] A TCC histology can also demonstrate areas of a variant subtype within a tumor, including micropapillary, squamous, glandular, or sarcomatoid differentiation. These are considered variants of TCC, and stage for stage, they do not portend a worse prognosis,[44,45] likely with the exception of sarcomatoid carcinoma, which presents with a higher stage and more distant metastases than conventional TCC.[46] Pure adenocarcinoma of the bladder may also arise in the embryonal remnant of the urachus on or above the bladder dome. Other adenocarcinomas may closely resemble intestinal adenocarcinoma and must be distinguished from direct spread to the bladder from an intestinal primary by careful clinical evaluation. Rarely, these demonstrate a signet ring cell or clear cell histology.

## Primary Tumors of the Bladder

The differential diagnosis of TCC usually does not pose a diagnostic difficulty for experienced pathologists, but tumors that are grade 1 and invasive are occasionally difficult to distinguish from von Brunn nests.[47] Also, rarely, an invasive TCC may be overdiagnosed when the glandular component of a nephrogenic adenoma is mistaken for TCC with glandular differentiation or for a pure adenocarcinoma. When invasion of the lamina propria has occurred, the pathologist must report whether muscularis propria is present in the submitted tissue and whether there is invasion of the muscularis propria. If muscularis propria is not present in the submitted tissue, this should be noted by the pathologist. Identification of invasion of the muscularis propria by the tumor may occasionally be difficult, because it may be confused with involvement of the muscularis mucosa, which is in the lamina propria.[48] More than two-thirds of newly diagnosed cases of bladder tumors are exophytic papillary TCCs that are confined to the epithelium (stage Ta) or invade only into the lamina propria (stage T1). These tumors are generally managed endoscopically and, in some cases, with the addition of intravesical therapy (discussed in the following paragraphs). Approximately one-half to two-thirds of patients with such tumors have a recurrence or a new TCC in the bladder within 5 years.

Bladder tumors are also classified by their cytologic characteristics as low grade (G1) or high grade (G2, G3).[43] Low-grade tumors may also be referred to as papillary tumors of low malignant potential (PNLMP). Tumor grade is clinically more significant for noninvasive tumors because nearly all of the invasive neoplasms are high grade at diagnosis. Papillary carcinomas of low grade are considered to be relatively benign tumors that histologically resemble the normal urothelium. They show only very slight pleomorphism or loss of polarity and rarely progress to a higher stage. On the contrary, CIS is cytologically synonymous with high-grade disease and carries a high risk of progression to invasive disease. Primary CIS (stage Tis) that presents without a concurrent exophytic tumor constitutes only 1% to 2% of newly detected cases of bladder cancer, but CIS is found accompanying more than half of bladders presenting with multiple papillary tumors. CIS, in this instance, is either adjacent to or involves mucosal sites remote from papillary lesions.[49] CIS is believed to be an important precursor of invasive cancer and, if untreated, will develop into muscularis propria–invasive disease within 5 years from the initial diagnosis in more than 50% of patients.

## Upper Tract Tumors

Like bladder tumors, 90% of upper tract tumors are TCCs with similar morphology.[50] Squamous cell carcinomas account for most of the remaining carcinomas, with adenocarcinoma representing, at most, 1% of upper tract malignancies. The cytologic characteristics for the classification of TCC by grade are the same for upper tract TCCs as they are for those in the bladder.

## Molecular Tumor Markers

Because the natural history of superficial urothelial tumors is that of recurrence, an area of controversy is if tumors that occur at separate sites or at separate times in the urothelial tract are derived from the same clone or are polyclonal in origin. A report by Sidransky et al.[51] demonstrated the clonality of multiple bladder tumors from different sites. Miyao et al.[52] showed concordant genetic alterations in asynchronous tumors from individual patients. These studies suggest that urothelial TCCs appearing at different times and sites can be derived from the same neoplastic clone. Moreover, many studies have reported an increasing frequency of specific genetic abnormalities in bladder tumors of more advanced stages.[53–56] Many tumor suppressor gene modifications, including those of *p53*, *pRB*, *p16*, *p21*, thrombospondin-1, glutathione, and factors controlling the expression and function of the epidermal growth factor receptor (EGFR), have been shown in retrospective analyses to be adverse prognostic factors in patients with TCC after various treatments.[58–62] However, even in the most intensively studied tumor suppressor gene in advanced TCC, the *p53* gene, retrospective analyses give. There is conflicting retrospective data on the association of *p53* mutation status and responsiveness to chemotherapy or radiation[59,60] led to a phase III trial that randomized 114 postcystectomy patients with p53 alteration to three cycles of adjuvant methotrexate, vinblastine, doxorubicin, and cisplatin (MVAC) or observation. Neither p53 status nor MVAC adjuvant chemotherapy impacted the risk of recurrence.[57]

The enthusiasm engendered by the development of novel biologic agents targeted against tumor-specific growth factor pathways or against angiogenesis has been fortified by positive studies in a variety of solid tumors. Two classes of agents that have received great attention are inhibitors of EGFR, including EGFR1 and EGFR2 (or HER2/neu), and inhibitors of vascular endothelial growth factor (VEGF) or its receptors. Ample preclinical evidence has shown that (1) many, if not most, bladder tumors express products of the EGFR family, (2) overexpression correlates with an unfavorable outcome, and (3) inhibition of these pathways may have an antitumor effect.[64–69]

Evidence suggests that *p53*, *p16*, and *pRB* altered expression are of no prognostic significance in patients treated with chemoradiation, but that overexpression of *HER2* correlated with a significantly inferior complete response rate. The recently closed Radiation Therapy Oncology Group (RTOG) 0524 protocol evaluated the addition of trastuzumab to chemoradiation for Her2 overexpressing tumors. EGFR overexpression, which occurred in only 19% of the patients, was associated with improved disease-specific survival.[70]

Another potential therapeutic avenue is the inhibition of angiogenesis. Several studies have correlated elevated VEGF levels or cyclooxygenase-2 (COX-2) expression with disease recurrence or progression, often as an independent prognostic factor by multivariate analysis.[69,71]

Preclinical data support the concept that COX-2 inhibitors may inhibit the development of non–muscle-invasive bladder cancer. A randomized, double-blind, placebo-controlled trial sought to determine whether celecoxib, a COX-2 inhibitor, could reduce the time-to-recurrence of superficial tumors. No benefit was observed in patients receiving daily celecoxib.[72]

The major challenge for clinical and translational investigators is to design appropriate trials that will identify which molecular tumor markers will be prognostic of outcome *and* also be predictive of whether a patient will do better treated by surgery, radiation, chemotherapy, molecular targeted therapy, or a combination of these. An example of recent encouraging results include the identification of MRE11, a protein involved in DNA damage double-strand break repair, as a predictive marker of disease specific survival following radiation or chemoradiation for muscle invasive bladder cancer.[73,74] Only when such molecular biomarkers are validated and incorporated into clinical decision making will

physicians be able to make better treatment choices on behalf of their patients.

## CANCER OF THE BLADDER

Cancers of the bladder can be grouped into three general categories by their stages at presentation: (1) those that do not invade the muscularis propria, (2) muscularis propria–invasive cancers, and (3) metastatic cancers. Each differs in clinical behavior, primary management, and outcome. When treating non–muscularis-invasive tumors, the aim is to prevent recurrences and progression to a stage that is life threatening. With muscularis propria–invasive disease, the main issue is to determine which tumors require cystectomy, which can be successfully managed by bladder preservation using combined modality therapy, and which tumors, by virtue of a high metastatic potential, require an integrated systemic chemotherapeutic approach from the outset. Combination chemotherapy is the standard for treating metastatic disease. Despite reports of complete responses (CR) in more than 40% of cases, the duration of response and overall cure rates remain low.

### Clinical Presentations and Staging

Bladder cancer is rarely incidentally discovered at autopsy. Indeed, almost all cases show symptoms in the premortem period. The most common presentation is gross painless hematuria. Unexplained urinary frequency and irritative voiding symptoms should alert one to the possibility of CIS of the bladder or, less commonly, muscularis propria–invasive cancer.

#### Workup

The workup of suspected bladder cancer should include urine cytology, a cystoscopy, and an upper tract study. The preference for the upper tract study is a renal computed tomography (CT) urogram because both ureters and renal pelves as well as the relevant lymph nodes and the kidney parenchyma can be particularly well visualized.

Careful staging is important, because treatment depends on the initial stage of the disease. The clinical stage of the primary tumor is determined by transurethral resection of the bladder tumor (TURBT). This resection should include a sample of the muscularis propria for appropriate diagnosis, particularly if the tumor appears sessile or high grade. Once the specimen has been resected, the base of the resected area should be separately biopsied. Any suspicious areas in the remainder of the bladder should be biopsied, and many advocate additional selected biopsies of the bladder mucosa and a prostatic urethral biopsy as well. Urethral biopsies are clearly indicated in patients with risk factors for urethral involvement, as previously discussed, and in those who have persistent positive cytologies in the absence of a demonstrated bladder lesion. Patients who have T1, G3 tumors on biopsy without muscularis propria in the specimen require a second biopsy in order to obtain muscularis propria to reduce the risk of understaging. Indeed, the authors rebiopsy all patients with T1, G3 disease, because it has been shown that even if muscularis propria is in the initial specimen, a significant number of patients will be upstaged (T2) on the second biopsy.

5-Alpha amino levulinic acid installation into the bladder, resulting in porphyrin-induced fluorescence of vascular lesions when viewed with blue light, and narrow band imaging, which increases the contrast between vascular lesions and normal mucosa, have been recommended by some to increase the yield of positive biopsies. Several studies have shown a slight advantage to these techniques in reducing disease recurrence, but it remains difficult to differentiate inflammatory lesions from urothelial carcinomas with either technique, and not all well-designed clinical trials have shown a benefit.[75–78]

## Staging

The primary bladder cancer is staged according to the depth of invasion into the bladder wall or beyond (Table 39.1).[70,79] The urothelial basement membrane separates non–muscularis propria bladder cancers into Ta (noninvasive) and T1 (invasive) tumors. Stage T2 and higher T-stage tumors invade the muscularis propria, the true muscle of the bladder wall. If the tumor extends through the muscle to involve the full thickness of the bladder and into the serosa, it is classified as T3. If the tumor involves contiguous structures such as the prostate, the vagina, the uterus, or the pelvic sidewall, the tumor is classified as stage T4 (nonstromal invasive urothelial tumors of the prostate are not classified as T4, because the prognosis in this group is quite good). In a fragmented TURBT specimen, in contrast to a cystectomy specimen, it is relatively infrequent for the pathologist to be able to make an accurate assessment as to the depth of invasion of the tumor into the muscularis propria. Thus, the primary pathologic substages of the TNM (tumor, nodes, metastasis) staging system shown in Table 39.1, such as pT2a and pT2b, cannot be determined from TURBT specimens. Of note, significant rates of clinical–pathologic stage discrepancy and clinical (TURBT) understaging have been described.[138] CT scans or magnetic resonance images (MRI), even those done prior to the TURBT, are not reliable for staging of

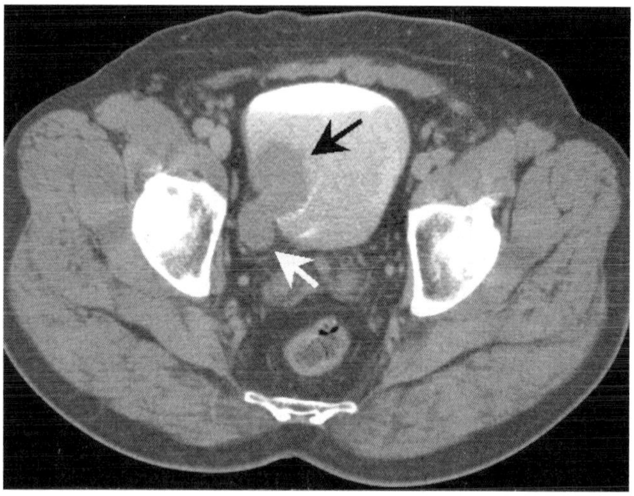

**Figure 39.1** A computed tomography scan of a patient with a muscularis propria–invasive bladder cancer performed before a transurethral tumor resection, unequivocally showing an extravesical extension of tumor (stage T3). The tumor projecting into the bladder lumen (*black arrow*); portion of the tumor extending into the ureter outside the bladder (*white arrow*).

### TABLE 39.1

**American Joint Committee on Cancer 2009 TNM Bladder Cancer Staging**

**Primary Tumor (T)**

| | |
|---|---|
| Tis | Carcinoma in situ |
| Ta | Noninvasive papillary tumor |
| T1 | Tumor invades the lamina propria, but not beyond |
| T2 | Tumor invades the muscularis propria |
| pT2a | Tumor invades superficial muscle (inner half) |
| pT2b | Tumor invades deep muscle (outer half) |
| T3 | Tumor invades perivesical tissue |
| pT3a | Microscopically |
| pT3b | Macroscopically (extravesical mass) |
| T4 | Tumor invades any of the following: prostatic stroma, uterus, vagina, pelvis, or abdominal wall |
| T4a | Tumor invades prostate, uterus, vagina |
| T4b | Tumor invades pelvic or abdominal wall |

**Regional Lymph Nodes (N)**

| | |
|---|---|
| NX | Regional lymph nodes cannot be assessed |
| N0 | No regional lymph node metastasis |
| N1 | Metastasis in a single lymph node in primary drainage region |
| N2 | Metastasis in multiple lymph nodes in primary drainage region |
| N3 | Common iliac lymph node involvement |

**Distant Metastasis (M)**

| | |
|---|---|
| MX | Distant metastasis cannot be assessed |
| M0 | No distant metastasis |
| M1 | Distant metastasis |

Used with the permission of the American Joint Committee on Cancer (AJCC), Chicago, Illinois. The original source for this material is the *AJCC Cancer Staging Manual*, Seventh Edition (2010) published by Springer Science and Business Media LLC, www.springer.com, page 500.

the primary tumor. Neither scan can differentiate a Ta/T1 tumor from a T2/T3 tumor because neither can visualize the depth of invasion of the primary tumor into the bladder wall. These scans are helpful, however, when they show unequivocal tumor extension outside the bladder (stage T3) (Fig. 39.1). CT scans or MRIs following a TURBT also are not reliable for staging of the primary tumor because either surgically induced edema in the resected portion of the bladder wall or postsurgical extravesical inflammatory stranding may be confused with extravesical tumor extension. For this reason, it is preferable and recommended to perform a staging CT or MRI prior to TURBT.

Patients who have documented muscularis propria–invasive bladder cancer require an additional set of studies: a chest x-ray or CT scan, liver function studies, creatinine and electrolytes level studies, and a CT evaluation of the pelvic and retroperitoneal lymph nodes. A bimanual examination is also performed at the time the tumor is transurethrally resected to evaluate for possible extravesical extension of the tumor and to determine mobility of the pelvic contents. An MRI lymphangiography, using a lymphotropic iron nanoparticle administered intravenously, shows potential.[80] Nodes that appear to be enlarged on a CT may be differentiated by this technique as to whether they are inflammatory or malignant. The sensitivity and specificity of the test are quite high.

If there is a history of functional bowel abnormality, a barium study of the segment of bowel to be used for the diversion should be performed. It is the authors' practice when using colon in the reconstruction of the urinary tract to obtain a barium enema or colonoscopy so that there are no surprises at the time of surgery. Finally, patients with muscularis propria–invasive bladder cancer must have a prostatic urethra and bulbous urethra biopsy to determine whether an orthotopic bladder may be placed or whether the procedure should encompass the urethra—that is, a cystoprostato-urethrectomy in males or a cystourethrectomy and anterior exenteration in females.

## Treatment of Non–Muscularis Propria–Invasive Bladder Cancer (Ta, Tis, T1)

Of patients with bladder cancer, 70% have disease that does not involve the muscularis propria at presentation. Approximately 15% to 20% of these patients will progress to stage T2 disease or greater over time. Of those presenting with Ta or T1 disease, 50% to 70% will have a recurrence following initial therapy. Low-grade tumors

(G1 or G2) and low-stage (Ta) disease tend to have a lower recurrence rate at about 50% and a 5% progression rate, whereas high-risk disease (G3, T1 associated with CIS, and multifocal disease) has a 70% recurrence rate and a 30% to 50% progression rate to stage T2 disease or greater. Less than 5% of patients with non–muscularis propria–invasive bladder cancer will develop metastatic disease without developing evidence of muscularis propria invasion (stage T2 disease or greater) of the primary lesion.

Patients who are at significant risk for developing progressive or recurrent disease following TURBT are generally considered candidates for adjuvant intravesical drug therapy. This includes those with multifocal CIS, CIS associated with Ta or T1 tumors, any G3 tumor, multifocal tumors, and those whose tumors rapidly recur following TURBT of the initial bladder tumor. A number of drugs have been used intravesically, including bacillus Calmette-Guérin (BCG), interferon (IFN) and BCG, thioTEPA, mitomycin C, doxorubicin, and gemcitabine. Complications generally include frequency, dysuria, and irritative voiding symptoms. Over the long term, bladder contracture may occur with these agents. Other complications, which are specific for each drug, are as follows: BCG administration may result in fever, joint pain, granulomatous prostatitis, sinus formation, disseminated tuberculosis, and death; thioTEPA may cause myelosuppression; mitomycin C may cause skin desquamation and rash; and doxorubicin may cause gastrointestinal upset and allergic reactions. The proposed benefit of intravesical chemotherapy is to lessen the rate of recurrences and reduce the incidence of progression. Unfortunately, it cannot be clearly stated that any of these drugs accomplish these goals over the long term.

The use of electromotive installation as an adjunct to intravesical therapy remains controversial. A randomized trial sought to clarify the benefit of electromotive installation of mitomycin. Patients were randomized to TURBT alone (n = 124), immediate post-TURBT mitomycin (n = 126), or pre-TURBT electromotive mitomycin (n = 124). Trial results demonstrated that intravesical electromotive installation of mitomycin before TURBT reduced recurrence and improved the disease-free interval compared with intravesical mitomycin after TURBT and TURBT alone.[81]

Intravesical BCG therapy is typically initiated with an induction course of 6 weekly instillations, followed by a cystoscopic evaluation 1 month after induction. In cases in which CIS is present or suspected, only a biopsy can differentiate this from inflammatory change secondary to treatment. For those who respond to induction, maintenance BCG therapy for up to 3 years is a standard of care, although patients frequently discontinue therapy early due to bladder toxicity.[82]

A European Organisation for Research and Treatment of Cancer (EORTC) phase III trial in over 1,300 patients sought to evaluate whether a third of a dose versus a full dose and a 1-year treatment versus a 3-year treatment could suffice.[83] The trial thus had four different doses and schedules of BCG maintenance therapy. No meaningful differences in toxicity, progression, or survival were observed across dose and schedules. However, the recurrence rate was lowest in high-risk patients treated with the full dose therapy for 3 years, supporting current treatment recommendations.

A number of studies have compared one intravesical chemotherapeutic agent with another. For the most part, BCG in these comparisons has a slight advantage in reducing recurrences.[84] However, when the follow-up is more than 5 years, it appears that there is minimal overall effect at reducing the recurrence rate when compared with no treatment. BCG and epirubicin are the most commonly used agents in this setting and both are considered effective for the treatment of superficial bladder cancer. However, superiority of one over the other is unknown. A meta-analysis of over 1,100 patients treated with either drug reported that intravesical BCG was more efficacious, although also more toxic.[85]

BCG failure is a clinical concern and a treatment dilemma with limited truly effective nonsurgical options. The precise definitions of BCG failure are well outlined by the 2005 International Consensus Panel on T1 bladder cancer and include four subtypes of BCG failure.[86] BCG refractory T1 disease should be of paramount concern and raises the concern for understaged diseases. Options for further intravesical treatment after BCG failure include BCG plus IFNα-2B, gemcitabine, valrubicin, docetaxel, and other novel agents.[85–92] Unfortunately, however, no single agent has yet proven to be more reliably or durably effective than another, and a true consensus on continued intravesical treatment in this setting remains to be determined.

Approximately 70% of patients with high-grade disease will experience recurrence whether or not they are treated with intravesical therapy. Moreover, there is no well-documented evidence that the use of these agents prevents disease progression, for example, from stage Ta/T1 disease to stage T2 or greater disease. One-third of patients who are at high risk for disease progression (those with G3, T1 disease) will progress to stage T2 or greater disease whether or not they are treated with BCG.[93] One-third of patients at 5 years who have disease progression and undergo a cystectomy die of metastatic disease. Thus, approximately 15% of patients with superficial disease at high risk for disease progression (CIS with associated Ta or T1 disease, rapidly recurrent disease, or G3 disease), irrespective of treatment modality, will die of their disease.[94] If definitive therapy (cystectomy) is performed when the disease is found to progress into the muscularis propria (T2 or greater), there is no difference in cure rate when these patients are compared with those who present primarily with T2 or greater disease. These statistics have encouraged some to perform a preemptive cystectomy in those patients at high risk for progression before muscularis propria invasion is documented. Ten-year cancer-specific survivals of 80% are given as justification for this approach, as compared with 50% in patients in whom the cystectomy is performed when the disease progresses to involve the muscularis propria.[95] Unfortunately, this approach subjects approximately two-thirds of these patients who are included in the 80% cancer-specific survival figure to a needless cystectomy, making it questionable as to whether there is in fact any survival advantage whatsoever. Although cystectomy remains the gold standard for recurrent BCG refractory T1 disease, there is an open protocol RTOG 0926 evaluating chemoradiation for such patients who opt for an attempt at bladder preservation or are otherwise not good cystectomy candidates.[96]

## Treatment of Muscularis Propria–Invasive Disease

### Surgical Approaches

The standard of care for squamous cell carcinoma, adenocarcinoma, TCC, and sarcomatoid or spindle cell carcinoma that invade the muscularis propria of the bladder is a bilateral pelvic lymph node dissection and a cystoprostatectomy, with or without a urethrectomy in the male. In the female, an anterior exenteration is performed, which includes the bladder and urethra (the urethra may be spared if uninvolved and an orthotopic bladder reconstruction is performed), the ventral vaginal wall, and the uterus. A radical cystectomy may be indicated in non–muscularis propria–invasive bladder cancers when G3 disease is multifocal or associated with CIS or when bladder tumors rapidly recur, particularly in multifocal areas following intravesical drug therapy. When the prostate stroma is involved with TCC or when there is concomitant CIS of the urethra, a cystoprostatourethrectomy is the treatment of choice.[97] If the urethra needs to be removed, the type of urinary reconstruction is limited to an abdominal urinary diversion. In selected circumstances in the male, the neurovascular bundles coursing along the lateral side of the prostate caudally and adjacent to the rectum more cephalad may be preserved, sometimes preserving potency. Partial cystectomies may rarely be performed in selected patients, thus preserving bladder function and affording in the properly selected patient the same cure rate as a radical cystectomy.[98] Patients who are candidates for such procedures must have focal disease located far enough away from the ureteral orifices and bladder neck to achieve at least a 2-cm margin around the tumor and a margin sufficient around the ureteral orifices and bladder neck to reconstruct the bladder. Practically, this limits partial cystectomies to those patients who have small tumors located in the dome of the bladder and in whom random bladder biopsies show no evidence of CIS or other bladder tumors.

## Survival

The probability of survival from bladder cancer following a cystectomy is determined by the pathologic stage of the disease. Survival is markedly influenced by the presence or absence of positive lymph nodes. Some have argued that the number of positive nodes impacts survival in that, when resected, there is a potential for cure provided there are less than four to eight positive nodes.[99,100] Positive perivesical nodes have a less ominous prognosis when compared with involvement of iliac or para-aortic nodes. Pathologic type may also impact outcome, but in most series, survival is more dependent on pathologic stage than on the cell type of the cancer. Most large series of survival statistics following treatment include all patients regardless of cell type. These series are generally constituted as to histologic type as follows: TCC, 85% to 90%; combination of TCC and either squamous cell or adenocarcinoma, 6%; pure squamous cell carcinoma, 3%; pure adenocarcinoma, 3%; small-cell and sarcomatoid or spindle cell carcinoma, 2% (Table 39.2).

## Types of Urinary Diversion

Urinary diversions may be divided into continent and incontinent. Incontinent urinary diversions or conduits involve the use of a segment of ileum or colon and, less commonly, a segment of jejunum. The distal end is brought to the skin, and the ureters are implanted into the proximal end. The patient wears a urinary collection appliance. The advantages of a conduit (ileal or colonic) are its simplicity and the reduced number of immediate and long-term

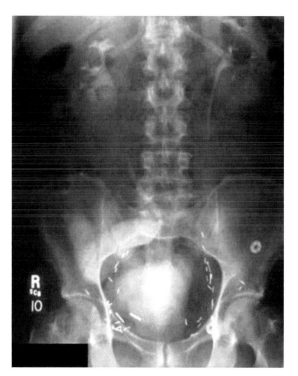

**Figure 39.2** An intravenous urogram of a patient with an orthotopic bladder after a radical cystoprostatectomy. The orthotopic bladder was constructed of the right colon and distal ileum.

postoperative complications. In most series, 13% of patients who undergo a cystectomy and urinary diversion of this type will have a significant complication that impacts on hospital stay or recovery. Generally, the distal ileum is used for the urinary conduit or reservoir; however, if it has been irradiated or is otherwise involved, one may select the right colon or a short segment of jejunum. The latter is the least desirable choice because electrolyte problems may be significant. On occasion, during exenterative surgery when an end colostomy is created, a segment of distal bowel is used, thus obviating the need for an intestinal anastomosis.

Continent diversions may be divided into two types: abdominal and orthotopic. Abdominal diversions require a continence valve, whereas an orthotopic neobladder depends on the urethral sphincter for continence. The reservoir is made of bowel that is fashioned into a globular configuration. In the abdominal type of continent diversion, the stoma is brought through the abdominal wall to the skin. The patient catheterizes the pouch every 4 hours. Orthotopic urinary diversions entail the use of bowel brought to the urethra, thus allowing the patient to void by Valsalva (Fig. 39.2). Patients must have the facility to catheterize themselves, because it is mandatory in the abdominal continent diversion and occasionally necessary in the orthotopic reconstruction. The advantage of continent diversions is the avoidance of a collection device. The advantage of an orthotopic bladder over all other types of continent diversions is that it rehabilitates the patient to normal voiding through the urethra, often without the need for intermittent catheterization or the need to wear a collection device. Postoperative and long-term complications of continent diversion are increased over the conduit types of diversions. Indeed, in some series, postoperative complications range from 13% to 30%. Long-term metabolic complications are also increased.

## Complications of Cystectomy and Urinary Diversion

The complications of all types of urinary diversion may be divided into three groups: metabolic, neuromechanical, and surgical.

## TABLE 39.2

**Survival After Radical Cystectomy According to Pathologic Stage at 10 Years**

| Pathologic Stage | Disease-Specific Survival (%) | Overall Survival (%) |
|---|---|---|
| pTa, Tis, T1 with high risk of progression | 82 | — |
| Organ confined, negative nodes (pT2, pN0) | 73 | 49 |
| Non–organ confined (pT3–4a or pN1–2) | 33 | 23 |
| Lymph node positive (any T, pN1–2) | 28, 34 | 21 |

From Gschwend JE, Dahm P, Fair WR. Disease specific survival as endpoint of outcome for bladder cancer patients following radical cystectomy. *Eur Urol* 2002;41:440–448; Stein JP, Cai J, Groshen S, et al. Risk factors for patients with pelvic lymph node metastases following radical cystectomy with en bloc pelvic lymphadenectomy: concept of lymph node density. *J Urol* 2003;170:35–41; Stein JP, Lieskovsky G, Cote R, et al. Radical cystectomy in the treatment of invasive bladder cancer: long-term results in 1,054 patients. *J Clin Oncol* 2001;19:666–675; Dalbagni G, Genega E, Hashibe M, et al. Cystectomy for bladder cancer: a contemporary series. *J Urol* 2001;165:1111–1116; Grossman HB, Natale RB, Tangen CM, et al. Neoadjuvant chemotherapy plus cystectomy compared with cystectomy alone for locally advanced bladder cancer. *N Engl J Med* 2003;349:859–866; and Zehnder P, Studer UE, Skinner EC, et al. Super extended versus extended pelvic lymph node dissection in patients undergoing radical cystectomy for bladder cancer: a comparative study. *J Urol* 2011;186:1261–1268.

**Metabolic Complications of Urinary Intestinal Diversion.** When the intestine is interposed in the urinary tract, there is the potential for a number of metabolic complications.[104] These may involve electrolyte abnormalities and altered drug metabolism, which may result in altered sensorium, infection, osteomalacia, growth retardation, calculi both within the reservoir as well as in the kidney, short bowel syndrome, cancer, and altered bile metabolism.

Depending on the segment used, different specific electrolyte abnormalities may occur. When the ileum and colon are used, hyperchloremic metabolic acidosis may result; when jejunum is used, hypochloremic or hyperkalemic metabolic acidosis may follow.

Hypokalemia is more common when the colon is used, whereas hypocalcemia is more common when the ileum and colon are used, and hypomagnesemia is more common when the ileum and the colon are used.

The most pervasive detrimental effect created by all urinary intestinal diversions is due to acidosis. Acidosis may result in electrolyte abnormalities, osteomalacia, growth retardation, altered sensorium, altered hepatic metabolism, renal calculi, and abnormal drug metabolism. In general, patients with normal renal function as well as normal hepatic function are less prone to acidosis and its complications.

Treatment for the metabolic acidosis is straightforward and can be accomplished with bicarbonate or with Bicitra solution, which is sodium citrate and citric acid. Polycitra, which is a combination of potassium citrate, sodium citrate, and citric acid, may also be employed. It has the advantage of supplying potassium, which, on occasion, is deficient. Chlorpromazine and nicotinic acid have been used to block the chloride bicarbonate exchanger, and thus lessen the potential for the acidosis.

Decreased renal function is seen in a majority of patients in the decade following a radical cystectomy, and choice of diversion does not predict the decline. Postoperative hydronephrosis, pyelonephritis, and uretero-enteric strictures represent factors that, if addressed, may mitigate the loss of function.[105]

Patients with conduits may have a 3% to 4% incidence of renal calculi over the long term. Those with reservoirs have up to a 20% incidence of calculi within the reservoir. The pathogenesis may be a metabolic alteration or infection, whereas reservoir stones are most commonly due to a surgical foreign body or mucus serving as a nidus.

There is a high incidence of bacteriuria in patients with either conduits or pouches, and the incidence of sepsis is 13%. There appears to be diminished antibacterial activity of the intestinal mucosa, with the immunoglobulins, which are normally secreted by the mucosa, being altered. In addition to this, when the bowel is distended, there can be a translocation of bacteria from the lumen into the bloodstream.

Because the intestine is interposed in the urinary tract, drugs that are eliminated unchanged from the body through the kidney and have the potential to be reabsorbed by the gut can in fact result in significant alterations in metabolism of that drug. Patients with a urinary diversion, when given systemic chemotherapy, have a higher incidence of complications and are more likely to have their chemotherapy limited when compared with patients without diversion who receive the same drugs and dose.[106]

The loss of the distal ileum may result in vitamin $B_{12}$ malabsorption, which then manifests itself as anemia and neurologic abnormalities. Bile salt malabsorption may occur and result in diarrhea. Loss of the ileocecal valve may result in diarrhea with bacterial overgrowth of the ileum and malabsorption of vitamin $B_{12}$ and fat-soluble vitamins A, D, E, and K. Loss of the colon may result in diarrhea and bicarbonate loss.

**Neuromechanical Complications.** Neuromechanical complications may be of two types: atonic, resulting in an atonic segment with urinary retention, and hyperperistaltic contractions. The latter is relevant in continent diversions, as this may result in incontinence and a low-capacity reservoir.

**Surgical Complications.** There are a number of complications that occur following any major surgical procedure, which include thrombophlebitis, pulmonary embolus, wound dehiscence, pneumonia, atelectasis, myocardial infarction, and death. Complications specific to cystectomy and urinary diversion are divided into short term and late. The short-term complications include acute acidosis (16%), urine leak (3% to 16%), bowel obstruction or fecal leak (10%), and pyelonephritis (5% to 15%). The longer term complications include ureteral or intestinal obstruction (15%), renal deterioration (15%), renal failure (5%), stoma problems (15%), and intestinal stricture (10% to 15%).[107,108]

The morbidity of salvage cystectomy for a recurrence following bladder sparing chemoradiation has also been described and appears acceptable when compared to primary cystectomy series.[109]

### Selective Bladder-Preserving Approaches

The treatment options for muscularis propria–invasive bladder tumors can broadly be divided into those that remove the bladder and those that spare it. In the United States, a radical cystectomy with pelvic lymph node dissection remains the standard method used to treat patients with this tumor. Several reports from North America and Europe have described long-term results using multimodality treatment of muscularis propria–invading bladder cancer, with appropriate safeguards for early cystectomy should this treatment fail. For bladder-conserving therapy to be more widely accepted, this treatment approach must have a high likelihood of eradicating the primary tumor, must preserve good organ function, and must not result in compromised patient survival. It does appear that, for selected patients, bladder sparing therapy with salvage cystectomy reserved for tumor recurrence represents a safe and effective alternative to immediate radical cystectomy.[110]

Successful bladder-preserving approaches have evolved during the past 3 decades. They began with the use of radiation therapy but expanded when the National Bladder Cancer Group first demonstrated the safety and efficacy of cisplatin as a radiation sensitizer in patients with muscle-invasive bladder cancer that was unsuitable for cystectomy.[111] The long-term survival with stage T2 tumors (64%) and stage T3 to T4 tumors (22%) was encouraging. This was validated by the National Cancer Institute–Canada randomized trial of radiation (either definitive or precystectomy) with or without concurrent cisplatin for patients with T3 bladder cancer, which showed a significant improvement in long-term survival with pelvic tumor control (67% versus 47%) in the patients who were assigned cisplatin.[112] Additional single-institution studies showed that the combination of a visibly complete TURBT followed by radiation therapy or radiation therapy concurrent with chemotherapy safely improved local control.[113,114] These findings led the RTOG to develop protocols for bladder preservation beginning with a TURBT of as much of the tumor as is safely possible, followed by the combination of radiation with concurrent radiosensitizing chemotherapy. One key to the success of such a program is the selection of patients for bladder preservation on the basis of the initial response of each individual patient's tumor to therapy. Thus, bladder conservation is reserved for those patients who have a clinical CR to concurrent chemotherapy and radiation. A prompt cystectomy is recommended for those patients whose tumors respond only incompletely or who subsequently develop an invasive tumor (Fig. 39.3). Up to 30% of the patients entering a potential bladder-preserving protocol with trimodality therapy (initial TURBT followed by concurrent chemoradiation) will ultimately require a salvage radical cystectomy.

For over 2 decades, the Massachusetts General Hospital (MGH), the RTOG, and several centers in Europe have evaluated in phase II and III protocols concurrent chemoradiation plus neoadjuvant or adjuvant chemotherapy (Table 39.3). Radiosensitizing drugs studied in these series, either singly or in various combinations, include cisplatin, carboplatin, paclitaxel, 5-fluorouracil (5-FU), mitomycin C,

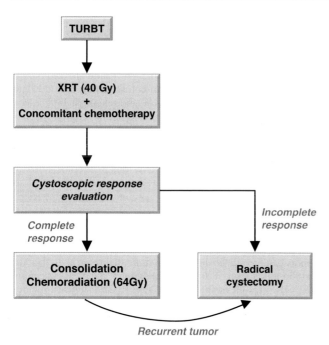

**Figure 39.3** Schema for trimodality treatment of muscularis propria–invasive bladder cancer with selective bladder preservation. XRT, radiation therapy.

and gemcitabine.[113] The first RTOG study of patients treated with once-daily radiation treatment and concurrent cisplatin yielded a 5-year survival of 52% (42% with intact bladder).[115] RTOG studies 8802 and 8903 used methotrexate, cisplatin, and vinblastine (MCV) chemotherapy as neoadjuvant treatment.[116] In the latter study, the neoadjuvant therapy was tested in a randomized fashion.[117] No improvement was seen in survival or in local tumor eradication as a result of neoadjuvant therapy, although the trial was closed early and underpowered to give a definitive answer. The toxicity of the MCV arm was considerable, with only 67% of patients able to complete the planned treatment. The use of contemporary neoadjuvant

chemotherapy (dose-dense methotrexate, vinblastine, adriamycin, cisplatin [ddMVAC] or gemcitabine and cisplatin [GC]) regimens with appropriate supportive therapy in well-selected bladder-sparing patients may warrant further investigation.

Other studies from Paris and Germany have reported their large experience with bladder sparing.[118,119] The CR rate in the German study was 72%, and local control of the bladder tumor after the CR without a muscle-invasive relapse was maintained in 64% of the patients at 10 years. The 10-year disease-specific survival was 42%, and more than 80% of these survivors preserved their bladder. This series reported the sequential use of radiation with no chemotherapy (126 patients), followed by concurrent cisplatin (145 patients), then concurrent carboplatin (95 patients), and finally concurrent cisplatin with 5-FU (49 patients). The CR rates in these four protocols were 51%, 81%, 64%, and 87%, respectively.[120,121] The 5-year actuarial survival with an intact bladder in these studies was 38%, 47%, 41%, and 54%, respectively. These results strongly suggest that radiochemotherapy, when given concurrently, is superior to radiation therapy alone; that carboplatin is less radiosensitizing than cisplatin; and that cisplatin plus 5-FU may be superior to cisplatin alone.

The RTOG protocols have subsequently explored both twice-daily radiation therapy and novel radiosensitization using cisplatin with or without 5-FU or paclitaxel.[62,122, 123,124] Complete response and bladder preservation rates are consistently high, with no one regimen clearly superior.[62]

Gemcitabine has been also tested in bladder-treatment protocols. In a phase I trial from the University of Michigan, 23 patients, mostly T2, were treated with gemcitabine and concurrent daily radiation. At a median follow-up of 5.6 years, an impressive 91% CR rate was observed, and the 5-year actuarial estimates of survival include a bladder-intact survival of 62%, an overall survival of 76%, and a disease-specific survival of 82%.[125] A phase II study from the United Kingdom of 50 patients treated with concurrent weekly gemcitabine and hypofractionated radiation reported an 88% complete endoscopic response rate, a 3-year overall survival of 75%, and cancer-specific survival of 82%.[126] Twice weekly low-dose gemcitabine was recently evaluated as a radiosensitizer with daily radiation in protocol RTOG 0712.

Cisplatin is not always an ideal drug for bladder cancer patients, because it may cause impaired renal function in many. A British group observed high response rates using the combination of 5-FU

TABLE 39.3

**Results of Multimodality Treatment for Muscle-Invading Bladder Cancer**

| Series (Ref.) | Multimodality Therapy Used | Number of Patients | 5-Year Overall Survival (%) | 5-Year Survival with Intact Bladder (%) |
|---|---|---|---|---|
| RTOG 8512, 1993[115] | External-beam radiation with cisplatin | 42 | 52 | 42 |
| RTOG 8802, 1996[116] | TURBT, MCV, external-beam radiation with cisplatin | 91 | 51 | 44 (4 y) |
| RTOG 8903, 1998[117] | TURBT with or without MCV, external-beam radiation with cisplatin | 123 | 49 | 38 |
| University of Paris, 1998[118] | TURBT, 5-FU, external-beam radiation with cisplatin | 120 | 63 | N/A |
| Erlangen, 2002[119] | TURBT, external-beam radiation, cisplatin, carboplatin, or cisplatin and 5-FU | 415 (cisplatin, 82; carboplatin, 61; 5-FU/cisplatin, 87) | 51 | 42 |
| RTOG 9906, 2009[122] | TURBT, TAX plus CP plus XRT; adjuvant CP plus GEM | 80 | 56 | 47 |
| MGH, 2012[130] | TURBT, external-beam radiation and cisplatin *with or without* 5-FU or TAX; neoadjuvant or adjuvant chemotherapy | 348 | 52 | 42 |

MCV, methotrexate, cisplatin, vinblastine; 5-FU, 5-fluorouracil; N/A, not available; TAX, paclitaxel; CP, cisplatin; GEM, gemcitabine.

and mitomycin C with pelvic radiotherapy.[127] These results led to the phase III Bladder Cancer 2001 (BC2001) trial, in which 360 patients with muscle-invasive bladder cancer were randomized to either radiotherapy alone or to radiotherapy with concomitant 5-FU and mitomycin C chemotherapy. Local–regional disease-free survival was superior for those patients receiving chemotherapy (67% versus 54% at 2 years; hazard ratio [HR] 0.68, $p = 0.03$ with median follow-up of 70 months). Survival at 5 years was higher with chemoradiotherapy (48% versus 35%), but did not reach statistical significance (HR 0.82; $p = 0.16$).[128]

## Predictors of Outcome

A common feature of all the RTOG protocols was early bladder tumor response evaluation and the selection of patients for bladder conservation on the basis of their initial response to TURBT combined with chemotherapy and radiation.[130] Bladder conservation was reserved for those who had a complete clinical response at the midpoint in therapy (after a radiation dosage of 40 Gy). Complete responders to induction therapy then received consolidation with additional chemotherapy and radiation to a total tumor dose of 64 to 65 Gy. Incomplete responders were advised to undergo a radical cystectomy, as were patients whose invasive tumors persisted or recurred after treatment. The current schema for trimodality treatment of muscle-invading bladder cancer is provided in Figure 39.3. Other tumor presentations associated with successful bladder-sparing therapy include: solitary T2 or early T3 tumors (typically <6 cm in size), no tumor-associated hydronephrosis, tumors allowing a visibly complete TURBT, invasive tumors not associated with extensive carcinoma in situ, and urothelial carcinoma histology (because alternative histologies have not been rigorously evaluated in bladder sparing protocols).

In the MGH series,[130] the median follow-up for all surviving patients was 7.7 years. Of patients, 72% (78% with stage T2) had CR to induction therapy. The 10-year actuarial overall survival was 35% (T2, 43%; T3–T4a, 27%) and the 10-year disease-specific survival was 59% (T2, 67%; stage T3–T4a, 49%) (Figs. 39.4 and 39.5). The clinical stage and achieving a CR were significantly associated with both overall survival and disease-specific survival. A nomogram predicting response has been developed from this data.[129] The use of neoadjuvant chemotherapy with MCV, however, was not associated with survival or incidence of metastases, although this may warrant further investigation in the modern era.

The 10-year disease-specific survival rate for the 102 patients (29%) undergoing a cystectomy was 44%, illustrating the very

important contribution of prompt salvage cystectomy. The 10-year disease-specific survival with an intact bladder was 45% (T2, 52%; T3–T4a, 36%). No patient required a cystectomy due to bladder morbidity. The overall survival and disease-specific survival for all 348 patients and for some clinically important subgroups are shown in Table 39.4. The value of complete TURBT in bladder-sparing therapy is demonstrated in this report. Of the 348 patients followed, 227 underwent a complete TURBT and 116 had an incomplete TURBT. Patients who underwent a complete TURBT had improved CR, overall survival, disease-specific survival, and lower rates of cystectomy (22% versus 42%) compared to those with an incomplete TURBT. In a review of the patients who were complete responders after induction therapy, 55% developed no further bladder tumors, 29% subsequently developed a superficial occurrence, and 16% developed an invasive tumor.[132] Most patients with superficial recurrence were treated successfully by TURBT and intravesical chemotherapy. For these individuals, the overall survival was comparable to those who had no failure. However, one-quarter of these patients ultimately required a salvage cystectomy.

Notably, age is not a contraindication to successful bladder sparing therapy, and indeed, results are favorable in patients aged 75 years or older.[130] This is an important consideration given that the elderly generally appear to be undertreated for invasive bladder cancer in the United States.[131] Bladder-sparing chemoradiation remains a good option for those patients who are not cystectomy candidates and, often, such patients would be treated with daily radiation and appropriate concurrent chemotherapy without a break.

## Radiation Treatment

The most common approach with external-beam irradiation reported from North America and Europe involves the treatment of the pelvis to include the bladder, the prostate (in men), and often, the low external and internal iliac lymph nodes for a total dose of 40 to 45 Gy in 1.8- to 2.0-Gy fractions during 4 to 5 weeks. Subsequently, the target volume is reduced to deliver a final boost dose of 20 to 25 Gy in 15 fractions to the primary bladder tumor. Some protocols call for partial bladder radiation as the boost volume if the location of the tumor in the bladder can be satisfactorily identified by the use of cystoscopic mapping, selected mucosal biopsies, and imaging information from CT or MRI. Figure 39.6 is an isodose color wash of a partial bladder boost in a three-dimensional–conformal plan. Plans using conventional fractionation that result in a whole bladder dose of 50 to 55 Gy and a bladder tumor volume dose of 65 Gy in combination with concurrent

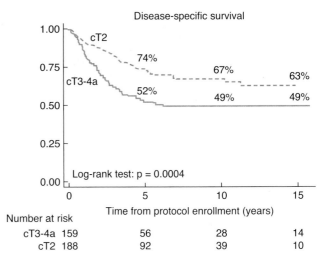

**Figure 39.5** Massachusetts General Hospital Selective Bladder Preservation Series 1986 to 2002 disease-specific survival reported by intention to treat.

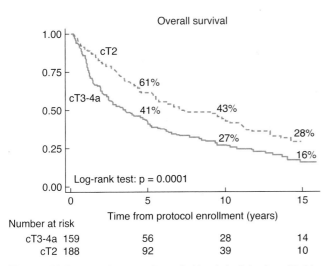

**Figure 39.4** Massachusetts General Hospital Selective Bladder Preservation Series 1986 to 2002 overall survival reported by intention to treat.

### TABLE 39.4

## Survival Outcomes by Patient and Tumor Characteristics: Massachusetts General Hospital

| Patient Group | n | Overall Survival (%) | | | | Disease-Specific Survival (%) | | | |
|---|---|---|---|---|---|---|---|---|---|
| | | 5 Year | 10 Year | 15 Year | P value | 5 Year | 10 Year | 15 Year | P value |
| All patients | 348 | 52 ± 5.3[a] | 35 ± 5.6[a] | 22 ± 5.6[a] | | 64 ± 5.8[a] | 59 ± 6.2[a] | 57 ± 6.6[a] | |
| **Age at Entry (y)** | | | | | | | | | |
| <75 | 262 | 54 | 39 | 27 | 0.004 | 65 | 59 | 58 | 0.59 |
| >75 | 86 | 45 | 23 | 2.9 | | 63 | 60 | 52 | |
| *Sex* | | | | | | | | | |
| Female | 91 | 55 | 37 | 17 | 0.72 | 64 | 55 | 55 | 0.59 |
| Male | 257 | 51 | 35 | 24 | | 64 | 60 | 58 | |
| **Clinical Stage** | | | | | | | | | |
| T2 | 188 | 61 | 43 | 28 | 0.0001 | 74 | 67 | 63 | 0.0004 |
| T3–T4a | 159 | 41 | 27 | 16 | | 52 | 49 | 49 | |
| **Hydronephrosis** | | | | | | | | | |
| No | 289 | 55 | 39 | 24 | 0.0004 | 68 | 63 | 61 | 0.0005 |
| Yes | 58 | 34 | 17 | 10 | | 44 | 38 | 38 | |

[a] 95% confidence interval.
*Source:* Efstathiou JA, Spiegel DY, Shipley WU, et al. Long-term outcomes of selective bladder preservation by combined-modality therapy for invasive bladder cancer: the MGH experience. *Eur Urol* 2012;61:705–711.

cisplatin-containing chemotherapy have been widely used. The available information suggests that higher doses per fraction may lead to a higher rate of significant late complications. Data looking at toxicity from urodynamic and quality-of-life studies indicate that lower dose per fraction irradiation given once or twice a day concurrent with chemotherapy results in excellent long-term bladder function and low rates of late pelvic toxicity.[133,134]

Because the bladder is not a fixed organ, its location and volume can vary considerably from day to day. This results in a number of

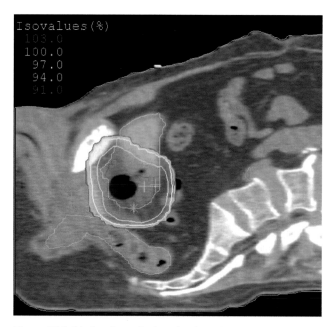

**Figure 39.6** Display of a sagittal section through the three-dimensional (3-D) data set, with dose displayed in color wash, for a patient with bladder cancer treated with a partial bladder tumor boost with 3-D conformal radiotherapy. Note sparing of the anterior, non–tumor bearing portion of bladder.

logistic problems to ensure adequate coverage of the bladder. Studies have identified substantial movement of the bladder during the course of external-beam radiation therapy, and as a result of these findings, many have recommended that the bladder be emptied when simulated and prior to each treatment to maximize reproducibility and avoid a geographic miss. Forms of image-guided delivery (including daily cone-beam CT and fiducials) have also been employed for accurate localization. Another acceptable approach often employed in the United Kingdom, is for radiation to be delivered to 55 Gy in 20 fractions or 64 Gy in 32 fractions to the whole bladder without a tumor boost and without fields to specifically cover the pelvic lymph nodes.[135]

Brachytherapy is another technique to deliver a higher dose of radiation to a limited area of the bladder within a short period. This approach has been reported from institutions in the Netherlands, Belgium, and France. It is reserved for patients with solitary bladder tumors and as part of combined modality therapy with transurethral resection and external-beam radiation therapy as well as interstitial radiation therapy. External-beam doses of 30 Gy are used in combination with an implant tumor dose of 40 Gy. These groups report that for patients with solitary clinical stage T2 to T3a tumors less than 5 cm in diameter, local control rates at 5 to 10 years range from 72% to 84% with disease-specific survivals of approximately 75%.[136]

## Comparison of Treatment Outcomes of Contemporary Cystectomy Series with Contemporary Selective Bladder-Preserving Series

Comparing the results of selective bladder-preserving approaches with those of radical cystectomy series is confounded by selection bias and the discordance between clinical (TURBT) staging and pathologic (cystectomy) staging. Clinical staging will understage the extent of disease 40% of the time with regard to penetration into the muscularis propria or beyond when compared to pathologic staging.[137,138] The University of Southern California and Memorial Sloan-Kettering Cancer Center have reported their large cystectomy experience,[102,136,139] and the national phase III protocol by Southwest Oncology Group (SWOG), Eastern Cooperative Oncology Group, and Cancer and Leukemia Group B (CALGB)

**TABLE 39.5**

## Muscle-Invasive Bladder Cancer: Survival Outcomes in Contemporary Series

| Series (Ref.) | Stages | Number of Patients | Overall Survival (%) | |
|---|---|---|---|---|
| | | | 5 Year | 10 Year |
| **Cystectomy** | | | | |
| University of Southern California, 2001[101] | pT2–pT4a | 633 | 48 | 32 |
| Memorial Sloan-Kettering, 2001[102] | pT2–pT4a | 181 | 36 | 27 |
| SWOG/ECOG/CALGB,[a,b] 2003[103] | cT2–cT4a | 303 | 49 | 34 |
| **Selective Bladder Preservation (Chemoradiation)** | | | | |
| University of Erlangen,[a] 2002[119] | cT2–cT4a | 326 | 45 | 29 |
| MGH,[a] 2012[130] | cT2–cT4a | 348 | 52 | 35 |
| RTOG,[a] 1998[117] | cT2–cT4a | 123 | 49 | — |
| BC2001,[a] 2012[128] | cT2–4a | 182 | 48 | |

[a] These series include all patients by their intention to treat.
[b] Fifty percent of patients were randomly assigned to receive three cycles of neoadjuvant MVAC (methotrexate, vinblastine, doxorubicin, cisplatin).
ECOG, Eastern Cooperative Oncology Group; CALGB, Cancer and Leukemia Group B; RTOG, Radiation Therapy Oncology Group, Bladder Cancer 2001 (BC2001) trial.

has also reported valuable prospective data.[103] The overall survival rates from these contemporary cystectomy series are comparable to those reported from single-institution and cooperative group results using contemporary selective bladder-preserving approaches with trimodality therapy and prompt salvage cystectomy for the minority of patients who recur (Table 39.5). An attempt to compare cystectomy to bladder-sparing therapy in a randomized fashion in the United Kingdom failed to accrue.

### Bladder-Preservation Treatments with Less than Trimodality Therapy

It has been argued that trimodality therapy might represent excessive treatment for many patients with invasive bladder cancer and that comparable results could be obtained by TURBT, either alone or with chemotherapy. Herr[140] reported the outcome of 432 patients initially evaluated by repeat TURBT for muscle-invasive bladder tumors. In that series, 99 patients (23% of the original 432 patients) initially treated conservatively without immediate cystectomy had a 34% rate of progression to a recurrent muscle-invading tumor at 20 years. In series combining TURBT and MVAC chemotherapy, only 50% of those found to have a clinical CR proved to be tumor-free at cystectomy.[141] By comparison, one of the clearest examples of the improved success of trimodality treatment was reported in the study from the University of Paris.[142] TURBT followed by concurrent cisplatin, 5-FU, and accelerated radiation was used by this group initially as a precystectomy regimen. In the first 18 patients, all of whom demonstrated no residual tumor on cystoscopic evaluation and rebiopsy (a CR) but who all underwent a cystectomy, none had any tumor in the cystectomy specimen (100% had a pathologic CR). Comparing approaches by TURBT plus MVAC chemotherapy alone with trimodality therapy, the 5-year survival rates are comparable (50%), but the preserved bladder rate for all patients studied ranged from 20% to 33% when radiation therapy was not used and from 41% to 45% when radiation therapy was used.[142] Thus, trimodality therapy increases the probability of surviving with an intact bladder by 30% to 40% compared with the results reported with TURBT and chemotherapy alone.

Herr[143] reported on 63 patients who had achieved a complete clinical response to neoadjuvant chemotherapy with a cisplatin-based regimen, who then refused to undergo a planned cystectomy. He reported that the most significant predictor of improved survival was complete resection of the tumor before starting chemotherapy. Over 90% of surviving patients had small low-stage invasive tumors that were completely resected. Thus, he concluded, selected patients with T2 bladder cancers may do well after a transurethral resection and chemotherapy.

## Systemic Chemotherapy with Radical Therapy

### Neoadjuvant Chemotherapy

The advantage of neoadjuvant chemotherapy is its potential to downsize and downstage tumors and to attack occult metastatic disease early, especially given the frequent postoperative complications and prolonged recovery that can delay or derail plans for adjuvant chemotherapy. Moreover, although trials described as follows suggest a survival advantage for neoadjuvant chemotherapy, there have been no contemporary studies supporting a benefit with adjuvant chemotherapy. The disadvantages of neoadjuvant therapy include the inherent difficulties in assessing response, the fact that clinical rather than pathologic criteria must be relied on, the debilitating effects of chemotherapy in some patients, increasing the risks of surgery and possibly complicating or delaying full recovery from surgery, and the possibility of the deleterious effects of the delay in cystectomy or radiation associated with neoadjuvant chemotherapy.[144]

Although downstaging of the primary tumor has been demonstrated, randomized studies using single-agent neoadjuvant chemotherapy have failed to demonstrate a survival benefit. Studies in patients with measurable metastatic disease clearly showed the superiority of MVAC over single-agent cisplatin on survival, inspiring further studies of multiagent neoadjuvant therapy.[145]

The study by Grossman et al.[143] randomly assigned patients with muscularis propria–invasive bladder cancer (stage T2 to T4a) to radical cystectomy alone or three cycles of MVAC followed by radical cystectomy. During an 11-year period, 317 patients were enrolled. The authors reported that MVAC can be given before radical cystectomy, but the side effects are appreciable. One-third of patients had severe hematologic or gastrointestinal reactions, but, on the positive side, there were no drug-related deaths and the chemotherapy did not adversely affect the performance of surgery. The authors concluded:

1. The survival benefit associated with MVAC appeared to be strongly related to downstaging of the tumor to pT0. Of the chemotherapy-treated patients, 38% had no evidence of cancer at cystectomy, as compared with 15% of patients in the cystectomy-only group. In both groups, improved survival was associated with the absence of residual cancer in the cystectomy specimen.

2. The median survival was 77 months for the chemotherapy-treated patients compared with 46 months for the cystectomy-only group.

3. The 5-year actuarial survival was 43% in the cystectomy group, which was not significantly different from 57% in the chemotherapy-treated group.

Stratification by tumor stage indicated greater improvement in median survival with chemotherapy in subjects with T3–T4a disease (65 versus 24 months, chemotherapy versus observation) than in subjects with T2 disease (105 versus 75 months). The authors point out that their study is different from seven previous negative studies that used either single-agent cisplatin (demonstrated to be inferior to MVAC in measurable metastatic disease) or a two-drug combination. They also acknowledged problems of interpretation created by slow accrual and a lack of pathologic review.

The Medical Research Council and the EORTC performed a prospective randomized trial of neoadjuvant cisplatin, methotrexate, and vinblastine in patients undergoing cystectomy or full-dose external-beam radiotherapy for muscularis propria–invasive bladder cancer.[146,147] In the initial report with a median follow-up of 7.4 years, the difference in 5-year survival between those who received chemotherapy (49%) and those who did not (43%) just reached clinical significance with a probability value of 0.048.[147] However, the survival benefit did not reach the prespecified study goal. Long-term follow-up of the study with median follow-up of 8 years and more death events demonstrated that systemic chemotherapy plus local treatment improved overall 10-year survival by 6% and reduced the risk of bladder cancer death by 17% compared to local treatment alone. For patients whose local treatment included a cystectomy, the use of cisplatin, methotrexate, and vinblastine (CMV) resulted in a 26% reduction in the risk of death compared to surgery alone.[148] Based on their interpretation of the data as presented, Sharma and Bajorin[149] now recommend neoadjuvant chemotherapy, although others are concerned that the "number needed to treat" is very high.

A third randomized trial was the Nordic Cystectomy Trial 1.[150] Patients were treated with two cycles of neoadjuvant doxorubicin and cisplatin. All patients received 5 days of radiation followed by cystectomy. A subgroup analysis was performed and showed a 20% difference in disease-specific survival at 5 years in patients with T3 and T4 disease, but there was no difference in stages T1 and T2, nor a difference when all entered patients were compared.

The Nordic Cystectomy Trial 2 included only stage T3 or T4a patients in an attempt to confirm the positive results in Nordic 1 in this subgroup of patients.[151] This trial eliminated radiation therapy and substituted methotrexate for doxorubicin in order to lower toxicity. In 317 patients studied, no survival benefit was noted in the chemotherapy arm. The authors concluded that despite substantial downstaging, no survival benefit was seen with neoadjuvant chemotherapy after 5 years of follow-up, although the choice of chemotherapy was unconventional by contemporary standards.

Raghavan et al.[152] published a meta-analysis of all completed randomized trials of neoadjuvant chemotherapy for invasive bladder cancer (2,688 patients). They concluded that single-agent neoadjuvant chemotherapy is ineffective and should not be used; current combination chemotherapy regimens improve the 5-year survival by 5%, which reduces the risk of death by 13% compared with the use of definitive local treatment alone (from 43% to 38%).

Additional meta-analyses have been published[144,153-155] that showed a 4% to 6% absolute increase in 5-year survival. Many phase II studies are now investigating alternative neoadjuvant combinations including cisplatin/gemcitabine and dose-dense or accelerated MVAC, and time will tell whether any have superiority.[156-162]

In the 2014 National Comprehensive Cancer Network *Clinical Practice Guidelines in Oncology: Bladder Cancer*, neoadjuvant chemotherapy is a category 1 recommendation for localized stage T2–T4a disease. According to the National Cancer Data Base in the United States, only 11.6% of patients underwent any perioperative chemotherapy, with most in the adjuvant setting.[162] In the future, gene profiling may identify those most likely to respond to chemotherapy.[163]

## Adjuvant Chemotherapy

The advantage of adjuvant, as opposed to neoadjuvant, chemotherapy is that pathologic staging allows for a more accurate selection of patients. This approach facilitates the separation of patients in stage pT2 from those in stages pT3 or pT4 or node-positive disease, all at a high risk for metastatic progression.

Adjuvant chemotherapy has been studied in two major clinical settings: (1) following bladder-sparing chemoirradiation and (2) following a radical cystectomy. In the former case, there is no guidance from pathologic staging, but experience has shown that up to 50% of those with invasive cancers have, in truth, a systemic disease.[164] Respecting this, the RTOG studies have added adjuvant chemotherapy at first with MCV, later using cisplatin plus gemcitabine, and more recently adding paclitaxel.[165] The results thus far do not indicate whether adjuvant chemotherapy is affecting survival.

The place of adjuvant chemotherapy after cystectomy has been studied more thoroughly, but again, the results are not clear. Investigators generally agree that in the face of positive nodes, and even with negative nodes and high pathologic stage of the primary tumor, adjuvant chemotherapy is likely to be important in improving survival. In reviewing existing reports of adjuvant trials in bladder cancer, there are five randomized trials using adjuvant chemotherapy.[166-170] Three studies found no difference between adjuvant chemotherapy and cystectomy alone, but all three were seriously flawed in design or accrual.[149] Two of the five studies[169,170] showed a survival benefit for cystectomy and adjuvant chemotherapy over cystectomy alone, but both are subject to criticism for both method considerations and small accrual.

Nonetheless, in a follow-up report by Stockle et al.[171] an analysis of 166 patients, including the 49 initially randomized patients, a difference was noted in the 80 patients who received adjuvant chemotherapy as compared with 86 patients who underwent cystectomy alone. The extent of nodal involvement proved important, and when patients were stratified by the number of nodes involved, adjuvant chemotherapy was most effective in patients with N1 disease.

In an important review of the current status of adjuvant chemotherapy in muscle-invasive bladder cancer, the Advanced Bladder Cancer Meta-Analysis Collaboration examined 491 patients from six trials, representing 90% of all patients randomized in cisplatin-based combination chemotherapy trials. They concluded that there is insufficient evidence on which to base reliable treatment decisions, and they recommended further research.[172]

More recent studies have used different adjuvant chemotherapy regimens or molecular stratification. A randomized trial performed in Italy randomized patients after cystectomy either to four courses of gemcitabine plus cisplatin (n = 102) or to the same treatment at time of relapse (n = 92). There was no difference in the 5-year overall survival across treatment arms. However, due to poor accrual, the study was insufficiently powered to detect a survival difference.[173]

As described earlier, p53 alteration status was hypothesized to be both prognostic for recurrence after cystectomy and predictive for a survival benefit conferred by adjuvant chemotherapy. A phase III trial separated patients based on p53 status, with all p53-negative patients followed with observation alone. Patients with p53 alteration (n = 114) were randomized postcystectomy to three cycles of adjuvant MVAC or observation. Neither p53 status nor MVAC adjuvant chemotherapy impacted risk of recurrence.[57]

Gallagher et al.[174] studied adjuvant, sequential chemotherapy in a nonrandomized design, using as a basis the improvement in survival in breast cancer when sequential adjuvant chemotherapy was used. In this study and others similarly designed,[175,176] adjuvant, sequential chemotherapy for patients with high-risk uro-thelial cancer did not appear to improve disease-specific survival over that observed with surgery alone.

Dreicer,[161] in reviewing the published literature, made the case for adjuvant chemotherapy as the standard of care given the lethality of radical cystectomy alone in muscle-invasive bladder cancer, but he acknowledges that "suboptimal trial design, insufficient numbers of patients, and lack of standardization of the chemotherapy regimens used have plagued adjuvant studies."

## Combined Modality Treatment of Local–Regionally Advanced Disease

The place of combined modality therapy for advanced disease has not been settled. Several series have suggested an improvement in long-term survival in selected patients undergoing resection of persistent cancer deposits after MVAC or CMV.[164,177]

In our experience, carefully selected patients with locally advanced unresectable bladder cancer, including some patients with pelvic nodal masses, may experience long-term survival with the combination of chemotherapy and radiation. To be selected for this combined modality treatment, patients must have (1) an excellent performance status, (2) locally advanced measurable disease, (3) normal kidney function tests, and (4) no evidence of distant metastases beyond the common iliac lymph nodes. The initial treatment consists of four to six cycles of combination chemotherapy. If a significant regression of tumor is achieved, radiation treatment is administered in combination with radiosensitizing chemotherapy. These patients were carefully selected, but in the majority of patients so treated, excellent tumor shrinkage and long-term survival were achieved in patients who would otherwise have been expected to succumb rapidly if treatment had consisted of chemotherapy alone.

## Quality of Life After Cystectomy or Bladder Preservation

Evaluating the quality of life in long-term survivors of bladder cancer has been difficult, and only recently have attempts been made to assess this in an objective and quantitative fashion.[134,178–191] A number of problems arise in the interpretation of the published studies. Tools to assess quality-of-life variables were developed early for common prostate and gynecologic cancers, but until very recently no such instruments existed for bladder cancer. The instruments in use for bladder cancer have thus been adaptations of uncertain validity. The published studies are all cross-sectional and patients have follow-ups of varying lengths. This matters in a surgical series in which functional outcome improves with time and in a radiation series in which it may deteriorate. Despite these limitations, some conclusions can now be drawn.

A radical cystectomy causes changes in many areas of quality of life, including urinary, sexual, and social function, daily living activities, and satisfaction with body image.[166–171,192] During the past decade, researchers have concentrated on the relative merits of continent and incontinent diversions. Available data have been mixed with some groups, surprisingly, reporting few differences between the quality of life of those with an ileal conduit and those with continent diversions. Hart et al.[182] have compared outcome in cystectomy patients who have either ileal conduits, cutaneous Koch pouches, or urethral Koch pouches. Regardless of the type of urinary diversion, the majority of patients reported good overall quality of life, little emotional distress, and few problems with social, physical, or functional activities. Problems with their diversions and with sexual function were most commonly reported. After controlling for age, no significant differences were seen among urinary diversion subgroups in any quality-of-life area. It might be anticipated that those receiving the urethral Koch

diversions would be the most satisfied, and the explanation why this is not so is unclear. It may be that the subgroups were too small to detect differences, but perhaps it is more likely that each group adapts in time to the specific difficulties presented by that type of diversion. Somani et al.[184] reviewed 40 published studies that evaluated overall quality of life, reporting on 3,645 patients. Only two studies reported a better quality of life for those who had neobladder and only two reported a better body image.[184] Another prospective study reported by Mansson et al.[185] suggested that there may be a large cultural component to the response with big differences seen between Egyptian and Swedish men followed prospectively through trials of chemotherapy and cystectomy.

Porter and Penson[183] attempted a systematic review of the literature, testing the premise that continent diversions result in improved health-related quality-of-life outcomes. They concluded that, whatever our assumptions, there is no literature to support the use of one urinary diversion over another. Reviews by Gerharz et al.[187] and Somani et al.[184] came to the same conclusion. It appears that women have more problems with continent diversions, particularly the need to catheterize, than do men.[186]

Zietman et al.[188] have performed a study on patients treated with chemoradiation for muscle-invasive bladder cancer. Patients underwent a urodynamic study and completed a quality-of-life questionnaire with a median time from therapy of 6.3 years. This long follow-up is sufficient to capture the majority of late radiation effects. Seventy-five percent of patients had normally functioning bladders by urodynamic studies. Reduced bladder compliance, a recognized complication of radiation, was seen in 22%, but in only one-third of these was it reflected in distressing symptoms. The questionnaire showed that bladder symptoms were uncommon, especially among men, with the exception of control problems. These were reported by 19%, with 11% using incontinence products (all women). Distress from urinary symptoms was half as common as their prevalence. Bowel symptoms occurred in 22% with only 14% recording any level of distress. The majority of men retained sexual function. Global health-related quality of life was high. A study reported by Herman et al.[189] showed that when low doses of gemcitabine are used as an alternative radiation-sensitizer to cisplatin, then treatment is also very tolerable. Thus, the great majority of patients treated by trimodality therapy retain good bladder function.

Two cross-sectional questionnaire studies, one from Sweden and one from Italy, have compared the outcome following radiation with the outcome following cystectomy.[190,191] The questionnaire results for urinary function following radiation were very similar to those recorded in the MGH study. More than 74% of patients reported good urinary function. Both studies compared bowel function in irradiated patients with that seen in patients undergoing cystectomy. In both, the bowel symptoms were greater for those receiving radiation than for those receiving cystectomy (10% versus 3% and 32% versus 24%, respectively), but in neither was this statistically significant.

Data on the assessment of sexual function are limited to men. The majority in the MGH series report adequate erectile function (full or sufficient for intercourse). These findings are in line with those obtained in the Swedish and Italian series in which three times as many men retained useful erections as compared with cystectomized controls.

A Bladder Cancer Index has now been developed and validated.[193] It has been shown to have high internal and retest consistency and can be used regardless of local treatment type and across the genders. This is the first such tool developed and it holds great promise for comparative treatment studies in the future.

## Metastatic Bladder Cancer

An estimated 12,500 deaths per year in the United States are due to metastatic bladder cancer.[194] Through lymphatic and hematogenous means, bladder cancer metastasizes to distant organs, most commonly the lungs, bone, liver, and brain. The prognosis of metastatic bladder cancer, as with other metastatic solid tumors, is poor, with a median survival on the order of only 12 months. Nevertheless, since the discovery that platinum-containing agents have significant antitumor effect in bladder cancer, there has been great interest in the use of chemotherapy for advanced disease.

Compared with other solid-tumor malignancies, transitional cell cancer is chemosensitive. In phase II clinical trials, radiographic response rates may be as high as 70% to 80%, and in phase III clinical trials, response rates are often on the order of 50%. Moreover, a small but substantial minority of responding patients manifest a CR, and among these patients some long-term, durable responses are observed. Overall, however, the duration of response in TCC is short, with a median of 4 to 6 months, and therefore, the impact of chemotherapy on survival has been disappointing. As newer targeted agents come into clinical practice, the hope is that their incorporation into treatment regimens will lengthen the duration of response and, ultimately, will translate into a real change in survival.

## Cisplatin

In 1976, a series of 24 patients with bladder cancer treated with single-agent cisplatin was reported.[195] The investigators observed eight partial responses in addition to four minor responses. Subsequent studies confirmed the activity of cisplatin in TCC, although the response rate to single-agent cisplatin has been lower than that of cisplatin-containing combination therapy.[196,197] Thus, most subsequent studies have explored combination regimens.

## Cisplatin-Based Combination Chemotherapy

The standard chemotherapy regimen for advanced bladder cancer for more than a decade was MVAC.[198,199] MVAC is administered in 28-day cycles, with starting doses of methotrexate 30 mg/m$^2$ (days 1, 15, and 22), vinblastine 3 mg/m$^2$ (days 2, 15, and 22), doxorubicin 30 mg/m$^2$ (day 2), and cisplatin 70 mg/m$^2$ (day 2). Another commonly used regimen has been CMV, which omits the doxorubicin and has somewhat less toxicity.[200] The MVAC regimen has superior activity to cisplatin alone[196,197] and to other cisplatin-containing regimens.[201] The response rate to MVAC is 40% to 65%,[197,198,202] and there is improved progression-free and overall survival compared with either single-agent cisplatin or cisplatin, cyclophosphamide, and doxorubicin. Complete response is seen in 15% to 25% of patients, with an expected median survival of 12 months (Table 39.6).[196–201]

On the negative side, MVAC is associated with substantial toxicity, and most patients require dose adjustment at some point in their treatment. Toxic effects of MVAC in notable numbers of patients include neutropenia, anemia, thrombocytopenia, stomatitis, nausea, and fatigue.[136,149,202] The rate of chemotherapy-induced fatality among patients with metastatic disease may be as high as 3%, most often due to neutropenic sepsis.[202]

The doublet of gemcitabine and cisplatin showed encouraging results in phase II studies, with response rates of 42% to 66% and CR rates of 18% to 28%.[203,204] Primary toxicity was hematologic and was generally easily managed, with rare hospitalizations for febrile neutropenia and no toxic deaths. Based on these encouraging results, GC was compared with MVAC in a multicenter phase III study.[202,205] MVAC was administered as previously described, and GC was administered in 28-day cycles with gemcitabine 1,000 mg/m$^2$ (days 1, 8, and 15) and cisplatin 70 mg/m$^2$ (day 2). In the study, 405 patients were randomized to one of the two treatment arms, and the two groups exhibited similar characteristics. Median survival was 14 months with GC and 15.2 months with MVAC, which were statistically comparable.[205] Patients treated with GC, however, had significantly less toxicity and improved tolerability. Patients receiving GC gained more weight, reported less fatigue, and had better performance status than patients who received MVAC. As a result of this study, GC is generally considered the current standard of care for metastatic bladder cancer.

## Taxane- and Platinum-Containing Regimens

The addition of taxanes to cisplatin-based regimens has been the subject of numerous phase II trials in bladder cancer (Table 39.7). The doublets of cisplatin and paclitaxel and cisplatin and docetaxel appear to have response rates comparable to that of GC.[211–214] Trials with carboplatin suggest that this agent has good activity, although likely not the same level of activity as cisplatin.[207,221]

Many patients with bladder cancer cannot receive cisplatin due to medical comorbidities. The EORTC reported a randomized phase III study comparing an historic standard of care in Europe, the three-drug regimen of methotrexate, carboplatin, and vinblastine (M-CAVI), to the doublet gemcitabine and carboplatin in patients who were felt to be unfit for cisplatin-based therapy. All had previously untreated locally advanced or metastatic urothelial cancer. Severe toxicity was greater in patients receiving the three-drug regimen. Responses were greater in the two-drug regimen, but this did not translate into a difference in survival between the two arms. The authors recommended gemcitabine plus carboplatin as the

## TABLE 39.6

### Standard Cisplatin-Containing Regimens for Transitional Cell Carcinoma

| Regimen | | | Response | | | |
|---|---|---|---|---|---|---|
| Agents (Ref.) | | Schedule | Composite Number of Assessable Patients | Complete Response (%) | Response Rate (%) | Median Survival (Mo) |
| MVAC[197,198,200] | Methotrexate | 30 mg/m$^2$ d 1, 15, 22 | 374 | 12–35 | 39–65 | 12.5–14.8 |
| | Vinblastine | 3 mg/m$^2$ d 2, 15, 22 | | | | |
| | Doxorubicin | 30 mg/m$^2$ d 2 | | | | |
| | Cisplatin | 70 mg/m$^2$ d 2 | | | | |
| CMV[213] | Cisplatin | 70 mg/m$^2$ d 2 | 104 | 10 | 36 | 7 |
| | Methotrexate | 30 mg/m$^2$ d 1, 8 | | | | |
| | Vinblastine | 4 mg/m$^2$ d 1, 8 | | | | |
| GC[214] | Gemcitabine | 1000 mg/m$^2$ d 1, 8, 15 | 203 | 12 | 49 | 13.8 |
| | Cisplatin | 70 mg/m$^2$ d 2 | | | | |

CMV, cisplatin, methotrexate, vinblastine.

**TABLE 39.7**

**Phase II Trials of Taxane-Containing Chemotherapy Regimens**

| Regimen | Composite Number of Patients | Response Rate (%) | Median Survival (Mo) | Reference |
|---|---|---|---|---|
| Carboplatin/paclitaxel | 104 | 21–65 | 8.5–9.5 | 206, 207, 209 |
| Cisplatin/paclitaxel | 52 | 50 | 10.6 | 211 |
| Cisplatin/docetaxel | 129 | 52–60 | 8.0–13.6 | 212–214 |
| Cisplatin/gemcitabine/paclitaxel | 61 | 78 | 15.8 | 168, 215 |
| Carboplatin/gemcitabine/paclitaxel | 49 | 68 | 14.7 | 216 |
| Cisplatin/gemcitabine/docetaxel | 35 | 66 | 15.5 | 217 |
| Gemcitabine/paclitaxel | 94 | 54–60 | 14.4 | 218–220 |

new standard of care based on a better safety profile in this patient population.[208]

A phase III trial compared MVAC with carboplatin and paclitaxel.[209] The study failed to reach its accrual goal, with only 85 patients randomized, although no significant differences in efficacy were seen. It is of note that the MVAC group exhibited a trend toward higher response rate (36% versus 28%), progression-free survival (8.7 versus 5.2 months), and overall survival (15.4 versus 13.8 months).

To date, there has been no consensus regarding those patients who should not receive cisplatin-based chemotherapy. A review of trial eligibility shows marked variation across studies. To address this concern, criteria for trials for "cisplatin-ineligible" patients were reviewed, and a set of criteria for all future studies was proposed by an international group of investigators.[210]

The complete omission of platinum has been studied as well. The doublet of gemcitabine and paclitaxel appears to have good activity, with phase II studies suggesting that this regimen has response rates and survival comparable to GC, with minimal toxicity.[218–220,222] Gemcitabine with paclitaxel may be a reasonable regimen to consider in patients unfit for platinum therapy. Gemcitabine and docetaxel demonstrated a response rate of 33% and median survival of 12 months in a trial of 27 patients with advanced TCC.[223]

### Triplet Chemotherapy

Because of the activity of each of these agents in TCC, investigators then asked whether triplet combinations of platinum, taxanes, and gemcitabine might have increased activity over the doublets. In phase II trials, three such combinations, including cisplatin/gemcitabine/paclitaxel,[168] carboplatin/gemcitabine/paclitaxel,[224] and cisplatin/gemcitabine/docetaxel,[217] demonstrated high CR rates of 28% to 32%, and overall response rates of 66% to 78%, although the number of patients with visceral metastases was relatively low. A second study of carboplatin/gemcitabine/paclitaxel showed a more modest response rate of 43% and overall survival of 11 months in a more typical population of metastatic TCC.[216] A triplet of paclitaxel, cisplatin, and infusional high-dose 5-FU with leucovorin has also been studied. The response rate was 75%, with 28% CRs, and a median overall survival of 17 months. Significant toxicity included frequent myelosuppression, gastrointestinal disturbances, infections, and two treatment-related deaths.[225]

A randomized phase III trial compared the standard GC regimen with GC plus paclitaxel (PCG).[215] Preliminary results and updated data are available. Despite a response rate that was superior in the three drug arm (55.5% versus 43.6%, $p = 0.0031$) and a median overall survival that was slightly longer in patients receiving the third drug (15.8 months versus 12.7 months), the HR for survival did not achieve statistical significance (HR, 0.85; $p = 0.075$). Thus, the standard of care remains the doublet of gemcitabine plus cisplatin.[226]

### Biologic Agents

The enthusiasm engendered by the development of novel biologic agents targeted against tumor-specific growth factor pathways or angiogenesis has been fortified in recent years by positive studies in a variety of solid tumors. Two classes of agents that may be of interest in TCC are inhibitors of EGFR, including EGFR1 and EGFR2 (HER2/neu), and inhibitors of VEGF or its receptors. There is ample preclinical evidence that many bladder tumors express members of the EGFR family, that overexpression may correlate inversely with prognosis, and that inhibition of these pathways may have an antitumor effect.[63–69] A number of groups are conducting studies with inhibitors of EGFR1 and HER2/neu in the treatment of advanced bladder cancer. Similarly, the utility of angiogenesis inhibitors in TCC is currently being explored in a cooperative group trial in metastatic TCC studying GC with or without the addition of bevacizumab.

### Second-Line Therapy and Beyond

There is no U.S. Food and Drug Administration (FDA)-approved therapy or regimen for second-line chemotherapy for progressive bladder cancer. One phase III trial randomized 370 patients with advanced TCC who had received prior platinum-based chemotherapy 2:1 to single-agent vinflunine or best supportive care. Median survival favored the vinflunine population (6.9 versus 4.6 months), but the difference was not statistically significant ($p = 0.287$).[226] These findings were confirmed at longer follow-up.[228] The lack of benefit combined with adverse effects have not led to broad approval of vinflunine worldwide or approval by the FDA in the United States. In practice, treatment beyond first-line chemotherapy typically employs doublet regimens described previously, single-agent chemotherapy, or clinical trials, where available.

## CANCERS OF THE RENAL PELVIS AND URETER

The majority of tumors of the upper urinary collecting system are TCCs. However, these are uncommon, with fewer than 3,000 cases diagnosed annually in the United States. The incidence has remained constant, but there has recently been a slight stage migration toward a higher proportion of earlier stage tumors.[229] Because of the challenge in gaining access to them, initial diagnosis and staging are less accurate than for cancer of the bladder. Histologically, 90% of upper tract tumors are TCC. Squamous cell carcinoma accounts for nearly all of the remainder. There is a predilection for these tumors to arise in the renal pelvis; primary tumors of the ureter occur only half as frequently as do tumors of the renal pelvis.[230] Men develop upper tract TCC two to three times more often than women, with the peak age of development of these tumors in the 7th and 8th decades of life.[211] Women, however, are more likely than men to have a more advanced and higher grade tumor at nephroureterectomy.[231] As discussed in the first section of this chapter, the majority of these tumors arise as a result of, or at least in association with, environmental exposures and stresses.[7–13,25]

## Clinical Presentation, Diagnosis, and Staging

Gross hematuria is the presenting symptom in 75% to 95% of all patients who present with tumors of the renal pelvis and ureter. Hematuria may be accompanied by colicky flank pain if the tumor or blood clots cause obstruction of the upper urinary tract. Patients often describe the passage of vermiform clots, which are unusual in bleeding from a lower tract source. Hydronephrosis may also be a presenting sign. Urinary cytology is an important part of the workup for an upper tract tumor. Voided urine cytology, however, has only 10% to 40% sensitivity in the detection of low-grade TCC lesions. Cytology is far more useful for high-grade tumors, for which the sensitivity may be as high as 70%.[232,233]

Improvements in endoscopic technology allow the urologist to view directly and to obtain tissue in many of the TCCs of the upper tract. A pathologic confirmation may be obtained prior to treatment. Also, the grade may be a useful predictor of advanced stage disease.[234,235]

Historically, intravenous urography was the mainstay of a radiographic evaluation of upper tract tumors, but now, in most major centers, a CT urogram is preferred (Fig. 39.7).[236] An MRI urography may also be useful in patients when sensitivity to iodinated contrast prevents the use of that agent.[237,238] When a patient is found or judged to have a TCC more aggressive than a G1 stage I tumor, additional staging of the patient is indicated, including CT scans of the chest, abdomen, and pelvis. Because standard therapy is radical excision of the kidney and the ipsilateral ureter, an evaluation of the total remaining renal function prior to a proposed nephrectomy is indicated. Isotope renal scanning can accurately estimate the function of the uninvolved kidney.

The current American Joint Committee on Cancer TNM staging for tumors of the upper urinary tract is shown in Figure 39.8 and in Table 39.8. The staging is determined by the extent of invasion by the primary tumor and by microscopic evaluation of the regional lymph nodes.

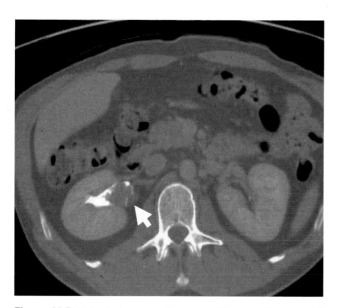

**Figure 39.7** Abdominal computed tomographic scan of a stage T3 transitional cell carcinoma of the right renal pelvis, with intravenous contrast showing a large filling defect in the right renal pelvis (*arrow*).

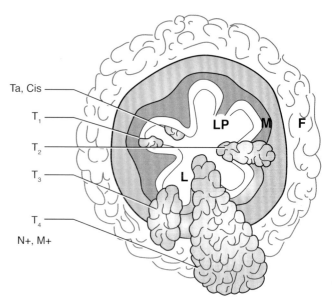

**Figure 39.8** Schematic diagram of the American Joint Committee on Cancer TNM (tumor, necrosis, metastasis) staging of cancers of the renal pelvis; LP, lamina propria; M, muscularis propria; F, peripelvic fat; L, lumen.

## Surgical Treatment

The standard surgical treatment for patients with transitional cell cancer of the upper urinary tract of all grades and stages is radical nephroureterectomy. This involves a complete removal of the kidney with its surrounding perirenal fat contained within Gerota fascia and en bloc removal of the ureter down to, and including, the portion of ureter within the urinary bladder (the ureteral orifice and the intramural ureter).[239] A retroperitoneal lymph node dissection along the ipsilateral great vessel (the vena cava for right-sided tumors; the aorta for left-sided tumors) is performed for more complete surgical staging, especially for higher grade and invasive cancers (Fig. 39.9). A lymphadenectomy and complete bladder cuff excision may not be necessary in cases of upper tract TCC, particularly at a low stage and grade.[240] When TCC of the renal pelvis invades the renal vein or the vena cava, an extensive surgical procedure, including thrombus extraction or partial vena cava dissection, may be required. A nephroureterectomy may be performed via open or laparoscopic surgical techniques. Common open approaches employ either a single extended midline abdominal incision or nephrectomy via a thoracoabdominal incision and a separate incision in the lower abdomen to accomplish the distal ureterectomy with a cuff of the contiguous urinary bladder.

Open surgical approach had long been the standard of treatment for the majority of patients with tumors of the renal pelvis and ureter, although morbidity may be reduced by using a laparoscopic technique.[241,242] The operative time and blood loss with the laparoscopic technique may be substantially less and the hospital stay shorter than those of an open surgical technique. With proper technique in resecting the distal ureter, laparoscopic or robotic-assisted nephroureterectomy is equally oncologically effective.[243,244] Invasive TCC may seed the abdomen if spilled, allowing tumor implantation, and this has led to concern among surgical oncologists about the laparoscopic approach. One group has reported three cases of laparoscopic port-site recurrence; however, in all three of these cases, the tumor was spilled from the operative specimen, allowing growth of the tumor tissue at the trocar sites.[245]

In patients in whom radical excision of the tumor would result in severe renal insufficiency that required dialysis (such as patients with a solitary kidney or in a patient with substantially diminished renal function), other surgical therapies may be considered. Endoscopic resection techniques have been developed and shown to be effective when done selectively and in experienced hands.[246] Endoscopic ablation via laser or electrocautery may be used to treat small tumors of the ureter and renal collecting system. However, the success of focal resection can be thwarted by the multicentricity of these tumors and the common concurrent existence of CIS.[247] Furthermore, although small, low-grade tumors can often be effectively treated endoscopically, high-grade tumors are often understaged by endoscopic assessment only, and therefore, may be treated inadequately without nephroureterectomy.[248]

Percutaneous endoscopic surgery of renal pelvic and calyceal TCC with access via the flank has been developed as a treatment option in highly select patients who have poor renal function or who medically could not withstand an open surgical procedure.[249] Using standard endoscopic tools, it is possible to resect tumors in the fashion similar to that which is used for bladder tumors. All limited resection endoscopic procedures require vigilant follow-up with an endoscopic reevaluation on a regular schedule because recurrence is quite common. In one study, 33% of patients ultimately required nephroureterectomy and 11% of patients died of TCC.[250]

Although endoscopic management of high-grade tumors can result in undertreatment and poorer oncologic outcomes, a

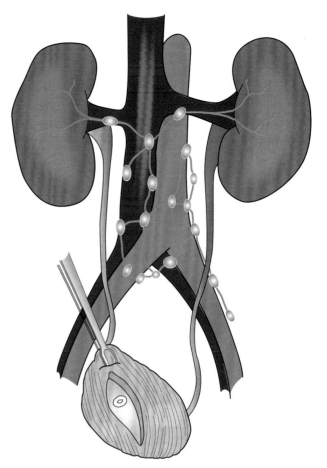

**Figure 39.9** Diagram of the kidneys, ureters, bladder, and retroperitoneal lymph nodes to demonstrate that a nephroureterectomy for upper tract transitional cell carcinoma requires a complete excision of the distal ureter, including the portion within the wall of the bladder. The bladder here is open to reveal the distal ureter, which tunnels within the wall of the bladder.

## TABLE 39.8

**American Joint Committee on Cancer 2009 TNM Staging of Renal Pelvis and Ureter Cancers: Definition of TNM**

**Primary Tumor (T)**

| | |
|---|---|
| TX | Primary tumor cannot be assessed |
| T0 | No evidence of primary tumor |
| Ta | Papillary noninvasive carcinoma |
| Tis | Carcinoma in situ |
| T1 | Tumor invades subepithelial connective tissue |
| T2 | Tumor invades the muscularis |
| T3 | (For renal pelvis only) Tumor invades beyond muscularis into peripelvic fat or the renal parenchyma |
| T3 | (For ureter only) Tumor invades beyond muscularis into periureteric fat |
| T4 | Tumor invades adjacent organs or through the kidney into the perinephric fat |

**Regional Lymph Nodes (N)[a]**

| | |
|---|---|
| NX | Regional lymph nodes cannot be assessed |
| N0 | No regional lymph node metastasis |
| N1 | Metastasis in a single lymph node 2 cm or less in greatest dimension |
| N2 | Metastasis in a single lymph node more than 2 cm but not more than 5 cm in greatest dimension or multiple lymph nodes; none more than 5 cm in greatest dimension |
| N3 | Metastasis in a lymph node, more than 5 cm in greatest dimension |

**Distant Metastasis (M)**

| | |
|---|---|
| MX | Distant metastasis cannot be assessed |
| M0 | No distant metastasis |
| M1 | Distant metastasis |

[a] Laterality does not affect the N classification.
Used with the permission of the American Joint Committee on Cancer (AJCC), Chicago, Illinois. The original source for this material is the *AJCC Cancer Staging Manual*, Seventh Edition (2010) published by Springer Science and Business Media LLC, www.springer.com, page 493.

kidney-sparing approach to appropriately selected isolated ureteral tumors using surgical resection is becoming a more accepted alternative to nephroureterectomy with similar oncologic outcomes.[251,252] This involves segmental resection of the ureter incorporating the tumor and the entire ureter distally, including the ureteral orifice/bladder cuff, and appropriate lymphadenectomy. Because recurrences and urothelial atypia are usually distal in the ureter to the index lesion, it is reasonable to spare the kidney without undue risk of recurrent disease. Surgically, it is possible to remove approximately half of the distal ureter and reimplant it in the bladder. For upper ureteral tumors, replacement of the ureter with a segment of the ileum may be considered. Although segmental resection is becoming more accepted for mid and distal ureteral tumors, radical nephroureterectomy does remain the gold standard, especially for tumors in the proximal ureter and tumors with extensive ureteral involvement.

### Results of Surgical Therapy

The success rate of surgical procedures is primarily influenced by the pathologic stage of the disease at the resection (Table 39.9). Tumors lower in the urinary tract have a better prognosis when matched by stage with tumors higher in the ureter and pelvis.[254] Within the upper tract, the location of the tumor in the ureter versus the renal pelvis does not seem to affect the prognosis.[255,256] In a report with a long follow-up from the University of Texas Southwestern Medical Center, of 252 patients treated surgically for upper tract TCC, disease-specific and overall survival were strongly influenced by the pathologic stage of the primary tumor.[253] The

**TABLE 39.9**

**Five-Year Disease-Specific Survival by Primary Tumor Pathologic Stage After Surgical Resection of Transitional Cell Carcinoma of the Upper Urinary Tract**

| Tumor Stage | Number of Patients | Percentage (%) |
|---|---|---|
| pTa/pTis | 38 | 100 |
| pT1 | 99 | 92 |
| pT2 | 34 | 73 |
| pT3 | 53 | 41 |
| pT4 | 19 | 0 |

From Hall MC, Womack S, Sagalowsky AI, et al. Prognostic factors, recurrence, and survival in transitional cell carcinoma of the upper urinary tract: a 30-year experience in 252 patients. *Urology* 1998;52:594–601, with permission

5-year actuarial disease-specific survival rates by primary tumor pathologic stage were 100% for noninvasive tumors (Ta and Tis), 92% for pathologic stage T1, 73% for pathologic stage T2, and 41% for pathologic stage T3. There were no long-term survivors for those with stage T4 tumors (Table 39.9). The type of open surgical procedure used (nephroureterectomy in 77% of the patients compared with a kidney-sparing approach used in 17%) was evaluated by a univariate and multivariate analysis. Patients undergoing nephroureterectomy were found to have a significantly improved recurrence-free and disease-specific survival on multivariate analysis but not on the univariate analysis. However, as discussed previously, in other more recent series, patients with ureteral cancers who were appropriately selected for kidney-sparing resections did not have a poorer outcome.

### Adjuvant Topical Therapy Following Local Excision Only

In cases in which endoscopic resection is performed, topical immunotherapy or topical chemotherapy may be important in preventing or delaying local tumor recurrence. BCG appears to be useful in treating carcinomas of the upper tract that are stage Tis.[247] Adriamycin given prophylactically following conservative resection of upper tract TCCs, using an antegrade infusion, also has been judged to be of some benefit in reducing recurrence.[257] The risk of systemic absorption of BCG or the chemotherapeutic agents is substantially higher than in treatment of the bladder and should be considered in therapeutic decision making.

### Adjuvant Combined-Modality Therapy: Advanced Primary Tumors

The most appropriate treatment for invasive transitional cell cancers of the upper urinary tract is nephroureterectomy. Despite aggressive surgery, cure rates are low when the disease has spread beyond the muscularis, with 5-year survival rates varying between zero and 34%.[257–262] Whether these low survival rates can be improved by adjuvant therapy depends on the pattern of failure and the efficacy of the available treatment. Metastatic relapse appears to predominate over local relapse when systemic cisplatin-based chemotherapy has been used, extrapolating from the experience with locally advanced bladder cancer. The true rate of local–regional failure is, however, unknown because many of the published series are old and employed pre-CT methods of intra-abdominal evaluation. The available data suggest an overall local–regional failure of 2% to 27%, although these figures may be underestimated.[263–265] Cozad et al.[266] report local failure rates of 50% in stage T3 disease,

rising to 60% if the tumors were high grade. Brookland and Richter[267] have reported local–regional recurrence in 45% and 62%, respectively. Most series report a close association between local failure and distant metastasis, although whether the association is causal or simply synchronous cannot be determined from the small numbers in the series.

Radiation has been employed as an adjuvant therapy with mixed results reported in the literature (Table 39.10). Several small phase II studies have suggested a local control and perhaps survival advantage for adjuvant radiation.[267–273] One study reported no benefit, although their treated population was diluted with 30% early stage patients. Another study showed no advantage to radiation, but the radiation doses given were inadequate. In others, chemotherapy was given in addition. Therefore, it is difficult to determine the true benefit of adjuvant radiation, if any. However, in a recent retrospective report by Chen et al.,[273] a survival advantage was seen in patients with T3/T4 disease of the renal pelvis or ureter receiving postoperative radiation with a median dose of 50 Gy to the tumor bed.

At the MGH, a more aggressive approach has been taken during the past 20 years in which patients with high-risk disease were treated first with adjuvant radiation alone and then more recently with concomitant radiation-sensitizing chemotherapy and, if tolerable, further combination chemotherapy.[271] Although the authors' series of 31 patients is nonrandomized and small, local failure was lower if chemotherapy was combined with radiation and the survival rate at 5 years was higher (see Table 39.10). Kwak et al.[272] also suggested that cisplatin-based adjuvant chemotherapy may reduce the rate of relapse and death from disease at 5 years. The small size of these two series and the biases inherent in this kind of retrospective review make it difficult to draw conclusions.

Very little published data exist to guide physicians managing patients with a local relapse following a nephroureterectomy. If the relapse is bulky and metastases are present elsewhere, then palliation with chemotherapy would be the most appropriate course. When the relapse appears isolated and the patient relatively vigorous, consideration can be given to an aggressive approach that holds out the chance for cure. The first step would be to downsize and perhaps improve the respectability of the recurrence using external radiation to a modest preoperative dose of 30 to 45 Gy along with sensitizing chemotherapy. An attempt could then be made at resection or debulking and, if the facility were available, intraoperative radiation could then be given directly onto the tumor bed or onto an unresectable mass, with the bowel and other critical organs displaced out of the field. Such an approach allows for the delivery of high doses of radiation to the target without the risk of bowel injury that is present when managing such disease using external radiation treatment alone (Fig. 39.10).

### Advanced Transitional Cell Carcinoma of the Upper Tract

Most patients with upper tract TCC have superficial disease, with a favorable prognosis.[274,275] However, patients with disease that invades beyond the muscularis propria have a significantly worse prognosis. The most consistent prognostic variables for the outcome of patients with upper tract TCC, including renal pelvic and ureteral carcinomas, are tumor stage and grade.[276–279] Molecular markers are being studied, and a poor outcome may be predicted by overexpression of $p53$ and a higher Ki-67 labeling index.[280–282]

In a series of 252 patients with mostly localized disease, relapse occurred in 67 patients (27%) after a median of 12 months.[265] Survival was highly stage specific, with 5-year disease-specific survival of 92% for T1, 73% for T2, 41% for T3, and zero for T4. In a series of 126 patients with nonmetastatic but more advanced renal pelvic or ureteral tumors, relapsed disease was noted in 81 patients (64%) after a median of 9 months.[268] Overall, 5- and 10-year survival rates

**TABLE 39.10**

**Larger Published Series Using Surgery with or without Adjuvant Radiation for Carcinoma of the Upper Urinary Tract**

| Method/Study (Ref.) | Number of Patients | Median Dose (Gy) | Local–Regional Failure % (Absolute) | Overall 5-Year Survival (%) |
|---|---|---|---|---|
| **Surgery with Radiotherapy** | | | | |
| Ozsahin et al.[268] | 45 | 50 | 38 (17/45) | 21 |
| Maulard-Durdux et al.[269] | 26[a] | 45 | 19 (5/26) | 49 (T2, 60%; T3, 19%) |
| Catton et al.[270] | 86[b] | 35 | 34 (29/86) | 43 (T3N0, 45%; N+, 15%) |
| Brookland and Richter[267] | 11 | 50 | 9 (1/11) | 27 |
| Cozad et al.[266] | 9 | 50 | 11 (1/9) | 44 |
| Czito et al.[271] | 31 | 47 | 23 (7/31) | 39 (67% in combined-modality group) |
| Chen[273] | 67 | 50 | 22 (15/67) | 50 |
| **Surgery Only** | | | | |
| Ozsahin et al.[268] | 81 | | 65 (53/81) | 33 |
| Cozad et al.[266] | 17[c] | | 53 (9/17) | 24 |
| Brookland and Richter[267] | 11 | | 45 (5/11) | 17 |
| Chen[273] | 66 | | 35 (23/66) | 45 |

[a] Thirty percent stage T2.
[b] Twenty-seven percent stage T1 to T2.
[c] All stages ≥T3.

were 29% and 19%, respectively. The most common sites of distant metastases were liver, bone, or lung. Utilization of postoperative radiation therapy did not impact on local or distant relapse. Factors that influenced survival outcomes in a multivariate analysis were initial tumor stage, residual postsurgery tumor, and the location of the initial tumor, with renal pelvic cancer being more favorable than ureteral cancer. The role of adjuvant chemotherapy in reducing relapse has not been explored in randomized fashion in this uncommon disease.

The biology of upper tract TCC is considered to be identical to that of bladder TCC. Consequently, the chemotherapy regimens recommended for advanced or metastatic upper tract TCC are the same as that for bladder cancer, as previously described. Standard treatment is cisplatin-based combination therapy, such as gemcitabine and cisplatin or methotrexate, vinblastine, doxorubicin, and cisplatin. As with bladder cancer, upper tract TCC is highly responsive to chemotherapy but has a short median duration of response.

Coronal pretreatment

Coronal posttreatment

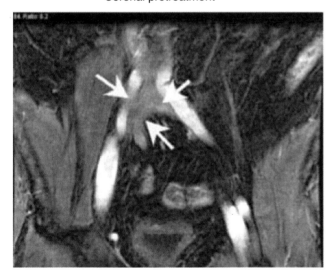
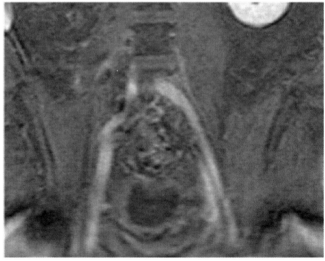

**Figure 39.10** Sequential coronal MRI of a patient with an unresectable ureteral tumor mass. The mass shown on the MRI on the **left** (*arrows*) was at the bifurcation of the aorta; it was initially judged unresectable because of involvement of the vessels. A partial resection, however, became possible as part of a combined-modality treatment approach that included preoperative conformal external-beam radiation. Intraoperative electron-beam radiation was given to the entire tumor bed after resection. On the **right** is the repeat MRI 1 year after treatment without any visible tumor.

# REFERENCES

1. Siegal R, Naishadham D, Jemal A. Cancer statistics 2013. *CA Cancer J Clin* 2013;63:11–30.
2. Maralani S, Wood DP Jr, Grignon D, et al. Incidence of urethral involvement in female bladder cancer: an anatomic pathologic study. *Urology* 1997;50: 537–541.
3. Erckert M, Stenzl A, Falk M, et al. Incidence of urethral tumor involvement in 910 men with bladder cancer. *World J Urol* 1996;14:3–8.
4. Munoz JJ, Ellison LM. Upper tract urothelial neoplasms: incidence and survival during the last 2 decades. *J Urol* 2000;164:1523–1525.
5. Oldbring J, Glifbert I, Mikulowski P, et al. Carcinoma of the renal pelvis and ureter following bladder carcinoma: frequency, risk factors and clinicopathological findings. *J Urol* 1989;141:1311–1313.
6. Rabbani F, Perrotti M, Russo P, et al. Upper-tract tumors after an initial diagnosis of bladder cancer: argument for long-term surveillance. *J Clin Oncol* 2001;19:94–100.
7. Hurle R, Losa A, Manzetti A, et al. Upper urinary tract tumors developing after treatment of superficial bladder cancer: 7-year follow-up of 591 consecutive patients. *Urology* 1999;53:1144–1148.
8. Toncheval DI, Antanossova SY, Gergov TD, et al. Genetic changes in uroepithelial tumors of patients with Balkan endemic nephropathy. *J Nephrol* 2002;15:387–393.
9. Nortier JL, Martinez MC, Schmeiser HH, et al. Urothelial carcinoma associated with the use of a Chinese herb (*Aristolochia fangchi*). *N Engl J Med* 2000;342:1686–1692.
10. Grollman AP, Shibutani S, Moriya M, et al. Aristolochic acid and the etiology of endemic (Balkan) nephropathy. *Proc Natl Acad Sci U S A* 2007;104: 12129–12134.
11. Jelaković B, Karanović S, Vuković-Lela I, et al. Aristolactam-DNA adducts are a biomarker of environmental exposure to aristolochic acid. *Kidney Int* 2012;81:559–567.
12. Hranjec T, Kovac A, Kos J, et al. Endemic nephropathy: the case for chronic poisoning by Aristolochia. *Croat Med J* 2005;46:116–125.
13. Yang MH, Chen KK, Yan CC, et al. Unusually high incidence of upper urinary tract urothelial carcinoma in Taiwan. *Urology* 2002;59:681–687.
14. Chen CH, Dickman KG, Moriya M, et al. Aristolochic acid-associated urothelial cancer in Taiwan. *Proc Natl Acad Sci U S A* 2012;109:8241–8246.
15. Lai MN, Wang SM, Chen PC, et al. Population-based case-control study of Chinese herbal products containing aristolochic acid and urinary tract cancer risk. *J Natl Cancer Inst* 2010;102:179–186.
16. Soloman DA, Kim JS, Bondaruk J, et al. Frequent truncating mutations of STAG2 in bladder cancer. *Nat Genet* 2013;45:1428–1430.
17. Guo G, Sun X, Chen C, et al. Whole-genome and whole-exome sequencing of bladder cancer identifies frequent alterations in genes involves in sister chromatid cohesion and segregation. *Nat Genet* 2013;45:1459–1463.
18. Balbas-Martinez C, Sagrera A, Carrillo-de-Santa-Pau E, et al. Recurrent inactivation of STAG2 in bladder cancer is not associated with aneuploidy. *Nat Genet* 2013;45:1464–1469.
19. Shinohara N, Koyanagi T. Ras signal transduction in carcinogenesis and progression of bladder cancer: molecular target for treatment? *Urol Res* 2002;30:273–278.
20. Primdahl H, von der Masse H, Sorenson FB, et al. Immunohistochemical study of the expression of cell cycle regulating proteins at different stages of bladder cancer. *J Cancer Res Clin Oncol* 2002;128:295–301.
21. Olesen SH, Thykjaer T, Orntoft TN. Mitotic checkpoint genes hBuB1, hBuB1B, hBuB3 and TTK in human bladder cancer, screening of mutations and loss of heterozygosity. *Carcinogenesis* 2001;22:813–815.
22. Feldman AS, Tang Z, Kirley S, et al. Expression of CABLES, a cell cycle regulatory gene is lost in invasive transitional cell carcinoma of the bladder. *J Urol* 2003;169:188.
23. Sgambato A, Migaldi M, Faraglia B, et al. Cyclin D1 expression in papillary superficial bladder cancer: its association with other cell cycle-associated proteins, cell proliferation and clinical outcome. *Int J Cancer* 2002;97:671–678.
24. Santos LL, Amaro T, Pereira SA, et al. Expression of cell-cycle regulatory proteins and their prognostic value in superficial low-grade urothelial cell carcinoma of the bladder. *Eur J Surg Oncol* 2003;29:74–80.
25. Bianco FJ Jr, Gervasi DC, Tiguert R, et al. Matrix metalloproteinase-9 expression in bladder washes from bladder cancer patients predicts pathological stage and grade. *Clin Cancer Res* 1998;4:3011–3016.
26. Zeegers MP, Goldbohm RA, van den Brandt PA. A prospective study on active and environmental tobacco smoking and bladder cancer risk (The Netherlands). *Cancer Causes Control* 2002;13:83–90.
27. Moyer VA. Screening for bladder cancer: US Preventive Services Task Force recommendation statement. *Ann Intern Med* 2011;133:246–251.
28. Mohr DN, Offord KP, Owen RA, et al. Asymptomatic microhematuria and urologic disease: a population-based study. *JAMA* 1986;256:224–229.
29. Mishriki SF, Nabi G, Cohen NP, et al. Diagnosis of urologic malignancies in patients with asymptomatic dipstick hematuria: prospective study with 13 years' follow-up. *Urology* 2008;71:13–16.
30. Messing EM, Madeb R, Young T, et al. Long-term outcome of hematuria home screening for bladder cancer in men. *Cancer* 2006;107:2173–2179.
31. Stampfer DS, Carpinito GA, Rodriguez-Villanueva J, et al. Evaluation of NMP22 in the detection of transitional cell carcinoma of the bladder. *J Urol* 1998;159:394–398.
32. Oeda T, Manabe D. The usefulness of urinary FDP in the diagnosis of bladder cancer: comparison with NMP22, BTA and cytology. *Nippon Hinyokika Gakkai Zasshi* 2001;92:1–5.
33. Eissa S, Swellam M, Sadek M, et al. Comparative evaluation of the nuclear matrix protein, fibronectin, urinary bladder cancer antigen and voided urine cytology in the detection of bladder tumors. *J Urol* 2002;168:465–469.
34. Ichikawa T, Nakayama Y, Yamada D, et al. Clinical evaluation of basic fetoprotein in bladder cancer. *Nippon Hinyokika Gakkai Zasshi* 2000;91:579–583.
35. Strefford JC, Lillington DM, Steggall M, et al. Novel chromosome findings in bladder cancer cell lines detected with multiplex fluorescence in situ hybridization. *Cancer Genet Cytogenet* 2002;135:139–146.
36. Utting M, Werner W, Dahse R, et al. Microsatellite analysis of free tumor DNA in urine, serum, and plasma of patients: a minimally invasive method for the detection of bladder cancer. *Clin Cancer Res* 2002;8:35–40.
37. Ito H, Kyo S, Kanaya T, et al. Detection of human telomerase reverse transcriptase messenger RNA in voided urine samples as a useful diagnostic tool for bladder cancer. *Clin Cancer Res* 1998;4:2807–2810.
38. Boman H, Hedelin H, Holmang S. Four bladder tumor markers have a disappointingly low sensitivity for small size and low grade recurrence. *J Urol* 2002;167:80–83.
39. Lokeshwar VB, Habuchi T, Grossman HB, et al. Bladder tumor markers beyond cytology: international consensus panel on bladder tumor markers. *Urology* 2005;66:35–63.
40. Lotan Y, Roehrborn CG. Sensitivity and specificity of commonly available bladder tumor markers versus cytology: results of a comprehensive literature review and meta-analysis. *Urology* 2003;61:109–118.
41. Young RH. Pathology of carcinomas of the urinary bladder. In: Vogelzang NJ, Scardino PT, Shipley WU, Coffey DS, eds. *Comprehensive Textbook of Genital Urinary Oncology*, 2nd ed. Philadelphia: Lippincott Williams & Wilkins; 2000:310.
42. Reuter VE. Pathology of bladder cancer: assessment of prognostic variables in response to therapy. *Semin Oncol* 1990;17:524–532.
43. Epstein JI, Amin MB, Reuter VE, et al. The World Health Organization/International Society of Urological Pathology consensus classification of urothelial (transitional cell) neoplasms of the urinary bladder. *Am J Surg Pathol* 1998;22:1435–1448.
44. Fairey AS, Daneshmand S, Wang L, et al. Impact of micropapillary urothelial carcinoma variant histology on survival after radical cystectomy. *Urol Oncol* 2014;32:110–116.
45. Willis DL, Porten SP, Kamat AM. Should histologic variants alter definitive treatment of bladder cancer? *Curr Opin Urol* 2013;23:435–443.
46. Wang J, Wang FW, Lagrange CA, et al. Clinical features of sarcomatoid carcinoma (carcinosarcoma) of the urinary bladder: analysis of 221 cases. *Sarcoma* 2010; 2010:pii: 454792.
47. Young RH, Oliva E. Transitional cell carcinomas of the urinary bladder that may be underdiagnosed: a report of four invasive cases exemplifying the homology between neoplastic and nonneoplastic transitional cell legions. *Am J Surg Pathol* 1996;20:1448.
48. Younes M, Sussman J, Truc LD. The usefulness of the level of the muscularis mucosae in the staging of invasive transitional cell carcinoma of the urinary bladder. *Cancer* 1990;66:543–548.
49. Farrow GM. Pathology of carcinoma in situ of the urinary bladder and related lesions. *J Cell Biochem* 1992;161:39–43.
50. Melamed MR, Reuter VE. Pathology and staging of urothelial tumors of the kidney and ureter. *Urol Clin North Am* 1993;20:333–347.
51. Sidransky D, Frost P, Von Eschenbach A, et al. The clonal origin of bladder cancer. *N Engl J Med* 1992;326:737–740.
52. Miyao N, Tsai YC, Lerner SP, et al. Role of chromosome IX in human bladder cancer. *Cancer Res* 1993;53:4066–4070.
53. Williams SG, Buscarini M, Stein JP. Molecular markers for diagnosis, staging and prognosis of bladder cancer. *Oncology* 2001;15:1461–1470.
54. Markl IDC, Salem CE, Jones PA. Molecular biology of bladder cancer. In: Volgelzang NJ, Scardino PT, Shipley WU, Coffey DS, eds. *The Comprehensive Textbook of Genitourinary Oncology*, 2nd ed. Philadelphia: Lippincott Williams & Wilkins; 2000:298.
55. Raghavan D. Molecular targeting and pharmacogenomics in the management of advanced bladder cancer. *Cancer* 2003;97:2086–2089.
56. Cordon-Cardo C. Molecular alterations associated with bladder cancer initiation and progression. *Scand J Urol Nephrol Suppl* 2008;218:154–165.
57. Stadler WM, Lerner SP, Groshen S, et al. S Phase II study of molecularly targeted adjuvant therapy in locally advanced urothelial cancer of the bladder based on p53 status. *J Clin Oncol* 2011;29:3443–3449.
58. Colquhoun CL, Jones GDD, Al-Moneef M, et al. Improving and predicting radiosensitivity in muscle invasive bladder cancer. *J Urol* 2003;169:1983–1992.
59. Cote RJ, Esrig D, Groshen S, et al. p53 and the treatment of bladder cancer. *Nature* 1997;385:123–125.
60. Sarkis A, Bajorin D, Reuter V, et al. Prognostic value of p53 nuclear over expression in patients with invasive bladder cancer treated with neoadjuvant MVAC. *J Clin Oncol* 1995;13:1384–1390.
61. Rodel C, Grabenbauer GG, Rodel F, et al. Apoptosis, p53, bcl-2, Ki-67 in invasive bladder carcinoma: possible predictors for response to radiochemotherapy and successful bladder preservation. *Int J Radiat Oncol Biol Phys* 2000; 46:1213.

62. Smith ND, Rubinstein JN, Eggener SE, et al. The p53 tumor suppressor gene and nuclear protein: basic science review and relevance in the management of bladder cancer. *J Urol* 2003;169:1219–1228.

63. Al-Sukhun S, Hussain M. Current understanding of the biology of advanced bladder cancer. *Cancer* 2003;97:2064–2075.

64. Neal DE, Sharples L, Smith K, et al. The epidermal growth factor receptor and the prognosis of bladder cancer. *Cancer* 1990;65:1619–1625.

65. Wood DP Jr, Fair WR, Chaganti RS. Evaluation of epidermal growth factor receptor DNA amplification and mRNA expression in bladder cancer. *J Urol* 1992;147:274–277.

66. Lipponen P, Eskelinen M. Expression of epidermal growth factor receptor in bladder cancer as related to established prognostic factors, oncoprotein (c-erbB-2, p53) expression and long-term prognosis. *Br J Cancer* 1994;69: 1120–1125.

67. Mellon JK, Lunec J, Wright C, et al. C-erbB-2 in bladder cancer: molecular biology, correlation with epidermal growth factor receptors and prognostic value. *J Urol* 1996;155:321–326.

68. Ciardiello F, Caputo R, Bianco R, et al. Antitumor effect and potentiation of cytotoxic drugs activity in human cancer cells by ZD-1839 (Iressa), an epidermal growth factor receptor-selective tyrosine kinase inhibitor. *Clin Cancer Res* 2000;6:2053–2063.

69. Jimenez RE, Hussain M, Bianco FJ Jr, et al. Her-2/neu over-expression in muscle-invasive urothelial carcinoma of the bladder: prognostic significance and comparative analysis in primary and metastatic tumors. *Clin Cancer Res* 2001;7:2440–2447.

70. Chakravarti A, Winter K, Wu CL, et al. Expression of the epidermal growth factor receptor and Her-2 are predictors of favorable outcome and reduced complete response rates, respectively, in patients with muscle-invading bladder cancers treated by concurrent radiation and cisplatin-based chemotherapy: a report from the Radiation Therapy Oncology Group. *Int J Radiat Oncol Biol Phys* 2005;62:309–317.

71. Lautenschlaeger T, George A, Klimowicz AC, et al. Bladder preservation therapy for muscle-invading bladder cancers on Radiation Therapy Oncology Group trials 8802, 8903, 9506, and 9706: vascular endothelial growth factor B overexpression predicts for increased distant metastasis and shorter survival. *Oncologist* 2013;18:685–686.

72. Sabichi AL, Lee JJ, Grossman HB, et al. A randomized controlled trial of celecoxib to prevent recurrence of nonmuscle-invasive bladder cancer. *Cancer Prev Res (Phila)* 2011;4:1580–1589.

73. Choudhury A, Nelson LD, Teo MT, et al. MRE11 expression is predictive of cause-specific survival following radical radiotherapy for muscle-invasive bladder cancer. *Cancer Res* 2010;70:7017–7026.

74. Laurberg JR, Brems-Eskildsen AS, Nordentoft I, et al. Expression of TIP60 (tat-interactive protein) and MRE11 (meiotic recombination 11 homolog) predict treatment-specific outcome of localised invasive bladder cancer. *BJU Int* 2012;110:E1228–E1236.

75. Daniltchenko DI, Riedl CR, Sachs MD, et al. Long-term benefit of 5-aminolevulinic acid fluorescence assisted transurethral resection of superficial bladder cancer: 5-year results of a prospective randomized study. *J Urol* 2005;174:2129–2133

76. Denzinger S, Burger M, Walter B, et al. Clinically relevant reduction in risk of recurrence of superficial bladder cancer using 5-aminolevulinic acid-induced fluorescence diagnosis: 8-year results of prospective randomized study. *Urology* 2007;69:675–679.

77. Naselli A, Introini C, Timossi L, et al. A randomized prospective trial to assess the impact of transurethral resection in narrow band imaging modality on non-muscle-invasive bladder cancer recurrence. *Eur Urol* 2012;61:908–913.

78. Stenzl A, Penkoff H, Dajc-Sommerer E, et al. Detection and clinical outcome of urinary bladder cancer with 5-aminolevulinic acid-induced fluorescence cystoscopy: A multicenter randomized, double-blind, placebo-controlled trial. *Cancer* 2011;117:938–947.

79. American Joint Committee on Cancer. *Cancer Staging Manual*, 7th ed. New York: Springer-Verlag; 2008.

80. Harisinghani MG, Barentsz J, Hahn PF, et al. Noninvasive detection of clinically occult lymph-node metastases in prostate cancer. *N Engl J Med* 2003;348:2491–2499.

81. Di Stasi SM, Valenti M, Verri C, et al. Electromotive instillation of mitomycin immediately before transurethral resection for patients with primary urothelial non-muscle invasive bladder cancer: a randomised controlled trial. *Lancet Oncol* 2011;12:891–899.

82. Lamm DL, Blumenstein BA, Crissman JD, et al. Maintenance bacillus Calmette-Guerin immunotherapy for recurrent TA, T1 and carcinoma in situ transitional cell carcinoma of the bladder: a randomized Southwest Oncology Group Study. *J Urol* 2000;163:1124–1129.

83. Oddens J, Brausi M, Sylvester R, et al. Final results of an EORTC-GU cancers group randomized study of maintenance bacillus Calmette-Guérin in intermediate- and high-risk Ta, T1 papillary carcinoma of the urinary bladder: one-third dose versus full dose and 1 year versus 3 years of maintenance. *Eur Urol* 2013;63:462–472.

84. Bohle A, Jocham D, Bock PR. Intravesical bacillus Calmette-Guerin versus mitomycin C for superficial bladder cancer: a formal meta-analysis of comparative studies on recurrence and toxicity. *J Urol* 2003;169:900.

85. Shang PF, Kwong J, Wang ZP, et al. Intravesical BCG vs epirubicin for Ta and T1 bladder cancer. *Cochrane Database Syst Rev* 2011;(5):CD006885.

86. Nieder AM, Brausi M, Lamm D, et al. Management of stage T1 tumors of the bladder: International Consensus Panel. *Urology* 2005;66:108–125.

87. O'Donnell MA, Krohn J, DeWolf WC, et al. Salvage intravesical therapy with interferon-alpha 2b plus low dose bacillus Calmette-Guerin is effective in patients with superficial bladder cancer in whom bacillus Calmette-Guerin alone previously failed. *J Urol* 2001;166:1300–1304.

88. Rosevear HM, Lightfoot AJ, Birusingh KK, et al. Factors affecting response to bacillus Calmette-Guerin plus interferon for urothelial carcinoma in situ. *J Urol* 2011;186:817–823.

89. Steinberg G, Bahnson R, Brosman S, et al. Efficacy and safety of valrubicin for the treatment of bacillus Calmette-Guerin refractory carcinoma in situ of the bladder. The Valrubicin Study Group. *J Urol* 2000;163:761–767.

90. Addeo R, Caraglia M, Bellini S, et al. Randomized phase III trial on gemcitabine versus mytomicin in recurrent superficial bladder cancer: evaluation of efficacy and tolerance. *J Clin Oncol* 2010;28:543–548.

91. Skinner EC, Goldman B, Sakr WA, et al. 1666 SWOG S0353 phase II trial of intravesical gemcitabine in patients with non-muscle invasive bladder cancer who recurred following at least two prior courses of BCG. *J Urol* 2012;187:e673.

92. Laudano MA, Barlow LJ, Murphy AM, et al. Long-term clinical outcomes of a phase I trial of intravesical docetaxel in the management of non-muscle-invasive bladder cancer refractory to standard intravesical therapy. *Urology* 2010;75:134–137.

93. Shahin O, Thalmann GN, Rentsch C, et al. A retrospective analysis of 153 patients treated with or without intravesical bacillus Calmette-Guerin for primary state T1 grade 3 bladder cancer: recurrence, progression and survival. *J Urol* 2003;169:96–100.

94. Davis JW, Sheth SI, Doviak MJ, et al. Superficial bladder carcinoma treated with bacillus Calmette-Guerin: progression-free and disease specific survival with minimum 10-year followup. *J Urol* 2002;167:494–500.

95. Yiou R, Patard JJ, Benhard H, et al. Outcome of radical cystectomy for bladder cancer according to the disease type at presentation. *BJU Int* 2002;89:374–378.

96. Gray PJ, Shipley WU, Efstathiou JA, et al. Recent advances and the emerging role for chemoradiation in nonmuscle invasive bladder cancer. *Curr Opin Urol* 2013;23:429–434.

97. McDougal WS. Urethrectomy. In: McDougal WS, ed. *Rob and Smith's Operative Surgery, Urology*, 4th ed. London: Butterworth; 1983:526.

98. Knoedler JJ, Boorjian SA, Kim SP, et al. Does partial cystectomy compromise oncologic outcomes for patients with bladder cancer compared to radical cystectomy? A matched case-control analysis. *J Urol* 2012;188:1115–1119.

99. Gschwend JE, Dahm P, Fair WR. Disease specific survival as endpoint of outcome for bladder cancer patients following radical cystectomy. *Eur Urol* 2002;41:440–448.

100. Stein JP, Cai J, Groshen S, et al. Risk factors for patients with pelvic lymph node metastases following radical cystectomy with en bloc pelvic lymphadenectomy: concept of lymph node density. *J Urol* 2003;170:35–41.

101. Stein JP, Lieskovsky G, Cote R, et al. Radical cystectomy in the treatment of invasive bladder cancer: long-term results in 1,054 patients. *J Clin Oncol* 2001;19:666–675.

102. Dalbagni G, Genega E, Hashibe M, et al. Cystectomy for bladder cancer: a contemporary series. *J Urol* 2001;165:1111–1116.

103. Grossman HB, Natale RB, Tangen CM, et al. Neoadjuvant chemotherapy plus cystectomy compared with cystectomy alone for locally advanced bladder cancer. *N Engl J Med* 2003;349:859–866.

104. McDougal WS. Metabolic complications of urinary intestinal diversion. *J Urol* 1992;147:1199–1208.

105. Eisenberg M, Thompson R, Frank I, et al. Long-term renal function outcomes after radical cystectomy. *J Urol* 2014;191:1–7

106. Srinivas S, Mahalati K, Freiha FS. Methotrexate tolerance in patients with ileal conduits and continent diversions. *Cancer* 1998;82:1134–1136.

107. Chahal R, Sundaram SK, Iddenden R, et al. A study of the morbidity, mortality and long-term survival following radical cystectomy and radical radiotherapy in the treatment of invasive bladder cancer in Yorkshire. *Eur Urol* 2003;43: 246–257.

108. Shabsigh A, Korets R, Vora KC, et al. Defining early morbidity of radical cystectomy for patients with bladder cancer using a standardized reporting methodology. *Eur Urol* 2009;55:164–174.

109. Eswara JR, Efstathiou JA, Heney NM, et al. Complications and long-term results of salvage cystectomy after failed bladder sparing therapy for muscle invasive bladder cancer. *J Urol* 2012;187:463–468.

110. Gakis G, Efstathiou J, Lerner SP, et al. ICUD-EAU International Consultation on Bladder Cancer 2012: Radical cystectomy and bladder preservation for muscle-invasive urothelial carcinoma of the bladder. *Eur Urol* 2013;63:45–57.

111. Shipley WU, Prout GR Jr, Einstein AB, et al. Treatment of invasive bladder cancer by cisplatin and radiation in patients unsuited for surgery. *JAMA* 1987;258:931–935.

112. Coppin CM, Gospodarowicz MK, James K, et al. Improved local control of invasive bladder cancer by concurrent cisplatin and preoperative or definitive radiation. The National Cancer Institute of Canada Clinical Trials Group. *J Clin Oncol* 1996;14:2901–2907.

113. Shipley WU, Prout GR Jr, Kaufman SD, et al. Invasive bladder carcinoma. The importance of initial transurethral surgery and other significant prognostic factors for improved survival with full-dose irradiation. *Cancer* 1987;60:514–520.

114. Dunst J, Sauer R, Schrott KM, et al. Organ-sparing treatment of advanced bladder cancer: a 10-year experience. *Int J Radiat Oncol Biol Phys* 1994;30: 261–266.

115. Tester W, Porter A, Asbell S, et al. Combined modality program with possible organ preservation for invasive bladder carcinoma: results of RTOG protocol 85-12. *Int J Radiat Oncol Biol Phys* 1993;25:783–790.

116. Tester W, Caplan R, Heaney J, et al. Neoadjuvant combined modality program with selective organ preservation for invasive bladder cancer: results of Radiation Therapy Oncology Group phase II trial 8802. *J Clin Oncol* 1996;14:119–126.

117. Shipley WU, Winter KA, Kaufman DS, et al. Phase III trial of neoadjuvant chemotherapy in patients with invasive bladder cancer treated with selective bladder preservation by combined radiation therapy and chemotherapy: initial results of Radiation Therapy Oncology Group 89-03. *J Clin Oncol* 1998;16:3576–3583.

118. Housset M, Dufour B, Durdux C, et al. [Concurrent radio-chemotherapy in infiltrating cancer of the bladder: a new therapeutic approach.] *Cancer Radiother* 1998;2:67s–72s.

119. Rodel C, Grabenbauer GG, Kuhn R, et al. Combined-modality treatment and selective organ preservation in invasive bladder cancer: long-term results. *J Clin Oncol* 2002;20:3061–3071.

120. Rodel C, Grabenbauer GG, Kuhn R, et al. Organ preservation in patients with invasive bladder cancer: initial results of an intensified protocol of transurethral surgery and radiation therapy plus concurrent cisplatin and 5-fluorouracil. *Int J Radiat Oncol Biol Phys* 2002;52:1303.

121. Rodel C, Grabenbauer GG, Kuhn R, et al. Invasive bladder cancer: organ preservation by radiochemotherapy. *Front Radiat Ther Oncol* 2002;36:118–130.

122. Kaufman DS, Winter KA, Shipley WU, et al. Phase I-II RTOG study (99-06) of patients with muscle-invasive bladder cancer undergoing trans–urethral surgery, paclitaxel, cisplatin, and twice-daily radiotherapy followed by selective bladder preservation or radical cystectomy and adjuvant chemotherapy. *Urology* 2009;73:833–837.

123. Shipley WU, Kaufman DS, Tester WJ, et al. Overview of bladder cancer trials in the Radiation Therapy Oncology Group. *Cancer* 2003;97:2115–2119.

124. Mitin T, Hunt D, Shipley WU, et al. Transurethral surgery and twice-daily radiation plus paclitaxel-cisplatin or fluorouracil-cisplatin with selective bladder preservation and adjuvant chemotherapy for patients with muscle invasive bladder cancer (RTOG 0233): a randomised multicentre phase 2 trial. *Lancet Oncol* 2013;14:863–872.

125. Oh KS, Soto DE, Smith DC, et al. Combined-modality therapy with gemcitabine and radiation therapy as a bladder preservation strategy: long-term results of a phase I trial. *Int J Radiat Oncol Biol Phys* 2009;74:511–517.

126. Choudhury A, Swindell R, Logue JP, et al. Phase II study of conformal hypofractionated radiotherapy with concurrent gemcitabine in muscle-invasive bladder cancer. *J Clin Oncol* 2011;29:733–738.

127. Hussain SA, Stocken DD, Peake DR, et al. Long-term results of a phase II study of synchronous chemoradiotherapy in advanced muscle invasive bladder cancer. *Br J Cancer* 2004;90:2106–2111.

128. James ND, Hussain SA, Hall E, et al. Radiotherapy with or without chemotherapy in muscle-invasive bladder cancer. *N Engl J Med* 2012;366:1477–1488.

129. Coen JJ, Paly JJ, Niemierko A, et al. Nomograms predicting response to therapy and outcomes after bladder-preserving trimodality therapy for muscle-invasive bladder cancer. *Int J Radiat Oncol Biol Phys* 2013;86:311–316.

130. Efstathiou JA, Spiegel DY, Shipley WU, et al. Long-term outcomes of selective bladder preservation by combined-modality therapy for invasive bladder cancer: the MGH experience. *Eur Urol* 2012;61:705–711.

131. Gray PJ, Fedewa SA, Shipley WU, et al. Use of potentially curative therapies for muscle-invasive bladder cancer in the United States: results from the National Cancer Data Base. *Eur Urol* 2013;63:823–829.

132. Zietman AL, Grocela J, Zehr E, et al. Selective bladder conservation using transurethral resection, chemotherapy, and radiation: management and consequences of Ta, T1, and Tis recurrence within the retained bladder. *Urology* 2001;58:380–385.

133. Horwich A, Dearnaley D, Huddart R, et al. A randomised trial of accelerated radiotherapy for localised invasive bladder cancer. *Radiother Oncol* 2005;75:34–43.

134. Efstathiou JA, Bae K, Shipley WU, et al. Late pelvic toxicity following bladder-sparing therapy in patients with invasive bladder cancer: analysis of RTOG 89-03, 95-06, 97-06, 99-06. *J Clin Oncol* 2009; 27:4055–4061.

135. Turner SL, Swindell R, Bowl N, et al. Bladder movement during radiation therapy for bladder cancer: implications for treatment planning. *Int J Radiat Oncol Biol Phys* 1997;39:355–360.

136. Aluwini S, van Rooij PH, Kirkels WJ, et al. Bladder function preservation with brachytherapy, external beam radiation therapy, and limited surgery in bladder cancer patients: long-term results. *Int J Radiat Oncol Biol Phys* 2014;88:611–617.

137. Wijkstrom H, Norming U, Lagerkvist M, et al. Evaluation of clinical staging before cystectomy in transitional cell bladder carcinoma: a long-term follow-up of 276 consecutive patients. *Br J Urol* 1998;81:686–691.

138. Gray PJ, Lin CC, Jemal A, et al. Clinical-pathologic stage discrepancy in bladder cancer patients treated with radical cystectomy: results from the National Cancer Data Base. *Int J Radiat Biol Phys* 2014;88:1048–1056.

139. Zehnder P, Studer UE, Skinner EC, et al. Super extended versus extended pelvic lymph node dissection in patients undergoing radical cystectomy for bladder cancer: a comparative study. *J Urol* 2011;186:1261–1268.

140. Herr HW. Transurethral resection of muscle-invasive bladder cancer: 10-year outcome. *J Clin Oncol* 2001;19:89–93.

141. Scher H, Shipley W, Herr H. *Cancer of the Bladder*, 5th ed. Philadelphia: JB Lippincott; 1997.

142. Housset M, Maulard C, Chretien Y, et al. Combined radiation and chemotherapy for invasive transitional-cell carcinoma of the bladder: a prospective study. *J Clin Oncol* 1993;11:2150–2157.

143. Herr HW. Outcome of patients who refuse cystectomy after receiving neoadjuvant chemotherapy for muscle-invasive bladder cancer. *Eur Assoc Urol* 2008;54:126–132.

144. Black PC, Brown GA, Grossman HB, et al. Neoadjuvant chemotherapy for bladder cancer. *World J Urol* 2006;24:531–542.

145. Vogelzang NJ. Neoadjuvant MVAC: the long and winding road is getting shorter and straighter [editorial]. *J Clin Oncol* 2001;19:4003–4004.

146. Hall RR. Neoadjuvant cisplatin, methotrexate, and vinblastine chemotherapy for muscle-invasive bladder cancer: a randomized controlled trial. *Lancet* 1999;354:533–540.

147. Hall RR. Updated results of a randomized controlled trial of neoadjuvant cisplatin, methotrexate and vinblastine chemotherapy for muscle invasive bladder cancer. *Proc Am Soc Clin Oncol* 2002;21:178.

148. International Collaboration of Trialists. International phase III trial assessing neoadjuvant cisplatin, methotrexate, and vinblastine chemotherapy in muscle-invasive bladder cancer. Long-term results of the BA06 30894 trial. *J Clin Oncol* 2011;29:2171–2177.

149. Sharma P, Bajorin D. Controversies in neoadjuvant and adjuvant chemotherapy for muscle-invasive urothelial cancer and clinical research initiatives in locally advanced disease. *Am Soc Clin Oncol* 2003;1092:478.

150. Malmstrom PU, Rintala E, Wahlqvist R, et al. Five-year follow-up of a prospective trial of radical cystectomy and neoadjuvant chemotherapy: Nordic Cystectomy Trial I. The Nordic Cooperative Bladder Cancer Study Group. *J Urol* 1996;155:1903.

151. Sherif A, Rintala E, Mestad O, et al. Neoadjuvant cisplatin-methotrexate chemotherapy for invasive bladder cancer. Nordic Trial 2. *Scand J Urol Nephrol* 2002;36:419–425.

152. Raghavan D, Quinn D, Skinner DG, et al. Surgery and adjunctive chemotherapy for invasive bladder cancer. *Surg Oncol* 2002;11:55–63.

153. Advanced Bladder Cancer Overview Collaboration. Neoadjuvant chemotherapy for invasive bladder cancer. *Cochrane Database Syst Rev* 2005;2:CD005246.

154. Winquist E, Waldron T, Segal R, et al., eds. *Use of Neoadjuvant Chemotherapy in Transitional Cell Carcinoma of the Bladder*. Practice Guideline Report #3-2-2 (Version 2.2005). Toronto: Cancer Care Ontario; 2012.

155. Winquist E, Waldron T, Segal R, et al. Neoadjuvant chemotherapy in transitional cell carcinoma of the bladder: a systematic review and meta-analysis. *J Urol* 2004;171:561–569.

156. Milowsky MI, Stadler WM, Bajorin DF. Integration of neoadjuvant and adjuvant chemotherapy and cystectomy in the treatment of muscle-invasive bladder cancer. *BJU Int* 2008;102:1339–1344.

157. Dash A, Pettus JA 4th, Herr HW, et al. A role for neoadjuvant gemcitabine plus cisplatin in muscle-invasive urothelial carcinoma of the bladder: a retrospective experience. *Cancer* 2008;113:2471–2477.

158. Yafi FA, Kassouf W. Is neoadjuvant chemotherapy with gemcitabine plus cisplatin beneficial in patients with muscle-invasive bladder cancer? *Expert Rev Anticancer Ther* 2009;9:747–752.

159. Sonpavde G, Goldman BH, Speights VO, et al. Quality of pathologic response and surgery correlate with survival for patients with completely resected bladder cancer after neoadjuvant chemotherapy. *Cancer* 2008;115:4101.

160. Weight CJ, Garcia JA, Hansel DE, et al. Lack of pathologic down-staging with neoadjuvant chemotherapy for muscle-invasive urothelial carcinoma of the bladder: a contemporary series. *Expert Rev Anticancer Ther* 2009;9:792–799.

161. Dreicer R. Chemotherapy for muscle-invasive bladder cancer in the perioperative setting: current standards. *Urol Oncol* 2007;25:72–75.

162. Donat SM. Integrating perioperative chemotherapy into the treatment of muscle-invasive bladder cancer: strategy versus reality. *J Natl Compr Canc Netw* 2009;7:40–47.

163. Takata R, Katagiri T, Kanehira M, et al. Predicting response to methotrexate, vinblastine, doxorubicin and cisplatin neo-adjuvant chemotherapy for bladder cancers through genome-wide gene expression profiling. *Clin Cancer Res* 2005;11:2625.

164. Prout GR Jr, Griffin PP, Shipley WU. Bladder carcinoma as a systemic disease. *Cancer* 1979;43:2532–2539.

165. Bellmunt J, Guillem V, Paz-Ares L, et al. Phase I–II study of paclitaxel, cisplatin and gemcitabine in advanced transitional-cell carcinoma of the urothelium. *J Clin Oncol* 2000;18:3247–3255.

166. Studer UE, Bacchi M, Biedermann C, et al. Adjuvant cisplatin chemotherapy following cystectomy for bladder cancer: results of a prospective randomized trial. *J Urol* 1994;152:81–84.

167. Bono AV, Benvenuti C, Reali L, et al. Adjuvant chemotherapy in advanced bladder cancer. Italian Uro-Oncologic Cooperative Group. *Prog Clin Biol Res* 1989;303:533–540.

168. Freiha F, Reese J, Torti FM. A randomized trial of radical cystectomy versus radical cystectomy plus cisplatin, vinblastine and methotrexate chemotherapy for muscle invasive bladder cancer. *J Urol* 1996;155:495–499.

169. Skinner DG, Daniels JR, Russell CA, et al. The role of adjuvant chemotherapy following cystectomy for invasive bladder cancer: a prospective comparative trial. *J Urol* 1991;145:459–464.

170. Stockle M, Meyenburg W, Wellek S, et al. Advanced bladder cancer (stages pT3b, PT4a, pN1 and pN2): Improved survival after radical cystectomy and 3 adjuvant cycles of chemotherapy results of a controlled prospective study. *J Urol* 1992;148:302–306.

171. Stockle M, Meyenburg W, Wellek S, et al. Adjuvant polychemotherapy of nonorgan-confined bladder cancer after radical cystectomy revisited: long-term results of a controlled prospective study and further clinical experience. *J Urol* 1995;153:47–52.

172. Advanced Bladder Cancer (ABC) Meta-analysis Collaboration. Adjuvant chemotherapy in invasive bladder cancer: a systematic review and meta-analysis of individual patient data Advanced Bladder Cancer (ABC) Meta-analysis Collaboration. *Eur Urol* 2005;48(2):189–199.

173. Cognetti F, Ruggeri EM, Felici A, et al. Adjuvant chemotherapy with cisplatin and gemcitabine versus chemotherapy at relapse in patients with muscle-invasive bladder cancer submitted to radical cystectomy: an Italian multicenter phase III trial. *Ann Oncol* 2012;23:695–700.

174. Gallagher DJ, Milowsky MI, Bajorin DF. Advanced bladder cancer: status of first-line chemotherapy and the search for active agents in the second-line setting. *Cancer* 2008;113;1284–1293.

175. Calabro F, Sternberg CN. Neoadjuvant and adjuvant chemotherapy in muscle-invasive bladder cancer. *Eur Urol* 2009;55:303–358.

176. Monzo Gardiner JI, Herranz Amo F, Cabello Benavente R, et al. Response to adjuvant chemotherapy after radical cystectomy in patients with infiltrative bladder: analysis of 397 cases. *Arch Esp Urol* 2009;62:275–282.

177. Miller RS, Freiha FS, Torti FM. Surgical Resection of residual tumor mass following chemotherapy for advanced transitional cell carcinoma. *Oncol Muchen Sympomed* 1994;3:370.

178. Boyd SD, Feinberg SM, Skinner DG, et al. Quality of life survey of urinary diversion patients: comparison of ileal conduits versus continent Koch urinary reservoirs. *J Urol* 1987;138:1386–1389.

179. Mansson A, Johnson G, Mansson W. Quality of life after cystectomy: comparison between patients with conduit and those with caecal reservoir urinary diversion. *Br J Urol* 1988;62:240–245.

180. Raleigh ED, Berry M, Monite JE. A comparison of adjustments to urinary diversions: a pilot study. *J Wound Ostomy Continence Nurs* 1995;22:58–63.

181. Bjerre BD, Johansen C, Steven K. Health related quality of life after cystectomy: bladder substitution compared with ileal conduit diversion. A questionnaire survey. *Br J Urol* 1995;75:200–205.

182. Hart S, Skinner EC, Meyerowitz BE, et al. Quality of life after radical cystectomy for bladder cancer in patients with an ileal conduit, or cutaneous or urethral Kock pouch. *J Urol* 1999;162:77–81.

183. Porter MP, Penson DF. Health related quality of life after radical cystectomy and urinary diversion for bladder cancer: a systematic review and critical analysis of the literature. *J Urol* 2005;173:1318–1322.

184. Somani BK, Gimlin D, Fayers P, et al. Quality of life and body image for bladder cancer patients undergoing radical cystectomy and urinary diversion—a prospective cohort study with systematic review of the literature. *Urology* 2009;74:1138–1143.

185. Mansson A, Al Amin M, Malmstrom PU, et al. Patient-assessed outcomes in Swedish and Egyptian men undergoing radical cystectomy and orthotopic bladder substitution—a prospective comparative study. *Urology* 2007;70:1086–1090.

186. Bartsch G, Daneshmand S, Skinner E, et al. Urinary functional outcomes in female neobladder patients. *World J Urol* 2014;32:221–228.

187. Gerharz EW, Mansson A, Hunt S, et al. Quality of life after cystectomy and urinary diversion: an evidence based analysis. *J Urol* 2006;174:1729–1736.

188. Zietman AL, Sacco D, Skowronski U, et al. Organ-conservation in invasive bladder cancer treated by trans-urethral resection, chemotherapy, and radiation: results of a urodynamic and quality of life study on long-term survivors. *J Urol* 2003;170:1772–1776.

189. Herman JM, Smith DC, Montie J, et al. Prospective quality of life assessment in patients receiving concurrent gemcitabine and radiotherapy as a bladder preservation strategy. *Urology* 2004;64:69–73.

190. Caffo O, Fellin G, Graffer U, et al. Assessment of quality of life after cystectomy or conservative therapy for patients with infiltrating bladder carcinoma. *Cancer* 1996;78:1089–1097.

191. Henningsohn L, Wijkstrom H, Dickman PW, et al. Distressful symptoms after radical radiotherapy for urinary bladder cancer. *Radiother Oncol* 2002;60: 215–225.

192. Millikan R, Dinney C, Swanson D, et al. Integrated therapy for locally advanced bladder cancer: final report of a randomized trial of cystectomy plus adjuvant M-VAC versus cystectomy with both preoperative and postoperative M-VAC. *J Clin Oncol* 2001;19:4005–4013.

193. Gilbert SM, Dunn RL, Hollenbeck BK, et al. Development and validation of the Bladder Cancer Index: a comprehensive, disease specific measure of health related quality of life in patients with localized bladder cancer. *J Urol* 2010;183:1764–1769.

194. Jemal A, Murray T, Samuels A, et al. Cancer statistics, 2003. *CA Cancer J Clin* 2003;53:5–26.

195. Yagoda A, Watson RC, Gonzalez-Vitale JC, et al. Cis-dichlorodiammineplatinum(II) in advanced bladder cancer. *Cancer Treat Rep* 1976;60:917–923.

196. Saxman SB, Propert KJ, Einhorn LH, et al. Long-term follow-up of a phase III intergroup study of cisplatin alone or in combination with methotrexate, vinblastine, and doxorubicin in patients with metastatic urothelial carcinoma: a cooperative group study. *J Clin Oncol* 1997;15:2564–2569.

197. Loehrer PJ Sr, Einhorn LH, Elson PJ, et al. A randomized comparison of cisplatin alone or in combination with methotrexate, vinblastine, and doxorubicin in patients with metastatic urothelial carcinoma: a cooperative group study. *J Clin Oncol* 1992;10:1066–1073.

198. Sternberg CN, Yagoda A, Scher HI, et al. Methotrexate, vinblastine, doxorubicin, and cisplatin for advanced transitional cell carcinoma of the urothelium. Efficacy and patterns of response and relapse. *Cancer* 1989;64:2448–2458.

199. Sternberg CN, Yagoda A, Scher HI, et al. Preliminary results of M-VAC (methotrexate, vinblastine, doxorubicin and cisplatin) for transitional cell carcinoma of the urothelium. *J Urol* 1985;133:403–407.

200. Harker WG, Meyers FJ, Freiha FS, et al. Cisplatin, methotrexate, and vinblastine (CMV): an effective chemotherapy regimen for metastatic transitional cell carcinoma of the urinary tract. A Northern California Oncology Group study. *J Clin Oncol* 1985;3:1463–1470.

201. Logothetis CJ, Dexeus FH, Finn L, et al. A prospective randomized trial comparing MVAC and CISCA chemotherapy for patients with metastatic urothelial tumors. *J Clin Oncol* 1990;8:1050–1055.

202. von der Maase H, Hansen SW, Roberts JT, et al. Gemcitabine and cisplatin versus methotrexate, vinblastine, doxorubicin, and cisplatin in advanced or metastatic bladder cancer: results of a large, randomized, multinational, multicenter, phase III study. *J Clin Oncol* 2000;18:3068–3070.

203. Kaufman D, Raghavan D, Carducci M, et al. Phase II trial of gemcitabine plus cisplatin in patients with metastatic urothelial cancer. *J Clin Oncol* 2000;18:1921–1927.

204. Moore MJ, Winquist EW, Murray N, et al. Gemcitabine plus cisplatin, an active regimen in advanced urothelial cancer: a phase II trial of the National Cancer Institute of Canada Clinical Trials Group. *J Clin Oncol* 1999;17: 2876–2881.

205. Roberts JT, von der Maase H, Sengelov L, et al. Long-term survival results of a randomized trial comparing gemcitabine/cisplatin and methotrexate/vinblastine/doxorubicin/cisplatin in patients with locally advanced and metastatic bladder cancer. *Ann Oncol* 2006;17:v118.

206. Johannsen M, Sachs M, Roigas J, et al. Phase II trial of weekly paclitaxel and carboplatin chemotherapy in patients with advanced transitional cell cancer. *Eur Urol* 2005;48:246–251.

207. Vaishampayan UN, Faulkner JR, Small EJ, et al. Phase II trial of carboplatin and paclitaxel in cisplatin-pretreated advanced transitional cell carcinoma: a Southwest Oncology Group study. *Cancer* 2005;104:1627–1632.

208. De Santis M, Bellmunt J, Mead G, et al. Randomized phase II/III trial assessing gemcitabine/carboplatin and methotrexate/carboplatin/vinblastine in patients with advanced urothelial cancer "unfit" for cisplatin-based chemotherapy: phase II—results of EORTC study 30986. *J Clin Oncol* 2009: 5634–5639.

209. Dreicer R, Manola J, Roth BJ, et al. Phase III trial of methotrexate, vinblastine, doxorubicin, and cisplatin versus carboplatin and paclitaxel in patients with advanced carcinoma of the urothelium. *Cancer* 2004;100:1639–1645.

210. Galsky MD, Hahn NM, Rosenberg J, et al. Treatment of patients with metastatic urotherlial cancer unfit for cisplatin-based chemotherapy. *J Clin Oncol* 2011;29:2432–2438.

211. Dreicer R, Manola J, Roth BJ, et al. Phase II study of cisplatin and paclitaxel in advanced carcinoma of the urothelium: an Eastern Cooperative Oncology Group Study. *J Clin Oncol* 2000;18:1058–1061.

212. Sengelov L, Kamby C, Lund B, et al. Docetaxel and cisplatin in metastatic urothelial cancer: a phase II study. *J Clin Oncol* 1998;16:3392–3397.

213. Dimopoulos MA, Bakoyannis C, Georgoulias V, et al. Docetaxel and cisplatin combination chemotherapy in advanced carcinoma of the urothelium: a multicenter phase II study of the Hellenic Cooperative Oncology Group. *Ann Oncol* 1999;10:1385–1388.

214. Garcia del Muro X, Marcuello E, Guma J, et al. Phase II multicentre study of docetaxel plus cisplatin in patients with advanced urothelial cancer. *Br J Cancer* 2002;86:326–330.

215. Bellmunt J, von der Maase H, Mead GM, et al. Randomized phase III study comparing paclitaxel/cisplatin/gemcitabine and gemcitabine/cisplatin in patients with locally advanced or metastatic urothelial cancer without prior systemic therapy: EORTC 30987/intergroup study. *Proc Am Soc Clin Oncol* 2007;25:1107–1113.

216. Hainsworth JD, Meluch AA, Litchy S, et al. Paclitaxel, carboplatin, and gemcitabine in the treatment of patients with advanced transitional cell carcinoma of the urothelium. *Cancer* 2005;103:2298–2303.

217. Pectasides D, Glotsos J, Bountouroglou N, et al. Weekly chemotherapy with docetaxel, gemcitabine and cisplatin in advanced transitional cell urothelial cancer: a phase II trial. *Ann Oncol* 2002;13:243–250.

218. Meluch AA, Greco FA, Burris HA 3rd, et al. Paclitaxel and gemcitabine chemotherapy for advanced transitional-cell carcinoma of the urothelial tract: a phase II trial of the Minnie pearl cancer research network. *J Clin Oncol* 2001;19:3018–3024.

219. Sternberg CN, Calabro F, Pizzocaro G, et al. Chemotherapy with an every-2-week regimen of gemcitabine and paclitaxel in patients with transitional cell carcinoma who have received prior cisplatin-based therapy. *Cancer* 2001;92:2993–2998.

220. Kaufman DS, Carducci MA, Kuzel T, et al. Gemcitabine (G) and paclitaxel (P) every two weeks (GP2w): a completed multicenter phase II trial in locally advanced or metastatic urothelial cancer. *Proc Am Soc Clin Oncol* 2002;21:767a.

221. Dogliotti L, Carteni G, Siena S, et al. Gemcitabine plus cisplatin versus gemcitabine plus carboplatin as first-line chemotherapy in advanced transitional cell carcinoma of the urothelium: results of a randomized phase 2 trial. *Eur Urol* 2007;52:134–141.

222. Michaelson MD, Kaufman DS, Oh WK. Transitional cell carcinoma of the upper uroepithelial tract. *Clin Adv Hematol Oncol* 2003;1:102–104.

223. Gitlitz BJ, Baker C, Chapman Y, et al. A phase II study of gemcitabine and docetaxel therapy in patients with advanced urothelial carcinoma. *Cancer* 2003;98:1863–1869.

224. Hussain M, Vaishampayan U, Du W, et al. Combination paclitaxel, carboplatin, and gemcitabine is an active treatment for advanced urothelial cancer. *J Clin Oncol* 2001;19:2527–2533.

225. Lin CC, Hsu CH, Huang CY, et al. Phase II trial of weekly paclitaxel, cisplatin plus infusional high dose 5-fluorouracil and leucovorin for metastatic urothelial carcinoma. *J Urol* 2007;177:84–89.

226. Bellmunt J, von der Maase H, Mead GM, et al. Randomized phase III study comparing paclitaxel/cisplatin/gemcitabine and gemcitabine/cisplatin in patients with locally advanced or metastatic urothelial cancer without prior systemic therapy: EORTC Intergroup Study 30987. *Clin Oncol* 2012;30: 1107–2213.

227. Bellmunt J, Theodore C, Demkov T, et al. Phase III trial of vinflunine plus best supportive care compared with best supportive care alone after a cisplatin containing regimen in patients with advanced transitional cell carcinoma of the urothelial tract. *J Clin Oncol* 2009;27:4454–4461.

228. Bellmunt J, Fougeray R, Rosenberg J, et al. Long-term survival results of a randomized phase III trial of vinflunine plus best supportive care versus best supportive care alone in advanced urothelial carcinoma patients after failure of platinum-based chemotherapy. *Ann Oncol* 2013;24:1466–1472.

229. David KA, Mallin K, Milowsky M. et al. Surveillance of urothelial carcinoma: stage and grade migration, 1993-2005 and survival trends, 1993-2000. *Cancer* 2009;115:1435–1447.

230. Grabstald H, Whitmore WF, Melamed MR. Renal pelvic tumors. *JAMA* 1971;218:845–854.

231. Lughezzani G, Sun M, Perrotte P, et al. Gender related differences in patients with stage I to III upper tract urothelial carcinoma: results from the SEER database. *Urology* 2010;75:321–327.

232. Walsh IK, Keane PF, Ishak LM, et al. The BTA stat test: a tumor marker for the detection of upper tract transitional cell carcinoma. *Urology* 2001;58:532–535.

233. Skacel M, Fahmy M, Brainard JA, et al. Multitarget fluorescence in situ hybridization assay detects transitional cell carcinoma in the majority of patients with bladder cancer and atypical or negative urine cytology. *J Urol* 2003;169: 2101–2105.

234. Brown GA, Mati SF, Busby JE, et al. Ability of clinical grade to predict final pathologic stage in upper urinary tract transitional cell carcinoma: implications for therapy. *Urology* 2007;70:252–256.

235. Lughezzani G, Burger M, Margulis V, et al. Prognostic factors in upper urinary tract urothelial carcinomas: a comprehensive review of the current literature. *Eur Urol* 2012;62:100–114.

236. O'Malley ME, Hahn PF, Yoder IC, et al. Comparison of excretory phase, helical computed tomography with intravenous urography in patients with painless haematuria. *Clin Radiol* 2003;58:294–300.

237. Jung P, Brauers A, Nolte-Ersting CA, et al. Magnetic resonance urography enhanced by gadolinium and diuretics: a comparison with conventional urography in diagnosing the cause of ureteric obstruction. *BJU Int* 2000;86:960–965.

238. Lee KS, Zeikus E, DeWolf WC, et al. MR urography versus retrograde pyelography/ureteroscopy for the exclusion of upper urinary tract malignancy. *Clin Radiol* 2010;65:185–192.

239. Heney NM, Nocks BN. The influence of perinephric fat involvement on survival in patients with renal cell carcinoma extending into the inferior vena cava. *J Urol* 1982;128:18–20.

240. Lughezzani G, Jeldre C, Isbarn H, et al. A critical appraisal of the lymph node dissection at nephroureterectomy for upper tract urothelial carcinoma. *Urology* 2010;75:118–124.

241. El Fettouh HA, Rassweiler JJ, Schulze M, et al. Laparoscopic radical nephroureterectomy: results of an international multicenter study. *Eur Urol* 2002;42:447–452.

242. Gill IS, Sung GT, Hobart MG, et al. Laparoscopic radical nephroureterectomy for upper tract transitional cell carcinoma: the Cleveland Clinic experience. *J Urol* 2000;164:1513–1522.

243. Matin SF, Gill IS. Recurrence and survival following laparoscopic radical nephroureterectomy with various forms of bladder cuff control. *J Urol* 2005;173:395–400.

244. Ambani SN, Weizer AZ, Wolf JS Jr, et al. Matched comparison of robotic vs laparoscopic nephroureterectomy: an initial experience. *Urology* 2014; 83:345–349.

245. Ong AM, Bhayani SB, Pavlovich CP. Trocar site recurrence after laparoscopic nephroureterectomy. *J Urol* 2003;170:1301.

246. Daneshmand S, Quek ML, Huffman JL. Endoscopic management of upper urinary tract transitional cell carcinoma: long-term experience. *Cancer* 2003;98:55–60.

247. Okubo K, Ichioka K, Terada N, et al. Intrarenal bacillus Calmette-Guerin therapy for carcinoma in situ of the upper urinary tract: long-term follow-up and natural course in cases of failure. *BJU Int* 2001;88:343–347.

248. Cutress ML, Stewart GD, Tudor EC, et al. Endoscopic versus laparoscopic management of noninvasive upper tract urothelial carcinoma: 20-year single center experience. *J Urol* 2013;189:2054–2060.

249. Goel MC, Mahendra V, Roberts JG. Percutaneous management of renal pelvic urothelial tumors: long-term followup. *J Urol* 2003;169:925–929.

250. Thompson RH, Krambeck AE, Lohse CM, et al. Endoscopic management of upper tract transitional cell carcinoma in patients with normal contralateral kidneys. *Urology* 2008;71:713–717.

251. Jeldres C, Lughezzani G, Sun M, et al. Segmental ureterectomy can safely be performed in patients with transitional cell carcinoma of the ureter. *J Urol* 2010;183:1324–1329.

252. Colin P, Ouzzane A, Pignot G, et al. Comparison of oncological outcomes after segmental ureterectomy or radical nephroureterectomy in urothelial carcinomas of the upper urinary tract: results from a large French multicentre study. *BJU Int* 2012;110:1134–1141.

253. Hall MC, Womack S, Sagalowsky AI, et al. Prognostic factors, recurrence, and survival in transitional cell carcinoma of the upper urinary tract: a 30-year experience in 252 patients. *Urology* 1998;52:594–601.

254. Van der Poel HG, Antonini N, Van Tinteren H, et al. Upper urinary tract cancer: location is correlated with prognosis. *Eur Urol* 2005;48:438–444.

255. Isbarn H, Jeldres C, Shariat SF, et al. Location of the primary tumor is not an independent predictor of cancer specific mortality in patients with upper urinary tract urothelial carcinoma. *J Urol* 2009;182:2177.

256. Holmäng S, Johansson SL. Urothelial carcinoma of the upper urinary tract: comparison between the WHO/ISUP 1998 consensus classification and the WHO 1999 classification system. *Urology* 2005;66:274–278.

257. See WA. Continuous antegrade infusion of adriamycin as adjuvant therapy for upper tract urothelial malignancies. *Urology* 2000;56:216–222.

258. Rubenstein MA, Walz BJ, Bucy JG. Transitional cell carcinoma of the kidney: 25 year experience. *J Urol* 1978;119:595–597.

259. Reitelman C, Sawczuk IS, Olsson CA, et al. Prognostic variables in patients with transitional cell carcinoma of the renal pelvis and proximal ureter. *J Urol* 1987;138:1144–1145.

260. Heney NM, Nocks BN, Daly JJ, et al. Prognostic factors in carcinoma of the ureter. *J Urol* 1981;125:632–636.

261. Kirkali Z, Moffat LE, Deane RF, et al. Urothelial tumors of the upper urinary tract. *Br J Urol* 1989;64:18–24.

262. Booth CM, Cameron KM, Pugh RCB. Urothelial carcinoma of the kidney and ureter. *Br J Urol* 1980;52:430–435.

263. Mufti GR, Gove JRW, Badenoch DF, et al. Transitional cell carcinoma of the renal pelvis and ureter. *Br J Urol* 1989;63:135–140.

264. Das AK, Carson CC, Bolick D, et al. Primary carcinoma of the upper urinary tract (effect of primary and secondary therapy on survival). *Cancer* 1990;66:1919–1923.

265. Vahlensieck W Jr, Sommerkamp H. Therapy and prognosis of carcinoma of the renal pelvis. *Eur Urol* 1989;16:286–290.

266. Cozad SC, Smalley SR, Austenfeld M, et al. Transitional cell carcinoma of the renal pelvis or ureter: patterns of failure. *Urology* 1995;46:796–800.

267. Brookland RK, Richter MP. The postoperative irradiation of transitional cell carcinoma of the renal pelvis and ureter. *J Urol* 1985;133:952–955.

268. Ozsahin M, Zouhair A, Villa S, et al. Prognostic factors in urothelial renal pelvis and ureter tumours: a multicentre Rare Cancer Network study. *Eur J Cancer* 1999;35:738–743.

269. Maulard-Durdux C, Dufour B, Hennequin C, et al. Postoperative radiation therapy in 26 patients with invasive transitional cell carcinoma of the upper urinary tract: no impact on survival? *J Urol* 1996;155:115–117.

270. Catton CN, Warde P, Gospodarowicz MK, et al. Transitional cell carcinoma of the renal pelvis and ureter: outcome and patterns of relapse in patients treated with postoperative radiation. *Urol Oncol* 1996;2:171–176.

271. Czito B, Zietman AL, Kaufman DS, et al. Adjuvant combined modality therapy in locally advanced upper urinary tract malignancies. *J Urol* 2004; 172:1271.

272. Kwak C, Lee SE, Jeong IG, et al. Adjuvant systemic chemotherapy in the treatment of patients with invasive transitional cell carcinoma of the upper urinary tract. *Urology* 2006;68:53–57.

273. Chen B, Zeng ZC, Wang GM, et al. Radiotherapy may improve overall survival of patients with T3/T4 transitional cell carcinoma of the renal pelvis or ureter and delay bladder tumour relapse. *BMC Cancer*. 2011;11:297.

274. Guinan P, Volgelzang NJ, Randazzo R, et al. Renal pelvic transitional cell carcinoma. The role of the kidney in tumor-node-metastasis staging. *Cancer* 1992;69:1773–1775.

275. Seaman EK, Slawin KM, Benson MC. Treatment options for upper tract transitional-cell carcinoma. *Urol Clin North Am* 1993;20:349–354.

276. Huben RP, Mounzer AM, Murphy GP. Tumor grade and stage as prognostic variables in upper tract urothelial tumors. *Cancer* 1988;62:2016–2120.

277. Charbit L, Gendreau MC, Mee S, et al. Tumors of the upper urinary tract: 10 years of experience. *J Urol* 1991;146:1243–1246.

278. Corrado F, Ferri C, Mannini D, et al. Transitional cell carcinoma of the upper urinary tract: evaluation of prognostic factors by histopathology and flow cytometric analysis. *J Urol* 1991;145:1159–1163.

279. Guinan P, Vogelzang NJ, Randazzo R, et al. Renal pelvic cancer: a review of 611 patients treated in Illinois 1975–1985. Cancer Incidence and End Results Committee. *Urology* 1992;40:393–399.

280. Terrell RB, Cheville JC, See WA, et al. Histopathological features and p53 nuclear protein staining as predictors of survival and tumor recurrence in patients with transitional cell carcinoma of the renal pelvis. *J Urol* 1995;154: 1342–1347.

281. Masuda M, Iki M, Takano Y, et al. Prognostic significance of Ki-67 labeling index in urothelial tumors of the renal pelvis and ureter. *J Urol* 1996;155: 1877–1881.

282. Rey A, Lara PC, Redondo E, et al. Overexpression of p53 in transitional cell carcinoma of the renal pelvis and ureter. Relation to tumor proliferation and survival. *Cancer* 1997;79:2178–2185.

# 40 Genetic Testing in Urinary Tract Cancers

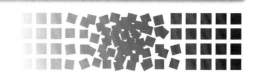

Gayun Chan-Smutko

## INTRODUCTION

Cancers of the urinary tract include renal cell carcinoma (RCC) and transitional cell carcinoma, or urothelial carcinoma (UC). About 64,770 cases of invasive cancer of the kidney and renal pelvis, 74,510 cases of urinary bladder cancer, and 2,860 cases of cancer of the ureter and other urinary organs are expected to be diagnosed in men and women in the United States in 2012.[1] The lifetime risk of cancer of the kidney and renal pelvis is 1.6%, with an average age at diagnosis (based on statistics from 2005 to 2009) of 64 years.[2] A family history of RCC is associated with a 2.2- to 2.8-fold increased risk for developing RCC.[3] Most cases of RCC are sporadic, and approximately 4% are due to a hereditary susceptibility.

RCC is a heterogeneous disease, which has been divided into the following subtypes based on the World Health Organization 2004 classification system: Clear cell (80%), papillary types 1 and 2 (10%), chromophobe (5%), collecting duct (1%), and RCC unclassified (4% to 6%). Additional rarer types that collectively account for <2% of RCCs have been described as well.[4] The molecular pathways driving tumorigenesis in hereditary syndromes such as von Hippel-Lindau (VHL) disease, Birt-Hogg-Dubé (BHD) syndrome, hereditary leiomyomatosis and RCC, and hereditary papillary renal cell carcinoma (HPRCC) have provided greater insight into the molecular mechanisms behind the four major subtypes of RCC. This understanding has led to targeted therapies aimed at specific molecular pathways such as the hypoxia-inducible factor (HIF) pathway. This review is devoted primarily to the discussion of renal neoplasms in the adult population and their associated hereditary syndromes (Table 40.1). Genetic testing for susceptibility to urothelial cancers of the upper urinary tract is also presented.

## GENETIC SUSCEPTIBILITY TO RENAL CELL CARCINOMA

### von Hippel-Lindau Disease

VHL disease is an autosomal dominant condition that affects approximately 1 in 36,000 live births worldwide. The VHL gene is located on the short arm of chromosome 3 (3p25) and is the only known susceptibility locus associated with the condition. It is a well-studied tumor suppressor gene that demonstrates loss of heterozygosity in RCCs of patients with VHL disease and sporadic clear cell RCC as well.

VHL disease is a multisystem condition, and an affected individual is at risk to develop any of the following lesions: (1) hemangioblastoma of the cerebellum, spine, or retina; (2) papillary cystadenoma of the epididymis, the adnexal organs, or the endolymphatic sac; (3) adrenal pheochromocytoma and occasionally extra-adrenal paraganglioma; (4) pancreatic cysts, serous cystadenomas, and neuroendocrine tumors (NET); and (5) multiple and/or bilateral RCC and cysts.

Although the penetrance of VHL disease is 100%, where individuals will develop at least one associated lesion by their sixth decade of life, the expressivity is highly variable even among individuals sharing the same gene mutation. The disease is phenotypically categorized into type 1 and type 2 based on risk for developing pheochromocytoma, with the latter further divided into three subtypes (2A, 2B, and 2C) based on risk for developing RCC. The genotype/phenotype correlations within each type are described in Table 40.2.

### Renal Lesions

RCCs of patients with VHL disease are of exclusively clear cell histology. The lifetime risk for developing RCC is 25% to 45%, and when renal cysts are included, the risk rises to 60%.[5] Renal cysts and RCCs develop at an earlier age in patients with VHL in comparison to sporadic counterparts, with an average age of 39 years (range, 16 to 67 years).[5] Cystic lesions are typically asymptomatic; however, complex cysts must be monitored closely with computed tomography (CT) or magnetic resonance imaging as they will harbor a visibly solid RCC component. RCC will often arise from noncystic parenchyma as well.

### Nonrenal Clinical Features

With the exception of RCC and pancreatic NETs, the malignancy risk with VHL-associated tumors is very low. Renal lesions and hemangioblastoma of the cerebellum, spine, or retina are common presenting lesions in VHL. The risk for developing a single hemangioblastoma of the spine, cerebellum, and brainstem is 60% to 80%, and the average age is 33 years (range, 9 to 73 years),[5] although most patients can develop multiple lesions at any point in their lifetime. Patients may remain completely asymptomatic, especially during periods of no growth or slow growth. Surgical resection is delayed until onset of symptoms.

Retinal hemangioblastomas (retinal angiomas) are usually multifocal and bilateral. These hypervascular tumors can lead to retinal detachment and vision loss. Retinal hemangioblastomas have been observed in 25% to 60% of patients with an average age of 25 years (range, 1 to 67 years). Approximately 5% of lesions are seen younger than 10 years, making genetic testing of at-risk children essential as affected children should undergo annual retinal examinations beginning at birth. Pheochromocytoma has also been observed in young children and can present as a hypertensive crisis. The average age at presentation is 30 years (range, 5 to 58 years), and the risk is 10% to 20%.[5]

Pancreatic manifestations include multiple simple cysts and serous cystadenomas (47% and 11%, respectively), which follow a benign course and are almost always asymptomatic in patients. Pancreatic NETs are less common (15%); however, approximately 2% undergo malignant transformation.[6] A NET tends to be indolent and is seldom the initial presenting lesion; however, close monitoring is indicated for timing of surgical resection. A less common manifestation of VHL is a papillary cystadenoma of the endolymphatic sac, or inner ear, which is extremely rare in the general population but more prevalent in VHL disease (~11%). Papillary cystadenomas may also arise in the epididymis in men and less commonly in the adnexal organs in women.

TABLE 40.1

**Genetic Susceptibility to Renal Cell Carcinoma**

| Syndrome | Acronym | Gene(s) | Phenotype | RCC Type | Genetic Testing Sensitivity |
|---|---|---|---|---|---|
| von Hippel-Lindau syndrome | VHL | *VHL* | Hemangioblastoma (cerebellum, spine, retina), pheochromocytoma, papillary cystadenoma (pancreas, epididymis, adnexal organs, endolymphatic sac pancreatic NET, and cysts) | Clear cell | Nearly 100%[a] |
| Birt-Hogg-Dubé syndrome | BHD | Folliculin, *FLCN* | Fibrofolliculoma, trichodiscoma, acrochordon, lung cysts, spontaneous pneumothorax | 50% chromophobe/ oncocytic hybrid, 34% chromophobe, 9% clear cell, 5% oncocytoma, 2% papillary | ~88%[20] |
| Hereditary leiomyomatosis and RCC | HLRCC | *FH* | Cutaneous leiomyoma, uterine leiomyoma | Papillary type 2 | ~93%[25] |
| Hereditary papillary RCC | HPRCC | *MET* | No additional features | Papillary type 1 | Not well established as families are rare |
| Hereditary paraganglioma/ pheochromocytoma | HPGL | *SDHB*, possibly *SDHD* and *SDHC* | Pheochromocytoma and paraganglioma | Not well defined, but clear cell and papillary types reported | Unknown in families with RCC and no paraganglioma or pheochromocytoma |

RCC, renal cell carcinoma; NET, neuroendocrine tumor.
[a] Stolle C, Glenn G, Zbar B, et al. Improved detection of germline mutations in the von Hippel–Lindau disease tumor suppressor gene. *Hum Mutat* 1998;12:417–423.

## von Hippel-Lindau Molecular Genetics

The *VHL* gene was cloned by Latif et al.[7] in 1993 and is the most well studied of the familial RCC syndromes. Loss of *VHL* function has been demonstrated to cause RCC formation in VHL disease as well as in the majority of sporadic clear cell RCCs.[8,9] The *VHL* gene encodes the pVHL protein, which in normoxic conditions forms a complex with elongin B, elongin C, Cullin 2, and Rbx1. The VHL complex targets HIF-1α and HIF-2α for ubiquitin-mediated degradation. The HIF-1α and HIF-2α genes, along with HIF-3α, encode the α subunit of the HIF heterodimer. In hypoxic conditions, the VHL complex does not interact with HIF-1α and HIF-2α, leading to an accumulation of these subunits and downstream transcription of HIF-dependent genes. Loss of VHL protein

function in renal tumors simulates low tissue oxygen levels, or "pseudohypoxia," where HIF-1α and HIF-2α accumulate, causing upregulation of many genes involved in tumorigenesis such as vascular endothelial growth factor (proangiogenesis), epidermal growth factor receptor (cell proliferation and survival), and glucose transporter 1 (regulation of glucose uptake).

## von Hippel-Lindau Genetic Testing

Genetic testing of the VHL gene is available on a clinical basis and involves full-gene sequencing and large gene rearrangement analysis. When both methods are used, the mutation detection rate is nearly 100% in patients with a clinical diagnosis of VHL.[10] Approximately 80% of patients have a parent with VHL, and ~20% represent de

TABLE 40.2

**von Hippel-Lindau Genotype Phenotype Correlations**

| VHL Phenotype | Pheo | RCC | HB | Predominant Mutation Type |
|---|---|---|---|---|
| Type 1 | Rare or absent | High | High | Large deletions, nonsense, frameshift |
| Type 2A | High | Rare | High | Missense |
| Type 2B | High | High | High | Missense |
| Type 2C (uncommon) | High | Absent | Absent | Missense |

*Note:* The majority of type 1 mutations are partial or complete deletions and protein truncating (nonsense and frameshift), whereas 96% of type 2 mutations are missense. Missense mutations that disrupt amino acid residues on the surface of the VHL protein confer a higher Pheo risk than missense mutations that disrupt protein structure.
VHL, von Hippel-Lindau; Pheo, pheochromocytoma; RCC, renal cell carcinoma; HB, hemangioblastoma.
From Maher ER, Webster AR, Richards FM, et al. Phenotypic expression in von Hippel–Lindau disease: Correlations with germline VHL gene mutations. *J Med Genet* 1996;33:328–332; and Ong KR, Woodward ER, Killick P, et al. Genotype–phenotype correlations in von Hippel–Lindau disease. *Hum Mutat* 2007;28:143–149.

novo cases where neither parent carries the mutation. Genetic testing is recommended for a proband with a personal and family history of VHL, as the identification of causative mutations aids in determining disease subtype (see Table 40.2). Disease subtype information along with a careful, detailed family history aids in guiding screening and surveillance of patients with VHL. In simplex cases, where a patient has two or more VHL-associated lesions and a negative family history, genetic testing is recommended to establish a diagnosis. When a mutation is identified in a proband, at-risk family members should be offered predictive testing. Since young children with VHL are known to be at risk for retinal lesions and pheochromocytoma, genetic testing should be offered any time after birth.

## Birt-Hogg-Dubé Syndrome

In 1977, Drs. Birt, Hogg, and Dubé first described a multigenerational kindred showing autosomal dominant transmission of fibrofolliculomas with trichodiscomas and acrochordons.[11] The phenotype was later expanded beyond dermatologic manifestations to include lung cysts and pneumothorax and renal tumors.[12] The number of families with BHD syndrome described in the literature to date is small, and therefore, the exact incidence is unknown. Inherited mutations in the folliculin (*FLCN*) gene are associated with BHD syndrome.

## Renal Lesions

An individual with BHD syndrome is at increased risk of developing multiple and bilateral renal tumors, frequently of more than one histologic type even within the same renal unit, and at younger ages compared with the general population. The lifetime risk is in the range of 27% to 45%,[13,14] and the wide range may be a reflection of ascertainment bias introduced when families are recruited predominantly through dermatology clinics versus urology. The most common tumor pathology found in patients is a hybrid oncocytic RCC, which contains a mixture of oncocytic and chromophobe cells. Furthermore, radical nephrectomy specimens of patients have demonstrated oncocytosis where tiny nodules of cells similar to the larger hybrid tumors are diffusely scattered throughout the renal parenchyma. A retrospective study by Pavlovich et al.[15] examined 130 tumor specimens from 30 patients (25 males, 5 females) in 19 different BHD families. The authors found that hybrid oncocytic (50%) and chromophobe (34%) were the more common histologic findings, followed by clear cell (9%), benign oncocytoma (5%), and papillary (2%). The average age at first tumor was 50.7 years, and patients averaged 5.3 tumors each (range, 1 to 28). Other studies reporting histologic subtypes of BHD syndrome–related renal tumors have similar findings.

## Nonrenal Manifestations

Skin findings associated with BHD syndrome are benign and consist of fibrofolliculoma, trichodiscoma (which are histologically and clinically indistinguishable from angiofibroma), perifollicular fibroma, and acrochordons. Fibrofolliculoma is highly specific for BHD syndrome, whereas trichodiscomas and acrochordons are not. Onset for skin lesions is typically at older than 25 years, and a dermatologic diagnosis of BHD syndrome can be made on the basis of the presence of five or more facial or truncal papules with at least one histologically confirmed fibrofolliculoma.

Approximately 83% to 89% of patients with BHD syndrome will have multiple pulmonary cysts[14,16,17] identified upon chest CT. The lifetime risk of spontaneous pneumothorax is 24% to 32%,[14,18] and the majority of patients have their first event by age 50 years. The presence of lung cysts is strongly associated with risk of pneumothorax,[17] but the mechanism behind this is not known. A possible association between BHD syndrome and parotid oncocytoma has also been reported in a small number of cases.[14]

## FLCN Molecular Genetics

The *FLCN* gene is located on chromosome 17p11.2 and was cloned by Nickerson et al.[12] in 2002. The gene has 14 exons and encodes the protein folliculin. The role of *FLCN* and tumorigenesis has not been fully established, but animal studies and loss of heterozygosity studies in renal tumors provide some evidence that it is a tumor suppressor gene. Folliculin binds with folliculin-interacting proteins (FNIP1 and FNIP2) and then binds AMP-activated protein kinase, which is part of the cellular energy and nutrient sensing system. AMP-activated protein kinase also helps regulates mTOR activity (mTORC1 and mTORC2). Studies of renal tumors from heterozygous BHD knockout mice and renal tumors from patients with BHD syndrome show mTOR activation. Therapeutic agents inhibiting mTOR activity in sporadic chromophobe tumors are currently under investigation and may have implications for patients with BHD syndrome–related renal tumors.[19]

The mutation detection rate for *FLCN* clinical testing is approximately 89%, and nearly all of the mutations described to date have been truncating point mutations (frameshift and nonsense). Splice-site mutations have also been reported in a small number of BHD families, and one missense mutation in a patient with bilateral renal tumors has been reported as well.[20] A mutational hotspot in a polycytosine tract in exon 11 has been suggested.[14]

## Hereditary Papillary Renal Cell Carcinoma

HPRCC is inherited in an autosomal dominant manner with reduced penetrance where patients with HPRCC are at risk of developing multiple and/or bilateral papillary RCCs at a young age. The phenotype is limited to the risk of papillary RCC alone, particularly papillary type 1, although the distinction between type 1 and type 2 is not always made on initial pathology review.

Germ-line mutations in the *c-met* or *MET* proto-oncogene on chromosome 7q31.2 have been associated with HPRCC.[21] This is a comparatively uncommon condition, and few families with a *MET* mutation have been reported to date. Missense mutations found in HPRCC families occur in exons 16, 17, 18, and 19 of the *MET* proto-oncogene, which encodes the tyrosine-kinase domain of the protein product. These mutations have been shown to be activating or gain-of-function mutations, unlike most hereditary cancer susceptibility syndromes, which are associated with loss-of-function mutations in tumor suppressor genes. Papillary tumors obtained from patients with HPRCC typically show duplication of chromosome 7, as do their sporadic counterparts.[22] Furthermore, HPRCC-associated tumors show nonrandom duplication of the chromosome 7 copy harboring the mutation *MET* allele,[22,23] suggesting that overexpression of *MET* may lead to cellular proliferation, although the exact mechanism has not yet been elucidated.

Analysis by Lindor et al.[24] of 59 apparently sporadic patients with papillary type 1 tumors, including 13 cases with multifocal or bilateral disease, found no germ-line mutations in *MET*. This suggests differing etiology in sporadic versus papillary type 1 cancers. The rarity of the disease and low likelihood of identifying mutation carriers in isolated cases poses a challenge for genetic counseling of these patients. In the setting of a positive family history, *MET* genetic testing should be offered to patients with papillary type 1 RCC. A negative genetic test result, however, does not exclude the possibility of a hereditary susceptibility.

## Hereditary Leiomyomatosis and Renal Cell Carcinoma

Susceptibility to papillary type 2 RCC has been associated with hereditary leiomyomatosis and RCC (HLRCC) syndrome demonstrating autosomal dominant transmission. Most individuals with HLRCC-associated renal lesions present with unilateral, solitary tumors; however, bilateral and multifocal disease has also been observed.[25] The tumors tend to be highly aggressive with poor prognosis, which has implications for screening and early detection in at-risk patients. Although papillary type 2 is the predominant histology, collecting duct RCC and mixed cystic, papillary, and tubulopapillary RCC have also been reported. The incidence of RCC in individuals with HLRCC is approximately 25% to 40%.[25,26]

Cutaneous leiomyomatosis and uterine leiomyomatosis are additional features of the disease. Leiomyomas of the skin appear as firm skin-colored to light brown papules and can be distributed anywhere along the trunk, extremities, head, or neck. Uterine leiomyomas (fibroids) are common in the general population; however, HLRCC-associated burden tends to be greater in women with HLRCC. Compared with the general population, the average age at onset is younger where many women become symptomatic before the age of 30 years, significantly impacting their childbearing years. The fibroids tend to be multiple (ranging from 1 to 15 in one series of 22 women from 16 families studied) and large (1 to 8 cm), often requiring myomectomy or hysterectomy for treatment.[25] Not all individuals with HLRCC will have cutaneous manifestations, although it is worthwhile to note that the presence of cutaneous leiomyomas has a strong concordance with uterine leiomyoma. A very small number of cases have been reported of cutaneous and uterine leiomyosarcoma in HLRCC families. The fumarate hydratase gene, or *FH*, is the only gene associated with the disease to date. Fumarate hydratase functions in the Krebs cycle to convert fumarate to malate. Alteration of the *FH* gene results in accumulation of fumarate, which inhibits HIF-a prolyl hydroxylase enzymes (HPH). HIF-a is hydroxylated by HPH in normoxic conditions, but when HPH is inhibited, HIF-a levels rise, leading to increased transcription of downstream genes involved in tumorigenesis.[19]

## Hereditary Paraganglioma and Pheochromocytoma Associated with SDHB

Several genes have been implicated in hereditary paraganglioma with and without pheochromocytoma, such as the succinate dehydrogenase complex genes (*SDHB*, *SDHD*, and *SDHC*), as well as *TMEM127*, *SDHAF2*, *VHL*, *MEN2*, and others.

Earlier reports of families with mutations in *SDHB* also noted renal tumors in a minority of these families with a paraganglioma/pheochromocytoma phenotype.[27] Different renal tumor histologic findings have been reported including clear cell, chromophobe, carcinoma not classifiable, papillary type 2, or oncocytoma.[27–31] Gill et al.[32] examined five renal tumors from four families with an *SDHB* mutation and suggest that *SDHB*-associated renal tumors share common morphologic features such as bubbly eosinophilic cytoplasm with intracytoplasmic inclusions and indistinct cell borders.

Genetic testing of *SDHB* should be considered in patients presenting with early-onset and/or multifocal/bilateral RCC and a family history of paraganglioma or pheochromocytoma. Testing can also be considered in familial RCC especially in multigeneration and early-onset families, although there are not enough data at this time to suggest whether many *SDHB* carriers will be identified in the absence of known paraganglioma or pheochromocytoma. Ricketts et al.[29] studied a cohort of 68 patients with RCC and no evidence of syndromic RCC susceptibility and identified three *SDHB* mutation carriers (4.4%). One had a personal history of RCC at 24 years and a positive family history; two had a history of bilateral disease, one at the age of 30 years and the other at the age of 38 years; none of the three cases had a personal or family history of paraganglioma or pheochromocytoma.[29]

## GENETIC SUSCEPTIBILITY TO UROTHELIAL CANCERS

### Hereditary Nonpolyposis Colorectal Cancer, or Lynch Syndrome

Hereditary nonpolyposis colorectal cancer, or Lynch syndrome, is an inherited syndrome characterized by an increased risk for carcinoma of the colon, uterus, stomach, ovary, pancreas, and upper urinary tract. Inherited mutations in the DNA mismatch repair genes (*MLH1*, *MSH2*, *MSH6*, and *PMS2*) are associated with the syndrome.

Upper urinary tract cancers are the third most common cancer in Lynch syndrome, with a 5% to 6% lifetime risk. The associated cancers are mainly UCs of the ureter and renal pelvis with a relative risk of 22 times higher than that of the general population and a median age at onset of 56 years, or 10 to 15 years earlier.[33] Upper urinary UC may be the initial presenting feature in some patients from Lynch families. Most of the reported cases are in families with *MSH2* mutations, but have been observed in smaller number of *MLH1* and *MSH6* families as well. Bladder UC has been reported in patients with Lynch syndrome, with some studies reporting a relative risk similar or slightly higher to that of the general population.[34] In a cohort of Dutch families with Lynch syndrome, the relative risk of bladder cancer compared with the Dutch population was higher: 4.2 for men and 2.5 for women. *MSH2* mutation carriers in this cohort showed an even higher risk of 7 for men and 5.8 for women.[35]

Upper urinary tract cancers may be an underrecognized entity in Lynch syndrome, particularly in the urology specialty setting. Patients with UC of the ureter and renal pelvis may warrant a referral to genetics for risk assessment when presenting at young ages and/or synchronous or metachronous disease. Family history positivity for upper urinary tract cancers and other Lynch-associated tumors should be an indication for referral as well.

## INDICATIONS FOR GENETIC TESTING

One or more of the indicators listed in the following should prompt a referral for evaluating a patient for genetic susceptibility to RCC. Possible entry points for the patient include a diagnosis of RCC, pheochromocytoma or paraganglioma, spontaneous pneumothorax, bilateral cystic kidneys, cystic pancreas, or suspicious cutaneous lesions. A proposed guide to making a differential diagnosis is depicted in Figure 40.1.

- Syndromic features: A thorough medical history and physical examination may provide supporting evidence of syndromic features. Review of available radiology examinations is warranted. Patients with suspicious cutaneous lesions should be referred to dermatology for biopsy and histologic confirmation.
- Personal diagnosis of RCC: Even in the absence of known family history, early-onset (<40 years) and/or presence of multifocal or bilateral lesions warrants referral.
- Family history: Obtaining and reviewing pathology reports on renal tumors from family members is essential. Patients should be queried for a positive family history of related tumors such as pheochromocytoma, skin findings, and colon cancer.

## GENETIC TESTING AND COUNSELING

Genetic testing for *VHL*, *FLCN*, *MET*, *FH*, and *SDHB* is clinically available for approximately $1,000 to $1,200 per gene, although the per-gene cost is anticipated to decrease as the cost of sequencing technologies decreases and more multigene panels are offered.

## Approach to diagnosis of familial RCC

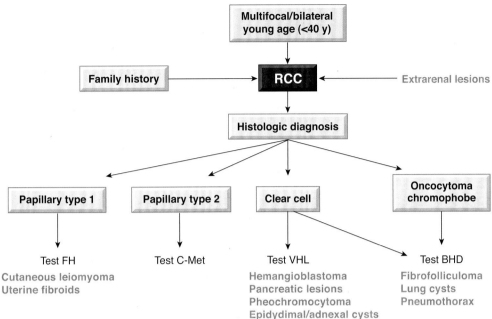

**Figure 40.1** Proposed approach for evaluation and testing for inherited susceptibility to RCC. Family history, age at onset, extrarenal lesions, and renal histology guide testing. RCC, renal cell carcinoma; FH, fumarate hydratase; VHL, von Hippel-Lindau; BHD, Birt-Hogg-Dubé.

Lynch syndrome testing is also available; however, it is a genetically heterogeneous disease, and tumor screening with microsatellite instability analysis and immunohistochemistry of the DNA mismatch repair genes can help guide germline testing (see "Colon Nonpolyposis" section of this book). A summary of the mutation detection rates for each gene can be found in Table 40.1. Testing sensitivity is predictably highest in syndromic cases with uncommon tumors that are highly specific for the syndrome such as hemangioblastoma (VHL) and fibrofolliculoma (BHD). Genetic testing is still warranted in less suspicious cases as a positive test result in a patient (i.e., germline mutation) prompts close monitoring in a rational, targeted manner. This includes screening for new renal tumors and nonrenal manifestations such as pheochromocytoma and paraganglioma. High-risk, aggressive papillary type 2 tumors are associated with HLRCC and warrant prompt intervention. Early detection and monitoring of nonpapillary type 2 renal lesions provide the patient and physician with information on disease burden, tumor size, and doubling time. Because patients with hereditary conditions such as VHL are at high risk of developing multiple RCC over their lifetime, close surveillance provides necessary clinical information for timing surgical intervention and increases the likelihood that nephron-sparing approaches can be used.

When a deleterious mutation is identified, at-risk family members should be offered predictive genetic testing. Genetic counseling regarding the natural history of the condition, the risk of carrying the mutation, age-appropriate screening, and the limitations of genetic testing is essential. In the case of BHD, HPRCC, and HLRCC, there is no consensus for a minimum age at which genetic testing should be considered. Timing of testing of asymptomatic relatives may be guided by ages at onset within the family. Each first-degree relative of a mutation carrier has an empiric risk of 50%. A negative test effectively rules out the disease and spares the individual from unnecessary imaging and screening. A positive test prompts close monitoring, such as regular imaging of the kidneys with CT or magnetic resonance imaging. With respect to limitations, it is important for patients to understand that a positive test result does not predict which tumors they will develop over their lifetime, age at onset of tumors, or severity of their disease.

VHL disease represents an exception where genetic testing should be offered anytime after a child is born. When a child tests negative for the familial VHL mutation, he/she is spared unnecessary screening; a child who carries the mutation must begin annual retinal examinations within the first year of life, with additional imaging examinations of the abdomen and brain around the onset of puberty. Multiple cases of retinal hemangioblastomas (angioma) in young children have been reported, and the morbidity of undiagnosed retinal tumors is high. Similarly, childhood-onset pheochromocytoma is also known to be associated with VHL and hereditary paraganglioma/pheochromocytoma syndromes.

Predictive testing of minors in their teenage years should be treated with a greater sensitivity to the minor's intellectual and emotional capacity. Some parents include their child on the decision to test, depending on the age and emotional maturity of their child. This helps maintain trust between the child and the parent, and lays a foundation for greater comprehension of the test result and the implications, whether the results are positive or negative. In the setting of genetic predisposition counseling, the concept of risk and the struggle to cope with risk information is a tenuous position for any adult patient. This is no less stressful for a teenager and his/her parents demanding elevated sensitivity and awareness from the provider and genetic counselor caring for the family.

Not including an older child in the testing decision is also the parents' prerogative; however, the health-care provider or genetic counselor working with the family should help parents consider the potential ramifications of initiating testing without the child's knowledge. Questions to consider include when and how they would disclose the results to their child in an age-appropriate way. When we consider a teenaged minor who is intellectually capable of giving assent for genetic testing, the process of obtaining the minor's assent involves the health-care professional who, together with the parents, provides age-appropriate information about the genetic disease, what is involved in carrying out the test, and how results will be disclosed. Parents may wish to test their teenage minor without his/her knowledge primarily because they are hoping for a "good news" scenario of a negative test result where both the teen and the parents can be worry-free. When parents request testing for their teenager without his/her knowledge, the provider should help parents anticipate that they may be putting their child's trust in them (and their child's trust in the medical community) at risk, particularly if it results in a positive diagnosis.

The role of the genetic counselor and health-care provider is to support the patient and family with a focus on improving their understanding of their disease and on helping the family find a common language with which to communicate their fears, concerns, and needs. Families often benefit from participating in multidisciplinary practices staffed by a combination of medical oncology, advanced practice nursing, genetic counseling, urosurgery, and other practitioners.[36] These disease specialty clinics are geared toward meeting the medical and informational needs of the patient and family, which are expected to evolve with age and with major life transitions.

# SUMMARY

The genetic basis of heritable susceptibility to cancers of the urinary tract is a complex problem composed of many different genes and molecular pathways. Careful inspection of family medical history, tumor histology, and physical findings such as cutaneous lesions provide the opportunity for a stepwise approach to genetic risk assessment of the patient with cancer. Genetic testing of cancer susceptibility genes has downstream implications for surveillance and treatment of disease, and identification of causative mutations provides valuable information for patients and their at-risk family members. Genetic counseling of patients and their family members allows for enhanced understanding of the disease and treatment.

## REFERENCES

1. Siegel R, Naishadham D, Jemal A. Cancer statistics. *CA Cancer J Clin* 2012; 62:10–29.
2. National Cancer Institute. SEER Stat Fact Sheets: Kidney and Renal Pelvis Cancer. SEER Web site. http://seer.cancer.gov/statfacts/html/kidrp.html#risk. Accessed May 2, 2012.
3. Clague J, Lin J, Cassidy A, et al. Family history and risk of renal cell carcinoma: Results from a case-control study and systematic meta-analysis. *Cancer Epidemiol Biomarkers Prev* 2009;18:801–807.
4. Deng FM, Melamed J. Histologic variants of renal cell carcinoma: Does tumor type influence outcome? *Urol Clin North Am* 2012;39:119–132.
5. Lonser RR, Glenn GM, Walther M, et al. von Hippel–Lindau disease. *Lancet* 2003;361:2059–2067.
6. Charlesworth M, Verbeke CS, Falk GA, et al. Pancreatic lesions in von Hippel–Lindau disease? A systematic review and meta-synthesis of the literature. *J Gastrointest Surg* 2012;16:1422–1428.
7. Latif F, Tory K, Gnarra J, et al. Identification of the von Hippel–Lindau disease tumor suppressor gene. *Science* 1993;260:1317–1320.
8. Gnarra JR, Tory K, Weng Y, et al. Mutations of the VHL tumour suppressor gene in renal carcinoma. *Nat Genet* 1994;7:85–90.
9. Shuin T, Kondo K, Torigoe S, et al. Frequent somatic mutations and loss of heterozygosity of the von Hippel–Lindau tumor suppressor gene in primary human renal cell carcinomas. *Cancer Res* 1994;54:2852–2855.
10. Schimke RN, Collins DL, Stolle CA. Von-Hippel Lindau Syndrome. GeneReviews at GeneTests: Medical Genetics Information Resource (website) http://www.genetests.org. Updated December 22, 2009. Accessed April 11, 2012.
11. Birt AR, Hogg GR, Dube WJ. Hereditary multiple fibrofolliculomas with trichodiscomas and acrochordons. *Arch Dermatol* 1977;113:1674–1677.
12. Nickerson ML, Warren MB, Toro JR, et al. Mutations in a novel gene lead to kidney tumors, lung wall defects, and benign tumors of the hair follicle in patients with the Birt–Hogg–Dube syndrome. *Cancer Cell* 2002;2: 157–164.
13. Pavlovich CP, Grubb RL 3rd, Hurley K, et al. Evaluation and management of renal tumors in the Birt–Hogg–Dube syndrome. *J Urol* 2005;173: 1482–1486.
14. Schmidt LS, Nickerson ML, Warren MB, et al. Germline BHD-mutation spectrum and phenotype analysis of a large cohort of families with Birt–Hogg–Dube syndrome. *Am J Hum Genet* 2005;76:1023–1033.
15. Pavlovich CP, Walther MM, Eyler RA, et al. Renal tumors in the Birt–Hogg–Dube syndrome. *Am J Surg Pathol* 2002;26:1542–1552.
16. Zbar B, Alvord WG, Glenn G, et al. Risk of renal and colonic neoplasms and spontaneous pneumothorax in the Birt–Hogg–Dube syndrome. *Cancer Epidemiol Biomarkers Prev* 2002;11:393–400.
17. Toro JR, Pautler SE, Stewart L, et al. Lung cysts, spontaneous pneumothorax, and genetic associations in 89 families with Birt–Hogg–Dube syndrome. *Am J Respir Crit Care Med* 2007;175:1044–1053.
18. Houweling AC, Gijezen LM, Jonker MA, et al. Renal cancer and pneumothorax risk in Birt–Hogg–Dube syndrome; an analysis of 115 FLCN mutation carriers from 35 BHD families. *Br J Cancer* 2011;105:1912–1919.
19. Singer EA, Bratslavsky G, Middelton L, et al. Impact of genetics on the diagnosis and treatment of renal cancer. *Curr Urol Rep* 2011;12:47–55.
20. Toro JR, Wei MH, Glenn GM, et al. BHD mutations, clinical and molecular genetic investigations of Birt–Hogg–Dube syndrome: A new series of 50 families and a review of published reports. *J Med Genet* 2008;45:321–331.
21. Schmidt L, Duh FM, Chen F, et al. Germline and somatic mutations in the tyrosine kinase domain of the MET proto-oncogene in papillary renal carcinomas. *Nat Genet* 1997;16:68–73.
22. Fischer J, Palmedo G, von Knobloch R, et al. Duplication and overexpression of the mutant allele of the MET proto-oncogene in multiple hereditary papillary renal cell tumours. *Oncogene* 1998;17:733–739.
23. Zhuang Z, Park WS, Pack S, et al. Trisomy 7–harbouring non-random duplication of the mutant MET allele in hereditary papillary renal carcinomas. *Nat Genet* 1998;20:66–69.
24. Lindor NM, Dechet CB, Greene MH, et al. Papillary renal cell carcinoma: Analysis of germline mutations in the MET proto-oncogene in a clinic-based population. *Genet Test* 2001;5:101–106.
25. Wei MH, Toure O, Glenn GM, et al. Novel mutations in FH and expansion of the spectrum of phenotypes expressed in families with hereditary leiomyomatosis and renal cell cancer. *J Med Genet* 2006;43:18–27.
26. Gardie B, Remenieras A, Kattygnarath D, et al. Novel FH mutations in families with hereditary leiomyomatosis and renal cell cancer (HLRCC) and patients with isolated type 2 papillary renal cell carcinoma. *J Med Genet* 2011;48: 226–234.
27. Vanharanta S, Buchta M, McWhinney SR, et al. Early-onset renal cell carcinoma as a novel extraparaganglial component of SDHB-associated heritable paraganglioma. *Am J Hum Genet* 2004;74:153–159.
28. Henderson A, Douglas F, Perros P, et al. SDHB-associated renal oncocytoma suggests a broadening of the renal phenotype in hereditary paragangliomatosis. *Fam Cancer* 2009;8:257–260.
29. Ricketts C, Woodward ER, Killick P, et al. Germline SDHB mutations and familial renal cell carcinoma. *J Natl Cancer Inst* 2008;100:1260–1262.
30. Ricketts CJ, Forman JR, Rattenberry E, et al. Tumor risks and genotype–phenotype–proteotype analysis in 358 patients with germline mutations in SDHB and SDHD. *Hum Mutat* 2010;31:41–51.
31. Srirangalingam U, Walker L, Khoo B, et al. Clinical manifestations of familial paraganglioma and pheochromocytomas in succinate dehydrogenase B (SDH-B) gene mutation carriers. *Clin Endocrinol (Oxf)* 2008;69:587–596.
32. Gill AJ, Pachter NS, Chou A, et al. Renal tumors associated with germline SDHB mutation show distinctive morphology. *Am J Surg Pathol* 2011; 35:1578–1585.
33. Rouprêt M, Yates DR, Comperat E, et al. Upper urinary tract urothelial cell carcinomas and other urological malignancies involved in the hereditary nonpolyposis colorectal cancer (Lynch syndrome) tumor spectrum. *Eur Urol* 2008;54:1226–1236.
34. Crockett DG, Wagner DG, Holmäng S, et al. Upper urinary tract carcinoma in Lynch syndrome cases. *J Urol* 2011;185:1627–1630.
35. van der Post RS, Kiemeney LA, Ligtenberg MJ, et al. Risk of urothelial bladder cancer in Lynch syndrome is increased, in particular among MSH2 mutation carriers. *J Med Genet* 2010;47:464–470.
36. VHL Alliance. A list of VHL specialty clinics in the United States and other countries. www.vhl.org. Accessed September 3, 2014.

# 41 Molecular Biology of Prostate Cancer

Felix Y. Feng, Arul M. Chinnaiyan, and Edwin M. Posadas

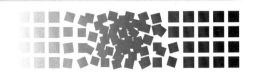

## INTRODUCTION

Prostate cancer is the most common malignancy and the second leading cause of cancer death in men in the United States.[1] It also poses a global problem, with recent significant increases in incidence outside the Western world.[2] This malignancy is marked by extremely clinical and biological heterogeneity, which creates the opportunity for resistant clones to emerge, leading to eventual relapse and disease progression, and thus presenting problems for both patients and their physicians.

A major limitation in the management of this disease has been in the nomenclature used to describe the nature of each patient's underlying disease. The currently employed staging system and the histopathologic scores established by Gleason reflect neither our current understanding of prostate cancer biology, nor the implications of this biology for outcomes and management. There has remained a need to further refine the pathologic classification of prostate cancers to account for the various families of molecular aberrations that exist within this disease. It is hoped that this refinement of classification may allow for more precise or "personalized" management of prostatic adenocarcinomas.

Systemic therapy for this disease begins with the reduction of circulating testosterone levels by medical or surgical castration. In most cases, this results in clinical benefit. However, progression to castration-resistant prostate cancer (CRPC) eventually occurs. A number of effective CRPC therapies have recently emerged. Regretfully, none are curative and all have a limited benefit, as shown in clinical trials. Refining our understanding of the molecular nature of this disease will hopefully lead to better characterization and, ultimately, more effective assignment of treatments to improve outcomes for patients.

## OVERVIEW OF THE GENOMIC LANDSCAPE OF PROSTATE CANCER

The advent of next-generation sequencing technology has significantly broadened our understanding of the genomic landscape of prostate cancer. Recent studies have characterized the complete prostate cancer genome from 75 patients and have reported on the exomes of hundreds of additional cases.[3–7] In combination with gene expression and copy number data previously interrogated from thousands of tumors, these studies provide a relatively comprehensive profile of the prostate cancer genome and transcriptome. Like other epithelial tumors, prostate cancers harbor genomic lesions, such as amplifications and deletions; point mutations; and translocations, as well as transcriptional changes leading to overexpression of oncogenes and underexpression of tumor suppressor genes.

Subsets of tumors have been shown to harbor recurrent amplifications and deletions ranging from focal alternations (one to a few genes) to others that span entire chromosomal arms (Fig. 41.1). These alterations tend to increase in prevalence with higher grade and stage. The most common deletions occur on chromosomes 8p,

10q, and 13q, and include genes such as NKX3-1, PTEN, and RB1. Metastatic tumors harbor amplifications of chromosome X and 8q, which include the androgen receptor (AR) and MYC oncogenes (see Fig. 41.1). Although the prostate cancer genome exhibits an overall low mutation rate (~1 per MB), the landscape of prostate cancer can also be defined by copy number and mutational alterations along several key oncogenic and tumor suppressor pathways, which are commonly involved when the individual genes in each pathway are considered collectively. Three of these pathways—the AR pathway, the phosphatidylinositol 3-phosphate kinase (PI3K)/AKT pathway, and the retinoblastoma (RB) pathway—are altered in more than one-third of primary cancers and in the vast majority of metastatic lesions.[3–7] Frequent alterations in these pathways suggest that, in prostate cancer, different individual genes in the pathway may be targeted to activate or suppress a common pathway lesion (Fig. 41.2).

In addition to pathway-based analyses, prostate cancer can be defined by recurrent lesions of single genes. Approximately 50% of prostate-specific antigen (PSA)-screened prostate cancers harbor gene fusions involving E26 transformation specific (ETS) transcription factors, which represent oncogenic drivers.[8,9] Strikingly, ETS fusions and certain other lesions, such as mutation of the E3 ubiquitin ligase SPOP and fusions involving RAF, appear to be mutually exclusive, suggesting a framework for molecular subtyping of prostate cancer.[5,10,11] The sections that follow further describe the altered pathways and recurrent genetic lesions most validated in prostate cancer.

## ANDROGEN RECEPTOR BIOLOGY AND THERAPY

### Introduction to the Androgen Receptor

AR has remained one of the most important and most studied proteins in prostate cancer. The dependence of most prostate cancers on AR activation has served as a basis for important therapeutic approaches, such as luteinizing hormone releasing hormone (LHRH) analogs, antiandrogens, and androgen biosynthesis inhibitors.

AR is a 110-kb steroid receptor transcription factor, located on Xq12.[12] Upon binding to an androgen, AR mediates the transcription of a number of genes involved in survival and differentiation of prostate epithelial cells, starting at development of the normal gland. Expression of AR is high in the luminal epithelial cells but lower in the basal epithelial cells that define glandular structure.[13]

In conjunction with NKX3.1 and FOXA1, AR plays a critical role in normal prostate organogenesis and disease progression.[14] NKX3.1 is an AR-regulated prostatic tumor suppressor gene that is located on chromosome 8p and present through development.[15] It is the earliest marker of organogenesis and is involved with ductal morphogenesis and secretory function.[16] Mutations are infrequent in human cancers, but loss of heterozygosity in 8p becomes more frequent during cancer progression, with 86% loss in prostate cancers (see Fig. 41.1).[17] Loss of NKX3.1 has been associated with

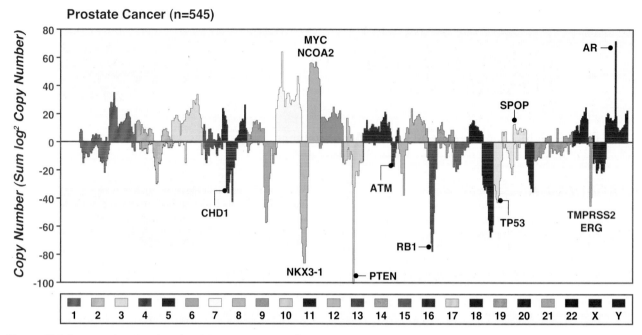

**Figure 41.1** Copy number alterations found in prostate cancer. Genomewide copy number profiles were plotted from four publicly available datasets including 545 prostate cancers, using the Oncomine Powertools DNA Copy Number Browser (Life Technology). Each chromosome is color coded (see legend), and the locations of key genes harboring recurrent copy number gains/losses or mutations are labeled. The y axis indicates the sum of the log2 copy number for each segmented sample, as plotted in genomic order.

activation of the TMPRSS2-ERG gene fusion, which promotes tumorigenesis.[18] *FOXA1* is a member of the forkhead transcription factor family that opens compacted chromatin to facilitate AR recruitement.[19] It is known to play a pivotal role in AR and steroid receptor function.[20] It is now recognized that mutation and overexpression of FOXA1 can promote progression to CRPC (see Fig. 41.2).[3,5]

Polymorphisms of *AR* as well as *CYP17* and *SRD5A2* are low penetrant risk factors for prostate cancer development in some but not all studies.[21] AR-pathway alterations exist in 60% of primary tumors and nearly 100% of metastatic tumors. *NCOA2* (also called *SRC2*) is the most commonly altered member of this pathway (see Fig. 41.2) and is an AR coactivator that potentiates transcriptional output. Several other AR coactivators, including *NCOA1, TNK2,* and *EP300*, are upregulated in metastatic disease, whereas AR corepressors, including *NRIP1, NCOR1,* and *NCOR2*, are downregulated (see Fig. 41.2).

## Targeting Androgen Receptor Activity: GnRH-Targeting Therapies and Androgen Biosynthesis Inhibitors

The inhibition of androgen synthesis has been used a means of suppressing AR activity. Gonadotropin-releasing hormone-luteinizing hormone (GnRH) agonists or antagonists represent the first-line approach for inhibiting androgen synthesis (Fig. 41.3). These therapies work by suppressing the hypothalamic–pituitary–gonadal axis by eventually causing luteinizing hormone (LH) levels to fall, thereby minimizing testicular production of testosterone and its subsequent conversion to dihydrotestosterone (DHT) by 5-alpha reduction. DHT is the most potent activator of AR and binds to the AR, resulting in translocation to the nucleus and activation of transcription (see Fig. 41.3).

These strategies, although initially highly effective, are often overcome during tumor progression. Alternative sources of DHT and alternative means of AR activity have been identified as mechanisms of resistance. GnRH-targeting agents have no impact on

nongonadal androgen synthesis (i.e., suppression of adrenocorticotropic hormone [ACTH] and, hence, adrenal androgen synthesis) (see Fig. 41.3). The adrenal glands can synthesize adequate levels of androgens to promote cancer growth. CYP17 is a key P450 enzyme in the androgen biosynthesis pathway that generates dehydroepiandrosterone (DHEA) and androstenedione in the adrenal glands. These weak androgens can be further converted into testosterone or alternative steroid substrates that are reduced to DHT.[22,12] This step is recognized as a particular bottleneck in androgen production. The specific inhibition of CYP17 decreases androgen synthesis, with less effect on the production of other essential steroids. Abiraterone acetate is a pregnenolone derivative that is a high-affinity, irreversible inhibitor of CYP17, and results in decreased adrenal androgen synthesis. At higher doses, this agent inhibits other DHT synthetic pathways such as 3β-hydroxysteroid dehydrogenase.[23]

Intratumoral androgens may be increased in CRPC.[24] Measurements of intratumoral androgens showed that CRPC tumors have more testosterone than primary tumors in untreated men.[25] Expression profiling studies comparing CRPC with primary tumors have shown that androgen synthesis enzymes are upregulated in CRPC.[26,27] Patient samples at all stages of disease contain an abundance of AKR1C3 and SRD5A1, which are necessary for the conversion of androstenedione to DHT. However, the samples lacked high expression of enzymes necessary for de novo steroidogenesis.[28] These data suggest that autocrine androgen synthesis may allow tumors to grow despite low serum androgen levels, but that this process may, in part, be dependent on adrenal precursors.

## Targeting Androgen Receptor Activity: Antiandrogens

Antiandrogens compete with endogenous androgens for the ligand binding pocket of AR (see Fig. 41.3). Older agents promote translocation of AR from the cytoplasm into the nucleus and DNA binding, but induce conformational changes that prevent optimal transcriptional activity. In the United States, there have been

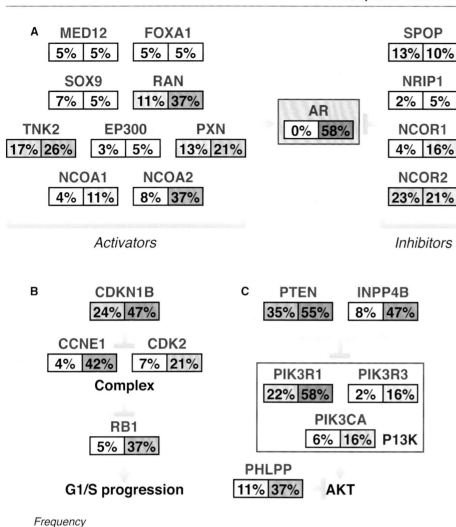

**Figure 41.2** Alterations in common pathways dysregulated in prostate cancer. The androgen receptor *(AR)* **(A)**, retinoblastoma **(B)**, and phosphatidylinositol 3-kinase *(PI3K)* **(C)** pathways are altered in more than one-third of primary cancers and in the vast majority of metastatic lesions. This schematic depicts alteration frequencies for individual genes and for the entire pathway in primary and metastatic tumors. Alterations are defined as those having significant up- or downregulation compared with normal prostate samples, or by somatic mutations, and are interpreted as activation *(red)* or inactivation *(blue)* of protein function. (Figure adapted from the 9th edition of Devita, Hellman, and Rosenberg's *Cancer: Principles and Practice of Oncology.*)

three historic nonsteroidal antiandrogens (NSAA): flutamide, bicalutamide, and nilutamide. Each has been associated with an antiandrogen withdrawal effect, whereby treated patients experiencing disease progression on treatment derive clinical benefit when the antiandrogen is stopped.[29] Although this was initially believed to be related to AR mutation, later studies have shown this is due to AR activation by these NSAAs.[30,31]

Newer NSAAs have now been developed that lack agonist effects on the AR. Enzalutamide (MDV3100) was approved by the U.S. Food and Drug Administration (FDA) in 2012.[32] Other next-generation NSAAs are in development, including ARN-509.

Finally, new approaches are being taken to inhibit AR at the amino terminus.[33] As opposed to interrupting ligand binding, agents such as EPI-001 interfere with transcriptional activity of AR. These agents are still in early development, but appear very promising because they display activity even when the ligand-binding domain of AR has been altered.

## Alterations in the Androgen Receptor During Prostate Cancer Progression

Prostate cancers eventually progress to a more lethal state: castration resistance. The time to development of resistance and the molecular pathways to CRPC differ from patient to patient. Progression of CRPC is usually accompanied by the restoration of PSA secretion, indicating a reactivation of AR activity in these cases.[12]

Gene amplification and increased protein expression represent the most common mechanisms of means of reactivating AR signaling in the face of castration therapy. These changes allow cancer cells to respond to subphysiologic concentrations of androgen.[34] AR mutations are detected in up to 10% of CRPC cases and allow for activation by alternative ligands.[35] Overexpression of AR is seen in approximately 30% of cases of CRPC.[36] Alternative splicing of AR mRNA can lead to a truncated protein missing the ligand-binding domain. These increase in number in the face of many second-line NSAAs.[37,38] Some of these variants have constitutive transcriptional activity in the absence of androgens. Overexpression of these variants can confer castration resistance in preclinical models.[39] More recent studies show that these variants impact sensitivity to taxanes[40] and even next-generation antiandrogens such as enzalutamide.[41]

## ADDITIONAL PATHWAYS FREQUENTLY ALTERED DURING DISEASE PROGRESSION

### The Phosphatidylinositol 3-Phosphate Kinase (*PI3K*) Pathway

Progression to CRPC is characterized by gain of function in *AR* and activation of the phosphatidylinositol 3-phosphate kinase

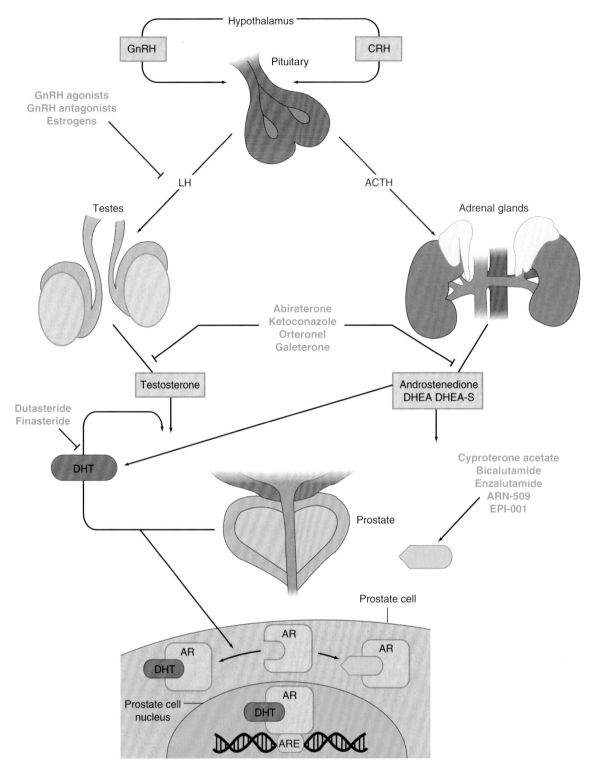

**Figure 41.3** The androgen-signaling axis and its inhibitors. Testicular androgen synthesis is regulated by the gonadotropin-releasing hormone-luteinizing hormone (GnRH–LH) axis. Pharmacologic inhibitors are labeled in *red* at respective steps. GnRH-driven activity can be inhibited by both GnRH agonists and antagonists, as well as estrogens. Adrenal androgen synthesis is regulated by the corticotrophin-releasing hormone (CRH)–adrenocorticotropic hormone (ACTH) axis. CYP17 is a critical enzyme in androgen synthesis inhibited by abiraterone, orteronel, and galeterone. CYP17 inhibitors decrease synthesis of androgen from the adrenal glands, testes, and (in advanced disease) the tumors themselves. 5-Alpha reductase inhibitors prevent reduction of testosterone and other androgen intermediates to DHT. Antiandrogens such as enzalutamide and ARN-509 block activation of AR by inhibiting the binding of androgens to androgen receptors. DHEA-S, dehydroepiandrosterone sulfate; ARE, androgen-response element.

(PI3K) pathway. Cross-talk between these pathways has been proposed[42,43] because a loss of *PTEN* and subsequent PI3K activation is associated with repression of androgen responsive genes. Conversely, AR inhibition results in the upregulation of PI3K activity.[42,43] As such, combination therapy with PI3K and AR inhibition are currently being evaluated in clinical trials.

The PI3K signaling cascade is one of the most commonly altered pathways in human malignancy. *PTEN* is a tumor suppressor that deactivates PI3K signaling. *PTEN* deletions are present in nearly 30% of primary prostate cancers, and inactivating mutations of *PTEN* occur in another 5% to 10%; both are more common in advanced disease (see Fig 41.2).[3,5,7,44,45] Functional studies across multiple preclinical model systems of prostate cancer consistently reinforce the role of *PTEN* in suppressing tumorigenesis and prostate cancer progression.[46,47] Dysregulation of *PTEN* represents a poor prognostic factor. There is significant evidence that *PTEN* deletion is associated with higher stage, higher Gleason grade, and higher rates of progression, recurrence after therapy, and disease-specific mortality.[48,49]

Amplification and point mutations in *PIK3CA*, encoding a catalytic subunit of PI3K, also result in overactivation of the pathway and are enriched in metastatic versus localized prostate cancer (see Fig 41.2).[3,50] Activating *PIK3CA* lesions and inactivation of *PTEN* are usually mutually exclusive, supporting a similar endpoint in driving downstream signaling.

Recent studies have also identified the presence of rarer events that affect PI3K signaling. These lesions include the rearrangement of *MAGI2*, the deletion of *PHLPP1*, mutations in *GSK3B*, and point mutations and genomic deletions of *CDKN1B*.[3,4,44,47,51] Recurrent alterations in multiple nodes along the PI3K pathway emphasize its critical importance in the pathogenesis of prostate cancer and support the rationale for therapies targeting this pathway.

## The Retinoblastoma Pathway

Another tumor suppressor pathway that is frequently inactivated in epithelial malignancies is the RB pathway (see Fig. 41.2). The p130 RB protein regulates cell cycle progression by binding to E2F family members and repressing E2F-mediated gene transcription. RB is inactivated via phosphorylation by cyclin-dependent kinases (CDK), resulting in E2F-mediated cell cycle progression.[52] The absence of RB signaling results in aberrant cell cycle progression and tumor proliferation.

Similar to *PTEN* deletion, the loss of *RB* is enriched in prostate cancer metastases compared to primary disease (see Fig. 41.2).[53] Within preclinical prostate cancer models, the inactivation of RB confers castration-resistant tumor growth via E2F1-mediated activation of AR gene transcription.[53] RB status is currently being explored as a stratification variable for treatment strategies on ongoing clinical trials.

# E26 TRANSFORMATION SPECIFIC (ETS) GENE FUSIONS AND THE MOLECULAR SUBTYPES OF PROSTATE CANCER

## E26 Transformation Specific (ETS) Gene Fusions

In addition to pathway-based analyses, prostate cancer can be defined by recurrent lesions of single genes. The most common molecular abnormality in prostate cancer is a gene fusion involving an ETS transcription factor.[8,9] These genetic rearrangements, found in approximately 50% of prostate cancers, occur when genes encoding an ETS transcription factor are translocated downstream of the regulatory, usually androgen-responsive, element of a second gene.[8,9,54] These fusions result in AR-driven overexpression of an ETS transcription factor, causing transcriptional dysregulation of downstream oncogenic pathways, increased invasion, and carcinogenesis in preclinical models of prostate cancer.[8,9,54,55] The most prevalent ETS gene rearrangement involves either chromosomal deletion or insertion of chromosome 21, resulting in fusion of the 5' untranslated region of the androgen-regulated gene *TMPRSS2* with the ETS family member *ERG*. Over 90% of ETS rearrangements involve *ERG*, whereas the remaining ETS fusions include *ETV1* (chromosome 7), *ETV5* (chromosome 3), or *ETV4* (chromosome 17) as common 3' partners (Fig. 41.4). Although *TMPRSS2* is the most common 5' partner for *ERG*, over 10 androgen-regulated genes, including *SLC45A3* and *NDRG1*, have been identified as 5' fusion partners in ETS rearrangements (see Fig. 41.4).

Several studies have investigated the prognostic value of ETS fusion status, with conflicting results likely stemming from the heterogeneity of study cohorts, screening practices, and management

CANCERS OF THE GENITOURINARY SYSTEM

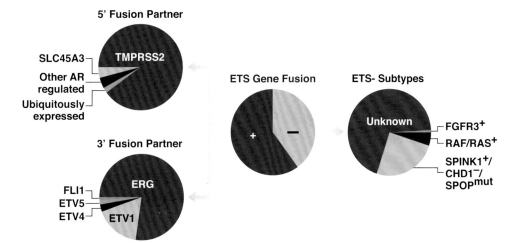

**Figure 41.4** The molecular subtypes of prostate cancer subtypes. The approximate distribution of prostate cancer subtypes, as defined by driving molecular lesions, is presented for PSA-screened Caucasian populations. Approximately 50% to 60% of all prostate cancers harbor ETS gene fusions *(central pie chart)*. ETS gene fusions are nearly mutually exclusive with other alterations, such as *FGFR3* fusions, *RAF* fusions, *SPOP* mutations, *CHD1* deletions, and SPINK1 overexpression *(right pie chart)*. The predominant 5' fusion partner in ETS fusions is the androgen-regulated promoter of the TMPRSS2 gene *(top left pie chart)*. The primary 3' fusion partner is ERG, though other genes encoding ETS transcription factors, such as ETV1, ETV4, ETV5, and FLI1, are involved at lower frequencies *(bottom left pie chart)*.

strategies, as well as the variability in tumor sampling, disease multifocality, and measured clinical outcomes. In the context of non–PSA-screened populations managed conservatively, population-based studies have demonstrated a significant association between ETS fusion status and adverse clinicopathologic predictors, metastases, or disease-specific mortality.[56,57,58] However, in the context of patients treated with radical prostatectomy, the prognostic impact of ETS fusions is uncertain, with some studies demonstrating an association between ETS fusion status and features of aggressive prostate cancer, and other studies finding no such associations. The largest report, a prospective cohort study involving over 1,100 patients treated with radical prostatectomy, found that ETS related gene (ERG) rearrangement or overexpression was associated with tumor stage, but not recurrence or mortality.[59] Overall, ETS fusions are associated with poorer prognosis in population-based studies of watchful waiting cohorts, but are of uncertain prognostic value in radical prostatectomy patients.

## The Molecular Subtypes of Prostate Cancer

Although the prognostic value of ETS fusions remains unclear, the molecular characterization of prostate cancer often begins with the determination of ETS fusion status, by either fluorescence in situ hybridization or immunohistochemical approaches. Transcriptomic, genomic, and epigenetic profiling studies have demonstrated that ETS fusion-positive prostate cancers are biologically distinct from ETS fusion-negative disease.[4,60] For example, certain lesions, such as deletions or mutations of the PTEN or TP53 tumor suppressors, are significantly enriched in ETS-positive cancers.[4,44,61] Strikingly, other alterations, such as RAF fusions, SPOP mutations, CHD1 deletions, and SPINK1 overexpression, occur exclusively in ETS-negative cancers,[3,5,62] (Fig. 41.4) providing evidence that these alterations define distinct biologic subsets of prostate cancer and may provide a framework for defining molecular subtypes of prostate cancer.[3,10,11] The potential subtypes are described in the following paragraphs.

Gene fusions and known activating mutations in RAF and RAS family members have also been identified in approximately 1% to 2% of all prostate cancers (see Fig. 41.4).[3,5,11] RAF encodes for a serine/threonine-specific protein kinase, and RAS encodes for a GTPase. RAF-RAS[+] tumors are exclusively negative for ETS fusions, SPOP mutations, CHD1 deletions, and SPINK1 overexpression. Both RAF and RAS serve as signaling intermediates in the mitogen activated protein kinase (MAPK) pathway, and activation of RAF and RAS may enhance the transcriptional activity of the androgen receptor.[63] Of note, activating events in the RAF/RAS/MAPK pathway may be targetable by existing kinase inhibitors.

SPOP mutations represent the most prevalent point mutations in localized prostate cancer, occurring at a frequency of 10% to 15%.[3,4] SPOP codes for the substrate-recognition component of a Cullin3-based E3-ubiquitin ligase. Recurrent mutations are located exclusively within the region of SPOP, which forms the substrate-binding cleft, suggesting that they prevent substrate binding.[3,64] Previous studies have suggested that SPOP substrates include AR and its coactivator SRC-3,[65,66] and that SPOP mutations result in increased androgen signaling. SPOP-mutant prostate cancers have a distinct genomic profile; in addition to occurring only in ETS-negative cases, SPOP mutations are also mutually exclusive with TP53 mutations/deletions, and generally lack PI3K pathway alterations. Additionally, SPOP mutations are significantly associated with deletions of the CHD1 gene, which is a DNA binding protein that functions in remodeling chromatin states. Of note, cases with CHD1 deletions are significantly enriched in the number of genomic rearrangements that they harbor, compared to other prostate cancers.[67,68] Thus, SPOP mutations and CHD1 deletions appear to define a distinct ETS fusion–negative subtype of prostate cancer.

SPINK1 is a secreted protease that is overexpressed in approximately 10% of prostate cancers.[62] Although SPINK1 overexpression is present in only ETS fusion–negative cases, SPINK1 overexpression can co-occur with SPOP mutations and CHD1 deletions, suggesting that multiple aberrations can define this subset of ETS-negative prostate cancer (see Fig. 41.4). SPINK1 interacts with epidermal growth factor receptor (EGFR) to mediate its neoplastic effects, suggesting that SPINK1-positive prostate cancers may be targeted via EGFR inhibition.[69]

Lastly, a recent study has identified a potential new subset of ETS-negative prostate cancers, defined by the presence of a fibroblast growth factor receptor (FGFR) fusion, in which the FGFR2 gene is translocated downstream of an androgen-regulated promoter, resulting in androgen-driven overexpression of FGFR2.[70] Although these FGFR fusions are rare, they have, to date, not been found to co-occur with the other subtypes described previously. In total, results described previously suggest the presence of molecular subtypes of prostate cancer, several of which are mutually exclusive and represent biologically distinct diseases. As the biology underlying these subtypes is elucidated and as therapeutic approaches are further investigated for each subtype, the hope is that physicians will eventually be able to utilize a simple molecular barcode (i.e., ETS/SPINK1/SPOP/CHD1/RAS-RAF/FGFR status) to better personalize therapy.

## EMERGING AREAS IN PROSTATE CANCER BIOLOGY AND THERAPY

Our growing understanding of prostate cancer biology has opened a variety of potential therapeutic venues (Fig. 41.5) These opportunities range from kinase inhibition to immunotherapy, which impact both the tumor and microenvironment.

### Kinase Targeting in Castration-Resistant Prostate Cancer

Multiple kinase signaling pathways beyond those listed previously have been implicated in CRPC. Examples of these pathways and targets include mesenchymal epithelial transition factor (MET) and the Src-family kinases (SFKs). MET is a transmembrane receptor tyrosine kinase activated by hepatocyte growth factor that plays a crucial role in the development of the normal prostate as well as in the progression of cancer. Activation of MET has been associated with increased proliferation, survival, motility, invasiveness, and angiogenesis in several tumor models, as well as clinical aggressiveness.[71,72] AR blockade also appears to promote the expression of MET.[73] These findings have led to a series of clinical studies exploring the utility of MET as a therapeutic target for CRPC with agents such as cabozantinib (see Fig. 41.5).

SFKs have also been implicated in the progression to CRPC. SRC, FYN, and Lck-Yes novel tyrosine kinase (LYN) have all been associated with prostate cancer progression.[74,75] In particular, SRC has been implicated as playing a role in tumorigenesis,[76] whereas FYN and LYN have been implicated in the progression of metastatic and castration-resistant disease.[74,77] Initial therapeutic trials with SFK inhibitors such as dasatinib have been difficult to interpret because the appropriate means of manipulating SFK biology in CRPC remain under investigation (see Fig. 41.5).

### Targeting Chromatin Regulatory Pathways in Castration-Resistant Prostate Cancer

Recent studies have demonstrated that chromatin regulation and remodeling leads to disease progression across a wide range of human cancers. Overexpression of the Enhancer of Zest Homolog 2 (EZH2) gene, which encodes a histone methyltransferase,

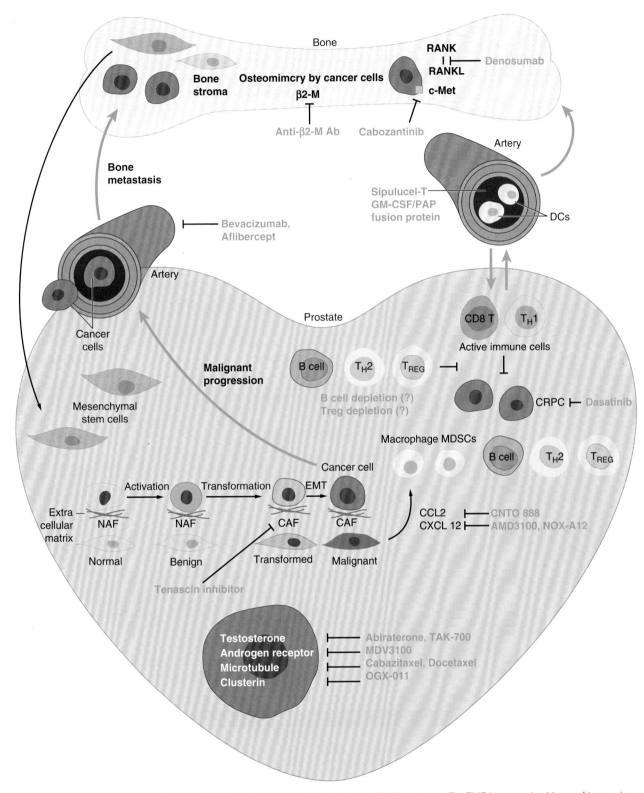

**Figure 41.5** The tumor microenvironment (TME) and agents targeting the tumor–TME interaction. The TME is a complex biome of interactions between the prostate cancer tumor cell and various environmental components, including cancer-associated fibroblasts (CAF) and mesenchymal stem cells (MSC) in the local prostatic stroma, as well as bone stromal cells and MSCs in the metastatic TME in areas such as bone. The TME also includes neovasculature and the immune microenvironment. Inhibitors are shown in *red* at respective sites of action. Events in the TME that promote metastasis include osteomimicry by cancer cells, transformation of normal fibroblasts to protumorigenic/prometastatic CAFs, and alternations of endothelial cell function allowing for vascular invasion and hematogenous dissemination of tumor cells. β2-M, beta-2 microglobulin; DC, dendritic cells; EMT, epithelial-to-mesenchymal transition; NAF, normal fibroblast; RANKL, receptor-activated nuclear factor κB (Ligand); Treg, T-regulatory cells.

is associated with aggressive and metastatic disease in prostate cancer.[78] Studies have shown that EZH2 may function via silencing gene expression, or alternatively, by activating AR and other transcription factors.[79,80] EZH2 inhibitors are currently being developed as a potential therapeutic strategy for advanced prostate cancer.

## Tumor Microenvironment

It has become increasingly clear that the tumor microenvironment (TME) plays a crucial role in disease initiation and progression.[81–83] Reactive stroma, including fibroblasts, endothelial cells, osteoblasts, osteoclasts, and mesenchymal stem cells, have been associated with prostate cancer development and tumorigenesis (see Fig. 41.5).[84,85] Studies of human prostate cancers have revealed a loss of transforming growth factor beta type receptor 2 (TGFβRII) in cancer-associated fibroblasts. In a murine model, stromal TGFβRII knockout alone results in the development of spontaneous prostate cancers.[86]

The TME has become an target for newer therapies because host stromal cells do not exhibit the same high level of genetic instability as the tumor.[87] Considerable work has been done in the area of angiogenesis. A greater emphasis is now placed on stromal and mesenchymal cells and their influence on epithelial differentiation and even the prostate cancer cell of origin.[88,89] As an example, osteoclast inhibition with bisphosphonates and receptor-activated nuclear factor κB (RANKL) inhibitors has been shown to yield clinical benefit. With the emergence of therapies active on the immune microenvironment, this field is continues to expand (see Fig. 41.5).

## Immunotherapy

Unlike other forms of anticancer therapy, immune-based treatments have the capacity to adapt to changes in the tumor. This biological advantage bears particular importance given the emerging recognition of progressive temporal-spatial heterogeneity and chromoplexy in cancer.[6,90] The dendritic cell–based therapy, sipuleucel-T, was the first successful demonstration of immunotherapy in prostate cancer. This relatively nontoxic treatment used prostate alkaline phosphatase as a primary target and provided a survival benefit for men with asymptomatic metastic CRPC (mCRPC).[91] A number of alternative immunotherapy strategies have gone into advanced development, such as the PSA-directed prime and boost vaccinia/fowlpox ProstVac approach developed by the National Cancer Institute (NCI).[92] This approach uses PSA as an antigen and employs three costimulatory molecule transgenes: *B7.1*, *ICAM-1*, and *LFA-3*. CTLA-4 and suppression of the PD-L1/PD-1

interaction have also been identified as potentially useful immune strategies in metastatic CRPC.[93,94] Although these approaches have great appeal, there remains an absence of biomarkers to measure the degree of benefit that such therapies may provide.

## Neuroendocrine Prostate Cancer

The use of more potent suppressors of AR activation has raised concerns over neuroendocrine prostate cancer. There is growing concern that AR suppression may foster the development of this particularly aggressive subtype of prostate cancer. The approach to these cancers has been hampered by a lack of consensus on nomenclature. The term *neuroendocrine* has been used to describe those cancers that are pure small-cell carcinomas to those clearly differentiated with biochemical features suggesting some level of neuroendocrine differentiation (e.g., expression of synaptophysin or chromogranin A).

Small-cell carcinoma composes only 0.5% to 2% of all primary tumors.[95] This is a pathologic diagnosis histologically marked by small round cells with no glandular architecture. Molecularly, this disease is characterized by the deletion of *RB1*,[96] increased MET and RANKL activation,[97] and amplification of *AURKA* and *MYCN*.[98] Non–small-cell neuroendocrine cancers are also clinically identified. The importance of these findings and their impact on therapeutic approaches remains an area where research is needed.

## Noncoding RNAs

Recent data from the ENCODE sequencing consortium has suggested that, although up to 70% of the genome is transcribed into RNA, only 1.5% of the genome represents protein-coding genes.[99] Thus, the majority of the RNA in each cell represents *noncoding* RNAs. Of all the different noncoding RNA species, genes encoding long noncoding RNAs (lncRNAs) are most similar to protein-coding genes, based on common features, such as transcription by RNA polymerase II, polyadenylation, the presence of multiple exons, similar splicing patterns, and similar epigenetic signatures.[100] Recent sequencing efforts have resulted in the discovery of lncRNAs that are enriched in prostate cancer compared to normal tissue. These differentially expressed lncRNAs include prostate cancer associated transcript 1 (PCAT-1), which downregulates BRCA2 to confer *BRCAness* and sensitivity to PARP1 inhibitors in preclinical models of prostate cancer,[101] as well as second chromosome locus associated with prostate 1 (SChLAP1), which promotes metastases by antagonizing the Switch/Sucrose NonFermentable (SWI-SNF) epigenetic complex.[102] As RNA targeting strategies improve, it is likely that future biomarker and therapeutic strategies will begin to focus on these noncoding RNA elements.

# REFERENCES

1. Siegel R, Ma J, Zou Z, et al. Cancer statistics, 2014. *CA Cancer J Clin* 2014;64:9–29.
2. Jemal A, Bray F, Center MM, et al. Global cancer statistics. *CA Cancer J Clin* 2011;61:69–90.
3. Barbieri CE, Baca SC, Lawrence MS, et al. Exome sequencing identifies recurrent SPOP, FOXA1 and MED12 mutations in prostate cancer. *Nat Genet* 2012;44:685–689.
4. Berger MF, Lawrence MS, Demichelis F, et al. The genomic complexity of primary human prostate cancer. *Nature* 2011;470:214–220.
5. Grasso CS, Wu YM, Robinson DR, et al. The mutational landscape of lethal castration-resistant prostate cancer. *Nature* 2012;487:239–243.
6. Baca SC, Prandi D, Lawrence MS, et al. Punctuated evolution of prostate cancer genomes. *Cell* 2013;153:666–677.
7. Weischenfeldt J, Simon R, Feuerbach L, et al. Integrative genomic analyses reveal an androgen-driven somatic alteration landscape in early-onset prostate cancer. *Cancer Cell* 2013;23:159–170.
8. Tomlins SA, Rhodes DR, Perner S, et al. Recurrent fusion of TMPRSS2 and ETS transcription factor genes in prostate cancer. *Science* 2005;310:644–648.
9. Kumar-Sinha C, Tomlins SA, Chinnaiyan AM. Recurrent gene fusions in prostate cancer. *Nat Rev Cancer* 2008;8:497–511.
10. Rubin MA, Maher CA, Chinnaiyan AM. Common gene rearrangements in prostate cancer. *J Clin Oncol* 2011;29:3659–3668.
11. Palanisamy N, Ateeq B, Kalyana-Sundaram S, et al. Rearrangements of the RAF kinase pathway in prostate cancer, gastric cancer and melanoma. *Nat Med* 2010;16:793–798.
12. Feldman BJ, Feldman D. The development of androgen-independent prostate cancer. *Nat Rev Cancer* 2001;1:34–45.
13. Knudsen BS, Vasioukhin V. Mechanisms of prostate cancer initiation and progression. *Adv Cancer Res* 2010;109:1–50.
14. Abate-Shen C, Shen MM, Gelmann E. Integrating differentiation and cancer: the Nkx3.1 homeobox gene in prostate organogenesis and carcinogenesis. *Differentiation* 2008;76:717–727.
15. Gurel B, Ali TZ, Montgomery EA, et al. NKX3.1 as a marker of prostatic origin in metastatic tumors. *Am J Surg Pathol* 2010;34:1097–1105.
16. Bhatia-Gaur R, Donjacour AA, Sciavolino PJ, et al. Roles for Nkx3.1 in prostate development and cancer. *Genes Dev* 1999;13:966–977.

17. Bova GS, Carter BS, Bussemakers MJ, et al. Homozygous deletion and frequent allelic loss of chromosome 8p22 loci in human prostate cancer. *Cancer Res* 1993;53:3869–3873.

18. Thangapazham R, Saenz F, Katta S, et al. Loss of the NKX3.1 tumor suppressor promotes the TMPRSS2-ERG fusion gene expression in prostate cancer. *BMC Cancer* 2014;14–16.

19. Kaestner KH. The FoxA factors in organogenesis and differentiation. *Curr Opin Genet Dev* 2010;20:527–532.

20. Augello MA, Hickey TE, Knudsen KE. FOXA1: master of steroid receptor function in cancer. *Embo J* 2011;30:3885–3894.

21. Nelson WG, De Marzo AM, Isaacs WB. Prostate cancer. *N Engl J Med* 2003; 349:366–381.

22. Chang KH, Li R, Papari-Zareei M, et al. Dihydrotestosterone synthesis bypasses testosterone to drive castration-resistant prostate cancer. *Proc Natl Acad Sci U S A* 2011;108:13728–13733.

23. Li R, Evaul K, Sharma KK, et al. Abiraterone inhibits 3beta-hydroxysteroid dehydrogenase: a rationale for increasing drug exposure in castration-resistant prostate cancer. *Clin Cancer Res* 2012;18:3571–3579.

24. Mostaghel EA, Page ST, Lin DW, et al. Intraprostatic androgens and androgen-regulated gene expression persist after testosterone suppression: therapeutic implications for castration-resistant prostate cancer. *Cancer Res* 2007;67: 5033–5041.

25. Montgomery RB, Mostaghel EA, Vessella R, et al. Maintenance of intratumoral androgens in metastatic prostate cancer: a mechanism for castration-resistant tumor growth. *Cancer Res* 2008;68:4447–4454.

26. Holzbeierlein J, Lal P, LaTulippe E, et al. Gene expression analysis of human prostate carcinoma during hormonal therapy identifies androgen-responsive genes and mechanisms of therapy resistance. *Am J Pathol* 2004;164:217–227.

27. Stanbrough M, Bubley GJ, Ross K, et al. Increased expression of genes converting adrenal androgens to testosterone in androgen-independent prostate cancer. *Cancer Res* 2006;66:2815–2825.

28. Hofland J, van Weerden WM, Dits NF, et al. Evidence of limited contributions for intratumoral steroidogenesis in prostate cancer. *Cancer Res* 2010;70: 1256–1264.

29. Kelly WK, Scher HI. Prostate specific antigen decline after antiandrogen withdrawal: the flutamide withdrawal syndrome. *J Urol* 1993;149:607–609.

30. Tran C, Ouk S, Clegg NJ, et al. Development of a second-generation antiandrogen for treatment of advanced prostate cancer. *Science* 2009;324: 787–790.

31. Chen CD, Welsbie DS, Tran C, et al. Molecular determinants of resistance to antiandrogen therapy. *Nat Med* 2004;10:33–39.

32. Scher HI, Fizazi K, Saad F, et al. Increased survival with enzalutamide in prostate cancer after chemotherapy. *N Engl J Med* 2012;367:1187–1197.

33. Myung JK, Banuelos CA, Fernandez JG, et al. An androgen receptor N-terminal domain antagonist for treating prostate cancer. *J Clin Invest* 2013; 123:2948–2960.

34. Waltering KK, Helenius MA, Sahu B, et al. Increased expression of androgen receptor sensitizes prostate cancer cells to low levels of androgens. *Cancer Res* 2009;69:8141–8149.

35. Taplin ME, Balk SP. Androgen receptor: a key molecule in the progression of prostate cancer to hormone independence. *J Cell Biochem* 2004;91:483–490.

36. Linja MJ, Savinainen KJ, Saramaki OR, et al. Amplification and overexpression of androgen receptor gene in hormone-refractory prostate cancer. *Cancer Res* 2001;61:3550–3555.

37. Giubellino A, Bullova P, Nolting S, et al. Combined inhibition of mTORC1 and mTORC2 signaling pathways is a promising therapeutic option in inhibiting pheochromocytoma tumor growth: in vitro and in vivo studies in female athymic nude mice. *Endocrinology* 2013;154:646–655.

38. Yuan X, Cai C, Chen S, et al. Androgen receptor functions in castration-resistant prostate cancer and mechanisms of resistance to new agents targeting the androgen axis. *Oncogene* 2014;33:2815–2825.

39. Dehm SM, Schmidt LJ, Heemers HV, et al. Splicing of a novel androgen receptor exon generates a constitutively active androgen receptor that mediates prostate cancer therapy resistance. *Cancer Res* 2008;68:5469–5477.

40. Thadani-Mulero M, Portella L, Sun S, et al. Androgen receptor splice variants determine taxane sensitivity in prostate cancer. *Cancer Res* 2014;74: 2270–2282.

41. Li Y, Chan SC, Brand LJ, et al. Androgen receptor splice variants mediate enzalutamide resistance in castration-resistant prostate cancer cell lines. *Cancer Res* 2013;73:483–489.

42. Carver BS, Chapinski C, Wongvipat J, et al. Reciprocal feedback regulation of PI3K and androgen receptor signaling in PTEN-deficient prostate cancer. *Cancer Cell* 2011;19:575–586.

43. Mulholland DJ, Tran LM, Li Y, et al. Cell autonomous role of PTEN in regulating castration-resistant prostate cancer growth. *Cancer Cell* 2011;19: 792–804.

44. Taylor BS, Schultz N, Hieronymus H, et al. Integrative genomic profiling of human prostate cancer. *Cancer Cell* 2010;18:11–22.

45. Cairns P, Okami K, Halachmi S, et al. Frequent inactivation of PTEN/MMAC1 in primary prostate cancer. *Cancer Res* 1997;57:4997–5000.

46. Carver BS, Tran J, Gopalan A, et al. Aberrant ERG expression cooperates with loss of PTEN to promote cancer progression in the prostate. *Nat Genet* 2009;41:619–624.

47. Chen M, Pratt CP, Zeeman ME, et al. Identification of PHLPP1 as a tumor suppressor reveals the role of feedback activation in PTEN-mutant prostate cancer progression. *Cancer Cell* 2011;20:173–186.

48. McMenamin ME, Soung P, Perera S, et al. Loss of PTEN expression in paraffin-embedded primary prostate cancer correlates with high Gleason score and advanced stage. *Cancer Res* 1999;59:4291–4296.

49. Krohn A, Diedler T, Burkhardt L, et al. Genomic deletion of PTEN is associated with tumor progression and early PSA recurrence in ERG fusion-positive and fusion-negative prostate cancer. *Am J Pathol* 2012;181:401–412.

50. Sun X, Huang J, Homma T, et al. Genetic alterations in the PI3K pathway in prostate cancer. *Anticancer Res* 2009;29:1739–1743.

51. Lapointe J, Li C, Giacomini CP, et al. Genomic profiling reveals alternative genetic pathways of prostate tumorigenesis. *Cancer Res* 2007;67:8504–8510.

52. Udayakumar T, Shareef MM, Diaz DA, et al. The E2F1/Rb and p53/MDM2 pathways in DNA repair and apoptosis: understanding the crosstalk to develop novel strategies for prostate cancer radiotherapy. *Semin Radiat Oncol* 2010;20:258–266.

53. Sharma A, Yeow WS, Ertel A, et al. The retinoblastoma tumor suppressor controls androgen signaling and human prostate cancer progression. *J Clin Invest* 2010;120:4478–4492.

54. Tomlins SA, Laxman B, Dhanasekaran SM, et al. Distinct classes of chromosomal rearrangements create oncogenic ETS gene fusions in prostate cancer. *Nature* 2007;448:595–599.

55. Tomlins SA, Laxman B, Varambally S, et al. Role of the TMPRSS2-ERG gene fusion in prostate cancer. *Neoplasia* 2008;10:177–188.

56. Attard G, de Bono JS, Clark J, et al. Studies of TMPRSS2-ERG gene fusions in diagnostic trans-rectal prostate biopsies. *Clin Cancer Res* 2010;16:1340; author reply.

57. Demichelis F, Fall K, Perner S, et al. TMPRSS2:ERG gene fusion associated with lethal prostate cancer in a watchful waiting cohort. *Oncogene* 2007; 26:4596–4599.

58. Lin DW, Newcomb LF, Brown EC, et al. Urinary TMPRSS2:ERG and PCA3 in an active surveillance cohort: results from a baseline analysis in the Canary Prostate Active Surveillance Study. *Clin Cancer Res* 2013;19:2442–2450.

59. Pettersson A, Graff RE, Bauer SR, et al. The TMPRSS2:ERG rearrangement, ERG expression, and prostate cancer outcomes: a cohort study and meta-analysis. *Cancer Epidemiol Biomarkers Prev* 2012;21:1497–1509.

60. Borno ST, Fischer A, Kerick M, et al. Genome-wide DNA methylation events in TMPRSS2-ERG fusion-negative prostate cancers implicate an EZH2-dependent mechanism with miR-26a hypermethylation. *Cancer Discov* 2012;2:1024–1035.

61. Demichelis F, Setlur SR, Beroukhim R, et al. Distinct genomic aberrations associated with ERG rearranged prostate cancer. *Genes Chromosomes Cancer* 2009;48:366–380.

62. Tomlins SA, Rhodes DR, Yu J, et al. The role of SPINK1 in ETS rearrangement-negative prostate cancers. *Cancer Cell* 2008;13:519–528.

63. Bakin RE, Gioeli D, Sikes RA, et al. Constitutive activation of the Ras/mitogen-activated protein kinase signaling pathway promotes androgen hypersensitivity in LNCaP prostate cancer cells. *Cancer Res* 2003;63:1981–1989.

64. Lindberg J, Klevebring D, Liu W, et al. Exome sequencing of prostate cancer supports the hypothesis of independent tumour origins. *Eur Urol* 2013;63: 347–353.

65. Geng C, He B, Xu L, et al. Prostate cancer-associated mutations in speckle-type POZ protein (SPOP) regulate steroid receptor coactivator 3 protein turnover. *Proc Natl Acad Sci U S A* 2013;110:6997–7002.

66. An J, Wang C, Deng Y, et al. Destruction of full-length androgen receptor by wild-type SPOP, but not prostate-cancer-associated mutants. *Cell Rep* 2014;6:657–669.

67. Baca SC, Prandi D, Lawrence MS, et al. Punctuated evolution of prostate cancer genomes. *Cell* 2013;153:666–677.

68. Liu W, Lindberg J, Sui G, et al. Identification of novel CHD1-associated collaborative alterations of genomic structure and functional assessment of CHD1 in prostate cancer. *Oncogene* 2012;31:3939–3948.

69. Ateeq B, Tomlins SA, Laxman B, et al. Therapeutic targeting of SPINK1-positive prostate cancer. *Sci Transl Med* 2011;3:72ra17.

70. Wu YM, Su F, Kalyana-Sundaram S, et al. Identification of targetable FGFR gene fusions in diverse cancers. *Cancer Discov* 2013;3:636–647.

71. Knudsen BS, Gmyrek GA, Inra J, et al. High expression of the Met receptor in prostate cancer metastasis to bone. *Urology* 2002;60:1113–1117.

72. Zhang S, Zhau HE, Osunkoya AO, et al. Vascular endothelial growth factor regulates myeloid cell leukemia-1 expression through neuropilin-1-dependent activation of c-MET signaling in human prostate cancer cells. *Mol Cancer* 2010;9–9.

73. Verras M, Lee J, Xue H, et al. The androgen receptor negatively regulates the expression of c-Met: implications for a novel mechanism of prostate cancer progression. *Cancer Res* 2007;67:967–975.

74. Jensen AR, David SY, Liao C, et al. Fyn is downstream of the HGF/MET signaling axis and affects cellular shape and tropism in PC3 cells. *Clin Cancer Res* 2011;17:3112–3122.

75. Varkaris A, Katsiampoura AD, Araujo JC, et al. Src signaling pathways in prostate cancer. *Cancer Metastasis Rev* 2014;33(2–3):595–606.

76. Cai H, Smith DA, Memarzadeh S, et al. Differential transformation capacity of Src family kinases during the initiation of prostate cancer. *Proc Natl Acad Sci U S A* 2011;108:6579–6584.

77. Park SI, Zhang J, Phillips KA, et al. Targeting SRC family kinases inhibits growth and lymph node metastases of prostate cancer in an orthotopic nude mouse model. *Cancer Res* 2008;68:3323–3333.

78. Varambally S, Dhanasekaran SM, Zhou M, et al. The polycomb group protein EZH2 is involved in progression of prostate cancer. *Nature* 2002;419:624–629.

79. Xu K, Wu ZJ, Groner AC, et al. EZH2 oncogenic activity in castration-resistant prostate cancer cells is Polycomb-independent. *Science* 2012;338:1465–1469.

80. Asangani IA, Ateeq B, Cao Q, et al. Characterization of the EZH2-MMSET histone methyltransferase regulatory axis in cancer. *Mol Cell* 2013;49:80–93.

81. Barron DA, Rowley DR. The reactive stroma microenvironment and prostate cancer progression. *Endocr Relat Cancer* 2012;19:R187–R204.

82. Kiskowski MA, Jackson RS 2nd, Banerjee J, et al. Role for stromal heterogeneity in prostate tumorigenesis. *Cancer Res* 2011;71:3459–3470.

83. Chung LW, Baseman A, Assikis V, et al. Molecular insights into prostate cancer progression: the missing link of tumor microenvironment. *J Urol* 2005;173:10–20.

84. Camacho DF, Pienta KJ. Disrupting the networks of cancer. *Clin Cancer Res* 2012;18:2801–2808.

85. Msaouel P, Nandikolla G, Pneumaticos SG, et al. Bone microenvironment-targeted manipulations for the treatment of osteoblastic metastasis in castration-resistant prostate cancer. *Expert Opin Investig Drugs* 2013;22:1385–1400.

86. Bhowmick NA, Chytil A, Plieth D, et al. TGF-beta signaling in fibroblasts modulates the oncogenic potential of adjacent epithelia. *Science* 2004;303:848–851.

87. Josson S, Sharp S, Sung SY, et al. Tumor-stromal interactions influence radiation sensitivity in epithelial- versus mesenchymal-like prostate cancer cells. *J Oncol* 2010;2010.

88. Goldstein AS, Witte ON. Does the microenvironment influence the cell types of origin for prostate cancer? *Genes Dev* 2013;27:1539–1544.

89. Wang R, Sun X, Wang CY, et al. Spontaneous cancer-stromal cell fusion as a mechanism of prostate cancer androgen-independent progression. *PLoS One* 2012;7:e42653.

90. Gerlinger M, Rowan AJ, Horswell S, et al. Intratumor heterogeneity and branched evolution revealed by multiregion sequencing. *N Engl J Med* 2012;366:883–892.

91. Kantoff PW, Higano CS, Shore ND, et al. Sipuleucel-T immunotherapy for castration-resistant prostate cancer. *N Engl J Med* 2010;363:411–422.

92. Kantoff PW, Schuetz TJ, Blumenstein BA, et al. Overall survival analysis of a phase II randomized controlled trial of a Poxviral-based PSA-targeted immunotherapy in metastatic castration-resistant prostate cancer. *J Clin Oncol* 2010;28:1099–1105.

93. Sfanos KS, Bruno TC, Meeker AK, et al. Human prostate-infiltrating CD8+ T lymphocytes are oligoclonal and PD-1+. *Prostate* 2009;69:1694–1703.

94. Kwek SS, Cha E, Fong L. Unmasking the immune recognition of prostate cancer with CTLA4 blockade. *Nat Rev Cancer* 2012;12:289–297.

95. Palmgren JS, Karavadia SS, Wakefield MR. Unusual and underappreciated: small cell carcinoma of the prostate. *Semin Oncol* 2007;34:22–29.

96. Tan S, Sood A, Rahimi H, et al. Rb loss is characteristic of prostatic small cell neuroendocrine carcinoma. *Clin Cancer Res* 2014;20:890–903.

97. Chu GC, Zhau HE, Wang R, et al. RANK- and c-Met-mediated signal network promotes prostate cancer metastatic colonization. *Endocr Relat Cancer* 2014;21:311–326.

98. Beltran H, Rickman DS, Park K, et al. Molecular characterization of neuroendocrine prostate cancer and identification of new drug targets. *Cancer Discov* 2011;1:487–495.

99. Bernstein BE, Birney E, Dunham I, et al. An integrated encyclopedia of DNA elements in the human genome. *Nature* 2012;489:57–74.

100. Prensner JR, Chinnaiyan AM. The emergence of lncRNAs in cancer biology. *Cancer Discov* 2011;1:391–407.

101. Prensner JR, Chen W, Iyer MK, et al. PCAT-1, a long noncoding RNA, regulates BRCA2 and controls homologous recombination in cancer. *Cancer Res* 2014;74:1651–1660.

102. Prensner JR, Iyer MK, Sahu A, et al. The long noncoding RNA SChLAP1 promotes aggressive prostate cancer and antagonizes the SWI/SNF complex. *Nat Genet* 2013;45:1392–1398.

# 42 Cancer of the Prostate

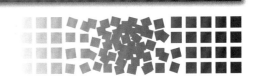

Howard I. Scher, Peter T. Scardino, and Michael J. Zelefsky

## INTRODUCTION

The approach to prostate cancer diagnosis and treatment has changed dramatically across the spectrum of the illness. Recognizing the need to reduce overdiagnosis and overtreatment of clinically insignificant cancers, new diagnostic algorithms have become available to identify which men have a higher likelihood of having a clinically significant cancer and benefit from early detection and early treatment. New clinical and biologic biomarkers are being validated to determine, once localized prostate cancer is diagnosed, which tumors can be optimally treated using an active surveillance (AS) approach that closely monitors the cancer—based on the likelihood that the tumor will or has metastasized, putting the patient at risk for an impaired quality of life (QOL) and a shortened life expectancy. The techniques of surgery have evolved and more patients are being treated with robot-assisted approaches with the aims of reducing morbidity and shortening hospital stays without compromising cancer control. The ability to deliver higher doses of radiation safely has improved disease control rates without compromising long-term QOL. The past 4 years have also seen unparalleled progress in the treatment of castration-resistant metastatic tumors, as five agents with different mechanisms of action were proven to prolong life. At the same time that more patients and physicians recognize there are effective treatments for metastatic disease, these agents are also being tested earlier in minimal disease settings where they have the potential to provide even greater benefit.

In contrast to other tumor types, the paradigm of early detection leading to increased cure rates must be cautiously applied to prostate cancer. The widespread use of prostate-specific antigen (PSA)-based detection strategies has resulted, unfortunately, in increased treatment of clinically insignificant cancers, to the point where the morbidity and mortality associated with making a diagnosis and the therapy utilized to treat it can exceed that of the cancer itself. The high prevalence of prostate cancer in the general population, coupled with a natural history that can range from a few years to decades, mandates a different framework than that provided by the more traditional tumor, node, and metastasis (TNM) staging. There are also many prostate cancers from which a relapse after primary treatment does not require any intervention because the probability is low that the cancer will become metastatic, symptomatic, or lethal.

Many of these issues are addressed by describing the spectrum of the disease as a series of clinical states, ranging from prediagnosis to the lethal metastatic castration-resistant phenotype (Fig. 42.1).[1] Each state represents a milestone in the disease that is easily recognizable by patients and physicians, enabling them to define therapeutic objectives based on the manifestations present at a particular point in time or the likelihood that specific disease manifestations might occur in the future. The utility of specific diagnostic tests needed to maximally inform a treatment decision for a specific context of use at a particular point in time is considered analogously; in short, how the performance and the result of the test guide management. This chapter will refer throughout to this clinical states model.

## INCIDENCE AND ETIOLOGY

### Incidence and Mortality

In 2014, some 233,000 men in the United States are expected to be diagnosed with prostate cancer and 29,480 to die of the disease,[2] accounting for 14% of all new cancers in men and women[3] and 11% of male cancer deaths.[4] Over the past decade, men in the United States had a 15.4% chance of being diagnosed with prostate cancer and a 2.7% chance of dying of it.[2] Worldwide, there were an estimated 899,100 new cases and 258,100 deaths from prostate cancer in 2008.[5] Histologic cancers, found in the prostate at autopsy in men who die of other causes, are even more common, and their age-adjusted frequency varies relatively little from country to country, about 2.4-fold.[6] In contrast, the mortality rate from prostate cancer varies by 10.8-fold among different countries, suggesting different mechanisms of carcinogenesis and progression, and supporting the concept of distinct "indolent" and "aggressive" forms of the disease.[6–8] There are significant age, ethnic, racial, geographic, and familial differences in incidence and mortality rates.[9]

### Risk Factors

#### Age

Clinically detected prostate cancer is rare before age 40, but then the incidence increases with age faster than that of any other cancer, and continues to rise through the ninth decade of life. Histologic evidence of invasive cancer can be found in the prostates of men as early as the third decade of life, and its prevalence increases dramatically with age to reach 50% to 60% by age 90. As life expectancy increases throughout the world, morbidity and mortality from prostate cancer will impose increasing burdens in developing countries.[5]

#### Family History and Genetic Susceptibility

A family history of prostate cancer increases the risk that a man will develop the disease. The level of risk when a family member is affected is similar in breast and prostate cancers. Men with a first-degree relative with prostate cancer have a 2- to 3-fold increased risk, and those with two or more first-degree relatives affected have a 5- to 11-fold increased risk compared with the general population.[10] Nevertheless, familial factors have been thought to play a role in only 11% of prostate cancers, although studies of twins suggest that inherited factors may be involved in as many as 42% of all cases.[11] While over 70 risk alleles (single nucleotide polymorphisms [SNP]) have been associated with prostate cancer in genome-wide association studies, few are associated with the risk of aggressive or lethal cancer. Many such SNPs are in genes that code for PSA or related kallikreins, blood levels of which are widely used for diagnosis.[12] For these SNPs, the increased risk is for a diagnosis of prostate cancer, not metastases or death from the disease. Several high-penetrance mutated genes have been identified, such

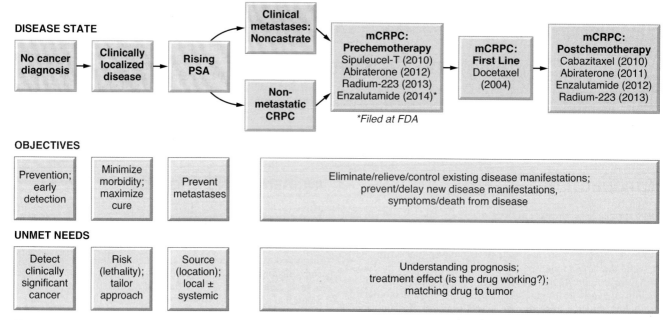

**Figure 42.1** Clinical states model of prostate cancer progression. *Green boxes* indicate castration-resistant prostate cancer (CRPC) and *blue* indicate noncastrate disease. PSA, prostate-specific antigen; mCA RPC, metastatic castration-resistant prostate cancer. (Modified from Scher HI, Heller G. Clinical states in prostate cancer: towards a dynamic model of disease progression. *Urology* 2000;55:323–327.)

as HOX13B, which are more common in patients with early-onset and familial disease, but this variant is rare (occurring in 0.1% of the population) and it is not associated with the lethal form of the disease.[13] In contrast, men who carry BRCA2 mutations are more likely to develop early-onset prostate cancer, which is more likely to be aggressive and lethal.[14]

### Race and Ethnicity

The incidence and frequency of diagnosed clinical cancers are similar in most Western countries, with the highest age-adjusted mortality rates in Scandinavia and significantly lower rates in non-Western countries. Both genetic susceptibility and exposure to causative environmental factors contribute to these variations.

Men of African ancestry in the United States and Caribbean have the highest incidence of prostate cancer in the world, with striking differences in incidence (1.8-fold) and mortality (2.4-fold) relative to American men of European descent. African American men are diagnosed at a younger age and have higher tumor burdens within each stage category,[15] a two-fold higher frequency of metastatic disease at presentation,[16] and lower survival rates.[17] Incidence and mortality rates are significantly lower for Americans of Asian descent and somewhat lower for those of Hispanic descent.

Environmental factors also affect mortality risk.[7] Asians who immigrate to the United States have a higher incidence of and mortality from the disease than in their countries of origin, which increases with each succeeding generation, but remains below the rates in men of African or European descent.[18]

### Other Risk Factors

Diet, Supplements, and Lifestyle Factors. The increased incidence and mortality from prostate cancer evident in immigrants moving from low- to high-risk countries supports an important role for environmental in addition to genetic risk factors. Many epidemiologic studies support an association between high fat intake and breast, colon, and prostate cancer incidence and mortality.[19,20] Adult obesity has been associated with aggressive prostate cancer, adverse outcomes after therapy, and increased mortality.[11,21,22] The risk of death from prostate cancer has been reported to increase

15% to 20% for each 5 kg/m² increase in body mass index (BMI).[23] Among men diagnosed with prostate cancer, the risk of death from the disease is significantly associated with increased BMI (1.5-fold for overweight men and 2.7-fold for obese men).[24] Physical activity may reduce the risk of mortality from prostate cancer; the data are inconsistent for development of the disease, but convincing once the diagnosis has been established.[25] Smoking has not been shown to alter incidence rates, but it may be associated with the risk of prostate cancer death, especially when assessed in men after diagnosis.[25]

Despite many indications that certain micronutrients, minerals, and vitamins have a protective effect on the development of prostate cancer or mortality from the disease, firm evidence is sparse. In the large Selenium and Vitamin E Cancer Prevention Trial (SELECT), vitamin E and selenium, alone or in combination, failed to reduce the incidence of prostate cancer. In fact, men who took vitamin E alone may have had a greater risk of the disease,[26] although there is some suggestion that aggressive, potentially lethal cancer may be reduced among smokers taking vitamin E supplements.[27] There is no evidence that ingestion of calcium or administration of vitamin D affects incidence or mortality from prostate cancer. Diets rich in tomato-based products, which contain high amounts of carotenoids and lycopene, may reduce the risk of advanced prostate cancer.[28,29]

Alcohol use, blood group, body hair distribution, sexual activity, urban versus rural residence, and vasectomy do not affect risk.[30] There are no data supporting a viral origin of prostate cancer.[31]

### Prevention

While the evidence is incomplete and there are no large intervention trials addressing the role of diet and exercise in preventing prostate cancer, it is reasonable to recommend a low-fat diet, regular exercise, and maintenance of a normal BMI as likely having a modest effect in reducing the risk of developing prostate cancer. More evidence suggests there may be some benefit for such lifestyle changes after the diagnosis of prostate cancer is established.[11,21,22]

Finasteride, a competitive inhibitor of type II 5α-reductase (5αRI) that blocks the conversion of testosterone to dihydrotestosterone (DHT) within prostatic cells, is a safe and effective drug that reduces the size of the prostate and relieves voiding symptoms in men with benign prostatic hyperplasia (BPH). Hence, it was logical to test the hypothesis that finasteride, or other 5αRIs, could prevent prostate cancer. The Prostate Cancer Prevention Trial (PCPT) randomly assigned 18,882 men, age 55 years or older, who had a normal digital rectal examination (DRE) and PSA, to receive finasteride or placebo over a 7-year period.[32] Finasteride reduced by 25% the risk of detecting prostate cancer on biopsy (either end-of-study biopsy or one ordered during study "for cause"). Toxicity was low, but there were more high-grade cancers (Gleason score ≥7) in the finasteride group.[33] Many subsequent analyses strongly suggested that the small increase in high-grade cancers was probably a detection artifact resulting from the 20% shrinkage of the prostate by the drug,[34] and there were no differences in long-term survival in either arm.[35]

In a separate randomized trial (REDUCE), the dual 5αRI dutasteride also reduced the detection rate of cancer by 23%.[36] However, the US Food and Drug Administration (FDA) conducted an extensive review of the data from the PCPT trial and a reanalysis of the biopsy specimens from the REDUCE trial after Gleason grades were reassigned using contemporary criteria.[37] The FDA reviewers agreed that while both 5αRIs reduced the risk of a prostate cancer diagnosis, the effect was seen only among low-grade cancers (Gleason score ≤6), and there was a small (0.5%) but significant absolute increase in the risk of the highest-grade cancers (Gleason score 8 to 10). The FDA concluded that the tradeoff for using a 5αRI in healthy, asymptomatic men would be the occurrence of one additional high-grade cancer for every three or four low-grade cancers (of uncertain clinical potential) prevented, and recommended against the approval of these drugs for chemoprevention of prostate cancer.[34]

Other agents, such as statins, metformin, and resveratrol, may have protective effects,[38] but to demonstrate their benefit will require studies focusing on populations at high risk of developing clinically significant cancers.[38] PSA levels at midlife hold great promise for identifying men most likely to benefit from aggressive prevention strategies (see "Prostate-Specific Antigen: A Powerful Tool For Risk Stratification").

## ANATOMY AND PATHOLOGY

The prostate is an exocrine organ weighing 20 g to 25 g, which consists of lobular tubuloalveolar glands that secrete fluid through ducts that empty into the prostatic urethra. The fluid comprises

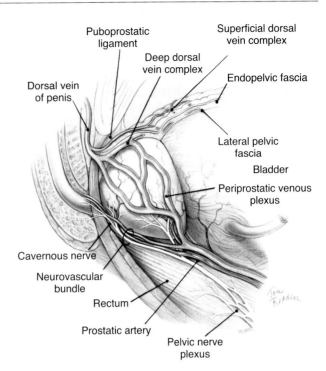

**Figure 42.2** Lateral view of normal anatomy of the pelvis. (Redrawn from Ohori M, Scardino PT. Localized prostate cancer. *Curr Probl Surg* 2002;39: 833–957.)

the bulk of seminal emissions and is rich in PSA. The prostate is located deep in the pelvis between the bladder and the external urinary sphincter, anterior to the rectum and below the pubis (Fig. 42.2).[39] The cavernous nerves, which control blood flow to the penis and hence erectile function, run from the pelvic plexus lateral to the rectum along the posterolateral prostate and external urinary sphincter to enter the corpora cavernosa. Because the prostate is located at this critical anatomic juncture, cancers of the prostate and the treatment of these cancers place urinary, sexual, and bowel function at risk.

The prostate has three anatomic zones and an anterior fibromuscular stroma (Fig. 42.3). The central zone surrounds the ejaculatory

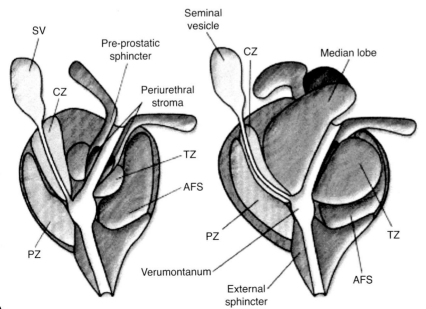

**A**    **B**

**Figure 42.3** Zonal anatomy of the prostate. **(A)** Young male with minimal transition zone hypertrophy. Note that preprostatic sphincter and periejaculatory duct zone (central zone of McLean) are clearly defined. **(B)** Older male with transition zone hypertrophy, which effaces the preprostatic sphincter and compresses the periejaculatory duct zone. SV, seminal vesicle; CZ, central zone; PZ, peripheral zone; TZ, transition zone; AFS, anterior fibromuscular stroma. (From McLaughlin PW, Troyer S, Berri S, et al. Functional anatomy of the prostate: implications for treatment planning. *Int J Radiat Oncol Biol Phys* 2005;63:479, with permission.)

ducts, the transition zone surrounds the urethra, and the peripheral zone makes up the bulk of the normal gland. The posterior peripheral zone lies against the rectum and is the area that is palpable by DRE. These zonal boundaries are indistinct in the prostate of a normal postpubescent male, but as men age the transition zone enlarges from nonmalignant growth (BPH). The frequency of malignancy in the different zones is disproportionate to the glandular tissue present. Very few cancers originate in the central zone, and only 15% originate in the transition zone; most originate in the peripheral zone.

## Patterns of Spread

Localized prostate cancer is typically multifocal, in 85% of patients. Most cancers arise near the capsule in the peripheral zone; the surrounding capsule is invaded early and frequently, in up to 80% of cancers detected clinically. Local extension occurs through the capsule (termed "focal" or "established" extracapsular extension [ECE], depending on extent, when observed in a radical prostatectomy [RP] specimen), but may also extend through defects in the capsule where the neurovascular structures and ejaculatory ducts enter the gland, or in the region of the bladder neck. Local invasion can progress to involve the seminal vesicles or the bladder, or to invade the levator muscles. Rarely does tumor invade through Denonvilliers' fascia to reach the rectal wall. Lymphatic dissemination can involve the hypogastric, obturator, external iliac, presacral, common iliac, or retroperitoneal nodes, with no consistent sentinel landing zone. Hematogenous spread most commonly involves the bones of the axial skeleton and, less commonly, the lung, liver, and other soft tissue organs. The predilection for bone seems to result from a unique bidirectional interaction between tumor cells and the marrow stroma.

## Histopathology

Two main growth-related diseases develop in the prostate: BPH, which affects both the epithelial and mesenchymal components, and cancer.[40] There is no direct etiologic relationship between BPH and cancer; they are related only by their close anatomic site of origin and high incidence in men over 40 years of age. More than 95%

of malignant tumors of the prostate are adenocarcinomas that arise in acinar and proximal ductal epithelium. Grossly, carcinoma appears as pale yellow or gray flecks of tissue coalesced into a firm, poorly defined mass that is difficult to distinguish from surrounding normal tissue. Adenocarcinomas are often multifocal, heterogeneous, and follow a papillary, cribriform, comedo, or acinar pattern. Immunohistochemistry may assist the diagnosis when atypical areas, suspicious for carcinoma, are present in a biopsy sample, particularly in the differentiation of high-grade prostatic intraepithelial neoplasia (PIN) and atypical adenomatous hyperplasias from low-grade carcinoma. A hallmark of prostate cancer is the loss of basal cells, highlighted by negative staining for basal cell markers (high molecular weight/basal-specific cytokeratin) and p63, and positive staining for alpha-methyl-CoA racemase, which is upregulated in cancer.[41]

## Pathogenesis

Prostate cancers develop from the accumulation of genetic alterations that result in an increase in cell proliferation relative to cell death, arrest differentiation, and confer the ability to invade, metastasize, and proliferate in a distant site. Histologic changes can be found in the prostates of men in their 20s, yet the diagnosis is typically made three to four decades later, which suggests that the development of the disease is a multistep process resulting from a variety of genetic and epigenetic alterations.[42] The accumulation of changes acting synergistically seems to be more critical than the order in which the alterations occur. Identifying and understanding the events has implications for control of the disease at the earliest stages of transformation, for progression to an invasive tumor, for prognostication, and for points of therapeutic attack. Men who are castrated or who become hypopituitary before the age of 40 rarely develop prostate cancer.[43] The evolution of the tumor is heavily influenced by hormonal factors; it is also influenced by environmental, infectious/inflammatory factors, and given the long history once the diagnosis is established, the response to specific treatments.

## Premalignant Lesions

The phenotypic alterations that occur during prostate carcinogenesis and progression are shown in Figure 42.4. The earliest precursor lesion is the subject of debate, as is the cell type that

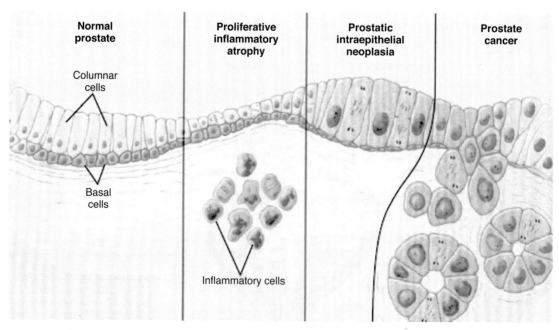

**Figure 42.4** Proliferative inflammatory atrophy is hypothesized to be a precursor to prostatic intraepithelial neoplasia, which in turn is the precursor of prostate cancer. (From Nelson WG, De Marzo AM, Isaacs WB. Prostate cancer. *N Engl J Med* 2003;349:366, with permission.)

is actually transformed. Recognizable changes begin with proliferation of cells within glands, termed PIN, often found adjacent to areas of proliferative inflammatory atrophy.[44] PIN is defined by the presence of cytologically atypical or dysplastic epithelial cells within architecturally benign-appearing acini, and is subdivided into low- and high-grade. Only high-grade PIN is considered a precursor for some invasive carcinomas.[45,46] Because high-grade PIN develops preferentially in the peripheral zone where most cancers originate, it precedes the development of cancer by 10 years or more,[47] and prostates with extensive high-grade PIN tend to have multifocal tumors. With subsequent loss of the basal cell layer surrounding prostatic glands and the development of anaplastic cellular morphology with nuclear pleomorphism and prominent nuclei, the tumor invades the basement membrane, spreads locally, and begins to metastasize. Not all lesions progress to invasive prostatic cancer during the lifetime of the host. Foci of small atypical acini that display some but not all features diagnostic of adenocarcinoma are referred to as atypical small acinar proliferation, a significant predictor of invasive cancer on subsequent prostate biopsy.[48,49] Atypical adenomatous hyperplasia, on the other hand, is not considered a malignant precursor lesion.

## Gleason Grade

For adenocarcinomas, the degree of differentiation has prognostic significance and pathologists judge biopsy specimens using the Gleason grading system, which assesses the architectural details of malignant glands under low to medium magnification.[50–52] Cytologic features under high magnification are not considered.[53,54] Five distinct patterns of growth from well- to poorly differentiated were originally described by Gleason using a scale from 1 to 5 (Fig. 42.5). Pattern 1 tumors were considered the most differentiated with discrete glandular formation, while pattern 5 lesions were the most undifferentiated with strands of disorganized, free-floating cells and complete loss of the glandular architecture. Prostate cancers tend to be heterogeneous, with two or three patterns occurring within a typical prostate. So the final Gleason *score* is the sum of the grades of the primary (largest) and secondary patterns, ranging from 2 (1 + 1) to 10 (5 + 5).

The prognostic importance of Gleason's scoring system has been difficult to improve on, but the system has been modified several times, most recently by a consensus of expert pathologists, to reflect current data and best practices.[55,56] In biopsy specimens, patterns 1 and 2 are almost never recognized, so Gleason 3 + 3 = 6 cancers are the earliest, most well-differentiated tumors currently reported by pathologists. Careful reassessment of the histologic criteria for assigning Gleason pattern 3 has resulted in reclassification

of many grade 3 cancers as grade 4, and some grade 4 variants are now considered grade 3. As a result, there has been "grade inflation" over the last decade, and the prognosis for both Gleason 3 + 3/well-differentiated cancers and for 3 + 4/moderately differentiated cancers is better than in historical series.

If three Gleason patterns are seen within a single biopsy, the accepted approach is to designate the largest area as the primary grade and the highest grade as the secondary grade to arrive at a score. So a biopsy with a large area of pattern 3, a smaller area of pattern 4, and an even smaller area of pattern 5 would be designated 3 + 5 = 8. Multiple cores are typically taken during each biopsy session, and the Gleason score assigned to the patient is the score of the highest single core. In contemporary biopsy series, 25% to 50% of tumors are low-grade (Gleason 3 + 3 = 6 or less), 40% to 70% are intermediate grade (Gleason 3 + 4 or 4 + 3 = 7), and 5% to 10% are high grade (Gleason 8 to 10).[55]

The Gleason grading system is also used to assign grade in RP specimens, with some modifications. When the pathologist inspects all areas of cancer within the prostate, it is not unusual to identify more than two Gleason patterns.[57] The original system ignored patterns that represented <5% of the cancer, but the presence of a small amount of high-grade tumor has subsequently been shown to worsen prognosis. The current recommendation is to report a tertiary grade (i.e., 3 + 4 = 7 with tertiary 5).[40] Transition zone cancers tend to have lower Gleason grades than peripheral zone cancers of comparable size, and they are less likely to extend to the seminal vesicles or lymph nodes (LN).[58] Despite its apparent complexity, the Gleason grading system has proven reliable and reproducible, it is strongly associated with prognosis, and it is accepted worldwide.

## Other Histologic Types

Although other tumors and histologic variants of adenocarcinoma rarely develop within the prostate, the most notable include ductal carcinomas (now considered a variant of poorly differentiated adenocarcinoma), small cell or neuroendocrine tumors, and transitional cell carcinomas. Pure ductal carcinomas comprise <1% of prostate cancers, but ductal elements are present in ~5%. These tumors are biologically similar to high-grade prostate adenocarcinomas, are clinically aggressive, and are associated with lower PSA levels than comparable adenocarcinomas.[59] Small cell or neuroendocrine tumors of the prostate typically comprise small, round, undifferentiated cells.[60] Distinguishing these tumors from lymphomas or round cell sarcomas can be difficult without immunohistochemical analysis.[40] Neuroendocrine cells can be found in almost all adenocarcinomas, but they do not affect the biology of the tumor unless they are a large component, in which case the tumors tend to metastasize early and have a poor prognosis. The presence of neuroendocrine cells may raise serum levels of neuroendocrine markers such as chromogranin-A, and the tumors should be treated with immediate chemotherapy as well as androgen ablation (androgen deprivation therapy [ADT]). Transitional cell carcinoma of the prostate is most frequently associated with and may be an extension of bladder cancer. When found in isolation, as a primary tumor on prostate biopsy without an associated bladder cancer, transitional cell carcinoma may be confined to periurethral ducts, but often invades stroma. Treatment may require cystoprostatectomy. Malignant mesenchymal tumors make up <0.3% of prostatic neoplasms, of which rhabdomyosarcomas are most common in younger patients and leiomyosarcomas in older patients. Carcinosarcomas are defined by the coexistence of adenocarcinomas of the epithelial cells, along with malignant mesenchymal elements that have differentiated into identifiable chondrosarcoma, osteosarcoma, myosarcoma, liposarcoma, or angiosarcoma.[61] These tumors may be found in previously irradiated patients and are highly resistant to therapy. Metastatic tumors to the prostate include lymphomas, leukemias, adenocarcinomas of the lung, melanoma, seminoma, and malignant rhabdoid tumors, whereas tumors of the bladder and colon may sometimes involve the gland by direct extension.

## Gleason Pattern

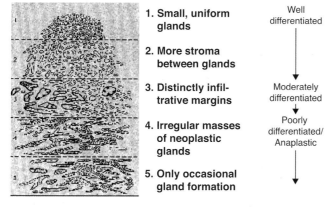

1. **Small, uniform glands** — Well differentiated

2. **More stroma between glands**

3. **Distinctly infiltrative margins** — Moderately differentiated

4. **Irregular masses of neoplastic glands** — Poorly differentiated/Anaplastic

5. **Only occasional gland formation**

**Figure 42.5** Gleason histologic grading of prostate cancer demonstrating progressive loss of glandular formation with increasing score. (Adapted from Gleason DF. Histologic grade, clinical stage, and patient age in prostate cancer. *NCI Monogr* 1988:15.)

# SCREENING

## Screening and Early Detection

The clinical states model (see Fig. 42.1) can also be applied to men without a cancer diagnosis by considering an individual's need for screening or other diagnostic tests designed to detect cancer on the likelihood that he already has or will develop a clinically significant prostate cancer. Operationally, a "clinically significant" cancer can be defined as one that, left untreated, would lead to symptoms, metastases, or a premature death from cancer—but for each individual, these risks must be balanced against his competing risks of noncancer-related morbidity and mortality, and the risk of suffering harm from overtreatment or unnecessary treatment.

PSA level and DRE are commonly used for screening and early detection, although both are limited by low specificity: only one-quarter of men with an abnormal DRE or a PSA level >3 ng/ml are found to have cancer on biopsy.[62,63]

## Prostate-Specific Antigen: A Powerful Tool for Risk Stratification

PSA is a 28 kDa protein of the kallikrein family, a group of serine proteases whose genes are found on chromosome 19q13. PSA is abundant in seminal fluid, at concentrations up to 3 mg/ml, a million times higher than in serum.[64] The enzymatic activity of PSA induces liquefaction of seminal fluid and the release of mobile spermatozoa. PSA is synthesized in the ductal and acinar epithelium and is secreted into the lumina of the prostate gland. PSA is organ-specific but not cancer-specific; normal prostatic tissue (and BPH) produces more PSA per gram than cancer, and well-differentiated cancer produces more PSA than poorly differentiated cancer.[65] Under pathologic conditions, PSA is thought to reach the circulation through the disrupted epithelial basement membranes. Circulating levels of PSA are inherently variable, fluctuating spontaneously by 15% from year to year.[66] When cancer is present, each gram of tumor raises the serum PSA level above background by approximately 3 ng/ml, whereas each gram of BPH contributes an average of only 0.3 ng/ml. Thus, there is considerable overlap in values between patients with cancer and those with benign conditions such as BPH and prostatitis. Acute urinary retention, urethral catheterization, urinary tract infection, and prostatic manipulation by needle biopsy, or transurethral resection of the prostate (TURP) may raise serum PSA levels dramatically. Performance of DRE does not.

A commonly used threshold for a normal PSA level in adult men is 4.0 ng/ml. But there is no "normal" level; the risk of cancer rises directly with PSA levels as a continuum.[67] PSA levels in healthy men vary with age. The population median PSA at age 45 to 50 is 0.6 ng/ml (interquartile range, 0.4 to 1.0), at age 60 the median is 1.1 (interquartile range, 0.6 to 2.0), and at age 70, 1.6 (interquartile range, 0.9 to 2.6).[68–70]

PSA levels at midlife predict with remarkable accuracy the risk that a man will develop advanced prostate cancer or die of the disease.[68,70,71] For example, in the Malmö Preventive Medicine cohort of 60-year-old men followed to age 85, stored blood samples from 1981 were retrieved and analyzed for PSA. Ninety percent of deaths from prostate cancer were in men in the top quartile of PSA levels (>2 ng/ml). In contrast, the risk of death from prostate cancer was only 0.2% by age 85 for those with a PSA below median (<1.1 ng/ml) at age 60.[70] PSA levels in men as young as 44 to 50 years were also prognostic, with 81% of advanced cancers diagnosed within 30 years occurring in men with PSA levels above the median (0.65 ng/ml).[68]

In fact, PSA levels at midlife are more informative than family history or ethnicity (Table 42.1), and can be used to stratify the intensity of screening over the next two to three decades of life, an approach that could substantially reduce false-positive test results without delaying detection of potentially lethal cancers.[17,72]

**TABLE 42.1**

**Proportion of Prostate Cancer Deaths in Men Defined as at High Risk by Family History, Race, or Prostate-Specific Antigen in Middle Age**

| Risk Factor (scenario) | % High Risk/ % Death | Risk Group Size/ No. Risk Group Deaths |
|---|---|---|
| Prostate-specific antigen | 10/44 | 4.4 |
| Family history | 10/14 | 1.4 |
| African American | 12.6/28 | 2.2 |

Adapted from Vertosick EA, Poon BY, Vickers AJ. Relative value of race, family history and prostate-specific antigen as indications for early initiation of prostate cancer screening. *J Urol* 2014 [Epub ahead of print], with permission.

## Prostate-Specific Antigen for Screening

Although PSA has proved to be a valuable test for early detection, prognosis, and monitoring the response to therapy, its use for population-based screening for prostate cancer remains controversial. The widespread adoption of PSA testing in the United States shifted the stage at diagnosis away from metastases in 20% of patients in the 1980s to 5% in the 1990s, with a corresponding increase in frequency of early-state cancers that are potentially curable with surgery or radiation. Over the last two decades, the age-adjusted mortality rate for prostate cancer in the United States has declined by 42% from its peak in 1992, a more rapid decline than in any other country.[2] In the largest randomized trials, PSA screening reduced the risk of dying from prostate cancer by 21% to 44% (29% to 56% among men actually screened).[71,73] With long-term follow-up, the number needed to screen to prevent one prostate cancer death declined from 1,410 at 9 years to 293 at 14 years, and is estimated in models to be 98 over the lifetimes of men screened at ages 55 to 69.[63,71,74] The number of men who need to be diagnosed or treated (40% were managed expectantly on AS) was estimated to be 48 at 9 years, but falls to 12 at 14 years and 5 over the lifetime of men screened.[63,71,74] These numbers compare favorably with other screening programs. With mammography screening from age 50 to 70, 111 to 235 women need to be screened and 10 to 14 diagnosed to avert one death from breast cancer.[75–77] For colorectal cancer screening, 850 need to be screened with flexible sigmoidoscopy to prevent one colorectal cancer death.[78]

Nevertheless, PSA has low specificity: three of four men who have a biopsy for a PSA >3 ng/ml are not found to have cancer,[63] and 10% to 56% of those in whom cancer is found would probably have lived out their lives with no symptoms from the disease, and are therefore considered "overdetected."[79] An additional consideration is that the prostate biopsy itself carries a risk of bleeding and infection in 3% to 4% of those undergoing the procedure, which increases with the number of cores obtained. In cases where "saturation" biopsies are performed, in which upwards of 24 to 30 cores are sampled in the same session, the risk is higher and mortalities have resulted. Most cancers detected have been treated immediately with radical surgery or radiation,[80] with substantial risk of adverse effects on bowel, urinary, and sexual function.

In screening large populations, the lack of specificity of PSA leads to overdiagnosis, the discovery of incidental, clinically insignificant cancers that pose little or no immediate threat to life or health,[81] which often leads to overtreatment with accompanying morbidities that may be permanent and compromise QOL. With rare exceptions, low-risk cancers managed expectantly, as well as intermediate-risk cancers in older men, have a good prognosis when carefully observed on an "AS" protocol, rather than proceeding to immediate treatment.[82–86] AS is treatment that is designed to detect changes in the cancer that indicate it has become more aggressive and therefore requires more definitive intervention(s).

But most men with low-risk prostate cancer are treated, especially in the United States,[80] with all the attendant risks of bothersome side effects and altered QOL. These findings led the US Preventive Services Task Force (USPSTF) to conclude that "there is moderate or high certainty that this service has no net benefit or that the harms outweigh the benefits" (grade D recommendation).[87] Rather than screening all men or no men, a risk-adapted approach is clearly preferable (see "Clinical States Model").

## Screening Trials

Two large, prospective randomized trials of screening for prostate cancer have been published, with conflicting results.[79,88] Both studies were recently updated.[89,90] The European Randomized Study of Screening for Prostate Cancer (ERSPC) compared screening with PSA every 2 to 4 years to no screening in a core group of 162,243 men age 55 to 69 years in seven European countries. At a median of 9 years, prostate cancer was diagnosed more often in the screened (8.2%) than in the control (4.8%) group (relative risk [RR] = 1.63), while the risk of dying of prostate cancer was reduced by 20% (RR = 0.80; $p$ = 0.04). The number of men needed to be screened to prevent one death from prostate cancer was 1,410 (1,068 among those actually screened), comparable to the data for breast cancer and colorectal cancer screening.[75–78] However, the number needed to diagnose to prevent one death

was high, 48, probably because the full impact of prostate cancer on mortality was not manifest within 9 years, and because some of the cancers detected were indolent. With further follow-up, the reduction in prostate cancer mortality at a median of 11 years was 21% in the screening arm ($p$ <0.0001), and 29% among those actually screened. The number needed to be screened fell to 1,055 and the number needed to diagnose to 37.

The Göteborg randomized population-based prostate cancer screening trial was planned and initiated independently of the ERSPC in 1995, although the investigators subsequently agreed to include a subset of participants in the ERSPC. In Göteborg, 20,000 men ages 50 to 64 were randomly assigned to be screened with PSA every 2 years up to age 69, or to a control group with no screening. After a median of 14 years, cancer was detected in 12.7% of the screened group and 8.2% of the controls (RR = 1.64), and the risk of death from prostate cancer was reduced by 44% (RR = 0.56; $p$ <0.002) in the screening group (56% among the 76% who were actually screened at least once, RR = 0.44) (Fig. 42.6). At 14 years, the number needed to be screened fell to 293, while the number needed to diagnose to prevent one death from prostate cancer was only 12. (Forty percent of the men diagnosed with cancer were monitored expectantly and not treated.)[74]

In contrast, screening with PSA and DRE in a US cohort did not reduce mortality from prostate cancer.[88,89] The Prostate, Lung, Colorectal and Ovarian Cancer (PLCO) Screening Trial enrolled 76,685 men ages 55 to 74 in a prospective randomized trial from 1993–2001, comparing annual PSA for 6 years and DRE for 4 years

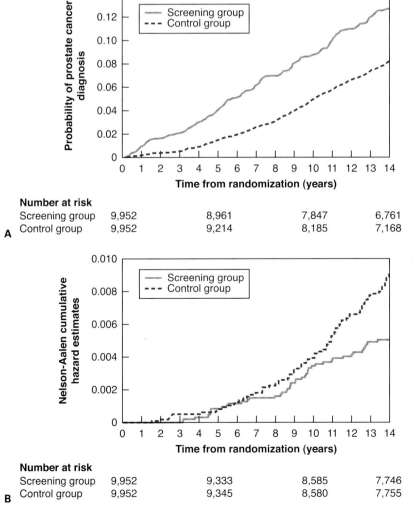

**Figure 42.6 (A)** Cumulative incidence of prostate cancer in the screening group and in the control group. **(B)** Cumulative risk of death from prostate cancer using Nelson-Aalen cumulative hazard estimates. (From Hugosson J, Carlsson S, Aus G, et al. Mortality results from the Goteborg randomised population-based prostate-cancer screening trial. *Lancet Oncol* 2010;11:725–732, with permission.)

with opportunistic screening. At the most recent (13-year) follow-up, the cancer detection rate was slightly higher (RR = 1.12) in the screened arm, but there was no difference in the risk of dying of prostate cancer.

The difference in outcomes of the US and European trials largely stems from the very different contexts in which the trials were conducted. The American trial was initiated in the 1990s, when PSA screening had already become widespread in the United States. In fact, 44% of the PLCO study subjects had had at least one PSA test before randomization, which would have excluded many men with potentially lethal cancers. The mortality rate from prostate cancer in both arms of the PLCO trial (1.7 and 2 per 10,000 person-years in the control and screened arms) was much lower than in the ERSPC (3.9 and 3.2, respectively), suggesting a heavily prescreened population. Many men (45% to 85%) in the PLCO control arm had at least one PSA test after randomization, compared with <20% in the ERSPC control arm, further diluting the potential for a difference between the arms.

## Screening Recommendations

The USPSTF's recent recommendation against screening[87,91] has been understandably criticized as based on a one-time analysis of a rapidly changing field.[92] The USPSTF justifiably raised concerns about the high level of overdetection and overtreatment inherent in PSA screening, which can lead to the immediate risks of harm from invasive prostate biopsies and subsequent radical therapy when cancer is found. But the potential harms from PSA screening can be greatly reduced by risk-adjusting screening so that it focuses on men at high risk of otherwise dying of prostate cancer; incorporating into screening newer, more specific biomarkers; and avoiding radical treatment of low-risk cancers.[93] In a recently published computer simulation model of PSA screening, prostate cancer mortality was reduced by 28% over the lifetime of men screened annually from ages 55 to 69. Over the lifetime of this population of 1,000 men, only 98 men would need to be screened and five cancers detected (three treated and two managed expectantly) to prevent one death from prostate cancer.[94]

In response to the changes in the USPSTF recommendations, a number of professional organizations have revised their guidelines for prostate cancer screening. The American Society of Clinical Oncology recommends that men with a life expectancy >10 years have a discussion with their physician about whether screening for prostate cancer is appropriate, including a clear statement that screening may save lives but is associated with harms, including complications from unnecessary biopsies, surgery, or radiation treatments. Men with a shorter life expectancy should not be screened.[95] The American Urological Association recommends that men ages 55 to 69 years engage in shared decision making with their physicians and proceed based on each man's values and preferences. For men younger than 55 years at higher risk (e.g., African American men, or those with a positive family history), the decision about screening should be individualized.[96]

The American Cancer Society recommends that men have an opportunity to make an informed decision with their health-care providers about whether to be screened. This decision should be made after the patients have received information about the uncertainties, risks, and potential benefits of screening; men should not be screened unless they have received this information. The American Cancer Society further recommends that discussion about screening should take place at age 50 for men who are at average risk of prostate cancer and are expected to live at least 10 more years, and at age 45 for men at high risk of developing prostate cancer (e.g., African American men and those with a first-degree relative diagnosed with prostate cancer at an early age [<65 years]). This discussion should occur at age 40 for men at even higher risk, that is, those with more than one first-degree relative who had prostate cancer at an early age.[97]

# DIAGNOSIS, RISK ASSESSMENT, AND STATE ASSIGNMENT

## Signs and Symptoms

The most common symptoms arising from the prostate in men over 40 years are bladder outlet obstruction, including hesitancy; nocturia; incomplete emptying; and a diminished urinary stream. The occurrence of these symptoms, although more commonly related to BPH, should prompt a careful DRE and a PSA determination. The acute development of pelvic or perineal pain, erectile dysfunction, or hematuria should prompt further evaluation of the prostate. Today, men rarely present with symptoms of metastatic disease such as bone pain, pathologic fracture, anemia, or pancytopenia from bone marrow replacement, or disseminated intravascular coagulation.

## Digital Rectal Examination

The physical examination should focus on a thorough DRE of the prostate, although palpable nodes can sometimes be detected in the inguinal or supraclavicular areas. Special attention should be paid to detect areas of induration within the prostate, extension through the capsule, or involvement of the seminal vesicles. If there is bladder outlet obstruction, the bladder may be palpable. Although not uniformly accurate or reproducible, DRE results are associated with pathologic stage and prognosis, and are the principal basis for assigning the clinical T stage of the cancer.[98]

## Prostate-Specific Antigen and Related Biomarkers

PSA levels are best considered as a continuum: the higher the level, the greater the likelihood that any cancer, or high-grade cancer, will be found on biopsy. The most commonly used threshold for recommending a biopsy is 3 ng/ml.[72] A level this high is found in only 5% to 10% of men age 45 to 69 years. As PSA levels vary,[66] a rise in PSA to a newly "elevated" level should be verified 2 to 3 months later, after the patient has been evaluated by a medical history, DRE, and appropriate laboratory tests to exclude causes other than cancer for the "rise." The likelihood of finding cancer is about 15% to 20% in men with a normal DRE and a PSA level between 2.5 to 4 ng/ml. Among men with a PSA level of 4 to 10 ng/ml, 20% to 30% will have cancer. If the PSA level is >10 ng/ml, 60% of men will have cancer on biopsy. Many of these cancers will be low risk and can be managed conservatively without radical therapy.

Higher circulating PSA levels prior to treatment are associated with larger, more extensive cancers, although there may be a wide range of levels within any clinical T, N, or M category.[99,100] Although poorly differentiated cancers produce less PSA per gram than well-differentiated cancers, higher PSA levels indicate a more extensive cancer and a poorer prognosis across all Gleason scores. Rare, highly aggressive, poorly differentiated cancers are found in men with low PSA levels (<2 ng/ml), but patients with these cancers usually present with rapidly progressive voiding symptoms and palpably abnormal DRE.

PSA levels rise with age because of age-related increases in prostate volume due to BPH. Adjusting the upper limit of normal for age, PSA should be <2.5 ng/ml for men age 40 to 49 years, <3.5 for men aged 50 to 59, <4.5 for men aged 60 to 69, and <6.5 for men aged 70 to 79.[101] The utility of *age-specific PSA levels* has been challenged in screening trials because sensitivity is lost for a small increase in specificity in older men.[102]

PSA levels can also be adjusted for the volume of the prostate gland. *PSA density* (PSAD) is the ratio of PSA to gland volume, measured in ng/ml per cm³.[103] As more PSA is released into the serum by cancer (3 ng/g) than by BPH (0.3 ng/g),[104] PSAD can help to discriminate cancer from BPH. Because DRE correlates poorly with gland volume, an imaging study (transrectal ultrasound [TRUS] or magnetic resonance imaging [MRI]) is required to measure PSAD accurately, so PSAD is generally useful only in men who have had an ultrasound during a biopsy. PSAD has proved to be more valuable in prognosis than in detection, where it has been largely replaced by the *free/total PSA ratio*. The percent-free PSA in serum is higher in men with BPH than in men with cancer and can be used to discriminate cancer from BPH. Percent-free PSA values <10% are more indicative of cancer in men with values in the 4 to 10 ng/ml range.[62,105]

PSA levels rise more rapidly over time in men with cancer than in those without cancer, even within the normal range.[106] The rate of change, termed *PSA velocity*, may indicate the presence of cancer, but normal biologic variations in PSA levels over time create many more false positives and lessen the accuracy of the calculated results.[107] Once a man's PSA level is known, PSA velocity contributes no additional information to predict the presence of a cancer,[107] except in the rare case of an unusually aggressive, high-grade cancer that produces little PSA.

## Panels of Kallikrein Markers

The major limitation of PSA for screening and early detection of prostate cancer is the high proportion of false-positive tests: 70% to 80% of men with a PSA >3 ng/ml and a normal DRE do not have cancer on biopsy. The specificity of PSA testing can be increased substantially at any given level of sensitivity by incorporating additional kallikreins into a panel of markers. There are two commercially available panels: the 4Kscore test (OPKO Lab, Nashville, TN) and the *phi* (Prostate Health Index; Beckman Coulter, Brea, CA). To baseline measurements of PSA and free-PSA levels the 4Kscore adds "intact" PSA and hK2, and the *phi* adds -2(pro) PSA.[108–111] All three of these kallikreins are elevated in cancer, relative to BPH. Both the 4Kscore and *phi* panels increase specificity, reducing the indication for biopsy among men with an elevated PSA level. In published studies, the number of biopsies was reduced by 40% to 50% while missing few high-grade cancers. The 4Kscore preserves sensitivity for high-grade (Gleason ≥7) cancer while reducing the number of negative biopsies and biopsies finding only low-grade (Gleason ≤6), small-volume cancer.[110,111]

## Urinary Molecular Biomarkers

Prostatic fluid may contain shed cells from prostate cancer that can be recognized by measuring the level of RNA for prostate cancer antigen-3 (PCA-3) relative to that for PSA in urinary sediment using reverse transcription–polymerase chain reaction technology. Urinary PCA-3 has been approved by the FDA to determine the likelihood of cancer in men with an elevated PSA level and a previously negative biopsy,[112] but is also useful in comparable men with no previous biopsy to avoid unnecessary biopsies. The test requires collection of urine after a prostatic massage by DRE, and the levels of PCA-3 do not reflect the volume, grade, and extent of cancer,[113] limiting its clinical utility, especially when the goal is to avoid biopsy in men with only low-risk cancers. Other urinary assays for molecular markers are being explored, including one for the TMPRSS fusion gene, which may be more prognostic than PCA-3.[113]

## Biopsy

Because prostate cancer is rarely curable when it causes symptoms, and rises in incidence with age, detection has focused on evaluating asymptomatic men between the ages of 50 and 70. The principal indications for biopsy are either an abnormal DRE or, more commonly, an elevated PSA level. Any palpable induration

**TABLE 42.2**

**Probability of a Positive Prostate Biopsy Based on the Results of the Digital Rectal Examination and Serum Prostate-Specific Antigen Level**

| DRE Status (%) | PSA (ng/ml) | | | |
|---|---|---|---|---|
| | 0–2 | 2–4 | 4–10 | >10 |
| DRE− | 1 | 15 | 25 | >50 |
| DRE+ | 5 | 20 | 45 | >75 |

PSA, prostate-specific antigen; DRE, digital rectal examination; DRE−, normal findings on the digital rectal examination; DRE+, findings on digital rectal examination suspicious for prostate cancer.
Modified from Thompson IM, Pauler DK, Goodman PJ, et al. Prevalence of prostate cancer among men with a prostate-specific antigen level < or = 4.0 ng per milliliter. *N Engl J Med* 2004;350:2239–2246; Catalona W, Richie J, deKernion JB, et al. Comparison of prostate specific antigen concentration versus prostate specific antigen density in the early detection of prostate cancer. *J Urol* 1994;152:2031–2036.

should be evaluated further, but only about a third of men with an abnormal DRE prove to have prostate cancer. Similarly, a normal DRE does not exclude the presence of cancer. The likelihood that cancer will be found on biopsy depends on the results of the DRE and PSA test (Table 42.2).[67,114]

The diagnosis of prostate cancer is typically established by TRUS-guided transrectal needle biopsy. TRUS is most useful for identifying the regions within the prostate for needle biopsy and for determining prostate volume; it is not used routinely for screening. When cancers are seen on TRUS, they are typically hypoechoic relative to normal prostate tissue, but the sensitivity of detection is low and MRI has proven to be more accurate and is the preferred imaging modality for identifying suspicious lesions for TRUS-guided biopsies within the prostate.

A needle biopsy of the prostate is usually performed transrectally with an 18-gauge needle mounted on a spring-loaded gun directed by ultrasound. Any palpable abnormality on DRE should be targeted for biopsy using finger guidance. In addition, abnormal areas visible on TRUS or MRI should be sampled, along with a total of at least 10 systematic biopsies of the prostate taken from the left and right apex, middle, and base of the peripheral zone. Each core or group of cores from a single region should be identified separately as to location and orientation so that the pathologist can report the extent and grade of cancer in each region and the presence of any perineural invasion or extraprostatic extension. Higher Gleason scores are strongly associated with larger tumor volume, extension outside the prostate, probability of metastases, and duration of response to therapy.[115,116] Biopsy results are used not only to assign a Gleason score to the cancer, but also to assess the volume and extent of the cancer by determining the number and percent of cores involved by cancer,[117,118] the amount of cancer in each core, and the total length of cancer in all cores. Each of these features adds important additional staging and prognostic information.[119–122]

Because patient selection for AS is critically dependent on the results of the prostate biopsy, some investigators have suggested more extensive biopsy strategies to better assess the true extent of cancer within the prostate. Transperineal "mapping" biopsies use a brachytherapy template, with needle cores taken at 5 mm to 10 mm intervals throughout the gland.[123] These template biopsies more accurately reflect the grade and extent of cancer. One study collected a median of 46 individual cores and found bilateral cancer in 55% of patients and an increased Gleason score in 23%. However, the risk of acute urinary retention, hematuria, and erectile dysfunction are increased with mapping biopsy, compared with standard transrectal needle biopsy. Further experience is needed before extensive mapping biopsies can be recommended as routine. Today, more attention is being focused on targeted biopsies of suspicious lesions seen on MRI.[124]

## Imaging for Diagnosis and Staging

The overwhelming majority of men diagnosed with prostate cancer today do not have metastases at the time of diagnosis, so imaging studies to detect metastases are usually not indicated. Neither bone scans nor computed tomography (CT) are helpful for patients with clinically localized cancer unless they have a poorly differentiated tumor (Gleason score 8 to 10) or a PSA >20 ng/ml.[125] Consequently, most patients diagnosed with a clinically localized prostate cancer need no further studies to rule out metastases. Patients with very aggressive tumors (PSA >20 ng/ml and biopsy Gleason score >7), advanced local lesions (T3-4), or symptoms suggestive of metastatic disease should have imaging studies, including a bone scan and a CT of the chest, abdomen, and pelvis.

### Magnetic Resonance Imaging

With current magnet strengths of 3 Tesla (3T), a multiparametric MRI, which provides T1- and T2-weighted images as well as diffusion-weighted and contrast images, permits excellent visualization of the prostate and surrounding tissues and the pelvic LN (in which case CT imaging of the pelvis is unnecessary).[126] The endorectal coil is helpful for enhanced visualization of the internal anatomy of the prostate when the magnetic strength is ≤1.5T, but magnetic resonance spectroscopy is rarely used today despite early promising results. On T1-weighted images, the prostate should appear homogenous and low intensity; cancers are not visible, but high-intensity areas resulting from recent biopsy should be noted to avoid misinterpreting corresponding low-intensity areas on T2 images as malignant lesions. On T2-weighted images, cancers can be recognized by their low signal intensity relative to the normal peripheral zone.

Diffusion-weighted imaging is a promising MRI technique that takes advantage of the known variability of random movements of water molecules observed between normal tissues and tumors. The rate of diffusion of water molecules is more restricted within tumors than in normal tissues and allows for an important metric known as the apparent diffusion coefficient. In one study

comparing MRI with combined MRI and diffusion-weighted MRI, the sensitivity and specificity were 86% and 84%, respectively.[127] Dynamic contrast-enhancement MRI may also identify malignant lesions within the prostate.[128] In one study, the combination of T2-weighted imaging and dynamic contrast-enhancement MRI findings had sensitivity and specificity rates of 77% and 91% for detecting tumor foci that measured 0.2 cm³, but these values improved to 90% and 88%, respectively, when detecting tumors >0.5 cm³.[129–131]

Opinions vary regarding the value of MRI in routine staging and imaging of the prostate, and a wide range in specificity and sensitivity has been reported for the detection of extraprostatic extension and seminal vesicle invasion (SVI). In general, multiparametric MRI permits excellent visualization of the prostate and is more sensitive than DRE, TRUS, and CT for identifying extraprostatic extension and SVI (Fig. 42.7). MRI also allows accurate estimates of the size and shape of the prostate, the proximity of cancer to the neurovascular bundles and the urethral sphincter, the presence of a large anterior tumor that may be invading the anterior fibromuscular stroma or bladder neck, and the length of the membranous urethral sphincter, making MRI a valuable adjunct to the preoperative evaluation of patients with apparently localized prostate cancer.[132]

### Computed Tomography

CT scans of the abdomen and pelvis are ordered far too frequently in the initial evaluation of men with prostate cancer, as they have limited capability to detect cancer within the prostate or the presence of extraprostatic extension or SVI. CT scans can detect LN metastases within the pelvis, but these can be detected equally well with pelvic/prostatic MRI, which provides more information about the primary tumor.

### Bone Scan

A radionuclide bone scan is the standard imaging study used to identify the presence of osseous metastases,[130] but is not generally indicated in patients with clinically localized cancer because true positive results are much less common than false positives. In patients with a baseline PSA level <10 ng/ml, a bone scan identifies metastases in <1% of men who have no symptoms of bone pain.

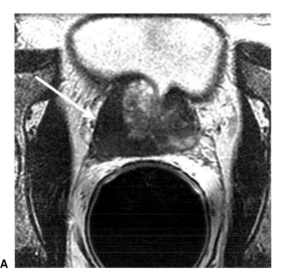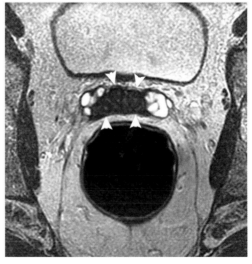

**Figure 42.7** Clinical stage T2a prostate cancer. On the transverse image **(A)**, the patient was noted to have a dominant tumor at the right base with loss of normal contour and irregular bulging consistent with extracapsular extension (*arrow*). Image **(B)** indicates the evidence of seminal vesicle involvement (*arrowheads*) demonstrating mild enlargement of the seminal vesicles and low signal intensity tissue replacing normal thin walls and obliterating the lumen. (From Hricak H, Choyke PL, Eberhardt SC, et al. Imaging prostate cancer: a multidisciplinary perspective. *Radiology* 2007;243:28, with permission of the Radiological Society of America.)

For patients with PSA levels between 10 ng/ml and 50 ng/ml or >50 ng/ml, the probability of a positive bone scan is 10% and 50%, respectively.[131] Bone scans are frequently used to assess the response to hormonal therapy and chemotherapy in men with metastatic disease.

## Risk Assessment

### Characterization of the Local Tumor

A thorough evaluation of the extent of the local tumor should include a diagram of the area of induration and a recording of the clinical T stage, which reflects the size, location, and extent of the cancer (determined by DRE and imaging), histologic grade (Gleason score) in the biopsy specimen, baseline serum PSA level, and systematic biopsy results. These factors are used to predict pathologic stage, assist in treatment planning, and determine prognosis.

### Tumor, Node, and Metastasis Classification

At the time of initial diagnosis, prostate cancers are staged using the TNM classification developed by the American Joint Committee on Cancer and the Union for International Cancer Control.[50–52,133,134] We recommend the use of the seventh edition published in 2010[51] (Table 42.3). With the TNM system, designations for the primary tumor, regional nodes, and distant metastases are noted separately. A distinct category, T1c, is used to describe cancers that are neither palpable nor visible, but were detected by

a biopsy performed after an abnormal PSA test or for other reasons. Cancers that are not palpable but visible on imaging such as TRUS or MRI are classified appropriately along with palpable cancers in the T2-4 categories. However, the TNM system does not fully reflect prognosis because it does not include PSA levels, Gleason grade, or the extent of cancer in the biopsy specimen.

### Staging Tables and Risk Groups

While individual prognostic factors can be informative, combining multiple factors together produces more accurate estimates of pathologic stage and prognosis. Partin et al.[135] developed a nomogram reported as a series of staging tables (Partin tables) that combine clinical tumor stage, biopsy Gleason grade, and PSA to predict pathologic stage. The accuracy of these tables has been widely validated.[136]

As pathologic stage is only a proxy for prognosis, a classification scheme has been developed to predict the risk of recurrence after treatment of the primary tumor using the same key prognostic factors (clinical stage, Gleason grade, and PSA).[137] The D'Amico classification, now adopted by the American Urological Association, assigns patients to one of three logical (rather than empirical) risk groups according to their clinical T stage, Gleason grade, and PSA.[137] Although it is intuitive to group patients into such risk-group categories, each "group" actually contains a heterogeneous population.[138] For example, patients with a clinical stage T1c, Gleason grade 3 + 3, and PSA 9.9 ng/ml would be classified as low risk, but if the PSA were 10.1 ng/ml, the same patient would be considered intermediate risk. Using categorical values

**TABLE 42.3**

**Comparison of the 1992, 1997, 2002, and 2010 American Joint Committee on Cancer/International Union Against Cancer Tumor, Node, Metastasis Staging System**

| Stage | 1992[50] | 1997[52] | 2002[133] | 2010[51] |
|---|---|---|---|---|
| TX | Primary tumor cannot be assessed | | | |
| T0 | No evidence of primary tumor | | | |
| T1 | Clinically inapparent, not palpable or visible by imaging | | | |
| T1a | Incidental histologic finding, ≤5% of resected tissue | | | |
| T1b | Incidental histologic finding, >5% of resected tissue | | | |
| T1c | Tumor identified by needle biopsy, for any reason (e.g., elevated PSA) | | | |
| T2 | Palpable or visible tumor, confined within the prostate[a] | | | |
| T2a | ≤ Half one lobe | One lobe | ≤ Half one lobe | ≤ Half one lobe |
| T2b | One lobe | Both lobes | One lobe | > Half one lobe, not both |
| T2c | Both lobes | No T2c classification | Both lobes | Both lobes |
| T3 | Tumor extends through prostate capsule[b] | | | |
| T3a | Unilateral ECE | ECE, unilateral or bilateral | | ECE, unilateral or bilateral |
| T3b | Bilateral ECE | Seminal vesicle involvement | | Seminal vesicle involvement |
| T3c | Seminal vesicle involvement | No T3c classification | | No T3c classification |
| T4 | Tumor is fixed or invades adjacent structures | | | Tumor is fixed or invades adjacent structures other than seminal vesicles, such as external sphincter, rectum, bladder, levator muscles, and/or pelvic wall |
| T4a | Invades bladder neck, external sphincter, or rectum | | | No T4a classification |
| T4b | Invades levator muscles or fixed to pelvic sidewalls | | | No T4b classification |

PSA, prostate-specific antigen; ECE, extracapsular extension.
[a] Tumor found in one or both lobes by needle biopsy, but not palpable or reliably visible by imaging, is classified as T1c.
[b] Invasion into the prostatic apex or into (but not beyond) the prostatic capsule is classified not as T3 but as T2.
Modified from Beahrs OH, Henson DE, Hutter RVP, et al. *American Joint Committee on Cancer. AJCC Cancer Staging Manual.* 4th ed. Philadelphia, PA: Lippincott-Raven; 1992; Edge S, Byrd DR, Compton CC, et al. *American Joint Committee on Cancer. AJCC Cancer Staging Manual.* 7th ed. New York: Springer; 2010; Fleming ID, Cooper JS, Henson DE, et al. *American Joint Committee on Cancer. AJCC Cancer Staging Manual.* 5th ed. Philadelphia: JB Lippincott; 1997; Greene FL, Page DL, Fleming ID, et al. *American Joint Committee on Cancer. AJCC Cancer Staging Manual.* 6th ed. New York: Springer; 2002; and Ohori M, Wheeler TM, Scardino PT. The New American Joint Committee on Cancer and International Union against Cancer TNM classification of prostate cancer. *Cancer* 1994;74:104–114.

(e.g., PSA 10 to 20 ng/ml) rather than continuous values, and assigning a patient to an increased risk group if any single variable is high (e.g., tumor stage cT2c, Gleason 8 to 10, or PSA >20 ng/ml), is inherently inaccurate. Predictions are much more accurate when nomograms are used to combine individual prognostic factors into a single prognostic score assigned to an individual patient. Consequent comparisons of the results of different treatments are also more accurate when patients are more precisely matched.

## Nomograms

Nomograms now widely available to predict prognosis in men with prostate cancer combine clinical and pathologic prognostic factors as continuous rather than categorical variables.[139] The prognosis or probability of recurrence after definitive therapy of an apparently localized prostate cancer depends on the clinical stage and grade of the cancer, the number or percent of positive biopsy cores, as well as the PSA level before treatment. Nomograms have proved highly useful in clinical practice and have been developed for external beam radiation therapy (EBRT)[140] and brachytherapy as well as surgery.[141] These nomograms may provide clues about the relative efficacy of different treatment modalities in patients with comparable tumors. All these nomograms are available at http://www.mskcc.org/cancer-care/prediction-tools (accessed June 13, 2014).

## Molecular Profiles

Genomic testing has recently been introduced to characterize the level of aggressiveness of prostate cancer, and, as in breast cancer,[142–144] can help to guide treatment decisions.[145] There are currently two commercially available genomic tests for risk-stratification of prostate cancer, the Cell Cycle Progression assay (Prolaris, Myriad Genetic Laboratories Inc., Salt Lake City, UT) and the Genomic Prostate Score assay (Oncotype DX, Genomic Health, Redwood City, CA).[146–149] Both these tests use reverse transcription–polymerase chain reaction techniques to assay the expression level of a panel of genes that reflect the biologic activity of the cancer relative to the level of housekeeper genes. The Cell Cycle Progression-Prolaris assay was developed on a cohort of men with a wide spectrum of prostate cancer managed conservatively; the molecular profile added significantly to the ability of standard clinicopathologic features (stage, grade, PSA, and extent of cancer in biopsy specimens) to predict time to death from prostate cancer.[147] When needle biopsy specimens from men who were candidates for AS were assayed with Genomic Prostate Score-Oncotype DX, the assay independently predicted the risk of adverse pathology (extraprostatic extension or Gleason grade 4 + 3 or greater) in RP specimens. Both tests can successfully assay expression profiles from as little as 1 mm of cancer in an 18-g needle core obtained as long as 10 to 15 years previous to the assay, and both show a wide range of expression levels, and therefore prognoses, within any clinicopathologic risk group.

The clinical utility of these molecular profiles is under active investigation; today, the assays are largely used to recommend AS in men with low- or intermediate-risk, low-volume cancer and favorable expression profiles. Assay results tend to be concordant with the clinicopathologic risk classification in approximately 45% of patients, whereas it is higher or lower in the remaining 55%. In a recent study, 14% of patients considered low risk and suitable for AS were reclassified as higher risk patients for whom active intervention was warranted, and 7% of those with clinically aggressive tumors were reclassified as low-risk and suitable for AS by the Cell Cycle Progression-Prolaris assay.[150]

## Pathologic Stage

Several other indices have been developed that improve the biologic characterization of a given tumor. Pathologic stage, determined by examining the RP specimen, predicts recurrence much more accurately than clinical stage.[151] Independent prognostic factors include the level of invasion through the capsule of the prostate, SVI, LN metastases, and positive surgical margins, as well as the Gleason score in the RP specimen and the preoperative serum PSA level. Some investigators have considered tumor volume an important prognostic factor, but others have found that it has no independent prognostic significance. Stephenson et al.[152] combined these independent prognostic factors into postoperative nomograms to predict biochemical recurrence (BCR)[153] 10 years after RP and 15-year cancer-specific survival.[139,154] These nomograms are more accurate than the preoperative nomogram, because they incorporate the final Gleason grade and pathologic stage as well as preoperative PSA.[154]

## Stage Assignment

### Clinical States Model

Given the range of prognoses among men within each of the TNM-defined stages at diagnosis, a risk-adapted approach to diagnosis and treatment is mandated. To facilitate this approach, a model was developed that divides the disease continuum from prediagnosis to advanced metastatic disease into a series of clinical states. Each state represents a distinct clinical milestone defined by the status of the tumor in the primary site, the presence or absence of metastatic disease on imaging, whether the testosterone levels in the blood are in noncastrate or castrate (<50 ng/dl) range, and prior therapy. This model differs from staging algorithms in that it applies to both the newly diagnosed, untreated patient and to the patient who has received treatment as his disease evolves. Unmet needs in diagnosis, defining treatment objectives, and assessing outcomes vary by clinical state (see Fig. 42.1). Applied clinically to men without a cancer diagnosis, this approach accommodates the need to assess an individual's cancer based on the risk of harboring or developing clinically significant disease.

In the clinical states model, an individual is assigned to only one state and he remains in that state until his disease has progressed. He can only move forward, never back, even if his disease has been eradicated completely. Each assessment is considered a new evaluation in which the patient's symptoms and overall tumor status are reviewed, and the decision to offer treatment, and the specific form of treatment, are based on the current state of the disease or the future risk posed by the cancer relative to comorbid conditions.

For example, the rising PSA states include patients who have a rising PSA following treatment of the primary tumor with either surgery or radiation, an indication that the disease has recurred. Issues for these patients include whether the recurrence is systemic or limited to the prostate bed (following surgery) or the prostate itself (following radiation). A more important consideration is whether any treatment is needed, based on the likelihood in the long term that the cancer will cause symptoms, local or distant, or shorten a patient's life. Patients with rising PSA who are considered to have disease in the prostate bed (or the prostate itself) are discussed in the sections of this chapter that review the primary treatment modalities for prostate cancer. Treatment objectives and the means to assess outcomes vary by clinical state and will be considered separately. The more rapidly the disease is progressing or the more advanced the disease state, the greater the need for treatment.

## Principles of Treatment and Assessing Outcomes

Treatment is offered with therapeutic intent that considers (1) why the treatment should be administered, (2) the potential benefits it can provide relative to potential morbidity, and (3) financial cost. Changing established practice paradigms requires demonstrating that a new therapy or approach provides incremental clinical benefit relative to a previous standard (if one exists) or to a suitable control in prospective randomized trials. Clinical benefit in regulatory terms represents an improvement in the way a patient functions or feels, or in how long he survives.[155] Examples of clinical benefits include prolonging life, relieving pain or other symptoms, and/or reducing toxicity relative to an established standard. It is also important to demonstrate that a new approach, whether it is a therapeutic procedure or a drug, is safe and well tolerated in an elderly population.

### Assessing Treatment Effects

It has long been recognized that the most common manifestations of prostate cancer, which include disease in the primary site, a rising PSA, and metastasis to bone, are not evaluable by the traditional measures of tumor regression used to monitor disease status in other solid malignancies (Response Evaluation Criteria In Solid Tumors [RECIST] 1.1).[156] Changes in nodal and visceral sites that can be assessed reliably using RECIST occur less often. To address this unmet need, the Prostate Cancer Working Group (PCWG2) was formed to develop guidelines for clinical trial design in castration-resistant prostate cancer (CRPC) that also apply to earlier disease states.[157]

In the clinical states framework, treatment objectives are divided into early outcomes representing the control, relief, or elimination of disease manifestations present when a treatment is being considered or initiated, and later outcomes representing the delay or prevention of future manifestations. Existing manifestations may include disease limited to the prostate (localized disease), a biochemical recurrence following local treatment (rising PSA), or cancer in the extrapelvic LN, bone, or viscera with or without a rising PSA (clinical metastases). Potential manifestations that might be delayed or prevented from occurring include growth in the primary site, BCR, growth in an existing site, new sites of spread, pain, or other complications of progressive osseous disease described as skeletal-related events (SRE),[158] and death from disease. SREs, first used in the regulatory filing of zoledronate, include fractures, pain requiring a change in therapy, epidural disease, and/or surgery to bone.[159]

"Control/relieve/eliminate" outcomes representing "response" are reported individually by the change in each disease manifestation present—PSA level, soft tissue disease, bone disease, and/or symptoms when treatment was started—rather than by grouped categorizations, such as complete and partial remission, that include all sites of disease. For example, a key PSA-based outcome for patients treated with RP is the proportion of patients who achieve an undetectable PSA level postoperatively, whereas for patients with CRPC treated with a systemic approach, a waterfall plot showing the percent change from baseline for each patient treated, or the proportion of patients achieving a defined degree of decline (e.g., ≥50%), is more informative. "Delay/prevent" outcomes focusing on time-to-event progression are also measured individually. For a patient with localized disease, outcomes from surgery or radiation include a response measure that demonstrates whether the disease was eliminated completely (e.g., a negative biopsy of the prostate at a certain time after radiotherapy) or time-to-event outcomes that include time to PSA recurrence, metastases, symptoms, or death from disease. This approach to evaluating outcomes enables the physician to focus on the specific therapeutic objective for a single patient or group of patients in a given disease state, rather than on changes in other, less-relevant measures, and at the same time enables clinical trial investigators to explore the relation between changes in individual disease manifestations and other measures of clinical benefit such as overall survival.

## MANAGEMENT BY CLINICAL STATES

### Clinically Localized Disease

The clinical course of newly diagnosed prostate cancer is difficult to predict. Men with similar clinical stage, serum PSA levels, and biopsy features can have markedly different outcomes. Although prostate cancer is unequivocally lethal in some patients, most men die with, rather than of, their cancer. The challenge to physicians is to identify those men with aggressive, localized prostate cancer with a natural history that can be altered by definitive local therapy, while sparing the remainder the morbidity of unnecessary treatment. Not all men with clinically localized prostate cancer require or benefit from therapy. Depending on the characteristics of their cancer, their age, and comorbidities, some men would benefit greatly by aggressive treatment, whereas others would suffer harm.

Well-established prognostic factors for clinically localized prostate cancer include age, PSA level, clinical stage based on DRE and imaging, Gleason grade, and extent of the cancer on biopsy. Prognosis can be estimated more accurately by combining these risk factors into nomograms[99] that calculate the probability of a clinically important endpoint, such as freedom from BCR 10 years after surgery[153] or cancer-specific survival 15 years after surgery.[139]

### Active Surveillance

AS is a planned treatment of monitoring a patient with a potentially curable prostate cancer based on the likelihood that the cancer will progress, delaying active treatment until signs of progression to a more aggressive, potentially lethal cancer are detected. AS attempts to avoid the adverse effects of treatment in the majority of men, intervening with curative therapy for selected men only for specific indications. AS is now widely recommended for most men with low-risk cancer, based on the lack of survival benefit of immediate surgery versus observation at 12 years in the PIVOT trial[160] and the low risk of prostate cancer death at 10 years in large phase 2 studies of AS.[84] In this and other AS trials, the risk of progression or treatment for men with low-risk cancer is about 20% to 40% within 5 years and 35% to 60% within 10 years, depending on the initial eligibility criteria and the indications for delayed intervention.

A recommendation for AS assumes that the risk posed by the cancer at diagnosis can be assessed accurately, that progression can be identified by regular monitoring, and that deferring treatment until it is necessary will offer cancer control and survival rates similar to immediate treatment. Achieving all of these goals has not yet been realized. Standard assessment at diagnosis includes PSA, clinical stage, Gleason grade, and extent of cancer in biopsy results. This limited evaluation underestimates the grade and extent of the cancer in 15% to 25% of patients.[161] A multiparametric MRI of the prostate can detect large, more aggressive cancers in some patients, and these findings can be confirmed by biopsies targeting the suspicious lesions.[162] Alternatively, one can depend on annual repeat biopsies[163] or PSA velocity[84] to detect progression in time for effective intervention. In either case, patients under AS must accept frequent, regular, detailed evaluations of the status of their cancer for as long as they are healthy and young enough to be candidates for definitive therapy. Patients under AS are generally monitored every 6 months with DRE and measurement of free and total PSA, with repeat imaging and biopsy every 2 to 3 years after the baseline evaluation. The goal is to detect progression of the cancer while cure is still possible.

#### Outcomes of Active Surveillance with Selective Delayed Intervention

There are few reports of long-term outcomes of AS for localized prostate cancer. Klotz et al.[84] conducted a prospective phase 2 study of AS in men with low-risk cancer (or those over 70 with Gleason 7 [3 + 4] and PSA <15 ng/ml). The indications for intervention were a short PSA doubling time (PSADT) or grade progression on repeat biopsy. At 8 years, overall survival was 85% and disease-specific and metastasis-free survival 99%. Some 25%

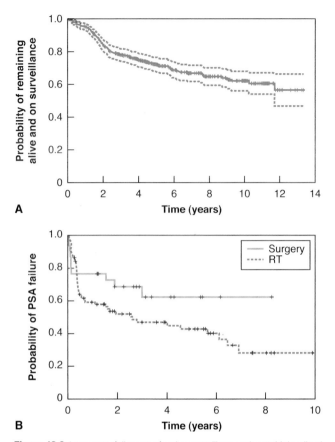

**A**

**B**

**Figure 42.8** Long-term follow-up of active surveillance cohort with localized prostate cancer. **(A)** Likelihood of remaining alive and on surveillance in 450 patients. *Green lines* indicate 95% confidence intervals. **(B)** Prostate-specific antigen (PSA) failure in 117 patients treated with surgery or radiation after a period of surveillance. RT, radiotherapy. (From Klotz L, Zhang L, Lam A, et al. Clinical results of long-term follow-up of a large, active surveillance cohort with localized prostate cancer. *J Clin Oncol* 2010;28:126–131, with permission.)

of patients were treated within 5 years, and 40% by 10 years (Fig. 42.8). Delayed intervention was associated with a relatively low rate of cancer control, raising concerns that treatment for men with a short PSADT (<2 years) was too late.

Carter et al.[96] observed a cohort of 769 men with very-low-risk prostate cancer and low PSA density (<0.15) from 1 to 15 years after diagnosis with DRE, measurements of total and free PSA every 6 months, and an annual surveillance biopsy. Treatment was recommended based on biopsy changes (any Gleason pattern 4 or 5, more than two cores that were positive for cancer, or >50% of any one core that was involved with cancer) or if a patient requested a change in management, but not for changes in PSA alone. A total of 41% of patients had been treated at 5 years, and 59% at 10 years, and the median time to treatment was 6.5 years. Cancer control after delayed therapy was excellent. The large number of men who required delayed intervention suggested that many tumors were underestimated at baseline, and the high cure rates at delayed intervention call into question the clinical significance of the criteria for delayed intervention. Many physicians now recommend more comprehensive initial evaluation of candidates for AS with multiparametric MRI and/or early confirmatory biopsies.[164]

These and other studies confirm that in appropriately selected men, AS is associated with an extremely low rate of progression to metastatic disease and/or death, and that the majority of patients do not require intervention over the first decade. Further follow-up

is necessary to determine the long-term risk of progression. The National Comprehensive Cancer Network recommends AS as the appropriate initial management strategy for patients with low-risk cancer and a life expectancy <10 years, as well as for patients with very low-risk cancer and a life expectancy <20 years.[125]

## Radical Prostatectomy

The modern anatomic technique for RP was developed nearly 35 years ago and has proven safe and effective in many large cohort studies and randomized clinical trials. The retropubic technique originally described by Walsh[165] for open surgery is equally suitable for laparoscopic and robot-assisted RP. Initially focused on patients with early-stage, organ-confined cancers, RP with pelvic LN dissection (PLND) is now recommended primarily for patients with aggressive cancers (intermediate- and high-risk), whereas low-risk tumors are generally managed with AS (see previous discussion). Because of the risk inherent in major surgery, RP should be reserved for patients without serious systemic comorbidity. Although the risk of recurrence after RP rises with higher clinical stage, Gleason grade, and serum PSA level, no absolute cutoff values exclude a patient as a candidate.

**Surgical Technique.**   The goals of modern RP are to remove the entire cancer with negative surgical margins, minimal blood loss, no serious perioperative complications, and complete recovery of continence and potency. Achieving these goals requires careful surgical planning. Because no single test provides a reliable estimate of the size, location, and extent of the cancer, we rely on the results of DRE, serum PSA levels, and a detailed analysis of the amount and grade of cancer in each individually labeled biopsy core, along with multiparametric MRI. The results are used to plan the steps necessary to remove the cancer completely and to assess the likelihood that one or both of the neurovascular bundles will have to be resected partially or fully to minimize the risk of a positive surgical margin. The retropubic procedure is performed either through a suprapubic incision (open RP) or using a minimal access (laparoscopic or robot-assisted laparoscopic) approach. The operation should be exactly the same internally, regardless of the method of access.

### Selecting Patients for Pelvic Lymph Node Dissection

Cancer that has spread to the pelvic LN carries a worse prognosis than when the nodes are negative, enhancing accurate staging. However, the therapeutic benefit of PLND is uncertain. Overall rates of pelvic LN metastases found at RP vary from 2% to 35% depending on the extent of the node dissection, whether the cancer was discovered after screening, and the stage and grade of the cancer.[166] Men with low-risk screen-detected cancer are rarely found to have nodal metastases (0.5% to 2%),[166–168] so PLND is generally unnecessary, but it may be indicated if imaging studies or intraoperative findings suggest a more advanced cancer. The limited PLND commonly performed today, especially with robot-assisted RP, has underestimated the rate of nodal metastases.[169] In men with intermediate-risk prostate cancer, LN metastases are found in 5% (screen-detected) to 20%, whereas in men with high-risk cancer, the rates are 20% to 50%, respectively, when a full or extended PLND is performed.[166,170–173] The incidence of LN metastases increases with increasing PSA, clinical stage, and Gleason score.[168] Our current practice is to restrict PLND at the time of RP to men with a ≥2% risk of positive nodes according to a contemporary nomogram.[174] Even so, controversy persists concerning the role of PLND in patients with prostate cancer.

### Limited Versus Extended Pelvic Lymph Node Dissection

No prospective studies have demonstrated the optimal anatomic limits of a PLND for prostate cancer. However, lymphatic drainage of the prostate is known to be highly variable and involves regions not sampled during an external iliac–only PLND.[166] Some surgeons resect only the external iliac LN unless imaging suggests abnormal LN in other regions, whereas other surgeons routinely perform a more extensive dissection that includes the obturator, external iliac, and hypogastric areas.[175] No sentinel LN has been identified in prostate cancer. The more extensive the PLND, the greater the number of LN removed, and the greater the number of positive nodes.[166,168,171–173] Nevertheless, the total number of positive LN is one in 50% of patients, two in 30%, and three or more in only 20% of patients who have an extended LN dissection.[166] A PLND that includes the external iliac, hypogastric, and obturator node packets is feasible in both open and minimally invasive RP, and carries no greater risk than a PLND limited to the external iliac nodes alone.

### Therapeutic Benefit of Pelvic Lymph Node Dissection

Evidence from several surgical series of patients undergoing RP demonstrates a potential therapeutic benefit of extended PLND, particularly in men with only one or two positive nodes and Gleason score ≤7 in cancer identified in the RP specimen (Fig. 42.9).[170–172,176–178] In a series of patients with positive LN treated at Johns Hopkins Hospital, men who had an extended PLND were less likely to develop BCR at 5 years, compared with men who underwent a limited PLND when 15% or fewer of the removed LN were involved.[170] In the Memorial Sloan Kettering Cancer Center (MSKCC) series, 25% to 30% of patients with positive nodes remained free of BCR 10 years after surgery with no additional therapy.[179]

### Radical Prostatectomy: Surgical Approach

RP is one of the most complex operations performed by urologists. The outcomes—cancer control, urinary continence, and erectile function—are exquisitely sensitive to fine details in surgical technique. No surgeon achieves perfect results, and outcomes vary dramatically among individual surgeons.[180,181] Technical refinements have resulted in lower rates of urinary incontinence and higher rates of recovery of erectile function, less blood loss and fewer transfusions, shorter hospital stays, and lower rates of positive surgical margins. Laparoscopic and robot-assisted RP promised better cancer control and functional recovery, but numerous studies have confirmed that the only consistent advantages of "minimally invasive" surgery are shorter hospital stays and fewer blood transfusions.[182] A thorough understanding of periprostatic anatomy and

vascular control by contemporary surgeons further increases the probability of a successful RP with reduced morbidity.

### Open Radical Prostatectomy

*Acute Postoperative Complications.* Refinements in anesthesia, perioperative care, and surgical technique have decreased blood loss, length of hospital stay, complications, and mortality after open surgery.[183] The mortality rate ranges from 0.16% to 0.66% in modern series, rising with increasing age and comorbidity. Deep venous thrombosis and pulmonary embolism occur in approximately 2% of cases, with little evidence that anticoagulants or sequential pneumatic compression are preventive. Early ambulation and shorter hospital stays are likely responsible for the lower rate of thromboembolic events. Routine perioperative anticoagulation is not used because of the increased risks of bleeding and lymphocele. Rectal injuries are uncommon. Standardized treatment pathways have been shown to decrease the cost of radical retropubic prostatectomy without compromising quality of care. Hospital stays now average 2 days for open RP and 1 day for robot-assisted RP.

### Robot-Assisted Radical Prostatectomy

Surgeons have demonstrated that robot-assisted RP (RALP) can be performed with excellent results in the hands of experienced surgeons. The initial enthusiasm for RALP was based on the idea that less bleeding and a magnified surgical image would markedly improve patient outcomes, which has not been borne out in carefully performed population-based studies.[182,184,185] Open RP and RALP each have a number of theoretical advantages and disadvantages (Table 42.4).[186] No prospective randomized trials have yet compared the two techniques, and it is now clear that variations in outcomes among individual surgeons are much greater than variations between technologic approaches.[181] Hu et al.[184] have suggested that the rapid increase in utilization of minimally invasive RP despite insufficient data demonstrating superiority over the well-established open operation may be a reflection of a society and a health-care system enamored of a new technology that has increased health-care costs but has yet to uniformly realize marketed or potential benefits during early adoption. As with open surgical techniques, laparoscopic RP and RALP outcomes, including surgical margin status, continence, and potency, reflect surgical technique (the actions and expertise of the surgeon) more than surgical approach. Current data suggest that the best way to improve outcomes after RP is to have the procedure performed by a skilled surgeon, regardless of the approach he or she uses.[181,187]

### Cancer Control with Radical Prostatectomy

*Benefits of Surgery Relative to Active Surveillance.* The most compelling evidence that selected patients with prostate cancer benefit from active treatment compared with watchful waiting comes from the Scandinavian randomized trial (SPCG-4) of 695 unscreened men with clinically localized prostate cancer.[188,189] Over 23 years of follow-up, RP (compared with watchful waiting) reduced the risk of death from any cause by 29% and risk of death from prostate cancer by 44% (an absolute difference of 11%). The need for subsequent ADT was reduced by 51%, and clinical local recurrence was reduced by 66%. At 18 years of follow-up, the number needed to treat to prevent one death from prostate cancer was eight overall and four in men under age 65. This elegant study firmly documents the overall benefit of RP in patients with clinically localized prostate cancer diagnosed in the absence of systematic screening.[188,189]

In a population of men subjected to widespread PSA screening, the benefit of surgery for prostate cancer was tested in the Prostate Cancer Intervention Versus Observation Trial (PIVOT).[160] This

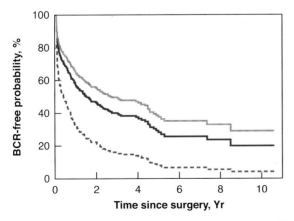

**Figure 42.9** Probability of freedom from biochemical recurrence (BCR) by number of positive nodes. *Orange line,* one positive node; *blue line,* two positive nodes; *red line,* three or more positive nodes. (From Touijer KA, Mazzola CR, Sjoberg DD, et al. Long-term outcomes of patients with lymph node metastasis treated with radical prostatectomy without adjuvant androgen-deprivation therapy. *Eur Urol* 2014;65:20–25, with permission.)

## TABLE 42.4

### Advantages and Disadvantages of Various Surgical Approaches to Radical Prostatectomy

| Claims by Minimally Invasive Surgeons: Advantages | Rebuttal by Open Surgeons |
|---|---|
| Magnification improves visualization | Magnification achieved with surgical loupes |
| Less blood loss | Transfusion rates are similar |
| Improved visualization permits more precise dissection of the prostatic apex and neurovascular bundles | Outcomes fail to demonstrate any advantage in terms of continence and potency |
| Less pain and quicker recovery | Postoperative pain and recovery are comparable |
| Watertight anastomosis allows earlier catheter removal | No difference noted in most large series |
| **Claims by Open Surgeons: Disadvantages** | **Rebuttal by Minimally Invasive Surgeons** |
| Lack of proprioception compromises cancer control | Positive margin rates are equivalent |
| Complication rates are lower with open surgery | Complication rates with laparoscopic surgery decrease with experience |
| Mobilization of the neurovascular bundles with electrocautery compromises potency | Potency rates are similar |
| Significant learning curve | Proctoring reduces learning curve |
| Longer operative time | No rebuttal |
| Increased cost | No rebuttal |

trial was conducted in the United States and randomly assigned 731 men with clinically localized prostate cancer to RP or observation. The mean age was 67, the median PSA level was 7.8 ng/ml, and approximately three-quarters of the men had a biopsy as a consequence of an elevated PSA; half had no palpable tumor (cT1c) and 70% had low-grade (Gleason ≤6) cancer on biopsy. With a median of 10 years of follow-up, 48% of the patients had died, but only 7% had died from prostate cancer. There were no differences in overall or cancer-specific mortality between the two arms of the trial. But there were clear indications that RP reduced the risk of dying of cancer in the subset of men who had aggressive cancers, including those whose PSA was >10.0 ng/ml and those with high-risk cancers.

Taken together, these two trials indicate that most men with cancers detected without screening and those with screen-detected intermediate- and high-risk cancers have less risk of metastases and of death from prostate cancer when treated with early RP than with observation alone. In contrast, men with screen-detected low-risk cancer can be managed safely with AS and do not need immediate surgery or radiotherapy. Life expectancy should be considered in the choice of immediate therapy or AS, as the risks of RP increase and benefits decline progressively with age and comorbidity.[190] A UK-based trial (ProtecT) is currently assessing treatment versus no treatment in a PSA-screened population in >1,500 patients.[191]

Progression rates after RP depend on the clinical stage, biopsy Gleason score, and serum PSA level before surgery, as well as pathologic findings in the surgical specimen. After RP, the PSA level should become undetectable. Cancer control, as measured by freedom from BCR, is excellent after RP and is reproducible among many large series (Table 42.5).[179, 192–196] Of 12,086 patients treated with RP between 1966 and 2003, 69% to 84% were free of progression at 5 years, and 47% to 78% at 10 years.[179, 192–196]

Fifteen-year outcomes have been reported after RP based on preoperative and pathologic factors (Table 42.6). Bianco, Scardino, and Eastham[179] calculated the risk of recurrence in 1,743 consecutive patients with clinical stage T1-T3, N0 or X, M0 cancer treated with RP and followed with serum PSA levels for a mean of 72 months (range, 1 month to 240 months). Failure after RP was defined as a rising serum PSA >0.2 ng/ml, clinical evidence of local or distant recurrence, or the initiation of adjuvant radiotherapy or

## TABLE 42.5

### Freedom from Prostate-Specific Antigen Progression After Radical Retropubic Prostatectomy

| Group (Ref.) | No. of Patients | Clinical Stage | Years of RP | PSA Nonprogression (%) | | |
|---|---|---|---|---|---|---|
| | | | | **Five-Y** | **Ten-Y** | **Fifteen-Y** |
| Han et al.[193] | 2,091[a] | T1c-2NX | 1982–1999 | 84 | 72 | 61 |
| Trapasso et al.[195] | 601[b] | T1-3NX | 1987–1992 | 69 | 47 | — |
| Zincke et al.[196] | 3,170[c] | T1-2NX | 1966–1991 | 70 | 52 | 40 |
| Roehl et al.[192] | 3,478[c] | T1-3NX | 1983–2003 | 80 | 68 | — |
| Hull et al.[194] | 1,000[d] | T1-2NX | 1983–1998 | 78 | 75 | — |
| Bianco, Scardino, and Eastham[179] | 1,746[e] | T1-3NX | 1983–2003 | 82 | 77 | 75 |

PSA, prostate-specific antigen; RP, radical prostatectomy.
[a] Progression defined as a serum PSA ≥0.2 ng/ml.
[b] Progression defined as a serum PSA >0.4 ng/ml.
[c] Progression defined as a serum PSA >0.3 ng/ml.
[d] Progression defined as a serum PSA ≥0.4 ng/ml.
[e] Progression defined as a serum PSA ≥0.4 ng/ml before 1996 and ≥0.2 ng/ml afterward.

TABLE 42.6

**Actuarial 5-, 10-, and 15-Year (Prostate-Specific Antigen–Based) Nonprogression Rates (%) After Radical Retropubic Prostatectomy for Clinically Localized Prostate Cancer According to Preoperative and Pathologic Factors**

| | Johns Hopkins University[a] | | | MSKCC SPORE in Prostate Cancer Database[b] | | |
|---|---|---|---|---|---|---|
| | **Five-Y** | **Ten-Y** | **Fifteen-Y** | **Five-Y** | **Ten-Y** | **Fifteen-Y** |
| No. of patients | 2,404 | 2,404 | 2,404 | 4,037 | 4,037 | 4,037 |
| BCR | 412 | 412 | 412 | 630 | 630 | 630 |
| BCR-free (%) | 84 | 74 | 66 | 82 | 75 | 73 |
| **Actuarial Nonprogression Rate (95% CI) by Preoperative Serum PSA (ng/ml)** | | | | | | |
| ≤4 | 94 (92–96) | 91 (87–93) | 67 (34–86) | 92 (89–95) | 89 (85–93) | 86 (80–92) |
| >4 and ≤10 | 89 (86–91) | 79 (74–83) | 75 (69–80) | 87 (85–89) | 80 (77–83) | 78 (74–81) |
| >10 and ≤20 | 73 (68–78) | 57 (48–64) | 54[c] (44–63) | 75 (72–78) | 68 (64–71) | 66 (62–70) |
| >20 | 60 (49–69) | 48 (36–59) | 48 (36–59) | 58 (54–62) | 52 (47–57) | 50 (43–56) |
| **Actuarial Nonprogression Rate (95% CI) by Clinical Stage** | | | | | | |
| cT1ab | 90 (83–95) | 85 (76–91) | 75 (58–86) | 90 (85–95) | 85 (79–92) | 83 (76–90) |
| cT1c | 91 (88–93) | 76 (48–90) | 76[c] (48–90) | 88 (86–90) | 79 (73–85) | NA |
| cT2a | 86 (83–88) | 75 (71–79) | 66 (59–72) | 85 (82–88) | 77 (71–83) | 75 (70–80) |
| cT2b | 75 (70–79) | 62 (56–68) | 50 (41–58) | 74 (70–79) | 69 (64–75) | 69 (64–75) |
| cT2c | 71 (61–79) | 57 (45–68) | 57 (45–68) | 71 (68–75) | 64 (59–68) | 62 (57–67) |
| cT3 | 60 (45–72) | 49 (34–63) | NA | 54 (44–64) | 51 (40–62) | NA |
| **Actuarial Nonprogression Rate (95% CI) by Specimen Gleason Sum** | | | | | | |
| 2–4 | 100 | 100 | 100 | 100 | 100 | 100 |
| 5 | 98 (96–99) | 94 (90–96) | 86 (78–92) | 92 (90–94) | 89 (86–92) | 88 (84–92) |
| 6 | 95 (93–97) | 88 (83–92) | 73 (59–82) | 91 (89–93) | 83 (80–86) | 81 (78–85) |
| 7 (All) | 73 (69–76) | 54 (48–59) | 48 (41–56) | 77 (75–79) | 70 (66–74) | 67 (63–72) |
| 3 + 4 | 81 (77–84) | 60 (53–67) | 59 (51–65) | 82 (79–84) | 74 (69–79) | 72 (62–82) |
| 4 + 3 | 53 (44–61) | 33 (22–43) | 33 (22–43) | 60 (50–70) | 53 (44–64) | 53 (44–64) |
| 8–10 | 44 (36–52) | 29 (22–37) | 15 (5–28) | 41 (35–47) | 33 (24–42) | NA |
| **Actuarial Nonprogression Rate (95% CI) by Pathologic Stage** | | | | | | |
| Organ confined | 97 (95–98) | 93 (90–95) | 84 (77–90) | 93 (92–94) | 89 (87–91) | 87 (85–89) |
| EPE+, GS <7, SM− | 97 (94–98) | 93 (89–96) | 84 (70–92) | 92 (89–94) | 89 (84–94) | 86 (79–92) |
| EPE+, GS <7, SM+ | 89 (80–94) | 73 (61–82) | 58 (41–71) | 74 (64–84) | 65 (54–76) | 65 (54–76) |
| EPE+, GS ≥7, SM− | 80 (75–85) | 61 (52–68) | 59 (50–67) | 76 (66–86) | 68 (61–75) | 65 (56–74) |
| EPE+, GS ≥7, SM+ | 58 (49–66) | 42 (32–52) | 33 (23–44) | 60 (53–67) | 55 (44–66) | 55 (44–66) |
| SV+, LN− | 48 (38–58) | 30 (19–41) | 17 (5–35) | 44 (38–50) | 31 (24–38) | 28 (19–37) |
| LN+ | 26 (19–35) | 10 (5–18) | 0 | 25 (18–32) | 15 (5–25) | 0 |
| Negative margins | NA | NA | NA | 87 (86–88) | 81 (79–83) | 79 (76–82) |
| Positive margins | NA | NA | NA | 66 (63–69) | 56 (52–60) | 54 (49–59) |

MSKCC SPORE, Memorial Sloan Kettering Cancer Center Specialized Programs of Research Excellence; BCR, biochemical recurrence; CI, confidence interval; PSA, prostate-specific antigen; NA, not applicable; EPE, extraprostatic extension; GS, Gleason sum; SM, surgical margin; SV, seminal vesicles; LN, lymph node.
[a] Single surgeon series. From Han M, Partin AW, Pound CR, et al. Long-term biochemical disease-free and cancer-specific survival following anatomic radical retropubic prostatectomy. The 15-year Johns Hopkins experience. *Urol Clin North Am* 2001;28:555–565.
[b] Includes 1,092 radical prostatectomies performed by a single surgeon.
[c] Fourteen-year data.

hormonal treatment. At 5 years 84% of patients, at 10 years 78%, and at 15 years 73% were free of progression (see Table 42.5).

Of particular interest are patients with high-grade cancers (Gleason sum 7 to 10). Of patients with Gleason 3 + 4 = 7 cancers in the RP specimen, 68% were free of progression at 15 years. When the tumor was Gleason 4 + 3 = 7, 51% were free of progression at 15 years.[179] Even patients with Gleason sum 8 to 10 cancers fared well, with 27%

free of progression at 10 years. These progression rates are substantially lower than the 15-year cancer mortality rates reported for patients with Gleason sum 7 to 10 cancers managed with watchful waiting.[197]

Once the prostate is removed, the most powerful prognostic factor is the pathologic stage (see Table 42.6). When the cancer is confined to the prostate (defined as cancer not extending into the periprostatic soft tissue), 92% to 98% of patients remain free of progression at 5 years and 88% to 96% remain free 10 years after RP.[194] Focal penetration through the capsule into the periprostatic soft tissue alone, in the absence of SVI, results in a 73% 10-year nonprogression rate. Established (extensive) penetration through the prostatic capsule into the periprostatic soft tissue, in the absence of SVI, results in a 42% 10-year nonprogression rate. Even some patients with SVI (pT3cN0) can be cured with surgery, with 30% being free of disease recurrence at 10 years (see Table 42.6).

The slow clinical progression of prostate cancer after RP has led to the widespread use of PSA recurrence as the primary end point for evaluating treatment outcome. However, doing so ignores the fact that the prognosis of men in the rising PSA state is highly variable, and that the rising PSA by itself does not necessarily mean that a patient will develop metastatic disease, develop symptoms, or die of his cancer. For many, the threat posed to a man's duration and quality of survival is limited at best.

Reports of long-term, prostate cancer–specific survival rates after RP have clearly shown that many patients with PSA recurrence live out their lives free of cancer.[179,193,194,196,198] The long-term risk of prostate cancer–specific mortality (PCSM) after RP for patients treated in the era of widespread PSA screening has

recently been estimated based on a multi-institutional cohort of 12,677 patients treated with RP between 1987 and 2005.[139] Fifteen-year PCSM and all-cause mortality were 12% and 38%, respectively. The estimated PCSM ranged from 5% to 38% for patients in the lowest and highest quartiles of nomogram-predicted risk of PSA-defined recurrence (Table 42.7). Only 4% of contemporary patients had a predicted 15-year PCSM of >5%.

Clearly, few patients will die from prostate cancer within 15 years of RP, despite the presence of adverse clinical features. It is not known whether this favorable prognosis is related to the effectiveness of RP (with or without secondary therapy) or to the low lethality of cancers detected by early screening. Although year of surgery, biopsy Gleason grade, and PSA level are associated with PCSM risk, an individual patient's risk cannot be predicted on the basis of clinical features alone. Further research is needed to identify novel markers specifically associated with the biology of lethal prostate cancer.

### High-Risk Prostate Cancer

Monotherapy is often believed to be inadequate for high-risk cancers, and some clinicians are reluctant to consider RP in high-risk

### TABLE 42.7

**Risk of Prostate Cancer–Specific Mortality at 10 and 15 Years After Radical Prostatectomy[a]**

| Variable | Patients[b] No. | Patients[b] % | Events[b] No. | Events[b] % | Ten-Y PCSM % | Ten-Y PCSM 95% CI | Fifteen-Y PCSM % | Fifteen-Y PCSM 95% CI |
|---|---|---|---|---|---|---|---|---|
| **Nomogram-Predicted 5-y PFP (%)** | | | | | | | | |
| 76–99 | 8,555 | 73 | 51 | 26 | 1.8 | 1.2–2.4 | 5 | 3–7 |
| 51–75 | 2,228 | 19 | 75 | 38 | 6 | 4–7 | 15 | 10–21 |
| 26–50 | 656 | 6 | 40 | 21 | 9 | 6–12 | 16 | 9–22 |
| 1–25 | 209 | 2 | 29 | 15 | 15 | 9–22 | 38 | 19–56 |
| **Risk Group** | | | | | | | | |
| PSA <10, Gleason score 6, T1c or T2a | 5,200 | 46 | 14 | 7 | 0.9 | 0.3–1.5 | 2 | 0.3–4 |
| PSA 10–20, Gleason score 7, T2b | 4,184 | 37 | 64 | 32 | 4 | 2–5 | 10 | 6–14 |
| PSA >20, Gleason score 8–10, T2c-T3 | 1,962 | 17 | 121 | 61 | 8 | 7–10 | 19 | 14–24 |
| **Pretreatment PSA (ng/ml)** | | | | | | | | |
| <4 | 2,285 | 18 | 18 | 9 | 2 | 1–4 | 4 | 1–7 |
| 4–10 | 7,574 | 61 | 75 | 37 | 3 | 2–4 | 9 | 5–12 |
| 10.1–20 | 1,874 | 15 | 50 | 24 | 4 | 3–6 | 11 | 6–15 |
| 20.1–50 | 726 | 6 | 62 | 30 | 10 | 7–12 | 22 | 15–30 |
| **1992 TNM Clinical Stage** | | | | | | | | |
| T1ab | 174 | 2 | 4 | 2 | 2 | 0–4 | 6 | 0–12 |
| T1c | 6,413 | 56 | 28 | 14 | 2 | 1–3 | 6 | 5–7 |
| T2a | 2,520 | 22 | 42 | 21 | 3 | 2–4 | 7 | 4–10 |
| T2b | 1,461 | 13 | 57 | 29 | 5 | 3–7 | 14 | 9–19 |
| T2c | 714 | 6 | 38 | 19 | 7 | 4–9 | 12 | 8–17 |
| T3 | 254 | 2 | 28 | 14 | 15 | 9–21 | 38 | 22–54 |
| **Biopsy Gleason Score** | | | | | | | | |
| 2–6 | 7,454 | 65 | 78 | 40 | 2 | 1–3 | 6 | 4–8 |
| 7 | 3,292 | 29 | 55 | 28 | 5 | 3–7 | 17 | 8–26 |
| 8–10 | 702 | 6 | 61 | 32 | 16 | 11–20 | 34 | 23–46 |

PCSM, prostate cancer–specific mortality; CI, confidence interval; PFP, progression-free probability; PSA, prostate-specific antigen; TNM, tumor, node, metastasis.
[a] Values were based on a previously validated nomogram, risk groups, clinical stage, pretreatment PSA, and biopsy Gleason score.
[b] Percentages refer to proportion of total in each category.
From Stephenson AJ, Kattan MW, Eastham JA, et al. Prostate cancer-specific mortality after radical prostatectomy for patients treated in the prostate-specific antigen era. *J Clin Oncol* 2009;27:4300–4305, with permission.

## TABLE 42.8

**Estimates of 5- and 10-Year Progression-Free Probability in Men Undergoing Radical Prostatectomy for High-Risk Prostate Cancer**

| High-Risk Definition | BCR/No. of Patients | Five-Y PFP (95% CI) | Ten-Y PFP (95% CI) |
|---|---|---|---|
| Biopsy Gleason 8–10 | 109/274 | 53 (46,60) | 42 (38,56) |
| Preoperative PSA ≥20 | 121/275 | 56 (50,62) | 47 (40,54) |
| 1992 TNM stage T3 | 62/144 | 49 (39,58) | 41 (29,53) |
| PSA ≥20 or ≥T2c or GS ≥8 | 299/957 | 68 (65,71) | 59 (55,63) |
| Nomogram 5-y PFP ≤50% | 180/391 | 53 (47,57) | 43 (36,49) |
| PSA ≥20 or ≥T3 or GS ≥8 | 234/605 | 57 (53,62) | 50 (44,55) |
| PSA ≥15 or ≥T2b or GS ≥8 | 466/1,752 | 73 (71,75) | 65 (62,68) |
| PSA velocity >2 ng/ml/y | 161/952 | 80 (77,83) | 74 (70,78) |

BCR, biochemical relapse; PFP, progression-free probability; CI, confidence interval; PSA, prostate-specific antigen; TNM, tumor, node, metastasis; GS, Gleason score.
From Yossepowitch O, Eggener SE, Bianco FJ Jr, et al. Radical prostatectomy for clinically localized, high risk prostate cancer: critical analysis of risk assessment methods. *J Urol* 2007;178:493–499, with permission.

## TABLE 42.9

**Estimated 10-Year Disease-Specific Mortality After Radical Prostatectomy for Patients with High-Risk Cancer by Various Definitions**

| High-Risk Definition | Ten-Y DSM (95% CI) |
|---|---|
| Biopsy Gleason 8–10 | 12 (7–19) |
| Preoperative PSA ≥20 | 9 (6–13) |
| 1992 TNM stage T3 | 11 (7–19) |
| PSA ≥20 or ≥T2c or GS ≥8 | 7 (5–9) |
| Nomogram 5-y PFP ≤50% | 8 (6–12) |
| PSA ≥20 or ≥T3 or GS ≥8 | 8 (6–11) |
| PSA ≥15 or ≥T2b or GS ≥8 | 5 (4–7) |
| PSA velocity >2 ng/ml/y | 3 (2–6) |

DSM, disease-specific mortality; CI, confidence interval; PSA, prostate-specific antigen; TNM, tumor, node, metastasis; GS, Gleason score; PFP, progression-free probability.
From Yossepowitch O, Eggener SE, Serio AM, et al. Secondary therapy, metastatic progression, and cancer-specific mortality in men with clinically high-risk prostate cancer treated with radical prostatectomy. *Eur Urol* 2008;53:950–959, with permission.

patients. However, there are no standardized criteria to define high-risk before definitive treatment. Among 4,708 patients undergoing RP, high-risk patients were identified based on eight established definitions, and their pathologic characteristics and PSA outcomes were examined (Table 42.8). Depending on the definition used, high-risk patients composed 3% to 38% of the study population. Among patients defined as high-risk, 22% to 63% of tumors proved to be confined to the prostate on pathologic examination. Although high-risk patients had a 1.8- to 4.8-fold increased hazard of PSA relapse, their 10-year relapse-free probability after RP alone was 41% to 74% (see Table 42.8).[199] Disease-specific survival at 12 years was between 78% to 94% (Table 42.9).[200] Of the high-risk patients who relapsed, 25% (across all definitions) relapsed more than 2 years after surgery, and in 26% to 39% the PSADT at recurrence was ≥10 months. These results show that the commonly used definitions of high risk have the potential to deny patients potentially curative treatment. New criteria are needed to identify those patients who need the integration of systemic therapy to improve outcomes beyond what can be achieved with monotherapies directed to the prostate itself.[201]

### Impact of the Surgeon on Outcomes After Radical Prostatectomy

Recent research has focused on the ways in which surgical volume and the individual surgeon influence results after RP. Begg et al.[202] used the Surveillance, Epidemiology, and End Results–Medicare-linked database to evaluate health-related outcomes after RP. The rates of postoperative complications, late urinary complications (strictures or fistulas 31 days to 365 days after the procedure), and long-term incontinence (>1 year after the procedure) were inferred from the Medicare claims records of 11,522 patients who underwent RP between 1992 and 1996. These rates were analyzed in relation to hospital volume and surgeon volume (the number of procedures performed at individual hospitals and by

individual surgeons, respectively). Neither hospital volume nor surgeon volume was significantly associated with surgery-related death. Significant trends in the relation between volume and outcome were observed with respect to postoperative complications and late urinary complications. Postoperative morbidity was lower in very-high-volume hospitals than in low-volume hospitals (27% versus 32%; $p = 0.03$) and was also lower when the prostatectomy was performed by very-high-volume surgeons than when it was performed by low-volume surgeons (26% versus 32%; $p < 0.001$). The rates of late urinary complications followed a similar pattern. Results for long-term preservation of continence were less clear-cut. In a detailed analysis of the 159 surgeons who performed a high or very high volume of procedures, wide surgeon-to-surgeon variations in clinical outcomes were observed, and these variations were much greater than would have been predicted on the basis of chance or observed variations in the case mix. These findings suggest that, in general, high-volume surgeons have superior results compared with low-volume surgeons, in terms of early postoperative morbidity and urinary complications after RP. However, the much better than anticipated outcomes among the highest-volume surgeons suggest that individual surgical technique also influences clinical outcomes.

Individual patient data from four institutions was used to study the association between a surgeon's prior experience and BCR after RP (the principal reason that patients visit an oncologic surgeon).[181] This relationship has often been termed the *learning curve* and probably reflects differences in surgical skill. A retrospective cohort study of consecutive patients treated from 1987 to 2003 was conducted at four academic, tertiary referral centers in the United States. In this study, 7,850 patients with localized prostate cancer received no neoadjuvant therapy and underwent open radical retropubic prostatectomy by 1 of 73 different surgeons.[179] For each patient, surgeon experience was coded as the total number of RPs conducted by the surgeon prior to the incident case, and cancer control was defined as a corroborated rising PSA level >0.4 ng/ml. The study demonstrated that cancer control improved with increasing surgeon experience (Fig. 42.10), and this relationship[181] remained highly significant ($p < 0.001$) after adjustment for tumor characteristics and year of surgery. The learning curve for cancer control after radical retropubic prostatectomy was steep but did not begin to plateau until a surgeon had completed approximately 250 prior operations. Five-year probability of BCR was 17.8% for patients treated by surgeons in the early phase of their career (10 prior operations),

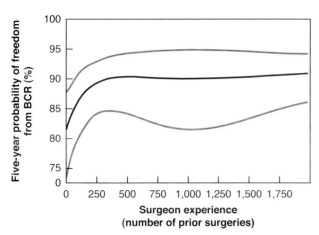

**Figure 42.10** The surgical learning curve for cancer control after radical prostatectomy. Predicted probability (*purple curve*) and 95% confidence intervals (*orange curves*) for freedom from biochemical recurrence (BCR) at 5 years after radical prostatectomy are plotted against increasing surgeon experience. Probabilities are for a patient with typical cancer severity (mean prostate-specific antigen level, pathologic stage, and grade) treated in 1997 (approximately equal numbers of patients were treated before and after 1997). (From Vickers AJ, Bianco FJ, Serio AM, et al. The surgical learning curve for prostate cancer control after radical prostatectomy. *J Natl Cancer Inst* 2007;99:1171–1177, with permission.)

compared with 10.9% when surgeons had performed 250 operations (absolute risk difference, 6.9%; 95% confidence interval [CI] = 4.3% to 9.5%) (see Fig. 42.10). We saw no evidence that patient risk attenuates the learning curve: there was a statistically significant association between BCR and surgeon experience in all analyses. The relative risk for a patient receiving treatment from a surgeon with 10 rather than 250 prior RP was 2.5, 1.8, and 1.3 for low-, medium-, and high-risk patients, respectively.

## Radiotherapy for Localized Prostate Cancer

Radiotherapy given by external beam or brachytherapy techniques is a second treatment option for men with clinically localized prostate cancers. With the availability of sophisticated treatment planning systems and image-guided approaches, there have been significant advances in radiotherapy enabling higher doses to be delivered more safely, and concomitant improvements in disease-free survival outcomes. Intensity-modulated external beam radiotherapy (IMRT) has become a standard mode of treatment delivery and has facilitated the application of higher radiation dose levels of ≥80 Gy, with lower risks of late rectal and urinary toxicities. Such treatments coupled with image guidance have enabled the routine use of tighter margins, incorporating less normal tissue within the high-dose region and leading to further decrements in late toxicities. Brachytherapy using permanent or temporary radioactive implants within the prostate alone or combined with IMRT is another commonly used radiotherapeutic approach. This approach has also improved with more accurate image guidance and intraoperative real-time planning for brachytherapy, resulting in more highly conformal dose distributions, which in turn has resulted in better outcomes and lower toxicity rates, relative to what has been previously reported. In some cases, ADT is used in several contexts: to improve local eradication of locally advanced tumors by reducing tumor size, to eliminate tumor clonogens inherently resistant to radiotherapy by impairing DNA repair pathways, and/or reducing prostate volumes by 30% to 40%, which improves the ability to deliver maximal radiation dose levels without exceeding the tolerance for the surrounding normal tissue. Hormone therapy also has a favorable effect on micrometastatic disease that may be present at the time of diagnosis in men with high-risk tumors.

Although there are no randomized trials comparing modern, sophisticated high-dose EBRT to brachytherapy for the treatment of localized prostate cancer, there are several criteria used to help select the most appropriate form of therapy for the patient. For patients with low-risk disease in whom AS may not be considered—owing to PSA velocity, the presence of a dominant lesion on imaging studies, or a larger volume of disease determined by biopsy—high-dose IMRT alone (in the range of 80 Gy) or brachytherapy alone are excellent treatment options.

Larger prostate volumes, the presence of urinary obstructive symptoms, and medical comorbidities may influence the selection away from a brachytherapy-based treatment. In contrast, brachytherapy may be the preferred choice for patients without these factors because of its excellent ablative capabilities (leading to long-term PSA relapse-free survival outcomes) and its convenience (as a treatment accomplished in a single outpatient setting). For patients with intermediate- and higher-risk disease, combined modality treatments including brachytherapy and supplemental IMRT are preferred to allow for the delivery of a high and concentrated dose of radiation to the prostate. Ultrahypofractionated EBRT regimens have generated increasing interest as another therapeutic option for patients with localized disease; however, the long-term results of this approach are not available, and the results of ongoing trials are awaiting more mature follow-up.

### External Beam Radiotherapy

#### Intensity-Modulated Radiotherapy and Image-Guided Techniques

IMRT, a type of conformal radiotherapy (CRT), has become a standard mode of treatment planning for patients with localized prostate cancer and takes advantage of inverse-planning methods to optimize dose distribution. Inverse planning is part of a mathematical optimization algorithm that creates a treatment plan based on predefined, desired dose-distribution parameters for the target and dose constraints imposed on the normal tissues. The highly conformal radiation beam is produced with the ability to vary the intensities of the X-rays from each treatment field over the entire cross-section of the beam.

More recently, image-guided approaches have enhanced IMRT delivery. Acquisition of CT images or kilovoltage images on the treatment machine immediately before the radiation treatment allows for visualization of the target and correction of its position, which can fluctuate on a daily basis, related to bladder or rectal filling. Linac-based kilovoltage image guidance systems have become commercially available; they possess capabilities for kilovoltage two-dimensional projection imaging (radiographs), fluoroscopy, and three-dimensional cone beam CT, and are thus ideally suited for monitoring inter- and intrafractional motion. The use of image-guided radiotherapy and enhanced target localization could lead to a further reduction of safety margins and a decrease in morbidity related to ultrahypofractionated regimens. A recent retrospective report demonstrated reduced urinary-related treatment toxicities and improved tumor control outcomes among patients with clinically localized prostate cancer treated with image-guided approaches, compared with patients not treated with image-guided therapy.[203] Among a cohort of patients treated to dose levels of 86.4 Gy, the incidence of late grade 2 urinary toxicities was 20% for those treated with daily image guidance, compared with 10% for patients treated with daily image guidance and target positional corrections ($p = 0.02$)

#### Definition of Target Volume

The multifocal nature of prostate cancer and the well-documented risk of microscopic ECE, even for patients with early clinical stages of disease, are important considerations that influence the design of the target volume for radiation treatment planning. The clinical target volume (CTV) includes the entire prostate gland and immediate periprostatic tissues, as well as the seminal vesicles, as visualized on CT. For patients with low-risk disease with unremarkable imaging studies, the CTV may exclude the seminal vesicles, owing to the low likelihood of disease involvement. The planning target volume places an additional margin around the CTV to take into account patient setup uncertainties and organ motion. With the use of image-guided approaches, the margin can be safely reduced to 5 mm to 6 mm around the CTV, except at the prostate-rectal interface, where an even tighter margin (3 mm to 5 mm) is used.

## Role of Dose Escalation in Patients with Clinically Localized Disease

Findings from several randomized phase 3 trials (Table 42.10)[204–208] and the long-term results of single-institution studies[209–212] demonstrate a significant improvement in treatment outcomes with higher radiation doses in patients with clinically localized disease. As shown in Table 42.10, these studies have generally demonstrated a 10% to 20% improvement in 5- to 10-year PSA survival outcomes when higher doses of 78 Gy to 80 Gy are applied, compared with dose levels of 70 Gy, and such benefits have been observed for low-, intermediate-, and high-risk cohorts. Although overall survival benefits have not been demonstrated with dose escalation, improvements in distant metastases–free survival are emerging with longer follow-up, suggesting that survival benefits will be seen as these studies mature. In one report, a reduction in death due to prostate cancer was noted at 10 years for intermediate- and high-risk patients treated with doses of 78 Gy, compared with those treated at 70 Gy.[213]

For patients with intermediate- and especially high-risk disease, doses beyond 80 Gy may be required to achieve optimal tumor control outcomes. To do so requires ultra-high-dose IMRT, which constrains the dose delivered to normal tissues, such as the bladder and the rectum. In a recent update of the long-term outcomes of ultra-high-dose IMRT at MSKCC, 1,002 patients treated with 86.4 Gy, using a five- to seven-field IMRT technique, had 7-year PSA-relapse-free survival rates of 99%, 86%, and 68% for low-, intermediate-, and high-risk patients, respectively. The incidence of distant metastases for these respective risk groups was 0.5%, 6%, and 18% at 7 years, and incidence of grade 3 rectal and urinary toxicities was 0.7% and 2.2%. The median follow-up was 5.5 years.[214]

## Sequelae of External Beam Radiotherapy

Complication rates after EBRT vary as a function of the dose, the volume of normal tissues irradiated at particular dose levels, and the treatment field. Acute symptoms typically appear during the third week of treatment and resolve within days to weeks after its completion. Acute intestinal symptoms, especially those associated with whole pelvic irradiation, are most commonly relieved with dietary manipulations. Otherwise, medications such as loperamide hydrochloride (Imodium; McNEIL-PPC, Inc., Fort Washington, PA) or diphenoxylate hydrochloride and atropine sulphate (Lomotil; Pfizer, New York, NY) are appropriate to relieve symptoms. Internal and external hemorrhoids, which may become inflamed during the course of therapy, are often best treated with sitz baths and hydrocortisone suppositories. Patients may also experience changes in the consistency of their bowel movements or an increase in mucous discharge. Acute urinary symptoms are treated with phenazopyridine hydrochloride (Pyridium; Warner Chilcott, Rockaway, NJ), nonsteroidal anti-inflammatory agents, or alpha-blockers, such as tamsulosin hydrochloride (Flomax; Boehringer Ingelheim Pharmaceuticals, Inc., Ridgefield, CT). Alpha-blockers have been reported to be significantly more effective than nonsteroidal anti-inflammatory agents, resulting in significant resolution of urinary symptoms in 66% of patients and moderate improvement in 22%.[215]

## TABLE 42.10

### Phase 3 External Beam Radiotherapy Dose Escalation Studies

| Study (Ref.) | No. of Patients | Median Follow-Up | Treatment Arms | PSA Relapse-Free Survival Outcome | P Value |
|---|---|---|---|---|---|
| Beckendorf et al.[204]/ GETUG 06 | 306 | 5 y | 80 Gy vs. 70 Gy | At 5 y: Overall results<br>High dose, 72%<br>Low dose, 61% | 0.039 |
| Al-Mamgani et al.[205] | 669 | 70 mo | 78 vs. 68 Gy (neoadjuvant short-term and long-term ADT used in two participating institutions for high-risk patients) | At 7 y: Intermediate- and high-risk patients<br>High dose, 54%<br>Low dose, 47% | <0.04 |
| Kuban et al.[206] | 301 | 8.7 y | 78 vs. 70 Gy (no ADT given) | At 8 y: Overall results<br>High dose, 78%<br>Low dose, 59%<br>At 8 y: PSA >10 ng/ml<br>High dose, 78%<br>Low dose, 39% | 0.004<br><br><br><0.001 |
| Zietman et al.[207] | 393 | 8.9 y | 79.2 Gy equivalent vs. 70.2 Gy equivalent (dose delivered with combination of protons/photons) | At 10 y: Overall results<br>High dose, 83%<br>Low dose, 68%<br>At 10 y: Low-risk patients<br>High dose, 93%<br>Low dose, 72% | <0.001<br><br><br><0.001 |
| Dearnaley et al.[208]/ MRC-RT01 | 843 | 10 y | 74 vs. 64 Gy 30-CRT (3–6 mo neoadjuvant + concurrent ADT administered) | At 10 y: Low-risk patients<br>High dose, 55%<br>Low dose, 43% | 0.0003 |

PSA, prostate-specific antigen; GETUG, Genitourinary Tumor Group; ADT, androgen deprivation therapy; MRC, Medical Research Council; CRT, conformal radiotherapy.

Late rectal toxicities attributed to radiotherapy typically manifest 12 months to 18 months after completion of treatment and may persist for several years thereafter; the development of rectal complications after 5 years is rare. Late rectal toxicities may include rectal bleeding, mucous discharge, and mild incontinence of stool. The more-severe toxicities, including ulcer development and fistula formation, are observed in ≤1% of patients. Grade 2 rectal bleeding can be effectively treated with steroid suppositories, sitz baths, and an increase in dietary fiber. Because of the increased risk of further trauma to the rectal mucosa and the risk of fistula formation, deep rectal biopsies and cauterization procedures should be avoided unless absolutely necessary. For radiation-induced proctitis not responsive to conservative measures, argon-beam plasma laser coagulation can decrease the frequency of rectal bleeding episodes.[216] Hyperbaric oxygen treatments, at a pressure of 2.4 atmospheres for a median of 36 sessions (90 minutes per session), may be helpful; in one study, they were associated with a complete resolution of rectal bleeding in 48% of patients and a reduction in bleeding episodes in 28% of patients.[217] It is assumed that hyperbaric oxygen improves the delivery of oxygen to ischemic rectal mucosa, promoting angiogenesis and advancing mucosal healing and fibroblast proliferation.

Late urinary toxicities include chronic urethritis, which occurs in approximately 10% to 15% of patients, and urethral strictures, which occur in 2% to 3%. Hemorrhagic cystitis is uncommon with conformal radiation techniques, which reduce the dose to the bladder. Current treatment approaches for hemorrhagic cystitis include intravesical formalin therapy and selective embolization of the hypogastric arteries. For patients refractory to such measures, hyperbaric oxygen therapy can be considered for radiation-induced hemorrhagic cystitis. In one report, 49 of 57 patients (86%) experienced complete resolution or marked improvement of hematuria following hyperbaric oxygen treatment.[218]

Whereas any form of radiotherapy can increase the risk of developing a secondary cancer, the incidence after prostate radiotherapy appears to be lower than expected. One report comparing the risks of secondary cancers among patients treated with RP, EBRT, and brachytherapy did not find the therapeutic intervention to be a significant predictor of secondary cancer at 10-year follow-up.[219] Longer follow-up will be required to determine whether any significant differences eventually develop between the treatment arms. Nonetheless, given the risk of secondary cancer with any form of radiotherapy, close monitoring is important. Colonoscopy every 5 years and careful evaluation of patients who present with hematuria after radiotherapy are recommended to rule out the possibility of a secondary bladder cancer.

IMRT is also associated with a reduced risk of rectal-related toxicities after high-dose radiotherapy. In the initial cohort of patients treated with 81 Gy, late rectal and urinary complications were significantly reduced with IMRT relative to conventional three-dimensional CRT (Fig. 42.11). In 561 patients treated with IMRT (81 Gy) at MSKCC,[220] the 8-year actuarial likelihood of developing grade 2 rectal bleeding was 1.6% with no grade 4 events and late grade 2 and 3 (urethral strictures) urinary toxicities were 9% and 3%, respectively. Among patients who were potent before IMRT, 49% developed erectile dysfunction.[220]

Factors predictive of late urinary toxicities after high-dose IMRT included a lower baseline urinary symptom score (International Prostate Symptoms Score) ($p = 0.006$) and an increased maximal dose beyond the prescribed dose to the bladder trigone region ($p = 0.003$).[221] When high-dose radiotherapy is used, efforts should be made to restrict the high-dose region from receiving >15% to 20% of the prescription doses for the urethra and, in particular, for the bladder neck and the region of the bladder trigone. These and other data indicate that patients with significant urinary symptoms before treatment may be better served by surgery, rather than radiotherapy.

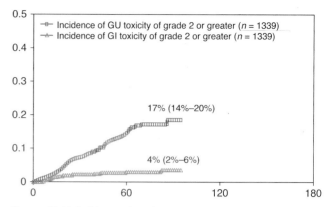

**Figure 42.11** Incidence of grade 2 or greater genitourinary (GU) and gastrointestinal (GI) toxicities for patients receiving intensity-modulated radiation therapy only for patients treated at Memorial Sloan Kettering Cancer Center. *X-axis* represents months from completion of treatment. *Y-axis* represents the percentage incidence of toxicity.

## Potency Preservation with External Beam Radiotherapy

The reported rates of impotence at 3 years or longer after EBRT ranges widely from 36% to 68%,[222] a reflection of the differences in methodologies used to assess this end point and the heterogeneity of the EBRT patient population. Factors such as advanced age and the presence of medical comorbidities (coronary artery disease, diabetes, and use of antihypertensive medications) can have a profound effect on erectile function. Besides erectile dysfunction, aspects of sexual dysfunction that occur after radiotherapy include decreased volume of ejaculate, absence of ejaculate, decreased intensity of orgasm, and decreased libido.

## Hypofractionated External Beam Radiotherapy

The administration of larger doses for each treatment fraction has potential radiobiologic advantages (hypofractionated radiotherapy) that can result in a greater degree of cell kill.[223,224] One approach is stereotactic body radiosurgery, which has been used increasingly during the last several years. Unfortunately, most reports to date are uncontrolled single-center series of selected patients which, despite recognized limitations, are showing promising results using PSA-based outcomes.[225–227] These treatments are delivered with a linear accelerator mounted with an image-guided device to achieve greater precision of the dose delivery. With tight margins used, high doses per fraction allow completion of the course of therapy in 1 week. A pooled analysis of 1,100 patients treated from 2003 to 2011 at eight institutions was recently reported.[228] The median dose delivered for these patients was 36.25 Gy in five fractions. The median follow-up was 3 years; the 5-year PSA-relapse-free survival rates were 95%, 84%, and 81% for low-, intermediate-, and high-risk patients, repsectively. Stereotactic radiosurgery appears promising, but this form of treatment cannot be considered an established form of radiotherapy delivery, and ongoing studies will define its role better in the years ahead.

## The Role of Proton Therapy for Localized Prostate Cancer

Recently, there has been increasing interest in the use of proton therapy for clinically localized disease because of the known physical advantages of this charged particle—namely, the Bragg peak—by which the majority of the energy of the beam is deposited at the end of its track, creating a rapid falloff of dose beyond the target. The result is that exit dose beyond the target volume is eliminated, providing the potential to achieve greater sparing of normal tissues with dose escalation. Theoretically, physical advantages of the proton beam may also translate into a reduced risk of second malignancies, owing to the reduced exposure of normal tissues to the radiation beam relative to photon therapy. A series by Mendenhall et al.[229] examined the 5-year clinical outcomes of 211 prospectively treated patients who received proton therapy using an image-guided approach. Low-risk patients received 78 Gy, intermediate-risk 78 Gy to 82 Gy, and high-risk 78 Gy with concomitant docetaxel followed by ADT; the 5-year PSA-relapse-free survival rates were 99%, 99%, and 76%, respectively. The incidence of grade 3 rectal and urinary toxicities was 1% and 5.4%, respectively, comparable if not superior to those with high-dose IMRT. Randomized trials to confirm these findings are ongoing, including a multi-institutional trial comparing 80 Gy versus a similar dose of protons for low- and intermediate-risk patients; the end point is 2-year QOL and late toxicities.

Reports addressing the question of whether protons are associated with reduced long-term toxicities relative to high-dose photon therapy are conflicting. One recent study of 1,242 patients treated with either proton therapy at doses of 76 Gy to 82 Gy or IMRT at doses of 75.6 Gy to 79.4 Gy showed similar QOL scores for the bowel, urinary incontinence, urinary irritative symptoms, and sexual domains at the last follow-up evaluation. Further exploration of specific function outcomes showed that patients treated with proton therapy had less frequent bowel movements and rectal urgency, compared with patients treated with IMRT.[230] However, an analysis of the relative toxicities of IMRT and proton therapy in patients with localized prostate cancer based on the Surveillance, Epidemiology, and End Results–Medicare-linked database showed that IMRT was associated with fewer gastrointestinal (GI)-related toxicities and hip fractures, whereas proton therapy was associated with a lower risk of erectile dysfunction.[231] It is anticipated that future improvements in intensity-modulated proton therapy will also improve the conformality of the proton beam, resulting in fewer complications with proton dose escalation. To date, however, there is no established evidence that proton therapy provides superior tumor control outcomes, compared with well-delivered high-dose IMRT or image-guided radiotherapy, for the treatment of prostate cancer.

## Prostate Brachytherapy

Excellent long-term tumor control can be achieved with brachytherapy, and the approach is considered a standard treatment intervention associated with outcomes comparable to those with prostatectomy and EBRT for patients with clinically localized disease.[232–237] By category, low-risk disease is managed with seed implantation alone (i.e., monotherapy), whereas intermediate- and selected high-risk disease is managed with a combination of brachytherapy (low-dose-rate [LDR] permanent interstitial implantation or high-dose-rate [HDR] brachytherapy via after-loading catheters) and EBRT. Whether the addition of EBRT is necessary in all patients with intermediate-risk prostate cancer is being studied in a phase 3 randomized trial (Radiation Therapy Oncology Group [RTOG] 0232).

### Technical Aspects of Prostate Brachytherapy

Transperineal ultrasound-guided approaches have facilitated image-guided placement of the seeds and are credited with improved long-term outcomes and reduced treatment-related complications. These approaches have further improved the accuracy and consistency of the dose delivery to the target, with a concomitant reduction of dose to the urethra and rectum. The use of adjunctive intraoperative CT scanning to verify the actual deposited seed coordinates may eliminate the need for postimplantation assessments and may allow for opportunities, if necessary, to correct suboptimal implanted regions within the gland before the reversal of anesthesia. Close collaboration between the radiation oncologist and the medical physicist in

the design of the pre- or intraoperative treatment plan is critical for a successful outcome.

The two most commonly used radioisotopes for permanent seed brachytherapy are iodine-125 ($^{125}$I) and palladium-103 ($^{103}$Pd). The half-life of $^{125}$I is 60 days, with a mean photon energy of 27 KeV and an initial dose rate of 0.07 Gy/h. In contrast, the half-life of $^{103}$Pd is 17 days, with a mean photon energy of 21 KeV and an initial dose rate of 0.19 cGy/h. The active periods for $^{125}$I and $^{103}$Pd are 10 months and 3 months, respectively. When $^{125}$I is used, the typical prescription dose is 144 Gy; 125 Gy is routinely used for $^{103}$Pd.

The quality of the implant and dose distributions are routinely evaluated using CT scans obtained on the day of the implant or 30 days later. Postimplantation CT scans are used to generate dose-volume histograms, which allow detailed analysis of the radiation dose distribution relative to the prostate and surrounding normal tissues. Dosimetric parameters include V100 for the target (volume of the prostate receiving 100% of the prescription dose), D90 of the target (dose delivered to 90% of the prostate), and the average and maximum rectal and urethral doses.[238]

Table 42.11 summarizes the published biochemical control outcomes after LDR interstitial seed implantation, according to prognostic risk groups.[235,237,239–243] The size of the prostate gland should preferably be <60 cm$^3$ and optimally <50 cm$^3$. In larger gland sizes, the pubic arch may interfere with needle placement reaching the anterolateral portions of the gland, resulting in inadequate dose coverage of the target volume. Larger glands require more seeds and activity to achieve coverage of the gland with the prescription dose, which may result in an increase in the central urethral doses and potentially increase the risk of urinary morbidity.[244] The size of the prostate can be effectively addressed with combined androgen-blockade therapy. An approximately 30% reduction in volume is commonly observed after 3 months of ADT. For patients who have imaging findings consistent with gross ECE or SVI not detected on rectal examination, monotherapy is not sufficient, and supplemental EBRT should be considered.

Patients with a significant degree of urinary obstructive symptoms are more prone to develop prolonged morbidity after brachytherapy and would be better suited to other treatment interventions. A previous TURP may increase the risk of urinary morbidity after seed implantation[245]; brachytherapy should be performed with caution in such patients. Careful attention to dose-volume considerations to the periurethral region and the area of the TURP defect should reduce the likelihood of long-term morbidities.

Seed implantation may be a more suitable intervention for patients with bilateral hip replacements, in whom CT-based treatment planning is technically difficult because of the substantial artifact created by the prosthesis, precluding adequate visualization of the target volume. Ultrasound-based seed implantation would be an appropriate alternative for such patients, as artifacts would not pose a difficulty with this imaging modality. In most cases, patients with hip prostheses are able to tolerate the extended dorsal lithotomy position for adequate perineal exposure during seed implantation. Patients with small bowel in close proximity to the prostate volume are also better suited to brachytherapy, owing to the lower doses to the bowel expected with brachytherapy. Brachytherapy may be safe for patients with a history of inflammatory bowel disease, a condition that represents a relative contraindication for EBRT. Of 24 patients with a history of inflammatory bowel disease who were treated with brachytherapy, none experienced grade 3 or higher rectal toxicities (median follow-up, 4 years), but late grade 2 rectal bleeding (19%) was significantly higher than among patients without a history of inflammatory bowel disease.[246]

Transient urinary morbidity related to radiation-induced urethritis or prostatitis represents the most common side effect following seed implantation. Symptoms include urinary frequency, urgency,

## TABLE 42.11

**Prostate-Specific Antigen Relapse-Free Survival Outcomes for Low-Dose–Rate Brachytherapy**

| Study (Ref.) | No. of Patients | Median Follow-Up (y) | Treatment | Five-Y Biochemical Outcome According to Risk Group | Comments |
|---|---|---|---|---|---|
| Stock et al.[239] | 1,377 | 4.2 | MT/CMT | Low, 94%<br>Intermediate, 89.5%<br>High, 78% | Interactive real-time planning |
| Zelefsky et al.[237] | 2,693 | 5.2 | MT | Low, 82%<br>Intermediate, 70%<br>High, 48% | D90 ≥130 Gy<br>8-y PSA control, 93%<br>D90 <130 Gy<br>8-y PSA control, 76% |
| Guedea et al.[240] | 1,050 | 2.5 | MT | Low, 93%<br>Intermediate, 88%<br>High, 80% | — |
| Khaksar et al.[241] | 300 | 4 | MT | Low, 96%<br>Intermediate, 89%<br>High, 93% | — |
| Zelefsky et al.[242] | 367 | 5.3 | MT | Low, 96%<br>Intermediate, 89% | Real-time intraoperative planned implants |
| Sylvester et al.[243] | 232 | 9.4 | CMT | Low, 86%<br>Intermediate, 80%<br>Unfavorable, 68% | — |
| Potters et al.[235] | 1,449 | 7 | MT/CMT | Low, 89%<br>Intermediate, 78%<br>Unfavorable, 63% | |

MT, monotherapy; CMT, combined-modality therapy (implant + external beam); D90, the dose received by 90% of the prostate; PSA, prostate-specific antigen.

and dysuria, which usually peak 1 to 3 months after the implant procedure and gradually resolve during the subsequent months. The incidence of urinary symptoms persisting after 1 year is 15% to 25%; the risk of urethral strictures ranges from 1% to 12%. The incidence of grade 3 and 4 rectal or urinary toxicities, including urinary or rectal incontinence, is ≤1% (Table 42.12).[239,242,247–255]

The incidence of grade 2 rectal toxicity after prostate brachytherapy ranges from 2% to 5%[247,256,257]; grade 3 or 4 rectal toxicity is unusual (<2%). These results are similar to late toxicities observed after high-dose EBRT. Meticulous attention to needle and seed placement, as well as to the intraoperative dose-volume histogram data on normal tissue, should reduce rectal doses and lower risks of toxicity to minimal levels.

### Erectile Function After Brachytherapy

Impotence rates after prostate brachytherapy and EBRT are likely underestimated in the literature. With longer follow-up, observations and responses from patient surveys indicate that approximately 40% to 50% of patients maintain erectile function after prostate brachytherapy.[258,259] Preimplant erectile-function score and the dose to 50% of the proximal crura of the penis have been shown to be significant predictors of erectile dysfunction.[258]

Excellent responses have been observed with sildenafil citrate in the treatment of impotence after brachytherapy and EBRT. In one report,[259] 80% of patients responded to the medication. With long-term follow-up, 37% of patients discontinued use of the medication. Similar responses have been reported for patients who developed erectile dysfunction after EBRT and were treated with sildenafil citrate. There has been increasing interest in the use of sildenafil before the development of erectile dysfunction to reduce the risk of erectile dysfunction after treatment. The RTOG randomized patients to receive sildenafil following radiotherapy but before the development of erectile dysfunction and found no demonstrable benefit.[260] However, a recent randomized trial from MSKCC showed improvements in sexual function parameters 12 months and 24 months after therapy among patients treated with prophylactic sildenafil, compared with those who received placebo.[261]

### Combined Brachytherapy and External Beam Radiotherapy

Combined brachytherapy and EBRT is considered to be a more suitable treatment option than implantation alone for patients with unfavorable intermediate- or high-risk disease. The combined approach effectively delivers an increased dose of radiation that has been estimated to have a biologic equivalent that well exceeds a 100-Gy dose of EBRT. Conventional or conformal-based techniques are used to deliver 45 Gy to 50 Gy of EBRT to the prostate and periprostatic tissues. If an LDR boost is used, the brachytherapy prescription dose is 90 Gy to 100 Gy for [103]Pd implants and 110 Gy for [125]I implants. In the absence of clinical trials comparing HDR brachytherapy boosts with LDR boosts or establishing the optimal sequence of therapy (brachytherapy boost preceding EBRT or vice versa) or the preferred isotope to be used for combined-modality therapy, there is no definitive evidence demonstrating the superiority of a particular treatment strategy over another.

The phase 3 trial RTOG 0232 is comparing permanent-source brachytherapy as monotherapy with EBRT followed by brachytherapy for patients with intermediate-risk prostate cancer. The study is ongoing but no longer recruiting patients. The primary end point of this study is survival; secondary end points include PSA-relapse-free survival, distant metastases–free survival, and QOL. Eligibility criteria for this study include clinical stage T1c–T2b and either Gleason score <7 with a PSA level of 10 ng/ml to 20 ng/ml, or Gleason score of 7 with a PSA level <10 ng/ml. The American Urological Association voiding symptom score should be ≤15, and prostate volume should be <60 g.

**TABLE 42.12**

**Late Toxicity Outcomes After Prostate Brachytherapy**

| Study (Ref.) | No. of Patients | Median Follow-Up (y) | Genitourinary | Gastrointestinal |
|---|---|---|---|---|
| Stock et al.[239] | 325 Incontinence, 1% | 7 | Grade 3, 2% (urethral stricture) | Grade ≤2, 24% Grade 3–4, 0% |
| Waterman and Dicker[248] | 98 | 3 | | Grade 2, 10% |
| Merrick et al.[247] | 1,186 | 4.3 | Grade 3, 3.6% Urethral stricture | |
| Gelblum et al.[249,250] | 825 | 4 | Grade 3, 4.7% 17% post TURP developed incontinence | Grade 1, 9% Grade 2, 6.6% Grade 3, 0.5% |
| Bottomley et al.[251] | 667 | 2.5 | Acute retention, 14.5% Late retention, 1% Urethritis at 6 months, 13.5% Urethritis at 24 months, 2.5% | Grade 4, <1% |
| Lee et al.[252] (RTOG 0019) | 138 | 4 | Late ≥ grade 3 gastrointestinal/ genitourinary, 15% (combined-modality therapy) | |
| Shah et al.[253] | 135 | 3.5 | | Diarrhea, 7.3% Urgency, 6.5% Bleeding, 7.3% |
| Keyes et al.[254] | 805 | 3.3 | AUR: IPSS 0–5, 8% IPSS 10–15, 15% IPSS >16, 21% | |
| Albert et al.[255] | 201 | 2.8 | Radiation-cystitis Monotherapy, 0% Combined-modality therapy, 5% | Grade 3 Monotherapy, 8% Combined-modality therapy, 30% |
| Zelefsky et al.[242] | 367 | 5.2 | Grade 2, 19% Grade 3, 4% | Grade 2, 7% Grade 3, 1% |

TURP, transurethral resection of the prostate; RTOG, Radiation Therapy Oncology Group; AUR, acute urinary retention; IPSS, International Prostate Symptom Score.

## High-Dose-Rate Brachytherapy

HDR brachytherapy has been used in combination with EBRT for the treatment of prostate cancer.[262–266] Patients undergo ultrasound-guided transperineal placement of afterloading catheters in the prostate. After CT-based treatment planning, several high-dose fractions, ranging from 4 Gy to 6 Gy each, are administered during an interval of 24 hours to 36 hours using [192]Ir, followed by supplemental EBRT directed to the prostate and periprostatic tissues at a dose of 45 Gy to 50.4 Gy using conventional fractionation. The results of a randomized trial[267] comparing hypofractionated EBRT at 55 Gy in 20 fractions with EBRT at 35.75 Gy in 13 fractions followed by an HDR brachytherapy boost of 17 Gy in two fractions delivered over 24 hours showed a 7-year likelihood of biochemical control of 66% in the combined-modality group versus 48% in the EBRT group ($p = 0.04$).

HDR brachytherapy offers several potential advantages over other techniques. Taking advantage of an afterloading approach, the radiation oncologist and physicist can more easily optimize the delivery of radiotherapy to the prostate, reducing the potential for underdosage ("cold spots"). This technique also reduces radiation exposure to the radiation oncologist and others involved in the procedure, compared with that from permanent interstitial implantation. Finally, HDR brachytherapy boosts may be radiobiologically more efficacious in terms of tumor cell kill for patients with increased tumor bulk or adverse prognostic features, compared with LDR boosts using [125]I or [103]Pd.

## Selecting the Optimal Radiotherapeutic Approach for Localized Disease Adapted for Risk Group

For patients with low-risk disease who have significant volume of disease (≥50% cores involved by cancer on the diagnostic biopsy), increasing PSA velocity, or a dominant lesion noted on MRI, a treatment intervention would be often indicated. For such patients, brachytherapy as monotherapy or IMRT at dose levels of 80 Gy would be appropriate and associated with biochemical outcomes of approximately 90% at 10 years. In these cases, brachytherapy is preferred over IMRT, given the convenience of a single treatment accomplished in an outpatient setting. Patients with significant urinary obstructive symptoms or other medical comorbidities may be better suited to IMRT. Patients with enlarged prostate glands of 60 ml to 90 ml are best treated with ADT to reduce the size of the gland before brachytherapy which in most cases, will result in a 30% volume reduction in 3 to 4 months.

For patients with intermediate- or high-risk disease, doses higher than 80 Gy may be necessary to achieve further improvement in local tumor control. In the absence of randomized trials comparing the efficacy of various forms of radiotherapy to deliver high dose levels for patients with intermediate- and high-risk disease, it has been our preference to recommend for these patients brachytherapy in combination with image-guided EBRT. In a recent study from MSKCC comparing intermediate-risk patients treated with brachytherapy combined with supplemental

IMRT versus IMRT alone to levels of 86.4 Gy, the 7-year actuarial prostate PSA-relapse-free survival rates were 81.4% versus 92.0% ($p$ <0.001) and distant metastases–free survival rates were 93.0% versus 97.2% ($p$ = 0.04) for IMRT alone versus brachytherapy combined with IMRT, respectively. Multivariate analysis demonstrated that brachytherapy combined with IMRT boost was associated with better PSA-relapse-free survival (hazard ratio [HR] = 0.40; 95% CI = 0.24 to 0.66; $p$ <0.001) and better distant metastases–free survival (HR = 0.41 [0.18 to 0.92]; $p$ = 0.03). The trade-off was a higher rate of acute urinary grade 2 symptoms in the combined treatment arm, which in most cases gradually resolved with time. Late toxicity outcomes were 4.6% versus 4.1% for grade 2 GI toxicity ($p$ = 0.89), 0.4% versus 1.4% for grade 3 GI toxicity ($p$ = 0.36), 19.4% versus 21.2% for grade 2 genitourinary toxicity ($p$ = 0.14), and 3.1% versus 1.4% for grade 3 genitourinary toxicity ($p$ = 0.74) for the IMRT versus the combination RT groups, respectively.

## Androgen Deprivation Therapy and Radiotherapy

ADT has been used as part of a combined modality approach with radiation, and randomized trials have demonstrated improved outcomes, including an overall survival benefit for this combination, compared with radiotherapy alone. The uses include neoadjuvant and concurrent; neoadjuvant, concurrent, and adjuvant; and concurrent and adjuvant. It is routinely recommended for patients with high-risk disease and selected patients with intermediate-risk disease when used in combination with EBRT. Reported trials, however, vary in the total dose of radiation used to the primary site, whether pelvic radiation was utilized, as well as the duration and timing of ADT. The end points also vary from PSA recurrence alone, whether a biopsy of the gland was performed to assess for local disease control, to the documentation of metastatic disease or death. For many, follow-up is simply too short to draw definitive conclusions. Recognizing these caveats, outcomes and indications for use in practice are summarized.

### Randomized Trials for High-Risk Disease

Table 42.13[268–270] summarizes the outcomes of randomized trials comparing radiotherapy alone to radiotherapy combined with ADT for patients with locally advanced high-risk prostate cancer. These trials have consistently demonstrated improved outcomes when ADT is combined with EBRT and the administered dose is ≥70 Gy (see Table 42.10).

Several trials have used adjuvant hormonal therapy for various durations after EBRT and demonstrated long-term disease-free survival benefits. In another important randomized trial, the European Organization for Research and Treatment of Cancer (EORTC) 22863, node-negative patients with clinical stage T3 disease or T1–T2 patients with high-grade disease received adjuvant ADT on the first day of radiotherapy (prescribed dose of 70 Gy) and continued for 3 years. Improved outcomes were observed for all parameters, including absolute survival (median follow-up, 9 years).[271] The 10-year overall survival was 58% versus 40% for patients treated with ADT plus EBRT and EBRT alone, respectively ($p$ = 0.0004). In addition, the 10-year PCSM rates for these respective cohorts of patients were 10% and 30% ($p$ <0.0001).

The duration of ADT was addressed in RTOG 92-02, the first ADT trial performed with baseline PSA information available, which randomized patients with clinical T2–T4 disease with PSA baseline levels <150 ng/ml to receive either neoadjuvant and concurrent ADT for a total of 4 months or the same therapy plus an additional 24 months of adjuvant ADT for a total of 28 months. The prescribed radiation dose levels used in this study ranged from 65 Gy to 70 Gy. At a median follow-up of 5.8 years, the results showed that all outcomes were improved for patients who received 28 months with the exception of overall survival. A subset analysis,

however, showed a 10% overall survival advantage for patients with Gleason scores of 8 to 10 who were treated with the longer course of ADT.[272]

RTOG 94-13 evaluated two sequencing regimens of adjuvant ADT as well as the role of pelvic radiotherapy in the setting of treatment with ADT in patients with T2c–T4 disease or those with an estimated LN risk ≥15%. The radiation dose administered was 70.2 Gy in 39 fractions. Patients were randomized to receive either 4 months of ADT before and during radiotherapy or 4 months of ADT as adjuvant therapy following the completion of EBRT. Patients were also randomized to receive either whole-pelvic radiotherapy or treatment directed to the prostate only. Neoadjuvant and concurrent ADT in conjunction with whole-pelvic radiotherapy was associated with a trend for an improved progression-free survival (PFS) compared to the other study arms (48% PFS for neoadjuvant ADT and whole-pelvic radiotherapy versus 40% for prostate only radiotherapy and adjuvant ADT; $p$ = 0.065).[273]

### Randomized Trials for Intermediate-Risk Disease

Recent studies have explored the role of ADT for patients with earlier stages of disease. D'Amico et al.[274] reported the results of a randomized trial comparing 70 Gy of three-dimensional CRT alone or a similar dose of radiotherapy combined with 6 months of ADT (initiated 2 months before radiotherapy). Of note, most of the patients included in this study had intermediate-risk disease—namely, pretreatment PSA levels 10 ng/ml to 40 ng/ml or Gleason score >7 with T1–T2 disease. Overall 5-year (median follow-up, 4.5 years) survival advantage was demonstrated for the combination-therapy regimen, compared with radiotherapy alone (88% versus 78%; $p$ = 0.04). RTOG 9408[269] compared radiation alone with radiation plus 4 months of ADT (starting 2 months before radiation) in 1,979 patients with stage T1b, T1c, T2a, or T2b prostate cancer and a PSA level ≤20 ng/ml. The total EBRT dose was 66.6 Gy, 46.8 Gy delivered to the pelvis (prostate and regional LN), followed by 19.8 Gy to the prostate (see Table 42.13). Low-risk disease was defined as a Gleason score ≤6, PSA level ≤10 ng/ml, and clinical stage T2a or lower; intermediate-risk disease was defined as a Gleason score of 7, Gleason score ≤6 and PSA level from 10 ng/ml to 20 ng/ml, or clinical stage T2b; and high-risk disease was defined as a Gleason score of 8 to 10. The 10-year overall survival (median follow-up, 9.1 years) was 62% for EBRT + ADT, compared with 57% for EBRT alone ($p$ = 0.03). The addition of ADT decreased 10-year PCSM from 8% to 4% ($p$ = 0.001). The reduction in risk was primarily observed in intermediate-risk patients; no significant reductions in mortality were noted among low-risk patients. Conclusions from this trial are limited by the dose of radiation administered, which was far lower than contemporary standards. Nevertheless, this study provides further level I evidence that short-course ADT is associated with a survival benefit when combined with subtherapeutic doses of EBRT. A subsequent trial in a similar patient population showed that 8 months of ADT was not superior to 3 months of therapy. This multi-institutional phase 3 study from Canada[275] randomized 378 patients to receive either 3 months or 8 months of total androgen blockade. Conventional radiotherapy at 66 Gy was initiated within 2 weeks of completion of the ADT regimen. In this trial, 31% of the patients were considered to have high-risk disease; the remaining patients had low- or intermediate-risk disease. No differences in any of the end points, including BCR-free survival, were observed.

The various trials have used different sequences to deliver ADT, and the eligibility criteria have not been consistent. Nevertheless, some broad conclusions can be drawn regarding the optimal integration of ADT with radiotherapy. For patients with high-risk cancers, and in particular high-grade cancers, ADT is indicated and adjuvant courses of hormonal therapy that extend ≥2 years

## TABLE 42.13

### Randomized Trials Involving Hormone Therapy and Radiation Therapy for Locally Advanced Prostate Cancer

| Trial | Eligibility | Arms | LF (%) | DM (%) | bNED (%) | DFS (%) | OS (%) |
|---|---|---|---|---|---|---|---|
| RTOG 85-31 | T3 (15%) or T1-2, N+ or path T3 and (+) margin or (+) SV | RT (HT at failure) vs. RT + AHT indefinite | 10-y: 38 vs. 23 (p <0.0001) | 10-y: 39 vs. 24 (p <0.0001) | 10-y: 9 vs. 31 (p <0.0001) | 10-y: 23 vs. 37 (p <0.0001) | 10-y: 39 vs. 49 (p = 0.002) |
| EORTC 22863 | T3-4 (89%) or T1-2 WHO 3 | RT vs. RT + CAHT 3 y | 5-y: 16.4 vs. 1.7 (p <0.0001) | 5-y: 29.2 vs. 9.8 (p <0.0001) | 5-y: 45 vs. 76 (p <0.0001) | 5-y: 40 vs. 74 (p <0.0001) | 5-y: 62 vs.78 (p = 0.0002) |
| RTOG 86-10 | Bulky T2b, T3-4, N+ allowed | RT vs. RT + NHT (TAB) 3.7 mo | 8-y: 42 vs. 30 (p = 0.016) | 8-y: 45 vs. 34 (p = 0.04) | 8-y: 3 vs. 16 (p <0.0001) | 8-y: 69 vs. 77 (p = 0.05) | 8-y: 44 vs. 53 (p = 0.10) |
| RTOG 92-02 | T2c-4 w/PSA <150, N+ allowed | RT + NHT (TAB) 4 mo vs. RT + NHT + AHT × 28 mo | 5-y: 12.3 vs. 6.4 (p = 0.0001) | 5-y: 17 vs. 11.5 (p = 0.0035) | 5-y: 45.5 vs. 72 (p <0.0001) | 5-y: 28.1 vs. 46.4 (p <0.0001) | 5-y: 78.5 vs. 80 (p = 0.73) |
| RTOG 94-13 | T2c-4 w/Gleason ≥6, or >15% risk of N+ | WP + NHT, WP + AHT, PO + NHT, PO + AHT | 4-y: 9.1 WP vs. 8.0 PO (p = 0.78) | 4-y: 8.2 WP vs. 6.6 PO (p = 0.54) | 4-y: 69.7, 63.3, 57.2, 63.5 (p = 0.048) | 4-y: 59.6, 48.9, 44.3, 49.8 (p = 0.008) | 4-y: 84.7 vs. 84.3 (p = 0.94) |
| Brigham and Women's Hospital[274] | PSA ≥10, Gleason ≥7, T1-T2b | RT 70 Gy 30-CRT vs. RT + 6 mo ADT | NS | NS | | 5-y: 82 vs. 57 (p = 0.002) | 5-y: 88 vs.78 (p = 0.04) |
| RTOG 94-08[269] | PSA ≥20, Gleason any, T1b-T2b | RT 66.6 Gy vs. RT + 4 mo ADT | NS | 10-y: 8 vs. 6 (p = 0.04) | 10-y (biochemical failure): 41 vs. 26 (p <0.001) | 10-y (disease-specific mortality): 8 vs. 4 (p = 0.001) | 10-y: 57 vs 62 (p = 0.03) |

LF, local failure; DM, distant metastasis; bNED, biochemical failure-free survival; DFS, disease-free survival; OS, overall survival; RTOG, Radiation Therapy Oncology Group; SV, seminal vesicle; RT, radiation therapy; HT, hormone therapy; AHT, adjuvant HT; EORTC, European Organisation for Research and Treatment of Cancer; WHO, World Health Organization; CAHT, concurrent adjuvant HT; NHT, neoadjuvant HT; TAB, total androgen blockade; PSA, prostate-specific antigen; WP, whole pelvis; PO, prostate only; CRT, conformal RT; ADT, androgen deprivation therapy; NS, not significant.

Adapted from D'Amico AV. Radiation and hormonal therapy for locally advanced and clinically localized prostate cancer. *Urology* 2002;60:32–37; D'Amico AV, Manola J, Loffredo M, et al. 6-month androgen suppression plus radiation therapy vs radiation therapy alone for patients with clinically localized prostate cancer: a randomized controlled trial. *JAMA* 2004;292:821–827. Jones CU, Hunt D, McGowan DG, et al. Radiotherapy and short-term androgen deprivation for localized prostate cancer. *N Engl J Med* 2011;365:107–118; Lee AK. Radiation therapy combined with hormone therapy for prostate cancer. *Semin Radiat Oncol* 2006;16:20–28.

appear to be associated with disease-free survival improvements compared to shorter courses. The preliminary results of the EORTC phase 3 trial 22961,[276] comprising 970 patients with locally advanced prostate cancer who were randomized to receive either 6 months or 3 years of ADT in conjunction with 70 Gy of EBRT, show that biochemical control and PFS were shorter for patients treated with the 6-month ADT regimen than for those treated with the longer course. No differences in survival have been noted so far between the two treatment arms. These data suggest that, for high-risk patients, longer courses of ADT may be critical in the setting of subtherapeutic doses of EBRT (i.e., 70 Gy). One cannot extrapolate from the published randomized trials whether 2-year or longer courses for high-risk disease are necessary when using modern dose escalated radiotherapy in the range of 78 Gy to 80 Gy. Nevertheless, longer courses of ADT are routinely used in clinical practice for high-risk patients in combination with dose-escalated radiotherapy. For patients with lower Gleason scores but with larger-volume disease, or for select patients with intermediate-risk disease, a shorter course of 6 months may be sufficient to provide a significant clinical benefit. In a meta-analysis of studies using various durations of ADT in conjunction with radiotherapy, a two-fold reduction in prostate cancer mortality was observed among patients treated with longer courses of ADT.[277]

As all of the previously mentioned trials used doses of radiotherapy ≤70 Gy, the role of ADT in the setting of an escalated dose of radiotherapy (≥75.6 Gy) remains uncertain. Higher doses of radiotherapy have been shown to improve local tumor control and may obviate the need for ADT. Nevertheless, in the absence of a randomized trial in this setting, it remains uncertain whether ADT should be avoided in the treatment of high-risk patients. Retrospective data from MSKCC showed that, among intermediate-risk patients treated with high-dose IMRT, short-course ADT (6 months) was associated with improved PSA-relapse-free survival, distant metastases–free survival, and PCSM, compared with high-dose radiotherapy alone.[278] The 10-year incidence of distant metastases and PCSM rates were 6.5% and 2.4%, respectively, for patients treated with high-dose IMRT and ADT compared to 12.3% and 5%, respectively, for patients treated with IMRT alone (p <0.001).

Definitive trials addressing the role of ADT in combination with brachytherapy are lacking, but its use is supported by basis extrapolating the results of randomized trials of patients treated with EBRT. Several reports[262,279,280] have suggested that, in the setting of brachytherapy (LDR or HDR brachytherapy boosts), ADT may be less beneficial than EBRT, whereas others[239] have suggested a benefit for higher-risk patients. It is possible that the primary role of ADT is to act as a radiosensitizer of EBRT when lower radiation doses, such as 70 Gy, are used. When higher radiation doses were used, or with the incorporation of brachytherapy boosts, several retrospective reports found no benefit of hormone therapy, except in high-grade, high-risk patients. In the absence of randomized trials in this setting, it is reasonable to recommend the use of ADT in high-risk patients, even when higher radiation doses are used. Many reports have not confirmed the role of ADT in conjunction with brachytherapy for intermediate-risk disease. The phase 3 RTOG 0815 trial will address the role of short-course ADT for intermediate-risk patients who receive dose-escalated radiotherapy and brachytherapy as well; 1,520 patients will be randomized to receive either 6 months of ADT with high-dose radiotherapy or radiotherapy alone. High-dose radiotherapy will be administered either at 79.2 Gy in conventional fractionation or as combined brachytherapy with EBRT.

## Morbidities for Androgen Deprivation Therapy and Radiotherapy

Finally, there is a growing awareness that the use of ADT in conjunction with radiation therapy is not without cost, as outcomes suggest an increased risk of subsequent congestive heart failure

or myocardial infarction. Although most of the previously cited randomized trials did not report an increase in cardiac-related events, a meta-analysis of patients with unfavorable-risk prostate cancer with moderate to severe medical or cardiac-related comorbidities showed no survival difference between the two groups due to a relative increase in noncancer-related deaths in the ADT-treated group.[281] In a report of 12,792 men treated with brachytherapy, the use of a 4-month course of ADT was associated with an increased risk of all-cause mortality among those with a history of coronary artery disease–induced heart failure or myocardial infarction.[282] The effect of longer courses of ADT in patients with moderate or severe comorbidities is unclear. These data suggest that the use of ADT among favorable-risk patients, in whom its oncologic benefit is unproven, should be carefully considered (particularly in those with severe cardiac comorbidities), owing to its potential morbidity.[283] Future, well-designed prospective studies will be needed to elucidate these issues.

## Adjuvant Radiation Therapy for High-Risk Patients After Radical Prostatectomy

### Adjuvant Radiotherapy

### Randomized Studies

The long-term (median follow-up, 14 years) results of Southwest Oncology Group (SWOG) trial 8794, which included 425 patients with high-risk localized disease who were randomized to receive either 60 Gy to 64 Gy to the prostatic fossa or only observation, have demonstrated a survival benefit of adjuvant radiotherapy in high-risk patients after RP.[284] The 10-year distant metastases–free survival and overall survival rates were 71% and 74% for the adjuvant radiotherapy arm, compared with 61% and 66% for the observation arm, respectively (p = 0.01; HR = 0.71 and 0.72, respectively). The differences between the treatment groups were detected only after 10 years, highlighting the importance of long-term follow-up in these patients (Fig. 42.12).

EORTC 22911 included 1,005 patients with positive surgical margins or pT3 (ECE and SVI) disease; these patients were randomized to receive either adjuvant EBRT (50 Gy to the prostatic

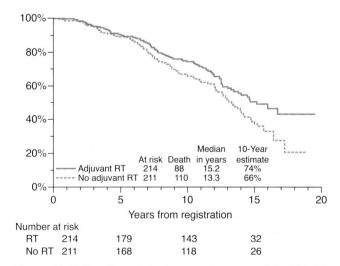

| | At risk | Death | Median in years | 10-Year estimate |
|---|---|---|---|---|
| Adjuvant RT | 214 | 88 | 15.2 | 74% |
| No adjuvant RT | 211 | 110 | 13.3 | 66% |

Number at risk

| | | | | |
|---|---|---|---|---|
| RT | 214 | 179 | 143 | 32 |
| No RT | 211 | 168 | 118 | 26 |

**Figure 42.12** Overall survival advantage demonstrated for high-risk postoperative patients receiving adjuvant radiation therapy (RT) versus observation in the Southwest Oncology Group 8794 trial. (From Thompson IM, Tangen CM, Paradelo J, et al. Adjuvant radiotherapy for pathological T3N0M0 prostate cancer significantly reduces risk of metastases and improves survival; long-term followup of a randomized clinical trial. *J Urol* 2009;181:956–962, with permission.)

fossa and periprostatic tissue plus a 10-Gy to 14-Gy boost to the prostatic fossa only) or no immediate treatment.[285] A published update of this study (median follow-up, 10.6 years) showed that adjuvant radiotherapy improved the biochemical PFS rate from 40.1% to 60.6% (*p* <0.0001); the 10-year rate of locoregional relapse was 7.3% for the adjuvant radiotherapy group and 16.6% for the control group. There was no difference in prostate cancer mortality (HR = 0.78; *p* = 0.34): 10-year prostate cancer mortality was 3.9% for the adjuvant irradiation group versus 5.4% for the observation group.[286]

The results of adjuvant radiation therapy trials show improvements in shorter term end points, including PSA PFS and locoregional relapse free survival, as anticipated. A meaningful improvement in PCSM has not been shown. Noteworthy as well is that PCSM rate in the nonadjuvant radiation therapy group was only 5.4%,[286] reinforcing that preventing a BCR alone does not necessarily translate into a significant survival benefit and that deferring treatment until the disease has declared itself as being more aggressive is an option.

Similar results were observed in a phase 3 trial from Germany (ARO 96-02) which randomized 388 patients with pathologic T3 prostate cancer with undetectable postoperative PSA levels to receive either adjuvant radiotherapy or observation. The 10-year PFS was 56% for the adjuvant radiotherapy group and 35% for the observation group (*p* <0.0001) with no survival benefit.[287]

These trials provide evidence that adjuvant postprostatectomy radiotherapy reduces the risk of BCR and in one trial, an improvement in distant metastases–free survival. Yet it remains unproven that deferring radiotherapy until manifestation of an early biochemical relapse would compromise the outcome of patients, compared with subjecting all high-risk patients to salvage radiotherapy. To address this issue, the RADICALS (NCT00541047) trial is randomizing patients to receive either immediate radiotherapy or salvage radiotherapy on detection of PSA during follow-up observations. In this trial, patients with positive margins after RP or pathologic stage T3 disease with a postoperative PSA ≤0.2 ng/ml would be randomized to receive early adjuvant radiotherapy or deferred radiotherapy on manifestation of a PSA relapse (defined as a detectable and rising PSA >0.1 ng/ml or three consecutive rising PSA values). The primary end point of this study is distant metastases–free survival. A second randomization will evaluate the role of ADT with salvage radiotherapy and will randomize patients to be treated with RT alone versus RT with concomitant/adjuvant ADT for 6 months; a third arm will be treated with RT and concomitant/adjuvant RT for 24 months. For this second randomization, the primary end point is disease-free survival.

## The Clinical State of Rising Prostate-Specific Antigen

### Management of the Patient with Rising Prostate-Specific Antigen After Definitive Local Therapy

The most frequent manifestation of a potential relapse after definitive local therapy is a rise in PSA with no detectable disease on imaging. Here, the need is to determine whether the PSA rise is from a locally recurrent tumor or micrometastatic disease outside the pelvis, and, once determined, to assess whether an intervention is needed to prevent morbidity or mortality from cancer.

The former may benefit from additional local therapy, whereas the latter would require a systemic approach. Patients who develop a rising PSA following RP may be candidates for potentially curative salvage radiation, particularly those who have an undetectable PSA after surgery and develop the rising PSA later (see "Salvage Radiotherapy for the Patient with Rising Prostate-Specific Antigen After Prostatectomy"). Patients who develop a rising PSA after radiation therapy may be candidates for salvage RP, salvage cryotherapy, or

brachytherapy, assuming the sole source of the PSA is the gland itself. Here we consider salvage local therapy. Systemic options are considered later.

### Salvage Therapies

### Salvage Radiotherapy for the Patient with Rising Prostate-Specific Antigen After Prostatectomy

Numerous nonrandomized studies have shown improved biochemical control outcomes with salvage EBRT, yet the overall PSA-relapse-free survival outcome at ≥5 years is approximately 50%.[288–292] Prognostic factors associated with relapse include surgical Gleason score, the presence of SVI, absolute preradiotherapy PSA level, and preradiotherapy PSADT. Improved outcomes are achieved with salvage radiotherapy when preradiotherapy PSA values are ≤0.5 ng/ml.[290]

At MSKCC, 285 patients with increasing PSA levels after prostatectomy[291] were treated with either salvage three-dimensional CRT or IMRT. The median dose delivered to the prostate fossa was 70.2 Gy. Neoadjuvant and concurrent ADT were used in 31% of treated patients. The 7-year (median follow-up, 5 years) PSA-relapse-free survival and distant metastases–free survival rates were 37% and 77%, respectively. Multivariate analysis demonstrated that predictors of postradiotherapy failure included the presence of vascular invasion, negative surgical margins, presalvage PSA level >0.4 ng/ml, and radiotherapy alone (i.e., without ADT). Patients treated without any adverse prognostic features had a 5-year PSA-relapse-free survival of 70%, compared with 30% for those with any adverse feature. In a multi-institutional cohort of 472 patients treated with salvage radiotherapy for a BCR after prostatectomy,[292] the overall PSA-relapse-free survival at 5 years (median follow-up, 4 years) was 73%. Variables significant as predictors of biochemical tumor control included Gleason score, surgical margin status, and preradiotherapy PSA level. Although it is difficult to compare retrospective series, it would appear that this latter multi-institutional cohort comprised a more favorable group with fewer adverse pathologic features.

The efficacy of salvage EBRT alone for clinically palpable local disease or imaging evidence of disease within the prostatic bed is suboptimal in part due to the inability to deliver full therapeutic doses of radiation safely.[293,294] Here, ADT can be used to improve local tumor eradication by reducing the size of a mass, by the concurrent elimination of tumor clonogens inherently resistant to radiotherapy, or both. The 30% to 40% size reduction also increases the ability to deliver maximal radiation dose levels without exceeding the tolerance for the surrounding normal tissue. As such, it is our policy that neoadjuvant and concurrent ADT should be considered in patients with palpable local recurrence, imaging evidence of recurrent disease, especially if biopsy proven, or an immediate detectable PSA after surgery, extrapolating from randomized trials showing the benefit of ADT in patients treated with the prostate intact. Further studies are needed in this setting.

There is limited information on the role of ADT in combination with salvage radiotherapy in the postprostatectomy setting. RTOG 0534 is accruing patients with an increasing PSA level after prostatectomy to receive either radiotherapy alone to the prostate bed, radiotherapy to the prostate bed plus 4 to 6 months of ADT, or radiotherapy to the pelvis and prostate bed plus 6 months of ADT. The previously mentioned RADICALS study incorporates a second randomization of all patients that will explore the role of ADT in the setting of salvage or adjuvant therapy.

The American Society for Radiation Oncology and American Urological Association guidelines recommend that, among patients with adverse pathologic features after prostatectomy (such as positive surgical margins and SVI), adjuvant radiotherapy should be used to reduce the risk of biochemical failures and clinical progression, although its impact on overall survival is unclear. The level of evidence grade was C. The guidelines also recommend that salvage radiotherapy should be offered to patients with an increasing PSA level or with evidence of local recurrence in the absence of metastatic disease. The recommended definition of biochemical failure after surgery is a detectable or rising PSA level >0.2 ng/ml, with a second confirmatory increase >0.2 ng/ml. Once documented, earlier administration of salvage radiotherapy is appropriate, as disease control is improved when salvage radiotherapy is administered at lower PSA levels.[295]

### Salvage Therapy for Locally Recurrent Disease After Radiation

Patients with persistent disease in the prostate after radiation therapy can be considered for salvage local therapies including a salvage RP, brachytherapy, or cryosurgery. Patient selection requires a performance status of 80 or more, histologic confirmation of disease in the gland, and no evidence of metastatic disease by imaging.

Salvage RP is technically challenging. Reported short-term and long-term complication rates exceed those of standard RP, but with appropriate patient selection and surgical expertise, the procedure has become less hazardous. Despite these advances, complications including bladder-neck contractures and anastomotic strictures have continued to be problematic.[296] Urinary incontinence rates remain high and in an MSKCC series,[152] only 74% (95% CI = 54% to 94%) recover urinary control and 20% require a sling procedure or artificial urinary sphincters. The 15-year nonprogression rate was 29% and the 15-year cancer-specific survival rate was 64% after salvage RP. The 5-year actuarial nonprogression rate was 86% for patients with organ-confined cancer (pT2N0), 61% for those with ECE, and 48% for those with SVI.

### Salvage Brachytherapy

Initial efforts to use brachytherapy in the salvage setting were restricted because of concerns about treatment-related complications. Improvements in imaging, dosimetry, and approaches (including HDR brachytherapy) have significantly lowered the risks of treatment-related complications to an acceptable level. After recurrent disease in the prostate is documented histologically, preferred candidates include those with no clinical or radiologic evidence of distant disease, adequate urinary function, age and overall health indicative of a >5- to 10-year life expectancy, prolonged disease-free interval (>2 years) from primary radiotherapy, and a long PSADT (>6 to 9 months) at the time of recurrence. Salvage brachytherapy should be avoided in patients with evidence of SVI recurrence and extracapsular disease, as these patients are poorly treated in the conventional setting.

Therapeutic approaches include permanent interstitial seed implantation,[297–299] with reported 5- to 10-year PSA-relapse-free survival rates ranging from 10% to 53%. In a second series of 37 patients with a median follow-up of 86 months, 10-year PSA-relapse-free survival and cause-specific survival rates were 54% and 96%, respectively. Improved biochemical tumor control was associated with a presalvage PSA level of ≤0.6 ng/ml in multivariate analysis.[297] In another report, 69 patients were treated with salvage permanent seed implantation using [103]Pd with a planned D90 dose of 100 Gy as monotherapy of whom 90% received concurrent ADT. With a median follow-up of 5 years, 5-year PSA-relapse-free survival rates were 86%, 75%, and 66% for patients with low-, intermediate-, and high-risk disease, respectively. Grade 3 urinary toxicity was observed in 9% of patients.[298]

In 52 patients treated with salvage HDR brachytherapy after radiotherapy failure delivering 36 Gy in six fractions using two TRUS-guided HDR prostate implants, separated by 1 week, the 5-year PSA-relapse-free survival was 51% (median follow-up, 60 months). The incidence of grade 3 urinary toxicity was 2%,

and that of grade 2 rectal toxicity was 4%.[300] A prospective phase 2 protocol at MSKCC assessed the safety and efficacy of salvage HDR brachytherapy after EBRT failure in 42 patients; the median dose was 81 Gy. The 5-year PSA-relapse-free survival and distant metastasis–free survival rates were 69% and 82%, respectively. Late grade rectal toxicity was 8%; grade 2 urethral toxicity was 7%. One patient developed urinary incontinence.[301]

Caution and meticulous treatment planning are necessary when considering repeat irradiation, especially in the setting of previous high-dose EBRT. Given the radiation dose previously delivered to the prostate and nearby normal tissue structures, side effects can manifest, including chronic urinary retention, hematuria, rectal ulcers, rectal bleeding, and permanent sexual dysfunction. Yet in the absence of randomized trials, the nonrandomized published studies suggest salvage brachytherapy as potentially less toxic relative to salvage RP.

### Salvage Cryotherapy

With the development of second- and third-generation probes, real-time TRUS for intraoperative monitoring, thermocouplers, and urethral warmers, cryotherapy is potentially less toxic and a feasible alternative for salvage local therapy after radiation failure. Case selection criteria include a prostate volume between 20 g to 30 g. The procedure is not advised for patients in whom the gland is ≥60 g. Patients with a prior TURP have an increased risk of urethral sloughing and urinary retention. Reported biochemical disease-free survival rates range from 34% to 98%.[302–307] Reported long-term complications include erectile dysfunction (77% to 100%), rectal pain (10% to 40%), urinary incontinence (4% to 20%), urinary retention (0% to 7%), and urethral sloughing (0% to 5%).[302–307] Rectourethral fistulas, the most serious complication following cryotherapy, are relatively uncommon (0% to 4%).

A second series of 187 patients with local follow-up[306] showed that patients with precryotherapy PSA levels <4 ng/ml had 5- and 8-year (mean follow-up, 49 months) BCR-free survival rates of 56% and 37%, respectively, whereas those with precryotherapy levels ≥10 ng/ml had 5- and 8-year BCR-free survival rates of only 1% and 7%, respectively. A total of 17% of patients overall had a positive four-quadrant prostate biopsy after salvage cryotherapy.

## Advanced Prostate Cancer: Rising Prostate-Specific Antigen and Clinical Metastases— Noncastrate and Castrate

The core principle of treatment of advanced prostate cancer is to deplete androgens or inhibit signaling through the androgen receptor (AR). The approach was first described in the 1940s by Huggins and Hodges,[308] who showed that surgical removal of the testes or the administration of exogenous estrogen could induce tumor regressions, reduce the level of acid phosphatase in the blood, and palliate symptoms of the disease.[308,309] Both remained the standard of care until the luteinizing hormone–releasing hormone (LHRH) agonists were introduced in the 1980s.[310,311] The palliative role of surgical adrenalectomy for disease that was progressing following orchiectomy was first described in 1945,[312] later replaced by the first-generation enzymatic inhibitors of adrenal steroid biosynthesis (aminoglutethimide and ketoconazole).[313,314] Nonsteroidal antiandrogens were introduced in the 1980s.[315,316] All these agents lower androgen levels, with the exception of the nonsteroidal antiandrogens that block the binding of androgens to the AR.

The "combined androgen blockade" era followed, during which various hormone combinations were explored in an attempt to increase the degree of AR signaling inhibition and thereby response. The first combined a LHRH agonist with flutamide,[317] others with adrenal androgen synthesis inhibitors; none of these meaningfully improved survival.[318,319]

Other approaches to treating advanced prostate cancer include cytotoxic agents, biologic agents, and immunotherapy. In 1996, the first cytotoxic drug, mitoxantrone, was approved for the palliation of pain secondary to progressive osseous disease based upon a trial that was not specifically designed to show a survival benefit.[320] But it was not until 2004 that the first systemic therapy, docetaxel, was shown to prolong the lives of men with progressive CRPC,[321,322] setting a new benchmark for drug approvals that has not been exceeded by any docetaxel-based combination, several of which have proved inferior to docetaxel alone (Table 42.14).[322–337]

Efforts were also focused on better understanding of the biology of the disease. This effort has led to the approval of six new treatments with diverse mechanisms of action since 2010. Five were shown to prolong life (see Table 42.14), including a biologic agent (sipuleucel-T),[323] a cytotoxic (cabazitaxel),[325] a bone-seeking alpha-emitting radionuclide (radium-223),[326] and two hormonal agents, the CYP17 inhibitor abiraterone acetate that inhibits androgen biosynthesis in combination with prednisone and a next-generation antiandrogen, enzalutamide, which is mechanistically unique from the first-generation compounds.[327,328] The sixth agent, denosumab, a monoclonal antibody that binds the cytokine RANKL (receptor activator of nuclear factor-κB ligand), was shown to reduce the morbidity associated with skeletal metastases relative to a previously established standard (zoledronate).[338]

Taken together, the results of these new treatments showed that survival could be prolonged by targeting different aspects of the malignant process in addition to direct targeting of the tumor, and demonstrated the complexity of measuring success for these new agents. Separately, the success of hormonal agents that inhibit the AR and AR signaling confirmed that prostate cancers progressing despite castrate levels of testosterone are not uniformly hormone-refractory; instead, they are more accurately described as castration-resistant.

## Efficacy End Points

Prostate cancer treatment outcomes are reported based on the changes in individual disease manifestations that are present when therapy is initiated and the prevention of development of subsequent manifestations. The appropriateness of one metric over another depends on the class and mechanism of the drug or therapy being used, the disease state of the patients being treated, and the clinical benefit or outcome the therapy is expected to achieve. Measurements of PSA levels alone are not sufficient to gauge efficacy for several classes of agents. For example, AR and AR signaling inhibitors may, in some patients, produce declines in PSA without affecting tumor growth. Conversely, bone-seeking radiopharmaceuticals may relieve pain without decreasing PSA levels. A drug that inhibits cell proliferation without inducing an apoptotic effect may lead to a prolonged period of disease stability or "nonprogression," preventing disease manifestations such as the development of new metastatic lesions or pain that were expected to occur. Such a drug might be beneficial independent of its effect on PSA. In contrast, a hormonal agent or cytotoxic drug that

**TABLE 42.14**

**(A) Phase 3 Trials of Single Agents Leading to Regulatory Approval in Castration-Resistant Prostate Cancer. (B) Completed or Ongoing Phase 3 Studies Examining Docetaxel-Based Combinations in the First-Line Treatment of Metastatic Castration-Resistant Prostate Cancer**

| Trial: Therapy (Approved Date) | N | Disease State | Comparator | HR | OS | P Value |
|---|---|---|---|---|---|---|
| **(A) Phase 3 Trials of Single Agents Leading to Regulatory Approval** | | | | | | |
| IMPACT: Provenge vaccine (2010)[323] | 512 | Prechemotherapy Asymptomatic | Placebo | 0.775 | 25.8 vs. 21.7 | 0.032 |
| COU-AA-302: Abiraterone acetate (2013)[324] | 1,088 | Prechemotherapy | Placebo Prednisone | 0.75 | NYR vs. 27.2 | 0.01 |
| TAX327: Docetaxel (2004)[322] | 1006 | First-line | Mitoxantrone Prednisone | 0.76 | 18.9 vs. 16.5 | 0.009 |
| TROPIC: Cabazitaxel (2010)[325] | 755 | Postchemotherapy Symptoms | Mitoxantrone Prednisone | 0.70 | 15.1 vs. 12.7 | <0.0001 |
| COU-AA-301: Abiraterone acetate (2011)[327] | 1195 | Postdocetaxel | Placebo Prednisone | 0.646 | 14.8 vs. 10.9 | <0.0001 |
| AFFIRM: Enzalutamide (2012)[328] | 1199 | Postdocetaxel | Placebo | 0.631 | 18.4 vs. 13.6 | <0.0001 |
| ALYMPTA: Alpharadin (2013)[326] | 922 | Pre- and postsymptomatic | Placebo | 0.695 | 14.0 vs. 11.2 | 0.00085 |
| **(B) Phase 3 Trials with Docetaxel-Based Combinations** | | | | | | |
| CALGB 90401: Docetaxel ± bevacizumab[329] | 1,050 | First-line | Placebo | 0.091 | 22.6 vs. 21.5 | 0.181 |
| VENICE: Docetaxel ± aflibercept[330] | 1,224 | First-line | Placebo | 0.94 | 22.1 vs. 21.2 | 0.38 |
| SWOG S0421: Docetaxel ± atrasentan[331] | 994 | First-line | Placebo | 1.04 | 17.8 vs. 17.6 | 0.64 |
| ENTHUSE: Docetaxel ± zibotentan[332] | 1,052 | First-line | Placebo | 1.00 | 20.0 vs. 19.2 | 0.963 |
| READY: Docetaxel ± dasatinib[333] | 1,380 | First-line | Placebo | 0.99 | 21.5 vs. 21.2 | 0.90 |
| VITAL-2: Docetaxel ± GVAX[334] | 408 | First-line Symptomatic | Placebo | 1.70 | 12.2 vs. 14.1 | 0.0076 |
| MAINSAIL: Docetaxel ± lenalidomide[335] | 1,059 | First-line | Placebo | 1.53 | 17.7 vs. NYR | 0.0017 |
| ASCENT: Docetaxel ± calcitriol[336] | 953 | First-line | Placebo | 1.42 | 17.8 vs. 20.2 | 0.002 |
| SYNERGY: Docetaxel ± custirsen[337] | 1,022 | First-line | Placebo | 0.93 | 23.4 vs. 22.2 | 0.207 |

HR, hazard ratio; OS, overall survival (mo); NYR, not yet reached.

does not produce a decline in PSA is likely to be inactive. Examples of agents that provide clinical benefit without PSA declines include the delay and prevention benefit of zoledronate[159] and denosumab[338] on SREs, and separately, the survival benefit shown for sipuleucel-T[323] and radium-223.[326]

It is for these reasons that the PCWG2 recommended focusing less on whether a treatment was "working" and more on when it was "not working," and to carefully consider the potential significance of an apparent adverse change in PSA before stopping therapy.[157] Rather than discontinue treatment based on a PSA change alone, it is preferable to wait until there is evidence of radiographic or clinical progression. Figure 42.13 shows examples where (1) a significant initial rise in PSA or (2) a slow rise following an initial decline did not associate with radiographic or clinical progression for a considerable period of time (2 years and 3.5 years, respectively, in Fig. 42.13).[339] In each case, reliance on the PSA change alone to guide management would have resulted in the premature discontinuation of therapy and denied the patient durable disease control.

## Noncastrate Prostate Cancer (Rising Prostate-Specific Antigen and Noncastrate Metastases)

### Hypothalamic-Pituitary-Gonadal Axis

The regulation of androgen production begins with LHRH being secreted from the hypothalamus, which acts on the pituitary gland to release follicle-stimulating hormone, which acts on Sertoli cells, and luteinizing hormone (LH), which acts on Leydig cells to control androgen synthesis and spermatogenesis in the testes (Fig. 42.14).[340]

Bilateral orchiectomy is an inexpensive standard treatment that reliably reduces testosterone levels to the "castrate" range (<50 ng/dl). Estrogens inhibit the production of LHRH, which decreases the release of follicle-stimulating hormone and LH, and reduces androgen levels in a dose-dependent manner. A dose of diethylstilbesterol (DES), 3 mg/d, generally achieves castrate testosterone levels.

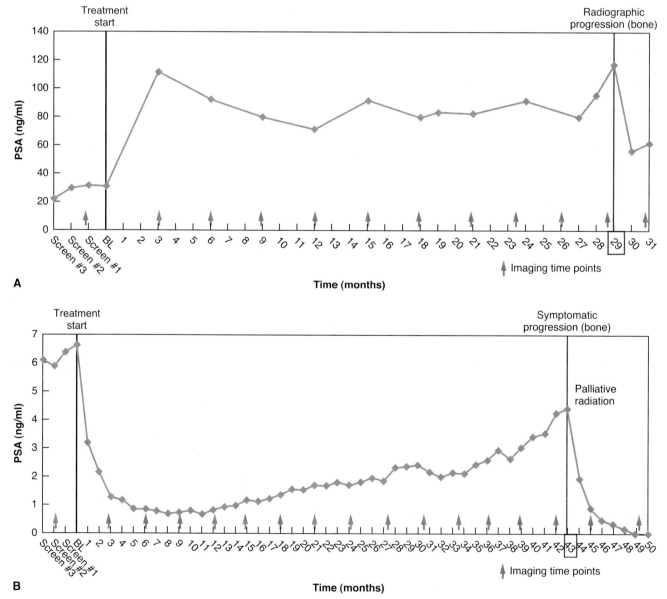

**Figure 42.13** Prostate-specific antigen (PSA) rise alone is not sufficient reason to discontinue treatment; there must also be radiographic or clinical evidence of progression. **(A)** An initial rapid rise in PSA, with subsequent decline above baseline on a second value, in a patient who remained biochemically, radiographically, and clinically stable for 22 months on abiraterone acetate. **(B)** A slow rise in PSA after an initial rapid decline, with no evidence of radiographic or clinical progression for 28 months while receiving enzalutamide. (From Scher HI, Morris MJ, Basch E, et al. End points and outcomes in castration-resistant prostate cancer: from clinical trials to clinical practice. *J Clin Oncol* 2011;29:3695–3704, with permission.)

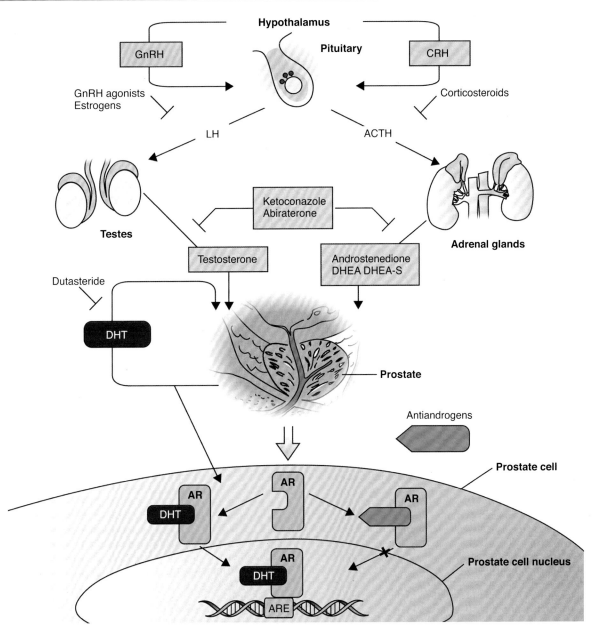

**Figure 42.14** The androgen-signaling axis and its inhibitors. Testicular androgen synthesis is regulated by the gonadotropin-releasing hormone (GnRH)–luteinizing hormone (LH) axis, whereas adrenal androgen synthesis is regulated by the corticotrophin-releasing hormone (CRH)-adrenocorticotropic hormone (ACTH) axis. GnRH agonists and corticosteroids inhibit stimulation of the testes and adrenals, respectively. Abiraterone inhibits CYP17, a critical enzyme in androgen synthesis. Bicalutamide, flutamide, and nilutamide competitively inhibit the binding of androgens to androgen receptors; enzalutamide also blocks the translocation of the ligand bound AR complex to the nucleus and from binding to DNA. DHEA, dehydroepiandrosterone; DHEA-S, dehydroepiandrosterone sulphate; DHT, dihydrotestosterone; AR, androgen receptor; ARE, androgen-response element. (Adapted from Chen Y, Clegg NJ, Scher HI. Anti-androgens and androgen-depleting therapies in prostate cancer: new agents for an established target. *Lancet Oncol* 2009;10:981–991, with permission.)

LHRH agonists produce an initial rise in LH that increases testosterone levels, followed 1 to 2 weeks later by downregulation of LH receptors that results in a medical castration.[310,311] The initial rise in testosterone can flare the disease, precipitating or exacerbating symptoms such as pain, obstructive uropathies, and spinal cord compromise. These agents were first approved on the basis of trials showing an improved safety profile compared with oral estrogens, most notably the reduction in cardiovascular-related events such as edema, thrombosis and thromboembolism, myocardial infarction, and stroke.[341–343] Several are approved for use in the United States, including leuprolide acetate (Lupron, given intramuscularly [AbbVie, North Chicago, IL]; Eligard, given subcutaneously [TOLMAR Pharmaceuticals, Inc., Fort Collins, CO]; Viadur, implanted subcutaneously [Bayer HealthCare Pharmaceuticals Inc.,

Montville, NJ]), goserelin acetate (Zoladex, given subcutaneously in the abdominal wall [AstraZeneca, London, England]), triptorelin pamoate (Trelstar, given intramuscularly [Actavis Pharma, Inc., Parsippany, NJ]), and histrelin acetate (Vantas, implanted subcutaneously [Endo Pharmaceuticals Inc., Dublin, Ireland]). These drugs are available as daily or monthly injections, and 3-, 4-, 6-, or 12-month depot injections.

In contrast, LHRH antagonists produce castrate levels of testosterone in 48 hours without the initial rise (Fig. 42.15), making them a compelling choice for the initial treatment of patients with symptoms. At present, degarelix, available as monthly subcutaneous injections, is the only LHRH antagonist that is approved in the United States. Reported outcomes suggest a comparable to slightly improved efficacy relative to the agonists/antagonists discussed

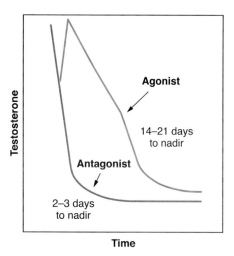

**Figure 42.15** Testosterone levels following treatment with a luteinizing hormone–releasing hormone agonist and antagonist. Nadir is achieving castrate range.

previously.[344] The tradeoff is the need for monthly injections and a higher frequency of injection-site reactions.

## Antiandrogens

Antiandrogens block the binding of testosterone to the AR (see Fig. 42.14). There are two types: the steroidal type I agents such as cyproterone acetate have progestational properties that suppress LH levels and lower serum testosterone; these are not widely used. The nonsteroidal type II agents bind to the AR and act as competitive antagonists for ligands that might otherwise bind and activate the ligand-dependent transcriptional activity of the receptor. The three first-generation type II agents approved are flutamide, which has a short half-life requiring multiple daily doses, and bicalutamide and nilutamide, which have weekly half-lives and are administered once daily. All three were approved initially in combination with a LHRH analog: flutamide to prevent the flare that can result from the initial rise in testosterone that occurs with LHRH analogs,[345,346] bicalutamide (50 mg daily) on the basis of an improved safety profile relative to flutamide,[347] and nilutamide in combination with surgical orchiectomy based on greater efficacy relative to orchiectomy alone.[348] Type II agents given as monotherapy do not inhibit LH synthesis in the hypothalamus or pituitary, and circulating testosterone levels rise. None of these antiandrogens are approved as monotherapy in the United States, although bicalutamide 150 mg is approved in the European Union.[349]

## Enzymatic Inhibitors of Androgen Synthesis

All steroidal hormones are derived from pregnenolone and subsequently metabolized via several CYP450 class enzymes. Within the adrenal gland, CYP17 mediates the synthesis of weak androgens dehydroepiandrosterone (DHEA) and androstenedione (Fig. 42.16), whereas in the testes, the presence of 17-keto reductase generates testosterone that can be further converted to DHT in peripheral tissues by 5α-reductase. Ketoconazole is a nonspecific P450 inhibitor that, at a dose of 1,200 mg/d, produces castrate levels of testosterone in 24 hours through inhibition of adrenal and testicular steroidogenesis. The effect is not durable, limiting the drug's use as first-line treatment. It was useful for patients who presented with acute spinal cord compression or disseminated intravascular coagulation, when LHRH analogs are contraindicated and the risk of hemorrhage from surgery is significant.[314]

## Toxicities of Androgen Deprivation Therapy

The adverse effects associated with ADT include those associated with the hypogonadal state and others that are unique to the specific drugs utilized. Symptoms associated with castration, whether medical or surgical, can be grouped under the "androgen deprivation syndrome," and include hot flashes, a decrease in libido, erectile dysfunction, impotence, fatigue, anemia, weight gain and alterations in fat metabolism, loss of muscle mass and weakness, bone loss, a decrease in mental acuity, mood swings, personality changes, memory loss, depression, and insomnia. Consequently, to relieve patients' anxiety and minimize stress, it is essential to inform them of the goals of treatment and the potential adverse events that may occur. Many of the adverse effects of ADT can be relieved by exercise.[350–352] Table 42.15 shows the frequency and methods of amelioration. Hot flashes occur in more than 80% of patients at any time, even during sleep, and may last for several seconds or an hour or more. They are bothersome in about 25% of cases, and if significant, can be reduced in frequency and intensity with estrogens at doses as low as 0.3 mg/d by patch[353] or progestins (e.g., megestrol acetate or medroxyprogesterone acetate).[354]

Erectile dysfunction and loss of libido are almost universal. Penile and testicular size may diminish and facial and body hair decrease, but male-pattern baldness may improve. Fatigue, in part related to anemia, is also frequent, as 90% of men on ADT show a decrease in hemoglobin of 10%, and 25% show a decrease of 18% or more.[355] Weight gain is also frequent (most of which is fat, as lean body mass decreases) and exceeded 6 kg on average at 12 months in one study.[356] Other factors contributing to weight gain include an increase in appetite and sedentary lifestyle.

Metabolic changes include an increase in cholesterol in 10% of patients, increase in triglycerides in 26%, and incident diabetes,[357] a consequence of insulin resistance. It is uncertain whether glucose intolerance results from an increase in weight or adiposity, a decrease in exercise tolerance, or a combination of these or other factors.

Osteopenia and osteoporosis are well documented, and in one prospective trial bone mass decreased by 2% to 5% after 1 year of ADT, leading to an increased rate of fracture,[358] although few fractures occur in patients treated for <1 year (Fig. 42.17).[359] Changes in bone can be monitored by bone densitometry and bone turnover markers such as urinary N-telopeptide (a breakdown product of collagen), bone-specific alkaline phosphatase, and osteocalcin.[360] Bone loss and fracture rates can be reduced by bisphosphonates such as zoledronate[361] or denosumab, blocking osteoclast maturation, function, and survival,[362,363] and toremifene, a selective estrogen receptor modulator.[364] Supplemental calcium (1,000 mg/d to 1,500 mg/d) and vitamin D (400 international units) daily are also advised to prevent bone loss, but data to support their use are limited. Integral parts of the maintenance of bone integrity are exercise, reduction in caffeine, and smoking cessation.

Other adverse effects of ADT include depression, mood swings, emotional lability, decreased mental acuity, and memory loss.[365] Psychological tests for cognitive dysfunction suggest that certain aspects of spatial reasoning and spatial ability,[366] along with memory and attention, can be impaired by ADT.[367]

Cardiovascular issues are also a concern, given the multiplicity of risk factors that are worsened by ADT, including weight gain, increased adipose tissue, decreased exercise tolerance, hyperlipidemia, decreased insulin sensitivity, and glucose intolerance. The literature on the effects of ADT on cardiovascular mortality shows that this remains an area of controversy. A recent advisory panel from the American Heart Association concluded that links between ADT and cardiovascular mortality remain controversial, and that there is no reason at present to initiate cardiac testing in patients with cardiovascular disease before initiation of ADT.[368,369]

## Antiandrogen Toxicity

Antiandrogens do not lower serum androgens, and as a result, there is less loss of libido, fewer hot flashes, and potency may be spared, while muscle and bone mass are retained. Unique toxicities relative to testosterone-lowering approaches include GI events such as

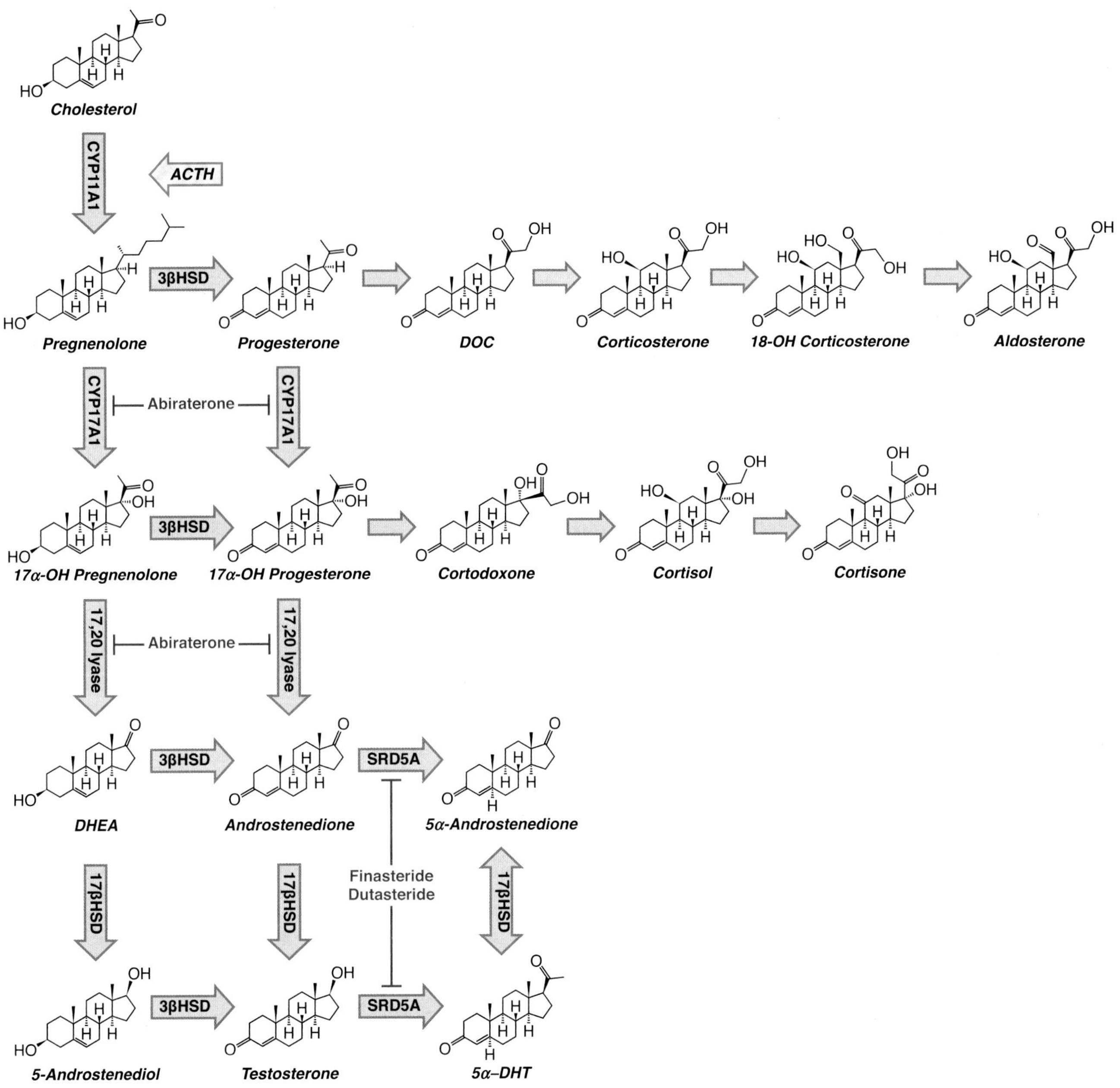

**Figure 42.16** The effects of abiraterone acetate on steroid biosynthesis. ACTH, adrenocorticotropic hormone; DOC, 11-deoxycorticosterone; DHEA, dehydroepiandrosterone; DHT, dihydrotestosterone.

elevations in hepatic enzymes, stomach upset and diarrhea,[347] and pulmonary complications such as fibrosis; these toxicities are a rare class effect of the first-generation antiandrogens,[370] which occur most frequently with nilutamide. Gynecomastia and/or breast tenderness may also develop, which, if severe, might require a reduction mammoplasty. Prophylactic breast irradiation can reduce the frequency and severity of these effects.[350,351]

## Contemporary Management

For the patient with metastatic disease and/or symptoms, or the patient in the rising PSA state for whom treatment is advised based on the absolute level of PSA or PSA kinetics, standard practice is to initiate therapy and monitor the disease with serial PSA measurements and imaging as appropriate until there are signs that the disease has started to progress, at which point it is considered "castration-resistant." In most patients, this is manifested first by a rise in PSA despite castrate (<50 ng/dl) levels of testosterone.

Androgen deprivation and/or blockade produces declines in PSA, regression of measurable tumor masses if present, and a period of clinical quiescence or stability in which PSA levels and tumor size does not change, followed in a variable period of time by a rise in PSA, tumor proliferation, and clinically detectable changes on imaging. Applying the control/relieve–delay/prevent metric, approximately 60% to 70% of patients with an abnormal PSA will show a normalization to a value of ≤4 ng/ml, 30% to 50% of measurable tumor masses will regress by ≥50%, 30% to 40% of bone scans will improve while the majority remain stable, and >60% of patients with symptoms will show palliation, be the symptoms urinary or osseous in origin.

The complete elimination of disease in any site with ADT is rare, be it in bone or the prostate itself, although in many cases, LN disease that was present when hormone therapy is initiated does not recur. When ADTs are used as neoadjuvant therapy prior to surgery for upwards of 8 months, <5% of prostates removed subsequently are pathologically free of tumor,[371] which suggests that hormone therapy

**TABLE 42.15**

**Adverse Effects of Androgen Deprivation, Approximate Frequency, and Potential Therapeutic Options for Amelioration[a]**

| Effect | Approximate Frequency | Potential Corrective Actions |
|---|---|---|
| Libido loss | Universal | None known |
| Erectile dysfunction | Universal | None known |
| Hot flashes | 50%–80% | Venlafaxine, estrogens, progestins |
| Muscle loss | Common, duration-dependent | Exercise |
| Weight gain | Common | Exercise/diet |
| Facial/body hair loss | Very common | None known |
| Fatigue | Not defined | Exercise |
| Emotional lability | Not defined | None known |
| Depression | 0%–30% | Various antidepressants |
| Cognitive dysfunction | Not defined | None known |
| Gynecomastia | Up to 20% | Preemptive radiation |
| Breast tenderness | Not defined | Aromatase inhibitors |
| Osteoporosis | Common, duration-dependent | Exercise/bisphosphonates |
| Anemia | 5%–13% | Erythropoietin not recommended |
| Hyperlipidemia | 10% | Diet, statins |
| Diabetes | 0.8%/year increase | Exercise, oral agents |
| Myocardial infarction | 0.25%/year increase | Treatment of risk factors |
| Coronary heart disease | 1%/year increase | Treatment of risk factors |

[a] A number of events are poorly defined in frequency as a consequence of a lack of controlled studies, quantitative assessments, and/or agreed on definitions.

alone does not cure the disease. Prognosis varies by the disease state, grade of the tumor, rapidity of growth, and extent of disease when hormone therapy was started. Adverse features from multiple series include a high Gleason score (8 to 10), low performance status, bone pain, low hemoglobin, high alkaline phosphatase, low testosterone level, and extensive as opposed to minimal disease.[372,373] The number of metastases[344] or percentage of the skeleton involved by tumor[345] is also prognostic. In one series, 2-year survival times were 94%, 71%,

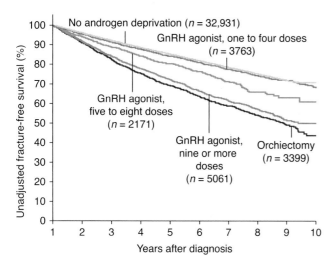

**Figure 42.17** Fracture rate as a function of time after androgen deprivation therapy in men older than age 68 in the United States. Number of doses is the number administered within 12 months after diagnosis. GnRH, gonadotropin-releasing hormone. (From Shahinian VB, Kuo YF, Freeman JL, et al. Risk of fracture after androgen deprivation for prostate cancer. *N Engl J Med* 2005;352:154, with permission.)

61%, and 40% for men with 0 to 5, 6 to 10, 19, and ≥20 lesions, respectively.[374,375] Using a different classification, patients with minimal disease (involvement confined to the axial skeleton [pelvis and/or spine] and/or LN) and extensive disease (disease in long bones, skull or ribs, and/or viscera) had median PFS of 46 months and 16 months, respectively, and overall survival times of 51 months and 27.5 months, respectively.[376]

Prognosis can be estimated in part by the degree and rapidity of response determined by the posttreatment PSA nadir and the timing of the nadir. In a trial enrolling 1,345 patients, failure to achieve a PSA nadir of ≤4 ng/ml within 7 months was associated with a median survival of 13 months, whereas those with a nadir between 0.2 to 4.0 ng/ml had a median survival of 44 months, and patients with a nadir ≤0.2 ng/ml had a median survival of 75 months.[377] With respect to the timing of the nadir, those who achieved a nadir in <6 months had a median survival of 4.5 years versus 7.8 years for those with a nadir after 6 months from the start of treatment.[378]

Unfortunately, more contemporary natural history studies for patients with metastatic disease are lacking, in part because fewer men are presenting with metastatic disease, and because this approach has been the standard of care for over seven decades, fewer randomized trials are being conducted. As a result, comparing different treatments outside of dedicated trials is difficult due to the different methods used to determine and define disease extent, the posttreatment monitoring schema, and how outcomes were reported, leaving several basic questions in management incompletely resolved.

*Is one form of monotherapy that suppresses testosterone levels superior to another?* No. All single-therapy hormonal interventions that lower serum testosterone levels to castrate levels had similar overall survival times after 2 years of treatment.[379] An EORTC study, powered for a 13% difference around the medians, showed similar outcomes between DES 1 mg and orchiectomy.[380] In a meta-analysis of 10 randomized controlled trials that included

LHRH agonists/antagonists, orchiectomy, DES, or choice of DES or orchiectomy, outcomes were similar.

*Is more complete androgen suppression superior?* Geller et al.[381] were the first to document elevated DHT levels in patients treated by orchiectomy, a finding validated later when more sensitive and specific mass spectroscopy–based assays became available,[382] and the demonstration of persistent PSA and TMPRSS2:ERG expression in posthormone treated RP specimens indicating continued AR signaling.[383,384] This led to trials testing the hypothesis that more complete androgen suppression using a combination of an antiandrogen (flutamide, bicalutamide, or nilutamide) to inhibit adrenal androgens with a LHRH agonist/antagonist or orchiectomy would provide greater benefit.[317] Adrenal androgens can contribute 5% to 45% of the residual androgens present in tumors after surgical castration alone. Early results were promising,[385] but subsequent meta-analyses have been conducted showing that the first-generation antiandrogens did not add significantly to the antitumor effects of surgical castration.[319,341,386,387] One, summarizing 27 randomized trials with 8,275 patients, showed a 2% difference in mortality at 5 years: 72.4% for monotherapy versus 70.4% for the combined approach[386]; a second meta-analysis limited to trials of a nonsteroidal antiandrogen showed a 2.9% difference: 75.3% versus 72.4% at 5 years.[341] Other combinations explored to effect more complete androgen suppression included low-dose DES and megestrol acetate; an LHRH analog and ketoconazole plus hydrocortisone; an LHRH analog, antiandrogen and ketoconazole, plus hydrocortisone or aminoglutethimide and hydrocortisone.[387] None proved meaningfully superior.

*When should hormone therapy be initiated? Early versus late?* This question is difficult to answer because of methodologic differences in the trials designed to address it. The differences include the clinical state of the patient group studied, whether the primary tumor has been treated and how (no treatment, surgery, or radiation including dose and treatment field), the specific hormones used, the duration they were administered, and the patient follow-up including the frequency of visits and the specific clinical, laboratory, and imaging assessments performed. Critical to the discussion as well is the "trigger" used to start treating patients randomized to the "no immediate treatment" arm of the study, which range from a predefined degree or level of PSA rise alone, the documentation of metastases, or the development of symptoms. Further confounding the issue is that in some studies, a significant proportion of patients in the "no immediate treatment" group were never treated.

A complete review of all of the trials designed to assess this question is beyond the scope of this chapter. In general, randomized trials that address this question show "early" hormone therapy delays the time to metastases and symptoms, but the effect on overall survival is less clear. A key consideration in formulating a recommendation for patients at a particular point in the illness is to balance the likelihood that a patient would require treatment based on the development of metastatic disease or symptoms and when, with the likelihood that no treatment would ever be required based on these same metrics.

Trials in patients who did not receive treatment of the primary tumor were reported by the Veterans Administration Research Service Cooperative Urological Research Group, the Medical Research Council (MRC), and the Early Prostate Cancer Trials Group. The Veterans Administration Research Service Cooperative Urological Research Group trials enrolled 1,900 patients staged primarily by DRE and showed that DES or orchiectomy could delay the development of metastatic disease in patients with locally advanced stage C tumors,[388,389] although overall survival was worse due to cardiovascular complications. There was also no overall survival benefit for patients with metastatic disease.

The MRC PR03 trial randomized 998 patients with locally advanced or asymptomatic metastatic prostate cancer to "immediate" treatment (orchiectomy or LHRH analog) or to the same treatment deferred until there was an "indication." The trigger to initiate treatment was "clinically significant progression," which was as frequent locally as metastatic. The trial showed that patients treated with early therapy were less likely to require a TURP or develop ureteral obstruction, progress from M0 to M1 disease (P <0.001, two-tailed), to develop pain (P <0.001), or to die of prostate cancer relative to those in whom therapy was "deferred." Even so, survival times were similar between the two groups. An important caveat limiting the extrapolation of the results to the question of "early" versus "late" was that half of the men who died in the deferred arm never received therapy.[390]

The Early Prostate Cancer Trials Group trial (n = 985) randomized men with T0-4N0-2M0 prostate cancer who were not candidates for local therapy to immediate or to deferred treatment until symptomatic progression was documented. The results showed an increased risk of death in the deferred arm (HR = 1.25; 95% CI = 1.05 to 1.48), which remained after adjusting for baseline factors. Notable was that only 49.7% of men in the deferred arm began anticancer therapy during the median 7.8-year follow-up period, suggesting that a significant proportion of men on the immediate arm were overtreated. The median time to treatment for those who required it, however, was 3.2 years. Deaths were equally balanced between prostate cancer (n = 193, 18.8% of the population) and cardiovascular disease (n = 185) (Fig. 42.18).[391]

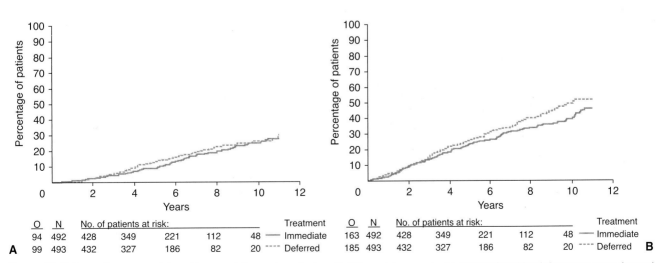

**Figure 42.18** Immediate versus deferred hormonal therapy in patients with M0 prostate cancer who either refused local therapy or were deemed unsuitable for local therapy. **(A)** Prostate cancer–specific mortality. **(B)** Non-prostate cancer mortality. (From Studer UE, Whelan P, Albrecht W, et al. Immediate or deferred androgen deprivation for patients with prostate cancer not suitable for local treatment with curative intent: European Organisation for Research and Treatment of Cancer [EORTC] Trial 30891. *J Clin Oncol* 2006;24:1868, with permission.)

### Rising Prostate-Specific Antigen (Extrapelvic Disease)

For the patient presumed to have microscopic nodal or more distant disease that would not respond or which cannot be addressed by additional treatment to the primary site, the optimal timing of ADT initiation is controversial. The first issue is to determine the risk of developing metastatic disease and in what time frame. One series that addressed this question included 1997 RP-treated patients, of whom 315 (15%) developed a rising PSA and were followed with annual imaging and PSA assessment until metastatic disease was documented. Of these patients, metastatic disease was subsequently documented in 103 at a median actuarial time of 8 years, of whom 44 (44%, or 2% of the 1997) died of disease.[392] Factors associated with the development of metastasis included the grade of the primary tumor, the time interval between the start of the treatment to the date of first recurrence, the absolute PSA value, and the rate that it was rising, typically expressed in terms of the PSADT.[393] In a separate study, virtually all cancer-related deaths occurred in men who had PSADT ≤6 months, independent of whether the patient received radiation or surgery as primary treatment.[394] In practice, many physicians consider treating patients when the PSADT is ≤12 months, although there remains no absolute PSA level mandating that treatment be started.

*Strategies to Reduce the Toxicities Associated with Androgen Deprivation Therapy.* Now, with the widespread use of PSA-based detection and monitoring, fewer men are diagnosed with or develop symptoms of advanced prostate cancer. For these individuals, the tolerance of castration is less than for men who receive treatment to relieve the symptoms of urinary obstruction or bone pain from osseous spread. This, coupled with the adverse events that can occur with longer use, has led to the evaluation of noncastrating approaches in an effort to improve patient tolerance without compromising efficacy.

*Antiandrogen Monotherapy.* Several randomized trials have compared antiandrogens alone to conventional testosterone-lowering forms of castration. Bicalutamide 50 mg daily, the dose approved for use in combination with an LHRH analog, was inferior to surgical orchiectomy.[395] Bicalutamide 150 mg, which produces a higher frequency of PSA normalization than does the 50 mg dose (97% versus 73% of cases), showed mixed results: inferiority to castration for patients with metastatic disease but equivalence for patients with M0 disease (rising PSA values with no detectable metastases on imaging studies).[396] Another approach is to begin with the antiandrogen alone and add a testosterone-lowering therapy when PSA levels rise. Unfortunately, only 30% of patients treated in this fashion respond to the addition of the LHRH analog.[397] Nevertheless, some patients may be willing to accept this risk

rather than experience the impotence and other adverse effects of testosterone-lowering treatment, as long as symptoms of disease are controlled.

*Intermittent Androgen Depletion/Blockade.* A second approach that is now used widely is intermittent androgen deprivation (IAD). It evolved somewhat empirically in the era of estrogen therapy, pre-PSA, when it was recognized that patients in whom therapy was stopped for noncancer-related reasons would often respond when the treatment was resumed to control the disease.[398] The central hypothesis, based on studies in murine tumors, is that by minimizing the exposure time to a castrate environment, the sensitivity to subsequent androgen depletion would be retained.[399,400] An additional advantage is the potential for an improved QOL during the "off" intervals.

Applied today, the approach is considered for patients who respond well to ADT, typically defined as a PSA nadir ≤4 ng/ml for those with metastatic disease, and is restarted when PSA levels return to a predetermined level (typically 10 ng/ml to 20 ng/ml). Multiple phase 3 trials have been reported that differ in the patient population treated (BCR only, metastatic disease only, or both), the type and duration of treatment (3 months to 8 months), the criteria for discontinuation and for restarting it, and the primary end point. Most report a time to progression measure but do not use the same criteria. Few are powered for survival. Several large randomized trials have been reported recently: none showed the intermittent approach to be superior to continuous therapy in terms of cancer control, but most show a better QOL during the off intervals, which patients prefer.

In one trial enrolling 1,386 patients, median survival in the intermittent versus continuous arms was 8.8 years and 9.1 years, respectively, with more prostate cancer deaths in the intermittent arm and more deaths from other causes, including cardiovascular events, in the continuous arm. In this trial, a slight increase in cancer-related deaths in the intermittent arm was counterbalanced by an increase in nonprostate cancer deaths in the continuous arm.[401]

In the largest trial reported to date, 3,040 men with noncastrate metastatic disease were enrolled, of whom 1,535 met the criteria for discontinuation. The trial was designed as a noninferiority study to show that the intermittent approach was no more than 20% inferior to continuous therapy. No significant different in survival was observed overall, but for the subset of men with disease limited to the axial skeleton and no visceral disease at presentation, the median survival was 7.1 years for continuous therapy and 5.1 years for the intermittent group (HR = 1.23; 95% CI = 1.02 to 1.48); the study did not exclude IAD to be inferior.[402] Three meta-analyses were recently reported based on 8 trials enrolling a total of 4,664 patients,[403] nine trials of 5,508 patients,[404] and 13 trials

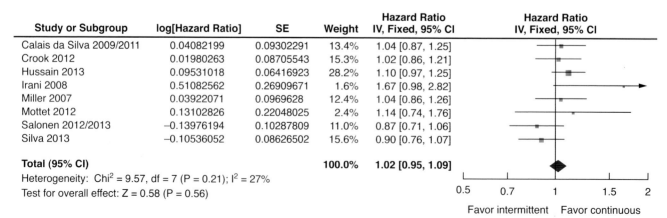

| Study or Subgroup | log[Hazard Ratio] | SE | Weight | Hazard Ratio IV, Fixed, 95% CI | Hazard Ratio IV, Fixed, 95% CI |
|---|---|---|---|---|---|
| Calais da Silva 2009/2011 | 0.04082199 | 0.09302291 | 13.4% | 1.04 [0.87, 1.25] | |
| Crook 2012 | 0.01980263 | 0.08705543 | 15.3% | 1.02 [0.86, 1.21] | |
| Hussain 2013 | 0.09531018 | 0.06416923 | 28.2% | 1.10 [0.97, 1.25] | |
| Irani 2008 | 0.51082562 | 0.26909671 | 1.6% | 1.67 [0.98, 2.82] | |
| Miller 2007 | 0.03922071 | 0.0969628 | 12.4% | 1.04 [0.86, 1.26] | |
| Mottet 2012 | 0.13102826 | 0.22048025 | 2.4% | 1.14 [0.74, 1.76] | |
| Salonen 2012/2013 | −0.13976194 | 0.10287809 | 11.0% | 0.87 [0.71, 1.06] | |
| Silva 2013 | −0.10536052 | 0.08626502 | 15.6% | 0.90 [0.76, 1.07] | |
| **Total (95% CI)** | | | **100.0%** | **1.02 [0.95, 1.09]** | |

Heterogeneity: Chi² = 9.57, df = 7 (P = 0.21); I² = 27%
Test for overall effect: Z = 0.58 (P = 0.56)

0.5     0.7     1     1.5     2
Favor intermittent     Favor continuous

**Figure 42.19** Overall survival with intermittent versus continuous androgen deprivation in prostate cancer. This figure is licensed under a Creative Commons Attribution 4.0 license. (From Botrel TE, Clark O, dos Reis RB, et al. Intermittent versus continuous androgen deprivation for locally advanced, recurrent or metastatic prostate cancer: a systematic review and meta-analysis. *BMC Urol* 2014;14:9.)

of 6,419 men[405] (Fig. 42.19). All showed no difference in overall survival, two showed no significant differences in disease-specific survival,[403,405] and one showed more deaths with IAD offset by more prostate cancer deaths with continuous therapy.[404] IAD was superior with respect to overall QOL and sexual function with significantly reduced costs.

While some controversy remains whether a patient will accept the tradeoff of a potentially higher risk of a prostate cancer death in return for time off therapy, it is important to recognize that the approach should only be considered for patients who respond well to ADT. In the recently reported SWOG study, only 1,535 of the 3,040 enrolled patients (51%) reached the defined PSA nadir of $\leq 4$ ng/ml.[402]

## Castration-Resistant Disease: Metastatic and Nonmetastatic

A rising PSA despite castrate levels of testosterone represents the transition to a castration-resistant (CRPC) state, which is lethal for most men. Clinically, there are several phenotypes: nonmetastatic that includes a rising PSA or disease limited to the prostate or prostate bed, and metastatic which includes the patterns of osseous disease and no soft tissue disease, nodal spread and no bone or visceral spread, and visceral spread with or without osseous disease. In some cases, the pattern of spread is observed with no increase in PSA. Symptoms may or may not be present. Disease in other sites, including the adrenal glands, omentum, kidney, pancreas, or brain, is rare. Which pattern develops in a patient is influenced in part by the extent of disease at the time ADT was first initiated. The patient who initially received hormones for a rising PSA alone is likely to relapse with a rising PSA and negative imaging studies—the nonmetastatic-CRPC state. A therapeutic objective for these patients is to prevent the development of bone metastases, the likelihood of which is highly variable between patients. In the placebo arm of one metastasis prevention study evaluating denosumab, the median time to metastasis was 25.2 months,[406] whereas in a second evaluating zoledronate, only one-third of patients had evidence of radiologic spread after 2 years of follow-up.[407] In Smith et al.,[408] men with a PSADT of $\leq 6$ months had a median time to first bone metastases of 18.5 months.

In both trials, overall risk of developing visible metastases by imaging was most informed by the PSA level at baseline and the PSADT: men with higher PSA levels and faster PSADT had a shorter time to first bone metastasis. In contrast, the patient who first receives hormones for symptomatic osseous disease is more likely to develop recurrent symptoms and is at higher risk of death from prostate cancer. Considered by site of spread based on trials enrolling patients with progressing metastatic CRPC, 85% to 90% have osseous disease, 20% to 40% have measurable pelvic or retroperitoneal nodal disease, and 5% to 10% have visceral (lung and liver) spread.[409–411]

A unique pattern of spread being recognized with increasing frequency is one in which new metastases, predominantly in the lung or viscera, develop in the absence of a PSA rise. Histologically on repeat biopsy, these tumors may be pure small cell/neuroendocrine lesions similar to what is seen in other sites, or are classified more broadly as "anaplastic" tumors.[409,410] These entities, when documented, are generally treated with platinum-containing chemotherapy regimens similar to what is used in small cell tumors that occur in the lung. The responses are similar: rapid improvements of short duration.[412]

### Patient Management

Patients with progressive disease with castrate levels of testosterone should continue LHRH agonist/antagonist therapies recognizing that no randomized trials have prospectively addressed this issue. Although not direct evidence, the survival benefits seen with the recently approved agents that inhibit AR signaling would

suggest that allowing testosterone levels to rise may adversely affect outcome. A retrospective analysis of 341 patients treated on four trials of secondary therapies suggested an improved survival for continuous androgen suppression when corrected for other factors,[413] but another did not.

The first consideration is to document castrate levels of testosterone. In rare cases, approximately 1% in prospective trials, LHRH analogs do not effect complete testosterone suppression.[414] The second is whether the patient has been on long-term antiandrogen therapy in combination with an LHRH analog or surgical orchiectomy, and if so, whether to discontinue the antiandrogen (continuing LHRH analog therapy) and to monitor the patient for a withdrawal response. The withdrawal response, consistent with the conversion of an antagonist to an agonist, was first reported in 1993 with flutamide discontinuation and later shown to occur with bicalutamide, nilutamide, cyproterone acetate, estrogens, glucocorticoids, and progestational agents.[415,416] The onset of the withdrawal response, when it occurs, is directly related to the half-life of the drug: early for flutamide with its short half-life and 6 weeks to 8 weeks for agents such as bicalutamide, which has a 7-day half-life. The disease flare that can occur with megestrol acetate prescribed to increase appetite is consistent with an agonist effect.[397,417–419]

Previously, if no withdrawal response was observed, patients were often treated with a different antiandrogen to which they had not been exposed, with limited benefit. The approaches included estrogens such as oral DES at a dose of 1 mg/d to 3 mg/d,[420] Premarin (1.25 mg three times daily; Wyeth Pharmaceuticals Inc., Philadelphia, PA),[421] estramustine, the first agent with a formal indication in this setting,[422] and various parenteral formulations.[423] All provided PSA decline rates in the 24% to 42% range, although durable responses were rare.[422,424] Attempts to reduce the thromboembolic risk of estrogens by using transdermal estrogen delivery systems have been made; however, efficacy in these trials has generally been less than anticipated.[425,426]

Ketoconazole, 600 to 1,200 mg/d in combination with hydrocortisone to minimize adrenal insufficiency, produces PSA declines by $\geq 50\%$ in up to 71% of patients,[427] the response correlating with higher serum androgen levels at baseline.[428] Absorption requires an acidic environment and so it is typically taken with juice. Proton-pump inhibitors and $H_2$ antagonists potentially interfere with absorption. Caution is urged with ketoconazole use as it is a potent inhibitor of CYP3A4. Cancer progression is associated with rises in androstenedione and DHEA sulfate,[429] implying that steroidogenic compensatory mechanisms contribute to escape from ketoconazole.

Prednisone 10 mg daily was shown to palliate symptoms of the disease in one-third of patients by Tannock et al.[430] in the pre-PSA era. Based on this, prednisone became an integral part of the "control" arms of many phase 3 trials in this disease. Similar results have been reported with hydrocortisone 30 mg/d to 40 mg/d and low-dose dexamethasone 0.5 mg to 2 mg daily in the PSA era, with reported decline rates ranging from 16% to 59% of patients.[431] These agents also lower serum androgen levels and, in a recent phase 3 trial in which patients were treated with prednisone 10 mg daily plus placebo, median survival times increased with each quartile increase in baseline serum androgen levels. PSA levels at baseline strongly associated with survival ($p < 0.0001$) in bivariate and multivariable analyses.[432]

### Cytotoxic Therapy

*Mitoxantrone.* Building on the palliative benefits observed with prednisone alone, its combination with mitoxantrone 12 mg/m² every 3 weeks suggested superiority to prednisone monotherapy. The definitive phase 3 trial enrolling 160 patients, small by today's standard, used a primary end point of pain palliation assessed with a patient-reported outcome scale and measuring daily analgesic consumption.[320] The trial was not designed nor was it powered to show a survival benefit. The results showed that a higher proportion of patients treated with the combination had a decrease in pain (29% versus 12%) and overall palliative response (38% versus 21%). Consistent with the findings was a decrease in analgesic consumption, improved bowel function, and increased patient mobility. Disease control shown by the duration of pain relief among mitoxantrone responders was 43 weeks versus 18 weeks for the control group. Similar results were obtained in a second trial,[433] leading to the approval of mitoxantrone and prednisone for the treatment of CRPC in 1996 and establishing the regimen as the first cytotoxic-containing standard and the standard to which other treatments would be compared. Common toxicities with mitoxantrone at doses of 12 mg/m² every 3 weeks included nausea (61%), fatigue (39%), alopecia (29%), and anorexia (25%). Grade 3/4 neutropenia is reported in approximately 20% of patients, but febrile neutropenia is relatively unusual (2% of patients). Cardiac function is a concern; decreased cardiac function was reported in 5% to 7% of patients.

*Docetaxel.* Two pivotal trials were reported in 2004 showing that docetaxel plus prednisone could palliate symptoms, delay progression, and definitively prolong life relative to mitoxantrone and prednisone. TAX327 compared docetaxel 75 mg/m² every 3 weeks for up to 10 cycles (group 1), docetaxel 30 mg/m² weekly for 5 cycles (group 2), or mitoxantrone 12 mg/m² every 3 weeks for 10 cycles (group 3). Prednisone (10 mg daily) was added to all regimens. The primary end point was overall survival; secondary end points included changes in pain, PSA, and overall QOL. Median survival for the respective arms was 18.9 months, 17.4 months, and 16.5 months, respectively, which led to the approval of docetaxel plus prednisone for "androgen-independent (hormone-refractory)" disease. The 2.4-month difference in median survival (18.9 months versus 16.5 months) for the every-three-week docetaxel versus the mitoxantrone schedule established the every-three-week regimen as the de facto standard.[322]

SWOG 99-16 randomized 770 patients to estramustine (280 mg orally three times daily on days 1 to 5), docetaxel (60 mg/m² every 3 weeks), and dexamethasone (60 mg every 3 weeks) versus mitoxantrone and prednisone (5 mg twice a day) to a maximum of 12 cycles with no crossover at progression. The primary end point was overall survival. PSA declines, soft tissue response, and PFS were secondary end points. Here again, a 2-month difference in median survival was observed for docetaxel/estramustine (17.5 months versus 15.6 months), representing a 20% reduction in mortality (HR = 0.8). A higher incidence of neutropenia and fever, nausea, vomiting, and vascular events with docetaxel/estramustine was noted despite the lower dose of docetaxel. The results further supported docetaxel 70 mg/m² every 3 weeks as the standard regimen.[321]

With docetaxel established as the first-line cytotoxic standard, drug development efforts focused on three discrete clinical contexts: the prechemotherapy space, the first-line cytotoxic chemotherapy space to build on the results of docetaxel, and the postchemotherapy space for which there was no standard of care at the time. Notable is that none of the docetaxel-based combination trials showed an improvement over single-agent therapy, whereas, in several trials, outcomes were inferior with the combination arm (see Table 42.14).[329–337]

Cabazitaxel is a next-generation taxane with an improved therapeutic index relative to docetaxel that is noncross-resistant with the parent compound in selected contexts.[434] Following successful early phase trials showing antitumor activity in docetaxel-refractory metastatic CRPC, a randomized phase 3 trial comparing cabazitaxel plus prednisone (n = 377) to mitoxantrone plus prednisone (n = 378) was developed in this setting. At the final analysis, median survival and median PFS for the cabazitaxel and mitoxantrone cohorts was 15.1 months and 12.7 months (HR =0.70; 95% CI = 0.59 to 0.83; *p* <0.0001) and 2.8 months and 1.4 months (HR = 0.74; 95% CI = 0.64 to 0.86; *p* <0.0001), respectively.[325] In 2010, the FDA

approved cabazitaxel plus prednisone for the treatment of metastatic CRPC previously treated with a docetaxel-containing regimen.

Further progress was not achieved until there was a more complete understanding of the biology of the disease. Through profiling studies of prostate cancers representing different clinical states, a series of oncogenic changes in the AR signaling pathway were identified that showed CRPC remained hormone driven, while serving as points for therapeutic attack. These changes included amplification of a wild-type AR gene, overexpression of the enzymes involved in androgen synthesis, and alterations in the ligand-binding domain and co-activator/co-repressor protein interactions leading to promiscuous activation by other steroid hormones and antiandrogens.[435] Consistent with the upregulation of the androgen biosynthetic machinery, and with the development of mass spectroscopy based assays for serum and tissue androgens,[436] came the demonstration that intratumoral androgen levels in metastatic CRPC tumor samples could exceed those present in the prostates of men in a eugonadal state.[437] This finding, coupled with overexpression of the receptor itself, enabled an intracrine signaling mechanism to sustain growth.

Abiraterone acetate plus prednisone: The cytochrome P450 (17) inhibitor abiraterone was developed to inhibit testicular and adrenal androgen production,[438] and shown in a series of three dose-escalating studies to achieve androgen suppression in both noncastrate and castrate men.[439] A subsequent phase 1 trial in men with CRPC who had not received chemotherapy showed a sustained decrease in testosterone to the 1 ng/dl to 2 ng/dl range as well as a reduction in estradiol, DHEA, and androstenedione, confirming the dependence of CRPC on ligand-activated AR signaling. Antitumor effects included significant declines in PSA, tumor regressions, and favorable changes in circulating tumor cell number. Adverse clinical and laboratory events consistent with mineralocorticoid excess including hypertension, fluid retention, and hyperkalemia were identified, which could be reduced by eplerenone or prednisone.[440] A second phase 1 trial showed similar results in the same patient group and established a dose of 1,000 mg daily for phase 2 investigations.[441]

Phase 2 trials of abiraterone acetate alone[442] or abiraterone acetate plus prednisone[443] in postchemotherapy-treated CRPC followed based on the hypothesis that the decision to treat a patient with chemotherapy would not change the underlying biology of the disease significantly, and that if efficacy were shown, the track to approval would be shorter because the prognosis of these patients was inferior to that of patients who had not received prior chemotherapy. The unmet need for effective therapy was also greater in this population because there was no standard of care that had been shown to prolong life. Two phase 2 trials followed, one that excluded prior ketoconazole exposure[442] and one which did not[443]; both trials showed significant activity leading to the definitive phase 3 trial, Cougar AA-301, comparing the combination of abiraterone acetate (1,000 mg daily) plus prednisone (5 mg twice a day) to placebo plus prednisone (5 mg twice a day). The primary end point was overall survival, and secondary end points were radiographic PFS (rPFS), PSA response, time to PSA progression, and changes in QOL. Superiority of the combination relative to the placebo combination with respect to overall survival was shown in both interim (median 14.8 months versus 10.9 months; HR = 0.65; 95% CI = 0.54 to 0.77; *p* <0.001) and final (15.8 months versus 11.2 months; HR = 0.74; 95% CI = 0.64 to 0.86) analyses. The drug was approved in 2011 for postchemotherapy-treated CRPC.[327,444]

Subsequently, there was an abiraterone phase 3 trial in chemotherapy-naïve patients that used a coprimary end point of rPFS and overall survival. Notably, the rPFS end point included the PCWG2 definition of bone scan progression, which enabled 72% (166 of 229) of patients with apparent progression on a first follow-up to continue treatment because no additional new lesions were documented on the confirmatory scan. In the final analysis with a median follow-up period of 27.1 months, rPFS was

8.3 months in the placebo arm and not yet reached in the abiraterone arm (HR = 0.43; 95% CI = 0.35 to 0.52; $p$ <0.0001). Improvement in overall survival (35.3 months versus 30.1 months; HR = 0.78; 95% CI = 0.66 to 0.95; $p$ = 0.0151) did not reach the prespecified statistical efficacy boundary but was supported by significant improvements in time-to-opiate-use and time-to-cytotoxic-chemotherapy end points.[324,445] Abiraterone plus prednisone gained expanded approval for chemotherapy-naïve metastatic CRPC in 2012.[324]

### Next-Generation Antiandrogens

Enzalutamide (previously MDV3100) was rationally designed with the aim of developing an antiandrogen active in prostate cancers with overexpressed AR, a setting in which the tumor is both resistant and growth is stimulated by bicalutamide, consistent with an antagonist-agonist conversion.

In the phase 1/2 enzalutamide clinical trial that enrolled patients with pre- and postchemotherapy CRPC treated with a variety of dose levels, there were PSA declines of ≥50% in 71% and 37% of patients who were prechemotherapy or postchemotherapy treated, respectively, along with soft tissue regressions, and a posttherapy conversion of circulating tumor cell counts from unfavorable to favorable in 49% (25 of 51) of patients.[446] The results led to the phase 3 AFFIRM trial in which 1,199 men with progressive postchemotherapy-treated CRPC were randomized in a 2:1 ratio to enzalutamide 160 mg daily ($n$ = 800) or placebo ($n$ = 399). The primary end point was overall survival and at the first interim analysis, a statistically significant reduction in mortality was seen (HR = 0.63; 95% CI = 0.53 to 0.74; $p$ <0.001), with a median overall survival of 18.4 months (95% CI = 17.3 to not yet reached) for enzalutamide versus 13.6 months (95% CI = 11.3 to 15.8) in the placebo group. All secondary end points favored enzalutamide including rPFS (8.3 months versus 2.9 months; HR = 0.40; $p$ <0.001), the time to the first SRE (16.7 months versus 13.3 months; HR = 0.69; $p$ <0.001), and QOL response rate (43% versus 18%; $p$ <0.001). The results led to FDA approval in 2012.[328]

More recently, the results of the prechemotherapy enzalutamide trial PREVAIL were reported; PREVAIL randomized 1,717 patients with prechemotherapy CRPC to enzalutamide 160 mg daily or placebo using the coprimary end points of rPFS and overall survival. This study was stopped by the data and safety monitoring board after 540 deaths based on the superiority of enzalutamide in delaying radiographic progression or death (HR = 0.19; 95% CI = 0.15 to 0.23; $p$ <0.001) and risk of death (HR = 0.71; 95% CI = 0.60 to 0.84; $p$ <0.001) relative to placebo. The benefit of enzalutamide was consistent for all secondary end points including rate of ≥50% PSA decline (78% versus 3%;), overall soft tissue response (59% versus 5%), time to PSA progression (HR = 0.17), time to initiation of cytotoxic chemotherapy (HR = 0.35), and time to first SRE (HR = 0.72) ($p$ <0.001 for all comparisons).[447] These results have been submitted to the FDA, and an expanded indication is pending.

New antiandrogens in development include ARN-509 and galeterone. ARN-509 was more potent than enzalutamide in preclinical models,[448] has shown significant activity in a phase 1 trial,[449] and is now in phase 3 testing in nonmetastatic CRPC (NCT01946204). Galeterone (previously TOK-001) has multiple effects, including blocking and degrading AR,[450] and will be entering phase 3 testing shortly.

## Targeting the Tumor Microenvironment

### Immunotherapy

Sipuleucel-T (Provenge; Dendreon Corporation, Seattle, WA) is an autologous active cellular immunotherapy that includes an acid phosphatase specific, replication-competent adenovirus that is cotransfected with granulocyte macrophage–colony-stimulating

factor. Mononuclear cells are harvested by leukopheresis, transfected with the viral construct, and maintained in culture under an adequate number of the defined mononuclear cell fraction has developed to enable re-infusion to the patient. A phase 1 dose-ranging study showed that injection of the primed cells into the prostates of patients with recurrent disease after radiation therapy was safe, and declines in PSA were observed that correlated with the administered dose of the virus.[451]

A randomized phase 3 trial in which patients received either primed and unprimed mononuclear cells was then performed; the trial failed to meet the primary end point of PFS,[452] but with longer follow-up, an overall survival benefit was observed.[453] A pivotal trial was then designed in which 512 patients with asymptomatic or minimally symptomatic metastatic CRPC were randomized to three doses of the biologic product or autologous cells that had been treated similarly but not exposed to the granulocyte macrophage–colony-stimulating factor/prostatic acid phosphatase fusion protein. The results showed a significant improvement in survival for the immunized patients (HR = 0.77; 95% CI = 0.61 to 0.97; $p$ = 0.02), median 25.8 months in the sipuleucel-T arm and 21.7 months in the control arm. Adverse reactions were primarily related to the infusion of the activated cells and included chills (53%), fatigue (41%), fever (31%), back pain (30%), nausea (21%), joint aches (20%), and headaches (18%). Most of these reactions had resolved within 2 days of infusion. Grade 3–4 events were <3% for each of these conditions. No improvement in PFS or response rate was seen in the large randomized trial, suggesting either that these parameters were not accurately measured or that slower kinetics of the disease were manifest after progression was initially measured. FDA approval was granted in 2010.[324]

PROSTVAC (Bavarian Nordic, Kvistgaard, Denmark) is a vaccinia and fowlpox immunization approach that includes the gene sequence for PSA and three costimulatory molecules (B7-1, ICAM-1, and LFA-3) collectively designated as TRICOM. In the phase 1 trial, patients received the recombinant vaccinia virus vaccine first, which was followed by a booster injection with recombinant fowlpox virus; all patients generated an immune response to vaccinia.[454] A randomized phase 2 trial was then performed with a primary end point of PFS, which showed no difference between the groups, but 3 years post study, 30% (25 of 82) of the vaccine-treated versus 17% (7 of 40) of the placebo-treated patients were alive (median survival 25.1 months versus 16.6 months; HR = 0.56; 95% CI = 0.37 to 0.85).[453] A phase 3 trial is ongoing.

Ipilimumab: Cytotoxic T-lymphocyte antigen-4 is a T-cell co-inhibitory and immune checkpoint molecule expressed by activated and regulatory T cells that plays a critical role in maintaining immune homeostasis and peripheral tolerance to self-antigens. In preclinical studies, cytotoxic T-lymphocyte antigen-4 blockade augmented T cell–mediated immune responses against tumors. This led to the development of ipilimumab, a fully humanized immunoglobulin G₁ monoclonal antibody to cytotoxic T-lymphocyte antigen-4 in malignant melanoma, renal cell carcinoma, prostate cancer, and other tumors. Two phase 3 trials demonstrated an overall survival benefit in malignant melanoma leading to FDA approval, and of particular note is the durable, complete remission of over 4 years in approximately 20% to 25% of patients.[455,456] Antitumor activity was shown in a phase 1/2 trial of ipilimumab alone or in combination with EBRT in prostate cancer,[457] which led to a phase 3 trial in patients with CRPC who had received prior treatment with docetaxel of radiation therapy alone versus radiation therapy plus ipilimumab.[458] This study failed to meet the primary overall survival end point but did show evidence of activity at later time points. A second trial in prechemotherapy treated CRPC has fully accrued.

There are two randomized, double-blind, phase 3 registration trials in metastatic CRPC, which have fully accrued. One trial, comparing the efficacy of ipilimumab versus placebo in asymptomatic or minimally symptomatic patients with chemotherapy-naïve metastatic CRPC (NCT01057810), fell short of the primary end point. Results from preclinical studies and early clinical trials suggest synergistic effect of ipilimumab and next-generation drugs targeting the AR signaling axis, cytotoxics and other immune modulators (poxvirus).

Cabozantinib (previously XL-184) is an orally bioavailable tyrosine kinase inhibitor with potent activity against MET and vascular endothelial growth factor receptor 2 shown in preclinical bone metastatic CRPC models to inhibit osteoblasts and osteoclasts function. In the clinic, the drug produced dramatic improvements in radionuclide bone scans which were associated with relief of pain. In a subsequent phase 2 randomized discontinuation study (nonrandomized extension),[459] 122 patients with postdocetaxel CRPC with measurable disease received cabozantinib 100 mg daily for 12 weeks and were then randomized based on response: subjects with response by modified RECIST criteria continued open-label cabozantinib, subjects with progressive disease discontinued therapy, and subjects with stable disease were randomized to either placebo or continued cabozantinib (primary end point: PFS). The results showed improvements on bone scan in 68% of patients, including complete resolution in 12%, declines in total alkaline phosphatase and plasma cross-linked C-terminal telopeptide of type I collagen of ≥50% in 57% of patients, and 67% showed reductions in pain. Notable was that improvements in pain and changes in PSA were in 40% of patients.

A subsequent nonrandomized extension was conducted in 85 patients evaluable for bone scan response, and 51 (60%) had a partial resolution, 24 (28%) stable disease, 5 (6%) progressive disease, and 5 (6%) discontinued prior to follow-up scan. Measurable disease was reduced in 21/30 patients (70%). Of the 33 patients with a Brief Pain Inventory score ≥4, 16 (49%) had pain reduction durable for ≥6 weeks; 46% had decreased narcotic use, including 27% who discontinued use completely.

The results led to the design of two, currently ongoing, phase 3 trials of cabozantinib in patients with metastatic CRPC who have progressed on docetaxel-containing chemotherapy and abiraterone or enzalutamide. In COMET-1 (NCT01605227), the effect of cabozantinib on overall survival is being compared to prednisone. COMET-2 (NCT01522443) explores the effect of cabozantinib versus mitoxantrone plus prednisone on pain response and bone scan response.

Tasquinimod (formerly ABR-215050) is a quinoline carboxamide that binds to the immunomodulatory protein S100A9 with antiangiogenic activity in xenograft models through a vascular endothelial growth factor–independent mechanism.[460–462] A randomized placebo-controlled phase 2 trial of 201 men with chemotherapy-naïve CRPC showed improvement in median PFS (7.6 months versus 3.3 months; HR = 0.57; 95% CI = 0.39 to 0.85; $p = 0.0042$)[463] and a trend toward improvement in median overall survival (33.4 months versus 30.4 months; $p = 0.49$).[464] The results led to a phase 3 trial (10TASQ10) in men with asymptomatic to mildly symptomatic metastatic CRPC. Other ongoing studies include the phase 1 CATCH trial combining tasquinimod and cabazitaxel in postchemotherapy metastatic CRPC (NCT01513733) and a phase 2 trial evaluating the drug as a maintenance therapy for men with metastatic CRPC who are not progressing after first-line docetaxel-based therapy (NCT01732549).

## PALLIATION

### Bone-Directed Therapy

The high propensity for prostate cancers to metastasize to the skeleton puts patients at a high risk for significant morbidity from SREs. This can be complicated further by the bone loss associated with ADT itself, and the frequent use of corticosteroids for antitumor effects, to reduce the toxicities of anticancer agents such as the taxanes and CYP17 inhibitors, and for palliation of pain or symptoms related to neurologic compromise. Targeting the bone microenvironment can provide palliation of symptoms, delay SREs, and prolong life.

### Targeting Growth Factors and Cytokines

Bisphosphonates localize to the bone tumor interface and inhibit osteoclast activity to reduce bone turnover. The bisphosphonate zoledronate is the only FDA-approved agent for CRPC with bone metastases. In randomized trials, zoledronate (4 mg intravenously every 3 to 4 weeks) reduced the frequency of SREs (defined as pathologic fractures, radiation to bone, spinal cord compression, and/or surgery to bone) by 25% (33% with zoledronate versus 44%; $p = 0.021$). Time to first SRE was prolonged, whereas skeletal morbidity rate and the proportion of patients with an individual SRE were lowered. There was no effect on overall survival.[159] Bisphosphonates are also used in patients with prostate cancer to reduce the risk of osteoporosis, exacerbated by ADT, that increases the susceptibility to fracture or collapse of a vertebra in nontumor-bearing areas.[159] Nephrotoxicity can occur with these agents, and doses must be adjusted on the basis of renal function.

Denosumab is a monoclonal antibody that binds RANKL, inhibiting osteoclast function. Initial trials showed a decrease in bone loss and reduction in fracture rate for patients on ADT.[465] A subsequent phase 3 trial enrolled 1,904 patients and compared denosumab (120 mg subcutaneous monthly) to zoledronate (4 mg every 3 weeks). The primary end point, delay in time to first SRE, showed a benefit in favor of denosumab (20.7 months versus 17.1 months; HR = 0.82; $p < 0.001$ for noninferiority and $p = 0.008$ for superiority). The denosumab arm had a slightly higher frequency of serious adverse events (63% versus 60%), Common Terminology Criteria for Adverse Events grade 3-4 adverse events (72% versus 66%; $p = 0.01$), and grade ≥3 hypocalcemia (5% versus 1%). There was no significant difference in the rate of serious adverse events, disease progression, or overall survival. The frequency of osteonecrosis of the jaw was similar (2% versus 1%). This relatively rare but serious side effect seems associated with bisphosphonate or denosumab use in combination with dental disease, dental surgery (e.g., tooth extraction), oral trauma, periodontitis, poor dental hygiene, glucocorticoid use, or chemotherapy use.[338]

Denosumab 120 mg every 4 weeks was also shown to delay the development of bone metastases relative to placebo in patients with nonmetastatic CRPC at a high risk of bone metastases (baseline PSA ≥8 ng/ml or PSADT ≤10 months). In this trial, bone metastasis–free survival was increased by a median of 4.2 months (median 29.5 months, 95% CI = 25.4 to 33.3 for denosumab versus 25.2 months, 95% CI = 22.2 to 29.5 for placebo). Denosumab also prolonged the time to first bone metastasis. Osteonecrosis was observed in 5% of patients receiving denosumab. Although statistically significant, denosumab's effect upon bone metastases was deemed insufficient for FDA approval.[406]

### Pain

Optimal palliation of pain requires careful attention to the pain frequency, pattern, and precipitating factors. It also requires early performance of appropriate diagnostic studies to establish an etiology.

Critical for pain management is a low threshold for recommending an MRI if there should be any of the following: back pain suggestive of neurologic compromise of the spinal cord or cauda equina; diplopia, dysarthria, difficulty swallowing, or facial weakness suggestive of involvement of the base of the skull; or numbness in the jaw or chin suggestive of mental nerve compromise that may interfere with eating.[466] If neurologic encroachment is documented in any of these areas, radiotherapy should be administered on an urgent basis to preserve function and to maximize the chance of recovery. Corticosteroids are also administered to provide more immediate palliation, and to reduce the risk of further compromise secondary to swelling that can occur after radiotherapy is initiated.[467] An MRI can also be recommended for patients with extensive bony disease in the absence of symptoms, as one series showed occult cord compromise in 11% of patients, which involved multiple locations in several patients.[468] Metastases to the base of the skull leading to cranial nerve palsies can also severely compromise function unless diagnosed and treated expeditiously.

For one or more painful lesions that can be encompassed by a single or regional radiation port, EBRT offers excellent palliation. A variety of fractionation schemes and administered daily doses have been studied: 30 Gy administered as 300 cGy in 10 fractions is considered standard, although randomized trials have shown a single administered dose of 8 Gy in 1 fraction to be equivalent but not as durable. Patients treated with 30 Gy are less likely to require repeat treatment (18% versus 9%). High-dose hypofractionation regimens have also been studied, including 20 Gy or 24 Gy as a single dose, or 500 cGy to 800 cGy in three separate doses. A limitation of EBRT is that the disease is often diffuse and that lacking some form of systemic control, patients often experience recurrence in a relatively short interval after a first lesion is treated. In such cases of patients with recurrence of painful lesions outside of radiated areas, a systemic approach is preferred. Retreatment of a site previously irradiated is also necessary in approximately 25% of cases.[469–471]

### Radiopharmaceuticals

Therapies to control more diffuse pain include those directed at the tumor/bone interface with little effect on tumor, those directed at specific cytokines and growth factors produced by tumor cells and the host that contribute to the progression and survival of prostate cancer cells in the skeleton, and those directed at the tumor itself.

Bone-seeking radiopharmaceuticals are taken up rapidly at the tumor/bone interface with maximal deposition at the site of maximal bone turnover. The distribution of the isotope through the tumor is uncertain, making dosimetry difficult to calculate, but estimates are that the administered dose to the tumor itself is typically below that achieved with EBRT. Three such agents are currently approved in the United States on the basis of phase 3 trials.[326,472–474]

Strontium-89 is a low-energy beta-emitter with a long (50-day) half-life. It was approved on the basis of a trial enrolling patients with symptomatic skeletal metastasis randomized to EBRT alone or EBRT plus the radiopharmaceutical, showing patients treated with strontium were less likely to have pain in new metastatic sites.[474]

Samarium ($^{153}$Sm) lexidronam,[475,476] with a 2.9-day half-life, relies on the diphosphonate moiety for targeting, while the radionuclide simultaneously emits gamma energies that can be imaged and short-range beta energies that can be therapeutic. Technetium (99mTc) methyl diphosphonate bone imaging can identify tumors with high uptake.

$^{153}$Sm-EDTMP exhibits pharmacokinetic, toxicity, and pain response using an escalating dose schedule in treatment of metastatic bone cancer. This agent was approved on the basis of a trial that randomized patients to radioactive ($^{153}$Sm) versus nonradioactive ($^{152}$Sm) drug, showing a reduction in both opioid analgesic consumption and improvement in patient-reported visual analog scales and pain descriptor scales. The most common side effects were pain flare in approximately 10% of cases that could last for several days and myelosuppression which varies with the extent of disease and with the amount of bone marrow that has received radiation in the past.[472,477] $^{153}$Sm lexidronam has also been safely administered on a repetitive basis in combination with docetaxel.[478]

As beta-emitters, both strontium-89 and $^{153}$Sm lexidronam have a penetration energy up to 2.4 mm in bone that disrupts normal hematopoiesis leading to myelosuppression and anemia. Tumor cell kill results from the inability to repair single-strand DNA breaks induced by the agent.

Radium-223 dichloride (radium-223) is a high linear energy transfer radiation that has a very short (<0.1 mm) range and induces double-strand DNA breaks, rendering cellular repair mechanisms ineffective. Exposure of the surrounding tissues is minimized. After activity was shown in a phase 1 trial,[479] a phase 3, randomized, double-blind, placebo-controlled study was completed that enrolled, in a 2:1 ratio, 922 patients with symptomatic bone metastases and no visceral disease who had either received, were not eligible to receive, or declined docetaxel. Patients were randomized to receive six injections of radium-223 (at a dose of 50 kBq per kg of body weight intravenously) or matching placebo; one injection was administered every 4 weeks. The primary end point was overall survival. Secondary end points included time to the first symptomatic SRE; time to bone-specific alkaline phosphatase progression, response, and normalization; PSA progression; and changes in several biochemical measures. Relative to placebo, radium-223 significantly improved overall survival (median, 14 months versus 11.2 months; HR = 0.66; 95% CI = 0.58 to 0.83; two-sided $p$ = 0.00007). Assessments of all main secondary efficacy end points also showed a benefit for radium-233 compared with placebo, including the time to first SRE, which was prolonged from a median 9.8 months for placebo to 15.6 months (HR = 0.66; 95% CI = 0.52 to 0.83). Notable was that the drug was associated with low myelosuppression rates and fewer adverse events.[326]

## FUTURE DIRECTIONS

The key to prostate cancer diagnosis and management is the assessment of risk based on the continuous reassessment of the disease at the current point in time and projecting the likelihood of disease-specific events in the future. Now, advances in our understanding of prostate cancer biology have changed diagnostic and treatment paradigms and improved the outcomes for patients across the clinical spectrum of the disease. The diagnostic algorithms used to detect disease are increasingly incorporating biologic determinants to better enable the detection of clinically significant cancers rather than all cancers. Many of the prognostic models used to define the metastatic and lethal potential of a tumor are also including molecular measures in addition to the standard clinicopathologic measures such as T stage (plagued by interobserver variability), PSA (lacks sensitivity and specificity), and Gleason score based on morphology. All prognostic models aim to ensure that only those tumors with the potential to cause symptoms, metastasize, or shorten patient survival are treated, while recognizing that for the tumors that are not treated, close monitoring using an AS approach is the "treatment."

Technologic advances in surgery and radiation therapy have resulted in better cancer control rates, particularly for "high-risk" patients, with fewer and lesser short- and long-term morbidities. In these cases, the focus of treatment centers on two objectives: control of the primary tumor and of metastatic disease. A range of biomarkers are in development to better inform prognosis (who needs treatment), prediction (what type of treatment), treatment efficacy (if it is working), and regulatory approval (providing clinical benefit). Missing in many biomarker studies is clinical utility—showing the incremental information provided by the "test" relative to what is currently available, a key factor in whether a test will be used in practice.

The same needs apply to patients who have experienced recurrence after primary therapy: to determine the likelihood that a tumor can be cured if still localized, independent of whether the primary treatment was surgery or radiation, and if not still localized, to guide the need for a systemic intervention based on the likelihood that metastatic disease might develop and when. Equally important is that we have learned that prostate cancer in an individual is more than one disease that can have different drivers of growth in different tumors as well as within one individual site of disease. The heterogeneity increases even further with the increasing number of drugs to which the cancer has been exposed. To address this will require the continued characterization of disease biology. However, the necessary repeated tissue- or blood-based diagnostics to do so are presently not part of routine clinical practice.

Unfortunately, the field is still plagued by the use of end points of convenience that occur early as opposed to end points that take longer to observe but which more accurately reflect clinical benefit. Few reports include a clearly defined statistical design, and those that do rarely define a level of improvement to justify the development of a large-scale definitive trial to generate the evidence required to change practice standards.

The recent approval of several life-prolonging therapies as well as agents that reduce morbidity is particularly encouraging. However, it also presents an additional challenge because the use of effective treatments *after* a patient has been treated on a clinical trial reduces the trial's ability to show a survival benefit for an experimental drug. The failure to show a survival benefit in the phase 3 trials in CRPC with the Cyp 17 inhibitor orteronel[480] and custirsen,[481] an antisense molecule that reduces the levels of the antiapoptotic protein clusterin, are recent examples. The latter represents another docetaxel-based combination that failed to show a survival benefit relative to docetaxel alone. Yet, both agents showed promising effects in phase 2 studies[482–484] and show that it is essential to carefully consider the regulatory path to approval for any prostate cancer drug. Critical here is the discovery, validation, and qualification of predictive biomarkers of sensitivity. Such biomarkers will enable the enrollment of patients most likely to respond to the treatment being evaluated and will supply trial end points short of survival that could potentially lead to regulatory approvals.

A challenge now is to design trials that show how to maximize patient benefit with the available agents, used alone in sequence or in combination, and to understand cross-resistance and synergies. Strategies to improve outcomes with AR and AR signaling inhibitors include the development of new antiandrogens such as ARN-509 and galeterone (previously TOK-001). An analysis of the posttherapy PSA patterns of patients treated with AR and AR signaling inhibitors shows that a proportion of tumors are intrinsically resistant, a proportion show a pattern consistent with acquired resistance, and others show durable response followed later by progression.[485] Studies in preclinical models have associated intrinsic

resistance with reciprocal feedback between the AR and phosphatidylinositol kinase signaling pathways,[486] and AR splice variants,[487] in particular the AR-V7 variant,[488] whereas acquired resistance has been associated with an acquired mutation in the ligand-binding domain of the AR at position 876L.[489] Cooptation of the AR by the glucocorticoid receptor[490] and a number of new agents and combinations are being evaluated in the clinic based on activity demonstrated in these models.

The efficacy seen with newer agents in late-stage disease also suggests that the time is now to shift our paradigm from palliation to cure by evaluating available life-prolonging therapies in noncastrate settings with low disease burdens. Several trials exploring combinations of ADT and radiation therapy have been completed and have shown significant survival improvements. Such has not been the case with trials of ADT and RP as, to date, only one trial that enrolled patients with node-positive disease following RP showed a survival improvement.[491] More recently, another trial, CHAARTED, showed that early use of docetaxel in combination with standard ADT conferred a 13.6-month improvement in median survival for patients with high-grade, high-volume, noncastrate disease.[492] Two ongoing randomized trials are awaited that will evaluate a similar combination in the high-risk neoadjuvant setting (NCT00430183) and in patients with a rising PSA with rapid PSADT (NCT01813370). An important consideration in the design of such studies is to demonstrate that the "experimental" treatment proposed has sufficient activity to justify large-scale testing. Here, neoadjuvant studies are particularly important because they ensure that adequate amounts of tumor material are available for analysis.[493] One promising approach reported recently was a randomized trial in which abiraterone acetate and prednisone in combination with leuprolide acetate was shown to provide a higher pathologic complete response rate relative to leuprolide acetate alone.[494] To test this further, the trial in patients with a rising PSA and rapid PSADT is comparing degarelix in combination with abiraterone acetate and prednisone to degarelix alone, with the end point of an undetectable PSA (NCT01813370). Trials of this type can be useful to support larger-scale studies to address whether even greater benefit can be provided to patients with potentially lethal disease if treated early, an approach that has been shown to be effective in many cancer types.

# REFERENCES

1. Scher HI, Heller G. Clinical states in prostate cancer: towards a dynamic model of disease progression. *Urology* 2000;55:323–327.
2. American Cancer Society. Cancer facts and figures 2014. http://www.cancer.org /research/cancerfactsstatistics/cancerfactsfigures2014/. Accessed May 29, 2014.
3. SEER Program. SEER stat fact sheets: prostate cancer. http://seer.cancer.gov/ statfacts/html/prost.html. Accessed May 29, 2014.
4. Prostate.net. Prostate cancer statistics. http://www.prostate.net/prostate-cancer /prostate-cancer-statistics/. Accessed May 29, 2014.
5. Center MM, Jemal A, Lortet-Tieulent J, et al. International variation in prostate cancer incidence and mortality rates. *Eur Urol* 2012;61:1079–1092.
6. Sakr WA, Grignon DJ, Crissman JD, et al. High grade prostatic intraepithelial neoplasia (HGPIN) and prostatic adenocarcinoma between the ages of 20-69: an autopsy study of 249 cases. *In Vivo* 1994;8:439–443.
7. Haenszel W, Kurihara M. Studies of Japanese migrants. I. Mortality from cancer and other diseases among Japanese in the United States. *J Natl Cancer Inst* 1968;40:43–68.
8. Scardino PT, Weaver R, Hudson MA. Early detection of prostate cancer. *Hum Pathol* 1992;23:211–222.
9. Kosary CL, Ries LAG, Miller BA, et al. *SEER cancer incidence public-use database, 1970-1980.* Bethesda, MD: National Cancer Institute; 1998.
10. Smith JR, Freije D, Carpten JD, et al. Major susceptibility locus for prostate cancer on chromosome 1 suggested by a genome wide search. *Science* 1996;274:1371–1374.
11. Wilson KM, Giovannucci EL, Mucci LA. Lifestyle and dietary factors in the prevention of lethal prostate cancer. *Asian J Androl* 2012;14:365–374.
12. Scardino PT. Prostate cancer: improving PSA testing by adjusting for genetic background. *Nat Rev Urol* 2013;10:190–192.
13. Ewing CM, Ray AM, Lange EM, et al. Germline mutations in HOXB13 and prostate-cancer risk. *N Engl J Med* 2012;366:141–149.
14. Gallagher DJ, Gaudet MM, Pal P, et al. Germline BRCA mutations denote a clinicopathologic subset of prostate cancer. *Clin Cancer Res* 2010;16:2115–2121.
15. Demark-Wahnefried W, Strigo T, Catoe K, et al. Knowledge, beliefs, and prior screening behavior among blacks and whites reporting for prostate cancer screening. *Urology* 1995;46:346–351.
16. Polednak AP, Flannery JT. Black versus white racial differences in clinical stage at diagnosis and treatment of prostatic cancer in Connecticut. *Cancer* 1992;70:2152–2158.
17. Vertosick EA, Poon BY, Vickers AJ. Relative value of race, family history and prostate-specific antigen as indications for early initiation of prostate cancer screening. *J Urol* 2014 [Epub ahead of print]. doi: 10.1016/j.juro.2014.03.032
18. Cook LS, Goldoff M, Schwartz SM, et al. Incidence of adenocarcinoma of the prostate in Asian immigrants to the United States and their descendants. *J Urol* 1999;161:152–155.
19. Bosland MC, Oakley-Girvan I, Whittemore AS. Dietary fat, calories, and prostate cancer risk. *J Natl Cancer Inst* 1999;91:489–491.
20. Correa P. Epidemiological correlations between diet and cancer frequency. *Cancer Res* 1981;41:3685–3690.
21. Allott EH, Masko EM, Freedland SJ. Obesity and prostate cancer: weighing the evidence. *Eur Urol* 2013;63:800–809.
22. Muller RL, Gerber L, Moreira DM, et al. Obesity is associated with increased prostate growth and attenuated prostate volume reduction by dutasteride. *Eur Urol* 2013;63:1115–1121.
23. Cao Y, Ma J. Body mass index, prostate cancer-specific mortality, and biochemical recurrence: a systematic review and meta-analysis. *Cancer Prev Res (Phila)* 2011;4:486–501.
24. Ma J, Li H, Giovannucci E, et al. Prediagnostic body-mass index, plasma C-peptide concentration, and prostate cancer-specific mortality in men with prostate cancer: a long-term survival analysis. *Lancet Oncol* 2008;9:1039–1047.

25. Kenfield SA, Stampfer MJ, Giovannucci E, et al. Physical activity and survival after prostate cancer diagnosis in the health professionals follow-up study. *J Clin Oncol* 2011;29:726–732.

26. Klein EA, Thompson IM Jr, Tangen CM, et al. Vitamin E and the risk of prostate cancer: the Selenium and Vitamin E Cancer Prevention Trial (SELECT). *JAMA* 2011;306:1549–1556.

27. Peters U, Littman AJ, Kristal AR, et al. Vitamin E and selenium supplementation and risk of prostate cancer in the Vitamins and lifestyle (VITAL) study cohort. *Cancer Causes Control* 2008;19:75–87.

28. Giovannucci E, Ascherio A, Rimm EB, et al. Intake of carotenoids and retinol in relation to risk of prostate cancer. *J Natl Cancer Inst* 1995;87:1767–1776.

29. Giovannucci E, Rimm EB, Liu Y, et al. A prospective study of tomato products, lycopene, and prostate cancer risk. *J Natl Cancer Inst* 2002;94:391–398.

30. Demark-Wahnefried W, Halabi S, Paulson DF. Serum androgens: associations with prostate cancer risk and hair patterning. *J Androl* 1998;19:631.

31. Paprotka T, Delviks-Frankenberry KA, Cingoz O, et al. Recombinant origin of the retrovirus XMRV. *Science* 2011;333:97–101.

32. Thompson IM, Goodman PJ, Tangen CM, et al. The influence of finasteride on the development of prostate cancer. *N Engl J Med* 2003;349:215–224.

33. Scardino PT. The prevention of prostate cancer—the dilemma continues. *N Engl J Med* 2003;349:297–299.

34. Theoret MR, Ning YM, Zhang JJ, et al. The risks and benefits of 5alpha-reductase inhibitors for prostate-cancer prevention. *N Engl J Med* 2011;365:97–99.

35. Thompson IM Jr, Goodman PJ, Tangen CM, et al. Long-term survival of participants in the prostate cancer prevention trial. *N Engl J Med* 2013;369:603–610.

36. Andriole GL, Bostwick DG, Brawley OW, et al. Effect of dutasteride on the risk of prostate cancer. *N Engl J Med* 2010;362:1192–1202.

37. US Food and Drug Administration. FDA Drug Safety Communication: 5-alpha reductase inhibitors (5-ARIs) may increase the risk of a more serious form of prostate cancer. June 9, 2011. Accessed May 21, 2014. http://www.fda.gov/Drugs/DrugSafety/ucm258314.htm.

38. Schmitz-Drager BJ, Schoffski O, Marberger M, et al. Risk adapted chemoprevention for prostate cancer: an option? *Recent Results Cancer Res* 2014;202:79–91.

39. Ohori M, Scardino PT. Localized prostate cancer. *Curr Probl Surg* 2002;39:833–957.

40. Epstein JI, Algaba F, Allsbrook WC Jr, et al.Tumors of the prostate. In Eble NJ, Suater G, Epstein JI, et al., eds. *World Health Organization Classification of Tumors. Pathology and Genetics of Tumors of the Urinary System and Male Genital Organs.* Lyon, France: IARC Press; 2004:159–216.

41. DeMarzo AM, Nelson WG, Isaacs WB, et al. Pathological and molecular aspects of prostate cancer. *Lancet* 2003;361:955–964.

42. Nelson WG, De Marzo AM, Isaacs WB. Prostate cancer. *N Engl J Med* 2003;349:366–381.

43. Montie JE, Pienta KJ. Review of the role of androgenic hormones in the epidemiology of benign prostatic hyperplasia and prostate cancer. *Urology* 1994;43:892–899.

44. De Marzo AM, Marchi VL, Epstein JI, et al. Proliferative inflammatory atrophy of the prostate: implications for prostatic carcinogenesis. *Am J Pathol* 1999;155:1985–1992.

45. Bostwick DG. Prospective origins of prostate carcinoma. Prostatic intraepithelial neoplasia and atypical adenomatous hyperplasia. *Cancer* 1996;78:330–336.

46. Bostwick DG, Brawer MK. Prostatic intra-epithelial neoplasia and early invasion in prostate cancer. *Cancer* 1987;59:788–794.

47. Sakr WA. Prostatic intraepithelial neoplasia: a marker for high-risk groups and a potential target for chemoprevention. *Eur Urol* 1999;35:474–478.

48. De Marzo AM, Platz EA, Epstein JI, et al. A working group classification of focal prostate atrophy lesions. *Am J Surg Pathol* 2006;30:1281–1291.

49. Schlesinger C, Bostwick DG, Iczkowski KA. High-grade prostatic intraepithelial neoplasia and atypical small acinar proliferation: predictive value for cancer in current practice. *Am J Surg Pathol* 2005;29:1201–1207.

50. Beahrs OH, Henson DE, Hutter RVP, et al. *American Joint Committee on Cancer. AJCC Cancer Staging Manual.* 4th ed. Philadelphia, PA: Lippincott-Raven, 1992.

51. Edge S, Byrd DR, Compton CC, et al. *American Joint Committee on Cancer. AJCC Cancer Staging Manual.* 7th ed. New York: Springer, 2010.

52. Fleming ID, Cooper JS, Henson DE, et al. *American Joint Committee on Cancer. AJCC Cancer Staging Manual.* 5th ed. Philadelphia: JB Lippincott, 1997.

53. Gleason DF. Classification of prostatic carcinomas. *Cancer Chemother Rep* 1966;50:125–128.

54. Gleason DF, Mellinger GT. Prediction of prognosis for prostatic adenocarcinoma by combined histological grading and clinical staging. *J Urol* 1974;111:58–64.

55. Epstein JI. Prognostic significance of tumor volume in radical prostatectomy and needle biopsy specimens. *J Urol* 2011;186:790–797.

56. Epstein JI, Allsbrook WC Jr, Amin MB, et al. The 2005 International Society of Urological Pathology (ISUP) Consensus Conference on Gleason grading of prostatic carcinoma. *Am J Surg Pathol* 2005;29:1228–1242.

57. Aihara M, Wheeler TM, Ohori M, et al. Heterogeneity of prostate cancer in radical prostatectomy specimens. *Urology* 1994;43:60–66.

58. Noguchi M, Stamey TA, Neal JE, et al. An analysis of 148 consecutive transition zone cancers: clinical and histological characteristics. *J Urol* 2000;163:1751–1755.

59. Morgan TM, Welty CJ, Vakar-Lopez F, et al. Ductal adenocarcinoma of the prostate: increased mortality risk and decreased serum prostate specific antigen. *J Urol* 2010;184:2303–2307.

60. Nadal R, Schweizer M, Kryvenko ON, et al. Small cell carcinoma of the prostate. *Nat Rev Urol* 2014;11:213–219.

61. Ginesin Y, Bolkier M, Moskovitz B, et al. Carcinosarcoma of the prostate. *Eur Urol* 1986;12:441–442.

62. Catalona WJ, Richie JP, Ahmann FR, et al. Comparison of digital rectal examination and serum prostate specific antigen in the early detection of prostate cancer: results of a multicenter clinical trial of 6,630 men. *J Urol* 1994;151:1283–1290.

63. Siegel R, Ma J, Zou Z, et al. Cancer statistics, 2014. *CA Cancer J Clin* 2014;64:9–29.

64. Lilja H, Piironen TP, Rittenhouse HG, et al. Value of molecular forms of prostate-specific antigen and related kallikreins, hk2, in diagnosis and staging of prostate cancer. In Vogelzang NA, Scardino PT, Shipley WU, et al. *Comprehensive Textbook of Genitourinary Oncology.* 2nd ed. Philadelphia: Lippincott Williams & Wilkins; 2000:638–650.

65. Aihara M, Lebovitz RM, Wheeler TM, et al. Prostate specific antigen and gleason grade: an immunohistochemical study of prostate cancer. *J Urol* 1994;151:1558–1564.

66. Eastham JA, Riedel E, Scardino PT, et al. Variation of serum prostate-specific antigen levels: an evaluation of year-to-year fluctuations. *JAMA* 2003;289:2695–2700.

67. Thompson IM, Pauler DK, Goodman PJ, et al. Prevalence of prostate cancer among men with a prostate-specific antigen level < or =4.0 ng per milliliter. *N Engl J Med* 2004;350:2239–2246.

68. Lilja H, Cronin AM, Dahlin A, et al. Prediction of significant prostate cancer diagnosed 20 to 30 years later with a single measure of prostate-specific antigen at or before age 50. *Cancer* 2011;117:1210–1219.

69. Orsted DD, Bojesen SE, Kamstrup PR, et al. Long-term prostate-specific antigen velocity in improved classification of prostate cancer risk and mortality. *Eur Urol* 2013;64:384–393.

70. Vickers AJ, Cronin AM, Bjork T, et al. Prostate specific antigen concentration at age 60 and death or metastasis from prostate cancer: case-control study. *BMJ* 2010;341:c4521.

71. Orsted DD, Nordestgaard BG, Jensen GB, et al. Prostate-specific antigen and long-term prediction of prostate cancer incidence and mortality in the general population. *Eur Urol* 2012;61:865–874.

72. MSKCC Prostate Cancer: Screening Guidelines. Accessed May 6, 2014. http://www.mskcc.org/cancer-care/adult/prostate/screening-guidelines-prostate.

73. Ulmert D, Cronin AM, Bjork T, et al. Prostate-specific antigen at or before age 50 as a predictor of advanced prostate cancer diagnosed up to 25 years later: a case-control study. *BMC Med* 2008;6:6.

74. Hugosson J, Carlsson S, Aus G, et al. Mortality results from the Goteborg randomised population-based prostate-cancer screening trial. *Lancet Oncol* 2010;11:725–732.

75. Gotzsche PC, Nielsen M. Screening for breast cancer with mammography. *Cochrane Database Syst Rev* 2009:CD001877.

76. Independent UK Panel on Breast Cancer Screening. The benefits and harms of breast cancer screening: an independent review. *Lancet* 2012;380:1778–1786.

77. Paci E, Euroscreen Working Group. Summary of the evidence of breast cancer service screening outcomes in Europe and first estimate of the benefit and harm balance sheet. *J Med Screen* 2012;19:5–13.

78. Elmunzer BJ, Hayward RA, Schoenfeld PS, et al. Effect of flexible sigmoidoscopy-based screening on incidence and mortality of colorectal cancer: a systematic review and meta-analysis of randomized controlled trials. *PLoS Med* 2012;9:e1001352.

79. Schroder FH, Hugosson J, Roobol MJ, et al. Screening and prostate-cancer mortality in a randomized European study. *N Engl J Med* 2009;360:1320–1328.

80. Cooperberg MR, Cowan JE, Hilton JF, et al. Outcomes of active surveillance for men with intermediate-risk prostate cancer. *J Clin Oncol* 2011;29:228–234.

81. Hugosson J, Aus G, Lilja H, et al. Results of a randomized, population-based study of biennial screening using serum prostate-specific antigen measurement to detect prostate carcinoma. *Cancer* 2004;100:1397–1405.

82. Bellardita L, Rancati T, Alvisi MF, et al. Predictors of health-related quality of life and adjustment to prostate cancer during active surveillance. *Eur Urol* 2013;64:30–36.

83. Cooperberg MR, Broering JM, Carroll PR. Time trends and local variation in primary treatment of localized prostate cancer. *J Clin Oncol* 2010;28:1117–1123.

84. Klotz L, Zhang L, Lam A, et al. Clinical results of long-term follow-up of a large, active surveillance cohort with localized prostate cancer. *J Clin Oncol* 2010;28:126–131.

85. Taneja SS. Re: active surveillance for low-risk prostate cancer worldwide: the PRIAS study. *J Urol* 2013;189:1322.

86. Tosoian JJ, Trock BJ, Landis P, et al. Active surveillance program for prostate cancer: an update of the Johns Hopkins experience. *J Clin Oncol* 2011;29:2185–2190.

87. Moyer VA, U.S. Preventive Services Task Force. Screening for prostate cancer: U.S. Preventive Services Task Force recommendation statement. *Ann Intern Med* 2012;157:120–134.

88. Andriole GL, Crawford ED, Grubb RL 3rd, et al. Mortality results from a randomized prostate-cancer screening trial. *N Engl J Med* 2009;360:1310–1319.

89. Andriole GL, Crawford ED, Grubb RL 3rd, et al. Prostate cancer screening in the randomized Prostate, Lung, Colorectal, and Ovarian Cancer Screening Trial: mortality results after 13 years of follow-up. *J Natl Cancer Inst* 2012;104:125–132.

90. Schroder FH, Hugosson J, Roobol MJ, et al. Prostate-cancer mortality at 11 years of follow-up. *N Engl J Med* 2012;366:981–990.

91. Chou R, Croswell JM, Dana T, et al. Screening for prostate cancer: a review of the evidence for the U.S. Preventive Services Task Force. *Ann Intern Med* 2011;155:762–771.

92. Carlsson S, Vickers AJ, Roobol M, et al. Prostate cancer screening: facts, statistics, and interpretation in response to the US Preventive Services Task Force Review. *J Clin Oncol* 2012;30:2581–2584.

93. Vickers AJ, Roobol MJ, Lilja H. Screening for prostate cancer: early detection or overdetection? *Annu Rev Med* 2012;63:161–170.

94. Heijnsdijk EA, Wever EM, Auvinen A, et al. Quality-of-life effects of prostate-specific antigen screening. *N Engl J Med* 2012;367:595–605.

95. Basch E, Oliver TK, Vickers A, et al. Screening for prostate cancer with prostate-specific antigen testing: American Society of Clinical Oncology Provisional Clinical Opinion. *J Clin Oncol* 2012;30:3020–3025.

96. Carter HB, Albertsen PC, Barry MJ, et al. Early detection of prostate cancer: AUA Guideline. *J Urol* 2013;190:419–426.

97. American Cancer Society. Can prostate cancer be found early? Updated March 12, 2014. Accessed June 6, 2014. http://www.cancer.org/cancer/prostatecancer/detailedguide/prostate-cancer-detection.

98. Stamey TA, Sozen S, Yemoto CM, et al. Classification of localized untreated prostate cancer based on 791 men treated only with radical prostatectomy: common ground for therapeutic trials and TNM subgroups. *J Urol* 1998;159: 2009–2012.

99. Kattan MW, Eastham JA, Stapleton AM, et al. A preoperative nomogram for disease recurrence following radical prostatectomy for prostate cancer. *J Natl Cancer Inst* 1998;90:766–771.

100. Pound CR, Partin AW, Epstein JI, et al. Prostate-specific antigen after anatomic radical retropubic prostatectomy. Patterns of recurrence and cancer control. *Cancer* 1997;79:528–537.

101. Oesterling JE, Jacobsen SJ, Chute CG, et al. Serum prostate-specific antigen in a community-based population of healthy men: establishment of age-specific reference ranges. *JAMA* 1993;270:860–864.

102. Petteway J, Brawer MK. Age specific versus 4.0 ng/ml as a PSA cutoff in the screening population: impact on cancer detection (abstract). *J Urol* 1995;153:465A.

103. Benson MC, Whang IS, Pantuck A, et al. Prostate specific antigen density: a means of distinguishing benign prostatic hypertrophy and prostate cancer. *J Urol* 1992;147:815–816.

104. Stamey T, Yang N, Hay A, et al. Prostate-specific antigen as a serum marker for adenocarcinoma of the prostate. *N Engl J Med* 1987;317:909–916.

105. Ohori M, Scardino PT. Early detection of prostate cancer: the nature of cancers detected with current diagnostic tests. *Semin Oncol* 1994;21:522–526.

106. Carter HB, Epstein JI, Chan DW, et al. Recommended prostate-specific antigen testing intervals for the detection of curable prostate cancer. *JAMA* 1997;277:1456–1460.

107. O'Brien MF, Cronin AM, Fearn PA, et al. Pretreatment prostate-specific antigen (PSA) velocity and doubling time are associated with outcome but neither improves prediction of outcome beyond pretreatment PSA alone in patients treated with radical prostatectomy. *J Clin Oncol* 2009;27:3591–3597.

108. Loeb S, Sokoll LJ, Broyles DL, et al. Prospective multicenter evaluation of the Beckman Coulter Prostate Health Index using WHO calibration. *J Urol* 2013;189:1702–1706.

109. Catalona WJ, Partin AW, Sanda MG, et al. A multicenter study of [-2]pro-prostate specific antigen combined with prostate specific antigen and free prostate specific antigen for prostate cancer detection in the 2.0 to 10.0 ng/ml prostate specific antigen range. *J Urol* 2011;185:1650–1655.

110. Christensson A, Bruun L, Bjork T, et al. Intra-individual short-term variability of prostate-specific antigen and other kallikrein markers in a serial collection of blood from men under evaluation for prostate cancer. *BJU Int* 2011; 107:1769–1774.

111. Vickers AJ, Gupta A, Savage CJ, et al. A panel of kallikrein marker predicts prostate cancer in a large, population-based cohort followed for 15 years without screening. *Cancer Epidemiol Biomarkers Prev* 2011;20:255–261.

112. Heidenreich A, Abrahamsson PA, Artibani W, et al. Early detection of prostate cancer: European Association of Urology recommendation. *Eur Urol* 2013;64:347–354.

113. Dijkstra S, Mulders PF, Schalken JA. Clinical use of novel urine and blood based prostate cancer biomarkers: a review. *Clin Biochem* 2014;47:889–896.

114. Catalona W, Richie J, deKernion JB, et al. Comparison of prostate specific antigen concentration versus prostate specific antigen density in the early detection of prostate cancer. *J Urol* 1994;152:2031–2036.

115. Epstein JI, Pound CR, Partin AW, et al. Disease progression following radical prostatectomy in men with Gleason score 7 tumor. *J Urol* 1998;160:97–100.

116. Gleason DF. Histologic grade, clinical stage, and patient age in prostate cancer. *NCI Monogr* 1988;15–18.

117. Porten SP, Whitson JM, Cowan JE, et al. Changes in prostate cancer grade on serial biopsy in men undergoing active surveillance. *J Clin Oncol* 2011;29:2795–2800.

118. Whitson JM, Porten SP, Hilton JF, et al. The relationship between prostate specific antigen change and biopsy progression in patients on active surveillance for prostate cancer. *J Urol* 2011;185:1656–1660.

119. D'Amico AV, Whittington R, Malkowicz SB, et al. Clinical utility of the percentage of positive prostate biopsies in defining biochemical outcome after radical prostatectomy for patients with clinically localized prostate cancer. *J Clin Oncol* 2000;18:1164–1172.

120. Epstein JI, Walsh PC, Carmichael M, et al. Pathologic and clinical findings to predict tumor extent of nonpalpable (stage T1c) prostate cancer. *JAMA* 1994;271:368–374.

121. Goto Y, Ohori M, Arakawa A, et al. Distinguishing clinically important from unimportant prostate cancers before treatment: value of systematic biopsies. *J Urol* 1996;156:1059–1063.

122. Ohori M, Suyama K, Maru N, et al. Prognostic significance of systemic needle biopsy findings. *J Urol* 2000;163:287A.

123. Barqawi AB, Rove KO, Gholizadeh S, et al. The role of 3-dimensional mapping biopsy in decision making for treatment of apparent early stage prostate cancer. *J Urol* 2011;186:80–85.

124. Rastinehad AR, Baccala AA Jr, Chung PH, et al. D'Amico risk stratification correlates with degree of suspicion of prostate cancer on multiparametric magnetic resonance imaging. *J Urol* 2011;185:815–820.

125. Mohler JL, Kantoff PW, Armstrong AJ, et al. NCCN Guidelines: Prostate cancer, version 2.2014. *J Natl Compr Canc Netw* 2014;12:686–718.

126. Vargas HA, Akin O, Shukla-Dave A, et al. Performance characteristics of MR imaging in the evaluation of clinically low-risk prostate cancer: a prospective study. *Radiology* 2012;265:478–487.

127. Yoshimitsu K, Kiyoshima K, Irie H, et al. Usefulness of apparent diffusion coefficient map in diagnosing prostate carcinoma: correlation with stepwise histopathology. *J Magn Reson Imaging* 2008;27:132–139.

128. Futterer JJ, Engelbrecht MR, Huisman HJ, et al. Staging prostate cancer with dynamic contrast-enhanced endorectal MR imaging prior to radical prostatectomy: experienced versus less experienced readers. *Radiology* 2005;237: 541–549.

129. Villers A, Puech P, Mouton D, et al. Dynamic contrast enhanced, pelvic phased array magnetic resonance imaging of localized prostate cancer for predicting tumor volume: correlation with radical prostatectomy findings. *J Urol* 2006;176:2432–2437.

130. Hricak H, Choyke PL, Eberhardt SC, et al. Imaging prostate cancer: a multidisciplinary perspective. *Radiology* 2007;243:28–53.

131. Lin K, Szabo Z, Chin BB, et al. The value of a baseline bone scan in patients with newly diagnosed prostate cancer. *Clin Nucl Med* 1999;24:579–582.

132. Sciarra A, Barentsz J, Bjartell A, et al. Advances in magnetic resonance imaging: how they are changing the management of prostate cancer. *Eur Urol* 2011;59:962–977.

133. Greene FL, Page DL, Fleming ID, et al. *American Joint Committee on Cancer. AJCC Cancer Staging Manual.* 6th ed. New York: Springer, 2002.

134. Ohori M, Wheeler TM, Scardino PT. The New American Joint Committee on Cancer and International Union against Cancer TNM classification of prostate cancer. *Cancer* 1994;74:104–114.

135. Partin AW, Mangold LA, Lamm DM, et al. Contemporary update of prostate cancer staging nomograms (Partin Tables) for the new millennium. *Urology* 2001;58:843–848.

136. Eifler JB, Feng Z, Lin BM, et al. An updated prostate cancer staging nomogram (Partin tables) based on cases from 2006 to 2011. *BJU Int* 2013;111:22–29.

137. D'Amico AV, Whittington R, Malkowicz SB, et al. Biochemical outcome after radical prostatectomy, external beam radiation therapy, or interstitial radiation therapy for clinically localized prostate cancer. *JAMA* 1998;280:969–974.

138. Mitchell JA, Cooperberg MR, Elkin EP, et al. Ability of 2 pretreatment risk assessment methods to predict prostate cancer recurrence after radical prostatectomy: data from CaPSURE. *J Urol* 2005;173:1126–1131.

139. Stephenson AJ, Kattan MW, Eastham JA, et al. Prostate cancer-specific mortality after radical prostatectomy for patients treated in the prostate-specific antigen era. *J Clin Oncol* 2009;27:4300–4305.

140. Kattan MW, Zelefsky MJ, Kupelian PA, et al. Pretreatment nomogram for predicting the outcome of three-dimensional conformal radiotherapy in prostate cancer. *J Clin Oncol* 2000;18:3352–3359.

141. Kattan MW, Potters L, Blasko JC, et al. Pretreatment nomogram for predicting freedom from recurrence after permanent prostate brachytherapy in prostate cancer. *Urology* 2001;58:393–399.

142. Paik S, Shak S, Tang G, et al. A multigene assay to predict recurrence of tamoxifen-treated, node-negative breast cancer. *N Engl J Med* 2004;351: 2817–2826.

143. Paik S, Tang G, Shak S, et al. Gene expression and benefit of chemotherapy in women with node-negative, estrogen receptor-positive breast cancer. *J Clin Oncol* 2006;24:3726–3734.

144. Albain KS, Barlow WE, Shak S, et al. Prognostic and predictive value of the 21-gene recurrence score assay in postmenopausal women with node-positive, oestrogen-receptor-positive breast cancer on chemotherapy: a retrospective analysis of a randomised trial. *Lancet Oncol* 2010;11:55–65.

145. Holt S, Bertelli G, Humphreys I, et al. A decision impact, decision conflict and economic assessment of routine Oncotype DX testing of 146 women with node-negative or pNImi, ER-positive breast cancer in the U.K. *Br J Cancer* 2013;108:2250–2258.

146. Cuzick J, Berney DM, Fisher G, et al. Prognostic value of a cell cycle progression signature for prostate cancer death in a conservatively managed needle biopsy cohort. *Br J Cancer* 2012;106:1095–1099.

147. Shore N, Concepcion R, Saltzstein D, et al. Clinical utility of a biopsy-based cell cycle gene expression assay in localized prostate cancer. *Curr Med Res Opin* 2014;30:547–553.

148. Bishoff JT, Freedland SJ, Gerber L, et al. Prognostic utility of the cell cycle progression score generated from biopsy in men treated with prostatectomy. *J Urol* 2014;192:409–414.

149. Klein EA, Cooperberg MR, Magi-Galluzzi C, et al. A 17-gene assay to predict prostate cancer aggressiveness in the context of Gleason grade heterogeneity, tumor multifocality, and biopsy undersampling. *Eur Urol* 2014 [Epub ahead of print]. doi: 10.1016/j.eururo.2014.05.004.

150. Cuzick JM, Stone S, Fisher G, et al. Validation of an RNA cell cycle progression (CCP) score for predicting prostate cancer death in a conservatively managed needle biopsy cohort. *J Clin Oncol* 2014;32:Abstr 5059.

151. Stephenson AJ, Scardino PT, Eastham JA, et al. Postoperative nomogram predicting the 10-year probability of prostate cancer recurrence after radical prostatectomy. *J Clin Oncol* 2005;23:7005–7012.

152. Stephenson AJ, Scardino PT, Bianco FJ Jr, et al. Morbidity and functional outcomes of salvage radical prostatectomy for locally recurrent prostate cancer after radiation therapy. *J Urol* 2004;172:2239–2243.

153. Stephenson AJ, Scardino PT, Eastham JA, et al. Preoperative nomogram predicting the 10-year probability of prostate cancer recurrence after radical prostatectomy. *J Natl Cancer Inst* 2006;98:715–717.

154. Eggener SE, Scardino PT, Walsh PC, et al. Predicting 15-year prostate cancer specific mortality after radical prostatectomy. *J Urol* 2011;185:869–875.

155. Food and Drug Administration. *Guidance for Industry: Clinical Trial Endpoints for the Approval of Cancer Drugs and Biologics.* May 2007. Accessed May 21, 2014. http://www.fda.gov/downloads/Drugs/.../Guidances/ucm071590.pdf.

156. Eisenhauer EA, Therasse P, Bogaerts J, et al. New response evaluation criteria in solid tumours: revised RECIST guideline (version 1.1). *Eur J Cancer* 2009;45:228–247.

157. Scher HI, Halabi S, Tannock I, et al. Design and end points of clinical trials for patients with progressive prostate cancer and castrate levels of testosterone: recommendations of the Prostate Cancer Clinical Trials Working Group. *J Clin Oncol* 2008;26:1148–1159.

158. Smith MR. Bisphosphonates to prevent skeletal complications in men with metastatic prostate cancer. *J Urol* 2003;170:S55–S57.

159. Saad F, Gleason DM, Murray R, et al. A randomized, placebo-controlled trial of zoledronic acid in patients with hormone-refractory metastatic prostate carcinoma. *J Natl Cancer Inst* 2002;94:1458–1468.

160. Wilt TJ, Brawer MK, Jones KM, et al. Radical prostatectomy versus observation for localized prostate cancer. *N Engl J Med* 2012;367:203–213.

161. Berglund A, Garmo H, Tishelman C, et al. Comorbidity, treatment and mortality: a population based cohort study of prostate cancer in PCBaSe Sweden. *J Urol* 2011;185:833–839.

162. Vargas HA, Akin O, Afaq A, et al. Magnetic resonance imaging for predicting prostate biopsy findings in patients considered for active surveillance of clinically low risk prostate cancer. *J Urol* 2012;188:1732–1738.

163. Liu D, Lehmann HP, Frick KD, et al. Active surveillance versus surgery for low risk prostate cancer: a clinical decision analysis. *J Urol* 2012;187:1241–1246.

164. Mullins JK, Bonekamp D, Landis P, et al. Multiparametric magnetic resonance imaging findings in men with low-risk prostate cancer followed using active surveillance. *BJU Int* 2013;111:1037–1045.

165. Walsh PC. Anatomic radical prostatectomy: evolution of the surgical technique. *J Urol* 1998;160:2418–2424.

166. Godoy G, von Bodman C, Chade DC, et al. Pelvic lymph node dissection for prostate cancer: frequency and distribution of nodal metastases in a contemporary radical prostatectomy series. *J Urol* 2012;187:2082–2086.

167. Burkhard FC, Bader P, Schneider E, et al. Reliability of preoperative values to determine the need for lymphadenectomy in patients with prostate cancer and meticulous lymph node dissection. *Eur Urol* 2002;42:84–90.

168. Schumacher MC, Burkhard FC, Thalmann GN, et al. Is pelvic lymph node dissection necessary in patients with a serum PSA<10ng/ml undergoing radical prostatectomy for prostate cancer? *Eur Urol* 2006;50:272–279.

169. Feifer AH, Elkin EB, Lowrance WT, et al. Temporal trends and predictors of pelvic lymph node dissection in open or minimally invasive radical prostatectomy. *Cancer* 2011;117:3933–3942.

170. Allaf ME, Palapattu GS, Trock BJ, et al. Anatomical extent of lymph node dissection: impact on men with clinically localized prostate cancer. *J Urol* 2004;172:1840–1844.

171. Bader P, Burkhard FC, Markwalder R, et al. Is a limited lymph node dissection an adequate staging procedure for prostate cancer? *J Urol* 2002;168:514–518, discussion 518.

172. Heidenreich A, Varga Z, Von Knobloch R. Extended pelvic lymphadenectomy in patients undergoing radical prostatectomy: high incidence of lymph node metastasis. *J Urol* 2002;167:1681–1686.

173. Touijer K, Rabbani F, Otero JR, et al. Standard versus limited pelvic lymph node dissection for prostate cancer in patients with a predicted probability of nodal metastasis greater than 1%. *J Urol* 2007;178:120–124.

174. Cagiannos I, Karakiewicz P, Eastham JA, et al. A preoperative nomogram identifying decreased risk of positive pelvic lymph nodes in patients with prostate cancer. *J Urol* 2003;170:1798–1803.

175. Touijer KA, Ahallal Y, Guillonneau BD. Indications for and anatomical extent of pelvic lymph node dissection for prostate cancer: practice patterns of uro-oncologists in North America. *Urol Oncol* 2013;31:1517–1521.

176. Touijer KA, Mazzola CR, Sjoberg DD, et al. Long-term outcomes of patients with lymph node metastasis treated with radical prostatectomy without adjuvant androgen-deprivation therapy. *Eur Urol* 2014;65:20–25.

177. Carlsson SV, Tafe LJ, Chade DC, et al. Pathological features of lymph node metastasis for predicting biochemical recurrence after radical prostatectomy for prostate cancer. *J Urol* 2013;189:1314–1318.

178. von Bodman C, Godoy G, Chade DC, et al. Predicting biochemical recurrence-free survival for patients with positive pelvic lymph nodes at radical prostatectomy. *J Urol* 2010;184:143–148.

179. Bianco FJ Jr, Scardino PT, Eastham JA. Radical prostatectomy: long-term cancer control and recovery of sexual and urinary function ("trifecta"). *Urology* 2005;66:83–94.

180. Vickers A, Savage C, Bianco F, et al. Cancer control and functional outcomes after radical prostatectomy as markers of surgical quality: analysis of heterogeneity between surgeons at a single center. *Eur Urol* 2011;59:317–322.

181. Vickers AJ, Bianco FJ, Serio AM, et al. The surgical learning curve for prostate cancer control after radical prostatectomy. *J Natl Cancer Inst* 2007;99:1171–1177.

182. Gandaglia G, Sammon JD, Chang SL, et al. Comparative effectiveness of robot-assisted and open radical prostatectomy in the postdissemination era. *J Clin Oncol* 2014;32:1419–1426.

183. Eastham J, Scardino PT. Radical prostatectomy. In Campbell MF, Walsh PC, eds. *Campbell's Urology.* 7th ed. Philadelphia: W.B. Saunders; 1998;2547–2564.

184. Hu JC, Gu X, Lipsitz SR, et al. Comparative effectiveness of minimally invasive vs open radical prostatectomy. *JAMA* 2009;302:1557–1564.

185. Lowrance WT, Elkin EB, Jacks LM, et al. Comparative effectiveness of prostate cancer surgical treatments: a population based analysis of postoperative outcomes. *J Urol* 2010;183:1366–1372.

186. Lepor H. Open versus laparoscopic radical prostatectomy. *Rev Urol* 2005;7:115–127.

187. Murphy DG, Bjartell A, Ficarra V, et al. Downsides of robot-assisted laparoscopic radical prostatectomy: limitations and complications. *Eur Urol* 2010;57:735–746.

188. Bill-Axelson A, Holmberg L, Garmo H, et al. Radical prostatectomy or watchful waiting in early prostate cancer. *N Engl J Med* 2014;370:932–942.

189. Bill-Axelson A, Holmberg L, Ruutu M, et al. Radical prostatectomy versus watchful waiting in early prostate cancer. *N Engl J Med* 2005;352:1977–1984.

190. Vickers A, Bennette C, Steineck G, et al. Individualized estimation of the benefit of radical prostatectomy from the Scandinavian Prostate Cancer Group randomized trial. *Eur Urol* 2012;62:204–209.

191. Lane JA, Hamdy FC, Martin RM, et al. Latest results from the UK trials evaluating prostate cancer screening and treatment: the CAP and ProtecT studies. *Eur J Cancer* 2010;46:3095–3101.

192. Roehl KA, Han M, Ramos CG, et al. Cancer progression and survival rates following anatomical radical retropubic prostatectomy in 3,478 consecutive patients: long term results. *J Urol* 2004;172:910–914.

193. Han M, Partin AW, Zahurak M, et al. Biochemical (prostate specific antigen) recurrence probability following radical prostatectomy for clinically localized prostate cancer. *J Urol* 2003;169:517–523.

194. Hull GW, Rabbani F, Abbas F, et al. Cancer control with radical prostatectomy alone in 1,000 consecutive patients. *J Urol* 2002;167:528–534.

195. Trapasso JG, deKernion JB, Smith RB, et al. The incidence and significance of detectable levels of serum prostate specific antigen after radical prostatectomy. *J Urol* 1994;152:1821–1825.

196. Zincke H, Oesterling JE, Blute ML, et al. Long-term (15 years) results after radical prostatectomy for clinically localized (stage T2c or lower) prostate cancer. *J Urol* 1994;152:1850–1857.

197. Lu-Yao GL, Albertsen PC, Moore DF, et al. Outcomes of localized prostate cancer following conservative management. *JAMA* 2009;302:1202–1209.

198. Han M, Partin AW, Pound CR, et al. Long-term biochemical disease-free and cancer-specific survival following anatomic radical retropubic prostatectomy. The 15-year Johns Hopkins experience. *Urol Clin North Am* 2001;28:555–565.

199. Yossepowitch O, Eggener SE, Bianco FJ Jr, et al. Radical prostatectomy for clinically localized, high risk prostate cancer: critical analysis of risk assessment methods. *J Urol* 2007;178:493–499.

200. Yossepowitch O, Eggener SE, Serio AM, et al. Secondary therapy, metastatic progression, and cancer-specific mortality in men with clinically high-risk prostate cancer treated with radical prostatectomy. *Eur Urol* 2008;53:950–959.

201. Chang AJ, Autio KA, Roach M 3rd, et al. High-risk prostate cancer-classification and therapy. *Nat Rev Clin Oncol* 2014;11:308–323.

202. Begg CB, Riedel ER, Bach PB, et al. Variations in morbidity after radical prostatectomy. *N Engl J Med* 2002;346:1138–1144.

203. Zelefsky MJ, Kollmeier M, Cox B, et al. Improved clinical outcomes with high-dose image guided radiotherapy compared with non-IGRT for the treatment of clinically localized prostate cancer. *Int J Radiat Oncol Biol Phys* 2012;84:125–129.

204. Beckendorf V, Guerif S, Le Prise E, et al. 70 Gy versus 80 Gy in localized prostate cancer: 5-year results of GETUG 06 randomized trial. *Int J Radiat Oncol Biol Phys* 2011;80:1056–1063.

205. Al-Mamgani A, van Putten WL, Heemsbergen WD, et al. Update of Dutch multicenter dose-escalation trial of radiotherapy for localized prostate cancer. *Int J Radiat Oncol Biol Phys* 2008;72:980–988.

206. Kuban DA, Tucker SL, Dong L, et al. Long-term results of the M. D. Anderson randomized dose-escalation trial for prostate cancer. *Int J Radiat Oncol Biol Phys* 2008;70:67–74.

207. Zietman AL, Bae K, Slater JD, et al. Randomized trial comparing conventional-dose with high-dose conformal radiation therapy in early-stage adenocarcinoma of the prostate: long-term results from Proton Radiation Oncology Group/American College of Radiology 95-09. *J Clin Oncol* 2010;28:1106–1111.

208. Dearnaley DP, Jovic G, Syndikus I, et al. Escalated-dose versus control-dose conformal radiotherapy for prostate cancer: long-term results from the MRC RT01 randomised controlled trial. *Lancet Oncol* 2014;15:464–473.

209. Eade TN, Hanlon AL, Horwitz EM, et al. What dose of external-beam radiation is high enough for prostate cancer? *Int J Radiat Oncol Biol Phys* 2007;68: 682–689.

210. Kupelian P, Kuban D, Thames H, et al. Improved biochemical relapse-free survival with increased external radiation doses in patients with localized prostate cancer: the combined experience of nine institutions in patients treated in 1994 and 1995. *Int J Radiat Oncol Biol Phys* 2005;61:415–419.

211. Lyons JA, Kupelian PA, Mohan DS, et al. Importance of high radiation doses (72 Gy or greater) in the treatment of stage T1-T3 adenocarcinoma of the prostate. *Urology* 2000;55:85–90.

212. Zelefsky MJ, Fuks Z, Hunt M, et al. High dose radiation delivered by intensity modulated conformal radiotherapy improves the outcome of localized prostate cancer. *J Urol* 2001;166:876–881.

213. Kuban DA, Levy LB, Cheung MR, et al. Long-term failure patterns and survival in a randomized dose-escalation trial for prostate cancer. Who dies of disease? *Int J Radiat Oncol Biol Phys* 2011;79:1310–1317.

214. Spratt DE, Pei X, Yamada J, et al. Long-term survival and toxicity in patients treated with high-dose intensity modulated radiation therapy for localized prostate cancer. *Int J Radiat Oncol Biol Phys* 2013;85:686–692.

215. Zelefsky MJ, Ginor RX, Fuks Z, et al. Efficacy of selective alpha-1 blocker therapy in the treatment of acute urinary symptoms during radiotherapy for localized prostate cancer. *Int J Radiat Oncol Biol Phys* 1999;45:567–570.

216. Sebastian S, O'Connor H, O'Morain C, et al. Argon plasma coagulation as first-line treatment for chronic radiation proctopathy. *J Gastroenterol Hepatol* 2004;19:1169–1173.

217. Dall'Era MA, Hampson NB, Hsi RA, et al. Hyperbaric oxygen therapy for radiation induced proctopathy in men treated for prostate cancer. *J Urol* 2006;176:87–90.

218. Corman JM, McClure D, Pritchett R, et al. Treatment of radiation induced hemorrhagic cystitis with hyperbaric oxygen. *J Urol* 2003;169:2200–2202.

219. Zelefsky MJ, Pei X, Teslova T, et al. Secondary cancers after intensity-modulated radiotherapy, brachytherapy and radical prostatectomy for the treatment of prostate cancer: incidence and cause-specific survival outcomes according to the initial treatment intervention. *BJU Int* 2012;110: 1696–1701.

220. Zelefsky MJ, Chan H, Hunt M, et al. Long-term outcome of high dose intensity modulated radiation therapy for patients with clinically localized prostate cancer. *J Urol* 2006;176:1415–1419.

221. Ghadjar P, Zelefsky MJ, Spratt DE, et al. Impact of dose to the bladder trigone on long-term urinary function after high-dose intensity modulated radiation therapy for localized prostate cancer. *Int J Radiat Oncol Biol Phys* 2014;88:339–344.

222. van der Wielen GJ, Mulhall JP, Incrocci L. Erectile dysfunction after radiotherapy for prostate cancer and radiation dose to the penile structures: a critical review. *Radiother Oncol* 2007;84:107–113.

223. Higgins GS, McLaren DB, Kerr GR, et al. Outcome analysis of 300 prostate cancer patients treated with neoadjuvant androgen deprivation and hypofractionated radiotherapy. *Int J Radiat Oncol Biol Phys* 2006;65:982–989.

224. Kupelian PA, Thakkar VV, Khuntia D, et al. Hypofractionated intensity-modulated radiotherapy (70 gy at 2.5 Gy per fraction) for localized prostate cancer: long-term outcomes. *Int J Radiat Oncol Biol Phys* 2005;63:1463–1468.

225. Anwar M, Weinberg V, Chang AJ, et al. Hypofractionated SBRT versus conventionally fractionated EBRT for prostate cancer: comparison of PSA slope and nadir. *Radiat Oncol* 2014;9:42.

226. Katz AJ, Santoro M, Ashley R, et al. Stereotactic body radiotherapy for organ-confined prostate cancer. *BMC Urol* 2010;10:1.

227. King CR, Brooks JD, Gill H, et al. Long-term outcomes from a prospective trial of stereotactic body radiotherapy for low-risk prostate cancer. *Int J Radiat Oncol Biol Phys* 2012;82:877–882.

228. King CR, Freeman D, Kaplan I, et al. Stereotactic body radiotherapy for localized prostate cancer: pooled analysis from a multi-institutional consortium of prospective phase II trials. *Radiother Oncol* 2013;109:217–221.

229. Mendenhall NP, Hoppe BS, Nichols RC, et al. Five-year outcomes from 3 prospective trials of image-guided proton therapy for prostate cancer. *Int J Radiat Oncol Biol Phys* 2014;88:596–602.

230. Hoppe BS, Michalski JM, Mendenhall NP, et al. Comparative effectiveness study of patient-reported outcomes after proton therapy or intensity-modulated radiotherapy for prostate cancer. *Cancer* 2014;120:1076–1082.

231. Sheets NC, Goldin GH, Meyer AM, et al. Intensity-modulated radiation therapy, proton therapy, or conformal radiation therapy and morbidity and disease control in localized prostate cancer. *JAMA* 2012;307:1611–1620.

232. Grimm PD, Blasko JC, Sylvester JE, et al. 10-year biochemical (prostate-specific antigen) control of prostate cancer with (125)I brachytherapy. *Int J Radiat Oncol Biol Phys* 2001;51:31–40.

233. Merrick GS, Butler WM, Wallner KE, et al. Monotherapeutic brachytherapy for clinically organ-confined prostate cancer. *W Virginia Med J* 2005;101: 168-171.

234. Morris WJ, Keyes M, Spadinger I, et al. Population-based 10-year oncologic outcomes after low-dose-rate brachytherapy for low-risk and intermediate-risk prostate cancer. *Cancer* 2013;119:1537–1546.

235. Potters L, Morgenstern C, Calugaru E, et al. 12-year outcomes following permanent prostate brachytherapy in patients with clinically localized prostate cancer. *J Urol* 2005;173:1562–1566.

236. Zelefsky MJ, Chou JF, Pei X, et al. Predicting biochemical tumor control after brachytherapy for clinically localized prostate cancer: The Memorial Sloan-Kettering Cancer Center experience. *Brachytherapy* 2012;11:245–249.

237. Zelefsky MJ, Kuban DA, Levy LB, et al. Multi-institutional analysis of long-term outcome for stages T1-T2 prostate cancer treated with permanent seed implantation. *Int J Radiat Oncol Biol Phys* 2007;67:327–333.

238. Nag S, Bice W, DeWyngaert K, et al. The American Brachytherapy Society recommendations for permanent prostate brachytherapy postimplant dosimetric analysis. *Int J Radiat Oncol Biol Phys* 2000;46:221–230.

239. Stock RG, Stone NN, Cesaretti JA, et al. Biologically effective dose values for prostate brachytherapy: effects on PSA failure and posttreatment biopsy results. *Int J Radiat Oncol Biol Phys* 2006;64:527–533.

240. Guedea F, Aguilo F, Polo A, et al. Early biochemical outcomes following permanent interstitial brachytherapy as monotherapy in 1050 patients with clinical T1-T2 prostate cancer. *Radiother Oncol* 2006;80:57–61.

241. Khaksar SJ, Laing RW, Henderson A, et al. Biochemical (prostate-specific antigen) relapse-free survival and toxicity after 125I low-dose-rate prostate brachytherapy. *BJU Int* 2006;98:1210–1215.

242. Zelefsky MJ, Yamada Y, Cohen GN, et al. Five-year outcome of intraoperative conformal permanent I-125 interstitial implantation for patients with clinically localized prostate cancer. *Int J Radiat Oncol Biol Phys* 2007;67:65–70.

243. Sylvester JE, Grimm PD, Blasko JC, et al. 15-Year biochemical relapse free survival in clinical Stage T1-T3 prostate cancer following combined external beam radiotherapy and brachytherapy; Seattle experience. *Int J Radiat Oncol Biol Phys* 2007;67:57–64.

244. Keyes M, Miller S, Mirvan V, et al. Acute and late urinary toxicity in 606 prostate brachytherapy patients—The BC Cancer Agency experience. American Brachytherapy Society 2007 Annual Meeting. *Brachytherapy* 2007;6:91.

245. Kollmeier MA, Stock RG, Cesaretti J, et al. Urinary morbidity and incontinence following transurethral resection of the prostate after brachytherapy. *J Urol* 2005;173:808–812.

246. Peters CA, Cesaretti JA, Stone NN, et al. Low-dose rate prostate brachytherapy is well tolerated in patients with a history of inflammatory bowel disease. *Int J Radiat Oncol Biol Phys* 2006;66:424–429.

247. Merrick GS, Butler WM, Wallner KE, et al. Risk factors for the development of prostate brachytherapy related urethral strictures. *J Urol* 2006;175:1376–1380.

248. Waterman FM, Dicker AP. Probability of late rectal morbidity in 125I prostate brachytherapy. *Int J Radiat Oncol Biol Phys* 2003;55:342–353.

249. Gelblum DY, Potters L. Rectal complications associated with transperineal interstitial brachytherapy for prostate cancer. *Int J Radiat Oncol Biol Phys* 2000;48:119–124.

250. Gelblum DY, Potters L, Ashley R, et al. Urinary morbidity following ultrasound-guided transperineal prostate seed implantation. *Int J Radiat Oncol Biol Phys* 1999;45:59–67.

251. Bottomley D, Ash D, Al-Qaisieh B, et al. Side effects of permanent I125 prostate seed implants in 667 patients treated in Leeds. *Radiother Oncol* 2007; 82:46–49.

252. Lee WR, Bae K, Lawton C, et al. Late toxicity and biochemical recurrence after external-beam radiotherapy combined with permanent-source prostate brachytherapy: analysis of Radiation Therapy Oncology Group study 0019. *Cancer* 2007;109:1506–1512.

253. Shah JN, Wuu CS, Katz AE, et al. Improved biochemical control and clinical disease-free survival with intraoperative versus preoperative preplanning for transperineal interstitial permanent prostate brachytherapy. *Cancer J* 2006; 12:289–297.

254. Keyes M, Schellenberg D, Moravan V, et al. Decline in urinary retention incidence in 805 patients after prostate brachytherapy: the effect of learning curve? *Int J Radiat Oncol Biol Phys* 2006;64:825–834.

255. Albert M, Tempany CM, Schultz D, et al. Late genitourinary and gastrointestinal toxicity after magnetic resonance image-guided prostate brachytherapy with or without neoadjuvant external beam radiation therapy. *Cancer* 2003;98:949–954.

256. Snyder KM, Stock RG, Hong SM, et al. Defining the risk of developing grade 2 proctitis following 125I prostate brachytherapy using a rectal dose-volume histogram analysis. *Int J Radiat Oncol Biol Phys* 2001;50:335–341.

257. Zelefsky MJ, Yamada Y, Cohen GN, et al. Intraoperative real-time planned conformal prostate brachytherapy: post-implantation dosimetric outcome and clinical implications. *Radiother Oncol* 2007;84:185–189.

258. Merrick GS, Butler WM, Wallner KE, et al. Erectile function after prostate brachytherapy. *Int J Radiat Oncol Biol Phys* 2005;62:437–447.

259. Merrick GS, Butler WM, Lief JH, et al. Efficacy of sildenafil citrate in prostate brachytherapy patients with erectile dysfunction. *Urology* 1999;53:1112–1116.

260. Pisansky TM, Pugh SL, Greenberg RE, et al. Tadalafil for prevention of erectile dysfunction after radiotherapy for prostate cancer: the Radiation Therapy Oncology Group [0831] randomized clinical trial. *JAMA* 2014;311:1300–1307.

261. Zelefsky MJ, Shasha D, Branco RD, et al. Prophylactic sildenafil citrate improves selected aspects of sexual function in men treated by radiotherapy for prostate cancer. *J Urol* 2014;192:868–874.

262. Galalae RM, Martinez A, Mate T, et al. Long-term outcome by risk factors using conformal high-dose-rate brachytherapy (HDR-BT) boost with or without neoadjuvant androgen suppression for localized prostate cancer. *Int J Radiat Oncol Biol Phys* 2004;58:1048–1055.

263. Demanes DJ, Rodriguez RR, Schour L, et al. High-dose-rate intensity-modulated brachytherapy with external beam radiotherapy for prostate cancer: California endocurietherapy's 10-year results. *Int J Radiat Oncol Biol Phys* 2005;61:1306–1316.

264. Deger S, Boehmer D, Roigas J, et al. High dose rate (HDR) brachytherapy with conformal radiation therapy for localized prostate cancer. *Eur Urol* 2005;47:441–448.

265. Yamada Y, Bhatia S, Zaider M, et al. Favorable clinical outcomes of three-dimensional computer-optimized high-dose-rate prostate brachytherapy in the management of localized prostate cancer. *Brachytherapy* 2006;5:157–164.

266. Phan TP, Syed AM, Puthawala A, et al. High dose rate brachytherapy as a boost for the treatment of localized prostate cancer. *J Urol* 2007;177:123–127.

267. Hoskin PJ, Rojas AM, Bownes PJ, et al. Randomised trial of external beam radiotherapy alone or combined with high-dose-rate brachytherapy boost for localised prostate cancer. *Radiother Oncol* 2012;103:217–222.

268. D'Amico AV. Radiation and hormonal therapy for locally advanced and clinically localized prostate cancer. *Urology* 2002;60:32–37.

269. Jones CU, Hunt D, McGowan DG, et al. Radiotherapy and short-term androgen deprivation for localized prostate cancer. *N Engl J Med* 2011;365:107–118.

270. Lee AK. Radiation therapy combined with hormone therapy for prostate cancer. *Semin Radiat Oncol* 2006;16:20–28.

271. Bolla M, Van Tienhoven G, Warde P, et al. External irradiation with or without long-term androgen suppression for prostate cancer with high metastatic risk: 10-year results of an EORTC randomized study. *Lancet Oncol* 2010;11:1066–1073.

272. Hanks GE, Pajak TF, Porter A, et al. Phase III trial of long-term adjuvant androgen deprivation after neoadjuvant hormonal cytoreduction and radiotherapy in locally advanced carcinoma of the prostate: the Radiation Therapy Oncology Group Protocol 92-02. *J Clin Oncol* 2003;21:3972–3978.

273. Roach M 3rd, DeSilvio M, Lawton C, et al. Phase III trial comparing whole-pelvic versus prostate-only radiotherapy and neoadjuvant versus adjuvant combined androgen suppression: Radiation Therapy Oncology Group 9413. *J Clin Oncol* 2003;21:1904–1911.

274. D'Amico AV, Manola J, Loffredo M, et al. 6-month androgen suppression plus radiation therapy vs radiation therapy alone for patients with clinically localized prostate cancer: a randomized controlled trial. *JAMA* 2004; 292:821–827.

275. Crook J, Ludgate C, Malone S, et al. Report of a multicenter Canadian phase III randomized trial of 3 months vs. 8 months neoadjuvant androgen deprivation before standard-dose radiotherapy for clinically localized prostate cancer. *Int J Radiat Oncol Biol Phys* 2004;60:15–23.

276. Bolla M, van Tienhoven G, de Reijke TM, et al. Concomitant and adjuvant androgen deprivation (ADT) with external beam irradiation (RT) for locally advanced prostate cancer: 6 months versus 3 years ADT—Results of the randomized EORTC Phase III trial 22961. *J Clin Oncol* 2007;25:5014.

277. Sasse AD, Sasse E, Carvalho AM, et al. Androgenic suppression combined with radiotherapy for the treatment of prostate adenocarcinoma: a systematic review. *BMC Cancer* 2012;12:54.

278. Zumsteg ZS, Spratt DE, Pei I, et al. A new risk classification system for therapeutic decision making with intermediate-risk prostate cancer patients undergoing dose-escalated external-beam radiation therapy. *Eur Urol* 2013; 64:895–902.

279. Merrick GS, Butler WM, Wallner KE, et al. Androgen deprivation therapy does not impact cause-specific or overall survival in high-risk prostate cancer managed with brachytherapy and supplemental external beam. *Int J Radiat Oncol Biol Phys* 2007;68:34–40.

280. Zumsteg ZS, Zelefsky MJ. Short-term androgen deprivation therapy for patients with intermediate-risk prostate cancer undergoing dose-escalated radiotherapy: the standard of care? *Lancet Oncol* 2012;13:e259–e269.

281. Nguyen PL, Je Y, Schutz FA, et al. Association of androgen deprivation therapy with cardiovascular death in patients with prostate cancer: a meta-analysis of randomized trials. *JAMA* 2011;306:2359–2366.

282. Nguyen PL, Chen MH, Beckman JA, et al. Influence of androgen deprivation therapy on all-cause mortality in men with high-risk prostate cancer and a history of congestive heart failure or myocardial infarction. *Int J Radiat Oncol Biol Phys* 2012;82:1411–1416.

283. Nanda A, Chen MH, Braccioforte MH, et al. Hormonal therapy use for prostate cancer and mortality in men with coronary artery disease-induced congestive heart failure or myocardial infarction. *JAMA* 2009;302:866–873.

284. Thompson IM, Tangen CM, Paradelo J, et al. Adjuvant radiotherapy for pathological T3N0M0 prostate cancer significantly reduces risk of metastases and improves survival: long-term followup of a randomized clinical trial. *J Urol* 2009;181:956–962.

285. Bolla M, van Poppel H, Collette L, et al. Postoperative radiotherapy after radical prostatectomy: a randomised controlled trial (EORTC trial 22911). *Lancet* 2005;366:572–578.

286. Bolla M, van Poppel H, Tombal B, et al. Postoperative radiotherapy after radical prostatectomy for high-risk prostate cancer: long-term results of a randomised controlled trial (EORTC trial 22911). *Lancet* 2012;380:2018–2027.

287. Wiegel T, Bartkowiak D, Bottke D, et al. Adjuvant radiotherapy versus wait-and-see after radical prostatectomy: 10-year follow-up of the ARO 96-02/AUO AP 09/95 trial. *Eur Urol* 2014 [Epub ahead of print]. doi: 10.1016/j.eururo .2014.03.011

288. Stephenson AJ, Scardino PT, Kattan MW, et al. Predicting the outcome of salvage radiation therapy for recurrent prostate cancer after radical prostatectomy. *J Clin Oncol* 2007;25:2035–2041.

289. Katz MS, Zelefsky MJ, Venkatraman ES, et al. Predictors of biochemical outcome with salvage conformal radiotherapy after radical prostatectomy for prostate cancer. *J Clin Oncol* 2003;21:483–489.

290. Pfister D, Bolla M, Briganti A, et al. Early salvage radiotherapy following radical prostatectomy. *Eur Urol* 2014;65:1034–1043.

291. Goenka A, Magsanoc JM, Pei X, et al. Long-term outcomes after high-dose postprostatectomy salvage radiation treatment. *Int J Radiat Oncol Biol Phys* 2012;84:112–118.

292. Briganti A, Karnes RJ, Joniau S, et al. Prediction of outcome following early salvage radiotherapy among patients with biochemical recurrence after radical prostatectomy. *Eur Urol* 2013 [Epub ahead of print]. doi: 10.1016/j.eururo.2013.11.045.

293. Choo R, Hruby G, Hong J, et al. (IN)-efficacy of salvage radiotherapy for rising PSA or clinically isolated local recurrence after radical prostatectomy. *Int J Radiat Oncol Biol Phys* 2002;53:269–276.

294. Macdonald OK, Schild SE, Vora SA, et al. Salvage radiotherapy for palpable, locally recurrent prostate cancer after radical prostatectomy. *Int J Radiat Oncol Biol Phys* 2004;58:1530–1535.

295. Valicenti RK, Thompson I Jr, Albertsen P, et al. Adjuvant and salvage radiation therapy after prostatectomy: American Society for Radiation Oncology /American Urological Association guidelines. *Int J Radiat Oncol Biol Phys* 2013;86:822–828.

296. Eastham JA, Kattan MW, Rogers E, et al. Risk factors for urinary incontinence after radical prostatectomy. *J Urol* 1996;156:1707–1713.

297. Burri RJ, Stone NN, Unger P, et al. Long-term outcome and toxicity of salvage brachytherapy for local failure after initial radiotherapy for prostate cancer. *Int J Radiat Oncol Biol Phys* 2010;77:1338–1344.

298. Vargas C, Swartz D, Vashi A, et al. Salvage brachytherapy for recurrent prostate cancer. *Brachytherapy* 2014;13:53–58.

299. Lahmer G, Lotter M, Kreppner S, et al. Protocol-based image-guided salvage brachytherapy. Early results in patients with local failure of prostate cancer after radiation therapy. *Strahlenther Onkol* 2013;189:668–674.

300. Chen CP, Weinberg V, Shinohara K, et al. Salvage HDR brachytherapy for recurrent prostate cancer after previous definitive radiation therapy: 5-year outcomes. *Int J Radiat Oncol Biol Phys* 2013;86:324–329.

301. Yamada Y, Kollmeier MA, Pei X, et al. A Phase II study of salvage high-dose-rate brachytherapy for the treatment of locally recurrent prostate cancer after definitive external beam radiotherapy. *Brachytherapy* 2014;13:111–116.

302. Bahn DK, Lee F, Silverman P, et al. Salvage cryosurgery for recurrent prostate cancer after radiation therapy: a seven-year follow-up. *Clin Prostate Cancer* 2003;2:111–114.

303. Chin JL, Pautler SE, Mouraviev V, et al. Results of salvage cryoablation of the prostate after radiation: identifying predictors of treatment failure and complications. *J Urol* 2001;165:1937–1941.

304. Donnelly BJ, Saliken JC, Ernst DS, et al. Role of transrectal ultrasound guided salvage cryosurgery for recurrent prostate carcinoma after radiotherapy. *Prostate Cancer Prostatic Dis* 2005;8:235–242.

305. Finley DS, Pouliot F, Miller DC, et al. Primary and salvage cryotherapy for prostate cancer. *Urol Clin North Am* 2010;37:67–82.

306. Ng CK, Moussa M, Downey DB, et al. Salvage cryoablation of the prostate: followup and analysis of predictive factors for outcome. *J Urol* 2007;178: 1253–1257.

307. Pisters LL, Leibovici D, Blute M, et al. Locally recurrent prostate cancer after initial radiation therapy: a comparison of salvage radical prostatectomy versus cryotherapy. *J Urol* 2009;182:517–525.

308. Huggins C, Hodges CV. Studies on prostatic cancer. I. The effect of castration, of estrogen and of androgen injection on serum phosphatases in metastatic carcinoma of the prostate. *Cancer Res* 1941;1:293–297.

309. Huggins C, Stevens RE Jr, Hodges CV. Studies on prostatic cancer. II. The effect of castration on advanced carcinoma of the prostate gland. *Arch Surg* 1941;43:209–223.

310. Schally AV, Redding TW, Comaru-Schally AM. Inhibition of prostate tumors by agonistic and antagonistic analogs of LH-RH. *Prostate* 1983;4:545–552.

311. Tolis G, Ackman D, Stellos A, et al. Tumor growth inhibition in patients with prostatic carcinoma treated with luteinizing hormone-releasing hormone agonists. *Proc Natl Acad Sci U S A* 1982;79:1658–1662.

312. Huggins C, Scott WW. Bilateral adrenalectomy in prostatic cancer. *Ann Surg* 1945;122:1031–1041.

313. Sanford EJ, Drago JR, Rohner TJ Jr, et al. Aminoglutethimide medical adrenalectomy for advanced prostatic carcinoma. *J Urol* 1976;115:170–174.

314. Trachtenberg J, Halpern N, Pont A. Ketoconazole: a novel and rapid treatment for advanced prostatic cancer. *J Urol* 1983;130:152–153.

315. Neri RO. Antiandrogens. *Adv Sex Horm Res* 1976;2:233–262.

316. Peets EA, Henson MF, Neri R. On the mechanism of the anti-androgenic action of flutamide (alpha-alpha-alpha-trifluoro-2-methyl-4'-nitro-m-propionotoluidide) in the rat. *Endocrinology* 1974;94:532–540.

317. Labrie F, Dupont A, Giguere M, et al. Advantages of the combination therapy in previously untreated and treated patients with advanced prostate cancer. *J Steroid Biochem* 1986;25:877–883.

318. Maximum androgen blockade in advanced prostate cancer: an overview of 22 randomised trials with 3283 deaths in 5710 patients. Prostate Cancer Trialists' Collaborative Group. *Lancet* 1995;346:265–269.

319. Caubet JF, Tosteson TD, Dong EW, et al. Maximum androgen blockade in advanced prostate cancer: a meta-analysis of published randomized controlled trials using nonsteroidal antiandrogens. *Urology* 1997;49:71–78.

320. Tannock IF, Osoba D, Stockler MR, et al. Chemotherapy with mitoxantrone plus prednisone or prednisone alone for symptomatic hormone-resistant prostate cancer: a Canadian randomized trial with palliative end points. *J Clin Oncol* 1996;14:1756–1764.

321. Petrylak DP, Tangen CM, Hussain MH, et al. Docetaxel and estramustine compared with mitoxantrone and prednisone for advanced refractory prostate cancer. *N Engl J Med* 2004;351:1513–1520.

322. Tannock IF, de Wit R, Berry WR, et al. Docetaxel plus prednisone or mitoxantrone plus prednisone for advanced prostate cancer. *N Engl J Med* 2004;351:1502–1512.

323. Kantoff PW, Higano CS, Shore ND, et al. Sipuleucel-T immunotherapy for castration-resistant prostate cancer. *N Engl J Med* 2010;363:411–422.

324. Ryan CJ, Smith MR, de Bono JS, et al. Abiraterone in metastatic prostate cancer without previous chemotherapy. *N Engl J Med* 2013;368:138–148.

325. de Bono JS, Oudard S, Ozguroglu M, et al. Prednisone plus cabazitaxel or mitoxantrone for metastatic castration-resistant prostate cancer progressing after docetaxel treatment: a randomised open-label trial. *Lancet* 2010;376:1147–1154.

326. Parker C, Nilsson S, Heinrich D, et al. Alpha emitter radium-223 and survival in metastatic prostate cancer. *N Engl J Med* 2013;369:213–223.

327. de Bono JS, Logothetis CJ, Molina A, et al. Abiraterone and increased survival in metastatic prostate cancer. *N Engl J Med* 2011;364:1995–2005.

328. Scher HI, Fizazi K, Saad F, et al. Increased survival with enzalutamide in prostate cancer after chemotherapy. *N Engl J Med* 2012;367:1187–1197.

329. Kelly WK, Halabi S, Carducci M, et al. Randomized, double-blind, placebo-controlled phase III trial comparing docetaxel and prednisone with or without bevacizumab in men with metastatic castration-resistant prostate cancer: CALGB 90401. *J Clin Oncol* 2012;30:1534–1540.

330. Tannock IF, Fizazi K, Ivanov S, et al. Aflibercept versus placebo in combination with docetaxel/prednisone for first-line treatment of men with metastatic castration-resistant prostate cancer (mCRPC): Results from the multinational phase III trial (VENICE). *J Clin Oncol* 2013;31:Abstr 13.

331. Quinn DI, Tangen CM, Hussain M, et al. SWOG S0421: Phase III study of docetaxel (D) and atrasentan (A) versus docetaxel and placebo (P) for men with advanced castrate resistant prostate cancer (CRPC). *J Clin Oncol* 2012;30:Abstr 4511.

332. Fizazi KS, Higano CS, Nelson JB, et al. Phase III, randomized, placebo-controlled study of docetaxel in combination with zibotentan in patients with metastatic castration-resistant prostate cancer. *J Clin Oncol* 2013;31:1740–1747.

333. Araujo JC, Trudel GC, Saad F, et al. Overall survival (OS) and safety of dasatinib/docetaxel versus docetaxel in patients with metastatic castration-resistant prostate cancer (mCRPC): Results from the randomized phase III READY trial. *J Clin Oncol* 2013;31:Abstr LBA8.

334. Small E, Demkow T, Gerritsen WR, et al. A phase III trial of GVAX immunotherapy for prostate cancer in combination with docetaxel versus docetaxel plus prednisone in symptomatic, castration-resistant prostate cancer (CRPC). 2009;Abstr 7.

335. Petrylak DP, Fizazi K, Sternberg CN, et al. A phase III study to evaluate the efficacy and safety of docetaxel and prednisone (DP) with or without lenalidomide (LEN) in patients with castrate-resistant prostate cancer (CRPC): the MAINSAIL trial. *Ann Oncol* 2012;23:Abstr LBA24.

336. Scher HI, Jia X, Chi K, et al. Randomized, open-label phase III trial of docetaxel plus high-dose calcitriol versus docetaxel plus prednisone for patients with castration-resistant prostate cancer. *J Clin Oncol* 2011;29:2191–2198.

337. Oncogenex Pharmaceutical, Inc. OncoGenex announces top-line survival results of phase 3 SYNERGY trial evaluating custirsen for metastatic castrate-resistant prostate cancer. Accessed June 25, 2014. http://ir.oncogenex.com/releasedetail.cfm?ReleaseID=842949.

338. Fizazi K, Carducci M, Smith M, et al. Denosumab versus zoledronic acid for treatment of bone metastases in men with castration-resistant prostate cancer: a randomised, double-blind study. *Lancet* 2011;377:813–822.

339. Scher HI, Morris MJ, Basch E, et al. End points and outcomes in castration-resistant prostate cancer: from clinical trials to clinical practice. *J Clin Oncol* 2011;29:3695–3704.

340. Chen Y, Clegg NJ, Scher HI. Anti-androgens and androgen-depleting therapies in prostate cancer: new agents for an established target. *Lancet Oncol* 2009;10:981–991.

341. Bennett CL, Tosteson TD, Schmitt B, et al. Maximum androgen-blockade with medical or surgical castration in advanced prostate cancer: A meta-analysis of nine published randomized controlled trials and 4128 patients using flutamide. *Prostate Cancer Prostatic Dis* 1999;2:4–8.

342. The Leuprolide Study Group, Garnick MB, Glode LM. Leuprolide versus diethylstilbestrol for metastatic prostate cancer. *N Engl J Med* 1984;311:1281–1286.

343. Cassileth BR, Soloway MS, Vogelzang NJ, et al. Patients' choice of treatment in stage D prostate cancer. *Urology* 1989;33:57–62.

344. Klotz L, Boccon-Gibod L, Shore ND, et al. The efficacy and safety of degarelix: a 12-month, comparative, randomized, open-label, parallel-group phase III study in patients with prostate cancer. *BJU Int* 2008;102:1531–1538.

345. Labrie F, Dupont A, Belanger A, et al. Flutamide eliminates the risk of disease flare in prostatic cancer patients treated with a luteinizing hormone-releasing hormone agonist. *J Urol* 1987;138:804–806.

346. Schulze H, Senge T. Influence of different types of antiandrogens on luteinizing hormone-releasing hormone analogue-induced testosterone surge in patients with metastatic carcinoma of the prostate. *J Urol* 1990;144:934–941.

347. Schellhammer PF, Sharifi R, Block NL, et al. Clinical benefits of bicalutamide compared with flutamide in combined androgen blockade for patients with advanced prostatic carcinoma: final report of a double-blind, randomized, multicenter trial. Casodex Combination Study Group. *Urology* 1997;50:330–336.

348. Bertagna C, De Gery A, Hucher M, et al. Efficacy of the combination of nilutamide plus orchidectomy in patients with metastatic prostatic cancer. A meta-analysis of seven randomized double-blind trials (1056 patients). *Br J Urol* 1994;73:396–402.

349. Schellhammer PF. An evaluation of bicalutamide in the treatment of prostate cancer. *Expert Opin Pharmacother* 2002;3:1313–1328.

350. Ahmadi H, Daneshmand S. Androgen deprivation therapy: evidence-based management of side effects. *BJU Int* 2013;111:543–548.

351. Flaig TW, Glode LM. Management of the side effects of androgen deprivation therapy in men with prostate cancer. *Expert Opin Pharmacother* 2008;9:2829–2841.

352. Holzbeierlein JM, Castle EP, Thrasher JB. Complications of androgen-deprivation therapy for prostate cancer. *Clin Prostate Cancer* 2003;2:147–152.

353. Gerber GS, Zagaja GP, Ray PS, et al. Transdermal estrogen in the treatment of hot flushes in men with prostate cancer. *Urology* 2000;55:97–101.

354. Morrow PK, Mattair DN, Hortobagyi GN. Hot flashes: a review of pathophysiology and treatment modalities. *Oncologist* 2011;16:1658–1664.

355. Strum SB, McDermed JE, Scholz MC, et al. Anaemia associated with androgen deprivation in patients with prostate cancer receiving combined hormone blockade. *Br J Urol* 1997;79:933–941.

356. Diamond TH, Higano CS, Smith MR, et al. Osteoporosis in men with prostate carcinoma receiving androgen-deprivation therapy: recommendations for diagnosis and therapies. *Cancer* 2004;100:892–899.

357. Basaria S, Muller DC, Carducci MA, et al. Hyperglycemia and insulin resistance in men with prostate carcinoma who receive androgen-deprivation therapy. *Cancer* 2006;106:581–588.

358. Basaria S, Lieb J 2nd, Tang AM, et al. Long-term effects of androgen deprivation therapy in prostate cancer patients. *Clin Endocrinol (Oxf)* 2002;56:779–786.

359. Shahinian VB, Kuo YF, Freeman JL, et al. Risk of fracture after androgen deprivation for prostate cancer. *N Engl J Med* 2005;352:154–164.

360. Smith MR. Treatment-related osteoporosis in men with prostate cancer. *Clin Cancer Res* 2006;12:6315s–6319s.

361. Saad F, Higano CS, Sartor O, et al. The role of bisphosphonates in the treatment of prostate cancer: recommendations from an expert panel. *Clin Genitourin Cancer* 2006;4:257–262.

362. Hanley DA, Adachi JD, Bell A, et al. Denosumab: mechanism of action and clinical outcomes. *Int J Clin Pract* 2012;66:1139–1146.

363. Smith MR, Egerdie B, Hernandez Toriz N, et al. Denosumab in men receiving androgen-deprivation therapy for prostate cancer. *N Engl J Med* 2009;361:745–755.

364. Smith MR, Morton RA, Barnette KG, et al. Toremifene to reduce fracture risk in men receiving androgen deprivation therapy for prostate cancer. *J Urol* 2013;189:S45–S50.

365. Pirl WF, Siegel GI, Goode MJ, et al. Depression in men receiving androgen deprivation therapy for prostate cancer: a pilot study. *Psychooncology* 2002;11:518–523.

366. Nelson CJ, Lee JS, Gamboa MC, et al. Cognitive effects of hormone therapy in men with prostate cancer: a review. *Cancer* 2008;113:1097–1106.

367. Salminen EK, Portin RI, Koskinen A, et al. Associations between serum testosterone fall and cognitive function in prostate cancer patients. *Clin Cancer Res* 2004;10:7575–7582.

368. Conteduca V, Di Lorenzo G, Tartarone A, et al. The cardiovascular risk of gonadotropin releasing hormone agonists in men with prostate cancer: an unresolved controversy. *Crit Rev Oncol Hematol* 2013;86:42–51.

369. Levine GN, D'Amico AV, Berger P, et al. Androgen-deprivation therapy in prostate cancer and cardiovascular risk: a science advisory from the American Heart Association, American Cancer Society, and American Urological Association: endorsed by the American Society for Radiation Oncology. *CA Cancer J Clin* 2010;60:194–201.

370. Bennett CL, Raisch DW, Sartor O. Pneumonitis associated with nonsteroidal antiandrogens: presumptive evidence of a class effect. *Ann Intern Med* 2002;137:625.

371. Gleave ME, Goldenberg SL, Chin JL, et al. Randomized comparative study of 3 versus 8-month neoadjuvant hormonal therapy before radical prostatectomy: biochemical and pathological effects. *J Urol* 2001;166:500–506.

372. Glass TR, Tangen CM, Crawford ED, et al. Metastatic carcinoma of the prostate: identifying prognostic groups using recursive partitioning. *J Urol* 2003;169:164–169.

373. Sylvester RJ, Denis L, de Voogt H. The importance of prognostic factors in the interpretation of two EORTC metastatic prostate cancer trials. European Organization for Research and Treatment of Cancer (EORTC) Genito-Urinary Tract Cancer Cooperative Group. *Eur Urol* 1998;33:134–143.

374. Noguchi M, Kikuchi H, Ishibashi M, et al. Percentage of the positive area of bone metastasis is an independent predictor of disease death in advanced prostate cancer. *Br J Cancer* 2003;88:195–201.

375. Soloway MS, Hardeman SW, Hickey D, et al. Stratification of patients with metastatic prostate cancer based on extent of disease on initial bone scan. *Cancer* 1988;61:195–202.

376. Eisenberger MA, Blumenstein BA, Crawford ED, et al. Bilateral orchiectomy with or without flutamide for metastatic prostate cancer. *N Engl J Med* 1998;339:1036–1042.

377. Hussain M, Tangen CM, Higano C, et al. Absolute prostate-specific antigen value after androgen deprivation is a strong independent predictor of survival in new metastatic prostate cancer: data from Southwest Oncology Group Trial 9346 (INT-0162). *J Clin Oncol* 2006;24:3984–3990.

378. Choueiri TK, Xie W, D'Amico AV, et al. Time to prostate-specific antigen nadir independently predicts overall survival in patients who have metastatic hormone-sensitive prostate cancer treated with androgen-deprivation therapy. *Cancer* 2009;115:981–987.

379. Seidenfeld J, Samson DJ, Hasselblad V, et al. Single-therapy androgen suppression in men with advanced prostate cancer: a systematic review and meta-analysis. *Ann Intern Med* 2000;132:566–577.

380. Robinson MR, Smith PH, Richards B, et al. The final analysis of the EORTC Genito-Urinary Tract Cancer Co-Operative Group phase III clinical trial (protocol 30805) comparing orchidectomy, orchidectomy plus cyproterone acetate and low dose stilboestrol in the management of metastatic carcinoma of the prostate. *Eur Urol* 1995;28:273–283.

381. Geller J, Albert JD, Nachtsheim DA, et al. Comparison of prostatic cancer tissue dihydrotestosterone levels at the time of relapse following orchiectomy or estrogen therapy. *J Urol* 1984;132:693–696.

382. Titus MA, Schell MJ, Lih FB, et al. Testosterone and dihydrotestosterone tissue levels in recurrent prostate cancer. *Clin Cancer Res* 2005;11:4653–4657.

383. Mostaghel EA, Page ST, Lin DW, et al. Intraprostatic androgens and androgen-regulated gene expression persist after testosterone suppression: therapeutic implications for castration-resistant prostate cancer. *Cancer Res* 2007;67:5033–5041.

384. Ryan CJ, Smith A, Lal P, et al. Persistent prostate-specific antigen expression after neoadjuvant androgen depletion: an early predictor of relapse or incomplete androgen suppression. *Urology* 2006;68:834–839.

385. Labrie F, Dupont A, Belanger A. Complete androgen blockade for the treatment of prostate cancer. *Important Adv Oncol* 1985:193–217.

386. Prostate Cancer Trialists' Collaborative Group. Maximum androgen blockade in advanced prostate cancer: an overview of 22 randomized trials with 3283 deaths in 5710 patients. *Lancet* 1995;346:265–269.

387. Schmitt B, Bennett C, Seidenfeld J, et al. Maximal androgen blockade for advanced prostate cancer. *Cochrane Database Syst Rev* 2000:CD001526.

388. Blackard CE. The Veterans' Administration Cooperative Urological Research Group studies of carcinoma of the prostate: a review. *Cancer Chemother Rep* 1975;59:225–227.

389. Byar DP, Corle DK. Hormone therapy for prostate cancer: results of the Veterans Administration Cooperative Urological Research Group studies. *NCI Monogr* 1988:165–170.

390. Walsh PC. Immediate versus deferred treatment for advanced prostatic cancer: initial results of the Medical Research Council trial. The Medical Research Council Prostate Cancer Working Party Investigators Group. *Br J Urol* 1997;79: 235–246.

391. Studer UE, Whelan P, Albrecht W, et al. Immediate or deferred androgen deprivation for patients with prostate cancer not suitable for local treatment with curative intent: European Organisation for Research and Treatment of Cancer (EORTC) Trial 30891. *J Clin Oncol* 2006;24:1868–1876.

392. Pound CR, Partin AW, Eisenberger MA, et al. Natural history of progression after PSA elevation following radical prostatectomy. *JAMA* 1999;281:1591–1597.

393. Antonarakis ES, Feng Z, Trock BJ, et al. The natural history of metastatic progression in men with prostate-specific antigen recurrence after radical prostatectomy: long-term follow-up. *BJU Int* 2012;109:32–39.

394. Zhou P, Chen MH, McLeod D, et al. Predictors of prostate cancer-specific mortality after radical prostatectomy or radiation therapy. *J Clin Oncol* 2005; 23:6992–6998.

395. Iversen P, Tveter K, Varenhorst E. Randomised study of Casodex 50 MG monotherapy vs orchidectomy in the treatment of metastatic prostate cancer. The Scandinavian Casodex Cooperative Group. *Scand J Urol Nephrol* 1996;30:93–98.

396. Iversen P, Tyrell CJ, Kaisary AV, et al. Casodex (bicalutamide) 150-mg monotherapy compared with castration in patients with previously untreated nonmetastatic prostate cancer: results from two multicenter randomized trials at a median follow-up of 4 years. *Urology* 1998;51:389–396.

397. Scher HI, Liebertz C, Kelly WK, et al. Bicalutamide for advanced prostate cancer: the natural versus treated history of disease. *J Clin Oncol* 1997;15:2928–2938.

398. Klotz LH, Herr HW, Morse MJ, et al. Intermittent endocrine therapy for advanced prostate cancer. *Cancer* 1986;58:2546–2550.

399. Bruchovsky N, Rennie PS, Coldman AJ, et al. Effects of androgen withdrawal on the stem cell composition of the Shionogi carcinoma. *Cancer Res* 1990;50:2275–2282.

400. Sato N, Gleave ME, Bruchovsky N, et al. Intermittent androgen suppression delays progression to androgen-independent regulation of prostate-specific antigen gene in the LNCaP prostate tumour model. *J Steroid Biochem Mol Biol* 1996;58:139–146.

401. Crook JM, O'Callaghan CJ, Duncan G, et al. Intermittent androgen suppression for rising PSA level after radiotherapy. *N Engl J Med* 2012;367:895–903.

402. Hussain M, Tangen CM, Berry DL, et al. Intermittent versus continuous androgen deprivation in prostate cancer. *N Engl J Med* 2013;368:1314–1325.

403. Tsai HT, Penson DF, Makambi KH, et al. Efficacy of intermittent androgen deprivation therapy vs conventional continuous androgen deprivation therapy for advanced prostate cancer: a meta-analysis. *Urology* 2013;82:327–333.

404. Niraula S, Le LW, Tannock IF. Treatment of prostate cancer with intermittent versus continuous androgen deprivation: a systematic review of randomized trials. *J Clin Oncol* 2013;31:2029–2036.

405. Botrel TE, Clark O, dos Reis RB, et al. Intermittent versus continuous androgen deprivation for locally advanced, recurrent or metastatic prostate cancer: a systematic review and meta-analysis. *BMC Urol* 2014;14:9.

406. Smith MR, Saad F, Coleman R, et al. Denosumab and bone-metastasis-free survival in men with castration-resistant prostate cancer: results of a phase 3, randomised, placebo-controlled trial. *Lancet* 2012;379:39–46.

407. Smith MR, Eastham J, Gleason DM, et al. Randomized controlled trial of zoledronic acid to prevent bone loss in men receiving androgen deprivation therapy for nonmetastatic prostate cancer. *J Urol* 2003;169:2008–2012.

408. Smith MR, Saad F, Oudard S, et al. Denosumab and bone metastasis-free survival in men with nonmetastatic castration-resistant prostate cancer: exploratory analyses by baseline prostate-specific antigen doubling time. *J Clin Oncol* 2013;31:3800–3806.

409. Beltran H, Tomlins S, Aparicio A, et al. Aggressive variants of castration-resistant prostate cancer. *Clin Cancer Res* 2014;20:2846–2850.

410. Epstein JI, Amin MB, Beltran H, et al. Proposed morphologic classification of prostate cancer with neuroendocrine differentiation. *Am J Surg Pathol* 2014;38:756–767.

411. Pond GR, Sonpavde G, de Wit R, et al. The prognostic importance of metastatic site in men with metastatic castration-resistant prostate cancer. *Eur Urol* 2014;65:3–6.

412. Aparicio AM, Harzstark AL, Corn PG, et al. Platinum-based chemotherapy for variant castrate-resistant prostate cancer. *Clin Cancer Res* 2013;19:3621–3630.

413. Taylor CD, Elson P, Trump DL. Importance of continued testicular suppression in hormone-refractory prostate cancer. *J Clin Oncol* 1993;11:2167–2172.

414. Crawford ED, Sartor O, Chu F, et al. A 12-month clinical study of LA-2585 (45.0 mg): a new 6-month subcutaneous delivery system for leuprolide acetate for the treatment of prostate cancer. *J Urol* 2006;175:533–536.

415. Kelly WK, Slovin S, Scher HI. Steroid hormone withdrawal syndromes. Pathophysiology and clinical significance. *Urol Clin North Am* 1997;24:421–431.

416. Scher HI, Kelly WK. Flutamide withdrawal syndrome: its impact on clinical trials in hormone-refractory prostate cancer. *J Clin Oncol* 1993;11:1566–1572.

417. Oh WK, Manola J, Bittmann L, et al. Finasteride and flutamide therapy in patients with advanced prostate cancer: response to subsequent castration and long-term follow-up. *Urology* 2003;62:99–104.

418. Crombie C, Raghavan D, Page J, et al. Phase II study of megestrol acetate for metastatic carcinoma of the prostate. *Br J Urol* 1987;59:443–446.

419. Courtney KD, Taplin ME. The evolving paradigm of second-line hormonal therapy options for castration-resistant prostate cancer. *Curr Opin Oncol* 2012;24:272–277.

420. Smith DC, Redman BG, Flaherty LE, et al. A phase II trial of oral diethylstilbestrol as a second-line hormonal agent in advanced prostate cancer. *Urology* 1998;52:257–260.

421. Pomerantz M, Manola J, Taplin ME, et al. Phase II study of low dose and high dose conjugated estrogen for androgen independent prostate cancer. *J Urol* 2007;177:2146–2150.

422. Aggarwal R, Weinberg V, Small EJ, et al. The mechanism of action of estrogen in castration-resistant prostate cancer: clues from hormone levels. *Clin Genitourin Cancer* 2009;7:E71–E76.

423. Kitahara S, Umeda H, Yano M, et al. Effects of intravenous administration of high dose-diethylstilbestrol diphosphate on serum hormonal levels in patients with hormone-refractory prostate cancer. *Endocr J* 1999;46:659–664.

424. Estramustine phosphate in prostate cancer. Seminar. *Urology* 1984;23:1–88.

425. Bland LB, Garzotto M, DeLoughery TG, et al. Phase II study of transdermal estradiol in androgen-independent prostate carcinoma. *Cancer* 2005;103: 717–723.

426. Kandola S, Anyamene N, Payne H, et al. Transdermal oestrogen therapy as a second-line hormonal intervention in prostate cancer: a bad experience. *BJU Int* 2007;99:53–55.

427. Small EJ, Baron AD, Fippin L, et al. Ketoconazole retains activity in advanced prostate cancer patients with progression despite flutamide withdrawal. *J Urol* 1997;157:1204–1207.

428. Ryan CJ, Halabi S, Ou SS, et al. Adrenal androgen levels as predictors of outcome in prostate cancer patients treated with ketoconazole plus antiandrogen withdrawal: results from a cancer and leukemia group B study. *Clin Cancer Res* 2007;13:2030–2037.

429. Small EJ, Halabi S, Dawson NA, et al. Antiandrogen withdrawal alone or in combination with ketoconazole in androgen-independent prostate cancer patients: a phase III trial (CALGB 9583). *J Clin Oncol* 2004;22:1025–1033.

430. Tannock I, Gospodarowicz M, Meakin W, et al. Treatment of metastatic prostatic cancer with low-dose prednisone: evaluation of pain and quality of life as pragmatic indices of response. *J Clin Oncol* 1989;7:590–597.

431. Montgomery B, Cheng HH, Drechsler J, et al. Glucocorticoids and prostate cancer treatment: friend or foe? *Asian J Androl* 2014;16:354–358.

432. Ryan CJ, Molina A, Li J, et al. Serum androgens as prognostic biomarkers in castration-resistant prostate cancer: results from an analysis of a randomized phase III trial. *J Clin Oncol* 2013;31:2791–2798.

433. Kantoff PW, Halabi S, Conaway M, et al. Hydrocortisone with or without mitoxantrone in men with hormone-refractory prostate cancer: results of the Cancer and Leukemia Group B 9182 study. *J Clin Oncol* 1999;18:2506–2513.

434. Bouchet BP, Galmarini CM. Cabazitaxel, a new taxane with favorable properties. *Drugs Today (Barc)* 2010;46:735–742.

435. Scher HI, Sawyers CL. Biology of progressive, castration-resistant prostate cancer: directed therapies targeting the androgen-receptor signaling axis. *J Clin Oncol* 2005;23:8253–8261.

436. Tamae D, Byrns M, Marck B, et al. Development, validation and application of a stable isotope dilution liquid chromatography electrospray ionization /selected reaction monitoring/mass spectrometry (SID-LC/ESI/SRM/MS) method for quantification of keto-androgens in human serum. *J Steroid Biochem Mol Biol* 2013;138:281–289.

437. Montgomery RB, Mostaghel EA, Vessella R, et al. Maintenance of intratumoral androgens in metastatic prostate cancer: a mechanism for castration-resistant tumor growth. *Cancer Res* 2008;68:4447–4454.

438. Barrie SE, Potter GA, Goddard PM, et al. Pharmacology of novel steroidal inhibitors of cytochrome P450(17) alpha (17 alpha-hydroxylase/C17-20 lyase). *J Steroid Biochem Mol Biol* 1994;50:267–273.

439. O'Donnell A, Judson I, Dowsett M, et al. Hormonal impact of the 17alpha-hydroxylase/C(17,20)-lyase inhibitor abiraterone acetate (CB7630) in patients with prostate cancer. *Br J Cancer* 2004;90:2317–2325.

440. Attard G, Reid AH, Yap TA, et al. Phase I clinical trial of a selective inhibitor of CYP17, abiraterone acetate, confirms that castration-resistant prostate cancer commonly remains hormone driven. *J Clin Oncol* 2008;26:4563–4571.

441. Ryan CJ, Smith MR, Fong L, et al. Phase I clinical trial of the CYP17 inhibitor abiraterone acetate demonstrating clinical activity in patients with castration-resistant prostate cancer who received prior ketoconazole therapy. *J Clin Oncol* 2010;28:1481–1488.

442. Reid AH, Attard G, Danila DC, et al. Significant and sustained antitumor activity in post-docetaxel, castration-resistant prostate cancer with the CYP17 inhibitor abiraterone acetate. *J Clin Oncol* 2010;28:1489–1495.

443. Danila DC, Morris MJ, de Bono JS, et al. Phase II multicenter study of abiraterone acetate plus prednisone therapy in patients with docetaxel-treated castration-resistant prostate cancer. *J Clin Oncol* 2010;28:1496–1501.

444. Fizazi K, Scher HI, Molina A, et al. Abiraterone acetate for treatment of metastatic castration-resistant prostate cancer: final overall survival analysis of the COU-AA-301 randomised, double-blind, placebo-controlled phase 3 study. *Lancet Oncol* 2012;13:983–992.

445. Rathkopf DE, Smith MR, de Bono JS, et al. Updated interim efficacy analysis and long-term safety of abiraterone acetate in metastatic castration-resistant prostate cancer patients without prior chemotherapy (COU-AA-302). *Eur Urol* 2014 [Epub ahead of print]. doi: 10.1016/j.eururo.2014.02.056.

446. Scher HI, Beer TM, Higano CS, et al. Antitumour activity of MDV3100 in castration-resistant prostate cancer: a phase 1-2 study. *Lancet* 2010;375:1437–1446.

447. Beer TM, Armstrong AJ, Rathkopf DE, et al. Enzalutamide in metastatic prostate cancer before chemotherapy. *N Engl J Med* 2014;371:424–433.

448. Clegg NJ, Wongvipat J, Joseph JD, et al. ARN-509: a novel antiandrogen for prostate cancer treatment. *Cancer Res* 2012;72:1494–1503.

449. Rathkopf DE, Morris MJ, Fox JJ, et al. Phase I study of ARN-509, a novel anti-androgen, in the treatment of castration-resistant prostate cancer. *J Clin Oncol* 2013;31:3525–3530.

450. Stein MN, Patel N, Bershadskiy A, et al. Androgen synthesis inhibitors in the treatment of castration-resistant prostate cancer. *Asian J Androl* 2014;16:387–400.

451. Small EJ, Fratesi P, Reese DM, et al. Immunotherapy of hormone-refractory prostate cancer with antigen-loaded dendritic cells. *J Clin Oncol* 2000;18:3894–3903.

452. Small EJ, Schellhammer PF, Higano CS, et al. Placebo-controlled phase III trial of immunologic therapy with sipuleucel-T (APC8015) in patients with metastatic, asymptomatic hormone refractory prostate cancer. *J Clin Oncol* 2006;24:3089–3094.

453. Kantoff PW, Schuetz TJ, Blumenstein BA, et al. Overall survival analysis of a phase II randomized controlled trial of a Poxviral-based PSA-targeted immunotherapy in metastatic castration-resistant prostate cancer. *J Clin Oncol* 2010;28:1099–1105.

454. DiPaola RS, Plante M, Kaufman H, et al. A phase I trial of pox PSA vaccines (PROSTVAC-VF) with B7-1, ICAM-1, and LFA-3 co-stimulatory molecules (TRICOM) in patients with prostate cancer. *J Transl Med* 2006;4:1.

455. Hodi FS, O'Day SJ, McDermott DF, et al. Improved survival with ipilimumab in patients with metastatic melanoma. *N Engl J Med* 2010;363:711–723.

456. Robert C, Thomas L, Bondarenko I, et al. Ipilimumab plus dacarbazine for previously untreated metastatic melanoma. *N Engl J Med* 2011;364:2517–2526.

457. Slovin SF, Higano CS, Hamid O, et al. Ipilimumab alone or in combination with radiotherapy in metastatic castration-resistant prostate cancer: results from an open-label, multicenter phase I/II study. *Ann Oncol* 2013;24:1813–1821.

458. Kwon ED, Drake CG, Scher HI, et al. Ipilimumab versus placebo after radiotherapy in patients with metastatic castration-resistant prostate cancer that had progressed after docetaxel chemotherapy (CA184-043): a multicentre, randomised, double-blind, phase 3 trial. *Lancet Oncol* 2014;15:700–712.

459. Smith DC, Smith MR, Sweeney C, et al. Cabozantinib in patients with advanced prostate cancer: results of a phase II randomized discontinuation trial. *J Clin Oncol* 2013;31:412–419.

460. Dalrymple SL, Becker RE, Isaacs JT. The quinoline-3-carboxamide anti-angiogenic agent, tasquinimod, enhances the anti-prostate cancer efficacy of androgen ablation and taxotere without effecting serum PSA directly in human xenografts. *Prostate* 2007;67:790–797.

461. Gupta N, Ustwani OA, Shen L, et al. Mechanism of action and clinical activity of tasquinimod in castrate-resistant prostate cancer. *Onco Targets Ther* 2014;7:223–234.

462. Isaacs JT, Pili R, Qian DZ, et al. Identification of ABR-215050 as lead second generation quinoline-3-carboxamide anti-angiogenic agent for the treatment of prostate cancer. *Prostate* 2006;66:1768–1778.

463. Pili R, Haggman M, Stadler WM, et al. Phase II randomized, double-blind, placebo-controlled study of tasquinimod in men with minimally symptomatic metastatic castrate-resistant prostate cancer. *J Clin Oncol* 2011;29:4022–4028.

464. Armstrong AJ, Haggman M, Stadler WM, et al. Long-term survival and biomarker correlates of tasquinimod efficacy in a multicenter randomized study of men with minimally symptomatic metastatic castration-resistant prostate cancer. *Clin Cancer Res* 2013;19:6891–6901.

465. Smith MR, Saad F, Egerdie B, et al. Effects of denosumab on bone mineral density in men receiving androgen deprivation therapy for prostate cancer. *J Urol* 2009;182:2670–2675.

466. McDermott RS, Anderson PR, Greenberg RE, et al. Cranial nerve deficits in patients with metastatic prostate carcinoma: clinical features and treatment outcomes. *Cancer* 2004;101:1639–1643.

467. Loblaw A, Mitera G. Malignant extradural spinal cord compression in men with prostate cancer. *Curr Opin Support Palliat Care* 2011;5:206–210.

468. Venkitaraman R, Sohaib SA, Barbachano Y, et al. Detection of occult spinal cord compression with magnetic resonance imaging of the spine. *Clin Oncol (R Coll Radiol)* 2007;19:528–531.

469. Falkmer U, Jarhult J, Wersall P, et al. A systematic overview of radiation therapy effects in skeletal metastases. *Acta Oncol* 2003;42:620–633.

470. Hartsell WF, Scott CB, Bruner DW, et al. Randomized trial of short- versus long-course radiotherapy for palliation of painful bone metastases. *J Natl Cancer Inst* 2005;97:798–804.

471. Kaasa S, Brenne E, Lund JA, et al. Prospective randomised multicenter trial on single fraction radiotherapy (8 Gy x 1) versus multiple fractions (3 Gy × 10) in the treatment of painful bone metastases. *Radiother Oncol* 2006;79:278–284.

472. Anderson P, Nunez R. Samarium lexidronam (153Sm-EDTMP): skeletal radiation for osteoblastic bone metastases and osteosarcoma. *Expert Rev Anticancer Ther* 2007;7:1517–1527.

473. Gartrell BA, Saad F. Managing bone metastases and reducing skeletal related events in prostate cancer. *Nat Rev Clin Oncol* 2014;11:335–345.

474. Porter AT, McEwan AJ, Powe JE, et al. Results of a randomized phase-III trial to evaluate the efficacy of strontium-89 adjuvant to local field external beam irradiation in the management of endocrine resistant prostate cancer. *Int J Radiat Oncol Biol Phys* 1993;25:805–813.

475. Farhanghi M, Holmes RA, Volkert WA, et al. Samarium-153-EDTMP: pharmacokinetic, toxicity and pain response using an escalating dose schedule in treatment of metastatic bone cancer. *J Nucl Med* 1992;33:1451–1458.

476. Collins C, Eary JF, Donaldson G, et al. Samarium-153-EDTMP in bone metastases of hormone refractory prostate carcinoma: a phase I/II trial. *J Nucl Med* 1993;34:1839–1844.

477. Sartor O, Reid RH, Hoskin PJ, et al. Samarium-153-Lexidronam complex for treatment of painful bone metastases in hormone-refractory prostate cancer. *Urology* 2004;63:940–945.

478. Autio KA, Pandit-Taskar N, Carrasquillo JA, et al. Repetitively dosed docetaxel and (1)(5)(3)samarium-EDTMP as an antitumor strategy for metastatic castration-resistant prostate cancer. *Cancer* 2013;119:3186–3194.

479. Nilsson S, Larsen RH, Fossa SD, et al. First clinical experience with alpha-emitting radium-223 in the treatment of skeletal metastases. *Clin Cancer Res* 2005;11:4451–4459.

480. Dreicer R, Jones R, Oudard S, et al. Results from a phase 3, randomized, double-blind, multicenter, placebo-controlled trial of orteronel (TAK-700) plus prednisone in patients with metastatic castration-resistant prostate cancer (mCRPC) that has progressed during or following docetaxel-based therapy (ELM-PC 5 trial). *J Clin Oncol* 2014;32;Abstr 7.

481. OncoGenex Pharmaceuticals, Inc. OncoGenex Announces Top-Line Survival Results of Phase 3 SYNERGY Trial Evaluating Custirsen for Metastatic Castrate-Resistant Prostate Cancer [press release]. April 28, 2014. Accessed June 20, 2014. http://ir.oncogenex.com/releasedetail.cfm?ReleaseID=842949.

482. Dreicer R, MacLean D, Suri A, et al. Phase I/II trial of orteronel (TAK-700)—an investigational 17,20-lyase inhibitor—in patients with metastatic castration-resistant prostate cancer. *Clin Cancer Res* 2014;20:1335–1344.

483. Petrylak D, Gandhi JG, Clark WR, et al. A phase I/II study of safety and efficacy of orteronel (TAK-700), an oral, investigational, nonsteroidal 17,20-lyase inhibitor, with docetaxel and prednisone (DP) in metastatic castration-resistant prostate cancer (mCRPC): Updated phase II results. *J Clin Oncol* 2013;31:Abstr 59.

484. Saad F, Hotte S, North S, et al. Randomized phase II trial of Custirsen (OGX-011) in combination with docetaxel or mitoxantrone as second-line therapy in patients with metastatic castrate-resistant prostate cancer progressing after first-line docetaxel: CUOG trial P-06c. *Clin Cancer Res* 2011;17:5765–5773.

485. Rathkopf D, Scher HI. Androgen receptor antagonists in castration-resistant prostate cancer. *Cancer J* 2013;19:43–49.

486. Carver BS, Chapinski C, Wongvipat J, et al. Reciprocal feedback regulation of PI3K and androgen receptor signaling in PTEN-deficient prostate cancer. *Cancer Cell* 2011;19:575–586.

487. Sprenger CC, Plymate SR. The link between androgen receptor splice variants and castration-resistant prostate cancer. *Horm Cancer* 2014;5:207–217.

488. Antonarakis ES, Lu C, Luber B, et al. AR-V7 and resistance to enzalutamide and abiraterone in prostate cancer. *N Engl J Med* 2014 [Epub ahead of print].

489. Balbas MD, Evans MJ, Hosfield DJ, et al. Overcoming mutation-based resistance to antiandrogens with rational drug design. *Elife* 2013;2:e00499.

490. Arora VK, Schenkein E, Murali R, et al. Glucocorticoid receptor confers resistance to antiandrogens by bypassing androgen receptor blockade. *Cell* 2013;155:1309–1322.

491. Messing EM, Manola J, Sarosdy M, et al. Immediate hormonal therapy compared with observation after radical prostatectomy and pelvic lymphadenectomy in men with node-positive prostate cancer. *N Engl J Med* 1999;341:1781–1788.

492. Sweeney C, Chen YH, Carducci MA, et al. Impact on overall survival (OS) with chemohormonal therapy versus hormonal therapy for hormone-sensitive newly metastatic prostate cancer (mPrCa): An ECOG-led phase III randomized trial. *J Clin Oncol* 2014;32;Abstr LBA2.

493. McKay RR, Choueiri TK, Taplin ME. Rationale for and review of neoadjuvant therapy prior to radical prostatectomy for patients with high-risk prostate cancer. *Drugs* 2013;73:1417–1430.

494. Taplin ME, Montgomery RB, Logothetis C, et al. Effect of neoadjuvant abiraterone acetate (AA) plus leuprolide acetate (LHRHa) on PSA, pathological complete response (pCR), and near pCR in localized high-risk prostate cancer (LHRPC): Results of a randomized phase II study. *J Clin Oncol* 2012;30:Abstr 4521.

# 43 Cancer of the Urethra and Penis

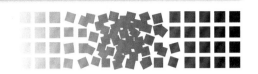

Edouard J. Trabulsi and Leonard G. Gomella

CANCERS OF THE GENITOURINARY SYSTEM

## INTRODUCTION

Penile and urethral carcinomas are uncommon malignancies, with a peak incidence in the 6th decade of life. Often overshadowed by more common genitourinary cancers, penile and urethral cancers represent difficult challenges for the treating physician. Squamous cell carcinoma is the most frequent type of cancer in the penis and the urethra. Carcinoma of the penis is a slow-growing tumor with a usually well-defined pattern of dissemination. This orderly spread allows definitive local–regional management of the primary tumor in most cases. In contradistinction, urethral carcinoma in men and women tends to invade locally and metastasize to regional nodes early. Depending on the site of the urethra involved and disease extent, a multimodal treatment approach may be required to treat this aggressive tumor.[1]

## CANCER OF THE MALE URETHRA

Carcinoma of the male urethra is uncommon. Chronic irritation and infection are the strongest risk factors. The incidence of urethral stricture in men with development of urethral cancer ranges from 24% to 76%, and most of these strictures involve the bulbomembranous urethra, also the most frequent site of cancer.[2] Human papillomavirus-16 (HPV-16) likely has a causative role in the development of squamous cell carcinoma of the urethra.[3] No racial predisposition has been noted.

The onset of malignancy in a patient with a longstanding urethral stricture disease is often insidious, and a high index of suspicion is needed to diagnose these tumors early. The new onset of urethrorrhagia or urethral stricture in a man without a history of trauma or venereal disease should raise the possibility of urethral carcinoma. A palpable urethral mass associated with obstructive voiding symptoms is the most common presenting symptom.[4] Pain associated with a periurethral abscess or urethral fistula may be the harbinger of a male urethral cancer.

### Pathology

Overall, 80% of male urethral cancers are squamous cell, 15% are urothelial (transitional cell), and approximately 5% are adenocarcinomas or undifferentiated tumors.[5] The anatomic location of urethral cancer largely determines the histologic type. Carcinomas of the prostatic urethra are urothelial in 90% and squamous in 10%; conversely, carcinomas of the penile urethra are squamous in 90% and urothelial in 10%. Adenocarcinomas of the urethra arise from metaplasia of mucosa or from periurethral glands, but direct invasion of rectal adenocarcinoma must be ruled out. Adenocarcinoma has the same prognosis, stage for stage, as the other histologies.[4]

The bulbomembranous urethra is most commonly involved (60%), followed by the penile urethra (30%) and the prostatic urethra (10%).[4] The incidence of urethral involvement associated with carcinoma of the bladder has been estimated to be approximately 6%,[6] and urethral recurrences after radical cystectomy occur in 4% to 17%.[7]

Male urethral cancer may spread locally to involve the corpus spongiosum or may metastasize to regional nodes. The lymphatics of the anterior urethra drain into the superficial and deep inguinal lymph nodes and occasionally to the external iliac nodes. The lymphatics from the posterior urethra drain into the external iliac, obturator, and hypogastric nodes. Palpable inguinal nodes are found in approximately 20% and almost always suggest metastatic disease, in contrast to penile cancer, where 50% of palpable nodes are inflammatory. Bulbomembranous urethral cancer in particular spreads to the urogenital diaphragm, prostate, perineum, and scrotum. Hematogenous spread is rare except in advanced disease and in primary transitional cell carcinoma of the prostatic urethra.

### Evaluation and Staging

The 2010 American Joint Committee on Cancer (AJCC) tumor, node, metastasis (TNM) staging system[8] is based on the depth of invasion of the primary tumor and the presence or absence of regional lymph node involvement and distant metastasis (Table 43.1). The 2010 AJCC system subdivides T1 lesions into T1a (no lymphovascular invasion or poorly differentiated tumors) and T1b (the presence of lymphovascular invasion or poorly differentiated histology); prostatic invasion is now reclassified as T4 disease (previously T3). Examination under anesthesia is useful to evaluate the local extent of disease. Cystoscopy and transurethral or needle biopsy of the lesion, and of the prostate if indicated, are also performed at the time of examination under anesthesia. A complete blood count and serum chemistry analysis coupled with urine culture and cytology are routinely obtained. Cytology is particularly helpful in patients with transitional cell carcinoma. A computed tomography (CT) scan with contrast is useful in local staging with magnetic resonance imaging (MRI) scan with gadolinium the ideal staging modality for evaluating local soft tissue, lymph node, and bone involvement.[9]

### Treatment

Surgery is the mainstay of treatment of carcinoma of the male urethra. In general, anterior urethral cancers are more amenable to surgical extirpation, and the prognosis is better than that of posterior urethral tumors, which are more often associated with extensive local invasion and distant metastasis.[10] Radiation therapy is reserved for patients with early-stage lesions of the anterior urethra who refuse surgery. Although it preserves the penis, radiation may cause urethral stricture or chronic penile edema and may not prevent new tumor occurrence. Multimodal treatment combining chemotherapy and radiation therapy with surgical excision for locally advanced urethral carcinomas has yielded promising results (disease-free survival 60% in one series).[11] The median survival without treatment or with palliation is approximately 3 months.

#### Site-Specific Treatment

**Carcinoma of the Distal Urethra.** Superficial tumors (Ta, Tis, and T1) are usually treated with transurethral resection and fulguration with close follow-up. Tumors invading the corpus

## TABLE 43.1

**American Joint Committee on Cancer Tumor, Node, Metastasis Classification System for Urethral Cancer**

### Stage Grouping

| | | | |
|---|---|---|---|
| 0a | Ta | N0 | M0 |
| 0is | Tis | N0 | M0 |
| | Tis (prostatic urethra) | N0 | M0 |
| | Tis (prostatic ducts) | N0 | M0 |
| I | T1 | N0 | M0 |
| II | T2 | N0 | M0 |
| III | T1 | N1 | M0 |
| | T2 | N1 | M0 |
| | T3 | N0 | M0 |
| | T4 | N1 | M0 |
| IV | T4 | N0 | M0 |
| | T4 | N1 | M0 |
| | Any T | N2 | M0 |
| | Any T | Any N | M1 |

From American Joint Committee on Cancer. *AJCC Cancer Staging Manual.* 7th ed. New York: Springer-Verlag; 2010, with permission.

spongiosum (T2) and localized to the distal half of the penis are best treated with a partial penile amputation with a 2-cm margin proximal to the visible or palpable tumor. If infiltrating tumor is confined to the proximal penile urethra or involves the entire urethra, total penectomy is indicated. Isolated reports of penile-sparing surgery (urethrectomy with corpora cavernosa sparing) have a high incidence of failure.[12] Ilioinguinal node dissection is indicated only in the presence of palpable adenopathy. Prophylactic groin dissection has no proven role in this site.

**Carcinoma of the Bulbomembranous Urethra.** Early superficial tumors (Ta, Tis, and T1) can be treated with transurethral fulguration or segmental resection with end-to-end anastomosis; however, such cases are rare. Invasive tumors (T2, T3) are best treated with radical cystoprostatectomy with en bloc penectomy and pelvic lymphadenectomy. Despite this aggressive approach, the prognosis remains dismal, with a 5-year disease-free survival of 26% in patients with invasive bulbomembranous carcinomas.[13] Isolated reports of penile preservation surgery for invasive bulbomembranous cancers have used adjuvant radiation therapy (45 Gy) and concurrent chemotherapy with 5-fluorouracil (5-FU) and mitomycin C with acceptable results.[14]

**Carcinoma of the Prostatic Urethra.** Primary carcinoma arising from the prostatic urethra is rare. Adenocarcinomas and urothelial carcinomas are found. Although superficial lesions (Tis-pu, Tis-pd, T1) can be managed by transurethral resection, such tumors are rare. Invasive urothelial carcinoma of the prostatic stroma (T2) carries a poor prognosis despite aggressive surgical therapy. Extravesical extension of disease has a worse prognosis than intraurethral disease, with a higher chance of nodal involvement and a 5-year survival rate of only 32%.[15]

Advanced carcinoma (T3-4N1 to N3) of the prostatic urethra is best treated with a combination of neoadjuvant chemotherapy (methotrexate sodium, vinblastine sulfate, doxorubicin hydrochloride [Adriamycin, Pharmacia S.p.A, Milan, Italy], and cisplatin [MVAC]) with consolidation surgery or irradiation. One series of five patients (with T2-4N0M0 lesions) treated with neoadjuvant

MVAC chemotherapy had a complete response rate of 60%.[16] MVAC chemotherapy preoperatively was ineffective against nonurothelial carcinoma.

### Radiation and Multimodal Therapy

Radiation therapy alone has poor results in male urethral carcinoma. Patients who receive radiation therapy followed by salvage surgery seem to fare worse than with surgery in an integrated fashion. The most common approach has been external-beam radiotherapy of 50 to 60 Gy with best results for *distal* urethral lesions. Multimodal therapy with chemoradiation has shown the efficacy of 5-FU, mitomycin C, and cisplatin with radiation for squamous cell carcinoma of the urethra.[17,18]

## CARCINOMA OF THE FEMALE URETHRA

Carcinoma of the urethra is the only genitourinary neoplasm that is more common in women than in men (four-to-one ratio). The peak incidence is in the sixth decade, more commonly in white women. Chronic irritation, recurrent urinary tract infections, and a host of proliferative lesions (caruncles, papillomas, polyps) are predisposing factors, and HPV may play a role. Leukoplakia of the urethra is considered a premalignant condition. In females, the urethra is approximately 4 cm long, mostly buried in the anterior vaginal wall, and divided into the distal one-third (anterior urethra) and the proximal two-thirds (posterior urethra). The most common presenting symptom (greater than 50%) is urethrorrhagia. Urinary frequency, obstructive voiding, a foul-smelling discharge, and a palpable urethral mass are other modes of presentation. Initially, it may be difficult to distinguish fungating tumors of the urethra from those of the vagina or vulva.

Spread of urethral carcinoma follows the anatomic subdivision: lymphatics of the anterior urethra drain into the superficial and deep inguinal nodes and the posterior urethra into the external iliac, hypogastric, and obturator nodes. At presentation, one-third of patients have inguinal lymph node metastases and 20% have pelvic node involvement. Palpable inguinal nodes in patients with urethral cancer invariably contain metastatic carcinoma. The most common sites of distant spread are the lungs, liver, and bone.[19]

An epidemiologic survey of female urethral cancer identified over 700 women in the Surveillance, Epidemiology, and End Results database.[20] No other study approaches this one in number of patients analyzed. The median overall survival in this large cohort was 42 months, with 5- and 10-year overall survival rates of 43% and 32%, respectively. The median cancer-specific survival was 78 months, and the 5- and 10-year cancer-specific survival was 53% and 46%, respectively. On multivariate analysis of nonmetastatic patients, variables predicting for worse cancer-specific survival were African-American race, stage T3 through T4 tumors, node-positive disease, nonsquamous cell histology, and advanced age.

### Pathology

Stratified squamous epithelium lines the distal two-thirds of the female urethra, and transitional epithelium (urothelium) lines the proximal one-third. The majority (60%) of neoplasms of the female urethra are squamous cell carcinomas. Less common types are urothelial carcinoma (20%), adenocarcinoma (10%), undifferentiated tumors (8%), and melanoma (2%). Clear cell carcinoma is a distinctive clinical entity that has generated considerable interest with respect to its prognosis and relationship to urethral diverticulae.[21] Histology does not affect the prognosis, and all are treated similarly. In general, anterior urethral carcinomas are low grade and stage; carcinomas involving the proximal or entire urethra are of a higher grade and stage.

## Evaluation and Staging

The workup for women with suspected urethral carcinoma includes a pelvic examination under anesthesia, cystourethroscopy, and biopsy. Radiographic evaluation includes a chest x-ray and CT of the pelvis and abdomen. MRI is particularly useful for staging of female urethral carcinoma. Although the 2010 AJCC TNM staging includes female urethral cancer,[8] the practical usefulness is limited. Clinically, it is more useful to stage, treat, and prognosticate female urethral cancers by stratifying patients based on anatomic location (anterior versus posterior urethra versus entire urethra) and clinical stage (low stage versus high stage).[22]

## Treatment

The anatomic location and stage of the tumor are the most significant prognostic factors predicting local control and survival. Treatment is based on the stage at the time of initial presentation, with low-stage distal urethral tumors having a better prognosis than high-stage proximal urethral tumors. In one series, the 5-year disease-specific survival was 46%, with 89% survival for low-stage tumors and 33% for high-stage disease.[23]

Local surgical excision is often sufficient in selected patients with low-stage distal urethra carcinoma. With proximal urethra and for bulky locally advanced tumors, more aggressive treatment with an anterior pelvic exenteration is often needed (en bloc total urethrectomy, cystectomy, pelvic lymphadenectomy, hysterectomy with salpingectomy, removal of the anterior vaginal wall). Bulky proximal urethral tumors that invade the pubic symphysis may require resection of the pubic symphysis and inferior rami. Anterior exenteration alone has been reported to produce a 5-year survival rate of <20% in patients with invasive carcinoma of the female urethra.[24] Radiation therapy (brachytherapy alone or with external-beam radiation) is an alternative to surgery in low-stage urethral carcinoma with cure rates up to 75%. The reported doses have ranged from 50 to 60 Gy for brachytherapy alone and 40 to 45 Gy external-beam radiation to the whole pelvis followed by a brachytherapy boost of 20 to 25 Gy over 2 to 3 days. Proximal urethral tumors with bladder neck invasion and bulky tumors require combined external-beam and brachytherapy. Large primary tumor bulk and treatment with external radiation alone (no brachytherapy) were independent adverse prognostic factors. Brachytherapy reduced the risk of local recurrence, possibly as a result of the higher radiation dose.[25] Complications from radiation therapy occur in about 20% and include urethral strictures and stenosis, urethrovaginal fistulas, incontinence, and bowel obstruction.

Combined modality treatment with neoadjuvant chemotherapy and preoperative radiation therapy, followed by surgery, is recommended for advanced female urethral carcinoma. A 55% survival rate has been reported with advanced urethral carcinoma treated with radiotherapy plus surgery, as compared with a rate of 34% with radiation alone.[26] Although long-term results from multimodal therapy are not yet available, combination chemotherapy, radiation, and surgery is believed essential for local control and cure with larger or locally advanced urethral cancer.[23] The prognosis for women with carcinoma of the urethra is poor, regardless of the treatment modality used, and the median time to local recurrence for invasive carcinoma is 13 months.

## Distal Urethral Carcinoma

Small superficial (Ta, Tis, and T1) tumors of the distal female urethra can be removed surgically with little risk of urinary incontinence. Spatulation of the urethra and approximation to the adjacent vagina preserve urinary continence and prevent meatal stenosis. For small invasive tumors of the distal urethra (T2), brachytherapy alone is an excellent therapeutic option.

## Proximal Urethral Carcinoma

Proximal female urethral carcinomas tend to be more aggressive and bulky. For advanced (T3 and T4) lesions, a multimodal approach is preferred. Surgery consists of a radical cystourethrectomy or an anterior exenteration, depending on the extent of the disease. Radiation therapy with a combination of brachytherapy and external-beam irradiation is usually required. Neoadjuvant chemotherapy with 5-FU and mitomycin C has been noted to enhance the therapeutic ratio of radiation therapy.

# CANCER OF THE PENIS

Carcinoma of the penis is an uncommon malignancy in Western countries, representing 0.4% of male malignancies and 3.0% of all genitourinary cancers. Penile cancer constitutes a major health problem in many countries in Asia, Africa, and South America, where it may comprise up to 10% of all malignancies. The incidence of penile cancer has been declining in many countries, partly because of increased attention to personal hygiene.[27] It most commonly presents in the sixth decade but may occur in men younger than 40 years. Analysis of the Surveillance, Epidemiology, and End Results database data shows no racial difference in the incidence of penile cancer among African American men and white men, but significant disparities exist in the mortality of invasive penile carcinoma in the United States.[28] Significantly lower rates of invasive penile cancer are seen in Asian American men and significantly higher rates are seen in Hispanic American men. Regional and socioeconomic differences are also noted, with higher rates in the southern area of the United States and in lower socioeconomic populations.

## Etiology

Penile cancer is associated with phimosis and poor local hygiene, with phimosis found in more than half the patients. The irritative effect of smegma, a byproduct of bacterial action on desquamated epithelial cells in the preputial sac, is well known, although definitive evidence of its role in carcinogenesis is lacking. Neonatal circumcision as practiced by religious groups virtually eliminates the occurrence of penile carcinoma. While circumcision can reduce the risk of various sexually transmitted diseases such as HIV, and possibly HPV and herpes virus, delaying circumcision until puberty or adult circumcision does not have the same benefit with respect to penile cancer.[29]

HPV infection, particularly HPV-16, has been implicated in the development of invasive penile cancer, as has the number of sexual partners.[29] HPV infection accounts for about half of penile cancers, with HPV-16 and -18 the predominant subtypes.[30,31] Evidence now indicates that penile cancer has two primary etiologies: approximately half are related to HPV infection, with the other half related to inflammatory conditions such as phimosis, chronic balanitis, and lichen sclerosis.[32] The use of tobacco products is an independent risk factor.[33] Thus, avoidance of tobacco products and HPV infection, penile hygiene, and neonatal circumcision represent important preventive strategies against penile cancer. Vaccination of younger men against HPV is controversial but may change the incidence and burden of this disease.[34,35]

## Symptoms

Local symptoms and signs often draw attention to penile cancer. The clinical spectrum of penile cancer is varied: subtle areas of erythema or induration to a frankly ulcerated, fungating, foul-smelling mass. Penile cancer is commonly associated with concomitant infection, with infection playing an important role in the pathogenesis and ultimately in the presentation of the disease. Pain usually is not a prominent feature and is not proportional to the extent of local destruction. The lesion primarily involves the prepuce and glans, often under a tight phimotic ring. In late stages, involvement and destruction of the shaft of the penis or urethra are seen. Urethral obstruction is rare. Instead, erosion of the urethra with multiple fistulas ("watering-can perineum") may be seen. Rarely, inguinal ulceration may be the presenting symptom, with the primary tumor concealed within a phimotic preputial sac.

Patients with penile cancer, more than with other types of cancer, delay seeking medical attention. Historically, up to 50% of patients delayed more than 1 year in seeking medical help; contemporary series, especially from the United States, fail to show such a trend.

## Pathology

More than 95% of penile carcinomas are squamous cell. Nonsquamous cell carcinomas consist of melanomas, basal cell carcinomas, lymphomas, and sarcomas. Nearly 18% of patients with acquired immunodeficiency syndrome–related Kaposi sarcoma have penile involvement.[36]

Squamous cell carcinomas are graded using Broder classification. Low-grade tumors (grades I and II), typically confined to the prepuce and glans penis, constitute nearly 80% of penile cancers. Most lesions that involve the shaft of the penis are high grade (grade III), with grade and stage often correlated. The incidence of lymph node metastases from squamous cell carcinoma of the penis is related to histologic grade. Verrucous carcinoma, a particularly exuberant variant of squamous cell carcinoma, has low potential for lymph node spread and a good prognosis. Another important predictor of lymph node metastases and, hence, prognosis is the presence of vascular invasion.[37]

## Premalignant Lesions

The description of early and premalignant lesions has been complicated by the rarity of the disease and a proliferation of eponyms.

### Leukoplakia

Leukoplakia is characterized by the presence of solitary or multiple whitish plaques involving the glans or prepuce in the setting of chronic or recurrent balanoposthitis. Surgical excision in the form of circumcision or local wedge resection is usually curative.

### Balanitis Xerotica Obliterans

Balanitis xerotica obliterans (BXO) is an inflammatory condition of the glans and prepuce of unknown cause; it is a form of lichen sclerosis isolated to the penis. BXO is a scaly, indurated, whitish plaque that produces significant phimosis and meatal stenosis. Although selected reports suggest an association with penile cancer, treatment remains controversial and consists of topical steroids and surgical excision. Meatoplasty may be required, with early circumcision the most effective treatment for BXO.[38]

### Buschke-Löwenstein Tumor

The Buschke-Löwenstein tumor is a large exophytic mass involving the glans penis and prepuce; it is a giant condyloma acuminatum that has a good prognosis and does not metastasize. Except for unrestrained local growth, this lesion has malignant features. A viral etiology has been proposed, with identification of HPV-6 and -11 in some tumors. Treatment consists of local conservative resection. Recurrence is common. Systemic interferon-α therapy combined with neodymium: yttrium aluminum garnet (Nd:YAG) laser therapy is successful in some cases. Radiation therapy is contraindicated because rapid malignant degeneration has been described.

## Diagnosis and Staging

The workup for penile cancer begins with physical examination of the genitalia and inguinal nodes to ascertain local extent of the

### TABLE 43.2

**American Joint Committee on Cancer Tumor, Node, Metastasis Classification System for Penile Cancer**

**Stage Grouping**

| | | | |
|---|---|---|---|
| 0 | Tis | N0 | M0 |
| | Ta | N0 | M0 |
| I | T1a | N0 | M0 |
| II | T1b | N0 | M0 |
| | T2 | N0 | M0 |
| | T3 | N0 | M0 |
| IIIa | T1-3 | N1 | M0 |
| IIIb | T1-3 | N2 | M0 |
| IV | T4 | Any N | M0 |
| | Any T | N3 | M0 |
| | Any T | Any N | M1 |

From American Joint Committee on Cancer. *AJCC Cancer Staging Manual.* 7th ed. New York: Springer-Verlag; 2010, with permission.

lesion and the presence of inguinal adenopathy. Nodal status is the most significant prognostic variable predicting survival. Approximately 50% of patients with penile cancer present with palpable inguinal nodes. Only half of these patients will have metastatic disease, with the remainder having inflammatory adenopathy secondary to infection of the primary lesion. Conversely, 20% of patients with clinically negative groin examination are found to have metastases on prophylactic node dissection. The most common distant metastatic sites are the lung, bone, and liver. The AJCC system (seventh edition) for staging penile cancer uses the TNM classification to determine the stage of the primary tumor and the extent of nodal metastases (Table 43.2).[8] After biopsy confirmation of the lesion, no further radiologic workup is generally needed in patients with early-stage disease and the absence of inguinal adenopathy on examination or other worrisome symptoms. Ultrasound and gadolinium-enhanced MRI are recommended for high-grade and high-stage lesions suspected of involving the corporal bodies, especially if partial penectomy is contemplated. Abdominal and pelvic CT scanning is recommended in obese patients to evaluate the inguinal nodes. In patients with known inguinal metastases, CT-guided biopsy of enlarged pelvic nodes, if positive, may be an indication for neoadjuvant chemotherapy. The role of positron emission tomography scan in the staging of penile cancer is unclear, with conflicting data.[39–41]

## Treatment

Treatment of penile carcinoma depends on the local extent of the primary neoplasm and the regional lymph node status. For the primary lesion, a 2-cm proximal margin of resection is recommended. If an adequate margin can be obtained, a partial penectomy offers excellent local control. Leaving the patient with adequate penile length for hygienic upright micturition and sexual intercourse is the goal. Thus, depending on the extent of the primary tumor, resection may include a partial or total penectomy, with local recurrence rare.[42]

In advanced cases (T4), more aggressive resections (emasculation, hemipelvectomy, hemicorpectomy) have been reported with mixed results. Although surgery is the mainstay for treatment of the primary lesion, radiation therapy can be considered for a select group of patients. Radiation therapy allows preservation of the penis, obviating the psychosocial and physical morbidity caused by partial or total penectomy. External-beam and brachytherapy techniques have been used for treatment of the primary cancer. Circumcision is generally recommended before radiation therapy is initiated. This allows for further evaluation of the tumor extent and reduces morbidity associated with radiation (swelling, maceration, secondary infection), all of which may eventually result in secondary phimosis. Local control and penile preservation rates approaching 70% at 10 years have been reported for carefully selected early (T1 to T2) lesions.[43] Treatment of more advanced penile cancers has a much higher risk of local recurrence and progression to nodal and systemic disease.[44] Thus, radiation therapy, although cosmetically attractive, has disadvantages, and the number of patients for whom this treatment is appropriate is small.

Of paramount importance in treatment is consideration of the lymphatic drainage of the penis. The inguinal lymph nodes constitute the first echelon of drainage. Superficial and deep inguinal nodes are involved in a stepwise manner. Bilateral drainage occurs as a result of free anastomoses and crossover at the base of the penis. Therefore, the pattern of nodal metastasis is not limited to one side. The superficial inguinal nodes are located in the deep portion of Camper fascia above the deep fascia of the thigh (fascia lata). The superficial lymphatics drain into the deep inguinal lymphatics, which surround the femoral vessels deep to the fascia lata. Secondary drainage is to the iliac nodes, although direct drainage to these nodes (skip metastasis) can occur rarely.

Five-year disease-free survival rates for palpably negative adenopathy (cN0) or low volume palpable groin disease (cN1) are similar and favorable at 93% and 84%, respectively, with a markedly worse survival for palpably bulky disease (cN2 or cN3) of 32% and 0%, respectively.[45] When stratified by pathologic stage, low volume nodal involvement (pN1) had favorable and similar 5-year disease-free survival rates when compared to pathologically negative nodes (pN0) at 93% and 90%, respectively. Pathologically confirmed bulky adenopathy (pN2 and pN3) had very poor long-term outcomes with 5-year disease-free survival rates of 31% and 0%, respectively.

Based on the rarity of advanced penile carcinoma in the Western world, there is growing awareness that these men may receive better outcomes if they are directed to tertiary care centers with expertise in penile carcinoma and inguinal lymphadenectomy. In the United Kingdom, the National Institute for Clinical Excellence published guidelines in 2002 that included the treatment of penile carcinoma and advocated the creation of regional multidisciplinary teams.[46] These guidelines have increased the rate of penis-preserving procedures and inguinal lymphadenectomy, with decreased mortality.[47]

## Treatment of Primary Lesion

Surgery for penile carcinoma ranges from circumcision, conservative local resection, laser ablation, and Mohs micrographic surgery to partial and total penectomy. Radiation therapy can be used in selected patients with early superficial lesions.

### Carcinoma In Situ (Tis).

Penile squamous cell carcinoma in situ, also known as erythroplasia of Queyrat, is a red, velvety, well-marginated lesion of the glans penis or the prepuce of uncircumcised men. After confirmatory biopsy, a conservative approach that spares penile anatomy and function is preferred. Preputial lesions are adequately treated with circumcision. Topical 5-FU cream and imiquimod have been used with excellent cosmetic results for glandular and meatal lesions (imiquimod 5% cream for 5 days per week for 4 to 6 weeks or 5-FU 5% cream every other day for 4 to 6 weeks). A prospective study of carbon dioxide and Nd:YAG lasers has shown good local tumor control and satisfactory cosmetic results.[48] Mohs micrographic surgery has been described as a less-deforming alternative, with local control rates up to 86% in selected patients with early penile cancer.[49] Radiation therapy can often eradicate these lesions with minimal morbidity.

### Verrucous Carcinoma (Ta).

Penile verrucous carcinoma is characterized by aggressive local growth and a low metastatic potential. Partial or total penectomy is usually overtreatment, and conservative therapeutic approaches are favored. Laser ablation or Mohs micrographic surgical technique has yielded acceptable results. Intra-aortic infusion with methotrexate has been reported with reasonable results.[50] Radiation therapy is contraindicated as it has been shown to cause subsequent rapid malignant degeneration and metastases.

### Invasive Penile Cancer (T1, T2, T3, and N1).

Distal penile lesions, in which a serviceable penis for upright micturition and sexual function can be achieved, are best treated with a partial penectomy. Extensive lesions that approach the base of the penis usually require total penectomy with corporal body excision and perineal urethrostomy. Local recurrence after a partial penectomy in properly selected cases is rare. Most relapses occur within the first 12 to 18 months after penectomy, and salvage surgery is beneficial.

The effectiveness of radiation therapy in the treatment of penile cancer is hindered by a lack of uniformity of radiation treatment in terms of type of delivery and doses. Radiation therapy is effective for local control of small, 2- to 4-cm, T1 and T2 lesions but also for more advanced T-stage tumors. Local recurrence is higher in those with T3 and T4 tumors, but a significant percentage can be salvaged by adjuvant surgical resection.[51] Before treatment, patients should have a circumcision to allow direct inspection and staging of the tumor and to facilitate management of the acute side effects of radiation. External-beam and brachytherapy techniques have been used. External-beam radiotherapy can be delivered by a direct field method that uses a low-energy photon beam or an electron beam applied directly to the tumor, with a safety margin of 2 cm beyond the visible and palpable extent of the tumor. This approach is suitable only for very superficial tumors (Tis and T1). For T2 and T3 lesions, a parallel opposed field method is used. Using this approach, the entire thickness of the penis can be irradiated by encasing the lesion in a wax mold to ensure uniform dosage and to negate the skin-sparing effects of supervoltage beams with a total dose of 60 Gy recommended. A 65% to 80% local success rate has been reported with radiation therapy for small T1 and T2 tumors.[43] Brachytherapy involves placement of radioactive material (usually iridium-192 wire) within the tumor (interstitial brachytherapy) or molded around the tumor (plesio-brachytherapy) and is limited to T1 and T2 tumors. This form of therapy is not suitable for patients with bulky tumors, deeply infiltrating tumors, and obese patients with a short penis. Radiation therapy as primary treatment for invasive penile carcinoma has significant disadvantages: acute effects of skin edema, maceration, and dysuria may persist for 6 to 8 weeks. Telangiectasia and fibrosis are found in more than 90% of cases. The most serious late effects are urethral fistula, meatal stenosis, and penile necrosis. Postradiation fibrosis, scar, and necrosis may be difficult to distinguish from recurrent cancer. Infection is very often associated with penile cancer and reduces the therapeutic efficacy of radiation while increasing the risk of penile necrosis. Thus, in summary, radiation therapy for primary penile cancer should be considered only in a select group of patients: young patients with small (2 to 4 cm) superficial lesions of the distal penis who wish to maintain penile integrity, patients who refuse surgery, and patients with inoperable cancer or those unsuitable for major surgery.

### Advanced Penile Cancer (T4, N2-3, and M1).

Large proximal shaft tumors require a total penectomy with a perineal urethrostomy. For extensive, proximal tumors with invasion of adjacent structures, total emasculation (total penectomy, scrotectomy, and orchiectomy) is recommended. In extreme cases, a hemipelvectomy or even a hemicorporectomy has been described. Multimodal therapy with chemoradiation and salvage surgery has also been used in this setting.

## Management of Regional Lymph Nodes

The presence and extent of inguinal lymph node metastases are the most important prognostic factors in penile cancer. Although 50% of patients with a penile lesion have clinically palpable inguinal nodes at presentation, in more than half of these the adenopathy is inflammatory. A 4- to 6-week course of antibiotics (e.g., first- or second-generation cephalosporin) after treatment of the primary lesion is recommended. Persistent palpable adenopathy after antibiotic therapy should be biopsied. Unlike many other genitourinary malignancies that require systemic chemotherapy, once lymph node metastases are discovered, inguinal metastases from penile cancer are potentially curable by lymphadenectomy alone. Inguinal lymphadenectomy therefore should be performed at the earliest suspicion of metastases.

### Clinical Node Negative (N0).

Although there is no controversy in the literature regarding management of the patient with clinically positive inguinal lymph nodes after a course of antibiotics, considerable controversy surrounds the management of the clinically N0 patient. Approximately 20% of these clinically negative groins harbor occult lymphatic metastases on prophylactic lymph node dissection. Stated another way, approximately 80% of patients with clinically negative groins would be subjected to the morbidity of inguinal lymph node dissection without benefit. To resolve this dilemma, a risk-based approach to management of the clinically negative groin has been recommended in most contemporary series. Analysis of histopathologic data from the primary penile cancer allows stratification of patients into high- and low-risk groups for lymph node metastases.[52]

*Low-Risk Group.* Patients with carcinoma in situ (Tis), verrucous carcinoma (Ta), and T1 tumors who have grade 1 or 2 tumor histology have a <10% chance of developing lymph node metastases and are best served by surveillance and a low incidence of lymphovascular invasion, a risk for nodal metastasis.[37]

*High-Risk Group.* Patients with invasive penile cancer (T2 and T3) with grade 3 tumors and the presence of vascular invasion have a >50% incidence of inguinal lymph node metastases in various series. Vascular invasion is strongly correlated with lymph node metastases. In pT2 patients, the incidence of lymph node metastases was found to be 75% in the presence of vascular invasion and only 25% when vascular invasion was absent.[52] In this cohort of patients, a prophylactic lymphadenectomy is reasonable.

The timing of surgery in the clinically negative groin has been debated in the past. Most contemporary series favor *early adjunctive* lymphadenectomy, especially in the high-risk group, over surveillance and *delayed therapeutic* lymphadenectomy. Sentinel lymph node biopsy, originally described by Cabanas,[53] is no longer recommended in view of the high false-negative rate. Intraoperative lymphatic mapping using dynamic scintigraphy with technetium-labeled sulfur colloid have decreased the false-negative rate considerably.[54] Other approaches that use sentinel lymph node biopsy have also been advocated, including measurement of the size of the micrometastatic sentinel lymph node to determine whether to perform lymphadenectomy.[55] Sentinel node biopsy remains controversial, with recent studies demonstrating a much lower false negative rate,[56,57] but further data are required.[58] Lymphotropic nanoparticle-enhanced MRI has been investigated to detect micrometastasis but awaits validation.[59]

Inguinal lymph node dissection superficial to the fascia lata has been found to be adequate for the N0 patient. Superficial inguinal lymph node dissection should include a frozen section, and if positive, a modified complete dissection should be carried out. Creation of thicker skin flaps, control of infection, and preservation of the areolar fat superficial to the Scarpa fascia have greatly decreased the complications of flap necrosis, scrotal and extremity edema, lymphocele, and lymphorrhea.

*Prediction Models.* Ficarra et al.[60] and Kattan et al.[61] have developed predictive nomograms to help determine an individual patient's risk of nodal involvement and cancer-specific survival. One nomogram to predict the probability of lymph node involvement uses eight clinical and pathologic variables (tumor thickness, growth pattern, grade, lymphovascular invasion, corpora cavernosal involvement, spongiosal involvement, urethral involvement, palpable lymph nodes).[60] Not surprisingly, clinically suspicious inguinal lymph nodes are a powerful predictor of pathologic nodal involvement. For cancer-specific survival of patients who undergo surgery for squamous cell carcinoma of the penis, two separate nomograms were created, depending on whether clinical or pathologic staging of inguinal lymph nodes was used.[61] These nomograms may guide patients and clinicians alike on the appropriate treatment and can potentially avoid the risks of lymph node dissection in low-risk patients.

### Clinical Node Positive (N1, N2, or N3).

The modified inguinal lymph node dissection as described by Catalona[62] has replaced the standard complete inguinal lymphadenectomy as the procedure of choice with clinically persistent nodes after antibiotics. It involves a smaller incision, limited field of inguinal dissection, and preservation of the saphenous vein in an effort to reduce the morbidity of the standard procedure while adhering to standard oncologic principles. Unlike superficial dissection, the deep nodes within the fossa ovalis are also removed. In the face of synchronous unilateral N+ disease, it is standard practice to proceed with a bilateral lymph node dissection in view of the high incidence of bilateral drainage. The exception to this rule is the patient with a clinically negative groin in whom metachronous unilateral inguinal lymphadenopathy develops sometime after treatment of the primary tumor. In these patients, a unilateral dissection of the clinically positive groin usually suffices. The value of pelvic lymphadenectomy in the presence of positive inguinal lymph nodes is for the purposes of staging and identifying patients who would be candidates for adjuvant chemotherapy and had little therapeutic efficacy (5-year survival with pelvic lymph node metastases is <5%).

Patients with advanced nodal disease or bulky fixed inguinal nodes (N3) may require neoadjuvant radiation or chemotherapy before any surgery. Groin lymph nodes adherent to or fungating through the skin require wide excision with myocutaneous flaps to cover the skin defect. The published literature unequivocally favors surgical resection as superior to radiation therapy for the treatment of inguinal lymph nodes. Clinical evaluation of the groin is difficult because of postradiation tissue changes, and the inguinal area tolerates radiation rather poorly. Radiation therapy can be used as a palliative measure in patients with fixed inoperable inguinal nodes or in those with advanced unresectable penile cancer in which the primary and the ilioinguinal region can be treated with radiation therapy.

## Role of Chemotherapy and Multimodality Therapy

The role of chemotherapy in the management of penile carcinoma is evolving, and the exact role of chemotherapy has not been established. Data suggest that penile cancer is sensitive to chemotherapy.[63] Besides the use of 5-FU in the treatment of superficial penile cancer, single-agent chemotherapy with cisplatin, methotrexate, and bleomycin has modest activity in advanced penile cancer. The combination of methotrexate, bleomycin, and cisplatin is more active than cisplatin alone but is associated with marked toxicity. Anti–epidermal growth factor receptor therapy may also hold some promise in this disease.[64]

The Southwest Oncology Group reported on the largest prospective clinical trial in patients with penile cancer.[65] In 40 evaluable patients treated with a combination of methotrexate, bleomycin, and cisplatin, an overall response of 32.5% and a complete response of 12.5% were observed. The median response duration was 16 weeks, and the median survival was 28 weeks. Toxicity was formidable, with 11% treatment-related mortality, and 17% of the remaining patients experiencing life-threatening toxicity. Another prospective trial from a UK consortium reported on 29 patients treated with three 21-day cycles of TPF (docetaxel 75 mg/m$^2$ and cisplatin 60 mg/m$^2$ on day 1 and 5-FU 750 mg/m$^2$ per day days 1 to 5) in patients with locally advanced or metastatic penile cancer. The objective response rate was 28.5% and 1-year overall survival rate was 55%, demonstrating activity of this regimen in advanced penile cancer. There was significant toxicity, however, with neutropenic fever in 25% and dose delays or reductions in nearly half

of patients.[66] Multimodality therapy, using a combination of chemotherapy and surgery or chemotherapy and radiation, has been used in isolated reports of advanced penile cancer. Small series in men with fixed, unresectable inguinal nodes had neoadjuvant vincristine, bleomycin, and methotrexate before surgery with some long-term responses.[67] Another small series of patients who underwent surgical resection after neoadjuvant chemotherapy for unresectable penile squamous cell were treated with several different chemotherapy combinations, including bleomycin, methotrexate, cisplatin; ifosfamide, paclitaxel, cisplatin; or paclitaxel/carboplatin with some responses.[68] Clearly, more tolerable and active regimens are needed for unresectable or metastatic penile cancer.

## REFERENCES

1. Tefilli MV, Gheiler EL, Shekarriz B, et al. Primary adenocarcinoma of the urethra with metastasis to the glans penis: successful treatment with chemotherapy and radiation therapy. *Urology* 1998;52:517–519.
2. Sharp DS, Angermeier KW. Surgery of penile and urethral carcinoma. In: Wein AJ, ed. *Campbell-Walsh Urology*. 9th ed. Philadelphia: WB Saunders; 2007:993.
3. Wiener JS, Liu ET, Walther PJ. Oncogenic human papillomavirus type 16 is associated with squamous cell cancer of the male urethra. *Cancer Res* 1992;52:5018–5023.
4. Russell AH, Dalbagni G. Cancer of the urethra. In: Vogelzang NJ, Scardino PT, Scardino WU, et al., eds. *Comprehensive Textbook of Genitourinary Oncology*. 3rd ed. Philadelphia: Lippincott Williams & Wilkins; 2006:883.
5. Grabstald H. Proceedings: Tumors of the urethra in men and women. *Cancer* 1973;32:1236–1255.
6. Erckert M, Stenzl A, Falk M, et al. Incidence of urethral tumor involvement in 910 men with bladder cancer. *World J Urol* 1996;14:3–8.
7. Sherwood JB, Sagalowsky AI. The diagnosis and treatment of urethral recurrence after radical cystectomy. *Urol Oncol* 2006;24:356–361.
8. American Joint Committee on Cancer. *AJCC Cancer Staging Manual*. 7th ed. New York: Springer-Verlag; 2010.
9. Ryu JA, Kim B. MR imaging of primary urethral lymphoma in a man. *AJR* 2003;181:600–601.
10. Zeidman EJ, Desmond P, Thompson IM. Surgical treatment of carcinoma of the male urethra. *Urol Clin North Am* 1992;19:359–372.
11. Gheiler EL, Tefilli MV, Tiguert R, et al. Management of primary urethral cancer. *Urology* 1998;52:487–493.
12. Davis JW, Schellhammer PF, Schlossberg SM. Conservative surgical therapy for penile and urethral carcinoma. *Urology* 1999;53:386–392.
13. Dalbagni G, Zhang ZF, Lacombe L, et al. Male urethral carcinoma: analysis of treatment outcome. *Urology* 1999;53:1126–1132.
14. Christopher N, Arya M, Brown RS, et al. Penile preservation in squamous cell carcinoma of the bulbomembranous urethra. *BJU Int* 2002;89:464–465.
15. Shen SS, Lerner SP, Muezzinoglu B, et al. Prostatic involvement by transitional cell carcinoma in patients with bladder cancer and its prognostic significance. *Hum Pathol* 2006;37:726–734.
16. Scher HI, Yagoda A, Herr HW, et al. Neoadjuvant M-VAC (methotrexate, vinblastine, doxorubicin and cisplatin) for extravesical urinary tract tumors. *J Urol* 1988;139:475–477.
17. Oberfield RA, Zinman LN, Leibenhaut M, et al. Management of invasive squamous cell carcinoma of the bulbomembranous male urethra with co-ordinated chemo-radiotherapy and genital preservation. *Br J Urol* 1996;78:573–578.
18. Licht MR, Klein EA, Bukowski R, et al. Combination radiation and chemotherapy for the treatment of squamous cell carcinoma of the male and female urethra. *J Urol* 1995;153:1918–1920.
19. Srinivas V, Khan SA. Female urethral cancer—an overview. *Int Urol Nephrol* 1987;19:423–427.
20. Champ CE, Hegarty SE, Shen X, et al. Prognostic factors and outcomes after definitive treatment of female urethral cancer: a population-based analysis. *Urology* 2012;80:374–381.
21. Tiguert R, Ravery V, Madjar S, et al. [Acute urinary retention secondary to clear cell adenocarcinoma of the urethra]. *Prog Urol* 2001;11:70–72.
22. Sailer SL, Shipley WU, Wang CC. Carcinoma of the female urethra: a review of results with radiation therapy. *J Urol* 1988;140:1–5.
23. Dalbagni G, Zhang ZF, Lacombe L, et al. Female urethral carcinoma: an analysis of treatment outcome and a plea for a standardized management strategy. *Br J Urol* 1998;82:835–841.
24. Grabstald H, Hilaris B, Henschke U, et al. Cancer of the female urethra. *JAMA* 1966;197:835–842.
25. Milosevic MF, Warde PR, Banerjee D, et al. Urethral carcinoma in women: results of treatment with primary radiotherapy. *Radiother Oncol* 2000;56:29–35.
26. Narayan P, Konety B. Surgical treatment of female urethral carcinoma. *Urol Clin North Am* 1992;19:373–382.
27. Yeole BB, Jussawalla DJ. Descriptive epidemiology of the cancers of male genital organs in greater Bombay. *Indian J Cancer* 1997;34:30–39.

28. Hernandez BY, Barnholtz-Sloan J, German RR, et al. Burden of invasive squamous cell carcinoma of the penis in the United States, 1998–2003. *Cancer* 2008;113:2883–2891.
29. Maden C, Sherman KJ, Beckmann AM, et al. History of circumcision, medical conditions, and sexual activity and risk of penile cancer. *J Natl Cancer Inst* 1993;85:19–24.
30. Miralles-Guri C, Bruni L, Cubilla AL, et al. Human papillomavirus prevalence and type distribution in penile carcinoma. *J Clin Pathol* 2009;62:870–878.
31. Backes DM, Kurman RJ, Pimenta JM, et al. Systematic review of human papillomavirus prevalence in invasive penile cancer. *Cancer Causes Control* 2009;20:449–457.
32. Chaux A, Cubilla AL. The role of human papillomavirus infection in the pathogenesis of penile squamous cell carcinomas. *Sem Diagn Pathol* 2012;29:67–71.
33. Harish K, Ravi R. The role of tobacco in penile carcinoma. *Br J Urol* 1995;75:375–377.
34. Bosch FX, Broker TR, Forman D, et al. Comprehensive control of human papillomavirus infections and related diseases. *Vaccine* 2013;31:G1–G31.
35. Flaherty A, Kim T, Giuliano A, et al. Implications for human papillomavirus in penile cancer. *Urol Oncol* 2014;32:53.e1–e8.
36. Grossman HB. Premalignant and early carcinomas of the penis and scrotum. *Urol Clin North Am* 1992;19:221–226.
37. Lopes A, Hidalgo GS, Kowalski LP, et al. Prognostic factors in carcinoma of the penis: multivariate analysis of 145 patients treated with amputation and lymphadenectomy. *J Urol* 1996;156:1637–1642.
38. Depasquale I, Park AJ, Bracka A. The treatment of balanitis xerotica obliterans. *BJU Int* 2000;86:459–465.
39. Scher B, Seitz M, Reiser M, et al. 18F-FDG PET/CT for staging of penile cancer. *J Nucl Med* 2005;46:1460–1465.
40. Graafland NM, Leijte JA, Valdes Olmos RA, et al. Scanning with 18F-FDG-PET/CT for detection of pelvic nodal involvement in inguinal node-positive penile carcinoma. *Eur Urol* 2009;56:339–345.
41. Leijte JA, Graafland NM, Valdes Olmos RA, et al. Prospective evaluation of hybrid 18F-fluorodeoxyglucose positron emission tomography/computed tomography in staging clinically node-negative patients with penile carcinoma. *BJU Int* 2009;104:640–644.
42. Korets R, Koppie TM, Snyder ME, et al. Partial penectomy for patients with squamous cell carcinoma of the penis: the Memorial Sloan-Kettering experience. *Ann Surg Oncol* 2007;14:3614–3619.
43. Crook JM, Haie-Meder C, Demanes DJ, et al. American Brachytherapy Society-Groupe Europeen de Curietherapie-European Society of Therapeutic Radiation Oncology (ABS-GEC-ESTRO) consensus statement for penile brachytherapy. *Brachytherapy* 2013;12:191–198.
44. Crook JM, Jezioranski J, Grimard L, et al. Penile brachytherapy: results for 49 patients. *Int J Radiat Oncol Biol Phys* 2005;62:460–467.
45. Marconnet L, Bouchot O, Culine S, et al. [Treatment of lymph nodes in epidermoid carcinoma of the penis: review of literature by the Committee of Cancerology of the French Association of Urology-External Genital Organs Group (CCAFU-OGE)]. *Prog Urol* 2010;20:332–342.
46. National Institute for Clinical Excellence. *Improving Outcomes in Urological Cancers: The Research Evidence*. London: National Institute for Health and Clinical Excellence; 2002.
47. Bayles AC, Sethia KK. The impact of Improving Outcomes Guidance on the management and outcomes of patients with carcinoma of the penis. *Ann R Coll Surg Engl* 2010;92:44–45.
48. Windahl T, Andersson SO. Combined laser treatment for penile carcinoma: results after long-term followup. *J Urol* 2003;169(6):2118–2121.
49. Mohs FE, Snow SN, Larson PO. Mohs micrographic surgery for penile tumors. *Urol Clin North Am* 1992;19:291–304.
50. Sheen MC, Sheu HM, Huang CH, et al. Penile verrucous carcinoma successfully treated by intra-aortic infusion with methotrexate. *Urology* 2003;61:1216–1220.
51. Krieg R, Hoffman R. Current management of unusual genitourinary cancers. Part 1: Penile cancer. *Oncology* 1999;13:1347–1352.
52. Slaton JW, Morgenstern N, Levy DA, et al. Tumor stage, vascular invasion and the percentage of poorly differentiated cancer: independent prognosticators

for inguinal lymph node metastasis in penile squamous cancer. *J Urol* 2001;165:1138–1142.

53. Cabanas RM. An approach for the treatment of penile carcinoma. *Cancer* 1977;39:456–466.

54. Jakub JW, Pendas S, Reintgen DS. Current status of sentinel lymph node mapping and biopsy: facts and controversies. *Oncologist* 2003;8:59–68.

55. Kroon BK, Nieweg OE, van Boven H, et al. Size of metastasis in the sentinel node predicts additional nodal involvement in penile carcinoma. *J Urol* 2006;176:105–108.

56. Leijte JA, Hughes B, Graafland NM, et al. Two-center evaluation of dynamic sentinel node biopsy for squamous cell carcinoma of the penis. *J Clin Oncol* 2009;27:3325–3329.

57. Jensen JB, Jensen KM, Ulhoi BP, et al. Sentinel lymph-node biopsy in patients with squamous cell carcinoma of the penis. *BJU Int* 2009;103:1199–1203.

58. Loughlin KR. Is sentinel node biopsy indicated in penile cancer? *Nat Clin Pract Urol* 2007;4:80–81.

59. Tabatabaei S, Harisinghani M, McDougal WS. Regional lymph node staging using lymphotropic nanoparticle enhanced magnetic resonance imaging with ferumoxtran-10 in patients with penile cancer. *J Urol* 2005;174: 923–927; discussion 927.

60. Ficarra V, Zattoni F, Artibani W, et al. Nomogram predictive of pathological inguinal lymph node involvement in patients with squamous cell carcinoma of the penis. *J Urol* 2006;175:1700–1704; discussion 1704–1705.

61. Kattan MW, Ficarra V, Artibani W, et al. Nomogram predictive of cancer specific survival in patients undergoing partial or total amputation for squamous cell carcinoma of the penis. *J Urol* 2006;175:2103–2108; discussion 2108.

62. Catalona WJ. Modified inguinal lymphadenectomy for carcinoma of the penis with preservation of saphenous veins: technique and preliminary results. *J Urol* 1988;140:306–310.

63. Trabulsi EJ, Hoffman-Censits J. Chemotherapy for penile and urethral carcinoma. *Urol Clin North Am* 2010;37:467–474.

64. Necchi A, Nicolai N, Colecchia M, et al. Proof of activity of anti-epidermal growth factor receptor-targeted therapy for relapsed squamous cell carcinoma of the penis. *J Clin Oncol* 2011;29:e650–e652.

65. Haas GP, Blumenstein BA, Gagliano RG, et al. Cisplatin, methotrexate and bleomycin for the treatment of carcinoma of the penis: a Southwest Oncology Group study. *J Urol* 1999;161:1823–1825.

66. Bahl A, Nicholson S, Harland SJ, et al. Phase II trial of docetaxel, cisplatin, 5-fluorouracil (TPF) in locally advanced and metastatic squamous cell carcinoma (SCC) of the penis (CRUK/09/001). *J Clin Oncol* 2012;20:326.

67. Pizzocaro G, Piva L. Adjuvant and neoadjuvant vincristine, bleomycin, and methotrexate for inguinal metastases from squamous cell carcinoma of the penis. *Acta Oncol* 1988;27:823–824.

68. Bermejo C, Busby JE, Spiess PE, et al. Neoadjuvant chemotherapy followed by aggressive surgical consolidation for metastatic penile squamous cell carcinoma. *J Urol* 2007;177:1335–1338.

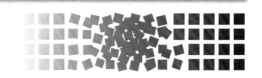

# 44 Cancer of the Testis

Lance C. Pagliaro and Christopher J. Logothetis

## INTRODUCTION

Testicular cancers are the most common malignant neoplasm affecting men ages 15 to 35 years. Approximately 90% of testicular cancers are germ cell tumors, which can be broadly classified as seminoma or nonseminomatous germ cell tumors (NSGCT). Male extragonadal germ cell tumors are also discussed in this chapter. Analogous germ cell and sex cord stromal tumors in women are not included here, but in many cases the male and female counterparts share a common biology and therapeutic approach.

## INCIDENCE AND EPIDEMIOLOGY

In the United States, 8,820 new cases of testicular cancer per year is estimated for 2014.[1] This figure greatly underestimates the prevalence of testicular cancer survivors. This is because the cancer-specific survival rate for testicular cancer with standard treatment is >95%.[2] The incidence varies among geographic areas, being highest in Scandinavia, Switzerland, and Germany, and lowest in Africa and Asia.[3] Although testicular germ cell tumors are most common among adolescent and young adult men, they can potentially occur in males of any age or genetic background. For reasons that have yet to be discovered, the incidence of testicular germ cell tumors has increased over the preceding 30 years in the United States and United Kingdom.[4]

### Risk Factors

Men whose family history includes a first-degree relative with testicular germ cell tumor or who have a personal history of cryptorchidism are at increased risk of developing germ cell tumor.[5,6] Testicular cancer survivors are also at increased risk of a second primary cancer in the contralateral testicle.[7] These risk factors suggest a genetic or developmental etiology for testicular germ cell tumors. No postnatal environmental risk factors have yet been identified.[8]

In the United States, testicular cancer is rare among African Americans and most common among Caucasian men.[9] This racial disparity in testicular cancer diagnosis and its geographic distribution suggest a genetic linkage with the Caucasian phenotype, but no high penetrance allele has yet been identified.[4] Testicular germ cell tumors are commonly accompanied by intratubular germ cell neoplasia (ITGCN). It is thought that all adult germ cell tumors, with the exception of spermatocytic seminoma, arise from ITGCN.[10] The widely accepted theory is that ITGCN begins in utero.[11] The multifocality of ITGCN suggests a field effect within the testicle and provides a mechanistic explanation for cases of bilateral testicular cancer.

Men without a history of testicular cancer are occasionally found to have ITGCN on testicular biopsy or orchiectomy that was performed for other reasons. The incidental finding of testicular microlithiasis on ultrasound may also provide evidence of ITGCN in an otherwise healthy man.[12,13] The risk of testicular cancer for such individuals has not been determined, but they should be counseled regarding a potential increased risk and to report any new testicular symptoms.[14]

## INITIAL PRESENTATION AND MANAGEMENT

### Symptoms and Signs

Testicular swelling is the most common presenting complaint and in most cases is detected by the patient himself. Patients may also report a pressure-like sensation, heaviness, or mild-to-moderate testicular pain. This will sometimes be confused with orchitis or epididymitis and treated initially with antibiotics. Acute or severe pain is rarely caused by testicular cancer and suggests a different etiology such as testicular torsion. Testicular ultrasound should be obtained as soon as a neoplasm is suspected, and it will appear as one or more hypoechoic lesions within the testicle. Ultrasound distinguishes a solid from cystic mass, and intratesticular from intrascrotal/extratesticular location. A solid intratesticular mass on ultrasound is presumed to be a neoplasm and is an indication for radical inguinal orchiectomy.[15]

Approximately half of patients present with a testicular mass and no clinical evidence of metastasis (clinical stage I). Others present with metastatic disease that may also be symptomatic. Primary tumors can be small and asymptomatic, even in the presence of metastatic disease, and occasionally they "burn out" leaving only a fibrotic scar (burned-out primary). Metastases can be the source of clinical symptoms on presentation in such cases, and include back pain, shortness of breath, cough, gynecomastia, hemoptysis, and weight loss.[16] Ultrasound of the testicles is helpful in establishing the diagnosis even if there is no palpable testicular mass.[15] The detection of elevated serum tumor markers can also be helpful when an occult testicular primary or extragonadal germ cell tumor is suspected.[17]

### Diagnosis

Radical inguinal orchiectomy is the standard diagnostic and therapeutic procedure for a solid intratesticular mass.[18] Transscrotal orchiectomy or biopsy is specifically contraindicated because of the risk of tumor cell seeding of the inguinal and pelvic lymphatic drainage. Biopsy is also of limited value because testicular germ cell tumors are heterogeneous. Removal of the entire organ is necessary to properly identify the histologic type(s) present and to select the appropriate therapy. It is reasonable to perform needle biopsy of a metastatic site in cases of occult testicular primary, burned-out primary, or extragonadal germ cell tumor; although, the results of needle biopsy must always be interpreted with caution due to sampling error. The pattern of serum tumor marker elevation is also informative about the likely cell types present (seminoma or nonseminoma), as discussed in the next section.[17]

## HISTOLOGY

Male germ cell tumors are broadly classified as seminoma and NSGCT (Table 44.1).[19,20] Patients with pure seminoma are

## TABLE 44.1

**World Health Organization Histologic Classification of Testicular Germ Cell Tumors**

**Germ Cell Tumors**
  Intratubular germ cell neoplasia, unclassified
  Other types

**Tumors of One Histologic Type (Pure Forms)**
  Seminoma
    Seminoma with syncytiotrophoblastic cells
  Spermatocytic seminoma
    Spermatocytic seminoma with sarcoma
  Embryonal carcinoma
  Yolk sac tumor
  Trophoblastic tumors
    Choriocarcinoma
    Trophoblastic neoplasms other than choriocarcinoma
  Teratoma
    Dermoid cyst
    Monodermal teratoma
    Teratoma with somatic type malignancies

**Tumors of More Than One Histologic Type (Mixed Forms)**
  Mixed embryonal carcinoma and teratoma
  Mixed teratoma and seminoma
  Choriocarcinoma and teratoma/embryonal carcinoma
  Others

*Source:* Eble JN, Sauter G, Epstein JI, et al., eds. *Pathology and Genetics of Tumours of the Urinary System and Male Genital Organs.* Lyon, France: IARC Press; 2004.

managed differently than patients with NSGCT or mixed histology tumors, although mixed tumors may have a component of seminoma. In that sense, when we refer to seminoma as a clinical diagnosis it is meant as pure seminoma, whereas seminoma as a histologic pattern may also be present in mixed NSGCT.

## Seminoma

The microscopic appearance of seminoma is characterized by sheets of neoplastic cells with abundant cytoplasm, round, hyperchromatic nuclei and prominent nucleoli (Fig. 44.1). A prominent lymphocytic infiltrate is common, such that it is sometimes confused with lymphoma until the surface immunophenotype has been determined. Most seminomas do not produce serum tumor markers, but the presence of syncytiotrophoblastic giant cells in a minority of cases accounts for modest elevations of serum human chorionic gonadotropin (hCG).[21] Seminomas never produce alpha-fetoprotein (AFP), and patients whose tumors have the histologic appearance of seminoma and whose serum AFP is elevated should be considered to have a mixed NSGCT, even if a nonseminomatous histologic pattern cannot be identified.[22] Exceptions are cases in which there is another explanation for the elevated AFP, such as liver disease or a chronic nonspecific elevation.

Immunohistochemistry is usually positive for placental alkaline phosphatase (PLAP), negative for CD30, AFP, and epithelial membrane antigen, and either negative or weak/focally positive for cytokeratin.[23]

Histologic variations of seminoma such as "anaplastic" or "atypical" seminoma are of no known clinical relevance. Spermatocytic seminoma, however, is the one variant of seminoma that has a different natural history and is even of uncertain relation to other germ cell tumors. Spermatocytic seminoma usually occurs in older individuals and has low metastatic potential.[24] Orchiectomy is the only treatment required. Unlike all other germ cell tumors, spermatocytic seminoma is not associated with ITGCN.

## Nonseminomatous Histologies

Germ cell tumors may be composed of a single histology or multiple histologic patterns.[19] Through poorly understood processes of mutation and differentiation, a single clone beginning as ITGCN can develop into an undifferentiated neoplasm (seminoma), or to a primitive zygotic neoplasm (embryonal carcinoma).[25] Further differentiation from embryonal carcinoma results in somatically differentiated tumors (teratoma) or extraembryonal-differentiated tumors (yolk sac and choriocarcinoma).[26] Nonseminomatous histologies are found in 55% of germ cell tumors. Male germ cell tumors that contain any histologic cell type other than seminoma or syncytiotrophoblasts are collectively referred to as NSGCT.

### Embryonal Carcinoma

Embryonal carcinoma is the most undifferentiated type of germ cell tumor and is thought to be pluripotent. Cells are characterized by indistinct borders and scant cytoplasm, which can be arranged in solid sheets or in glandular or tubular structures (Fig. 44.2). On immunohistochemical staining, embryonal carcinoma can be positive for cytokeratin, CD30, PLAP, AFP, and hCG. Modest elevations of serum AFP and/or hCG can be seen, and frequently it is marker-negative. Lactate dehydrogenase (LDH) concentration in the serum is an important prognostic factor in metastatic embryonal carcinoma that is marker negative.

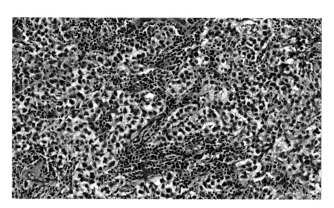

**Figure 44.1** Seminoma, classic type, with neoplastic cells (*arrow*) and the typical accompanying lymphocytic infiltrate (*arrowhead*). (Source: Rao B, Pagliaro LC. Testicular germ cell tumors. In: Silverman PM, ed. *Oncologic Imaging: A Multidisciplinary Approach.* Philadelphia: Elsevier; 2012:335–357.)

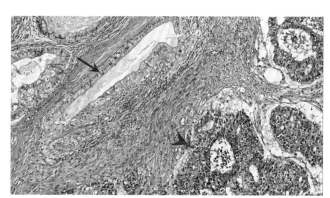

**Figure 44.2** Mixed nonseminomatous germ cell tumor comprised of teratoma (*arrow*) and embryonal carcinoma (*arrowhead*). (Source: Rao B, Pagliaro LC. Testicular germ cell tumors. In: Silverman PM, ed. *Oncologic Imaging: A Multidisciplinary Approach.* Philadelphia: Elsevier; 2012:335–357.)

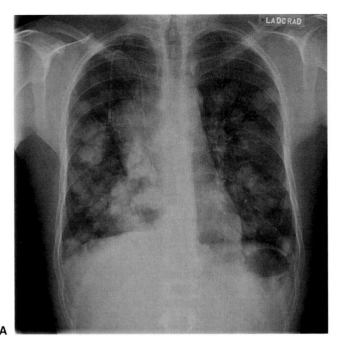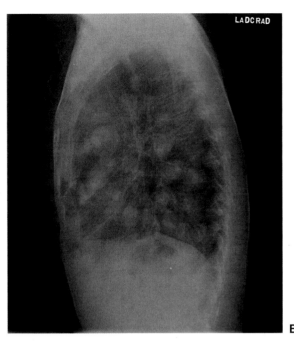

**Figure 44.3** Chest radiograph of a man with primary mediastinal choriocarcinoma and pulmonary metastases.

### Choriocarcinoma

Choriocarcinoma is composed of both cytotrophoblasts and syncytiotrophoblasts.[27] The cells strongly express hCG. The clinical presentation of a choriocarcinoma-predominant or pure choriocarcinoma tumor often includes very high serum hCG levels, widespread hematogenous metastases, and tumor hemorrhage (Fig. 44.3). Syncytiotrophoblasts and syncytiotrophoblastic giant cells can be associated with other germ cell histologies, so the presence of cytotophoblasts is required for the diagnosis.

### Yolk Sac Tumor

Yolk sac tumor (endodermal sinus tumor) is commonly seen as a component of mixed NSGCT. Pure yolk sac tumors represent a significant proportion of mediastinal germ cell tumors, but are rarely seen in adult testicular cancer. Histologic patterns include papillary, solid, glandular, hepatoid, macrocystic, and microcystic types. Perivascular arrangements of epithelial cells can be seen in yolk sac tumor and are known as glomeruloid or Schiller-Duval bodies. Immunostains are diffusely positive for AFP and may also be positive for cytokeratin, SALL4, glipican-3, PLAP, and CD117. Yolk sac tumor is associated with high serum levels of AFP.

### Teratoma

Teratoma arises from a pluripotent malignant precursor (embryonal carcinoma or yolk sac tumor) and contains somatic cells from at least two germ cell layers (ectoderm, endoderm, or mesoderm). Teratoma is commonly seen as a component of adult mixed NSGCT (see Fig. 44.2). A small percentage (2% to 3%) of postpubertal male germ cell tumors appear to have teratoma as the only histologic type, but these are always assumed to harbor a minor component of pluripotent NSGCT and are treated the same as a mixed NSGCT.

Immature teratoma shows partial somatic differentiation, whereas mature teratoma has terminally differentiated tissues such as cartilage, skeletal muscle, or nerve tissue, and frequently forms cystic structures. Although these cells can resemble normal tissues, teratoma is a low-grade malignancy and if untreated will grow until it is unresectable. Moreover, teratomas can give rise to secondary somatic malignancy, such as rhabdomyosarcoma, poorly

differentiated carcinoma, or primitive neuroectodermal tumor.[28] These typically display the biology of their de novo counterparts and are treated accordingly.[29,30]

Teratoma does not produce elevated serum AFP or hCG. Patients with elevated serum AFP and/or hCG should be assumed to have a nonteratoma germ cell tumor component, unless the elevation can be otherwise explained.

## BIOLOGY

### Mechanism of Germ Cell Transformation

ITGCN is thought to derive from malignant transformation of primordial germ cells or gonocytes during fetal development.[31] Primordial germ cells migrate from the proximal epiblast (yolk sac) through the hindgut and mesentery to the genital ridge, and become gonocytes. The precise molecular events underlying transformation to ITGCN are not well understood. The most consistent genetic finding in germ cell tumors is a gain of material from chromosome 12p. The majority of NSGCT and seminomas contain i(12p), an isochromosome comprised of two fused short arms of chromosome 12. The remaining i(12p)-negative germ cell tumors also have a gain of 12p sequences in the form of tandem duplications that may be transposed elsewhere in the genome.

Gain of 12p sequences has been found in ITGCN, indicating that it is an early event in testicular cancer pathogenesis. The acquisition of i(12p) is not thought to be the initiating event, however, because it is preceded by polyploidization.[32] Overexpressed genes on 12p are likely to be important, and there are candidate genes on 12p including several that confer growth advantage (*KRAS2*, *CCND2* [cyclin D2]), and others that establish or maintain the stem cell phenotype (*NANOG*, *DPPA3*, *GDF3*). The exact genes that are critical to this step have not yet been identified.

Seminomas are usually hypertriploid, whereas NSGCT is more commonly hypotriploid.[33] Other chromosome regions were found to have nonrandom gains or losses in germ cell tumors with less frequency than 12p. Single gene mutations are uncommon in germ cell tumors. The most commonly mutated genes are *BRAF*, *KIT*, *KRAS*, *NRAS*, and *TP53*.[11] The KIT/kit ligand (*KITLG*) pathway

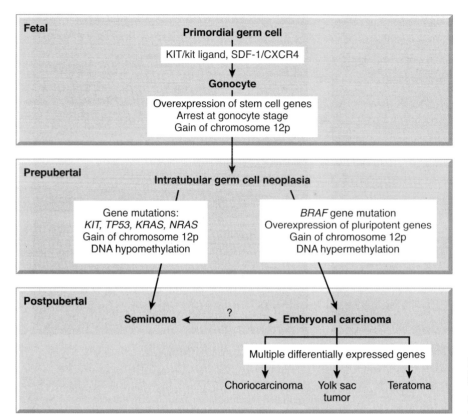

**Figure 44.4** Pathogenesis of testicular germ cell tumors. (Adapted from Sheikine Y, Genega E, Melamed J, et al. Molecular genetics of testicular germ cell tumors. *Am J Cancer Res* 2012;2:153–167.)

has special relevance for gonadal development. The biologic function of this pathway is broad and includes development of hematopoietic cells, melanocytes, and germ cells.[34] KITLG is essential for primordial germ cell survival and motility, as are the chemokine SDF-1 (CXCL12) and its receptor CXCR4.[11] Immunohistochemical markers found on primordial germ cells and gonocytes (PLAP, CD117 [KIT], OCT3/4 [POU5F1]) are also found on ITGCN, suggesting a transformation from these cells during fetal development (Fig. 44.4). The biallelic expression of imprinted genes in germ cell tumors has been reported, showing that they likely arose from primordial germ cells where the genomic imprinting is temporarily erased.[31]

Somatic mutations in KIT as well as increased copy number have been described in 9% of testicular germ cell tumors and 20% of seminomas.[4] The somatic alterations in KIT found in germ cell tumors are predicted to upregulate pathway activity. KITLG plays a role in determining skin pigmentation and has undergone strong selection in European and Asian populations. Difference in the frequency of risk alleles for KITLG between European and African populations may provide an explanation for the difference in germ cell tumor incidence between Caucasian and African Americans.

There is evidence that epigenetic regulation of gene expression plays a role in the pathogenesis of germ cell tumors. The DNA methylation patterns are different among histologic types. Global hypomethylation is more common in seminomas than in NSGCT.[31] In a study of 16 germ cell tumors, the methylation of CpG islands in NSGCT was similar to that observed in other tumor types, whereas it was virtually absent in seminomas.[35] Aberrant promoter methylation is generally associated with absent or downregulated expression of the methylated genes. This can result, for example, in the silencing of tumor suppressor genes.[31] Methylation has also been correlated with germ cell tumor differentiation. The more differentiated tumors (yolk sac tumor, choriocarcinoma, teratoma) were consistently hypermethylated, whereas seminoma and ITGCN were hypomethylated.[36] Some of the observed methylation patterns may reflect normal development rather than germ cell tumor pathogenesis.

## Pluripotency of Embryonal-Like Differentiation in Germ Cell Tumors

Embryonal carcinoma has a six-gene signature (DNMT3B, DPPA4, GAL, GPC4, POU5F1, TERF1), which was detected in three of five independent studies.[11] All six of these genes are involved in establishing and maintaining pluripotency. SOX2 encodes a transcription factor essential for maintaining self-renewal of embryonic stem cells and is upregulated in embryonal carcinoma. Two additional genes that encode transcription factors associated with stem cell pluripotency, NANOG and POU5F1, are upregulated in both seminoma and embryonal carcinoma.[26] Lineage differentiation takes place in NSGCT, mimicking the development of a normal zygote. Thus, embryonal carcinoma can be thought of as the transformed counterpart of embryonic stem cells, displaying self-renewal, pluripotency, and lineage differentiation.

## Familial Predisposition to Germ Cell Tumors

Approximately 1.4% of patients with newly diagnosed germ cell tumor report a family history of germ cell tumor.[34] First-degree male relatives of patients with testicular cancer have a 6- to 10-fold increased risk of developing testicular cancer. These observations point to the likely existence of a hereditary germ cell tumor subset. The inheritable effect is mild, and the most common number of affected relatives in a family is two. The age at diagnosis among familial cases is 2 to 3 years younger than sporadic cases, and there is a higher incidence of bilateral tumors.

The gr/gr deletion on chromosome Y, common among infertility patients and associated with a two- to threefold increased risk of testicular cancer, was studied as a candidate region for hereditary risk.[4] The frequency of gr/gr variant is low, however, such that it could only account for a small component of hereditary risk. Genome-wide association studies (GWAS) for testicular cancer have been hampered by relatively small sample sizes. Nevertheless, five loci of interest were identified in a GWAS study from the

United Kingdom, on chromosomes 1, 4, 5q31.3, 6, and 12p22, including confirmatory data for the chromosome 6 locus. The single nucleotide polymorphism (SNP) associations on chromosomes 1 and 4 were not convincingly replicated in an independent US study, whereas the associations on chromosomes 5 and 12 were confirmed. The strongest associated SNPs were at 12q22 within the *KITLG* gene, for which there is a >2.5 risk of disease per major allele. For the chromosome 5 and 6 loci, a 1.5-fold increased risk was identified per major allele. The loci on chromosome 5 implicate the gene *SPRY4*, which encodes an inhibitor of the mitogen-activated protein kinase pathway. The locus on chromosome 6 falls within the intron of *BAK1*, which promotes apoptosis. The location of a disease-associated SNP near or within a gene does not definitively implicate that gene, yet all three of the genes identified in GWASs are directly or indirectly associated with the KIT/KITLG pathway.[11] These genes may be responsible for an estimated 15% of genetic predisposition to germ cell tumors, whereas the genetic basis of the other 85% of familial aggregations remains unexplained.

## Cisplatin Sensitivity and Acquired Resistance in Adult Germ Cell Tumors

Exquisite sensitivity to chemotherapy distinguishes germ cell tumors from most other cancers. Levels of p53 protein are elevated in all germ cell tumors except teratoma.[31] To maintain genomic integrity, embryonic stem cells have a high sensitivity to DNA damage, suggesting that the high levels of wild-type p53 seen in germ cell tumors may be intrinsic to their germ cell nature. *TP53* gene mutations are uncommon in germ cell tumors, however, and the role of acquired *TP53* mutations in the emergence of chemotherapy resistance has not been established.[11] Moreover, levels of p53 protein assessed by immunohistochemistry were not associated with outcome. While mutations in *TP53* have been observed in about 7% of seminomas, its significance in germ cell tumors remains unclear.

Mutations of *BRAF* including V600E mutations have been detected in a small percentage of NSGCT. *BRAF* mutations were most prevalent in mediastinal primary tumors, late relapse, and cisplatin-resistant NSGCT, suggesting a role in chemoresistance. Further study is needed to define the prognostic significance of *BRAF* mutation and whether the V600E mutation can be therapeutically targeted. A high ratio of proapoptotic Bax to antiapoptotic Bcl-2 was found in invasive germ cell tumors and may explain the rapid apoptotic response to DNA-damaging drugs; however, the Bax:Bcl-2 ratio was not associated with treatment outcome.[31] Finally, the emergence of cisplatin resistance may be intimately associated with the expression of genes and pathways responsible for lineage differentiation in NSGCT, in other words, intrinsic to the germ cell biology rather than the result of specific mutations.

## IMMUNOHISTOCHEMICAL MARKERS

SALL4 is expressed in almost all germ cell tumors and has been reported to be positive in ITGCN, classic seminoma, spermatocytic seminoma, embryonal carcinoma, yolk sac tumor, choriocarcinoma, and teratoma.[37,38] OCT3/4 is variably expressed in ITGCN, classic seminoma, embryonal carcinoma, and yolk sac tumor. Spermatocytic seminoma, choriocarcinoma, and teratoma are usually negative for OCT3/4. CD117 (KIT) helps highlight ITGCN and classic seminoma. CD30, SOX2, and keratin are helpful in the diagnosis of embryonal carcinoma, whereas SALL4 and Glypican-3 are often positive in yolk sac tumor.[39] In tumors of unknown primary or those presenting as a retroperitoneal or mediastinal mass, SALL4, OCT3/4, CD117, SOX2, CD30, and low-molecular-weight keratins all may be useful in distinguishing germ cell tumors from non–germ cell tumors.

## STAGING

The most widely used system for staging testicular cancer is the tumor, node, metastasis classification endorsed by the American Joint Commission on Cancer and the International Union Against Cancer (Tables 44.2 and 44.3).[40] An important distinction for germ cell tumors is the inclusion of "S" classification (S0 to S3), signifying serum tumor marker elevation. There are three stage groupings of tumor, node, metastasis/serum tumor marker elevation classifications whereby, in general, stage I disease is confined to the testis, stage II is confined to the retroperitoneal lymph nodes with serum tumor markers in the good-prognosis range (S0 to S1), and stage III includes metastases that extend beyond the retroperitoneum or are extranodal in location. Stage III NSGCT also includes any patient with serum tumor markers in the intermediate- or poor-prognosis range (S2 to S3).

### Patterns of Metastasis

Testicular cancers can undergo both lymphatic and hematogenous dissemination. The lymphatics arising from the testicle accompany the gonadal vessels in the spermatic cord. Some follow the gonadal vessels to their origin while others diverge and drain into the retroperitoneum. The landing zone for metastasis from the right testicle is in the interaortocaval lymph nodes just inferior to the renal vessels (Fig. 44.5). The landing zone from the left testicle is in the para-aortic lymph nodes just inferior to the left renal vessels (Fig. 44.6). Large volume disease tends to progress in retrograde fashion to the aortic bifurcation and below, along the iliac vessels.[41]

#### Seminoma

Seminoma can spread extensively through the lymphatic system to include retroperitoneal, retrocrural, mediastinal, supraclavicular, and cervical lymph nodes, often in the absence of hematogenous metastasis.[42] Metastasis to lungs (stage IIIA) is common; metastasis to nonpulmonary organs (stage IIIB) is less common.[43] Serum tumor markers do not affect the stage (except in stage IS) or prognosis in seminoma. Hematogenous metastasis to extrapulmonary organs (e.g., bone) in seminoma carries an intermediate prognosis. There is no stage IIIC or poor-prognosis designation in seminoma.[44]

#### Nonseminomatous Germ Cell Tumors

Similar to seminoma, lymphatic spread is the most common and usually the earliest type of dissemination in NSGCT. Stage groupings depend on both the anatomic extent of disease and serum tumor markers.[40] Stage IIIB is distinguished from stage II or IIIA on the basis of tumor markers being in the intermediate-prognosis range (S2). Stage IIIC NSGCT carries a poor prognosis, and more often than seminoma it involves multiple organs such as liver and brain.[44]

Embryonal carcinoma, in some cases, exhibits hematogenous metastasis to lungs or nonpulmonary viscera without clinical involvement of retroperitoneal lymph nodes.[45] Computed tomography (CT) of the chest is necessary for complete staging workup of tumors that have a high percentage of embryonal carcinoma.

### Serum Tumor Markers

Serum tumor markers are an important part of the staging system for germ cell tumors. Three markers, namely AFP, hCG, and total LDH, are considered for establishing the correct prognostic classification (good, intermediate, or poor prognosis).[44] Markers should be assessed after orchiectomy and before the start of chemotherapy. Markers that are elevated prior to orchiectomy and then normalize appropriately have no prognostic significance. Markers that do not normalize in a patient without any other clinical evidence of metastatic disease are considered stage IS.[40] In the absence of residual disease, the expected half-life of postoperative serum tumor marker decline is 2 to 3 days for hCG and 5 to 7 days for AFP.

**TABLE 44.2**

## Definition of TNM

| TNM Category | Description |
|---|---|
| **Primary Tumor (T)** | |
| pTX | Primary tumor cannot be assessed. |
| pT0 | No evidence of primary tumor (e.g., histologic scar in testis). |
| pTis | Intratubular germ cell neoplasia (carcinoma in situ) |
| pT1 | Tumor limited to the testis and epididymis without vascular/lymphatic invasion. Tumor may invade into the tunica albuginea but not the tunica vaginalis. |
| pT2 | Tumor limited to the testis and epididymis with vascular/lymphatic invasion or tumor extending through the tunica albuginea with involvement of the tunica vaginalis. |
| pT3 | Tumor invades the spermatic cord with or without vascular/lymphatic invasion. |
| pT4 | Tumor invades the scrotum with or without vascular/lymphatic invasion. |

Note: Except for pTis and pT4, extent of primary tumor is classified by radical orchiectomy. TX may be used for other categories in the absence of radical orchiectomy.

| | |
|---|---|
| **Regional Lymph Nodes (N)** | |
| **Clinical** | |
| NX | Regional lymph nodes cannot be assessed. |
| N0 | No regional lymph node metastasis |
| N1 | Metastasis with a lymph node mass 2 cm or less in greatest dimension or multiple lymph nodes; none >2 cm in greatest dimension. |
| N2 | Metastasis with a lymph node mass >2 cm but not >5 cm in greatest dimension, or multiple lymph nodes, any one mass >2 cm but not >5 cm cm in greatest dimension. |
| N3 | Metastasis with a lymph node mass >5 cm in greatest dimension. |
| **Pathologic (pN)** | |
| pNX | Regional lymph nodes cannot be assessed. |
| pN0 | No regional lymph node metastasis |
| pN1 | Metastasis with a lymph node mass 2 cm or less in greatest dimension and ≤5 nodes positive; none >2 cm in greatest dimension. |
| pN2 | Metastasis with a lymph node mass >2 cm but not >5 cm in greatest dimension, or >5 nodes positive, none >5 cm, or evidence of extranodal extension of tumor. |
| pN3 | Metastasis with a lymph node mass >5 cm in greatest dimension. |
| **Distant Metastases (M)** | |
| M0 | No distant metastasis. |
| M1 | Distant metastasis |
| M1a | Nonregional nodal or pulmonary metastases |
| M1b | Distant metastasis other than to nonregional lymph nodes and lungs |
| **Serum Tumor Markers (S)** | |
| SX | Marker studies not available or not performed |
| S0 | Marker study levels within normal limits |
| S1 | LDH <1.5 × N[a] **AND** <br> hCG (mIU/mL) <5,000 **AND** <br> AFP (ng/mL) <1,000 |
| S2 | LDH 1.5–10 × N **OR** <br> hCG (mIU/mL) 5,000–50,000 **OR** <br> AFP (ng/mL) 1,000–10,000 |
| S3 | LDH >10 × N **OR** <br> hCG (mIU/mL) >50,000 **OR** <br> AFP (ng/mL) >10,000 |

TNM, tumor, node, metastasis; LDH, lactate dehydrogenase; hCG, human chorionic gonadotropin; AFP, α-fetoprotein; S, serum tumor markers.
[a] N indicates upper limit of normal for the LDH assay.
Used with the permission of the American Joint Committee on Cancer (AJCC), Chicago, Illinois. The original source for this material is the Edge SB, Byrd DR, Compton CC, et al., eds. *AJCC Cancer Staging Manual*, 7th ed. New York: Springer Science and Business Media LLC; 2010: 471–472.

| | | | | |
|---|---|---|---|---|
| **TABLE 44.3** | | | | |
| **Stage Grouping** | | | | |
| **Group** | **T** | **N** | **M** | **S**$^a$ |
| **Stage 0** | pTis | N0 | M0 | S0 |
| **Stage I** | pT1–4 | N0 | M0 | SX |
| IA | pT1 | N0 | M0 | S0 |
| IB | pT2 | N0 | M0 | S0 |
| | pT3 | N0 | M0 | S0 |
| | pT4 | N0 | M0 | S0 |
| IS | Any pT/Tx | N0 | M0 | S1–3 |
| **Stage II** | Any pT/Tx | N1-3 | M0 | SX |
| IIA | Any pT/Tx | N1 | M0 | S0 |
| | Any pT/Tx | N1 | M0 | S1 |
| IIB | Any pT/Tx | N2 | M0 | S0 |
| | Any pT/Tx | N2 | M0 | S1 |
| IIC | Any pT/Tx | N3 | M0 | S0 |
| | Any pT/Tx | N3 | M0 | S1 |
| **Stage III** | Any pT/Tx | Any N | M1 | SX |
| IIIA | Any pT/Tx | Any N | M1a | S0 |
| | Any pT/Tx | Any N | M1a | S1 |
| IIIB | Any pT/Tx | N1–3 | M0 | S2 |
| | Any pT/Tx | Any N | M1a | S2 |
| IIIC | Any pT/Tx | N1–3 | M0 | S3 |
| | Any pT/Tx | Any N | M1a | S3 |
| | Any pT/Tx | Any N | M1b | Any S |

$^a$ Measured after orchiectomy.
Used with the permission of the American Joint Committee on Cancer (AJCC), Chicago, Illinois. The original source for this material is the Edge SB, Byrd DR, Compton CC, et al., eds. *AJCC Cancer Staging Manual*, 7th ed. New York: Springer Science and Business Media LLC; 2010: 471–472.

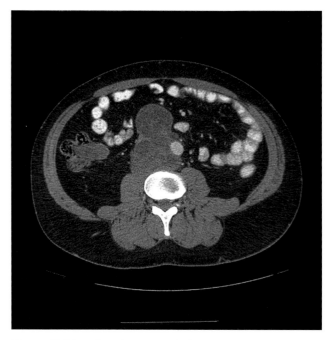

**Figure 44.5** Lymph node metastasis from nonseminomatous germ cell tumor of the right testicle. Postchemotherapy resection showed metastatic teratoma.

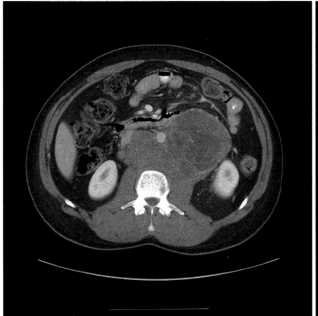
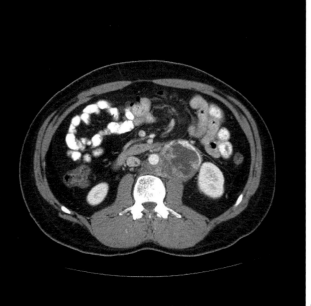

A         B

**Figure 44.6** Lymph node metastasis from nonseminomatous germ cell tumor of the left testicle **(A)** at diagnosis, and **(B)** upon completion of chemotherapy. Postchemotherapy resection showed metastatic teratoma with somatic transformation to primitive neuroectodermal tumor.

**TABLE 44.4**

**Germ Cell Tumor Risk Classification**

| Risk Group | Seminoma | Nonseminoma |
|---|---|---|
| Good | Any hCG<br>Any LDH<br>Nonpulmonary visceral metastases absent<br>Any primary site | AFP <1,000 ng/mL<br>hCG <5,000 mIU/mL<br>LDH <1.5 × ULN<br>Nonpulmonary visceral metastases absent<br>Gonadal or retroperitoneal primary site |
| Intermediate | Nonpulmonary visceral metastases present<br>Any hCG<br>Any LDH<br>Any primary site | AFP 1,000–10,000 ng/mL<br>hCG 5,000–50,000 mIU/mL<br>LDH 1.5–10.0 × ULN<br>Nonpulmonary visceral metastases absent<br>Gonadal or retroperitoneal primary site |
| Poor | Does not exist | Mediastinal primary site<br>Nonpulmonary visceral metastases present (e.g., bone, liver, brain)<br>AFP >10,000 ng/mL<br>hCG >50,000 mIU/mL<br>LDH >10 × ULN |

hCG, human chorionic gonadotropin; LDH, lactate dehydrogenase; AFP, α-fetoprotein; ULN, upper limit of normal range.
*Source:* International Germ Cell Consensus Classification: a prognostic factor-based staging system for metastatic germ cell cancers. International Germ Cell Cancer Collaborative Group. *J Clin Oncol* 1997;15:594–603.

Elevated AFP has special significance in seminoma because it is only produced by NSGCT. Germ cell tumors that histologically appear to be pure seminoma with elevated serum AFP are given the clinical diagnosis of NSGCT, and are treated as such.[22] HCG can be elevated in either seminoma or NSGCT, but has prognostic significance only for NSCGT.

Total LDH concentration prior to chemotherapy functions as a prognostic factor in NSGCT and helps to determine stage. In seminoma with bulky metastases, LDH can be markedly elevated but has no prognostic significance.

There are several potential causes of spurious elevation of tumor markers. AFP is not cancer specific; it may be elevated in the presence of liver disease or as a nonspecific chronic elevation. Stability of AFP over time suggests a benign etiology. HCG is cancer specific in men, but it is not specific to germ cell tumors. It can be associated with other neoplasms and with exposure to cannabis products. Patients should be questioned about the use of marijuana. A positive hCG test can also occur as a laboratory artifact in patients with low serum testosterone, owing to the increased secretion of luteinizing hormone and its sequence similarity to hCG.[46,47]

## Clinical Staging

The most commonly used methods for detecting metastatic disease are serum tumor markers and CT scan.[15] Positron emission tomography (PET) scan can be helpful in the staging evaluation of a seminoma patient by distinguishing hypermetabolic lymph node metastases from reactive lymph nodes. PET is not as useful in NSGCT, where CT scan with oral and intravenous contrast is the preferred technique for detecting retroperitoneal adenopathy.

## Pathologic Staging

The T classification is determined by pathology of the orchiectomy specimen.[40] The presence of lymphovascular invasion (LVI) or invasion through the tunica albuginea with involvement of the tunica vaginalis are pT2, invasion of the spermatic cord is pT3, and involvement of the scrotum constitutes pT4 (see Table 44.2).

Prophylactic retroperitoneal lymph node dissection (RPLND) is performed for surgical staging in some patients with clinical

stage I NSGCT. In such cases, if no metastatic germ cell tumor is found, the stage is pathologic stage I; when disease is found, it is designated pathologic stage II.

## Factors Affecting Outcome

In clinical stage I NSGCT, the presence of LVI (pT2) is associated with an approximately 50% risk of recurrence with surveillance alone. A high percentage of embryonal carcinoma has also been associated with high risk in some series, but embryonal carcinoma is often seen together with LVI and has not been validated as an independent risk factor.[48]

In clinical stage I seminoma, tumor size ≥4 cm is associated with approximately 30% risk of recurrence with surveillance alone. Involvement of rete testis has not been validated as a risk factor, although it is often mentioned.[49]

The classification of patients with metastatic germ cell tumors as good, intermediate, or poor prognosis, based on serum tumor markers and extent of disease, was proposed in 1997 by The International Germ Cell Cancer Collaborative Group (Table 44.4).[44] In this system, the presence or absence of nonpulmonary, extranodal metastasis was validated as an independent prognostic factor for progression-free survival. For NSGCT, the degree of marker elevation and mediastinal primary (versus testis or retroperitoneal primary) were also validated as prognostic factors. The threshold values for tumor markers (hCG, AFP, and LDH) have been incorporated into the American Joint Commission on Cancer/International Union Against Cancer staging system as the "S" classification. These prognostic groupings are used to make treatment decisions and are discussed in the following sections.

## MANAGEMENT OF CLINICAL STAGE I DISEASE

Virtually all patients with clinical stage I germ cell tumors survive (cancer specific survival 98% to 99%).[49] In general, patients managed with observation have the same life expectancy as those who receive adjuvant intervention. Treatment decisions must therefore be based on considerations of cost, burden of therapy, and patient preference.[48]

## Seminoma

Clinical stage I seminoma is grouped into high-risk and average-risk based on tumor size, but similar options exist for all patients with stage I seminoma, regardless of risk.[48,49] Stage I is a common presentation, accounting for approximately 70% of patients diagnosed with pure seminoma.

### Surveillance

The average risk of recurrence with surveillance for stage I seminoma is 15% to 20%. Recurrences are temporally distributed over a 10-year period.[50] High-risk tumors have a recurrence probability of 30% to 35%, whereas tumors <4 cm without rete testis involvement may have a risk as low as 12%.[51] Observation is heavily dependent on CT scanning because the region at highest risk is in the retroperitoneum, and most seminomas do not secrete tumor markers.

### Adjuvant Chemotherapy

Carboplatin is a simple and apparently safe form of adjuvant chemotherapy that is very similar in efficacy to prophylactic radiotherapy. In a randomized trial of carboplatin given as a single infusion (area under curve equals 7) versus radiotherapy to the para-aortic lymph nodes, there was no significant difference in progression-free survival (94.7% and 96%, respectively).[52,53] There was only one death from seminoma (N = 1,447) reported at a median follow-up of 6.5 years. Recurrences after adjuvant carboplatin were frequently retroperitoneal in location, meaning that follow-up CT scans are mandatory. There has been no reported evidence of second malignant neoplasms (SMN), and there have been fewer contralateral germ cell tumors reported in the patients treated with chemotherapy versus radiotherapy at medium-term follow-up. Two courses of carboplatin have also been shown to be effective in the adjuvant setting, and in its 2014 guidelines the National Comprehensive Cancer Network (NCCN) endorsed one or two courses as a standard of care for clinical stage I seminoma, regardless of the estimated risk of recurrence.[54] Observation is also standard and is the preferred option.

### Prophylactic Radiotherapy

Treatment of para-aortic lymph nodes to a dose of 20 Gy was associated with excellent local control approaching 100%. A randomized trial of 20 Gy versus 30 Gy showed no difference in rate of recurrence.[55] Omission of ipsilateral iliac lymph nodes from the treatment field resulted in less toxicity (infertility, gastrointestinal effects) and minimal loss of efficacy. The recurrence rate after prophylactic radiotherapy for clinical stage I seminoma is about 4%, and most of those patients survive with additional treatment (combination chemotherapy). Recurrences tend to occur below the radiation field (pelvic lymph nodes) or above it (lungs). Radiotherapy is contraindicated for patients with horseshoe kidney or inflammatory bowel disease.

Radiotherapy was once popularized because it reduced the number of CT scans that were necessary for follow-up, with a net reduction in the cost of treatment.[56] There is, however, a different type of cost with radiotherapy, and that is the risk of SMN.[57] Studies of testicular cancer survivors 20 or more years after treatment have revealed an increase in midline cancers such as gastrointestinal and genitourinary malignancies.[58] This has brought about a reassessment of prophylactic radiotherapy, specifically, whether it is warranted when 80% of seminoma patients will be treated unnecessarily, there is a risk of SMN, and there is no survival benefit. While it continues to be offered, the use of prophylactic radiotherapy for seminoma is declining.[59]

## Nonseminomatous Germ Cell Tumor

Clinical stage I NSGCT is broadly categorized as high risk and average risk. Although there are many differences in presentation, including tumor size, histology, and tumor marker pattern, only LVI has been validated as a risk factor. NSGCT with LVI has a recurrence rate of approximately 50% with observation.[60] Most recurrences are seen within 2 to 3 years of the orchiectomy.[50] The average risk is 30%, and most patients with LVI-negative ("good risk") stage I NSGCT probably have a risk of recurrence <30%. The risk of recurrence for LVI-negative stage I NSGCT with predominantly embryonal carcinoma histology, however, may be higher (30% to 50%).[61]

### Surveillance

Approximately two-thirds of relapses among patients on surveillance are in retroperitoneal lymph nodes and one-third occur in lungs or by marker elevation alone. Recurrences in nonpulmonary viscera are rare. Most relapses occur within 2 to 3 years of orchiectomy, and patients need to remain on follow-up for at least 5 years. The ability to cure systemic disease with cisplatin-based chemotherapy in those who relapse makes observation an attractive option. It avoids unnecessary therapy for about two-thirds of patients.

Criteria for selecting patients for observation have been suggested in the literature and in the NCCN guidelines.[54] Selection based on whether the patient is "reliable" (i.e., likely to be compliant with follow-up) was once the prevalent view, but this has been largely replaced by a more objective risk-adapted approach. Observation is the standard of care for patients with stage IA NSGCT. The alternative is nerve-sparing RPLND, which is an unnecessary procedure for the majority of these patients. There is no subgroup of stage IA for whom RPLND is preferred, but patients who choose observation should agree to be compliant with follow-up and to receive chemotherapy in the event of recurrence. Patients with stage IA embryonal carcinoma–predominant tumors are probably the least likely to benefit from RPLND because of the tendency for hematogenous spread and associated risk of recurrence in lungs.[61,62]

Most patients with LVI-negative, clinical stage I NSGCT are candidates for observation. There is less of a consensus on management of patients with pT2-pT4 tumors (including LVI-positive). A minority of patients with pT2 tumors may choose observation, but they must understand that the risk of recurrence is 50% and they should agree (as in stage IA) to comply with follow-up. The preferred treatment for LVI-positive or advanced T classification NSGCT is adjuvant chemotherapy.

### Adjuvant Chemotherapy

Primary chemotherapy for NSGCT consists of bleomycin, etoposide, and cisplatin (BEP) (Table 44.5).[63,64] There are several published studies using either one or two courses of adjuvant BEP or similar regimens in patients with clinical stage I NSGCT.[65–68] A phase II study by the Medical Research Council found 98% relapse-free survival after two courses of bleomycin, vincristine, and cisplatin, although chemotherapy-induced neurotoxicity (CIN) remained a problem.[68] Two courses of BEP are similarly effective in preventing recurrence with less CIN; however, etoposide causes transient myelosuppression and is associated with a low but real risk of treatment-induced leukemia. The toxicity of two courses of BEP makes it unacceptable for stage IA NSGCT, but reasonable for stage IB where the relapse rate on observation is 50%.[48] One limitation of adjuvant chemotherapy is the continuing risk of growing teratoma syndrome. Only RPLND can remove foci of teratoma from the retroperitoneum, where they may persist and grow following chemotherapy.[69]

One strategy for lowering the toxicity of adjuvant chemotherapy is by shortening treatment to one course of BEP. Two European studies provide data collected prospectively; in one study, patients were randomized to a single course of BEP or RPLND (none were observed), and in a second study, the patients with LVI-negative tumors were offered surveillance or one course of BEP, while

## TABLE 44.5

### Chemotherapy Regimens for Stage II/III Germ Cell Tumor

**Previously Untreated—Good Risk[a]**

| Etoposide | 100 mg/m$^2$ IV daily × 5 days |
| Cisplatin | 20 mg/m$^2$ IV daily × 5 days; *Four cycles administered at 21-day intervals* |

| Etoposide | 100 mg/m$^2$ IV daily × 5 days |
| Cisplatin | 20 mg/m$^2$ IV daily × 5 days |
| Bleomycin | 30 units IV weekly (e.g., days 1, 8, 15); *Three cycles administered at 21-day intervals* |

**Previously Untreated—Intermediate and Poor Risk**

| Etoposide | 100 mg/m$^2$ IV daily × 5 days |
| Cisplatin | 20 mg/m$^2$ IV daily × 5 days |
| Bleomycin | 30 units IV weekly (e.g., days 1, 8, 15); *four cycles administered at 21-day intervals* |

**Previously Treated—1st-Line Salvage Therapy**

| Ifosfamide | 1.2 g/m$^2$ IV daily × 5 days |
| Mesna | 400 mg/m$^2$ IV every 8 h × 5 days |
| Cisplatin | 20 mg/m$^2$ IV daily × 5 days |
| Vinblastine | 0.11 mg/kg IV days 1 and 2; *Four cycles administered at 21-day intervals* |

| Paclitaxel | 250 mg/m$^2$ IV by continuous infusion over 24 h on day 1 |
| Ifosfamide | 1.5 g/m$^2$ IV daily on days 2–5 |
| Cisplatin | 25 mg/m$^2$ IV daily on days 2–5 |
| Mesna | 500 mg/m$^2$ IV every 8 h on days 2–5; *Four cycles administered at 21-day intervals* |

IV, intravenous.
[a] Good risk regimens (BEP or EP) can also be used for stage I adjuvant or stage IS.

patients with LVI-positive tumors were offered one or two courses of adjuvant BEP.[66,67] Both of these studies showed a <5% recurrence rate after one course of BEP and an acceptably low rate of growing teratoma. The 2014 NCCN guideline endorses either one or two courses of adjuvant BEP for stage IB NSGCT.[54]

### Retroperitoneal Lymph Node Dissection

RPLND performed in clinical stage I NSGCT is done to accurately stage the patient (as pathologic stage I or stage II) and remove all viable disease. RPLND is curative for teratoma, which has been reported in 21% to 30% of cases with viable disease.[70] Mortality from RPLND is <1%; minor complications include prolonged ileus, wound infection, and lymphocele. Major complications (hemorrhage, ureteral injury, chylous ascites, pulmonary embolus, wound dehiscence, bowel obstruction) are rare. A notable long-term morbidity is sympathetic nerve damage leading to failure of ejaculaton.[71]

For optimal outcomes, RPLND should be performed at a referral center with an experienced surgeon. A bilateral infrahilar RPLND includes the precaval, retrocaval, paracaval, interaortocaval, retroaortic, preaortic, paraortic, and common iliac lymph nodes.

There are two types of nerve-sparing RPLND: the modified template RPLND and nerve-dissection bilateral RPLND.[70,72,73] The template dissection helps the surgeon avoid regions where the risk of metastasis may be less. The nerve-dissection technique identifies and preserves both sympathetic chains, postganglionic sympathetic fibers, and the hypogastric plexus, which are necessary for anterograde ejaculation. The reported incidence of retrograde ejaculation with this technique is <5%. Another innovation is the robot-assisted RPLND, in which robotic instruments are inserted through a series of trocar entry sites and controlled remotely by the surgeon.[74–76] Patients have less pain, shorter hospitalization time, rapid recovery, and smaller surgical scars.

The relapse rate following RPLND is variable. It may be as low as 4% with a low-risk patient and an experienced surgeon. Most series include patients who also received adjuvant chemotherapy, typically with two courses of BEP, for pathologic stage II disease. Thus, the success of RPLND comes at the expense of double therapy for some patients. The LVI-positive and other high-risk patients have higher reported failure rates (10% to 14%) with prophylactic RPLND alone.[62] The greatest advantage of RPLND is the early control of teratoma when it exists. The randomized trial of RPLND versus one course of BEP found a recurrence rate of 8.3% in the RPLND arm and 1.1% in the BEP arm.[66] With median follow-up of 4.7 years, only one patient had growing teratoma after BEP. Limitations of the study were that unilateral dissections were performed (nonstandard) and that the experience level of surgeons varied, as it was a community-based study. The low incidence (1% to 2%) of growing teratoma seen among patients on observation or adjuvant chemotherapy is lower than one would expect based on results of surgical staging, and this suggests that not all teratoma has the same potential for growth or malignant transformation.

## MANAGEMENT OF CLINICAL STAGE II (LOW TUMOR BURDEN)

The anatomic definition of stage II germ cell tumor is metastasis confined to retroperitoneal lymph nodes. For NSGCT, there is the further requirement that tumor markers be in the good-prognosis range (S0 to S1).[40] For both seminoma and NSGCT, the majority of these patients are cured with standard treatment.

### Seminoma

Seminoma is exquisitely sensitive to both chemotherapy and radiation. Radiotherapy to the retroperitoneum with a boost to the involved nodes is standard for disease with a transverse measurement of 3 cm or less.[77–79] The fields include the landing zone and proximal ipsilateral iliac lymph nodes (dog-leg field). Radiotherapy is curative in 80% to 90% of patients, with recurrence owing largely to occult disease outside the radiation field.[80] Nevertheless, prophylactic radiotherapy to the mediastinum or supraclavicular nodes is not recommended because of toxicity concerns.[81] There is an excellent rate of success with combination chemotherapy in the patients who do relapse after radiotherapy.[82]

For patients with bulky (>3 cm transverse dimension) retroperitoneal disease, primary treatment with cisplatin-based chemotherapy is standard.[54,82] As in the adjuvant setting, patients with horseshoe kidney or inflammatory bowel disease should not receive radiotherapy; chemotherapy is the primary treatment for such patients regardless of nodal size.

## Nonseminomatous Germ Cell Tumor (Low Tumor Burden)

### Stage IS

Serum tumor markers that do not normalize after radical orchiectomy are evidence of micrometastases. Treatment is with three courses BEP followed by surveillance.

### Pathologic Stage II after Retroperitoneal Lymph Node Dissection

In the case of low-volume metastatic NSGCT, a prophylactic RPLND may be curative without additional therapy.[69,83] Patients with fewer than six lymph nodes involved, no focus >2 cm, and without extranodal extension (pN1) have an estimated 10% to 20% risk of recurrence and can be managed with surveillance. Adjuvant chemotherapy with BEP or EP (two courses) is an option for selected patients based on their access to follow-up, psychological factors, and tumor histology. Although there is no strong evidence to support adjuvant decision making based on the histology, metastases with predominantly teratoma or yolk sac tumor may have lower post-RPLND risk of recurrence than those that have predominantly embryonal carcinoma or choriocarcinoma. Nevertheless, surveillance and treatment with three or four courses of chemotherapy at recurrence is likely to yield a similar overall survival as adjuvant treatment. Adjuvant chemotherapy should be recommended for patients with pN2-N3 disease.

### Clinical Stage IIA

Primary chemotherapy with three courses of BEP is the standard treatment for patients with enlarged retroperitoneal lymph nodes and elevated serum tumor markers (S1).[63] Patients with enlarged lymph nodes and normal serum tumor markers (N1, S0) may be appropriate for nerve-sparing bilateral RPLND or chemotherapy. A primary RPLND can be considered if the primary tumor contains teratoma and is not embryonal carcinoma–predominant, tumor markers are not elevated, and there is no back pain. Elevated tumor markers, back pain, or nodal size >2 cm suggest multifocal or unresectable disease, and chemotherapy is preferred.[84]

Embryonal carcinoma can be marker negative and also requires chemotherapy. If metastatic embryonal carcinoma is suspected on clinical grounds (enlarged retroperitoneal lymph nodes), chemotherapy is the treatment of choice, whether or not the markers are elevated.

## MANAGEMENT OF STAGE II WITH HIGH TUMOR BURDEN AND STAGE III DISEASE

Patients with metastatic germ cell tumor and high tumor burden are curable, but they can be critically ill at presentation. The chance of survival improves with early recognition of the diagnosis by medical providers, often on clinical grounds, and the prompt administration of chemotherapy. Whenever possible, patients with stage IIIC NSGCT should be treated by an experienced team at a tertiary care center.[85,86]

## Good Prognosis

The International Germ Cell Cancer Collaborative Group risk classification identifies a "good prognosis" subset with overall survival of 90% to 95% with standard therapy.[44] These patients include most of those with metastatic seminoma, including mediastinal seminoma, excluding only seminoma with nonpulmonary visceral metastasis; and NSGCT stages II and IIIA (metastasis confined to lymph nodes and lungs and tumor markers below the intermediate- [S2] or high-risk [S3] levels).[87] For good prognosis NSGCT, three courses of BEP results in normalization of tumor markers for the majority of patients.[63] Postchemotherapy surgery is necessary for some patients with NSGCT who have a residual mass, as this can harbor teratoma or other viable disease (see Fig. 44.6).[88]

An alternative to three courses of BEP, for the good prognosis patients only, is etoposide and cisplatin (EP) given for four courses.[89–91] For selected patients, the added risk of CIN and other complications from a fourth course of EP may be balanced by avoidance of the pulmonary toxicity risk of bleomycin. In practice, patients with seminoma are less tolerant of bleomycin because of older age, and four courses of EP is a reasonable standard for the majority of these patients.

## Intermediate and Poor Prognosis

The intermediate prognosis subset (stage IIIB) accounts for 25% of patients with metastatic germ cell tumors and has an overall survival of approximately 75% with standard therapy.[44] The poor prognosis group (stage IIIC) is exclusively NSGCT, accounts for 15% of metastatic germ cell tumors, and has 5-year progression-free survival of 45%. These include any patient with mediastinal primary NSGCT, nonpulmonary visceral metastasis, or tumor markers in the S3 range. Four courses of BEP is the standard primary treatment for stage IIIB and IIIC germ cell tumors.[92–94] Patients with seminoma with intermediate prognosis are unlikely to tolerate bleomycin, and addition of ifosfamide to etoposide and cisplatin (VIP) is a reasonable standard for these patients.[82] In NSGCT, VIP can also be used instead of BEP if there is an increased risk of bleomycin lung toxicity because of respiratory distress, age 50 years or older, smoking or other chronic respiratory disease, or anticipated major thoracic surgery.

## Personalized Strategy Based on Tumor Marker Decline

Serum tumor markers (AFP, hCG) virtually always decline during the initial two to three cycles of chemotherapy. Failure of either marker to normalize is a well-recognized feature of chemotherapy resistance.[95] The rate of tumor marker decline has also been studied as a predictor of poor outcome. For patients presenting with stage IIIC NSGCT, it is possible to identify a subgroup of about 25% who will do comparatively well, and a larger group of about 75% whose outcome with standard therapy is poor.[96] This observation led to a phase III clinical trial in which patients with stage IIIC NSGCT received BEP in the first cycle; based on the tumor marker decline in the first cycle, those with favorable decline remained on BEP (four courses total) and the rest were randomized (1:1) to BEP or an intensified regimen. Preliminary results of this study confirmed the superior progression-free and overall survival of the group with favorable decline compared to unfavorable decline (treated with BEP), and demonstrated a statistically significant improvement in progression-free survival for patients randomized to intensified treatment based on unfavorable marker decline.[97]

## Central Nervous System Metastases

Patients with brain metastasis are curable.[98] Imaging of the brain, preferably with magnetic resonance imaging, is appropriate at baseline for stage II or III disease. The initial management for most patients with asymptomatic brain metastases is with systemic chemotherapy. Responses tend to occur swiftly (Fig. 44.7), but there is a risk of intracranial hemorrhage. The risk of bleeding can be minimized by modifying the first cycle of chemotherapy (e.g., EP given for 3 days). Tumors with active bleeding may require craniotomy. Radiotherapy is useful for postchemotherapy consolidation of residual lesions in the brain. Gamma knife is preferable to whole brain radiotherapy in these patients with potentially long survival and risk of cognitive impairment.

The brain is a potential sanctuary site. This can manifest as a solitary recurrence in the brain shortly after the completion of chemotherapy, for which surgical resection may be curative.

## Choriocarcinoma Syndrome

Metastatic choriocarcinoma is characterized by rapid hematogenous spread.[27] It usually starts as a component of a mixed testicular NSGCT, but can then proliferate and dominate the clinical picture.[27] Choriocarcinoma syndrome is recognizable by very high serum hCG levels in the range of $10^5$ to $10^6$ mIU/mL, and occasionally over 1 million, a testicular mass (or mediastinal mass), diffuse lung metastases, involvement of nonpulmonary viscera (brain, liver), tumor hemorrhage (hemoptysis, hemoperitoneum, intracranial bleed), and hyperthyroidism. The hyperthyroidism occurs at very high levels of hCG because hCG has sequence similarity to thyroid stimulating hormone.[99,100]

Patients with choriocarcinoma syndrome have a high rate of mortality caused by complications such as hemorrhage or as a result of recurrent/refractory disease. At the time of diagnosis, however, the clinical condition rapidly stabilizes with the administration of chemotherapy. It is not recommended to use bleomycin for the first course in most cases because of high volume pulmonary metastases and the risk of pulmonary hemorrhage. To avoid destabilizing the patient, EP chemotherapy can be shortened to 3 days for the first course only. For subsequent courses, EP is not sufficient for stage IIIC NSGCT and either BEP or an ifosfamide-containing regimen should be given. Administration of a beta blocker during the first course alleviates symptoms of hyperthyroidism (hypertension, tachycardia).

A male patient with testicular mass or anterior mediastinal mass, serum hCG over 50,000 mIU/mL, and clinical picture of choriocarcinoma syndrome does not require orchiectomy or biopsy prior to the start of treatment. The clinical diagnosis of choriocarcinoma should be recognized and treated as a medical emergency. Immediate chemotherapy offers the best chance for survival. Resection of the involved testis should be performed between cycles when the patient has stabilized, or at the time of RPLND.

## Mediastinal Nonseminomatous Germ Cell Tumor

Extragonadal germ cell tumors are the result of arrested migration of germ cells along the urogenital ridge during embryogenesis. This aberrant germinal tissue is usually located along the craniocaudal axis in adult life, and malignant transformation can occur in both women and men. The most common presentation is in the anterior mediastinum of an adult man.[101] Patients with Klinefelter syndrome are at increased risk for mediastinal germ cell tumors.[102,103]

Mediastinal NSGCT is curable but at a lower rate than most testicular germ cell tumors.[104] The 3-year progression-free survival described in recent series was 48% to 54%.[105-108] The first-line chemotherapy is the same as other stage IIIC germ cell tumors, consisting of four courses of BEP for patients with good pulmonary function, and four courses of VIP for those who are unlikely to tolerate bleomycin. Some authors have advocated that VIP is the preferred regimen because most patients will undergo postchemotherapy thoracic surgery.[109] In a prospective multicenter study, however, 66 patients with mediastinal NSGCT were treated with bleomycin-containing regimens and excessive pulmonary complications were not seen.[97] Mediastinal primary tumors have a high incidence of viable germ cell malignancy, teratoma, and transformation to somatic malignancy in postchemotherapy resections, so surgical consolidation is essential.[105,110]

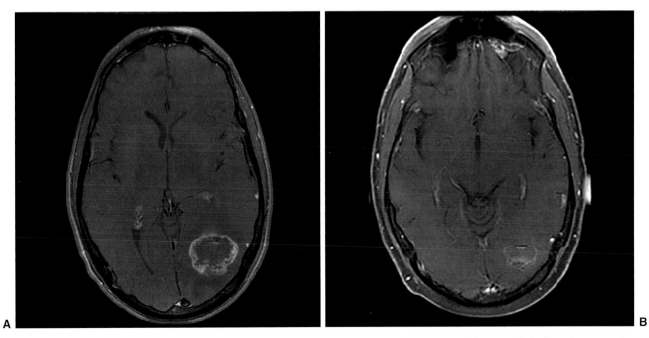

**Figure 44.7** Brain metastasis in a patient with testicular nonseminomatous germ cell tumor and clinical features of choriocarcinoma syndrome. Magnetic resonance images were acquired **(A)** at diagnosis and **(B)** after three cycles of cisplatin-based chemotherapy (9 weeks), using modified regimens to avoid thrombocytopenia.

## Management of Residual Mass

Patients with high tumor burden frequently have one or more sites of residual disease after chemotherapy and normalization of tumor markers. The management of a residual mass is critical to the curative management of germ cell tumors. There are different treatment considerations based on the setting of seminoma or NSGCT and the size of the lesion.

### Residual Nodal Size <1 cm

For either seminoma or NSGCT, a radiographic complete response does not require consolidative treatment. The size criterion for absence of residual mass in a site of lymph node metastasis is a transverse dimension <1 cm (on CT imaging). There is a potential benefit to some patients with NSGCT from the surgical consolidation of residual masses >0.5 cm and <1.0 cm, based on the possibility of teratoma.[69] By some estimates, as many as 20% of nodes <0.5 cm and 29% of nodes <1.0 cm harbor teratoma. As noted previously, however, the incidence of growing teratoma syndrome among patients observed without RPLND is lower (1% to 2%) and these can be detected on follow-up with CT imaging. Most are treated successfully, and RPLND for a residual mass <1 cm is the exception rather than the rule.

### Residual Mass >1 cm

A persistent mass in a nodal site after chemotherapy is of concern for residual germ cell malignancy in both seminoma and NSGCT, and for teratoma in NSGCT. The same applies for residual masses in extranodal organs.

For NSGCT, the standard management of a residual mass >1 cm in the retroperitoneum is a bilateral RPLND.[88] Modified template RPLND is not appropriate in this setting, as it may leave behind disease in 7% to 32% of cases. Robot-assisted RPLND is an option for some patients resulting in less short-term morbidity of the procedure compared to an open RPLND.[75] The principal long-term morbidity is retrograde ejaculation.[111] After the standard three or four courses of BEP, viable germ cell malignancy is found in only 15% of specimens. A total of 40% contain teratoma, and 45% contain only necrosis and fibrosis. There is no reliable method for determining preoperatively whether teratoma is present. Twenty-five to forty-five percent of patients with no teratoma in the primary tumor can still have teratoma in a residual mass. Biopsy is useless for ruling out the presence of teratoma because of sampling error. Complete excision is the standard of care. For the minority of patients with viable germ cell malignancy (other than teratoma) in a residual mass, the standard treatment is postoperative administration of two additional courses of chemotherapy. Residual teratoma requires no further therapy.

### Seminoma

Unlike NSGCT, seminoma does not produce teratoma. A residual mass is common, however, owing to the fibrotic reaction that occurs in the treated lymph nodes. Surgery is technically difficult and in most cases unnecessary. Patients with very high volume seminoma or residual mass >3 cm can suffer relapse from residual seminoma. The optimal consolidation for these patients is an unsettled question. Patients with residual mass <3 cm can remain on observation. For those with a mass >3 cm, radiotherapy is one means to reduce the risk of relapse. An overall survival benefit from postchemotherapy radiation has not been demonstrated. This may be in part due to the overall high survival rate for seminoma and the relatively small proportion of patients at risk for relapse after chemotherapy. The 2014 NCCN guidelines recommend surgery (RPLND), if technically feasible, for residual mass >3 cm with PET positivity.

## MANAGEMENT OF RECURRENT DISEASE

Patients in first relapse after BEP chemotherapy can be successfully salvaged in about 50% of cases. The relapse-free survival with high-dose chemotherapy and autologous stem cell transplant (HDC-ASCT) in one retrospective study was 60% (90 of 149 patients with recurrent/refractory NSGCT). Whether this was an improvement in outcome over conventional chemotherapy or a reflection of patient selection is unknown. A randomized trial for patients in first relapse with four courses of paclitaxel, ifosfamide, and cisplatin versus HDC-ASCT will hopefully answer this question.

### Conventional Dose Chemotherapy

Standard-dose regimens have resulted in a complete response rate of 35% to 70% in the second line without the use of HDC-ASCT. The most effective regimens for first recurrence after BEP have been combinations with ifosfamide and cisplatin.[112,113] Examples are vinblastine, ifosfamide, and cisplatin (VeIP), and paclitaxel, ifosfamide, and cisplatin, typically four courses with consolidation surgery (see Table 44.5).[114,115]

### High-Dose Chemotherapy and Stem Cell Transplant

In a retrospective study of patients treated at Indiana University from 1996 to 2004, 135 patients in first recurrence received one to two cycles of standard VeIP followed by two cycles of high-dose carboplatin plus etoposide ("tandem transplant").[116] At a median follow-up of 4 years, 94 of 135 (70%) remained continuously disease-free. This study included 61 patients who relapsed from a complete response (favorable), but excluded mediastinal NSGCT, late relapses, and other nongonadal primary sites (unfavorable). In a prospective trial from Memorial Sloan-Kettering Cancer Center, 81 patients received one to two cycles of paclitaxel plus ifosfamide followed by three cycles of high-dose carboplatin plus etoposide as first salvage.[117] At a median of 5 years, 56% remained free of disease. This study excluded patients with a testicular primary tumor who either had a prior complete response to first-line chemotherapy or a partial response with negative markers, but included patients with mediastinal NSGCT, late relapse, and other nongonadal primary sites.

### Second and Subsequent Relapse

Patients with recurrence after conventional second-line chemotherapy such as VeIP or TIP can be considered for HDC-ASCT.[116] Compared to the patients in first relapse, however, these patients have more chemotherapy sequelae such as CIN, renal insufficiency, and decreased performance status, leading to a high complication rate and mortality from HDC-ASCT. Conventional chemotherapy after second-line or HDC-ASCT is usually palliative. Regimens endorsed by NCCN guidelines include gemcitabine and oxaliplatin, gemcitabine and paclitaxel, gemcitabine/oxaliplatin/paclitaxel, and oral etoposide.[118–121]

Molecular targeted therapies do not yet have an established role in the treatment of germ cell tumors. There are two published studies of sunitinib in relapsed/refractory germ cell tumors.[122,123] A study from the Canadian Urologic Oncology Group and the German Testicular cancer study group found three confirmed and one unconfirmed partial responses (13%) among 32 patients with refractory germ cell tumors treated with sunitinib. Another study from Memorial Sloan-Kettering Cancer Center found no responses among 10 men with highly refractory germ cell tumors treated with sunitinib, although 4 patients had some decline in serum tumor markers. An inhibitor of cyclin-dependent kinase 4/6 showed activity in patients with unresectable teratoma, leading to clinical trials.[124] Patients with chemotherapy-refractory germ cell tumors should be encouraged to participate in clinical trials.

## Surgery after Salvage Chemotherapy

Residual lesions that persist after chemotherapy should be resected whenever feasible. There is often viable tumor in the setting of recurrent/refractory disease, even when tumor markers have normalized on chemotherapy.[125] When tumor markers decline to a plateau but do not normalize, surgery to remove all viable disease is a consideration. Surgical salvage is successful in about 20% of patients.[126,127] Patients with elevated AFP and normal hCG have better prognosis with surgery than patients with elevated or rising hCG. Adjuvant chemotherapy is not known to improve the outcome when surgery reveals viable germ cell malignancy after salvage chemotherapy.

## Late Recurrence Nonseminomatous Germ Cell Tumor

Most NSGCT recurrences after chemotherapy are seen within 2 to 3 years. Only about 2% of patients experience a relapse after 2 years. These late recurrences appear to be less sensitive to subsequent chemotherapy than the earlier recurrences.[128,129] Surgery can be curative in cases that are slowly growing and anatomically resectable. Treatment must be individualized. Although late recurrences are less chemosensitive as a group, complete responses have been described. Surgery should always be considered and integrated as a component of the overall treatment plan.

# TREATMENT SEQUELAE

Both chemotherapy and radiotherapy have long-term adverse effects on survivors of testicular cancer.[2,57,58,81] With posttreatment life expectancy of 40 years or more, the morbidity attributable to chronic and late effects of treatment can exceed that of the cancer itself.

## Cardiovascular Effects

One of the most significant delayed effects of chemotherapy is an increased risk of cardiovascular disease.[81] The risk of suffering a cardiac event is two- to seven-fold higher in survivors of testicular cancer who received cisplatin-based chemotherapy than the general population.[130,131] Other risk factors such as hyperlipidemia, obesity, and hypertension (metabolic syndrome) are also more common among survivors of testicular cancer. The health and longevity of survivors of testicular cancer can be maximized through early treatment of hypertension and hyperlipidemia, and by interventions such as diet, exercise, and tobacco cessation.

## Chemotherapy-Induced Neurotoxicity

Peripheral neurotoxicity is a common adverse effect of cisplatin. Approximately 20% to 40% of patients treated with neurotoxic chemotherapy drugs develop CIN, which can cause painful and permanent sensory disturbance. Drug therapy for CIN is only partially effective in relieving symptoms.[132] The mechanisms of CIN are not well understood, and they appear to include damage to neuronal cell bodies in dorsal root ganglia.[133] Circulating platinum levels remain elevated for many years after chemotherapy, and it is not known whether this also contributes to long-term morbidity.[134] The severity of CIN is influenced by the cumulative dose of cisplatin, exposure to other neurotoxic drugs (e.g., paclitaxel), and other medical conditions such as diabetes.

## Hypogonadism and Infertility

Chemotherapy can damage the germinal epithelium and increase the risk of abnormal sperm morphology, motility, and number. Oligospermia has been associated with prior radiotherapy for seminoma, presumably due to scatter radiation to the contralateral testis. It is also recognized that at the time of diagnosis, the percentage of men with germ cell tumor who are subfertile or infertile is greater than the general male population. Thus, sperm banking should be offered to all patients undergoing chemotherapy or radiotherapy, and to patients undergoing RPLND because they are at risk for retrograde ejaculation.

The risk of infertility from treatment is proportional to the type and duration of treatment. In a study of paternity following treatment, 71% of unselected survivors of testicular cancer were successful at 15 years. For treatment subgroups, successful paternity was 81% with surveillance, 77% after RPLND, 65% after radiotherapy, 62% after chemotherapy, and 38% after high-dose salvage chemotherapy. The risk to patients receiving fewer than four cycles of chemotherapy has not been studied, particularly in the adjuvant setting (one or two cycles), or with carboplatin in the setting of seminoma. While the risk of infertility may be lower in the adjuvant setting, these patients should receive fertility counseling and an opportunity for cryopreservation of semen.

Hypogonadism, or low testosterone, is also a common finding. Testicular dysfunction is more common among survivors of testicular cancer than the general male population. Persistent low testosterone in a patient who has completed therapy is an indication of a functional deficit in the contralateral testis. Testosterone replacement therapy can prevent complications such as weight gain, gynecomastia, erectile dysfunction, loss of libido, fatigue, depression, and osteoporosis.

## Ototoxicity

Cisplatin can result in permanent, bilateral sensorineural hearing loss in 19% to 77% of patients, and tinnitus in 19% to 42%.[135] The incidence and severity of ototoxicity is related to the cumulative dose and dose intensity of cisplatin.[136] The mechanism is thought to be through overproduction of reactive oxygen species in the cochlea, causing irreversible free radical–related apoptosis of outer hair cells, spiral ganglion cells, and the stria vascularis.[135] There may be genetic underpinnings to the susceptibility to ototoxicity from chemotherapy. There is no effective method for treating or preventing cisplatin-induced ototoxicity.[137]

## Psychosocial Functioning

There are potential short-term and long-term psychological consequences in the posttreatment period.[138] Anxiety and depression are common in the first 6 months, whereas most patients are well adjusted by 1 year. Certain patients (10% to 30%) continue to suffer moderate to severe nervousness, anxiety, or depression. Patients who have sexual difficulties, are unemployed, or have financial difficulties appear to be at greatest risk. Strain in relationships can be due to a perception of sexual dysfunction; however, some studies suggest that in married couples the patient is more concerned than the spouse, and divorce rates are no higher than the general population.[139]

## Second Malignant Neoplasms

Both radiotherapy and chemotherapy increase the risk of SMN later in life. Second malignancies can occur 20 years after treatment or later. An exception is acute leukemia, which occurs 2 to 4 years after chemotherapy. The risk of treatment-related leukemia is proportional to the cumulative dose of etoposide, and is estimated to be <0.5% for two courses (1,000 mg/m²), less than 1% for three or four courses (1,500 to 2,000 mg/m²), and as high as

6% for cumulative etoposide doses >3,000 mg/m². Chromosomal translocations involving 11q are characteristic of etoposide-related acute leukemia.[140]

Acute leukemia is also seen in a small percentage of patients with mediastinal NSGCT. While chemotherapy may be a contributing factor, the leukemia associated with mediastinal primary tumors has a separate etiology. Megakaryocytic leukemia has been described and may be more common in this setting.[141] Studies have identified the clonal marker i(12p) in leukemic cells, indicating that they are clonally descended from the primary germ cell tumor.[142,143] One hypothesis is that yolk sac tumor (a common histology among mediastinal germ cell tumors) retains the pluripotency of the normal yolk sac, which functions as a hematopoietic organ during embryogenesis.[144] This association has not been described in yolk sac tumor of testicular origin.

Second primary germ cell tumor of the contralateral testicle occurs in approximately 2% of survivors, and occasionally as a synchronous (bilateral) presentation. The risk of second germ cell tumor is present over the lifetime of the individual, making it especially important that the patient is counseled to report any testicular symptoms, and that long-term follow-up includes surveillance of the contralateral testicle. Prophylactic radiation of the contralateral testicle has been promoted in Europe as a means to reduce the risk, and surveillance alone is standard in the United States. Although adjuvant carboplatin for stage I seminoma appeared to reduce the incidence of second primary tumors, longer follow-up is needed to determine whether it is merely a delay in clinical presentation.[53]

## LONG-TERM FOLLOW-UP

The mandatory duration of follow-up for detection and management of recurrence of germ cell tumors is 5 years for NSGCT and 10 years for seminoma. There is wide consensus, however, that survivors of testicular cancer should have lifelong follow-up, whether it is at the primary treatment center or with a general internist who is knowledgeable about survivorship issues. Long-term follow-up is necessary for detection of late recurrences, second testicular primaries, and SMN. Survivors require management of cardiovascular effects and symptoms of neurotoxicity. Special care may be required for maintenance of sexual health, fertility issues, and psychosocial functioning.

## MIDLINE TUMORS OF UNCERTAIN HISTOGENESIS

Tumors of unknown primary site in young patients occasionally respond well to cisplatin-based chemotherapy. This can be the presentation of an extragonadal germ cell tumor. The diagnosis should be considered in relatively young patients in whom the tumor has predominantly midline distribution and histologic appearance of poorly differentiated carcinoma. Serum tumor markers may or may not be elevated. Molecular cytogenetic analysis for 12p genetic content can help to confirm the diagnosis, but is often inconclusive. Immunohistochemical markers SALL4, OCT3/4, CD117, SOX2, CD30, and low-molecular-weight keratins can also facilitate the diagnosis.

## OTHER TESTICULAR TUMORS

### Sex Cord/Gonadal Stromal Tumors

#### Leydig and Sertoli Cell Tumors

The most common sex cord stromal tumors in men are Leydig cell and Sertoli cell tumors (Table 44.6). These tumors are occasionally

**TABLE 44.6**

**World Health Organization Histologic Classification of Testicular Sex Cord/Gonadal Stromal Tumors**

Leydig cell tumor

Malignant Leydig cell tumor

Sertoli cell tumor
　Sertoli cell tumor lipid rich variant
　Sclerosing Sertoli cell tumor
　Large cell calcifying Sertoli cell tumor

Malignant Sertoli cell tumor

Granulosa cell tumor
　Adult type granulosa cell tumor
　Juvenile type granulosa cell tumor

Tumors of the thecoma/fibroma group
　Thecoma
　Fibroma

Sex cord/gonadal stromal tumor: Incompletely differentiated

Sex cord/gonadal stromal tumors, mixed forms

Malignant sex cord/gonadal stromal tumors

Tumors containing both germ cell and sex cord/gonadal stromal elements
　Gonadoblastoma
　Germ cell-sex cord/gonadal stromal tumor, unclassified

*Source:* Eble JN, Sauter G, Epstein JI, et al., eds. *Pathology and Genetics of Tumours of the Urinary System and Male Genital Organs.* Lyon, France: IARC Press; 2004.

metastatic, but the majority are benign. Treatment is radical orchiectomy. The risk of metastasis has been associated with vascular invasion, cellular atypia, tumor necrosis, infiltrative margins, increased mitotic rate, tumor size >5 cm, older age at presentation, increased proliferation index, and aneuploidy. The pattern of metastasis is initially to the retroperitoneal lymph nodes.[20,145,146]

Leydig and Sertoli cell tumors are associated with steroid hormone hypersecretion. Sertoli cell tumors may be accompanied by precocious puberty in boys. Patients with Leydig cell tumors may have decreased libido and gynecomastia, or virilization in prepubertal boys.

Chemotherapy and radiotherapy are not known to be effective for metastatic sex cord stromal tumors. There are several reports of treatment with mitotane, which was used because it is known to be effective in adrenocortical carcinoma, another steroid-producing tumor. Reported results with mitotane treatment of metastatic sex cord stromal tumors have been mixed, but it can be considered, especially for functional tumors with symptom of steroid hormone excess.

### Granulosa Cell Tumors

Granulosa cell tumors of the testicle are rare.[147] They resemble granulosa cell tumors of the ovary. Tumors secrete estrogen, and patients may present with gynecomastia. Treatment is radical orchiectomy, which is usually curative. Granulosa cell tumor (juvenile type) is the most common testicular neoplasm in neonates.

### Gonadoblastoma

Gonadoblastoma contains both germ cell and sex cord stromal elements.[20] It is associated with testicular dysgenesis and karyotypic anomalies. It has potential for metastasis of the germ cell component of the primary tumor.

## Mesothelioma

Mesothelioma of the tunica vaginalis can invade the testis and spermatic cord.[148] Treatment is radical orchiectomy with complete excision of the spermatic cord and hemiscrotum. RPLND should be considered in patients with LVI or invasion of the testicular parenchyma.

## Adenocarcinoma of the Rete Testis

Adenocarcinoma of the rete testis has a poor prognosis.[149] It is not responsive to radiotherapy or chemotherapy. Treatment is radical orchiectomy, and 30% to 50% of patients die within 1 year of metastatic disease. RPLND should be considered for selected patients and may be curative for low-volume metastatic disease.

## Epidermoid Cyst

Epidermoid cyst is often asymptomatic.[150] On palpation, it is firm and sharply demarcated, and it appears cystic on ultrasound. It is of uncertain relation to germ cell tumors and is not associated with ITGCN. Histologically, the cyst is lined with squamous epithelium and the adjacent testicular parenchyma is benign. The clinical course is benign. Treatment with enucleation of the tumor or radical orchiectomy is curative.

## Lymphoma

Lymphoma presents as painless enlargement of the testicle and may be bilateral.[20] It is the most common secondary malignancy of the testis in men older than 50 years. It typically occurs in the setting of advanced systemic disease, often accompanied by central nervous system or bone marrow involvement.

## Metastatic Carcinoma

Metastatic carcinoma is rarely confused with primary testicular cancer. It occurs most commonly in the setting of advanced disseminated disease. Treatment is determined by the type of primary tumor.

# REFERENCES

1. Siegel R, Ma J, Zou Z, et al. Cancer statistics, 2014. *CA Cancer J Clin* 2014;64:9–29.
2. Travis LB, Beard C, Allan JM, et al. Testicular cancer survivorship: research strategies and recommendations. *J Natl Cancer Inst* 2010;102:1114–1130.
3. Bray F, Ferlay J, Devesa SS, et al. Interpreting the international trends in testicular seminoma and nonseminoma incidence. *Nat Clin Pract Urol* 2006;3:532–543.
4. Rapley EA, Nathanson KL. Predisposition alleles for testicular germ cell tumour. *Curr Opin Genet Dev* 2010;20:225–230.
5. Dieckmann KP, Pichlmeier U. Clinical epidemiology of testicular germ cell tumors. *World J Urol* 2004;22:2–14.
6. Husmann DA. Cryptorchidism and its relationship to testicular neoplasia and microlithiasis. *Urology* 2005;66:424–426.
7. Schaapveld M, van dan Belt-Dusebout AW, Gietema JA, et al. Risk and prognostic significance of metachronous contralateral testicular germ cell tumours. *Br J Cancer* 2012;107:1637–1643.
8. Looijenga LH, Van Agthoven T, Biermann K. Development of malignant germ cells—the genvironmental hypothesis. *Int J Dev Biol* 2013;57:241–253.
9. McGlynn KA, Devesa SS, Sigurdson AJ, et al. Trends in the incidence of testicular germ cell tumors in the United States. *Cancer* 2003;97:63–70.
10. Hussain SA, Ma YT, Palmer DH, et al. Biology of testicular germ cell tumors. *Expert Rev Anticancer Ther* 2008;8:1659–1673.
11. Sheikine Y, Genega E, Melamed J, et al. Molecular genetics of testicular germ cell tumors. *Am J Cancer Res* 2012;2:153–167.
12. Tan MH, Eng C. Testicular microlithiasis: recent advances in understanding and management. *Nat Rev Urol* 2011;8:153–163.
13. Peterson AC, Bauman JM, Light DE, et al. The prevalence of testicular microlithiasis in an asymptomatic population of men 18 to 35 years old. *J Urol* 2001;166:2061–2064.
14. Coffey J, Huddart RA, Elliott F, et al. Testicular microlithiasis as a familial risk factor for testicular germ cell tumour. *Br J Cancer* 2007;97:1701–1706.
15. Rao P, Pagliaro LC. Testicular germ cell tumors. In: Silverman PM, ed. *Oncologic Imaging: A Multidisciplinary Approach.* Philadelphia: Elsevier; 2012:335–357.
16. Bosl GJ, Vogelzang NJ, Goldman A, et al. Impact of delay in diagnosis on clinical stage of testicular cancer. *Lancet* 1981;2:970–973.
17. Barlow LJ, Badalato GM, McKiernan JM. Serum tumor markers in the evaluation of male germ cell tumors. *Nat Rev Urol* 2010;7:610–617.
18. Richie JP. Surgical aspects in the treatment of patients with testicular cancer. *Hematol Oncol Clin North Am* 1991;5:1127–1142.
19. Chieffi P, Franco R, Portella G. Molecular and cell biology of testicular germ cell tumors. *Int Rev Cell Mol Biol* 2009;278:277–308.
20. Eble JN, Sauter G, Epstein JI, et al., eds. *Pathology and Genetics of Tumours of the Urinary System and Male Genital Organs.* Lyon, France: IARC Press; 2004.
21. Lempiäinen A, Sankila A, Hotakainen K, et al. Expression of human chorionic gonadotropin in testicular germ cell tumors. *Urol Oncol* 2014 (epub ahead of print).
22. Nazeer T, Ro JY, Amato RJ, et al. Histologically pure seminoma with elevated alpha-fetoprotein: a clinicopathologic study of ten cases. *Oncol Rep* 1998;5:1425–1429.
23. Chieffi P, Chieffi S, Franco R, et al. Recent advances in the biology of germ cell tumors: implications for the diagnosis and treatment. *J Endocrinol Invest* 2012;35:1015–1020.
24. Gigantino V, La Mantia E, Franco R, et al. Testicular and testicular adnexa tumors in the elderly. *Anticancer Drugs* 2013;24:228–236.
25. Almstrup K, Hoei-Hansen CE, Wirkner U, et al. Embryonic stem cell-like features of testicular carcinoma in situ revealed by genome-wide gene expression profiling. *Cancer Res* 2004;64:4736–4743.
26. Houldsworth J, Korkola JE, Bosl GJ, et al. Biology and genetics of adult male germ cell tumors. *J Clin Oncol* 2006;24:5512–5518.
27. Alvarado-Cabrero I, Hernandez-Toriz N, Paner GP. Clinicopathologic analysis of choriocarcinoma as a pure or predominant component of germ cell tumor of the testis. *Am J Surg Pathol* 2014;38:111–118.
28. Ehrlich Y, Beck SD, Ulbright TM, et al. Outcome analysis of patients with transformed teratoma to primitive neuroectodermal tumor. *Ann Oncol* 2010;21:1846–1850.
29. Rabbani F, Farivar-Mohseni H, Leon A, et al. Clinical outcome after retroperitoneal lymphadenectomy of patients with pure testicular teratoma. *Urology* 2003;62:1092–1096.
30. Donadio AC, Motzer RJ, Bajorin DF, et al. Chemotherapy for teratoma with malignant transformation. *J Clin Oncol* 2003;21:4285–4291.
31. Ma YT, Cullen MH, Hussain SA. Biology of germ cell tumors. *Hematol Oncol Clin North Am* 2011;25:457–471, vii.
32. Geurts van Kessel A, van Drunen E, de Jong B, et al. Chromosome 12q heterozygosity is retained in i(12p)-positive testicular germ cell tumor cells. *Cancer Genet Cytogenet* 1989;40:129–134.
33. Gilbert D, Rapley E, Shipley J. Testicular germ cell tumours: predisposition genes and the male germ cell niche. *Nat Rev Cancer* 2011;11:278–288.
34. Greene MH, Kratz CP, Mai PL, et al. Familial testicular germ cell tumors in adults: 2010 summary of genetic risk factors and clinical phenotype. *Endocr Relat Cancer* 2010;17:R109–R121.
35. Smiraglia DJ, Szymanska J, Kraggerud SM, et al. Distinct epigenetic phenotypes in seminomatous and nonseminomatous testicular germ cell tumors. *Oncogene* 2002;21:3909–3916.
36. Netto GJ, Nakai Y, Makayama M, et al. Global DNA hypomethylation in intratubular germ cell neoplasia and seminoma, but not in nonseminomatous male germ cell tumors. *Mod Pathol* 2008;21:1337–1344.
37. Emerson RE, Ulbright TM. Intratubular germ cell neoplasia of the testis and its associated cancers: the use of novel biomarkers. *Pathology* 2010;42:344–355.
38. Cao D, Li J, Guo CC, et al. SALL4 is a novel diagnostic marker for testicular germ cell tumors. *Am J Surg Pathol* 2009;33:1065–1077.
39. Wang F, Liu A, Peng Y, et al. Diagnostic utility of SALL4 in extragonadal yolk sac tumors: an immunohistochemical study of 59 cases with comparison to placental-like alkaline phosphatase, alpha-fetoprotein, and glypican-3. *Am J Surg Pathol* 2009;33:1529–1539.
40. American Joint Committee on Cancer. Testis. In: Edge SB, Byrd DR, Compton CC, eds. *AJCC Cancer Staging Manual.* 7th ed. New York: Springer-Verlag; 2010:471–472.
41. Dixon AK, Ellis M, Sikora K. Computed tomography of testicular tumours: distribution of abdominal lymphadenopathy. *Clin Radiol* 1986;37:519–523.
42. Tickoo SK, Hutchinson B, Bacik J, et al. Testicular seminoma: a clinicopathologic and immunohistochemical study of 105 cases with special reference to seminomas with atypical features. *Int J Surg Pathol* 2002;10:23–32.
43. Gholam D, Fizazi K, Terrier-Lacombe MJ, et al. Advanced seminoma—treatment results and prognostic factors for survival after first-line, cisplatin-based chemotherapy and for patients with recurrent disease: a single-institution experience in 145 patients. *Cancer* 2003;98:745–752.

44. International Germ Cell Consensus Classification: a prognostic factor-based staging system for metastatic germ cell cancers. International Germ Cell Cancer Collaborative Group. *J Clin Oncol* 1997;15:594–603.

45. Vugrin D, Chen A, Feigl P, et al. Embryonal carcinoma of the testis. *Cancer* 1988;61:2348–2352.

46. Germa JR, Arcusa A, Casamitjana R. False elevations of human chorionic gonadotropin associated to iatrogenic hypogonadism in gonadal germ cell tumors. *Cancer* 1987;60:2489–2493.

47. Morris MJ, Bosl GJ. Recognizing abnormal marker results that do not reflect disease in patients with germ cell tumors. *J Urol* 2000;163:796–801.

48. Pagliaro LC. Testicular cancer: when less is more. *Curr Oncol Rep* 2010; 12:271–277.

49. Beard CJ, Travis LB, Chen MH, et al. Outcomes in stage I testicular seminoma: a population-based study of 9193 patients. *Cancer* 2013;119:2771–2777.

50. Chung P, Parker C, Panzarella T, et al. Surveillance in stage I testicular seminoma—risk of late relapse. *Can J Urol* 2002;9:1637–1640.

51. Soper MS, Hastings JR, Cosmatos HA, et al. Observation versus adjuvant radiation or chemotherapy in the management of stage I seminoma: clinical outcomes and prognostic factors for relapse in a large US cohort. *Am J Clin Oncol* 2012.

52. Oliver RT, Mason MD, Mead GM, et al. Radiotherapy versus single-dose carboplatin in adjuvant treatment of stage I seminoma: a randomised trial. *Lancet* 2005;366:293–300.

53. Oliver RT, Mead GM, Rustin GJ, et al. Randomized trial of carboplatin versus radiotherapy for stage I seminoma: mature results on relapse and contralateral testis cancer rates in MRC TE19/EORTC 30982 study (ISRCTN27163214). *J Clin Oncol* 2011;29:957–962.

54. National Comprehensive Cancer Network. *NCCN Clinical Practice Guidelines in Oncology.* Fort Washington, PA: National Comprehensive Cancer Network: 2014.

55. Jones WG, Fossa SD, Mead GM, et al. Randomized trial of 30 versus 20 Gy in the adjuvant treatment of stage I testicular seminoma: a report on Medical Research Council Trial TE18, European Organisation for the Research and Treatment of Cancer Trial 30942 (ISRCTN18525328). *J Clin Oncol* 2005;23:1200–1208.

56. Sharda NN, Kinsella TJ, Ritter MA. Adjuvant radiation versus observation: a cost analysis of alternate management schemes in early-stage testicular seminoma. *J Clin Oncol* 1996;14:2933–2939.

57. Travis LB, Curtis RE, Storm H, et al. Risk of second malignant neoplasms among long-term survivors of testicular cancer. *J Natl Cancer Inst* 1997;89:1429–1439.

58. Travis LB, Fossa SD, Schonfeld SJ, et al. Second cancers among 40,576 testicular cancer patients: focus on long-term survivors. *J Natl Cancer Inst* 2005;97:1354–1365.

59. Nallu A, Mannuel HD, Hussain A. Testicular germ cell tumors: biology and clinical update. *Curr Opin Oncol* 2013;25:266–272.

60. Sturgeon JF, Moore MJ, Kakiashvili DM, et al. Non-risk-adapted surveillance in clinical stage I nonseminomatous germ cell tumors: the Princess Margaret Hospital's experience. *Eur Urol* 2011;59:556–562.

61. Afshar K, Lodha A, Costei A, et al. Recruitment in pediatric clinical trials: an ethical perspective. *J Urol* 2005;174:835–840.

62. Stephenson AJ, Bosl GJ, Bajorin DF, et al. Retroperitoneal lymph node dissection in patients with low stage testicular cancer with embryonal carcinoma predominance and/or lymphovascular invasion. *J Urol* 2005;174:557–560; discussion 560.

63. Williams SD, Birch R, Einhorn LH, et al. Treatment of disseminated germ-cell tumors with cisplatin, bleomycin, and either vinblastine or etoposide. *N Engl J Med* 1987;316:1435–1440.

64. Behnia M, Foster R, Einhorn LH, et al. Adjuvant bleomycin, etoposide and cisplatin in pathological stage II non-seminomatous testicular cancer. The Indiana University experience. *Eur J Cancer* 2000;36:472–475.

65. Swanson DA. Two courses of chemotherapy after orchidectomy for high-risk clinical stage I nonseminomatous testicular tumours. *BJU Int* 2005;95:477–478.

66. Albers P, Siener R, Krege S, et al. Randomized phase III trial comparing retroperitoneal lymph node dissection with one course of bleomycin and etoposide plus cisplatin chemotherapy in the adjuvant treatment of clinical stage I nonseminomatous testicular germ cell tumors: AUO trial AH 01/94 by the German Testicular Cancer Study Group. *J Clin Oncol* 2008;26:2966–2972.

67. Tandstad T, Dahl O, Cohn-Cedermark G, et al. Risk-adapted treatment in clinical stage I nonseminomatous germ cell testicular cancer: the SWENOTECA management program. *J Clin Oncol* 2009;27:2122–2128.

68. Dearnaley DP, Fossa SD, Kaye SB, et al. Adjuvant bleomycin, vincristine and cisplatin (BOP) for high-risk stage I non-seminomatous germ cell tumours: a prospective trial (MRC TE17). *Br J Cancer* 2005;92:2107–2113.

69. Stephenson AJ, Bosl GJ, Motzer RJ, et al. Retroperitoneal lymph node dissection for nonseminomatous germ cell testicular cancer: impact of patient selection factors on outcome. *J Clin Oncol* 2005;23:2781–2788.

70. Eggener SE, Carver BS, Sharp DS, et al. Incidence of disease outside modified retroperitoneal lymph node dissection templates in clinical stage I or IIA nonseminomatous germ cell testicular cancer. *J Urol* 2007;177:937–942; discussion 942–943.

71. Donohue JP, Thornhill JA, Foster RS, et al. Retroperitoneal lymphadenectomy for clinical stage A testis cancer (1965 to 1989): modifications of technique and impact on ejaculation. *J Urol* 1993;149:237–243.

72. Sheinfeld J. Mapping studies and modified templates in nonseminomatous germ cell tumors. *Nat Clin Pract Urol* 2007;4:60–61.

73. Carver BS, Shayegan B, Eggener S, et al. Incidence of metastatic nonseminomatous germ cell tumor outside the boundaries of a modified postchemotherapy retroperitoneal lymph node dissection. *J Clin Oncol* 2007;25:4365–4369.

74. Davol P, Sumfest J, Rukstalis D. Robotic-assisted laparoscopic retroperitoneal lymph node dissection. *Urology* 2006;67:199.

75. Williams SB, Lau CS, Josephson DY. Initial series of robot-assisted laparoscopic retroperitoneal lymph node dissection for clinical stage I nonseminomatous germ cell testicular cancer. *Eur Urol* 2011;60:1299–1302.

76. Steiner H, Peschel R, Janetschek G, et al. Long-term results of laparoscopic retroperitoneal lymph node dissection: a single-center 10-year experience. *Urology* 2004;63:550–555.

77. Classen J, Schmidberger H, Meisner C, et al. Radiotherapy for stages IIA/B testicular seminoma: final report of a prospective multicenter clinical trial. *J Clin Oncol* 2003;21:1101–1106.

78. Chung PW, Warde PR, Panzarella T, et al. Appropriate radiation volume for stage IIA/B testicular seminoma. *Int J Radiat Oncol Biol Phys* 2003;56:746–748.

79. Neill M, Warde P, Fleshner N. Management of low-stage testicular seminoma. *Urol Clin North Am* 2007;34:127–136; abstract vii–viii.

80. Chung PW, Gospodarowicz MK, Panzarella T, et al. Stage II testicular seminoma: patterns of recurrence and outcome of treatment. *Eur Urol* 2004;45:754–759; discussion 759–760.

81. van den Belt-Dusebout AW, de Wit R, Gietema JA, et al. Treatment-specific risks of second malignancies and cardiovascular disease in 5-year survivors of testicular cancer. *J Clin Oncol* 2007;25:4370–4378.

82. Fizazi K, Delva R, Caty A, et al. A risk-adapted study of cisplatin and etoposide, with or without ifosfamide, in patients with metastatic seminoma: results of the GETUG S99 multicenter prospective study. *Eur Urol* 2014;65:381–386.

83. Rabbani F, Sheinfeld J, Farivar-Mohseni H, et al. Low-volume nodal metastases detected at retroperitoneal lymphadenectomy for testicular cancer: pattern and prognostic factors for relapse. *J Clin Oncol* 2001;19:2020–2025.

84. Stephenson AJ, Bosl GJ, Motzer RJ, et al. Nonrandomized comparison of primary chemotherapy and retroperitoneal lymph node dissection for clinical stage IIA and IIB nonseminomatous germ cell testicular cancer. *J Clin Oncol* 2007;25:5597–5602.

85. Collette L, Sylvester RJ, Stenning SP, et al. Impact of the treating institution on survival of patients with "poor-prognosis" metastatic nonseminoma. European Organization for Research and Treatment of Cancer Genito-Urinary Tract Cancer Collaborative Group and the Medical Research Council Testicular Cancer Working Party. *J Natl Cancer Inst* 1999;91:839–846.

86. Thibault C, Fizazi K, Barrios D, et al. Compliance with guidelines and correlation with outcome in patients with advanced germ-cell tumours. *Eur J Cancer* 2014;50:1284–1290.

87. Moran CA, Suster S, Przygodzki RM, et al. Primary germ cell tumors of the mediastinum: II. Mediastinal seminomas—a clinicopathologic and immunohistochemical study of 120 cases. *Cancer* 1997;80:691–698.

88. Oldenburg J, Alfsen GC, Lien HH, et al. Postchemotherapy retroperitoneal surgery remains necessary in patients with nonseminomatous testicular cancer and minimal residual tumor masses. *J Clin Oncol* 2003;21:3310–3317.

89. Kondagunta GV, Bacik J, Bajorin D, et al. Etoposide and cisplatin chemotherapy for metastatic good-risk germ cell tumors. *J Clin Oncol* 2005;23:9290–9294.

90. Culine S, Kerbrat P, Kramar A, et al. Refining the optimal chemotherapy regimen for good-risk metastatic nonseminomatous germ-cell tumors: a randomized trial of the Genito-Urinary Group of the French Federation of Cancer Centers (GETUG T93BP). *Ann Oncol* 2007;18:917–924.

91. Bajorin DF, Sarosdy MF, Pfister DG, et al. Randomized trial of etoposide and cisplatin versus etoposide and carboplatin in patients with good-risk germ cell tumors: a multiinstitutional study. *J Clin Oncol* 1993;11:598–606.

92. Hinton S, Catalano PJ, Einhorn LH, et al. Cisplatin, etoposide and either bleomycin or ifosfamide in the treatment of disseminated germ cell tumors: final analysis of an intergroup trial. *Cancer* 2003;97:1869–1875.

93. Kaye SB, Mead GM, Fossa S, et al. Intensive induction-sequential chemotherapy with BOP/VIP-B compared with treatment with BEP/EP for poor-prognosis metastatic nonseminomatous germ cell tumor: a Randomized Medical Research Council/European Organization for Research and Treatment of Cancer study. *J Clin Oncol* 1998;16:692–701.

94. Motzer RJ, Nichols CJ, Margolin KA, et al. Phase III randomized trial of conventional-dose chemotherapy with or without high-dose chemotherapy and autologous hematopoietic stem-cell rescue as first-line treatment for patients with poor-prognosis metastatic germ cell tumors. *J Clin Oncol* 2007;25:247–256.

95. Beck SD, Patel MI, Sheinfeld J. Tumor marker levels in post-chemotherapy cystic masses: clinical implications for patients with germ cell tumors. *J Urol* 2004;171:168–171.

96. Fizazi K, Culine S, Kramar A, et al. Early predicted time to normalization of tumor markers predicts outcome in poor-prognosis nonseminomatous germ cell tumors. *J Clin Oncol* 2004;22:3868–3876.

97. Fizazi K, Pagliaro LC, Flechon A, et al. A phase III trial of personalized chemotherapy based on serum tumor marker decline in poor-prognosis germ-cell tumors: Results of GETUG 13 (meeting abstract). *J Clin Oncol* 2013;31.

98. Forquer JA, Harkenrider M, Fakiris AJ, et al. Brain metastasis from non-seminomatous germ cell tumor of the testis. *Expert Rev Anticancer Ther* 2007;7:1567–1580.

99. Goodarzi MO, Van Herle AJ. Thyrotoxicosis in a male patient associated with excess human chorionic gonadotropin production by germ cell tumor. *Thyroid* 2000;10:611–619.

100. Giralt SA, Dexeus F, Amato R, et al. Hyperthyroidism in men with germ cell tumors and high levels of beta-human chorionic gonadotropin. *Cancer* 1992;69:1286–1290.
101. Moran CA, Suster A. Primary germ cell tumors of the mediastinum: I. Analysis of 322 cases with special emphasis on teratomatous lesions and a proposal for histopathologic classification and clinical staging. *Cancer* 1997;80:681–690.
102. McNeil MM, Leong AS, Sage RE. Primary mediastinal embryonal carcinoma in association with Klinefelter's syndrome. *Cancer* 1981;47:343–345.
103. Nichols CR, Heerema NA, Palmer C, et al. Klinefelter's syndrome associated with mediastinal germ cell neoplasms. *J Clin Oncol* 1987;5:1290–1294.
104. Logothetis CJ, Samuels ML, Selig DE, et al. Chemotherapy of extragonadal germ cell tumors. *J Clin Oncol* 1985;3:316–325.
105. Rodney AJ, Tannir NM, Siefer-Radtke AO, et al. Survival outcomes for men with mediastinal germ-cell tumors: the University of Texas M. D. Anderson Cancer Center experience. *Urol Oncol* 2012;30:879–885.
106. Nichols CR, Saxman S, Williams SD, et al. Primary mediastinal nonseminomatous germ cell tumors. A modern single institution experience. *Cancer* 1990;65:1641–1646.
107. Fizazi K, Culine S, Droz JP, et al. Primary mediastinal nonseminomatous germ cell tumors: results of modern therapy including cisplatin-based chemotherapy. *J Clin Oncol* 1998;16:725–732.
108. Bokemeyer C, Nichols CR, Droz JP, et al. Extragonadal germ cell tumors of the mediastinum and retroperitoneum: results from an international analysis. *J Clin Oncol* 2002;20:1864–1873.
109. Radaideh SM, Cook VC, Kesler KA, et al. Outcome following resection for patients with primary mediastinal nonseminomatous germ-cell tumors and rising serum tumor markers post-chemotherapy. *Ann Oncol* 2010;21:804–807.
110. Moran CA, Suster S, Koss MN. Primary germ cell tumors of the mediastinum: III. Yolk sac tumor, embryonal carcinoma, choriocarcinoma, and combined nonteratomatous germ cell tumors of the mediastinum—a clinicopathologic and immunohistochemical study of 64 cases. *Cancer* 1997;80:699–707.
111. Baniel J, Foster RS, Rowland RG, et al. Complications of primary retroperitoneal lymph node dissection. *J Urol* 1994;152:424–427.
112. Loehrer PJ Sr, Einhorn LH, Williams SD. VP-16 plus ifosfamide plus cisplatin as salvage therapy in refractory germ cell cancer. *J Clin Oncol* 1986;4:528–536.
113. Motzer RJ, Cooper K, Geller NL, et al. The role of ifosfamide plus cisplatin-based chemotherapy as salvage therapy for patients with refractory germ cell tumors. *Cancer* 1990;66:2476–2481.
114. Loehrer PJ Sr, Gonin R, Nichols CR, et al. Vinblastine plus ifosfamide plus cisplatin as initial salvage therapy in recurrent germ cell tumor. *J Clin Oncol* 1998;16:2500–2504.
115. Kondagunta GV, Bacik J, Donadio A, et al. Combination of paclitaxel, ifosfamide, and cisplatin is an effective second-line therapy for patients with relapsed testicular germ cell tumors. *J Clin Oncol* 2005;23:6549–6555.
116. Einhorn LH, Williams SD, Chamness A, et al. High-dose chemotherapy and stem-cell rescue for metastatic germ-cell tumors. *N Engl J Med* 2007;357:340–348.
117. Feldman DR, Sheinfeld J, Bajorin DF, et al. TI-CE high-dose chemotherapy for patients with previously treated germ cell tumors: results and prognostic factor analysis. *J Clin Oncol* 2010;28:1706–1713.
118. Kollmannsberger C, Beyer J, Liersch R, et al. Combination chemotherapy with gemcitabine plus oxaliplatin in patients with intensively pretreated or refractory germ cell cancer: a study of the German Testicular Cancer Study Group. *J Clin Oncol* 2004;22:108–114.
119. Einhorn LH, Brames MJ, Juliar B, et al. Phase II study of paclitaxel plus gemcitabine salvage chemotherapy for germ cell tumors after progression following high-dose chemotherapy with tandem transplant. *J Clin Oncol* 2007;25:513–516.
120. Bokemeyer C, Oechsle K, Honecker F, et al. Combination chemotherapy with gemcitabine, oxaliplatin, and paclitaxel in patients with cisplatin-refractory or multiply relapsed germ-cell tumors: a study of the German Testicular Cancer Study Group. *Ann Oncol* 2008;19:448–453.
121. Cooper MA, Einhorn LH. Maintenance chemotherapy with daily oral etoposide following salvage therapy in patients with germ cell tumors. *J Clin Oncol* 1995;13:1167–1169.
122. Oechsle K, Honecker F, Cheng T, et al. Preclinical and clinical activity of sunitinib in patients with cisplatin-refractory or multiply relapsed germ cell tumors: a Canadian Urologic Oncology Group/German Testicular Cancer Study Group cooperative study. *Ann Oncol* 2011;22:2654–2660.
123. Feldman DR, Turkula S, Ginsberg MS, et al. Phase II trial of sunitinib in patients with relapsed or refractory germ cell tumors. *Invest New Drugs* 2010;28:523–528.
124. Vaughn DJ, Flaherty K, Lal P, et al. Treatment of growing teratoma syndrome. *N Engl J Med* 2009;360:423–424.
125. Eggener SE, Carver BS, Loeb S, et al. Pathologic findings and clinical outcome of patients undergoing retroperitoneal lymph node dissection after multiple chemotherapy regimens for metastatic testicular germ cell tumors. *Cancer* 2007;109:528–535.
126. Murphy BR, Breeden ES, Donohue JP, et al. Surgical salvage of chemorefractory germ cell tumors. *J Clin Oncol* 1993;11:324–329.
127. Eastham JA, Wilson TG, Russell C, et al. Surgical resection in patients with nonseminomatous germ cell tumor who fail to normalize serum tumor markers after chemotherapy. *Urology* 1994;43:74–80.
128. Carver BS, Motzer RJ, Kondagunta GV, et al. Late relapse of testicular germ cell tumors. *Urol Oncol* 2005;23:441–445.
129. Ronnen EA, Kondagunta GV, Bacik J, et al. Incidence of late-relapse germ cell tumor and outcome to salvage chemotherapy. *J Clin Oncol* 2005;23:6999–7004.
130. Meinardi MT, Gietema JA, van der Graaf WT, et al. Cardiovascular morbidity in long-term survivors of metastatic testicular cancer. *J Clin Oncol* 2000;18:1725–1732.
131. Huddart RA, Norman A, Shahidi M, et al. Cardiovascular disease as a long-term complication of treatment for testicular cancer. *J Clin Oncol* 2003;21:1513–1523.
132. Smith EM, Pang H, Cirrincione C, et al. Effect of duloxetine on pain, function, and quality of life among patients with chemotherapy-induced painful peripheral neuropathy: a randomized clinical trial. *JAMA* 2013;309:1359–1367.
133. Argyriou AA, Bruna J, Marmiroli P, et al. Chemotherapy-induced peripheral neurotoxicity (CIPN): an update. *Crit Rev Oncol Hematol* 2012;82:51–77.
134. Gietema JA, Meinardi MT, Messerschmidt J, et al. Circulating plasma platinum more than 10 years after cisplatin treatment for testicular cancer. *Lancet* 2000;355:1075–1076.
135. Travis LB, Fossa SD, Sesso HD, et al. Chemotherapy-induced peripheral neurotoxicity and ototoxicity: new paradigms for translational genomics. *J Natl Cancer Inst* 2014;106.
136. Rademaker-Lakhai JM, Crul M, Zuur L, et al. Relationship between cisplatin administration and the development of ototoxicity. *J Clin Oncol* 2006;24:918–924.
137. Oldenburg J, Kraggerud SM, Cvancarova M, et al. Cisplatin-induced long-term hearing impairment is associated with specific glutathione s-transferase genotypes in testicular cancer survivors. *J Clin Oncol* 2007;25:708–714.
138. Kaasa S, Aass N, Mastekaasa A, et al. Psychosocial well-being in testicular cancer patients. *Eur J Cancer* 1991;27:1091–1095.
139. Gritz ER, Wellisch DK, Wang HJ, et al. Long-term effects of testicular cancer on sexual functioning in married couples. *Cancer* 1989;64:1560–1567.
140. Kollmannsberger C, Beyer J, Droz JP, et al. Secondary leukemia following high cumulative doses of etoposide in patients treated for advanced germ cell tumors. *J Clin Oncol* 1998;16:3386–3391.
141. Nichols CR, Hoffman R, Einhorn LH, et al. Hematologic malignancies associated with primary mediastinal germ-cell tumors. *Ann Intern Med* 1985;102:603–609.
142. Chaganti RS, Ladanyi M, Samaniego F, et al. Leukemic differentiation of a mediastinal germ cell tumor. *Genes Chromosomes Cancer* 1989;1:83–87.
143. Ladanyi M, Samaniego D, Reuter VE, et al. Cytogenetic and immunohistochemical evidence for the germ cell origin of a subset of acute leukemias associated with mediastinal germ cell tumors. *J Natl Cancer Inst* 1990;82:221–227.
144. Orazi A, Neiman RS, Ulbright TM, et al. Hematopoietic precursor cells within the yolk sac tumor component are the source of secondary hematopoietic malignancies in patients with mediastinal germ cell tumors. *Cancer* 1993;71:3873–3881.
145. Di Tonno F, Tavolini IM, Belmonte P, et al. Lessons from 52 patients with leydig cell tumor of the testis: the GUONE (North-Eastern Uro-Oncological Group, Italy) experience. *Urol Int* 2009;82:152–157.
146. Giglio M, Medica M, De Rose AF, et al. Testicular sertoli cell tumours and relative sub-types. Analysis of clinical and prognostic features. *Urol Int* 2003;70:205–210.
147. Miliaras D, Anagnostou E, Moysides I. Adult type granulosa cell tumor: a very rare case of sex-cord tumor of the testis with review of the literature. *Case Rep Pathol* 2013;932986.
148. Plas E, Riedl CR, Pfluger H. Malignant mesothelioma of the tunica vaginalis testis: review of the literature and assessment of prognostic parameters. *Cancer* 1998;83:2437–2446.
149. Perimenis P, Athanasopoulos A, Speakman M. Primary adenocarcinoma of the rete testis. *Int Urol Nephrol* 2003;35:373–374.
150. Smith AK, Hansel DE, Klein EA. Epidermoid cyst of the testicle. *Urology* 2009;74:544.

Note: page locators followed by *f* and *t* indicate figure and table, respectively.

*i*